Osteolysis
  Osteomyelitis
  Osteoporosis
Granulomatous disease
Acidosis
Spurious
  Hyperalbuminemia

  Decreased
Eclampsia
Renal secondary
  hyperparathyroidism
Hypoalbuminemia
Hypomagnesemia
Hypoparathyroidism
Pancreatitis
Rhabdomyolysis
Dietary
  Hypovitaminosis D
  Excess dietary phosphorus
C-cell thyroid tumors
Malabsorption
Hypercalcitoninism
  Iatrogenic
Parathyroidectomy
Phosphate enemas
Intravenous phosphate
  administration
Alkalosis
Ethylene glycol
Spurious
  EDTA contamination
  Oxalate contamination

Chloride
  Increased
Dehydration
Metabolic acidosis
Bromide therapy

  Decreased
Gastric vomiting
Metabolic alkalosis

Cholesterol
  Increased
Cholestasis
Endocrine disease
  Hypothyroidism
  Hyperadrenocorticoidism
  Diabetes mellitus
Postprandial
Dietary
Nephrotic syndrome
Primary hyperlipidemia
  Idiopathic hypercholesterolemia
  Primary hyperchylomicronemia
    (cats)
  Lipoproteinlipase deficiency (cats)

  Decreased
Protein-losing enteropathy
Portosystemic shunt
Malassimilation
  Malabsorption
  Maldigestion
Lymphangiectasia
Starvation
Liver failure
Hypoadrenocorticism

Cholinesterase
  Decreased
Organophosphates
Carbamates

Cobalamin (B$_{12}$)
  Decreased
Bacterial overgrowth

Creatinine
  Increased
Azotemia
  Prerenal
  Renal
  Postrenal

  Decreased
Decrease muscle mass

Creatine kinase (CK)
  Increased
Muscle inflammation
  Immune mediated
  Eosinophilic myositis
  Masticatory muscle myositis
  Endocarditis
  Infectious
    Toxoplasmosis
    Neosporum caninum
  Nutritional
    Hypokalemia (polymyopathy)
    Taurine deficiency
  Trauma
    Exertional myositis
    Surgical
    Intramuscular injections
    Hypothermia
    Pyrexia
    Prolonged recumbency
    Post-infarct ischemia
    Cardiomyopathy
    Disseminated intravascular
      coagulation

Fibrinogen
  Increased
Inflammation
Pregnancy

  Decreased
Liver failure
Coagulopathies
Primary hypofibrinogenemia

Folate
  Increased
Bacterial overgrowth

Fructosamine
  Increased
Diabetes mellitus

  Decreased
Spurious
Hypoproteinemia
Anemia (false)

**Gamma glutamyltransferase
(GGT)**
  Increased
Cholestasis
  Intrahepatic
  Extrahepatic
Drugs (canine)
  Glucocorticoids
  Anticonvulsants
  Primadone
  Phenobarbital

  Decreased
Spurious
Hemolysis

Globulin
  Increased
Dehydration (albumin and total
  protein)

Inflammation
Gammopathy
  Monoclonal
    Plasma cell myeloma
    Ehrlichia
    Dirofilariasis
  Polyclonal
    Chronic inflammatory disease
    Feline infectious peritonitis
    Dental disease
    Dermatitis
    Inflammatory bowel disease
    Parasitic diseases
    Immune-mediated diseases
    Neoplasia

  Decreased
Neonatal
Immunodeficiency
  Congenital
  Acquired
Blood loss
Protein-losing enteropathy

Glucose
  Increased
Endocrine
  Acromegaly
  Diabetes mellitus
  Hyperadrenocorticism
Pancreatitis
Stress (cats)
Drugs
  Intravenous glucose administration
  Glucocorticoids
  Xylazine
  Progestagens (Ovaban and others)

  Decreased
Liver failure
Endocrine
  Hypoadrenocorticism
  Hypopituitarism
Starvation
Neoplasia
Hyperinsulinism
  Iatrogenic
  Insulinoma
  Idiopathic
    Puppies
    Toy breed dogs
Septicemia
Polycythemia
Leukemia
Glycogen storage disease
Artifact
  Delayed serum separation

Iron
  Increased
Hemolysis

  Decreased
Chronic blood loss
Dietary deficiency

Lactate dehydrogenase (LDH)
  Increased
Organ/tissue damage
Hemolysis
  In vivo
  In vitro
Hepatocytes
Muscle
Kidney
Spurious
  Failure to separate serum from
    RBCs

Lipase
  Increased
Pancreatic disease
  Pancreatitis
  Necrosis
  Neoplasia
  Enteritis
Renal disease
Glucocorticoids

Magnesium
  Decreased
Dietary
Diabetic Ketacidosis
Potential causes:
  gastrointestinal
    malabsorption
    chronic diarrhea
  renal
    glomerular disease
    tubular disease
  drugs
    diuretics
    Amphotericin B
  others

Phosphorus
  Increased
Reduced GFR
  Renal
    Acute
    Chronic
  Postrenal
Hemolysis
Hyperthyroidism
Neonates
Intoxication
  Hypervitaminosis D
  Jasmine ingestion
Dietary excess
Iatrogenic
  Phosphate enemas
  Intravenous phosphate
    administration
Osteolysis
Hypoparathyroidism
Spurious
  Delayed serum separation

  Decreased
Hyperparathyroidism
  Primary
  Nutritional secondary
Neoplasia
  PTH-like hormone
  C-cell thyroid tumors
Insulin therapy
Diabetic ketoacidosis
Dietary deficiency
Eclampsia
Hyperadrenocorticism

Potassium
  Increased
Renal failure
  Distal RTA
  Oliguric/anuric
Postrenal
  Obstruction
  Ruptured bladder
Spurious
  Breed idiosyncracy (Akitas)
  Leukemias
  Thrombocytosis
  Collection in potassium
    heparin
  Collection in potassium EDTA
Hypoadrenocorticism

TEXTBOOK OF VETERINARY INTERNAL MEDICINE

DISEASES OF THE DOG AND CAT

TEXTBOOK OF VETERINARY INTERNAL MEDICINE

DISEASES OF THE DOG AND CAT

Fifth Edition   **VOLUME 1**

STEPHEN J. ETTINGER, D.V.M.
California Animal Hospital, Los Angeles, California

EDWARD C. FELDMAN, D.V.M.
University of California, Davis, California

W.B. SAUNDERS COMPANY
A Division of Harcourt Brace & Company
Philadelphia   London   Toronto   Montreal   Sydney   Tokyo

W.B. SAUNDERS COMPANY
A Division of Harcourt Brace & Company

The Curtis Center
Independence Square West
Philadelphia, Pennsylvania 19106

Library of Congress Cataloging-in-Publication Data

Textbook of veterinary internal medicine: diseases of the dog and cat / [edited by]
Stephen J. Ettinger, Edward C. Feldman.—5th ed.

p.   cm.

ISBN 0–7216–7256–6 (2 vol. set)

1. Dogs—Diseases.   2. Cats—Diseases.   3. Veterinary internal medicine.
   I. Ettinger, Stephen J.   II. Feldman, Edward C.

SF991.T48 2000   636.7′0896—dc21   98–34212

TEXTBOOK OF VETERINARY INTERNAL MEDICINE: Volume 1 ISBN 0–7216–7257–4
Diseases of the Dog and Cat   Volume 2 ISBN 0–7216–7258–2
                                                       Set ISBN 0–7216–7256–6

Printed in the United States of America.

Last digit is the print number: 9   8   7   6   5   4   3   2   1

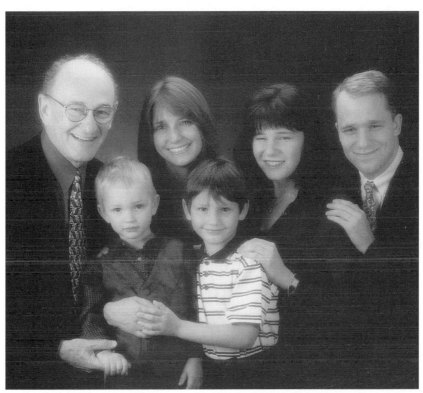

For my wife Pat and my children Nicole, Andrew,
Michael and Robert.
You are the treasures that I love!

Stephen J. Ettinger

Throughout life we are encouraged, trained, influenced, advised, and nurtured (consciously and unconsciously) by those with whom we interact. The "mentoring" of people to benefit their lives and their careers ranks among our highest vocations. During my veterinary career, I have been the recipient of unselfish, sincere, and well-thought-out counseling by many people, including my teachers, peers at many stages of my development, faculty colleagues, house officers, clients, students, children, and others. I would like to dedicate this work to those who have most influenced my professional life through positive mentoring, especially my brother Bernard Feldman and my good friends Stephen Ettinger and Richard Nelson. I also dedicate this publication to those veterinarians who are committed to life-long learning and who use this text in the pursuit of that goal.

All my love to my family for enduring my sense of obligation to this effort.

Edward C. Feldman

EDITORS

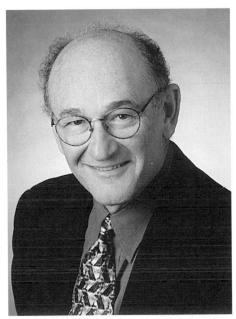

STEPHEN J. ETTINGER, DVM

California Animal Hospital, Los Angeles, California
Diplomate, American College of Veterinary Internal
Medicine (Internal Medicine and Cardiology)
*Weakness and Syncope; Coughing; Dietary Modifications
in Cardiac Disease; Electrocardiography; Diseases of the
Trachea; Canine and Feline Cardiomyopathy (CIS); Col-
lapsing Trachea (CIS); Congenital Heart Disease (CIS);
Canine Valvular Insufficiency and Congestive Heart Failure
(CIS)*

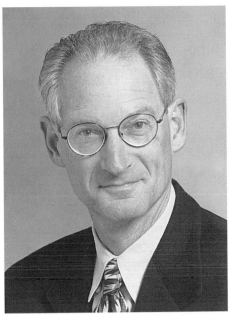

EDWARD C. FELDMAN, DVM

University of California, Davis, California
Diplomate, American College of Veterinary Internal
Medicine
*Disorders of the Parathyroid Glands; Hyperadrenocorti-
cism; Ovarian and Estrous Cycle Abnormalities; Cystic En-
dometrial Hyperplasia, Pyometra, and Infertility; o,p'-DDD
Treatment of Pituitary Cushing's (CIS); Diabetes Mellitus in
Dogs and Cats (CIS); Hyperthyroidism in Cats (CIS); Ste-
roid Therapy (CIS)*

CONTRIBUTORS

Zeineb Alhaidari, DVM, DECVD

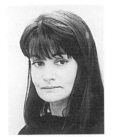

Dermatologist, Hospital Owner, Clinique Vétérinaire, Roquefort, Les Pins, France

Changes in Pigmentation

Jeanne A. Barsanti, DVM, MS, DACVIM (Med)

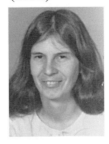

Professor, Department of Small Animal Medicine, The University of Georgia, Athens, Georgia

Dietary Considerations for Urinary Diseases

Clarke Atkins, DVM, DACVIM (Cardiol)

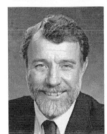

Professor of Medicine and Cardiology, College of Veterinary Medicine, North Carolina State University, Raleigh, North Carolina

Canine Heartworm Disease (CIS)

Joseph W. Bartges, DVM, PhD, DACVIM, DACVN

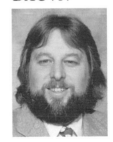

Associate Professor of Medicine and Nutrition, Department of Small Animal Clinical Sciences, College of Veterinary Medicine; Staff Internist and Nutritionist, Veterinary Teaching Hospital, The University of Tennessee, Knoxville, Tennessee

Discolored Urine; Dietary Considerations for Urinary Diseases; Canine Lower Urinary Tract Disorders; Disorders of Renal Tubules

Rodney S. Bagley, DVM, DACVIM (Neurol)

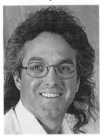

Associate Professor, Washington State University College of Veterinary Medicine, Pullman, Washington

Multifocal Neurologic Disease

John E. Bauer, DVM, PhD, DACVN

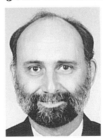

Professor, Department of Small Animal Medicine and Surgery, College of Veterinary Medicine, Texas A&M University, College Station, Texas

Hyperlipidemias

Margaret C. Barr, DVM, PhD

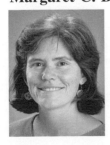

Assistant Professor, Department of Neuropharmacology, The Scripps Research Institute, La Jolla, California

FIV and FIV-Related Disease

Ellen N. Behrend, VMD, MS, DACVIM

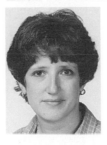

Assistant Professor, Department of Small Animal Medicine and Surgery, College of Veterinary Medicine, Auburn University, Auburn, Alabama

Polyphagia

David S. Biller, DVM, DACVR

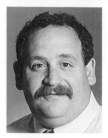

Associate Professor, Department of Clinical Sciences, and Radiologist, Veterinary Teaching Hospital, College of Veterinary Medicine, Kansas State University, Manhattan, Kansas

Mediastinal Disease

Stéphane Blot, DVM, PhD, DECVN

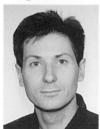

Maitre de Conférences, Head of Medical Neurology, Departement of Small Animal Internal Medicine, Ecole Nationale Vétérinaire d'Alfort, Maisons-Alfort, France

Disorders of the Skeletal Muscles

John D. Bonagura, DVM, MS, DACVIM (Cardiol, Int Med)

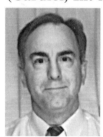

Gilbreath-McLorn Professor of Veterinary Cardiology, University of Missouri–Columbia, Columbia, Missouri

Echocardiography

Dawn Merton Boothe, DVH, PhD, DACVIM, DACVCP

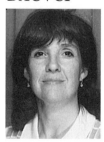

Associate Professor, Department of Veterinary Physiology and Pharmacology, and Veterinary Teaching Hospital; Director, Clinical Pharmacology Laboratory, College of Veterinary Medicine, Texas A&M University, College Station, Texas

Principles of Drug Therapy

Kyle A. Brayley, DVM, DACVIM (Int Med, Cardiol)

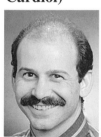

Veterinary Medical Specialists of Houston, The Animal Emergency Clinic, Houston, Texas

Diseases of the Trachea

Edward B. Breitschwerdt, DVM, DACVIM

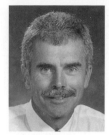

Professor of Medicine and Infectious Diseases, College of Veterinary Medicine, North Carolina State University, Raleigh; Adjunct Assistant Professor of Medicine, Duke University Medical School, Durham, North Carolina

The Rickettsioses

Ronald M. Bright, DVM, DACVS

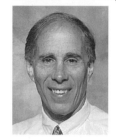

College of Veterinary Medicine, University of Tennessee, Knoxville, Tennessee

Rectoanal Disease

Marjory Brooks, DVM, DACVIM

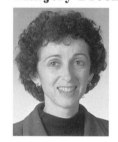

Associate Director, Comparative Coagulation Section, Diagnostic Laboratory, Department of Population Medicine and Diagnostic Science, College of Veterinary Medicine, Cornell University, Ithaca, New York

Coagulopathies and Thrombosis

Cathy A. Brown, VMD, PhD, DACVP

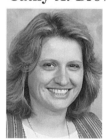

Assistant Professor, Diagnostic Laboratory, College of Veterinary Medicine, University of Georgia, Athens, Georgia

Dietary Considerations for Urinary Diseases

Scott A. Brown, VMD, PhD, DACVIM

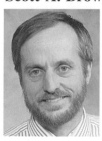

Associate Professor, Department of Physiology, and Department of Small Animal Medicine, Veterinary Medical Teaching Hospital, College of Veterinary Medicine, University of Georgia, Athens, Georgia

Dietary Considerations for Urinary Diseases

Susan E. Bunch, DVM, PhD, DACVIM

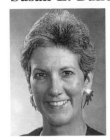

Professor of Medicine, College of Veterinary Medicine, North Carolina State University, Raleigh, North Carolina

Acute Hepatic Disorders and Systemic Disorders That Involve the Liver

Mary Beth Callan, VMD, DACVIM

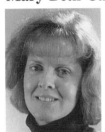

Assistant Professor of Medicine, Department of Clinical Studies, School of Veterinary Medicine, University of Pennsylvania, Philadelphia, Pennsylvania

Petechiae and Ecchymoses

Karen L. Campbell, DVM, MS, DACVIM, DACVD

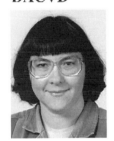

Professor, Veterinary Clinical Medicine, College of Veterinary Medicine, University of Illinois, Urbana, Illinois

External Parasites: Identification and Control

Paul J. Canfield, BVSc, PhD

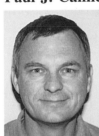

Associate Professor in Veterinary Pathology, Department of Veterinary Anatomy and Pathology, University of Sydney, New South Wales, Australia

Diagnostic Cytology of Skin Lesions

Andrea G. Cannon, DVM, DACVD

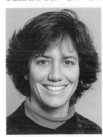

Private Practice, Animal Dermatology and Allergy, Modesto and Loomis, California

Scaling and Crusting Dermatoses

D. N. Carlotti, DVM, DECVD

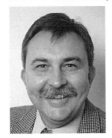

Cabinet de Dermatologie Veterinaire, Bordeaux-Merignac, France

Cutaneous and Subcutaneous Lumps, Bumps, and Masses

Anne E. Chauvet, DVM, DACVIM (Neurol)

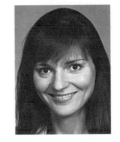

Clinical Instructor, Neurology/Neurosurgery, University of Wisconsin, Madison, Wisconsin

Shivering and Trembling

Brian Keith Collins, DVM, MS, DACVO

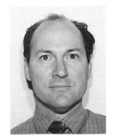

Owner, Animal Eye Specialists, Waukesha, Wisconsin

Neuro-Ophthalmology—Pupils That Teach

Brendan Corcoran, MVB, DPharm, PhD, MRCVS

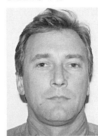

Senior Lecturer and Head of Cardiopulmonary Service, Department of Veterinary Clinical Studies, University of Edinburgh, Edinburgh, Scotland

Clinical Evaluation of the Patient With Respiratory Disease

Etienne Côté, DVM, DACVIM (Cardiol)

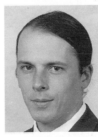

Resident in Internal Medicine, California Animal Hospital, Los Angeles, California; Current: Angell Memorial Hospital, Boston, Massachusetts

Over-the-Counter Pharmaceuticals; Electrocardiography; Antibiotics (CIS)

Susan M. Cotter, DVM, DACVIM (Int Med/Oncol)

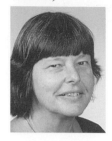

Professor of Medicine and Section Head of Small Animal Medicine, Tufts University School of Veterinary Medicine, North Grafton, Massachusetts

Non-regenerative Anemia

C. Guillermo Couto, DVM, DACVIM

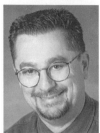

Department of Veterinary Clinical Sciences, College of Veterinary Medicine and Comprehensive Cancer Center, The Ohio State University, Columbus, Ohio

Non-neoplastic Disorders of the Spleen

Larry Cowgill, DVM, PhD, DACVIM

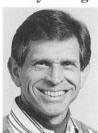

Professor, Department of Medicine and Epidemiology, School of Veterinary Medicine, University of California, Davis; Director, Companion Animal Hemodialysis Unit, Veterinary Medical Teaching Hospital, Davis, California

Acute Renal Failure

Autumn P. Davidson, DVM, DACVIM

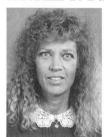

Associate Clinical Professor, University of California, Davis, Davis, California; Veterinarian, Guide Dogs for the Blind, Inc., San Rafael, California

Diseases of the Nose and Nasal Sinuses; Ovarian and Estrous Cycle Abnormalities; Birth Control Alternatives (CIS); Breeding Management of the Bitch (CIS); Whelping in the Bitch (CIS); Dystocia in the Bitch (CIS); Pyometra (CIS)

Susan Dawson, BVMS, PhD

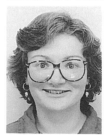

Lecturer, Faculty of Veterinary Science, University of Liverpool, Liverpool, England

FIP-Related Disease

Deborah G. Day, DVM, MS, DACVIM

Internist, Louisville Veterinary Specialty and Emergency Services, Louisville, Kentucky

Indications and Techniques for Liver Biopsy

Linda J. DeBowes, DVM, MS, DACVIM, DAVDC

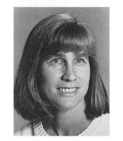

Associate Professor, College of Veterinary Medicine, Kansas State University, Manhattan, Kansas

Ptyalism; Dentistry: Periodontal Aspects

Terese C. DeManuelle, DVM, DACVD

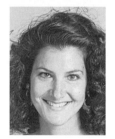

Dermatologist, Animal Allergy and Skin Clinic, Beaverton, Oregon; Adjunct Assistant Professor of Dermatology, Washington State University College of Veterinary Medicine, Pullman, Washington

Canine Demodicosis (CIS): Fleas and Flea Allergy Dermatitis (CIS); Food Hypersensitivity (CIS)

Robert C. DeNovo, Jr., DVM, MS, DACVIM

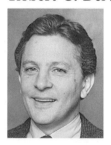

Associate Professor of Medicine, College of Veterinary Medicine, University of Tennessee, Knoxville, Tennessee

Rectoanal Disease

Stephen P. DiBartola, DVM, DACVIM

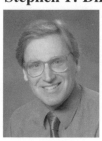

Professor of Medicine, Department of Veterinary Clinical Sciences, College of Veterinary Medicine, Ohio State University; Small Animal Clinician, OSU Veterinary Teaching Hospital, Columbus, Ohio

Clinical Approach and Laboratory Evaluation of Renal Disease; Glomerular Disease; Familial Renal Disease in Dogs and Cats

Ray Dillon, DVM, MS, DACVIM

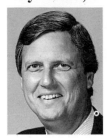

Jack O. Rash Professor of Medicine, Department of Small Animal Surgery and Medicine, College of Veterinary Medicine, Auburn University, Auburn, Alabama

Dirofilariasis in Dogs and Cats

Edward R. Eisner, DVM, DAVDC

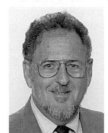

Hospital Director, Campus Veterinary Clinic and Denver Veterinary Dental Service, Denver, Colorado

Dentistry: Endodontic and Restorative Treatment Planning

Hans-Klaus Dreier, DVM

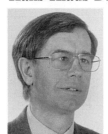

FTA für Kleintiere, Fachteirarzt–Ordination für Kleintiere, Baden, Austria

Vaginal and Preputial Discharge

Denise Ann Elliott, BVSc (Hons), DACVIM

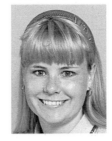

Department of Molecular Biosciences, School of Veterinary Medicine, University of California, Davis; Veterinary Medical Teaching Hospital, University of California, Davis, Davis, California

Acute Renal Failure; Ethylene Glycol Toxicity (Radiator Fluid) (CIS)

Kenneth J. Drobatz, DVM, DACVIM

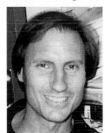

Associate Professor, Critical Care, Department of Clinical Studies, University of Pennsylvania School of Veterinary Medicine; Director, Emergency Service, Veterinary Hospital of the University of Pennsylvania, Philadelphia, Pennsylvania

Pleural Effusion

Annelie Eneroth, DVM

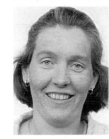

Doctor and PhD student, Department of Obstetrics and Gynaecology, Faculty of Veterinary Medicine, Swedish University of Agricultural Sciences, Uppsala, Sweden

Abnormalities in Pregnancy, Parturition, and the Periparturient Period

Robert DuFort, DVM, DACVIM

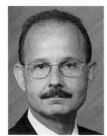

Chief, Internal Medicine, IDEXX Veterinary Services, West Sacramento, California

Abnormal Laboratory Findings (endsheets)

G.C.W. England, BVM, PhD, DVM, DVR, DVRep, FRCVS, DACT

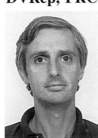

Professor of Veterinary Reproduction, Royal Veterinary College, University of London, Hatfield, Hertfordshire, England

Semen Evaluation, Artificial Insemination, and Infertility in the Male Dog

Joan Dziezyc, DVM, DACVO

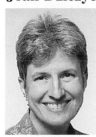

Associate Professor, Department of Small Animal Medicine and Surgery, Texas A&M University College of Veterinary Medicine, College Station, Texas

Red Eye

Bernard F. Feldman, DVM, PhD

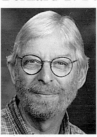

Professor of Veterinary Clinical Hematology and Biochemistry, Department of Biomedical Sciences and Pathobiology, Virginia-Maryland Regional College of Veterinary Medicine, Virginia Polytechnic Institute and State University, Blacksburg, Virginia

Platelets and von Willebrand's Disease; von Willebrand's Disease (CIS)

David G. Feldman, DVM, DACVIM

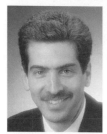

Internal Medicine, California Animal Hospital, Los Angeles, California

Subcutaneous Space Accumulation; Immune-Mediated Arthritis (CIS)

Angela E. Frimberger, VMD, DACVIM (Oncol)

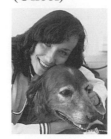

"Our Danny Cancer Fund" Postdoctoral Research Fellow, University of Massachusetts Cancer Center, Worcester, Massachusetts

Principles of Chemotherapy

William R. Fenner, DVM, DACVIM (Neurol)

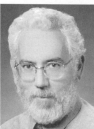

Professor, Veterinary Clinical Sciences, Ohio State University, Columbus, Ohio

Diseases of the Brain

Virgina Luis Fuentes, MA, VetMB, CertVR, DVC, MRCVS

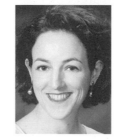

Visiting Lecturer, Veterinary Medical Teaching Hospital, University of Missouri–Columbia, Columbia, Missouri

Echocardiography

Delmar R. Finco, DVM, PhD, DACVIM

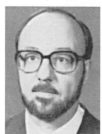

Professor, Department of Physiology, College of Veterinary Medicine, University of Georgia, Athens, Georgia

Dietary Considerations for Urinary Diseases

Rance M. Gamblin, DVM, DACVIM (Oncol)

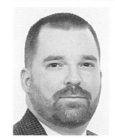

Staff Oncologist, Akron Veterinary Referral and Emergency Center, Akron, Ohio

Non-neoplastic Disorders of the Spleen

Theresa W. Fossum, DVM, MS, PhD, DACVS

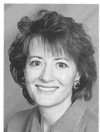

Associate Professor and Chief of Surgery, Department of Small Animal Medicine and Surgery, College of Veterinary Medicine, Texas A&M University, College Station, Texas

Pleural and Extrapleural Diseases; Diseases of the Gallbladder and Extrahepatic Biliary System

Rosalind Gaskell, BVSc, PhD

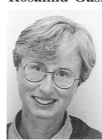

Professor, Faculty of Veterinary Science, University of Liverpool, Liverpool, England

FIP-Related Disease

Philip R. Fox, DVM, MSc, DACVIM and DECVIM (Cardiol), DACVECC

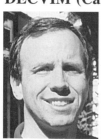

Director, Caspary Research Institute, The Animal Medical Center; Cardiologist, Department of Medicine, Bobst Hospital of The Animal Medical Center, New York, New York

Feline Cardiomyopathies; Peripheral Vascular Disease

Urs Giger, PD, DMV, MS, DACVIM, DECVIM

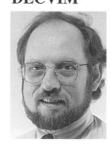

Charlotte Newton Sheppard Professor of Medicine and Chief, Section of Medical Genetics, School of Veterinary Medicine; Professor of Medicine, School of Medicine, University of Pennsylvania, Philadelphia, Pennsylvania; Professor of Small Animal Medicine, University of Zurich, Zurich, Switzerland

Clinical Genetics; Polycythemia; Regenerative Anemias Caused by Blood Loss or Hemolysis

Richard E. Goldstein, DVM, DACVIM

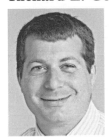

Veterinary Medical and Surgery Group, Ventura, California

Chronic Hepatitis in the Dog (CIS); Hepatic Lipidosis in Cats (CIS)

John-Karl Goodwin, DVM, DACVIM (Cardiol)

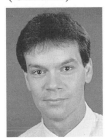

Adjunct Assistant Professor, College of Medicine, Department of Cardiology, University of Florida; Director, Staff Cardiologist, Veterinary Heart Institute, Gainesville, Florida

Pulse Alterations

Jacqueline L. Grandy, DVM

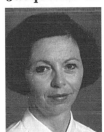

Research Associate, Department of Surgical and Radiological Sciences, School of Veterinary Medicine, University of California, Davis, Davis, California

Diseases of the Spinal Cord

Gregory F. Grauer, DVM, MS, DACVIM

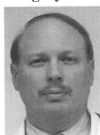

Professor and Section Chief, Small Animal Medicine, Department of Clinical Sciences, and Staff Internist, Veterinary Teaching Hospital, College of Veterinary Medicine and Biomedical Sciences, Colorado State University, Fort Collins, Colorado

Glomerular Disease

Deborah S. Greco, DVM, PhD, DACVIM

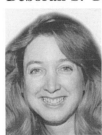

Associate Professor, Colorado State University, Fort Collins, Colorado

Cachexia

Craig E. Greene, DVM, MS, DACVIM (Internal Med and Neurol)

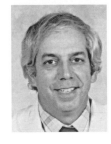

Professor, Department of Small Animal Medicine, College of Veterinary Medicine, University of Georgia, Athens, Georgia

Bacterial Diseases

Michael G. Groves, DVM, MPH, PhD, DACVPM (Epidemiol)

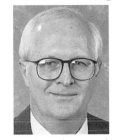

Professor and Department Head, Department of Epidemiology and Community Health, School of Veterinary Medicine, Louisiana State University; Director, Louisiana Veterinary Medical Diagnostic Laboratory, Department of Agriculture, Baton Rouge, Louisiana

Frequently Asked Questions About Zoonoses

W. Grant Guilford, BVSc, BPhil, PhD, DACVIM (Int Med)

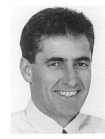

Head, Institute of Veterinary, Animal, and Biomedical Sciences, Massey University, Palmerston North, New Zealand

Melena and Hematochezia; Flatulence and Borborygmus; Adverse Reactions to Foods: Allergies Versus Intolerance; Flatulence (CIS); Gastric Dilatation–Volvulus (CIS)

Lynn Guptill-Yoran, DVM, PhD, DACVIM

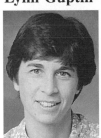

Assistant Professor, Purdue University, West Lafayette, Indiana

Hypothyroidism

Jens Häggström, DVM, PhD, DECVIM (Cardiol)

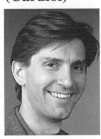

Assistant Professor, Department of Animal Physiology, Faculty of Veterinary Medicine, University of Agricultural Sciences, Uppsala, Sweden

Acquired Valvular Heart Disease

Edward J. Hall, MA, VETMB, PhD, DECVIM, MRCVS

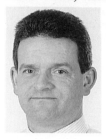

Lecturer in Small Animal Internal Medicine, Department of Clinical Veterinary Science, University of Bristol, Langford, Bristol, England

Diseases of the Small Intestine

Jean A. Hall, DVM, MS, PhD, DACVIM

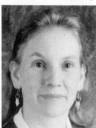

Assistant Professor, College of Veterinary Medicine, Oregon State University, Corvallis, Oregon

Diseases of the Stomach

Holly L. Hamilton, DVM, MS, DACVO

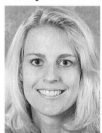

Assistant Professor, Veterinary Clinical Sciences, School of Veterinary Medicine, Louisiana State University, Baton Rouge, Louisiana

Acute Vision Loss

Marcella F. Harb-Hauser, DVM, DACVIM

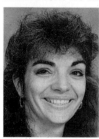

Private Practice, San Rafael, California

Managing PEG Tubes and Feeding Tubes (CIS)

Elizabeth M. Hardie, DVM, PhD

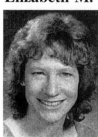

Professor, Small Animal Surgery, North Carolina State University College of Veterinary Medicine, Raleigh, North Carolina

Pain: Management

Kathleen S. Harrington, MS

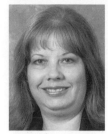

Veterinary Laboratory Specialist II, Department of Epidemiology and Community Health, School of Veterinary Medicine, Louisiana State University, Baton Rouge, Louisiana

Frequently Asked Questions About Zoonoses

Andreas H. Hasler, DMV, DACVIM, DECVIM-CA

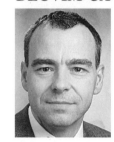

Tieraerztliches Überweisungszentrum, Tenniken, Switzerland

Polycythemia

Eleanor C. Hawkins, DVM, DACVIM

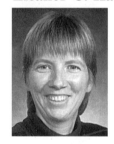

Associate Professor of Medicine, College of Veterinary Medicine, and Internist, Veterinary Teaching Hospital, North Carolina State University, Raleigh, North Carolina

Pulmonary Parenchymal Diseases

Joan C. Hendricks, VMD, PhD, DACVIM

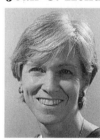

Professor and Chief, Section of Critical Care, Department of Clinical Studies, School of Veterinary Medicine, University of Pennsylvania, Philadelphia, Pennsylvania

Sleep Disorders

Ann E. Hohenhaus, DVM, DACVIM (Oncol, Int Med)

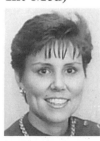

Chairman, Department of Medicine, and Head, George Jaqua Transfusion Medicine Service, The Bobst Hospital of the Animal Medical Center, New York, New York

Blood Banking and Transfusion Medicine

Johnny D. Hoskins, DVM, PhD, DACVIM

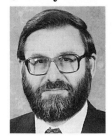

Professor Emeritus, Department of Veterinary Clinical Sciences, Louisiana State University, School of Veterinary Medicine, Baton Rouge, Louisiana

Neonatal and Pediatric Nutrition; Canine Viral Diseases; Congenital Defects of the Cat; Congenital Defects of the Dog

Katherine A. Houpt, VMD, PhD, DACVB

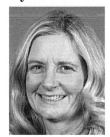

Professor of Physiology, College of Veterinary Medicine, Cornell University; Animal Behavior Clinic, Ithaca, New York

Behavioral Disorders

Lynn Rolland Hovda, DVM, MS, DACVIM

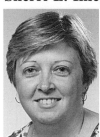

Director, Veterinary Toxicology, Prosar, St. Paul, Minnesota

Common Plant Toxicities

Sherri L. Ihle, DVM, MS, DACVIM

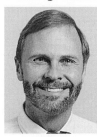

Associate Professor, Department of Companion Animals, Atlantic Veterinary College, University of Prince Edward Island, Charlottetown, Prince Edward Island, Canada

Failure to Grow

Peter J. Ihrke, VMD, DACVD

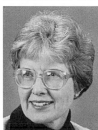

Professor of Dermatology, Department of Medicine and Epidemiology; and Chief, Dermatology Service, Veterinary Medicine Teaching Hospital, School of Veterinary Medicine, University of California, Davis; Adjunct Clinical Associate Professor, School of Medicine, Stanford University, Stanford, California

Pruritus

Karen Dyer Inzana, DVM, PhD, DACVIM (Neurol)

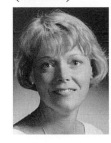

Associate Professor, Virginia-Maryland Regional College of Veterinary Medicine, Virginia Polytechnic Institute and State University, Blacksburg, Virginia

Peripheral Nerve Disorders

Frédéric Jacob, DVM

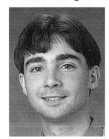

Resident, Internal Medicine and Clinical Nutrition, College of Veterinary Medicine, University of Minnesota, St. Paul, Minnesota

Chronic Renal Failure

Luc A.A. Janssens, DMV, PhD, DECVS, CVA

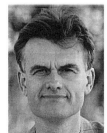

Private Practice, Antwerp, Belgium

Acupuncture in Small Animal Practice

Christine C. Jenkins, DVM, DACVIM

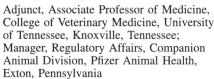

Adjunct, Associate Professor of Medicine, College of Veterinary Medicine, University of Tennessee, Knoxville, Tennessee; Manager, Regulatory Affairs, Companion Animal Division, Pfizer Animal Health, Exton, Pennsylvania

Dysphagia and Regurgitation

Albert E. Jergens, DVM, MS, DACVIM

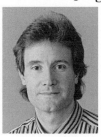

Staff Internist and Associate Professor, Department of Veterinary Clinical Sciences, Iowa State University College of Veterinary Medicine, Ames, Iowa

Diseases of the Large Intestine; Colitis (CIS); Non-Neoplastic Infiltrative Bowel Diseases (CIS)

Kenneth A. Johnson, MVSc, PhD, FACVSc, MRCVS, DACVS, DECVS

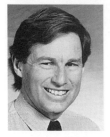

Professor of Companion Animal Studies, University of Bristol, Department of Clinical Veterinary Science, Langford, Bristol, United Kingdom

Skeletal Diseases

Lynelle Johnson, DVM, MS, DACVIM

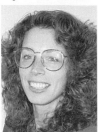

Research Assistant Professor, University of Missouri—Columbia, Department of Veterinary Biomedical Sciences, Columbia, Missouri

Diseases of the Bronchus

Susan E. Johnson, DVM, MS, DACVIM

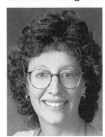

Associate Professor, Department of Veterinary Clinical Sciences, College of Veterinary Medicine, The Ohio State University; Internist, OSU Veterinary Teaching Hospital, Columbus, Ohio

Chronic Hepatic Disorders

Spencer A. Johnston, VMD, DACVS

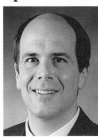

Associate Professor, Department of Small Animal Clinical Sciences, Virginia-Maryland Regional College of Veterinary Medicine, Virginia Polytechnic Institute and State University, Blacksburg, Virginia

Pain: Identification

Brent D. Jones, DVM

Associate Professor, Veterinary Medicine and Surgery, Veterinary Teaching Hospital, University of Missouri–Columbia, Columbia, Missouri

Constipation, Tenesmus, Dyschezia, and Fecal Incontinence

Brett Kantrowitz, DVM, DACVR

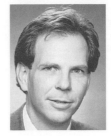

Veterinary Diagnostic Imaging, Ojai, California

Diseases of the Trachea

Bruce W. Keene, DVM, MSc, DACVIM (Cardiol)

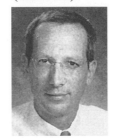

Associate Professor of Cardiology, College of Veterinary Medicine, North Carolina State University, Raleigh, North Carolina

Primary Myocardial Disease in the Dog

Rebecca Kirby, DVM, DACVIM, DACVECC

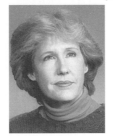

Adjunct Professor, University of Wisconsin, Madison, Veterinary Medical Teaching Hospital, Department of Surgery, Madison; Director of Education, Animal Emergency Center and Referral Services, Milwaukee, Wisconsin

Fluid Therapy, Electrolytes, and Acid-Base Control

Mark D. Kittleson, DVM, PhD, DACVIM (Cardiol)

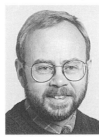

Professor, Department of Medicine and Epidemiology, School of Veterinary Medicine, and Associate Director, Small Animal Clinic, Veterinary Medical Teaching Hospital, University of California, Davis, Davis, California

Therapy of Heart Failure

Jeffrey S. Klausner, DVM, MS, DACVIM (Internal Med, Oncol)

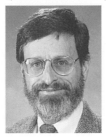

Professor and Interim Dean, College of Veterinary Medicine, University of Minnesota, St. Paul, Minnesota

Prostatic Diseases

Deborah W. Knapp, DVM, MS, DACVIM (Oncol)

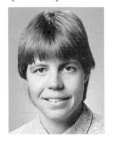

Associate Professor of Comparative Oncology, Department of Veterinary Clinical Sciences, Purdue University, West Lafayette, Indiana

Tumors of the Urogenital System and Mammary Glands; Canine Mammary Tumors (CIS)

Donald R. Krawiec, DVM, MS, PhD, DACVIM

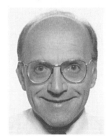

Staff Internist, North County Speciality Animal Hospital; Hospital Director, North County Emergency Animal Clinic/ Speciality Animal Hospital, San Marcos, California

Proteinuria

Philip Koblik, DVM, MS, DACVR

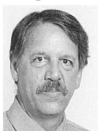

Professor, Department of Surgical and Radiological Sciences, School of Veterinary Medicine, University of California, Davis, Davis, California

Diseases of the Nose and Nasal Sinuses

John M. Kruger, DVM, PhD, DACVIM

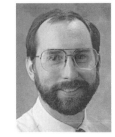

Associate Professor, Michigan State University College of Veterinary Medicine, East Lansing, Michigan

Feline Lower Urinary Tract Disorders

Gary J. Kociba, DVM, PhD, DACVP

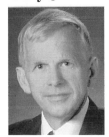

Professor, Veterinary Biosciences, The Ohio State University, and Clinical Pathologist, OSU Veterinary Teaching Hospital, Columbus, Ohio

Leukocyte Changes in Disease

Stephen A. Kruth, DVM, DACVIM

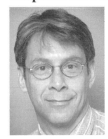

Professor and Chair, Department of Clinical Studies, Ontario Veterinary College, University of Guelph, Guelph, Ontario, Canada

Abdominal Distention, Ascites, and Peritonitis

Mark J. Kopit, DVM

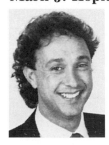

Director, Veterinary Diagnostic Service, Orange, California

Gagging

Gail A. Kunkle, DVM, DACVD

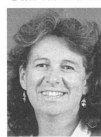

Professor, Department of Small Animal Clinical Sciences, and Service Chief, Dermatology, College of Veterinary Medicine, University of Florida, Gainesville, Florida

Alopecia

Susan A. Kraegel, DVM, DACVIM (Oncol)

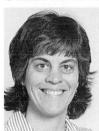

Oncologist, Special Veterinary Services, Berkeley, California

Tumors of the Skin; Chemotherapy (CIS); Lymphoma (CIS); Osteosarcoma (CIS); Vaccine-Induced Sarcoma in Cats (CIS)

Lisa K. Kurosky, DVM, DACVIM

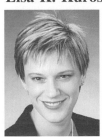

Associate Veterinarian, California Animal Hospital, Los Angeles, California

Abnormalities of Magnesium, Calcium, and Chloride

Margaret V. Root Kustritz, DVM, PhD, DACV (Theriogenol)

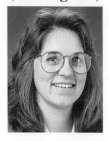

Assistant Clinical Specialist, Small Animal Reproduction, University of Minnesota, College of Veterinary Medicine, St. Paul, Minnesota

Early Spay and Neuter; Prostatic Diseases; Whelping in the Bitch (CIS)

Clarence Kvart, DVM, PhD

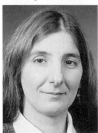

Associate Professor, Department of Animal Physiology, Faculty of Veterinary Medicine, University of Agricultural Sciences, Uppsala, Sweden

Acquired Valvular Heart Disease

Mary Anna Labato, DVM, DACVIM

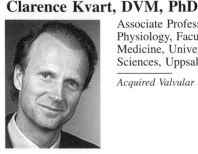

Clinical Associate Professor, Department of Clinical Sciences, and Staff Veterinarian, Foster Hospital for Small Animals, Tufts University School of Veterinary Medicine, North Grafton, Massachusetts

Cardiopulmonary Arrest and Resuscitation

India F. Lane, DVM, MS, DACVIM

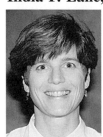

Assistant Professor and Clinical Internist, Department of Small Animal Clinical Sciences, University of Tennessee College of Veterinary Medicine, Knoxville, Tennessee

Urinary Obstruction and Functional Urine Retention

Michael R. Lappin, DVM, PhD, DACVIM

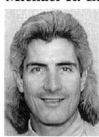

Associate Professor, Department of Clinical Sciences, College of Veterinary Medicine and Biomedical Sciences, Colorado State University, Fort Collins, Colorado

Protozoal and Miscellaneous Infections

Gérard Le Bobinnec, DVM, DECVIM (Cardiol)

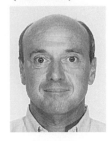

In charge of courses of Cardiology at the Veterinary School of Nantes, France

Electrocardiography

Richard A. LeCouteur, BVSc, PhD, DACVIM (Neurol)

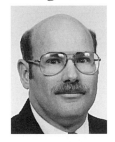

Professor, Department of Surgical and Radiological Sciences, School of Veterinary Medicine, University of California, Davis, Davis, California

Diseases of the Spinal Cord; Disc Disease (CIS)

George E. Lees, DVM, MS, DACVIM

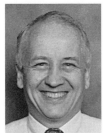

Professor of Internal Medicine, Small Animal Medicine and Surgery, College of Veterinary Medicine, Texas A&M University, College Station, Texas

Incontinence, Enuresis, Dysuria, and Nocturia

Alfred M. Legendre, DVM, DACVIM (Oncol)

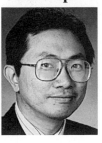

Professor of Medicine, University of Tennessee, Knoxville, Knoxville, Tennessee

Pneumonia (CIS); Feline Immunodeficiency Virus (CIS); Feline Leukemia Virus Vaccinations in Cats (CIS); Parvovirus in Dogs (CIS); Canine Distemper (CIS)

Chalermpol Lekcharoensuk, DVM

Research Associate, Department of Small Animal Clinical Sciences, College of Veterinary Medicine, University of Minnesota, St. Paul, Minnesota

Feline Lower Urinary Tract Disorders; Canine Lower Urinary Tract Disorders

Cynthia R. Leveille-Webster, BS, DVM, DACVIM

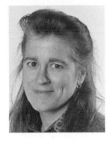

Assistant Professor, Tufts University School of Veterinary Medicine, North Grafton, Massachusetts

Laboratory Diagnosis of Hepatobiliary Disease

Julie K. Levy, DVM, PhD, DACVIM

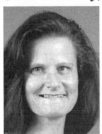

Assistant Professor, College of Veterinary Medicine, University of Florida, Gainesville, Florida

FeLV and Non-Neoplastic FeLV-Related Disease

Catharina Linde-Forsberg, DVM, PhD

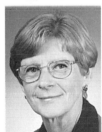

Associate Professor of Small Animal Reproduction, Department of Obstetrics and Gynaecology, Faculty of Veterinary Medicine, Swedish University of Agricultural Sciences, Uppsala, Sweden

Abnormalities in Pregnancy, Parturition, and the Periparturient Period

Gerald V. Ling, DVM

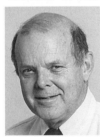

Professor, Department of Medicine and Epidemiology, School of Veterinary Medicine and Veterinary Medical Teaching Hospital, University of California, Davis, Davis, California

Bacterial Infections of the Urinary Tract; Chronic and/or Recurrent Urinary Tract Infections (CIS)

David Lipsitz, DVM, DACVIM (Neurol)

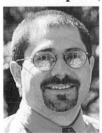

Clinical Assistant Professor, Department of Medical Sciences, University of Wisconsin—Madison, Madison, Wisconsin

Shivering and Trembling

Meryl P. Littman, VMD, DACVIM

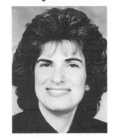

Associate Professor of Medicine, University of Pennsylvania School of Veterinary Medicine, Philadelphia, Pennsylvania

Hypertension

M. J. Lommer, DVM

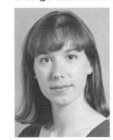

Clinician, Veterinary Medical Teaching Hospital, School of Veterinary Medicine, University of California, Davis, Davis, California

Dental Disease in Dogs and Cats (CIS)

Cheryl London, DVM, DACVIM (Oncol)

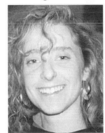

Assistant Professor, School of Veterinary Medicine, Department of Surgery and Radiological Sciences, University of California, Davis, Davis, California

Tumor Biology

Jody P. Lulich, DVM, PhD, DACVIM

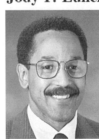

Associate Professor, College of Veterinary Medicine, University of Minnesota, St. Paul, Minnesota

Feline Lower Urinary Tract Diseases; Canine Lower Urinary Tract Disorders

Patricia J. Luttgen, DVM, MS, DACVIM (Neurol)

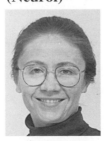

Neurological Center for Animals, Denver, Colorado

Diseases of the Ear

John M. MacDonald, DVM, DACVD

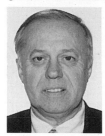

Professor, College of Veterinary Medicine, Auburn University, Auburn, Alabama

Glucocorticoid Therapy

Orla M. Mahony, MVB, MRCVS, DACVIM, DECVIM

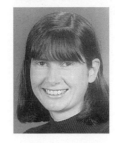

Clinical Assistant Professor, Department of Small Animal Clinical Sciences, Tufts University, School of Veterinary Medicine, North Grafton, Massachusetts

Bleeding Disorders: Epistaxis and Hemoptysis

Douglass K. Macintire, DVM, MS, DACVIM

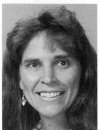

Associate Professor in Medicine and Co-Director, Critical Care Ward, Auburn University College of Veterinary Medicine, Auburn University, Alabama

Hypotension

Stanley L. Marks, BVSc, PhD, DACVIM (Int Med, Oncol), DACVN

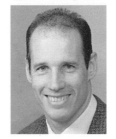

Assistant Professor, Department of Medicine and Epidemiology, and Chief, Nutrition Support Service, School of Veterinary Medicine, University of California, Davis, Davis, California

Enteral and Parenteral Nutritional Support

Jill Maddison, BVSc, PhD, FACVSc

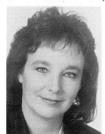

Senior Lecturer in Pharmacology, Department of Pharmacology, University of Sydney, New South Wales, Australia

Adverse Drug Reactions

Ian S. Mason, BVM, PhD, CSAD, DECVD, MRCVS

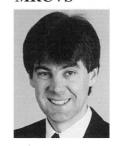

Principal, Veterinary Dermatology Consultants, Sunbury on Thames, Middlesex, United Kingdom

Erosions and Ulcerations

Bruce R. Madewell, VMD, MS, DACVIM

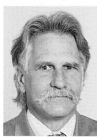

Professor, Department of Surgical and Radiological Sciences, and Chief, Oncology Service, Veterinary Medical Teaching Hospital, School of Veterinary Medicine, University of California, Davis, Davis, California

Tumors of the Skin

Kyle G. Mathews, DVM, MS, DACVS

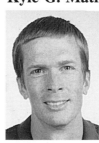

Assistant Professor, Small Animal Surgery, Department of Companion Animal and Special Species Medicine, North Carolina State University, College of Veterinary Medicine, Raleigh, North Carolina

Diseases of the Nose and Nasal Sinuses

Michael L. Magne, DVM, MS, DACVIM

Staff Internist, Animal Care Center of Sonoma County, Rohnert Park, California

Swollen Joints and Lameness

Brendan C. McKiernan, DVM, DACVIM

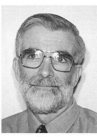

Staff Internist, Denver Veterinary Specialists, Wheat Ridge Veterinary Hospital, Wheat Ridge, Colorado

Sneezing and Nasal Discharge

Susan A. McLaughlin, DVM, MS, DACVD

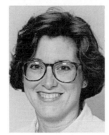

Associate Professor, Department of Small Animal Surgery and Medicine, College of Veterinary Medicine, Auburn University, Auburn, Alabama

Acute Vision Loss

W. Duane Mickelsen, DVM, MS, DACT

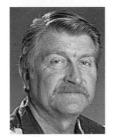

Professor (Emeritus), Theriogenology, Department of Veterinary Clinical Sciences, College of Veterinary Medicine, Washington State University, Pullman, Washington

Inherited and Congenital Disorders of the Male and Female Reproductive Systems

Mushtaq A. Memon, BVSc, PhD, DACT

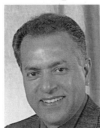

Associate Professor, Theriogenology, Department of Veterinary Clinical Sciences, College of Veterinary Medicine, Washington State University, Pullman, Washington

Inherited and Congenital Disorders of the Male and Female Reproductive Systems

James B. Miller, DVM, MS, DACVIM (Int Med)

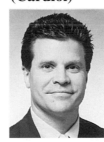

Professor, Department of Companion Animals, and Service Chief, Veterinary Teaching Hospital (Small Animal Medicine), Atlantic Veterinary College, University of Prince Edward Island, Charlottetown, Prince Edward Island, Canada

Hyperthermia and Hypothermia

Sandra Merchant, DVM, DACVD

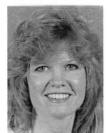

Department of Clinical Sciences, School of Veterinary Medicine, Louisiana State University, Baton Rouge, Louisiana

Canine Atopic Dermatitis (CIS); Otitis Externa (CIS)

Matthew W. Miller, DVM, MS, DACVIM (Cardiol)

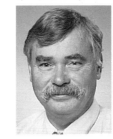

Associate Professor, Department of Small Animal Medicine and Surgery, College of Veterinary Medicine, Texas A & M University, College Station, Texas

Pericardial Disorders

Hein P. Meyer, DVM, PhD

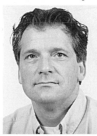

Assistant Professor, Internal Medicine and Nephrology of Companion Animals, Department of Clinical Sciences of Companion Animals, Faculty of Veterinary Medicine, University of Utrecht, Utrecht, The Netherlands

History, Physical Examination, and Signs of Liver Disease

Kathryn E. Michel, DVM, MS, DACVN

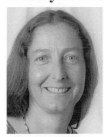

Clinical Assistant Professor of Nutrition, Department of Clinical Studies, School of Veterinary Medicine, University of Pennsylvania, Philadelphia, Pennsylvania

Nutritional Management of Gastrointestinal, Hepatic, and Endocrine Diseases

William E. Monroe, DVM, MS, DACVIM

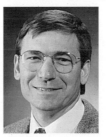

Associate Professor of Small Animal Medicine, Department of Small Animal Clinical Sciences, Virginia-Maryland Regional College of Veterinary Medicine, Virginia Polytechnic Institute and State University, Blacksburg, Virginia

Anorexia

Antony S. Moore, BVSc, MVSc, DACVIM (Oncol)

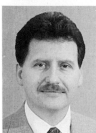

Associate Professor of Medicine/Oncology, Tufts University School of Veterinary Medicine, North Grafton, Massachusetts

Principles of Chemotherapy

Cecil P. Moore, DVM, MS, DACVO

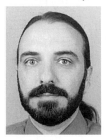

Professor and Acting Chairman, Department of Veterinary Medicine and Surgery; Chief, Ophthalmology Service, and Acting Director, Veterinary Medical Teaching Hospital, College of Veterinary Medicine, University of Missouri, Columbia, Missouri

Ocular Manifestations of Systemic Diseases

Helio Autran de Morais, DVM, PhD, DACVIM (Int Med, Cardiol)

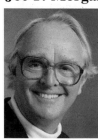

Associate Professor and Department Chair, Departamento de Clínicas Veterinárias, Universidade Estadual de Londrina; Internist/Cardiologist, Hospital Veterinário, Universidade Estadual de Londrina, Londrina, Paraná, Brazil

Pathophysiology of Heart Failure and Clinical Evaluation of Cardiac Function

Joe P. Morgan, DVM, DACVR

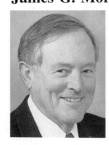

Professor Emeritus, Department of Surgical and Radiological Sciences, School of Veterinary Medicine, University of California, Davis, Davis, California

Joint Diseases of Dogs and Cats

James G. Morris, PhD, DACVN

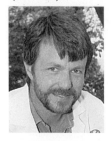

Professor, School of Veterinary Medicine, University of California, Davis, Davis, California

Nutrition of Healthy Dogs and Cats in Various Stages of Adult Life

Richard W. Nelson, DVM, DACVIM

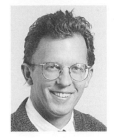

Professor, Department of Medicine and Epidemiology, School of Veterinary Medicine, University of California, Davis, Davis, California

Insulin-Secreting Islet Cell Neoplasia; Diabetes Mellitus

Steven S. Nicholson, DVM, DACVIM (Toxicol)

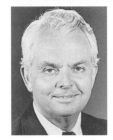

Associate Professor, Veterinary Toxicology, School of Veterinary Medicine, Louisiana State University, Baton Rouge, Louisiana

Toxicology

Carol Norris, DVM, DACVIM

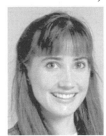

Clinician, Veterinary Medical Teaching Hospital, School of Veterinary Medicine, University of California, Davis, Davis, California

Feline Bronchitis ("Feline Asthma") (CIS); Immune-Mediated Hemolytic Anemia and Immune-Mediated Thrombocytopenia (CIS)

Gregory K. Ogilvie, DVM, DACVIM

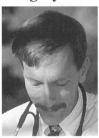

Professor, Medical Oncologist, and Internist, Head of the Medical Oncology Research Laboratory, College of Veterinary Medicine and Biomedical Sciences, Colorado State University, Fort Collins, Colorado

Paraneoplastic Syndromes; Complementary/ Alternative Cancer Therapy—Fact or Fiction?

Thierry Olivry, Dr-Vet, PhD, DACVD, DECVD

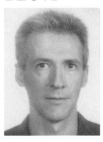

Assistant Professor of Dermatology, College of Veterinary Medicine, North Carolina State University, Raleigh; Adjunct Clinical Assistant Professor of Dermatology, School of Medicine, University of North Carolina, Chapel Hill, North Carolina

Scaling and Crusting Dermatoses

Patricia N. Olson, DVM, PhD, DACVT

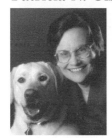

Director of Training Operations, Guide Dogs for the Blind, Inc., San Rafael, California

Early Spay and Neuter

Theresa Ortega, DVM, DACVIM

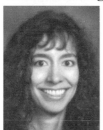

Veterinary Medical and Surgery Group, Ventura, California

Managing PEG Tubes and Feeding Tubes (CIS)

Carl A. Osborne, DVM, PhD, DACVIM

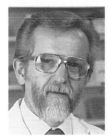

Professor, Department of Small Animal Clinical Sciences, College of Veterinary Medicine, University of Minnesota, St. Paul, Minnesota

Chronic Renal Failure; Feline Lower Urinary Tract Diseases; Canine Lower Urinary Tract Disorders; Urinary Stones: Cause; Treatment; Prevention (CIS); Does Your Cat Have Lower Urinary Tract Disease? (CIS)

Rodney L. Page, MS, DVM, DACVIM (Internal Med, Oncol)

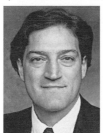

Professor of Medical Oncology, College of Veterinary Medicine, North Carolina State University, Raleigh, North Carolina

Soft Tissue Sarcomas and Hemangiosarcomas

Mark G. Papich, DVM, MS, DACVCP

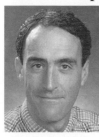

Associate Professor of Clinical Pharmacology and Clinical Pharmacologist and Supervisor of Clinical Pharmacology Laboratory, Veterinary Teaching Hospital, College of Veterinary Medicine, North Carolina State University, Raleigh, North Carolina

Antimicrobial Drugs

Joane M.L. Parent, DMV, MVetSc, DACVIM (Neurol)

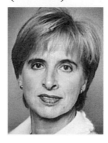

Professor, Department of Veterinary Clinical Studies, Ontario Veterinary College, University of Guelph, Guelph, Ontario, Canada

Ataxia, Paresis, and Paralysis

Niels C. Pedersen, DVM, PhD

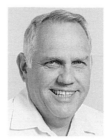

Professor, Department of Medicine and Epidemiology, School of Veterinary Medicine, University of California, Davis, Davis, California

Joint Diseases of Dogs and Cats

Yonatan Peres, DVM

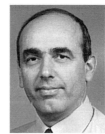

Clinician, Director, Veterinary Teaching Hospital, and Director, Emergency and Critical Care Unit, Hebrew University of Jerusalem, Koret School of Veterinary Medicine, Rehovot, Israel

Hyponatremia and Hypokalemia

Mark E. Peterson, DVM, DACVIM

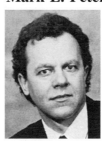

Head, Division of Endocrinology, Department of Medicine, Bobst Hospital; Associate Director, Caspary Research Institute, The Animal Medical Center, New York, New York

Hyperthyroidism

Jean-Paul Petrie, DVM, DACVIM (Cardiol)

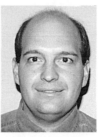

Department of Medicine, Bobst Hospital of The Animal Medical Center, New York, New York

Peripheral Vascular Disease

Tom R. Phillips, DVM, MS, PhD

Assistant Professor, Department of Neuropharmacology, The Scripps Research Institute, La Jolla, California

FIV and FIV-Related Disease

Ilana R. Reisner, DVM, DACVB

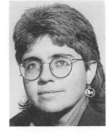

Private Practice, Animal Behavior Clinic, Ithaca, New York

Behavioral Disorders

Michael Podell, MSc, DVM, DACVIM (Neurol)

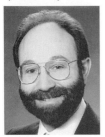

Associate Professor, Department of Veterinary Clinical Sciences, College of Veterinary Medicine; Member, Comprehensive Cancer Center, The James Cancer Hospital, The Ohio State University, Columbus, Ohio

Neurologic Manifestations of Systemic Disease; Seizures (CIS)

George P. Reppas, BVSc(Hons), DipVetPath

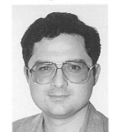

Registered Specialist Veterinary Pathologist, Horsley Park, New South Wales, Australia

Diagnostic Cytology of Skin Lesions

David J. Polzin, DVM, PhD, DACVIM

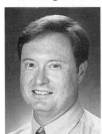

Professor, College of Veterinary Medicine, University of Minnesota, St. Paul, Minnesota

Chronic Renal Failure; Feline Lower Urinary Tract Diseases; Chronic Renal Failure (CIS)

Claudia E. Reusch, DMV, PhD, DECVIM-CA

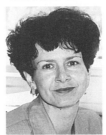

Professor for Internal Veterinary Medicine of Small Animals, Faculty of Veterinary Medicine, and Clinic Director, Clinic for Small Animal Internal Medicine, University of Zurich, Zurich, Switzerland

Hypoadrenocorticism

Beverly J. Purswell, DVM, PhD, DACVT

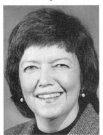

Associate Professor, Virginia-Maryland Regional College of Veterinary Medicine, Virginia Polytechnic Institute and State University, Blacksburg, Virginia

Vaginal Disorders

Daniel C. Richardson, DVM, DACVS

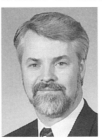

Adjunct Professor, Surgery, North Carolina State University, Raleigh, North Carolina, and Kansas State University, Manhattan, Kansas; Director of Research, Hill's Pet Nutrition, Inc., Topeka, Kansas

Developmental Orthopedic Disease of Dogs

Andrée D. Quesnel, DVM, DVSc, DACVIM (Neurol)

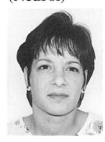

Assistant Professor, Faculté de Médecine Vétérinaire, University of Montreal, St. Hyacinthe, Québec, Canada

Seizures

Ad Rijnberk, DVM, PhD, DECVIM

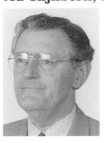

Professor of Companion Animal Medicine, Faculty of Veterinary Medicine, Utrecht, Utrecht, The Netherlands

Acromegaly; Diabetes Insipidus

Narda G. Robinson, DO, DVM

Affiliate Faculty, Department of Clinical Sciences, and Course Director for Acupuncture Training Programs, Colorado State University, College of Veterinary Medicine and Biomedical Sciences; Director of Complementary Medicine Service, Colorado State University Veterinary Teaching Hospital; Private practice in human acupuncture and osteopathic medicine, Fort Collins, Colorado

Complementary/Alternative Cancer Therapy—Fact or Fiction?

Kenita S. Rogers, DVM, MS, DACVIM

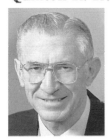

Associate Professor, Department of Small Animal Medicine and Surgery, College of Veterinary Medicine, and Staff Oncologist, Texas Veterinary Medical Center, Texas A&M University, College Station, Texas

Anemia

Quinton R. Rogers, PhD, DACVN

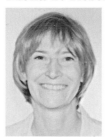

Professor, School of Veterinary Medicine, University of California, Davis, Davis, California

Nutrition of Healthy Dogs and Cats in Various Stages of Adult Life

Mona P. Rosenberg, DVM, DACVIM

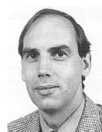

Veterinary Cancer Referral Group, Corona del Mar, California

Hemangiosarcoma in the Dog (CIS); Mast Cell Tumors in Dogs (CIS)

Sheri J. Ross, DVM, BSc

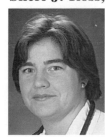

Resident in Internal Medicine and Clinical Nutrition, College of Veterinary Medicine, University of Minnesota, St. Paul, Minnesota

Chronic Renal Failure

Edmund J. Rosser, Jr., DVM, DACVD

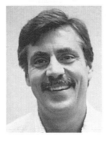

Professor of Dermatology, Michigan State University, College of Veterinary Medicine, Department of Small Animal Clinical Sciences, Veterinary Medical Center, East Lansing, Michigan

Pustules and Papules

Rod A. W. Rosychuk, DVM, DACVIM

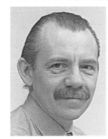

Assistant Professor, Department of Clinical Sciences, Colorado State University, Fort Collins, Colorado

Diseases of the Ear

Jan Rothuizen, DVM, PhD

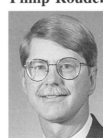

Associate Professor, Internal Medicine, and Hepatology of Companion Animals, Department of Clinical Sciences of Companion Animals, Faculty of Veterinary Medicine, University of Utrecht, Utrecht, The Netherlands

Jaundice; History, Physical Examination, and Signs of Liver Disease

Philip Roudebush, DVM, DACVIM

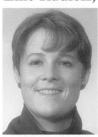

Adjunct Professor, College of Veterinary Medicine, Kansas State University, Manhattan, Kansas; Veterinary Fellow, Hill's Science and Technology Center, Topeka, Kansas

Adverse Reactions to Foods: Allergies Versus Intolerance

Elke Rudloff, DVM, DACVECC

Director of Medical Services, Animal Emergency Center and Referral Services, Milwaukee, Wisconsin

Fluid Therapy, Electrolytes, and Acid-Base Control

Rafael Ruiz de Gopegui, DVM, PhD

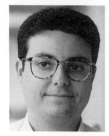

Assistant Professor, Department of Pathology and Animal Production, Veterinary Faculty, Autonomous University of Barcelona, Barcelona, Spain

Platelets and von Willebrand's Disease; von Willebrand's Disease (CIS)

John E. Saidla, DVM

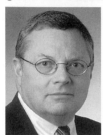

Senior Lecturer, College of Veterinary Medicine, and Chief, Dental Services, Veterinary Medicine Teaching Hospital, College of Veterinary Medicine, Cornell University, Ithaca, New York

Dentistry—Genetic, Environmental, and Other Considerations

Auke C. Schaefers-Okkens, DVM, PhD

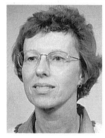

Assistant Professor, Theriogenology, Faculty of Veterinary Medicine, Department of Clinical Sciences of Companion Animals, University of Utrecht, Utrecht, The Netherlands

Estrous Cycle and Breeding Management of the Healthy Bitch

Michael Schaer, DVM, DACVIM, DACVECC

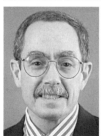

Professor of Internal Medicine and Associate Department Chairman; Service Chief, Small Animal Medicine, University of Florida College of Veterinary Medicine, Gainesville, Florida

Hyperkalemia and Hypernatremia

Bradley R. Schmidt, DVM, DACVIM (Oncol)

Animal Hospital Center, Highlands Ranch, Colorado

Tumors of the Urogenital and Mammary Glands

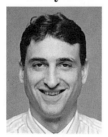

J. Catharine R. Scott-Moncrieff, MA, VetMB, MS, DACVIM

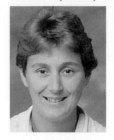

Associate Professor, Purdue University, West Lafayette, Indiana

Hypothyroidism; Canine Hypothyroidism (CIS)

Linda Shell, DVM, DACVIM (Neurol)

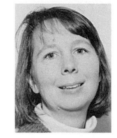

Professor, Virginia-Maryland Regional College of Veterinary Medicine, Virginia Polytechnic Institute and State University, Department of Small Animal Clinical Sciences, Blacksburg, Virginia

Altered States of Consciousness: Coma and Stupor

Kenneth W. Simpson, DVM, PhD, DACVIM

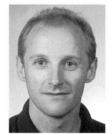

Assistant Professor of Medicine, Department of Clinical Sciences, College of Veterinary Medicine, Cornell University, Ithaca, New York

Diseases of the Small Intestine

D. David Sisson, DVM, DACVIM (Cardiol)

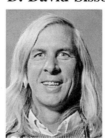

Director of the Cardiology Service, Associate Professor of Cardiovascular Medicine, College of Veterinary Medicine, University of Illinois, Urbana, Illinois

Congenital Heart Disease; Primary Myocardial Disease in the Dog; Pericardial Disorders

Mark M. Smith, VMD, DACVS, DAVDC

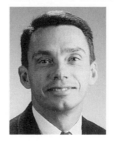

Professor, Department of Small Animal Sciences, Comparative Oral Research Laboratory, Virginia-Maryland Regional College of Veterinary Medicine, Virginia Polytechnic Institute and State University, Blacksburg, Virginia

Oral and Salivary Gland Disorders; Solar-Induced Squamous Cell Carcinoma in Cats (CIS)

Anthony A. Stannard (deceased), DVM, PhD, DACVD

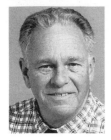

Late Chairman of Department of Medicine and Epidemiology and Professor of Veterinary Medicine-Dermatology, Department of Medicine, School of Veterinary Medicine, University of California, Davis, Davis, California

Scaling and Crusting Dermatoses

Rebecca L. Stepien, DVM, MS, DACVIM (Cardiol)

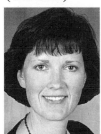

Clinical Assistant Professor, Department of Medical Sciences, University of Wisconsin School of Veterinary Medicine, and Clinical Cardiologist, University of Wisconsin Veterinary Medical Teaching Hospital, Madison, Wisconsin

Cyanosis

Rodney C. Straw, BVSc, DACVS

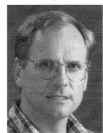

Honorary Reader, Companion Animal Clinical Sciences, School of Veterinary Science and Animal Production; Specialist in Surgical Oncology and Director, Animal Cancer Care Pty Ltd, University of Queensland, Brisbane, Australia

Bone and Joint Tumors

Peter F. Suter, DMV, DACVR

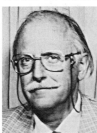

Professor Emeritus of Internal Medicine, Veterinary Medical Faculty, University of Zurich, Zurich, Switzerland

Peripheral Vascular Disease

Joseph Taboada, DVM, DACVIM

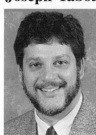

Professor and Director of Professional Instruction and Curriculum, School of Veterinary Medicine, Louisiana State University, Baton Rouge, Louisiana

Frequently Asked Questions About Zoonoses; Systemic Mycoses

Todd R. Tams, DVM, DACVIM

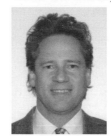

Chief Medical Officer, Veterinary Centers of America; Staff Internist, VCA West Los Angeles Animal Hospital, West Los Angeles, California

Diarrhea

Susan Meric Taylor, DVM, DACVIM

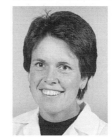

Professor of Small Animal Internal Medicine, Western College of Veterinary Medicine, University of Saskatchewon, Saskatoon, Saskatchewon, Canada

Polyuria and Polydipsia

Alain Théon, DVM, MS, DACVR-RO

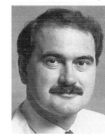

Associate Professor, School of Veterinary Medicine, Department of Surgical and Radiological Sciences, and Chief, Radiation Oncology Service, Veterinary Medical Teaching Hospital, University of California, Davis, Davis, California

Practical Radiation Therapy; Diseases of the Nose and Nasal Sinuses

William P. Thomas, DVM, DACVIM (Cardiol)

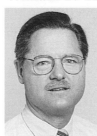

Professor of Cardiovascular Medicine, School of Veterinary Medicine, University of California, Davis, Davis, California

Congenital Heart Disease; Primary Myocardial Disease in the Dog

Donald E. Thrall, DVM, PhD, DACVR

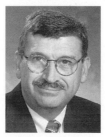

Professor of Radiology, College of Veterinary Medicine, North Carolina State University, Raleigh, North Carolina

Soft Tissue Sarcomas and Hemangiosarcomas

Grant H. Turnwald, BVSc, MS, DACVIM

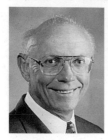

Professor of Small Animal Clinical Sciences and Associate Dean for Academic Affairs; Virginia-Maryland Regional College of Veterinary Medicine, Virginia Polytechnic Institute and State University, Blacksburg, Virginia

Dyspnea and Tachypnea

David C. Twedt, DVM, DACVIM

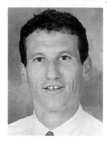

Professor, Small Animal Medicine, Department of Clinical Sciences, College of Veterinary Medicine and Biomedical Sciences and Veterinary Teaching Hospital, Colorado State University, Fort Collins, Colorado

Vomiting

David M. Vail, DVM, DACVIM (Oncol)

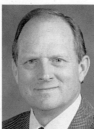

Associate Professor of Oncology, Department of Medical Sciences, School of Veterinary Medicine; Member, Comprehensive Cancer Center, University of Wisconsin, Madison, Madison, Wisconsin

Hematopoietic Tumors

Philip B. Vasseur, BS, DVM, DACVS

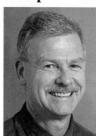

Professor, Department of Surgical and Radiological Sciences, School of Veterinary Medicine, and Chief, Small Animal Surgery Service, Veterinary Medical Teaching Hospital, University of California, Davis, Davis, California

Joint Diseases of Dogs and Cats

Anjop J. Venker–van Haagen, DVM, PhD

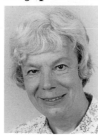

Associate Professor, Veterinary Ear, Nose, and Throat, University of Utrecht, Faculty of Veterinary Medicine, Utrecht, The Netherlands

Diseases of the Throat

John P. Verstegen, DVM, MSc, PhD

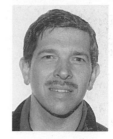

Agrege, Head of Small Animal Reproduction Department, University of Liege Veterinary College, Liege, Belgium; President of the European Veterinary Society for Small Animal Reproduction

Contraception and Pregnancy Termination; Feline Reproduction

F. J. M. Verstraete, DVM

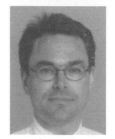

Associate Professor, School of Veterinary Medicine, Department of Surgery and Radiology, University of California, Davis, Davis, California

Dental Disease in Dogs and Cats (CIS)

Wendy A. Ware, DVM, MS, DACVIM (Cardiol)

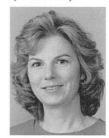

Associate Professor, Departments of Veterinary Clinical Sciences and Biomedical Sciences, College of Veterinary Medicine, and Staff Cardiologist, Veterinary Teaching Hospital, Iowa State University, Ames, Iowa

Abnormal Heart Sounds and Heart Murmurs

Robert J. Washabau, VMD, PhD, DACVIM

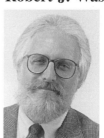

Associate Professor and Section Chief of Medicine, Department of Clinical Studies, School of Veterinary Medicine, University of Pennsylvania, Philadelphia, Pennsylvania

Diseases of the Esophagus; Gastrointestinal Endocrine Disease

David J. Waters, DVM, PhD

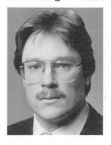

Associate Professor of Surgery and Comparative Oncology, Purdue University, Department of Veterinary Clinical Sciences, West Lafayette, Indiana

Tumors of the Urogenital System and Mammary Glands

A. D. J. Watson, BVSc, PhD, FRCVS

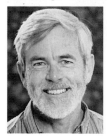

Associate Professor in Veterinary Medicine, Department of Veterinary Clinical Sciences, The University of Sydney; Consulting Specialist in Canine and Feline Medicine, University Veterinary Centre, University of Sydney, Sydney, Australia

Skeletal Diseases

Alice M. Wolf, DVM, DACVIM

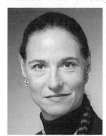

Professor, Department of Small Animal Medicine and Surgery, College of Veterinary Medicine, Texas A&M University, College Station, Texas

Other Feline Viral Diseases

Stephen D. White, DVM, DACVD

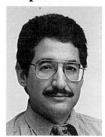

Professor, Department of Medicine and Epidemiology, School of Veterinary Medicine, University of California, Davis, Davis, California

The Skin as a Sensor of Internal Medical Disorders

Karen J. Wolfsheimer, DVM, PhD, DACVIM

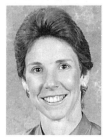

Adjunct Professor, Department of Physiology, Pharmacology, and Toxicology and Department of Clinical Sciences, School of Veterinary Medicine, Louisiana State University; Director, Endocrine Diagnostics and Consultation, Baton Rouge, Louisiana

Obesity

Michael D. Willard, DVM, MS, DACVIM

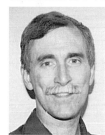

Professor of Small Animal Medicine and Surgery, College of Veterinary Medicine, and Staff Internist/Gastroenterologist, Texas Veterinary Medical Center, Texas A&M University, College Station, Texas

Diseases of the Large Intestine; Diseases of the Gallbladder and Extrahepatic Biliary System; Gastrointestinal Food Allergies (CIS), Megaesophagus (CIS)

Carole A. Zerbe, DVM, PhD, DACVIM

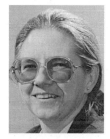

Assistant Professor, Department of Clinical Studies, School of Veterinary Medicine, University of Pennsylvania, Philadelphia, Pennsylvania

Gastrointestinal Endocrine Disease

David A. Williams, MA, VetMB, PhD, DACVIM

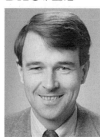

Professor and Head, Small Animal Medicine and Surgery, College of Veterinary Medicine, Texas A&M University, College Station, Texas

Exocrine Pancreatic Disease and Pancreatitis; Pancreatitis (CIS)

Steven C. Zicker, DVM, PhD, DACVN, DACVIM

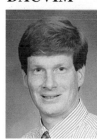

Adjunct Faculty, Kansas State University, Manhattan, Kansas; Veterinary Clinical Nutritionist, Hill's Pet Nutrition, Inc, Topeka, Kansas

Developmental Orthopedic Disease of Dogs

CALIFORNIA EDITORIAL STAFF

Marsha Feldman

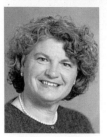

Administrative Coordinator

W.B. SAUNDERS STAFF

Al Beringer

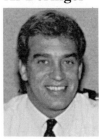

Director of Composition

Dave Kilmer

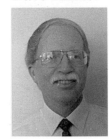

Developmental Editor

Catherine M. Stamato

Senior Editorial Assistant

Paul M. Fry

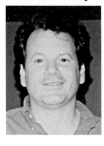

Senior Designer

Joan Nikelsky

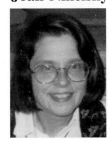

Proofreading Supervisor

Tom Stringer

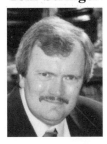

Copy Editing Supervisor

Raymond R. Kersey

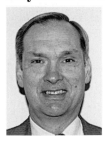

Editorial Manager, Veterinary Medicine

Frank Polizzano

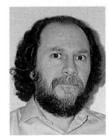

Senior Production Manager

Walt Verbitski

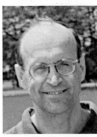

Illustrations Specialist

PREFACE *to the Fifth Edition*

"Life can only be understood backwards; but it must be lived forwards."

SØREN KIERKEGAARD

Each edition of this textbook becomes more difficult to organize as the wealth of knowledge increases while space limitations remain unchanged. We have maintained the book's size while significantly adding material. Recently identified biochemical, genetic, and molecular biologic data are incorporated. Older information is more concisely presented to allow the addition of new studies.

References are thorough but not encyclopedic. This allows the reader to completely review the source material. Many chapters refer to prior editions of the textbook's reference sources so as not to lengthen the book unnecessarily. From the reference sources, the reader is able to complete a full reference list if desired.

The field of veterinary internal medicine, like all other medical fields, is advancing rapidly, yet not every new article or procedure is useful or better than those of the past. The physical examination and history often provide enough information to make a diagnosis. The problem of continuous testing must be guarded against by rejecting complacency and reinforcing fundamental medical principles. It is not up to the veterinarian to decide what a pet owner should or should not do. We are professionally and ethically obliged to provide the client with options. The client brings their pet to us for professional care, not to be laden with additional guilt (although at times it might be appropriate). Louis Rukeyser, the investment advisor, suggests that people who add years do not necessarily add knowledge; some travel around the world and see nothing; others journey through life with all their biases intact. We hope that the reader who utilizes this book will do so profitably, learning from what others have contributed.

This fifth edition is again entirely rewritten and revised. We used the previous outline as a guide to design the new edition. We believe that the first section, Clinical Manifestations of Disease, is extremely useful to the student and practitioner. It is the essence of clinical medicine. It describes briefly but succinctly the approach to medical problems in a logical and sequential order. Although a good clinician can be trained without such an organized thought process, one may become academically wise but "exam room" lean. We have expanded this section to include virtually every condition likely to be encountered during an internal medical examination of the dog or cat. Each of these chapters has a decision-making tree to use in the evaluation of that clinical problem. This section is expanded from 50 to 63 chapters, including genetics, acute vision loss, pain management, an expanded dermatology section, behavioral considerations, and hematologic syndromes. Finding a subject is simplified by allowing the reader to go directly to an area of interest highlighted by the sub-section titles that include "urogenital," "neurologic," "skin and subcutaneous," and others. The relevance of abnormal laboratory tests is highlighted by listing their relationships directly on the inside covers of the book for faster reference.

Dietary Considerations of Systemic Problems is expanded from six to nine chapters, including sections on enteral support, basic nutritional guidelines, and adverse food reactions. Therapeutic Considerations in Medicine is expanded from eight to eleven chapters, to include toxicology, transfusion medicine, and blood banking. There are new chapters on acupuncture, alternative therapies, and holistic medicine as options for those wishing to explore the nontraditional. The reader is to decide for him/herself the value of these modalities; we intend neither to recommend nor to challenge but rather to offer relevant arguments to the reader as presented by qualified and thoughtful scientists.

The Infectious Disease section has expanded chapters on feline viral, mycotic, rickettsial, and protozoal diseases. Cancer, the ever present enigma in our society, has been expanded from six to nine chapters. Neoplastic diseases are also included within specific organ systems, and multisystemic information is also presented in this section. There are revised areas on tumor biology, chemotherapy principles, paraneoplastic conditions, hematopoietic tumors, skin tumors, and soft tissue masses.

Revised and updated sections on neurology, cardiovascular and respiratory diseases incorporate new diagnostic as well as therapeutic modalities, as does the expanded Eyes, Ears, Nose, and Throat section. The Gastrointestinal System section is lengthened again and includes several chapters on dentistry. Diseases of the Liver and Pancreas is now a complete and independent section. Endocrine and Reproductive sections include 20 chapters, 11 written by new authors while 5 of the 10 chapters in the Reproduction section are from European centers where the greatest advances have been made.

The Urinary System section has several new authors participating in this edition. Prostatic diseases are included in this section, and bacterial infections as well as lower urinary problems are updated with new data. Hematology and Immunology are emphasized. Regenerative and non-regenerative anemias, platelet disorders, coagulopathies, and white cell changes are discussed in that order. Non-neoplastic splenic diseases are also considered in this section. Joint and skeletal disorders of medical (nonsurgical) relevance are described, and surgery, where in order, is identified.

An entirely new section, designed for the practicing veterinarian, is the Client Information Series. We have asked authors to prepare one-page information sheets specifically geared to clients. Each of the 56 reports considers a major clinical area of internal medicine. We encourage you to copy and hand out these information sheets to your clients. Each is written in lay terms to help your clients better understand their pet's problem. The topics include a wide spectrum of common veterinary internal medicine conditions. We need to be made aware of the facility of these handouts in your practice.

As with past editions, the editors are most grateful to the

contributing authors. Incredible time and effort goes into producing even a short chapter. In many cases, the shorter the chapter the more difficult it is to write. One sign of a really fine writer and educator is to know how to abbreviate material and include relevant data at the same time.

We encourage your comments about the text. Your observations help us to improve and add to the value of this book. Neither natural talent, intelligence, nor a wonderful education guarantees success. A successful person needs the sensitivity to understand what other people want and the willingness to give it to them. Worldly success depends on pleasing others. No one will gain fame, recognition, or advancement just because he or she thinks it is deserved. Someone else has to think so also.

The editorial and production staffs at WB Saunders have again demonstrated skill and expertise in maneuvering this enormous work from inception to final publication. We wish to thank Mr. Dave Kilmer and his colleagues: Mr. Frank Polizzano, Ms. Cass Stamato, Mr. Tom Stringer, Mr. Ray Kersey, and their colleagues for their helpfulness and fine attention to detail. On the closer front, Ms. Marsha Feldman has assumed the responsibility of seeing that the details of production, written letters, and communication have been diligently adhered to. Without her help, this book would not have been published in a timely or effective manner. Both Drs. Ettinger and Feldman offer their day-to-day colleagues a sincere thank you. They have been helpful in making suggestions and corrections. Their words of encouragement when it looked like the book would never get done are very much appreciated.

We would like to end the preface to this twenty-fifth silver anniversary of the book by thanking you, our professional colleagues, for having supported this endeavor over the past four editions. Your support has given us reason to continue the effort; your encouragement has told us how to proceed and improve, and your generous welcome wherever we have traveled has made this the most worthwhile and professionally rewarding experience in our lives. We close by reminding you that Groucho Marx commented, "Outside of a dog, a book is a man's best friend. Inside of a dog it's too dark to read."

STEPHEN J. ETTINGER
EDWARD C. FELDMAN

CONTENTS

VOLUME 1

SECTION I
CLINICAL MANIFESTATIONS OF DISEASE

Section II
Dietary Considerations of Systemic Problems

Section III
Therapeutic Considerations in Medicine

SECTION IV

INFECTIOUS DISEASE

SECTION V

CANCER

SECTION VI
THE NERVOUS SYSTEM

SECTION VII
THE CARDIOVASCULAR SYSTEM

VOLUME 2

SECTION XI
DISEASES OF THE LIVER AND PANCREAS

SECTION XII
THE ENDOCRINE SYSTEM

SECTION XIII
THE REPRODUCTIVE SYSTEM

SECTION XIV
THE URINARY SYSTEM

SECTION XV
HEMATOLOGY AND IMMUNOLOGY

Section XVI
Joint and Skeletal Disorders

Appendices

Abnormal Laboratory Findings

Conditions Associated With Hematologic Change

Urinalysis Abnormalities ....Found on the inside covers

Robert M. DuFort

SECTION I

CLINICAL MANIFESTATIONS OF DISEASE

CHAPTER 1

CLINICAL GENETICS

Urs Giger

Clinical genetics is involved in the diagnosis, management, and control of hereditary disorders. Lifesaving advances in medicine and surgery have increased the chance of survival of animals with such defects and thus tend to raise their recognition. Inbreeding to preserve desirable traits in certain breeds favors the occurrence of recessively inherited diseases. Technologic advances now allow the recognition and characterization of clinicopathologic, biochemical, and molecular basis of many hereditary diseases. Specific genetic disorders are covered under individual organ systems. This chapter reviews the characteristic clinical features of hereditary diseases in small animals, the various modes of inheritance, diagnostic tests, management, and control of these diseases. The importance of genetic counseling is addressed, i.e., providing information for pet owners and breeders of animals afflicted with a hereditary disorder concerning the consequences of such a disorder and the ways in which it can be prevented in future generations.

FREQUENCY

Because of the increased awareness of genetic defects, the number of reported hereditary diseases in small animals is rapidly growing. Originally, diseases with apparent clinical manifestations affecting the appearance and gait of an animal were recognized. Thus, it is not surprising that skeletal malformations, skin and eye abnormalities, as well as neuromuscular defects were more frequently reported than disorders involving internal organs. Animals with recurrent or chronic infections or immune-mediated diseases may have a genetic defect that dysregulates their immune function. A variety of other genetic predispositions of certain animals, families, or breeds to develop disorders such as hip dysplasia, gastric torsion, and cancer have been clearly established.

At present, approximately 400 hereditary diseases in dogs and 150 disorders in cats have been adequately documented, and every year over a dozen new defects are being reported. These numbers are much higher than in food animals, where economic pressures rapidly eliminate and prevent investigation of diseased animals. In contrast, several thousand hereditary disorders have been accumulated in McKusick's *Catalog of Mendelian Inheritance in Man*. Thus, practically all diseases described in small animals have also been seen in humans and generally represent close homologues.

Although any genetic defect may occur in any animal, many have been documented only in a family or breed. In fact, in some breeds, the frequency of a particular disorder may be very high. This may be due to a founder effect in which one or more of the founders of a small ancestral group was a carrier or even affected, or as observed in several smaller breeds where a popular sire was later determined to be a carrier of a mutant gene. Unfortunately,

genetic disease frequencies are generally not available or are biased because of data collection. Large-scale screening programs and open registries have rarely been established. For instance, the prevalence of hip dysplasia may differ greatly depending on methods used to reach a diagnosis and whether a registry requires or only encourages recording of every examined animal. The Bernese Mountain Dog Club has established the first open registry for malignant histiocytosis, mast cell tumor, and hip and elbow dysplasia with Canine Genetics, Inc., Davis, CA.

Although many hereditary diseases occur rarely, and often in only one breed, all together they represent an important clinical problem. For the small animal practitioner, it can be a daunting, nearly impossible task to remember all these diseases. Recently, however, various resources became available to obtain genetic information. In addition to the list of hereditary diseases and associated breeds in the appendices of this book, there are other published lists organized by breed or disease. A list of genetic diseases in all species with references assembled by Frank W. Nicholas, known as *Mendelian Inheritance in Animals*, can be obtained online. The most comprehensive and updated searchable information is Donald F. Patterson's *Canine Genetic Disease Information System*, available on disk and in book format.

INHERITANCE

Genetic diseases are caused by chromosomal alterations or gene mutations. Disease-causing mutations are heritable changes in the sequence of genomic DNA that alter the structure and function of the coded protein. These changes include point mutations, deletions, and insertions in the DNA sequence that result in a missense or nonsense sequence. The molecular genetic defect is now known for more than a dozen hereditary disorders in small animals (Table 1–1). Among the disorders caused entirely or partly by genetic factors, three main types are recognized: chromosomal, single gene, and complex or multifactorial disorders. For approximately half of the disorders suspected to be of a genetic nature, however, the mode of inheritance remains unknown.

CHROMOSOMAL DISORDERS

The dog has 76 autosomes (38 pairs) and 2 sex chromosomes (78XX or 78XY), whereas the cat has 38XX or 38XY. The major human genome project has also allowed major progress in canine and feline gene mapping. Through physical and genetic mapping strategies, genes can now be assigned to and localized along a chromosome, and new genes can be identified.

Chromosomal disorders are caused by an excess or defi-

TABLE 1–1. EXAMPLES OF HEREDITARY DISORDERS CHARACTERIZED AT THE MOLECULAR LEVEL

DISORDER	BREED
Autosomal Recessive Disorders	
Band 4.1 deficiency (elliptocytosis)	Mixed breed dog
Cystinuria	Newfoundland
α-Fucosidosis	English springer spaniel
Globoid cell leukodystrophy	West Highland white and Cairn terrier
Gangliosidosis GM$_1$	Korat and domestic shorthair cat
Hyperlipidemia	Cats
Mucopolysaccharidosis I	Plothound
Mucopolysaccharidosis VI	Siamese, domestic shorthair cat
Mucopolysaccharidosis VII	Mixed breed dog
Glycogenosis IV	Norwegian Forest cat
Pyruvate kinase deficiency	Basenji, West Highland white terrier, Abyssinian, Somali
Phosphofructokinase deficiency	English springer spaniel, American cocker spaniel
von Willebrand's disease type 1	Doberman pinscher
von Willebrand's disease type 3	Scottish terrier, Manchester terrier
X-Chromosomal Recessive Disorders	
Hemophilia B	Terrier mix
	Labrador
Hypomyelination of CNS	English springer spaniel
Muscular dystrophy (Duchenne)	Golden retriever
	Rottweiler, German shorthair pointer,
	Domestic shorthair cat
Severe combined immunodeficiency	Basset hound
	Welsh corgi

ciency of genes contained in a chromosome or chromosomal segment. Understandably, such defects may result in severe, often lethal clinical syndromes. Although alterations of autosomes have only rarely been reported in small animals—some had syndromes with multiple defects—they are common in infants and are often responsible for fetal losses. In contrast, abnormalities involving the X and Y chromosomes leading to sex developmental disorders are well recognized. The best example is the tricolored (calico, tortoiseshell) male cat with testicular hypoplasia and an XXY chromosome set. However, not every sex developmental disorder is due to a defect in the sex chromosomes, e.g., XX-sex reversal.

SINGLE GENE TRAITS

A single gene defect is often called *Mendelian* and involves one mutant gene (allele) at a single locus. When an animal has a pair of identically mutant alleles, it is said to be homozygous (a homozygote), whereas when only one of the genes is mutated, it is said to be heterozygous (a heterozygote) at that gene locus. The pattern of inheritance depends mainly on two factors: (1) whether the mutation is located on an autosome (autosomal) or on the X chromosome (X-linked); and (2) whether the phenotype, the observable expression of a genotype as a disease trait, is dominant, i.e., expressed when only one chromosome of a pair carries the mutation, or recessive, i.e., expressed when both chromosomes of a pair carry the mutation. Thus, it is the phenotype rather than the mutant gene or protein that is dominant or recessive. Whereas in humans most diseases are dominantly inherited, recessive traits are favored by the common inbreeding practices in small animals.

AUTOSOMAL RECESSIVE INHERITANCE

Autosomal recessive inherited traits are most common in small animals. The parents of affected animals have to be carriers (heterozygotes), therefore, called obligate carriers. Typically one fourth of males and females in a litter are equally likely to be affected. Phenotypically normal offspring may be in a ratio of 2:1 either carriers (heterozygotes) or free of a mutant allele ("clear," homozygous normal). Although the parents could also be affected, diseased animals generally are not used for breeding.

X-LINKED RECESSIVE INHERITANCE

In X-linked recessively inherited disorders, males who are hemizygous for the X chromosome typically are affected. When heterozygous females (carriers) are mated to a normal male, half of their male offspring will be affected and half of their female offspring will be phenotypically normal carriers, whereas the other males and females will be "clear." The mutant X-chromosomal gene is never passed on from the sire to a male offspring, but is transmitted by an affected male to all its female offspring (obligate carriers). Affected females would occur only if a carrier female is mated with an affected male. Heterozygous females are usually unaffected, although some manifestations may occur because of X-chromosomal inactivation. In addition, an X-linked dominant trait may need to be considered but has been reported only in Samoyeds with a glomerulonephropathy. X-linked disorders should not be confused with sex-limited disorders, such as diseases related to the primary and secondary sex organs. Finally, Y-chromosomal diseases have not been reported in animals.

AUTOSOMAL DOMINANT INHERITANCE

In autosomal dominant traits, the disease appears in every generation. An affected animal generally has one affected parent unless this animal has a new mutation in the gamete of a phenotypically normal parent or when the disease is variably expressed (nonpenetrant in parent). Males and females are equally likely to transmit the disease to an offspring of either sex. Because affected animals are generally heterozygous, however, half of all offspring will be affected. Affected animals generally are not used in breeding programs. Furthermore, homozygous states of dominant traits are often lethal.

MITOCHONDRIAL INHERITANCE

Mitochondrial inheritance is a very rare and atypical mendelian inheritance of disorders involving the mitochondrial DNA. Because all mitochondrial DNA is transmitted from the ova, all offspring from an affected female, but none from an affected male, will be diseased. In humans several neuromuscular diseases are known to be associated with mutations in mitochondrial DNA, and in dogs some myopathies may be caused by a mitochondrial defect.

COMPLEX OR MULTIFACTORIAL INHERITANCE

A number of developmental disorders resulting in congenital malformations are caused by complex or multifactorial inheritance, as well as other disorders in adult animals. Rather than having one single gene error, several minor defects (polygenic) in the genetic information together with certain environmental factors can produce or predispose to a serious illness. Hip and other dysplasias as well as certain congenital heart defects (conotruncal defect) are examples, and the degree to which a trait (e.g., hip dysplasia) is genetically determined may greatly vary between breeds (heritability).

The hereditary nature of a particular disease may be suggested or established by a familial occurrence, breed predilection, breed studies, an established mode of inheritance, and/or an identified gene defect.

CLINICAL SIGNS

Gene defects can involve any gene or organ; therefore, the clinical signs of hereditary diseases are extremely variable and may mimic other acquired disorders. Some typical features, however, may raise our suspicion of a genetic disorder.

In contrast to infectious diseases, intoxications, and nutritional imbalances that generally affect an entire litter, hereditary diseases often involve only a few in a litter. Furthermore, the age of onset of clinical signs for a particular gene defect is rather specific and independent of environmental factors.

Most genetic defects cause clinical signs early in life. In fact, fetal resorptions, abortions, and stillborns may also be caused by genetic traits but are rarely determined. Most puppy and kitten losses occur during the first week of life, shortly after the maternal homeostatic system can no longer compensate for an endogenous defect. Some neonatal kitten losses have recently been attributed to blood type incompatibility: type A and AB kittens born to type B queens develop life-threatening neonatal isoerythrolysis when nursing and absorbing anti-A containing colostrum during the first day of life. Certain congenital malformations also may not be compatible with life, such as severe cleft palates and hernias. The term *congenital* only implies that the disease is present at birth, however, and does not necessarily mean it is hereditary.

A common presentation is failure to thrive. These animals lag behind their healthy littermates in their development; they do not gain weight at a normal rate and are generally lethargic. They are poor doers, often fade (hence the term *fading puppy* or *kitten syndrome*), and finally die. Failure to thrive should not be confused with growth retardation, which refers to a proportionally stunted growth that may or may not be associated with other clinical signs. In addition to these relatively unspecific clinical signs, some defects may cause specific clinical manifestations. Easy to recognize are malformations that involve any part of the skeleton and lead to disproportionate dwarfism, gait abnormalities, and/or facial dysmorphia. A large number of hereditary eye diseases have been described in dogs, some of which are not recognized until adulthood. Neuromuscular signs may vary from exercise intolerance to ataxia and seizures. Defects of many other internal organs are associated with unspecific clinical signs. Many disorders cause an isolated typical sign, whereas others produce a characteristic overall pattern of anomalies known as *syndromes.*

Clinical manifestations of hereditary diseases are extremely variable, ranging from benign to debilitating and lethal. They are usually chronic and progressive, i.e., once an animal shows signs it probably will not recover, and often cause death at an early age. A few hereditary defects, however, result in intermittent or recurrent problems, such as hereditary bleeding disorders and primary immunodeficiencies.

DIAGNOSTIC TESTS

Diagnostic tests generally are required to further support a genetic disorder in a diseased animal. Radiology and other imaging techniques may reveal skeletal malformations or cardiac anomalies, and ophthalmologic examination may further define an inherited eye disease, although some are not recognized before several years of age. Routine tests such as complete blood cell count, chemistry screen, and urinalysis may suggest some specific hematologic or metabolic disorders or rule out many acquired disorders. Furthermore, clinical function studies may more clearly define a gastrointestinal, liver, kidney, or endocrine problem. Histopathology and/or electron microscopy of a tissue biopsy from an affected animal or from the necropsy of a littermate or relative may give the first clue as to a genetic defect.

A few laboratories provide special diagnostic tests that allow a specific diagnosis of an inborn error of metabolism. Inborn errors of metabolism include all biochemical disorders due to a genetically determined, specific defect in the structure and/or function of a protein molecule. Aside from the classic enzyme deficiencies, genetic defects in structural protein receptors, plasma and membrane transport proteins, and other proteins covered by this definition will result in biochemical disturbances. The laboratories' approach is to detect the failing system or to determine the specific protein or gene defect. Disorders of intermediary metabolism typically produce a metabolic block in a biochemical pathway leading to product deficiency, accumulation of substrates, and production of substances via alternative pathways. The most useful specimen to detect biochemical derangements is urine because abnormal metabolites in the blood will be filtered through the glomeruli, but fail to be reabsorbed, as no renal transport systems exist for most abnormal metabolites.

Once the failing system has been identified, the defect can be determined at the protein level. These tests include the classic enzyme function tests as well as immunologic assays. Because most enzymes are present in abundant amounts, no major functional abnormalities are observed unless the enzyme activity is severely reduced, usually to less than 20 percent of normal value. Thus, homozygously affected animals have very low protein activity and/or quantities, often in the range of 0 to 5 percent. These tests may also be used to detect carriers (heterozygotes), who typically have intermediate quantities at the protein level (40 to 60 percent). Unfortunately, protein assays require submission of appropriate tissue or fluid under special conditions to specialized laboratories along with a control sample, and are labor intensive. The Section of Medical Genetics at the School of Veterinary Medicine of the University of Pennsylvania is one of the few places that performs such tests to diagnose known or investigate novel hereditary disorders.

The molecular genetic defect has been identified for several hereditary diseases, and thus DNA screening tests have been developed. These tests are mutation-specific and can therefore be used only in animals suspected of having the exact same gene defect. Small animals within the same or a closely related breed will likely have the same mutation for a particular disease, e.g., phosphofructokinase deficiency in English springer and American cocker spaniels. However, dogs and cats as well as unrelated breeds of a species with the same disorder will likely have different mutations, as shown with X-linked muscular dystrophy and erythrocyte pyruvate kinase deficiency in various dog breeds and cats.

DNA tests have several advantages over other biochemical tests. The test results are independent of the age of the animals; thus, the tests can be performed at birth or at least long before an animal is placed in a new home. DNA is very stable and only the smallest quantities are needed; hence, there are no special shipping requirements. DNA can be extracted from any nucleated cell, e.g., blood, buccal mucosa, hair follicle, semen, and even formalinized tissue. For instance, blood can be sent in an EDTA tube or a drop of blood can be applied to a special filter paper. Buccal swabs can be obtained with a special brush, although this method should not be used in nursing animals, or if absolutely necessary, only after flushing the oral cavity. The DNA segment of interest is amplified with appropriate primers and polymerase chain reaction. The mutant and/or normal allele are identified by DNA size difference directly on a gel in case of deletions or insertions or after restriction enzyme digestion for point mutations. These tests are generally simple, robust, and accurate as long as appropriate techniques and controls are used. Furthermore, they can be used not only for the detection of affected animals but also for carriers.

For a few inherited disorders, the defective gene remains unknown; however, a polymorphic DNA marker that is linked to the mutant allele has been discovered. Such linkage tests are available for copper toxicosis in Bedlington terriers and some forms of retinopathy and are accurate for a particular patient as long as there is a known affected animal in its family (informative family). At present, mutation-specific and linkage tests are available only for single gene defects in small animals; however, complex genetic traits may also soon be approached by these methods as they are for humans.

PROGNOSIS AND THERAPY

Because the clinical consequences of the many hereditary disorders vary greatly, it is not surprising that the prognosis for survival and quality of life ranges from excellent to grave. The clinical course and outcome for a particular defect are rather similar among affected animals. Some defects are recognized as an incidental finding, e.g., microcytosis in Akitas, whereas others are progressive and lead to severe organ dysfunction and death, e.g., lysosomal storage diseases.

At present, the therapeutic options in the treatment of hereditary diseases are limited and ethical principles need to be carefully considered. Although several structural malformations can be surgically corrected, such as cryptorchism, hernias, hepatic shunts, and a patent ductus arteriosus, these animals should not be shown or bred. In a few cases, a deficient protein, cofactor, substrate, or metabolite can be supplemented to correct the defect. For instance, vitamin B_{12} deficiency in cachectic and lethargic giant schnauzers and Border collies with an ileal receptor defect can be helped by monthly cobalamin injections. Pancreatic enzyme supplementation and daily insulin injections are used to manage animals with exocrine or endocrine pancreatic insufficiency, respectively. Fresh-frozen plasma is administered in the treatment of hereditary coagulopathies and von Willebrand's disease whenever animals excessively bleed. Other enzyme and protein replacements are also experimentally attempted.

Although kidney transplants have been established in clinical practice for chronic renal failure, they have not been applied in animals with hereditary (juvenile) renal disorders. Several hereditary disorders of hematopoietic cells have been experimentally corrected by bone marrow transplantation, e.g., pyruvate and phosphosfructokinase deficiency, cyclic hematopoiesis, and interleukin-2 (IL-2) receptor defects. Furthermore, bone marrow transplantation is being attempted to deliver functional cells or active proteins to other tissues including liver, bone, and brain, e.g., in lysosomal storage diseases. Finally, gene therapy, the integration of a functional gene into the patient's own defective cells, will likely be feasible in the twenty-first century. Experiments in rodent models have already provided encouraging results; however, the technology needs to be improved to achieve persistent and regulated gene expression in larger mammals including dogs and cats.

CONTROL

Much more important than the treatment of hereditary disorders is the control of these traits in breeding programs. Thus, in order to reduce the frequency or eliminate altogether a genetic defect, the further spread of the mutant gene has to be prevented in a family or entire breed. It is obvious that affected animals of any genetic disease should not be used for breeding. This approach is simple and effectively eliminates disorders with a dominant trait. For recessively inherited disorders, however, the elimination of affected animals is not sufficient to markedly reduce the prevalence of a defect within a breed or kennel/cattery. Although it might be safest not to breed any related animals of affected animals (as requested by the Swedish Kennel Club), this practice may, because of inbreeding and narrow gene pools in some breeds, eliminate all breeders in an entire kennel or cattery and may severely reduce the gene diversity of a breed. Thus, it will be pivotal to detect carriers (heterozygotes) and truly "clear" animals (homozygous normal). Obligate carriers can be readily identified for autosomal (both parents of affected) and X-linked recessive (mother of affected) disorders. As mentioned above, for some diseases, reliable carrier detection tests are available and many breeders know about them and inform the veterinarian. For instance, carriers have half-normal (~50 percent) enzyme activity by functional assays, or have a normal *and* mutant DNA sequence for the diseased gene on a DNA test. Breeders should, therefore, be encouraged to screen their animals before breeding for known genetic diseases whenever carrier tests are available. Unfortunately, many breeders mistrust these newer tests; either they were disappointed by the inaccuracy of early tests or they fear that the results may become public and would hurt their business. Thus, breeders need to be educated by well-informed veterinarians. If no carrier tests are available, a test mating between the dog in question and a known carrier or affected could be performed, and no affected or at least 5 and 11 healthy puppies/kittens, respectively, need to be produced to "clear" an animal. For many breeders, this approach is ethically unacceptable because it may produce affecteds. Furthermore, if a carrier needs to be used because of a narrow gene pool and many other desirable traits, it should be bred with a homozygously normal (clear) animal and all its offspring need to be tested. Only clear animals should be used in future breedings.

CHAPTER 2

HYPERTHERMIA AND HYPOTHERMIA

James B. Miller

All veterinarians have been taught that obtaining a body temperature is part of every physical examination. Too frequently the veterinarian associates any elevation in body temperature with true fever and that this "fever" is caused by an infectious agent. Hypothermia may be thought to be caused by environmental factors. This approach to hyperthermia and hypothermia can lead to improper diagnosis or therapy (or the lack of therapy).

THERMOREGULATION

The thermoregulatory center for the body is located in the region of the anterior hypothalamus (AH). Changes in ambient and core body temperatures are sensed by the peripheral and central thermoreceptors, and this information is conveyed to the AH. Thermoreceptors sensing that the body is below or above its normal temperature (normal "set point") will stimulate the AH to cause the body to increase heat production and reduce heat loss through conservation if the body is too cold or dissipate heat if the body is too warm (Fig. 2–1). Through these mechanisms, the dog and cat can maintain a narrow core body temperature range in a wide variety of environmental conditions.

HYPERTHERMIA

Hyperthermia is the term used to describe any increase in core body temperature above normal for that species. Hyperthermia is a result of the loss of equilibrium in the heat balance equation such that heat is produced or stored in the body at a rate that is in excess of heat lost through radiation, convection, or evaporation. The term fever is reserved for those hyperthermic animals where the set point in the AH has been "re-set" to a higher temperature. In hyperthermic states other than fever, the hyperthermia is not a result of the body attempting to raise its temperature, but is due to physiologic, pathologic, or pharmacologic intervention (Table 2–1).

TRUE FEVER

Exogenous Pyrogens. True fever may be initiated by infectious agents or their products, immune complexes, tissue inflammation or necrosis, and several pharmacologic agents. Collectively, these substances are called exogenous pyrogens (Table 2–2). Their ability to directly affect the thermoregulatory center is probably minimal, and their ac-

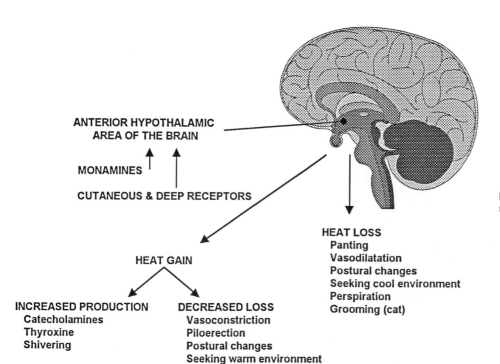

ANTERIOR HYPOTHALAMIC AREA OF THE BRAIN

MONAMINES

CUTANEOUS & DEEP RECEPTORS

HEAT GAIN

INCREASED PRODUCTION
Catecholamines
Thyroxine
Shivering

DECREASED LOSS
Vasoconstriction
Piloerection
Postural changes
Seeking warm environment

HEAT LOSS
Panting
Vasodilatation
Postural changes
Seeking cool environment
Perspiration
Grooming (cat)

Figure 2–1. Schematic representation of normal thermal regulation.

TABLE 2–1. CLASSIFICATION OF HYPERTHERMIA

True fever
    Production of endogenous pyrogens
Inadequate heat dissipation
    Heat stroke
    Hyperpyrexic syndromes
Exercise hyperthermia
    Normal exercise
    Hypocalcemic tetany (eclampsia)
    Seizure disorders
Pathologic or pharmacologic
    Lesions in or around the AH
    Malignant hyperthermia
    Hypermetabolic disorders
    Monoamine metabolism disturbances

TABLE 2–3. PROTEINS WITH PYROGENIC ACTIVITY

ENDOGENOUS PYROGEN	PRINCIPAL SOURCE
Cachectin/tumor necrosis factor–α (TNF-α)	Macrophages
Lymphotoxin/tumor necrosis factor–β (TNF-β; LT)	Lymphocytes (T and B)
Interleukin-1α (IL-1α) Interleukin-1β (IL-1β)	Macrophages and many other cell types
Interferon-α	Leukocytes (esp. monocyte-macrophages)
Interferon-β	Fibroblasts
Interferon-γ	T lymphocytes
Interleukin-6 (IL-6)	Many cell types
Macrophage inflammatory protein 1α Macrophage inflammatory protein 1β Interleukin-8 (IL-8)	Macrophages

Adapted from Beutler B, Beutler SM: The pathogenesis of fever. In Bennett JC, Plum F (eds): Cecil Textbook of Medicine, 20th ed. Philadelphia, WB Saunders, 1996, p 1535.

tion is to cause the release of endogenous pyrogens by the host.

Endogenous Pyrogens. In response to stimuli by an exogenous pyrogen, proteins released from cells of the immune system trigger the febrile response. Macrophages are the primary immune cell involved, although T and B lymphocytes play significant roles. These proteins are called endogenous pyrogens or fever-producing cytokines. Although interleukin-1 is considered the most important cytokine, at least 11 cytokines capable of initiating a febrile response have been identified (Table 2–3). Some neoplastic cells are also capable of producing cytokines. The cytokines travel via the bloodstream to the AH, where they bind to the vascular endothelial cells within the AH and stimulate the release of prostaglandins (primarily PGE_2 and possibly $PGE_{2\alpha}$). The set point is raised, and the core body temperature rises through increased heat production and conservation (Fig. 2–2).

INADEQUATE HEAT DISSIPATION

Heat Stroke. Heat stroke is a common form of inadequate heat dissipation. Exposure to high ambient temperatures may increase heat load at a faster rate than the body can dissipate. This is especially true in larger breeds of dogs and brachycephalic breeds. Heat stroke may occur rapidly in the dog, especially in closed environments with poor ventilation (e.g., inside a car with windows closed) even on only moderately hot days. Environmental temperatures inside a closed car exposed to the direct sun may exceed 120°F in less than 20 minutes even when the outside temperature is only 75°F. Death may occur in less than an hour, especially in the breed types described above. Heat stroke will not respond to antipyretics used in true fever. The patient must

TABLE 2–2. EXOGENOUS PYROGENS

Infectious agents	Infectious agents *Continued*
Bacteria (live and killed)	Virus
Gram-positive	Rickettsia
Gram-negative	Protozoa
Bacterial products	Nonmicrobial agents
Lipopolysaccharides	Soluble antigen-antibody complexes
Streptococcal exotoxin	Bile acids
Staphylococcal enterotoxin	Pharmacologic agents
Staphylococcal proteins	Bleomycin
Fungi (live and killed)	Colchicine
Fungal products	Tetracycline (cats)
Cryptococcal polysaccharide	Levamisol (cats)
Cryptococcal proteins	Tissue inflammation/necrosis

have total body cooling immediately if a fatal outcome is to be avoided. Total body cooling is best accomplished by water baths and rinses using cool, but not cold, water. If the water is too cold, there is a tendency for peripheral vasoconstriction, which will inhibit heat loss and slow the cooling process. Cool water gastric lavage or enemas have also been suggested. Cooling should be discontinued when body temperature approaches normal to avoid potential hypothermia. In addition to total body cooling, treatment for vascular collapse and shock should be instituted with severe hyperthermia (greater than 107°F) or when clinical judgment warrants its use. Intravenous crystalloid solutions given at shock doses and glucocorticoids may be indicated to prevent permanent organ damage and disseminated intravascular coagulopathy (DIC).

Hyperpyrexic Syndrome. Hyperpyrexic syndrome is associated with moderate to severe exercise in hot and humid climates. This syndrome may be more common in hunting dogs or dogs that "jog" with their owners. In humid environments, there is a tendency toward a zero thermal gradient for dry heat loss leading to a net heat gain. In addition, severe exercise may cause the cardiovascular system to supply skeletal muscles with adequate blood flow while compromising peripheral heat loss by not allowing proper vasodilatation in the skin. Many hunting dogs and dogs that run with their owners will continue to work/run until they become weak, begin to stagger, and then collapse. In suspected cases, owners should obtain a rectal thermometer and evaluate the dog's rectal temperature and the first sign the dog becoming weak or not wanting to continue. Owners should be instructed that rectal temperatures above 106°F require immediate total body cooling and that temperatures above 107°F are an immediate threat to permanent organ damage or death.

EXERCISE HYPERTHERMIA

Body temperatures slowly increase with sustained exercise, owing to increased heat production associated with muscular activity. Even when extreme heat and humidity are

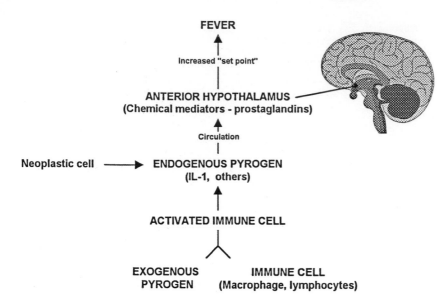

Figure 2–2. Schematic representation of the pathophysiology of fever.

not factors, dogs will occasionally reach temperatures that would require total body cooling. This is especially true in dogs that have not had significant exercise recently, are overweight, or have respiratory disease. Puppies presented for vaccinations have often been excited and active during the trip to the veterinarian. The animals' activity and probable release of catecholamines frequently result in elevation in body temperatures obtained on physical examination. These dogs will display features suggestive of attempting to dissipate excess body heat and are neither febrile nor ill.

Eclampsia results in extreme muscular activity that can lead to significant heat production resulting in severe hyperthermia. Total body cooling should be initiated in conjunction with specific eclampsia therapy if the patient is hyperthermic.

Seizure disorders due to organic, metabolic, or idiopathic causes are encountered frequently. Hyperthermia associated with severe muscular activity can be a feature, especially if the seizures are prolonged. The initial concern of the clinician should be to stop the seizures, but, when significant hyperthermia is present, total body cooling may be necessary.

PATHOLOGIC AND PHARMACOLOGIC HYPERTHERMIA

These types of hyperthermia encompass several disorders that lead to impairment of the heat balance equation. Lesions in the hypothalamus may obliterate the thermoregulatory center, leading to impaired response to both hot and cold environments. Malignant hyperthermia has been reported in the dog and cat that can cause a myopathy initiated by pharmacologic agents, including inhalation anesthetics (especially halothane) and muscle relaxants such as succinylcholine. The result is extreme muscle rigidity and production of excess body heat. Removal of the offending causative agent and total body cooling may prevent death. Hypermetabolic disorders may lead to hyperthermic states. Endocrine disorders such as hyperthyroidism and pheochromocytoma can lead to an increased metabolic rate and/or vasoconstriction resulting in excess heat production and decreased ability to dissipate heat. These conditions rarely lead to severe hyperthermia requiring total body cooling.

CLINICAL APPROACH TO THE HYPERTHERMIC PATIENT

When examining a dog or cat with an increased body temperature, an effort should be made to approach the problem in a logical manner (Fig. 2–3). A complete history and physical examination should be performed unless the problem is of an extreme nature (temperature greater than 106°F) and the patient is obviously attempting to dissipate heat (panting, postural changes) or comatose. In such cases, immediate total body cooling and supportive care should be initiated. In other cases, specific questions concerning previous injuries or infections, exposure to other animals, disease in other household pets, previous geographic environment, and previous or current drug therapy may be beneficial. Through this type of questioning and a complete physical examination, the clinician can frequently decide if the increase in temperature is true fever or not. Temperatures less than 106°F, unless prolonged, are usually not life-threatening, and antipyretics are not indicated. The highest percentage of true fevers in the dog and cat are probably caused by infectious agents or their products. The prevalence of the causative infectious agent varies depending on the area where the clinician practices and the previous travel environment of the dog or cat. The next most common cause of true fevers are immune-mediated diseases. Most immune-mediated diseases occur in young adults. Immune complexes are potent stimulators for the release of fever-producing cytokines and frequently lead to temperatures of 105 or 106°F. Neoplasia is not as common as immune-mediated disease in causing fever but should always be considered, especially in the older patient. Another, often overlooked cause of fever is tissue trauma. Mild fevers (103 to 104°F), 1 or 2 days post surgery, are common when there has been significant muscle trauma. Most of these patients do not have infections and probably should not be treated with antibiotics without additional evidence for their use.

Evaluating for infectious disease, immune-mediated disease, neoplasia, and causes of tissue trauma will usually lead to a final diagnosis even when there is no obvious cause for the fever.

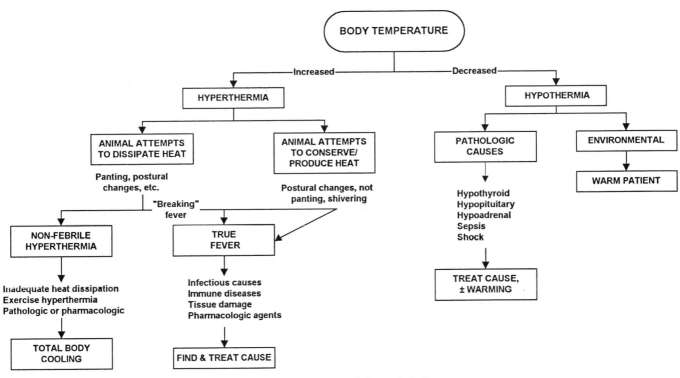

Figure 2–3. Algorithm for causes of changes in body temperature.

NONSPECIFIC THERAPY FOR FEVER

Mild to moderate increases in body temperature are rarely fatal and may be beneficial. Hyperthermia may inhibit viral replication, increase leukocyte function, and decrease the uptake of iron by microbes, the latter being necessary for growth and replication of many microbes. If a fever exceeds 107°F, a significant risk of permanent organ damage and the initiation of DIC exists. The benefits of nonspecific therapy versus its potential negative effects should be weighed.

Nonspecific therapy for true fever usually involves the use of inhibitors of prostaglandin synthesis. The compounds most commonly used are the nonsteroidal anti-inflammatory drugs (NSAIDs) including the salicylates (acetylsalicylic acid and sodium salicylate), ketoprofen, carprofen, and dipyrone. These products inhibit the chemical mediators of fever production and allow the normal thermoregulation. They do not block the production of endogenous pyrogens. These products are relatively safe, although acetylsalicylic acid is potentially toxic to cats and a reduced dosage and frequency of administration relative to the dog are recommended. Dipyrone may lead to bone marrow suppression, especially when given over a prolonged period. Carprofen has not been approved for use in cats and has been related to potentially severe liver problems in dogs on a rare occasion. Ketoprofen has been recommended only for short term use in cats.

Phenothiazines can be effective in alleviating true fever and appear to act on the thermoregulatory center and to cause peripheral vasodilatation. The sedative qualities and potential for hypotension caused by the phenothiazines should be considered before their use.

HYPOTHERMIA

Hypothermia is defined as a core body temperature below accepted normal values for that species. It can be further divided into three categories: accidental hypothermia, pathologic hypothermia, and purposeful hypothermia. With the exception of pathologic hypothermia, all other forms are approached and treated in a similar manner depending on the severity of the hypothermia.

Accidental hypothermia occurs as a spontaneous decrease in core body temperature that is independent of any disruption of the thermal regulatory center. Mild hypothermia is frequently seen in association with surgical procedures, especially when body cavities are opened for a prolonged period of time. Accidental hypothermia associated with exposure to cold or cold wet environments can frequently lead to severe hypothermia and possible death. At core temperatures of less than 94°F, the ability to generate heat through shivering is impaired or lost. As the body temperature continues to drop, there are decreases in heart rate, cardiac output, glomerular filtration, and blood pressure. There is also a significant decrease in metabolic rate of most tissues.

Pathologic hypothermia may be associated with disease processes that decrease metabolic rate or directly affect the thermal regulatory center. Endocrine diseases including hypothyroidism, hypopituitarism, and hypoadrenocorticism have been associated with mild hypothermia. Lesions in the hypothalamus may lead to hypothermia. Sepsis and shock may both lead to decreased body temperatures.

Purposeful hypothermia has been used in cardiac surgery to decrease tissue oxygen demand and allow the heart to be stopped for as long as 20 minutes without significant brain damage.

CLINICAL APPROACH TO HYPOTHERMIA

The degree of hypothermia is the most important factor when evaluating a patient with a low body temperature (see Fig. 2–3). Mild hypothermia (temperatures greater than

96°F) is not a significant threat to a dog or cat, and such animals may be "passively" rewarmed. This involves the prevention of further heat loss and the use of blankets. For more severe hypothermia, active rewarming is often indicated. The use of circulating warm water blankets, hot water bottles, heat lamps, and forced air hair dryers have all been used to rewarm hypothermic patients. Caution should be used with these types of rewarming because peripheral vasoconstriction in the patients make them susceptible to thermal burns. Warming the periphery alone may decrease the stimulus for the body to actively rewarm itself while the core temperature is still cold. Using warmed intravenous fluids or gastric and colonic lavage using warmed isotonic solutions has been advocated for core body warming.

If a dog or cat has no known reason for accidental hypothermia, the animal should be evaluated for pathologic conditions that lead to hypothermia. Evaluation for endocrine diseases, sepsis, or intracranial disease is indicated.

CHAPTER 3

WEAKNESS AND SYNCOPE

Stephen J. Ettinger

WEAKNESS

Weakness can be categorized as lassitude, fatigue, generalized muscle weakness (asthenia), faintness or syncope, and altered states of consciousness. This chapter deals only with lassitude, fatigue, asthenia, and syncope. The causes and significance of altered states of consciousness may be found in Chapters 42 and 103.

Lassitude and fatigue both refer to a lack of energy. Synonymous terms include lethargy and listlessness. *Lethargy* further identifies a state of drowsiness, inactivity, or indifference in which there are delayed responses to external (auditory, visual, or tactile) stimuli. Overstimulation is necessary to evoke a normal response in these animals. Lethargy may progress to obtundation, which is a dull indifference displayed by the animal while it is conscious. These conditions need to be distinguished from altered states of consciousness, such as stupor and coma, as well as from narcolepsy.

Generalized muscular weakness refers to a true loss of strength, either continuous or following repeated muscle contractions. This asthenia may proceed to paresis, motor paralysis, loss of sensation, and ataxia, but does so without a loss of consciousness.

Syncope refers to a sudden, transient loss of consciousness due to a deprivation of energy substrates, either oxygen or glucose, that briefly impairs cerebral metabolism. The differences between lassitude, fatigue, and asthenia are of degree; there are no clearly defined lines of distinction. These terms are not synonymous, and they do reflect progressive levels of disease or illness. Nevertheless, the owner usually ascribes clinical signs to "weakness." In cats, in which clinical signs are often hidden, it is not unusual for the pet to progress surreptitiously into more advanced stages of weakness.

History (Database). The initial portion of the minimum database required for the study of weakness or syncope begins with a thorough historical evaluation. Current problems, pertinent history and surgical procedures, and, whenever possible, a familial history should be obtained. The clinician should delve into past and current drug use as well as exposure to drugs, chemicals, or external parasites.

Physical Examination. The physical examination may identify the cause of weakness. Weight loss, ascites, or limb edema may suggest a specific problem. Palpably enlarged thyroid glands in a cat may explain marked weight loss and weakness. The odor of the breath may suggest uremia or oral, dental, pharyngeal, or esophageal lesions. Evaluation of the mucous membranes (anemia, cyanosis, jaundice, and venous return), and the pulse (cardiac disease, arrhythmias, anemia, hyperkinesis, or pulsus alternans) may aid the clinician. Enlarged lymph nodes suggest lymphosarcoma or regional adenopathy associated with neoplasia or a septic process. Auscultation of the heart and lungs may identify cardiac arrhythmias, murmurs, or abnormal respiratory sounds. Fever is associated with signs of generalized weakness in both dogs and cats (see Chapter 2). It is important to stress the enormous significance that the physical examination plays in the evaluation of the patient with signs of weakness and/or syncope.

Laboratory Tests. An animal with signs of weakness or syncope should be tested with a complete blood count, a blood glucose level, serum urea nitrogen or serum creatinine determination. Serum electrolyte and carbon dioxide concentrations should be measured. A complete urinalysis is also indicated. Further, serum chemistries, thyroid profiles, radiographs (abdomen and thorax), electrocardiography, and more specialized laboratory techniques may be indicated.

Most diseases at some point result in weakness. Figure 3–1 lists the categories and major causes of weakness usually recognized in small animal veterinary practice. This chapter does not discuss individual causes of weakness but rather emphasizes important concepts regarding its clinical diagnosis.

Anemia. Acute blood loss can cause syncope. Long-standing anemia is associated with more subtle weakness that may be intermittent and episodic. In chronic anemia, cardio-

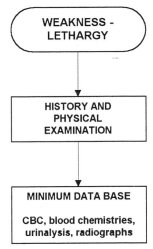

WEAKNESS - LETHARGY

↓

HISTORY AND PHYSICAL EXAMINATION

↓

MINIMUM DATA BASE

CBC, blood chemistries, urinalysis, radiographs

Rule out:

1. Anemia
2. Abdominal Effusions
3. Cardiovascular
4. Chronic Inflammation / Infections
5. Chronic Wasting Diseases
6. Drug Related
7. Electrolyte Disorders
8. Endocrine Disorders
9. Fever
10. Metabolic Dysfunction States
11. Neoplasia
12. Neurological Disorders
13. Neuromuscular / Polyneuropathies
14. Nutritional Disorders
15. Overactivity
16. Psychological Disorders
17. Pulmonary Diseases
18. Skeletal Diseases

Figure 3–1. Major causes of weakness in small animals.

megaly may be apparent radiographically, whereas in severe acute anemia there is a microcardia.

Anemia in the dog usually does not cause weakness until hemoglobin levels drop below 7 to 8 g/dL and the hematocrit levels are less than 22 to 25 per cent. In the cat, anemia may not be clinically apparent until hemoglobin levels drop to 4 or 5 g/dL and the hematocrit to 10 or 15 per cent. The differential diagnosis in acute and chronic blood loss includes the accelerated destruction of red blood cells as a result of hemolysis, and the loss of red cells by hemorrhage through the urinary or intestinal system, in the peritoneal or pleural fluid, in the subcutaneous tissue, or through the skin itself. Anemia may also be the result of insufficient production of red blood cells.

Ascites. Ascites is associated with weakness due to organ dysfunction, protein and nutritional losses, pain, and a compromised pulmonary state. The reader is referred to Chapter 39 for a discussion of the causes of acute and chronic accumulations of fluid in the abdominal cavity.

Cardiovascular Signs. Syncope may be the result of an acute decrease in cardiac output. In more chronic conditions of diminished cardiac output, both cardiac wasting and weakness can develop. Cardiac cachexia is associated with chronic cardiac disease (see Chronic Wasting). A reduction in cardiac output may be the result of hemodynamic consequences of a cardiac rhythm disturbance. Such hemodynamic consequences depend on the ventricular rate, the duration of the abnormal rate, the temporal relationship between the

atria and ventricles, the sequence of ventricular activation, the functional cardiac status, cardiac drug therapy, concomitant medical diseases, the degree of preservation of the motor system, and the level of anxiety. Tachycardia and bradycardia may cause signs of weakness and/or syncope as well as congestive heart failure and sudden death. Arrhythmias can reduce cerebral and coronary blood flow sufficiently to produce weakness or syncope (Chapter 114).

Bacterial endocarditis may be associated with signs of weakness, particularly when there is chronic infection or septicemia. Pericardial effusion, regardless of etiology, diminishes cardiac output and is a cause of weakness. Cats and dogs with pericardial effusion often have signs of severe weakness. Congestive heart failure occurs later in the illness. Unless congestive heart failure is incipient, valvular heart diseases and congenital heart diseases do not usually cause weakness. When heart failure does occur, the congestion and associated tissue hypoxia cause weakness. Clinical cardiomyopathies are usually associated with profound weakness.

Heartworm disease is associated with weakness when heart failure, renal involvement, or pulmonary dysfunction is present. Syncopal events, especially when associated with pulmonary hypertension, are likely. Other causes of pulmonary hypertension, including pulmonary emboli, must be considered in the diagnosis.

Chronic Inflammation or Infection. Among the nonspecific categories for clinical signs associated with weakness are conditions in which a fever or pain is present. Chronic diseases of inflammatory or infectious origin (e.g., liver, pancreas, prostate, skin, oral cavity, pulmonary, anal glands, ears, joints, bones, and muscles) all include weakness as a primary sign. In time, these diseases wear the patient (and the owner) down.

Chronic Wasting. Among the diseases that produce a loss of strength are those resulting in chronic wasting. Diseases of the liver terminating in cirrhosis, chronic cardiac cachexia, and chronic renal failure are examples. Interleukins and cytokines are substances produced (TNF-α) that are responsible for weakness.

Drug-Related Weaknesses. Drugs with beneficial therapeutic effects may also have adverse side effects. When patients fail to respond to medication or if the animal's condition deteriorates, it is reasonable to discontinue therapy and reevaluate the condition. Low-level toxemia, particularly chronic organophosphate or carbamate toxicity in cats, is reported to cause neuromuscular weakness without acute toxic signs. The veterinarian should know the adverse effects of drugs used. Individual variations also occur. Commonly used drugs that are associated with signs of weakness and lethargy include the glucocorticoids, barbiturates, antidiarrheals with sedatives, anticonvulsant preparations, antihistamines, tranquilizers, antibiotics, diuretic agents, vasodilators, antiarrhythmic preparations, and digitalis.

Electrolyte Disorders. Abnormalities of potassium, sodium (Chapters 61 and 62), chloride, calcium, magnesium (Chapter 63), and acid-base imbalances are related to clinical signs of weakness in dogs and cats. Specific signs of weakness are associated with hyper- and hyponatremia, -kalemia, and -calcemia. They are usually associated with diuretic therapy, excessive fluid administration, or hormonal imbalances. Acid-base imbalances are seen in many medical conditions as well as with drug therapy.

Hypocalcemia can be associated with the clinical signs of nervous excitability, tetany, and, in severe cases, convulsive seizures. Weakness is observed between periods of hyperexcitability. Hypocalcemia is typical of eclampsia, hypoparathyroidism, intestinal fluid loss with diarrhea, in hypoproteinemic states with decreased albumin levels, and when chronic renal failure occurs with increased serum phosphorus concentrations. Occasionally, hypocalcemia may be seen with paralytic ileus. The long-term treatment of hypocalcemia demands knowledge of the primary cause.

Hypercalcemic states associated with either primary or secondary hyperparathyroidism, multiple myeloma, bony metastasis, and various sites of either carcinoma or lymphoma have been described in both dogs and cats. The signs are variable but include depression, muscle weakness, and arrhythmias (Chapter 63).

Endocrine Disturbances. Weakness due to decreased neuromuscular excitability is a sign common to endocrine disturbances (see Section XII) including Cushing's syndrome, hypothyroidism, Addison's disease, hypoglycemia, hyperparathyroidism, hypoparathyroidism, pseudocyesis, the inappropriate secretion of antidiuretic hormone, and diabetes mellitus (both the ketoacidotic and hyperosmolar states).

Fever. The reader is referred to Chapter 2 for a complete discussion on the causes of hyperthermia and the differential diagnosis of weakness that occurs as a result.

Metabolic Dysfunction States. The diseases in this category are related to endocrine diseases, chronic infections and chronic wasting problems, and those identified as nutritionally related (see Nutritional Disorders). This includes conditions in which there is either decreased protein production or use of protein substances, decreased production or use of glucose, and primary or secondary dyslipoproteinemia, which may induce sluggishness or weakness. Lipoprotein disorders are discussed in Chapter 72. Conditions that cause secondary increases in lipid concentrations include diabetes mellitus, pancreatitis, myeloma, nephrosis, destructive liver disease, myxedema, dysgammaglobulinemia, glycogen storage disease, and pregnancy. Dietary indiscretions involving the excessive intake or metabolism of fats and carbohydrates are the most common causes of hyperlipoproteinemia.

Neoplastic Diseases. Neoplasia is frequently associated with episodic weakness resulting from an invasive or obstructive mass. Cancers may produce substances that cause or exacerbate clinical signs of weakness. Examples include the excessive production of neurotoxins, insulin, estrogen, steroids, epinephrine, parathormone, and thyroid hormones. In other cases, weakness results from acute episodes of bleeding due to rupture of a tumor (e.g., hemangiosarcoma) or secondary to bleeding disorders such as disseminated intravascular coagulopathy (DIC). Tumor emboli or thrombi that lodge in the lung, brain, or peripheral vessels may produce specific organ signs or severe weakness as a result of organ dysfunction. Chronic unidentified weakness is a cause for a thorough "tumor search."

Neurologic Disorders. There are many central and peripheral nervous system disorders that are associated with signs of episodic weakness. Infections within the brain or spinal canal resulting from viral, bacterial, fungal, and rickettsial diseases are responsible for episodes of neurologic weakness. Space-occupying lesions such as hydrocephalus, neoplasia, or granulomas produce signs of weakness. Injury or trauma to either the brain or peripheral nerves can cause weakness, along with motor and/or sensory dysfunction. Vascular accidents or strokes have similar effects.

Epilepsy (see Chapter 43) is likely to result in acute severe episodes of weakness and may be associated with chronic weakness as well. The drugs used to treat epileptic-type conditions also frequently cause lethargy and weakness.

Central or peripheral vestibulitis or involvement of the inner ear is likely to cause clinical signs associated with head tilt, occasional nausea, weakness, and ataxia. Instability of the atlanto-occipital or atlantoaxial joints as well as cervical nerve root disorders and cervical myelopathies are causes of weakness in small animals. Thoracic spinal cord problems are less common than thoracolumbar and sacral nerve root diseases such as intervertebral discs, myelopathies, infections, instabilities, and inflammations, which are causes of neurologic episodic weakness.

Polyneuropathies and Neuromuscular Diseases. Conditions such as tick paralysis, coonhound paralysis, and botulism are polyneuropathic diseases that can cause weakness. Other conditions causing generalized weakness include the administration of drugs such as phenytoin, excessive accumulation of heavy metals (such as lead), some nutritional disturbances (avitaminoses), endocrine disturbances (such as diabetes mellitus), and immune disorders such as lupus erythematosus and periarteritis.

Myasthenia gravis is a condition that blocks myoneural functions and is associated with severe episodic weakness. Polymyositis requires differentiation from the polyneuropathies and myasthenic states. Usually these conditions are differentiated on the basis of the neurologic examination, drugs that stimulate nerve terminals, and occasionally by electromyography. Complete laboratory analyses including muscle biopsies and chemical analyses may provide additional, specific, differentiating information, particularly with respect to the metabolic myopathies responsible for myoglobinuria or glycogen and lipid storage diseases. Myoglobinuria involves transient weakness, pain, and cramping, in contrast to chronic weakness with glycogen storage myopathies.

Nutritional Disorders. Primary nutritional disorders include inadequate diets that result in a starvation syndrome. Long-term nutritional deficiencies, either in general or specifically relating to individual vitamins, minerals, proteins, or carbohydrates, may result in generalized weakness. An owner's overindulgence of an animal's appetite may result in increased body weight and obesity, which prevents the animal from being able to exercise normally. In the "pickwickian syndrome," normal breathing is restricted and cor pulmonale with signs of respiratory distress and weakness occurs. Excessive caloric intake can induce hepatic lipidosis with hepatomegaly causing respiratory distress and weakness. Obesity limits normal activity, and this may be associated with weakness.

Any disease causing a secondary nutritional problem is likely to be an inciting cause of weakness. Examples include parasitism, protein-losing diseases, hepatoencephalopathy, cirrhosis, irritable bowel syndrome, chronic diarrhea, steatorrhea, chronic pancreatic insufficiency, lymphangiectasia, and neoplasia.

Poorly designed diets may be incomplete or may simply provide poor-quality nutrients resulting in dietary insufficiencies (e.g., taurine, potassium, and others). Nutritional osteodystrophy remains an uncommon problem in cats fed meat rich in phosphate but low in calcium, resulting in pathologic fractures and weakness. If underfed, animals performing high levels of work, such as hunting or working dogs, exhibit a starvation-like syndrome.

Overactivity, Overwork, and Psychologic Factors. This important category in human medicine is one that should not be overlooked in veterinary practice. The cause of the vast majority of cases of weakness and lethargy in humans is psychologic. Although psychologic causes probably account for a small percentage of dogs or cats with weakness or lethargy, one should not disregard signs of excessive stress. These may occur in animals being used for excessive racing or hunting, in those deprived of normal rest, and occasionally in animals stressed by owners with excessive expectations of their pet. In some instances, animals become shy to the noise of a gun, firecrackers, or thunder. These problems often result in fear and weakness. Altered states of consciousness, such as narcolepsy, must also be considered.

Aging pets—especially those experiencing recent blindness, deafness, or senility—may have weakness unexplained by physical examination or laboratory studies. Making the owner aware of such problems often helps them to understand their pet.

Pulmonary Diseases. Excessive weight results in restrictive pulmonary disease, respiratory distress, and weakness. Pulmonary emboli cause clinical signs associated with respiratory distress and weakness. This condition occurs not only with neoplastic diseases, but also occasionally as a result of inflammatory diseases involving other organs and the showering of the pulmonary tree. Chronic coughing and chronic pulmonary infection are likely to weaken an animal. Heartworm disease may cause malaise in the early phase of disease and is associated with pulmonary infarction and right ventricular enlargement as a result of migration of the heartworms to the pulmonary arteries. The disease occurs in animals severely parasitized as well as in those with only a few worms. The actual mechanism of this condition relates not only to the physical obstructive properties of the heartworms but also to the possible development of chemical abnormalities resulting from the heartworm infestation in the lungs. Other causes of pulmonary emboli include hyperadrenocorticism, nephrotic syndrome, bacterial endocarditis, immune-mediated hemolytic anemia, and cardiomyopathy.

SYNCOPE

Syncope or fainting refers to a sudden, yet transient loss of consciousness due to a deprivation of energy substrate, either oxygen or glucose, that briefly impairs the cerebral metabolism. In contrast to that of all other organs, the metabolism of the brain is entirely dependent on the perfusion of oxygen. The storage of high-energy phosphates in the brain is limited, and energy supply depends on the oxidation of glucose extracted from blood. Cessation of cerebral blood flow for as little as 10 seconds can lead to a loss of consciousness. A syncopal event is transient, and typically complete recovery occurs in seconds to minutes. Syncope should be considered a "symptom complex" rather than a primary disease.

Syncope includes the client-reported signs (at least they think these are occurring) of lightheadedness, vertigo, and "falling over" in their pet. It is usually a reversible clinical state, but if not reversed, it can result in death. Syncope may result from impaired cerebral circulation secondary to occlusive cerebrovascular disease, from a transient decrease in cardiac output, from diminished peripheral systolic pressure levels that are lower than those required to perfuse the brain, or from a shortage of energy substrates delivered to the brain through blood flow. Figure 3–2 and Table 3–1 identify the varying etiologies of syncope by categorizing the predominantly responsible physiologic mechanisms.

In small animals, syncope develops with generalized muscle weakness, progressing rapidly to ataxia, which may be followed by collapse and a brief period of loss of consciousness. Initially, the patient is motionless with relaxed skeletal muscles, but this may progress rapidly to uncoordinated muscular activity or jerks, giving the impression of seizure-like activity. Loss of control of muscle sphincters occurs in many cases, leading to involuntary urination and/or defecation. Often the animal cries out during the episode, and this release of central nervous activity is frequently misinterpreted by the owner as pain or fear. Recovery is usually rapid and complete, although the owner often reports that the episode is followed by a brief period of confusion. The differential diagnosis of syncope includes neurogenic seizures, narcolepsy, and catalepsy. Episodic weakness, acute hemorrhage, and diseases associated with reduced alertness also need to be distinguished from syncope.

Clinical Summary. With a complete history and physical examination, most cases of syncope can be identified without further study. Usually, all that is required would be an electrocardiogram and simple blood chemical analysis. In many cases, the clinician can identify the type and cause of syncope from the history. Postural hypotension requires ris-

TABLE 3–1. SYNCOPE

Decreased Cerebral Perfusion

Peripheral or neurogenic dysfunction (heart structurally normal)
  Vasovagal
  Postural hypotension
  Hyperventilation
  Carotid sinus sensitivity (vasodepressor type)
  Glossopharyngeal neuralgia associated with syncope
  Micturition syncope
Cardiac dysfunction (usually structurally abnormal)
  Obstruction to flow
    Aortic and pulmonary stenosis
    Myxomas
    Cardiac tamponade
    Dirofilariasis—severe
  Rhythm disturbances
    Heart block
    Tachyarrhythmia
  Cardiopulmonary dysfunction
    Low stroke volume
      Systolic dysfunction
      Diastolic dysfunction
    Pulmonary hypertension
    Pulmonary emboli
    Congenital heart disease (right-to-left shunt)
Myocardial infarction

Metabolic Disturbances

Anemia
Hepatic encephalopathy
Hyperkalemia
Hypoglycemia
Hypokalemia
Hypovolemia
Pheochromocytoma

Iatrogenic

Alpha-adrenergic blocking agents
Angiotensin-converting enzyme inhibitors
Antidepressants
Beta-blocking agents
Calcium channel blocking agents
Digitalis
Diuretics
Phenothiazine-related medications
Nitrates, vasodilators, etc.
Quinidine syncope

Miscellaneous

Tussive syncope
Pulseless disease
Syncope associated with swallowing

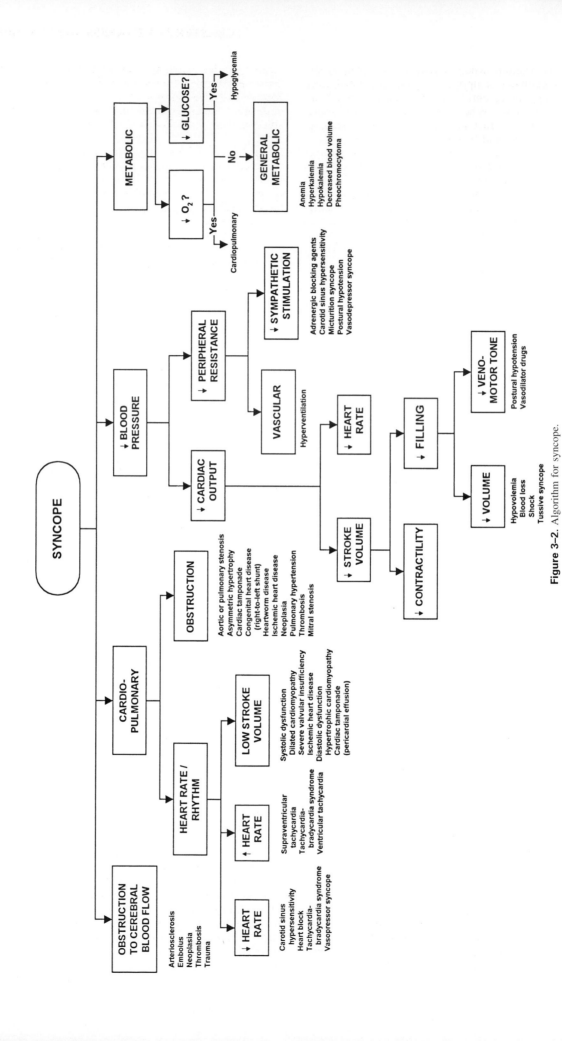

Figure 3–2. Algorithm for syncope.

ing to an upright position, whereas syncope occurring when the animal is recumbent or upright may be associated with hysterical fainting, hyperventilation, vasovagal, cardiac, or hypoglycemic episodes. When exercise precipitates the fainting attack, outflow tract obstruction, tachycardia, and postural hypotension should be considered.

Heart block should be considered when the dog or cat exercises and the heart rate is unable to increase sufficiently to maintain an adequate cardiac output for the patient's immediate needs. When fainting is continuously related to mealtime, the clinician should consider reactive or fasting hypoglycemic states. Antihypertensive agents, peripheral vasodilators, tranquilizers, nitrates, nitroglycerin, as well as diuretics, quinidine, and digitalis, are all possible causes for a syncopal episode.

Much can be determined by careful observation. Syncopal episodes are usually brief and transient. Premonitory signs do not precede syncope unless the patient feels generally weak or there is an arrhythmia occurring. In the rare case of cerebrovascular disease, the owner may report that the animal appears confused and has shown alterations in personality or mentation. Tussive syncope is preceded by bouts of hard, forceful coughing.

Auscultation of the heart, palpation of the pulses, and, when indicated, palpation of the bilateral cerebral pulses are required. Capillary refill time and the mucous membrane color should be evaluated. In some cases, further evaluation is necessary to identify the cause or type of fainting episode. Most of the clinical studies required can be performed with facilities available in a small animal veterinary practice. A full electrocardiogram is mandatory to detect atrial and ventricular arrhythmias. If the cause of syncope is still unknown, evaluation should be expanded to include an echocardiogram and 24-hour ambulatory electrocardiogram. While electrophysiologic testing via cardiac catheterization may be performed, ultrasonography is less risky and more commonly available. When blood pressure monitoring is available, indirect manometry for postural pressure measurements may yield valuable information in a small subset of patients.

Syncope in a Dog or Cat with a Normal Heart but with Peripheral Vascular Dysfunction. With peripheral or neurogenic dysfunction and a normal heart, the primary problem is either an abnormal reflex or a physiologic reflex initiated through a neuropsychiatric pathway. Neurocardiogenic (vasovagal or vasodepressor) syncope usually occurs in otherwise healthy individuals. In small animals, it appears to be associated with a sudden incident of either fright or extreme excitement. Often the pet has been immobile for a period of time leading up to the incident. Respiration usually increases, both in rate and depth, and the animal may appear weak and confused. The pupils dilate just prior to the loss of consciousness. Hemodynamically, there is peripheral arterial vasodilatation and venoconstriction. The cardiac output fails to rise despite a decrease in peripheral resistance and venoconstriction. Vagal overactivity results in bradycardia. This can be blocked with atropine in humans, but the fainting still occurs, suggesting that a decrease in the heart rate alone is not the cause.

Postural hypotension is also included in this category. Normal animals develop a slight fall in systolic blood pressure and a rise in diastolic pressure with only a slight increase in the heart rate upon rising. In contrast, those with postural hypotension develop a fall in both systolic and diastolic pressures with variable changes in the heart rate. Postural hypotension can be a complication of a number of

disease entities including diabetes mellitus, hypoadrenocorticism, and severe intravascular volume depletion due to disease or intensive diuresis. Drug therapy, including the broad category of beta-blocking agents, vasodilators, antihypertensives, and tranquilizers, is likely to induce similar side effects.

The hyperventilation syndrome belongs in the category of peripheral or neurogenic dysfunction. It is usually associated with anxious or hyperexcitable pets. The owner notes the patient's overbreathing, which, when continued, results in presyncopal symptoms up to and including a loss of consciousness. Such episodes may occur while the conscious animal is sitting, standing, or recumbent. Hyperventilation causes an overaeration of the alveoli and a subsequent fall in alveolar and arterial P_{CO_2} levels. Low P_{CO_2} levels have a profound effect on the vascular system and produce progressive cerebral arterial vasoconstriction along with peripheral vasodilatation. With stable or decreased perfusion pressure, there is a progressive decrease in oxygen delivery to the brain. The effects of hypoxia can be demonstrated on the electroencephalogram by diffuse slowing.

Carotid sinus sensitivity also belongs in the category of neurogenic dysfunction. The underlying reflex occurs as afferent impulses from the carotid sinuses are transmitted via the glossopharyngeal nerve to vasomotor and cardioinhibitory centers in the medulla. Vagal stimulation slows the heart by decreasing sinus and atrioventricular (A-V) nodal rates. This bradycardia and variable degree of A-V block decrease cardiac output and cerebral blood flow, and can cause cerebral anoxia. This chain of events can cause syncope. Atropine blocks this process, especially in brachycephalic dogs. Direct or indirect stimulation of the carotid sinus also causes sympathetic inhibition or vasodepressor effects that precipitate a fall in blood pressure. This syndrome is observed in pets in which neoplasms, inflammatory processes, or tight collars stimulate the carotid sinuses. Afferent impulses associated with pain in the ear, soft palate, or pharynx are transmitted centrally via the glossopharyngeal and vagal nerves and may also give rise to reflex hypotension and syncope (glossopharyngeal neuralgia). Syncope or, occasionally, severe dysrhythmia without syncope may be provoked by swallowing, usually in association with an esophageal tumor, diverticulum, or spasm, but syncope may occur without overt esophageal disease (deglutition syncope).

Syncope Due to Cardiac Dysfunction. A second major group of diseases resulting in decreased cerebral perfusion are those associated with cardiac dysfunction. Cardiac dysfunction for this purpose is divided into obstruction to blood flow, rhythm disturbances, cardiopulmonary dysfunction, and severely impaired myocardial contractility.

Subvalvular and valvular aortic stenosis are associated with syncope and a high incidence of sudden death. Exertional hypotension is a characteristic feature of virtually all forms of heart disease in which cardiac output is relatively fixed and fails to rise normally or declines during exertion. It is most characteristic of aortic stenosis and other forms of obstruction of left ventricular outflow in which cerebral ischemia occurs during exertion. Systemic vascular resistance ordinarily declines as a consequence of arteriolar dilatation secondary to the accumulation of vasodilator metabolites during exercise. Normally, compensation for this vasodilatation is via augmentation of cardiac output and arterial pressure. However, with outflow obstruction cardiac output rises proportionately less than vascular resistance falls and arterial pressure declines. The fixed, narrowed outflow tract is unable to accommodate the increased demands of cardiac output and oxygen requirements. In some pets, syncope occurs at rest. Animals with severe pulmonic stenosis with or without right-to-left shunts may similarly (but less commonly) suffer syncope upon exertion. Dogs or cats with atrial tumors may have syncope, as the pedunculated tumor intermittently obstructs the valve orifice. In severe dirofilariasis, the obstruction in the pulmonary arteries impairs blood flow to the lung. Ball valve thrombi in the atrium may similarly obstruct flow. Herniation of the appendage of the left atrium through an opening within the pericardium is a rare cause of syncope. Pedunculated LV and RV tumors cause recurrent syncopal attacks in dogs and cats.

In cardiac tamponade, pericardial effusion, and restrictive pericarditis, as well as all other forms of diastolic dysfunction, there is a delicate balance between the inflow of blood to the heart and the cardiac output. Sudden changes that decrease the return of blood to the heart or slow the rate may result in decreased cardiac output and, secondarily, syncope. In all cases associated with obstruction to the outflow of blood, ventricular dysrhythmias, or left ventricular failure following exercise should be considered as a possible cause of the syncope. Obstructive and restrictive cardiomyopathy in dogs and cats may reduce LV output enough to induce syncope. The heart rate increases, but the left ventricular volume is decreased and the result is a total reduction in cardiac output. Echocardiographic studies also suggest movement of the anterior (septal) mitral valve leaflet toward the ventricular septum during systole (SAM).

Rhythm disturbances causing syncope may include bundle branch blocks, bradyarrhythmias, and tachyarrhythmias. In heart block, the animal is characteristically alert when it regains consciousness. Often the animal appears unconcerned about the event and appears unaware that a problem existed. Transient heart block is a difficult diagnosis to establish without 24-hour continuous electrocardiographic monitoring. Stokes-Adams syncope refers to the syndrome associated with incomplete or complete A-V heart block and also includes sinus arrest, sinoatrial pause and block, and the sick sinus syndrome. In addition to syncope, there may be urinary and/or fecal incontinence as a result of a temporary loss of sphincter control. Seizure activity of a transient nature may also occur, necessitating a differential diagnosis from diseases of the central nervous system. Seizures are usually brief, may be tonic-clonic, tonic only, or the animal may be flaccid only but reported as having had a seizure.

Tachyarrhythmias result in decreased diastolic filling of the left ventricle, thereby resulting in a decreased cardiac output. Fainting may occur during the period of rapid heart beating or at the end of a paroxysm of atrial or ventricular tachycardia if asystole follows, the result of a physiologic condition called overdrive suppression.

In cardiopulmonary dysfunction, syncopal episodes usually occur with physical exertion or shortly thereafter. The duration of unconsciousness varies but is usually brief (1 to 2 minutes). Cyanosis is often present with this type of syncope. In congenital heart disease with shunting of blood from right to left, syncope is not uncommon owing to lowered blood Po_2 content causing cerebral anoxia. In the unusual occurrence of true myocardial infarction in dogs and cats, syncope may be due to left ventricular dysfunction or significant pain. Dogs and cats with severe myocardial disease have diminished cardiac reserve. Acute demands for additional cardiac output associated with exercise, excitement, or activity may result in a syncopal episode. Arrhythmias may similarly result in a short-term severe deficiency of blood flow, particularly newly developed atrial fibrillation.

Metabolic Disturbances Associated with Syncope. Syncopal episodes are associated with some metabolic disturbances. Hypoglycemia, hyperventilation with its associated alterations in physiologic parameters, calcium imbalances, and liver and renal dysfunction are other examples of metabolic disturbances that can cause fainting. Often the longer duration of the syncopal attack indicates a metabolic rather than a cardiac problem.

Iatrogenic Causes of Syncope. Iatrogenic causes of syncope must be considered whenever drugs are being administered. Digitalis intoxication associated with heart block, A-V dissociation, or a slow junctional rhythm is an example. Ventricular tachycardia and ventricular fibrillation can also result from digitalis intoxication. Potent diuretics, including the thiazides and furosemide, when given in excess, produce intravascular volume depletion that may contribute to or cause hypotension. Phenothiazine derivatives may produce a profound postural hypotension, resulting in disorientation and/or syncope when the patient suddenly rises. Peripheral vasodilating agents such as nitroglycerin and long-acting nitrates, beta blockade and calcium channel inhibitors, ACE inhibitors, and some antihypertension drugs may be associated with a fall in blood pressure, resulting in postural hypotension. Quinidine has the potential to produce arrhythmias and syncopal episodes.

Miscellaneous Causes of Syncope. Another category of syncopal episodes includes problems associated with coughing, lack of pulse, and swallowing. When attacks accompany paroxysms of coughing, *tussive syncope* is the result of an alteration in the normal circulation. Fainting occurs in the recumbent or standing subject, and consciousness is rapidly regained without serious sequelae. Coughing raises the intrathoracic pressure as well as cerebrospinal pressures. When the cerebrospinal fluid pressure is greater than the intracranial capillary perfusion pressures, there is a decrease in blood flow to the brain. The brain is then rapidly depleted of blood and oxygen, resulting in a syncopal attack. Therapy is directed toward the relief of the force and duration of the cough.

Pulseless disease is a cause of syncope when there are major obstructions to one or more major vessels supplying the head. The syncopal attack is usually precipitated by activity. Syncope associated with swallowing occurs with esophageal diverticula and other obstructive esophageal diseases. Various degrees of heart block develop upon initiation of the swallow reflex. The laryngeal nerves are sensitive to pressure, and these nerves are anatomically related to the carotid sinus. This disease should be considered a form of carotid sinus syncope, described earlier.

CHAPTER 4

ACUTE VISION LOSS

Susan A. McLaughlin and Holly L. Hamilton

Sudden apparent loss of vision in a dog or cat may be the chief or only presenting complaint. A wide range of lesions at various locations in the visual system can result in true blindness. The purpose of this chapter is to encourage complete ophthalmic evaluation and to provide guidelines for correlating ocular abnormalities with disease of other organ systems.

ABNORMALITIES RESULTING IN BLINDNESS

Blindness results from loss of vision in both eyes. Any lesion that interferes with the normal formation of an image on the retina, the transmission of that image to the visual cortex, or the final interpretation of the image by the visual cortex can result in blindness.

Lesions that result in opacification of the normally clear ocular media (cornea, aqueous humor, lens, and vitreous humor) prevent the formation of an image on the retina (Table 4–1). Diseases that affect the retina (Table 4–2) or the conducting pathway, consisting of the optic nerves, optic chiasm, optic tracts, lateral geniculate nuclei, and optic radiations (Table 4–3), interfere with the processing and transmission of the visual impulse to the brain. Finally, lesions in the visual cortex can prevent the interpretation of a normally

formed and transmitted image, resulting in blindness (Table 4–4).

ACUTE VISION LOSS VERSUS ACUTE RECOGNITION OF VISION LOSS

While certain systemic conditions may cause lesions in the eyes or central nervous system that result in acute loss of vision (e.g., diabetic cataracts, retinal detachment and vitreous hemorrhage due to hypertension, anoxia), many animals examined as a result of chief complaint of "sudden blindness" have problems that are neither acute nor systemic. These animals are brought to veterinarians because of an owner's sudden *recognition* of the vision loss. For example:

1. An animal that has lost vision slowly and compensated by memorizing its environment, such as a poodle with progressive retinal atrophy, undergoes an abrupt change in its environment.

2. An animal with unrecognized unilateral vision loss, such as a collie with retinal detachment due to collie eye anomaly or a cocker spaniel with chronic undiagnosed glaucoma, experiences acute disease in the other eye (e.g., the collie experiences a traumatic hyphema; the cocker spaniel develops acute glaucoma).

3. An animal with an ocular abnormality that causes partial visual impairment develops another abnormality that usually would result in only partial visual impairment; the two lesions together result in complete loss of vision (e.g., an elderly pug with pigmentary keratitis due to exophthalmos and lagophthalmos develops immature senile cataracts.)

A complete history and a thorough ophthalmic examination will help to differentiate these animals from those whose

TABLE 4–1. ABNORMALITIES CAUSING OPACIFICATION OF THE OCULAR MEDIA

Cornea

    Endothelial dystrophy
    Exposure keratitis
    Immune-mediated keratitis
    Keratoconjunctivitis sicca
    *Keratouveitis due to canine adenovirus I
    Lipid dystrophy
    Numerous genetic corneal dystrophies
    Scarring

Aqueous Humor

    *Fibrin (anterior uveitis)
    *Hyphema (trauma, blood dyscrasia, neoplasia)
    *Lipid

Cataracts

    Genetic
    *Metabolic (diabetes mellitus)
    Nutritional
    Toxic
    Traumatic

Vitreous Humor

    *Hemorrhage (trauma, systemic hypertension, retinal detachment, blood dyscrasia, neoplasia)
    *Hyalitis (numerous infectious diseases, penetrating injury)

  * Lesions that are most likely to result in the animal being presented with the complaint of acute vision loss.

TABLE 4–2. ABNORMALITIES RESULTING IN FAILURE OF THE RETINA TO PROCESS THE VISUAL MESSAGE

Retinopathies

    Central progressive retinal atrophy (retinal pigment epithelial dystrophy)
    Feline central retinal degeneration (taurine deficiency)
    Glaucoma
    Progressive retinal atrophy (includes rod-cone dysplasia, rod dysplasia, progressive rod-cone degeneration)
    *Sudden acquired retinal degeneration syndrome (SARD)

Retinal Detachment Syndromes

    Collie eye anomaly
    *Exudative/transudative retinal detachment (systemic hypertension, systemic mycoses, protothechosis, ehrlichiosis, toxoplasmosis, feline infectious peritonitis, canine distemper, immune-mediated disease)
    *Neoplasia
    Retinal dysplasia

  * Lesions that are most likely to result in the animal being presented with the complaint of acute vision loss.

17

*Canine distemper
Feline infectious peritonitis
*Granulomatous meningoencephalitis (GME, "reticulosis")
Hydrocephalus (optic radiations)
*Idiopathic (immune-mediated) optic neuritis
*Lead toxicity
*Neoplasia (particularly pituitary, meningioma, astrocytoma)
Optic nerve hypoplasia
*Systemic mycoses
Traumatic avulsion of optic nerves

* Lesions that are most likely to result in the animal being presented with the complaint of acute vision loss.

vision loss is the result of systemic disease. A minimum database should include evaluation of vision and pupillary light reflexes, measurement of intraocular pressures, and visual examination of the anterior and posterior segments of the eyes.

EVALUATION OF VISION

Objective measurements of vision, such as visually evoked cortical potentials or visual acuity testing, are still somewhat experimental in animals and are not widely available to most veterinarians. Clinical tests available to veterinarians for evaluation of vision are nonquantitative and nonstandardized. These fairly crude tests include negotiation of an obstacle course, detection of movement, the menace response, and the visual placing postural reaction (Fig. 4–1).

Obstacle Course. A simple obstacle course can be set up in an examination room or hallway using several fairly large, solid, but lightweight objects such as plastic wastebaskets. The animal is allowed to move freely, and its ability to avoid the obstacles is observed. We usually place the obstacles between the animal and the owner, have the owner call the animal's name (once or twice only, to reduce the probability of the animal following the sound), and watch the animal negotiate the maze. The obstacles can be rearranged for multiple trials in a constantly changing environment. If the room lights can be dimmed, comparative evaluation of day and night vision can be made. This test does not work well with cats, animals that are unable or unwilling to walk, or in demented, compulsively pacing animals.

TABLE 4–4. ABNORMALITIES RESULTING IN FAILURE TO INTERPRET THE VISUAL MESSAGE

*Canine distemper
Feline infectious peritonitis
*Granulomatous meningoencephalitis (GME, reticulosis)
*Heatstroke
Hepatoencephalopathy
Hydrocephalus
*Hypoglycemia
*Hypoxia
*Infarct (cerebral vascular accident)
*Neoplasia
*Postictal
Storage diseases
*Systemic mycoses
*Trauma (hemorrhage, edema)

* Lesions that are most likely to result in the animal being presented with the complaint of acute vision loss.

Motion Detection. An animal's ability to detect motion can be evaluated by dropping cotton balls or rolling a cylinder of tape through its visual field and observing eye or head movements as it follows the moving object. Care must be taken that the object does not create air currents or noise to which the blind animal may respond in a way that is mistaken for vision. Interpretation of this test is difficult in animals that are depressed or simply disinterested.

Menace Reaction. Menace testing involves advancing the hand or fist toward the eye such that the animal blinks or flinches in avoidance. This protective reaction is a learned response that should be present in dogs and cats older than 10 to 12 weeks of age, but it may be difficult to elicit a reliable response in some pets. In addition, severe dementia or severe cerebellar disease (e.g., tentorial herniation) will lessen or eliminate menace reaction.

Because blinking requires normal facial nerve and orbicularis oculi muscle function, the palpebral reflex should be evaluated before testing the menace response. If the animal is unable to blink, one may be able to observe retraction of the globe (cranial nerve VI and retractor bulbi muscle) and passive elevation of the third eyelid. As with motion detection, one must be careful not to create sounds or air currents that may evoke a menace reaction in a blind animal.

Visual Placing Postural Reaction. To test the visual placing postural reaction, the animal is suspended nearly horizontally, but with the forelimbs lower than the hindlimbs, and the forelimbs brought to the edge of a table. A sighted animal will elevate a foreleg and place it on the table's surface before the leg touches the table. A blind animal will not elevate its legs until they touch the table's edge.

PUPILLARY LIGHT REFLEXES AND ELECTRORETINOGRAPHY (see also Chapter 107)

Pupillary light reflexes and electroretinography do not test vision but may be helpful in localizing lesions. Testing the pupillary light reflex (PLR) requires a bright focal light source and a darkened room. Electroretinography requires specialized equipment and usually is available only at specialty practices or academic institutions.

Normal PLR depends on healthy retinas, optic nerves, optic chiasm, optic tracts, pretectal and accessory oculomotor (Edinger-Westphal) nuclei, oculomotor nerves (parasympathetic portion), and irises. The PLR is not significantly affected by lesions such as cataract or pigmentary keratitis, although opacification of the cornea or aqueous humor may prevent visualization of the response. Iris atrophy, a common finding in many older dogs and cats, will often cause a diminished PLR in animals with otherwise normal retinas and nerve pathways. Stimulation of the sympathetic nervous system can result in diminished PLR in animals that are nervous or frightened, such as dogs or cats with acute vision loss. Therefore, if the initial response is not normal, it should be reevaluated after the pet has had an opportunity to become accustomed to its surroundings.

Unfortunately, the PLR requires much less photoreceptor function than is required for normal vision. Animals with retinal detachment or extensive retinal degeneration may retain enough photoreceptor function to produce a fairly normal PLR. Thus, while the absence of PLR is significant, the presence of PLR does not rule out retinal disease.

Electroretinography records a mass electrical response of the retina to light stimulation. It primarily tests the function

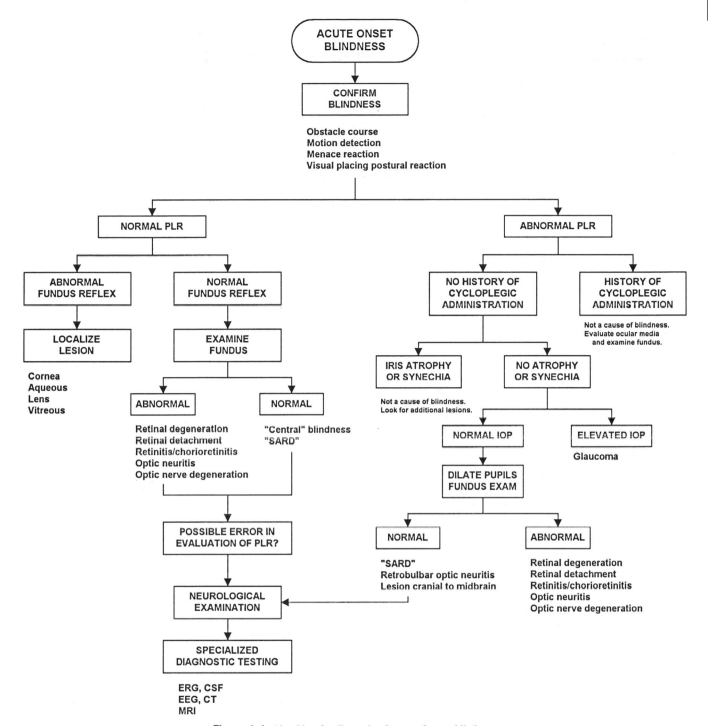

Figure 4–1. Algorithm for diagnosis of onset of acute blindness.

of the photoreceptors (rods and cones), although there is some contribution from cells of the inner nuclear layer (primarily Müller's cells), and the retinal pigment epithelium. In the dog, the electroretinogram (ERG) is fully developed by the eighth week of life. Electroretinography does not test the function of the nerve fiber layer of the retina, the optic nerve, or the other parts of the visual system involved in transmission or interpretation of the visual message. The most common use of the ERG in evaluation of acute vision loss is to differentiate between photoreceptor disease and diseases affecting the optic nerve and/or brain in animals that appear normal on ophthalmoscopic examination.

OTHER DIAGNOSTIC TESTS

Visually evoked cortical potentials (also called visually evoked responses) are electrical alterations in response to a visual stimulus that are recorded from the scalp over the occipital cortex. They require sophisticated equipment, and their significance is not well defined in animals.

Electroencephalography may be helpful in defining intracranial nervous system disease but is not universally available.

As indicated by the algorithm (see Fig. 4–1), other specialized tests such as serology, culture, cerebrospinal fluid analysis, computed tomography (CT) scans, and magnetic resonance imaging (MRI) may be required for definitive diagnosis of the patient with acute vision loss.

CHAPTER 5

PAIN: Identification

Spencer A. Johnston

Pain can be defined as the perception of an unpleasant sensation that originates from a specific body region. This perception is based not only on neuronal input, but also includes the interpretation of this input based on past experience and present state of mind. Although often considered to be bad, pain normally occurs only when there is actual or potential for tissue injury. It most frequently serves as a warning device so that the individual experiencing pain will avoid the potentially harmful stimulus. However, in instances of controlled injury, such as during surgery or medical intervention, the diagnosis and management of pain are more difficult.

Beyond being unpleasant, pain may have deleterious effects on other body systems by interfering with immune function, increasing tissue metabolism, or decreasing respiratory function. Although treatment of pain can be justified in terms of avoiding these deleterious effects, relief of pain is justification unto itself. In the words of Galen, "Divinum est sedare dolorem" (it is divine to allay pain).

PATHOPHYSIOLOGY

The basic anatomy and physiology of the structures necessary for pain perception are similar across species. Pain is initiated by the stimulation of nociceptors. These are free nerve terminals of afferent fibers that are present in nearly all tissues but are most numerous in those tissues that interact with the environment, such as the skin, muscles, and joints, versus the more protected tissues such as the viscera. These specialized receptors are specific for pain and are distinct from mechanoreceptors (which provide the sensations of touch, pressure, vibration, and proprioception) and non-nociceptive thermal receptors (that detect heat and cold). Nociceptors are innervated by two types of afferent nerves, myelinated Aδ and unmyelinated C fibers. Type Aδ fibers are fast-response fibers and are associated with nociceptors that respond to both mechanical and thermal injury. These are the type of fibers initially stimulated by an injury such as a pin prick. Type C fibers are associated with polymodal nociceptors that respond to mechanical, thermal, and chemical injury. Activation of type C receptors is associated with the dull, aching pain that occurs following the acute pain of a pin prick. Stimulation of type C fibers induces the release of inflammatory mediators and neurotransmitters in the dorsal horn of the spinal cord that enhance further pain perception, a phenomenon know as central sensitization.

One of the features that distinguishes nociceptors from other neural receptors is the lack of "fatigue" with continued stimulation. Stimulation of a nociceptor will result in an impulse being transmitted to the spinal cord as long as the nociceptor is being stimulated, and frequently results in increased sensitivity of the receptor to further stimulation. This differs from a touch receptor, where continuous stimulation will eventually result in receptor fatigue and extinction of the signal to the spinal cord, resulting in numbness. For this reason, relief of pain must occur either through correction of the underlying condition or through efforts to prevent the nociceptive impulse from reaching and ascending the spinal cord.

Pain is generally considered to have a somatic or visceral origin. Somatic pain, or that type of pain occurring from the musculoskeletal and other peripheral systems, is typically distinct and well localized. This is due to the mapping of the afferent Aδ and C fibers in the dorsal horn of the spinal cord, from which the impulse ascends to the thalamus and cerebral cortex, where integration and interpretation of the nociceptive input occurs. The density of nociceptive fibers and how they project onto the dorsal horn allow for specificity in localization. Visceral pain, or pain originating from the internal organs, is less well localized and is frequently described by humans as having a vague origin, or coming from deep within the body. Most visceral tissue does not respond to such damaging stimuli as cutting, crushing, or burning. Neoplastic deformation of many organs, such as the lungs and liver, does not seem to cause pain at all. However, some internal organs may be sensitive to other stimuli, such as distention, inflammation, and ischemia. For example, the gastrointestinal tract, urinary tract, and the gallbladder yield pain with both distention or inflammation. This pain is typically difficult to localize, most likely owing to the few nociceptors that are present in the abdominal viscera being distributed diffusely throughout the abdomen.

Peripheral pain typically becomes more localized with increasing intensity, whereas visceral pain generally becomes more diffuse. Furthermore, visceral pain but not somatic pain demonstrates the ability to summate; the greater the area involved (as in distention of the entire intestinal tract as compared with just a small portion of the duodenum), the greater the intensity of pain. The intensity of the stimulus necessary to cause a pain response may also be related to the surface area exposed to the stimulus. For example, a large amount of distention of an isolated region of the intestine may be necessary to elicit the same response as moderate distention of the entire intestine.

Although the viscera are relatively devoid of nociceptors, the peritoneum and pleura are rich with these structures, and frequently abnormalities of viscera that cause inflammation of the peritoneum or pleura will cause pain that may be quite severe. Additionally, referred pain may occur with visceral stimulation, whereby an afferent impulse from a visceral organ is superimposed on an afferent nerve branch from somatic tissue. The impulse then ascends to the dorsal horn and cerebral cortex, and is interpreted as originating from the somatic tissue. For this reason, pain originating from the urinary tract may be manifested as pain from the lumbar musculature.

RECOGNITION AND MEASUREMENT OF PAIN

It is clear that the perception of pain differs from nociception, or the neurologic activity of nociceptors. Despite simi-

lar levels of nociceptor activity, some animals are, like some humans, innately stoic, whereas others demonstrate pain readily. Although some species traits exist, there is frequently variation in an individual's response to painful stimuli, making interpretation by an observer difficult. Identification of all behaviors associated with pain is not practical. However, a common theme to nearly all behaviors associated with pain is an obvious change in behavior. Behavior changes associated with pain include either an aggressive or submissive posture, withdrawal from or lack of interest in the surrounding environment, loss of greeting behavior, depression, stupor, agitation, restlessness, changes in grooming habits, anorexia, insomnia, altered facial expression, and vocalization. Physical examination may include general findings, such as salivation, mydriasis, tachycardia, and tachypnea, or more specific findings that help to localize the origin of pain, such as edema, lameness, sensitivity to palpation and manipulation, and identification of areas of hyperalgesia (an exaggerated pain response to a noxious stimulus) or allodynia (pain produced by stimuli that would never normally do so). Body posture may be altered to protect an injured region, or an animal may refuse to lie down. When interpreting the significance of these clinical findings, consideration must be given to the patient's overall status and

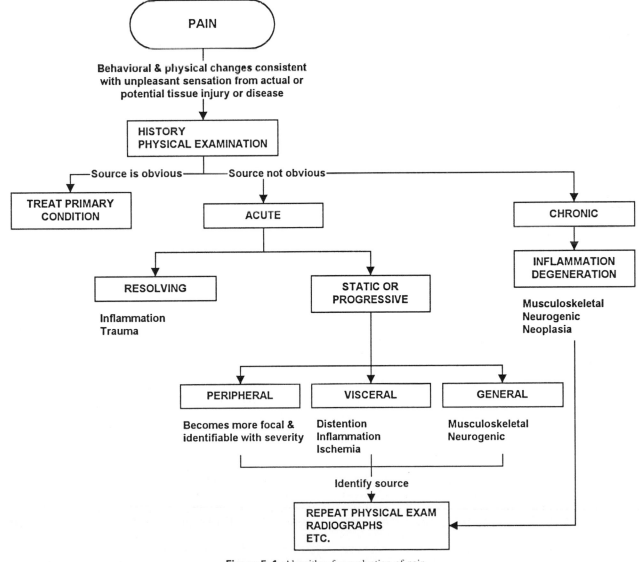

Figure 5–1. Algorithm for evaluation of pain.

ability to respond. Some patients may be too ill to display these behaviors, and absence of a response to an injury or disease state that would rationally be considered painful should not be interpreted as the patient being free from pain.

Identification of behaviors characteristic of acute pain may differ from those associated with chronic pain. Chronic pain is frequently associated with changes in behavior that can be observed by the owner, such as changes in routine, willingness to exercise or perform certain physical activities, appetite, sleep patterns, elimination habits, and overall demeanor. Physical examination findings are similar to those found with acute pain but may also include the result of disuse, such as muscle atrophy, or evidence of chronic tissue reactivity to an inflammatory process, such as hyperplasia or fibrosis.

Since interpretation of a pain response is subjective, attempts have been made to measure various physiologic parameters to quantitate pain. Mixed results have been obtained using this approach. Most frequently, subjective criteria for pain have not correlated with physiologic parameters such as heart and respiratory rate, blood pressure, or serum cortisol or catecholamine levels, although in certain studies trends may be noted. Unfortunately, application of specific criteria to individual animals for the diagnosis of pain is impractical. Rather, veterinarians should ask themselves whether the condition would be considered painful in a human being. The long held tenet that animals should experience pain following surgery in order to prevent them from destroying surgical fixation should be replaced with the notion that provision of analgesia will help to decrease stress and postoperative morbidity. Although complete ablation of pain may be the goal of analgesia, this rarely occurs. A more attainable goal for analgesia is to reduce pain and allow an animal to rest comfortably, recognizing that stimulation of an injured area often results in the perception of acute pain.

HISTORICAL FINDINGS

In animals, pain is usually associated with inflammation or tissue trauma. It is uncommon for an animal to be brought to a veterinarian with generalized pain but without any clue as to the source of the pain. Frequently, a history of trauma will provide a substantial basis for further diagnostic evaluation. Similarly, a history that rules out trauma allows the clinician to concentrate on other pathologic processes, such as degenerative, neurogenic, visceral, and neoplastic etiologies.

Since nociceptors do not fatigue, a history of acute onset of pain followed by recovery within a short period (days or less) is suggestive of trauma or inflammation that is resolving in the natural course of healing. Acute or chronic pain that worsens suggests progressive inflammation or tissue degeneration. Acute pain followed by chronic pain suggests partial resolution of injury or inflammation. Intermittent pain is usually associated with mild to moderate injury or disease exacerbated by periods of inflammation, often associated with use or other specific events. Severe generalized pain is often due to systemic inflammatory conditions involving the musculoskeletal or neurologic systems, such as myositis, inflammatory arthritis, or meningitis.

DIAGNOSTIC EVALUATION

Good observational and physical examination skills, which include thorough palpation and manipulation, will frequently allow the clinician to localize pain to a body region or system (Fig. 5–1). Once localized, more specialized diagnostic tests may then be performed to establish the primary cause of pain. Radiographic examination will frequently provide sufficient information to provide a diagnosis. Tissue aspiration and cytology or biopsy may provide information regarding inflammation or neoplasia. Other diagnostic tests are performed as indicated to confirm or rule out specific disease conditions.

If a diagnosis cannot be achieved through appropriate diagnostic testing for a specific condition, occasionally the only way to make a diagnosis is to wait for the disease condition to further manifest itself. Inflammatory conditions may naturally resolve; somatic pain conditions may become more localized; visceral conditions may summate and provide greater diagnostic clues; and radiographic changes may become more obvious. Observation of subtle behavioral changes during this time period may also greatly aid in diagnosing either the cause or the presence of pain.

CHAPTER 6

PAIN: Management

Elizabeth M. Hardie

Management of pain depends on the length of time pain has been present, the site from which the pain impulses arise, and the state of awareness of the animal.

ASPECTS OF PAIN

ACUTE VERSUS CHRONIC PAIN

Acute pain is associated with events such as an injury, surgery, a diagnostic manipulation, or a short-lived painful disease such as pancreatitis. Regardless, there is a sudden input of nociceptive (pain recognition) impulses to the central nervous system, followed by continuing impulses related to any ongoing injury or inflammation. If the nociceptive impulses reach the spinal cord, a "wind-up" phenomenon occurs, which results in the peripheral sensory fields enlarging and becoming more sensitive to input. Thus, whenever possible, the treatment goal in acute pain is to prevent these impulses from ever reaching the central nervous system. If this goal cannot be achieved, the goal is to modify central nervous system response to such impulses (Tables 6–1 and 6–2).

Chronic pain is defined as pain that has been present for over 3 months. Examples are osteoarthritis and cancer pain. Chronic pain is usually associated with a disease process that can be managed but not cured. Permanent changes in the central nervous system may reinforce the perception of pain and make treatment difficult. The goal of treatment is to provide modification of the pain sensation without exacerbation of the inciting disease. A useful concept in the treatment of chronic pain has been developed for cancer patients. Pain treatment occurs in "steps" up a ladder, and each step uses more potent pain control drugs.

SITE OF ORIGIN

The ability to manage pain depends greatly on the site of origin. If the injury/inflammation is localized to a region of the body from which nociceptive impulses can be blocked using local or epidural analgesia, the systemic reaction to pain can be eliminated. If body cavities or large amounts of tissue cranial to the pelvis are affected, prevention of a systemic stress response is not possible. The goal is then to make the patient more comfortable.

STATE OF AWARENESS

State of awareness determines whether or not there is cortical processing of the painful sensation. Thus anesthesia prevents the cortical response to pain, but does nothing to modify the peripheral and spinal processing of painful impulses. Similarly, sedatives may alter the perception of, or

response to, pain without modifying the transmission of nociceptive impulses. Since behavior is often used to assess pain, it is important to distinguish between the ability to feel pain, the body's response to pain, and conscious awareness of pain.

TECHNIQUES OF PAIN MANAGEMENT

LOCAL ANESTHETICS

Lidocaine and bupivicaine are used in acute pain to prevent nociceptive impulses from reaching the central nervous system. Mixing the drugs with epinephrine keeps the local anesthetic at the site and allows a longer duration of action with fewer systemic side effects. Lidocaine is used mainly for fast diagnostic or therapeutic procedures (catheter placement, bone marrow biopsy, suturing a laceration, removal of a skin mass) that require a quick onset of action and are not expected to result in ongoing pain. Bupivicaine is used when pain after the procedure is expected to be prolonged (tooth extraction, intercostal nerve block for flail chest). Infiltration techniques (injection into peripheral nerves supplying the painful site or infusion into cavities [thorax, joint]) may also be used.

EPIDURAL INJECTIONS

Drugs can be administered into the epidural space in order to modify spinal transmission of nociceptive impulses. Much lower doses of drug are needed with this route of administration versus systemic routes, decreasing the incidence of side effects. The most commonly used epidural drugs are morphine, bupivicaine, lidocaine, and medetomidine. Lipid-soluble drugs such as the local anesthetics and medetomidine have a predominately local effect and act on the caudal half of the animal. Morphine, a water-soluble drug, will distribute over several hours throughout the spinal canal. The duration of action depends on the drug, but a single epidural injection of 50 per cent morphine/50 per cent bupivicaine may last up to 18 hours.

Single epidural injections are used mainly for pain control during surgery and in the immediate postoperative period. Animals with ongoing painful conditions (pancreatitis, muscle trauma, large en-bloc tumor resections) are often managed best with indwelling epidural catheters that allow constant infusion of drugs at the spinal segments receiving impulses from the painful site. In particular, cats in pain are easier to manage with drugs administered through an epidural catheter, rather than systemically, because of the reduced side effects of the narcotics.

INTRAVENOUS AND INTRAMUSCULAR DRUGS

Systemically administered pain drugs are used to provide pain relief when the nociceptive impulses cannot be blocked

TABLE 6–1. EXAMPLES OF PAIN CONTROL DRUGS

CLASS	DRUG	DOSAGE	MAJOR TOXICITY/ COMMENTS
Local anesthetic	2% lidocaine with epinephrine (1:100,000)	1–5 mL/site, up to 7 mg/kg (dog) or 2 mg/kg (cat)	Seizures, hypotension, depression
Local anesthetic	0.5% bupivicaine with epinephrine (1:200,000)	1–5 mL/site, 0.5 mL/kg in joint, 1.5 mg/kg intrapleurally (dog), do not exceed 2 mg/kg in cat	Seizures, hypotension, depression
Epidural opioid	Preservative-free morphine	0.1–0.2 mg/kg (0.05 mg/kg if spinal)	Vomiting, urine retention, respiratory compromise
Epidural local anesthetic	0.25–0.5% bupivicaine with epinephrine	1 mL/5 kg (0.5 mL/kg if spinal)	Respiratory compromise, hind leg weakness
IV NSAID	Ketoprofen	2 mg/kg IV once	GI ulcers
IM alpha$_2$-agonist	Medetomidine	5–10 µg/kg IM, use with IM opioid	Bradycardia, respiratory depression
IV opioid	Morphine	0.1–0.5 mg/kg/hr IV (dog)	Respiratory depression, decreased GI motility, urinary retention
Transdermal opioid	Fentanyl, transdermal patch	25 µg/hr (cat) 10–20 kg dog, 50 µg/hr 20–30 kg dog, 75 µg/hr >30 kg dog, 100 µg/hr	12 hours to become effective, lasts 3 days, respiratory depression, decreased GI motility
Oral NSAID	Aspirin	10–25 mg/kg PO q 12 hr in food (dog) 10 mg/kg PO q 48–72 hr in food (cat)	GI irritation, ulcers, kidney damage
Oral NSAID	Carprofen	2 mg/kg PO q 12 hr (dog), limit to 2 days (cat)	Toxicity associated with chronic use in cats, idiosyncratic liver toxicity in dogs
Oral NSAID	Etodolac	5–15 mg/kg q 24 hr (dog)	Hypoproteinemia
Oral NSAID	Piroxicam	0.3 mg/kg PO q 24 hr, then q 48 hr in food (dog) Cancer dose: q 24 hr (dog)	GI irritation, ulcers, kidney damage, use misoprostol at high doses
Oral NSAID/weak opioid	Codeine 60 mg + acetaminophen 300 mg	1–2 mg/kg codeine PO q 6–8 hr (dog)	Acetaminophen is hepatotoxic
Oral opioid agonist/antagonist	Butorphanol	0.5–1 mg/kg PO q 6–8 hr (dog or cat)	Respiratory depression, decreased GI motility
Oral opioid	Morphine, oral sustained release	1.5–3 mg/kg PO q 12 hr (dog)	Respiratory depression, decreased GI motility
Oral tricyclic antidepressant	Amitriptyline	1–2 mg/kg PO q 12–24 hr (dog) 2.5–12.5 mg/cat PO q 24 hr	Sedation, nausea, cardiac conduction disturbances, dry eye, dry mouth, constipation

at the local or spinal level. They are also used to treat breakthrough pain, which is sudden pain associated with movement or periodic pain that escalates above the pain controlled by a baseline level of analgesia. Nonsteroidal anti-inflammatory drugs (NSAIDs), alpha$_2$-agonist drugs, and narcotics are common systemic agents.

Nonsteroidal anti-inflammatory drugs are most useful for surgical procedures such as superficial tumor removal, ovariohysterectomy, or minor orthopedic procedures. They must be used cautiously because hypotension can exacerbate their renal toxic effects and prolonged use may result in gastrointestinal side effects. Cats can often tolerate a single dose of these drugs but develop toxic effects with prolonged administration.

Alpha$_2$-agonist drugs are used primarily for sedation or anesthesia, but they also have pronounced analgesic effects. The cardiovascular side effects prevent their systemic use in high doses, but they are often useful in low doses, particularly in cats, as part of an analgesic "cocktail."

Narcotics are the most commonly used systemic pain control drugs. Butorphanol, a narcotic agonist-antagonist, is widely used but has short-lasting analgesic effects (less than 2 hours in the dog). Oxymorphone is a safe narcotic agonist,

providing analgesia for 3 to 4 hours, but it is expensive for use in larger animals and may cause excitement in cats. Morphine is inexpensive and can be administered as a constant-rate infusion in maintenance intravenous fluids. Buprenorphine, a partial opioid agonist, is used when constant supervision cannot be provided, since it provides analgesia for 6 to 8 hours. All narcotics are dosed to effect, because there is up to a fivefold variation in analgesic doses in normal individuals.

TRANSDERMAL DRUGS

Fentanyl, a narcotic agonist, is available in a skin patch that releases drug at a constant rate. These patches can be used to provide analgesia for both acute and chronic pain patients. Dogs and cats do not develop the respiratory depression that has resulted in the death of some people using patches; thus the patches are considered safe.

ORAL DRUGS

Oral drugs are used for treatment of dogs and cats with chronic pain and for transitioning acute pain patients off

TABLE 6–2. TREATMENT OF PAIN

I. Acute pain
  A. Postsurgical
    1. Premedication with opioid (oxymorphone) or alpha-blocker (medetomidine)
    2. Local nerve block before incision (intercostal block)
    3. Single epidural injection before incision (morphine)
    4. Local analgesia after surgery (infusion of bupivacaine through thoracostomy tube)
    5. Systemic analgesia after surgery (CRI of morphine for at least 12 hours)
    6. Taper to oral analgesics 24–48 hours after surgery (aspirin and codeine)
  B. Injury
    1. Systemic opioids to effect (oxymorphone)
    2. Transition to oral nonsteroidals (carprofen)
  C. Abdominal
    1. Place epidural catheter (CRI morphine/bupivacaine mixture)
    2. Systemic opioids for breakthrough pain

II. Chronic
  A. Neuropathic
    1. Oral tricyclic antidepressants (amitriptyline)
  B. Cancer
    1. Use World Health Organization multi-step treatment ladder
      a. Nonsteroidals (carprofen)
      b. Nonsteroidals plus weak opioids (acetaminophen and codeine)
      c. Strong opioids (fentanyl patches to effect, oral morphine)
    2. Adjuvant therapy (palliative radiation, acupuncture)

III. Osteoarthritis
  A. Environmental modification (ramps, padding)
  B. Weight control
  C. Controlled daily exercise
  D. Oral pain medications
    1. Dogs—nonsteroidals
    2. Cats—EOD aspirin, butorphanol, corticosteroids
  E. Chondroprotective agents

CRI = constant-rate infusion, EOD = every other day.

other forms of pain control. The common oral drugs are NSAIDs (aspirin only in the cat), NSAID-weak opioid combinations (dogs), narcotics, chondroprotective agents, and corticosteroids (cats).

NSAIDs are used for the treatment of inflammation associated with surgery or injury, osteoarthritis, and as the first step in the cancer pain treatment ladder. A variety of drugs (aspirin, carprofen, piroxicam, etodolac) can be used in the dog, although monitoring for side effects is critical. Aspirin is the only NSAID for which a safe chronic dosing regimen is known for the cat. The combination drugs (aspirin/codeine, acetaminophen/codeine) are used to transition surgical patients and as the intermediate step in the cancer pain treatment ladder. They can be used only in dogs.

Oral butorphanol is a useful chronic pain control drug in the cat, but it may produce sedative side effects. Oral morphine is used as the top step in the cancer pain control ladder in dogs, as are fentanyl skin patches in dogs and cats.

Corticosteroids are used for pain control in cats with end-stage arthritis. Chronic use of corticosteroids in arthritis may hasten the development of cartilage destruction, but at this stage of the disease, patient comfort is usually of primary concern.

Oral chondroprotective agents are often used in the treatment of osteoarthritis. To date, there is only anecdotal evidence of their efficacy in the chronic stages of this disease.

NEUROPATHIC PAIN

Neuropathic pain is pain that is the result of damage to or disease in nervous tissue. Examples include nerve root tumors, enlarging tumors that compress nerves, and idiopathic cystitis in cats. Neuropathic pain is often resistent to conventional pain therapy and is treated with tricyclic antidepressant drugs.

NONDRUG THERAPY

Acupuncture may be used to treat both acute and chronic pain. The mechanism of analgesia in acupuncture appears to involve stimulation of inhibitory interneurons in the spinal cord, as well as endogenous release of encephalins, endorphins, and opiates.

SUMMARY

Pain control is an integral part of patient management. Invasive diagnostic and therapeutic manipulations, surgery, and acutely painful medical conditions all require the use of analgesic drugs and techniques. In patients with chronic pain, the treatment plan is aimed at maintaining a good quality of life.

CHAPTER 7

THE SKIN AS A SENSOR OF INTERNAL MEDICAL DISORDERS

Stephen D. White

Knowledge of skin disease in small animals has so increased in recent years that it is difficult to describe a cutaneous condition that does *not* have some relation to internal medicine. Even the ubiquitous flea allergy dermatitis involves complex internal immunologic mechanisms. However, the purpose of this chapter is to discuss those diseases having cutaneous manifestations that should alert the clinician to further investigation of internal organ systems (Fig. 7–1).

CONGENITAL-HEREDITARY SYNDROMES (GENODERMATOSES)

These diseases are present at birth or noted shortly thereafter. Affected animals should not be bred.

Dermatomyositis. This disease has been reported primarily in collies and Shetland sheepdogs and their crosses, although other breeds have a sporadic incidence. As its name implies, the disease affects both the muscles and the skin. Cutaneous changes include crusts, ulcerations, vesicles, and/or alopecia around the mucocutaneous junctions, front legs, ear tips, and tail. Muscular atrophy may be generalized or selective, often affecting the temporal and masseter muscles. Clinical manifestations vary, with some dogs having only skin or muscular signs, while both systems are affected in others. Serum enzymes such as creatinine phosphokinase (CPK) are usually normal, and muscle involvement often may be proved only by biopsy or electromyography. Skin biopsies generally demonstrate perifollicular mononuclear inflammation and occasionally show intracellular edema of the basal cell layer of the epidermis with subepidermal clefts. The onset of clinical signs usually occurs before the age of 6 months. The severity of disease varies. Some dogs improve with age. Females should be spayed, as estrus may exacerbate clinical signs. Pentoxifylline, 10 mg/kg every 8 hours, is often effective in controlling the disease.

ENDOCRINOPATHIES

These diseases are probably the most common internal diseases associated with cutaneous manifestations.

Hypothyroidism. Cutaneous lesions may consist of total or partial alopecia; seborrhea; hyperpigmentation; thick, cool, or puffy skin; easy bruising; a dry, easily epilated hair coat; secondary pyoderma or dermatophytosis; and otitis externa. Pruritus may be present, particularly in association with pyoderma or seborrhea (see Chapter 151).

Hyperadrenocorticism. Cutaneous lesions in the dog include alopecia (usually truncal, but occasionally facial), hyperpigmentation, seborrhea, pyoderma, dermatophytosis or demodicosis secondary to immunosuppression, thin skin, comedones, easy bruising, and calcinosis cutis. Pruritus may be present in conjunction with pyoderma, seborrhea, demodicosis, or calcinosis cutis. Skin lesions may be the *only* abnormality noted by the client or the veterinarian, without polyuria, polydipsia, hepatomegaly, eosinopenia, or increased serum alkaline phosphatase (see Chapter 154). Hyperadrenocorticism in the cat may cause a bilateral nonpruritic alopecia, generalized demodicosis, and extremely thin fragile skin.

Sertoli Cell Tumor. Testicular Sertoli cell tumors in dogs may cause alopecia and feminization. Both seminomas and interstitial cell tumors may (rarely) cause the same clinical signs. The cause (at least in one third of dogs with Sertoli cell tumors) is the increased level of estrogen or estrogen-type hormones produced by the tumor. These dogs are occasionally pruritic with a papular eruption. Therapy consists of the removal of *both* testicles; not all tumors are palpable, and undescended testicles are at higher risk for neoplasia. A thorough presurgical evaluation is indicated (complete blood and platelet count, thoracic and abdominal radiographs), as bone marrow suppression and malignancy with metastases have been uncommonly reported.

Pheochromocytoma. Dogs with pheochromocytoma are usually brought to a veterinarian as a result of episodic weakness, panting, lethargy, collapse, or polyuria/polydipsia. This disease should be included in the differentiation of erythema without pruritus.

DISEASES INVOLVING INTERNAL ORGANS

Hepatic Disease. While hepatobiliary disease in humans often causes pruritus and other clinical signs, this seems to be relatively rare in small animals. Occasionally a cat with cholangiohepatitis or other liver disease is seen with a pruritic, generalized exfoliative dermatitis or with skin fragility similar to that reported in hyperadrenocorticism for this species. The etiology of this is not understood (see Chapter 140).

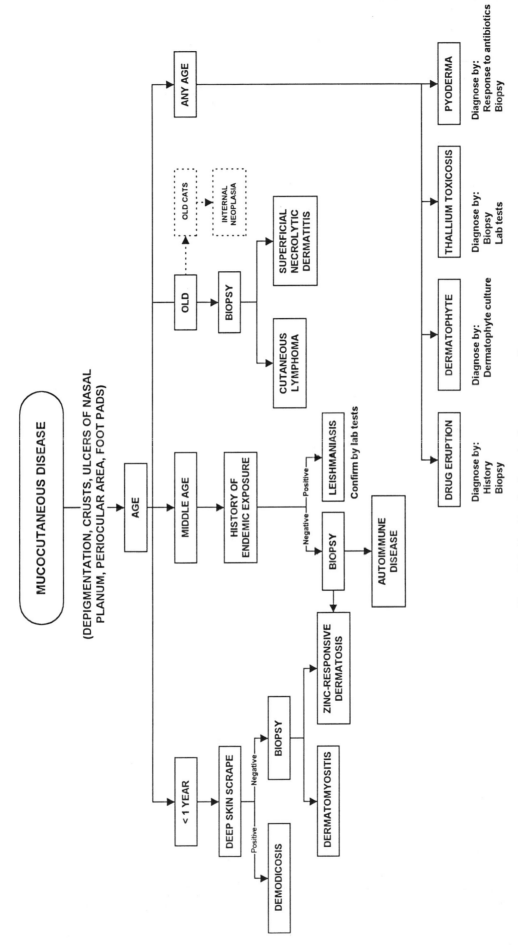

Figure 7–1. Algorithm for diagnosis of mucocutaneous disease.

A condition termed *superficial necrolytic dermatitis* (hepatocutaneous syndrome, epidermal metabolic necrosis, diabetic dermatosis) is being diagnosed with increased frequency in dogs, and has recently been reported in the cat. The cutaneous lesions include erythema, crusting, oozing, and alopecia of the face, genitals, and distal extremities, as well as hyperkeratosis and ulceration of the footpads. The skin disease may precede the onset of the signs of the internal disease. Histopathologic findings are diagnostic and include superficial perivascular-to-lichenoid dermatitis, with marked diffuse parakeratotic hyperkeratosis and striking inter- and intracellular edema limited to the upper half of the epidermis. Superficial dermatitis resembles the glucagonoma syndrome (necrolytic migratory erythema) of humans, which is usually associated with hyperglucagonemia and a glucagon-secreting alpha-cell neoplasm of the pancreas. Hyperglucagonemia has also been documented in dogs with this syndrome; however, dogs tend to have hepatic cirrhosis/parenchymal damage more commonly. Therapy is often unrewarding. The prognosis is slightly better if the underlying disease (drug-induced hepatopathy, removal of glucagonoma) and secondary skin infections (bacterial and/or yeast) can be treated.

Pancreatic Disease. Rarely, dogs with severe pancreatitis or pancreatic malignancy have had subcutaneous fat necrosis with erythema and draining tracts. It has been hypothesized that this is due to the increased concentrations of circulating lipase released from the inflamed pancreas (see Chapter 146). Cats with biliary or pancreatic malignancy have developed widespread alopecia and crusting of the footpads.

Renal Disease. Uremia has been reported to cause oral ulcerations with other signs of renal failure. The lesions are thought to be due to the toxic effects of urea and other waste products on the oral mucosa (see Chapter 169). Dysfunction of the renal tubules has been noted as a congenital syndrome in Vizslas and Lhasa apsos, with subsequent nodular calcium deposits in the skin and footpads.

A generalized *nodular dermatofibrosis* syndrome in German shepherds and occasionally other breeds associated with renal cystadenocarcinomas or cystadenomas has been reported. Histologic study of the nodules reveals dense collagen fibrosis. These nodules are most often found on distal extremities. Diagnosis of renal lesions is best performed by ultrasound. While the prognosis is serious, some dogs with benign renal cysts have survived for 5 years or longer after diagnosis.

Thymus. A rare exfoliative dermatitis has been described in older, usually "orange" cats. The disease has been associated with thymomas, usually diagnosed post mortem.

BACTERIAL INFECTIONS

Lyme Disease. Lyme disease is a tick-borne disorder of dogs and humans caused by the spirochete *Borrelia burgdorferi*. In the United States this disease is transmitted by the tick *Ixodes dammini*. Most afflicted dogs have been from the northeastern United States. Arthritis and fever are prominent signs. Early disease in humans is often characterized by an expanding annular lesion called erythema chronicum migrans, which may precede other "systems" involvement by days to months. This clinical sign has been documented in affected dogs in Europe.

FUNGAL INFECTIONS

Deep or Systemic Mycoses. Infections such as those caused by *Blastomyces dermatitidis, Histoplasma capsulatum, Cryptococcus neoformans,* and *Coccidioides immitis* may involve a number of organ systems. Cutaneous lesions may be varied, including nodules, plaques, draining tracts, alopecia, and seborrhea, and may be the first signs noted by the client (see Chapter 93).

PARASITIC DISEASES

Demodicosis. Generalized demodicosis is thought to occur in dogs with an underlying immunosuppressive disorder. In young dogs, this has been hypothesized to be a specific T-lymphocyte dysfunction. Older dogs with generalized demodicosis (or demodectic pododermatitis) may have hyperadrenocorticism, diabetes mellitus, hypothyroidism, or internal neoplasia. A thorough diagnostic evaluation, including a complete blood count, serum biochemical profile, thoracic and abdominal radiographs, and adrenal evaluation tests, are indicated. Therapy consists of the miticidal dip amitraz; ivermectin and milbemycin also have been used, although they are not approved for this use in the United States. Immunostimulants have not been effective. Older dogs with demodicosis have a poorer chance of cure but usually may be adequately controlled with intermittent amitraz dips and resolution of any underlying disease. Generalized demodicosis in cats is rare, but when present is usually in association with diabetes mellitus, feline leukemia virus infection, feline immunodeficiency virus, or hyperadrenocorticism.

Leishmaniasis. This protozoal disease has been reported in dogs in the United States both from an endemic focus in Oklahoma (species undetermined) and in dogs that have spent time in the Mediterranean area (*Leishmania donovani*). The disease may initially cause skin lesions. Alopecia, erythema, and especially scaling and ulceration of the ears and mucocutaneous junctions may occur. These dogs often have hyperproteinemia, hyperglobulinemia, nonresponsive anemia, and proteinuria. Diagnosis is by demonstration of the organism, most commonly identified in lymph nodes, bone marrow, or synovial fluid samples, by histology or culture, or by serum titers. Therapy consists of subcutaneous antimony compounds (meglumine) and oral allopurinol. Corticosteroids are indicated in cases of renal disease. Practitioners in the United States with a suspected or confirmed case should contact the public health authorities, as the dog may serve as a reservoir of human disease via vectors (*Phlebotomus* or *Lutzomyia* sand flies). The disease probably cannot be directly transmitted from dog to human (see Chapter 87). Antimonial compounds are available in the United States only through the Centers for Disease Control and Prevention in Atlanta, Georgia.

NUTRITIONAL DISEASE

Pansteatitis. Etiology is a deficiency of vitamin E and its antioxidant property. The deficiency is either due to an inadequate diet or a relative deficiency associated with the consumption of highly unsaturated fatty acids that destroy vitamin E. It has been reported only in cats, usually those eating diets containing red fish or excessive cod liver oil. Affected cats are usually depressed, febrile, anorectic, and sore or painful on palpation of the skin or abdomen. Subcutaneous and abdominal fat may feel firm or lumpy. Draining tracts may be present. Diagnosis is based on history and biopsy. Yellow to orange-brown fat nodules may be seen grossly that, when formalin-fixed, fluoresce yellow-orange under ultraviolet light. Histology shows fat necrosis and septal panniculitis, with a pink-yellow material seen within fat vacuoles and macrophages. This substance is termed ceroid and is believed to be an intermediate product of lipids. Abdominal and omental fat is frequently involved. Therapy consists of a proper diet, oral vitamin E (alphatocopherol), 25 to 75 IU every 12 hours, and corticosteroids for their anti-inflammatory and appetite-stimulating effects (prednisolone 0.5 mg/lb every 12 hours). Despite these measures, the author has seen cats with this disease that have failed to improve.

IMMUNE-MEDIATED DISORDERS

Systemic Lupus Erythematosus (SLE). Cutaneous lesions vary greatly and often include crusts, ulcers, or depigmentation affecting the mucocutaneous junctions and footpads. However, erythema, seborrhea, panniculitis, and vasculitis have all been reported. These lesions may be exacerbated by exposure to sunlight. Other clinical signs that may be noted are anemia, proteinuria, and polyarthritis. The etiology probably involves the deposition of antibody-antigen complexes in various tissues with subsequent activation of the complement cascade. Approximately 10 per cent of people with SLE-related dermatopathy do not have a positive antinuclear antibody (ANA) test, but do have anticytoplasmic antibodies. Simliar antibodies are occasionally found in dogs with SLE (see Chapter 184).

Erythema Multiforme. Erythema multiforme (EM) is an acute eruption of the skin and mucous membranes. It is characterized in human being by annular ("target") lesions. While these have been observed in animals, more commons signs are mucocutaneous vesicles, ulcers, maculae, and/or urticarial plaques. The lesions may be self-limiting. The lesions are usually secondary to another disease; in dogs, erythema multiforme has been reported in association with staphylococcal folliculitis and (most commonly) drug eruption. Severe mucocutaneous generalized EM (erythema multiforme major) often requires corticosteroids at immunosuppressive dosages.

Toxic Epidermal Necrolysis (TEN). This is a rare vesiculobullous and ulcerative disease of the skin and mucosa of dogs and cats. It is characterized by an acute onset of pyrexia, anorexia, lethargy, and/or depression, and a multifocal or generalized vesiculobullous eruption. The outer layer of skin adjacent to lesions may be easily rubbed away (positive Nikolsky's sign). Pain is moderate to severe. Histopathology includes intracellular edema (hydropic degeneration) of the basal epidermal cells, full-thickness epidermal necrosis, and minimal dermal inflammation. Dermoepidermal separation may be present. It is important to realize that TEN often seems to be associated with drug eruption. Therapy involves treating the underlying disease, symptomatic and supportive therapy, and corticosteroids.

CHAPTER 8

ALOPECIA

Gail A. Kunkle

Alopecia is the partial or complete lack of hair in areas where it is normally present. It occurs because either the hair has been lost from the follicle or there is failure of hair production. Alopecia can be partial or generalized, diffuse or focal. Whenever one is evaluating a dog or cat for alopecia, it is essential that the veterinarian consider the range of haircoat and hair density varieties relative to breed before an absolute diagnosis of alopecia is made.

Once it has been clearly determined that alopecia is present, factors such as the history, the distribution of the alopecia, and the clinical signs are most helpful in formulating a differential diagnosis. This differential then leads one to prioritize possible diagnostic tests that will aid in defining the cause of the alopecia.

The major cause of alopecia in both the dog and the cat is self-trauma associated with pruritus. The hair may be physically damaged from licking or scratching, or it may be more easily removed with trauma because of secondary infection within the hair follicle.

PATHOPHYSIOLOGIC MECHANISMS OF ALOPECIA

It is important to remember that most forms of alopecia have a significant component of pruritus with its associated inflammation. The inflammatory mediators often present within or surrounding the follicle can produce hair loss. In some infiltrative diseases, such as neoplasia or autoimmune skin disease, the hair follicle may be destroyed or damaged, resulting in subsequent absence of hair.

There are noninflammatory causes of alopecia. These include some of the congenital primary follicular diseases in which agenesis is responsible for the lack of hair. In other inherited conditions, the follicular abnormality is dysplasia. Endocrine, nutritional, and metabolic factors; systemic diseases; and occasionally drugs can cause follicular arrest or atrophy as noninflammatory alopecias.

HISTORY

The most important initial aspect of the history is to determine if the alopecia is acquired or if it has been present since birth. Most alopecias are acquired, and those congenital alopecias generally are easy to define and characterize with history, breed, and confirmation by skin biopsy. There are some inherited alopecias that are tardive in appearance and may not be visually present at birth. The breed, age of onset, and pattern of distribution should be helpful in defining these cases.

The history of distribution and speed of progressing alopecia can sometimes be helpful in narrowing the diagnosis. Slower progression of alopecia is more indicative of a systemic problem such as an endocrinopathy or metabolic imbalance. Hair loss from some anatomic areas such as the dorsal neck or tail is suggestive of hormonal imbalances.

CLINICAL SIGNS

Signalment

The signalment of the patient provides useful information for narrowing the list of differential diagnoses for alopecia.

There are some breeds and coat colors that are more prone to the development of conditions that may result in alopecia, so attention to breed is important. If there is a young age of onset, ectoparasites, infectious agents, and early signs of allergy must receive differential consideration. If the animal is middle aged to older at the onset of clinical signs, assessment of immune-mediated, metabolic, endocrine, and neoplastic conditions is needed. Of course, many dermatologic conditions in animals begin in early years and by middle age a plethora of problems are present. These often necessitate a step-by-step approach to diagnosis, initially requiring treatment of secondary problems and gradually working toward the primary diagnosis.

Physical Findings

The physical examination findings from an alopecic dog or cat are critical. A thorough physical examination should precede the integumentary examination and any abnormalities recorded. The cutaneous examination should initially take into consideration whether the distribution of the lesions is (1) localized *(differentials: demodicosis, dermatophytosis, bacteria, alopecia areata, injection reaction, cicatricial alopecia);* (2) multifocal or diffuse but patchy *(differentials: demodicosis, dermatophytosis, superficial pyoderma, color dilute alopecia, follicular dysplasia, dermatomyositis);* or (3) symmetrical, generalized, or diffuse *(differentials: demodi-*

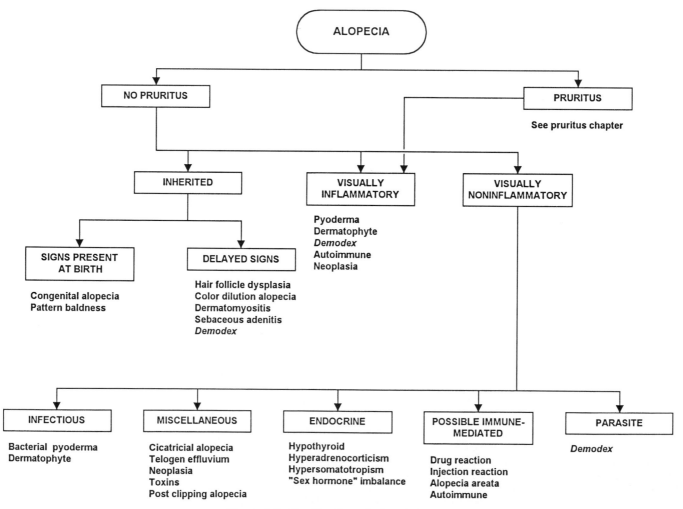

Figure 8–1. Algorithm for evaluation of alopecia.

cosis, dermatophytosis, superficial pyoderma, endocrinopathies, pattern baldness, follicular dysplasia, congenital alopecia, telogen effluvium, color dilution alopecia, and epidermotropic lymphoma).

One should note if the hair is shiny and contains unbroken hairs, both primary and undercoat hairs typical of the breed. The distal ends of the hair should be unbroken. The portion of the hair that extrudes from the follicle should be examined thoroughly for inflammation. It is necessary to completely examine the skin for signs of any primary or secondary eruptions. Signs and location of self-trauma are helpful in narrowing the list of pruritic diseases.

DIAGNOSTICS

The diagnostic tests selected for each case of alopecia will be dictated by the differential diagnosis list and the needs of the client (Fig. 8–1). Initially the dog or cat should be evaluated for secondary infection and treated while other diagnostic test results are pending or being considered. Cytology, cultures, and skin scrapings are part of the minimum database of almost all cases of alopecia in both dogs and cats. The spectrum of diagnostic tests needed for the pruritic patient is likely to be larger than those tests necessary for the nonpruritic patient, although some endocrinopathies can be quite complex and time consuming to diagnose.

OUTCOME

The prognosis of complete return of the haircoat to the normal state is highly dependent on the definitive diagnosis. If the cause relates to lack of proper hair growth and the factors responsible can be fully corrected, it is likely that the pet will grow a normal haircoat. If inflammation has been a chronic, deep, or a significant part of the process that induced the alopecia, there may be permanent changes such as fibrosis and destruction of the hair follicle. In these cases, only a moderate regrowth of hair may result.

For some owners, the aesthetics of the lack of hair in their pet can be the most difficult aspect of alopecia. It is important that the veterinarian educate the client that alopecia can be a hallmark of a serious systemic condition but that lack of hair alone is mostly a cosmetic problem rather than a life-threatening one.

CHAPTER 9

PRURITUS

Peter J. Ihrke

Pruritus may be defined as the sensation that elicits the desire to scratch. We infer pruritus in animals by either observing self-trauma or noting the erythema, excoriations, lichenification, and alopecia that result from self-mutilation. Pruritus may be manifested by licking, chewing, rubbing, hair removal, irritability, and even personality change (lack of tolerance, aggressive behavior). Pruritus is one of the most common owner complaints in veterinary practice. Since self-traumatized skin from any cause may appear similar, pruritic skin diseases can be diagnostically challenging and frustrating.

PATHOPHYSIOLOGY

The skin functions as an "external nervous system" providing continuous sensory input to the central nervous system through a finely arborized network of free nerve endings responsible for the sensations of touch, temperature, pain, and pruritus. In humans, "sensory spots" or "itch points" coincide with areas of increased density of free nerve endings. The sensations of pruritus and pain are carried centrally by nonmyelinated slow conducting C fibers and, to a lesser extent, along myelinated A delta fibers. Myelinated ganglion cell axons carry the message of itch from free nerve endings to neurons located in the posterior horn of the spinal cord. Axons of second-order neurons transmit the message across the midline to the lateral spinothalamic tract and upward to the thalamus. Thalamic neurons then carry the signal to the post-central gyrus of the cerebral cortex, where the message is interpreted as the sensation of pruritus.

Pruritus commonly stimulates self-trauma. The mechanisms by which scratching relieves itching are not known. Scratching may disturb the amplified, reverberating spinal circuits that perpetuate the sensation of itch. More severe self-trauma may substitute pain for pruritus. Severe self-trauma characterized by deep excoriations is more common in cats than in dogs.

Diffusible chemical mediators induce the sensation of itch. Endogenous mediators that have been implicated include histamine; peptides (mucunain, endopeptidases, bradykinin, substance P, vasoactive intestinal polypeptide, neurotensin, secretin, enkephalins, endorphins); proteases (trypsin, chymotrypsin, mast cell chymase, fibrinolysin, kallikrein, cathepsins, plasmin, leukopeptidases); prostaglandins; leukotrienes (especially LTB_4); monohydroxy fatty acids; and opioid peptides. Proteolytic enzymes are thought to be the most important mediators of pruritus in dogs, cats, and humans. Leukotrienes also play an important role. The hypothesized role of histamine has diminished as the importance of other mediators is recognized. Bacterial and fungal endopeptidases may initiate pruritus. Chemical mediators present in arthropod saliva, venom, body fluids, and on poisonous hairs or spines include proteolytic enzymes, histamine, paederin, cantharidin, apamin, mellitin, histidine decarboxylase, kinins, serotonin, endopeptidases, and proteinases.

A "gate theory" has been hypothesized to explain how central factors can amplify or reduce the sensation of pruritus. Stress or anxiety may amplify pruritus in humans by releasing opioid peptides. Boredom or sensations such as pain, heat, cold, or touch also can alter the perception of pruritus. Factors such as skin temperature, skin dryness, and low humidity can heighten the sensitivity of the skin to pruritic stimuli.

The concepts of *threshold phenomenon* and *summation of effect* are important in understanding and managing pruritus. A certain pruritic load may be tolerated in an animal without initiating clinical signs but a small increase in that load provoke clinical signs. The itch threshold often is reduced at night in humans and animals when other sensory inputs are diminished. *Summation of effect* occurs when additive pruritic stimuli from coexistent skin diseases raise an animal above threshold. As an example, pruritus from mild flea allergy is additive to pruritus from other skin diseases during flea season, thus exacerbating and perpetuating itch-scratch cycles.

DIAGNOSIS OF PRURITUS

Signalment, history, physical examination, diagnostic testing, and, occasionally, response to therapy are the cornerstones of diagnosis. Since many pruritic skin diseases are visually similar, clinical history coupled with knowledge of signalment predilections may offer more direct clues to the diagnosis than physical examination.

SIGNALMENT

Age. Age provides critical information for prioritizing differential diagnoses. Some skin diseases occur more commonly in young animals, while other dermatoses are seen more frequently in middle-aged or elderly animals. As examples, scabies and demodicosis are pruritic skin diseases seen more commonly in young dogs. Similarly, atopic dermatitis, food allergy, and pyoderma occur more commonly in adult animals.

Breed. Breed predilections for skin diseases are becoming increasingly available (see appendices). Some skin diseases are even breed-specific. As examples, golden retrievers, Dalmatians, and many small terrier breeds are at increased risk for the development of atopic dermatitis. The West Highland white terrier is at increased risk for secondary *Malassezia* dermatitis, and the Chinese Shar Pei seems predisposed to atopic dermatitis, food allergy, pyoderma, and demodicosis.

Sex. Sex predilections are not common in pruritic skin diseases. However, pruritus may be seen with Sertoli cell tumors, male feminizing syndromes, and canine female hyperestrogenism.

HISTORICAL FINDINGS

General History

General history should be sought referable to diet, environment, use, home skin care, recent exposures, other household pets, and the presence or absence of pruritus in other animals or people in the environment. These data are helpful in prioritizing differential diagnoses.

Diet. Food allergy or intolerance can cause pruritus in both dogs and cats. However, it frequently coexists with other allergic skin diseases such as atopic dermatitis and flea allergy dermatitis. In addition, lipid-deficient diets may exacerbate canine seborrhea.

Environment and Exposure. The likelihood of contagious pruritic ectoparasitic skin diseases is affected by environmental exposure. Flea allergy, canine and feline scabies, and less common ectoparasitic skin diseases are all seen more frequently in animals permitted to roam free. Feline scabies is endemic to certain geographic areas. Recent exposures to other animals such as the acquisition of a new pet or sheltering a stray animal increase the likelihood of contagious disease. Grooming establishments, kennels, and veterinary practices offer additional opportunities for contagion.

Other Household Pets. Pruritus or lack of pruritus in other animals may offer clues. However, even though dogs and cats share the cat flea as a common ectoparasite, flea allergy is much more common in dogs. A seemingly unaffected indoor/outdoor cat is often the source of flea acquisition in indoor dogs with flea allergy dermatitis. Although uncommon, asymptomatic carriers of canine scabies do exist because clinical disease requires hypersensitivity.

Human Contacts. A pruritic papular rash in an owner with a pruritic pet may suggest zoonotic infestation with canine or feline scabies mites or cheyletiellosis. Annular, erythematous lesions may suggest dermatophytosis.

Specific History

Specific history relates to the current pruritic skin disease. The initial site of skin lesions, onset and progression, intensity of pruritus, seasonality or other pattern (predictability), and response or lack of response to previous therapy may be important in establishing a diagnosis.

Site, Onset, and Progression. Knowledge of the initial sites of skin lesions may be useful if the disease has generalized before veterinary care is sought. For example, canine scabies often begins on the margins of the ear pinnae before generalizing. Rapid-onset pruritus should increase suspicion for ectoparasitic diseases as well as adverse drug reactions. Pruritus of insidious onset is more suggestive of slowly progressive, chronic skin diseases such as atopic dermatitis, food allergy, pyoderma, and seborrhea.

Intensity. Most animals do not exhibit pruritus in the examination room. Canine and feline scabies, canine flea allergy dermatitis, and feline food allergy are notable exceptions. Frequency and intensity of pruritus may be inferred from asking the owner how many times the animal will scratch (or chew, or lick) if left to its own devices while the owner is in the room.

Seasonality or Pattern (Predictability). Atopic dermatitis and flea allergy dermatitis are seasonal diseases in many areas of the world. *Malassezia* dermatitis may occur more frequently during months of higher humidity. Cyclical pruritus without seasonality can sometimes signify contact dermatitis associated with change of environment. Psychogenic pruritus may began as a predictable, attention-getting device. Pruritus seen with food allergy should be continuous unless the diet is changed.

Response to Previous Therapy. Response or lack of response to previous medications, particularly corticosteroids and antibiotics, may offer additional clues. Although allergic diseases all respond to corticosteroids to varying degrees, food allergy may be less responsive to corticosteroids than atopic dermatitis or flea allergy dermatitis. Prior diminished pruritus in response to antibiotics in dogs often is overlooked and indicates the likelihood of pyoderma.

PHYSICAL FINDINGS

A thorough, general physical examination is mandatory for any animal with skin disease. Skin disease may be seen secondary to internal medical disorders (see Chapter 7). Proper lighting is of paramount importance. Examination of the skin, mucocutaneous junctions, oral cavity, ears, genitals, and lymph nodes should be emphasized. The clinician should observe the animal for general demeanor and signs of pruritus while taking the history. Objective signs of pruritus include excoriations and broken or barbed hairs with a dry, lusterless hair coat. In the dog, worn incisors (buccal surface) and canine teeth (mesial surface) most frequently indicate chronic flea allergy dermatitis.

Pruritus may occur with or without primary skin lesions.

If present, primary skin lesions such as papules or pustules may be helpful in establishing a diagnosis. Coexistent alopecia may offer additional clues (see Chapter 8). Unfortunately, self-trauma often leads to the obliteration of initial, more diagnostic primary skin lesions, substituting excoriations, lichenification, and alopecia. The concept of "a rash that itches" indicates primary skin lesions that are itchy, and "an itch that rashes" indicates that pruritic patients traumatize themselves. Ectoparasitic skin diseases, pyoderma, and seborrhea are among the more common pruritic skin diseases where primary skin lesions are identified. Conversely, primary lesions are much less common in atopic dermatitis and food allergy. The distribution of lesions, presence or absence of bilateral symmetry, and major foci of pruritus can be valuable aids to diagnosis. Primary or secondary lesions, if present in a particular site, may be highly suggestive of specific diseases (Tables 9–1 and 9–2).

DIAGNOSTIC PLAN

Diagnostic plans should be formulated based on prioritization of differential diagnoses utilizing signalment, history,

TABLE 9–1. PRURITIC CANINE DERMATOSES

DISEASE	SITE	LESIONS
Flea allergy dermatitis A, E, F	Bilaterally symmetric, dorsal lumbosacral, caudal thighs, groin, axilla, caudal half of body	Papules, macules, alopecia, erythema, lichenification, hyperpigmentation, excoriations, fibropruritic nodules
Canine scabies A	Ventrum, ear margins, face, elbows, partially bilaterally symmetric	Macules, papules, erythema, alopecia, crusts, excoriations, alopecia
Demodicosis A	Periorbital, commisures of mouth, forelegs, generalized	Alopecia, erythema, crusts, follicular plugging, hyperpigmentation, secondary pyoderma
Pyoderma A	Groin, axilla, ventrum, interdigital webs, generalized, pressure points	Pleomorphic, pustules, crusted papules, erythema, alopecia, target lesions, coalescing collarettes, hyperpigmentation
Atopic dermatitis A, F	Face, periorbital, ears, caudal carpi and tarsi, feet, (dorsum), otitis externa, axilla, generalized	Erythema, alopecia, excoriations, lack of primary lesions, lichenification, hyperpigmentation
Malassezia dermatitis A, E, F	Ventral neck, groin, skinfolds, face, feet, ventrum	Erythema, exudative or dry, alopecia, hyperpigmentation, lichenification
"Seborrhea" A, E, F	Generalized, ears, preen body	Pleomorphic, scales, crusts, alopecia, erythematous plaques
Acral lick dermatitis A	Anterior carpal, metacarpal, radial, metatarsal, tibial regions; tail, stifle, hip	Firm, alopecic plaque, central irregular ulcer, hyperpigmented halo
Food allergy B	Face, feet, ears, generalized	Pleomorphic, erythema, alopecia, excoriations, lack of primary lesions
Contact dermatitis B	Hairless areas, feet (ventrum), genitals, groin, axilla, generalized	Erythema, exudation, lichenification, hyperpigmentation, papules
Drug eruptions B	Anywhere, localized or generalized, face, ears, scrotum	Pleomorphic, erythema, papules, coalescing target lesions
Endoparasitic migration in puppies C	Face, feet, generalized	Erythema, alopecia, excoriations, lack of primary lesions
Cheyletiellosis B, E	Dorsum of thorax, generalized	Large scales, crusts, alopecia, erythema
Chiggers B, E, F	Ventrum, legs, anywhere	Erythema, scales, crusts, papules, alopecia
Superficial necrolytic dermatitis C	Footpads, face, mucocutaneous junctions, genitals, groin	Adherent crusts, ulcers, excoriations, erythema, fissured pads
Psychogenic pruritus C	Carpi, tarsi, feet (one or more, especially forelegs), perianal, generalized	Erythema, alopecia, excoriations, lack of primary lesions
Pediculosis C, E, F	Dorsum, generalized	Scales, crusts, alopecia, papules
Tail-dock neuroma C	Previously docked tail	Erythema, excoriations, alopecia
Rhabditic dermatitis D, E, F	Ventrum, legs, groin	Erythema, papules, alopecia, crusts, scales
Subcorneal pustular dermatosis D	Generalized, especially face and ears	Pleomorphic, papules, pustules, vesicles, crusts, alopecia
Sterile eosinophilic pustulosis D	Generalized, ventrum	Erythema, papules, pustules, alopecia, scales, crusts, collarettes

A = common; B = less common; C = uncommon; D = rare or controversial; E = regional; F = seasonal.

TABLE 9–2. PRURITIC FELINE DERMATOSES

DISEASE	SITE	LESIONS
Flea allergy dermatitis A	Neck, dorsum, lumbosacral, caudal and medial thighs, groin, ears, generalized	"Miliary dermatitis," erythema, alopecia, eosinophilic plaques
Eosinophilic plaque A, E, F	Ventral abdomen, medial thighs, anywhere	Raised, ulcerated, erythematous alopecic plaques, seen secondary to allergy (primarily flea allergy dermatitis)
Otodectic acariasis A	Ears, head, neck, rarely generalized	Otitis externa, excoriations, "miliary dermatitis"
Food allergy A	Head, neck, ears, generalized	Erythema, excoriations, alopecia, lack of primary lesions, "miliary dermatitis"
Self-induced pruritic hair loss (atopic dermatitis, food allergy, flea allergy) B	Bilaterally symmetric, caudal and lateral thighs, ventral abdomen, perineum	Alopecia, hair stubble, erythema, papules, underlying skin can be normal
Self-induced psychogenic hair loss B	Bilaterally symmetric, stripe(s) on dorsal thorax, caudal and lateral thighs, ventral abdomen, perineum, forelegs	Alopecia, hair stubble, normal underlying skin
Cheyletiellosis B, E	Dorsum of thorax, generalized	Large scales, crusts, seborrhea, "miliary dermatitis"
Mosquito-bite hypersensitivity C, E, F	Bilaterally symmetric, dorsal muzzle, planum nasale, periorbital, pinnae, paw pad margins	Papules, crusts, alopecia, erosion, exudation
Pediculosis C, E, F	Dorsum, generalized	Scales, crusts, alopecia
Feline scabies C, E	Head, ears, neck, generalized, partially bilaterally symmetric	Erythema, papules, crusts, excoriations, alopecia
Dermatophytosis with pruritus C	Head, neck, ears, generalized	Erythema, alopecia, hair stubble, "miliary dermatitis," hyperpigmentation
Atopic dermatitis B, F	Head, neck, ears, generalized	"Miliary dermatitis," erythema, excoriations, alopecia
Drug eruptions	Anywhere, localized or generalized, ears, face	Pleomorphic, erythema, papules, coalescing target lesions
Pemphigus foliaceus D, E?, F?	Bilaterally symmetric, face, planum nasale, ears, interdigital webs, nipples, generalized	Crusts, vesicopustules, alopecia

A = common; B = less common; C = uncommon; D = rare or controversial; E = regional; F = seasonal.

and physical findings. Diagnostic procedures are selected based on the most likely differential diagnoses. The algorithm in Figure 9–1 offers an overview of possible diagnostic plans.

Skin Scrapings. Multiple skin scrapings should be performed on all pruritic dogs and cats. The affected area is gently clipped, and a Number 10 scalpel blade dipped in mineral oil is used to scrape in the direction of hair growth perpendicular to the skin surface. The acquired debris is dispersed on a slide, a coverslip is applied, and the specimen is examined microscopically using low light. Demodectic mites usually are readily demonstrable (except in some cases of chronic pododemodicosis and in the Chinese Shar Pei). Scabies mites are documented in less than half of affected dogs, underscoring the need for trial therapy in suspected cases. Dry scrapings may be stained as smears to look for *Malassezia pachydermatis*.

Smears, Tape Preparations. Affected skin, intact pustules, or exudates should be smeared, stained with a rapid stain such as Diff-Quik, and examined microscopically for the presence of bacteria, *Malassezia* organisms, and inflammatory cells. Clear tape preparations also may demonstrate *Cheyletiella* mites or *Malassezia pachydermatis*.

Fecal. Fecal examination may document endoparasite infestation in pruritic puppies and may reveal mites in any animal.

Skin Biopsy. Skin biopsy is an especially valuable diagnostic tool if primary skin lesions free of self-traumatic excoriations are present. If only self-traumatic lesions are present, definitive diagnosis is less likely but results may aid in prioritizing or ruling out various differential diagnoses.

Fungal Culture. Most dogs and cats with dermatophytosis are not pruritic. However, fungal culture may be warranted because many cases of dermatophytosis are not visually distinctive.

Elimination Diets. Animals suspected of having food allergy or food intolerance as a cause of pruritus should be fed a home-cooked diet consisting of one protein and one carbohydrate source for 8 to 12 weeks. Although less ideal, alternatively, many newer limited antigen diets are now available. Commercial restricted diets are recommended for long-term maintenance. There is nothing specifically "hypoallergenic" about any food source. Foods are selected simply based on lack of previous exposure. Whitefish, rabbit, venison, pork, cottage cheese, or tofu mixed with either potatoes or rice are commonly employed in the dog. Mutton, lamb, and chicken are no longer as useful as they were previously, owing to frequent current usage in commercial dry dog foods. Cats may be given rabbit, venison, pork, or mutton.

Intradermal Skin Testing. Substantial training is required to select appropriate candidates suspected of having atopic dermatitis, choose antigens, develop and maintain a reproducible technique, and interpret results. Consequently, skin testing is most effective when practiced by dermatologists or other clinicians with a strong interest in dermatology.

ELISA and RAST Testing. In vitro testing for atopic dermatitis offers convenience and accessibility. Reproducibility of test results has increased dramatically over the past 5 years. However, problems still remain with antigen selection, grouped testing, and standardization of results.

Environmental Restriction. If allergic contact dermatitis is suspected, an animal may be housed in a markedly different environment (water-rinsed kennel) for 10 days.

Patch Testing. Suspected allergens are applied to the skin in an attempt to elicit delayed hypersensitivity. Results with new standardized closed patch tests recommended by

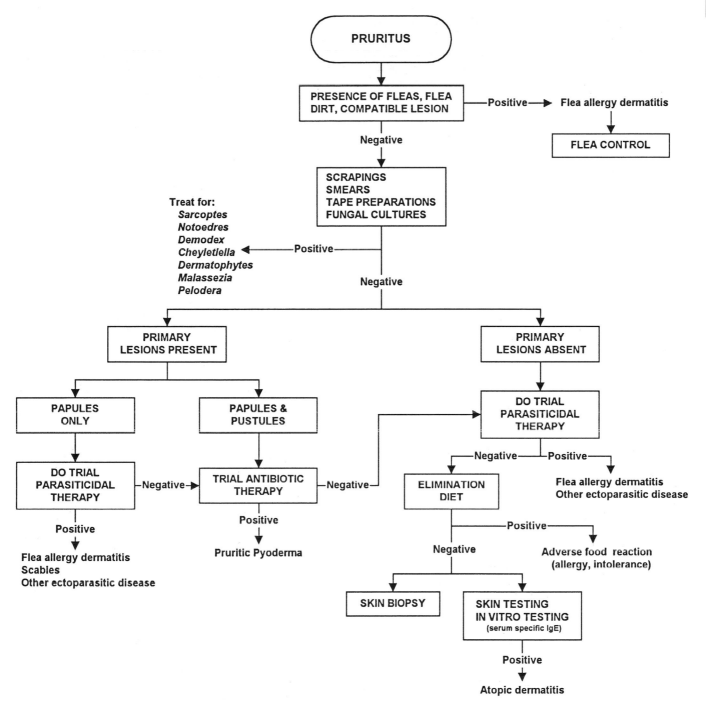

Figure 9–1. Algorithm for diagnosis and management of pruritus.

the International Contact Dermatitis Research Group have been encouraging. However, the process is expensive and labor-intensive.

Response to Trial Therapy. Trial therapy with parasiticidal agents is used routinely in suspected cases of scabies or flea allergy dermatitis. It is important to remember that flea allergy dermatitis is the most common cause of canine and feline pruritus. Since the lesions seen with canine superficial pyoderma may be markedly pleomorphic, trial use of antibiotics may be indicated in undiagnosed pruritic crusted papular dermatoses. While response to corticosteroids certainly is suggestive of underlying allergic disease, superficial pyoderma frequently will respond partially to corticosteroid therapy.

Cost Containment. Skin scrapings, fungal culture, smears, trial therapy for ectoparasites, and, surprisingly, skin biopsy are the most cost-effective diagnostic procedures for the pruritic animal.

GOALS OF THERAPY

Successful long-term management of a pruritic dog or cat usually requires definitive diagnosis. Repetitive parasiticidal therapy on a weekly basis for 3 or 4 weeks is required for the management of most contagious ectoparasitic diseases such as canine or feline scabies. However, management of flea allergy dermatitis is a lifelong endeavor encompassing control of fleas in the indoor and outdoor environment as well as control on the affected animal and all in-contact dogs and cats. Atopic dermatitis responds best to hyposensitization. If corticosteroids are used adjunctively for the long-term management of allergic skin disease, short-acting oral corticosteroids such as prednisone, prednisolone, or methyl-prednisolone are recommended on an alternate-day basis. Corticosteroids are contraindicated in the treatment of canine demodicosis and pyoderma. Many pruritic animals require long-term adjunctive topical management with shampoos and emollients or antipruritic rinses.

CHAPTER 10

CUTANEOUS AND SUBCUTANEOUS LUMPS, BUMPS, AND MASSES

D. N. Carlotti

Cutaneous and subcutaneous lumps, bumps, and masses include hematomas, abscesses, urticaria and angioedema, and pseudo-neoplasms and neoplasms.

CLINICAL AND HISTOPATHOLOGIC DEFINITIONS

A hematoma is a focal extravasation of blood with purpura (bruising) and pain, whereas an abscess is a localized collection of pus with pain, heat, and sometimes purpura. Urticaria is referred to as a group of wheals (sharply circumscribed, raised, edematous lesions) that appear and disappear rapidly. Angioedema is a large swelling in a distensible region such as the face and limbs.

Clinically, pseudo-neoplasms and neoplasms appear as nodules, plaques, and tumors. Ulceration always indicates a severe pathologic process. Pseudo-neoplasms include cysts, nevi, keratoses, granulomas, and pyogranulomas and other lesions. Pseudo-neoplasm is a better term than pseudo-tumor because the term *tumor* is clinical and should refer to a localized hypertrophy of a tissue or an organ, neoplastic or not. Cysts are epithelial lesions containing grayish keratinous material or serous material, such as apocrine cysts, which appear fluctuant, bluish, and well circumscribed. A hamartoma is a malformation formed by components of a normal organ arranged erroneously. A nevus is a cutaneous hamartoma that may arise from any skin component. Collagenous nevi are single or multiple nodules characterized histopathologically by large areas of collagen hyperplasia. In German shepherds, multiple collagenous nevi may appear, particularly on the limbs, in association with renal adenocarcinomas and uterine leiomyomas (nodular dermatofibrosis syndrome). Organoid (i.e., pilosebaceous) and epidermal nevi are variable in shape and may be linear. Vascular nevi are seen on the scrotum in dogs. Keratoses are solid, elevated, and circumscribed lesions characterized by a hyperproduction of keratin. They show up as greasy nodules and plaques (seborrheic keratoses), squamocrustous plaques (actinic keratoses, lichenoid keratoses on the ear pinnae), or cutaneous horns.

A granuloma is a circumscribed tissue reaction characterized by an organized infiltration of mononucleated phagocytes (histiocytes and macrophages) that may occur when foreign bodies, bacteria, fungi, parasites, or any material penetrates or deposits into the skin. If the "invader" is not destroyed by an acute inflammatory process, macrophages become epithelioid. A granuloma may persist until the cause has been eliminated. "Pyogranuloma" means granulomatous reaction with many neutrophils. Lesions of calcinosis circumscripta are pink-colored plaques located on pressure points or in the tongue that contain grayish material. Calcinosis cutis, seen in canine Cushing's disease, is characterized by hard erythematous plaques containing whitish material. Eosinophilic lesions in the cat are indolent ulcer, eosinophilic plaque, and collagenolytic granuloma (the latter often appearing linear). Nodular sterile panniculitis is characterized by deep nodules that fistulize, expressing an oily material. Canine juvenile cellulitis is characterized by facial swelling. Canine histiocytosis may be characterized by nodular lesions, particularly on the face, with a "clown nose" appearance.

Other various pseudo-neoplasms include acral lick dermatitis, idiopathic lichenoid dermatitis (coalescent plaques), feline plasma cell pododermatitis or stomatitis, and idiopathic focal mucinosis seen in Doberman pinschers.

ETIOLOGY AND PATHOPHYSIOLOGY

Hematomas are the result of trauma causing the rupture of blood vessels. They appear frequently after minor trauma in dogs with coagulopathies. Abscesses are the result of the collection of degenerated neutrophils and necrotic tissue cells when an infectious agent has penetrated into and under the skin. Usually a peripheral membrane forms from necrotic tissue and fibrin. Urticaria and angioedema are caused by immediate hypersensitivity reactions generated by insect bites (e.g., Hymenoptera); food; drugs; airborne allergens (atopy) as well as nonimmunologic stimuli such as contact with irritant material (weeds, e.g., *Urtica dioica,* insects such as *Thaumetopoea pityocampa* caterpillar); physical stimuli such as cold, heat, and sunlight; and even psychogenic factors. Cysts may be traumatic (epidermoid), hereditary (dermoid), follicular, or pilar (i.e. trichilemmal) caused by retention of material (keratin, glandular products) as a result of congenital or acquired loss of follicular orifices. Apocrine cysts are idiopathic. Nevi may be congenital, and the mechanism of their formation is unknown. However, nodular dermatofibrosis is due to an autosomal dominant gene. Keratoses are idiopathic except actinic keratoses and some cutaneous horns, which are associated with various skin neoplasms or FeLV infection in the cat.

Bacterial granulomas and pyogranulomas include canine furunculosis due to cocci such as *Staphylococcus intermedius,* botryomycosis (bacterial pseudomycetoma) due to various bacteria that may cause a granulomatous reaction, and nocardiosis and mycobacterioses (atypical mycobacterial infection, feline leprosy, tuberculosis, which is very rare). Fungal granulomas and pyogranulomas include kerions (inflammatory reaction to a dermatophyte) and pseudomycetomas caused by the subcutaneous development of a dermatophyte (*Microsporum canis* in cats, mainly), subcutaneous (intermediate) mycoses (sporotrichosis, pythiosis, mycetomas, phaeohyphomycosis, zygomycosis), and deep (systemic) mycoses (blastomycosis, coccidioidomycosis, histoplasmosis, aspergillosis, cryptococcosis, protothecosis, paecilomycosis, trichosporonosis). Endogenous or exogenous foreign bodies can cause granulomas. Endogenous foreign bodies are usually hair and keratin (leading to bacterial furunculosis), calcium (calcinosis circumscripta, idiopathic, and Cushing's disease), and lipids (xanthomas in case of hyperlipidemia in cats, associated with diabetes mellitus or hereditary). Exogenous foreign bodies include sutures and weed material. Parasitic granulomas include tick bites, canine dracunculosis, canine filariosis, canine leishmaniasis (the nodular form is seen more frequently in short-haired dogs such as the Boxer), feline toxoplasmosis, and canine cysticercosis. Arthropod bites (e.g., mosquitos, spiders) lead to eosinophilic furunculosis (particularly on the face in dogs and cats) with a granulomatous reaction. Some granulomas are idiopathic: lesions of the feline eosinophilic granuloma complex (although most of the cases are caused by flea allergy dermatitis, feline atopic dermatitis, or food allergy or intolerance), canine eosinophilic granuloma, sterile pyogranulomatous dermatosis, nodular sterile panniculitis (due to an inflammatory process of subcutaneous fat), canine juvenile cellulitis (perhaps viral), canine cutaneous histiocytosis (due to a proliferation of normal histiocytes), canine erythema nodosum–like, canine sterile sarcoidal granulomatous skin disease, and amyloidosis. Acral lick dermatitis is often a deep bacterial folliculitis and furunculosis, caused by constant licking attributed to an allergic pruritus or behavioral disorder. Lichenoid dermatitis may be idiopathic or an immune-mediated disease such as feline plasma cell prododermatitis and stomalitis sometimes associated with FeLV and/or FIV infection. Cutaneous and subcutaneous neoplasms include epithelial (epidermal and follicular), glandular (sebaceous, sweat, and hepatoid gland), mesenchymal (fibrocytic,

histiocytic, vascular), and melanocytic and round cell tumors (mast cell, histiocytic, lymphoma). Mammary neoplasms can be considered as subcutaneous. Most of the neoplasms have an unknown etiology. Viruses can cause specific tumors such as papillomas in dogs and fibrosarcomas and carcinomas in situ (Bowen's disease) in cats. Other causes include irritation, trauma, and actinic exposure. The latter is likely to be the cause of squamous cell carcinoma of the face and ears in the cat (particularly of white color). It is not clear whether repeated vaccinations can lead to fibrosarcomas in cats. Benign neoplasms can be harmful if they reach a large size and/or are located in particular areas (face, eyelids, external ear canal, mouth, feet, genitals, anus). Malignant neoplasms are invasive and will cause the necrosis of surrounding cells, leading to ulceration.

DIAGNOSIS

Diagnosis of cutaneous and subcutaneous lumps, bumps, and masses is based upon history, physical examination, and complementary aids (Fig. 10–1). Signalment of the animal may be of some importance. Neoplastic lesions occur mostly in adults and old dogs. However viral papilloma and histiocytoma (Langerhans' cell tumor) will be seen mainly in young animals. Intact male cats are prone to develop abscesses due to fighting. Mammary tumors and their cutaneous metastases occur in female dogs, whereas perianal gland tumors occur most frequently in the intact male. Most neoplasms, however, have no sex predilection. Breed predispositions are recognized for many superficial neoplasms. The Boxer is known to be predisposed to many of them, as it is for nodular leishmaniasis. The German shepherd is predisposed to keratinous cysts and nodular dermatofibrosis. Persian cats are predisposed to dermatophytic pseudomycetoma.

History of the lesions should be taken into account. Important points are the existence of previous similar lesions, association to general disease, known trauma, and rapidity of onset. Obviously, hematomas, abscesses, urticaria, and angioedema appear rapidly. Some lymphomas can develop rapidly. Feline eosinophilic plaques, urticaria and angioedema, some cases of calcinosis cutis, and mast cell tumors are pruritic. Hematomas, abscesses, and some tumors may be painful.

Physical examination should include evaluation of the lesions, local lymph nodes, and distant sites such as lungs. This strategy applies to most lumps, bumps, and masses, using the TNM approach (tumor, node, metastasis). The lesions should be characterized by localization, size, shape, pedunculated appearance, consistency, depth, and whether or not they are freely movable and/or ulcerated. For instance, feline collagenolytic granuloma and canine epidermal nerves can be linear; hematomas and most benign neoplasms are not attached to underlying tissues, whereas most of abscesses and malignant neoplasms are. Abscesses evolve from firm to fluctuant stages, while most pseudo-neoplasms and neoplasms are firm (except apocrine cysts and some angiomas/angiosarcomas). Benign neoplasms can be pedunculated. Feline indolent ulcer, eosinophilic plaques, some malignant neoplasms, and canine acral lick dermatitis ulcerate. Enlargement of local lymph nodes can be caused by inflammation (even in case of a neoplastic process) or metastasis. General lymph node enlargement can result from severe infections and lymphosarcoma. Metastasis can rarely be suspected clinically, except for cutaneous metastasis of mammary neoplasms and when an abnormal abdominal mass is palpated.

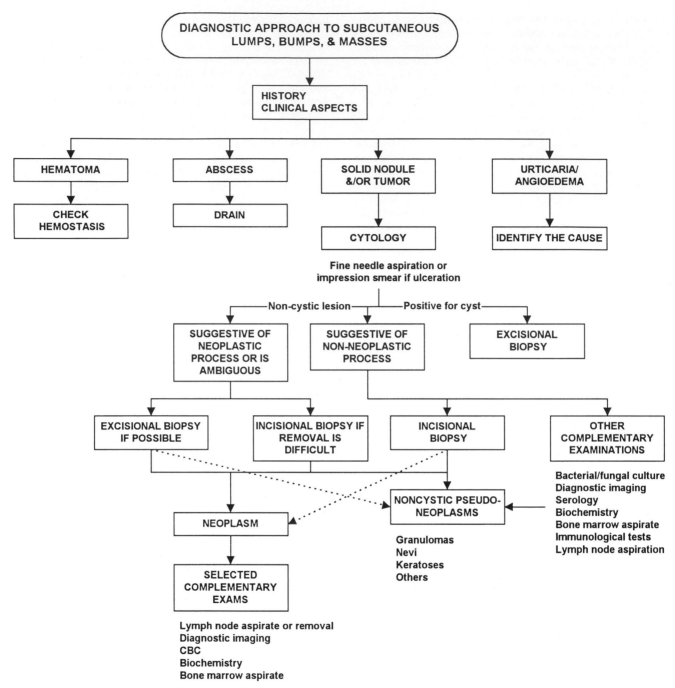

Figure 10–1. Algorithm for diagnostic approach to subcutaneous lumps, bumps, and masses.

Cytologic techniques usable for lumps, bumps, and masses are impression, scrape, swab, and fine-needle aspiration smears. There are no contraindications. Cytology allows rapid identification of cell types. Neoplasms are characterized by high cellularity and a homogeneous cell population. Cytologic criteria of malignancy include pleomorphism, high nucleocytoplasmic ratios, large nucleoli, and atypical mitoses. In many non-neoplastic lesions, the cytologic examination is highly suggestive of the diagnosis (e.g., pyoderma, fungal diseases, eosinophilic plaques). Fine-needle aspiration cytology of a local lymph node can help to differentiate an inflammatory reaction from malignancy.

Histopathology has a fundamental role in establishing specimens' diagnoses. Incisional biopsy specimens can be obtained with a scalpel or a punch, particularly when cytol-

ogy is ambiguous. Results aid in selecting appropriate medical therapy and/or surgery. The sample should be biopsied at the margin of the lesion to incorporate some normal-looking tissue, should not be larger than 1 cm, and should be put in 10 times its volume of 10 percent formalin. There is no contraindication for incisional biopsy because it does not increase risk of metastasis. The wound should be repaired, and the biopsy site should be removed by further surgery. General anesthesia may be required, and wound repair can be difficult. Excisional biopsy can also be performed, particularly when cytotogy is ambiguous, when the surgical removal of the lesion is easy, and when physical examination suggests a non-neoplastic or benign neoplastic lesion. If lesions are multiple, excisional biopsy of a typical mass should be considered. The removal of a lymph node for histopathologic analysis can be helpful and has no harmful consequence. Radiology and/or ultrasonography is useful in many instances, e.g., a lesion appearing to be attached to an underlying bone or suspicion of lung or abdominal metastasis.

PROGNOSIS

The prognosis of cutaneous and/or subcutaneous lumps, bumps, and masses is obviously linked to diagnosis, location of the lesion(s) and continuing evaluation (TNM). Establishing a prognosis based on physical examination only and clinical neglect, waiting for a possible enlargement of the lesion(s), are unacceptable errors.

TREATMENT

Treatment should be based upon diagnosis and prognosis. Medical treatment of urticaria/angioedema, hematomas, and abscesses is almost always successful. The result of treatment of granulomatous pseudo-neoplasms can lead to complete cure, particularly when a bacterial or superficial fungal agent has been identified. Surgical excision of cysts, nevi, keratoses, feline plasma cell podal lesions, and benign neoplasms is usually successful. Treatment for malignancies is rarely curative, but long remissions can be obtained, particularly if the owners wish to cooperate.

CHAPTER 11

EROSIONS AND ULCERATIONS

Ian S. Mason

Erosions and ulcers are defects in the cutaneous epithelium with a variety of causes. Erosions are defined as superficial breaks in the continuity of epithelia, but the basement membrane remains intact. Erosions usually heal without scarring. In contrast, ulcers are deeper epithelial defects that extend through the basement membrane into the underlying dermis. Ulcers heal slowly, and there is usually residual scarring.

It may be difficult to distinguish between ulcers and erosions except on histology. In some diseases, ulcers and erosions occur concurrently, representing different points on a continuum of disease. Other diseases may exhibit only one or another of these two types of lesions.

Ulcers and erosions may arise as a result of a range of causes with very different pathomechanisms (Table 11–1). Trauma, including self-trauma associated with pruritus, may lead to eroded and ulcerated lesions. Infectious diseases, bacterial or fungal, can lead to defects in the epithelial surface. In canine skin, bullae and vesicles are thin walled and rupture promptly after formation; they may leave residual erosions and ulcers. Chemical and physical factors such as urine scalding, irritant contact dermatitis, and thermal injury may also be responsible for defects in cutaneous continuity.

Erosive and ulcerative diseases in dogs and cats may affect the mucous membranes with or without concurrent cutaneous involvement. Animals with oral disease are usually brought to the clinician because of halitosis, dysphagia, or both.

Two important points need to be made regarding this group of diseases: Firstly, clinicians are quick to suspect autoimmune and immune-mediated diseases when examining dogs or cats with erosions and ulcerations. In fact, these diseases are uncommon or rare. There are a large number of causes of these lesions (Table 11–1); many of these are far more common than the immune-mediated and autoimmune group. Secondly, histology is an extremely valuable tool in the diagnosis of these lesions.

APPROACH TO THE DIAGNOSIS

In view of the broad spectrum of possible diseases involved in ulcerative and erosive diseases, the diagnostic approach must be carefully planned and thorough (Fig. 11–1).

A detailed history may yield important diagnostic clues. Certain obese or short-legged breeds of dogs are predisposed to intertriginous (or body fold) pyoderma and urine scalding. Older animals are more susceptible to metabolic and neoplastic disorders. Determining whether pruritus is present and at which stage it developed is pivotal to the diagnosis. If pruritus is present and developed early in the course of the disease, it is likely that this is primarily a pruritic disease due to hypersensitivity or ectoparasitism and the ulcers and erosions are simply caused by self-trauma. Cases with a late onset of pruritus are more difficult to assess, as secondary microbial infection of primary lesions may induce pruritus. Sun-exposed animals, especially those with poorly pigmented skin, may develop solar injuries and neoplasia. Concurrent systemic signs may indicate that the ulceration is due to metabolic disease or is a result of a drug eruption (assuming the animal has received therapy for these clinical signs).

TABLE 11–1. DIFFERENTIAL DIAGNOSIS OF ULCERS AND EROSIONS AFFECTING SKIN AND MUCOUS MEMBRANES

Canine Diseases

Infectious
  Bacterial pyoderma
    Surface
      Intertrigo
      Acute moist dermatitis (pyotraumatic dermatitis)
    Deep
      Folliculitis/furunculosis (including pyotraumatic folliculitis)
  Oral bacterial infections (aerobic/anaerobic)
  Fungal
    Yeast infections (*Malassezia pachydermatis, Candida* spp.)
    Systemic/subcutaneous
  Parasitic
    Demodicosis

Metabolic
  Calcinosis cutis (hyperadrenocorticism)
  Uremia/renal failure
  Necrolytic migratory erythema/metabolic epidermal necrosis

Neoplastic
  Squamous cell carcinoma
  Epitheliotropic lymphoma

Physical, chemical
  Solar injury
  Thermal injury (freeze or burn)
  Drug reactions
  Urine scald

Immune-mediated/autoimmune
  Discoid lupus erythematosus
  Pemphigus group
  Bullous pemphigoid
  Uveo-dermatologic syndrome
  Epidermolysis bullosa aquisita
  Miscellaneous autoimmune subepidermal vesiculobullous diseases

Miscellaneous
  Dermatomyositis
  Toxic epidermal necrolysis/erythema multiforme
  Idiopathic ulceration of collies
  Arthropod bites

Feline Diseases

Infectious
  Viral
    Calici and herpes
  Bacterial
    Atypical mycobacteriosis
  Fungal
    Subcutaneous and systemic mycoses
      Cryptococcosis
      Sporotrichosis

Metabolic
  Uremia/renal disease

Neoplastic
  Squamous cell carcinoma
  Fibrosarcoma
  Lymphoma

Physical/chemical
  Thermal
  Drug reactions

Immune-mediated/autoimmune
  Pemphigus foliaceus
  Toxic epidermal necrolysis/erythema multiforme

Miscellaneous/idiopathic
  Indolent ulcer
  Eosinophilic plaque
  Arthropod bites
  Idiopathic ulceration of dorsal neck

Physical examinations, both general and dermatologic, will greatly aid the establishment of a list of possible causes as well as enabling the clinician to identify any concurrent systemic disease. The distribution of lesions may be extremely helpful (Table 11–2). Involvement of the mucous membranes may indicate that uremia/renal failure; viral, bacterial, or yeast infection; certain immune-mediated disorders (bullous pemphigoid, pemphigus vulgaris); or epitheliotropic lymphoma is present.

The diagnosis of ulcerative and erosive diseases may be difficult. Initial diagnostic tests such as cytologic examination of impression smears and microscopy of skin scrapings are useful. However, the majority of causes will be identified by histology and therefore, as previously noted, biopsy specimens should be taken early in the development of this group of diseases.

INFECTIOUS CAUSES OF EROSIONS AND ULCERS

VIRAL DISEASES

Feline calicivirus and herpesvirus infections are usually associated with signs of upper respiratory tract disease and conjunctivitis. However, they may, rarely, exhibit cutaneous ulceration, typically on the feet. A tentative clinical diagnosis of calicivirus and herpesvirus can usually be made on grounds of history and physical examination.

BACTERIAL DISEASE

Pyoderma and other bacterial diseases may be difficult to recognize as a cause of erosive and ulcerated lesions. Such infections are highly pleomorphic. If there is any doubt as to whether the lesions are the result of bacterial infection, biopsy material should be taken for histopathology. Concurrent systemic antimicrobial therapy may be indicated before the histology report is returned. In some instances, histopathology will indicate that the lesions are bacterial in origin but clinically, little improvement will have occurred following antimicrobial therapy. In such instances, it is likely that the infection was secondary. A second biopsy sampling is indicated following antibacterial therapy in order to allow examination of tissue that does not have secondary infection.

Surface bacterial infections in dogs are characterized by erosion. Intertrigo (skinfold pyoderma) affecting lip, vulvar, facial, tail, or body folds is usually recognized. Impression cytology and culture of the folds may reveal evidence of bacterial infection, usually *Staphylococcus intermedius,* but *Malassezia pachydermatis* may also be involved. Pyotraumatic dermatitis ("hot spots" or acute moist dermatitis) is another form of canine surface pyoderma that is readily recognized clinically. However, in some cases, the infection is deeper than would appear on clinical examination (this is termed pyotraumatic folliculitis); the distinction between these two forms is made by histopathology and may be significant because glucocorticoid therapy is contraindicated in the deeper form.

Deep pyoderma in dogs may be characterized by erosion and ulceration. Examples include nasal pyoderma and German shepherd dog pyoderma. These may be confused with immune-mediated disorders. Histopathology and antimicrobial therapy are indicated early in the investigation of this disease as previously noted. Aerobic and anaerobic bacterial infection may affect the mucous membranes. Such infections are often secondary to dental disease, immunosuppression

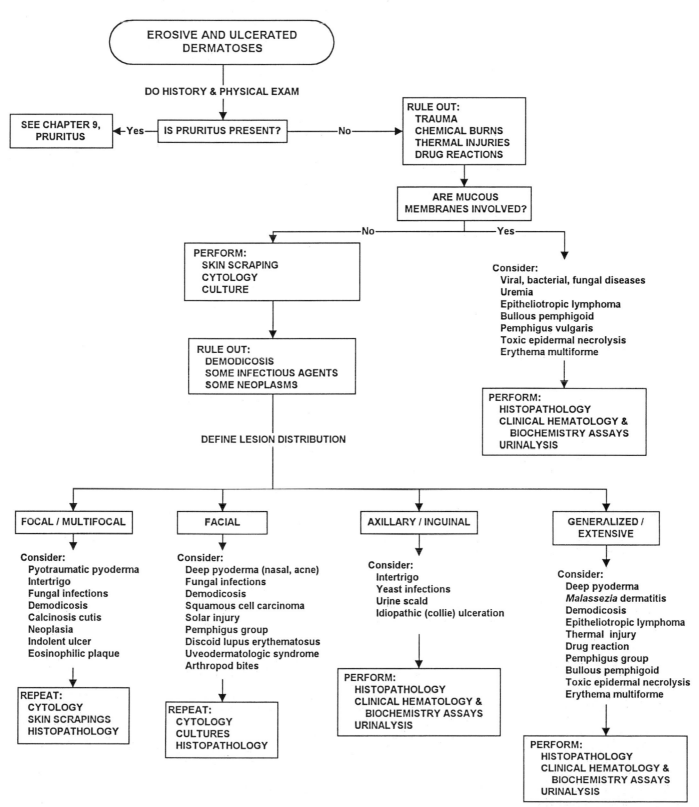

Figure 11–1. Algorithm for evaluation of erosive and ulcerated dermatoses.

TABLE 11–2. DISTRIBUTION OF ULCERS AND EROSIONS AS A DIAGNOSTIC CLUE

Focal/Multifocal

Pyoderma (principally pyotraumatic dermatitis or folliculitis) (D)
Intertrigo (D)
Systemic/subcutaneous mycosis (D, C)
Demodicosis (D)
Calcinosis cutis (D)
Neoplasia (D, C)
Indolent ulcer (C)
Eosinophilic plaque (C)

Facial

Deep pyoderma (D)
Systemic/subcutaneous mycosis (D, C)
Demodicosis (D)
Squamous cell carcinoma (C)
Solar injury (D, C)
Pemphigus foliaceus/erythematosus (D, C)
Discoid lupus erythematosus (D)
Uveo-dermatologic syndrome (D)
Dermatomyositis (D)
Arthropod bites (D, C)

Mucocutaneous

Viral infection (calici/herpes) (C)
Bacteria (aerobic/anaerobic) (D, C)
Fungal (*Malassezia pachydermatis, Candida* spp.) (D)
Uraemia (D, C)
Epitheliotropic lymphoma (D)
Bullous pemphigoid (D)
Pemphigus vulgaris (D)
Toxic epidermal necrosis/erythema multiforme (D, C)

Axillary/Inguinal

Intertrigo (D)
Fungal (*Malassezia pachydermatis, Candida* spp.) (D)
Urine scald (D)
Idiopathic ulceration of collies (D)

Generalized/Extensive

Deep pyoderma (D)
Malassezia dermatitis (D)
Demodicosis (D)
Epitheliotropic lymphoma (D)
Thermal injury (D, C)
Drug reaction (D, C)
Pemphigus group (D, C)
Bullous pemphigoid (D)
Toxic epidermal necrolysis/erythema multiforme (D, C)

D, disease can affect dogs; C, disease can infect cats.

and other systemic disease. Opportunist or atypical mycobacterial infections may occur when feline skin is inoculated with soil or water harbouring the usually free-living organism via traumatic injury. Affected cats exhibit chronic nonhealing wounds and ulcers with draining tracts. Systemic signs are usually absent.

FUNGAL DISEASE

In recent years infection of the skin surface associated with the yeast *Malassezia pachydermatis* has been recognized as an important problem. Ulceration is not a feature, but the affected skin may be eroded. Lesions usually occur in intertriginous regions, particularly in predisposed breeds (bassett hounds, West Highland white terriers, English cocker spaniels, dachshunds, and poodles). The lesions are characterized by intense erythema, a yellow waxy crust, and malodor. Dermatophytosis may lead to eroded and ulcerated

lesions in dogs and cats. Diagnosis is based on cytology, culture, and response to antifungal therapy.

Subcutaneous and systemic fungal infections are far less common. Impression smears and histopathology are indicated. Therapy is dependent on the organism involved.

OTHER CAUSES OF EROSIONS AND ULCERS

PARASITIC INFESTATIONS

Infestation with mites such as *Sarcoptes scabiei* or *Cheyletiella* spp. may lead to self-induced erosions and ulcers. Severe cases of demodicosis may, less commonly, lead to ulceration. Skin scrapings are diagnostic (and mandatory).

METABOLIC DISEASE

Calcinosis cutis is caused by accumulation of calcium in the skin, usually as a result of hyperadrenocorticism (spontaneous or iatrogenic). Ulcers may develop over these mineral plaques. Histopathology is diagnostic. Treatment of the underlying systemic disease is usually curative.

Hepatic cirrhosis or pancreatic adenocarcinoma may lead to cutaneous ulceration that particularly affects the feet and perineum of older dogs. This disease has a range of synonyms, including hepatocutaneous syndrome, necrolytic migratory erythema, and metabolic epidermal necrosis.

Uremia due to renal failure may lead to oral ulceration. Signs of systemic disease are usually present (anorexia, depression, dehydration, etc.). Halitosis is a feature. Urinalysis along with clinical biochemistry and hematology is usually diagnostic.

NEOPLASIA

Squamous cell carcinoma is a common feline neoplasm particularly affecting the extremities of white or lightly pigmented cats (e.g., ear tips and planum nasale). White English bull terriers also appear to be predisposed. The prevalence of squamous cell carcinoma is increased in geographic regions that enjoy much sunshine, especially if the animal is allowed to range freely outdoors. Waterproof, strong sun protection cream should be applied to animals at risk. Ideally, access to sunshine should be restricted.

Epitheliotropic lymphoma leads to nodular, scaling, eroded, and erythematous skin lesions in older dogs. Airedale terriers appear to be predisposed. Oral lesions (erythema, erosion) occur in the majority of cases. The prognosis is grave, with therapy having little impact on survival time. Most affected animals are dead within 6 months of the diagnosis being made. Diagnosis of cutaneous neoplasia is by histopathology, although cytology of fine-needle aspirates and impression smears may be helpful.

PHYSICAL AND CHEMICAL DISEASES

Such diseases can usually be diagnosed on the basis of history: exposure to extreme cold or scalding; recent treatments or, in the case of urine scalding, on the basis of clinical examination. Solar-induced disease may be more difficult to diagnose because the onset is chronic and some manifestations of solar dermatoses may resemble other erosive and ulcerative diseases.

IMMUNE-MEDIATED/AUTOIMMUNE

Although this group is ascribed much significance by clinicians, these diseases are uncommon or rare. Lesions arise when tissue is damaged as a result of an inappropriate immunologic response. In autoimmune disease, antibodies directed against a tissue component elicit an inflammatory response that may lead to cleavage of the epidermis from the underlying dermis (e.g., bullous pemphigoid, epidermolysis bullosa aquisita) or splitting within the epidermis itself (e.g., the pemphigus group). In some diseases, the precise pathologic mechanism is unknown (e.g., discoid lupus erythemato-

sus). The differentiation of the different immune-mediated diseases is important and is customarily made by histopathology. The different diseases respond to different forms of therapy. There is a risk that a benign disease may be treated too aggressively with immune-suppressive agents if a definitive diagnosis is not obtained.

MISCELLANEOUS DISEASES

Dermatomyositis is an hereditary disorder, primarily affecting the face and distal limbs of rough and Shetland collie pups, leading to alopecia, erosions, ulceration, and scarring. It is possible that it shares aspects of its pathogenesis with the idiopathic ulceration that is seen in the same breeds, although the lesions in the latter disorder tend to affect the ventral abdomen and groin and usually occur later in life.

CHAPTER 12

PUSTULES AND PAPULES

Edmund J. Rosser, Jr.

The most common causes of pustules and papules are bacterial skin diseases. Bacterial skin diseases of the dog will be reviewed. Pyoderma is extremely rare in cats.

CUTANEOUS BACTERIOLOGY

Bacteria that are isolated from the skin of the dog are commonly divided into three categories: resident organisms, transient organisms, and common pathogenic organisms. Resident bacterial organisms can be routinely and repeatedly isolated and cultured from the surface of the skin or haircoat of the dog and normally live in harmony with the host without causing clinical disease. The resident bacteria of canine skin include coagulase-negative staphylococci (*Staphylococcus epidermidis, S. cohnii, S. saprophyticus, S. hominis, S. haemolyticus, S. capitis, S. warneri, S. xylosus, S. simulans, and S. sciuri*); coagulase-positive staphylococci (*S. intermedius*); *Micrococcus* sp.; alpha-hemolytic streptococci; and *Acinetobacter* sp. The resident bacteria of canine hair and nasal mucosa are coagulase-positive staphylococci (*S. intermedius*). Transient bacterial organisms are not routinely or repeatedly cultured from the skin and haircoat of the dog. Under normal circumstances, these organisms do not multiply on the dog but occasionally become pathogens by secondary invasion. They include *Escherichia coli, Proteus mirabilis, Pseudomonas aeruginosa, Corynebacterium* sp., and *Bacillus* sp.

Primary pathogenic organisms are capable of tissue invasion and creating disease. They are usually coagulase-positive staphylococci (*S. intermedius, S. aureus, S. hyicus*), and

S. intermedius is the most common isolate from canine skin infections.

PATHOPHYSIOLOGY

As previously stated, the bacteria *Staphylococcus intermedius* is a normal resident of healthy canine skin and also serves as the most common causative organism in superficial and deep pyodermas. These skin infections can be classified as primary or secondary. Secondary infections are undoubtedly the most common and are easily recognized by the tendency of an infection to be recurrent. Recurrence is the result of an underlying disease process allowing *Staphylococcus intermedius* to become an opportunist and invade the stratum corneum and/or hair follicle. Underlying disease processes may alter the skin directly as a result of local trauma, irritants, or scratching from parasitic and other pruritic skin diseases (see Chapter 9). Alternatively, the disease may act systemically to decrease resistance to cutaneous infections as in metabolic and immune-mediated skin diseases (see Chapter 7). Primary skin infections are so classified because once they are appropriately treated, they do not recur. However, it seems most likely that some transient insult occurs affecting the skin that allows *Staphylococcus intermedius* to become a temporary opportunist and pathogen.

In either primary or secondary pyodermas, *Staphylococcus intermedius* begins by overcolonizing the surface of the skin and invading either the stratum corneum (as in impetigo) or the hair follicle (as in superficial folliculitis). In cases of impetigo, the invasion of the stratum corneum results in the formation of primarily nonfollicular pustules (i.e., the pustules do not have a hairshaft in the center), which rupture and often form crusts and epidermal collarettes. The lesions are usually nonpruritic and tend to be associated with minimal inflammation. In cases of superficial folliculitis, the invasion of the hair follicle results in the formation of follicular papules and pustules (i.e., hairshafts are present in the center of the lesions) that also rupture and often form crusts and epidermal collarettes. The lesions are usually pruritic and associated with inflammation and erythema. The older lesions often evolve into annular areas of alopecia and hyperpigmentation.

Deep pyodermas invariably begin as a superficial folliculitis. The infection travels into the deeper portions of the hair follicle and subsequently ruptures the hair follicle into the surrounding dermis, causing a furunculosis. The infection may continue to invade deeper dermal and subcutaneous tissues, resulting in cellulitis.

CLINICAL FEATURES

A pustule is defined as a small, elevated, purulent, fluid-filled cavity in the epidermis that is less than 0.5 cm in diameter. The base of the pustule is often erythematous. Pustules are most commonly associated with a superficial pyoderma. A papule is defined as a small elevated skin lesion up to 0.5 cm in diameter caused by the infiltration of inflammatory cells. They are usually pinkish or reddish in color. When they are oriented around a hair follicle, they usually indicate a superficial bacterial folliculitis. They are also commonly observed in cases of scabies and flea allergy (see Chapter 7). The presence of pustules and papules due to a bacterial infection is frequently associated with concurrent pruritus, owing to the production of proteolytic enzymes by the bacteria present in these lesions (primarily *Staphylococcus intermedius*). These lesions may then rupture spontaneously, or be altered in their appearance as a result of pruritus-induced self-trauma. Therefore, these primary lesions may be transient, leaving behind only the presence of secondary lesions such as erosions, crusts, epidermal collarettes, posttraumatic alopecia, and excoriations. As the disease becomes more chronic in nature, additional skin changes may develop, such as hyperpigmentation and lichenification.

SUPERFICIAL PYODERMAS

IMPETIGO (PUPPY PYODERMA)

Impetigo is most often observed in young dogs before puberty. This infection is considered to be an opportunistic or secondary pyoderma most frequently associated with poor nutrition, dirty environment, viral infections, ectoparasites, and intestinal parasitism. The disease is associated with the formation of superficial pustules that do not involve hair follicles and affects the inguinal, ventral abdominal, and, occasionally, the axillary regions. Minimal erythema is noted, and the puppy is usually nonpruritic. Impetigo is often an incidental owner finding or is noticed on routine physical examination.

SUPERFICIAL FOLLICULITIS

A folliculitis is an inflammation of the hair follicle that can be caused by bacteria (staphylococcal folliculitis), fungi (dermatophyte folliculitis), and parasites (demodicosis, pelodera dermatitis).

History and Physical Findings

Superficial folliculitis begins with the presence of pustules and papules initially affecting the inguinal and ventral abdominal regions. The papules and pustules are oriented around hair follicles, and the dog is usually pruritic. As the disease progresses, epidermal collarettes form with varying degrees of central hyperpigmentation and marginal erythema, and additional areas affected may include the axillary regions and ventrolateral thorax. When the truncal skin is affected, the haircoat often takes on a "moth-eaten" appearance (especially in short-coated breeds of dogs).

DEEP FOLLICULITIS AND FURUNCULOSIS

Furunculosis is an inflammation of hair follicles with subsequent follicular rupture extending into the surrounding dermis and subcutaneous tissue.

HISTORY AND PHYSICAL FINDINGS

The lesions initially observed include papules, pustules, and epidermal collarettes followed by the presence of exudation, crust formation, and deep draining tracts. As the process of folliculitis and furunculosis continues and the lesions coalesce, areas may become nodular and indurated, or a cellulitis may develop. Another lesion occasionally observed in these dogs is a hemorrhagic bulla. The lesions are usually first noticed in inguinal, ventral abdominal, and axillary regions as a superficial folliculitis. However, when the underlying disease process is not treated, deep folliculitis and furunculosis may develop. With this complication, involvement of the entire ventrum or a generalized process may ensue. Occasionally the lesions are most severe over the pressure and wear areas of the body such as the elbows and lateral aspects of the stifle, hip, and chest region. In most cases, the lesions seem to be pruritic or painful.

Signs of systemic involvement may be evident, including anorexia, depression, weight loss, lethargy, and fever. This is often the indication of the development of bacteremia and/or septicemia. A peripheral lymphadenopathy is also a common finding.

RECURRENT PYODERMAS

HISTORY AND PHYSICAL FINDINGS

Recurrent pyodermas may present as either a superficial folliculitis and/or a deep folliculitis and furunculosis. Invariably, a recurrent pyoderma has some underlying reason for reappearing. Therefore, the underlying problem should be identified and treated. One should first make certain that a recurrent pyoderma is not iatrogenic in nature. Iatrogenic recurrent pyodermas may be due to previously inadequate drug therapy including inappropriate antibiotic selection; inadequate dosage, frequency, and duration of antibiotic therapy; and the chronic use of corticosteroids as an adjunct to the treatment of a pyoderma.

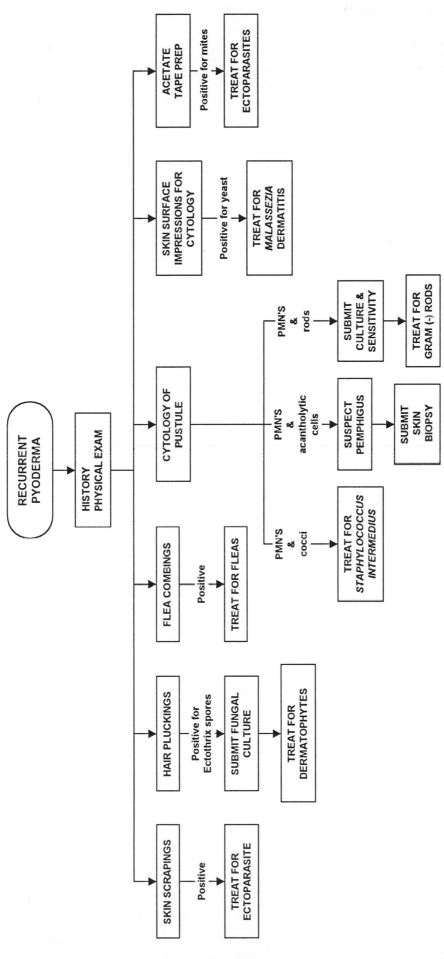

Figure 12–1. Algorithm for diagnosis and treatment of recurrent pyoderma. (From Rosser EJ, Littlewood J: Companion Animal Dermatology, Series I, Module 1, Practice Resource Manual. Guelph, Ontario, Lifelearn Inc, pp 4–15.)

TABLE 12–1. SYSTEMIC ANTIBIOTICS RECOMMENDED IN THE TREATMENT OF STAPHYLOCOCCAL PYODERMAS

ANTIBIOTIC	RECOMMENDED ORAL DOSAGE
Oxacillin	22 mg/kg q8h
Erythromycin	11 mg/kg q8h
Cephalexin	22 mg/kg q8h, or 33 mg/kg q12h
Cefadroxil	22 mg/kg q8–12h
Trimethoprim/sulfadiazine	30 mg/kg q12h
Ormetoprim/sulfadimethoxine	55 mg/kg on day 1, then 27.5 mg/kg q24h
Amoxicillin/clavulanate	14 mg/kg q12h

From Rosser EJ: Pyoderma. *In* Birchard SJ, Sherding RG (eds): Saunders Manual of Small Animal Practice, 2nd ed. Philadelphia, WB Saunders, in press.

DIAGNOSTIC APPROACH

The first part of the diagnostic approach to a patient with a pyoderma is to recognize the various lesions that indicate its presence. One of the commonly misinterpreted lesions on dermatologic examination is the epidermal collarette, especially when its margins are erythematous. It is often thought to be an indication of a dermatophyte (ringworm) infection but is more commonly an indication of a superficial pyoderma. Also, the presence of papules in patients with pruritus is frequently thought to be associated with primary allergic skin diseases and is treated solely with a corticosteroid. However, in many cases, closer inspection reveals the presence of a pinpoint pustule on top of the papule, or a hairshaft exiting the center of the papule, which indicates the presence of a folliculitis. If one is uncertain as to whether or not the lesion present may be an indication of a bacterial skin disease, a skin biopsy should be performed.

In approaching an antibiotic-responsive but recurrent pyoderma, the first step is to systematically evaluate the dog for some of the more common causes of recurrence and should include the routine use of the following diagnostic tests: skin scrapings, flea combing, hair plucking and microscopic examination, skin surface impression cytology, cytology of pustules, and acetate (Scotch) tape preparations (Fig. 12–1). When these test results are negative and the cytology or culture of pustules and papules indicates the presence of a pyoderma, an appropriate antibiotic must be selected. The antibiotic is either empirically chosen (Table 12–1) or, preferably, based on the results of culture and sensitivity testing. The next step involves the use of the dog's response to therapy as an aid to the definitive diagnosis. In a majority of dogs with recurrent pyoderma, some degree of pruritus is

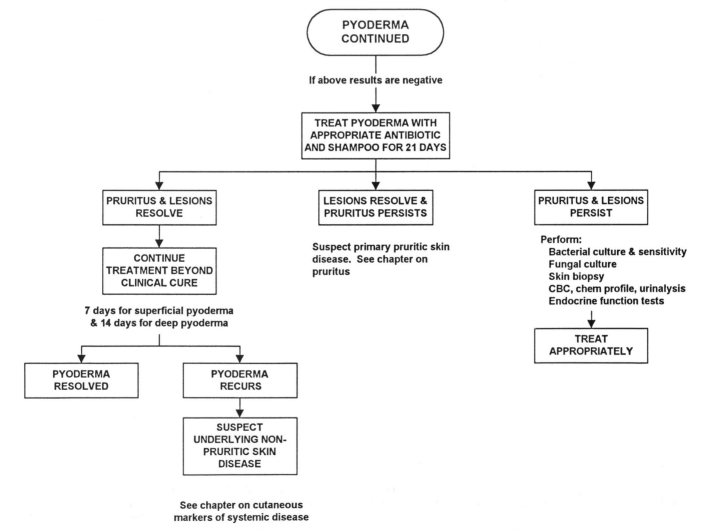

Figure 12–2. Algorithm for pyoderma continued. (From Rosser EJ, Littlewood J: Companion Animal Dermatology, Series I, Module 1, Practice Resource Manual. Guelph, Ontario, Lifelearn Inc, pp 4–15.)

present. However, at this stage of the work-up, the use of a corticosteroid (or any other antipruritic drug) needs to be avoided. The dog is then treated with *only* the appropriate antibiotic and shampoo therapy (benzoyl peroxide shampoo), for a period of 3 consecutive weeks, and then reevaluated (Fig. 12–2). This initial duration of therapy is usually adequate in cases of superficial folliculitis, but may need to be increased to 6 to 8 consecutive weeks in cases of deep folliculitis and furunculosis. If upon recheck examination the pyoderma has noticeably improved or resolved but the pruritus has persisted, the dog needs to be further evaluated for the presence of an underlying pruritic skin disease including flea allergy dermatitis, atopy, food allergy, scabies, demodicosis, allergic contact dermatitis, and seborrheic dermatitis. The owner should also be advised on the initial visit to observe the dog for the areas of the body where the pruritus

is persisting or most severe (i.e., the distribution pattern of pruritus) to assist the clinician in establishing the underlying differential diagnosis (see Chapter 9). However, if upon recheck examination the pyoderma has resolved and the dog has become nonpruritic in response to the antibiotic and shampoo therapy alone, it is necessary to establish whether the pyoderma is truly recurrent. The appropriate antibiotic and shampoo therapy should now be continued for a total treatment time of 8 weeks. After having this done, some patients with a previous history of a recurrent pyoderma will experience permanent resolution of their disease. If the pyoderma recurs after this treatment, the following diseases should be ruled out; hypothyroidism, Cushing's disease, diabetes mellitus, reproductive hormone imbalances, demodicosis, cheyletiellosis, staphylococcal hypersensitivity, and cell-mediated immunodeficiencies (see Chapter 7).

CHAPTER 13

SCALING AND CRUSTING DERMATOSES

Anthony A. Stannard, Andrea G. Cannon, and Thierry Olivry

Scaling and crusting are frequently encountered clinical signs in veterinary dermatology. Any superficial inflammatory process that involves the epidermis can and probably will be accompanied by scaling and/or crusting. Therefore, it is important to have a logical protocol for evaluating animals with crusting and/or scaling dermatoses. This discussion will be limited to those diseases in which scaling and/or crusting is the predominant lesion. For example, a dog with flea allergy dermatitis may exhibit scaling and excoriations, but the primary lesion/clinical sign is pruritus.

DEFINITIONS

The stratum corneum is formed as the keratinocytes differentiate, generate a cornified envelope, and undergo apoptosis. Corneocytes are produced and desquamated in a highly regulated and controlled manner such that there is almost no visible scale. In a normal dog, it takes about 21 days for a basal keratinocyte to become a corneocyte. Any alteration in epidermal kinetics (turnover time), disturbance of lipid production, or alterations in the humidity of the skin can produce visible scales. Scales can be either loose (e.g., dandruff) or adherent (e.g., elbow callosities).

Crusts are composed of serum, blood, and/or inflammatory cells that have admixed with corneocytes on the surface of the skin. Differentiating adherent scales and crusts may be difficult. Usually, this is accomplished by noting the color (crusts are generally red, brown to black) and what lies

under the "scab." Adherent scales are usually uniformly light in color and overlie a relatively normal epidermis. Crusts, by contrast, are not uniform and usually exhibit various shades of red, brown, and black. The underlying epidermis is frequently eroded or ulcerated.

SCALING DISEASES

CONGENITAL/HEREDITARY

Congenital (i.e., present at birth) and/or hereditary (i.e., with a genetic basis) diseases characterized by a defect in the formation of the cornified layer of the epidermis exhibit scaling as a major clinical sign and are classified as *cornification or keratinization defects. Primary seborrhea* has been used as a generic term to describe these disorders, but the authors prefer not to use this term because it implies excess sebum production.

Dogs or cats with a cornification defect are usually young and have an excess of scale, odor, with or without oiliness, and variable degrees of moderate pruritus. The scaling is predominantly truncal, but can be generalized. Unless there is a secondary pyoderma, lesions such as pustules and papules are usually not present. There are marked breed predilections, the classic example being "primary seborrhea of cocker spaniels." Other breeds reported in the literature include English springer spaniels, Bassett hounds, Dobermans, Labradors, Irish setters, miniature schnauzers, and

Chinese Shar Peis. The skin diseases seen in many of these breeds are characterized by a greasy and malodorous coat. Differential diagnoses include superficial pyoderma, *Malassezia* dermatitis, cheyletiellosis, scabies, dermatophytosis, demodicosis, hypothyroidism, and ichthyosis.

Treatments are focused on "normalizing" the keratinization process and alleviating clinical signs. Antiseborrheic shampoos such as coal tars (coal tars are toxic to cats), sulfur/salicylic acid, and selenium sulfide may control the clinical signs in mild cases. Some cocker spaniels, Labradors, and miniature schnauzers have responded to oral vitamin A therapy at 8000 to 10,000 IU twice daily, while others have required oral retinoid therapy (etretinate or isotretinoin). Cases that respond to vitamin A therapy have been referred to as *vitamin A–responsive dermatosis*. Additionally, these dogs are prone to secondary infections, which must be addressed because they exacerbate the signs.

West Highland white terriers have a unique clinical syndrome that is multifactorial and has been referred to as *epidermal dysplasia*. These dogs appear to have a cornification defect, concurrent allergic skin disease, pyoderma, and/or *Malassezia* dermatitis. Clinically, these dogs are extremely pruritic, greasy, alopecic, erythematous, malodorous, and scaly with severe lichenification and hyperpigmentation. The lesions usually start in the truncal region but tend to rapidly extend down the extremities and generalize. Diagnosis is primarily based on signalment, history, cytology, and clinical signs. Cytologic evidence of *Malassezia* or bacteria should lead to the initiation of oral antifungal (ketoconazole, 5 to 10 mg/kg once to twice daily) and/or oral antibacterial therapies as well as intensive topical therapies (coal tar, benzoylperoxide, or sulfur/salicylic acid shampoos every 2 to 3 days). If the pruritus persists after infection resolution, underlying allergic skin disease should be pursued. Although some dogs respond to antimicrobial therapy and/or management of allergic skin diseases, most require lifelong therapy to control their clinical signs.

Ichthyosis represents a group of hereditary, most commonly congenital, diseases of epidermal cornification and keratinization. They are characterized by generalized, severe, adherent scale and thickening of the pads. In humans, ichthyosis comprises a large group of hereditary disorders that are characterized by the severe accumulation of scale. In veterinary medicine, a number of ichthyoses have been reported, but the best described is a scaling disease similar to lamellar ichthyosis of humans. Lamellar ichthyosis has been reported in West Highland white terriers, Jack Russell terriers, King Charles Cavalier spaniels, terrier crosses, and in one litter of cats. The lesions are present at birth and increase in severity with age. Some dogs may not be presented to a veterinarian until early adulthood when the clinical signs have become more intense. Most of the body will be covered with adherent, tannish grey scale that may form cornified projections. Affected dogs may have secondary pyodermas and/or *Malassezia* dermatitis. The diagnosis is based on signalment, age of onset, clinical findings, and skin biopsy. Management of this disease involves frequent bathing (three to five times weekly) with mild antiseborrheic shampoos followed by a humectant or emollient rinse (Humilac [Allerderm], HyLyt*efa [DVM], or 75 per cent propylene glycol solution). Oral retinoids (isotretinoin at 1 to 2 mg/kg orally every 24 hours) have been effective in many cases. Clients should be counseled as to the chronic nature and possible genetic basis of this disease.

A cornification defect has been recognized in Persian cats (*hereditary primary seborrhea oleosa*). These cats present with a greasy scaling dermatitis with comedones and a curly matted haircoat. This disease appears to exhibit an autosomal recessive transmission based on limited pedigree analysis and test breeding. There does not appear to be a sex predilection. These cats have been controlled with topical "antiseborrheic" therapies (sulfur salicylic acid shampoos).

Sebaceous adenitis (SA) is a heritable skin disease that is marked by an inflammatory process centered on and destroying sebaceous glands. There are two forms of SA. One is a granulomatous disease that does not produce scaling or crusting and is seen in short-coated breeds such as the Vizsla. The second form, the scaly form, has been recognized in standard poodles, Akitas, and Samoyeds. Although the pathogenesis of SA is not known, in the standard poodle the trait appears to be inherited as autososmal recessive. Owing to the extreme scaling and response to oral retinoids or Vitamin A, SA has been theorized to be a defect in cornification/keratinization. The inflammatory attack on the sebaceous gland seen histologically has led to the theory that SA is an immune-mediated disease. Clinically, these dogs are first examined at 3 to 7 years of age with tightly adhered yellow to greyish scale and alopecia. The hair epilates easily and retains a waxy coat of scale around the base of the hair (*follicular cast*). These dogs often suffer from secondary pyodermas, which need to be treated concurrently. The treatment of SA is based on reducing scaling and rehydrating the epidermis. Frequent shampooing (every 2 to 3 days) with antiseborrheic shampoos (sulfur/salicylic acid, coal tar) followed by humectant or emollient rinses is the mainstay of therapy. Propylene glycol (75 per cent) applied once daily may help in more severe cases but can be objectionable to owners owing to the greasiness. Oral therapy may be needed in severe cases. Fatty acids, vitamin A (8000 to 10,000 IU twice daily) and oral retinoids (etretinate 1 mg/kg/day, isotretinoin 1 to 2 mg/kg q24h) have been used with variable success. Treatment with oral retinoids or vitamin A (vitamin A and retinoids should not be used in combination) should be continued for at least 1 month before evaluating effectiveness. If there is adequate improvement with oral vitamin A, the therapy is continued indefinitely. With retinoids, the dosage is reduced monthly with the goal of tapering the dose to the lowest dosage needed to control the disease. Clients should be counseled as to the chronic nature and potential genetic basis of this disease.

NUTRITIONAL/METABOLIC

Many metabolic diseases result in a scaling dermatosis characterized histologically by parakeratosis. The clinical manifestations are remarkably similar in these disorders with a spectrum of lesions from mild scaling to severe crusting with erosions and ulcerations. The lesions tend to affect the perioral or periocular regions, feet, and genitals. *Zinc-responsive dermatosis* comprises three syndromes. *Acrodermatitis* of bull terriers is a lethal autosomal recessive disease with decreased serum zinc levels and no response to zinc supplementation. In young rapidly growing large breed dogs, a *relative zinc deficiency* has been recognized. Adherent scale forms in these puppies over stress points, on the footpads, and nasal planum. The footpads and nasal planum may fissure and become secondarily infected. Dietary adjustments can resolve the problem, but a short course of zinc supplementation may hasten the response. In *Siberian huskies and Malamutes*, a scaly, crusted, alopecic dermatitis around the eyes, ears, mouth, scrotum, prepuce, or vulva with decreased serum zinc levels is recognized. The disease develops at 1 to 3 years of age with variable progression. Diagnosis is made based on signalment, dietary history, physical examination, and skin biopsy. Serum zinc levels may be helpful but are unreliable. Response to zinc supplementation may be ineffective in some dogs, especially Siberian huskies. Zinc is supplemented based on the amount of elemental zinc available; zinc sulfate (10 mg/kg/day), or zinc methionine (1.7 mg/kg/day) is most commonly used.

INFECTIOUS/PARASITIC

Cheyletiella spp. are highly contagious large mites that live in the stratum corneum on cats, dogs, rabbits, and humans. The mite causes a loose white scaling disorder along the dorsal midline with variable pruritus. Humans in contact with infected animals will often have a pruritic rash. The mite is an obligate parasite with a 21-day life cycle. All life stages occur on the host. Diagnosis is inconsistently made by demonstrating the characteristic mite or eggs using a combing or adhesive tape preparation. The disease is less common in areas where flea control is practiced because the mites are sensitive to common insecticides. Treatment involves aggressive "flea" control programs for the animals and the environment. Pyrethrins should be used for the household environment and all infected and in-contact animals for a period of 4 weeks. Recently, fipronil spray (Frontline Spray; Rhone Merieux) has been shown to be effective against *Cheyletiella* used at the label dose of 3 mL/kg applied to the coat every 3 weeks for a total of three treatments. Ivermectin can be used in cattery situations or in refractory cases at 200 to 300 µg/kg orally every week for three to four treatments.

Dermatophytosis is an infectious, zoonotic fungal disease caused by a keratinophilic fungi. The majority of cases in dogs and cats are caused by *Microsporum canis*, *Microsporum gypseum*, or *Trichophyton mentagrophytes*. These organisms live in the keratin of the hair follicles and exhibit an exothrix mode of hair invasion (live on the outside of the hair shaft). More rarely, dermatophytes may colonize the stratum corneum instead of the hair shafts. Kittens and Persians are most commonly affected. Cats can be asymptomatic carriers. Clinical signs are highly variable, but the most common are alopecia and scaling. The most important differential diagnoses are demodicosis and staphylococcal folliculitis. Positive fluorescence under a Wood lamp or demonstration of arthrospores or hyphae on trichogram supports a tentative diagnosis. Diagnosis is based on a positive fungal culture. Speciation of the dermatophyte is important in determining the mode of infection and for making environmental treatment recommendations aimed at resolving the infection and preventing transmission to other pets or humans. The disease in most healthy dogs and short-haired cats is self-limiting in 2 to 6 months. However, every case of dermatophytosis should be treated topically and long-haired cats should be clipped to reduce the risk of zoonotic transmission. Antimicrobial shampoos will remove scale, crusts, and infected hairs. Chlorhexidine, miconazole, and ketoconazole based shampoos are most frequently employed. Antifungal rinses such as chlorhexidine, miconazole, lime-sulfur, or enilconazole rinses may hasten recovery, while creams and lotions containing antifungal ingredients may be useful in localized lesions. Many affected animals and almost all cats require systemic therapy. Griseofulvin is the only approved drug for the treatment of dermatophytosis in

cats. *Griseofulvin* is a fungistatic drug that is not soluble in water and is absorbed better when administered with a high-fat meal. The recommended dosage of microsized griseofulvin in animals is 25 mg/kg of body weight orally twice daily, although doses as high as 60 mg/kg orally twice daily have been reported. Treatment should be continued 2 weeks beyond a negative fungal culture. Gastrointestinal side effects occur. (Neurotoxicosis has also been reported.) Severe neutropenic reactions have been reported in cats with feline immunodeficiency virus (FIV) receiving griseofulvin. Ideally, all cats should be FIV tested before administering griseofulvin. Griseofulvin is a known teratogen and should not be given to pregnant queens. *Ketoconazole, itraconazole, and fluconazole* have also been used in both human and veterinary medicine to treat dermatophytosis. Ketoconazole may not be as efficacious against *M. canis* as itraconazole and fluconazole. Itraconazole and fluconazole seem to be well tolerated by both cats and dogs. Both of these drugs are expensive and not licensed for use in the cat or dog.

While *bacterial infections* of the skin usually produce pustules, surface pyodermas or superficial spreading pyodermas may produce scaling and epidermal collarettes without pustules. Epidermal collarettes are circular areas of fine attached scale with a normal or hyperpigmented center. Diagnosis of a surface pyoderma is made based on clinical signs and cytology. Cytologic findings of bacteria and neutrophils, especially intracellular bacteria, lead to a diagnosis. These pyodermas respond well to topical antimicrobial shampoos and oral antibiotics.

In an older dog with severe erythroderma and generalized scaling, *cutaneous T-cell lymphoma* (CTCL) should be included in the list of differential diagnoses. The diagnosis is confirmed on skin biopsy. Treatment options are limited, and a veterinary oncologist or dermatologist should be consulted (Fig. 13–1).

CRUSTING DISEASES

In domestic animals the epidermis is thin and lesions such as pustules, vesicles, and bullae are transient. Therefore, crusts are often the only lesions found on physical examination (see Fig. 13–1).

Pyodermas, both superficial and deep, are one of the most common causes of crusting in the dog. In domestic animals, the epidermis is thin (1 to 2 cell layers) and pustules are short lived. Therefore, clinically, a crust or a crusted papule may be the only lesions seen. Pyoderma is common in dogs and uncommon in other species. The most common bacteria found in canine pyodermas is *Staphylococcus intermedius*. Diagnosis of pyoderma can be made by demonstrating intracellular bacteria on skin cytology, by culturing the organism, or by skin biopsy. Treatment should include baths with antimicrobial shampoos containing chlorhexidine, benzoyl peroxide, or ethyl lactate and systemic antibiotics. Potentiated penicillins, cephalosporins, and potentiated sulfas are the most commonly recommended antibiotics. For superficial pyodermas, treatment should be initiated for 2 to 4 weeks, whereas deep pyodermas should be treated for 4 to 6 weeks or 2 weeks beyond clinical resolution.

Malassezia dermatitis is often found in conjunction with pyoderma in dogs and needs to be treated concurrently. *Malassezia pachydermatis* is a nonmycelial, lipophilic yeast. *M. pachydermatis* is a commensal organism and can be an opportunistic pathogen. Infections with *M. pachydermatis* are usually secondary to allergic skin disease, keratinization/

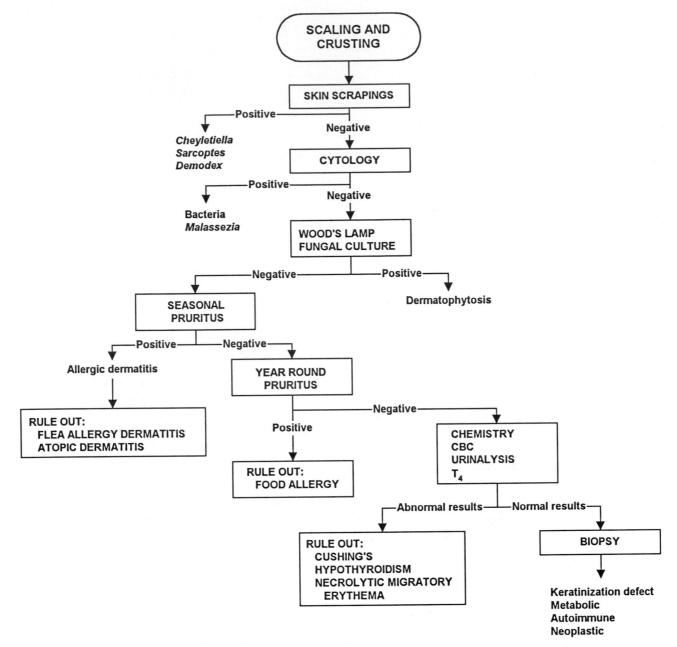

Figure 13–1. Algorithm for evaluation of scaling and crusting.

cornification defects, corticosteroids, or antibiotic therapy. The diagnosis of *Malassezia* dermatitis is based on clinical signs and skin cytology. On direct impression smears stained with Diff-Quik, the pathognomonic footprint or "peanut"-like organisms in sufficient numbers are diagnostic. Two organisms per high oil field with compatible clinical signs is considered suggestive of the diagnosis. Confirmation of the diagnosis requires response to antifungal therapy. Treatment in mild cases consists of frequent bathing with an antifungal shampoo such as Dermazole (Allerderm) or Nizoral (Janssen). In more severe cases, systemic therapy with ketoconazole (5 to 10 mg/kg orally twice a day) for 2 to 4 weeks may be needed in addition to topical therapy.

Sarcoptes scabei var. *canis* is a mite that is relatively host-specific for canines and lives within the stratum corneum. The mite does not survive long off of the host, only about 9 days. There are two forms of *scabies* seen in dogs. One form, sometimes referred to as *Norwegian scabies,* is charac-

terized by large numbers of mites that are readily identifiable on skin scrapings with little or no pruritus. In the more common form of scabies, the dogs are extremely pruritic and the mites are very difficult to identify. The lesions in scabies are yellowish, dry crusts with a macular papular eruption. The lesions usually occur on the ear margins, elbows, and ventrum, but can spread to affect the entire body. Humans in the household may be affected about 10 to 50 per cent of the time. Diagnosis is confirmed by demonstrating the distinctive sarcoptiform mite on microscopic examination of skin scrapings. If clinical suspicion is high but the mites are not found on multiple skin scrapings, a diagnosis may be obtained by response to appropriate therapy. Ivermectin is the treatment of choice for scabies. Ivermectin should not be used in collies, Shetland sheepdogs, Border collies, their crosses, or in dogs less than 16 weeks of age. Ivermectin is administered subcutaneously or orally at the dose of 200 to 250 μg/kg every 7 days for three to four treatments. Milbemycin oxime (Interceptor, Novartis Animal Health) has also been shown to be effective against sarcoptes and is potentially less toxic than ivermectin. Dogs are treated with 2 mg/kg of milbemycin oxime orally every 7 days for three doses. Weekly topical treatment with 5 per cent lime-sulfur dips or organophosphate (Paramite, Vet-Kem) dips for five to six dips are also effective. All in-contact dogs should be treated, as some dogs may act as inapparent carriers.

In dogs and cats, the most common autoimmune skin disease is *pemphigus foliaceus* (PF). PF forms pustules or vesicles that rupture and produce crusts. The lesions are most commonly found on the face, pinna, feet, and around the nipples (especially in cats), although the whole body can be involved. Diagnosis is based on skin biopsy. Biopsy of an intact pustule or vesicle is recommended. PF is treated with immunosuppressive doses of corticosteroids with or without azathioprine (in dogs), chlorambucil, or aurothioglucose. The disease can wax and wane, and response to therapy is variable. The side effects of the drugs must be weighed against the severity of the disease.

METABOLIC

Necrolytic migratory erythema (NME) (also known as superficial necrolytic dermatosis, metabolic epidermal necrolysis, hepatocutaneous syndrome) is a disease that is seen in middle-aged to older dogs that have concurrent liver disease,

glucagonomas, phenobarbital treatment, and mycotoxins. This rapidly advancing disease affects the skin as well as the liver. Clinically, affected dogs have crusting of the footpads, periorally, periocularly, and around the genitals. Diagnosis is based on skin biopsy, abdominal ultrasound, liver biopsy, and serum chemistries. The vast majority of dogs diagnosed with NME have the classic "honeycomb" patterns of the liver on abdominal ultrasound with increased serum liver enzyme activities and diagnostic histology of the liver and skin. Therapeutic attempts utilizing oral amino acid supplements, fatty acids, zinc supplementation, and antimicrobials have had limited success. However, one case of NME that was associated with a glucagonoma resolved after resection of the pancreatic tumor.

Many neoplastic skin diseases can be seen initially as a crusted lesion, for example, *squamous cell carcinoma (SCC)*, *Bowen's disease,* and *basal cell carcinoma.* SCC is a relatively common neoplasm of cats and dogs. SCC occurs most frequently in sun-damaged skin and may be preceded by actinic keratosis. SCC is seen more frequently in white animals and/or in sparsely haired regions such as the ears and inguinal region. Multicentric squamous cell carcinoma in situ or *Bowen's disease* is a rare type of premalignant SCC found in non–solar-exposed areas. *Basal cell carcinomas* are common in cats and uncommon in dogs. In cats, basal cell carcinomas occur most frequently on the face (nasal planum and eyelids). Treatment of these tumors include surgical removal, photodynamic therapy, cryosurgery, electrosurgery, hyperthermia, and radiotherapy.

CHAPTER 14

DIAGNOSTIC CYTOLOGY OF SKIN LESIONS

George P. Reppas and Paul J. Canfield

Veterinarians are discovering how useful and cost-effective cytology of skin lesions can be. Histology is the benchmark by which a definitive diagnosis is reached in dermatopathology. Cytology, however, is less expensive, less dangerous, and can achieve equivalent results, particularly for identification of microorganisms and round cell tumors. While cytology is not always diagnostic, the general disease process may be identifiable and further laboratory investigation or therapy can be directed with greater confidence. Moreover, the procedure is quick and minimally invasive.

The success with which cytology is implemented as a diagnostic procedure generally depends on three factors: collecting the most appropriate sample; preparing and staining the smears correctly; and examining and evaluating the smears systematically. It is only with practice, however, that veterinarians, with the assistance of a cytopathologist, will

realize the benefits and limitations of cytology and not be disappointed by their occasional nondiagnostic results.

COLLECTING THE MOST APPROPRIATE SAMPLE

Adequate restraint of the animal is of paramount importance in collecting a sample for cytology. Several methods are available for collection, but the one chosen will be dictated by the type and location of the skin lesion (Fig. 14–1). The objective is to obtain a representative cell population with little blood contamination. The essence of a good cytologic smear is one in which cells are arranged in monolayers with minimal damage. Thin smears (monolayers) will aid stain penetration and make cytologic examination of

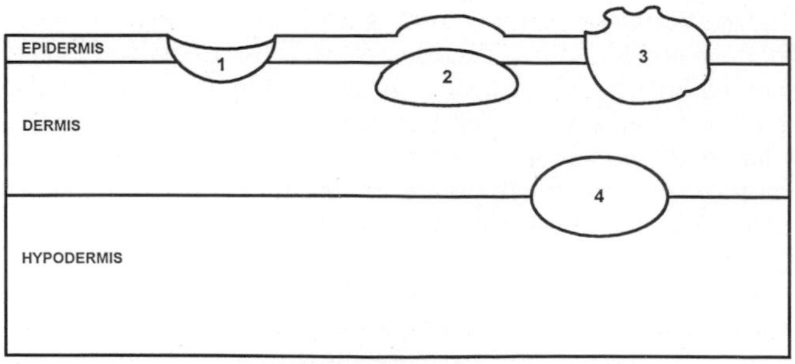

Figure 14–1. Schematic representation of location and type of cutaneous and subcutaneous lesions amenable to cytologic investigation: (1) crateriform lesion; (2) lesion with epidermal covering; (3) raised lesion without epidermal covering; (4) deep dermal/hypodermal lesion. Cytologic techniques applicable to each lesion include swabbing for lesions 1 and 3; impression smears for lesion 3; scraping for lesions 1 and 3; fine-needle aspiration for all lesions. (Modified with kind permission of FRISKIES Veterinary International.)

individual cells much easier. The equipment necessary to perform cytology is inexpensive and readily available.

Cotton-Tipped Swab Smears. This uncommon technique is reserved mainly for small ulcerative lesions of a crateriform nature or interdigital lesions where direct impression smears may not be possible. Samples are obtained with the use of a sterile swab, which can be moistened with a few drops of saline for use on dry lesions, and gently rolled onto a clean microscope slide to avoid unnecessary cellular distortion.

Impression Smears. This is a useful technique for obtaining cytologic samples from easily accessible, ulcerated but raised skin lesions, as well as from surgical biopsy specimens prior to their submission for histologic processing. Lesions or biopsies need to be cleaned using a saline-soaked swab to clear surface debris. This will inevitably cause bleeding, which should be controlled by applying firm pressure with a gauze swab until one is ready to make the impression smear.

Excisional surgical biopsy specimens can usually be cross-sectioned, blotted free of blood, and then the impression smears made. Impression smears are best made by "rolling" the slide onto the lesion's surface or vice versa.

Scraping. This technique is applicable to all ulcerated skin lesions. In contrast to the deep and vigorous scraping associated with ectoparasitic investigations, cytology employs a gentler scraping technique. Two to three gentle strokes, preferably with the blunt end of a sterile scalpel blade (size 22, 23, or 24) to minimize cell damage, should suffice. Ulcerated but previously cleaned surfaces of cutaneous lesions or the cut surfaces of incisional or excisional biopsies that have been blotted can be scraped. Scraping forcibly exfoliates cells from mesenchymal tumors, which normally fail to relinquish their cells freely upon impression smearing or swabbing.

A scraping technique adapted to investigating pustules of suspected autoimmune origin is known as Tzanck's method. It is specifically designed to reveal acanthocytes. A large pustule is almost totally sectioned with a sterile scalpel blade (size 22 to 24) and then inverted to allow its floor and the lower surface of the flap to be scraped.

Smears from scraping should be prepared by gently "buttering" the glass slide with the material accumulated on the edge of the scalpel blade.

Fine-Needle Aspiration (FNA). This is by far the most commonly used technique in cytology. Almost all types of

lesions can be sampled. The equipment required consists of a 21- to 25-gauge needle of 1-inch length and a 3-, 6-, or 12-mL syringe (depending on operator comfort and dexterity). A vacuum is applied to the attached syringe once the needle is firmly seated in the lesion. The vacuum should be released prior to needle redirection within a mass to avoid excess bleeding. The needle should be redirected two or three times to obtain a representative cell population. Aspiration should cease once material has been sighted within the hub of the needle or as soon as blood starts to fill the hub. The needle should then be withdrawn without applying vacuum, the syringe detached and filled with air, then re-attached to the needle and the air used to expel the contents of the needle onto a glass slide. Even if material is not obvious in the hub of the needle, the expelling process should be attempted, as diagnostic material may be present in the bore of the needle.

In some cases, it is advantageous to use the needle alone to collect a sample. The needle is embedded and redirected in a similar manner, but cells are collected by capillary action. Once withdrawn, the needle is attached to an air-filled syringe. Excellent results are obtainable using this technique for small round cell neoplasms, especially around the head (i.e., ears, muzzle, and eyelids).

Proper smear preparation from FNAs is crucial. Contents should be expelled as a drop, about 1 cm from one end of the slide. Usually there is enough material for making two slides. Gently place a second microscope slide on top of the expelled material at right angles to the first slide and gently pull the top slide to the other end of the bottom slide. This smear preparation technique is known as a squash preparation and is useful for viscid samples. Other techniques may also be used, depending on the nature of the sample. Samples that are fluid in consistency may be prepared using the blood smear technique. The latter produces a feathered edge to the smear. If one suspects a fluid sample to have low cellularity, the line smear may be employed. This begins like the blood smear but ends abruptly by lifting off the spreader slide as it nears the end of the smear. This results in a narrow line at the end of the smear in which many cells are concentrated. To facilitate rapidly locating this area during microscopic examination, one should use an etching marker to place an arrow on the slide next to the smear line. Other techniques may also be used to prepare smears. For example, the spray technique involves forcibly expelling the needle's contents across the glass slide at the lowest angle possible to produce a monolayer. With practice, one becomes familiar with the technique that best suits conditions at the time of cytologic examination.

STAINING SMEARS

The quality of smear staining is crucial in cytologic interpretation. Several types of cytologic stains are available, but in routine cytologic practice the easiest, quickest, and most cost-effective are the fast-staining Romanowsky-type stains (e.g., Diff-Quik). The main disadvantage of the Diff-Quik stain is that it does not appear to undergo the metachromatic reaction, which means that the granules of some mast cells do not stain. If such a problem is suspected, other stains including Wright's Giemsa or new methylene blue may be used. Inadequately stained Diff-Quik smears usually appear pink but can be restained by replacing them in the blue stain.

Several air-dried smears prepared differently should be evaluated, if possible. This will allow the clinician or cytopathologist to use further special stains such as a Gram stain for bacteria or wet India ink when looking for encapsulated fungal organisms (e.g., *Cryptococcus neoformans*). When sending samples to a cytopathologist for assessment, ensure that at least one smear is unstained. This will allow the cytopathologist to use a stain with which he/she is most familiar. If the delay in transit is expected to be greater than 18 to 24 hours, ensure that the smears, once air dried, are fixed in methanol.

EXAMINING AND EVALUATING CYTOLOGIC SMEARS

This begins at the lowest magnification (4× or 10× objectives). Here one attempts to assess the quality of the preparation by considering cellularity (numbers, size and shape of cells), contamination (erythrocytes and artifacts—e.g., squames), and staining uniformity. The most representative smear should be evaluated with the 40× and 100× objectives using a coverslip and immersion oil.

Essentially, cytologic interpretation depends on fulfilling two basic criteria: performing a detailed morphologic study of individual cells, and recognizing patterns in cell arrangement. Usually within cytologic smears of skin lesions, cells of four types may be found: erythrocytes, inflammatory cells, tissue cells, and neoplastic cells. Of these cell types, erythrocytes in small numbers are ubiquitous, while larger numbers may interfere with ability to read the slide. In addition to cells, acellular material (e.g., proteinaceous secretions) may be present. On the basis of cell types, presence of acellular material, and microorganisms, a lesion may be called *primary degenerative, primary inflammatory,* or *neoplastic* (Fig. 14–2). Further subclassification is possible but not always necessary for treatment purposes.

PRIMARY INFLAMMATORY SKIN LESIONS

The inflammatory cell type present usually defines the lesion. For example, neutrophils predominate in acute or ongoing active processes, while lymphocytes, plasma cells, and macrophages usually signify a more chronic process.

Neutrophils. Their abundance (>75 per cent of the cell population in the smear) usually indicates acute or ongoing active inflammation. A bacterial etiology should be suspected initially and neutrophils scanned for intracellular organisms. In many instances, bacterial toxin proliferation will result in neutrophil degeneration (karyolysis and loss of cytoplasmic margins). Further smears could be subjected to a Gram stain, while additional material could be submitted for culture. Nondegenerate neutrophils can characterize some bacterial infections of low toxicity but are generally associated with pathologic processes of a nonbacterial nature (e.g., trauma, foreign bodies, autoimmune skin disease, protozoal/parasitic infections like cryptococcal organisms and mites). They have a morphologically normal appearance, although some may exhibit natural aging changes such as pyknosis and cytoplasmic condensation.

Eosinophils. When eosinophils account for greater than 10 to 15 per cent of the total cell population, specific inflammatory conditions should be considered, i.e., allergy to parasites, subcutaneous mycoses, and collagenolytic disorders (e.g., eosinophilic granuloma complex). Tissue eosinophilia can also accompany mast cell neoplasia, particularly in the dog.

Lymphocytes and Plasma Cells. Numbers of 30 to 70 per cent usually indicate a strong immune response in chronic inflammation (e.g., feline pododermatitis). These cells may also characterize a variety of neoplasms that cause tissue damage and antigenic stimulation (e.g., squamous cell carcinomas). When lymphoid or plasma cells are present in large numbers (>70 per cent), neoplasia of the skin should also be considered.

Macrophages. These are present in inflammatory lesions when there is significant tissue debris, immune stimulation, or attraction by specific agents of disease (e.g., foreign bodies, free hair or keratin, fungi). They are large cells often with an eccentric, occasionally indented nucleus, and usually have a vacuolated cytoplasm that may contain phagocytosed material.

Macrophages usually account for 10 to 50 per cent of the cell population in chronic inflammation with the balance of cells being lymphocytes/plasma cells. When as many as 10 to 20 per cent of the cells are neutrophils, the term *active chronic inflammation* is often used. A specific form of chronic inflammation, called *granulomatous inflammation* is characterized by a macrophage population of greater than 50 per cent, most being in the form of epithelioid cells and/or multinucleate cells. When 10 to 20 per cent of the cells are neutrophils, the term *pyogranulomatous inflammation* is used. Both granulomatous and pyogranulomatous inflammation suggest the presence of a specific agent of disease such as mycobacteria or fungi.

PRIMARY DEGENERATIVE SKIN LESIONS

Within this category belong most fluid-filled (sialoceles, hematomas, seromas, hygromas), keratin-filled (epidermal or follicular cysts, certain benign tumors), and amorphous material occupying (mineralization—e.g., calcinosis circumscripta) skin lesions.

TABLE 14–1. CYTOLOGIC CRITERIA FOR MALIGNANCY*

General criteria
    Cellular pleomorphism (differences in size and shape)
    Anaplasia (poorly differentiated cells)
    Macrocytosis (≥21 μm)
    Hypercellularity (monomorphous cell population)
    Anisocytosis (uneven size of cells)

Cytoplasmic criteria
    Basophilia
    Vacuolation†

High nuclear to cytoplasmic ratio
    ≥1:1 or 1:2

Nuclear criteria
    Mitotic figures (especially abnormal mitotic figures)
    Multiple nuclei (especially trinucleate cells)
    Macrokaryosis (≥15 μm) (large nuclei)
    Anisokaryosis (uneven size of nuclei)
    Poikilokaryosis (differences in shape of nuclei)
    Nuclear molding
    Coarse chromatin pattern

Nucleolar criteria
    Multiple nucleoli (>2)
    Macronucleoliosis (≥5 μm) (large nucleoli)
    Anisonucleoliosis (uneven size of nucleoli)
    Poikilonucleoliosis (differences in shape of nucleoli)

*The importance of the listed criteria increases substantially as one progresses from the general to the nucleolar criteria.
†Not accepted by all cytopathologists.
Reproduced with kind permission of FRISKIES Veterinary International.

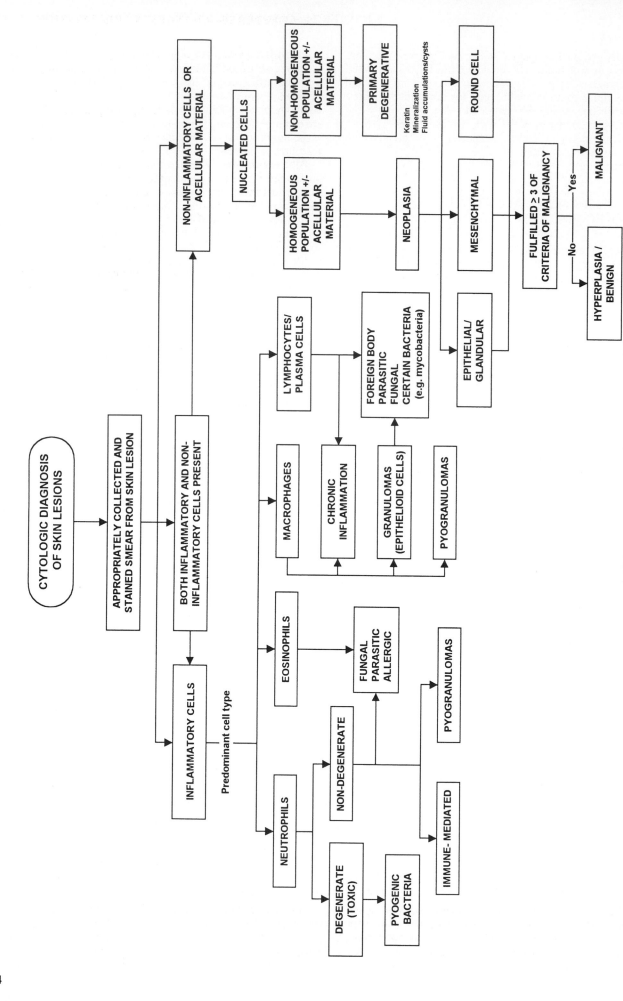

Figure 14–2. Algorithm for cytologic diagnosis of skin lesions.

NEOPLASTIC SKIN LESIONS

Cytologically, these are characterized by a homogeneous population of neoplastic cells. In many instances, there may also be a superimposed inflammatory component. Under such circumstances, dysplastic changes induced in some tissue cells by inflammation may mimic neoplastic changes. Once a general diagnosis of neoplasia is reached, the shape and arrangement of cells need to be considered so that further categorization of neoplastic skin lesions may be achieved.

Round Cell Neoplasms. These are the easiest tumors to recognize cytologically because they consist of round cells that exfoliate well as individual cells having distinct cytoplasmic membranes. This category includes mast cell tumors; canine cutaneous histiocytomas; cutaneous lymphoid neoplasia (mycoses fungoides, dermal lymphosarcoma); melanomas; transmissible venereal tumors; and solitary plasmacytomas.

Epithelial/Glandular Epithelial Neoplasms. These are generally characterized by round to square cells, usually with abundant cytoplasm that may be vacuolated in the case of glandular epithelium, having a tendency to adhere, form-ing clusters. Closer inspection of these clusters may reveal lines of cell-to-cell adherence. This category includes squamous cell carcinomas, basal cell and adnexal tumors as well as salivary gland tumors.

Mesenchymal (Spindle Cell) Neoplasms. These are characterized by spindle to angular cells that typically have cytoplasm trailing to one or both sides of the nucleus. Usually individual cells exfoliate, but clusters may occur. Apart from hemangiopericytomas, histopathology will need to be performed to provide the definitive diagnosis.

Recognition of Malignancy. Determining the prognosis of neoplastic lesions hinges upon recognizing malignancy. The hallmarks of malignancy are invasion and metastasis, both of which can only be assessed histologically. Cytology can be used to look for characteristics of malignancy (Table 14–1). These include variation in cell, nuclear, and nucleolar size and shape; numerous and abnormal mitoses; bizarre cells and nuclei; and high nuclear to cytoplasmic ratio. The certainty with which a diagnosis of malignancy can be made is directly proportional to the number of criteria of malignancy identified. Generally three to four criteria, preferably of nuclear or nucleolar origin, are regarded as the minimum number required for a diagnosis of malignancy to be made.

CHAPTER 15

CHANGES IN PIGMENTATION

Zeineb Alhaidari

Pigmentation changes are frequently seen in veterinary medicine, and they not only have potential cosmetic importance but also could imply medical or zootechnical consequences, as some of the possible etiologies are systemic diseases and/or genodermatoses. Evaluation of pigmentation changes necessitates developing a differential diagnosis. The term *leukoderma* refers to a loss of melanin pigmentation of the skin, and the term *leukotrichia* to a loss of melanin pigmentation of the hair. Similarly, *melanoderma* refers to an increased melanin pigmentation of the skin, and *melanotrichia* to an increased melanin pigmentation of the hair.

HYPOPIGMENTATION

HISTORY

Breed. There is a marked breed predilection for most noninfectious focal hypopigmentation disorders (Fig. 15–1).

- *Vitiligo,* an acquired focal depigmentation with a genetic basis, demonstrates a prevalence for rottweiler, Doberman pinscher, Newfoundland, and collie dogs, as well as the Siamese cat.
- The *uveo-dermatologic syndrome,* an autoimmune disorder targeting ocular and cutaneous melanocytes and resulting in uveitis and skin depigmentation, has been described mainly in northern breeds such as the Siberian husky, Samoyed, and Akita Inu.
- *Acquired idiopathic hypopigmentation of the nose,* an idiopathic gradual loss of nasal planum pigment, is widespread in some canine breeds such as the Labrador retriever, Siberian husky, Samoyed, poodle, and German shepherd.
- *Discoid lupus,* a presumed autoimmune photoaggravated disorder limited to the skin and concerning mainly the nose, affects mainly collies and German shepherds.
- *Dermatomyositis* is a genodermatosis described in the collie, Shetland sheepdog, and Beauceron shepherd breed. Crusting, ulceration, and depigmentation of the skin, affecting preferentially the face and extremities, are associated with varying degrees of muscle involvement.

Age of Onset. The age of onset often is helpful in the diagnosis of certain depigmenting disorders. An early age of onset usually suggests a genodermatosis. *Dermatomyositis* is classically first observed in 3- to 4-month-old puppies, with variably affected individuals in the litter. Symmetric unpig-

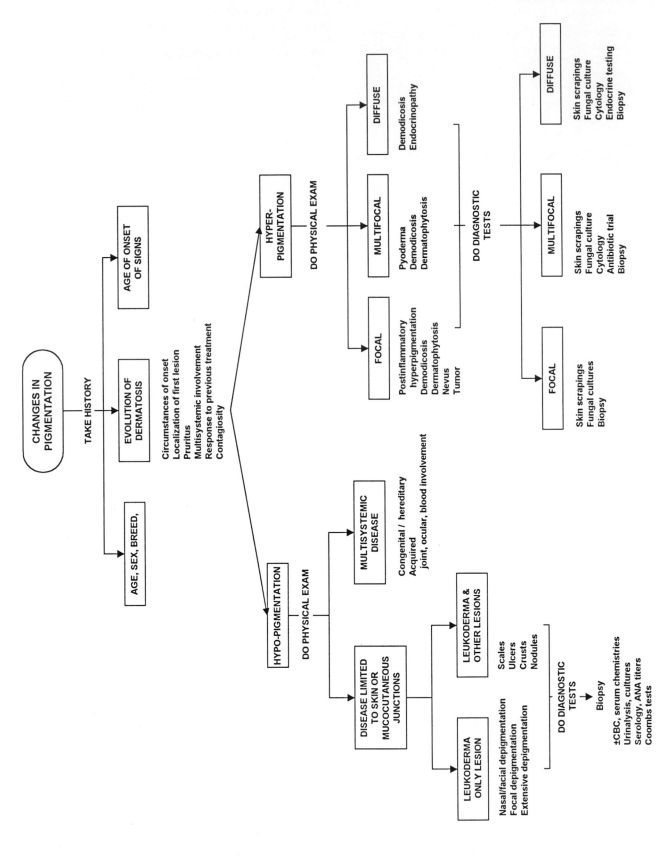

Figure 15–1. Algorithm for evaluation of changes in pigmentation.

mented macules involving the mucocutaneous junctions of the face in a young dog, aged 8 months to 3 years, are highly suggestive of *vitiligo*. *Discoid lupus*, which has a similar clinical appearance to vitiligo, also affects dogs of a similar age. The old animal is more prone to develop *bullous autoimmune dermatoses* and neoplastic disorders such as *epitheliotrophic lymphomas*.

Evolution. Evolution of the hypopigmentation should be carefully documented. Circumstances of onset should be investigated. Local trauma, including physical or chemical causes, must be considered as a potential etiology of melanocyte dysfunction or destruction. Any drug administration preceding the onset of symptoms should be noted. The nature and location of the initial lesion could be of major interest, especially in the differential diagnosis of nasal depigmentation. Unpigmented macules developing at the junction between the planum nasale and haired skin are highly suggestive of *bullous autoimmune diseases*. *Contact dermatitis* usually affects the rostral nares. Depigmentation developing on the floor of one nostril, and associated with a purulent discharge, is highly suggestive of *aspergillosis*. Since *lupus erythematosus* or *pemphigus erythematosus* lesions are exacerbated with sun exposure, seasonality of symptoms is an interesting observation. Reported concurrent clinical signs, such as lameness, can be indicative of *leishmaniasis* or *systemic lupus erythematosus*. Ocular involvement suggests *uveo-dermatologic syndrome, leishmaniasis,* or *systemic mycoses,* such as *cryptococcosis* or *blastomycosis.* Weight loss, fever, and anorexia can be manifestations of *neoplastic diseases, systemic lupus erythematosus, bullous autoimmune disorders, systemic mycoses,* or *leishmaniasis.*

PHYSICAL EXAMINATION

Physical examination is the second important step in the diagnosis of pigmentary changes. The physical evaluation should be complete in order to determine if the disease is limited to the skin or is multisystemic (see Fig. 15–1). If the disease is limited to the skin and if leukoderma and/or leukotrichia is the only skin lesion present, one has to consider the topography of the lesions. If the depigmentation is limited to the nose or facial mucocutaneous junctions, the persistence of normal nasal surface architecture favors a noninflammatory etiology, such as *vitiligo* or *acquired idiopathic hypopigmentation*. On the other hand, if the normal surface architecture has disappeared, an inflammatory dermatosis should be suspected. However, ultraviolet radiation associated with sunlight can induce an actinic dermatitis upon an initially uninflamed unpigmented lesion, with subsequent erythema, ulcers, crusts, and disappearance of cutaneous surface markings. If the unpigmented lesion is focal, a history of potential *trauma* should be investigated. Extensive acquired leukotrichia can follow an immunologic attack directed primarily against the hair follicles in *alopecia areata,* resulting in alopecia and occasional regrowth of white hairs. If leukoderma and/or leukotrichia is associated with other skin lesions such as scales, ulcers, or crusts, *leishmaniasis* or *autoimmune dermatoses* should be considered. Infiltrative lesions are usually good indicators of *systemic mycoses* or *tumors.*

As already stated, multisystemic involvement is seen in *leishmaniasis, systemic lupus erythematosus, systemic mycoses,* or *tumors.* Arthritis and glomerulonephritis are frequent features of both *systemic lupus erythematosus* and *leishmaniasis.* Hematologic disorders, such as hemolytic anemia, leu-

kopenia, and thrombocytopenia, can be associated with *systemic lupus erythematosus*. A regenerative anemia, leukopenia, and monocytosis frequently are present in *leishmaniasis*. In the *uveo-dermatologic syndrome,* uveitis and subsequent glaucoma usually precede the cutaneous manifestations. The eye is also a frequent target in *leishmaniasis* as well as in *systemic mycoses,* such as *cryptococcosis* and *blastomycosis.*

DIAGNOSTIC TESTS

Skin biopsy is the fundamental diagnostic procedure when faced with hypopigmentation (see Fig. 15–1). Specimens should be taken both from the center and from the margins of lesions, especially if the disease is active and spreading. Biopsies can demonstrate the presence or absence of an inflammatory infiltrate and the presence or absence of melanocytes. The presence or absence of melanocytes is difficult to ascertain, as special stains such as Fontana-Mason or dopa reaction cannot differentiate between nonfunctional and absent melanocytes, and the only available specific melanocyte surface marker is S100. If inflammatory infiltrates and melanocytes are absent, one can suspect either *vitiligo* or a *postinflammatory depigmentation* with complete destruction of melanocytes. If melanocytes are present, *acquired idiopathic hypopigmentation* can be suspected. Inflammatory infiltrates are associated with several depigmenting diseases. Of particular interest are lichenoid infiltrates, which are chiefly lymphocytic in *lupus erythematosus* and *epitheliotrophic lymphomas,* and granulomatous in *uveo-dermatologic syndrome.* Infectious agents such as leishmania, mycobacteria, or fungal organisms are sometimes demonstrated on histologic sections of inflamed unpigmented lesions. If a pyogranulomatous/granulomatous nodular to diffuse infiltrate is observed, special stains should be requested in an attempt to identify the presence of microorganisms.

Depending on biopsy results, diagnosis will be completed by other tests such as complete blood count, serum chemistry profile, urinalysis, cultures, serologic testing for leishmaniasis or systemic mycosis, antinuclear antibodies dosage, and Coombs' test.

HYPERPIGMENTATION

HISTORY

Breed. *Demodicosis* and most *endocrinopathies* occur more frequently in specific breeds. Doberman pinschers, Shar Peis, West Highland white terriers, Scottish terriers, Boston terriers, Great Danes, and Weimaraners are breeds known to have a high prevalence of *demodicosis*. Great Danes, Irish setters, Doberman pinschers, and Old English sheepdogs are predisposed to *hypothyroidism,* while poodles, Boxers, Boston terriers, beagles, and daschunds are predisposed to *hyperadrenocorticism.*

Age of onset is an important clue to the diagnosis of hyperpigmenting disorders. Infectious etiologies, such as *pyoderma, demodicosis,* or *dermatophytosis* should be suspected primarily in young animals, while older subjects are at risk for *endocrinopathies* or *tumors.*

The evolution of the hyperpigmentation should be carefully investigated. The age of onset and distribution of the initial lesions should be described. Any *trauma* can result in postinflammatory hyperpigmentation. Posttraumatic hyperpigmentation is observed more frequently in certain breeds such as the poodle (especially apricot or grey) or the Siamese cat. Scratching is a common cause of skin trauma. Thus, any chronic pruritic skin condition (e.g., *atopy, adverse food reactions, pyoderma,* Malassezia *dermatitis, sarcoptic mange*) potentially can result in lichenification and hyperpigmentation. This makes pruritus a criterion of primary importance in the differential diagnosis of hyperpigmentation. Response to previous therapeutic trials, including dosages and duration of therapy, should be reported. Spread to other animals in the environment, or to owners, increases the suspicion for contagious diseases such as *dermatophytosis* or *acariasis* (e.g., *scabies, cheyletiellosis*).

PHYSICAL EXAMINATION

When dealing with hyperpigmentation, the distribution of lesions is of major importance. If the lesion is solitary, the differential diagnosis should include *postinflammatory hyperpigmentation* (carefully review history), *demodicosis, dermatophytosis, nevus,* and *tumor.* If the lesions are multifocal and nummular with peripheral expansion, *pyoderma, demodicosis,* and *dermatophytosis* are primary suspects. In cases of diffuse nonpruritic hyperpigmentation, *demodicosis* and *endocrinopathies* should be considered.

DIAGNOSTIC TESTS

Multiple skin scrapings are mandatory in almost every dermatologic case. They can give a quick, inexpensive, and easy diagnosis of demodicosis, scabies, or cheyletiellosis, although the latter two mites can be difficult to demonstrate. To confirm or eliminate the diagnosis of dermatophytosis, Wood's lamp examinations, KOH examinations of hairs/scales, and fungal cultures should be performed in every case of focal, multifocal, or diffuse hyperpigmentation. Cytology is the third easy test to be used systematically when dealing with hyperpigmentation. It can reveal yeasts, such as *Malassezia pachydermatis,* or cocci. An initial antibiotic trial is indicated when dealing with multifocal nummular hyperpigmented lesions in dogs, as pyoderma in this species is very common. Antibiotics with well-known activity against staphylococci, including beta-lactamase–resistant penicillins, first-generation cephalosporins, macrolides and related molecules (i.e., lincomycin and clindamycin), potentiated sulfonamides, or fluoroquinolones, should be prescribed for 4 to 6 weeks before rechecking the dog. In cases with diffuse hyperpigmentation, a CBC, serum biochemistry panel, and urinalysis should be performed after the possibility of demodicosis has been excluded by skin scrapings. These diagnostic tests might provide helpful clues leading to the identification of specific underlying endocrinopathies. For example, a stress leukogram increases the suspicion of hyperadrenocorticism. Thyroid function can be evaluated by a basal T_4 concentration, endogenous TSH level, or TSH response test. Adrenal function can be evaluated utilizing ACTH stimulation, low-dose dexamethasone suppression, or urine cortisol: creatinine ratio tests. Sex hormone imbalances can be evaluated by basal estradiol and progesterone concentrations in female dogs and by hCG stimulation tests in male dogs. The last and least rewarding procedure when dealing with skin hyperpigmentation is skin biopsy. A biopsy generally gives only vague clues or eliminates certain possible etiologies. It can, however, in conjunction with history and physical examination, furnish a high suspicion index for specific diseases such as *seasonal flank alopecia.* Seasonal flank alopecia is a cyclic follicular dysplasia characterized clinically by recurrent symmetric hyperpigmented alopecic flank lesions and an unpredictable prognosis. Biopsies demonstrate follicular atrophy and infundibular hyperkeratosis, which extend into the ostia of the secondary follicles and sebaceous ducts, mimicking the appearance of a malformed foot.

As always in dermatology, a definitive etiologic diagnosis is a mandatory prerequisite to successful management. Pigmentation changes, including both hypopigmentation and hyperpigmentation, are no exceptions.

CHAPTER 16

EXTERNAL PARASITES: Identification and Control

Karen L. Campbell

External parasites can be causes of distress and disease. Some serve as vectors for rickettsial and bacterial infections, as intermediate hosts for other parasites, and as injectors of toxins causing severe local or systemic reactions. This chapter will be limited to a review of the ectoparasites of the phylum Arthropoda. The two classes of importance as ectoparasites are those of the classes Insecta and Arachnida.

INSECTA

The body of adult insects consists of a head, thorax, and abdomen. The thorax has three segments (fused in some species), six jointed legs, and up to four wings. Insects have a chitinous cuticle that serves as an ectoskeleton providing protection for the body and attachment sites for muscles.

The cuticle is molted at intervals to permit growth and metamorphosis. Some species, such as lice, undergo a simple metamorphosis. The instars (immature forms) resemble the adults except for being smaller and are called nymphs. Other insects, such as fleas and flies, undergo a complex metamorphosis with the juvenile instars appearing wormlike and called larvae, which pupate and transform into adult forms.

Only 3 of the 26 orders within the class Insecta are of veterinary importance. These are the fleas (Siphonaptera), the lice (Phthiraptera), and the flies (Diptera) (Table 16–1).

ORDER SIPHONAPTERA (FLEAS)

Adult fleas are wingless, laterally flattened insects that feed on the blood of animals. There are over 2000 species and subspecies; those most likely to affect dogs and cats are *Ctenocephalides felis, C. canis, Pulex irritans,* and *Echidnophaga gallinacea.*

Ctenocephalides organisms have both genal and pronotal combs, which are useful in taxonomic classification (Fig. 16–1). *Ctenocephalides felis* is the most common ectoparasite affecting dogs and cats. Its host range includes ferrets, domestic rabbits, urban raccoons, urban opossums, humans, and occasionally other domestic species such as calves and pigs. *C. felis* has a flatter head (head length is twice height), uniform length of spines on genal combs, and six notches with setae on the hind tibia; *C. canis* has a rounder head, shorter spine on the first genal "tooth," and eight notches with setae on the hind tibia. *Echidnophaga* (e.g., poultry sticktight fleas) and *Pulex* (e.g., human fleas) lack both genal and pronotal combs. *Echidnophaga* has an angular forehead, while that of *Pulex* is rounded.

The adult flea remains aboard its host feeding and reproducing until it dies or is removed by the animal's scratching or swallowing. Clinical signs vary with the number of fleas, the tolerance of the host, and the presence or absence of hypersensitivity to the flea saliva or flea whole body antigens. The finding of fleas or flea feces on the animal confirms a diagnosis of flea infestation. Hypersensitivity reactions can be documented via serum testing for anti-flea IgE antibodies or via intradermal skin tests.

Integrated pest management provides the most success in control of fleas. Areas to consider include removal of fleas from the pet, removal of fleas from the environment, and breaking the flea life cycle. Insect development inhibitors

TABLE 16–1. SCHEME FOR IDENTIFICATION OF ARTHOPOD ECTOPARASITES OF DOGS AND CATS

Adults with six legs, three body parts of head, thorax, and abdomen	**Class Insecta**
Adults wingless, laterally flattened	Order Siphonaptera (fleas)
Head with genal and pronotal combs	Genus *Ctenocephalides*
Flat head (length of head ≥ twice height of head)	*C. felis*
Round head (length of head < twice height of head)	*C. canis*
No combs on head, angular forehead	Genus *Echidnophaga*
No combs on head, rounded forehead	Genus *Pulex*
Adults wingless, flattened dorsoventrally, stout legs with claws	Order Phthiraptera (lice)
Long nose, sucking mouthparts	Suborder Anoplura
On dog	*Linognathus setosus*
Wide head, biting mouthparts	Suborder Mallophaga
On cat	*Felicola subrostratus*
On dog in United States (broad body)	*Trichodectes canis*
On dog in tropics (slender body)	*Heterodoxus spiniger*
Adults with one pair of wings	Order Diptera (flies)
Adults with eight legs, two body divisions (cephalothorax, abdomen), no antennae, simple eyes, and no wings	**Class Arachnida**
Flattened dorsoventrally, mouthparts of chelicera, hypostome, palp	Suborder Metastigmata (ticks)
Dorsal shield (scutum)	Family Ixodidae
Inornate scutum, anal groove forming an arch, lack festoons	Genus *Ixodes*
Inornate scutum, has festoons, basis capituli is hexagonal	Genus *Rhipicephalus*
Ornate scutum, has festoons, basis capituli is rectangular	Genus *Dermacentor*
Ornate scutum, has festoons, mouthparts are longer than basis capituli, the second palpal segment is twice as long as the third	Class Amblyomma
Soft bodied	Family Argasidae
Mite with respiratory pore in middle of body	Suborder Mesostigmata
Chelicerae long and stylet-like, 750–1000 μm body, long legs, red color after feeding, found near bird roosts or nests	Genus *Dermanyssus*
Mite without a respiratory pore	Suborder Astigmata
Round body 400–430 μm, terminal anus, short stubby legs with long unsegmented pedicels	Genus *Sarcoptes*
Round body 200–250 μm, dorsal anus, legs with medium length unsegmented pedicels	Genus *Notoedres*
Oval body 300–400 μm, terminal anus, anterior legs are long with short unsegmented pedicels and large suckers, rear legs have suckers in males and are rudimentary with whiplike setae in females	Genus *Otodectes*
430-520 μm elongated body, flaplike sternal extensions, terminal suckers on all legs, found "clasping" hairs on cats	Genus *Lynxacarus*
Mite with stigmata opening on the gnathosoma	Suborder Prostigmata
100–400 μm slender "cigar-shaped" body	Family Demodicidae
Found in hair follicles of dogs	Demodex canis
Found in hair follicles of cats, slender body	Demodex felis
Found in subcorneal location in cats, stubby body	Demodex unnamed species
400 μm oval body with large palpal claws, M-shaped gnathosomal mouthparts	Family Cheyletiellidae
Found on cats, cone-shaped sensory organ on genu I	*Cheyletiella blackei*
Found on dogs, heart-shaped sensory organ on genu I	*Cheyletiella yasguri*
Found on rabbits, globose-shaped sensory organ on genu I	*Cheyletiella parasitovorax*

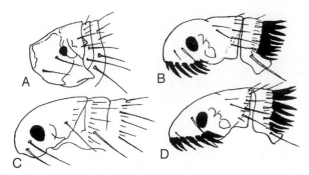

Figure 16–1. Identification of fleas of veterinary importance. *A, Echidnophaga gallinacea,* the "stick-tight" or poultry flea, lacks ctenidia and the frons (forehead) angles anteriorly. *B, Ctenocephalides canis,* the "dog" flea, has ctenidia and a head length less than twice its height; the first spine of the genal ctenidium is shorter than the second spine. *C, Pulex irritans,* the "human" flea, lacks ctenidia and the frons is rounded anteriorly. *D, Ctenocephalides felis,* the "cat" flea, has ctenidia and a head length that is twice its height; the spine of the first two ctenidium are equal in length. (From Urquhart GM, et al: Veterinary Parasitology. Essex, Longman Scientific & Technical, 1987.)

(IDIs) work by interfering with the synthesis of chitin or other substances necessary for the development and maturation of fleas. Chitin inhibitors include lufenuron (Program, Norvartis) and cyromazine. Lufenuron is given to dogs and cats orally once monthly or via subcutaneous injection (cats only) every 6 months. Insect growth regulators (IGRs) are juvenile hormone analogues that work by interfering with egg development and molting. The two most commonly available IGRs are methoprene (Precor) and pyriproxyfen (Nylar, McLauglin Gromley King Co.). These are found in sprays, foggers, and flea collars. These products do not kill adult fleas.

The initial elimination of fleas on pets can be accomplished with a variety of insecticide formulations and products. Formulations include shampoos, sprays, dips, foams, spot-ons, collars, powders, and oral systemics. Traditional ingredients include pyrethrins, pyrethroids, rotenone, citrus fruit derivatives (e.g. D-limonene), carbamates (e.g., carbaryl), and organophosphates. Two newer insecticides with excellent safety, efficacy, and prolonged residual activity are fipronil (Frontline and TopSpot, Merial Animal Health) and imidacloprid (Advantage, Bayer).

Killing of fleas in the environment is necessary during the initial phases of flea control. Mechanical removal (vacuuming, shampooing, laundering, etc.) should be combined with insecticidal treatments both indoors and outdoors with particular attention given to areas where pets sleep. Biologic control of fleas in yards can be achieved by the use of the nematode *Steinernema carpocapsa,* which is applied in a spray to shaded areas once monthly.

ORDER PHTHIRAPTERA (LICE)

Lice are highly host-specific with life cycles completed on the host. Most can survive only a day or two off of a host. The body is flattened dorsoventrally, wingless, and possesses stout legs and claws for clinging tightly to hair, fur, or feathers. A short pair of antennae are present, other sensory organs are poorly developed, and many of these organisms are blind. There are two suborders: the sucking lice *Anoplura,* and the biting lice *Mallophaga.*

The only species of sucking lice found on dogs is *Linognathus setosus,* the "long-nosed" louse (Fig. 16–2). These

lice are bluish-black, and their eggs are dark blue. They have powerful legs, each with a single large claw. These lice are relatively slow moving and easy to capture using flea combs or acetate tape. Biting lice have a relatively larger head than sucking lice, with mouthparts located ventrally. The claws are smaller than those of sucking lice. The only louse found on cats is *Felicola subrostratus.* The most common biting louse on dogs is *Trichodectes canis.* This louse is short, broad, and yellowish in color. A second biting louse, *Heterodoxus spiniger,* is only found in tropical and subtropical regions. *Heterodoxus* lice are more slender than *Trichodectes.* Biting lice can move rapidly. Lice of the two suborders have similar life cycles. During a life span of about a month, the female lays 200 to 300 operculate eggs ("nits"), which are glued to hairs. Transfer of lice from one host to another requires close physical contact between the animals or may occur via fomites (e.g., brushes). Lice are easily killed by insecticides used for flea control. Environmental treatment is not required; however, grooming tools should be cleaned.

ORDER DIPTERA (FLIES)

Diptera (flies) is one of the largest orders in the class Insecta with over 120,000 species. In some species the adults are parasitic on mammals, while in other species the larvae are parasitic. Diptera flies have only one pair of wings. Most are oviparous, laying small oval eggs in water, wet vegetation, animal feces, or in wounds on an animal. Adult flies may feed on blood, sweat, skin secretions, tears, saliva, urine, or feces. Diagnosis is made primarily on the basis of history, clinical signs, and observing and identifying flies feeding on the animal. Treatment involves identifying and removing sites where larvae develop, environmental applications of insecticides, and use of repellents and/or pyrethroids on the animal.

ARACHNIDA

Members of the class Arachnida are characterized by having the body divided into two parts: the cephalothorax and the abdomen. Adults have four pairs of legs, no wings, and have simple eyes with no antennae. The subclass of veterinary importance is Acari, which includes parasitic mites and ticks.

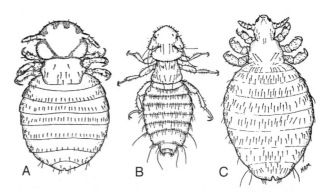

Figure 16–2. Identification of dog lice. *A, Trichodectes canis,* biting louse with wide head and short legs. *B, Heterodoxus spiniger,* biting louse with legs extending past width of abdomen. *C, Linognathus setosus,* sucking louse. (From Lapage G: Monnig's Veterinary Helminthology and Entomology, 5th ed. Baltimore, Williams & Wilkins, 1962.)

METASTIGMATA (TICKS)

There are two families of ticks: the Ixodidae (hard ticks) and the Argasidae (soft ticks). When animals are infested with a small number of ticks, manual removal can be accomplished by soaking the tick in alcohol and then grasping the head with small forceps or a hemostat and applying firm traction. With heavier infestations, the animal may be treated with a pyrethrin, pyrethroid, fipronil, or amitraz. An amitraz collar may be used to prevent tick attachment. Environmental control includes mowing and cutting of brush and grass and treating the areas with appropriate pesticides.

MESOSTIGMATA

Mesostigmata mites have respiratory pores (stigmata) in the middle of their bodies. The primary mite of this suborder of interest is the poultry mite *Dermanyssus gallinae*. *Dermanyssus* attacks poultry, wild birds, caged birds, dogs, cats, and people. It is 1.1 mm in size and is white, grey, or black prior to feeding and red when engorged with blood. Diagnosis is made by finding the mites in skin scrapings. Parasiticide sprays or dips will kill the mites; bird roosts and nests must be located and treated to prevent reinfestation.

ASTIGMATA

Astigmata mites lack stigmata, and respiration is through their integument. Astigmatids include the families Sarcoptidae, Knemidokoptidae, Psoroptidae, Listrophoroidae, Laminosiopties, Cytoditidae, Araridae, and Glyciphagidae.

Sarcoptes scabeii var. canis

Sarcoptes scabeii var. *canis* primarily affects dogs but can also cause disease in cats, foxes, and humans. The life cycle is completed on the host. Mites may survive for up to 21 days off the host. Adult mites are small (200 to 400 μm), oval, and white with two pairs of short legs. The pretarsi have long, unsegmented pedicels. The anus is at the posterior edge of the body. The mites initially affect relatively hairless areas of skin such as the ear pinnae and elbows of dogs. Diagnosis is based on history of a contagious, nonseasonal, intense pruritus, physical examination findings with typical lesion distribution, finding of mites or mite eggs or feces in superficial skin scrapings, demonstration of anti-mite IgE via serum tests or intradermal skin tests, or a presumptive diagnosis based on response to treatment trials. The only licensed method of treatment for canine scabies is repeated applications of a miticidal dip such as 2 per cent lime sulfur. Amitraz dips at a concentration of 250 ppm at 2-week intervals are also effective. Ivermectin and milbemycin oxime are highly effective but not approved for use in treatment of scabies.

Notoedres cati

N. cati primarily parasitizes cats but may also affect foxes, dogs, rabbits, and humans. Notoedric mange is highly contagious. The mites are smaller than *S. scabeii*, have medium-length unjointed sucker-bearing stalks on their legs, have more body striations, and have a dorsal anus in contrast to the terminal anus of *Sarcoptes*. Lesions first appear at the medial proximal edge of the ear pinnae and then spread to the upper ear, face, eyelids, neck, feet, and perineal region. The life cycle is identical to that of *Sarcoptes*. Mites are numerous in affected cats and easily diagnosed via skin scrapings of lesions. The only approved treatment in the United States is a 2 to 3 per cent lime sulfur dip. Alternative, but not approved, medications are ivermectin (0.3 mg/kg SQ) and amitraz dips (125 ppm).

Otodectes cynotis

O. cynotis, the ear mite, is a psoroptid mite (family Psoroptidae) that does not burrow but infests the external ear canal and adjacent skin of dogs, cats, foxes, and ferrets. Copious production of a dark "coffee grounds–like" cerumen is characteristic of otodectic otitis. Mites may be visualized through a magnifying otoscope or found on examination of material from ear swabs. Adult mites are white, with a terminal anus and four pairs of legs. All legs of the male bear short, unjointed stalks with suckers. On female mites, only the first two pairs of legs have stalks and the fourth pair of legs are rudimentary and do not extend beyond the body margin. Topical ceruminolytics should be used to remove cerumen and debris from the external ear canal. An otic acaricidal product should be used for 2 weeks beyond clinical cure. Treatment of the body with a parasiticidal product effective against fleas should eliminate mites outside of the ears. Systemic ivermectin has also been used with variable results.

Lynxacarus radovskyi

L. radovskyi is a hair-clasping fur mite of domestic cats. These mites have elongated bodies (430 to 520 μm long) with flaplike sternal extensions containing the first two legs and used to grasp the hair of the host. All the legs have terminal suckers. The mites cause little irritation in many cats and are sometimes found in large numbers attached to hairs along the back of the animal. Diagnosis is made by collecting mites from superficial skin scrapings or acetate tape preparations. Treatment with parasiticide sprays or dips is effective.

PROSTIGMATA

The suborder Prostigmata includes a diverse number of mites including free-living species, pilosebaceous mites, hair-clasping mites, and "chiggers" (Trombiculidae).

Family Demodicidae

Demodex spp. live as commensals in the skin of most mammals. Most species (including *D. canis* and *D. felis*) spend their entire life cycle in the hair follicles and sebaceous glands of their host. A few species (e.g., unnamed *Demodex* species of cats) are found burrowing within the epidermis. Dogs with a genetic susceptibility to demodicosis will have a juvenile onset of widespread lesions. Immunosuppression later in life may result in adult-onset demodicosis. Mites are usually easy to find from deep skin scrapings of affected areas. The mites have a characteristic "cigar-shape" with short, stubby legs. The unnamed species in cats, which burrows within the epidermis rather than in hair follicles, has a shorter "stubby" body. Four life stages can be identified: fusiform eggs, six-legged larvae, eight-legged nymphs, and eight-legged adults. Counts of each life stage should be recorded and followed during therapy. Localized infections in young dogs usually heal naturally; no treatment is required. Mite numbers should be monitored at monthly intervals; spreading of the lesions with an increased number of mites or an increase in the ratio of immature to adult mites may indicate a progression of the infection to a generalized form. An assessment of the general health of the animal and treatment of any secondary infections or concurrent diseases should be performed. The only approved miticidal treatment for demodicosis is dips with 250 ppm amitraz every 14 days; dips should be continued until multiple skin scrapings are negative and for an additional two to three treatments. If a favorable response is not seen, the frequency of the dips may be increased to every 7 days or an alternative treatment may be used. Daily administration of oral ivermectin at doses of 0.2 to 0.6 mg/kg is often effective but should never be used in an ivermectin-sensitive breed. Oral milbemycin at doses of 1 to 2 mg/kg/day has also been effective in the treatment of demodicosis. Dogs that have been treated for generalized demodicosis should be neutered following recovery. Adult-onset generalized demodicosis has a poorer prognosis.

D. cati usually affects the eyelids, periocular area, and head and neck of cats. The lesions are often self-limiting and may be treated with topical lime sulfur dips. Refractory cases or those with generalized lesions may be treated with amitraz dips at 125 ppm every 7 to 14 days or oral ivermectin. The unnamed species of *Demodex* in cats is more likely to be contagious and associated with pruritus, alopecia, or a ceruminous otitis externa. Most cases will respond favorably to weekly dips with 2 to 3 per cent lime sulfur.

Family Cheyletiella

Cheyletiella spp. are easily recognized by their big palpal claws, M-shaped gnathosomal mouthparts, and comblike tarsal appendages. The sensory organs on genu I may be used to identify different species (Fig. 16–3). *Cheyletiella* spp. go

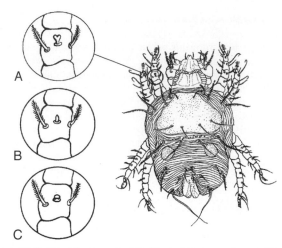

Figure 16–3. Identification of adult *Cheyletiella* spp. mites. *A,* The sense organ in *C. yasguri,* the species most commonly found on dogs, is heart shaped. *B,* The sense organ in *C. blakei,* the species most commonly found on cats, is conical in shape. *C,* The sense organ in *C. parasitovorax,* the species most commonly found on rabbits, is global shaped. (From Scott, DW, Miller W, Griffin C: Muller and Kirk's Small Animal Dermatology, 5th ed. Philadelphia, W. B. Saunders, 1995.)

freely from one host species to another and can also transiently affect humans. The mites move in pseudotunnels in epidermal debris. The entire life cycle is completed on the host with egg, larvae, nymph, and adult stages. The ova are smaller than louse nits and are attached to host hairs by fine fibrillar strands. Adult female mites may live up to 10 days in the environment. Superficial skin scrapings or acetate tape impressions may reveal mites or eggs. Mites may also be found in fecal flotations. Cheyletiellosis is easily treated with topical parasiticides. All in-contact dogs, cats, and rabbits should be treated. An environmental acaricidal spray approved for use in homes should also be used. Refractory cases may respond to oral ivermectin at a dose of 0.2 to 0.3 mg/kg repeated two or three times at 14-day intervals.

CHAPTER 17

SUBCUTANEOUS SPACE ACCUMULATIONS

David Feldman

DEFINITION AND ANATOMY

The subcutaneous space is bound superficially by the deep layers of the dermis and internally by fascial layers overlying muscles, tendons, and/or periosteum. The subcutaneous space exists in all areas of the body except the lip, eyelid, external ear, and anus—areas where functional constraints preclude its existence. In these areas, the dermis is bound directly to the fascia and musculature. Structures within the subcutaneous space include fat, blood and lymphatic vessels, lymphatic tissue, nerves, and anchoring fibrous bands that adhere the dermis to deeper fascial layers. These structures serve a number of vital functions, including thermogenesis, insulation, and protection from trauma. The subcutaneous space is expansile, owing to its loose connective tissue and elasticity of the overlying skin. Many disorders of the subcutaneous space simultaneously affect the skin and deeper tissues. Internal protrusions (inguinal hernia, bone tumor) may mimic a subcutaneous swelling.

PATHOGENESIS

Accumulations within the subcutaneous space may occur either by endogenous or exogenous mechanisms and can be solid or liquid (or both). Endogenous fluid accumulations may occur directly from small, deep dermal vessels that leak fluid and/or cellular material associated with inflammatory, traumatic, obstructive, degenerative, or oncotic conditions. Forces favoring extravasation of fluid from the vascular space to the interstitial space include increases in vascular hydrostatic pressure and decreases in vascular oncotic pressure. In contrast decreases in the colloid oncotic pressure of the plasma and increases in the interstitial fluid pressure (tissue tension) promote fluid movement into the vascular space. Normally, there is a small net force favoring the movement of fluid from the vascular to the interstitial space at the level of the precapillary arterioles. This fluid is then recycled away from the interstitial space back into the vascular compartment via lymphatics. Additional flow of lymph will accomodate limited additional tissue fluid build-up. When excessive tissue fluid accumulates, the lymphatics become overwhelmed and tissue edema results. Skin edema tends to accumulate in the subcutaneous space as a result of the presence of loose connective tissue. Depending upon the inciting cause, edema may be localized to the skin and subcutaneous space (e.g., trauma, angioedema) or may be distributed system-wide (e.g., congestive heart failure, hypoproteinemia).

A more thorough understanding of the pathophysiology of generalized peripheral edema requires the recognition of the primary or inciting cause (e.g., congestive heart failure, hypoproteinemia) and the consequences of decreased effective arterial blood volume. A complex cascade involving the renin-angiotensin-aldosterone system with subsequent salt and water retention, antidiuretic hormone activity, baroreceptor reflexes, and beta-adrenergic stimulation attempts to correct decreased effective arterial blood volume and blood pressure. If these regulatory mechanisms are unsuccessful in replacing the deficit, the retention of salt and water continues, and edema is exacerbated.

Edema may result from disrupted vascular endothelium via traumatic, inflammatory, thermal, or chemical mechanisms. In more extensive disease states (e.g., trauma), larger subcutaneous, muscular, periosteal, or intraosseous vessels may contribute to the fluid. Often, an exogenous insult results in endogenous production of subcutaneous material. Examples include traumatic injury and angioedema where blunt force and antigen exposure, respectively, result in endogenous fluid production.

Endogenous solid (or mixed solid/fluid) accumulations most commonly occur as a result of neoplastic, infectious, or sterile inflammatory disorders. Primary neoplasias are common within the subcutaneous space. Infectious granulomatous or pyogranulomatous lesions may begin after septicemia, although direct inoculation (foxtail, cat scratch) of an infectious agent is also possible. Sterile inflammatory conditions such as sterile nodular panniculitis (inflammation of subcutaneous fat) are either immune mediated or idiopathic. Exogenous causes of subcutaneous accumulations are usually iatrogenic or traumatic. Causes include foreign body penetration (either naturally occurring or surgically placed), excessive administration of intravenous fluids, and subcutaneous injections.

There are four possible mechanisms for the introduction of gas into the subcutaneous space. These include iatrogenic introduction of air (e.g., surgical procedures, subcutaneous injections), traumatic introduction of air (e.g., animal bites, projectile penetration), infectious processes (e.g., cellulitis with a gas-producing organism, draining fistulous tract), and extension from the respiratory tree. In the latter circumstance, air enters the mediastinal space through disruption of the subpleural respiratory tract tissue including pulmonary parenchyma, larger bronchi, and trachea. Air then progresses through the mediastinum and dissects through the fascial planes surrounding the musculature cranial to the thoracic inlet, eventually accumulating in the subcutis. Initiating events for this pathway include blunt trauma to the chest, excessive positive-pressure ventilation, and infections or neoplastic processes eroding a subpleural structure. With severe trauma, subcutaneous emphysema may occur from extension of a pneumothorax, with air dissecting directly through the disrupted parietal pleura and intercostal muscles. Finally, pleural air from a pneumothorax may inadvertently accumulate in the subcutaneous space with improper position of a thoracic drainage tube. This occurs when the holes within the tube are positioned both inside and outside of the thoracic cavity.

HISTORY AND PHYSICAL EXAMINATION

Most neoplastic conditions of the skin and subcutis are incidentally noted by the owner or veterinarian, although if metastatic, there may be signs associated with the primary site. Breed predilections for various neoplastic skin diseases are listed in the appendices. Most tumors are firm to the touch, although some may be more fluctuant, particularly lipomas and some mast cell tumors. Abscesses may be solid, fluctuant, or draining, depending on the infecting organism and stage of development. There may be a history of trauma, recent surgery, or infection elsewhere in the body. Fever and systemic illness may accompany an abscess. Generalized peripheral edema (anasarca) may be a symptom of congestive heart failure, hypoproteinemia syndromes, or vasculitis. Systemic signs associated with these disorders should be evident. Primary lymphedema and myxedema are usually cool and pitting.

Sinonasal, laryngeal, or tracheal surgery and thoracic drainage tube placement are procedures most commonly associated with subcutaneous emphysema. Occasionally, overzealous jugular venipuncture with trauma to the trachea may cause the condition. Tachypnea or cyanosis in the presence of subcutaneous emphysema suggests concurrent pneumothorax. Fever, redness, pain, and local heat would suggest a local abscess. If an anaerobic organism is present, subcutaneous gas could accumulate. A history of subcutaneous fluid administration or other injections may result in subcutaneous air, but the volume of this air is almost always clinically insignificant.

DIAGNOSIS

All clinically apparent subcutaneous accumulations are palpable; the specific diagnosis, therefore, typically involves

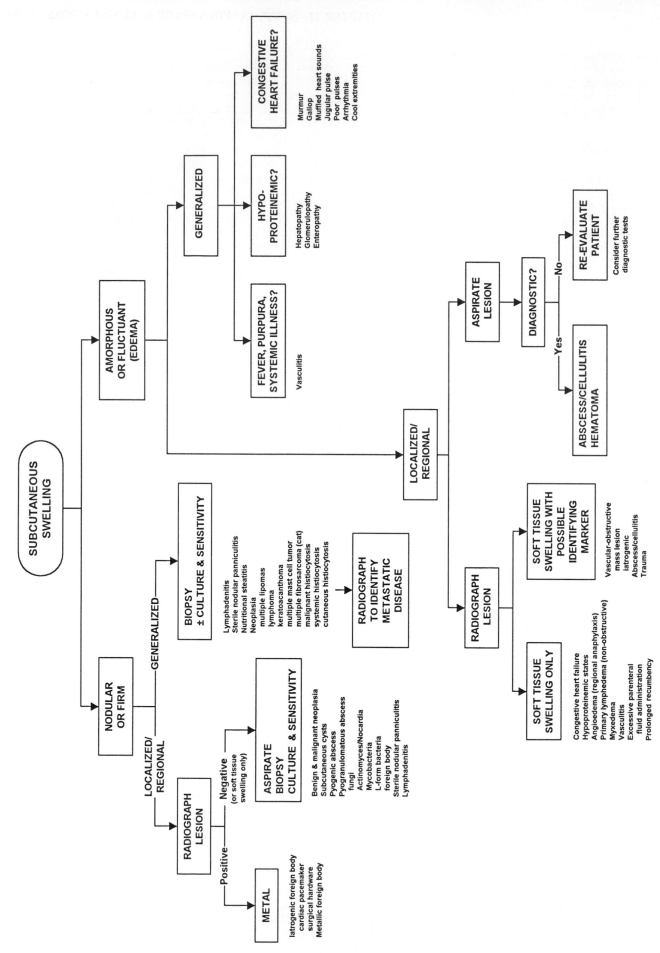

Figure 17-1. Algorithm for evaluation of subcutaneous swelling.

64

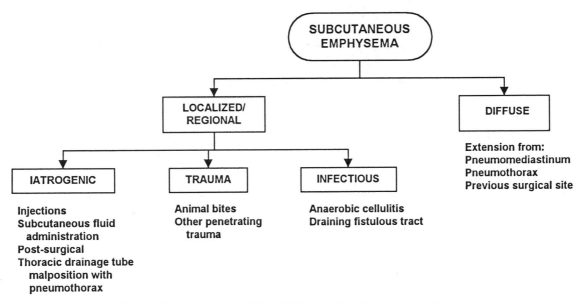

Figure 17–2. Algorithm of differential diagnosis for subcutaneous emphysema.

various aspiration or biopsy procedures, culture and sensitivity assays (when appropriate), and/or radiography or other imaging techniques (Fig. 17–1). All solid or defined subcutaneous masses can at a minimum be aspirated unless there is a clear contraindication (e.g., coagulopathy, overlying pyoderma). Some cancers (particularly soft tissue sarcomas) do not exfoliate well using fine-needle aspiration. Tru-Cut type specimens or surgical removal of the mass may be necessary for definitive diagnosis. Suspected or confirmed neoplastic disease processes require palpation and aspiration of regional lymph nodes as indicated.

Edematous tissue is rarely aspirated or biopsied to obtain a diagnosis. Searching for the cause of edema or swelling may involve palpation and radiographs for obstructive lesions (proximal to the edema). A complete blood count, serum chemistry analysis, and urinalysis would be useful for delineating causes of hypoproteinemia, abscess, and vasculitis. Serologic testing may be useful to further define causes of abscess and some cancers (e.g., FeLV, FIV, FeSV) and vasculitis (e.g., tick-borne diseases, ANA). Cardiac evaluation is warranted for suspected congestive heart failure. Coagulation tests (PT, PTT, PIVKA) would be useful if hematoma is suspected. Routine clinicopathologic testing and thyroid function testing are indicated if myxedema is suspected. Finally, evaluation of fluid "ins and outs" and respiratory, cardiac, and renal function is warranted in any animal on parenteral fluid therapy that develops edema (Fig. 17–1).

Any suspected infectious process should be cultured. Depending upon the clinical circumstance, aerobic, anaerobic, fungal, mycobacterial, or L-form bacterial cultures may be indicated. For fastidious or unusual bacterial infections, homogenized tissue culture may prove more rewarding. When suspecting atypical infectious diseases, it is paramount to procure the proper specimen and alert the laboratory for the proper culture medium.

Depending upon the disease state, routine radiographs may be useful in delineating causes of solid and fluid subcutaneous swellings. They are most helpful in evaluating trauma, edematous cardiac disease, metastatic cancer, foreign bodies, or obstructive masses in a limb. Specialized radiographic procedures are occasionally warranted. Ultrasonography may allow visualization of obstructive masses and can also evaluate renal, liver, and cardiac structure or function. Contrast fistulography can aid in the diagnosis of draining tracts. Lymphangiography can be useful in suspected cases of lymphedema. MRI or CT scanning is available but are rarely performed.

The diagnosis of subcutaneous emphysema is often evident by palpation (Fig. 17–2). A "crunchy" feeling or a feeling of cellophane-like material under the skin suggests the disorder. Radiography is confirmatory. Concurrent pneumothorax, pneumomediastinum, or evidence of surgical intervention or trauma may be apparent. Soft tissue swelling around a draining fistulous tract or anaerobic abscess may be evident.

TREATMENT

Treatment is specific for the underlying disorder. Malignant neoplasia should be removed with wide margins provided that obvious metastatic disease has not occurred. Adjuvant chemotherapy or radiation may be warranted. Benign neoplasia and some foreign bodies can often be left alone, provided that functional problems, abscessation, or ulceration have not occurred. Abscesses should be surgically drained and antibiotics, based on culture and sensitivity results, administered. Atypical infections (fungal disease, *Actinomyces, Nocardia,* mycobacteria, L-forms) require specific and often long-term antibiotic therapy for resolution. Lymphadenitis should resolve with resolution of the underlying cause.

The treatment of peripheral edema should resolve with successful treatment of the underlying cause. Symptomatic treatment of edema can involve postural elevation of a limb, cold compresses, pressure wraps, and judicious diuretic therapy. Diuretics must be used with care, particularly in conditions not related to congestive heart failure, as effective circulating arterial volume may be further diminished. Life-threatening peripheral edema (angioedema) may need to be managed with parenteral epinephrine, corticosteroids, antihistamines, and tracheal intubation. In addition to support wraps, diuretics, glucocorticoids, and surgical options, the drug rutin may prove useful in some cases of primary lymph-edema. Finally, discontinuation of fluid therapy and loop diuretic administration are warranted in any animal edematous from excessive parenteral fluid administration.

Treatment of subcutaneous emphysema, if associated with a "leak" in the respiratory tree, will resolve with resolution of the leak. Resolution may be spontaneous or may require surgery (e.g., tracheal tear).

CHAPTER 18

RED EYE

Joan Dziezyc

A "red eye" is the ophthalmologists' term for an eye that has dilated conjunctival, ciliary, and/or scleral vessels. Many ocular problems will cause a red eye. The most important differential diagnoses for a red eye include conjunctivitis, keratitis, uveitis, glaucoma, and scleritis/episcleritis.

The following sections deal with diagnosis only.

INITIAL EXAMINATION

As with any ocular disease, the behavior of the dog or cat on examination is important. Can the animal see? Vision can be evaluated by dropping cotton balls a few feet from the animal. These can be dropped on the side, to evaluate each eye. Does the patient follow the cotton balls with eye or head movement? Vision testing can also be performed by allowing the animal to walk around the room after obstacles are placed on the floor (maze test).

The next part of the examination should be done from a slight distance. Are the eyes, eyelids, and orbital areas symmetric? Room lights should be dimmed and a penlight held several feet from the animal's eyes. Compare the size of the pupils after obtaining a faint tapetal reflex. The room lights should be turned back on and the pupils examined again for symmetry. Pupils should be the same size. If the pupils are not symmetric, one should entertain the possibility that an intraocular problem is present. The algorithm (Figs. 18–1 and 18–2) starts with evaluation of pupil symmetry for this reason. The room lights can again be dimmed and a close penlight examination performed. It is easiest to perform a complete examination if one works from the outside to the inside: eyelids, conjunctiva/sclera, cornea, anterior chamber, iris, and center of lens. Only after pupillary dilation can the entire lens and fundus be examined.

CONJUNCTIVITIS

Conjunctivitis is one of the more frustrating diseases in small animal ophthalmology. It tends to be a diagnosis of exclusion: a red eye with no other findings. Conjunctivitis is by definition inflammation of the conjunctiva. Sometimes there is conjunctival edema (chemosis). Often there is a mucoid or mucopurulent discharge.

Conjunctival vessels are dilated, but not scleral vessels. Distinguishing dilated conjunctival from scleral vessels can be important. Conjunctival vessels are moveable; scleral vessels are not. Conjunctival vessels will blanch with topical phenylephrine; scleral vessels do not. If both conjunctival and scleral vessels are dilated, probably this animal does *not* have conjunctivitis; rather intraocular disease is causing the reddened conjunctiva.

A Schirmer tear test (STT) should always be the first test performed in cases of red eye with a mucoid or mucopurulent discharge. Most cases of chronic conjunctivitis in dogs are caused by keratoconjunctivitis sicca (KCS). This disease is the result of lowered lacrimal gland secretions. Some common causes of KCS in dogs are hereditary predisposition (possibly immune mediated), administration of sulfa and various other drugs, denervation of the lacrimal gland, and distemper.

There are no known causes of primary infectious conjunctivitis in dogs, unlike cats. There are certainly infectious systemic diseases that cause reddened conjunctiva, but no known primary pathogens. Bacterial culture of a dog's conjunctiva is usually unrewarding because even normal canine conjunctiva can host many different species of bacteria. A conjunctival scraping or snip biopsy may be more rewarding and is easily performed under topical anesthesia.

Feline herpesvirus 1 and *Chlamydia psittaci* are the two most common infectious causes of conjunctivitis in cats. These may also be associated with upper respiratory infection. *Mycoplasma* spp. may also be implicated in feline conjunctivitis. Feline herpes can also cause corneal ulcers or corneal stromal disease; *Chlamydia* cannot. Feline herpes polymerase chain reaction (PCR) is a fairly new and sensitive test for this disease.

Eyelid disease can be a cause of chronic conjunctivitis. Blepharitis can be associated with reddened conjunctiva. If the relationship of the globe to the eyelids is not ideal, there can be excess exposure of conjunctiva to dust and debris. Dogs with ectropion often have reddened conjunctiva. If the globe is smaller than normal, either as a congenital problem (microphthalmos) or acquired (phthisis bulbi), eyelids will not fit well and conjunctivitis will result. Entropion can cause a chronic conjunctivitis, tearing, and often chronic corneal ulceration.

If the conjunctivitis is not caused by KCS or eyelid

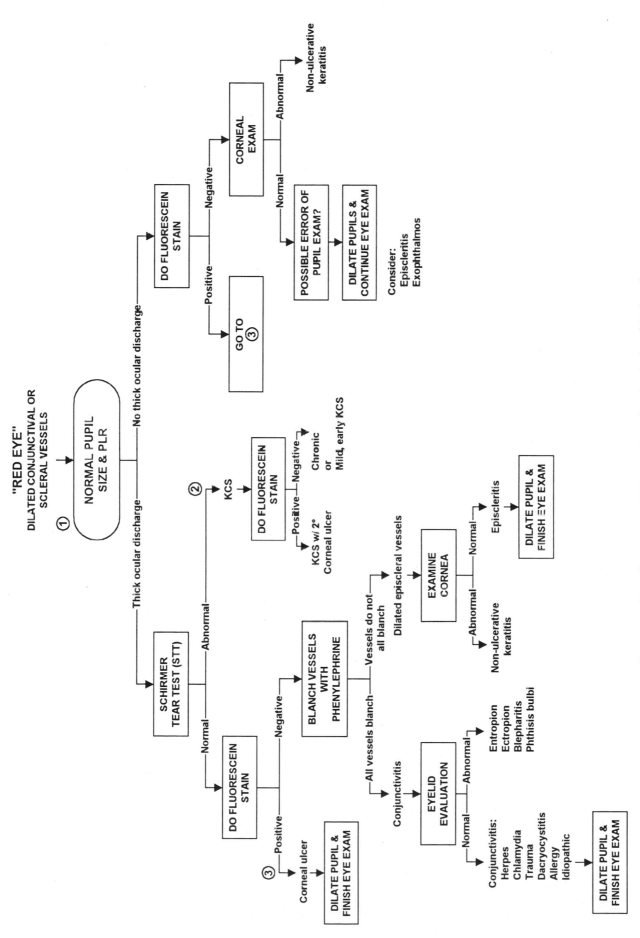

Figure 18–1 (part 1). Algorithm of differential diagnosis and evaluation of "red eye."

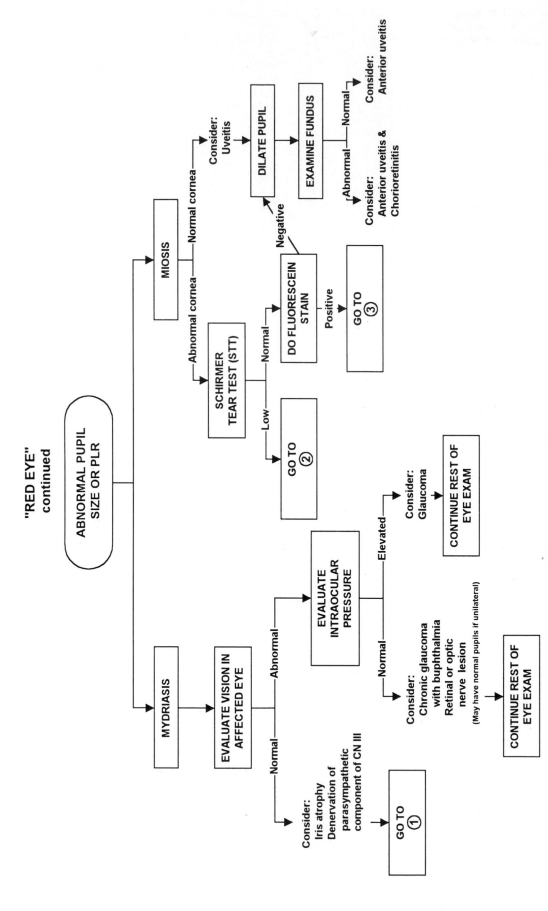

Figure 18–2 (part 2). Algorithm of differential diagnosis and evaluation of "red eye."

disease, one can postulate allergic conjunctivitis (not well defined in dogs and must be bilateral), irritation (dogs who ride with their heads out of windows), and idiopathic.

KERATITIS

Corneal ulcers are the most common cause of corneal disease in dogs and cats. Ulcers usually cause significant pain with conjunctival and sometimes scleral vessel dilatation. Definitive diagnosis is made when the cornea stains positively with fluorescein. STTs should always be evaluated prior to the fluorescein stain test if there is a history of an ocular discharge.

Corneal ulcers are usually secondary to some type of trauma, but the actual circumstances are usually unknown. Trauma from entropion, ectopic cilia, or a trapped foreign body can also be possible, so a good eyelid examination is essential.

Stimulation of corneal nerves can cause uveitis, so sometimes a miotic pupil can be seen with corneal ulcers. In cases of deep ulcers, inflammatory cells (hypopyon) or fibrin can be seen in the anterior chamber. Never will a corneal ulcer alone cause a dilated (mydriatic) pupil. If a mydriatic pupil is seen with corneal edema and a cornea ulcer, it is likely that the dog or cat has glaucoma with an ulcer secondary to the corneal edema.

Nonulcerative keratitis can be seen as a cause of red eye. This tends to be a catch-all category, like conjunctivitis. STTs should always be evaluated in a case of "odd" keratitis. This category includes pannus, nodular fasciitis, nodular granulomatous episclerokeratitis, pigmentary keratitis, and tumors in dogs; and stromal herpes keratitis, eosinophilic keratitis, and tumors in cats. Corneal and conjunctival scrapings or biopsies can often help make a diagnosis.

UVEITIS

Uveitis is inflammation of the vascular layer of the eye: iris, ciliary body, and choroid. Anterior uveitis involves the iris and ciliary body; posterior uveitis involves the choroid and clinically cannot be distinguished from retinitis. Hence posterior uveitis is usually described as chorioretinitis.

The hallmark of uveitis is a miotic (constricted) pupil. No other eye disease, with the exception of Horner's syndrome, will cause a miotic pupil. Horner's syndrome is usually associated with other clinical signs, but not a "red eye." Inflammatory mediators such as prostaglandins are released in uveitis, and these will cause muscles to constrict (pupillary sphincter muscle constriction = miosis, ciliary muscle constriction = pain). Normally there is a blood-eye barrier akin to the blood-brain barrier. With the release of inflammatory mediators, this barrier no longer exists. Uveitis causes the normal clear aqueous to become cloudy with protein (aqueous flare), white cells (hypopyon), red cells (hyphema), or fibrin. Corneal edema may be seen, but it is usually mild. Conjunctival, ciliary, and scleral vessels dilate, leading to a "red eye." In the fundus, cells and edema can be seen leading to elevated white lesions in the nontapetum,

hypo-reflective lesions in the tapetum, and retinal detachments.

If a dog or cat has acute unilateral uveitis, it can be treated empirically. However, if the uveitis is bilateral or chronic, infectious causes of uveitis should be suspected. Systemic disease can present first as a uveitis, either unilateral or bilateral. Consult a list of infectious diseases that are possible in your geographic area.

GLAUCOMA

Glaucoma is increased pressure in the eye caused by decreased drainage of aqueous. This is usually a hereditary problem in dogs but can also be seen secondary to chronic uveitis in dogs and cats. Hereditary glaucoma is usually observed in middle-aged dogs, and while it is a bilateral disease, both eyes may not develop increased pressures simultaneously.

The hallmark of glaucoma is a mydriatic (dilated) pupil. Usually there is no direct or indirect pupillary response in a glaucomatous eye, and the eye is blind. Diffuse corneal edema is usually present ranging from mild to dense. Whenever the cornea is diffusely edematous, consider the possibility of glaucoma. An edematous cornea should be stained with fluorescein dye, but do not be confused by a faint stippling of fluorescein dye uptake on an edematous cornea due to disruption of the epithelial cell integrity. Also consider the possibility of a corneal ulcer being self-induced by a dog or cat rubbing a painful eye. Primary corneal ulcers are usually edematous only where epithelium is missing; if the entire cornea is edematous, consider other problems, especially glaucoma. Dilated conjunctival and scleral vessels are also present; again, severity ranges from dog to dog. In chronic glaucoma, all the above signs are present, with the addition of buphthalmia (enlarged eye), optic nerve cupping, and some degree of retinal degeneration.

Time is of the essence in treating acute glaucoma. Even 24 hours of elevated intraocular pressure may be enough to cause permanent destruction of the optic nerve.

A tonometer is often necessary to confirm a diagnosis of glaucoma, and is certainly necessary to medically manage a case. If one does not have a tonometer and glaucoma is strongly suspected, begin treating with antiglaucoma drugs and refer the patient to someone with a tonometer. There are numerous drugs available to treat glaucoma, as well as several surgical procedures that work well in dogs.

EPISCLERITIS/SCLERITIS

Scleritis is an uncommon disease in dogs involving swelling and inflammation of the sclera. Most commonly seen is diffuse episcleritis where the sclera is diffusely swollen. On first glance it seems to be chemosis, but normal conjunctiva can be seen overlying the swollen episclera. Sometimes a faint halo of corneal edema is seen adjacent to the limbus, and retinal edema can occasionally be seen adjacent to the ora ciliaris retinae. The cause is unknown, but an immune-mediated disease is postulated.

CHAPTER 19

OBESITY

Karen J. Wolfsheimer

Obesity has been arbitrarily defined as a body weight 10 to 20 per cent above the ideal weight for that breed, sex, and species. Obesity, the major nutritional disease affecting dogs and cats, has been estimated to affect 25 to 40 per cent of canine and feline pets. Risk factors for obesity have not been well evaluated in dogs and cats. In one study, certain factors were associated with obesity in cats, including apartment dwelling, inactivity, middle age, male gender, neutering, and mixed breeding. Overweight cats were more likely to be fed prescription diets versus grocery store cat food. Genetic risk factors, which have been well recognized in people and laboratory animal models, are less well defined in dogs and cats. Certain dog breeds, including the Labrador retrievers, cocker spaniels, dachshunds, beagles, collies, Shetland sheepdogs, basset hounds, and terriers, tend to be obese, suggesting a genetic component to obesity. Breed incidence of endocrine diseases causing obesity should be considered as well. Pure breed cats, such as the Siamese and Abyssinian, have been found to be leaner than mixed breed cats.

The role of gonadectomy in the development of obesity in dogs and cats still remains unclear. In one study, ovariohysterectomy resulted in a decrease in maintenance energy requirements in adult cats. Other studies in cats have demonstrated an increase in falciform ligament fat and body weight in neutered cats (neutered at 7 weeks or 7 months of age), as compared with intact control cats. Ovariohysterectomized beagles showed no difference in subcutaneous fat, measured by ultrasound, when compared with control bitches, although they demonstrated an initial increase in food intake and weight gain. Other studies in dogs showed no effect on food intake, weight gain, or subcutaneous back fat depth regardless of age at neutering (7 weeks vs. 7 months of age).

Obesity has been reported to be more common in older dogs. However, one study showed that aged dogs actually showed a decrease in body condition using a body condition scoring system. Physical activity and lean body mass may decrease with age, resulting in lower energy requirements, so that if energy intake did not decrease appropriately, an increase in body fat and body weight could occur.

Sedentary lifestyles of contemporary pets and their owners may play a role in the development of obesity. Inactivity has been shown to be a significant risk factor for obesity in studies performed in both dogs and cats.

PATHOPHYSIOLOGY

Obesity develops as a result of disturbed nutrient ingestion and/or disturbed energy expenditure. Disturbed nutrient ingestion can be mediated by alterations in appetite, which is controlled, in part, by the hypothalamus and paraventricular nucleus. The lateral hypothalamus contains the hunger center, while the ventrolateral hypothalamus contains the satiety center. Differences in biochemical activity or metabolism in these centers may be responsible for differences in appetite. Appetite is influenced by various neurotransmitters, such as serotonin, norepinephrine, and dopamine. Other factors influencing appetite by modulating these neurotransmitters include dietary composition (fat, glucose, and amino acids), palatability, visualization of food, gastric distention, and stress.

Parasympathetic nervous activity (vagus) and sympathetic nervous activity play roles in the control of energy intake, storage, and oxidation in adipose tissue, liver, and muscle. Parasympathetic activity is increased in obesity, while sympathetic activity is decreased. The decrease in sympathetic activity seen in obesity can be reversed via adrenalectomy. Corticotropin-releasing factor increases with adrenalectomy and has been demonstrated to decrease food intake.

Daily energy expenditure is composed of resting metabolic rate (RMR) (60 to 70 per cent), the thermal effect of food- or diet-induced thermogenesis (10 to 20 per cent), and the thermal effects of exercise (20 to 30 per cent). RMR represents the requirement for maintaining the body at a homeothermic temperature. Therefore, in dogs and cats subjected to extremes in environmental temperatures, RMR and, thus, maintenance energy requirements may vary significantly. When RMR is adjusted for lean body mass, the variation among individuals can be as high as 20 per cent. Obesity is usually characterized by an increase in RMR as a result of an increase in fat-free mass as well as the increase in fat mass. Diet-induced thermogenesis consists of the energy expended digesting, absorbing, and processing nutrients.

The effects of exercise on energy expenditure include the energy cost of exercise per se, as well as its effect on diet-induced thermogenesis and RMR. Exercise may increase the thermogenic effects of food acutely, or as a chronic phenomenon associated with training. The increase in diet-induced thermogenesis is small compared with overall energy expenditure.

METABOLIC CONDITIONS ASSOCIATED WITH OBESITY

Hypothyroidism. In dogs with hypothyroidism, a reduced RMR contributes to decreased energy expenditure. Thyroid hormone normally increases RMR as a result of increasing activity of sodium-potassium-adenosine triphosphatase. Thyroid hormone also has a permissive effect on the sympathetic activity involved with diet-induced thermogenesis in adipose tissue. If there is a lack of thyroid hormone, a continued constant energy intake along with a decreased energy expenditure can result in obesity.

Hypothyroidism is a relatively infrequent cause of obesity in otherwise healthy dogs. Studies of thyroid function in non-hypothyroid healthy obese dogs have given conflicting results.

Hyperadrenocorticism. The obesity associated with hyperadrenocorticism is manifested as an increase in fat storage. Common sites for fat distribution are in the abdomen and the lumbar tail head region. An increase in glucocorticoids decreases corticotropin-releasing factor via negative feedback to the hypothalamus so that polyphagia can occur.

Pancreatic Beta-Cell Neoplasia and Insulin Therapy. Hyperinsulinemia is commonly recognized in association with pancreatic beta-cell neoplasia (insulinoma). Insulin increases food intake, probably because of a decrease in blood glucose concentration. Insulin is significantly anabolic. Chronically overdosed diabetic pets and those with insulin-secreting tumors are frequently obese.

Hypersomatotropism. Excessive concentrations of growth hormone (GH) can result in increases in soft tissue mass (mostly connective tissue) and bone mass, which often makes the animal look obese without an increase in body fat mass. However, because polyphagia is a side effect of GH, cats and dogs can have increases in body fat mass if caloric intake is excessive.

Hypogonadism Associated With Neutering. See earlier discussion of risk factors.

MEDICAL CONDITIONS POTENTIALLY AGGRAVATED BY OBESITY

Arthritis. An association between obesity and an increased risk for locomotor problems, including arthritis, has been shown in dogs. Obesity may contribute to arthritis by increasing forces across the joint and thus cause cartilage destruction.

Circulatory Disorders. Obesity increases the risk for circulatory disorders, including congestive heart failure, by increasing perfusion requirements of an expanded fat mass. This may cause an expanded blood volume, increased stroke volume, and increased cardiac output. Myocardial hypertrophy and increased cardiac muscle mass are accompanied by cardiac dilatation and an increased danger of congestive heart failure. Left ventricular hypertrophy may increase the risk of cardiac arrhythmia.

Chronic Respiratory Conditions. In obese animals, pulmonary volume restrictions, owing to intrathoracic fat deposits, as well as the cranial displacement of the diaphragm by abdominal fat, can cause a decrease in lung capacity. Excessive fat also requires an increase in oxygen demand and cardiac output. This increased demand can complicate preexisting lung disease.

Diabetes Mellitus. Hyperinsulinemia associated with insulin resistance has been shown to occur in some obese dogs and cats. This insulin resistance can aggravate glucose intolerance in animals already predisposed to diabetes. Most diabetic dogs have type 1 diabetes (an absolute insulin deficiency). However, even type 1 diabetics can experience insulin resistance if coexisting conditions such as obesity or hyperadrenocorticism exist. A significant number of diabetic cats may have type 2 diabetes (a relative insulin deficiency). In this case, insulin secretion is variable and insulin resistance may play a significant role in glucose intolerance. In the diabetic cat, decreases in caloric intake and subsequent decreases in body weight may improve glucose control, decrease insulin requirements, or even negate the need for exogenous insulin and/or oral hypoglycemic agents.

Hypertension. Obesity has been shown to cause hypertension in dogs in experimental conditions. Mild increases

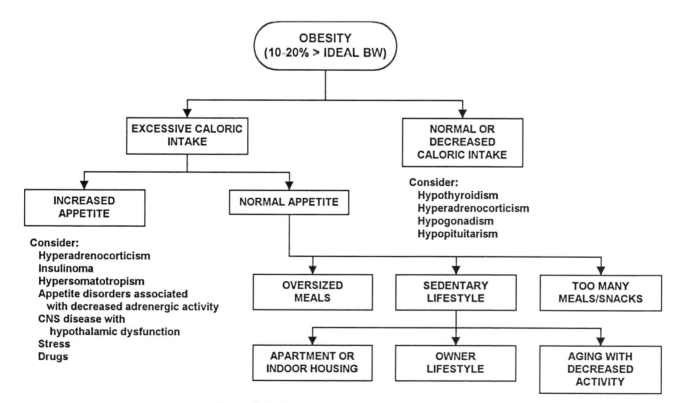

Figure 19–1. Algorithm for identifying causes for obesity.

or decreases in body weight have been shown to increase/decrease mean arterial blood pressure in dogs. Hypertension in obese dogs is seen in association with hyperinsulinemia, insulin resistance, increased sodium retention, and increased sympathetic nervous system activity. The incidence of obesity-induced hypertension in clinical practice has not been well evaluated in either pet dogs or cats.

Other Diseases. The role of obesity in the pathogenesis of neoplasias and decreased immune resistance to infectious diseases in dogs and cats has not been well documented. Hepatic lipidosis, in association with marked anorexia in cats, has often been seen in obese cats, but can also be seen in lean cats. The association between obesity and hepatic lipidosis is unclear. While caloric restriction has been incriminated as a precipitating event, some experimental studies failed to produce clinical signs or biochemical abnormalities typical of hepatic lipidosis.

EVALUATION OF THE OBESE PATIENT
(Fig. 19–1)

History. It is important to take a complete history of diet, including food composition (both meals and snacks), quantity of diet, and frequency of feeding. Based on information given by the client and available commercial feed composition, the clinician should be able to calculate the caloric intake and approximate fat, carbohydrate, and protein intake. This information will be helpful in deciding if excessive caloric intake is a major contributing factor to the pet's obesity. The owner's opinion as to the pet's degree of appetite may be helpful in determining the cause of obesity. Determination of lifestyle is also important in evaluating the patient's relative energy expenditure. Factors to consider include apartment living or predominant indoor housing, owner lifestyle, owner body appearance, and decreased activity associated with aging.

The presence of historical polyuria/polydipsia may alert the clinician to underlying metabolic disorders contributing to or complicating obesity. A drug history is important, since there are certain drugs, such as corticosteroids, phenobarbital, cyproheptadine, and benzodiazepines, that may increase appetite. Questions about changes in the household or other stressful events may be helpful, since stress can cause overeating.

Physical Examination/Determination of Obesity. The physical examination remains the most practical means of assessing body condition. Measuring body weight is inexpensive, easy, and useful. Ideal body weight may be difficult to determine because lean body mass and body fat content vary among and within breeds. Body condition scoring systems have been derived for both the dog and cat. Scales of 1 to 5 and 1 to 9 have been used, with 1 being cachectic and either 5 or 9 being extremely obese. These systems are based on rib palpation with degree of fat cover, waist observation, and/or abdominal tucking or inguinal fat. Calculation of body mass index (BMI) has been utilized to evaluate body mass in cats.

More objective techniques utilized in the cat include ultrasound measurement of inguinal fat apron, subcutaneous back fat in the lumbar region, and radiographic measurement of falciform fat in the lateral recumbency. Ultrasound measurement of inguinal apron fat has yielded inconsistent results. Ultrasound measurement of subcutaneous fat in the midlumbar region, between the third and fifth lumbar vertebrae, has shown to correlate well with determination of total body fat content by both carcass rendering and dual energy x-ray absorptiometry (DEXA) in dogs. The use of ultrasound has potential application because of the availability of ultrasound in private practice.

Obtaining a Minimum Database. When evaluating a significantly obese patient, it is ideal to obtain a minimum database consisting of a CBC, chemistry panel, and urinalysis. This is especially true if the patient is morbidly obese or a geriatric patient, or if physical examination findings, other than obesity, are abnormal. Evaluation of serum lipid profiles in healthy obese dogs has shown increased total triglyceride concentrations, while total cholesterol concentrations were not different from normal dogs. Elevations in both cholesterol and triglyceride concentrations can be observed with hypothyroidism and hyperadrenocorticism. Mild to severe hyperglycemia might be seen with hyperadrenocorticism or hypersomatotropism. Appropriate endocrine diagnostic testing would be indicated if physical, historical, and laboratory findings suggested an underlying endocrinopathy. Fasting hypoglycemia might be seen with a patient with insulinoma, warranting the measurement of concomitant fasting insulin concentrations.

CHAPTER 20

CACHEXIA

Deborah S. Greco

Weight loss greater than 10 per cent of initial body weight is significant and warrants investigation. As weight loss becomes more severe, emaciation may ensue as a result of catabolism of body protein and fat. Emaciation (weight loss usually greater than 20 percent of body weight) is characterized by prominence of the skeleton. *Cachexia* is the end stage of emaciation and may be associated with severe weakness, anorexia, and mental depression. Weight loss resulting in cachexia can be caused by increased energy demands (hypermetabolism), inadequate nutrient assimilation

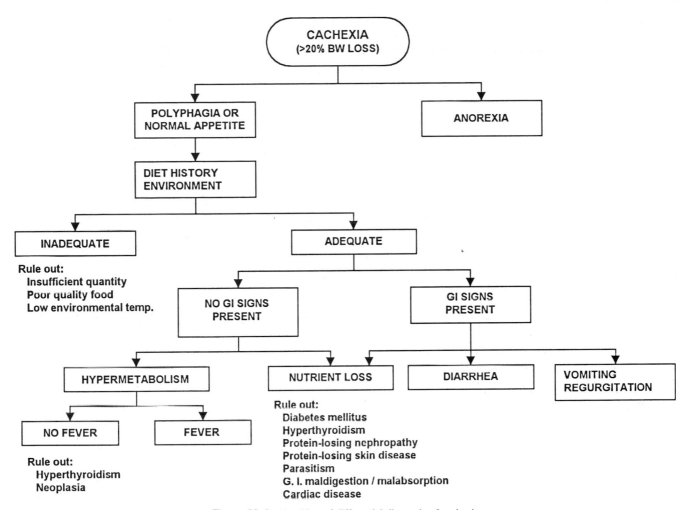

Figure 20–1. Algorithm of differential diagnosis of cachexia.

(anorexia, regurgitation, maldigestion, malabsorption), inadequate energy intake (insufficient quantity or poor quality of food), or increased loss of nutrients or fluid (proteinuria, glucosuria, dehydration).

HISTORICAL FINDINGS

A complete history should be collected; however, particular attention should be focused on the following: *appetite, diet,* the presence of *gastrointestinal signs,* and *environmental factors.*

Cachexia associated with polyphagia suggests malassimilation, excessive nutrient loss, hypermetabolism, inadequate feeding, or adverse environmental conditions. Cachexia may be caused by increased metabolic or environmental energy demands that are not being met by the pet's diet. Hypermetabolic states such as hyperthyroidism, pregnancy, lactation, congestive heart failure, fever, chronic infections, rapid growth, excessive physical activity, and neoplasia should be considered. Malassimilation (maldigestion, malabsorption) or excessive nutrient loss (diabetes mellitus, protein-losing nephropathy) can cause cachexia despite increased caloric intake.

Cachexia associated with malnutrition can be identified by a complete and detailed dietary history. Historical information on the exact quantity and type of food offered, dietary supplements, and variations in food should be one of

the first steps in determining the cause of cachexia. A thorough dietary history includes calculation of the animal's caloric needs and careful questioning as to the amount and frequency of feeding. Some owners may not be aware that they are feeding low calorie diets or that they may be underestimating the energy needs of their pet. Poor quality food can also be a problem. Owners who wish to save money by purchasing inexpensive pet food or who buy in bulk and allow the food to spoil can be identified by careful questioning. Inadvertent malnutrition may be caused by feeding health food or vegetarian diets with insufficient calories to carnivorous pets such as cats and dogs.

Cachexia associated with anorexia may indicate infectious, inflammatory, neoplastic, toxic, neurologic, or metabolic abnormalities. Broad categories of causes for anorexia include pseudoanorexia (dental disease, temporomandibular myositis, etc.), primary anorexia (CNS disorders), and secondary anorexia (metabolic, toxic, etc.).

Cachexia may be associated with gastrointestinal disease that causes inadequate nutrient uptake. Signs include anorexia, regurgitation, and vomiting.

PHYSICAL FINDINGS

A complete physical examination should be performed with particular attention focused on *body weight,* the presence or absence of *fever, gastrointestinal system,* and *organ size* and *shape*. *Cachexia associated with fever* can be due to (1) infectious (bacterial, viral, etc.), (2) inflammatory (immune, pancreatitis, etc.), (3) neoplastic, or (4) toxic (drugs, etc.) causes. Depending on the site and extent of involvement, infectious agents may cause cachexia via either fever or anorexia. Chronic bacterial or fungal infections including bacterial endocarditis, sepsis, pyometra, rickettsial diseases, systemic mycoses, and deep abscesses may cause cachexia. In cats, chronic viral infections, such as feline infectious peritonitis and feline leukemia virus, are common causes of emaciation and cachexia. Lastly, neoplastic disorders may directly (gastrointestinal neoplasia) or indirectly (lymphoma) affect assimilation of nutrients, appetite, and metabolic state resulting in "cancer cachexia." The diagnostic approach to hyperthermia and fever is described in Section I, Chapter 6.

Cachexia without fever may be caused by metabolic disorders such as renal, hepatic, and cardiac disease that may affect both appetite (usually decreased) and energy demands (increased). Renal failure can cause cachexia via anorexia (uremic ulcers), vomiting (gastric ulcers), malassimilation of nutrients, and increased nutrient loss (proteinuria). Cardiac cachexia results from intestinal and hepatic congestion that results in anorexia and malassimilation of nutrients.

Cachexia associated with nutrient loss can be secondary to urinary loss (protein, glucose), or gastrointestinal (parasitism, protein-losing enteropathy) disease. Gastrointestinal disease (without diarrhea) can result in cachexia via loss of nutrients (parasitism), via impaired absorption of nutrients (malabsorption, protein-losing enteropathy), or via maldigestion of nutrients (exocrine pancreatic insufficiency). Renal losses of nutrients (protein, glucose) as a result of protein-losing nephropathies (glomerulonephritis, amyloidosis) or from glucosuria (diabetes mellitus) are potential causes of cachexia.

DIAGNOSTIC PLAN

The diagnostic approach to weight loss is outlined in Figure 20–1. Historical and physical examination findings will usually determine which category of cachexia should be pursued (anorexia, polyphagia) or which body systems are involved (gastrointestinal, renal, etc). A minimum database consisting of a complete blood count, serum chemistry profile, urinalysis, fecal (cytology, parasite) examination, thoracic and abdominal radiography, and thyroid (T4) concentrations should be collected.

Serologic (viral, rickettsial, fungal, dirofilariasis, rickettsial, ANA, etc.) tests may be included in the minimum database. In cats, viral titers (FeLV, FIV) may be submitted to rule out feline leukemia and immunodeficiency viruses. Special studies such as contrast radiology, echocardiography, or ultrasonography may be indicated after the minimum database has excluded some of the many differential diagnoses. Finally, exploratory laparotomy, biopsies, and other more invasive diagnostic procedures may be necessary to determine the exact etiology of the cachexia.

CHAPTER 21

FAILURE TO GROW

Sherri L. Ihle

Growth is defined as the normal increase in size of an individual. In dogs and cats, growth occurs during the first 6 to 24 months of life. When an animal does not increase in size at the normal rate or to a normal extent, a "failure to grow" is identified. The owner of the affected pet may notice the problem and bring the animal to the veterinarian, or the animal's small size may be first noticed during a routine physical examination. In veterinary medicine, determination of normal growth is sometimes difficult, because breed sizes vary and mixed breed pets predominate. Comparing littermates, when possible, can be helpful in assessing the individual's growth rate and pattern.

PATHOPHYSIOLOGY

Growth is influenced by genetic, hormonal, metabolic, and nutritional factors. To meet its full genetic potential, an animal must have growth hormone (somatotropin) to stimulate insulin-like growth factor–I (IGF-I) production, which in turn stimulates skeletal growth, protein synthesis, and cell proliferation. Full IGF-I activity requires the concurrent presence of thyroid hormone. The animal must also consume sufficient calories and nutrients; digest, absorb, and retain the nutrients; transport the nutrients to the necessary tissues; and be able to use the nutrients for metabolic maintenance and growth. A defect in any of the above processes can disrupt, delay, or stop normal growth (Table 21–1; Fig. 21–1).

Genetic Abnormalities of Bone Growth. An inherited endochondral ossification defect in chondrodystrophic animals results in angular limb deformities and subnormal height.

Deficient Nutrient Intake. Gastrointestinal parasitism, resulting in a "relative" deficiency in nutrition, is the most common cause of reversible retarded growth in puppies and kittens. If an insufficient amount of food or food of poor quality is consumed, nutrients will be not be available to provide substrates and energy for tissue growth. Vomiting or regurgitation, owing to esophageal (ring anomalies) or gastric (pyloric stenosis) disorders, results in insufficient food reaching the intestines for digestion and absorption. Maldigestion or malabsorption can result in decreased uptake of nutrients. Renal, hepatic, cardiac, inflammatory, and hypoadrenal disease can suppress the appetite. Absorption and transport of nutrients from the intestines to other tissues can also be inadequate with cardiac disease.

Increased Caloric or Nutrient Loss. Fever can result in increased caloric loss as body heat. In diabetes mellitus, glucose is lost in the urine. Protein and salts can also be lost in the urine in animals with glomerular and renal tubular disease, respectively. Several intestinal disorders can result in protein-losing enteropathy. As previously described, parasitism is the most common cause of "lost" nutrients.

Abnormal Metabolism. Carbohydrate metabolism can be altered in inflammatory disease, renal disease, and hepatic disease. Protein production can also be decreased with hepatic disease. Hypothalamic or pituitary aplasia or neoplasia (e.g., craniopharyngioma) can result in low growth hormone and IGF-I concentrations. Hypothyroidism can decrease the activity of growth hormone. Since insulin has a positive effect on IGF-I production, insulin deficiency due to diabetes mellitus or malnutrition can slow growth. Cortisol excess, whether endogenous or exogenous, can inhibit secretion of growth hormone.

HISTORICAL FINDINGS

As previously mentioned, the animal with subnormal growth may be brought to a veterinarian for that problem,

TABLE 21–1. CAUSES OF GROWTH FAILURE IN DOGS AND CATS

Small Stature and Poor Body Condition

Dietary problem
  Underfeeding
  Poor-quality diet
Cardiac disorder
  Congenital anomaly
  Endocarditis
Hepatic dysfunction
  Portosystemic vascular anomaly
  Hepatitis
  Glycogen storage disease
Esophageal disease
  Megaesophagus
  Vascular ring anomaly (e.g., persistent right aortic arch)
Gastrointestinal disease
  Parasites
  Inflammatory bowel disease
  Obstruction (e.g., foreign body, intussusception)
  Histoplasmosis
  Exocrine pancreatic insufficiency
Renal disease
  Renal failure (congenital or acquired)
  Glomerular disease
  Pyelonephritis
Inflammatory disease
Hormonal disease
  Diabetes mellitus
  Hypoadrenocorticism

Small Stature and Good Body Condition

Chondrodystrophy
Hormonal disease
  Congenital hypothyroidism
  Congenital hyposomatotropism (pituitary dwarfism)
  Hyperadrenocorticism

or small body size may be noted during a routine examination. In either case, the owner of the dog or cat should be questioned as to the size of the pet's parents and littermates. If the parents and littermates were also at the lower end of the range of breed size, small stature may not be worrisome. However, if the pet is noticeably smaller than its littermates, the problem should be investigated. When the family history is unknown, the pet's size should be compared with others in the breed. For the mixed breed dog, the predominant breed should be determined based on physical characteristics, and that breed's average size should be the standard for comparison.

Duration of the Problem. Determining whether the animal's growth has been slow since birth or whether it was normal and then suddenly seemed to stop can be helpful. In the former case, congenital defects should be strongly considered, whereas in the latter case, acquired disorders must also be considered.

Diet. A detailed nutritional history should be obtained as to type of food, amount of food consumed, appetite, and feeding schedule. A less palatable or poor quality diet may not be eaten well or may be poorly utilized by the animal. A poor appetite despite the feeding of a palatable, high-quality food suggests the presence of a systemic illness causing inappetence or anorexia. Conversely, if the animal is always hungry and internal parasites have been ruled out or so-treated, underfeeding (owing to inadequate owner knowledge of the pet's nutritional needs) or a disorder causing increased nutrient loss (e.g., exocrine pancreatic insufficiency, diabetes mellitus, intestinal disease) should be considered.

Concurrent Clinical Signs. The owner should also be questioned about the presence or absence of other clinical signs, which may help define the cause of the problem. Regurgitation usually indicates a pharyngeal or esophageal problem (ring anomaly). Vomiting suggests a gastrointestinal problem (pyloric stenosis) or systemic illness (e.g., renal disease, hepatic disease, hypoadrenocorticism). Diarrhea or voluminous stools may be seen with disorders causing maldigestion (e.g., exocrine pancreatic insufficiency) or malabsorption (e.g., severe parasitism, inflammatory bowel disease, histoplasmosis). If polyuria is present, diabetes mellitus, renal disease, or hepatic dysfunction should be considered. Seizures, episodic abnormal behavior, vomiting, and/or diarrhea may be signs of hepatic dysfunction, such as a portosystemic shunt. Exercise intolerance or syncope can suggest a congenital cardiac abnormality. Poor response to housebreaking measures or obedience training, or lack of normal puppy play activities, can suggest the mental dullness of congenital hypothyroidism or the encephalopathy of hepatic failure. Glucocorticoid therapy for an unrelated problem may have slowed the pet's growth. Although the absence of these historical findings does not eliminate these disorders as possible problems, their presence can guide the diagnostic plan.

PHYSICAL EXAMINATION FINDINGS

Although some animals examined as a result of poor growth will have no other clinical abnormalities, in many animals a thorough physical examination can provide valuable clues as to the organ system(s) responsible for the problem. The animal's general appearance and body condition should be assessed. A short animal with a poor body condition is more likely to have a nutritional, metabolic, or

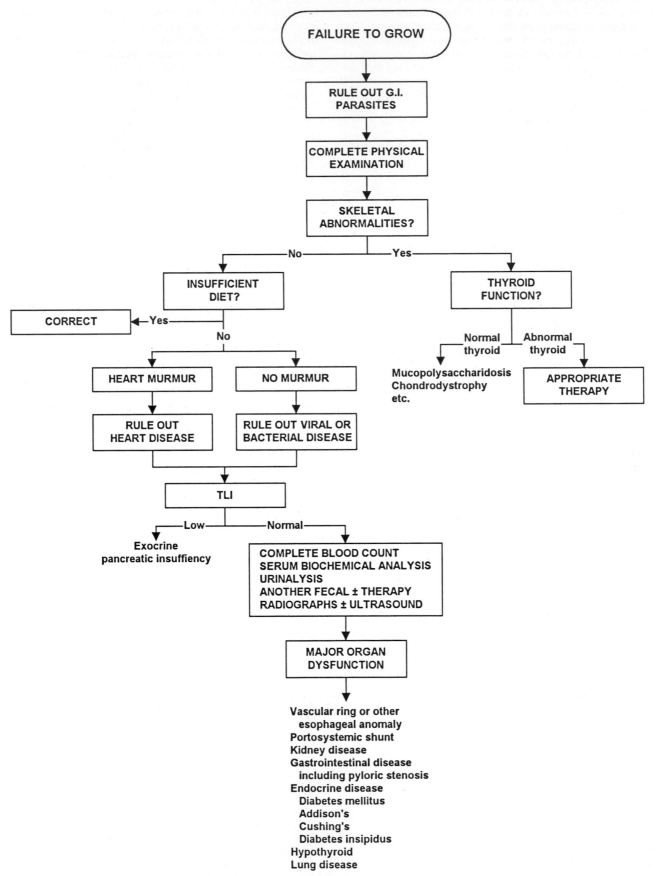

Figure 21–1. Algorithm for diagnostic evaluation of the dog or cat with failure to grow.

cardiac abnormality, whereas a short animal with a good body condition is likely to have a hormonal problem or to be chondrodysplastic (see Table 21–1). Chondrodysplastic animals and many animals with congenital hypothyroidism will also have an abnormal skeletal conformation (e.g., angular limb deformities). Symmetric truncal alopecia, the prolonged presence of a soft puppy haircoat, or thin scaly skin suggests a thyroid deficiency, growth hormone deficiency, or cortisol excess. Mental dullness can be seen with hypothyroidism or hepatic encephalopathy. Hepatic failure can also result in cortical blindness.

The head and neck should be examined for pale mucous membranes (anemia of chronic disease), icterus (hepatic disease), oral pain (dysphagia), and lymphadenopathy (inflammatory disease). The thorax should be carefully auscultated for a murmur (congenital cardiac disease) or bradycardia (hypoadrenocorticism). On abdominal palpation, enlarged or shrunken kidneys can indicate a renal problem, and hepatomegaly can suggest hepatic disease or dysfunction. Thickened bowel walls may be felt in the presence of inflammatory bowel disease, or a mass lesion may be palpated in the pet with a foreign body or intussusception.

DIAGNOSTIC PLAN

Decisions concerning the initial diagnostic plan should be based on the animal's body condition and any abnormalities identified from the history and physical examination (see Fig. 21–1). Food consumption should always be evaluated (see Historical Findings). If food intake is in question, a brief *feeding trial* can provide information on appetite and caloric consumption in relation to change in body weight. Multiple *fecal examinations* and possible deworming should be performed to eliminate severe parasitism as the cause of malnutrition. If the animal has been given a medication that may have slowed growth, the medication should be discontinued, if possible, and subsequent growth monitored. A *complete blood count* should be evaluated for anemia, inflammation, or eosinophilia. Results of a *serum biochemical profile* can suggest renal, hepatic, or gastrointestinal disease; diabetes mellitus; hypoadrenocorticism; hyperadrenocorticism; or hypothyroidism. A *urinalysis* may show proteinuria, isosthenuria, hyposthenuria, glucosuria, or inflammatory sediment. *Radiographs* can be used to detect a cardiopulmonary abnormality, organomegaly, a small liver or kidneys, or an intestinal foreign body. *Ultrasonography* may help to further characterize radiographic abnormalities and detect structural abnormalities within an organ. An *electrocardiogram* may be helpful in assessing serum electrolyte abnormalities (in an emergency) as well as congenital cardiac abnormalities. *Radiographic contrast studies* can be used to characterize congenital cardiac abnormalities, to identify portosystemic vascular anomalies, and to detect partial gastrointestinal obstructions. *Hepatic function tests* can identify the need for further investigation of the liver. *Gastrointestinal function tests* can be used to identify occult gastrointestinal disease and characterize the maldigestion or malabsorption. *Biopsy* may be needed if gastrointestinal, hepatic, or renal disease is identified. *Hormonal tests* can be used to detect hypothyroidism, hyperadrenocorticism, and hypoadrenocorticism; an assay for growth hormone is not currently available on a commercial basis, but an IGF-I assay is available for the dog.

TREATMENT

Treatment of the animal that exhibits growth failure varies widely based on the underlying pathology. Some disorders can be managed medically, and others require surgical correction.

CHAPTER 22

SWOLLEN JOINTS AND LAMENESS

Michael L. Magne

Arthritis is generally classified as either noninflammatory or inflammatory (Table 22–1). Noninflammatory joint disease is essentially synonymous with degenerative joint disease and is characterized by degenerative changes in joint cartilage, absence of inflammation in the synovium or synovial fluid, and lack of systemic signs such as leukocytosis or fever. Inflammatory joint diseases are classified as either infectious (septic) or immune-mediated (nonseptic) and are typically characterized by inflammatory changes in the synovium and synovial fluid as well as systemic signs such as fever, leukocytosis, and malaise. Immune-mediated polyarthritis can be further classified as erosive or nonerosive based on the presence or absence of joint cartilage destruction and typical bone erosion visible on radiograph. In many dogs and some cats, immune-mediated arthritis may merely be a symptom of another underlying disease, and clinical signs of the primary disease may predominate. For practical purposes, arthritis is usually considered as either monarticular

TABLE 22–1. CLASSIFICATION OF ARTHRITIS

I. Noninflammatory
    A. Degenerative joint disease
II. Inflammatory
    A. Infectious (septic)
    B. Immune-mediated (nonseptic)
        1. Erosive
            a. Canine rheumatoid arthritis
            b. Feline progressive polyarthritis
        2. Nonerosive
            a. Idiopathic
            b. Systemic lupus erythematosus
            c. Chronic infections
            d. Lymphocytic-plasmacytic synovitis
            e. Neoplasia-associated
            f. Other disease (IBD, CAH, etc.)

when a single joint is involved or polyarticular when more than one, and sometimes many, joints are involved. The term(s) oligo- or pauciarticular, referring to involvement of two to five joints, has little practical clinical utility and is rarely used. Immune-mediated polyarthritis is the most common form of polyarthritis seen in companion animals and is the focus of this chapter.

Erosive polyarthritis in dogs is similar to human rheumatoid arthritis, including the progressive, destructive, and deforming course of disease; radiographic appearance of affected joints; histopathology; and the presence of rheumatoid factor. Thus, in dogs, the term "rheumatoid arthritis" is generally accepted. A similar feline disease is referred to as chronic progressive polyarthritis, which is often associated with systemic viral infections such as feline leukemia virus or syncytia-forming virus. Feline progressive polyarthritis occurs in two forms, a severely erosive form similar to rheumatoid arthritis, referred to as the deforming type, and a more common, nondeforming type referred to as proliferative.

Immune-mediated nonerosive polyarthritis is the most common polyarticular disease in dogs. It appears to be the result of a type III immune response in which antigen-antibody complexes are deposited in the synovial membrane, which incites the inflammatory cascade. Synovial inflammation results from recruitment of macrophages, neutrophils, complement, and other inflammatory mediators into the synovium. Although most dogs have an idiopathic form of the disease, an immune-mediated polyarthritis may also be diagnosed with chronic infectious diseases, systemic lupus erythematosus (SLE), lymphocytic-plasmacytic synovitis, drug reactions, malignant disease, or other immunologically mediated disorders such as inflammatory bowel disease or chronic active hepatitis.

EROSIVE POLYARTHRITIS

Canine rheumatoid arthritis (CRA) occurs most commonly in small breed dogs as a chronic, progressive deforming polyarthritis. Although most common in dogs 2 to 6 years of age, it has been reported in older dogs as well as those less than 1 year of age. More distal weight-bearing joints (carpus and tarsus joints) are typically the first and most severely affected; early in the course of disease, the polyarthritis can be migratory, and "shifting limb lameness" may be noted. Discomfort or pain on rising or ambulation is common and is often easily localized to hot, painful swellings of the joints and periarticular tissues. Other common

signs include persistent or cyclic fever, anorexia, malaise, lymphadenopathy, splenomegaly, and muscle wasting. As the disease progresses, significant joint deformity can occur.

Feline progressive polyarthritis occurs exclusively in male cats with onset of signs usually occurring between 1 and 5 years of age. Distal joints are most commonly affected, but clinical manifestations differ between two common forms. The proliferative form occurs as an acute polyarthritis with the typical symptoms of fever, malaise, painful and stiff gait, joint effusion, peripheral lymphadenopathy, and generalized muscle wasting. These initial signs are usually followed, within several weeks, by periosteal new bone formation resulting in palpable exostoses. Deforming feline polyarthritis is less common and occurs in older male cats. Severe subchondral bone lysis as well as joint deformity, instability, and luxation characterize this form of the disease. The clinical course is often insidious, lacking an acute febrile stage, but is relentlessly progressive and eventually crippling.

NONEROSIVE POLYARTHRITIS

Regardless of underlying etiology, the signs in dogs with immune-mediated nonerosive polyarthritis are similar and include cyclic fever, malaise, anorexia, and varying degrees of lameness or weakness. A stiff or stilted gait is characteristic although not invariably present, and in some dogs, overt signs of joint disease such as effusion, pain, or heat may be subtle or absent. Distal joints, especially the carpus and tarsus, are most commonly affected, and physical examination results may range from normal-appearing to grossly hot, swollen, and painful joints. With chronicity, subtle signs of joint discomfort and synovial thickening may be the only findings. Many dogs demonstrate generalized hyperalgesia, often elicited with manipulation of the back or neck, owing to involvement of the vertebral articulations. Much like CRA, peripheral lymphadenopathy and generalized muscle wasting can be profound. Idiopathic polyarthritis is typically seen in dogs less than 5 to 6 years of age and is without sex predisposition. Breed predisposition has been suggested for German shepherds, Doberman pinschers, collies, spaniels, retrievers, terriers, and poodles.

Systemic lupus erythematosus (SLE) is reportedly more common in females and in German shepherds, collies, Shetland sheepdogs, beagles, and poodles but has no apparent age predilection. Protein-losing nephropathy (glomerulonephritis), hemolytic anemia, thrombocytopenia, vasculitis, cutaneous or mucocutaneous lesions, myelopathy, meningitis, myopathy, and subcutaneous edema may be seen concurrently with polyarthritis in dogs with SLE. Diagnosing any of these conditions in a dog with nonerosive polyarthritis is strong support for a diagnosis of SLE versus the more common diagnosis of idiopathic immune-mediated polyarthritis.

Lymphocytic-plasmacytic synovitis has been reported most commonly in German shepherds and other large breed dogs. The stifle joint is most commonly affected, and patients usually have significant degenerative joint disease and rupture of the anterior cruciate ligaments. Diagnostic confirmation is usually achieved by biopsy and histopathology of the abnormal-appearing synovium taken at the time of surgery for repair of the ruptured ligaments. Although drug-induced polyarthritis in dogs or cats appears to be rare, administration of trimethoprim-sulfadiazine has been associated with immune-mediated disorders, including polyarthritis, in dogs, and a genetic predisposition in Doberman pinschers to develop an allergic drug reaction to sulfadiazine has been postulated.

CLINICOPATHOLOGIC EVALUATIONS

Arthrocentesis and synovial fluid analysis are essential, and should be the first step in establishing a diagnosis of polyarthritis (Fig. 22–1). Often, only small or minute quantities of synovial fluid can be obtained, but several drops are usually adequate for a cytologic diagnosis as well as bacterial culture. Arthrocentesis of multiple joints is recommended, because a sample from a single joint may be nondiagnostic. Arthrocentesis is simple and requires little time, and dogs are usually not anesthetized or sedated for this procedure. Joints are "tapped" after a surgical clip and scrub, using 25-gauge needles for carpus and tarsus joints and 22-gauge needles for stifle and elbow. Normal synovial fluid is clear, colorless, viscous, and tenacious, although slight blood contamination from traumatic collection is not uncommon. Inflammatory joint fluid is often discolored, cloudy, or flocculent and exhibits decreased viscosity. Cytologically, the presence of neutrophils is the key characteristic in distinguishing inflammatory joint disease. Neutrophils are typically absent in normal joint fluid and present in small numbers in degenerative joint disease. Inflammatory synovial fluid is characterized by a predominance of neutrophils, both relative and absolute. Normal joints contain mononuclear cells, which average less than 3000 to 5000 cells/μL. Typical inflamed joints contain greater than 5000 neutrophils/μL. If the clinician creates his or her own slide, the cell count/μL can be estimated by multiplying the average number of cells seen in each high-power field by 1000. Although not performed routinely, usually owing to small sample size, other, less important evaluations of synovial fluid can be performed, including measurement of protein and glucose content and the mucin clot test. Briefly, increased protein (normal < 1.0 g/dL) content occurs with any inflammation, but greatly increased levels (>5.0 g/dL) are highly suggestive of joint infection. Synovial fluid glucose decreases with inflammation and is extremely low in septic arthritis. The mucin clot test indirectly measures hyaluronic acid polymerization, which is reduced with inflammatory disease. Culture of synovial fluid has been routinely performed by some clinicians, although negative culture results are the invariable result and should be viewed with caution. Some dogs, for example, those with subacute bacterial endocarditis or discospondylitis, may require culture of blood or urine for accurate diagnosis.

Serologic testing of the polyarthritis patient may be helpful, not only in establishing definitive diagnosis, but also in differentiating immune-mediated from chronic infectious

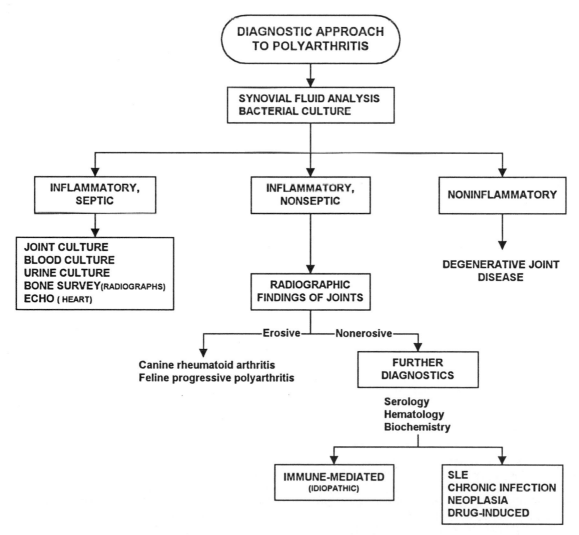

Figure 22–1. Algorithm for diagnostic approach to polyarthritis.

disease. Rheumatoid factor is found in up to 70 per cent of dogs with erosive polyarthritis, although false-positives can occur, both in healthy dogs and in dogs with other inflammatory diseases, e.g., SLE, idiopathic polyarthritis, or lymphocytic-plasmacytic synovitis. Antinuclear antibody (ANA) testing is often performed in an effort to confirm immune-mediated disease; however, it must be cautioned that positive ANA titers are found in many dogs with non–immune-mediated diseases including infections (subacute bacterial endocarditis, systemic fungal disease), inflammatory conditions, and neoplasia. Therefore, positive ANA test results are nonspecific. Dogs with nonerosive polyarthritis are treated the same, regardless of ANA result. Lupus erythematosus (LE) cell preparations are not routinely recommended, owing to significant test limitations. Depending on the clinical presentation as well as geographic location, serologic testing for diseases such as dirofilariasis, rickettsial infections, borreliosis, and systemic fungal infections may be appropriate. As previously mentioned, feline progressive polyarthritis is thought to perhaps be a viral-induced disease; essentially all affected cats are infected with feline syncytia-forming virus, and approximately two thirds will test positive for the feline leukemia virus.

Radiographic evaluation of affected joints is frequently performed, primarily to distinguish erosive from nonerosive disease. Findings of significant joint erosion or destruction are highly suggestive of septic or rheumatoid arthritis. Radiographic changes in nonerosive polyarthritis are usually minimal and often limited to soft tissue swelling and joint distention. Periarticular periosteal bone proliferation, thickening of periarticular soft tissue due to fibrosis, and degenerative joint disease may be observed in chronic cases, but such changes obviously lack specificity. The proliferative form of feline polyarthritis is radiographically characterized by periarticular soft tissue swelling, periarticular periosteal new bone proliferation, and perhaps subchondral bone lysis and narrowing of the affected joint. Deforming feline polyarthritis shows extensive bone destruction and joint deformity.

Ultrasonography may be helpful, in some dogs and cats, for diagnosing other diseases, particularly bacterial endocarditis or occult visceral neoplasia.

Hematology and biochemical profiling are most helpful in determining the presence of other primary disease, such as SLE, in which the polyarthritis is but one of a myriad of abnormalities. Findings of anemia, thrombocytopenia, positive Coombs' test, and proteinuria due to glomerulopathy in the patient with polyarthritis are consistent with an SLE diagnosis. It would be typical for a dog with immune-mediated polyarthritis to have mild to severe fever. These dogs also commonly have neutrophilia, called the "leukemoid response" or "reaction." The neutrophilia can be mild (15,000 to 25,000 neutrophils/μL), or it can be quite marked (30,000 to 100,000 neutrophils/μL). Hyperglobulinemia is not uncommon in patients with polyarthritis, and in certain patients, protein electrophoresis may be helpful in differentiating inflammatory from neoplastic disease.

UROGENITAL

CHAPTER 23

VAGINAL AND PREPUTIAL DISCHARGE

Hans-Klaus Dreier

VAGINAL DISCHARGE

Vaginal discharge of varying quantity, color, and consistency may occur in dogs with normal or diseased genital tracts. Vaginal discharge may also be seen in ovariohysterectomized animals. Vaginal discharge normally occurs during proestrus, estrus, parturition, and the postpartum period. However, vaginal discharges at other times are often a sign of disease. This chapter describes the wide variety of findings relevant to the most important conditions in which vaginal discharge appears. Table 23–1 provides an overview of possible causes of vaginal discharge.

The presence of an unexpected or abnormal vaginal discharge requires a thorough gynecologic or obstetric examination, with special emphasis on vaginoscopy. The appearance of the vaginal discharge and inspection of the abdomen (Table 23–2) provide the initial assessment of physiologic and pathologic conditions that may explain a vaginal discharge. In the course of a thorough inspection of the vulva, the extent of edema and inflammation (Table 23–3), as well as the presence of a putrid odor, should be noted before the vaginal discharge is collected on a white cotton swab and examined for color and consistency (Tables 23–4 and 23–5). Vaginal discharge appears in various colors—from transparent to pale serosanguineous to greyish-white or yellow to different kinds of green, sanguineous red, brown, and even black. In some cases (e.g., in abortion), two distinct colors can be found. The consistency of vaginal discharge varies from serous to mucous. In some cases, it contains flakes, coagula, or tissue debris. Tissue, e.g., material from a macerating fetus or from necrosis of placental sites, can turn a discharge to a crumbly sludge. In general, the steps described

TABLE 23–1. POTENTIAL CAUSES OF VAGINAL DISCHARGE

I. Pregnant bitch
  A. Pregnancy
    1. Hypoluteoidism
    2. Abortion
    3. Fetal maceration
    4. Hemorrhage related to pregnancy
  B. Parturition
    1. Normal
    2. Insufficient cervix dilatation
    3. Uterine inertia
    4. Retained placenta
    5. Torsion of uterus
    6. Uterine prolapse
  C. Postpartum period
    1. Normal involution
    2. Delayed uterine involution
    3. Postpartum infection
    4. Postpartum hemorrhage
    5. Necrosis of placental sites
    6. Subinvolution of placental sites

II. Non-pregnant intact bitch
  A. Proestrus
    1. Normal proestrus
    2. Cycle without ovulation
    3. Prolonged proestrus
    4. Granulosa thecal cell tumor
    5. Vaginal prolapse
  B. Estrus
    1. Normal
    2. Mating injury
  C. Diestrus
    1. Endometritis
    2. Pyometra
    3. Mucometria
  D. Miscellaneous
    1. Vaginitis secondary to a stricture
    2. (Pseudo)hermaphroditism
    3. Vaginal tumor
    4. Uterine tumor
    5. Foreign body
    6. Urovagina

III. Ovariohysterectomized (OVH) bitch
  A. 1–4 weeks post-OVH
    1. Stump hemorrhage
    2. Coagulopathy
    3. Foreign body
  B. Months to years post-OVH
    1. Vaginitis secondary to vaginal stricture
    2. Foreign body
    3. Tumor
    4. Uterine stump infection
    5. Ovarian remnant syndrome (proestrus)

TABLE 23–2. INSPECTION OF THE ABDOMEN IN CASES OF VAGINAL DISCHARGE

MARKED ENLARGEMENT	SLIGHT ENLARGEMENT	"HOLLOW" ABDOMEN	NORMAL-SIZED ABDOMEN
Pregnancy >35–40 days	Pregnancy <35 days	Early postpartum period	Estrus
Late abortion	Pseudopregnancy	Necrosis of placental sites	Metestrus
Fetal maceration	Hypoluteoidism		Subestrus
Hemorrhage: due to whelp	Abortion		Prolonged proestrus
Insufficient cervix dilatation	Small number of fetuses		Mating injury
Torsion of the uterus	Single fetus pregnancy		Endometritis
Closed pyometra	One-uterus-horn-gravidity		Cystic glandular hyperplasia endometria
Open pyometra	Insufficient cervix dilatation		Urovagina
Uterine tumor	Retained placenta		
	Delayed uterine involution		
	Granulosa thecal cell tumor		
	Uterine tumor		
	Open pyometra		

TABLE 23–3. APPEARANCE OF THE VULVA WITH VAGINAL DISCHARGE (POSSIBLE PHYSIOLOGIC AND PATHOLOGIC CAUSES)

EDEMA			EDEMA + INFLAMMATION	NONEDEMATOUS
Marked	*Moderate*	*Mild*		
Proestrus	Estrus	Diestrus	Juvenile vaginitis	Vaginal stricture
Silent cycle	Silent cycle	Endometritis	Endometritis	Endometrial cystic glandular hyperplasia
Cycle without ovulation	Cycle without ovulation	Accessory ovaries	Open pyometra	Vaginal tumor or polyp
Prolonged proestrus	1st week of diestrus	Residual ovary	Uterine "stump" pyometra	Subinvolution of placental site
Granulosa thecal cell tumor	Pregnancy	Postpartum period	(Pseudo)hermaphroditism	Vaginal foreign body
Accessory ovaries	Hypoluteoidism	Closed pyometra	Foreign body	
Residual ovary	Abortion	Fetal maceration		
Parturition	Hemorrhage: due to whelp	Insufficient cervix dilatation		
Uterine inertia	Accessory ovaries	Delayed uterine involution		
Torsion of the uterus	Residual ovary	Postpartum period infection		
Retained placenta	(Pseudo)hermaphroditism	Necrosis of placental sites		
(Pseudo)hermaphroditism				

TABLE 23–4. COLORS OF VAGINAL DISCHARGE IN THE NONPREGNANT ANIMAL UNDER PHYSIOLOGIC AND PATHOLOGIC CONDITIONS

BLOODY	PALE SEROSANGUINEOUS	RED-BROWN	
Pyometra	Pyometra	Pyometra	
Proestrus (l)	Estrus (l)	Abortion (l, m)	
Mating injury (l, c)	Accessory ovaries (l)	Diestrus (1st week) (m)	
Prolonged proestrus (l, c)	Residual ovary (l)	Prolonged proestrus (l)	
Granulosa thecal cell tumor (l)	Foreign body	Subestrus (l, m)	
Stump hemorrhage (l, c)	Vaginal stricture	Accessory ovaries (l)	
Accessory ovaries (l)		Residual ovary (l)	
Residual ovary (l)		Foreign body	
Foreign body		Vaginal stricture	
Vaginal stricture			

GREYISH-WHITE	BROWN-RED	GREY-GREEN YELLOW	WATERY
Pyometra	Open pyometra (l, m)*	Pyometra	Pyometra
Diestrus (m)	Uterine "stump" pyometra (l, m)*	Juvenile vaginitis (m)	Urovagina (l)
Vaginal tumor (m)	Foreign body	Endometritis (m)	Foreign body
Pseudopregnancy (m)	Vaginal stricture	Uterine "stump" pyometra (m)*	Vaginal stricture
Uterine "stump" tumor (m)		Foreign body (m)	
Uterine "stump" pyometra (m)*		Vaginal stricture	
Accessory ovaries (m)			
Residual ovary (m)			
Foreign body			
Vaginal stricture			

Consistency of the discharge is indicated by the following letters: l = liquiform; m = mucoid; c = contains coagula; * = putrid odor.

thus far will lead to a tentative diagnosis, which may be confirmed or disproved by vaginoscopic inspection.

Before a vaginoscope (or pediatric proctoscope) is introduced, the skin lateral and dorsal to the vulva should be gently stroked with a finger to test for "tail deviation." The flexing and raising of the tail and lifting of the vulva will occur only when a dog is in late "proestrus" or "estrus" phases of the ovarian cycle. There are abnormal conditions of estrogen secretion (typically with the "ovarian remnant syndrome" or rarely with granulosa thecal tumor of the ovary) when this response may also be noted. In addition, digital examination of the vaginal vault should also be completed prior to utilizing a vaginoscope. Digital examination is the most effective and reliable method of diagnosing a vaginal stricture. Congenital vaginal strictures are the most common cause of vaginal discharge in spayed dogs.

Vaginoscopic inspection of the vaginal vault is an indispensable and easily performed diagnostic procedure in dogs that do not have a stricture. It may explain the cause of a vaginal discharge. Usually the nonanesthetized and nonsedated dog is allowed to remain in a standing position when examined. The procedure is usually quick and not painful. A variety of vaginoscopes can be used. These include scopes that are 13 and 18 cm long, 6 and 20 mm in diameter. The scope should have a fiberoptic light source. One may want to have long "alligator" forceps for retrieving foreign bodies as well as long culture swabs for bacteriologic evaluation or for cytologic examinations.

The lubricated and warmed vaginoscope is introduced close to the dorsal commissure (avoid the clitoral fossa) and advanced in a nearly vertical direction through the vestibule up to the pelvic floor. Then the speculum is tilted cranially by approximately 90 degrees and gently pushed forward with slight rotation into the vagina. Resistance of vaginal mucosa to introduction of the scope may be of diagnostic value. High progesterone levels coinciding with high estrogen levels (estrus) render the mucosa resistant to vaginoscopy. If high estrogen levels are accompanied by low proges-

TABLE 23–5. COLOR AND CONSISTENCY OF VAGINAL DISCHARGE DURING PREGNANCY, PARTURITION, AND THE POSTPARTUM PERIOD UNDER PHYSIOLOGIC AND PATHOLOGIC CONDITIONS

GREYISH-WHITE YELLOWISH	BLOODY OR RED-BROWN	BLACK AND GREEN PARTLY BROWN (IN)
Pregnancy (m)	Hypoluteoidism (m)	Abortion (l, m)
	Fetal maceration (m, d)*	
	Hemorrhage due to pregnancy (l, m, c)	
	Parturition (l)	
	Torsion of the uterus (l)	
	Postpartum hemorrhage (m, l)	
	Subinvolution of placental sites (m)	

CLEAR TO GREYISH-WHITE FLAKES	GREEN	GREY AND RED-BROWN (IN)
Onset of delivery (m)	Parturition (l, m)	Delayed uterine involution (l)
	Insufficient cervix dilatation (l, m)	Necrosis of placental sites (d)*
	Uterine inertia (l)	Postpartum infection (l, m)
	Retained placenta (l)	

(IN) indicates non-homogeneous coloring. Consistency of the discharge is indicated by the following letters: l = liquiform; m = mucoid; d = contains debris; c = coagula. * = putrid odor.

terone levels, as in proestrus, resistance is only moderate. If the vaginoscope is smoothly introducible, this suggests that the dog is spayed, in anestrus, or is under the influence of high estrogen levels or high progesterone levels. Mechanical obstacles usually prevent vaginoscopy. When the speculum is in position, the stylet is withdrawn, and any adhering discharge is "rolled off" on a piece of absorbent white paper for additional examination.

Vaginoscopic inspection allows visualization of patterns characteristic of different physiologic and pathologic conditions (Tables 23–6 and 23–7). Therefore, it is imperative that the examiner be familiar with these patterns in order to identify the conditions they characterize. The most important features of these patterns are color of vagina and cervix, mucosal profile (vaginal folds), and color and consistency of the discharge. At the same time, specific cytologic and bacteriologic sampling from the cranial part of the vagina can be performed through the scope under direct vision. The most important findings are summarized in Table 23–8.

The final step in the clinical investigation of causes for vaginal discharge is palpation of the uterus. This is difficult and requires practice. The examiner stands or sits lateral to the bitch. The bitch should be standing on the examination table. Both hands are placed flat on the abdomen inside the knees. One hand is pressed into the abdomen, and the other one palpates the size and consistency of the uterus against the resistance. The ovaries usually escape palpation unless they are tumorous or highly cystic. Ideal palpation conditions are afforded by the flabby abdominal wall immediately after parturition. Findings related to causes of vaginal discharge appear in Table 23–9. Examination of the mammary glands is carried out with the bitch in a supine position. In assessing

TABLE 23–6. INSPECTION OF THE VAGINA AND CERVIX IN THE NONPREGNANT BITCH IN CASES OF VAGINAL DISCHARGE

PHYSIOLOGIC OR PATHOLOGIC STATE	VAGINOSCOPIC FINDINGS
Proestrus	Color: pale pink
	High-grade edema, deep folds
	Bloody discharge
Estrus	Color: anemic
	Edematous folds
	Fleshwater discharge
Diestrus	Color: rosy pink
Closed pyometra	Longitudinal folds
	Greyish-white discharge
Open pyometra	Color: pale pink, cyanotic
	No mucosal profile
	Brown-red or greyish-green–yellow discharge
Acute endometritis	Color of cervix: red
	Color of vagina: rosy pink
	Longitudinal folds
	Greyish-green–yellow discharge
Prolonged proestrus, granulosa thecal cell tumor	Color: anemic
	Constricted vaginal lumen
	Bloody discharge
Urovagina	Color: red
	Vagina tilted cranioventrally
	Pondlike liquid accumulation in cranial vagina
Mating injury	Color: anemic
	Red wound
	Wall of urinary bladder visible
	Mesometrium visible
	Bloody discharge
Foreign body	Color: rosy pink
	Grey-green–yellow discharge

TABLE 23–7. VAGINAL DISCHARGE: INSPECTION OF THE VAGINA AND CERVIX IN PREGNANCY, PARTURITION, AND IN THE POSTPARTUM PERIOD

PHYSIOLOGIC OR PATHOLOGIC STATE	VAGINOSCOPIC FINDINGS
Pregnancy	Color: pale pink
	Edema
	Greyish-white or yellow discharge
Hypoluteoidism	Color: pale pink
	Edema
	Bloody red-brown discharge
Abortion, fetal maceration	Color: red
	Open cervix
	Abnormal colored placenta + fetus
No or insufficient cervix dilatation	Color: pale pink
	Closed cervix
	Green discharge
Parturition	Color: pale pink
	Marked edema
	Open cervix
	Fetal sac
	Fetus
	Green discharge
Torsion of the uterus	Color: red
	Open cervix
	Strong labor
	No fetal sac or fetus
	Bloody discharge
Uterine inertia, retained placenta	Color: pale pink
	Edema
	Open cervix
	Flabby fetal sac, fetus and/or placenta
	Green discharge
Early postpartum period	Color: pale pink
	Numerous petechiae and hematomas
	Bloody brown-red discharge + tissue debris
Delayed uterine involution, necrosis of placental sites, postpartum infection	Color: pale pink, cyanotic
	Greyish–red-brown discharge
Hemorrhage due to pregnancy, subinvolution of placental sites	Color: pale pink
	Bloody discharge
Late postpartum period	Color: rosy pink
	No mucosal profile, dorsal vaginal fold
	Less greyish-white discharge

the mammae, note should be taken on the number and symmetry of the mammary glands, size, inflammation, necrosis, abscesses, tumors, and the number and appearance of the teats. Confirmation, modification, or refutation of any clinical diagnosis will require laboratory studies (hematology, endocrinology, serology, and chromosome examination) as well as radiographs and/or ultrasonography.

PREPUTIAL DISCHARGE

A history of preputial discharge should prompt a thorough physical examination. Small amounts of greyish-white or greyish-yellow preputial discharge are normal in the dog. Excessive preputial discharge is found in connection with balanoposthitis, irritation by hypersexual behavior, prostatic hypertrophy, prostatitis, trauma and injuries (sometimes connected with fracture of the os penis), inflammation by foreign bodies, tumors of the penis, and feminine pseudohermaphroditism.

The order in which the foregoing list is arranged roughly reflects the frequency of causes on the European continent, where preventive castration is not as widely accepted by pet owners as in the United States and, therefore, prostatic disorders are common.

TABLE 23–8. VAGINAL DISCHARGE: CELL CONTENT OF VAGINAL SMEAR UNDER PHYSIOLOGIC AND PATHOLOGIC CONDITIONS

	PBC	IMC	SFC	AC	RBC	WBC	BAC	CD	MUC	SP
Very early proestrus	+	+	−	−	+	+	−	−	+	−
Early proestrus	+	+	−	−	+	(+)	−	−	(+)	(+)
Late proestrus	−	(+)	+	+	+	−	(+)	(+)	−	(+)
Estrus	−	−	+	+	(+)	−	(+)	(+)	−	(+)
Diestrus	+	+	−	−	−	+	−	−	+	(+)
Pregnancy	+	+	−	−	−	+	−	−	+	−
Endometritis	+	+	+	+	+	+	+	+	+	−
Pyometra with closed cervix	+	+	−	−	−	+	−	−	+	−
Pyometra with open cervix	+	+	(+)	−	+	+	+	+	+	−
Prolonged proestrus	−	−	+	+	+	−	+	+	−	−
Granulosa thecal cell tumor	−	−	+	+	+	−	+	+	−	−

RBC = red blood cells; PBC = parabasal cells; WBC = white blood cells; IMC = intermediate cells; BAC = bacteria; SFC = superficial cells; CD = cell debris; MUC = mucus; SP = sperm; AC = anuclear cells.
+ = present, (+) = sometimes present, − = absent.

The history should be directed at determining duration, intensity, and color of the discharge; signs of pain; and altered sexual behavior. Castration history is useful for the exclusion of prostatic hypertrophy. The examination for causes of preputial discharge (Table 23–10) should begin with an inspection of the prepuce and the surrounding area for remnants of the discharge (confirmation of the owner's observation), hypoplasia and edema of the prepuce, or swelling of the penis. Hypoplasia is found in feminine pseudohermaphroditism; in this case, diagnostics should follow the scheme provided for vaginal discharge in this chapter. Edema of the prepuce points to traumatic or inflammatory disease; a nonedematous prepuce relates the discharge to prostatic hypertrophy, prostatitis, balanoposthitis, or a tumor of the penis. Swellings of the penis are found after severe trauma (fracture of the os penis) and, particularly, with tumors.

As a next step in the andrologic examination, palpation of the prepuce, penis, scrotum, and testicles is helpful in diagnosing tumors of the penis, fractures of the os penis, foreign bodies (palpation painful and often can be continued only under anesthesia), and other conditions that may have led to the discharge. After retraction of the prepuce using caution to identify impediments such as adhesions, phimosis, paraphimosis, or a persistent frenulum, the color of the discharge, the glans penis, and preputial mucosa can be evaluated. The color of the discharge is sanguineous in cases of trauma, injuries of penis and prepuce, and prostatic hypertrophy. Greyish-yellow colored discharge is found with balanoposthitis, foreign bodies, and prostatitis. The mucosa of the penis and prepuce should be inspected for signs of inflammation, lesions, and tumors. In case of balanoposthitis, the mucosa is ruggedly swollen and shows an intensive red color. Balanoposthitis usually starts from the bulbus penis and, in severe cases, extends to the glans. The replication fold at the bulbus should be thoroughly inspected for holes where foreign bodies may have penetrated the mucosa.

As a final step, particularly if the inspection of the penis and prepuce provides no pathologic findings except the discharge and if the dog is at an advanced age and has not been castrated, the prostate gland should be evaluated for hypertrophy and/or inflammation. Rectal palpation of the prostate allows for differentiation between prostatitis, in which palpation is highly painful for the animal, and hypertrophy, in which no pain reaction is elicited. These diagnoses should be complemented by diagnostic imaging (x-ray, ultrasound) as well as hematologic, endocrinologic, and serologic examination.

TABLE 23–9. FINDINGS RELATED TO CAUSES OF VAGINAL DISCHARGE USING ABDOMINAL PALPATION

Abdominal palpation is not painful

Uterus is not enlarged
  Proestrus
  Estrus
  Diestrus
Uterus is enlarged
  Regular uterine swellings
    Pregnancy, 25–30 days
    Hypoluteoidism, 4–5 weeks
  Irregular uterine swellings
    Abortion
    Pyometra
    Uterine tumors
  Tubular
    Pregnancy >40 days
    Pyometra

Abdominal palpation is painful

Uterus is not enlarged
  Endometritis
Uterus is enlarged
  Pyometra + peritonitis
  Torsion of the uterus
  Necrosis of the placental sites

TABLE 23–10. CAUSES OF EXCESSIVE (PATHOLOGIC) PREPUTIAL DISCHARGE

Castrated

No preputial edema present
  Balanoposthitis
  Tumor
Preputial edema present
  Trauma
  Foreign body

Not castrated

Preputial edema present
  Trauma
  Foreign body
No preputial edema present
  Balanoposthitis
  Tumor
Discharge + prostate pain reaction
  Prostatitis
Discharge + prostate not painful
  Prostatic hypertrophy

CHAPTER 24

POLYURIA AND POLYDIPSIA

Susan Meric Taylor

Increased thirst and urine production are common presenting complaints in small animal patients. Polyuria (PU) is defined as a daily urine output of greater than 50 mL/kg body weight per day, while polydipsia (PD) is defined as fluid intake exceeding 100 mL/kg body weight per day. The discovery of significantly increased fluid intake or urine production in an individual dog or cat should prompt a systematic diagnostic evaluation to determine the cause of PU/PD.

NORMAL PHYSIOLOGY

Water consumption and urine production are normally controlled by interactions between the kidney, the pituitary gland, and the hypothalamus. Changes in plasma osmolality and blood volume are the most important factors regulating thirst and antidiuretic hormone (ADH) secretion

Thirst. Plasma osmolality is normally maintained within narrow limits, and hyperosmolality (secondary to dehydration) will stimulate osmoreceptors in the anterior hypothalamus to enhance a sense of thirst. Nonosmotic factors stimulating thirst include fever, pain, drugs, and significant decreases in extracellular fluid volume or arterial blood pressure detected by baroreceptors within the cardiac atria and aortic arch.

ADH Secretion. ADH is synthesized in the hypothalamus, transported to the posterior pituitary gland, and released via the same osmotic and hemodynamic factors that stimulate thirst. Other factors that stimulate ADH secretion include nausea, hypoglycemia, stress, pain, fever, exercise, angiotensin, and certain drugs. ADH promotes renal conservation of fluids through the production of concentrated urine.

ETIOLOGY

The list of disorders causing PU and PD in dogs and cats is short, and making a specific diagnosis can be straightforward (Table 24–1; Fig. 24–1). The first problems to rule out are "incontinence" and "frequency." These problems can be confused with "polyuria," are common, and may be caused by lower urinary tract infection/inflammation, calculi, cancer, neurologic disorders, or anatomic defects (to name a few). Once these problems are ruled out, one can initiate an evaluation of polyuria.

DISORDERS CAUSING OSMOTIC DIURESIS

When the concentration of a solute present in the glomerular filtrate exceeds the proximal tubular capacity for reabsorption, passive water reabsorption is impaired. Even in the presence of ADH, urine cannot be concentrated, resulting in an osmotic or solute diuresis. Marked glucosuria causes an osmotic diuresis and secondary PD in *diabetes mellitus* and *primary renal glucosuria*. Postrenal obstruction may cause a dramatic increase in serum urea nitrogen, and a *postobstructive diuresis* once the obstruction is relieved. In dogs and cats with *chronic renal failure,* nephron loss results in a progressive inability of the tubules to reabsorb fluid and solutes, resulting in osmotic diuresis and decreased renal medullary tonicity (urine specific gravity usually 1.008 to 1.020).

ADH DEFICIENCY

Central Diabetes Insipidus (CDI). CDI is an uncommon condition resulting from a complete or partial deficiency in ADH synthesis or secretion (see Chapter 148). Most affected dogs and cats have an idiopathic syndrome, although almost 50 per cent of older dogs with CDI have a pituitary tumor. Rarely, CDI is due to head trauma or a congenital lesion. Various drugs including phenytoin, ethanol, and glucocorticoids inhibit ADH release, resulting in CDI. Release of ADH will be decreased in some dogs with hyperadrenocorticism. Clinical and laboratory features of ADH deficiency are unremarkable or indicative of mild

TABLE 24–1. DIFFERENTIAL DIAGNOSES FOR POLYURIA AND POLYDIPSIA

Primary Polyuria
  Osmotic diuresis
    Diabetes mellitus
    Primary renal glucosuria, Fanconi's syndrome
    Postobstructive diuresis
  ADH deficiency—central diabetes insipidus
    Idiopathic
    Trauma-induced
    Neoplastic
    Congenital
  Renal insensitivity to ADH—nephrogenic diabetes insipidus
    Primary nephrogenic diabetes insipidus
    Secondary nephrogenic diabetes insipidus
      Renal insufficiency/failure
      Pyelonephritis
      Pyometra
      Hypercalcemia
      Hypokalemia
      Hyperadrenocorticism
      Hyperthyroidism
      Hypoadrenocorticism
      Hepatic insufficiency
      Renal medullary solute washout
      Drugs/diet

Primary Polydipsia
  Psychogenic (behavioral)
  Encephalopathy
  Neurologic
  Fever
  Pain

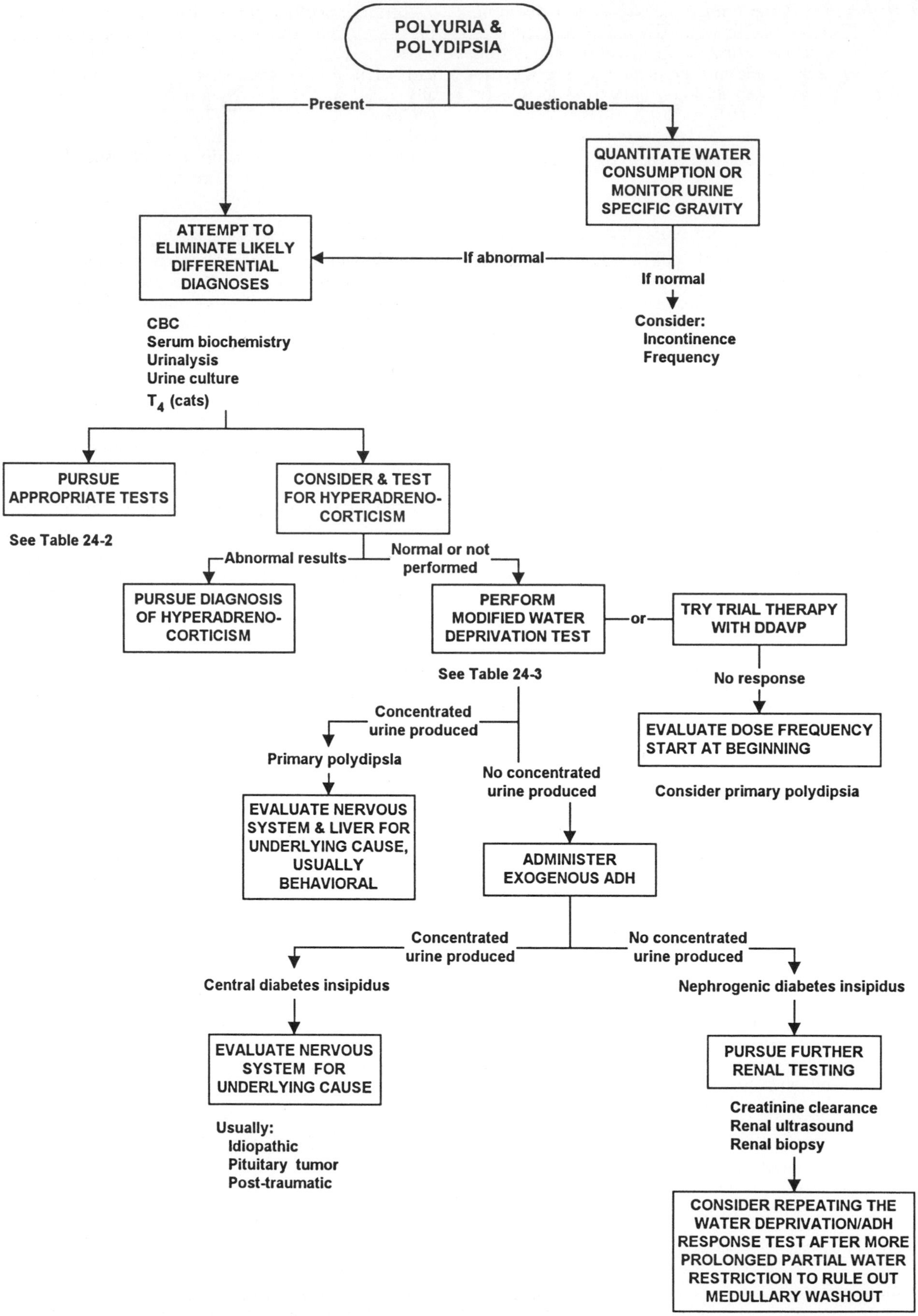

Figure 24–1. Algorithm for diagnostic evaluation of polyuria and polydipsia.

dehydration, which is the primary cause of the polydipsia, or severe dehydration due to water restriction coupled with an inability to concentrate urine. Dogs with CDI due to a growing intracranial neoplasm may exhibit central nervous system signs. Diagnosis depends on response to water deprivation and ADH response testing (Table 24–2).

INABILITY TO RESPOND TO ADH: NEPHROGENIC DIABETES INSIPIDUS

Nephrogenic diabetes insipidus (NDI) is a disorder caused by renal tubules that are insensitive to ADH, with kidneys failing to concentrate urine despite appropriate pituitary ADH release.

Primary Nephrogenic Diabetes Insipidus

Primary NDI is an extremely rare congenital structural or functional defect of the kidney. Renal function testing and biopsy may be warranted in patients with primary NDI.

Secondary Nephrogenic Diabetes Insipidus

Renal insensitivity to ADH is most often secondary to one of numerous metabolic conditions or a side effect from administration of certain drugs. Many of the acquired forms of NDI are potentially reversible with correction of the underlying illness.

Renal Insufficiency/Failure. Renal disease is one of the most common causes of PU/PD in dogs and cats. Inability to concentrate or dilute urine adequately is seen as an early sign of renal insufficiency (urine specific gravity usually 1.008 to 1.020). Diagnosis in a dog or cat that is not yet azotemic requires elimination of other causes of NDI and documentation of decreased glomerular filtration rate (GFR) and renal abnormalities on ultrasound or biopsy. As renal insufficiency progresses and GFR is decreased by 75 per cent or more, retention of solutes (urea, creatinine, phosphate) occurs, resulting in signs of uremia including inappetence, weight loss, and vomiting.

Pyelonephritis. Infection and inflammation of the renal pelvis can destroy the countercurrent mechanism in the renal medulla resulting in dilute urine and PU/PD. Pyelonephritis is best diagnosed by urine sediment examination and culture together with contrast dye studies of the renal pelvis or renal ultrasonography.

Pyometra. Pyometra may be associated with polyuria due to *Escherichia coli* endotoxin deposition in the tubules causing injury and interference with sodium and chloride reabsorption, resulting in a loss of medullary hypertonicity.

Hypercalcemia. Hypercalcemia directly impairs the ability of the renal tubules to respond to ADH, inactivating transport of sodium and chloride into the renal medullary interstitium and inhibiting ADH-mediated water reabsorption. Eventually calcium precipitation in the renal tubules will occur if hyperphosphatemia is also present, causing renal failure with azotemia and isosthenuria. Clinical signs of

TABLE 24–2. DIAGNOSTIC TESTS SUPPORTING DIFFERENTIAL DIAGNOSES FOR POLYURIA AND POLYDIPSIA

DIAGNOSIS	DIAGNOSTIC TESTS SUPPORTING DIAGNOSIS
Diabetes mellitus	Persistent hyperglycemia and glucosuria ± ketonuria
Renal glucosuria	Normal serum glucose with glucosuria; evaluate for aminoaciduria; renal ultrasound, intravenous urogram, and biopsy to characterize
Central diabetes insipidus	Normal or increased plasma osmolality, hyposthenuria, no response to water deprivation, responds to exogenous ADH; do tests to eliminate intracranial disease
Nephrogenic diabetes insipidus	Normal to increased plasma osmolality, no response to water deprivation or exogenous ADH; do tests to eliminate secondary causes of NDI, especially renal insufficiency
Renal insufficiency/failure	Isosthenuric urine, may have increased BUN and creatinine; abnormal creatinine clearance; renal ultrasound, intravenous urogram, and renal biopsy may reveal underlying process
Pyelonephritis	Fever, renal pain, inflammatory CBC, inflammatory urine sediment, positive urine culture; intravenous urogram and renal ultrasound
Pyometra	Vaginal discharge and/or palpable uterine enlargement; CBC inflammatory ± left shift; abdominal radiographs and ultrasound confirm
Hypercalcemia	Increased serum calcium concentration; test to search for underlying process: rectal examination, thoracic and abdominal radiographs, lymph node cytology/biopsy, bone marrow cytology, parathyroid hormone assay, PTHrP assay, ACTH stimulation test
Hypokalemia	Decreased serum potassium concentration; increased fractional excretion of potassium
Hyperadrenocorticism	Physical and clinicopathologic findings support diagnosis; diagnosis requires ACTH stimulation test, low-dose dexamethasone suppression test
Hyperthyroidism	Physical and clinicopathologic findings support diagnosis; increased serum T_4 concentration, cytology of cervical mass (dog); T_3 suppression test (cats)
Hypoadrenocorticism	Historical and physical findings support diagnosis; low serum Na:K ratio; ACTH stimulation test required for diagnosis
Hepatic insufficiency/portosystemic shunt	May have icterus or ascites; laboratory findings can include decreased albumin and BUN, increased liver enzymes; serum bile acids fasting and postprandially, ammonia tolerance test confirm liver disease; abdominal ultrasound, portal angiography, surgery, and liver biopsy may reveal underlying process
Renal medullary solute washout	Inadequate urine concentration with water deprivation; no further concentration when exogenous ADH is administered; re-evaluate modified water deprivation test/ADH response after more prolonged gradual water restriction and salt supplementation
Primary polydipsia	Low plasma osmolality, hyposthenuria, responds to water deprivation; do tests to eliminate underlying cause (hepatic encephalopathy, brain disease)

hypercalcemia may be subtle and include PU/PD, anorexia, inappetence, and weakness. Hypercalcemia most commonly occurs as a paraneoplastic syndrome but may also occur in association with renal failure, hyperparathyroidism, hypoadrenocorticism, or hypervitaminosis D. The diagnosis is made by documenting an increase in serum calcium concentration.

Hypokalemia. Severe hypokalemia (<3.5 mEq/L) may render the terminal portion of the nephron less responsive to ADH and may also interfere with normal pituitary release of ADH.

Hyperadrenocorticism. More than 80 per cent of dogs with hyperadrenocorticism exhibit PU/PD. This may be the only sign reported, although other clinical and laboratory features are usually present. Polyuria is most commonly due to a decrease in central release of ADH, although interference with the action of ADH at the renal tubule and loss of renal medullary tonicity from increased renal blood flow have been reported.

Hyperthyroidism. Hyperthyroidism may cause PU/PD through direct stimulation of excessive drinking or by decreasing medullary tonicity through increased renal blood flow. Chronic renal failure is also common in older hyperthyroid cats.

Hypoadrenocorticism. Urine is rarely concentrated in dogs with hypoadrenocorticism despite normal renal function and significant hypovolemia. Chronic renal sodium wasting due to mineralicorticoid deficiency results in medullary solute washout. The diagnosis is confirmed by demonstrating inadequate or absent response to exogenous ACTH.

Hepatic Failure. Dilute urine is common in dogs and cats with chronic liver disease. The exact cause of the PU is not known but may involve loss of medullary tonicity due to decreased urea production from ammonia, delayed clearance of endogenous aldosterone and cortisol, hypokalemia, and encephalopathic polydipsia. Most dogs and cats with severe liver failure have other clinical signs, including failure to grow, cachexia, episodic CNS disturbances, gastrointestinal problems, and ascites (see Table 24–2).

Renal Medullary Solute Washout. Renal medullary solute washout can occur to some degree with any disorder causing polyuria as increased tubular flow and volume decreases the reabsorption of sodium and urea. Loss of renal medullary hypertonicity will result in decreased ability to concentrate urine even with water deprivation, dehydration, or exogenous ADH administration. When renal medullary washout is suspected, it is important to restore medullary hypertonicity before performing a water deprivation/ADH response test in order to obtain interpretable results. This can be accomplished through gradual water restriction without dehydration and supplementation of the diet with sodium chloride in phase I of the modified water deprivation/ADH response test (Table 24–3).

Drugs/Diet. Many drugs and dietary changes have the potential to cause PU and PD. A thorough history must be obtained. Diuretics, anticonvulsants, synthetic levothyroxine, and glucocorticoids may cause PU/PD. Low-protein diets may result in renal medullary washout and primary polyuria, whereas high-salt diets may cause increased thirst and secondary polyuria.

PRIMARY (PSYCHOGENIC) POLYDIPSIA (PP)

Compulsive drinking may occur as a learned behavior in some dogs placed in exercise-restrictive environments or subjected to stress. A neoplastic or traumatic lesion in the thirst center of the hypothalamus could also result in compulsive polydipsia. Polyuria occurs secondary to the polydipsia. Urine is hyposthenuric (1.001 to 1.005), and plasma osmolality is decreased (285 to 295 mOsm/kg). Psychogenic polydipsia is diagnosed after excluding other common causes for PU/PD, finding no evidence of organic brain disease or hepatic dysfunction, and demonstrating that the dog can concentrate urine after gradual water deprivation and dehydration (see Table 24–3). Treatment of psychogenic polydipsia includes behavior modification and partial water restriction.

TABLE 24–3. PROTOCOL FOR THE MODIFIED WATER DEPRIVATION/ADH RESPONSE TEST*†

PHASE I. PREPARATION—to decrease renal medullary solute washout. This phase should be initiated 5 days (120 hours) before water deprivation begins.
  A. Days 5, 4, and 3 preceding water deprivation: limit water intake to 55 ml/lb (120 mL/kg)/day in small allotments.
  B. Day 2 preceding the test: limit water to 40 ml/lb (90 mL/kg)/day in small allotments.
  C. 24 hours prior to water deprivation: limit water intake to 30 ml/lb (60 mL/kg)/day in small allotments.
  D. Beginning on day 5 preceding water deprivation, lightly salt all meals.
  E. Withdraw all food 12 hours prior to initiating water deprivation.

PHASE II. WATER DEPRIVATION—to dehydrate the patient, stimulate endogenous ADH release, and monitor ability to concentrate urine.
  A. In the morning:
    1. Completely empty the bladder.
    2. Obtain exact body weight.
    3. Obtain serum osmolality.
    4. Obtain BUN, PCV, total protein.
    5. Check urine specific gravity and/or osmolality.
    6. Withdraw and withhold all food and water.
  B. Every hour:
    1. Completely empty the bladder.
    2. Check exact body weight.
    3. Check CNS status, clinical hydration, BUN, PCV, total protein.
    4. Check urine specific gravity and/or osmolality.

C. Phase II is ended when:
    1. Patient has lost >5% of body weight or appears clinically dehydrated. Whenever possible, dehydration should be documented by a measured increase in serum osmolality.
    2. Patient becomes ill or depressed.
    3. Patient produces concentrated urine (>1.030 dogs, >1.035 cats).

PHASE III. RESPONSE TO EXOGENOUS ADH—ADH is administered to an already dehydrated patient and urine concentration is measured. Response indicates inadequate endogenous ADH release.
  A. Completely empty the bladder.
  B. Continue withholding food and water.
  C. Administer aqueous vasopressin IM (0.25 U/lb [0.5 U/kg], maximum 5 U).
  D. Every 30 minutes for 120 minutes:
    1. Completely empty the bladder.
    2. Check urine specific gravity and/or osmolality.
    3. Check CNS status, clinical hydration, BUN, PCV, total protein.

PHASE IV. END OF TEST—slowly reintroduce the patient to water to prevent overdrinking.
  A. Offer small amounts of water (10 mL/lb [20 mL/kg]) every 30 minutes for 2 hours.
  B. Continue to monitor hydration, CNS status.
  C. After 2 hours return to ad lib water.

---

*Phases I and II are contraindicated in patients that are clinically dehydrated or that have not been evaluated for diabetes mellitus or the common etiologies of secondary NDI.
†Modified with permission from Feldman EC, Nelson RW (ed): Canine and Feline Endocrinology and Reproduction, 2nd ed. Philadelphia, WB Saunders, 1996.

DIAGNOSTIC APPROACH TO THE PATIENT WITH PU/PD

Confirm/Quantify. When an owner suspects increased urination or thirst, it is likely that PU/PD is truly present. If the history is inconclusive, it is advisable to have the owners *measure the water* the dog is drinking at home for 3 to 5 days. *Measuring urine specific gravity* may help confirm that the pet is polyuric.

Evaluate for Common Causes of PU/PD. Perform a careful *physical examination* and routine diagnostic tests to rule out the most common causes of PU/PD (see Fig. 24–1; Table 24–2). Recommended initial diagnostic tests include a *complete blood cell count*, a *urinalysis,* and a *serum biochemistry profile*. In an adult cat, *serum thyroxine* should also be measured. *Culture of a urine sample* obtained by cystocentesis should also be considered, even if the urinary sediment is not remarkable.

Abdominal radiographs and/or *ultrasound* may be warranted to evaluate liver, kidney, uterus, and adrenals. Tests of the pituitary-adrenal axis (*ACTH stimulation, low-dose dexamethasone suppression*) should be considered as part of the initial plan for adult dogs with PU/PD. Physical findings or initial laboratory results may provide a diagnosis or prompt further diagnostic testing including thoracic radiographs, lymph node aspiration, bone marrow biopsy, and liver function tests. After completion and review of the history, physical examination, and preliminary test results, most of the common differential diagnoses for PU/PD will have been identified or ruled out (see Fig. 24–1, Tables 24–1 and 24–2). In those cases in which a diagnosis has not been found, the less common differential diagnoses of PP, NDI, and CDI should be investigated.

Evaluation of Urine Specific Gravity. Consistently isosthenuric urine (1.008 to 1.015) is most often seen with renal insufficiency but may also be found in patients with partial CDI or NDI, particularly if water has been withheld. Hyposthenuria (<1.005) is seen in dogs and cats with complete CDI, primary or secondary NDI, PP, hyperadrenocorticism, or, uncommonly, liver failure.

Measurement of Plasma Osmolality. Dogs and cats with CDI and primary or secondary NDI have increased thirst as a result of increased serum osmolality caused by the obligatory loss of water in their urine. Plasma osmolality will usually be slightly high in these dogs or cats (300 to 315 mOsm/kg), and low (275 to 285 mOsm/kg) in patients with primary polydipsia. Plasma osmolality can be used to document hydration status during a water deprivation test.

Modified Water Deprivation/ADH Response Test. This test is designed to determine whether a dog or cat can release endogenous ADH in response to dehydration and whether the kidneys can respond to the ADH (see Table 24–3; Fig. 24–1). This test is most useful to differentiate between CDI, NDI, and PP. Some veterinarians choose to have the pet undergo trial treatment with synthetic ADH (DDAVP) at home rather than using the water deprivation test. Trial treatment is less expensive, less dangerous, and as reliable and specific in making a diagnosis.

Hyperadrenocorticism and all other causes of secondary NDI should be eliminated before performing a water deprivation test. Phase I will restore renal medullary hypertonicity in animals with renal medullary solute washout. Phase 2 involves dehydrating the animal and monitoring urine concentration. Phases 1 and 2 should not be performed in animals that are already clinically dehydrated or have a plasma osmolality greater than 320 mOsm/kg. If the animal becomes dehydrated without forming concentrated urine, exogenous ADH is administered to determine whether the kidneys can respond to ADH (phase 3). Whenever NDI is diagnosed, it is important to be certain once again that all of the causes of acquired secondary NDI have been systematically evaluated and eliminated.

CHAPTER 25

INCONTINENCE, ENURESIS, DYSURIA, AND NOCTURIA

George E. Lees

Urination (micturition) is the discharge or passage of urine. Urination normally is a conscious act under voluntary control. *Urinary incontinence* refers to lack of voluntary control over the passage of urine. *Enuresis* is involuntary passage of urine that occurs during sleep. *Nocturia* is excessive urination at night and usually is a sign of polyuria. *Dysuria* refers to urination that is painful or difficult. Specific signs of dysuria include increased frequency (pollakiuria), urgency, hesitancy, and stranguria.

GENERAL PATHOPHYSIOLOGY

Animals with disorders of micturition have signs correlating with the phase of micturition that is abnormal. Storage phase disorders typically produce urinary incontinence. Voiding phase disorders usually produce a degree of incomplete bladder emptying and urinary retention, but incontinence may also occur. Urinary incontinence has neurogenic and non-neurogenic causes.

Neurogenic Disorders. Neurologic lesions that disrupt upper motor neuron segments of the micturition reflex impair voluntary control of urination and produce a spastic neuropathic bladder. Because lower motor neurons are intact, detrusor contraction can occur. However, contractions are not coordinated with relaxation of urethral sphincters; voiding is involuntary and incomplete.

Neurologic lesions disrupting lower motor neuron segments of the micturition reflex preclude detrusor contraction and produce a flaccid neuropathic bladder. Bladder capacity is greater than normal. The bladder fills until intravesical pressure exceeds outlet resistance, and urine flow is determined by sphincter tone. When urethral tone is minimal, small increments of intravesical pressure produce some discharge of urine. When urethral tone is maintained, urine flow may not occur until intravesical pressure is substantially increased.

Non-neurogenic Disorders. Anatomic anomalies of the lower urinary tract may cause urinary incontinence. Ectopic ureters or other, less common, developmental abnormalities may permit urine to bypass normal sphincters or to flow through abnormal channels or openings. Acquired abnormalities of the lower urinary tract that cause incontinence are inflammatory or infiltrative diseases of the bladder or urethra. Chronic cystitis, urethritis, neoplasia, urolithiasis, and prostatic diseases may cause such problems.

A functional disorder exists when the bladder and urethra are structurally normal but fail to perform normally. The most common cause of incontinence is urethral sphincter mechanism incompetence, which is characterized by inability to keep the outlet closed during storage. Insufficiency of outlet resistance permits urine flow, while intravesical pressure remains normally low during bladder filling. Incontinence is sometimes caused by detrusor instability, which is characterized by failure of the bladder to remain relaxed during filling.

Diseases of the urinary bladder that increase stimulation of the micturition reflex may cause urge incontinence. Voiding is normal, but the storage phase is shortened. An intense urge to urinate may occur so rapidly that it cannot be controlled, and urination may appear involuntary.

Many lower urinary tract disorders cause excessive outlet resistance during voiding efforts. Obstruction of urine flow typically produces dysuria, stranguria, and urinary retention rather than incontinence. Nonetheless, partial obstruction may permit urine leakage as bladder pressure rises. Such paradoxic (obstructive) incontinence may be due to luminal or wall lesions.

Complications of Urinary Incontinence. The most common complication of urinary incontinence is development of urinary tract infection. Disorders that cause incontinence commonly impair urinary tract defenses against infection. When bladder overdistention occurs, disruption of tight junctions between smooth muscle fibers may lead to further detrusor malfunction.

Animals with urinary incontinence often require extensive nursing care and tremendous owner patience. Euthanasia may be requested if the problem is not controlled.

HISTORICAL FINDINGS AND THEIR MEANINGS

The signalment may suggest possible causes of incontinence. Young animals are more likely to have congenital lesions, whereas older animals are more likely to have acquired disorders. Some congenital abnormalities are known for their breed predilection.

A description of the problem's onset and progression should be obtained. The animal's urination pattern should be carefully reviewed. Polyuria, nocturia, pollakiuria, stranguria, and dysuria may be mistaken for incontinence. Whether urination is ever voluntary should be established. Ability to voluntarily initiate and maintain urination suggests the micturition reflex is intact and that the detrusor contracts when stimulated. When urine fills the bladder properly, absence of a micturition reflex suggests a neurogenic disorder. When an animal has intermittent dribbling of urine, stranguria, and incomplete bladder emptying, excessive outlet resistance is suggested. Neurogenic disorders may also produce intermittent urine dribbling. Leakage of urine during recumbency or sleep is suggestive of urethral sphincter mechanism incompetence. Continuous dribbling of urine may be produced by a variety of anatomic or functional abnormalities.

History may include traumatic events leading to nerve or spinal cord injuries. Prior abdominal or urogenital surgery might cause lower urinary tract damage leading to incontinence.

PHYSICAL FINDINGS AND THEIR MEANINGS

A complete physical examination should be performed, with special attention to the nervous and urogenital systems. The neurologic examination is the key to detection of neurogenic disorders of micturition because neurologic lesions rarely affect only the bladder and urethra. The bulbospongiosus and perineal reflexes, anal tone, and sensation over the caudal portion of the back and tail should be evaluated. When these are normal, sacral reflexes and pudendal nerve function probably are intact.

Non-neurogenic causes of incontinence often are identified by abdominal palpation combined with digital rectal palpation (perineal hernia, urethral abnormality) and examination of the vagina and/or external genitalia. The bladder should be palpated before and after urination. Finding that the bladder is large, distended, and thin walled suggests that it is flaccid and hyporeflexive. Finding that the bladder is small, contracted, and thick walled suggests that it is spastic and hyperreflexive. The bladder should be compressed manually to test outlet resistance and induce bladder emptying, if possible. Easily expelling urine with such compression suggests decreased outlet resistance. Difficult or unsuccessful manual expression of the bladder suggests normal or increased outlet resistance.

The animal's urination efforts should be observed to assess voluntary control and whether the detrusor contracts in concert with sphincter relaxation. Postmicturition residual urine volume is measured by urethral catheterization (normal values are 0.2 to 0.5 mL/kg). Excessive residual urine volume indicates incomplete voiding. Passing the catheter also helps to detect abnormalities causing urethral obstruction.

DIAGNOSTIC PLAN (Fig. 25–1)

Results of a *routine hemogram* and *serum biochemistry* tests generally do not indicate the cause of incontinence, but they aid assessment of the animal's overall physiologic status. Metabolic problems (e.g., azotemia, electrolyte distur-

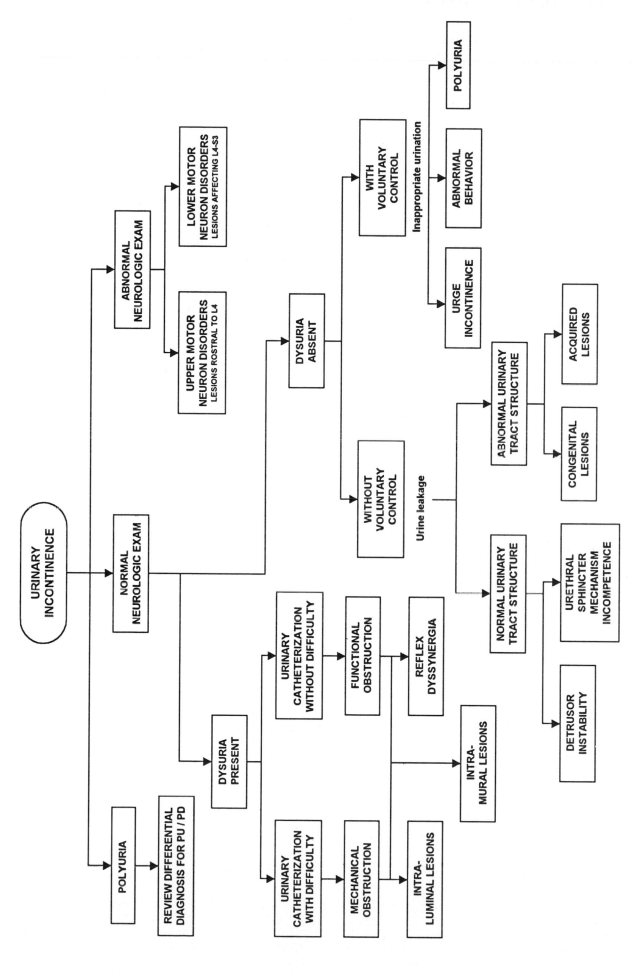

Figure 25–1. Algorithm for diagnostic approach to urinary incontinence.

bances, and acid-base imbalances caused by urethral obstruction) may require immediate medical attention or modify prognosis. Causes of polyuria may be suggested by certain laboratory test results.

When investigating urinary incontinence, *urinalysis* findings are especially important. Specific gravity less than or equal to 1.015 would be consistent with polyuria. Finding hematuria, proteinuria, and/or pyuria suggests presence of pathologic lesions in the urinary tract. Discovery of significant bacteriuria indicates presence of urinary tract infection. Bacteria may be seen during examination of urine sediment, but results of a *urine culture* are more reliable for evaluation of bacteriuria.

When a neurogenic disorder is indicated by deficits found during a neurologic examination, additional diagnostic evaluations are guided by the location and suspected cause(s) of the underlying neurologic disease. Diagnostic imaging of the portion(s) of the spinal column that might be affected usually is needed. Imaging techniques that can be used include survey spinal radiographs, myelography, computed tomography, and magnetic resonance imaging.

Detection and morphologic characterization of pathologic lesions in the urinary tract also are accomplished by diagnostic imaging. Because survey radiography is not highly sensitive for detection of many urinary lesions, *ultrasonography* is preferred for noninvasive imaging of urinary tract organs. In animals with incontinence or dysuria, ultrasonography is particularly helpful for evaluation of the urinary bladder and the prostate gland. When ureteral ectopia is suspected, ultrasonography may reveal an abnormal diameter or course of the ureter in the wall of the bladder neck and proximal urethra. Additionally, animals with ectopic ureters sometimes have upper tract anomalies (e.g., unilateral renal agenesis) that the ultrasound examination may detect. Ultrasonography is not as useful distal to the bladder neck, but detection of acquired urethral lesions can be accomplished by physical examination and/or urethral catheterization. When a developmental anomaly of the lower urinary tract is suspected, *endoscopy* is the best diagnostic technique. Animals with this problem mostly are young female dogs, and an endoscopic evaluation of the vaginal tract, urethra, and bladder (including presence of ureteral openings and urine flow into the trigone) is the most accurate way to determine whether these portions of the urogenital tract are structurally normal.

When ultrasonography and endoscopy are unavailable, or when these evaluations yield equivocal results, contrast radiographic studies can be used to seek for structural urinary abnormalities that might be contributing to urinary incontinence or dysuria. Radiographic imaging of ureters usually is accomplished with an *excretory urogram.* To evaluate the urethra and bladder, *positive contrast urethrography* or *vaginourethrography* and *double-contrast cystography* are the most informative studies.

When palpation or diagnostic imaging reveals an infiltrative lesion (e.g., neoplasm) in the bladder or urethra, specimens for cytologic or histologic evaluation can be obtained using *bladder wash* and/or *catheter biopsy* techniques. If available, endoscopy also can be used for this purpose.

Urodynamic studies measure pressure, volume, and flow in the bladder and urethra. Urodynamic tests described for dogs or cats include *urethral pressure profile* (which has been performed using several methods), *cystometrogram,* and *simultaneous cystometry and uroflowmetry. Electromyography* of urethral or anal sphincters also can be recorded during urodynamic tests. Urodynamic testing is available in only a few centers; therefore, details regarding the procedures and interpretation of results are omitted here. However, urodynamic testing usually is not needed for management of clinical cases. Valid functional assessments can be based on clinical observations of pressure and flow relationships.

GOALS OF TREATMENT

Two principles guide management of patients with urinary incontinence. First, priority should be given to alterations requiring immediate care, such as maintaining a nonobstructed urethra, and correcting fluid deficits, electrolyte disturbances, acid-base imbalances, and azotemia. Second, normal micturition should be restored as soon as possible, regardless of the cause. Delays in treating disorders of micturition may lead to severe complications.

When structural abnormalities contribute to incontinence, surgical correction usually is indicated. Surgery also may be needed for paradoxic (obstructive) incontinence. When the cause of excessive outlet resistance is functional, however, medical management usually is indicated. Pharmacologic agents are used to treat incontinence when urinary tract infection, structural abnormalities, and mechanical types of excessive outlet resistance have been excluded as possible causes. Specific recommendations for pharmacotherapy of disorders of micturition appear elsewhere.

OUTCOME

Prognosis for animals with structural anomalies and those with sphincter mechanism incompetence is fair to good. Animals with paradoxic incontinence are divided into two groups. Those with mechanical outlet obstruction usually regain normal function if they are treated promptly. However, prognosis often is poor for those with functional obstruction. For neurogenic disorders, prognosis for recovery of lower urinary tract function usually is the same as the prognosis for the underlying neurologic disease.

CHAPTER 26

URINARY OBSTRUCTION AND FUNCTIONAL URINE RETENTION

India F. Lane

During urine storage, the urinary bladder must remain relaxed and accommodate filling while the outlet maintains adequate resistance to prevent leakage. During voiding, the bladder must contract with sufficient force and duration to empty completely while the outlet relaxes and allows free flow of urine. Disorders of urine storage usually lead to urinary incontinence, whereas disruption of normal voiding leads to incomplete emptying and *urine retention*. Failure of emptying is due to either failure of detrusor contractile function (*bladder hypocontractility or detrusor atony*), inappropriate outlet resistance (*anatomic obstruction or functional obstruction*), or both. The diagnostic approach to urine retention is designed to elucidate the functional status of the bladder and the urethral outlet.

Consequences of dysfunctional voiding depend on the chronicity of the problem and the degree of urine retention. Postrenal azotemia, metabolic acidosis, and hyperkalemia can be life-threatening consequences of acute complete urinary obstruction. Rupture of the urinary tract also is possible. With prolonged partial or intermittent obstruction, renal dysfunction, hydronephrosis, hydroureter, and detrusor atony result from elevated intraluminal pressure. Urinary tract infections are common and readily ascend to the upper urinary tract.

COMMON CAUSES OF URINE RETENTION

FAILURE OF DETRUSOR CONTRACTILE FUNCTION

Detrusor dysfunction usually develops as a sequela to neurologic dysfunction or urinary bladder overdistention (Table 26–1). In suprasacral spinal cord lesions, motor and sensory pathways of the micturition reflex are disrupted while striated (external) sphincter tone is preserved or exaggerated. The bladder is firmly distended and often difficult to express (the *upper motor neuron* bladder). With time, bladder function may return via a sacral reflex, but voiding is usually involuntary, incomplete, and incoordinated with outlet relaxation (*detrusor-urethral dyssynergia*). With damage to the sacral cord segments or the pelvic and pudendal nerves, motor and most sensory bladder functions are lost, as is contractility of the striated muscle sphincter. Smooth (internal) sphincter tone may be preserved and fixed, allowing partial continence. The bladder is usually large and flaccid and variably expressible. Bladder atony also is a frequent component of *dysautonomia*, a rare disease of cats in the United Kingdom and of dogs in the United States. Neurogenic disorders rarely affect the urinary tract alone; other deficits can usually be detected on neurologic examination.

Acute or chronic *overdistention* due to neurogenic dysfunction or obstruction may disrupt neural and muscular transmission within the detrusor muscle, exacerbating atony. Disorders associated with generalized mucle weakness can also affect bladder function.

INAPPROPRIATE OUTLET RESISTANCE

Anatomic outlet obstruction is the most common cause of urinary obstruction in dogs and cats. This problem is usually

TABLE 26–1. CAUSES OF URINE RETENTION

Bladder Dysfunction

Neurogenic
  Suprasacral cord lesion
  Sacral cord lesion
  Pelvic nerve or pelvic plexus injury
  Dysautonomia
Myogenic
  Overdistension
    Obstruction
    Pain, inactivity, confinement
    Polyuria
  Disorders causing muscle weakness
  Peripheral neuropathy
  Viral disease
  Radiation injury
  Aging
  Anticholinergic/antispasmodic agents
  Idiopathic

Inappropriate Outlet Resistance

Physical obstruction
  Urolithiasis
  Mucoprotein plugs (cats)
  Bladder neck or urethral neoplasia
  Prostatic disease (usually neoplasia)
  Trauma, surgery, hemorrhage
  Inflammation/edema
  Urethral stricture
  Extraluminal compression
  Bladder prolapse or retroflexion
Functional obstruction
  Suprasacral or brain stem lesions
  Idiopathic detrusor–urethral dyssynergia
  Functional bladder neck obstruction
  Urethral spasticity
    Posturethral obstruction
    Inflammation
    Urethral or periurethral surgery
    Alpha-agonist agents

Other

Oliguria/anuria
Rupture of the urinary tract

a result of urolithiasis, urethral plugs, neoplasia, or large prostatic cysts or abscesses. *Functional urethral obstruction* can develop as a result of neurogenic or nonneurogenic causes (see Table 26–1). Urethral sphincter spasticity (smooth or striated muscle) most often develops following urethral inflammation or painful stimuli. Idiopathic functional obstructive disorders are observed in people and occasionally encountered in dogs. Functional obstructive disorders are clinically similar to anatomic obstruction, but no obstructive lesion or neurologic lesion can be found. Diagnosis is best provided by micturition studies that document impaired urine flow or inappropriate sphincter activity during periods of bladder contraction.

APPROACH TO URINE RETENTION
(Fig. 26–1)

Presenting complaints may include failure to urinate, pollakiuria, hematuria, stranguria, interrupted voiding, weak urine stream, urinary incontinence, recurrent urinary tract infection, abdominal distention, or abdominal pain. With prolonged complete obstruction, signs of postrenal uremia may predominate, including lethargy, dehydration, shock, and vomiting. With either detrusor dysfunction or partial outlet obstruction, urine leakage may be observed as the bladder becomes overdistended and intravesicular pressure exceeds outlet resistance (so-called *paradoxic or overflow incontinence*).

Historical information should include details regarding age, reproductive status, prior neurologic disease, trauma or surgery (especially involving the urinary tract, caudal abdomen, pelvis, or external genitalia), water intake, and voiding patterns. Previous urinary tract infections, episodes of urolithiasis, other systemic illnesses, and medications administered should be recorded.

During a general *physical examination*, the external genitalia should be examined for evidence of injury, abnormal conformation, masses, or urine scald. An attempt should be made to assess *bladder size and tone* prior to and following voluntary urination. The hallmark of urine retention disorders is a large urinary bladder. A *digital rectal examination* should be performed to assess anal tone, the pelvic canal, lumbosacral sensitivity, the prostate gland (males), and the pelvic urethra. A *digital vaginal examination* (female dogs) also allows palpation of the vaginal tract and urethral orifice for uroliths or obstructive masses.

A cursory *neurologic examination* should be included during the physical examination to evaluate mental status, gait, strength, hindlimb proprioception, tail carriage, and perineal sensation. The sacral reflex arc can be further assessed by gently squeezing the bulbus glandis or vulva, which should elicit a visible contraction of the anal spincter. Additional neurologic evaluation (radiography, electromyography, myelography) is warranted if deficits are observed.

Ideally, *voiding should be observed directly,* noting the animal's posture, ability to initiate voiding, urine stream, comfort or discomfort, and residual bladder size. When no urination is observed, urine retention within the bladder must be differentiated from oligoanuria or rupture of the urinary tract. With anatomic outlet obstruction, animals usually strain to urinate and may produce an attenuated urine stream

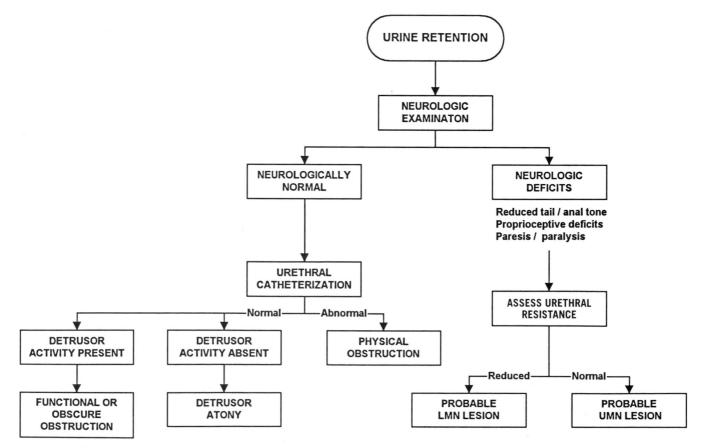

Figure 26–1. Algorithm for the diagnostic approach to urine retention in small animals. UMN = upper motor neuron; LMN = lower motor neuron.

or a few drops of bloody urine after prolonged effort. In some types of functional obstruction, urination may be initiated adequately; however, the urine stream is abruptly tapered or terminated, leaving a large residual volume. With primary bladder dysfunction, the dog or cat may or may not attempt to void voluntarily; the urine stream produced is often slow and weak. If the bladder remains distended after voiding, gentle attempts to express the urinary bladder can be made in order to assess outlet resistance. With excessive outlet resistance, the bladder is usually distended, firm, painful, and difficult to express. With primary detrusor atony or lower motor neuron disorders, the bladder may be large, flaccid, and readily expressible because outlet resistance is expected to be low. Manual bladder expression is difficult in normal male dogs and cats and in uncooperative animals. Caution is advised to avoid rupture of the urinary tract.

Urinary catheterization is a useful method of assessing residual urine volume (normally 0.2 to 0.4 mL/kg in dogs) and patency of the urethra and bladder neck. In general, a small-diameter, soft, flexible urinary catheter should be advanced gently into the urethra, feeling carefully for resistance or friction. In functional obstructive disorders or primary detrusor atony, an appropriately sized catheter should advance easily in the resting state. Exceptions include small or eccentric lesions that may be bypassed with little difficulty; small, loose uroliths may be pushed back into the bladder without apparent resistance. In animals with prostatic disease or fluctuant cysts or masses, the urethra may be collapsed but easily traversed with a polypropylene catheter. Ultrasonography or contrast urethrography may be required to completely rule out anatomic obstruction.

A complete *urinalysis and urine culture* is indicated when urine retention is found. Hematuria and pyuria may support urinary tract trauma due to urolithiasis or neoplasia, or may indicate secondary bacterial infection. Results of a *hemogram and serum biochemical profile* may rule in or rule

out metabolic causes of muscle weakness, provide clues to polyuric disorders, and detect severity of postrenal azotemia.

Survey radiography may be sufficient for identification of radiopaque uroliths, lumbosacral disease, pelvic trauma, and pelvic and caudal abdominal masses. *Ultrasonography* is a valuable tool for assessment of the kidneys, ureters, bladder, bladder neck, and prostate gland; calculi, cysts or abscesses, soft tissue masses, and blood clots are readily observed. *Contrast cystourethrography* may be helpful in outlining the bladder neck and urethra. Optimum studies are obtained by retrograde injection of contrast material against a moderately full urinary bladder. *Retrograde vaginourethrography* is useful for imaging the entire urethra in female dogs. *Voiding cystourethrograms* using sequential radiographs or fluoroscopic assistance are especially helpful in the identification of bladder neck obstruction or functional obstructive disorders but are difficult to perform well in dogs and cats.

Urodynamic procedures are available at some veterinary teaching hospitals. Cystometry and urethral pressure profilometry record objective measurements of bladder compliance, capacity and contractility, and urethral pressure and length. Hypercompliant, flaccid bladders can be documented, as well as urethral hypertonicity, urethral spasms, or focal high-pressure zones. External urethral sphincter activity can be isolated with the addition of electromyography. Unfortunately, most routine urodynamic evaluations are completed in a resting state, do not differentiate between neurogenic and myogenic disorders, and are better suited for evaluation of storage disorders than voiding disorders. Uroflowmetry and micturition studies have been described in dogs and cats but require additional expertise.

TREATMENT OF URINE RETENTION

Compressive neurologic lesions should be surgically addressed, physical obstructions should be removed or reposi-

TABLE 26-2. PHARMACOLOGIC AGENTS USED IN THE MANAGEMENT OF VOIDING DISORDERS

AGENT	ACTIONS	DOSAGES	ADVERSE EFFECTS	CONTRAINDICATIONS
Agents Used to Increase Bladder Contractility				
Bethanechol	Parasympathomimetic	Dog: 5–25 mg/dog PO q8h Cat: 1.25–5.0 mg/cat PO q8h	Vomiting, cramping Ptyalism, anorexia	Urethral obstruction, GI disease, hyperthyroidism
Metoclopramide	Dopamine antagonist	Dog: 0.2–0.5 mg/kg PO q8h Cat: 0.2–0.5 mg/kg PO q8h	CNS effects	GI obstruction
Cisapride	Enhanced acetylcholine release	Dog: 0.5 mg/kg PO q8–24h Cat: 2.5–5 mg/cat PO q8h	Diarrhea, abdominal pain	GI obstruction
Agents Used to Decrease Urethral Resistance				
Phenoxybenzamine	Alpha-antagonist; urethral smooth muscle relaxation	Dog: 0.25 mg/kg PO q12–24h OR 2.5–20 mg/dog PO q12–24h Cat: 1.25–7.5 mg/cat PO q12–24h	Hypotension, GI upset, tachycardia	Cardiac disease, glaucoma Diabetes mellitus, renal failure
Prazosin	Alpha-antagonist: urethral smooth muscle relaxation	Dog: 1 mg/15 kg PO q8h Cat: 0.5 mg/cat PO q8h? OR 0.03 mg/kg IV	As for phenoxybenzamine	As for phenoxybenzamine
Baclofen	Skeletal muscle relaxant	Dog: 1–2 mg/kg PO q8h Cat: Not recommended	Weakness, pruritus GI upset	
Dantrolene	Skeletal muscle relaxant	Dog: 1–5 mg/kg PO q8–12h Cat: 0.5–2 mg/kg PO q8h OR 1.0 mg/kg IV	Weakness, GI upset, sedation, hepatotoxicity	Cardiopulmonary disease
Diazepam	Benzodiazepine; Skeletal muscle relaxant	Dog: 2–10 mg/dog PO q8h Cat: 1–2.5 mg/cat PO q8h OR 0.5 mg/kg IV	Sedation, polyphagia, paradoxic excitement, hepatotoxicity	Hepatic disease, pregnancy

tioned with surgical or nonsurgical means, and metabolic derangements should be corrected by appropriate fluid therapy or pharmacologic means. The urinary bladder should be kept small by intermittent or indwelling urethral catheterization. Urinary tract infections should be identified and treated with appropriate antimicrobials, preferably after normal voiding has been restored.

Bladder and urethral function can be manipulated by pharmacologic means (Table 26–2), regardless of whether the etiology is neurogenic or myogenic. *Cholinergic agents* have been used to promote bladder emptying in atonic bladders, although the success of orally administered agents is unreliable. Bethanechol chloride is most commonly utilized in small animals. Initial dosages should be low and gradually increased to effect. Adverse effects include salivation, defecation, abdominal cramping, vomiting, and anorexia. Parenteral administration of bethanechol may be effective in refractory cases, but should be avoided because adverse cholinergic effects are common with this route. Other smooth muscle prokinetic agents, such as metoclopramide or cisapride, may be effective in increasing bladder contrac-

tility, but their efficacy is not documented. *Alpha-adrenergic antagonists* may be administered to reduce smooth muscle sphincter resistance in the urethra, whereas central or direct muscle relaxants are used to reduce striated muscle tone of the striated urethral sphincter.

OUTCOME

As treatment and recovery progress, residual volume should be assessed by observation of voiding, urinary bladder palpation, and periodic urinary catheterization. In most dogs and cats, medications can be slowly withdrawn after adequate voiding function has been sustained for several days. The prognosis for return to function is good for acute reversible neurologic lesions, acute detrusor atony due to overdistention, and acute functional obstruction associated with resolving obstructive or irritative disease. The prognosis is less favorable for dogs and cats with chronic detrusor atony or idiopathic functional obstructive disorders. Complete voiding function may not return, and long-term treatment may be required.

CHAPTER 27

DISCOLORED URINE

Joseph W. Bartges

NORMAL URINE

Normal urine is typically transparent and yellow or amber upon visual inspection. Primarily two pigments impart the yellow coloration: urochrome and urobilin. Urochrome is a sulfur-containing oxidation product of the colorless urochromagen. Urobilin is a degradation product of hemoglobin. Because the 24-hour urinary excretion of urochrome is relatively constant, highly concentrated urine will be amber in color, whereas dilute urine may be transparent or light yellow in color. The intensity of the color is in part related to the volume of urine collected and the concentration of urine produced; therefore, it should be interpreted in the context of knowing the specific gravity. Caution must be used not to overinterpret the significance of urine color as part of a complete urinalysis. Significant disease may exist when urine is normal in color. Abnormal urine color may be caused by the presence of several endogenous or exogenous pigments. Although the abnormal color indicates a problem, it provides relatively nonspecific information. Causes of abnormal coloration should be investigated with appropriate laboratory tests and examination of the urine sediment. Detection of abnormal urine color should prompt questions related to diet, administration of medications, environment, and collection technique. Knowledge of the urine color may also be important in interpreting calorimetric test results because it may induce interference with the test.

DISCOLORED URINE

Urine color that is anything other than yellow or amber is abnormal. There are many potential causes of discolored urine (Table 27–1). The most common abnormal urine color in dogs and cats is red, brown, or black, which may be caused by hematuria, hemoglobinuria, myoglobinuria, and bilirubinuria (Fig. 27–1).

PALE YELLOW URINE

Urine that is pale yellow or clear in appearance may be normal or may be indicative of a polyuric state. Urine may be appropriately dilute if it is associated with recent consumption or administration of fluids, consumption of a diet containing low quantities of protein or high quantities of sodium chloride, or administration of diuretics. Urine would be considered to be inappropriately concentrated if it were dilute in the presence of dehydration. Diseases that may be associated with persistently inappropriately concentrated urine include diabetes mellitus, diabetes insipidus, hyperadrenocorticism, hyperthyroidism, and renal failure. If urine is pale yellow or clear, the urine specific gravity is often less than 1.015. A simple test to determine whether polyuria is persistent is to determine the urine specific gravity of a sample collected in the morning. Other tests should include

TABLE 27–1. POTENTIAL CAUSES OF DISCOLORED URINE

URINE COLOR	CAUSES	URINE COLOR	CAUSES
Yellow or amber	Urochromes Urobilin	Yellow-brown or green-brown	Bile pigments
Deep yellow	Highly concentrated urine Quinicrine* Nitrofurantoin* Phenacetin* Riboflavin (large quantities)* Phenolsulfonphthalein (acidic urine)	Brown to black (brown or red-brown when viewed in bright light in thin layer)	Melanin Methemoglobin Myoglobin Bile pigments Thymol* Phenolic compounds* Nitrofurantoin* Nitrites* Naphthalene* Chlorinated hydrocarbons* Aniline dyes* Homogentisic acid*
Blue	Methylene blue Indigo carmine and indigo blue dye* Indicans* *Pseudomonas* infection* Water-soluble chlorophyll* Toluidine blue* Triamterene* Amitriptyline* Anthraquinone*	Colorless	Very dilute urine (diuretics, diabetes mellitus, diabetes insipidus, overhydration)
Green	Methylene blue Dithiazanine Indigo blue* Evan's blue* Biliverdin Riboflavin* Thymol* Phenol* Triamterene* Amitriptyline* Anthraquinone*	Milky white	Lipid Pus Crystals
Red, pink, red-brown, red-orange, or orange	Hematuria Hemoglobinuria Myoglobinuria Porphyrinuria Congo red Phenolsulfonphthalein (following alkalinization) Neoprontosil Warfarin (orange)* Food pigments (rhubarb, beets, blackberries)* Carbon tetrachloride* Phenazopyridine Phenothiazines* Diphenylhydantoin* Bromsulphalein (following alkalinization) Chronic heavy metal poisoning (lead, mercury)* Rifampin* Emodin* Phenindione* Eosin*	Brown	Methemoglobin Melanin Sulfasalazine* Nitrofurantoin* Phenacetin* Naphthalene* Sulfonamides* Bismuth* Mercury* Feces (rectal–urinary tract fistula) Fava beans* Rhubarb* Sorbitol* Metronidazole* Methocarbamol* Anthracin cathartics* Clofazimine* Primaquine* Chloroquine* Furazolidone*
Orange-yellow	Highly concentrated urine Excess urobilin Bilirubin Phenazopyridine Sulfasalazine* Fluorescein sodium* Flutamide* Quinicrine* Phenacetin*		

*Only observed in human beings.

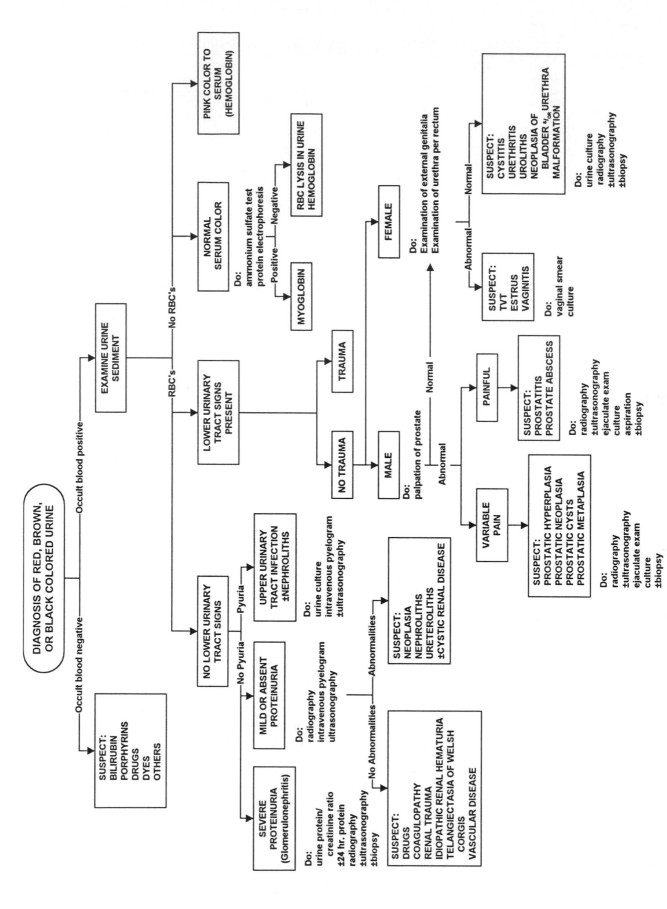

Figure 27–1. Algorithm for diagnosis of red, brown, or black colored urine.

TABLE 27–2. PROBABLE LOCALIZATION OF GROSS HEMATURIA

Hematuria Throughout Micturition

R/O		Renal disorder
	DX	Abdominal palpation; survey and contrast radiography; ultrasonography; biopsy; exploratory surgery
R/O		Diffuse bladder lesions
	DX	Abdominal palpation; examination of urine sediment; survey and contrast radiography; ultrasonography; catheter biopsy; cystoscopy and biopsy; exploratory surgery
R/O		Focal ventral or ventrolateral bladder lesions in active patients
	DX	Rectal and abdominal palpation; survey and contrast radiography; ultrasonography; catheter biopsy; aspiration biopsy; exploratory surgery
R/O		Severe prostatic or urethral lesions
	DX	Rectal and abdominal palpation; survey and contrast radiography; ultrasonography; catheter biopsy; exploratory surgery
R/O		Hemoglobinuria
	DX	Examination of urine sediment for red blood cells; hemogram
R/O		Systemic clotting defect
	DX	Clotting profile, platelet count; evaluation of other body systems for hemorrhage

Hematuria Independent or at the Beginning of Micturition

R/O		Urethral lesions
	DX	Rectal and abdominal palpation; comparison of analysis of urine samples collected by voiding and cystocentesis; survey and contrast radiography; catheter biopsy; exploratory surgery
R/O		Genital disease
	DX	Abdominal, rectal, and vaginal palpation; vaginal cytology; comparison of analysis of urine samples collected by voiding and cystocentesis; survey and contrast radiography; ultrasonography; endoscopy; exploratory surgery

Hematuria at End of Micturition

R/O		Focal ventral or ventrolateral lesions in inactive patients
	DX	Abdominal palpation; examination of urine sediment; survey and contrast radiography; ultrasonography; catheter biopsy; cystoscopy and biopsy; exploratory surgery
R/O		Renal disorder with intermittent hematuria in inactive patient
	DX	Abdominal palpation; survey and contrast radiography; biopsy; exploratory surgery; ultrasonography

serum biochemical analysis and a complete urinalysis. Additional testing may include measurement of serum thyroxine concentration, adrenal function testing, or monitoring specific gravity after several days of vasopressin administration.

RED, BROWN, OR BLACK URINE

The presence of red, brown, or black urine suggests blood, hemoglobin, myoglobin, or bilirubin (see Fig. 27–1). A positive occult blood reaction is obtained when urine contains any of these substances. The discoloration of urine may also result in false-positive reactions on other urine dipstick pads. Analysis of urine sediment will reveal the presence of red blood cells if the discoloration is due to hematuria. If gross hematuria is present, localization may be aided by where in the urine stream the hematuria is observed (Table 27–2). If no red blood cells are present on urine sediment examination, hemoglobin, myoglobin, or bilirubin should be suspected. Examination of plasma color will aid in differentiating these. If the discolored urine is due to myoglobin, the plasma will be clear because myoglobin in plasma is not bound

significantly to a carrying protein, resulting in filtration of myoglobin by the glomerulus. If the plasma is pink, it is suggestive of hemoglobin. If the plasma is yellow, it is suggestive of bilirubin. Hyperbilirubinemia may result from liver disease, posthepatic obstruction, or hemolysis. Hemoglobinemia is indicative of intravascular hemolysis resulting from immune-mediated, parasite-mediated, or drug-mediated destruction of red blood cells.

MILKY WHITE URINE

Milky white colored urine may be due to the presence of pus, lipid, or crystals. The more concentrated the urine sample is, the more opaque it may appear. The presence of pus secondary to a bacterial urinary tract infection is the most common cause of milky white urine. Lipiduria may be observed in healthy animals but is frequently observed in cats affected with hepatic lipidosis. Crystalluria if heavy and present in a concentrated urine sample may also result in a milky white urine color. Microscopic examination of urine sediment will aid in the differentiation of these causes.

CHAPTER 28

PROTEINURIA

Donald R. Krawiec

NORMAL PROTEINURIA

Proteinuria is a common and sometimes serious abnormality in dogs and cats. Proteinuria in cats is almost always associated with lower urinary tract disease; in dogs, renal proteinuria is not uncommon. Some amount of protein is commonly present in normal urine. Protein found in quantities less than 30 mg/kg/day has been determined to be normal, but because 24-hour urine collections are rarely performed, this information is not useful. Urine protein concentrations are easily determined by using urine dipsticks. Urine dipsticks are more sensitive for identifying albumin than globulin and may have false-positive or false-negative reactions. Nevertheless, they are commonly used as a screening test. The importance of urine protein concentration varies according to specific gravity. Under most circumstances, urine protein concentrations of 100 mg/dL or less in an otherwise normal concentrated urine are usually not significant. However, if urine is hyposthenuric, any amount of proteinuria may be abnormal. Protein found in normal urine may be derived from filtered plasma protein not reabsorbed by the proximal tubule; from Tamm-Horsfall proteins, which are produced from tubular segments distal to the descending limb of Henle; or from secretory globulins, which may be produced in any portion of the urinary tract.

IDENTIFYING ABNORMAL PROTEIN CONTENT IN URINE

Urine protein concentration is determined by quantifying the amount of protein in a volume of urine. Urine protein concentration is usually expressed in grams per deciliter. This determination may provide some information concerning the amount of protein in urine but may not accurately reflect daily loss. Quantifying 24-hour urine protein loss accurately determines whether abnormal amounts of protein are being lost in urine. Urine protein content may be identified by performing urine protein-creatinine ratios.

Urine protein-creatinine ratios (U-P/Cr) are now routinely accepted as accurate and reproducible methods of determining normal or abnormal urine protein content. Creatinine excretion is dependent on glomerular filtration. If creatinine excretion for a given glomerular filtration rate is constant, then changes in the protein-creatinine ratio are due to changes in urine protein excretion. To perform this assay, a random urine sample is collected, and the protein and creatinine concentrations are determined. The ratio is calculated by dividing the creatinine value into the protein value, both measured in milligrams per deciliter.

There is some disagreement in the literature about what constitutes a normal or questionable ratio. The generally accepted abnormal ratio is greater than 1 in dogs and 0.7 in cats. Any value less than 1 is usually considered normal, and values between 1 and 3 are unlikely to be due to

glomerular disease or the glomerular problem is not yet worrisome. Ratios greater than 1 but less than 5 are reportedly more likely to be caused by prerenal proteinuria. Ratios greater than 5 but less than 13 may be due to either renal glomerular disease or postrenal inflammation. Ratios greater than 13 are most likely due to renal glomerular disease. Renal amyloidosis seems to cause the highest U-P/Cr. However, this assay cannot be used to differentiate immune-mediated glomerulonephritis from renal amyloidosis.

In most instances, U-P/Cr is used by veterinarians to make a presumptive diagnosis of protein-losing glomerular disease. However, the most common cause of proteinuria is urinary tract infection. Any time an abnormal U-P/Cr is identified, a urine culture should be performed to rule out infection as the cause. If the urine culture is negative in a dog or cat with an abnormal U-P/Cr, a normal plasma protein concentration, and no hemoglobinemia, a tentative diagnosis of glomerular disease can be made. A renal cortical biopsy is required to confirm glomerular disease as well as to differentiate immune-mediated glomerulonephritis from amyloidosis.

Factors that may influence the accuracy of U-P/Cr include exercise, diet, hemorrhage, and inflammation. It has been determined that the time of day has no influence on the U-P/Cr accuracy. Likewise, it seems that urine can be collected by cystocentesis, catheterization, or free catch without affecting accuracy. Dietary protein has the potential for slightly increasing the glomerular filtration rate and U-P/Cr. Hemorrhage into the urinary tract due to either poor collection technique or trauma increases the U-P/Cr. This increase is proportional to the degree of hemorrhage. Urinary tract inflammation also increases the U-P/Cr. Exercise has been shown to cause an increase in urine protein content in humans. Although it is generally believed that exercise has a similar effect on dog and cat urine protein excretion, it is not known whether the magnitude of change is significant.

ABNORMAL PROTEINURIA

Abnormal proteinuria may occur from prerenal, primary, or postrenal causes. Prerenal proteinuria occurs when excess small-molecular-weight proteins circulate through the kidney. Excess myeloma proteins, hemoglobin, and myoglobin are excreted in urine. Functional proteinuria may be considered a variant of prerenal proteinuria. Functional proteinuria is proteinuria derived from the kidney but in the absence of kidney disease. Strenuous exercise, fever, stress, and heart failure have all been associated with functional proteinuria. Functional and prerenal proteinuria is usually associated with a U-P/Cr of less than 5.

Renal proteinuria may occur as a result of acute or chronic damage to the nephron. However, acute tubular necrosis, acute or chronic renal failure, polycystic disease, or Fanconi's syndrome may result in mild proteinuria. Renal amyloidosis and glomerulonephritis are classic causes of renal

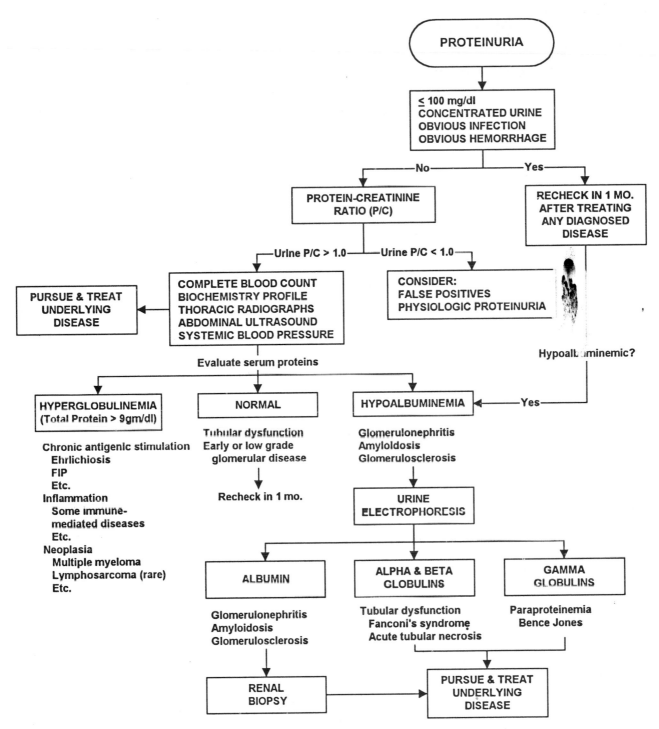

Figure 28–1. Algorithm for clinical evaluation of proteinuria.

proteinuria. In general, glomerular disease and pyelonephritis are the only abnormalities that produce appreciable, clinically significant renal proteinuria, and glomerular disease is the only renal proteinuria condition that induces hypoalbuminemia.

Postrenal proteinuria is caused by diseases of the ureter, urinary bladder, or urethra. In general, postrenal proteinuria is caused by infection, hemorrhage, or neoplasia in these areas.

DIAGNOSTIC APPROACH

The diagnostic approach to dogs and cats with abnormal proteinuria begins with an accurate history and thorough physical examination (Fig. 28–1). The goal is to localize the problem as accurately as possible. The history should identify whether the animal has signs of lower urinary tract inflammation that would cause postrenal proteinuria. Historical signs of systemic disease might be associated with a renal disorder. The animal should be evaluated for previous illnesses that might result in a chronic inflammatory condition. Chronic inflammation may be associated with glomerular disease.

The physical examination should include abdominal palpation to evaluate the kidney and bladder, as well as a digital rectal examination to evaluate the prostate. It should also include an ophthalmoscopic examination. Tortuous and dilated blood vessels, retinal hemorrhage or detachment, and hyphema may occur secondary to systemic hypertension, which can also cause glomerular disease. Physical exam findings that might be suggestive of a chronic inflammatory condition are important, because such disorders might lead to secondary glomerular disease.

Any animal suspected of having lower urinary tract disease or systemic illness should have a urinalysis performed.

Animals that are systemically ill should also have a complete blood count and serum biochemistry. Animals with abnormal proteinuria should also have a urine culture.

In certain conditions, survey and contrast abdominal radiographs, abdominal ultrasonography, or renal biopsy may be performed. Treatment and prognosis depend on the underlying cause of the abnormal proteinuria (see Fig. 28–1).

GASTROINTESTINAL-ABDOMINAL

CHAPTER 29

ANOREXIA

William E. Monroe

A good appetite for food is generally associated with health. Anorexia is loss of appetite for food, which is generally associated with illness. Reduced food consumption is a common manifestation of disease that is readily observable by pet owners and usually prompts them to seek veterinary attention. Anorexia may range from partial to complete, which may reflect the severity or cause of disease.

PATHOPHYSIOLOGY

The control of hunger and satiety involves a complex, multifaceted physiologic system. Not all the specific areas of the brain that may be involved with satiety and hunger have been identified, but the hypothalamus and caudal hindbrain (particularly the solitary nucleus) appear to be important. Satiety is associated with the absorptive phase when metabolic fuels are supplied by nutrients assimilated in the gastrointestinal tract. Hunger is associated with the postabsorptive phase when energy is derived from nutrients that are mobilized from body stores of triglyceride, glycogen, and protein.

The actual control of food intake is complex. Positive and negative sensory input such as palatability, texture, and quantity of recently consumed food affects appetite. Gastric and duodenal distention, as well as nutrient content of the gastrointestinal tract, affects satiety. Plasma concentration of nutrients, such as glucose and fatty acids, influences hunger by affecting peripheral (liver and gastrointestinal) and central (hypothalamic) nutrient-specific receptors. Whole body nutrient reserves, particularly the amount of adipose tissue, also influence appetite. The metabolic activity of tissues such as the liver also appears to be important to satiety. A decrease in the oxidation of metabolic fuels by the liver leads to hunger, and an increase in oxidation to satiety. Numerous hormones and peptides such as insulin, cholecystokinin, and glucagon inhibit food intake, whereas aldosterone, corticosterone, and insulin appear to stimulate appetite, depending on the circumstance. The neuropeptide serotonin

is an important stimulator of satiety, affecting both central (hypothalamic) and peripheral (perhaps pyloric) receptors. It is perhaps the final messenger leading to satiety. Learned behaviors and circadian rhythms play a modulating role in the control of appetite, which may override other physiologic signals for hunger and satiety.

Fear, pain, stress, trauma, organic disease, and neoplasia are all pathogenic events that may lead to anorexia. Ingestion of exogenous toxins or accumulation of endogenous toxins (uremia, hepatic disease), dehydration, and gastric overdistention may inhibit food intake via oxytocin or vasopressin producing parvocellular neurons in the paraventricular nucleus (PVN) of the hypothalamus. The reduction of food intake appears to be associated with decreased gastric motility initiated by the release of oxytocin or vasopressin by PVN neurons that project to the dorsomotor nucleus of the vagus. Cytokines, such as interleukin-1, tumor necrosis factor, and interferon, have negative effects on appetite, which may be important mechanisms for anorexia associated with infection, inflammation, and neoplasia. An increased concentration of tryptophan in the brain and peripherally appears to be important in the development of anorexia secondary to disease such as neoplasia, with the effects mediated by increased serotonin production centrally. Serotonin may be a final messenger in anorexia associated with disease, as well as in physiologic satiety. Any disorder that reduces cerebral arousal can also reduce food consumption. Gastroparesis may play an important role in the cause of anorexia seen in animals with diseases such as cancer or metabolic disorders.

The pathophysiologic consequences of acute starvation have not been studied extensively in hospitalized small animal patients. Malnutrition, however, has deleterious effects on all body systems. In human patients and some animal models, immune function appears to be affected early (within 48 hours) during acute starvation. Hospitalized, diseased human patients who are malnourished have higher rates of complications and infection, longer hospital stays, and increased risk of mortality than do those patients who are not malnourished. It is probably safe to assume that hospitalized veterinary patients suffer similar effects from malnourishment.

HISTORICAL FINDINGS

Environmental or psychologic factors that an owner may not perceive as significant (fear, dominance) may lead to anorexia. The addition of animals that are threatening or aggressive may interfere with eating. A new baby or other persons who make an animal feel threatened or ignored, or a change of housing, may also affect appetite. Changing the diet to one that is less palatable may also lead to anorexia or a reduced appetite.

Animals lacking a sense of smell (anosmia) may have difficulty finding their food. Pets with oral, pharyngeal, or cranial pain or dysfunction may show an interest in food but cannot eat. Pets with retrobulbar abscesses, masticatory myositis, mandibular fractures, maxillary or nasal fractures or masses, oral foreign bodies, periodontal disease, or broken or loose teeth may attempt to eat but stop, cry out, or drop food. Some may exhibit no interest in eating. There may be a history of trauma, feeding of bones, chewing on sticks or other potential sources of self-trauma, or an oral foreign body that inhibits eating. Dogs with neurologic dysfunction, such as trigeminal neuritis or other swallowing disorders, may attempt to eat with their tongues but drop food and be unable to consume sufficient quantities.

The historical findings in animals that do not eat because of systemic disease are variable and depend on the disease present. In general, animals that are anorexic because of systemic disease have no interest in food. Pain, lameness, motor dysfunction, urination abnormalities, vomiting, diarrhea, coughing, and dyspnea may all be signs of disease that leads to anorexia. Animals with neurologic disease resulting in decreased eating because of reduced cerebral arousal may have a history of behavioral changes or stupor.

PHYSICAL FINDINGS

Animals that are anorexic because of psychologic causes such as environmental stress or unpalatable diet usually appear normal on physical examination. Bite or fight wounds may be present in pets that are not eating because of another dominant animal or excessive competition.

To determine if an animal is having trouble finding food because of poor sense of smell, the pet can be blindfolded and aromatic food placed near its nose. If there is no sniffing behavior, the animal may not be able to smell. Observing the animal walk around the examination room where other animals have been may also reveal if it has a sense of smell. Most cats and dogs in such an environment exhibit sniffing behavior.

An animal that is unable to eat because of pain or dysfunction of the oral area may resist and cry out when the mouth is opened for examination. Fractures, soft tissue trauma, neoplasia, craniomandibular arthritis or osteoarthropathy, masticatory myositides, and retrobulbar masses may all be associated with pain when attempting to open the mouth. Abnormalities of the face, mandible, nose, mouth, or skull may be apparent. Evidence of dental disease such as severe plaque and calculus, loose or broken teeth, or pain or exudation when applying pressure to or tapping on the teeth may be noted. Ulcers, wounds, stomatitis, gingivitis, masses, or

foreign bodies such as sticks, rocks, or bones may be noted when examining the mouth and pharynx. If nasal disease is the cause of poor appetite, nasal swelling, epistaxis, mucopurulent discharge, masses, or ulceration of the mucocutaneous junctions of the nares may be seen. Exophthalmos is often noted with retrobulbar abscesses or tumors and masticatory myositides. Trigeminal neuritis or trauma to the jaw may be associated with a dropped jaw and inability to eat.

Physical examination abnormalities associated with systemic diseases causing anorexia are as varied as the potential causes of disease. Fever, pallor, jaundice, abdominal pain, spinal or limb pain, abnormally small or large organ size, ocular abnormalities, abdominal distention from fluid accumulation, dyspnea, muffled heart and lung sounds, adventitial breath sounds, cardiac murmurs, masses, or swellings are all signs of disease that may lead to anorexia.

DIAGNOSTIC PLAN

With psychologic causes of anorexia, the history is the most important diagnostic tool (Fig. 29-1). The importance of a thorough history and physical examination cannot be overemphasized. Pets that are anorexic, particularly those that seem interested in food but are unable or refuse to eat, should receive a thorough oral, dental, and cranial examination. If the dog or cat is uncooperative, sedation or anesthesia may be necessary. In addition to the more routine physical examination procedures, the spine should be carefully palpated for pain (e.g., discospondylitis), and a careful rectal examination should be performed in all dogs—male, female, or neutered—to assess the prostate, detect the presence of other masses, or detect unreported abnormalities such as hematochezia or perineal hernia. A thorough ocular examination should be performed, including fundic examination after pupil dilatation. Systemic diseases such as feline infectious peritonitis, lymphoma, deep mycoses, toxoplasmosis, canine distemper, and rickettsial infections may have characteristic ocular changes.

Pets without a history of a psychologic cause of anorexia and that have no abnormalities noted on the physical examination should have a minimal database performed that includes a complete blood count, heartworm test, tests for feline leukemia virus and feline immunodeficiency virus in cats, serum chemistry analysis, and urinalysis, including microscopic examination of the sediment. These tests may aid in the diagnosis of inflammatory, degenerative, endocrine, metabolic, neoplastic, or toxic disorders that can lead to anorexia. If systemic disease seems the probable cause of anorexia, further diagnostic testing should be directed toward abnormalities identified by the history, physical examination, or minimal database. For cases in which no historical, physical, or database abnormalities can be found, thoracic and abdominal radiographs or ultrasonography may reveal evidence of occult disorders such as masses, gastrointestinal foreign bodies, or pericardial, pleural, or abdominal fluid. If no abnormalities are noted with those procedures, a gastrointestinal radiographic contrast study or endoscopy may be indicated to identify otherwise inapparent neoplasia or other infiltrative gastrointestinal diseases.

GOALS OF TREATMENT

The first goal of therapy for anorexia is to correct the underlying cause. The animal should be supported with

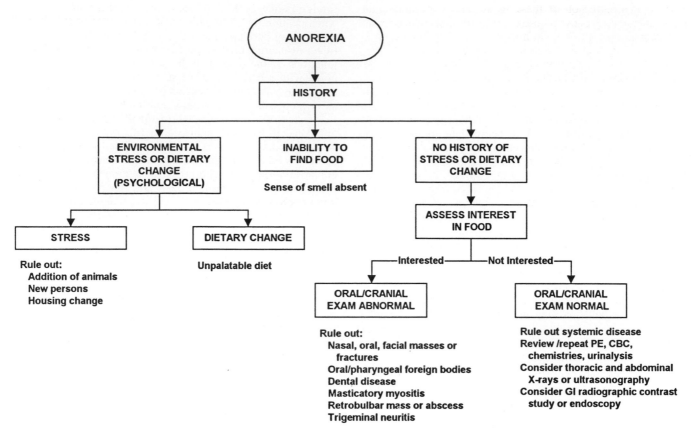

Figure 29–1. Algorithm for evaluation of anorexia.

fluids and appropriate electrolyte therapy until the diagnosis is made and definitive treatment initiated. If an animal is anorexic for more than 3 to 5 days, it should receive nutritional support in the form of enteral or parenteral feeding (see Chapter 71). Drug therapy to stimulate appetite has generally focused on agents affecting central nervous system control of feeding, such as benzodiazepines and cyproheptadine (serotonin antagonist). Recently, megestrol acetate has been useful for stimulating appetite in human patients with cancer. The efficacy of gastrokinetic agents such as metoclopramide and cisapride for stimulating eating in anorexic animals has not been determined, although limited studies in selected human patients have yielded positive results.

CHAPTER 30

POLYPHAGIA

Ellen N. Behrend

Polyphagia is the consumption of food in excess of normal caloric need. Hunger, satiety, and eating behavior are primarily controlled by specific regions within the central nervous system (CNS), but many factors affect the function of these areas. Thus, polyphagia can be classified as primary (a CNS abnormality) or secondary (a systemic problem affecting the CNS). Secondary polyphagia is by far more common and is usually accompanied by clinical signs of the underlying disease. Determining whether weight gain or loss has occurred should be the first step in formulating a list of differential diagnoses and a diagnostic plan.

PHYSIOLOGY

Eating behavior is controlled by the hypothalamus. The lateral nuclei of the hypothalamus represent the "feeding center," as stimulation of these areas causes an animal to eat, and their destruction results in severe, fatal anorexia. Conversely, the ventromedial nuclei are the "satiety center" because stimulation of these areas causes a refusal to eat even highly appetizing food, and their ablation leads to excessive eating and obesity. The feeding center appears to be constantly active unless inhibited by the satiety center, e.g., postprandially.

Other neural and non-neural factors play a regulatory role. Lesions of the amygdala or paraventricular nuclei can increase appetite. Non-neural factors such as decreased serum concentrations of glucose, amino acids, or lipid metabolites result in hunger by stimulating neural centers. Eating behavior can also be enhanced by increased utilization of nutrients, i.e., an increased metabolic rate. Conversely, insulin, glucagon, and cholecystokinin secreted in response to a meal decrease hunger via the CNS. Leptin, a polypeptide released from adipose tissue, may also help create a sense of satiety.

Thus, control of appetite is complex, working to maintain energy stores and body weight through an interplay of central and peripheral stimuli. Pathology that affects the CNS can increase appetite even in the presence of normal energy stores (primary polyphagia). Secondary polyphagia exists when hunger is stimulated by non-neural factors to restore or maintain energy reserves. This arises in response to an increased metabolic rate or decreased nutrient supply (Table 30–1). An augmented metabolic rate can be physiologic (e.g., pregnancy) or pathologic (e.g., hyperthyroidism). Diabetes mellitus is an unusual cause of decreased nutrient supply. Owing to an inability to respond to insulin or to a lack thereof, the body does not recognize glucose and reacts to a perceived hypoglycemia. Secondary polyphagia can also be a side effect of certain drugs (see Table 30–1).

HISTORY AND PHYSICAL EXAMINATION

Change in body weight is an important component in differentiating the various causes of polyphagia (see Table 30 1; Fig. 30–1). Primary or drug-induced polyphagia typically results in weight gain because excess nutrients are ingested. Physiologic polyphagia can result in weight gain (e.g., pregnancy, growth) or maintenance of weight (e.g., lactation, cold environment, increased exercise). If pathologic, secondary polyphagia is more commonly associated with weight loss, because the nutrient supply usually does not meet physiologic demand. Some disorders, such as acromegaly, hypoglycemia due to insulinoma, sudden acquired retinal degeneration syndrome (SARDS), and hyperadrenocorticism (Cushing's syndrome), result in weight gain. A dog or cat in the early stage of any disorder, however, may have no weight change.

Certain causes of polyphagia may be diagnosed on the basis of history. The possibility of exposure to a cold environment, increased exercise, and, for intact females, pregnancy and lactation should be ascertained. Polyphagia is commonly associated with use of anticonvulsants and glucocorticoids but has been observed with other medications (see Table 30–1). Psychogenic polyphagia has been noted after introduction of a more palatable diet or in response to a traumatic event, most commonly introduction of a new pet into the household. Feeding of a low-calorie diet may also be diagnosed on the basis of a complete dietary history.

An animal with primary polyphagia due to destruction of the satiety center may have a history of trauma or clinical

TABLE 30–1. CAUSES OF POLYPHAGIA

Primary Polyphagia	Secondary Polyphagia
Destruction of satiety center	Physiologic increased metabolic rate
Trauma	Cold temperature
Mass lesion (e.g., neoplasia)	Lactation
Infection	Pregnancy
Psychogenic	Growth
	Increased exercise
Drug-Induced Polyphagia	Pathologic increased metabolic rate
Glucocorticoids	Hyperthyroidism
Anticonvulsants	Acromegaly
Antihistamines	Decreased energy supply
Progestins	Diabetes mellitus
Benzodiazepines	Malassimilation syndromes
Amitraz	Pancreatic exocrine insufficiency
Reported Specific Cases Associated With Polyphagia	Infiltrative bowel disease
	Parasites
Feline infectious peritonitis	Lymphangiectasia
Lymphocytic cholangitis (feline)	Decreased intake
Spongiform encephalopathy (feline)	Megaesophagus (congenital)
	Low-calorie diet
	Hypoglycemia
	Unknown
	Hyperadrenocorticism
	Portosystemic shunt/ hepatoencephalopathy
	Sudden acquired retinal degeneration syndrome (SARDS)

signs associated with CNS disease. Perturbation of hypothalamic control of the pituitary can lead to reproductive, thyroidal, and/or adrenal hypofunction and associated clinical signs. Signs caused by diffuse or multifocal CNS disease depend on the affected areas. A complete neurologic examination should be performed, as well as a fundic examination with evaluation of the optic nerve.

Historical findings associated with secondary polyphagia are variable. Dogs and cats with diabetes mellitus, acromegaly, Cushing's, SARDS, and hyperthyroidism usually have a history of polyuria and polydipsia. Feline acromegaly is seen in middle-aged to older males and spontaneous canine acromegaly almost exclusively in intact bitches. In dogs of either sex, progestin administration can lead to reversible acromegaly, and use of this medication should be historically evident. It should also be noted that progestin administration in dogs and cats can increase appetite without causing acromegaly. Owners may note inspiratory stridor or a change in body conformation, such as increased interdental spaces, skin folds, or size of the head in acromegalic animals. A multitude of historical abnormalities can be associated with Cushing's syndrome, including abdominal enlargement, persistent panting, failure to regrow hair after clipping, lethargy, and muscle weakness. Animals with SARDS typically have the presenting complaint of sudden-onset blindness. Hyperthyroidism commonly leads to increased activity, especially in cats, but can be associated with depression and lethargy.

Multiple causes of hypoglycemia exist, but insulinoma is the most likely to cause polyphagia. Dogs (cats are diagnosed much less frequently) with insulinoma may exhibit signs due to severe hypoglycemia such as weakness, trembling, ataxia, disorientation, and, possibly, grand mal seizures. Pancreatic exocrine insufficiency (PEI) is most commonly diagnosed in dogs younger than 2 years of age, with a predisposition in the German shepherd. Rarely, PEI has been diagnosed in older dogs, usually due to chronic

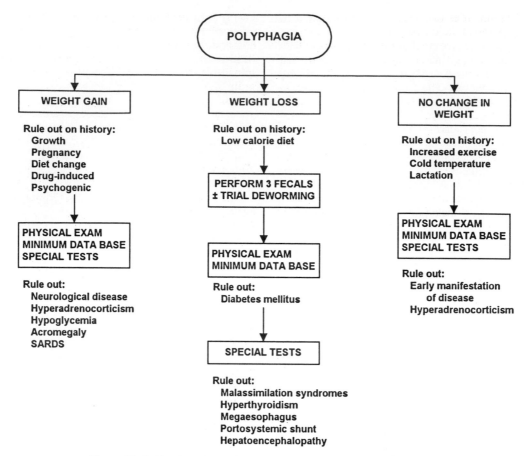

Figure 30–1. Algorithm for differential diagnosis and evaluation of polyphagia.

pancreatitis. Malassimilation syndromes and PEI generally cause large-volume, malodorous, soft stools. Acquired esophageal disease often leads to anorexia, but animals with congenital megaesophagus may be polyphagic and typically have a history of regurgitation. Although anorexia is more common in animals with a portocaval shunt, polyphagia has been reported in approximately 10 per cent of cases. Depression, vomiting, weight loss, polydipsia, and neurologic signs may also be noted. Polyphagia is rare in dogs with hepatoencephalopathy; other clinical findings are caused by hepatic failure and may be similar to those of an animal with a portosystemic shunt.

Physical examination findings in polyphagic animals vary, depending on the underlying disease. If it is unclear from the history, pregnancy can potentially be diagnosed by abdominal palpation, and lactation by inspection of the mammae. Animals with hyperthyroidism may have a palpable thyroid nodule, and a significant number of hyperthyroid cats have tachycardia or a gallop rhythm. Hyperadrenocorticism can have a variety of physical examination findings, including abdominal and hepatic enlargement, muscle wasting, and bilaterally symmetric alopecia or areas of poor hair regrowth. Although not noted by an owner, the physical changes associated with acromegaly can be documented on physical examination; a degenerative polyarthropathy may also be present. Examination findings in a dog with SARDS may be unremarkable, because in the early stages of the disease, the retinas appear normal on fundic examination.

Animals with PEI, insulinoma, megaesophagus, hepatoencephalopathy, portosystemic shunt, or malassimilation syndrome may have no abnormal physical findings other than the associated weight change. In rare cases, polyneuropathies may accompany insulinoma. Aspiration pneumonia may be present in animals with megaesophagus. Neurologic abnormalities may be detected in an animal with a portosystemic shunt; ascites is diagnosed in a minority of cases, and icterus is rare. Neurologic findings associated with hepatoencephalopathy may be episodic, and other examination findings vary with the cause of liver disease. Depending on the cause of malassimilation, the intestines may feel thickened. Lymphangiectasia may lead to ascites.

Occasionally, polyphagia may be a clinical sign for a disease with which it is not usually associated. For example, a cat with feline infectious peritonitis was reported to be polyphagic, as were 18 cats in Great Britain with lymphocytic cholangitis. Other historical and clinical signs may be present, depending on the cause.

DIAGNOSTIC PLAN

The first step in diagnosis is to ascertain what change, if any, has occurred in the animal's weight (see Fig. 30–1). After as many differential diagnoses as possible have been ruled out on the basis of history, further testing is warranted. In all cases, a minimal database including serum biochemistry profile, complete blood count, and urinalysis should be submitted.

For dogs and cats with weight gain, pregnancy must be ruled out by abdominal ultrasonography during early gestation or by radiography in later stages. To diagnose primary polyphagia, a complete neurologic examination should be performed, any abnormalities localized, and appropriate tests obtained. A cerebrospinal fluid analysis or diagnostic imaging such as radiography, computed tomography (CT), or magnetic resonance imaging (MRI) may be necessary. Hypoglycemia due to insulinoma can often be diagnosed by measuring the serum and insulin concentration after a fast long enough for the blood glucose to fall below 60 to 70 mg/dL (usually 4 to 6 hours). The diagnosis of SARDS can be made on the basis of appropriate history, physical examination findings, a database that rules out other causes, and, if necessary, an electroretinogram. Although certain changes in the minimal database are typical of Cushing's syndrome, they do not confirm the diagnosis, and further adrenal tests are warranted (see Chapter 154). Diagnosis of acromegaly can be difficult owing to lack of a commercial assay for growth hormone, but measurement of insulin-like growth factor-1 may be helpful (see Chapter 147). Conformational changes can provide evidence of an acromegalic syndrome if the dog is an intact female or has received progestin therapy. Acromegalic cats usually have insulin-resistant diabetes mellitus, and imaging of the pituitary (CT or MRI) usually reveals a tumor.

If weight loss is associated with polyphagia, the minimal database should be preceded by three fecal examinations. If these are negative, the database does not provide the diagnosis, and the animal is stable, trial therapy with parasiticides may be warranted. If deworming does not resolve the problem, additional tests need to be done. Hyperthyroidism can often be diagnosed on the basis of a single serum thyroxine measurement, but other tests may be required (see Chapter 150). Malassimilation syndromes cover myriad differential diagnoses (see Table 30–1). Depending on the suspected

cause, measurement of serum folate or cobalamin, assessment of fat absorption, or biopsy by either endoscopy or exploratory surgery may also be considered. For verification of PEI, serum trypsin-like immunoreactivity should be determined. Thoracic radiographs with a positive contrast esophagram should be used to diagnose megaesophagus. Determination of pre- and postprandial serum bile acid concentrations documents hepatic dysfunction, but a biopsy may be required to document the cause of hepatic failure. Ultrasonography may be used to identify a portocaval shunt.

If the disease is in the early stages, weight change may not have occurred, so the list of differentials may be difficult to narrow. However, a good history and physical examination eliminate many possibilities. Although animals with Cushing's syndrome may not have a weight change, abdominal enlargement may create the impression of weight gain.

MANAGEMENT

The management of polyphagia depends on the cause. Physiologic causes of polyphagia are transient. If drug-induced, the polyphagia may be temporary, as is usually seen with anticonvulsants. If polyphagia persists, the medication can be discontinued, or food intake should be limited to that necessary to satisfy caloric requirements. Polyphagia due to dietary factors can be managed as needed. Psychogenic polyphagia may be corrected by removing the instigating element, if possible, or by behavioral therapy (e.g., paying more attention to the animal). In cases of SARDS, polyphagia is usually self limited. For all other conditions, appropriate therapy should be initiated to resolve the underlying disease.

CHAPTER 31

PTYALISM

Linda J. DeBowes

Ptyalism refers to the excessive production of saliva. Pseudoptyalism is the dribbling or drooling of saliva that has accumulated in the oral cavity. The purpose of this chapter is to review those disorders that result in excessive salivation or drooling of saliva from the oral cavity.

GENERAL PATHOPHYSIOLOGY

The salivary nuclei located in the brain stem are excited by taste and tactile stimuli from the tongue and other areas of the mouth. Higher centers in the central nervous system (CNS) also have excitatory or inhibitory input into the salivary nuclei. When the salivary nuclei are stimulated, the formation and secretion of saliva increase. Oral lesions and CNS disorders may stimulate increased production of saliva.

Pharyngeal and esophageal diseases may also stimulate salivary secretions. Inflamed gastric mucosa may stimulate the salivary glands to produce excessive volumes of saliva. Excessive salivation may not be clinically obvious if the saliva is being swallowed. The predominant clinical sign may be excessive swallowing instead of excessive salivation. The repeated swallowing of foamy saliva results in an accumulation of air in the stomach and increased belching.

Saliva is continuously secreted into the oral cavity from the salivary glands. Anatomic abnormalities may cause saliva to drip from an animal's lips even when secretion is normal. If the normal amount of secreted saliva is not swallowed, the accumulated saliva drools from the mouth. Drooling is associated with diseases that interfere with normal swallowing because of an inability to swallow or an unwillingness to swallow owing to pain.

HISTORICAL FINDINGS AND THEIR MEANINGS

Age and Breed. Congenital anomalies (e.g., megaesophagus and portosystemic shunt) should be considered in young animals with hypersalivation. An increased incidence of congenital portosystemic shunt has been reported in certain pure breed dogs (e.g., Yorkshire terriers, Australian cattle dogs, Maltese terriers, Irish wolfhounds, miniature schnauzers). Puppies and kittens are more likely to have ingested a foreign body, bitten an electric cord, or ingested caustic compounds or toxins. Constant or intermittent drooling may be present at an early age in dogs or cats with conformational abnormalities of the jaw or lips. Severe retrognathism may result in a significant amount of drooling. Giant breeds, especially the Newfoundland and Saint Bernard, are prone to excessive drooling.

Diet. Excessive salivation and other signs of hepatic encephalopathy may be precipitated by a diet high in protein. A dog or cat with excessive salivation secondary to painful oral lesions may refuse to eat.

Eating Behavior. If excessive salivation is the result of oral pain, a dog or cat may change its eating behavior. With oral or dental pain, the animal may take a bite of food and then release it because of pain on chewing, or it may hold the head in unusual positions while attempting to eat. With a unilateral lesion, the animal may not chew on the affected side. A change in food preference to avoid eating dry (hard) foods may occur when painful oral lesions are present.

Anorexia and Weight Loss. Partial or complete anorexia may occur with acute or chronic oral lesions and with systemic diseases. Cats with severe oral ulcerative inflammatory disease often stop eating. Disorders of the intestinal tract may also lead to anorexia and weight loss.

Medications and Topical Products. Adverse reactions, including hypersalivation, can occur with the oral administration of cholinergic drugs (e.g., bethanechol) or anticholinesterase drugs (e.g., pyridostigmine). Parasite control products that contain cholinesterase inhibitors (e.g., organophosphate, carbamate) may result in cholinergic signs (e.g., ptyalism) if an overdose is given. Pyrethrin and pyrethroid insecticides may also cause ptyalism. Mild to severe hypersalivation is the most immediate sign in cats with D-limolene toxicosis (citrus oil insecticide). Ivermectin toxicity in dogs may cause increased salivation as well as other neurologic signs. Cats administered fluids containing a benzoic acid derivative (e.g., benzyl alcohol) as a preservative have developed clinical signs including hypersalivation, neurologic changes, and death. Oral ulceration may occur along with cutaneous lesions in animals with drug eruption or toxic epidermal necrolysis (see Chapter 7).

Environment. The environmental history is important to determine whether there is a known or potential exposure to products that may be caustic or toxic. Household cleaning products (e.g., cationic detergents, fabric softeners, disinfectants, phenol/phenolic compounds, pine oil disinfectants, bleaches) may cause irritation to the tissues in the oral cavity. Dogs and cats may ingest these directly or while grooming themselves. Chewing on house plants (e.g., dieffenbachia, poinsettia, Christmas tree) may cause oral inflammation with increased salivation. Illicit drugs (e.g., amphetamines, cocaine, opiates) and toxins resulting in CNS stimulation may cause excessive salivation. Caffeine toxicosis causes ptyalism as well as other signs of CNS stimulation. Many insecticides contain boric acid, which stimulates excess salivation. Increases in environmental temperature result in increased salivation in dogs and cats, especially dogs. Foreign bodies (e.g., bones, needles) may become lodged in the mouth, oropharynx, or esophagus and cause ptyalism. Dogs and cats may bite on electric cords, damaging tissue and causing oral pain, and excessive salivation.

Cats are especially sensitive to venom from black widow spiders. One of the clinical signs is excessive salivation. Increased salivation along with CNS signs also occurs with Gila monster and North American scorpion envenomation. Ptyalism is the most common clinical sign in dogs with pseudorabies. Pseudorabies should be considered in any dog that has acute ptyalism and has been exposed to swine.

Rubbing or Pawing at the Face or Mouth. Dogs with oral cavity problems (or hypocalcemia) may rub their muzzles on the ground. Dogs and cats may also paw at the face if they have pain or discomfort associated with the face or mouth.

Anesthesia. Reflux esophagitis is a potential complication of anesthesia. Signs of esophageal disease (e.g., hypersalivation, regurgitation) usually develop 1 to 4 days following the anesthetic procedure.

Swallowing Difficulty. Dysphagia should be confirmed by observing the dog or cat eating and drinking. Animals with problems swallowing may drool excessively. Rabies should be included in the differential diagnosis in any animal with difficulty swallowing.

Regurgitation. Regurgitation is a classic sign of esophageal disease, and animals with esophageal disease may salivate excessively. Regurgitation must be differentiated from vomiting. Hypersalivation, regurgitation, and vomiting are often noted soon after eating in cases of chronic reflux esophagitis.

Vomiting. Nausea, which is the first stage in the complex act of vomiting, may be accompanied by increased salivation and repeated attempts at swallowing.

Behavioral Changes. Dogs or cats with oral pain may have a change in their behavior. They may become aggressive and growl if disturbed or become more reclusive. Behavioral changes (e.g., aggression, depression) may be associated with hepatic encephalopathy, and ptyalism is a common clinical sign in cats with portosystemic shunts. Sudden behavior changes occur in rabid dogs or cats.

Hepatic Encephalopathy Signs. CNS signs, behavioral changes, and signs of hepatic failure (e.g., anorexia, weight loss, lethargy, polydipsia, polyuria, nausea, hypersalivation, vomiting, and diarrhea) should alert the clinician to the possibility of hepatic encephalopathy. Ptyalism is a common clinical sign in cats with portosystemic shunts. Signs of hepatic encephalopathy, which may be intermittent, may be precipitated by foods with a high level of protein or in association with gastrointestinal bleeding.

Seizures. Autonomic discharge may occur during a seizure, resulting in salivation, urination, and defecation. During a generalized seizure, an animal does not swallow saliva, and the chomping jaw action may exacerbate the drooling. Animals observed following a seizure may show evidence of increased salivation. Seizures may result from exposure to a number of toxins that also increase salivation (e.g., organophosphates).

PHYSICAL FINDINGS AND THEIR INTERPRETATION

Halitosis. Animals with ulcerated, infected, and necrotic oral lesions may have mild to severe halitosis. Esophageal disease may also result in halitosis if there is esophageal ulceration or necrosis or if food remains in the esophagus for prolonged periods. Gastric disorders are potential causes of halitosis.

Oral Cavity (see also Chapter 131)

Periodontal Disease. Dogs and cats may have severe gingival and oral mucosal inflammation in association with advanced periodontitis. Increased salivation may occur as a result of pain and inflammation.

Stomatitis. Inflammation and ulceration of the oral mucosa may cause significant discomfort, resulting in excessive salivation. Irritants, foreign bodies, trauma, periodontal disease, and other local factors may cause inflammation of the oral mucosa. Immune-mediated disease (e.g., pemphigus vulgaris) may cause ulcerative stomatitis with or without involvement of the mucocutaneous junctions. Systemic infections (e.g., feline immunodeficiency virus), toxins (e.g., thallium), and immunologic (e.g., neutropenia) or nutritional deficiencies may also cause inflammation in the oral cavity.

Oral Masses. Neoplasms, eosinophilic granulomas, and granulomatous lesions may be present in the oral cavity. Lesions that ulcerate and become painful may cause excessive salivation. They may also cause problems with swallowing if they are located in the caudal portion of the oral cavity or interfere with movement of the tongue. Ptyalism is a common clinical sign in dogs with tongue tumors. Tonsillar tumors or tumors in the pharyngeal region may cause dysphagia leading to excessive drooling. The saliva may be dark or blood tinged if the lesions become ulcerated or necrotic.

Glossitis. Lingual ulcers are painful and may result in excessive salivation. They may occur as a result of trauma (e.g., chemical irritants) to the tongue, systemic infections (viral), metabolic disorders (uremia), immune-mediated disease (e.g., pemphigus vulgaris), and tumors (e.g., squamous cell carcinoma). Lingual and palatal ulcers, along with an oculonasal discharge, may be present with herpesvirus and calicivirus infection in cats.

Base of Tongue. The base of the tongue should be examined for masses or evidence of a foreign body. Linear foreign bodies frequently get caught at the base of the tongue and may cut into the frenulum. Masses beneath the tongue may cause ptyalism secondary to pain; if there is difficulty in swallowing, the animal may drool.

Faucitis. Severe inflammation and ulceration of the glossopalatine arch are observed primarily in cats. Affected cats appear to be in pain and may be reluctant to have their mouths opened. They frequently have blood-tinged saliva dripping from their lips.

Blood-Tinged Saliva. Blood-tinged saliva indicates potential bleeding from the oral cavity, upper intestinal tract, or nasal passages. Hemoptysis may also cause blood-tinged saliva.

Ulcerations at Mucocutaneous Junctions. Immune-mediated skin disorders (e.g., pemphigus vulgaris) may cause ulceration at the mucocutaneous junctions. If ulcerative stomatitis is also present, an immune-mediated disease should be considered.

Facial Pain. A dog or cat with excessive salivation due to oral or pharyngeal disease may experience considerable pain and resist handling of the face and opening of the mouth.

Dysphagia. Animals that are drooling excessively should be evaluated for dysphagia, which may be caused by anatomic problems in the oral cavity or pharynx. The animal may be reluctant to attempt swallowing if swallowing causes pain. Neuromuscular dysfunction of cranial or pharyngeal muscles may also cause dysphagia (see Chapter 33).

Regurgitation. Regurgitation indicates an esophageal disorder. Ptyalism may also be a clinical sign of esophageal disease (e.g., foreign body, esophagitis) (see Chapter 135).

Cranial Nerve Deficits. Lesions of cranial nerves IX and X often cause dysphagia and a weak or absent gag reflex. Dysfunction of cranial nerve XII may also cause difficulty in swallowing. Animals with facial nerve paralysis may drool from the affected side.

Dropped Jaw. An animal with trigeminal nerve paralysis is unable to close its mouth and drools. The differential diagnosis should include idiopathic trigeminal nerve neuritis, trauma, and infectious disease (e.g., rabies).

Muscle Atrophy. Muscle atrophy may be secondary to cranial nerve deficits or diseases of the muscles (e.g., myositis) that result in a swallowing problem.

Lymph Nodes. Lymphadenopathy, especially enlarged retropharyngeal lymph nodes, may cause dysphagia.

Salivary Glands. Enlarged, painful, and firm salivary glands may indicate a salivary gland problem. In rare instances, ptyalism has been reported to be the result of salivary gland enlargement or necrosis.

DIAGNOSTIC PLAN

For an algorithm depicting a diagnostic plan, see Figure 31–1. A complete history should be obtained to determine whether clinical signs other than ptyalism are present. A complete physical examination should be performed to evaluate for systemic disease. The oral cavity and surrounding structures (e.g., salivary glands, lymph nodes, muscles) should be examined thoroughly. Cranial and cervical structures should be evaluated carefully for any change in size, symmetry, and pain. Sedation or anesthesia may be required if the animal is in too much pain or is difficult to examine. The animal should be observed while eating and drinking to evaluate for evidence of dysphagia. Rabies should be included as a differential diagnosis for any dog or cat with ptyalism and difficulty swallowing (see Chapter 88). The cranial nerves and muscles of mastication should be evaluated to determine whether a neuromuscular disorder causing dysphagia may be causing the drooling.

The source of excessive salivation or drooling may be apparent after careful examination of the oral cavity. The etiology of oral lesions may be revealed by the history (e.g., exposure to caustic or irritating materials), physical examination (e.g., foreign body, severe periodontal disease), or identification of a conformational problem (e.g., severe retrognathism) (see Chapter 131). Oral or cervical masses identified on physical examination should be evaluated either by fine-needle aspiration and cytology study or by biopsy and histopathologic study. Thoracic radiographs and evaluation of local lymph nodes are indicated when oral neoplasia is suspected. Exfoliative cytology of oral lesions may be beneficial in some cases (e.g., cryptococcosis). Culture of exudate from the oral cavity is generally unrewarding. Immune-mediated disease (e.g., pemphigus vulgaris) is evaluated by histologic and immunofluorescence examinations of skin and oral biopsies (see Chapter 131). Glossitis and oral inflammatory diseases of unknown etiology require a more complete diagnostic evaluation. If oral lesions are accompanied by signs of systemic disease, a minimal database (e.g., complete blood count, chemistry profile, urinalysis) should be collected so that the animal can be evaluated for systemic disease.

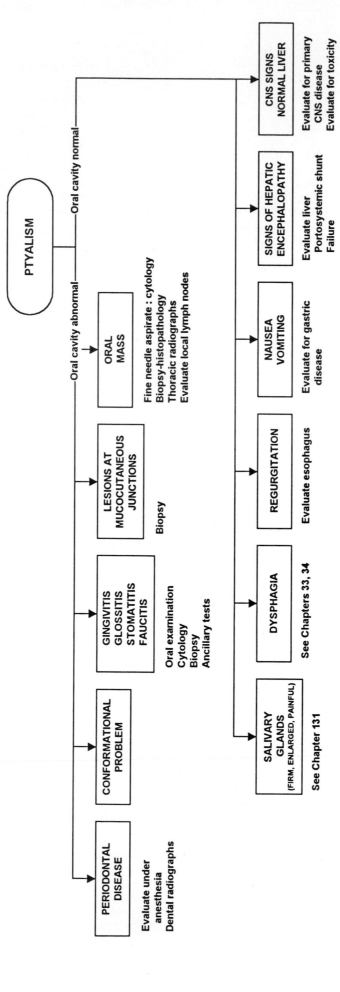

Figure 31–1. Algorithm for differential diagnosis of ptyalism.

CHAPTER 32

GAGGING

Mark J. Kopit

Gagging is a reflexive contraction of the constrictor muscles of the pharynx resulting from stimulation of the pharyngeal mucosa. It generally indicates that the neurologic pathways associated with the normal reflex are intact. Most neurologic disorders result in reduced gag reflex and a lack of gagging. Although gagging is commonly associated with other clinical signs, such as coughing, it can be the sole presenting complaint.

In many cases, gagging and retching are seen together. Retching is an involuntary and ineffectual attempt at vomiting and is caused by the same motor events that cause vomiting. It is associated with nausea. Expectoration is ejection of airway and laryngopharyngeal mucus or discharges and is not associated with nausea. It usually follows an episode of coughing such as that seen in animals with tracheobronchitis. Retching is discussed in Chapter 34.

Evaluation of gagging should include a thorough history and physical examination to obtain information about other historical data or problems that may relate to the complaint. Gagging may be related to a problem involving the nasal passage (causing postnasal pharyngeal discharge), pharynx, respiratory tract, or upper gastrointestinal tract. Atypical causes include pericardial effusion with ascites, middle ear neoplasia with extension of the mass into the pharynx, and familial progressive nephropathy.

HISTORY

The historical considerations that are important in evaluating a dog or cat with gagging relate to environmental circumstances and other clinical manifestations. Questions regarding sneezing; coughing; vomiting or regurgitation; salivation; appetite; activity level; overall strength; voice change; onset, duration, and progression of signs; environmental surroundings; foreign body exposure; potential for toxin exposure or ingestion; past medical problems; and relationship of all the foregoing to gagging need to be asked. Vaccine history, particularly rabies, must also be discussed.

PHYSICAL EXAMINATION

Physical examination of the oral cavity, pharyngeal and cervical palpation, thoracic auscultation, abdominal palpation, and evaluation of passage of air from the nares must all be completed. The examination may be continued with sedation or light anesthesia to perform complete tonsilar crypt, oropharyngeal, and laryngeal evaluations, as well as a thorough otoscopic examination. If the dog or cat is geriatric, is not in acute distress, and other systemic illness is suspected, a complete blood count, metabolic profile, urinalysis, and thyroid evaluation should be considered before chemical restraint.

A list of causes of gagging is presented in Table 32–1. The list has been subdivided by body region and morphologic versus functional causes. The algorithm presented in Figure 32–1 has been divided by other clinical signs present in the animal. There can be overlap of clinical signs among the different causes. In addition to the tests mentioned in the previous paragraph, radiography, computed tomography, or magnetic resonance imaging of the skull, pharynx, cervical region, thorax, and abdomen may be needed. Table 32–1 also has testing procedures that might aid in diagnosing the cause of gagging. Additional laboratory tests may include adrenocorticotropic hormone response testing, intravenous edrophonium (Tensilon) administration, acetylcholine receptor antibody determination, acetylcholinesterase level, bile acid clearance, histopathology, and nerve conduction testing. Other procedures to consider include rhinoscopy, bronchoscopy, esophagoscopy, gastroduodenoscopy, thoracic and abdominal sonography, barium swallow, upper gastrointestinal barium study, and fluoroscopy of the pharynx, esophagus, and stomach.

TABLE 32–1. DIFFERENTIAL DIAGNOSIS AND POTENTIAL DIAGNOSTIC TESTS FOR GAGGING DOGS OR CATS

I. Nasal sinus
   A. Cleft palate—complete oropharyngeal exam
   B. Nasal parasites—complete oropharyngeal exam, radiography of nasal passage, nasal aspirate cytology, visual exam of nasal passage (rostral and/or retrograde), CT/MRI scan, exploratory surgery of nasal sinus
   C. Nasal tumors—same as B plus histopathology
   D. Severe obstructive rhinitis—same as C
   E. Nasal foreign body—same as B plus foreign body retrieval

II. Pharynx (morphologic)
   A. Neoplasia—complete oropharyngeal exam, radiography of pharyngeal region, CT/MRI scan, fine-needle aspiration with cytology, core-needle biopsy with histopathology, exploratory surgery with histopathology
   B. Foreign body—same as A plus fistulogram
   C. Tonsilar enlargement—same as A
   D. Abscess—same as A
   E. Elongated soft palate—complete oropharyngeal exam
   F. Nasopharyngeal polyps—complete oropharyngeal and nasopharyngeal exams
   G. Canine necrotizing sialometaplasia—same as A
   H. Stylohyoid disarticulation—oropharyngeal exam, external and intraoral palpation of pharyngeal region, radiography of pharyngeal region

III. Pharynx (functional)
   A. Cricopharyngeal incoordination—oropharyngeal exam, radiographic barium swallow, fluoroscopic exam
   B. Cricopharyngeal achalasia—same as A
   C. Pharyngitis—oropharyngeal exam, mucosal cytology, culture and sensitivity, histopathology
   D. Neuromuscular disease
      1. Infectious disease (rabies)—history of exposure, vaccination history, clinical course, histopathology
      2. Hypocalcemia—serum calcium concentration, serum parathyroid level, reproductive status, parathyroid biopsy

IV. Respiratory tract
   A. Upper airway (morphologic)
      1. Foreign body—pharyngeal/laryngeal exam, radiography, CT/MRI scan, bronchoscopy
      2. Neoplasia—same as 1 plus cytology, histopathology
      3. Tracheal collapse—radiography, fluoroscopy, bronchoscopy
   B. Upper airway (functional)
      1. Laryngeal paralysis—pharyngeal/laryngeal exam
      2. Laryngitis—pharyngeal/laryngeal exam, cytology, culture and sensitivity, histopathology
      3. Tracheobronchitis—radiography, transtracheal aspiration cytology/culture, bronchoscopy cytology/culture/histopathology
   C. Lower airway (morphologic)
      1. Neoplasia—radiography, bronchoscopy cytology/histopathology, CT/MRI scan
      2. Parasitic granuloma—CBC, fecal exam, same as 1
   D. Lower airway (functional)
      1. Feline asthma—CBC, radiography, bronchoalveolar lavage
      2. Canine tracheobronchitis—history, physical exam, tracheal cytology
      3. Fungal pneumonitis—history, radiography, tracheal and bronchial cytology, serum fungal titers

V. Esophagus
   A. Morphologic
      1. Stricture—history, radiography barium swallow, fluoroscopy barium swallow, endoscopy
      2. Neoplasia—same as 1 plus CT/MRI scan
   B. Functional
      1. Esophagitis—history, radiography barium swallow, fluoroscopy barium swallow, endoscopy cytology/histopathology
      2. Megaesophagus—same as 1 plus acetylcholine receptor Ab titer, edrophonium HCl response test, EMG, cholinesterase level, TSH response test, ACTH response test, muscle biopsy, liver biopsy

VI. Stomach
   A. Acute gastritis—history, radiography upper GI barium series, endoscopic examination and biopsy
   B. Proximal gastric neoplasia—fecal occult blood, radiography upper GI barium series, endoscopic examination and biopsy

VII. Miscellaneous
   A. Pericardial effusion—thoracic radiography, ECG, echocardiography
   B. Neoplasm of middle ear—otoscopic exam, oropharyngeal exam, skull radiography, CT/MRI scan, histopathology
   C. Familial progressive nephropathy—signalment, biochemical profile, renal biopsy

CT = computed tomography; MRI = magnetic resonance imaging; CBC = complete blood count; EMG = electromyogram; TSH = thyroid-stimulating hormone; ACTH = adrenocorticotropic hormone; GI = gastrointestinal; ECG = electrocardiogram.

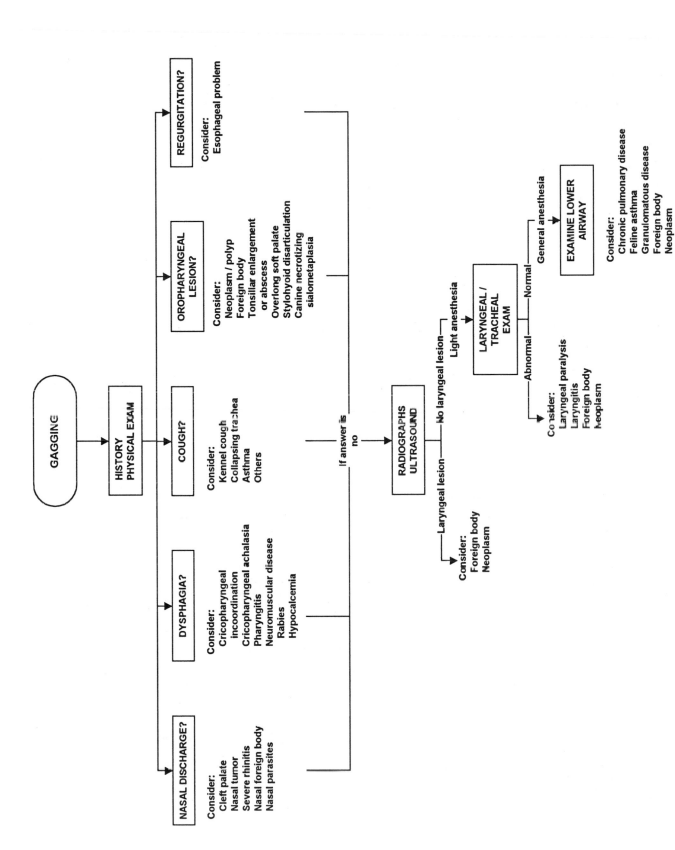

Figure 32–1. Algorithm for diagnostic management of gagging.

GAGGING

HISTORY
PHYSICAL EXAM

NASAL DISCHARGE?

Consider:
Cleft palate
Nasal tumor
Severe rhinitis
Nasal foreign body
Nasal parasites

DYSPHAGIA?

Consider:
Cricopharyngeal
incoordination
Cricopharyngeal achalasia
Pharyngitis
Neuromuscular disease
Rabies
Hypocalcemia

COUGH?

Consider:
Kennel cough
Collapsing trachea
Asthma
Others

**OROPHARYNGEAL
LESION?**

Consider:
Neoplasm / polyp
Foreign body
Tonsillar enlargement
or abscess
Overlong soft palate
Stylohyoid disarticulation
Canine necrotizing
sialometaplasia

REGURGITATION?

Consider:
Esophageal problem

If answer is
no

**RADIOGRAPHS
ULTRASOUND**

Laryngeal lesion

Consider:
Foreign body
Neoplasm

No laryngeal lesion

**LARYNGEAL /
TRACHEAL
EXAM**

Light anesthesia

Abnormal

Consider:
Laryngeal paralysis
Laryngitis
Foreign body
Neoplasm

Normal

General anesthesia

**EXAMINE LOWER
AIRWAY**

Consider:
Chronic pulmonary disease
Feline asthma
Granulomatous disease
Foreign body
Neoplasm

CHAPTER 33

DYSPHAGIA AND REGURGITATION

Christine C. Jenkins

Dysphagia and regurgitation are clinical manifestations of swallowing disorders. Differentiation between dysphagia and regurgitation may help to localize the anatomic site of disease. In some animals, however, regurgitation and dysphagia may coexist.

DYSPHAGIA

Dysphagia is defined as difficult or painful swallowing and occurs with obstructive or functional disorders of the oral cavity (oral dysphagia), pharynx (pharyngeal or cricopharyngeal dysphagia), or proximal esophagus (esophageal dysphagia).

CLINICAL SIGNS

Signs of dysphagia vary, depending on location and severity of the swallowing difficulty. Oral dysphagia is characterized by difficulty during prehension or mastication. Animals may chew on one side of the mouth, drop food, or make repeated attempts to prehend and chew food. Pharyngeal dysphagia may be evident during initial attempts to swallow a food bolus following normal prehension and mastication. Gagging and exaggerated swallowing efforts characterized by pronounced head movements such as throwing the head upward or side to side during attempts to swallow may be evident. Other signs of oral or pharyngeal dysphagia include pain, ptyalism, and anxiety or discomfort during eating and swallowing. Animals with esophageal dysphagia and those with pharyngeal dysphagia may have similar clinical signs. Regurgitation shortly after swallowing may occur with either. Animals with secondary aspiration pneumonia due to abnormal swallowing function may have respiratory signs with or without clinical signs of dysphagia (Table 33–1).

PHYSICAL EXAMINATION FINDINGS

Weight loss may be evident if a swallowing disorder is chronic or intermittent. Animals should be observed during eating to help identify which phase of swallowing is abnormal. If aspiration pneumonia is present as a sequela, fever, abnormal respirations, and harsh lung sounds may be evident (Fig. 33–1).

Dysphagic animals should undergo a complete oral examination to identify foreign objects, dental or periodontal disease, or oropharyngeal masses. This assessment may require sedation or general anesthesia. Animals should also have a complete neurologic examination with close attention to cranial nerve function. If rabies is a possible cause of dys-

phagia, oral examination and patient handling should be avoided or proper precautions should be taken.

RADIOGRAPHIC STUDIES

Survey radiographs of the oral cavity may be indicated in animals with signs of oral dysphagia to evaluate for foreign bodies, masses, and dental or temporomandibular joint disease. In animals showing signs of pharyngeal dysphagia, survey radiographs of the pharynx should be obtained to evaluate for masses, foreign bodies, or abnormal anatomic structures. Contrast studies using liquid barium or food may enhance the ability to identify morphologic abnormalities. Functional abnormalities such as cricopharyngeal dysphagia require dynamic imaging techniques such as contrast fluoroscopy to diagnose abnormal pharyngeal or proximal esophageal dysfunction during swallowing (see Fig. 33–1; Table 33–1).

TREATMENT

Elimination of the underlying cause of dysphagia is the goal of therapy, because these conditions usually progressively worsen. Foreign bodies should be removed, and masses should be removed or biopsied. Some animals with neurologic or neuromuscular disease may benefit from changing the amount, frequency, and consistency of food to facilitate consumption. Treatment of aspiration pneumonia with appropriate antibiotic therapy and by attempting to prevent further aspiration is essential.

REGURGITATION

Regurgitation is defined as passive retrograde passage of food and/or fluid from the esophagus into the oral and/or

---

TABLE 33–1. CAUSES OF DYSPHAGIA

Oral Dysphagia

Stomatitis
Dental or periodontal disease
Foreign body
Neoplasia
Neurologic

Pharyngeal Dysphagia

Cricopharyngeal achalasia or asynchrony
Foreign body
Neoplasia
Neurologic: rabies; brain stem lesion; cranial nerve X, XII dysfunction
Neuromuscular: myasthenia gravis, acute polyradiculoneuritis, polymyositis

114

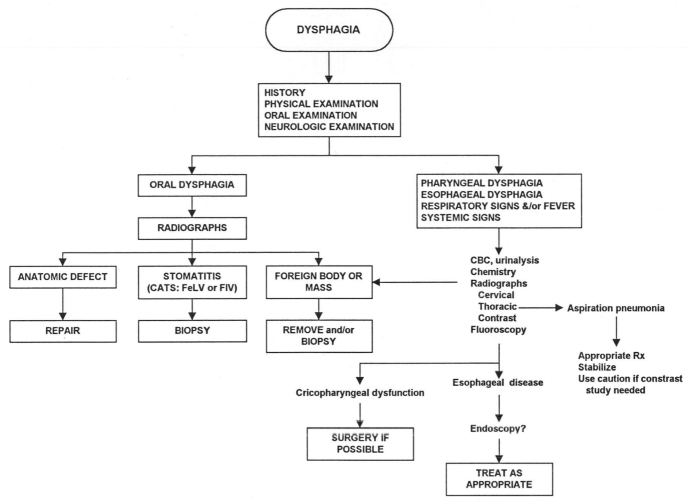

Figure 33–1. Algorithm for diagnosis of dysphagia. Note: Avoid handling of animals if rabies is possible.

nasal cavities. Regurgitation is usually indicative of esophageal dysfunction due to mechanical obstructive disease or functional (motility) abnormalities such as megaesophagus. It is important to differentiate regurgitation from vomiting. Vomiting usually occurs as a result of primary gastric, small intestinal, or numerous other problems. Vomiting, unlike regurgitation, requires abdominal effort.

CLINICAL SIGNS

Regurgitation is described as passive retrograde expulsion of gastric or esophageal contents. Regurgitated material may be composed of undigested or digested food that may or may not be tubular in shape; clear or frothy liquid with or without food may also be regurgitated. Regurgitation may occur shortly after eating or may be delayed for hours after eating. Systemic signs associated with regurgitation include weight loss, increased hunger, or, if aspiration pneumonia is present, dypsnea, fever, and/or cough. Respiratory signs may exist without apparent signs of regurgitation (Fig. 33–2).

PHYSICAL EXAMINATION FINDINGS

Decreased body weight may be noted if regurgitation is chronic. In some cases of severe megaesophagus, physical examination findings may include swelling of the ventral

neck due to esophageal distention and weight loss. Harsh lung sounds may be evident on thoracic auscultation if aspiration pneumonia is present. Neurologic examination is necessary to evaluate for possible neurologic or neuromuscular dysfunction that may occur in diseases such as myasthenia gravis, a condition commonly associated with regurgitation (Table 33–2).

RADIOGRAPHIC STUDIES

Survey cervical and thoracic radiographs are warranted to evaluate for esophageal foreign bodies, abnormal esophageal distention, and evidence of aspiration pneumonia. Radiography is also indicated to evaluate for underlying diseases, including thoracic neoplasia (e.g., thymoma) and mediastinal masses. Contrast radiography may be necessary to evaluate the shape and size of the esophagus. Contrast may also aid in identifying radiolucent foreign bodies, vascular ring abnormalities, masses, esophageal strictures, bronchoesophageal fistulas, and esophageal perforations. Fluoroscopic examination following feeding of contrast liquid or contrast mixed with food may help localize and identify an esophageal lesion or a motility disorder.

LABORATORY STUDIES

Regurgitation may be a sign of primary esophageal disease (e.g., megaesophagus) or motility disorders that can occur

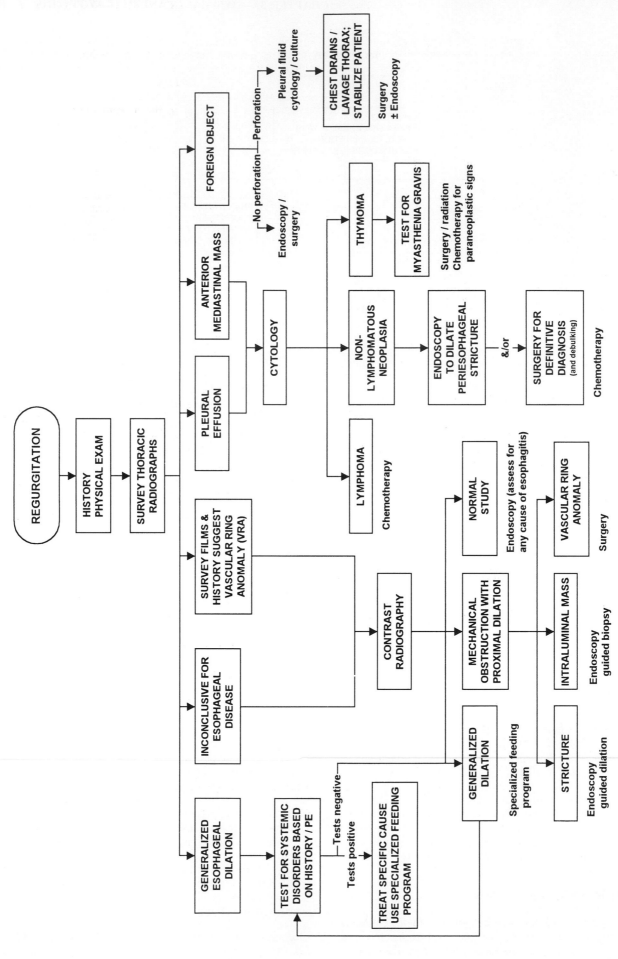

Figure 33–2. Algorithm for diagnosis of regurgitation.

TABLE 33-2. CAUSES OF REGURGITATION

Esophageal Diseases

Megaesophagus: primary (idiopathic) and secondary
Esophagitis
Motility disorder
Esophageal diverticulum
Esophageal obstruction: neoplasia, foreign body, stricture, vascular ring abnormality, granuloma

Alimentary Diseases

Pyloric outflow obstruction
Gastric dilatation volvulus
Hiatal hernia

Neuropathies

Peripheral: polyradiculoneuritis, dysautonomia, giant cell axonal neuropathy, polyneuritis, lead poisoning
Central: distemper, brain stem lesion, neoplasia, trauma

Neuromuscular Junction Abnormalities

Myasthenia gravis
Botulism
Tetanus
Anticholinesterase toxicity

Immune-mediated

Systemic lupus erythematosus
Polymyositis
Dermatomyositis

Endocrine

Hypothyroidism
Hypoadrenocorticism

secondary to numerous systemic diseases. Therefore, as part of the minimum database, a complete blood count, serum chemistries, and electrolytes should be evaluated to rule in or out metabolic diseases that can result in esophageal dysfunction. Based on the presence of suggestive clinical signs and abnormalities in the aforementioned blood tests, additional tests such as endocrine, immune, blood lead, or ACH-receptor antibodies may be indicated.

ANCILLARY TESTS

Endoscopic visualization of the entire esophagus may be required to diagnose foreign body, stricture, neoplasia, hiatal hernia, or reflux esophagitis. In some referral institutions, esophageal manometry is used to evaluate intraluminal pressures at the upper esophageal sphincter, esophageal body, and lower esophageal sphincter. Radiographic scintigraphy using a radioisotope mixed with food can also be used to measure esophageal transit time in animals with megaesophagus or esophageal hypomotility (see Fig. 33–2).

TREATMENT

Successful treatment of regurgitation requires elimination of the underlying cause. If regurgitation is caused by megaesophagus or primary esophageal diseases such as obstruction, prompt diagnosis and treatment are necessary to prevent further loss of normal esophageal function. In cases of aspiration pneumonia secondary to regurgitation, appropriate antibiotic therapy is warranted.

CHAPTER 34

VOMITING

David C. Twedt

Although vomiting has value to protect the animal from ingested noxious substances, the clinical importance stems from the large number of conditions that also cause it. Vomiting can result from a variety of disorders, including those of the gastrointestinal system and other abdominal conditions, systemic or metabolic disease, and drug toxicity, to name a few. Vomiting can result in serious consequences, including volume depletion, acid-base and electrolyte disturbance, esophagitis, aspiration pneumonia, and malnutrition.

PATHOPHYSIOLOGY

The act of vomiting can be divided into three components: nausea, retching, and vomiting. Nausea precedes retching and vomiting and is associated with an episode that defies complete definition in animals. Outward signs of nausea may include depression, shivering, hiding, yawning, and lip licking. Increased salivation and swallowing serve to lubricate the esophagus and neutralize gastric acid. There is also a reduction in gastric and esophageal motility but increased motility of the proximal small intestine, which often produces a reflux of duodenal contents into the stomach.

Retching is the second phase of vomiting and consists of forceful contractions of the abdominal muscles and diaphragm occurring with the glottis closed to produce negative intrathoracic pressure and positive abdominal pressure. These pressure changes are associated with movement of gastric contents into a dilated esophagus. It has been demonstrated in cats that during retching there is actually herniation of the abdominal esophagus and a portion of the gastric cardia into the thorax.

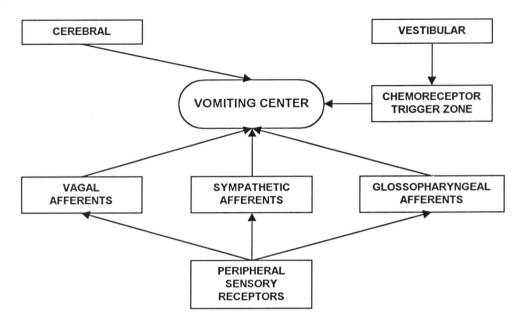

Figure 34–1. Pathways to the vomiting center.

Vomiting occurs as gastric contents are forcefully expelled out of the mouth. The driving force is contraction of the abdominal muscles and diaphragm causing intrathoracic pressure changes from negative during retching to positive during vomiting. As the vomitus passes through the pharyngeal cavity, the nasopharynx and glottis close to prevent aspiration.

Although vomiting is complex and poorly understood, it is best described as a reflex act that is initiated by stimulation of the conceptualized vomiting or emetic center located in the medulla oblongata of the brain. Activation of the vomiting center occurs either through a humoral pathway initiated by blood-borne substances or through various neural pathways leading to the vomiting center (Fig. 34–1). Adjacent to the vomiting center are areas for controlling respiration and salivation, which are also integrated in the vomiting process.

Neural stimulation of the vomiting center arises through afferent vagal, sympathetic, vestibular, and cerebrocortical pathways. Activation of peripheral receptors found throughout the body can stimulate these neural pathways. Particularly important are receptors located throughout the abdominal viscera, but especially those in the duodenum, which contains the highest concentration and has been referred to as the "organ of nausea." Disease or irritation of the gastrointestinal tract, other abdominal organs, or peritoneum can directly stimulate vomiting through vagal afferent pathways. Receptors in the kidneys, uterus, and urinary bladder send afferent impulses via sympathetic nerves and receptors located in the pharynx, and tonsillar fossae transmit impulses thorough afferent fibers of the glossopharyngeal nerve. There is also evidence that vagal receptors are located in the great vessels as they exit the heart, which may explain the common sign of vomiting observed in cats with heartworm disease.

Central nervous system (CNS) disease may directly stimulate the vomiting center through direct extension of inflammatory stimuli, hydrocephalus, or space-occupying lesions. Supramedullary receptors may also influence the reactivity of the vomiting center. For example, psychogenic vomiting appears to arise from the cerebral cortex and may occur as the result of fear, stress, or pain. Cyclic vomiting in the dog

has been associated with an autonomic or visceral epilepsy arising from the limbic region.

The vomiting center is stimulated indirectly via a humoral pathway by activating the chemoreceptor trigger zone (CRTZ) located in the area postrema. The blood-brain barrier is limited in this area, which allows the CRTZ to be exposed to chemical stimuli found in the circulation. Blood-borne substances stimulating the CRTZ include drugs (e.g., apomorphine, cardiac glycosides, and bacterial toxins) and uremic toxins; electrolyte, osmolar, and acid-base disorders, as well as a number of metabolic derangements, can also stimulate the CRTZ. There is evidence in the dog that vestibular

TABLE 34–1. COMMON CAUSES OF VOMITING

Metabolic/Endocrine Disorders	*Gastric Disorders*
Uremia	Gastritis
Hypoadrenocorticism	*Helicobacter*
Diabetes mellitus	Parasites
Hyperthyroidism	Ulceration
Hepatic disease	Neoplasia
Endotoxemia/septicemia	Foreign bodies
Hepatic encephalopathy	Dilatation-volvulus
Electrolyte disorders	Hiatal hernia
Acid-base disorders	Obstruction
	Motility disorders
Intoxicants	
Lead	*Small Intestinal Disorders*
Ethylene glycol	Inflammatory bowel disease
Zinc	Neoplasia
Strychnine	Foreign body
	Intussusception
Drugs	Parasites
Cardiac glycosides	Parvovirus
Erythromycin	Bacterial overgrowth
Chemotherapy agents	
Apomorphine	*Large Intestinal Disorders*
Xylazine	Colitis
Penicillamine	Obstipation
Tetracycline	Parasites
NSAIDs	
	Abdominal Disorders
Dietary	Pancreatitis
Indiscretion	Peritonitis
Intolerance	Neoplasia
Allergy	Hepatobiliary disease

stimulation passes through the CRTZ before activating the vomiting center. Motion sickness, inflammation of the labyrinth, or lesions in the cerebellum result in vomiting via this pathway.

CAUSES OF VOMITING

Because of the vast number of causes of vomiting, it may be best to classify them based on how they activate the vomiting center. A frequent misconception is that vomiting is invariably associated with gastrointestinal disease, but non-gastrointestinal disorders are commonly the cause of vomiting in small animals (Table 34–1).

CLINICAL APPROACH

A complete history is the first step in establishing the correct diagnosis in a vomiting animal. Signalment, history, and description of the vomiting episodes are required. From this information, one should confirm that the animal is truly vomiting and that the signs described are not associated with gagging, coughing, dysphagia, or regurgitation, all of which may appear to be similar. In some cases it may be difficult to differentiate the signs based on the history alone.

The signalment may be helpful. Young unvaccinated animals are more susceptible to infectious disease such as parvovirus or distemper; older animals generally call for a different set of differentials. Vaccination status, travel history, previous medical problems, and medication history should be determined. In particular, it should be noted whether nonsteroidal anti-inflammatory drugs (NSAIDs) have been used, because serious gastrointestinal ulceration may develop in conjunction with their use. The owner also should be questioned about the possibility of toxin or foreign body ingestion, which can invariably lead to vomiting. Questions should probe for other concurrent signs that may occur with systemic or metabolic disease. For example, polydipsia, polyuria, and weight loss are typical for vomiting associated with diabetic ketoacidosis or chronic renal failure.

The history should then focus on the actual vomiting episodes. Determine the duration, frequency, and relationship to eating or drinking, and obtain a complete physical description of the vomitus. A dietary history, including the type of diet or recent diet change, is important, because vomiting may be associated with an adverse reaction to food. Vomiting in the immediate postprandial period may suggest an adverse reaction to food or possibly simply overeating (e.g., a gluttonous cat vomiting meals shortly after eating improves when it is fed small frequent meals). Vomiting an undigested or partially digested meal more than 8 to 10 hours after eating, at which point the stomach should normally be empty, suggests a gastric outflow obstruction or a primary gastric hypomotility disorder. Gastric outflow obstructions occur from foreign bodies, mucosal hypertrophy, tumors, or polyps. Vomiting of a bile-tinged fluid, especially in the early morning hours, often results from enterogastric reflux syndrome.

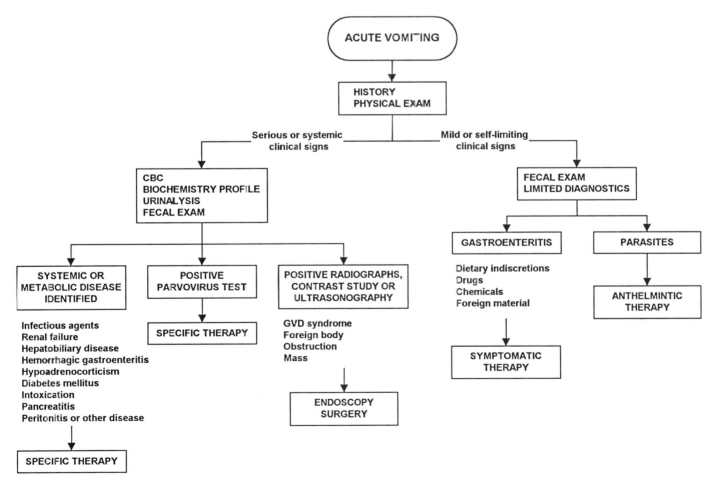

Figure 34–2. Algorithm for the diagnosis of acute vomiting.

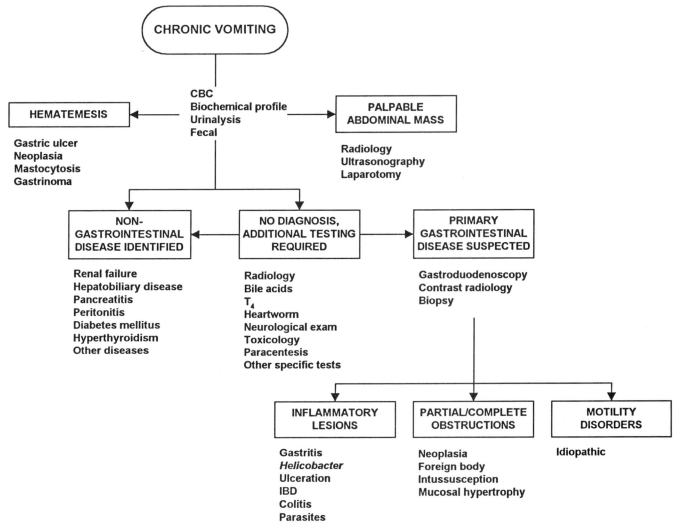

Figure 34–3. Algorithm for the diagnosis of chronic vomiting.

A description of the vomitus should note the amount, color, consistency, odor, and presence or absence of bile or blood. Undigested food suggests a gastric origin, and digested vomitus containing bile suggests an intestinal origin. Vomitus having a fecal odor suggests a low intestinal obstruction or small intestinal bacterial overgrowth. Bile in the vomitus implies that there is no pyloric outflow obstruction. The presence of blood in the vomitus—either fresh, bright-red blood or digested blood that has a "coffee grounds" appearance—indicates gastrointestinal erosion or ulceration. Hematemesis with metabolic-related ulcers such as hypoadrenocorticism or uremia, drug-induced ulceration, gastritis, and gastric neoplasia are possible etiologies.

Careful examination of the mouth and oral cavity may reveal icteric membranes, uremic breath and ulceration, or the presence of a linear foreign body located around the base of the tongue. String or similar material sometimes becomes caught under the tongue, with the remainder passing into the intestine and causing obstruction and plication.

The presence of a fever suggests an infectious or inflammatory process. Bradycardia or cardiac arrhythmias in a vomiting animal may be a sign of a metabolic disturbance such as hypoadrenocorticism. The abdomen should be carefully palpated for distention and tympany (e.g., gastric dilatation volvulus syndrome), effusion (e.g., peritonitis), masses or organomegaly (e.g., neoplasia, intussusception, or foreign body), and pain (e.g., peritonitis, pancreatitis, or intestinal obstruction). The presence of gas and fluid-filled intestines suggest obstruction, whereas plication of the bowel is characteristic of linear foreign body obstruction. A rectal examination provides characteristics of the colonic mucosa and feces. Melena suggests upper gastrointestinal bleeding, and the presence of foreign material in the feces supports a foreign body etiology. Animals with colitis or obstipation often vomit.

Finally, investigation of the CNS should be considered, especially when the cause of the vomiting is not obvious. Some animals with vestibular disease (e.g., nystagmus, head tilt, or ataxia) frequently vomit, which may be the primary clinical complaint. Other CNS diseases may be less obvious, necessitating a thorough neurologic evaluation. Occasionally dogs with intervertebral disk disease vomit because of pain or secondary intestinal ileus.

DIAGNOSTIC PLAN

Based on the history and physical examination, the animal should be classified as having either acute or chronic vomiting. The diagnostic and therapeutic approach differs considerably based on this clinical classification (Figs. 34–2 and 34–3).

If vomiting episodes are acute and of short duration, they may be self-limited and are frequently treated with symptomatic therapy. Most often acute vomiting is associated with gastroenteritis secondary to dietary indiscretions. A routine fecal examination for parasites should be performed in all animals with gastrointestinal signs to eliminate the possibility of parasitism. Investigation for environmental intoxicants is imperative. The first sign of ethylene glycol poisoning is acute vomiting, followed by renal failure. Young unvaccinated dogs should always be evaluated for parvovirus, because the disease frequently begins with vomiting before diarrhea appears. Radiographic studies may be necessary to confirm gastric dilatation volvulus syndrome, gastrointestinal foreign bodies, or obstructions. Severe acute vomiting or vomiting with concurrent systemic signs requires laboratory diagnostic evaluation and radiographic testing. Common systemic and metabolic diseases causing vomiting are usually identified with basic diagnostic testing.

Chronic vomiting, vomiting that has persisted for longer than 5 to 7 days, or vomiting that has failed to respond to symptomatic therapy requires an in-depth investigation. On the basis of the history, one should determine whether hematemesis is present. Hematemesis usually indicates gastric ulceration, and investigation should include NSAID therapy, gastric neoplasia, and systemic mastocytosis. Further investigation in an undiagnosed case of hematemesis involves determining serum gastrin concentrations (increased with gastrinomas). Animals with palpable masses require radiographic or ultrasonograhic studies and ultimately surgical exploration.

In the majority of chronic vomiting cases, routine laboratory tests and survey radiographs identify an etiology and direct appropriate therapy. If routine diagnostic testing fails to identify obvious disease, additional diagnostic testing is required. Evaluation of vomiting cats should include viral and heartworm serology and a thyroid evaluation to rule out hyperthyroidism. Adrenocortical testing for hypoadrenocorticism, bile acid testing for liver disease, toxologic testing (e.g., for lead poisoning), and neurologic examination should be considered under the appropriate clinical circumstances.

When there is a failure to identify non-gastrointestinal causes of chronic vomiting, the clinical focus should be directed to gastrointestinal causes. The diagnostic approach includes endoscopy, contrast radiology, ultrasonography, or laparotomy. Most frequently, inflammatory lesions are identified in an animal with gastrointestinal-associated chronic vomiting. Conditions such as gastritis possibly associated with *Helicobacter,* inflammatory bowel disease, or colitis are confirmed by biopsy, preferably obtained endoscopically. Cats in particular with inflammatory bowel disease may have vomiting as the major clinical sign. Conditions such as gastric antral pyloric mucosal hypertrophy, antral polyps, foreign bodies, or neoplasia can cause gastric outflow obstruction with gastric retention and vomiting. These gastric lesions are usually easily identified endoscopically. Obstructive intestinal lesions such as foreign bodies, intussusception, and neoplasia usually require radiographic contrast studies or ultrasonography for diagnosis. A diagnosis of gastrointestinal motility disorders should be considered only when there is a failure to identify inflammatory or obstructive gastrointestinal lesions. Specialized motility contrast studies and response to gastrointestinal prokinetic agents support that diagnosis.

CHAPTER 35

DIARRHEA

Todd R. Tams

Diarrhea is defined simply as passage of feces that contain an excess amount of water. This results in an abnormal increase in stool liquidity and weight. In some animals there may simply be an increase in frequency of defecation. The client's interpretation is often not as encompassing as the clinician's. To some, diarrhea indicates only profuse, watery stools. Variance from what is considered normal for an animal in terms of frequency and consistency should be considered potentially abnormal and worthy of discussion.

Although a variety of symptoms can be caused by intestinal disorders, diarrhea is the hallmark sign of intestinal dysfunction. It can result from primary intestinal disease (e.g., parasitism, inflammatory disorders, infectious problems, neoplasia), disorders of the liver or pancreas that affect normal intestinal digestive and absorptive processes, and

other factors or conditions that adversely affect intestinal function in some way (e.g., dietary indiscretion, adverse food reactions, drugs such as antibiotics and cardiac glycosides, systemic disorders such as renal failure and hypoadrenocorticism).

Diarrhea is often classified according to location of origin (small or large intestine), mechanism (osmotic, decreased solute absorption; secretory, hypersecretion of ions; exudative, increased permeability; and abnormal motility), and etiology. Most small animals with diarrhea can be successfully treated. Diarrhea that does not respond satisfactorily to routine care within a reasonable period, as determined by the animal's overall condition, frequency of clinical signs (increasing?), and presence of significant laboratory abnormalities, should be thoroughly investigated to determine the etiology before it becomes chronic and potentially nonresponsive to treatment. Intestinal biopsy is often required for diagnosis in animals with chronic, poorly responsive diarrhea.

Small bowel diarrhea is often characterized by an increased frequency of defecation with evacuation of larger than normal amounts of soft to watery stool. Dyschezia and tenesmus are not characteristics of a small bowel disorder and are apparent only if a large bowel disorder is present as well (this is an important point, probably indicating diffuse intestinal involvement). Urgency may be present in acute small bowel disorders or in those associated with cramping. Generally, rapid evacuation of a large volume of watery diarrhea ensues (as opposed to large bowel problems, in which only a small volume is passed). Undigested food indicates maldigestion, generally due to either exocrine pancreatic insufficiency (EPI) or rapid bowel transit time. Weight loss that occurs in conjunction with chronic diarrhea

is most often due to a significant disorder of malabsorption or maldigestion and may be associated with a guarded prognosis. Differentiation of small intestinal from large intestinal diarrhea is summarized in Table 35–1.

The presence of weight loss and inappetence in conjunction with chronic diarrhea suggests a significant small intestinal disorder (e.g., inflammatory bowel disease, lymphangiectasia, histoplasmosis, neoplasia) and should hasten the clinician's efforts toward making a definitive diagnosis. The combination of chronic diarrhea, weight loss, and increased appetite in cats suggests hyperthyroidism, inflammatory bowel disease, EPI (rare in cats), and occasionally lymphosarcoma (some cats with gastrointestinal lymphoma actually have an increased rather than a decreased appetite). This combination of signs in dogs is most consistent with EPI. Characteristics of diarrhea in animals with EPI include voluminous "cowpile"-consistency stools that are often rancid. Coprophagy is an ancillary sign that frequently occurs in

TABLE 35–1. DIFFERENTIATION OF SMALL INTESTINAL AND LARGE INTESTINAL DIARRHEA

PARAMETER	SMALL INTESTINE	LARGE INTESTINE
Feces		
Mucus	Rarely present	Frequently present
Hematochezia	Absent, except in hemorrhagic gastroenteritis syndrome	May be present, often appears as streaks of bright-red blood on surface of stool or admixed with loose stool
Volume	Increased	Normal to decreased
Quality of stool	Varies from nearly formed to quite watery; often appears soft formed ("cowpile"); undigested food or fat droplets or globules may be present, malodorous	Loose to nearly formed; mucus may be absent, present in small amounts, or constitute nearly the entire volume of material expelled; no undigested food
Shape	Variable—depends on amount of water in feces	May be normal or reduced in diameter (narrowed)
Steatorrhea	Present with maldigestive or malabsorptive disorders	Absent
Melena	May be present—appears as black, tarry stool	Absent
Color	Considerable variation—tan to dark brown, black (not always indicative of melena), grayish brown; may be altered by certain medications	Variable—usually brown; may be nearly clear (increased mucus) or laced with bright-red blood
Defecation		
Frequency	Usually increased to 2–4 times a day but may remain normal in some animals	Almost always increased; may be as frequent as 3–10 times a day (average 3–5); the combination of increased frequency of defecation and passage of decreased amounts of stool strongly suggests large intestinal involvement
Dyschezia	Absent	Frequent in dogs, less common in cats
Tenesmus	Absent	Frequent in dogs, less common in cats
Urgency	May be present in cases of acute severe enteritis, with rapid transit of large volumes of fluid through the gastrointestinal tract	Frequent; common reason for owner being awakened during the night to allow a dog outdoors to defecate; often causes restless or anxious behavior in well-trained house dogs as they await an opportunity to get outdoors
Associated Signs		
Weight loss	Usually occurs as disease becomes more chronic; occurs with both malabsorptive and maldigestive disease processes	Unusual; may occur in conjunction with severe colitis, diffuse neoplasia, or histoplasmosis; if both small and large bowel signs are present, any weight loss is more likely due to the small intestinal disease component
Vomiting	Common in animals with inflammatory bowel disorders and acute infectious disorders	May occur in 30–35% of animals with acute colitis; sometimes occurs before onset of abnormal stools
Appetite	Usually normal or decreased; may be cyclic, often decreasing in conjunction with flare-ups of symptoms; may be ravenous in some dogs with inflammatory bowel disease (especially Shar Peis); appetite may be increased in cats with inflammatory bowel disease or lymphoma (transiently in the latter)	Usually remains normal; may be decreased if disease is severe (neoplasia, histoplasmosis)
Halitosis	May be associated with maldigestive or malabsorptive diseases	Absent
Borborygmus	May be present	Absent
Flatulence	May be present	Absent
Fecal incontinence	Rare—associated only with severe enteritis and rapid transit of large volumes of watery diarrhea	May be present
"Scooting" or chewing at perianal area	Absent	Occasionally present; may be quite pronounced in some animals with proctitis

From Tams TR: Gastrointestinal symptoms. *In* Tams TR (ed): Handbook of Small Animal Gastroenterology. Philadelphia, WB Saunders, 1996, pp 44–45.

dogs with EPI. Weight loss and inappetence rarely occur in dogs and cats with intestinal disorders limited to the large bowel.

PHYSICAL EXAMINATION

Along with the history, physical findings help direct the clinician toward what specific tests, if any, should be done and how quickly a work-up should be expedited. Particular attention is paid to the animal's attitude, hydration, and posture. Depression and dehydration occurring in conjunction with acute diarrhea suggest an infectious or toxicity-related etiology. Careful evaluation for any signs of sepsis (fever or hypothermia, tachycardia, tachypnea, and signs of shock, which may include changes in mucous membrane color to brick red or pale, cool extremities and injected membranes) is conducted initially and at any indication that an animal's condition may be destabilizing again. Abnormal posture (e.g., arched back) may indicate abdominal pain. The neck is palpated in cats with diarrhea for evidence of an enlarged thyroid nodule (indicating hyperthyroidism). Body weight and overall physical stature are noted. The act of defecation, especially if there is a history of dyschezia or tenesmus, should be observed by the clinician whenever possible.

Abdominal palpation is done to examine for thickened bowel (inflammatory or neoplastic infiltration), intussusception, presence of a mass that could be causing partial intestinal obstruction with resultant diarrhea, and lymphadenopathy (benign or neoplastic). A rectal examination is always done in dogs to examine for increased mucosal sensitivity, presence of narrowing (e.g., infiltrative disease, stricture), foreign body, or mass effect and to obtain a fresh stool sample for gross examination.

DIAGNOSTIC PLAN

Specific diagnostic studies performed in animals with diarrhea are generally determined by the following considerations: (1) duration (acute vs. chronic [2 to 3 weeks or more]); (2) inappetence, weight loss, frequent vomiting, severe bloody diarrhea, listless behavior (expedite diagnostic efforts if any of these signs are present); (3) environmental history; (4) signalment; (5) localization of the diarrhea to either small or large bowel or both; (6) frequency of diarrhea (intermittent vs. chronic and persistent); and (7) physical examination findings. These considerations help the clinician determine whether a conservative step-by-step approach is feasible (e.g., diagnostic dietary trials, empiric treatment for parasites if screening fecal examinations are negative, treatment for mild acute colitis) or a more aggressive diagnostic effort is indicated.

Acute Diarrhea

Diet-induced problems, viral infections, and parasites are the major causes of acute diarrhea in dogs and cats. Because intestinal parasites may be a factor in any diarrheic state, fecal examinations (direct and flotation) should routinely be done. Multiple examinations may be required to identify *Giardia* and *Trichuris* infections. Examination of fresh saline smears may identify ova, larvae, or motile protozoan parasites. The most accurate practical flotation test for *Giardia* is zinc sulfate flotation. Zinc sulfate is also excellent for the detection of nematode parasites. A fecal enzyme-linked immunosorbent assay (ELISA) for *Giardia*-specific antigen is now available and can be done in-house or submitted to a commercial laboratory. This is an excellent screening test for *Giardia*.

Although diet-induced enteropathies are common, they are sometimes difficult to definitively diagnose. Acute diarrhea may result from overeating, a sudden change in diet (especially to a canned meat-based food), ingestion of spoiled food, food intolerance, or food allergy. The diagnosis is most likely to be made based on history, ruling out other causes, and response to treatment. Strict dietary trials with hypoallergenic diets are indicated for animals with more chronic signs.

Animals with such signs as depression, dehydration, and fever in conjunction with acute diarrhea, with or without blood, should be evaluated for systemic abnormalities. The minimum database always includes a complete blood count (CBC), looking for leukocytosis or leukopenia, presence or absence of left shift, and supportive evidence for dehydration (elevated packed cell volume [PCV] and total solids). In animals with hemorrhagic gastroenteritis, there may be a dramatic increase in PCV to levels as high as 70 to 75 per cent. This degree of increase in PCV contrasts with that in parvovirus infection and is the key to diagnosis of *hemorrhagic gastroenteritis*. If CBC results are not readily available, a blood smear should be examined for estimation of the white blood cell count. Serial blood counts may be necessary, because leukocytosis or leukopenia may be transient. A CBC may also suggest a possible diagnosis of hypoadrenocorticism (eosinophilia). Electrolyte analysis (including sodium and potassium), serial blood glucose assessments for evidence of sepsis, and urinalysis both for baseline evaluation of renal function and for serial urine specific gravity levels as an aid in monitoring hydration in animals with normal renal function should also be run.

Hemagglutination, hemagglutination inhibition, or ELISA tests are used to test for fecal shedding of viral antigen. In-office tests are available for detecting fecal shedding of parvovirus in acute cases and are probably more sensitive and specific than is hemagglutination. Fecal shedding of viral particles often decreases rapidly, however, so a negative result does not rule out infection. Fecal cultures to examine for *Salmonella* spp., *Campylobacter jejuni*, *Yersinia enterocolitica*, and *Shigella* are indicated in some situations (e.g., kennel outbreaks, animals recently obtained from pet stores or shelters, households in which more than one animal has diarrhea).

Chronic Diarrhea

Diarrhea that has not responded to conventional therapy within 2 or 3 weeks can be considered chronic and should be more thoroughly evaluated by using specific diagnostic tests (Fig. 35–1). Considerable expense may be involved, so it is always best to start by reviewing the history.

Small Intestinal Diarrhea

Chronic small intestinal diarrhea can be broadly categorized into three groups: maldigestive disease, malabsorptive disease, and functional disorders. A majority of canine and feline patients with chronic small intestinal diarrhea seen in clinical practice have malabsorptive-type problems, which have many causes. Maldigestive disease is principally caused by EPI

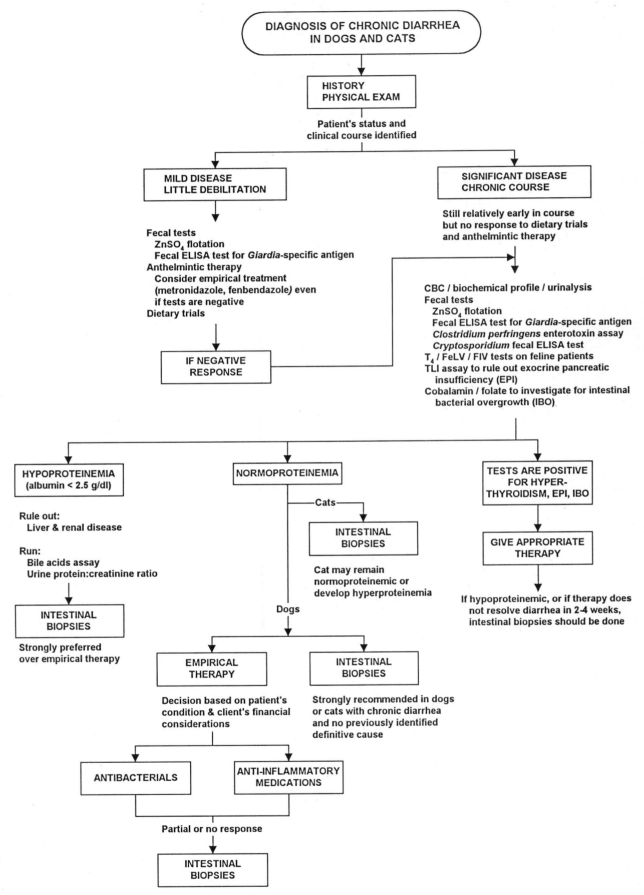

Figure 35–1. Algorithm for differential diagnosis of chronic diarrhea in dogs and cats. ZnSO₄ = zinc sulfate; CBC = complete blood count; ELISA = enzyme-linked immunosorbent assay; T₄ = thyroxine; FeLV = feline leukemia virus; FIV = feline immunodeficiency virus; TLI = trypsin-like immunoreactivity. (Adapted from Tams TR: Gastrointestinal symptoms. *In* Tams TR [ed]: Handbook of Small Animal Gastroenterology. Philadelphia, WB Saunders, 1996, p 55.)

Maldigestive Disease

EPI is uncommon in dogs and quite rare in cats. In the past EPI was greatly overdiagnosed, and many animals were needlessly and ineffectually placed on pancreatic enzyme replacement therapy. Much of the confusion was caused by the lack of a reliable and definitive test for EPI. Without question the most sensitive and specific test for EPI is the serum trypsin-like immunoreactivity (TLI) assay. This test simply involves obtaining a serum sample after fasting the animal for 12 to 18 hours. Serum TLI has been validated for use in both dogs and cats. Although EPI is an uncommon disease, it is recommended that a TLI test be run in dogs and cats with chronic diarrhea so that EPI can be definitively ruled out early in the course of diagnostic evaluation.

Malabsorptive Disease

Malabsorptive intestinal disease can be divided into protein-losing and non-protein-losing enteropathies. Use of this classification scheme helps the clinician determine to some extent the seriousness of the condition and thus aids in the decision regarding whether a detailed work-up, including intestinal biopsies, should be expedited as opposed to pursuing conservative therapeutic trials first (e.g., time-consuming strict dietary trials). In general, dogs with gastrointestinal signs and a total protein of less than 5.5 g/dL should undergo intestinal biopsy. Dogs with mild hypoproteinemia (5.5 to 5.9 g/dL) should be carefully monitored. Cats develop hypoproteinemia much less commonly than dogs. Hypoproteinemia usually indicates a significant degree of disease in cats, and intestinal biopsies should definitely be expedited if the intestine is considered to be the likely source of the problem.

Baseline tests, including CBC to identify leukocytosis (which suggests inflammatory disease), eosinophilia (eosinophilic enteritis, chronic previously undiagnosed endoparasitism), absolute lymphopenia (often observed in lymphangiectasia), and anemia (blood loss, anemia of chronic disease, nutrient malabsorption); biochemical profile (hypoalbuminemia, hypoproteinemia, abnormal liver enzymes, exclusion of metabolic disorders, and so forth); and urinalysis to evaluate renal function and check for proteinuria, should be run in all animals with chronic diarrhea. Even if a CBC and biochemical profile were run previously, soon after the onset of the diarrhea, it is often useful to repeat these tests, because those that were previously normal may be found to be abnormal.

Hypoproteinemia most often results from disorders of the small intestine (protein loss involves albumin or both albumin and globulin), liver (primarily hypoalbuminemia due to decreased production), and protein-losing glomerulonephropathy (primarily hypoalbuminemia). Although the combination of chronic diarrhea and hypoproteinemia is usually consistent with small intestinal disease, there may be concurrent disease in the liver or kidneys. It may therefore be necessary in some cases to evaluate these organs thoroughly (e.g., bile acid assay for liver function, urine protein–creatinine ratio to more accurately identify the degree of proteinuria).

Fecal cytology may be useful in evaluating animals with chronic diarrhea. Increased numbers of neutrophils appear with inflammatory small or large intestinal disease or secondary to invasive bacterial enteritis. Increased numbers of spores may be suggestive of *Clostridium perfringens* enterotoxicosis.

Dogs and cats with chronic diarrhea should routinely be tested for cryptosporidiosis (*Cryptosporidium parvum*). Although the incidence of this infectious disorder is unknown, it is certainly more common than has been recognized, and there is significant zoonotic potential associated with infection. Readily available tests for cryptosporidiosis include acid-fast stains on feces and a fecal ELISA test for *Cryptosporidium*-specific antigen (the latter test is available as an in-house test kit [Alexon] or through a commercial lab).

After baseline evaluation has been completed, the next step is to look for evidence of intestinal bacterial overgrowth and *C. perfringens* enterotoxicosis (see the section on Large Intestinal Diarrhea for a discussion of the latter disorder). The most accurate means of diagnosis is to obtain samples of duodenal fluid for both qualitative and quantitative analysis. This must be done using meticulous sterile technique either at laparotomy or with endoscopic instrumentation. Quantitative duodenal culture is expensive and cumbersome and is generally available only in academic institutions. The most practical method of testing for intestinal bacterial overgrowth is by measuring serum concentrations of vitamin B_{12} (cobalamin) and folate. These assays can be done in both dogs and cats.

At this stage, the next step is usually to perform intestinal biopsies. However, other procedures that might be indicated in some animals to aid in the decision-making process include contrast radiography and abdominal ultrasonography. Contrast studies of the small intestine may help identify segmental lesions, tumors, or foreign bodies. Accurate interpretation of mucosal lesions on contrast studies is very difficult. Whether a contrast study is done is usually determined by physical examination findings (suggestion of a mass or well-localized pain) and survey radiographs.

Ultrasound scanning of the intestinal tract provides an evaluation of peristalsis, wall thickness and diameter, lesion location, and appearance of luminal contents. Ultrasonography is particularly useful in the identification of obstruction and its various causes (e.g., masses, foreign objects, inflammatory disease, intussusception). Thickening of the bowel wall can occur in either inflammatory or neoplastic disease processes.

The definitive diagnostic step in many animals with chronic, nonresponsive diarrhea is to perform intestinal biopsies via either endoscopy or surgery. In a majority of cats and dogs with chronic diarrhea that exists with or without associated clinical signs (e.g., vomiting, appetite change, weight loss), a definitive diagnosis can be established based on endoscopic examination and biopsy. In most animals with chronic diarrhea, it is preferable to perform both upper and lower endoscopy, so that sections from both the small and the large intestine can be evaluated histologically to determine the extent of the disease process as accurately as possible. In addition, in a majority of dogs weighing more than 10 to 12 pounds, a pediatric endoscope can be advanced into the ileum via the colon by an experienced operator. Thus, complete colonoscopy followed by ileoscopy allows for more detailed evaluation of the small intestine (i.e., both upper and lower small intestine are examined and sampled for biopsy).

If an exploratory laparotomy is done to obtain intestinal biopsies, the entire bowel should be carefully evaluated. Focally abnormal areas should be biopsied (full-thickness samples), along with one or two normal areas. Many animals with chronic small bowel diarrhea have grossly normal intestine as observed at surgery, but biopsy samples must still be procured. Two or three full-thickness samples are obtained (duodenum and ileum, or duodenum, jejunum, and ileum). Any other tissue that appears abnormal (e.g., liver, pancreas, stomach, lymph nodes) should also be biopsied during exploratory laparotomy.

Large Intestinal Diarrhea

Large bowel disorders are common in dogs and cats. In mild cases, a diagnosis is often established based on fecal parasite examination (e.g., hookworms, coccidia, *Giardia*); positive response to empiric treatment for difficult-to-diagnose parasite problems (*Giardia* and whipworms); response to dietary trials (high-fiber diet, elimination diets); or response to empiric treatment for acute colitis. Diagnostic tests for chronic large bowel diarrhea principally involve:

1. Fecal cytology to look for increased numbers of *C. perfringens* spores and inflammatory cells (specifically neutrophils), which suggest bacterial or primary inflammatory disease.
2. Fecal culture if history or fecal cytology suggests the possibility of bacterial infectious disease (*Campylobacter, Salmonella*).
3. Reverse passive latex agglutination enterotoxin assay on stool to confirm a diagnosis of *C. perfringens* enterotoxicosis.
4. Colon biopsy via colonoscopy (preferred technique) or surgery.

Complete colonoscopy with examination of the rectum; descending, transverse, and ascending colon; cecum; and ileocolic orifice area is preferred. Although examination and biopsy of the descending colon with a rigid colonoscope are commonly diagnostic in animals with large bowel diarrhea, such problems as occult trichuriasis, in which whipworms may be grossly evident in the cecum but not in the descending colon; ileocolic or cecocolic intussusception; typhlitis; or neoplasia that is localized in the transverse or ascending colon may be missed unless a complete examination of the colon is done with a flexible endoscope. Another advantage of using a flexible endoscope is that ileoscopy may be accomplished in some animals after complete colonoscopy. Biopsy samples should always be obtained during colonoscopy, regardless of gross appearance.

MANAGEMENT

Treatment of diarrhea frequently involves dietary manipulation, specific anthelmintic therapy for parasite infections, antibacterial drugs for infectious disorders, and anti-inflammatory therapy for small and large intestinal inflammatory bowel disease. Symptomatic therapy for acute noncomplicated diarrhea includes bowel rest and dietary manipulation. If pharmacotherapy is deemed necessary, metronidazole is often the most indicated drug. It is emphasized that some animals with chronic diarrhea may have several disorders (e.g., inflammatory small bowel disease, *C. perfringens* enterotoxicosis, and intestinal bacterial overgrowth). A thorough work-up will lead to the diagnosis of each disorder, with subsequent development of a comprehensive treatment plan. The likelihood of more rapid resolution of symptoms is much greater when each existing problem is properly treated. Treatment of the various disorders that cause diarrhea is described in detail in the chapters pertaining to the gastrointestinal system.

CHAPTER 36

MELENA AND HEMATOCHEZIA

W. Grant Guilford

Melena describes black, tarry stools resulting from digested blood. Hematochezia refers to the presence of red blood on the stool. The presence of melena suggests large-volume hemorrhage from the upper gastrointestinal tract and is a warning sign of serious disease. Hematochezia is usually due to large bowel disease, in particular colitis. While often frightening to the client, hematochezia is less frequently associated with life-threatening diseases than melena.

ETIOPATHOGENESIS

Blackening of the stool occurs when enough hemoglobin is oxidized to hematin or other hematochromes within the intestinal lumen. It is the duration of blood within the lumen that determines its color, not its level of origin. It has been estimated that blood must be retained in the intestinal tract of humans for at least 8 hours for it to turn black. Black stools can result from lower small bowel or upper large bowel bleeding if transit time is sufficiently slow. This can occur when bleeding occurs proximal to an obstructive neoplasm. Transit time of blood in the gastrointestinal tract shortens as the volume of blood entering the tract increases. As a result of this phenomenon, large-volume upper gastrointestinal bleeds can result in feces containing fresh blood. Tarry stools result from bacterial breakdown of hemoglobin in the intestine. Melena will appear tarry only if there is a sufficiently large quantity of blood present.

Melena usually results from bleeding into the pharynx, esophagus, stomach, or upper small intestine (Table 36–1). Life-threatening volumes of blood can accumulate within the gastrointestinal tract, with little or no visible signs of external blood loss.

Fresh blood adherent to the feces (hematochezia) is strongly suggestive of lower large bowel hemorrhage. As mentioned previously, the usual cause is large bowel disease such as colitis, but neoplasia and coagulopathies, particularly platelet disorders, must be considered.

CLINICAL EXAMINATION

Age helps determine likelihood of gastrointestinal neoplasia. Chronicity of disease can assist diagnosis. Disorders due to gastrointestinal ischemia are most often acute, whereas neoplastic disorders usually have a more protracted course. The owner should be asked if nonsteroidal anti-inflammatory drugs or glucocorticoids have been administered. These drugs, particularly in combination, are a potent cause of gastroduodenal ulceration and melena in dogs. Most nonsteroidal drugs have the potential to produce ulceration. The

TABLE 36–1. CAUSES OF MELENA

Swallowed Blood

    Hemoptysis
    Nasal and oropharyngeal neoplasia

Esophagus

    Neoplasia

Stomach

    Severe gastritis
    Ulcers (drugs, stress, uremia, liver failure, mastocytosis, gastrinoma)
    Neoplasia (adenocarcinoma, leiomyosarcoma, lymphosarcoma)

Upper Small Intestine

    Severe duodenitis (enteritis, inflammatory bowel disease)
    Duodenal ulcers (drugs, stress, uremia, liver failure, mastocytosis, gastrinoma)
    Neoplasia (mast cell neoplasia, lymphosarcoma, adenocarcinoma)
    Severe hookworm burden

Lower Small Intestine and Large Bowel

    Neoplasia
    Polyps

Gastrointestinal Ischemia

    Shock
    Volvulus
    Intussusception
    Mesenteric avulsion
    Gastrointestinal infarction

Drug Administration

    Nonsteroidal anti-inflammatory drugs
    Glucocorticoids

Miscellaneous

    Coagulopathies (especially DIC)
    Gastrointestinal blood vessel malformations (varices, arteriovenous fistula)
    Severe acute pancreatitis
    Hemobilia
    Liver failure
    Rocky Mountain spotted fever
    Uremia
    Foreign bodies

Abridged from Strombeck DR, Guilford WG: Approach to clinical problems in gastroenterology. *In* Small Animal Gastroenterology, 2nd ed. Davis, CA, Stonegate Publishing, 1990, pp 56–89.

risk of glucocorticoid-induced ulceration is particularly high when dexamethasone is used in dogs undergoing surgery for spinal cord diseases. The risk of exposure to anticoagulant rodenticides should be assessed and the likelihood of trauma (that may have caused gastrointestinal avulsions or infarctions) determined.

The clinical manifestations of gastrointestinal bleeding depend on extent and rapidity of the hemorrhage. Signs range from mild weakness to collapse. Clinical signs usually pertain primarily to anemia and hypovolemia, but on occasion they may help localize the site of hemorrhage. Thus, concomitant regurgitation suggests esophageal or pharyngeal disease, cough raises the likelihood of hemoptysis, and jaundice and ascites imply liver disease. Hematemesis strongly suggests gastric or duodenal bleeding, but swallowed blood can cause vomiting. Concurrent signs of tenesmus, dyschezia, frequent defecation, and/or increased stool mucus suggest that hematochezia or melena is due to large bowel disease. The presence of behavioral abnormalities or marked depression in association with melena suggests the possibility of hepatic encephalopathy precipitated by the gastrointestinal hemorrhage.

The physical examination should include careful inspection of the nares and oropharynx for evidence of nasal or oropharyngeal sources of bleeding. Skin of the abdomen and mucous membranes should be evaluated for petechiation. Petechiation or ecchymosis supports suspicion of a coagulopathy such as thrombocytopenia or disseminated intravascular coagulation as cause of intestinal bleeding. Auscultation of the chest assists detection of lower respiratory diseases. Hemoptysis from lower respiratory diseases such as neoplasia is a rare cause of melena. Abdominal palpation may reveal abdominal pain or an abdominal mass suggestive of neoplasia.

DIAGNOSIS

The diagnostic evaluation of hematochezia is similar to that described for the evaluation of tenesmus, dyschezia, and diseases of the large bowel. A minimum database of complete blood count, serum biochemistry profile, urinalysis, and fecal flotation is necessary to detect thrombocytopenia, uremia, whipworms, and to assist in diagnosis of diseases such as sepsis, eosinophilic colitis, disseminated intravascular coagulation, and liver failure. All these disorders can cause hematochezia. Rectal scrapes are helpful for diagnosis of protozoal colitis, fungal colitis, and suppurative colitis due to enteropathogenic bacteria. Fecal culture may confirm bacterial colitis, and assay of fecal clostridial enterotoxin levels may support a role for *C. perfringens*. Survey radiographs help detect pelvic trauma, ileocolic intussusception, foreign bodies, and colonic or ileocecal neoplasia. Barium or air enemas may reveal large bowel disorders such as neoplasia, polyps, intussusceptions, and cecal inversion. Endoscopy is the procedure of choice for diagnosis of hematochezia and is usually required for the definitive diagnosis of colitis or large bowel neoplasia.

The first step in the diagnostic evaluation of melena is objective confirmation of the problem (Fig. 36–1). The classic appearance of melena is of coal-black, shiny, sticky, foul-smelling feces of tarlike consistency. On many occasions, however, feces will have some, but not all, of these classic features. For instance, there are a number of spurious reasons for black feces. Many normal animals consuming meat-based diets have black feces. Similarly, diets high in iron

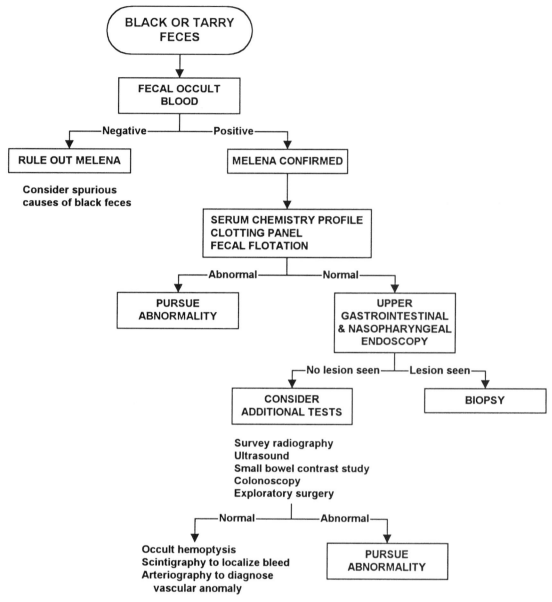

Figure 36–1. Algorithm for clinical evaluation of black or tarry feces.

can cause black feces, as can the use of some drugs such as salicylates, bismuth, and charcoal. Therefore, it may be important to confirm the presence of digested blood by use of tests for fecal blood, such as the orthotoluidine (Hematest) and guaiac (Hemoccult) tablet tests. Unfortunately, these tests can generate false-positive results and some of the spurious causes of black feces mentioned above will produce positive occult blood tests (for instance, salicylate use).

A complete blood count helps determine the severity and chronicity of the melena. The rapidity with which the hematocrit declines after gastrointestinal hemorrhage is variable depending on such factors as hydration status and preexisting anemia. Significant decline can occur within 1 to 2 hours. Microcytic, hypochromic anemias are common following chronic gastrointestinal blood loss. Reticulocytosis is usually present after a few days with the exception of those animals with iron-deficiency or neoplastic infiltrates in the bone marrow. Buffy coat examination for diagnosis of mast cell neoplasia and lymphoma can be a useful adjunct to the

complete blood count. Coagulation tests may be required if a bleeding problem is suspected.

The serum chemistry panel allows detection of renal and liver failure, which can result in melena. The serum urea:creatinine ratio rises after upper gastrointestinal hemorrhage. The rise in this ratio is due to the digestion and absorption of blood protein leading to the generation of urea. Lower bowel hemorrhage has little effect on serum urea nitrogen but may increase blood ammonia concentrations. Slight hyperbilirubinemia is common in humans after gastrointestinal hemorrhage. The hyperbilirubinemia results from the breakdown of large quantities of heme. A fecal flotation for hookworm should not be neglected.

The most valuable diagnostic procedure for localizing the site and cause of intestinal bleeding is upper gastrointestinal endoscopy. If no upper gastrointestinal lesions are found, the nasopharynx should be examined before the endoscope is withdrawn. Contrast radiography is usually of less value than endoscopy and does not provide a definitive (histologic) diagnosis. Exploratory surgery may be required, but because the mucosal surface of the gastrointestinal tract is not readily viewed during laparotomy, bleeding lesions can be missed. In difficult cases, scintigraphy using [99m]technetium-labeled red blood cells can be used to locate the site of bleeding. Arteriography may be required to diagnose vascular anomalies causing gastrointestinal hemorrhage.

TREATMENT

Treatment of hematochezia or melena depends predominantly on cause. If bowel disease is the suspected cause of the hematochezia, symptomatic management may include treatment trials with parasiticides effective against whipworms, sulfasalazine (the drug of choice for idiopathic coli-

tis), and sulfa drugs in young animals suspected of having coccidiosis. A dietary trial with a commercial hypoallergenic diet containing a fermentable fiber source (e.g., beet pulp) is also valuable. Alternatively, a homemade hypoallergenic diet to which has been added 1 to 6 teaspoons of a fermentable fiber such as Metamucil can be used. Symptomatic management of melena due to severe upper gastrointestinal hemorrhage can include crystaloids, colloids, and/or blood transfusions. Previous recommendations to lavage the stomach with cold solutions have been challenged on the basis that they may reduce blood clotting. Gavage with alpha-agonists such as norepinephrine is rarely necessary. Administration of inhibitors of gastric acid secretion (such as cimetidine or omeprazole) or sucralfate may be useful. Surgical resection of the bleeding lesion may be required.

CHAPTER 37

CONSTIPATION, TENESMUS, DYSCHEZIA, AND FECAL INCONTINENCE

Brent Jones

DEFINITIONS

Constipation is absent, infrequent, or difficult defecation associated with the retention of feces within the colon and rectum.

Obstipation is a condition of prolonged and intractable constipation resulting in severe impaction throughout the rectum and colon. Obstipated animals are unable to eliminate the impacted fecal mass.

Megacolon is a disorder characterized by recurrent constipation and obstipation associated with dilatation and hypomotility of the colon.

Tenesmus is a clinical sign characterizing an animal straining to defecate (alimentary) or urinate (urinary).

Dyschezia is difficult or painful evacuation of feces from the rectum and is usually associated with lesions in or near the anal region. Animals displaying dyschezia may vocalize as they attempt to defecate and may exhibit prolonged straining episodes.

Fecal incontinence is failure of voluntary control of the anal sphincters with involuntary passage of feces and flatus.

CONSTIPATION

PATHOPHYSIOLOGY

The colon of dogs and cats has the primary function of absorbing water and electrolytes from the passing ingesta.

The colon also functions as a storage facility for fecal material until it can be eliminated by the process of defecation and maintains an abundant growth of microbes that contribute to the digestive process. The colonic mucosa secretes mucus for lubrication and easier passage of fecal material. Segmental contractions in the colon mix ingesta and increase the absorption of water and electrolytes but decrease the actual movement of luminal contents through the colon. The primary propulsion of colonic material is a "mass movement" within the colon that occurs only a few times during the course of a day to propel feces into the rectum. Distention of an animal's rectal wall triggers the defecation process. The defecation reflex can be inhibited by cerebral input, allowing feces to be retained for an extended time. Therefore, pets that are house-trained can delay defecation until an appropriate place is found to defecate. Diet is the most important local factor in regulating colonic function. Adequate amounts of dietary fiber and fluid can prevent constipation. Dietary fiber helps stimulate colonic motility by increasing fecal output, reducing stool density, and increasing luminal bulk.

Any event that slows transit or obstructs colonic flow can eventually lead to constipation. Fecal material that has hardened in the colon can damage the colonic mucosa and may provoke secretion of fluid from the colon. These secretions may contain small amounts of blood and may appear as episodes of diarrhea. The secretions have little impact on softening the impacted fecal material and allowing it to pass. The many causes of constipation are grouped into several broad categories (Table 37–1).

HISTORICAL AND PHYSICAL FINDINGS

Constipated animals usually fail to defecate for several days. Tenesmus or frequent attempts to defecate may be

TABLE 37–1. CAUSES OF CONSTIPATION

Dietary

Ingested foreign material in feces (hair, bones, cat litter, rocks, garbage, plant material)
Inadequate water intake

Environmental/Behavioral

Dirty litter box
Hospitalization
Inactivity
Change in daily routine

Painful Defecation

Anal sac impaction or abscess
Perineal fistula
Perianal wound—cellulitis or abscess
Pseudocoprostasis
Myiasis

Rectocolonic Obstruction

Extraluminal
Prostatomegaly—tumor, cyst, prostatitis
Pelvic fracture or malunion
Perianal tumor
Perineal hernia
Pseudocoprostasis
Intraluminal
Foreign body
Rectocolonic stricture
Neoplasia
Atresia ani

Orthopedic

Spinal disease or injury
Injuries of the pelvis, hip joints, or pelvic limbs

Neurologic

Lumbosacral spinal cord diseases
Bilateral pelvic nerve injury
Dysautonomia (Key-Gaskell syndrome)
Idiopathic megacolon*

Fluid and Electrolyte Abnormalities

Dehydration
Hypokalemia
Hypercalcemia

Metabolic

Hypothyroidism
Hyperparathyroidism/pseudohyperparathyroidism
Pheochromocytoma

Drug-induced

Opiates
Anticholinergics
Antihistamines
Barium sulfate
Diuretics
Aluminum hydroxide antacids
Iron supplements
Phenothiazines
Kaolin-pectin
Vincristine

*Classification unknown.

noticed by the owner, resulting in veterinary consultation. Owners notice dogs assuming the defecation stance for extended periods or making attempts without producing feces. Owners might notice their cats spending an excessive amount of time in the litter box, vocalizing or demonstrating tenesmus while attempting to defecate, and changing position in the litter box several times, repeatedly attempting to defecate. Owners may notice liquid discharged during episodes of tenesmus. The liquid is a result of colonic mucosal irritation, and some owners may mistakenly believe that their pets have diarrhea. Other signs relating to constipation that owners observe include anorexia, lethargy, vomiting, dehydration, and a hunched up appearance resulting from abdominal discomfort.

Constipation is often a condition of older pets with limited activity. Some diseases leading to constipation tend to show up more commonly in certain breeds. Perianal fistulas in German shepherd dogs and perineal hernias in older male dogs are diseases associated with constipation. Idiopathic megacolon tends to affect adult male cats and is characterized by recurrent episodes of constipation. Manx cats and English bulldogs have an increased risk of sacral spinal deformity leading to constipation and fecal incontinence.

Owners of constipated pets should be questioned about diet, current drug therapy, and history of garbage or any other foreign body ingestion. Also, owners should be questioned about previous trauma or fractures, neuromuscular diseases, weight loss, and previous episodes of constipation.

Physical examination findings are usually nonspecific except for the obviously distended and firm colon. Animals that are chemically constipated or obstipated may become dehydrated, lethargic, and weak. Mucous membranes may be hyperemic, and the haircoat may appear dull. The animal may have a hunched appearance, and abdominal palpation may reveal a hard, irregular, tubular mass filling the entire length of the colon. A thorough physical examination is needed, giving special attention to the perineal area to rule out hernias, fistulas, anal sacculitis or abscess, or other diseases leading to difficult defecation. A digital rectal examination should be performed to assess the prostate; the presence of masses, pain, blood, pelvic canal obstruction, strictures, or other diseases affecting defecation; and anal sphincter tone. A neurologic examination should be performed to eliminate any underlying neurologic disease. Cats and dogs with constipation due to dysautonomia may have regurgitation resulting from megaesophagus, urinary and fecal incontinence, bradycardia, mydriasis, decreased lacrimation, or prolapse of the nictitating membrane.

DIAGNOSIS

Diagnosis of constipation is based on history and physical examination, with a goal of determining the underlying cause (Fig. 37–1). In addition to abdominal palpation, digital rectal examination, and neurologic examination, a complete blood count, serum biochemical profile, urinalysis, and thyroid function tests should be performed to rule out problems that may cause peripheral neuropathies or electrolyte imbalances.

Abdominal radiography and ultrasonography can help determine the extent of colonic impaction and may identify predisposing causes such as foreign material, abdominal masses, and pelvic or spinal lesions. Generalized and extreme colonic dilatation without any obstructive lesions supports a diagnosis of irreversible idiopathic megacolon. After the colon has been evacuated, contrast radiography with a barium enema or endoscopy, if available, can be used to

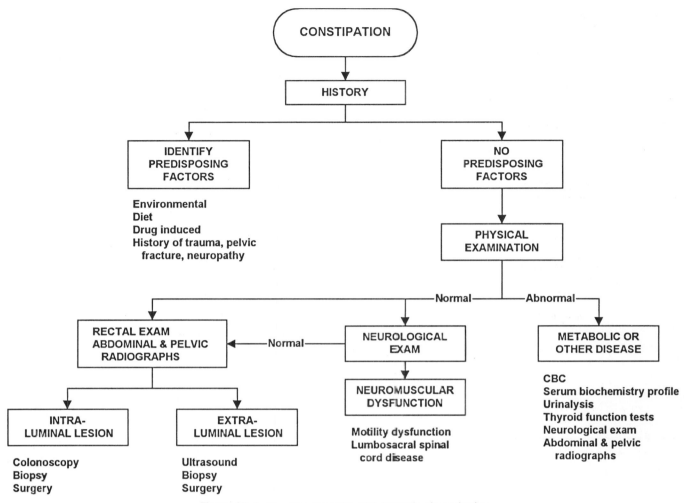

Figure 37–1. Algorithm for differential diagnosis of constipation.

identify intraluminal colonic masses or strictures. Endoscopically obtained biopsies may provide a histopathologic diagnosis.

TREATMENT AND OUTCOME

Treatment is based on the underlying cause and severity of constipation and includes correction of electrolyte imbalances, removal of the fecal mass, identification of the underlying cause, and prevention of recurrence. Simple or mild constipation without systemic signs can usually be treated on an outpatient basis with enemas or suppository laxatives (Table 37–2) to soften and lubricate the feces and stimulate defecation. A dosage of 5 to 10 mL/kg body weight of warm water or isotonic saline infused slowly using a red rubber feeding tube attached to an elevated 0.5 to 2 L enema bucket for dogs allows for a gentle infusion. Addition of emollient laxatives helps soften feces and stimulate colonic contractions. Sodium phosphate enemas are contraindicated (especially in cats and small dogs) for relieving fecal impactions because of the potential for fatal hyperphosphatemia, hypernatremia, hyperosmolarity, and hypocalcemia. Suppositories can also be given by the owner as needed to treat the constipation. Treatments for simple constipation may be needed for 2 to 3 days.

Severely constipated or obstipated animals require manual removal of the fecal mass in combination with colonic irriga-

tion. Before administering anesthesia, fluid and electrolyte imbalances should be corrected. A warm isotonic electrolyte solution infused into the colon and gentle transabdominal palpation are used to break up fecal impactions. The feces can then be milked to the distal rectum, where manual removal of the retained feces can be accomplished with a sponge or whelping forceps. Excessive trauma to the colon should be avoided, and it may be advisable to evacuate the colon manually in stages over 2 to 3 days. A colotomy may be indicated if manual evacuation is not therapeutic. For severe recurrent constipation or megacolon in cats that is unresponsive to medical therapy, subtotal colectomy is an effective alternative treatment.

PREVENTION

A fiber-supplemented diet or laxative medications are often sufficient to prevent constipation. Laxatives act on intestinal mucosal fluid transport and colonic motility and are classified by their mechanisms of action: bulk-forming, lubricant, emollient, osmotic, and stimulant (see Table 37–2). Underlying causes should be eliminated, if possible, by correcting any dietary, environmental, or drug-induced causes of constipation. Clean, fresh water should be available to encourage water intake. Surgical correction of anorectal diseases should be performed, and endocrine, spinal, or orthopedic disorders should be treated. Additional treatment pro-

TABLE 37–2. TREATMENT OF CONSTIPATION

TREATMENT	PRODUCT (MANUFACTURER)	DOSAGE
Enemas and Suppositories		
Enemas		
Warm tap water		5–10 mg/kg
Isotonic saline solution		5–10 mg/kg
Docusate sodium	Colace (Mead Johnson)	5–10 mL
Mineral oil	Many	1–2 mL/kg
Lubricant jelly	Many	5–10 mL
Sodium phosphate*	Fleet Children's Enema (Fleet)	1–2 mL/kg
Bisacodyl	Fleet Bisacodyl Enema (Fleet)	1 mL/kg
Rectal suppositories		
Glycerin	Many	1–2 pediatric suppositories
Docusate sodium	Colace (Mead Johnson)	1–2 pediatric suppositories
Bisacodyl	Dulcolax (Boehringer Ingelheim)	1–2 pediatric suppositories
Oral Cathartics		
Bulk-forming laxatives		
Coarse bran	Many	1–3 tsp q24h with food
Canned pumpkin	Many	1–3 tsp q24h with food
Psyllium	Metamucil (Procter & Gamble)	2 tsp/10 kg q24h with food
Lubricant laxatives		
White petrolatum	Laxatone (EVSCO)	1–2 mL PO q24h
Mineral oil†	Many	5–10 mL q24h
Emollient laxatives		
Docusate sodium	Colace (Mead Johnson)	50–100 mg PO q24h
Docusate calcium	Surfak (Hoechst-Roussel)	50–100 mg PO q24h
Osmotic laxatives		
Lactose	Milk	Add to diet to effect
Lactulose	Duphalac syrup (Reid-Rowell)	0.5–1 mL/kg PO q8–12h
	Cephulac (Merrell-Dow)	
Stimulant laxatives		
Bisacodyl	Dulcolax (Boehringer Ingelheim)	5 mg PO q24h
Castor oil‡	Emulsoil (Paddock)	5 mL PO (bowel prep)

*Do not use in cats or small dogs.
†Caution: May cause lipid aspiration and may interfere with absorption of fat-soluble vitamins; combination with docusate may cause undesirable absorption of mineral oil.
‡Used mainly to prepare the colon for radiography or endoscopy.
Modified from Sherding RG: Diseases of the intestines. *In* Sherding RG (ed): The Cat: Diseases and Clinical Management, 2nd ed. New York, Churchill Livingstone, 1994, pp 1211–1285; and DeNovo RC: Constipation, tenesmus, dyschezia, and fecal incontinence. *In* Ettinger SJ, Feldman EC (eds): Textbook of Veterinary Internal Medicine, 4th ed. Philadelphia, WB Saunders, 1995, pp 115–122.

tocols might include cisapride at a dosage of 2.5 mg by mouth every 8 hours for cats diagnosed with idiopathic megacolon. An alternative approach to treating constipation in the future might include direct electrical stimulation of the colon, but this presently is experimental.

TENESMUS AND DYSCHEZIA

PATHOPHYSIOLOGY

Tenesmus caused by disease of the alimentary tract must always be differentiated from tenesmus associated with urogenital disorders. Constipation, inflammatory, and obstructive diseases of the colon and rectum are indicated by alimentary tenesmus. Urethral obstruction, cystitis, vaginitis, neoplasia, and pregnancy are a few causes of urogenital tenesmus. Dyschezia in dogs and cats is more characteristic of rectal and anal diseases. Colorectal inflammation and ulceration stimulate the defecation reflex in dogs and cats. This reflex causes straining, painful defecation, urgency, and frequency and may be followed by mucus or fresh blood in the passed fecal material. Causes of tenesmus and dyschezia are listed in Table 37–3.

HISTORICAL AND PHYSICAL FINDINGS

An adequate history must be taken in order to differentiate tenesmus and dyschezia of alimentary origin from urogenital disease. Clients often assume that signs of tenesmus are associated with constipation. For example, male cat urethral blockage is often misinterpreted by clients as constipation. Tenesmus preceding defecation usually suggests constipation, whereas tenesmus following defecation suggests inflammation of the colonic or rectal mucosa. Continual tenesmus that is nonproductive of fecal material and is characterized by an abnormal squatting stance for defecation indicates the presence of an obstructive lesion. Normal squatting with tenesmus suggests an inflammatory lesion. Crying and whimpering during defecation may also be noted by the owner. Signs of anorexia, vomiting, and weight loss are more indicative of alimentary rather than urogenital tenesmus.

A thorough physical examination should be performed to determine the causes of tenesmus and dyschezia. The perineal area should be examined carefully to rule out a perineal hernia, perianal fistula, anal gland abscess, or pseudocoprostasis. The bladder should be palpated. A distended urinary bladder suggests obstruction, whereas a small painful bladder is consistent with cystitis. The abdominal palpation of hardened feces in a distended colon and rectum suggests constipation. A rectal examination should be performed to detect strictures, fistulas, and hardened feces; to evaluate the prostate and anal sac; and to detect any pelvic fractures or masses. A rough, irregular rectal mucosa palpated on rectal digital examination suggests an inflammatory or infiltrative bowel disease. The clinician should also carefully examine the penis or vagina for discharges, masses, calculi, and pain.

TABLE 37–3. CAUSES OF TENESMUS AND DYSCHEZIA

Colonic/Rectal Diseases

Constipation (see Table 37–1)
Colitis/proctitis
Neoplasia/polyps
Foreign body (bones, rocks, food wrappings)
Irritable bowel syndrome
Rectal abnormalities

Perineal/Perianal Diseases

Anal sac abscess
Anal sac neoplasia
Perineal hernia
Perianal fistula
Pseudocoprostasis

Urogenital Diseases

Cystitis, urethritis, vaginitis
Cystic or urethral calculi
Prostatomegaly (neoplasia, hyperplasia, abscess)
Parturition
Neoplasia of urethra, bladder, vagina
Vaginal cyst

Caudal Abdominal Cavity Disorders

Caudal abdominal cavity mass
Pelvis fracture/malunion

Modified from DeNovo RC: Constipation, tenesmus, dyschezia, and fecal incontinence. *In* Ettinger SJ, Feldman EC (eds): Textbook of Veterinary Internal Medicine, 4th ed. Philadelphia, WB Saunders, 1995, pp 115–122.

DIAGNOSIS

The diagnostic procedures for tenesmus and dyschezia are similar to those described for the evaluation of constipation. In addition to a thorough history and physical examination, rectal cytology could suggest the presence of an inflammatory or infectious disease (increased number of inflammatory cells). Complete blood count, serum biochemical profile, and urinalysis should be performed to assess metabolic status. Abdominal and pelvic radiographs can rule out disease processes such as constipation, prostatomegaly, megacolon, pelvic fractures, or malunion of pelvic bones following trauma. In addition, foreign bodies, neoplastic or granulomatous masses, and sublumbar lymphadenopathy may be identified by radiographs of the abdomen. Colonoscopy is frequently the most valuable diagnostic procedure for animals with tenesmus and dyschezia, and it can be performed using either a rigid proctosigmoidoscope or a flexible gastrointestinal endoscope. Rigid colonoscopy allows visualization of the anal canal, rectum, and left colon. The same structures plus the transverse and right colon can be examined with a flexible endoscope. In addition, a flexible endoscope can retroflex so that the internal anal mucosa can be examined. Biopsies can easily be obtained with either rigid or flexible colonoscopy.

If the cause of tenesmus and dyschezia has been localized to the urogenital system, additional diagnostic procedures should be performed. Urinary catheterization of the urethra and bladder determines patency. Urethroscopy, urinary tract contrast radiography, culture of urine and prostatic fluid, and biopsies of the urinary tract or prostate may be required.

TREATMENT AND OUTCOME

Treatment of tenesmus and dyschezia can usually be done on an outpatient basis. Clipping the hair around and thoroughly washing the perineal area often benefit animals with inflammation in the anal area. Enemas usually break up impacted fecal material. Topical corticosteroids and anesthetic medications (suppositories, creams, or ointments) can be administered to decrease inflammation of the anorectal area. If the anal glands are abscessed, they should be drained and flushed thoroughly with povidone-iodine solution. Anorectal diseases, such as perianal fistulas and perineal hernias, may require surgical correction to eliminate tenesmus and dyschezia. Tumors of the colon and rectum, rectal strictures, and anal sac carcinomas usually require surgery.

Medical therapy of animals with tenesmus and dyschezia due to inflammatory lesions of the colon and rectum is usually successful. Many of the underlying diseases causing these clinical signs can be surgically corrected, but there is always a risk of fecal incontinence and secondary complications with surgery. Animals with anal sac disease, perineal hernia, or wounds in and around the anorectal area have a better prognosis than those with strictures or neoplasia.

FECAL INCONTINENCE

Fecal incontinence can be broken down into two main categories: reservoir incontinence and sphincter incontinence. Animals afflicted with reservoir incontinence sense the urge to defecate and lose voluntary function of defecation. These animals show clinical signs of frequent tenesmus and the conscious ability to defecate. Animals with sphincter incontinence are unaware of fecal passage through the anal sphincter. These animals have episodes of involuntary expulsion and dribbling of feces from the anus. They also lack the conscious ability to assume the proper stance for defecating. Sphincter incontinence is usually a condition resulting from a neuromuscular disorder, although an anatomic disorder can cause non-neurogenic sphincter incontinence.

PATHOPHYSIOLOGY

Normal defecation in animals is maintained by several anatomic structures. The colon, rectum, and anal canal all contribute to fecal continence. Rectal coccygeal muscles surrounding the rectum and anal canal promote fecal propulsion via movement of the tail and perineum. In order for stool to pass through the anal canal, both the internal and external anal sphincters must relax. The internal sphincter, composed of smooth muscle, relaxes when the rectum becomes distended; this is known as the rectoanal distention reflex. The external anal sphincter, composed of skeletal muscle, contracts when the rectum is distended; this is the rectoanal contractile reflex. Defecation is a response to distention of the colon with fecal material. An animal's urge to defecate is triggered by tension receptors in the rectal wall. The signal is carried along parasympathetic pathways from the sacral spinal cord. The cerebral cortex receives these signals and can override the urge to defecate.

Reservoir fecal incontinence occurs when disease processes disrupt the normal capacity or compliance of the rectum. Inflammation, neoplasia, diarrhea, and constipation can lead to reservoir incontinence. Sphincter incontinence results mainly from neuromuscular damage. Insults causing damage to the pudendal nerves, sacral spinal cord, or levator ani and coccygeus muscles are a few examples of disorders causing neurogenic sphincter incontinence. Non-neurogenic sphincter incontinence can be caused by perineal trauma or perianal fistulas. Disorders causing fecal incontinence are listed in Table 37–4.

TABLE 37–4. CAUSES OF FECAL INCONTINENCE

Reservoir Incontinence
Colorectal disease
    Colitis
    Proctitis
    Neoplasia
Constipation
Diarrhea

Non-neurogenic Sphincter Incontinence
Perianal fistula
Traumatic injury
    Bite wound
    Laceration
    Gunshot wound
Iatrogenic
    Anal sac removal
    Perianal fistula repair
    Perineal hernia repair

Neurogenic Sphincter Incontinence
Cauda equina
    Compression vertebral malformation
    Congenital vertebral malformation
    Sacrococcygeal subluxation
    Lumbosacral instability
    Discospondylitis
    Neoplasia
    Vascular compromise
Central nervous system disease
    Spina bifida
    Trauma
    Degenerative myopathy
    Intervertebral disk extrusion
    Neoplasia
    Vascular compromise
    Meningomyelitis
    Fibrocartilaginous embolism
Peripheral neuropathies
    Trauma
    Drug-induced
    Infectious
    Dysautonomia

Miscellaneous
Aging
Behavior abnormality

HISTORICAL AND CLINICAL FINDINGS

Animals are brought to veterinarians after owners observe uncontrolled defecation or an increased frequency of defecation following exercise, barking, or rising from recumbency. Owners should be asked whether their pets are assuming the normal stance for defecation or if feces are dribbling out without apparent realization. If the pet is not assuming the normal stance for defecation, a neurologic disease is responsible. If the animal is a young or newly house-trained pet, a failure of house training may be the only problem. Owners should also be questioned about urinary incontinence, which suggests a neurologic disorder. The consistency of feces should be ascertained. If diarrhea is evident, reservoir incontinence caused by an inflammatory process is probably the cause. If the fecal material is normal in consistency, neurologic sphincter incontinence is suspected.

A thorough physical examination should be performed, including a complete visual inspection of the perineal region, as well as a digital rectal examination to evaluate anal tone. The presence of lesions such as strictures or masses can also be detected during a rectal examination, suggesting reservoir incontinence. The perineal region should be inspected for traumatic lesions and perianal fistulas, which would yield a diagnosis of non-neurogenic sphincter incontinence. A finding of excessive hardened feces on abdominal palpation of the colon suggests constipation. The bladder should be palpated for tone. An easily expressed bladder and a history of urinary incontinence point toward a neurologic disorder. A complete examination of the skin over the dorsal midline and on both pelvic limbs should be performed to detect any signs of trauma. Pain detected upon palpation of the dorsal midline suggests lumbosacral spinal cord lesion or disease.

A complete neurologic examination observing the gait, cranial nerves, myotactic reflexes, and postural reactions should be performed on all animals with suspected fecal incontinence. Decreased myotactic reflexes to an animal's pelvic limbs suggest a lesion of the lumbosacral spinal cord, cauda equina, myopathy, or a related neuropathy. The anal reflex is tested by touching the skin around the anus. An intact reflex is identified by constriction of the anus. The rectal-inflation reflex can be tested by placing air into the caudal rectum via a Foley catheter. An intact reflex is elicited if the animal's anus contracts. The pudendal-anal reflex should also be tested. Pressure is applied to the penis, and a reflex is displayed by contracture of the anus. These three reflexes allow for evaluation of the sacral spinal cord, pudendal nerves, and external anal sphincter.

DIAGNOSIS

A thorough history, physical examination, digital rectal examination, and complete neurologic examination often yield a diagnosis of fecal incontinence (Fig. 37–2). A complete blood count, biochemistry panel, and urinalysis are usually normal unless the animal has a lower urinary tract infection, which is often the case with urinary incontinence. A fecal flotation is diagnostic when diarrhea due to parasitism is suspected. Endoscopy of the colon and rectum, along with biopsies, can be helpful in cases of reservoir incontinence. Radiography of the lumbosacral spine can help rule out diseases of the vertebral column. Spinal cord diseases can also be diagnosed with myelograms, epidurograms, and

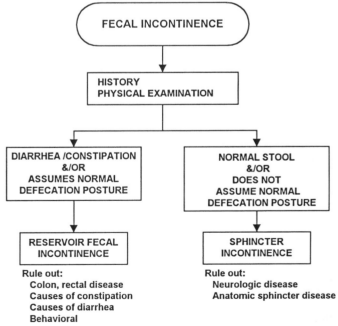

Figure 37–2. Algorithm for differential diagnosis of fecal incontinence.

diskography. Computed tomography and magnetic resonance imaging may be required for the diagnosis of certain spinal cord lesions. Electromyography to evaluate the muscles responsible for fecal continence may provide useful information. A lumbosacral tap to evaluate for infectious disease, inflammatory processes, neoplasia, and trauma can also be helpful.

TREATMENT AND OUTCOME

Treatment of fecal incontinence should be aimed at diagnosing and treating the underlying cause. Some cases of reservoir incontinence resolve following treatment, whereas neurologic disorders usually cannot be treated successfully. Owners should be aware of the greater risk of parasite exposure when caring for an animal with fecal incontinence.

Dietary therapy to reduce fecal production by increasing digestibility is an effective treatment for fecal incontinence. A low-residue diet such as cottage cheese and rice can reduce fecal volume. Opiate motility-modifying drugs such as diphenoxylate HCl (Lomotil) or loperamide HCl (Imodium) slow the passage time of fecal material by increasing segmental contractions. Therefore, these drugs increase the amount of water absorbed from the feces. It has been noted in humans that these drugs also increase anal sphincter tone. Phenylpropanolamine can be administered to improve sphincter tone but is not always effective. Fecal incontinence may be easily resolved following treatment of diarrhea caused by inflammation or parasitism.

Owners can make a pet an outdoor pet if it is healthy. Warm water enemas can be administered to evacuate feces from the colon. Animals may also respond to inflating air into the rectum via a Foley catheter. Other treatments to stimulate reflex defecation include pinching a toe on a hind limb or the tail to stimulate a mass reflex leading to defecation. Applying a warm washcloth to the perineal area can also stimulate the defecation reflex in some animals. Surgical procedures to correct causes of non-neurogenic sphincter incontinence, such as perianal fistulas, lead to a great improvement in fecal continence. Palliative surgery using fascial slings or silicone elastomer slings has been suggested for dogs with neurogenic sphincter incontinence.

Acknowledgment

The author acknowledges the assistance provided by Michael Little, DVM, in the preparation of this manuscript.

CHAPTER 38

FLATULENCE AND BORBORYGMUS

W. Grant Guilford

Flatulence refers to the anal passage of intestinal gas. Borborygmus is a rumbling noise caused by the propulsion of gas through the gastrointestinal tract. Borborygmus and flatulence more commonly affect dogs than cats and are most often observed in inactive dogs spending long periods indoors. They usually result from dietary intolerances but on occasion can herald more serious gastrointestinal disease, particularly of the small bowel or pancreas. Most owners accept flatulence in their pets as normal and are unconcerned about its consequences.

PATHOPHYSIOLOGY

The two most common sources of gastrointestinal gas are swallowed air and bacterial fermentation of nutrients such as carbohydrates. Additional sources are the chemical release of carbon dioxide from bicarbonates and diffusion of gas from the blood. The composition of gastrointestinal gas is primarily nitrogen, oxygen, hydrogen, methane, and carbon dioxide, all of which have no odor. Most of the intestinal nitrogen and oxygen is ingested in air and subsequently eliminated by eructation from the stomach and esophagus. In human beings, and probably in dogs and cats, hydrogen, carbon dioxide, and methane produced in the intestine constitute the bulk of flatus. Odoriferous, potentially volatile substances such as ammonia, hydrogen sulfide, indole, skatole, mercaptans, volatile amines, and short chain fatty acids constitute less than 1 per cent of intestinal gas.

The composition and volume of flatus are affected by the quantity and variety of nutrients eaten, as well as the type and abundance of bacterial flora. For instance, legumes contain large quantities of indigestible oligosaccharides. Unabsorbed oligosaccharides are fermented by clostridia and other bacteria to produce hydrogen, carbon dioxide, and methane. Variations in the metabolic capacity of bacteria may explain the different response to nonabsorbable carbohydrates in individual animals. Maldigestion due to exocrine pancreatic insufficiency or malabsorption resulting from small intestinal diseases often leads to excessive intestinal gas. It is notewor-

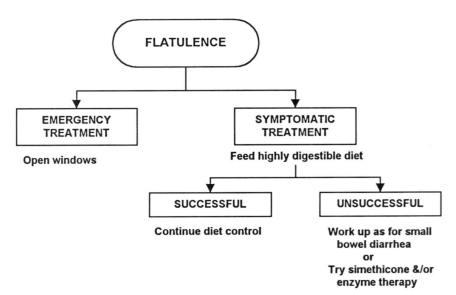

Figure 38–1. Algorithm for management of flatulence.

thy that the transit time for gas is considerably shorter than for liquids or solids. Furthermore, overdistention of the stomach or intestinal tract by gas can lead to considerable abdominal pain.

CLINICAL EXAMINATION FINDINGS

Historical findings of importance include the presence of concurrent abdominal pain, vomiting, or diarrhea, any of which suggests more serious gastrointestinal disease. The owner may report that the pet has a hunched posture, exhibits unsettled behavior, or adopts a praying position. These signs are common in dogs with irritable bowel syndrome and may result from excessive intestinal gas, motility disorders that disrupt the passage of gas through the bowel, or increased visceral sensitivity to bowel distention. The animal's temperament may be important. Excessive aerophagia in a nervous animal or greedy eater can increase gastric gas, although it is unclear whether ingested air contributes significantly to intestinal gas or flatus.

A complete dietary history is essential. In human beings, diets high in soybeans, whole wheat products, bran, lactose, and fats can cause gaseousness. Similar associations appear to occur in some dogs and cats. Spoiled food and diets high in protein or fat are particularly likely to yield odoriferous gases. Milk products can cause gaseousness in animals with lactase deficiency. With the exception of borborygmus, the physical examination of an animal with increased gaseousness is usually unremarkable unless concomitant gastrointestinal disease is present.

MANAGEMENT

The management of borborygmus and flatulence begins with changing the diet to one containing highly digestible protein and fat (Fig. 38–1). In addition, the diet should not contain excessive quantities of rapidly fermentable fiber. Suitable commercial products are available from most of the major manufacturers. Alternatively, the owner can prepare a homemade diet of highly digestible protein and carbohydrate sources such as cottage cheese and rice appropriately balanced with vitamins and minerals. Regular exercise is also beneficial, presumedly because exercise stimulates gastrointestinal motility and defecation. Reducing aerophagia by avoiding situations that provoke nervousness and by discouraging greedy eating, for instance, by ensuring that a dog does not have to compete for food, may also be helpful. In the rare event that dietary manipulation and regular exercise are not successful, consider an investigation similar to that for a dog with small bowel diarrhea (see Chapter 137). Alternatively, symptomatic pharmacologic management can be tried.

Pharmacologic management of excessive gaseousness relies on adsorbents, antifoaming agents, or digestive enzymes. Charcoal is the most commonly used adsorbent antiflatulent in people but is of questionable effectiveness and practicality. Simethicone (25 to 200 mg per dose, every 6 hours) is frequently used as a treatment for borborygmus, gaseous colic, and flatulence in human beings. It is an antifoaming agent that reduces surface tension, allowing bubbles to coalesce so that they may be more easily passed. It is not absorbed from the gastrointestinal tract and can be safely used in dogs and cats at or near the dose for human beings. Its effectiveness as an antiflatulent in dogs and cats is unknown. Antiflatulent enzyme supplements are claimed to assist the digestion of fermentable nutrients that are digested poorly by the gastrointestinal systems of monogastrics. Anecdotal reports suggest that these enzyme supplements can reduce the severity of flatulence in cats and dogs.

CHAPTER 39

ABDOMINAL DISTENTION, ASCITES, AND PERITONITIS

Stephen A. Kruth

Abdominal distention not caused by obesity or pregnancy may be a serious sign of disease and should be evaluated. The initial goal should be to determine if hepatomegaly, splenomegaly, or other mass is present, or if the predominant abnormality is the accumulation of fluid in the peritoneal cavity. Distinguishing between organ enlargement and the presence of an effusion can be accomplished through physical examination and abdominal radiography or ultrasonography.

When a mass or organomegaly is the predominant abnormality, a specific diagnosis can usually be achieved through needle biopsy. Appropriate management can then be pursued. When an effusion is present, the next step is to characterize it as a transudate, modified transudate, septic or nonseptic exudate, chyle, blood, or urine. If the effusion is a transudate or modified transudate, the animal is said to have ascites; if the effusion is an exudate, the animal has peritonitis. When caused by bile, urine, or pancreatitis, peritonitis is initially nonseptic. Septic peritonitis can be caused by leakage of intestinal contents, penetrating wounds, and foreign bodies, and a variety of organisms have been identified. The cause of the effusion should then be localized to an organ system (liver, right heart, small intestine, kidney, etc.), followed by diagnostic procedures chosen to identify a specific pathology (cirrhosis, right atrial hemangiosarcoma with tamponade, lymphangectasia, glomerulonephritis, etc.).

PATHOPHYSIOLOGY OF ABDOMINAL ORGAN ENLARGEMENT

Enlargement of the stomach or intestines is usually due to accumulation of gas and fluid in the lumen of the affected organ. Gas may accumulate as a consequence of aerophagia (usually secondary to respiratory disease), gastric dilatation, or ileus. Renal and/or urinary bladder enlargement can follow ureteral or urethral obstruction; bladder enlargement can also be associated with neurologic dysfunction. Enlargement of the liver can be a consequence of chronic passive congestion secondary to right heart failure, and torsion of the spleen can lead to splenic enlargement as a result of venous congestion. Gross organ enlargement is often due to infiltrative (usually neoplastic) conditions, which may cause diffuse or localized enlargement of the involved organ. However, less worrisome conditions such as hyperadrenocorticism can cause remarkable hepatomegaly and abdominal distention.

PATHOPHYSIOLOGY OF ABDOMINAL EFFUSIONS

The peritoneum is a serous membrane composed of mesothelial cells overlying a layer of collagen and elastic fibers, fat cells, reticulum cells, and macrophages. The parietal portion covers the transversalis fascia of the abdominal wall, and the visceral portion envelops the abdominal viscera. The peritoneal cavity formed by these two layers is almost nonexistent in normal animals, containing only a small amount of fluid that serves to lubricate the parietal and visceral peritoneal surfaces. This peritoneal fluid is constantly synthesized and reabsorbed; reabsorption is largely through lymphatic uptake, especially at the diaphragm. Lymph drains from the peritoneum to the sternal and mediastinal lymph nodes, cisterna chyli and thoracic duct, and omental lymphatics.

Two physiologic situations underlie the development of edematous or ascitic conditions. Firstly, *perturbation of the Starling forces* governing fluid movement across membranes occurs. Decreased *plasma colloidal osmotic pressure* associated with hypoalbuminemia, increased *capillary hydrostatic pressure*, and/or increased *permeability of the capillary endothelium* secondary to inflammation can all lead to the development of effusions. Secondly, the redistribution of extracellular fluid into the peritoneal cavity decreases the effective plasma volume, inducing *sodium and water retention* via a variety of neural, hormonal, and hemodynamic mechanisms. Fluid continues to be sequestered in the peritoneal cavity, without normalization of the plasma volume. The net effect is the perpetuation of the ascitic state.

In right-sided congestive heart failure, the increase in mean capillary hydraulic pressure increases the rate of fluid transfer from capillaries to the peritoneal space. Increased pre- and postcapillary resistance, decreased renin and aldosterone clearance, decreased oncotic pressure gradient, and decreased lymphatic flow in the thoracic duct contribute to the formation of the effusion.

Ascites secondary to chronic liver disease is a complex situation for which the mechanism of fluid accumulation is not completely known. The classic "underfill" theory suggests that a decrease in effective circulating volume occurs when fluid is sequestered in the abdominal cavity; critical imbalances of the Starling forces in hepatic sinusoids and splanchnic capillaries lead to increased lymph formation, exceeding the drainage capacity of the lymphatics. Concurrent hypoalbuminemia may contribute to contraction of the circulating volume and the development of ascites. Peripheral vasodilation due to an as yet unidentified vasodilator substance compounds the situation (and has been suggested to be an early event in the pathogenesis of sodium retention). Alternatively, the "overfill" theory suggests that liver disease directly stimulates renal retention of sodium and water by an unknown mechanism, leading to an increase in extracellular fluid volume, which (in the presence of preexisting hepatic venous outflow obstruction and portal hypertension) results in ascites. There is evidence that both underfill and overfill phenomena occur at different times in dogs with hepatic disease.

Erosion or occlusion of blood vessels or lymphatics by neoplasias such as hemangiosarcoma or lymphosarcoma can lead to the accumulation of blood or chyle in the peritoneal cavity. The most common cause of chylous ascites in dogs and cats is neoplasia. Rupture of blood vessels or lymphatics, ureters or bladder, or the biliary tree can all occur secondary to trauma.

CLINICAL SIGNS

Owner concerns for a dog or cat with ascites may include abdominal enlargement, perceived weight gain, decreased activity, inappetence, or increased respiratory rate. The rate of abdominal enlargement is extremely variable and may occur over a few days, regardless of the underlying cause. The history should include a review to assess for signs consistent with cardiac, renal, liver, and other organ systems. Abnormalities usually identified by abdominal palpation may include hepatomegaly, splenomegaly, or one or more mass lesions. Small amounts of fluid accumulation is associated with a "slippery" feel when the small bowel is palpated. A fluid wave can usually be appreciated with large volumes of effusion. Rapid breathing can be due to cranial displacement of the diaphragm by masses or fluid, causing restricted ventilation. Signs of abdominal pain may be present in peritonitis of any cause.

A careful general examination may reveal signs that will direct the diagnostic approach. For example, generalized lymphadenopathy would suggest lymphosarcoma and fine-needle aspiration of a peripheral lymph node may be diagnostic. Cardiovascular abnormalities such as murmurs, arrhythmias, weak femoral pulses, jugular distention, or pulsation are suggestive of right heart failure. Muffled heart sounds are consistent with pericardial effusion and tamponade. Jaundice is consistent with liver failure, and fever can be caused by inflammatory disorders.

DIAGNOSTIC APPROACH

Ultrasonographic examination of the abdomen is extremely useful for identifying organ enlargement, and alterations in organ echogenicity may be suggestive of specific disorders, such as neoplasia. Abdominal ultrasound is also helpful for demonstrating low-volume or localized effusions. After evaluating the animal's hemostatic ability, ultrasound-guided needle biopsies or fluid aspiration can be performed. Radiographic examination is less useful but is usually sufficient to differentiate between organomegaly, mass lesions, and effusions (Fig. 39–1).

When an effusion is present, a sample should be obtained

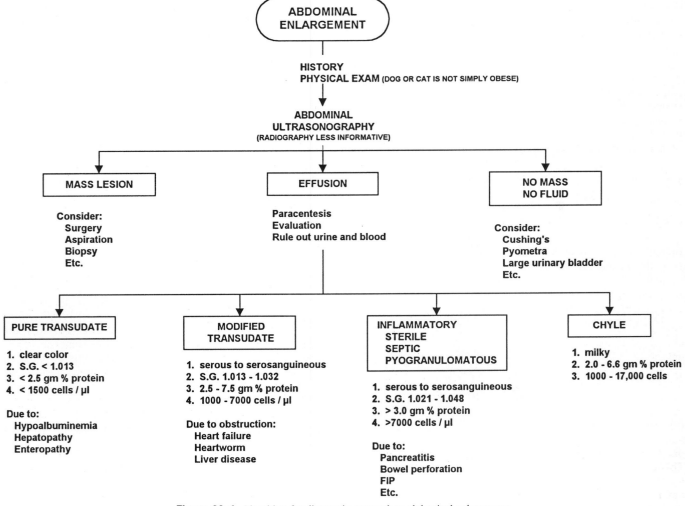

Figure 39–1. Algorithm for diagnostic approach to abdominal enlargement.

for cytology and biochemical evaluation. There are few contraindications for paracentesis other than advanced coagulopathies. Diagnostic paracentesis can be safely accomplished by aspirating the peritoneal cavity using a 22-gauge needle attached to a 12-mL syringe. Following aseptic skin preparation, the needle is placed through the ventral midline slightly caudal to the umbilicus, avoiding liver, spleen, and urinary bladder. The animal can be standing or in lateral recumbency, and local anesthesia is usually not necessary. Nondiagnostic aspirates may be obtained when significant amounts of blood are retrieved from the liver or spleen, or when only small amounts of effusion are present. Complications include laceration of the liver, spleen, or tumor, and bacterial contamination of the peritoneal cavity.

Smears of aspirated fluid should be made immediately and the fluid then split into EDTA and clot tubes. If the fluid is bloody, its packed cell volume should be determined and compared with that of peripheral blood. Blood obtained from the spleen or other organ will clot, wheras blood from abdominal hemorrhage will not clot. A sample should be saved for bacterial culture if indicated. Characterization of effusions is based upon the protein concentration and total cell count, as presented in the algorithm (see Fig. 39–1).

A CBC, serum biochemistry panel, and urinalysis are indicated for any animal with abdominal effusion. Animals with signs of right-sided heart failure should be evaluated with thoracic radiographs, echocardiography, ECG, and tested for heartworm. Any dog or cat that may have cancer or a mass should have thoracic radiographs evaluated for metastatic pulmonary disease. Masses or enlarged lymph nodes should be aspirated for cytologic evaluation. Animals with proteinuria should have a urine protein:creatinine ratio

determined, and ultrasonographic-guided renal biopsy considered.

MANAGEMENT OF ABDOMINAL EFFUSIONS

The management of ascites secondary to cardiac failure is based upon improving cardiac performance as dictated by the primary disorder and diuretic therapy. Ascites secondary to liver disease is also managed with diuretics, including the loop diuretic furosemide (initially 1 mg/kg two times per day, increasing as necessary) and the aldosterone antagonist spironolactone (initially 1 mg/kg twice a day, increasing as necessary). Both drugs can be administered concurrently to minimize electrolyte abnormalities. Total body sodium is increased in ascitic disorders, and a sodium-restricted diet is indicated. Large-volume paracentesis is indicated when animals are in respiratory distress, or when diuretic therapy has failed to mobilize the effusion.

The management of malignant effusions is dictated by the type of cancer and the clinical stage of the animal. Dogs with ruptured splenic or hepatic hemangiosarcoma may require immediate surgical intervention. Animals with uroabdomen or with bile-stained effusions usually need to be managed surgically.

Dogs and cats with exudative effusions associated with pancreatitis or bacterial peritonitis should also be considered as surgical candidates. Cats with the effusive form of feline infectious peritonitis (FIP) can be made more comfortable in the short term with large-volume paracentesis while medical management is considered.

NEUROLOGIC

CHAPTER 40

SHIVERING AND TREMBLING

David Lipsitz and Anne E. Chauvet

Shivering and trembling are terms that are often used interchangeably to describe involuntary rhythmic oscillations of a body or body parts. *Shivering* is characterized by involuntary high-frequency muscle contraction and relaxation. *Tremors* are involuntary repetitive rhythmic oscillations. Much confusion still exists regarding the classification of tremors in animals, with some authors describing resting versus action tremors while others compare local or generalized tremors. *Resting tremors*, which are classically seen in human beings with Parkinson's disease, are thought to be due in part to the loss of striatal neurons in the basal nuclei. This condition has not been reported in dogs and cats, and lesions that involve only the basal nuclei are uncommon. *Intention tremors* occur when movement is directed in a goal-oriented fashion. These tremors are often seen in ani-

mals with cerebellar disease involving the vermis or lateral cerebellar zones. They can be accentuated when an animal is tempted to eat or drink, but with careful observation they can be seen even in animals at rest as they try to maintain their head position. These animals may also have other cerebellar signs such as dysmetria, ataxia, nystagmus, etc. *Action tremors* appear when the muscles of a limb are actively contracted or by holding the limb in an outstretched manner and may increase when precision of movement is required.

PHYSIOLOGIC TREMORS AND SHIVERS

Although tremors are commonly referred to as movement disorders, at least two types of normal tremor occur in humans. One such type is a low-amplitude tremulous movement, not always clinically visible, that occurs even at rest. This tremor is thought to be secondary to cardiac activity causing passive vibration of body tissues and is called the ballistocardiographic tremor. Drugs with positive inotropic effects and other circumstances that increase cardiac activity, such as exercise, fright, stress, and thyrotoxicosis, can accentuate this physiologic tremor by enhancing peripheral beta-adrenergic activity. These tremors may be reduced by administration of a beta blocker, such as propranolol. The other form of physiologic tremor is a higher amplitude tremor of unknown etiology, as seen, for example, in the actively outstretched hand.

Shivering in animals is seen secondary to hypothermia and fear. The former is regulated by the hypothalamus, and the latter by the hypothalamus and the limbic system.

PATHOLOGIC TREMORS AND SHIVERS

Pathologic tremor syndromes in animals are not as well defined as those in people, but certain diseases and syndromes are recognized in veterinary medicine. These include infectious diseases, such as canine distemper. As with other neurologic disorders, a complete history and neurologic examination are essential in the evaluation of animals with tremors because certain congenital, inherited, metabolic, and toxic disorders are associated with tremor syndromes (Fig. 40–1).

CONGENITAL/INHERITED TREMOR SYNDROMES

Disorders of myelination have been reported in various breeds of dogs in which tremor is a major clinical sign. These include the Springer Spaniel (shaking pup), Chow Chow, Weimaraner, Samoyed, lurcher dog, Bernese Mountain dog, and Dalmatian. These disorders affect only the CNS and may be either hypomyelinating (majority of axons thinly myelinated) or dysmyelinating (majority of axons nonmyelinated and abnormal myelin). The pathophysiology of the tremors in these dogs is unknown but may be related to spontaneous (ectopic) excitation of naked axons as a result of increased extracellular potassium. The tremors are action tremors and worsen when the animals are excited or start to move and disappear with rest. The degree of tremor seems to correlate with the severity of the myelin deficit.

Hypomyelination in the shaking pup is a sex-linked recessive trait leading to a point mutation in the proteolipid protein (PLP) gene. Males develop signs at 10 to 12 days of age and show severe generalized tremors that continue throughout life. They are nonambulatory but when hand reared can live for several years. There is no treatment, and these animals do not improve with time. Female carriers may demonstrate variable degrees of tremor at the same age but are not as severely affected as the males and recover in 4 to 6 weeks. The entire CNS appears grossly nonmyelinated, and the majority of axons are thinly myelinated or nonmyelinated. Oligodendrocyte numbers are reduced and

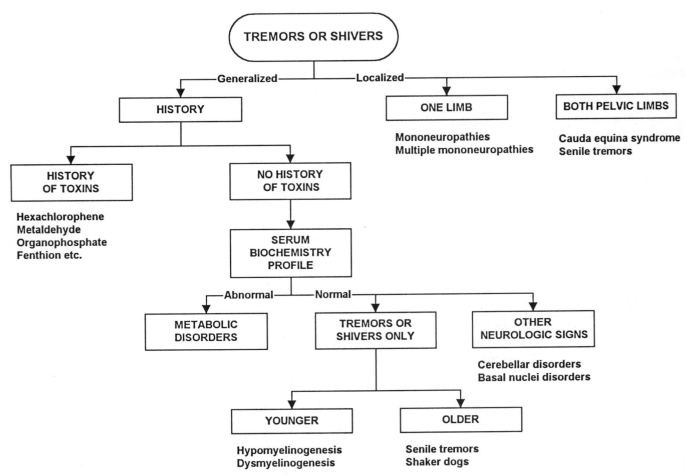

Figure 40–1. Algorithm for clinical evaluation of tremors or shivers.

demonstrate an obvious distention of the rough endoplasmic reticulum.

The abnormality reported in the Samoyed is similar to the *shaking pup* with a suspected sex-linked inheritance and an additional abnormality in maturation of the oligodendrocyte lineage.

The clinical and pathologic findings in the Chow Chow and Weimaraner are similar. Both are suspected to be autosomal recessive traits. The abnormality is first seen when the dogs begin to ambulate at 7 to 12 days of age. These dogs have severe tremors but are able to ambulate, unlike the shaking pup. The clinical signs plateau at 6 to 8 months of age and resolve by 1 year of age. The characteristic feature of these dogs is the hypomyelination of the lateral and ventral spinal columns' superficial tracts. Both breeds also show hypomyelination in the brain. A defect in migration of oligodendrocyte progenitors is suspected owing to the unique pattern of hypomyelination. Recovery in these dogs is most likely from myelination of axons by existing oligodendrocytes. The lurcher dogs and Bernese Mountain dogs are similar to the Weimaraner but do not have a paucity of oligodendrocytes as reported in the Weimaraner.

Lysosomal storage diseases result from a genetic defect in a specific metabolic enzyme pathway with accumulation of substrates in lysosomes of various cells. They usually have an autosomal recessive mode of inheritance and occur within the first few months of life. Tremors may be seen with these diseases, but other clinical signs such as ataxia, cerebellar signs, impaired vision, seizures, dementia, and behavior changes are also seen. These diseases are usually progressive and fatal. Diagnosis is based on breed, clinical signs, and determination of enzyme activity from brain, leukocytes, viscera, or skin fibroblast cultures.

METABOLIC DISEASES CAUSING TREMORS

Tremors may be a component of many metabolic encephalopathies. In human beings, a well-defined 8- to 10-Hz coarse, irregular tremor is most evident in the outstretched hand but can spread to other body parts. This detailed characterization has not been documented in animals, although tremors may be seen in many of the metabolic causes of brain dysfunction. These include hypocalcemia, hyperkalemia, hypoglycemia, hepatic encephalopathy, uremic encephalopathy, hyperthyroidism, hypothyroidism, hyperadrenocorticism, and hypoadrenocorticism. Diagnosis of these diseases is based on laboratory evaluation of metabolic function. Tremors usually resolve when the underlying metabolic abnormality has been corrected.

IDIOPATHIC TREMOR SYNDROME

An acute onset of generalized tremors in adult small breed white dogs such as the Maltese, West Highland White Terrier, and Poodle has been reported. These dogs may be referred to as "white shakers," but others have used the term idiopathic cerebellitis. This problem has been reported in other breeds. These tremors worsen with exercise and lessen or resolve at rest. Ocular tremors are often present. Paresis or ataxia is not a common finding but has been reported. The disease is nonprogressive after the first 2 to 3 days. Pathologic findings in several necropsied dogs are a mild, diffuse nonsuppurative meningoencephalitis. Possible etiologies of this disease include an immune-mediated or viral inflammatory disease. Speculation has centered around an immune reaction against tyrosine-producing cells, which are important in the production of many neurotransmitters. However, this is still speculative, as these dogs are not albinos. Treatment consists of immunosuppressive corticosteroid doses in tapering amounts, decreasing over a period of 2 to 3 months. Diazepam and propranolol may also be used in conjunction with the steroids. Clinical signs should dramatically resolve in several days with treatment. Some dogs are less responsive, and relapses can occur.

SENILE TREMORS

Tremors of the pelvic limbs or all four limbs are occasionally noted in older dogs. These tremors are exaggerated when the dogs move or stand and abate with rest. There are usually no other neurologic signs present, although sometimes weakness is evident. Underlying metabolic, musculoskeletal, or neurologic disease should be excluded. The pathophysiology of this tremor is unknown but may be similar to the senile form of essential tremor in people. The tremors usually do not cause the animal any clinical dysfunction. Propranolol may be tried in these cases, but clinical data to support this approach are lacking. If the tremors are localized to a single limb or the pelvic limbs, nerve root entrapment or spinal cord disease should be suspected.

TOXIN- AND DRUG-INDUCED TREMOR

Mycotoxins such as penitrem A found in moldy cheese or walnuts can cause severe tremors and seizures in dogs. Other toxins such as hexachlorophene, a chlorinated phenol used in many soaps and antiseptics, can lead to severe tremors in young animals after ingestion or absorption through mucous membranes. The cause of the tremors is intramyelinic edema and vacuolation of white matter in the CNS. The signs should resolve with time if the animals survive the initial phase. Tremors have also been associated with heavy metal poisoning such as lead, organophosphate toxicity, metaldehyde, and bromethalin.

Drugs such as droperidol/fentanyl, metoclopramide, and diphenhydramine can sometimes result in head tremors because of their presumed interference with neurotransmitters.

CHAPTER 41

ATAXIA AND PARESIS

Joane Parent

If an animal's mental status is normal, the combination of ataxia and paresis is caused by a problem within the spinal cord. Veterinarians must first recognize ataxia, then identify its type, and finally determine whether there is weakness. Weakness may be subtle in the early stages of spinal cord disease.

The gait of any animal examined with a complaint of difficulty walking must be critically evaluated. A complete neurologic examination should be performed, comprising six components: mental status, gait and posture, cranial nerve examination, postural reactions, spinal reflexes, and pain perception. Of these, the mental status and gait and posture are the most important. Abnormalities in mental status localize the lesion above the foramen magnum, i.e., in the brain. Brain conditions may be associated with gait abnormalities, but these animals usually have signs other than ataxia. This chapter is mainly concerned with spinal cord diseases and their effect on an animal's gait. Critical appraisal of gait requires that the animal be evaluated and walked in a reasonably large enclosure that has a nonslippery floor. Sidewalks and parking lots are usually adequate. Allow the animal some freedom to move around. Some abnormalities become more obvious with a shift in weight bearing or a change in direction and pace.

The complaint of an abnormal gait implies that more than one limb is affected. If only one limb is affected, an owners' complaint is usually that of "lameness." As the animal is observed walking, the veterinarian should attempt to answer the following questions: (1) is the gait abnormal? (2) are only the hind limbs, the limbs on one side, or the hind and front limbs affected? and (3) is there ataxia? If there is no ataxia, the disorder is muscular or orthopedic or involves the peripheral nervous system. Peripheral nervous system diseases do not result in ataxia. Ataxia is a concept that relates to the main axis, the vertebral column, and not to the limbs. As an example, limb amputation does not lead to ataxia. If ataxia is present, its type must be defined.

TYPES OF ATAXIA

The word *ataxia* has a Greek origin (*a* for negative, and *taxis* for order) and means a failure of muscular coordination or an irregularity of muscular action. It is always neurologic in origin. There are three types of ataxia: vestibular, cerebellar, and proprioceptive. The term *proprioceptive ataxia* is preferred over *sensory ataxia,* as the latter can encompass vestibular ataxia to some degree.

Vestibular ataxia is the easiest to recognize. The presence of a head tilt dominates the clinical picture. The head tilt is toward the side of the lesion (except in rare instances of paradoxic vestibular disorder). The vestibular ataxia is characterized by the animal leaning and falling toward the side of the lesion. Its severity correlates with the acuteness of the disease process and the concomitant presence of an abnormal nystagmus.

Proprioceptive ataxia is the most common form. It is also the most difficult to recognize clinically, especially in the early stages of the condition. The proprioceptive receptors situated in muscles, joints, and tendons convey to the brain instant information about the position of the body and limbs in space. This information is carried to the spinal cord via the peripheral nerves. In the spinal cord, it ascends to the brain by way of the reflex (spinocerebellar tracts) and conscious proprioceptive (fasciculi cuneatus and gracilis) pathways. The reflex pathways terminate in the cerebellum, and the conscious pathways end in the contralateral cerebrum. In the spinal cord, the proprioceptive fibers are large and situated in its periphery, making them more vulnerable to insult. As a result, proprioceptive ataxia is the first deficit to appear in spinal cord disease. The animal may veer as it stands with a wide base stance, or it may take longer strides and stumble. As ataxia progresses, "knuckling" becomes obvious while the animal is walking or performing the proprioceptive positioning reactions. Delayed or absent proprioceptive positioning is a severe sign of proprioceptive deficits. Proprioceptive ataxia is characteristically accompanied by weakness as a result of the concomitant involvement of the descending motor pathways or upper motor neurons. There is always a concomitant weakness in spinal cord disease, even in the early stages. With worsening of the disease, the upper motor neurons become more affected, and the paresis may evolve into paralysis. Proprioceptive ataxia may be present in brain diseases, but usually gait abnormalities are not prevailing features. With brain stem disorders, the predominant clinical feature is a decrease in consciousness (depression, stupor, or coma) plus a cranial nerve deficit. With unilateral cerebral disease (as is often the case), gait abnormalities are subtle or not observed. The postural reactions best show the abnormalities.

Cerebellar ataxia is ipsilateral with a unilateral lesion and bilateral with diffuse cerebellar disease. There are no proprioceptive deficits in animals with cerebellar disease, because the conscious proprioceptive pathways to the cerebrum are intact. The descending pathways, the upper motor neurons, are also intact, so there is no weakness. The cerebellum has a modulating effect on the upper motor neurons. Cerebellar lesions lead to a spastic, noncoordinated gait. Commonly there is hypermetria, i.e., exaggerated foot stepping. These animals have a characteristically bouncy gait.

CLINICAL SIGNS OF SPINAL CORD DISEASES

Spinal cord disorders characteristically result in bilateral deficits, with or without mild to marked asymmetry. The clinical signs associated with spinal cord disease, in order of appearance, include proprioceptive ataxia with mild paresis followed by moderate to severe ataxia with obvious paresis, paralysis, urinary incontinence, and absence of pain perception caudal to the lesion. Whereas the presence of ataxia and weakness localizes the problem to the spinal cord, the nature of the reflexes dictates the exact location along the spinal cord. The central core of the spinal cord is composed of grey matter. Damage to lower motor neuron cell bodies in the grey matter causes the reflexes and muscle tone to be decreased or absent. Diseases that affect the white matter result in normal to exaggerated reflexes and tone owing to the loss of inhibition from the upper motor neurons. Spinal cord lesions at the level of the lumbar enlargement result in decreased to absent reflexes and tone in the rear limbs. A lesion above the lumbar enlargement and below the second thoracic spinal segment results in normal to exaggerated reflexes and tone in the rear limbs. A lesion at the level of the cervical enlargement results in reflexes and tone that are normal to exaggerated in the hind limbs and decreased to absent in the front limbs. A lesion above the sixth cervical spinal segment results in reflexes and tone that are normal to exaggerated in all four limbs.

The lumbar enlargement is situated within the vertebrae L4 and L5. The spinal cord ends between vertebrae L6 and L7. The anatomic features within the vertebral canal at that level are the roots, ventral and dorsal. Diseases at the level of vertebrae L5, L6, and the lumbosacral junction behave like peripheral nervous system diseases. No ataxia is observed, although there may be proprioceptive deficits (knuckling) owing to involvement of the dorsal roots. Weakness and decreased to absent reflexes and tone are present.

DIFFERENTIAL DIAGNOSIS

Spinal cord diseases are divided into two main groups: painful and nonpainful. Pain may originate from bone, dorsal root ganglia, and meninges. The common orthopedic disorders include vertebral fracture-luxation, bony neoplasms, and infections such as discospondylitis and osteomyelitis. The most common disease with root pain is intervertebral disk disease. Aseptic meningitis is the only well-recognized cause of pain secondary to meningeal infiltration. Meningomyelitis may cause neck or back pain from the involvement of the meninges but not myelitis, as the parenchyma of the central nervous system has no sensory endings. The two most common nonpainful spinal cord diseases are fibrocartilaginous embolic myelopathy (acute) and degenerative myelopathy (chronic).

The history and signalment of the dog or cat are important considerations in determining a final diagnosis. Disk extrusion rarely if ever occurs in dogs younger than 1 year of age. Breeds with a corkscrewed tail have a higher incidence of vertebral malformations, with clinical signs appearing during the fast growth of the animal (5 to 9 months of age). Diseases localized on the lateral aspect of the canal, such as disk extrusion and invading nerve sheath tumors, have clinical signs that are slightly worse on the side of the lesion. Fibrocartilaginous embolic myelopathy results in profoundly asymmetric signs. Myelitis may produce similar signs. Fibrocartilaginous myelopathy is acute in onset and nonprogressive after the initial 12 hours, whereas degenerative myelopathy has an average of 2 months of progression at the first presentation.

PROGNOSIS

Prognosis is based on neurologic status and duration since the onset of clinical signs. If the disease is treatable, the animal examined within the first 5 days after onset, and pain perception is present, the prognosis for return to function is good. After 10 days, treatment is aimed primarily at stopping progression of the disease. There will be permanent deficits. Cervical lesions are usually not as severe as thoracolumbar lesions. Some purposeful movements are preserved, because paralysis is an uncommon clinical problem. Paralysis usually results in respiratory arrest caused by failure of the intercostal muscles and/or diaphragm, resulting in death. The prognosis is consequently better with cervical lesions, as urinary function and pain perception remain. Timely treatment is crucial for recovery. A diagnostic work-up that includes survey spinal radiographs, cerebrospinal fluid analysis, and myelography should be performed as early as possible. As a rule, recovery occurs in the opposite order of clinical signs, i.e., the last clinical sign to appear is the first to improve. Pain perception is the first function to return, and proprioception is the last.

CHAPTER 42

ALTERED STATES OF CONSCIOUSNESS: Coma and Stupor

Linda Shell

DEFINITIONS

Coma and stupor are pathologic abnormalities caused by an interruption in the structural, metabolic, and/or physiologic integrity of the cerebrum or brain stem. Coma is characterized by an unconscious state from which the animal cannot be aroused by any external stimuli, including those that are noxious. Stupor is clinically similar to coma except that the animal can be aroused with external stimuli but may quickly lapse back into its sleeplike state as soon as the stimuli are withdrawn. Stupor and coma are considered neurologic emergencies, and affected animals must be rapidly assessed with potential causes evaluated in order to begin specific treatment (Fig. 42–1). Serial examinations are necessary to detect changes in an animal's condition and to provide an accurate prognosis.

GENERAL PATHOPHYSIOLOGY

Pathophysiologic aspects such as cerebral edema, increased intracranial pressure, and herniation of brain tissue must be considered when a comatose or stuporous animal is being evaluated. Cerebral edema is the abnormal accumulation of fluid in brain parenchyma that increases intracranial pressure and reduces cerebral perfusion. Cellular hypoxia is exacerbated, causing further edema, possible brain enlargement, and herniation. Any increase in the volume of neural tissue, spinal fluid, or even blood can result in an increase in intracranial pressure because the skull is a nondistensible structure.

Brain Herniations. Four types of brain herniations (Table 42–1) have been described, but only two produce clinical signs of stupor and coma. In caudal transtentorial herniations, unilateral or bilateral portions of the temporal cortex (mainly the parahippocampal gyri) move ventral to the membranous tentorium cerebelli and compress the midbrain. Clinical signs of midbrain compression (Table 42–2) usually consist of decerebrate rigidity and coma, indicating interruption of descending motor tracts and reticular activating system input to the cerebral cortex, respectively. The presence of pupillary constriction suggests loss of sympathetic control as a result of hypothalamic or tectotegmentospinal tract involvement, whereas pupillary dilatation and/or ventrolateral strabismus suggests oculomotor nerve compression. If the herniation and attendant midbrain compression occur gradually, there may be no clinical signs.

Foramen magnum herniation occurs when the caudal cerebellar vermis moves through the foramen magnum, compressing the displaced cerebellum as well as the medulla oblongata. Injury to the respiratory center or pathways or to descending motor tracts results in apnea and tetraplegia. Depressed respiratory and cardiovascular function causes secondary dysfunction in the midbrain and cerebrum and leads to hypoxia-induced coma (see Table 42–2).

The most common causes of brain herniations in dogs are encephalitis, neoplasms, cranial trauma, and hydrocephalus. Herniations are also associated with anesthesia and/or cerebrospinal fluid aspiration in animals with underlying cerebral disease.

HISTORICAL AND EXAMINATION FINDINGS

The first step in managing a comatose or stuporous dog or cat is to identify and correct any life-threatening non-neural problem, such as hemorrhage, shock, or an obstructed airway. A quick but thorough history should ascertain the possibility of trauma, toxin, drug exposure, or any preexisting medical or neurologic sign or disorder. Respiratory and cardiac rates and rhythms should be carefully evaluated for cardiopulmonary disease, which could secondarily cause neurologic signs as a result of hypoxia. A complete neurologic examination should be performed (see Chapter 104), concentrating on level of consciousness, pupil size and response to light, eye movements, respiratory patterns, and skeletal motor responses.

Consciousness. Consciousness is maintained by the ascending reticular activating system (ARAS) located in the midbrain area; it projects diffusely to the cerebral cortex. Thus, diffuse cerebral disease or midbrain disease can cause stupor, coma, or other changes in consciousness (e.g., de-

TABLE 42–1. TYPES OF BRAIN HERNIATIONS

TYPE	STRUCTURE DISPLACED	STRUCTURE COMPRESSED	CLINICAL SIGNS
Caudal transtentorial	Portion of temporal cortex	Midbrain	Yes
Foramen magnum	Caudal cerebellar vermis	Medulla oblongata	Yes
Rostral transtentorial	Rostral cerebellar vermis	Temporal cortex	No
Cingulate gyrus	Cingulate gyrus	Contralateral cingulate gyrus	No

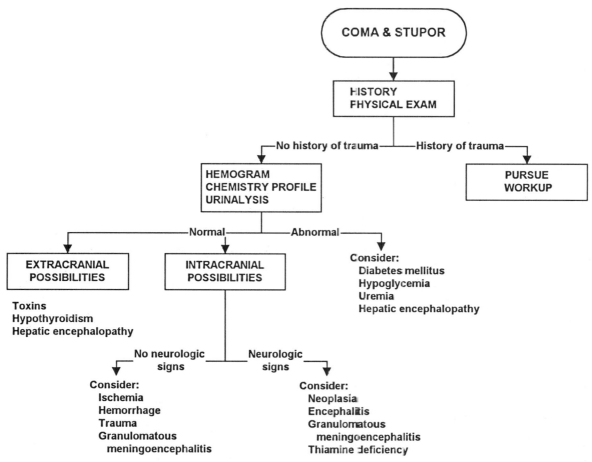

Figure 42–1. Algorithm for diagnostic approach to coma and stupor.

mentia, depressed mentation). Lesions of the medulla oblongata can also cause stupor or coma if the respiratory and cardiovascular centers are affected severely enough to produce hypoxia.

It can be difficult sometimes to separate coma from stupor based on physical appearance. The major difference is that stuporous animals can be aroused with external stimuli (loud sounds or a pinch of the toe with a pair of hemostats), whereas comatose animals do not respond to any external stimuli. As a general rule, a comatose condition has a less favorable prognosis than a stuporous one. However, animals can recover from a comatose state; therefore, trends in the level of consciousness often yield more valuable prognostic information than does the information obtained on one examination.

TABLE 42–2. LOCATION OF LESIONS CAUSING COMA

LOCATION	OTHER POSSIBLE CLINICAL SIGNS
Cerebrum	Seizures Normal or constricted pupils that respond to light Roving eye movements Cheyne-Stokes respirations
Midbrain	Hyperventilation Loss of oculocephalic response Negative caloric test Pinpoint or dilated pupils that do not respond to light
Medulla	Irregular respirations Cardiac arrhythmias

Pupil Size. When pupils are equal in size and respond normally to light and darkness, one can assume integrity of the retinae, optic nerves, optic chiasm, and rostral brain stem (see Chapter 107). Pupil size and reactivity to light can be normal in the comatose animal, but changes can help to localize the lesion and to assess prognosis (Table 42–3). As a general rule, lesions of the brain stem produce unilateral or bilateral pupil constriction or dilatation, whereas lesions of the cerebrum produce normal or constricted pupils that respond to both light and darkness. Pupils that are unresponsive to light imply a grave to hopeless prognosis.

Eye Movements. One can evaluate eye movements by moving the head rapidly from side to side as it is held fixed in a forward position. In the normal animal, several beats of horizontal nystagmus (fast phase toward the direction of head movement) are observed and disappear when the motion stops. This oculocephalic response requires the integrity of the vestibular nerves, brain stem, medial longitudinal fasciculus, and the cranial nerves that move the eyes (CN III, IV, and VI). If nystagmus continues after the head motion stops, a lesion in the vestibular system exists; and if the animal is comatose, a central vestibular disorder is likely to be present. If the oculocephalic response is absent in a comatose patient, severe brain stem injury is a likely diagnosis and the prognosis for return of brain function is poor.

The caloric test can confirm severe brain stem injury in the comatose patient. Infusion of warm or cold water into the ear canals should elicit nystagmus if the pathway for the oculocephalic response movements is intact. Cold water will induce nystagmus with the fast phase opposite the direction

TABLE 42–3. PUPILLARY REACTIONS IN THE STUPOROUS OR COMATOSE ANIMAL

PUPILS AT REST	RESPONSE TO LIGHT	RESPONSE TO DARKNESS	CAUSE OR SITE OF DYSFUNCTION
Equal and constricted	Constrict	Dilate	Metabolic disease
Equal and dilated	Constrict	Dilate	Sympathetic stimulation
Equal and dilated	No response	Fixed and dilated	Midbrain, optic chiasm, optic nerve II, oculomotor nerve III, retina
Unequal at rest (anisocoria)	Both constrict	Both dilate	Unilateral cerebral cortex lesion contralateral to larger pupil
Equal and constricted	Fixed	No response	Pons, ophthalmic injury with iridospasm, bilateral sympathetic denervation (Horner's syndrome)
Unequal, one fixed and dilated	Dilated pupil fixed; normal pupil constricts	Dilated pupil fixed; other dilates	Unilateral oculomotor nerve III

From Dayrell-Hart B, Klide AM: Intracranial dysfunction: Stupor and coma. Vet Clin North Am Sm Anim Pract 19(6):1214, 1989.

of the infused ear, whereas warm water will generate the fast phase toward the infused ear. Absence of nystagmus indicates a poor to hopeless prognosis.

Respiratory Character. Severe brain stem injury can result in apnea, irregular respirations, hyperventilation, or hypoventilation. If the medullary rhythmicity respiratory center is affected, respirations may be irregular and appear as gasps. Hyperventilation has been associated with lesions of the pneumotaxic center in the midbrain. Cheyne-Stokes respiration, characterized by hyperpnea alternating with apnea, is associated with bilateral cerebral hemispheric or diencephalic insults. A change in respiratory pattern suggesting one of the above conditions suggests a grave prognosis.

Skeletal Motor Responses. Comatose or stuporous animals do not have voluntary motor movements and are often tetraplegic because of injury to the descending motor tracts in the brain stem. Involuntary movements such as paddling may be associated with seizure activity. If opisthotonos or limb extensor rigidity develop, the prognosis becomes extremely grave. Decerebrate rigidity describes extensor rigidity in all four limbs resulting from a midbrain or pontine injury to the motor tracts that aid flexion; coma or stupor are present. It should not be confused with decerebellate rigidity associated with a rostral cerebellar lesion. With decerebellate rigidity, the hindlimbs are extended at times and flexed at others, and the level of consciousness should not be impaired if this is the only site of injury.

DIAGNOSTIC PLAN

There are numerous causes of stupor and coma (Table 42–4). Historical data and physical and neurologic examination findings are critical for ranking the possible causes. The majority of the disorders causing coma and stupor are discussed in Chapter 104.

Routine laboratory work (hemogram, serum chemistry profile, urinalysis) is indicated to evaluate possible metabolic causes of coma. Signs of inflammation or toxicity may be evident on the hemogram, whereas the blood chemistry profile and urinalysis may suggest metabolic and endocrine disorders. The lack of evidence of a toxic or metabolic disorder or of organ dysfunction outside the brain may lead one to investigate the possibility of primary brain disease. If metastatic neoplasia or systemic infection is a possibility, chest and abdominal radiographs should be considered. Likewise, skull radiographs may aid the diagnosis of cranial trauma when the history is unrewarding.

Two of the least invasive means of evaluating intracranial

disease are awake electroencephalography (EEG) and brain stem auditory evoked responses (BAER), both of which can be performed without sedation or anesthesia in most animals. The EEG is often helpful in establishing the possibility of an asymmetric cerebral mass lesion, encephalitis, hydrocephalus, cerebral edema, or brain death. The BAER offers a means of evaluating the brain stem and may be helpful in establishing the integrity of this area. Other diagnostic procedures such as spinal fluid analysis, skull radiographs, computed tomography, or magnetic resonance imaging (MRI) carry some degree of risk because of the necessity for anesthesia, which may enhance increases in intracranial pressure and subsequent herniation of the brain. Therefore, the benefit:risk ratio of such diagnostic procedures should be recognized.

Spinal fluid analysis in animals with neoplasia may show an increase in protein concentration. Increased numbers of

TABLE 42–4. CAUSES OF STUPOR AND COMA

Congenital or Familial Disorders

Hydrocephalus
Lysosomal storage disorders
Lissencephaly

Metabolic Disorders

Hepatic encephalopathy
Hypoadrenocorticism
Diabetes mellitus
Hypoglycemia
Hypothyroidism
Uremia
Hypoxia
Acid-base imbalance
Osmolality imbalance
Heat stroke
Hyperlipidemia

Nutritional Disorders

Thiamine deficiency (end stage)

Neoplasia

Primary lesions
Metastatic lesions

Inflammation

Canine distemper
Rabies
Rocky Mountain spotted fever
Ehrlichia
Feline infectious peritonitis
Fungal, protozoal, and bacterial infections
Granulomatous meningoencephalitis

Toxins/Drugs

Ethylene glycol
Lead
Barbiturates
Many others
Mushroom poisoning
Alcohol
Cannabinoids
Hallucinogens

Trauma

Cranial trauma

Vascular

Coagulopathies
Hypertension
Cardiomyopathy
Bacterial emboli
Feline ischemic encephalopathy
Ischemia

Other

Status epilepticus

cells suggest encephalitis. Occasionally, the etiology of the encephalitis can be determined by culture or by the type of cells found in the spinal fluid. Computed tomography and MRI can be rewarding in diagnosing brain tumors, hydrocephalus, and vascular injuries.

GOALS OF TREATMENT

Treatment of a comatose animal must be initiated at time of presentation and, therefore, is nonspecific at first and more specific as the cause becomes more apparent. First, establish a patent airway and ensure proper breathing and cardiac function. Second, place an intravenous catheter and collect blood samples prior to any treatments. Valuable preliminary information can be obtained while waiting on complete laboratory results if the following quick tests are performed: packed cell volume, total solids, blood urea nitrogen (via Azostix), blood glucose (via Dextrostix or Chemstrip bG), urine specific gravity, and urine dipstick.

If the animal is in shock, intravenous fluids are administered in appropriate volumes. Since excessive fluid administration can contribute to cerebral edema, it is wise to undercorrect for dehydration rather than overcorrect. The animal's head should be elevated to prevent excessive blood flow to the brain. The head should be maintained at a normal angle to the neck to avoid jugular compression, which can also increase intracranial pressure. Body temperature should be monitored and maintained within a normal range.

There are three main treatments for cerebral edema: corticosteroids, osmotic diuretics, and hyperventilation. Corticosteroids reduce the edema associated with brain tumors, but their benefit in cases of head trauma has been questioned. Although there is no standard dosage for corticosteroids to treat cerebral edema, dexamethasone can be dosed at 0.25 to 1 mg/lb (0.5 to 2 mg/kg) intravenously once followed by repeated divided doses daily or every other day until there are signs of improvement. Methylprednisolone sodium succinate can also be used at an initial dose of 15 mg/lb (30 mg/kg) intravenously followed by repeated doses of 3 to 7 mg/lb (15 mg/kg) at 2 and 6 hours after the initial dose. Because of corticosteroid-associated gastrointestinal ulceration and bleeding, injectable cimetidine should be considered.

Osmotic agents, such as mannitol, reduce intracranial pressure by decreasing brain water content. They are short lived in their therapeutic effect and should never be administered when the animal is hypovolemic. A 20 per cent solution of mannitol is usually administered intravenously at 0.25 to 1 g/lb (0.5 to 2 g/kg) and repeated every 4 to 6 hours. The use of mannitol in animals that have suffered head trauma is controversial because, if active brain hemorrhage is present, the reduction of intracranial pressure or the size of the brain may allow more hemorrhage to occur. In animals with focal neurologic signs suggesting a discrete area of hemorrhage, some clinicians prefer to use furosemide at 1 to 2 mg/lb (2 to 4 mg/kg) intravenously or intramuscularly instead of mannitol. Others use mannitol followed in 15 minutes with 0.5 mg/lb (1 mg/kg) furosemide to obtain a profound decrease in intracranial pressure.

Hyperventilation can also be used to treat increased intracranial pressure. By increasing Po_2 and reducing Pco_2 blood levels, cerebral blood flow and intracranial pressure are reduced. Disadvantages include the necessity for intubation and a short-lived effect. If blood gas analysis is available, the arterial Pco_2 should be maintained between 25 and 35 mmHg.

Seizures should be controlled with injectable diazepam at 0.25 to 0.5 mg/lb (0.5 to 1 mg/kg) intravenously or 1 mg/kg per rectum. Diazepam can be repeated at 5- to 10-minute intervals for a total of three doses. If seizures continue, a continuous intravenous infusion (5 to 20 mg per hour) in 0.9 per cent normal saline or 5 per cent dextrose can be administered. Injectable phenobarbital or pentobarbital (see Chapters 43 and 104) can also be used to control seizure activity.

Craniotomy is indicated to remove depressed fractures that are compressing the brain or to control hemorrhage from lacerated meningeal vessels.

Nursing care goals are to prevent hypostatic lung congestion by turning the dog or cat every 3 to 4 hours, to maintain fluid and electrolyte balances and proper nutrition, and to prevent decubital ulcer formation by keeping the animal on soft cage padding or a water bed. If the animal is not emptying its bladder, manual expression or catheterization should be performed three or four times daily. Eyes should be lubricated to prevent corneal drying and possible ulceration.

OUTCOME

The prognosis for the animal with coma or stupor is generally guarded until the underlying cause can be defined and appropriate treatment started. Serial neurologic examinations are necessary to give the owner an accurate prognosis. If no improvement is noted in 2 to 3 days despite appropriate treatments, the prognosis is extremely poor. Signs of deterioration include development of arrhythmias, loss of the oculocephalic response, and lack of pupil response to light. Should the animal's condition improve, the owner should be informed of possible sequalae such as permanent neurologic deficits and epilepsy.

CHAPTER 43

SEIZURES

Andrée D. Quesnel

A seizure is the clinical manifestation of an excessive discharge of hyperexcitable cerebrocortical neurons. Depending on the location and extent of the seizure discharge, the clinical appearance of seizures may vary. Without the use of electroencephalography, seizures can be classified only according to their clinical manifestations. Generalized seizures have a widespread onset within both cerebral hemispheres and manifest with loss of consciousness, recumbency, and generalized motor signs. Most generalized seizures manifest with violent motor activity that involves the whole body (convulsions), such as tonic (sustained) or clonic (repetitive) muscle contractions, limb paddling, and trembling. Jaw chomping and facial twitching are frequently observed. Signs of autonomic hyperactivity (e.g., pupillary dilatation, salivation, piloerection, micturition, defecation) are common. Rarely, the seizures may be atonic ("drop-attack") and must be differentiated from syncope and narcolepsy-cataplexy.

Partial seizures have a focal onset in one cerebral hemisphere and limited spreading within the brain. Their occurrence indicates the presence of a focal acquired structural brain lesion. Partial seizures may be simple or complex, depending on whether consciousness is disturbed. Simple partial seizures arise from and are confined to neocortical structures of one cerebral hemisphere. These do not cause consciousness alterations. Unilateral motor signs such as facial twitching, tonic or clonic movements of one or both limbs, and spasmodic turning of the head to one side are often observed and are contralateral to the side of the seizure focus.

In complex partial seizures, the spread of the seizure involves allocortical structures and often continues bilaterally. Consciousness is either impaired or completely lost. There may be contralateral or bilateral asymmetric or symmetric motor signs usually limited to some parts of the body. Bizarre stereotypic (e.g., circling) and behavioral activities (e.g., startling, growling, hissing, chasing and attacking imaginary or real objects, running in a panic) may also be observed, particularly in cats. Some seizures thought to be generalized may be complex partial. In these seizures, consciousness is impaired or lost, and there is bilateral motor activity that usually does not result in recumbency; there is, however, an arrest of the animal's ongoing activities (e.g., it stops if moving and may sit if standing). Motor signs are limited to bilateral facial twitching, jaw chomping, or lip smacking, sometimes with mild generalized trembling or spasms of the neck and front end. Occasionally, there may be decreased motor function that causes stumbling, crawling, or an inability to stand and walk. The dog or cat may still be aware and responsive to a various degree. Because these seizures are not manifested by complete loss of consciousness and generalized motor signs, the underlying neuronal discharge likely has a limited spreading within the brain, which is a feature of partial seizures. A third class of partial seizures includes those that secondarily evolve to generalized seizures. Secondary generalization may occur so quickly that no features of partial seizures may be observed clinically.

Another hallmark of partial seizures is an "aura." An aura is considered to be the initial portion of the seizure, experienced before consciousness is altered and for which memory is retained in people. It corresponds to the onset of a simple partial seizure before it evolves to a complex partial or a generalized seizure. In animals, it is most often manifested by behavioral changes within a few seconds or minutes of seizure onset (e.g., attention seeking or withdrawal, depression or agitation, pacing, whining, howling). Localized postictal motor deficits also indicate that a partial seizure has occurred. This is refered to as Todd's paralysis in human beings and consists of a transient (minutes to hours) localized loss of motor function that follows some partial seizures. It may be attributed to neuronal exhaustion or increased inhibition in the region of the seizure focus. It is observed contralaterally to the initial focus.

Seizures may occur as brief isolated events (usually lasting 2 minutes or less), cluster seizures (two or more over a 24-hour period), or status epilepticus (sustained or serial seizures lasting at least 30 minutes). They can be convulsive with generalized and violent motor activity (e.g., tonic-clonic generalized seizures) or nonconvulsive with milder and often subtle motor signs (e.g., partial seizures limited to facial twitching).

The term *epilepsy* should be restricted to seizure disorders with inactive intracranial causes. Primary (functional, asymptomatic) epilepsy is the result of functional cerebral disturbances for which there is no underlying cause other than a hereditary predisposition (e.g., canine idiopathic epilepsy). Secondary (structural, symptomatic) epilepsy is caused by acquired but inactive brain lesions (e.g., posttraumatic, postischemic, and postencephalitic gliosis). The term *cryptogenic epilepsy* may be used when there is evidence of a structural brain lesion (e.g., partial seizures), but this cannot be further documented and the etiology remains unknown.

GENERAL PATHOPHYSIOLOGY

The neuronal hyperexcitability that underlies the generation of seizures is the result of an imbalance between normal excitatory and inhibitory mechanisms. This may be due to an intracranial or extracranial disease process. Intracranial causes of seizures include primary brain disorders, either functional disturbances of neurons (e.g., idiopathic epilepsy) or structural brain lesions that irritate the surrounding neurons. Structural brain lesions can be active (e.g., neoplasms, encephalitides) or inactive (e.g., glial scars). Extracranial causes of seizures alter brain biochemical homeostasis in favor of excitation and may be exogenous (seizurogenic toxins) or endogenous (severe metabolic disturbances).

It is important to appreciate that seizures enhance the

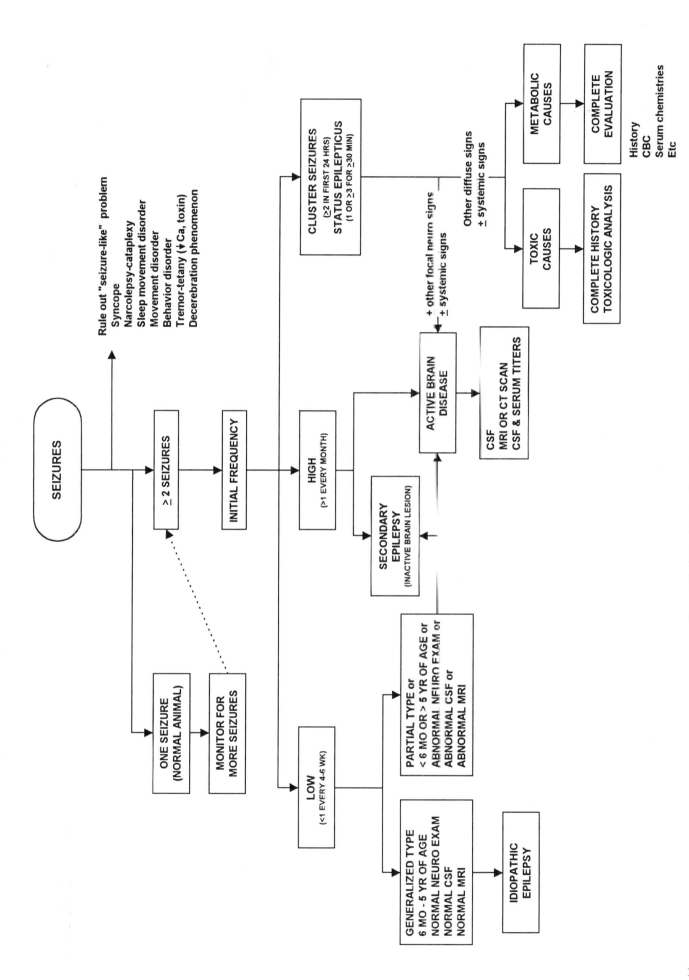

Figure 43–1. Algorithm for diagnostic approach to seizures.

likelihood of further seizures, regardless of their cause. The development of progressive and refractory seizure disorders correlates well with the cumulative number of seizures, especially when their frequency has been great and may occur relatively early in some cases. Such self-perpetuating phenomena may also be involved in acutely recurring seizures (cluster seizures and status epilepticus), which often become more difficult to control the longer the time from their onset. High-frequency seizures may recruit adjacent as well as remote areas of the brain into the epileptic discharge (kindling phenomenon) and may also produce neuronal damage. These factors likely contribute to the development of progressive and refractory seizure disorders. Early diagnostic and therapeutic procedures, especially aggressive antiepileptic drug therapy, are crucial for optimal seizure control in both acute and chronic seizure disorders.

DIAGNOSTIC APPROACH

HISTORICAL FINDINGS

Carefully scrutinizing the seizure history (age at the first seizure, seizure type, and initial frequency) often provides critical information about the underlying cause. This is overviewed in Figure 43–1.

In dogs, idiopathic epilepsy should be excluded if the first seizure did not occur between the age of 6 months and 5 years, if all seizures are not primarily generalized tonic-clonic, if aura or localized postictal motor deficits have been observed, or if the first few seizures occurred at less than 4-to 6-week intervals. Frequent seizures may develop with idiopathic epilepsy in large breeds (e.g., Border collie, Dalmatian, German shepherd, golden retriever, Siberian husky, Saint Bernard) but this usually occurs several months after the seizure onset. Another cause should be suspected in some breeds of dogs (e.g., Doberman pinscher, rottweiler, Newfoundland, brachycephalic breeds) and in cats, which are unlikely to suffer from idiopathic epilepsy.

PHYSICAL FINDINGS

Physical and fundic abnormalities may be related to seizures, thus revealing the existence of an infectious, metabolic, hypoxic (e.g., polycythemia), or neoplastic disease. On neurologic examination, particular attention should be paid to tests that evaluate the cerebral cortex, e.g., menace response, facial (nasal septum) sensation, and postural reactions (proprioceptive positioning and hopping). Subtle unilateral or bilateral but asymmetric deficits can be overlooked if the response obtained on both sides is not carefully compared. Such deficits indicate the presence of a structural lesion in the contralateral cerebral cortex or thalamus. The findings of neurologic deficits that cannot all be attributed to a focal cortical or thalamic lesion indicate multifocal central nervous system involvement, which is usually caused by infectious or noninfectious (immune-mediated) encephalitides.

DIAGNOSTIC PLAN

Once the seizure history has been scrutinized and the clinical examinations performed, the likelihood of an intra-

---

TABLE 43–1. EMERGENCY TREATMENT OF STATUS EPILEPTICUS AND CLUSTER SEIZURES

I. Immediately control the seizures
  A. Phase One: Give a diazepam (DZ) IV bolus of 0.5–1.0 mg/kg.
    1. If gross motor activity does not subside within 3–5 minutes, repeat the DZ bolus (can be repeated 2–3 times).
    2. Immediately start an IV infusion of DZ at the rate of 0.5–1.0 mg/kg/hour (to prevent seizure recurrence).
      a. Add the DZ to maintenance fluids in an in-line burette. Prepare only 1–2 hours of solution at a time (to minimize adsorption of DZ into the administration set plastic and its deactivation by light).
      b. When seizures have stopped for ≥ 4 hours, slowly decrease the infusion concentration (by 25% every 4–6 hours).
    3. If gross motor activity persists or if ≥ 2 seizures recur, continue to Phase Two.
  B. Phase Two
    1. Give a phenobarbital (PB) IV bolus of 2–5 mg/kg (can be repeated at 20-minute intervals, up to 2 times).
    2. Immediately add PB to the DZ infusion at the rate of 2–10 mg/hour.
    3. If sustained or high-frequency seizures persist or recur, continue to Phase Three.
  C. Phase Three
    1. Administer a pentobarbital IV bolus of 2–5 mg/kg (slowly over several minutes) to induce anesthesia (more may be needed).
      a. Intubate and provide oxygen supplementation.
      b. Monitor as for general anesthesia.
      c. Do not confuse paddling associated with recovery from pentobarbital anesthesia with recurrence of seizure activity.
    2. If further convulsive seizures occur, administer an additional bolus of pentobarbital and begin continuous infusion (5 mg/kg/hour) or proceed to inhalation (isoflurane) anesthesia.
II. Restore and maintain homeostasis.
  A. Maintain patent airway and administer oxygen, if necessary.
  B. Maintain body temperature between 38 and 40°C.
  C. Do not give glucose or calcium unless a deficiency is documented by laboratory testing (or is highly suspected and laboratory testing is not readily available).
  D. If seizures have been severe or if there are signs of cerebral edema, give methylprednisolone succinate (Solu-Medrol) 30 mg/kg IV or dexamethasone 0.25 mg/kg IV, unless it is contraindicated (e.g., infectious cause).
  E. Monitor for other potential complications (e.g., signs of increasing intracranial pressure, neurogenic pulmonary edema, cardiac arrhythmias).
III. Collect appropriate samples as soon as possible for hematology, biochemical profile, urology, and, in dogs or cats already on maintenance therapy, determination of serum antiepileptic drug concentration.
IV. Initiate or continue oral PB therapy.
  A. Give an initial loading dose of 5 mg/kg to conscious animals as soon as they can swallow, then continue with 2.5 mg/kg q12h.
  B. Continue usual PB administration in dogs or cats already on maintenance therapy; give IM if the oral route is not possible.
    1. Increase the dosage as soon as the PB serum concentration ([PB]$_s$) is known to be suboptimal (< 100–120 μmol/L or 23–28 μg/mL).
    2. If the [PB]$_s$ is already within the optimal range, add potassium bromide (KBr; 10–20 mg/kg q12h) to the dog oral daily regimen and DZ (0.5–1.0 mg/kg q12h) to the cat oral daily regimen. An oral loading dose of KBr 400–600 mg/kg, preferably divided in subdoses and administered with food over a 12- to 24-hour period, can be given to dogs to provide an immediate therapeutic serum concentration (10–15 mmol/L).
V. Continuously monitor vital signs and neurologic status and provide intensive supportive care to the stuporous or anesthetized dog or cat.

TABLE 43–2. GUIDELINES FOR MAINTENANCE ORAL ANTIEPILEPTIC DRUG THERAPY

I. Perform a complete blood count (CBC), biochemical profile, and urology study to establish pretreatment values.

II. First-choice antiepileptic drug: phenobarbital (PB).
   A. Initial dosage: 2 (1.0–2.5) mg/kg q12h. Increase the dosage by 50–100% in puppies (possibly in kittens also) because of their higher metabolic rate.
   B. Always measure trough PB serum concentration ($[PB]_s$) 2 weeks after initiation of therapy (after 1 week in immature animals) and adjust the dosage to reach an optimal $[PB]_s$ of 100–120 μmol/L (23–28 μg/mL). Use the formula: optimal $[PB]_s$ ÷ actual $[PB]_s$ × actual daily dose = optimal daily dose. Perform a CBC to detect rare but possible PB-induced blood dyscrasias (e.g., neutropenia, thrombocytopenia).
   C. Always measure $[PB]_s$ 2 weeks (1 week in immature animals) after any dosage modification (and adjust the dosage accordingly).
   D. If adequate seizure control (≤ 1 seizure/6–8 weeks) is not obtained or is no longer maintained despite an optimal $[PB]_s$, add a second drug to the treatment regimen; continue PB and maintain the $[PB]_s$ in the optimal range.

III. Second-choice antiepileptic drugs.
   A. Dogs: potassium bromide (KBr) 15 (10–20) mg/kg q12h.
      1. Measure serum KBr concentration ($[KBr]_s$) 6 weeks after initiation of therapy. If ≤ 10 mmol/L (100 mg/dL; 1000 μg/mL), increase the dosage by 25–50% to obtain an optimal $[KBr]_s$ of 15–20 mmol/L at steady state (reached 3 months after treatment initiation or modification).
      2. Measure $[KBr]_s$ at 6-week intervals until steady state is reached (and adjust the dosage accordingly).
      3. In some emergency situations, an oral loading dose of 400–600 mg/kg can provide an immediate therapeutic serum concentration (see Table 43–1.)
      4. The chloride content of the diet must be stable to avoid $[KBr]_s$ fluctuations (elimination of bromide is directly proportional to chloride intake).
      5. A lower dosage and closer monitoring of $[KBr]_s$ are advocated in animals with renal dysfunction.
   B. Cats: diazepam (DZ) 0.5–1.0 mg/kg q12h.
      1. Measure serum benzodiazepine concentration 5 days after onset of therapy and adjust the dosage (use the same formula as for PB) to reach a therapeutic range of 500–700 nmol/L (500–700 ng/mL).
      2. Evaluate liver enzymes at the same time to detect rare but possible idiosyncratic acute hepatic necrosis; if elevated, discontinue DZ and add KBr.

IV. Third-choice antiepileptic drugs.
   A. Dogs: felbamate 15–65 mg/kg q8h.
      1. Steady state is reached after the fourth oral dose, and therapeutic serum concentration is reported to be 15–100 μg/mL.
      2. CBC and liver enzyme monitoring are recommended as for PB therapy (felbamate is metabolized by the liver and causes enzyme induction).
   B. Cats: KBr 10–20 mg/kg/day (use the same guidelines as for dogs).

V. Client communication (verbal and written).
   A. Define the treatment goals and side effects and toxicity.
   B. Emphasize the importance of complying with drug administration regimens, of keeping a seizure calendar (date, duration, intensity), and of consulting as soon as seizure control is no longer achieved, as well as for any treatment modification.
   C. Insist on the importance of initial determinations of serum drug concentrations and periodic blood analysis (CBC, biochemistry, and serum antiepileptic drug concentration) every 6–12 months.
   D. Define emergency situations and establish an emergency plan.
   E. Recommend that intact females be spayed as soon as a diagnosis of epilepsy is made.

VI. For dogs known to have cluster seizures, provide injectable DZ to be administered per rectum at home: 1 mg/kg after the second seizure has occurred, to be repeated three to four times every 20 minutes. If this fails to abort the cluster seizures, emergency parenteral therapy is necessary.

VII. Drug interactions and contraindications.
   A. Do not administer drugs that lower the seizure threshold: acepromazine, xylazine ketamine, estrogens, tricyclic antidepressants (e.g., amitriptyline), and bronchodilators (e.g., aminophylline, terbutaline, theophylline).
   B. Do not administer drugs that interfere with the metabolism of PB (may result in a rapid accumulation of a toxic $[PB]_s$): chloramphenicol, cimetidine, ranitidine, and tetracyclines.

VIII. Only if no seizures have occurred for 6–12 months, consider slow weaning of antiepileptic drugs over a few months. If > 1 seizure/6–8 weeks occurs during or after antiepileptic drug weaning, resume therapy, probably for life.

---

or extracranial cause can often be established, and a rational diagnostic evaluation can be planned (see Figure 43–1). Despite extensive diagnostic investigation, an etiology is often difficult to establish in seizure disorders with intracranial causes. However, the main objective is not necessarily to reach a precise diagnosis, but rather to rule out conditions that would require or benefit from specific medical (e.g., encephalitides) or surgical (e.g., neoplasms) treatment. Once this has been done, symptomatic antiepileptic drug therapy is the only therapeutic option.

TREATMENT

Status epilepticus and cluster seizures, whether they are convulsive or nonconvulsive, are emergencies. Their management is outlined in Table 43–1.

Oral maintenance antiepileptic drug therapy should be initiated as soon as two consecutive seizures have occured within 6 weeks; this includes cluster seizures and status epilepticus, even at the first occurrence of seizures. Early, aggressive, and rational treatment is important. Guidelines for oral maintenance therapy are presented in Table 43–2. The goal of treatment is to reduce the seizure frequency to less than one single seizure every 6 to 8 weeks. Phenobarbital is the drug of first choice in dogs and cats because it is effective safe, and inexpensive. Although the therapeutic range is reported to be 65 to 175 μmol/L (15 to 40 μg/mL), levels below 100 μmol/L (23 μg/mL) are often insufficient to obtain and maintain adequate seizure control, and levels higher than 140 μmol/L (32 μg/mL) may cause hepatotoxicity.

Potassium bromide is the second-choice drug in dogs. Because it is not metabolized, it is the best drug for dogs with preexisting liver disease, as well as an alternative drug for dogs that develop hepatotoxicity or hypersensitivity reactions with phenobarbital (e.g., hyperactivity, pruritic dermatitis, neutropenia, thrombocytopenia). Side effects are similar to and add to those of phenobarbital (polydipsia and polyuria, polyphagia). Signs of bromide toxicity include sedation and hind limb paresis. These are usually seen with serum concentrations above 15 mmol/L (150 mg/dL; 1500 μg/mL), although many dogs tolerate levels up to 25 to 30 mmol/L. Some authors believe that bromide should be the initial drug for dogs because it is not hepatotoxic and its adverse effects are completely reversible once treatment is discontinued. Potassium bromide is also suitable for maintenance therapy in cats.

OUTCOME

Prognosis of seizure disorders depends mainly on the nature of the underlying cause and on the response to therapy. Idiopathic epilepsy often progresses to refractoriness despite adequate treatment in some large-breed dogs; this is much less frequent in small breeds. Although seizure disorders of cats are almost always the result of structural brain lesions, these are most often inactive or self-limited. Even if cats have severe seizures at some point during the course of the disease, these can most often be well controlled or even completely stopped with adequate therapy. Refractoriness to antiepileptic drug therapy appears to be less common in cats.

CHAPTER 44

SLEEP DISORDERS

Joan C. Hendricks

Sleep-associated problems in pet cats and dogs are uncommon owner complaints. Subjective disorders of sleep such as pathologic hypersomnolence and insomnia cannot be easily assessed by an owner or clinician. Slight to moderate disruption of daily behavior patterns that accompany many changes in sleep do not substantially alter an animal's ability to function as a pet. The disorders that prompt an owner to bring a pet for veterinary treatment tend to be those that dramatically change the animal's overt behavior, such as sleep-associated epilepsy or narcolepsy with cataplexy. Other disorders, such as sleep apnea or cardiac arrhythmias, can be triggered by sleep and may have profound consequences for an animal despite being overlooked by most owners. It is interesting to realize that relatively minor changes in sleep behavior may herald future manifestations of abnormal central nervous system (CNS) function.

Sleep is a complex physiologic state with two distinct stages in normal mammals. During the first of these, the animal seeks a quiet, secure resting place and takes a characteristic relaxed species-specific posture. A few minutes after closing its eyes and becoming immobile, changes in CNS activity occur in the electroencephalogram (EEG): the cerebral activity alters from the rapid, desynchronized neural firing patterns of waking to synchronous discharges that produce high-voltage, slow (approximately 5 to 12/second) wave activity. The pulse and respiratory rates slow, blood pressure decreases, and reflex arcs maintain homeostasis in autonomic systems. After a specific duration of uninterrupted slow-wave sleep (approximately 30 minutes in cats and dogs), behavioral and physiologic signs of a second stage appear. The observer notes a further relaxation of muscle tone, as a powerful postsynaptic inhibitory influence descends from the pontine brain stem along a ventral reticulospinal tract to the spinal motor neurons to produce postural muscle atonia. Several seconds to minutes after this atonia begins, volleys of distal small muscle twitching occur, producing rapid movements of the eyes, facial muscles, paws, and tail. Irregular respiration, heart rate, and blood pressure surges accompany these phasic bursts of small muscle movements. These small movements are the external manifestation of a highly activated brain: the flaccid musculature and lack of responsiveness belie a high rate of neural discharge throughout virtually all areas of the brain. During this second phase, most commonly known as rapid-eye movement, or REM, sleep, the autonomic systems are driven by cerebral and brain stem influences during the bursts of twitching activity, which override reflex control. REM lasts as long as 10 to 15 minutes in normal cats and dogs. In humans, this stage can last 20 to 35 minutes and represents the sleep period when almost all dreams occur.

Sleep is thus a complex CNS and somatic syndrome that normally has an orderly progression. The atonia of REM sleep has the important function of preventing overt movements during the sleep period when the cerebrum is highly active.

SLEEP-ASSOCIATED AGGRESSION

An abnormal behavior that seems to occur relatively commonly is sleep-associated aggression (Fig. 44–1). Owners report that a normally calm and friendly animal growls or attacks suddenly if disturbed while sleeping. Although owners may perceive this behavior as unpredictable and unprovoked, these attacks seem to be expressions of aggression, both dominance aggression related to the pet's sense of vulnerability upon arousal and territorial aggression related to defense of the resting place. No cases have been reported or documented in the literature in which animals displayed aggressive behavior directed at their owners while still asleep. Unfortunately, as this behavior is typically episodic and occurs in the home environment, it is difficult to observe directly. However, many or most dogs respond to behavioral approaches to treat aggression.

TRUE SLEEP DISORDERS

In general, true sleep disorders can be classified into two categories: those in which the CNS mechanisms of sleep are normal (see Fig. 44–1) but other CNS or physiologic abnormalities are unmasked or triggered by sleep, and those

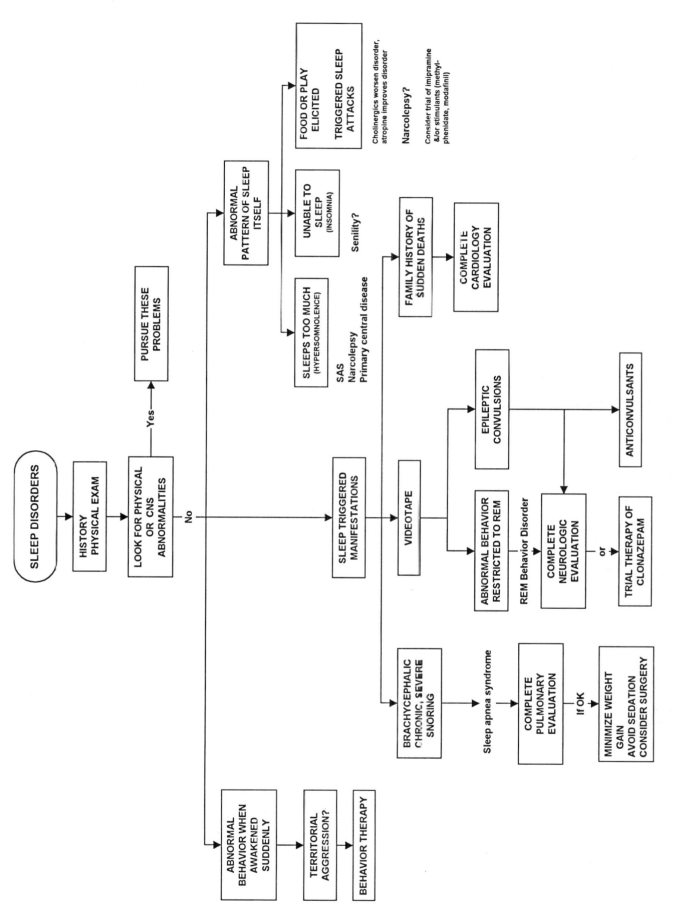

Figure 44–1. Algorithm for clinical evaluation of sleep disorders.

in which the CNS mechanisms of sleep itself are abnormal. The differential diagnosis of these problems is facilitated by knowing the physiology of sleep; augmenting a careful history with observation or, preferably, videotapes of behavior; and taking a rational approach to assessing the signs.

EXACERBATION OR UNMASKING OF ABNORMALITIES WITH SLEEP

Physiologic Abnormalities. Serious cardiovascular and respiratory disorders associated with sleep have been well documented in the literature and further studied in laboratory colonies of affected animals. Several families of German shepherds with histories of sudden cardiac death in apparently normal pups were identified. These dogs have an inherited predisposition to cardiac arrhythmias that are most common during sleep, especially during the REM stage. Abnormalities during standard clinical cardiac evaluation were relatively subtle, but ventricular tachycardia could be detected if pups were monitored by Holter monitors. Implanted pacemakers appear to have been successful in preventing sudden death in at-risk dogs. The mode of inheritance is complex, apparently either a polygenic or a dominant trait with incomplete penetrance. A colony of these dogs has been established, and studies of the underlying cellular abnormalities are in progress. In addition to the relevance of this basic research, it is significant that several families from widespread geographic regions were found to share a trait that can be transmitted by unaffected carriers. Thus, although the syndrome is well described in German shepherds descended from a single common ancestor, the possibility exists that similar abnormalities could occur in other families and in other canine breeds.

Sleep apnea has been described in English bulldogs. Even if they have normal arterial blood gases during waking, virtually all bulldogs exhibit episodes of apnea (pauses in breathing) and hypoxia during sleep, especially in REM sleep. These dogs normally compensate for their narrowed upper airways by augmenting the activity of upper airway dilating muscles during waking and much of non-REM sleep. However, during REM sleep, when muscle activity is reduced by normal atonia and reflexes are intermittently overridden by phasic cerebral influences, intermittent upper airway obstruction occurs. In laboratory studies, these pauses have been documented to occur at rates ranging from six per hour to over 100 per hour. The oxygen saturation can fall as low as 70 per cent but most commonly falls to 85 to 90 per cent from the normal 94 to 95 per cent. As is true for humans with sleep apnea, these dogs are hypersomnolent and exhibit obvious snoring. However, these signs in themselves do not usually present difficulties for owners or pets. Based on other experimental evidence, it is likely that the episodic drops in oxygen saturation lead to hypertension and cardiovascular consequences in both dogs and humans, but the clinical importance of these abnormalities for dogs has not been proved.

Although it is not clear whether sleep apnea alone warrants treatment, surgery is often performed in English bulldogs to relieve waking signs of upper airway obstruction, and this surgery appears to be partially effective in relieving obstructive sleep apnea as well. The usual treatment in humans is to prescribe a face mask to be worn nightly. This constant positive airway pressure mask forces air through the nares to the pharynx to maintain a patent airway; this is obviously not feasible in canine patients. Pharmacotherapy is being investigated, and at present, some approaches that alter serotonin appear to have promise.

As in the case of the sudden cardiac death syndrome of German shepherds, it seems likely that this type of disorder, well described in the laboratory in one breed, may exist in other predisposed animals. Any anatomic narrowing of the upper airway could lead to the same signs. Thus, brachycephalic conformation in any cat or dog, or an acquired narrowing caused by tumor or traumatic injury, could predispose to sleep apnea. Owners do not commonly complain of snoring, hypersomnolence, or gasping respiratory patterns in bulldogs, but they often describe these signs in response to direct questions. Similar signs have been described by owners of Shar Peis, pugs, beagles, and an obese, hypothyroid miniature poodle with obvious upper airway narrowing due to fat accumulation. In the latter case, treatment of the hypothyroidism resolved the profound sleepiness and sleep-induced apnea noted by the owners. This anecdotal evidence suggests that sleep apnea exists in several canine breeds. In addition, some owners of brachycephalic cats have described obvious snoring and irregular breathing, but none of these animals has been available for further laboratory assessment.

Diagnosis of sleep apnea requires continuous pulse oximetry and respiratory movement recordings, together with documentation of the sleep stage. This assessment can be noninvasive but is labor-intensive and impractical in a clinical setting. At present, the recommendation to a clinician who sees a pet with signs suggestive of sleep apnea is to treat the animal based largely on its waking signs.

CNS Abnormalities. Abnormal movements seen during sleep are often evidence of an underlying CNS disorder. The systematic changes in CNS activity that accompany normal sleep can unmask CNS disorders. Epilepsy from any cause, including idiopathic epilepsy, can be triggered by the rhythmic discharges of slow-wave sleep, although the seizures are rarely confined to sleep. Indeed, as part of the diagnostic work-up of human epilepsy, the EEG is recorded during slow-wave sleep in an effort to trigger the epileptic discharges. During the REM stage, abnormal movements can occur when the inhibitory pathway that normally produces atonia during REM sleep is disrupted. This pathway, which arises in the pons and descends in the spinal cord, can be interrupted by a number of brain stem or spinal cord abnormalities, including traumatic injuries. Interrupting this inhibitory pathway permits the expression of the ongoing cerebral activity. Humans with this disorder (REM behavior disorder, or RBD) report that the observed behaviors represent the motor behavior appropriate to their dream content. Thus, a patient may stand up and run, clutching an invisible object, while dreaming of playing football; or a patient may sit up and begin attacking his spouse and later describe that he was defending himself against a dream attacker. Dogs and cats with these disorders, which appear to be the most common sleep disorder in pets, judging by referrals, typically lift their heads and exhibit dramatic but intermittent paddling or locomotor activity during REM sleep. They can easily be aroused from these episodes, which occur during every REM period and can often be recognized by an experienced observer viewing videotapes of the behavior. Although many of these animals are completely normal at all other times, in some cases it is obvious that CNS damage is correlated with the disorder, as in the case of a kitten that suffered a traumatic injury to the cervical spinal cord before the onset of signs. Even individuals that have an unremarkable physical examination may have an underlying CNS disorder. In humans with RBD and no other abnormalities at diagnosis, 38 per cent developed overt Parkinson's disease an average of 3.7 years after the diagnosis of RBD. At the present time, the author has followed two cats with apparent congenital RBD for 10 or more years and observed no progression of signs. One of these cats eventually died and underwent a complete necropsy, and no gross or microscopic CNS abnormalities were identified. Clonazepam, a benzodiazepine tranquilizer, reduces the level of activity during RBD in the vast majority of humans and was partially effective in the two cats. Routine anticonvulsant agents are not effective, as they initially suppress REM sleep, with an eventual rebound of REM and recurrence of the behavior. Even if the disorder is not associated with other evidence of CNS disease, it can be life-threatening for cats and dogs, because some pets suffer urinary incontinence during the episodes, which is intolerable for some owners. In one cat treated for 8 years with clonazepam, the intensity of the behavior was reduced but not abolished. Withdrawing the clonazepam after 6 years resulted in an increase in motor behavior and related urination during REM, which was again partly controlled by reinstituting the treatment. Thus, chronic treatment is feasible in pets with this disorder, but no improvement of the underlying abnormality should be expected based on experience to date.

In summary, evidence of abnormal movements during sleep should be assessed in view of the possibility that these movements may reveal otherwise occult CNS disease. However, some individuals (only cats identified to date) appear to have a congenital abnormality of the REM motor inhibitory pathway, perhaps caused by a biochemical change in the neural systems that normally maintain atonia.

DISORDERS OF SLEEP MECHANISMS

Effects of Systemic Disease. Sleep itself is affected by many systemic disorders. Systemic changes in immune function may alter sleep. It is now clear that prostaglandin D and interleukin-1-beta produce the increase in sleep that occurs with many febrile illnesses, accounting for this common symptom. One specific condition that alters sleep in humans is infection with human immunodeficiency virus, and a recent study documented that cats with feline immunodeficiency virus show reduced sleep and disproportionately reduced REM sleep. The only owner complaints we receive regarding reduced sleep, or insomnia, involve elderly dogs who pace throughout the night. These dogs may be like humans with senile dementia, in whom the quantity and pattern of sleep become abnormal in association with increasing dementia. The opposite condition, increased sleep or pathologic hypersomnolence, can occur with sleep apnea and has also been described as an isolated idiopathic abnormality in humans and in one case report of a dog. However, the best described syndrome in which sleep mechanisms are abnormal is narcolepsy.

Narcolepsy. Narcolepsy is a fascinating but rare disease. Narcolepsy is well documented in humans and dogs. It has also been reported in a cat, a bull, and several horses. The abnormality appears to be in the CNS trigger mechanisms of the REM sleep state itself. The abnormalities that appear are caused by the sudden eruption of components of REM sleep, including unconsciousness, muscle atonia, and dream imagery, into wakefulness. Without the normal temporal insulation of non-REM sleep, such manifestations are disruptive to normal life. In animals, the sudden loss of muscle tone (cataplexy) is almost always the sign noted by owners. However, in one dog, a sleepy appearance led the owners to seek veterinary advice. Although some individual cases of human and canine narcolepsy are caused by organic brain disease, the vast majority have no obvious CNS abnormality. Several subtle changes in CNS pharmacology have been documented in canine narcoleptics. There is clearly an inherited form of the disease that has been best documented in a colony of Doberman pinschers.

The diagnostic process includes ruling out organic brain disease, and the diagnosis is best made when the behavior can be observed to be triggered by play or by food presentation, as is typical of canine narcoleptics. Fortunately, the disorder in dogs usually has only a moderate effect on their ability to lead normal lives, and in many cases it may be transient. In the colony of Doberman pinschers, the signs are maximal in pups at 4 to 7 months of age and then wane in severity. One case has been reported, however, in which the food-triggered cataplexy was so severe that complete anorexia resulted in a 20-kg weight loss, and long-term treatment was required. The biochemical control of muscle atonia is well characterized, but proven pharmacotherapeutic agents in dogs are limited to imipramine. Arousal-promoting agents can be used to relieve the hypersomnolence if necessary.

CHAPTER 45

BEHAVIORAL DISORDERS

Ilana R. Reisner and Katherine A. Houpt

Behavioral complaints by pet owners are rapidly increasing—not because there are new problems, but because people recognize that veterinary care includes treatment for behavior problems. Behavior problems, whether early and mild or chronic and severe, are common. By asking the right questions, clinicians can help make the ultimate difference in pet care.

CANINE BEHAVIOR PROBLEMS

Aggression

Dominance Aggression

Dominance aggression is extremely common and tends to occur in the following circumstances: (1) when the dog is protecting food, garbage, and certain objects (toys, stolen objects); (2) if disturbed while sleeping or resting, especially in socially significant areas such as furniture; (3) when a certain, closely bonded family member is approached or touched by other family members; (4) when the dog feels certain actions by owners "threaten" its social status (Fig. 45–1). This can include certain postures such as bending over the dog, prolonged staring, punishment, pulling by the leash or collar, or even petting. Because the stimulus can be subtle, dominance aggression is often described by owners as "unprovoked."

Dogs usually begin to exhibit serious aggression near the age of social maturity (1 to 3 years). Because the predisposition for dominance aggression tends to be inherited (with components of learned behavior), it cannot be completely "cured." However, aggression can often be controlled so that the dog becomes a good pet.

For understandable reasons, aggression directed toward children in the home is particularly upsetting to dog owners. Dogs targeting children may be motivated by dominance, but aggression due to fear (lack of familiarity or memory of pain) or even predation is also possible. Regardless of motivation for aggression, biting dogs should be removed from that environment, leashed, actively supervised, muzzled, or crated in the presence of small children. Predatory aggression presents a special problem because even pets with no history of dominance aggression may suddenly attack a small infant.

Treatment of dominance-related aggression includes avoidance of injury to owners, with active supervision or restraint as needed, particularly around children. The use of a basket-style muzzle is recommended in cases when dogs cannot be actively supervised, or when there is ongoing risk of biting. Owners are counseled to safely regain control of the dog by (1) active withdrawal of attention and affection; (2) use of a head collar (Gentle Leader, Premier Pet Products) and indoor lead; (3) obedience training to reestablish verbal control, using positive reinforcement; and (4) telling the dog to obey a command first before receiving anything it wants. Even mild aggression is potentially dangerous in a home with children. Because of the natural transgressions of children, prevention of problems (as distinct from treatment) should be emphasized in such homes. Punishment for aggressive behavior is unlikely to truly change the dog's motivation to bite; in some cases, it may worsen the aggression.

Pharmacologic intervention is sometimes indicated in cases of aggression. In all cases, but particularly when there is ongoing risk of injury, drugs should be used cautiously and with full disclosure of risks involved: there are no drugs approved specifically for aggressive behavior. For anxious aggressive dogs, anxiolytic drug therapy can be useful. Suggested drugs include (1) tricyclic antidepressants such as amitriptyline or clomipramine, (2) benzodiazepines such as alprazolam or clorazepate, and (3) buspirone (Table 45–1). Increasing brain serotonin with specific serotonin reuptake inhibitors may reduce aggression. Examples are fluoxetine and paroxetine.

Desensitization can be accomplished most safely using a basket muzzle. Dogs are less likely to be successfully desensitized to activities that startle them, such as being jumped on by a child or being woken abruptly.

In the treatment of any type of aggression, whether behavior modification is used alone or drugs are administered, it is critical to advise owners that the problem will not be cured, but only controlled (and quite often only partially). There is never a guarantee that biting will not recur; in fact, chances are often quite good that it will recur.

Territorial Aggression

Territorial aggression is directed at unfamiliar people. Aggressive barking, growling, and biting threats can be exhibited in the home, yard, car, or any area in which the dog has spent time. Males may be slightly more likely than females to exhibit territorial behavior, which, like dominance aggression, is usually first seen in socially mature dogs. Any breed can be presented, though some are clearly predisposed. Dogs that chase as well as threaten may also be exhibiting predatory aggression.

Territorially aggressive dogs are treated with a combination of increased physical control and desensitization to approaches by unfamiliar people. Instead of being tied to chains or allowed free time in the yard, dogs should be taken for supervised, on-lead walks. If any time is spent unsupervised in the yard, reliable fencing is critical; underground radiofrequency fences are potentially quite dangerous, because strongly motivated dogs will run through the shock and unsuspecting pedestrians may wander into the dog's turf. In the home, territorially aggressive dogs should always be on lead when visitors are entertained. This is a particularly severe problem in homes entered unannounced by children, or in situations in which the dog is alone when encountering visitors.

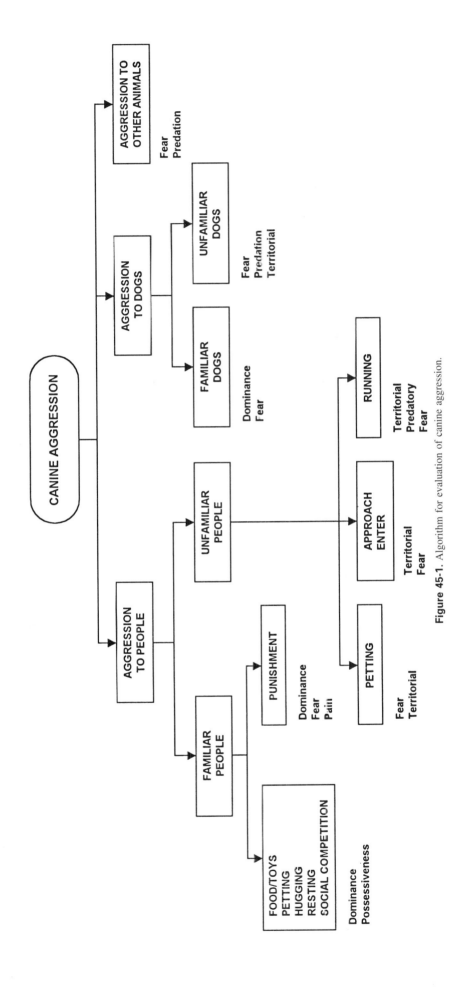

Figure 45-1. Algorithm for evaluation of canine aggression.

TABLE 45–1. SELECTED DRUGS USED TO TREAT BEHAVIOR PROBLEMS IN DOGS

GENERIC/TRADE NAME	DOSAGE	ROUTE	FREQUENCY	CLASS
Alprazolam (Xanax)	0.022 mg/kg	PO	prn up to q 8 hours	Benzodiazepine
Amitriptyline (Elavil)	2.2–4.4 mg/kg	PO	q 12 hours	Tricyclic antidepressant
Buspirone (BuSpar)	5–10 mg/dog	PO	q 12–8 hours	Anxiolytic
Clomipramine (Clomicalm, Anafranil)	3 mg/kg†	PO	q 12 hours	Tricyclic antidepressant
Clorazepate (Tranxene)	0.55–2.2 mg/kg‡	PO	prn up to q 8 hours	Benzodiazepine
Fluoxetine (Prozac)	5 mg/dog	PO	q 24 hours	Specific serotonin-reuptake inhibitor
Paroxetine (Paxil)	2.5–5 mg/dog	PO	q 24 hours	Specific serotonin-reuptake inhibitor

†Start at a low dose, e.g. 1 mg/kg for 2 weeks, then 2 mg/kg for 2 weeks, then 3 mg/kg.
‡Titrate to clinical sedation—dose may vary for individual dogs.

Territorially aggressive dogs should be conditioned to accept—even enjoy—the approach of house guests or pedestrians. Counter-conditioning trains the dog to sit or lie down quietly during approaches, door knocks, and other stimuli, first indoors and then outdoors.

Fear-Based Aggression

Defensive or fear-based aggression can be displayed toward either family members or unfamiliar people. Owners may elicit a fear-related growl or bite when punishing their pets. Without a detailed history of circumstances and postures assumed by the dog, such behavior may be difficult to distinguish from dominance-related aggression. Fearful dogs usually attempt to avoid threats and will bite primarily when cornered or otherwise directly confronted. Fear-based aggression may be displayed by either sex, at any age. All breeds are affected; severely fearful dogs can be either genetically predisposed or environmentally conditioned (or both). Poor early socialization can result in insecurity and defensiveness. There may be a significant component of fear in territorial aggression.

Treatment of fear-related aggression involves a combination of desensitization and counter-conditioning to the source of the fear. Severely fearful dogs may require anxiolytic medication during the training program (see Table 45–1). Fearful behavior should be neither reassured nor punished; instead, it should be ignored. Overt aggression should immediately be interrupted, then followed by obedience commands for which the dog can be praised.

Separation Anxiety

The manifestation of canine separation anxiety is variable, usually including destructiveness, elimination, and vocalization. The cause of the problem may be unclear. Prolonged separation, such as a vacation taken by owners, may precipitate a problem. Dogs adopted from shelters often exhibit separation anxiety, although it is unclear whether this is a cause or effect of having been surrendered into the shelter.

Diagnosis of separation anxiety is made when a dog exhibits agitation, salivation, destructiveness, elimination, and/or vocalization in the owner's absence. These behaviors typically occur within 30 minutes of the owner's departure. In addition, these dogs often appear anxious during departures and greetings.

Treatment involves a combination of anxiolytic drug therapy and desensitization to the owner's departure. Combination therapy is often helpful, for example, extended treatment with amitriptyline, plus clorazepate as needed, when the dog is alone.

Ideally the dog should not be left alone during the desensi-

tization period. If unavoidable, owners should try desensitizing to a "new" exit point, while leaving for work through the "old" door. Crating and confinement generally are contraindicated for dogs with separation anxiety. Owners should attempt to reduce the distinction between their presence and their absence; for example, lights and sound should be maintained when the dog is alone, and owners should discontinue greetings and good-byes, ignoring the dog instead. An attractive food-oriented toy is provided only during departures. All punishment should be avoided.

FELINE BEHAVIOR PROBLEMS

Inappropriate Elimination

Failure to use the litter box is the primary behavior problem of cats (Fig. 45–2). The most common medical cause of urinating outside the litter box is urinary tract infection and/or calculi. A urinalysis should be performed whenever an owner brings in a cat for spraying (depositing urine on vertical surfaces) or for urinating in an undesirable location. Medical problems must be treated successfully in order for behavioral problems to be resolved. Frequently, however, cats persist in urinating outside the box despite medical treatment because they may have learned to prefer the new substrate or location. Urine spraying may also be associated with urinary tract problems or impacted anal sacs. Defecation problems may be associated with either concurrent or historical constipation or diarrhea.

Once the type of elimination problem is determined and medical problems either identified or ruled out, careful questioning of the owner is necessary to determine what aspect of the litter box can be improved. The questions to be asked are: (1) Where does the cat eliminate? (2) Where is the litter box? (3) What type of box and litter are used? (4) How often is the litter scooped, and how often is it replaced?

The most common cause of inappropriate elimination is revealed by question 4: more frequent replacement of litter will solve many problems. The type of box can be a problem if it intensifies odors (covered box) or if it is difficult for the cat to jump into the box—a problem especially in older cats. The type of litter can be a problem if the owner has recently changed litters, but changing to a litter most cats prefer, such as sandy, clumping litter will encourage cats to use the box. Nonscented litter is preferred. The site of the litter box can be a problem if it has been changed recently or if the cat is old and unwilling to travel long or circuitous distances in the house. Many owners state that their cats are vindictive—urinating on their bed or shoes, especially while they are away on a trip or have just returned. This behavior could be nonspraying marking (marking on a horizontal

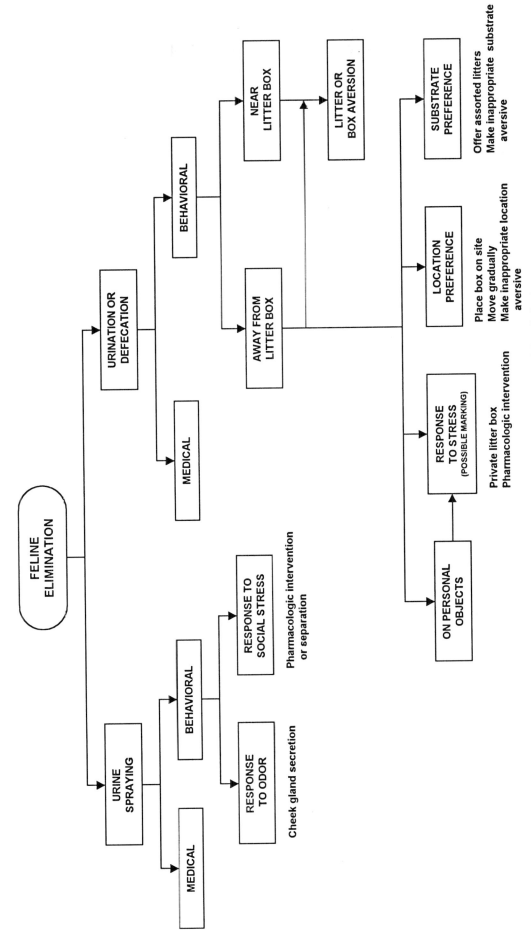

Figure 45-2. Algorithm for medical or behavioral management of feline elimination.

surface rather than spraying on a vertical surface) or elimination in a safe place that is associated with the owner.

The most efficient approach to nonspraying elimination problems is to provide several boxes, each with a different type of litter (clumping, nonclumping, clay-based or paper, etc.). The nonclumping litter should be discarded daily if the cat has used it at all. Clumping litter should be scooped daily and discarded every 2 weeks. Confinement is not necessary unless there are several cats in the household or if persistent elimination outside the box will force the owner to consider euthanasia. Litter depth should also be varied from one end of the box to the other to assess the cat's preference. Open, rather than covered, boxes are generally preferred. The soiled area can be covered with heavy plastic on which aversive odors are placed: strongly scented soap, citrus air fresheners. or camphor can be used.

Owners must be warned that punishment will not help, particularly if delivered a minute or more after the cat eliminated. In fact, even well-timed punishment is apt to make the cat more upset and, therefore, more likely to eliminate outside the box.

Provision of a second litter box (or more) often helps cats that inappropriately defecate. Cats apparently would prefer to defecate in one place and urinate in another. Defecation outside the litter pan is more frequently a problem of old cats and can be associated with constipation or other large bowel problems.

Urine Spraying

Urine spraying is more common in multiple cat households and can be difficult to solve if there is concurrent aggression. Spraying can be seen in intact and neutered male and female cats. It is important to distinguish spraying from elimination behavior. Spraying is usually (but not always) directed onto a vertical surface, and the amount of urine deposited is usually (but not always) small. Medical causes must be eliminated; 20 per cent of spraying cats have some urinary tract disorder. Psychoactive drugs are the most effective treatment for spraying because the stimuli that elicit spraying (e.g., other cats in the household) are probably going to persist (Table 45–2).

The drug of choice, based on efficacy and cost, has historically been diazepam, but reports of idiopathic hepatotoxicity have discouraged its use. Other drugs that have been used successfully are amitriptyline, buspirone, and paroxetine. The oral progestin megestrol acetate may also be effective, although long-term side effects are undesirable. Feline cheek gland secretions are applied to surfaces when cats rub. Synthetic components are available as a spray (Feliway, Abbott),

which, when applied to areas in which a cat has sprayed urine, decreases the rate of spraying by encouraging it to rub rather than spray.

Owners should be forewarned that pharmacologic treatment may have to be repeated the following year because urine spraying can be seasonal.

Aggression

Aggression to Cats

Dominance (Status-Related) Aggression (Fig. 45–3). A dominant cat will stare at and displace a subordinate cat from a resting place, from the owner's lap, or, less frequently, from food. Owners can try to reverse hierarchy by banishing the dominant cat to a room by itself and then gradually reintroducing it. In addition, the owner should give lap privileges only to the victim, feed it first, and punish with water, air, or a loud noise any staring or chasing by the dominant cat. In general, the dominant cat is usually confident and friendly, while the subordinate is more fearful (even in the absence of other cats). Treatment with buspirone may be useful for the subordinate and amitriptyline or paroxetine for the aggressor (see Table 45–2).

Territorial Aggression. Territorial aggression toward other household cats is characterized by ongoing unilateral aggression, often accompanied by vocalizing (caterwauling) and chasing. While some territorial cats may aggress only occasionally, others do not tolerate the proximity of other cats. This aggression may be directed specifically at only one member of a multiple cat household and, counterintuitively, may be seen in the most recently adopted cat toward resident cats. Territorially aggressive cats tend to seek out their targets, while cats exhibiting redirected or fear-based aggression may react only when the other cat appears. Treatment of territorial aggression is difficult; for severe problems, the best solution may be to place one cat in a new home. Long-term separation and drug therapy—avoiding use of potentially disinhibiting drugs such as benzodiazepines and buspirone—may be helpful.

Male cats are more likely to be involved in intraspecies aggression, attacking females as well as other males. Therefore, if clients insist on acquiring a second cat, they should be urged to get a female no matter what the sex of the first cat. A special type of territorial aggression occurs when one cat reenters the house after a trip or a visit to the veterinary hospital. Separation and odor exchange for a few days will generally resolve the problem: both cats may be rubbed with the same towel, concentrating on the cheeks and base of the tail, so that they smell alike.

TABLE 45–2. SELECTED DRUGS USED TO TREAT BEHAVIOR PROBLEMS IN CATS

GENERIC/TRADE NAME	DOSAGE	ROUTE	FREQUENCY	CLASS
Amitriptyline (Elavil)	5–10 mg/cat	PO	q 24 hours	Tricyclic antidepressant
Buspirone (BuSpar)	2.5–5 mg/cat	PO	q 12 hours	Anxiolytic
Clomipramine (Clomicalm, Anafranil)	0.5–1 mg/kg	PO	q 24 hours	Tricyclic antidepressant
Diazepam (Valium)	1–2.5 mg/cat‡	PO	q 12–8 hours	Benzodiazepine
Fluoxetine (Prozac)	5 mg/cat	PO	q 24 hours	Specific serotonin-reuptake inhibitor
Medroxyprogesterone acetate (Depo-Provera)	50–100 mg/cat	IM, SQ	q 4 months	Progestin
Megestrol acetate (Ovaban, Megace)	5–10 mg/cat†	PO	q 24 hours	Progestin
Paroxetine (Paxil)	2.5–5 mg/cat	PO	q 24 hours	Specific serotonin-reuptake inhibitor

†After 2 weeks, this dose should be reduced by half and after 4 weeks reduced again. Treatment should be discontinued after 6 weeks.
‡Sedation and ataxia should abate within several days.

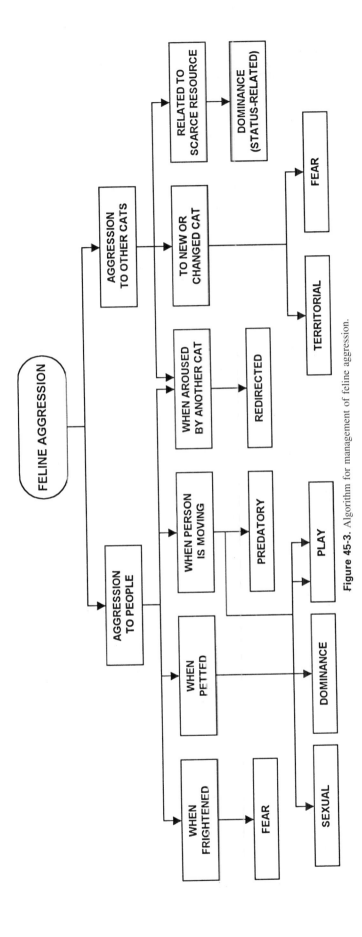

Figure 45-3. Algorithm for management of feline aggression.

Aggression Redirected to Cats. The causes of redirected aggression to cats are arousal or aggression in response to an inaccessible stimulus, usually another cat. The reactive cat vocalizes and swats or chases another household cat, often persisting after the initiating stimulus is identified and removed. A fearful reaction in the "victim," such as hissing or running away, may continue to elicit chasing and aggression. Such cats should be separated for a week or more while litter boxes and food bowls are exchanged. Drug therapy may be indicated, particularly to reduce anxiety in the attacked cat (see Table 45–2). The next step is to restrain the aggressor, either on a harness and leash or in a crate. The cats should be fed at opposite ends of a room and the dishes gradually moved closer together at each meal if there have been no signs of aggression.

Fear-Based Aggression. Fear-based aggression toward cats could be the result of redirected aggression (fear would be elicited in the victim cat) and is treated similarly. Cats exhibiting fearful postures and actions, such as hissing, crouching, switching the tail while crouching, ears flat, pupils dilated, and running away, may respond to anxiolytic drug therapy (see Table 45–2). Separation and gradual reintroduction of cats are helpful. During reintroduction sessions, the fearful cat should have greater access to the home so that self-confidence is regained.

Aggression to People

Dominance Aggression. Cats can exhibit dominance (or status-related) aggression toward people. A cat may stare at a person who is sitting in the its favored location, and, if the person fails to move, the cat will bite. Cats may not tolerate prolonged petting. They may rub against the owner excessively.

Owners should be advised to limit petting and to learn to anticipate a change in the cat's demeanor (for example, tail flicking as an indicator of agitation). Treatment consists of limiting the duration of rubbing by the cat (onto the owner), and even teaching the cat to sit or perform other activities on command. The owner should end petting sessions before the cat would normally do so; it is effective to end the session by standing up so that the cat falls passively to the floor. The owner can also hold the cat down in lateral recumbency for a few minutes daily.

Play Aggression. Play aggression, seen primarily in kittens and young cats, can be vigorous and cause injuries. Although it is usually outgrown, play aggression may persist. Treatment involves redirecting play to an appropriate outlet, such as a toy. As is true for all cat behavior problems, punishment should be indirect and unassociated with the owner. Examples of appropriate punishment are water guns, compressed air, and loud noises. Some cats will redirect vigorous play to a second young cat or kitten, but owners should be warned that risks of adopting a second cat may outweigh benefits, and that outcome is unpredictable.

Aggression Redirected to People. An aggressive response to an inaccessible stimulus may be redirected to humans. Cats may react aggressively to visual, auditory, or olfactory signs of other cats or any unfamiliar stimulus. As in the case of aggression redirected to other cats, such behavior appears to be fear or territory related. Attacks may be sudden and explosive, with or without vocalization (caterwauling). If possible, the initiating stimulus should be removed. Severely aggressive cats should be isolated from the owner in a dark room for several days. Food and light are brought by the owner for brief periods several times daily until there is no indication of anxiety or aggression. Drug therapy may be indicated in cases of refractory or severe aggression (see Table 45–2). Benzodiazepines and buspirone should be avoided because of the potential for disinhibition of aggressive behavior.

CARDIOTHORACIC

CHAPTER 46

COUGHING

Stephen J. Ettinger

Coughing is an expiratory effort against a closed glottis producing a sudden, noisy expulsion of air from the lungs, usually in an effort to free the lungs, bronchi, or trachea of excess secretion or foreign material (real or imagined). Coughing may be associated with respiratory distress but is not necessarily a sign of distress. The two should be separated. Animal handlers may confuse coughing with panting, forceful or labored breathing, wheezing, reverse sneezing, gagging, retching, or attempted vomiting. Occasionally, an animal may retch or vomit following a forceful bout of coughing. This should not be misinterpreted as a gastrointestinal problem. The presence of a terminal retch, either productive or nonproductive, is significant.

The cough reflex is the result of irritation (mechanical or chemical) at the level of the pharynx, larynx, tracheobronchial tree, and some of the smaller airways. Pathology of the pleura, pericardium, diaphragm, nose, and nasal sinuses less commonly stimulates coughing. Coughing is irritating to a dog or cat (and often to the owner) and may be so disturbing that it causes fatigue or exhaustion. It may also disseminate infectious disease organisms, aggravate existing inflammatory processes in the airways, or cause emphysema or pneumothorax by rupturing lung tissue.

The causes of coughing in small animals may be divided into the following major categories (Table 46–1): inflammatory, neoplastic, cardiovascular, allergic, traumatic, physical, and parasitic This division provides the clinician with a familiar grouping of etiologies for differentiating the coughing pet's problem.

DIAGNOSTIC APPROACH

General Approach. Diagnosis of the cause of a cough begins with a review of past and current medical problems

TABLE 46–1. CAUSES OF COUGHING IN DOGS AND CATS

Inflammatory

Pharyngitis
Tonsillitis
Tracheobronchitis
Chronic bronchitis
Bronchiectasis
Pneumonia—bacterial, viral, fungal
Granuloma
Abscess
Chronic pulmonary fibrosis
Collapsed trachea
Hilar lymph node enlargement
Secondary to esophageal dysfunction
Inhalation

Neoplastic

Primary
Mediastinal
Metastatic
Tracheal
Laryngeal
Ribs, sternum, muscle
Lymphoma

Cardiovascular

Left heart failure
Enlarged heart (especially left atrium)
Heart failure (pulmonary signs)
Pulmonary emboli
Pulmonary edema (vascular origin)

Allergic

Bronchial asthma
Eosinophilic pneumonitis
Eosinophilic pulmonary granulomatosis
Pulmonary infiltrate with eosinophilia (PIE)
Other immune states
Sinusitis (?)
Reverse sneeze (postnasal drip?)

Traumatic and Physical

Foreign body—esophageal, tracheal
Irritating gases
Trauma
Collapsed trachea
Hypoplastic trachea
Hepatomegaly
Inhalation—liquid, solid

Parasitic

Visceral larval migrans
Filaroides osleri (lungworm)
Aelurostrongylus (feline lungworm)
Paragonimus kellicotti (lung fluke—dog, cat)
Dirofilaria immitis (dog, cat)
Pneumocystis
Capillaria aerophilia (dog, cat)
Crenosoma vulpis (dog)
Filaroides milksi (dog)

(Fig. 46–1). Previous and current treatments are noted. A complete physical and radiographic examination of the thorax and cervical region should be considered. Radiographs are not necessary in every case but are indicated when there is failure to respond to symptomatic treatment. Auscultation of the heart for murmurs or arrhythmias and of the lungs for abnormal breath sounds is essential, as is palpation of the larynx, trachea, and thorax for deformities. A database consisting of complete blood count, fecal flotation, and heartworm examination (in endemic areas) should be considered. Specific testing of a serum chemistry profile, electrocardiogram, and bronchial washing, as well as culture, bronchoscopy, pleural tap, and blood gas analysis, may, in chronic or advanced cases, provide the clinician with specific information relevant to diagnosis and treatment.

Clinical expectations should be considered. For example, in young cats with ocular-nasal discharge, first rule out infectious disease: viral, bacterial, or parasitic. In older cats with coughing and wheezing and without discharge, asthmalike syndromes (pulmonary infiltrate with eosinophilia) or heartworm disease (in endemic areas) is more likely. Small dogs of middle to older age are likely to be afflicted with chronic obstructive lung disease, collapsing trachea, or chronic mitral valve disease; large- and giant-breed dogs of middle to older age develop congestive cardiomyopathy, laryngeal paralysis, or pneumonia. Brachycephalic canine breeds develop neoplasms and upper airway obstructive disease, whereas older female dogs are at risk for metastatic mammary gland cancers. All recently kenneled pets are at risk for infectious disease.

Nature of the Cough. Careful questioning regarding the nature of the cough should precede the physical examination. Specific information includes what time of day or night the cough occurs; what, if anything, initiates it; whether it is moist or dry, productive or nonproductive, and what it sounds like.

Nocturnal coughing may be associated with cardiac insufficiency, psychogenic problems, or collapsing trachea. Pulmonary edema, with a variety of etiologies, is also likely to result in nocturnal coughing. The cardiac cough is initially most prominent at night, but as the disease progresses it may be heard any time. A cough caused by pneumonia is likely to be worse initially during the day. Coughing, early in infectious processes, parasitic diseases, and allergic or neoplastic diseases, usually occurs in the daytime.

Coughing caused by tracheal irritation or trauma can be initiated by excitement, pulling on the collar, or just drinking water. A pet may also recognize, through experience, that paroxysmal coughing yields immediate attention, suggesting a psychogenic component. These coughing episodes occur both day and night but may be particularly stressful to the owner when the typical "goose-honk" sound of collapsing tracheal membranes occurs continuously.

Pneumonia, bronchitis, and bronchiectasis are initially daytime coughing syndromes that usually do not require stimulation to start, although excitement and pulling on the collar may bring about severe paroxysms of coughing. These conditions tend to be aggravated by exercise and excitement.

Dogs and cats with cardiac disease are likely to begin coughing without apparent cause. Following exercise, tracheal pressure, or excitement, they progressively experience paroxysms of coughing. However, cardiac coughing also occurs at rest, when pathophysiologic alterations in pulmonary interstitial fluid occur. These pathophysiologic changes result in an inability to breathe while in a recumbent position (orthopnea).

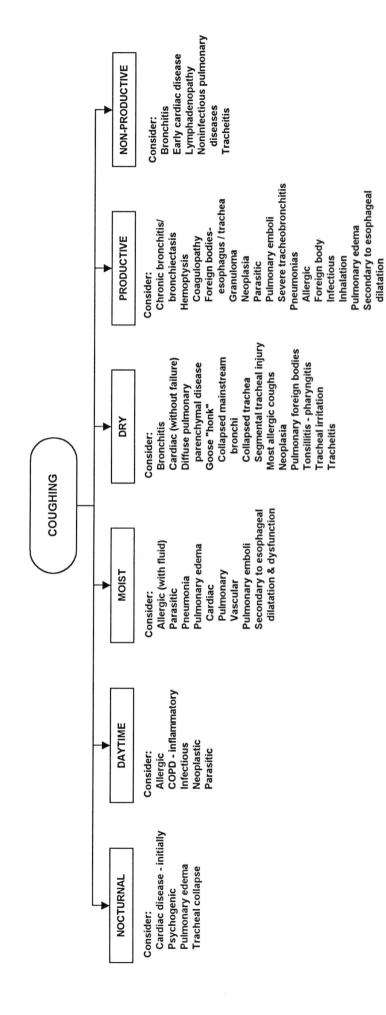

Figure 46–1. Algorithm for coughing based on clinical impression of the cough.

TABLE 46–2. ANTITUSSIVE AND BRONCHODILATOR-ANTITUSSIVE COMBINATION MEDICATIONS

GENERIC NAME AND PREPARATION	TRADE NAME	DOSAGE
Aminophylline 1 1/2 gr (100 mg) tablets		5 mg/lb q6–12h as needed
Theophylline (elixir 80 mg/tbsp: capsules 100 and 200 mg)	Elixophyllin, Theolixir	5 mg/lb q6–12h as needed
Oxtriphylline 400 or 600 mg sustained-action tablets	Choledyl SA	Similar to aminophylline; reported to cause fewer gastrointestinal problems
Theophylline with guaifenesin: 150 mg theophylline + 90 mg guaifenesin per capsule	Quibron	1 capsule q8–12h for larger dogs
Aminophylline with phenobarbital		1/2 to 1 tablet q6–12h with 1/4 or 1/2 gr phenobarbital
Theophylline 130 mg	Marax tablets	1/4 to 1 tablet q8–12h
Ephedrine HCl 25 mg		
Hydroxyzine 10 mg		
Hydrocodone bitartrate 5 mg	Hycodan	1/2 to 1 tablet (or teaspoon) q6–12h as needed; may increase dosage if sedative effect does not occur
Homatropine methylbromide 1.5 mg per tablet or per 5 cc		
Hydrocodone 5 mg per tablet	Tussionex	1/2 to 1 teaspoon q6–24h as needed; may increase dosage if sedative effect does not occur
Chlorpheniramine 8 mg per 5 cc		
Butorphanol tartrate 5, 10, 25 mg tabs	Torbutrol	0.25 mg/lb q6–12h; may cause sedation
Prednisone 2 mg per tablet	Temaril-P	1 tablet per 20 lbs q12h; good for allergic and noninfectious inflammatory coughing (e.g., tracheal collapse)
Trimeprazine 5 mg per tablet		
Guaifenesin 100 mg per tablet or per 5 cc	Robitussin-DM	Non-narcotic, over-the-counter preparation for temporary antitussive effect; dosage similar to that for adults and children
Dextromethorphan 15 mg		
Theophylline extentabs 100 mg	Theo-Dur	25 mg/kg once daily given usually at night

Coughing that develops during or shortly after eating suggests upper airway obstruction, laryngeal paralysis, or an esophageal disorder (e.g., megaesophagus or cricopharyngeal disease). Hemoptysis (coughing blood) may be related to pulmonary embolism (e.g., heartworms), neoplasia of the pulmonary system, severe tracheobronchitis, foreign body, granuloma, or coagulopathy.

Sound of the Cough. When attempting to determine the etiology of a cough, there is diagnostic value in describing its sound. Moist coughing suggests free alveolar or bronchial fluid. Soft, moist coughing suggests pneumonia, parasitic or allergic (with fluid) disease, pulmonary emboli, or pulmonary edema. Inhalation pneumonia has a characteristic gurgling component with respiration.

Dry coughing sounds invoke consideration of a cardiac origin (without cardiac failure), bronchitis, tracheobronchitis, tonsillitis, allergy, diffuse pulmonary parenchymal disease, or neoplasia without fluid accumulation. Physical deformities of the trachea are initially characterized by dry coughing. Metastatic neoplastic disease, tracheal irritation, and pulmonary foreign bodies cause a cough of similar quality unless there is fluid accumulating in the lower lung. Often these types of cough are associated with terminal nonproductive retching (i.e., nothing is brought up).

Coughing sounds that resemble a goose's honk are typically associated with collapsing tracheal membranes, hypoplastic trachea, collapsing main stem bronchi (also with sibilant rales), and segmental tracheal injury. These coughing episodes are usually dry.

Wheezing and rattling are noisy types of sounds often heard with bronchiectasis, chronic obstructive lung disease, and some allergies. The sounds represent passage of air through spastic airways that are narrowed by or obstructed with mucus or pus.

Terminal Retch. Coughing followed by a terminal retch is frequently encountered. It tends to be nonproductive in early cardiac disease, tracheitis, bronchitis, and irritating but noninfectious lesions of the pulmonary tract. In cardiac disease, it remains nonproductive until pulmonary edema develops, when the fluid is pink or blood-tinged. Earlier in the course of the disease, the owner may report attempts at gagging with only a small amount of white or clear phlegm produced. This is often the case in tracheitis and bronchitis before excessive fluid develops. When mucus, edema, mucopurulent debris, or hemorrhage accumulates in the pulmonary tree, there is likely to be expectoration following a coughing episode. The owner may relate that the material coughed up is swallowed rather than expectorated. Dogs and cats cannot spit.

Environmental Factors Related to Coughing. Urban animals are more likely to develop chronic respiratory disease as a result of environmental pollutants. Rural animals living outdoors may be susceptible to pneumonia, foreign bodies, or grass-related allergies. Indoor animals have a lower frequency of heartworm disease. Dogs and cats in contact with the intermediate hosts of parasites have a higher incidence of such diseases. Cats maintained indoors and kept isolated from other cats are less likely to experience upper respiratory viral or parasitic diseases.

The presence of a damp environment is a factor to consider in the history of animals suspected of having airway disease. Similarly, those experiencing coughing and living in a hot, dry region may have inflamed bronchial linings. Exposure to noxious gases (cigarette smoke) predisposes to irritation-related pulmonary diseases.

Environmental factors must be considered when evaluating a dog or cat with respiratory-related signs. Has there been a change in diet, environment, walking habits, or exercise? Dogs known to cough only with excitement or when pulling on a collar or leash are likely to have a collapsing trachea, the signs of which may be avoided by using a harness rather than a collar. Seasonal signs suggest allergy or irritation by specific elements (fleas). Obese animals and those with hepatomegaly are more likely to have restrictive lung disease, tracheal collapse, and coughing episodes.

TREATMENT GOALS

Knowledge of the history and environment may be useful in identifying the cause of a specific respiratory problem. The veterinarian may suggest modifications to reduce the frequency or severity of a cough. This does not negate the need for a thorough physical examination, but it facilitates the approach to diagnosis and treatment.

Drugs used to treat the coughing pet include antibiotics for infectious disease; corticosteroids for allergic conditions; cardiac agents such as digitalis, diuretics, and angiotensin-converting enzyme inhibitors for congestive heart failure; and antispasmodic or antitussive agents for inflammatory, noninfectious lung and tracheal problems. Some problems require specific therapy. Table 46–2 outlines antitussive agents generally used in veterinary practice. Any pet could benefit from a thorough evaluation when coughing is severe or when there is failure to respond to nonspecific symptomatic medication.

CHAPTER 47

DYSPNEA AND TACHYPNEA

Grant H. Turnwald

DEFINITIONS

The term *dyspnea* as used in people refers to the "sensation" of difficult breathing. Hence dyspnea is a subjective phenomenon and does not accurately define difficult breathing in animals. To use the term *dyspnea* (also called respiratory distress) in animals, an objective description is needed. Dyspnea or respiratory distress is an inappropriate degree of breathing effort, based on an assessment of respiratory rate, rhythm, and character. It is in the context of this definition that dyspnea is used in this chapter. Dyspnea may be exertional, paroxysmal, or continuous, depending on the cause and extent of the abnormality. *Tachypnea,* also known as polypnea, refers to an increased rate of breathing but need not be an indication of dyspnea. It is important to differentiate tachypnea associated with dyspnea from tachypnea associated with physiologic functions such as normal panting, exercise, hyperthermia, or anxiety. *Orthopnea* indicates difficulty breathing while in a recumbent position. Such animals typically assume a sitting or standing posture with elbows abducted and neck extended.

GENERAL PATHOPHYSIOLOGY

The major causes of dyspnea and tachypnea involve the respiratory, cardiac, hematologic, metabolic, and nervous systems (Table 47–1).

Respiratory Disorders. In obstructive respiratory disorders, there is obstruction at one or more airway sites. The obstruction may be endomural (e.g., mucus), mural (e.g., bronchospasm), or extramural (e.g., compression by thymic lymphosarcoma). From a functional standpoint, it is convenient to describe obstructive disease as either upper airway (above the thoracic inlet) or lower airway (below the thoracic inlet). Obstructive lesions tend to accentuate the normal dynamic decrease of airway diameter during inspiration (upper airway obstruction) and expiration (lower airway obstruction). Hence animals with upper airway obstructions are expected to have breathing patterns characterized by increased inspiratory effort and, depending on severity, tachypnea (see Table 47–1). Conversely, animals with lower airway obstructions can be expected to have increased expiratory effort, with or without tachypnea. Airway diameter in fixed obstructions (e.g., tracheal tumor) is relatively unchanged; thus if the obstruction is sufficient to cause dyspnea, animals will typically have inspiratory and expiratory dyspnea. In addition, coughing (see Chapter 46) is frequently present.

Restrictive respiratory disorders are those restricting expansion of the lungs. These disorders may involve the pulmonary parenchyma, chest wall, pleural cavity, diaphragm, peritoneal cavity, or peripheral nerves (see Table 47–1). In pleural disorders, an increase in inspiratory effort may be seen as an animal attempts to overcome restrictive lung disease. Depending on severity, animals with restrictive diseases typically have rapid, shallow breathing patterns. If pulmonary vascular disease (see Table 47–1) is of sufficient magnitude to cause dyspnea, both inspiratory and expiratory components of breathing are commonly increased.

Hemoglobin Disorders. In dogs or cats with reduced or altered hemoglobin states (see Table 47–1), dyspnea occurs when blood oxygen concentration falls below a critical value. The actual value of blood oxygen concentration for each animal varies and is greater in disorders with an acute onset. If dyspnea is present, the breathing pattern is typically increased in rate and depth.

Metabolic Disorders. In metabolic disorders with a marked decrease in arterial pH, an increase in rate and depth of breathing may occur. Severe hypokalemia in cats may be associated with muscle weakness (i.e., decreased breathing movements).

Nervous Disorders. The effect of brain disease on breathing depends on the anatomic distribution of the lesion. Tachypnea may be present; depth of breathing may be increased or decreased. Inappropriate breathing may also be associated with spinal cord or peripheral nerve disorders (see Section VI).

HISTORICAL FINDINGS AND SIGNIFICANCE

Signalment is important because some specific causes of dyspnea are most common in certain breeds or are age

TABLE 47–1. CAUSES OF DYSPNEA

Upper Airway Disorders

Nasal cavity*
  Stenotic nares
  Obstruction (infection, inflammation, neoplasia, trauma,
    bleeding disorders)
Pharynx, larynx
  Elongated or edematous soft palate
  Pharyngeal polyp (cat)
  Laryngeal edema, collapse, foreign body, inflammation,
    trauma, paralysis, spasm, neoplasia, vocal fold webbing
  Everted laryngeal saccules
Cervical trachea
  Collapse, stenosis
  Trauma, foreign body
  Neoplasia, osteochondral dysplasia
  Parasites (*Oslerus osleri*)

Lower Airway Disorders

Thoracic trachea (see cervical trachea)
  Extraluminal compression (lymphadenopathy, heart-based
    tumors, enlarged left atrium)
  Bronchial disease (allergic, infectious, parasitic, chronic
    obstructive pulmonary disease)

Pulmonary Parenchymal Disorders

Edema (cardiogenic, noncardiogenic)
Pneumonia (infectious, parasitic, inhalation)
Neoplasia
Allergy (allergic pneumonitis, including heartworm; eosinophilic
  granuloma; pulmonary infiltrates with eosinophilia)
Embolism (dirofilariasis, hyperadrenocorticism, disseminated
  intravascular coagulation)
Trauma, bleeding disorders

Pleural/Body Wall Disorders

Pneumothorax
Pleural effusion
Congenital body wall disorders (pectus excavatum)
Thoracic wall trauma
Thoracic wall neoplasia
Thoracic wall paralysis
Diaphragmatic hernia (congenital, acquired)

Mediastinal Disorders

Infection
Trauma, including pneumomediastinum
Neoplasia

Peritoneal Cavity Disorders

Organomegaly, obesity
Effusion
Gastric torsion

Hemoglobin Disorders

Anemia
Methemoglobinemia
Cyanosis

Miscellaneous

Central nervous system (brain, spinal cord)
Peripheral nerve, neuromuscular, muscular
Metabolic (acidemia; severe hypokalemia in cats)
Anxiety
Fear
Pain

*Only if the animal does not mouth breathe.

related. For example, brachycephalic (stenotic airway) syndrome occurs in brachycephalic dogs and short-faced cats; collapsed trachea occurs in older dogs of toy breeds; and acquired laryngeal paralysis occurs in older dogs of large breeds. Congenital disorders are more likely to be seen in animals younger than 1 year of age, whereas pulmonary metastases from neoplasias are most common in older animals. Association of dyspnea with other signs may be helpful (e.g., a change in phonation in laryngeal disorders, a "honking" cough in collapsed trachea). Geographic origin or location may be important (e.g., fungal diseases or dirofilariasis). Environmental history may be helpful in trauma and infectious disease. Obtaining vaccination status should be routine. Past medical history may reveal previous disorders leading to development of the current complaint. When investigating the current complaint, duration, progression, effect of treatment, and involvement of other body systems may assist in ascertaining the cause. Note that the owner may be unaware of dyspnea and may bring the dog or cat to the hospital for another problem (e.g., anorexia and weakness).

PHYSICAL FINDINGS

Physical examination of a dyspneic animal should include observation, palpation, auscultation, and possibly percussion. The dog or cat should be observed for any abnormal discharges, deformities, or other lesions and for the pattern of breathing. If possible, it is desirable to ascertain whether the dyspnea is inspiratory, expiratory, or both and whether there is an obstructive or restrictive breathing pattern. In flail chest (Chapter 130), there may be a paradoxic breathing movement, in that the chest wall collapses on the affected side during inspiration. The larynx and trachea should be carefully palpated, especially if upper airway obstruction is present. In cats, especially young cats, compressibility of the cranial mediastinum should be assessed; lack of compressibility is highly suggestive of a mass lesion. Auscultation may detect normal (including increased intensity of normal) or abnormal breath sounds such as crackles (diseases of small airways, less than 0.5 mm) and wheezes (diseases of larger airways, greater than 2 mm). There may also be stridor or abnormal cardiac sounds. The position of maximal intensity sounds assists in localizing the lesion. Detection of a "fluid line" in the thorax is suggested by muffled breath sounds ventrally and increased intensity of breath sounds dorsally. Heart sounds are generally increased with pleural fluid. Hyporesonance (dullness) on percussion suggests consolidation or fluid accumulation, and hyperresonance suggests pneumothorax.

DIAGNOSTIC PLAN

Some causes of dyspnea and tachypnea may be apparent on physical examination (e.g., stenotic nares or flail chest). Even if the cause is not apparent from the history and physical examination, it is usually possible to determine the following:

1. Respiratory rate and rhythm.
2. Whether the breathing pattern is predominantly inspiratory or expiratory, or whether both are prominent.
3. Whether the breath sounds are normal (including increased intensity of breath sounds) or abnormal (crackles, wheezes).

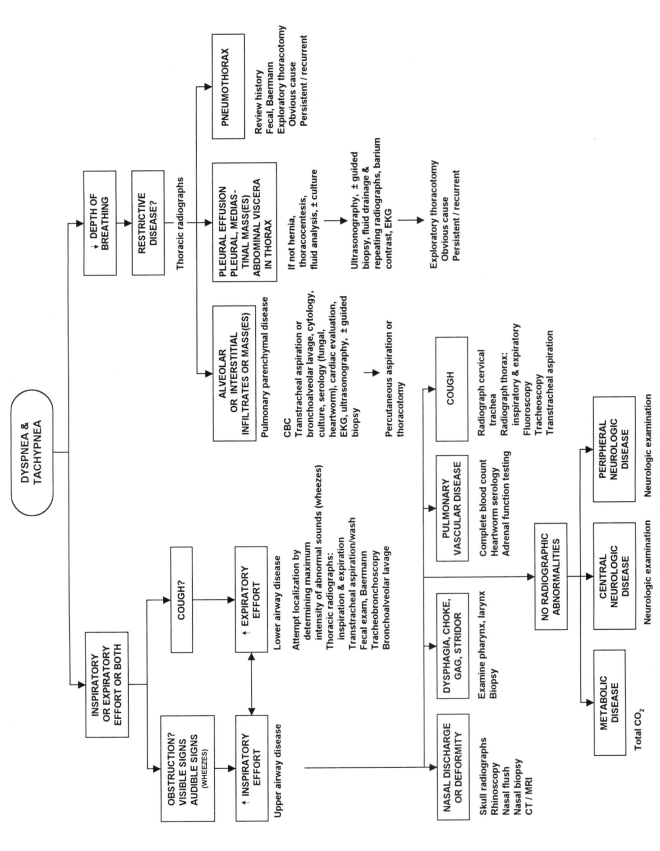

Figure 47–1. Algorithm for clinical diagnosis of dyspnea and tachypnea.

4. Whether the breathing pattern is restrictive or obstructive or has components of both patterns.

5. Presence and nature of coughing (see Chapter 46)

In nasal cavity disease, radiographs, computed tomography or magnetic resonance imaging scans are usually indicated early in the diagnostic evaluation and should be done before rhinoscopy and nasal biopsy (Fig. 47–1; see Chapter 123). Because results of nasal cultures for bacteria and fungi are difficult to interpret, they are not usually performed. In obstruction of the pharynx or larynx, the animal may need to be anesthetized to directly examine affected structures. If there are signs of obstructive disease, both inspiratory and expiratory radiographs should be taken of the trachea and lower airway. Although a collapsed trachea can be diagnosed by radiographs, it cannot be ruled out, even with inspiratory and expiratory films. If radiographs suggest evidence of airway disease and/or pulmonary parenchymal disease or a cough is present, transtracheal aspiration (TTA) may be worthwhile (see Fig. 47–1). Cytologic examination should be performed on a specimen of the aspirate, and another specimen placed in microbial transport medium and refrigerated. If there is cytologic evidence of inflammation, aerobic and possibly anaerobic culture should be performed. Endoscopy is useful in tracheal or bronchial disorders, particularly if obstructive disease (e.g., collapsed trachea) is present or suspected or if TTA analysis is not diagnostic. During endoscopy, specimens for culture, cytology, and histopathology may be useful. Bronchoalveolar lavage (see Chapter 128) may also be useful if TTA analysis is not diagnostic. Occasionally, fluoroscopy is performed on dogs or cats with obstructive disease to obtain a dynamic study.

If radiographic signs of heartworm disease are present, a Knott's or serologic (preferred) test is indicated. Although they do not usually provide a diagnosis, fecal flotation and Baermann's fecal analysis are inexpensive and noninvasive and, if positive definitively diagnose pulmonary and tracheal parasites (see Fig. 47–1). Serologic testing for pulmonary mycoses (except histoplasmosis) is useful in the dog if radiographic signs are compatible (see Chapter 93). If cardiac disease is suspected from clinical and/or radiographic signs, ultrasonography can be definitive.

If pleural effusion is present, thoracocentesis and fluid analysis are indicated. If the fluid is an exudate, aerobic and anaerobic cultures are usually indicated (except for effusive feline infectious peritonitis). If the fluid is a modified transudate, drainage and repeat radiographs may be indicated to further evaluate for cardiac disease, diaphragmatic hernia, mass, or foreign body. Ultrasonography is useful to detect pulmonary or mediastinal masses and to obtain ultrasound-guided biopsy. It is preferable to perform ultrasonography before removal of fluid. If diaphragmatic hernia is suspected but cannot be diagnosed by radiography or ultrasonography, a barium contrast study may be indicated in an attempt to demonstrate a portion of the gastrointestinal tract in the pleural cavity (see Fig. 47–1).

If the dog or cat has disseminated pulmonary parenchymal disease but a diagnosis has not been obtained by the aforementioned tests, percutaneous pulmonary biopsy may be diagnostic. Such aspiration can also be useful to diagnose neoplasia, particularly if samples can be obtained with ultrasound-guided biopsy equipment. If there is an increase in the rate and depth of breathing without obstruction or other evidence of bronchopulmonary disease, serum total carbon dioxide or bicarbonate concentrations can confirm or eliminate severe metabolic disorders (see Fig. 47–1). A serum chemistry profile, possibly urinalysis, and an arterial blood gas determination are indicated to further evaluate metabolic acidosis. Pulmonary vascular disease is usually apparent radiographically; occasionally, changes are not apparent despite severe dyspnea. In such cases, angiography or nuclear perfusion scans may be required. Rarely, exploratory thoracotomy and lung biopsy are necessary to establish a diagnosis.

In dogs or cats with decreased breathing movements, particularly if the respiratory rate is decreased, iatrogenic causes such as barbiturate overdose should be ruled out. Next, a neurologic examination should be performed (see Fig. 47–1). Ideally, the problem can be localized to brain disease causing depression of the respiratory center or to spinal cord, peripheral nerve, or muscle disease causing poor ventilation. In central disease, cerebrospinal fluid analysis would be indicated. If the neurologic disease is extracranial, it is necessary to distinguish upper motor neuron from lower motor neuron disease (see Chapters 104–106). Radiographs can be performed. If muscles are flaccid, lower motor neuron disease (e.g., myasthenia gravis, botulism, polyradiculoneuritis, tick paralysis) or myopathy is likely. Animals with lower motor neuron disease may have tachypnea.

A complete blood count is useful but rarely diagnostic. If bacterial bronchopneumonia is present, leukocytosis with a left shift and degenerate neutrophils may be evident. Eosinophilia is suggestive of pulmonary parasites, including dirofilariasis, allergic bronchitis or asthma, and pulmonary infiltrates with eosinophilia (see Chapter 128). In cats, eosinophilia is not helpful in predicting the predominant cell type in bronchial exudates. Gross appearance of blood (darker and browner than normal) and concurrent Heinz body anemia suggest methemoglobinemia.

GOALS OF TREATMENT

Goals of treatment of dyspnea and tachypnea are to identify the cause and to administer supportive, symptomatic, and, when indicated, specific treatment to alleviate the underlying disorder. Specific treatment requires a definitive diagnosis.

OUTCOME

The outcome of dyspnea and tachypnea varies according to the cause and duration of the disorder, as well as to the appropriateness of the treatment administered. The reader is referred to the appropriate chapter for expected outcomes of various causes of dyspnea and tachypnea. The majority of disorders are discussed in Section IX.

CHAPTER 48

ABNORMAL HEART SOUNDS AND HEART MURMURS

Wendy A. Ware

Heart sounds are created by turbulent blood flow and associated vibrations in adjacent tissue during the cardiac cycle. Transient heart sounds are sounds of short duration. The transient sounds normally heard in small animals are the first heart sound (S_1), associated with closure and tensing of the atrioventricular valves at the onset of systole, and the second heart sound (S_2), associated with closure of the aortic and pulmonic valves at the end of systole. Cardiac murmurs are longer sounds occurring during a normally silent part of the cardiac cycle.

TRANSIENT HEART SOUNDS

ALTERATIONS IN NORMAL TRANSIENT SOUNDS (S_1 AND S_2)

The intensity of S_1 and/or S_2 is affected by various factors. Causes of a loud S_1 include thin chest wall, high sympathetic tone, tachycardia, systemic arterial hypertension, and shortened P-R interval. Diminished intensity of S_1 can be caused by obesity, pericardial effusion, diaphragmatic hernia, dilated cardiomyopathy, hypovolemia (poor ventricular filling), and pleural effusion. A split or sloppy-sounding S_1 may be normal (especially in large dogs), may result from ventricular premature contractions, or may result from major intraventricular conduction disturbances (bundle branch blocks).

An increase in the intensity of S_2 can result from pulmonary hypertension of any cause. Normal (physiologic) splitting of S_2 can be heard in some dogs because of changes in stroke volume during respiration; increased venous return to the right heart and reduced filling of the left heart delay closure of the pulmonic valve during inspiration. Pathologic splitting of S_2 can result from delayed ventricular activation or prolonged right ventricular ejection secondary to ventricular premature contractions, right bundle branch block, ventricular or atrial septal defects, and pulmonary hypertension. Cardiac arrhythmias may cause variation in the intensity (or even an absence) of heart sounds.

ABNORMAL TRANSIENT SOUNDS

Gallop Sounds. The third (S_3) and fourth (S_4) heart sounds occur during diastole (Fig. 48–1) and are not normally audible. When an S_3 or S_4 sound is heard, the heart may sound like the galloping of a horse; hence the term gallop rhythm or gallop sounds. This can be confusing, because the presence or absence of an audible S_3 or S_4 has nothing to do with the heart's rhythm (i.e., electrical activation). The S_3 and S_4 are usually heard best with the bell of the stethoscope, because they are of lower frequency than S_1 and S_2.

The S_3, also known as an S_3 gallop or ventricular gallop, is associated with low-frequency vibrations occurring at the end of the rapid ventricular filling phase. An audible S_3 in a dog or cat usually indicates ventricular dilatation with myocardial failure. The extra sound can be loud or subtle and is best heard over the cardiac apex following S_2. This may be the only abnormality that can be auscultated in an animal with dilated cardiomyopathy. In dogs, an S_3 gallop may also be heard in advanced valvular heart disease and congestive heart failure.

The S_4 gallop, also called an atrial or presystolic gallop, is associated with low-frequency vibrations induced by blood flow into the ventricles during atrial contraction; it occurs just after the P wave of the electrocardiogram and before S_1. An audible S_4 in a dog or cat is usually associated with increased ventricular stiffness and hypertrophy (e.g., hypertrophic cardiomyopathy). At fast heart rates, differentiation between S_3 and S_4 is difficult. If both sounds are present, they may be superimposed; this is called a summation gallop.

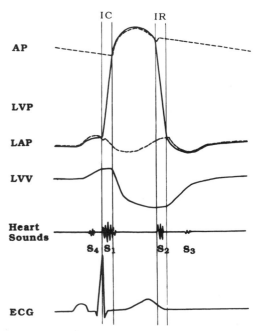

Figure 48–1. The cardiac cycle, depicting the relationships between great vessel, ventricular and atrial pressures, ventricular volume, heart sounds, and electrical activation. AP = aortic pressure; LVP = left ventricular pressure; LAP = left atrial pressure; LVV = left ventricular volume; ECG = electrocardiogram; IC = isovolumic contraction; IR = isovolumic relaxation. (From Ware WA: The cardiovascular examination. *In* Nelson RW, Couto CG [eds]: Small Animal Internal Medicine, 2nd ed. St. Louis, Mosby-Year Book, 1998.)

Other Transient Sounds. Several other brief sounds may be auscultated. The most common are systolic clicks. These are mid to late systolic sounds, usually heard best over the mitral valve area. Clicks have been associated with degenerative valvular disease (endocardiosis), mitral valve prolapse, and congenital mitral dysplasia. The sudden checking of a portion of the valve as it balloons toward the atrium during systole is thought to cause the clicks. A concurrent mitral insufficiency murmur may be present or may develop later. The click itself is not of great concern, although it should be differentiated from a split or gallop sound.

An early-systolic, high-pitched "ejection sound" at the left base may occur with valvular pulmonic stenosis or other diseases causing dilatation of a great artery. The sound is thought to arise from either the sudden checking of a fused pulmonic valve or the rapid filling of a dilated vessel during ejection. Rarely, restrictive pericardial disease causes an audible "pericardial knock." This diastolic sound is caused by the abrupt restriction of ventricular filling by the diseased pericardium; its timing is similar to that of an S_3.

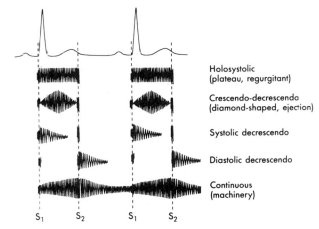

Figure 48–2. Murmur shapes and descriptions. The phonocardiographic shapes and timing of different murmurs are depicted, along with terms used to describe them. (From Ware WA: The cardiovascular examination. *In* Nelson RW, Couto CG [eds]: Small Animal Internal Medicine, 2nd ed. St. Louis, Mosby-Year Book, 1998.)

CARDIAC MURMURS

Cardiac murmurs are caused by turbulent blood flow in the heart or adjacent blood vessels. The development of turbulent blood flow (and resulting murmur intensity) is directly related to the velocity of blood flow and inversely related to blood viscosity. Thus, for example, a narrowed valve orifice (which increases blood flow velocity) and anemia (which decreases blood viscosity) are likely to cause turbulent blood flow and cardiac murmurs. Conversely, polycythemia (increased blood viscosity) may reduce turbulent flow associated with a right-to-left shunt so that no murmur is heard.

Murmurs can be described by their timing within the cardiac cycle (systolic or diastolic, or portions thereof), intensity (loudness), point of maximal intensity on the precordium, radiation over the chest wall, quality, and pitch. Systolic murmurs may occur in early (protosystolic), mid (mesosystolic), or late (telesystolic) systole or throughout systole (holosystolic). Diastolic murmurs generally occur in early diastole (protodiastolic) or throughout diastole (holodiastolic). Murmurs occurring at the very end of diastole are termed presystolic.

The intensity of a murmur is arbitrarily graded on a scale of I to VI (Table 48–1). Very loud cardiac murmurs are associated with palpable vibrations on the chest wall (a "precordial thrill"). The point of maximal intensity of a murmur is usually indicated by the hemithorax and intercostal space or valve area where it is loudest, or by the terms apex or base (e.g., left apex or over the mitral area). The point of maximal intensity usually corresponds to the anatomic origin of the murmur. The areas to which the murmur radiates can be extensive. The whole thorax as well as the

thoracic inlet and carotid arteries should be auscultated. A murmur's pitch and quality relate to its frequency components. "Noisy" or "harsh" murmurs contain mixed frequencies. "Musical" murmurs are of essentially one frequency with its overtones.

Murmurs can also be described by the shape that appears on a phonocardiogram. Figure 48–2 illustrates the shape and description of different murmur types. A plateau or regurgitant (holosystolic) murmur begins at about the time of S_1 and has a fairly uniform intensity throughout systole. Loud murmurs of this type may prevent distinction of S_1 and S_2 from the murmur. Atrioventricular valve insufficiency and interventricular septal defects commonly cause this type of murmur, as turbulent movement of blood occurs throughout ventricular systole. A crescendo-decrescendo or diamond-shaped murmur starts softly, builds intensity in mid-systole, then diminishes. S_1 and S_2 can be clearly heard before and after the murmur. This murmur is also called an ejection murmur because it occurs during ejection with ventricular outflow obstructions. A decrescendo murmur tapers down from its initial intensity over time; it may occur in systole or diastole. Continuous murmurs occur throughout systole and diastole.

Once a murmur is auscultated, it is most important to establish whether it occurs in systole or diastole, determine its point of maximal intensity, and grade its intensity.

CLINICAL ASSOCIATIONS OF ABNORMAL HEART SOUNDS

HISTORICAL AND PHYSICAL FINDINGS

Historical findings associated with abnormal cardiac sounds may be absent or may reflect underlying compromise of cardiac function. For example, exercise intolerance, weakness, or fainting may occur in animals with reduced cardiac output or hypoxemia. Likewise, tachypnea, dyspnea, cough, or abdominal distention may occur secondary to congestive heart failure. Occasionally, an owner notices a precordial thrill associated with a loud murmur.

A complete physical examination, including assessment of arterial pulses and jugular veins and palpation of the precordium (to detect the presence of a precordial thrill or

TABLE 48–1. GRADING OF CARDIAC MURMURS

Grade I	Very soft murmur; heard only in quiet surroundings after intently listening
Grade II	Soft murmur, but easily heard
Grade III	Moderate-intensity murmur
Grade IV	Loud murmur, but not accompanied by a precordial thrill
Grade V	Loud murmur with a palpable precordial thrill
Grade VI	Very loud murmur that can be heard with the stethoscope off the chest wall; accompanied by a precordial thrill

abnormal systolic impulse), is important in evaluating an animal with abnormal cardiac sounds.

CARDIAC AUSCULTATION

Because many heart sounds can be difficult to hear, patient cooperation and a quiet environment are important during auscultation. If possible, the animal should be standing, so that the heart is in its normal position. Panting should be quieted by holding the dog's mouth shut. Briefly placing a finger over one or both nostrils helps reduce respiratory noise further. Purring in cats can be discouraged by holding a finger over one or (briefly) both nostrils; other techniques include turning a water faucet on near the cat, holding an alcohol-soaked cotton ball near the cat's face, or gently compressing the larynx. The clinician must be aware of various artifacts that can interfere with cardiac auscultation. In addition to respiratory noises, shivering or muscle twitching, hair rubbing against the stethoscope, gastrointestinal sounds, and extraneous room noises can interfere. A good-quality stethoscope is also important for optimal auscultation. All areas of both sides of the chest should be carefully auscultated, with special attention to the areas overlying cardiac valves. The clinician should concentrate on the various heart sounds, correlating them to the events of the cardiac cycle (see Fig. 48–1) and listening for abnormal sounds in systole and diastole successively. It is important to understand these events and to identify the timing of systole and diastole in the animal. The precordial impulse occurs just after S_1 (systole), and the arterial pulse is felt between S_1 and S_2. Figure 48–3 outlines the more common associations of various abnormal heart sounds.

Abnormal Transient Sounds

The occurrence of a diastolic transient sound is suggestive of myocardial disease. As noted earlier, S_3 is most often associated with dilated cardiomyopathy, and S_4 is usually associated with hypertrophic cardiomyopathy (see Chapters 116 and 117). It is important to distinguish these diastolic (gallop) sounds from systolic transient sounds such as the mitral click (see the earlier discussion).

Systolic Murmurs

The murmur of mitral insufficiency is best heard at the left apex in the area of the mitral valve. It radiates well dorsally and often to the left base and right chest wall. Mitral insufficiency characteristically causes a plateau or regurgitant murmur (holosystolic in timing); however, in its early stages, the murmur may be protosystolic, tapering into a decrescendo configuration. Sometimes this murmur sounds like a musical "whoop." Mitral insufficiency can be caused by degenerative changes in the valve (endocardiosis), infectious endocarditis, diseases that cause left heart enlargement and distention of the valve annulus (e.g., dilated cardiomyopathy, patent ductus arteriosus), hypertrophic cardiomyopathy, and congenital malformations (see Chapters 112 and 113).

Systolic ejection murmurs are most often heard at the left base and are caused by ventricular outflow obstruction. The most common causes include congenital (sub)aortic or pulmonic stenosis and hypertrophic obstructive cardiomyopathy (causing dynamic left ventricular outflow obstruction because of excessive septal hypertrophy). Occasionally, tumors or other masses cause this type of murmur. Murmurs caused by ventricular outflow obstruction become louder as cardiac output or contraction strength increases. The murmur of subaortic stenosis is heard low on the left base and at the right base, because the murmur radiates up the aortic arch, which curves toward the right. This murmur also radiates up the carotid arteries and occasionally can be heard on the calvarium. The murmur of pulmonic stenosis is best heard high on the left base. "Relative" pulmonic stenosis occurs when the valve itself is normal but flow through the valve is greatly increased, as with a large left-to-right shunting atrial or ventricular septal defect.

Functional murmurs are nonpathologic, tend to be heard best at the left base, and are usually of soft to moderate intensity. They include innocent murmurs (no apparent cardiovascular cause), which are common in puppies, and physiologic murmurs (the heart is normal but an altered physiologic state exists). Physiologic murmurs have been associated with anemia, fever, high sympathetic tone, hyperthyroidism, peripheral arteriovenous fistula, hypoproteinemia, and athletic hearts.

Most murmurs heard over the right chest wall are holosystolic, plateau-shaped murmurs, with the exception of the murmur of subaortic stenosis, described earlier. The tricuspid insufficiency murmur sounds similar to that of mitral insufficiency and is loudest at the right apex, over the tricuspid valve. It may have a noticeably different pitch or quality from a concurrent mitral insufficiency murmur and often is accompanied by jugular vein pulsations. Tricuspid insufficiency can result from degenerative valve disease, acquired or congenital diseases that cause marked right heart enlargement and valve annulus distention, and congenital malformation of the valve. Tricuspid valve endocarditis is rare in dogs and cats.

Ventricular septal defect may cause a holosystolic murmur that usually is loudest at the right sternal border. This reflects the direction of the intracardiac shunt. Larger ventricular septal defects may also cause the murmur of relative pulmonic stenosis.

Diastolic Murmurs

Diastolic murmurs are uncommon in dogs and cats. They are usually associated with incompetence of a semilunar valve. Aortic insufficiency from bacterial endocarditis is the most frequent cause. Rarely, congenital or degenerative aortic valve disease occurs. Clinically significant pulmonic insufficiency is also rare. These diastolic murmurs begin at the time of S_2 and are best heard at the left base. They are decrescendo in configuration and extend a variable time into diastole, depending on the pressure difference between great vessel and ventricle. Some of these murmurs have a musical quality.

Continuous Murmurs

Continuous (also called "machinery") murmurs occur throughout the cardiac cycle. There is no interruption of the murmur at the time of S_2; rather, the intensity is often greater at that time. With slow heart rates, the murmur may taper off toward the end of diastole. Patent ductus arteriosus is the most common cause of a continuous murmur (see Chapter 112). This murmur is best heard high at the left base above the pulmonic valve area; the murmur tends to radiate cranially, ventrally, and to the right. The systolic component is usually louder and can be heard well all over the chest, whereas the diastolic component is more localized to the

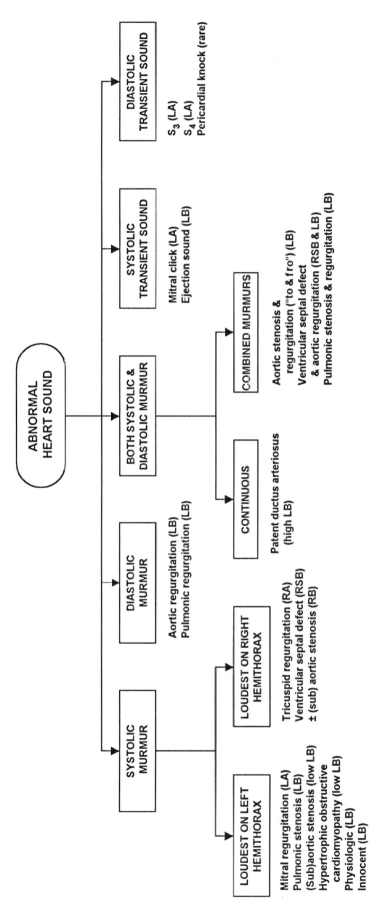

Figure 48-3. Algorithm for differentiating causes of various abnormal heart sounds and murmurs. The usual point of maximal intensity is noted in parenthesis. LA = left apex; LB = left base; RA = right apex; RB = right base; RSB = right sternal border.

left base in many cases. Careful auscultation is needed to distinguish a continuous murmur from concurrent systolic ejection and diastolic decrescendo murmurs.

Concurrent Systolic and Diastolic Murmurs

Sometimes a systolic ejection murmur and a diastolic decrescendo murmur occur in the same animal. These are called "to and fro" murmurs. The ejection murmur component tapers off in late systole, allowing the S₂ to be heard as a separate sound. The most common cause of "to and fro" murmurs is the combination of (sub)aortic stenosis and aortic insufficiency (from either infectious endocarditis or congenital malformation); rarely, stenosis and insufficiency of the pulmonic valve can also cause this type of murmur. Concurrent systolic and diastolic murmurs can also occur with a ventricular septal defect that causes loss of aortic root support and aortic insufficiency.

DIAGNOSTIC APPROACH

Once an abnormal heart sound has been identified, it is important to identify its cause. If structural cardiac disease is present, it is important to determine the underlying etiology and severity, as well as whether cardiac failure is present or imminent. Careful auscultation with an understanding of events during the cardiac cycle should permit identification of the most likely causes (see Fig. 48–3).

Other diagnostic tests can help further define the animal's abnormality. Electrocardiography may indicate an axis deviation and/or chamber enlargement pattern consistent with the underlying disease. Thoracic radiography should reveal significant chamber enlargement or great vessel abnormalities (e.g., poststenotic dilatation), changes in pulmonary vasculature, pulmonary parenchymal infiltrates suggestive of edema, or pleural fluid accumulation. Echocardiography is important in further evaluating structural and functional changes in the heart and proximal great vessels associated with the many diseases that cause abnormal heart sounds.

CHAPTER 49

PULSE ALTERATIONS

John-Karl Goodwin

INTRODUCTION AND DEFINITIONS

Assessment of arterial and venous pulse characteristics is an integral component of the physical examination. Arterial pulse qualities (rate, rhythm, symmetry, and strength) provide crucial information regarding the status of the cardiovascular system, specifically cardiac output and perfusion. Evaluation of venous pulse qualities (distention or pulsations) provides insight as to right-sided cardiac pressures and the status of venous return. Abnormalities of arterial and/or venous pulse characteristics are present in virtually all cardiovascular disease states. Detection of these changes often facilitates selection of additional diagnostics, enabling the clinician to make the proper diagnosis, and allows for monitoring of patient status and response to therapy.

Arterial and venous pulse characteristics should be evaluated in a systemic fashion, and the clinician should be familiar with the common abnormalities detected and their significance (Fig. 49–1). The intensity of the arterial pulse is determined by the difference between the systolic blood pressure and the diastolic blood pressure, termed the *pulse pressure*. An arterial pulse that is abnormally strong is termed *hyperkinetic,* bounding or water-hammer in quality. *Hypokinetic pulse* refers to a weak arterial pulse. An arterial pulse with a notably slow rise in pressure and decreased strength is termed *parvus et tardus pulse* and is characteristic of subaortic stenosis. A *pulse deficit* refers to the absence of an arterial pulse when corresponding heart sounds are auscultated. *Pulsus paradoxus* refers to a palpable or measurable variation in arterial pressure characterized by an exaggerated decrease in systolic and mean pressure during inspiration and is strongly suggestive of cardiac tamponade. In *pulsus alternans,* there is a cyclic attenuation of systolic pressure resulting in a weak pulse–normal pulse pattern. This pulse is associated with severe left ventricular dysfunction. The latter two pulse types may be difficult to document without instrumentation.

ARTERIAL PULSES

Assessment of the Arterial Pulse

The arterial pulse is most prominent and best evaluated at the femoral arteries (Fig. 49–2). The pulse rate and quality should be assessed by palpation of the proximal femoral arteries, close to their origin from the inguinal ring. It is important that both femoral arteries be palpated because differences in pulse quality between left and right femoral arteries may be present. The position of the animal during the examination is usually not important (e.g., standing vs. recumbent); however, the animal should be relatively still to ensure a proper examination. In addition to pulse pressure, body condition affects the perceived strength of the arterial pulse. Arterial pulses are usually more prominent in thin animals, whereas they may be difficult to palpate in obese

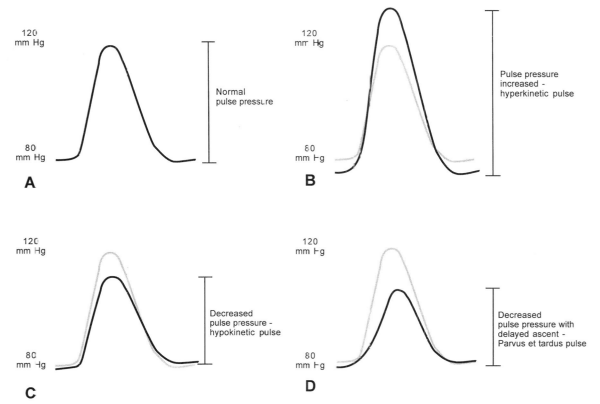

Figure 49–1. Schematic illustration of femoral artery pulse contours. *A*, Normal pulse—there is a rapid rise in pressure followed by a more gradual descent to diastolic pressure. The pulse pressure is indicated by the bar. *B*, Hyperkinetic pulse—elevation in systolic pressure and decrease in diastolic pressure have widened the pulse pressure, resulting in a strong or hyperkinetic pulse. *C*, Hypokinetic pulse—pulse pressure is reduced owing to decreased systolic pressure. *D*, Parvus et tardus pulse—this is a type of hypokinetic pulse characterized by a slow ascent and is typical for subaortic stenosis.

animals. The clinician should take into account the animal's body condition when assessing pulse strength.

To assess arterial pulse quality, the clinician should apply light pressure over the artery with the tips of two or three fingers. Sufficient digital pressure is needed to assess strength; however, excessive digital pressure will obliterate the pulsatile qualities and impair pulse evaluation.

Genesis of the Arterial Pulse

The major driving force of blood flow and arterial pressure is generated by the contractile force of the left ventricle and to a lesser extent by elastic recoil of the aorta. During systole, once left ventricular pressure exceeds aortic pressure, the aortic valve cusps open and ventricular ejection begins. Owing to the left ventricle's rapid force generation, the aortic pressure rises rapidly. As ventricular pressure declines and blood flows into the distal vasculature, aortic pressure decreases. During ventricular diastole, when left ventricular pressure drops below aortic pressure and aortic valve cusps close, diastolic blood pressure is maintained by elastic recoil of the aorta. Diastolic blood pressure gradually decreases as elastic recoil is consumed and blood flows distally. In peripheral arteries, where pulses are evaluated, systolic amplitude and pulse pressure are increased, and the rise in the pulse wave becomes steeper.

There are three physiologic factors important in determining arterial pressure: (1) heart rate, (2) peripheral vascular resistance, and (3) stroke volume. An increase in heart rate will result in an increase in diastolic arterial pressure, as there is less time for diastolic pressure to decline. This increase in diastolic pressure will result in a decrease in

pulse pressure and an increase in mean arterial pressure. Peripheral vascular resistance (PVR) is a function of vessel tone and arterial wall compliance. When PVR is increased, there is an increase in diastolic blood pressure and a corresponding decrease in pulse pressure. PVR is increased in older animals as a result of loss of arterial wall compliance and in animals with heart failure and elevated levels of the vasoactive compound angiotensin II. Likewise, a decrease in PVR will result in a decreased diastolic pressure and an increased pulse pressure. Anemic animals have reduced resistance resulting from decreased blood viscosity, and often have hyperkinetic pulses. When the amount of blood ejected by the left ventricle (stroke volume) increases, systolic pressure increases resulting in increases in pulse pressure and mean arterial pressure. Decreases in stroke volume (e.g., myocardial failure) often result in diminished pulse pressure (hypokinetic pulse) secondary to decreased systolic blood pressure and increased PVR.

Because the overall pulse strength is a function of the difference between peak systolic pressure and diastolic pressure, the pulse pressure (and therefore perceived pulse strength) will increase when diastolic pressure is decreased and systolic pressure is maintained. When there is significant aortic insufficiency or another source of diastolic pressure loss (such as patent ductus arteriosus), pulse pressure increases significantly and pulses become hyperkinetic, or bounding.

Arterial Pulse Alterations

Hypokinetic arterial pulses may be present whenever there is decreased left ventricular stroke volume. Common condi-

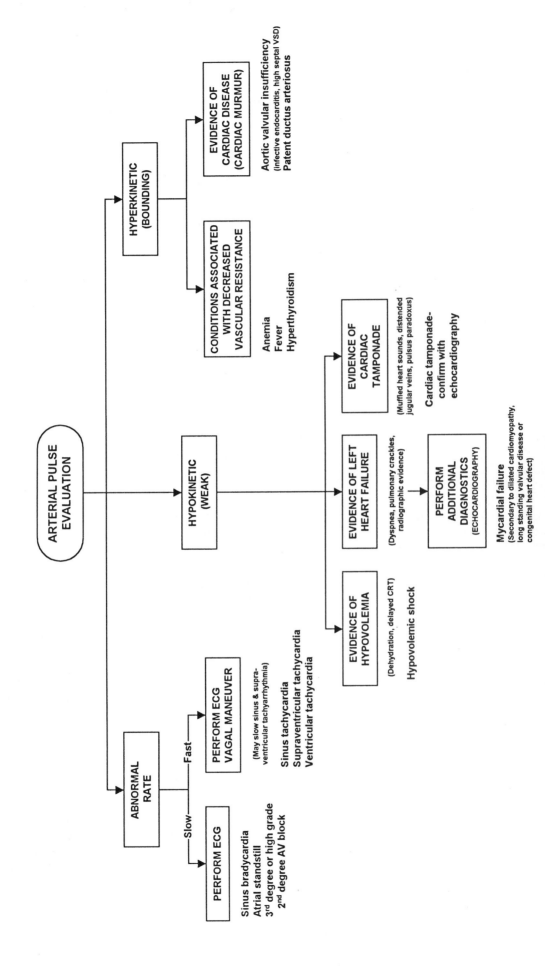

Figure 49–2. Algorithm for arterial pulse evaluation.

tions associated with reduced stroke volume include hypovolemia, left ventricular failure, and cardiac tamponade (see Section VII). Additionally, a compensatory tachycardia is usually present in these animals, further contributing to a loss of pulse pressure. In subaortic stenosis, arterial pulses are hypokinetic and also slow rising (parvus et tardus pulse) (see Fig. 49–2).

Hyperkinetic arterial pulses are most prominent in cases of aortic valvular insufficiency (infective endocarditis) and patent ductus arteriosus as a result of the extreme loss of diastolic pressure and increase in pulse pressure (see Chapter 112). These conditions are also associated with an increase in stroke volume that contributes to increased pulse pressures. Animals with significant aortic insufficiency have remarkably bounding pulses, in some cases to the point that the head and extremities jerk with each pulse (de Mussett's sign). Pulses can become hyperkinetic with mitral insufficiency as a result of volume overloading of the left ventricle and shortened ejection time associated with mitral regurgitation. When resistance is decreased, as in hyperthyroidism, fever, or anemia, pulses are often hyperkinetic.

Irregular Arterial Pulses and Pulse Deficits

In the normal animal, pulse rhythm is dependent on the rhythm of cardiac contractions, with a pulse for each complete cardiac cycle. When cardiac rhythm is irregular, as in normal sinus arrhythmia, the pulse rhythm will be correspondingly irregular. Pathologic alterations in cardiac rhythm may result in pulse deficits—the absence of a palpable arterial pulse when a first heart sound is auscultated. This occurs when an arrhythmia interrupts diastolic filling causing insufficient filling of the ventricle. If a premature contraction occurs before there is adequate ventricular filling, the resulting intraventricular pressure will be insufficient to open the aortic valve, and no ejection will occur. Since a much lower pressure is needed to result in atrioventricular valve closure, a first heart sound is heard. Following an isolated pulse deficit, the next pulse is often accentuated as a result of the increased stroke volume consequent to prolonged diastolic time and increased ventricular filling. It is imperative that electrocardiography be performed when pulse deficits are detected to document and characterize the arrhythmia. Irregular pulses and pulse deficits are present in atrial fibrillation owing to erratic ventricular ejection. Similar pulses occur when frequent atrial and/or ventricular premature contractions are present (see Chapter 114).

Pulsus Paradoxus and Pulsus Alternans

Pulsus paradoxus refers to a palpable or measurable variation in arterial pressure characterized by an exaggerated decrease in systolic, mean, and pulse pressure during inspiration. This pulse is strongly suggestive of cardiac tamponade (see Chapter 118). Detection of pulsus paradoxus may require instrumentation. Pulsus alternans may occur when there is severe left ventricular dysfunction (such as dilated cardiomyopathy) and is thought to be due to fluctuations in the contractile state of the left ventricle. When this pulse is present, a third heart sound is usually auscultatable.

Absent Arterial Pulsations

Systemic thromboembolism, a complication of feline cardiomyopathy, is often characterized by loss of arterial pulsations of the femoral arteries (see Chapter 117). Systemic thromboembolism may also occur secondary to coagulable states such as renal amyloidosis, hyperadrenocorticism, and infective endocarditis. Unilateral and bilateral femoral artery thromboembolism of an idiopathic nature has been observed in young to middle-aged Cavalier King Charles spaniels.

VENOUS PULSES

Assessment of the Venous Pulse

In most cases, adequate visualization of the jugular veins (from thoracic inlet to the angle of the jaw) requires clipping of overlying hair (Fig. 49–3). Subtle abnormalities of jugular venous flow are often missed if the hair has not been clipped. The animal should be standing or sitting for jugular venous examination. In normal animals, jugular pulsations should not extend more than one third the distance up the neck from the thoracic inlet. Pulsations from the underlying carotid arteries may mimic jugular venous pulsations—if pulsations continue despite light pressure at the thoracic inlet (occlusion of jugular vein), they are arterial in origin. Careful assessment for distention of jugular veins should always be performed when ascites is present—the presence of distended jugular veins is an indication of right-sided heart failure.

Components of the Normal Venous Pulse

Jugular venous pressures correlate with right atrial pressure; therefore, jugular distention occurs when right atrial pressure is increased, and jugular pulsations occur when tricuspid regurgitation is present. When jugular waveforms are analyzed, several components can be detected. The most prominent deflection is the A wave corresponding to right atrial contraction. During right atrial relaxation, a dip in pressure is noted (Z point). Immediately following the Z point, a second wave (C wave) corresponding to right ventricular isovolumetric contraction occurs. This wave is produced by bulging of the tricuspid valve into the right atrium and transmission of this pressure into the jugular veins. During right ventricular ejection, the tricuspid valve is displaced downward producing a prominent negative deflection, the X wave. Late in systole, a third positive deflection, the V wave, occurs resulting from increased blood volume and pressure within the right atrium. Immediately following the V wave, right atrial emptying occurs as a result of relaxation of the right ventricle producing a second prominent dip in jugular venous pressure, the Y wave. At slow heart rates, careful examination will usually reveal the three positive deflections (a, v, c) and two negative waves (x, y). Accentuation of jugular venous distention through the hepatojugular reflux may be accomplished by applying gentle pressure to the cranial abdomen for 30 to 60 seconds while observing the jugular veins. This technique results in increased venous return (increased right ventricular preload), which in the presence of underlying right heart disease will elevate right atrial pressure and impede jugular venous return.

Venous Pulse Alterations

Jugular venous distention and distention of peripheral veins are usually prominent in diseases causing significant

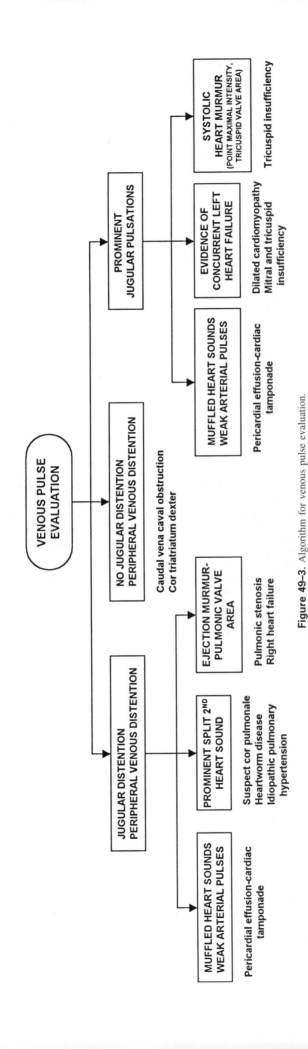

Figure 49–3. Algorithm for venous pulse evaluation.

increases in right ventricular diastolic pressure. Common examples include pericardial effusion, pulmonic stenosis, pulmonary hypertension, and cardiomyopathy. Tricuspid insufficiency secondary to degenerative valve disease may cause venous distention, as well as jugular pulsations (exaggerated V wave). Distention of caudal peripheral veins with normal jugular veins is suggestive of an obstructive lesion in the caudal vena cava, or cor triatriatum dexter—an abnormal septation within the right atrium obstructing caudal vena cava flow. The combination of weak arterial pulses and jugular venous distention is suggestive of cardiac tamponade (see Chapter 118).

CHAPTER 50

HYPERTENSION

Meryl P. Littman

Hypertension (HT), high systemic blood pressure (BP) associated with increased morbidity and mortality, is still being defined in dogs and cats. Most investigators agree that BP measurements (BPMs) in awake and untrained dogs and cats do not normally exceed 180/100 mmHg systolic/diastolic and that moderate to severe HT ($\geq$200/110 mmHg) is clinically significant, causes pathology, and should be treated.

Hypertension may be secondary to other diseases (usually renal, adrenal, or thyroid) or primary (essential or idiopathic), with no specific cause. End-organ (target-organ) damage occurs in tissues receiving blood at high BP. Because BP is not routinely measured, the prevalence of HT in dogs and cats is unclear.

BLOOD PRESSURE MEASUREMENT

Direct BPMs (DBPMs) can be done by arterial puncture with a needle or catheter connected to a pressure transducer and monitor. In a conscious, untrained animal, anxiety and/or pain from restraint and then needle insertion may increase the BPM. DBPMs are used mostly in critical care patients and in research. Telemetry (24-hour BPM) in colony animals shows BP to be very labile. Such monitoring has not been done in pets.

Indirect BPMs (IBPMs) are noninvasive, obtained with a cuff constricting a peripheral artery (on the leg or tail) using an ultrasonic (Doppler Flow Detector, Parks Electronics), oscillometric (Dinamap, Critikon), or photoplethysmographic (Finapres, Ohmeda) transducer distal to the cuff to detect blood flow or arterial wall motion. Cuff width should be 30 to 40 per cent of the limb's circumference (large cuffs falsely decrease BPM; small cuffs increase BPM). Correlations between DBPMs and IBPMs are generally good, although IBPMs may underestimate DBPMs by 8 to 14 mmHg. In a comparison of IBPM methods in anesthetized cats, the Doppler system on the leg was the most efficient, accurate, sensitive, and reproducible and the least expensive. The Doppler method can be used on animals of all sizes, but subjectivity for diastolic BPMs (when sounds are muffled) causes calculated mean arterial BP to be subjective as well. Average systolic BPM on 33 normal and conscious cats with the Doppler leg method was 118 mmHg. Some workers prefer to use the Dinamap system on dogs' tails, where the average BPM on 1903 normal and conscious dogs was 133/76 mmHg. Blood pressure was found to be higher in males, in older animals, in small breeds or sight hounds, and in obese animals.

Uncooperative or anxious animals may have falsely elevated BPMs (the "white-coat" effect). Repeated BPMs; acclimatization to the setting; minimal restraint, stress, or noise; averaging three to five BPMs; and discarding outliers help to establish a reliable BPM. IBPMs on pet dogs both in the hospital and at home showed no significant difference using the foreleg or the tail.

PATHOPHYSIOLOGY

Regulation of systemic BP involves complex relationships between central and peripheral adrenergic, renal, endocrine, and vascular systems. Essential HT is most common in humans; secondary HT appears to be most common in dogs and cats (Table 50–1).

Systemic BP is proportional to cardiac output (CO) and total peripheral resistance (TPR) (BP = CO × TPR); CO depends on heart rate and stroke volume (SV) and is related to total body water. Increased intracellular sodium chloride (NaCl) results in increased cytosolic Ca^{++}, leading to enhanced arteriolar tone and sensitivity to vasopressors (angiotensin II, catecholamines). Thus, increases in body NaCl can raise both SV and TPR. Steroids increase NaCl retention and angiotensinogen. Activation of the renin-angiotensin-aldosterone (RAA) system by renovascular or renal disease raises BP by increasing both SV and TPR; angiotensin II is a potent vasoconstrictor (increasing TPR), and aldosterone causes renal NaCl retention (increasing SV and TPR).

Increased TPR may be caused by raised arteriolar tone secondary to cytosolic Ca^{++}, vasopressors, or decreased vasodilators (e.g., vasodilatory prostaglandins or kinins from the renal medulla). Vascular remodeling (e.g., arteriosclerosis, atherosclerosis) may decrease arteriolar elasticity and cause increases in TPR.

TABLE 50–1. CAUSES AND MECHANISMS OF SECONDARY HYPERTENSION

Renal disease[*][†]— ↑ CO, ↑ TPR
    Glomerulonephritis, amyloidosis, glomerulosclerosis, chronic interstitial nephritis, pyelonephritis, polycystic renal disease, renal dysplasia
Hyperadrenocorticism[*]— ↑ CO, ↑ TPR
    Pituitary-dependent, adrenal neoplasia, iatrogenic
Hyperthyroidism[†]— ↑ HR
Pheochromocytoma— ↑ HR
Hyperaldosteronism— ↑ CO, ↑ TPR
Diabetes mellitus— ↑ TPR
Hyperkinetic heart syndrome— ↑ HR
    Anemia, hyperviscosity, polycythemia, fever, arteriovenous fistula
Renovascular disease— ↑ CO, ↑ TPR
    Renal arterial stenosis, thromboembolism, renal infarct
Intracranial disease (e.g., neoplasia)— ↑ CO, ↑ TPR
Hypothyroidism (atherosclerosis)— ↑ TPR
Coarctation of the aorta— ↑ CO, ↑ TPR
Hypercalcemia— ↑ TPR
Hyperestrogenism— ↑ CO, ↑ TPR
Pregnancy toxemia— ↑ CO, ↑ TPR
Licorice toxicity (mineralocorticoid)— ↑ CO, ↑ TPR

[*]Commonly found in dogs with clinically significant hypertension.
[†]Commonly found in cats with clinically significant hypertension.
CO = cardiac output; TPR = total peripheral resistance; HR = heart rate.

In a state of HT, the kidney excretes more NaCl and water (pressure diuresis). End-organ damage occurs when incoming blood at high BP causes exudation (by Starling's forces) of fluid (edema), plasma, or blood (hemorrhage). In vascular beds with autoregulation, spasm of arterioles in response to high BP protects the capillary bed. However, arteriolar damage (medial hypertrophy, arteriolosclerosis) and increased spasm may lead to hypoxia at the capillary bed, allowing for permeability changes (edema or hemorrhage) or infarcts. The end organs most sensitive to high BP include the eye, kidney, and cardiovascular and cerebrovascular systems (Fig. 50–1).

Increased TPR may induce concentric left ventricular hypertrophy (LVH) as the heart muscle works to overcome excess afterload. Arteries damaged by HT develop arteriosclerosis, which may increase TPR. Renal changes (nephrosclerosis, glomerulosclerosis) may alter the kidney's ability to excrete NaCl and water, activate the RAA system, and increase SV and TPR. Thus, HT may be self-perpetuating. Renal disease may be the cause of, the effect of, or coincident with HT. Research in dogs with HT shows resistance to severe damage to the kidneys even after years of untreated moderate HT.

HISTORICAL FINDINGS

Dogs and cats with moderate to severe HT are usually middle-aged or older. The LVH and higher BPMs seen in sight hounds appear to be functional, inbred, and not related to increased morbidity or mortality (although atherosclerosis with a high-fat diet is easier to induce). Breed predispositions for HT include those susceptible to renal disease or hyperadrenocorticism (Cushing's syndrome). Male dogs represented 77 per cent of 30 dogs with severe HT. Obesity is another risk factor.

Animals with HT have varied signs that are caused by the underlying disease or end-organ damage (see Fig. 50–1). Blindness and polyuria/polydipsia are most common.

PHYSICAL FINDINGS

A strong or bounding peripheral pulse does not prove HT but is an indication of the pulse pressure (the difference between the systolic and diastolic BP). The BP needs to be measured as discussed earlier. The most common findings in dogs and cats with moderate to severe HT include retinal hemorrhage, retinal detachment, small kidneys (cats), and low-grade mitral murmur (caused by LVH). Other findings may suggest an underlying cause of HT.

DIAGNOSTIC PLAN

Hypertension may be suspected because of historical, physical examination, laboratory, radiographic, or other findings suggestive of end-organ damage or of diseases known to cause secondary HT (Fig. 50–2). Repeated BPMs may be necessary to support the diagnosis of HT. When HT is confirmed, tests to find a cause and to stage end-organ damage help plan management and suggest prognosis.

The database, including complete blood count, biochemical profile, and urinalysis, may suggest renal failure (e.g., anemia, increased serum creatinine, blood urea nitrogen, phosphorus, isosthenuria, pyuria), Cushings syndrome (e.g., mature neutrophilia, lymphopenia, increased serum alkaline phosphatase, dilute urine, mild proteinuria), hyperthyroidism, or (much less common to rare) hyperaldosteronism (high Na^+, low K^+). Urine culture and sensitivity should be done if the urine sediment is active or if pyelonephritis or Cushing's syndrome is suspected. Proteinuria, low serum albumin, and high serum cholesterol may suggest glomerulonephropathy. The urine protein-creatinine ratio helps to quantify the extent of proteinuria. Thrombocytopenia or leukopenia may suggest an infectious or immune-mediated cause of proteinuria or azotemia. Serologic tests screen for immune-mediated disease or infections (e.g., tick-borne diseases, heartworm) causing proteinuria. Coagulation profile, nasal series, cerebrospinal fluid analysis, and/or brain scan may be indicated to help rule out other causes of epistaxis, retinal, or neurologic signs.

Chest and abdominal radiographs and abdominal ultrasonography may disclose neoplasia, abnormal kidney architecture, adrenal masses, ascites, or hepatomegaly associated with diseases that can cause HT secondarily. End-organ damage may also be detected (e.g., cardiomegaly or pleural effusion). Echocardiogram and electrocardiogram may show concentric LVH. In some cases, decompensation and heart failure may be found.

Tests for endocrine diseases include serum total and free thyroxine (T_4) concentrations or T_3 suppression test for hyperthyroidism; serum T_4 with serum thyroid-stimulating hormone assay for hypothyroidism; urine cortisol-creatinine ratio, low-dose dexamethasone suppression, and adrenocorticotropic hormone (ACTH) stimulation test for Cushing's syndrome (and abdominal ultrasonography, high-dose dexamethasone suppression test, or ACTH assay to discern adrenal neoplasia from pituitary-dependent Cushing's); and serum aldosterone assay in suspected cases of hyperaldosteronism. The diagnosis of pheochromocytoma may be supported by abdominal ultrasonography, a Regitine blocking test (if the alpha$_1$-adrenergic blocking agent phentolamine causes decreased BP by >35/25 mmHg), a clonidine suppression test (the alpha$_2$-agonist normally decreases BP centrally but not in pheochromocytoma), or high plasma or urinary catecholamines and metanephrines.

Renovascular HT (e.g., renal arterial stenosis) may be diagnosed by renal arteriogram and plasma renin activity tested on renal vein blood samples. Renal biopsy may support renal causes of HT. Glomerulosclerosis may be caused

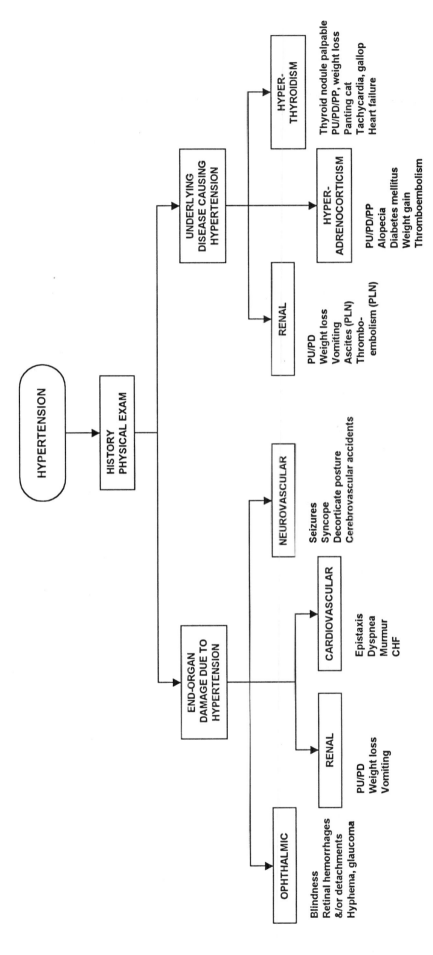

Figure 50–1. Algorithm for the differential diagnosis of hypertension.

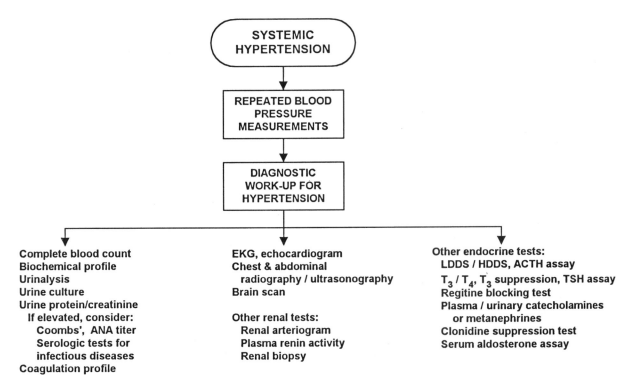

Figure 50–2. Algorithm for the initial evaluation of hypertension.

by damage from HT. Arterioles in other tissues may show damage from HT (e.g., medial hypertrophy, arteriosclerosis, onion-skinning, hyaline necrosis).

GOALS OF TREATMENT

Without morbidity and mortality data, it is not known whether treatment is warranted for the mild or borderline HT commonly noted in animals with renal disease or Cushing's syndrome (60 per cent), glomerulopathy (80 per cent), hyperthyroidism (87 per cent), or diabetes mellitus (51 per cent). If end-organ damage is apparent or if moderate to severe HT (BPM ≥200/110 mmHg) is identified, therapy is given to lower the BPM by 20 per cent or, if possible, to less than 160/100 mmHg. Control of HT is achieved with single or combination use of an angiotensin-converting enzyme inhibitor (to decrease TPR, CO) such as enalapril (Enacard, Vasotec, 0.5 mg/kg every 12 to 24 hours) or benazepril (Lotensin, 0.25 to 0.5 mg/kg every 12 to 24 hours), a calcium channel blocker (to lower TPR) such as amlodipine (Norvasc, 0.625 to 1.25 mg/cat every 24 hours; 0.5 to 1.0 mg/kg in dogs every 24 hours), and/or the cardioselective beta blocker (to lower the heart rate) atenolol (Tenormin, 2 mg/kg every 12 to 24 hours). Less commonly used drugs include diuretics (to lower CO and/or TPR) and alpha blockers (to lower TPR). Angiotensin-converting enzyme inhibitors (ACEIs) decrease TPR and SV by decreasing conversion of angiotensin I to angiotensin II, a potent vasoconstrictor that causes aldosterone release. The ACEI drugs also cause dilatation of the efferent renal arterioles and help decrease the progression of glomerulosclerosis by lowering glomerular filtration pressure. Amlodipine decreases cytosolic Ca^{++} in arterioles and heart muscle to cause a decrease in TPR and CO. Other drugs that lower TPR include alpha$_1$-adrenergic blockers and direct-acting vasodilators such as hydralazine. Beta-adrenergic blockers lower heart rate and CO and may also decrease the release of renin. Emergency hypertensive situations are rare in veterinary medicine but may occur (e.g., in acute renal crises). Aggressive intravenous therapy with nitroprusside or hydralazine may dangerously decrease renal perfusion.

Concurrent illness should be treated. Atenolol may be useful in hypertensive hyperthyroid cats; once euthyroid, they often do not require therapy for HT. Dogs with Cushing's syndrome and hypertension, however, may still need therapy for HT after the Cushing's is controlled. Steroids, alpha$_1$-adrenergic agonists (e.g., phenylpropanolamine for urinary incontinence), obesity, and high-salt diets (in case salt sensitivity exists) should be avoided.

Monitoring of BPMs, ocular examination, serum creatinine, and so forth are initially done every 1 to 2 weeks in outpatients and every 1 to 3 months in controlled cases. Vision may return with treatment if blindness was of 1 to 2 days' duration. Longer-duration blindness often does not respond, even with resolution of detachment or hemorrhage. Life expectancy is decreased in dogs presenting with azotemia, and in dogs or cats with neurologic or heart failure signs. Dogs with controlled essential HT may live many years without renal impairment. Elderly cats with HT and mild renal insufficiency and/or hyperthyroidism do well with treatment and may succumb to other geriatric diseases (e.g., malignancy) years later.

CHAPTER 51

HYPOTENSION

Douglass K. Macintire

Hypotension is defined as a mean systemic arterial blood pressure less than 60 to 70 mmHg and a systolic arterial blood pressure measurement less than 80 to 90 mmHg. Untreated hypotension can result in shock. The underlying defect common to all forms of shock is inadequate tissue perfusion resulting in diminished oxygen delivery to cells, altered cellular metabolism, cell death, and organ dysfunction.

Blood pressure should be monitored in animals that are critically ill, are receiving vasoactive drugs, have experienced trauma, or are under anesthesia. Animals with cardiac disease, renal disease, hypoadrenocorticism, severe dehydration, sepsis, anaphylaxis, and acidosis are at risk for hypotension. Serial monitoring of blood pressure in these critical patients can allow the astute clinician to detect alarming trends and institute appropriate resuscitative measures to restore perfusion before irreversible organ dysfunction occurs.

CLINICAL MANIFESTATIONS

The classic clinical signs of hypotension include cerebral depression, weak pulses, and tachycardia. Subjective measures used to clinically evaluate perfusion include mucous membrane color, capillary refill time, and pulse quality. As a general rule, when both metatarsal and femoral pulses are palpable, systolic blood pressure is assumed to be above 80 mmHg. When femoral pulses are weak and metatarsal pulses are absent, hypotension is present and systolic blood pressure may be less than 60 mmHg. With severe hypotension, autoregulation of the heart, brain, and renal perfusion beds fails. If perfusion is not restored to these vital organs, the patient's condition will decompensate into irreversable shock followed by death.

PATHOGENESIS

The three general causes of hypotension are decreased cardiac output, decreased blood volume, and decreased vascular tone (Table 51–1). Regardless of the underlying cause, certain compensatory mechanisms are activated in hypotensive animals that tend to maintain blood pressure in the normal range until severe compromise (>20 to 25 per cent loss of intravascular volume) occurs. As blood pressure falls, lack of stretch in the carotid sinus and aortic body baroreceptors initiates a neurohumoral response characterized by increased sympathetic nervous system activity, increased synthesis and secretion of adrenocorticotropic (ACTH) and antidiuretic hormones (ADH) from the pituitary, and enhanced release of cortisol and catecholemines from the adrenal glands. Receptors in the afferent arterioles and macula densa of the kidneys are also affected, leading to stimulation of the renin-angiotensin-aldosterone system.

The net effect of these mechanisms is an integrated response to maintain blood pressure and retain sodium and water. Initially, cardiac output is augmented by enhanced myocardial contractility, increased heart rate, and improved vasomotor tone. Arteriolar vasoconstriction in the skin, muscle, kidney, and gastrointestinal (GI) tract allows blood to be shunted centrally to the heart and brain. With severe hypovolemia or cardiac dysfunction, compensatory mechanisms become ineffective and organ function deteriorates. Evidence of poor perfusion is manifested by pale mucous membranes, weak pulses, tachycardia, and slow capillary refill time. Vicious cycles are initiated that contribute to organ failure. The heart requires more oxygen to function under stress conditions but has decreased coronary perfusion because of the short diastolic filling time associated with tachycardia. As heart function decreases, pulmonary edema and thrombosis may result. Acute renal failure can result from prolonged hypotension as renal blood flow and autoregulation are compromised. Impaired perfusion of the GI tract can lead to breakdown of the GI mucosal barrier with systemic absorption of bacteria and endotoxins. Impaired hepatic clearance and failure of the reticuloendothelial system contribute to continued circulation of vasoactive substances that can perpetuate shock. It is therefore important to recognize and correct hypotension *before* decompensation occurs.

DIRECT MEASUREMENT OF BLOOD PRESSURE

Systemic arterial blood pressure (SABP) can be measured either directly or indirectly. Direct measurement requires

TABLE 51–1. CAUSES OF HYPOTENSION

Cardiac Dysfunction	*Hypovolemia*
Impaired contractility	Hemorrhage
Cardiomyopathy	Trauma
Drug suppression—	Gastrointestinal losses
anesthetics, beta blockers	Excessive diuresis
Sepsis—release of myocardial	Hypoadrenocorticism
depressant factor	Pancreatitis
Impaired relaxation	Peritonitis
Feline hypertrophic	Burns
cardiomyopathy	Heatstroke
Valvular disease	
Mitral/tricuspid regurgitation	*Decreased Vascular Tone*
Aortic/pulmonic stenosis	Neurogenic
Impaired filling	Spinal cord trauma
Pericardial effusion,	Epidural anesthesia
restrictive pericarditis	Endotoxin release, sepsis
Pneumothorax	Anaphylaxis
Obstruction of venous return	Vasoactive drugs—phenothiazines,
Gastric dilatation-volvulus	ACE inhibitors, calcium
Thrombosis	channel blockers, nitroglycerin,
Neoplasia	nitroprusside, hydralazine
Arrhythmias/conduction defects	

placing either a needle or a catheter into an artery and connecting it to a transducer and oscilloscope. Direct measurement of SABP is considered the "gold standard" and provides accurate measurements even in hypotensive animals. Unfortunately, because special skills and equipment are required, the technique is most commonly employed in veterinary referral centers and research projects, rather than in routine practice.

The most common site for catheter placement for monitoring continuous direct SABP is the dorsal metatarsal artery, which lies in the groove between the second and third metatarsal bones. The catheter must be placed aseptically and should be flushed with heparinized saline by constant infusion or every 4 hours to prevent clotting. Many electrocardiographic monitors have a separate channel for blood pressure measurement. The typical pressure wave appears as a steep upstroke with a dicrotic notch. Complications with arterial catheter placement include infection, thrombosis, and hemorrhage if the catheter becomes dislodged. The dorsal metatarsal artery is easily compressed to control hemorrhage, but if other arteries such as the femoral or carotid are used, serious hemorrhage can result from catheter dislodgement, and close monitoring is required.

Measurement of central venous pressure (CVP) can provide an assessment of intravascular volume, cardiac function, and venous compliance. Hypotensive patients that are in need of intravenous fluid therapy will have low CVP readings, whereas hypotensive patients with myocardial failure will have high CVP readings. Serial measurements provide the most useful information, as they reflect trends and the patient's response to therapeutic interventions. Measurement of CVP requires placement of a catheter in the external jugular vein so that the tip rests in the cranial vena cava near the right atrium. The catheter is connected by extension tubing to a stopcock that is attached to a fluid administration set and a manometer. The level of the right atrium is approximated at the manubrium when the patient is in lateral recumbency or at the point of the scapula when it is sternal. This point is recorded as the zero point when the manometer is vertical. The CVP is measured by filling the manometer with fluid and then turning the stopcock off to the fluid port and allowing the pressure of the fluid in the manometer to equilibrate with the patient's CVP. Measurement of CVP provides valuable information about the hypotensive patient's ability to accommodate intravenous fluids in the presence of heart failure, renal dysfunction, systemic vasodilatation, or increased capillary permeability.

INDIRECT BLOOD PRESSURE MEASUREMENT

Noninvasive measurement of blood pressure can be accomplished using either an ultrasound flow detector (Parks Electronics, Aloha, OR) or an oscillometer (Dinamap, Critikon, Tampa, FL). With the Doppler method, a cuff is placed proximal to the transducer and inflated to 200 to 250 mmHg. The first sound heard as the pressure is gradually released from the cuff is the systolic blood pressure. Common locations for blood pressure measurement include the cranial tibial artery, the palmar and plantar arteries, and the tail. A disadvantage of the Doppler method is that it measures only systolic pressure, and mean blood pressure is more closely related to diastolic pressure. Advantages of the Doppler method are that it is inexpensive, easy to perform, and is usually sensitive enough to determine BP in small cats and dogs, as well as in mildly hypotensive animals.

The oscillometric method can be used to measure systolic, diastolic, and mean blood pressure. The machine can be set to cycle continuously, recording BP measurements at selected time intervals. Although the oscillometric method is easy and convenient, it is greatly affected by movement and often does not provide reliable readings in animals that have arrhythmias or are moving, shivering, or hypotensive.

With either indirect method, the cuff width should be 40 per cent of the limb circumference. Incorrect cuff size can give inaccurate readings. Unfortunately, with both indirect methods, locating an artery in a hypotensive animal can be frustrating. Indirect blood pressure measurement is best

TABLE 51–2. TREATMENTS FOR HYPOTENSION

For Volume Replacement

Crystalloid fluids (balanced electrolyte solution)
   40–90 mL/kg IV
Colloid fluids (blood, plasma, hydroxyethyl starch, dextran 70)
   10–20 mL/kg
Hypertonic saline (7.5% NaCl)
   4–6 mL/kg—follow with 10–20 mL/kg of balanced electrolyte fluid

For Positive Inotropic Support

Dobutamine
   Dogs: 5–20 µg/kg/min constant-rate infusion (CRI)
   Cats: 2.5–15 µg/kg/min CRI (may cause seizures)
Amrinone
   0.75 mg/kg IV bolus (slowly over 3–5 min) followed by 5–10 µg/kg/min CRI
Digoxin
   Dog: 0.22 mg/m² q 12 h PO
   Cat: 0.0312 mg/m² q 24 h PO
Dopamine (moderate dose)
   4–6 µg/kg/min CRI

For Vasopressor Effects

Norepinephrine 0.05–1 µg/kg/min CRI
Epinephrine 0.1–1.0 µg/kg/min CRI
Dopamine (high dose) 7–20 µg/kg/min CRI

For Ventricular Arrhythmias

Lidocaine
   Dogs: 2–4 mg/kg IV bolus, then 25–80 µg/kg/min CRI
   Cats: 0.25 mg/kg IV bolus, then 10 µg/kg/min CRI
Procainamide
   2 mg/kg bolus, repeated to maximum cumulative dosage of 20 mg/kg, then 10–40 µg/kg/min
Bretylium tosylate 10 mg/kg IV
Magnesium sulfate 50–100 mg/kg IV over 5–15 min

For Supraventricular Tachyarrhythmias (Nonresponsive to Volume Replacement)

Diltiazem 0.25 mg/kg IV slowly, repeated q 15 min to cumulative dose of 0.75 mg/kg
Verapamil 0.05–0.15 mg/kg IV, then 2–10 µg/kg/min
Esmolol 500 µg/kg IV, then 25–200 µg/kg/min CRI
Digoxin 0.0025 mg/kg IV, repeated q 30 min up to 4 doses

For Bradyarrhythmias

Atropine 0.02–0.04 mg/kg IV q 6 h
Transvenous pacemaker implantation

For Anaphylaxis

Epinephrine 0.01–0.02 mg/kg IV, IM, or SC
Prednisolone sodium succinate 10–25 mg/kg IV
Diphenhydramine HCl 0.5–1.0 mg/kg IV

For Enhancing Renal and Mesenteric Blood Flow

Dopamine (low dose)
   1–3 µg/kg/min CRI

For Refractory Septic Shock

Naloxone 30 µg/kg loading dose, then 60 µg/kg over 1 hour
Glucose-insulin-potassium infusion
   3 g glucose + 1 unit insulin + 0.5 mEq KCl per kg IV over 4–6 h

employed as a means to avoid hypotension in critical patients with potentially unstable cardiovascular function or in animals undergoing general anesthesia.

TREATMENT OF HYPOTENSION (Fig. 51–1)

Whenever the systolic BP is less than 90 mmHg or the mean BP is less than 60 mmHg, aggressive measures should be taken to restore perfusion. First and foremost, cardiovascular function should be assessed through auscultation, palpation of peripheral pulses, electrocardiography, and, if possible, measurement of CVP. Evidence of pulmonary edema (labored breathing, crackles and wheezes on auscultation, $CVP > 10$ cm H_2O) or cardiac arrhythmias are reasons to avoid intravenous fluids during initial treatment. Patients with cardiogenic shock generally require oxygen supplementation and positive inotropic support with dobutamine, dopa-

mine, or amrinone (Table 51–2). If there is evidence of pulmonary edema or increased CVP, a diuretic is indicated. Severe arrhythmias should be corrected. If patients with cardiogenic shock remain hypotensive despite these interventions, judicious fluid therapy can be administered while monitoring the CVP. Intravenous fluids are discontinued if the CVP exceeds 10 cm H_2O or rises more than 3 cm H_2O in 1 hour.

All animals with normal cardiac function should receive intravascular volume expansion as initial therapy for hypotension. The type of fluid chosen is somewhat controversial, although blood is indicated for hemorrhagic shock, crystalloid fluids are indicated for hypovolemia resulting from gastrointestinal or renal losses, and colloids are indicated in animals with hypotension secondary to increased vascular permeability or decreased oncotic pressure. Initial fluid rates should be 10 to 20 mL/kg for colloids and 40 to 90 mL/kg

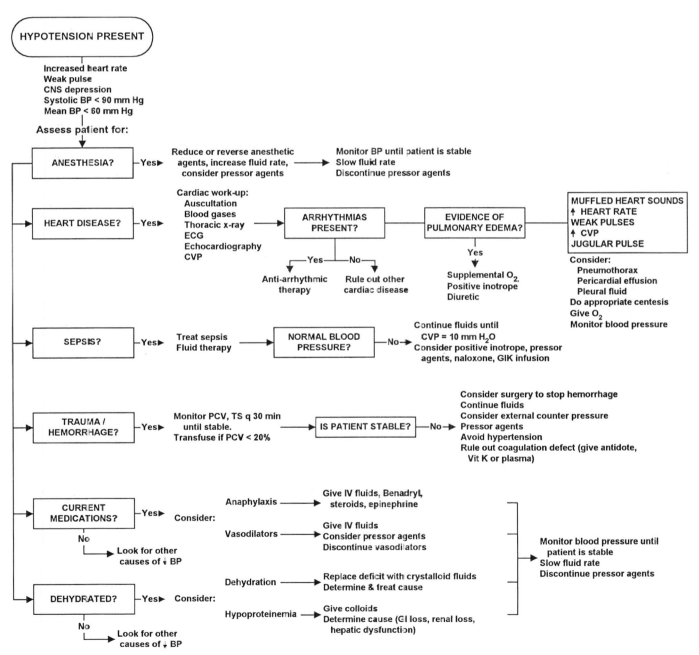

Figure 51–1. Algorithm for differential diagnosis and management of hypotension.

for crystalloids with the goal of achieving and maintaining an acceptable mean BP. Most hypotensive patients will improve with volume replacement. Nonresponsive patients may have ongoing hemorrhage, systemic vasodilatation, leaky capillaries, or irreversible shock and multiple organ failure. A blood transfusion should be given if the packed cell volume is less than 20 per cent (dog) or less than 15 per cent (cat). Septic animals are prone to myocardial depression, increased capillary permeability, and reduced systemic vascular resistance. They may benefit from positive inotropes, pressor agents, and administration of colloids. In experimental animals with endotoxic or hemorrhagic shock, naloxone was effective in reversing hypotension.

It is important to monitor blood pressure frequently in these critical patients to assess response to therapy. As soon as BP seems to be normalized, pressor agents should be gradually tapered to avoid excessive vasoconstriction of the renal and mesenteric arteries.

In summary, detection of hypotension in an unstable patient may be a harbinger of potential shock. Early recognition and reversal of hypotension may prevent the serious consequences associated with poor perfusion.

CHAPTER 52

PLEURAL EFFUSION

Kenneth J. Drobatz

The pleural space is normally a "potential space" between the visceral and parietal pleura. It usually contains only 3 to 5 mL of a low-protein fluid (1.5 g/dL) that provides lubrication during respiratory motion. In normal people, as much as 10 L of fluid will traverse the pleural space within a 24-hour period. This constant fluid flux is governed by the same Starling forces that determine net fluid flow across capillary walls, including intravascular and extravascular oncotic and hydrostatic pressures; capillary permeability; and lymphatic drainage. Pleural fluid may accumulate when capillary hydrostatic pressure or permeability is increased, intravascular oncotic pressure is decreased, or lymphatic drainage is impeded. The imbalance that causes fluid accumulation determines the fluid characteristics. Therefore, pleural effusion is not a disease entity itself, but a sign of an underlying disease.

CLINICAL RECOGNITION OF PLEURAL EFFUSION

Clinical signs associated with pleural effusion depend on the underlying disease process, the characteristics of the fluid, and the amount of the pleural fluid. The signs associated with the presence of pleural fluid are primarily respiratory. As the fluid accumulates within the pleural space, the expansion of the lungs becomes limited and tidal volume is decreased. Tachypnea is a physiologic compensation to maintain minute volume and adequate gas exchange and is the most common clinical sign associated with pleural effusion. In some animals, this pattern of shallow rapid breathing may be interrupted periodically by a prolonged and aggressive inspiration in an attempt to expand the lungs.

Auscultatable breath sounds are usually dull or muffled when a substantial amount of pleural fluid accumulates. Lung sounds are decreased ventrally with most pleural effusions, although in some chronic inflammatory conditions, fluid may become loculated, causing patchy areas of decreased breath sounds. Results of thoracic auscultation are usually symmetric, but asymmetry does occur in both dogs and cats when fluid accumulates unilaterally. The clinician should be aware that auscultatable lung sounds might seem normal when the muffling effect is counterbalanced by increased lung sounds associated with concurrent small airway or pulmonary parenchymal disease.

A thorough physical examination often provides clues to the underlying cause of the pleural effusion and should always be completed. Basic principles of emergency respiratory and cardiovascular system assessments should be adhered to in all patients. Animals with severe pulmonary and cardiovascular compromise and pleural effusion may succumb before the underlying cause is discerned if they are not first stabilized. The oral cavity should be evaluated for presence of masses or enlarged tonsils suggesting neoplasia. Horner's syndrome may indicate a thoracic mass. Uveitis concurrent with pleural effusion may be seen with systemic inflammation from neoplasia (particularly lymphosarcoma), feline infectious peritonitis, Rocky Mountain spotted fever, sepsis, or systemic fungal infections. Hyphema may suggest an underlying coagulopathy, trauma, or metastatic neoplasia. Thorough palpation of the neck region for lymphadenopathy or masses may indicate neoplasia or a thyroid nodule causing heart disease secondary to hyperthyroidism. Decreased cranial thoracic wall compliance in cats suggests a mediastinal mass. Observation of jugular pulses indicates increased central venous pressure that may be secondary to pericardial effusion, right-sided heart failure, heartworm caval syndrome, intracardiac thrombus or mass, or tricuspid insufficiency. Decreased arterial pulse intensity on inspiration (pulsus paradoxus) may be noted in about 50 per cent of dogs with pericardial effusion. Thorough palpation of the skeleton should be performed for masses, pain, or periosteal proliferation associated with primary bone tumors, metastatic tumors, or pulmonary neoplasia. Abdominal palpation of a mass suggests disseminated neoplasia. Abdominal pain may indicate peritonitis, pancreatitis, or neoplasia, any of which can be associated with pleural effusion. Paucity of palpable abdominal organs is sometimes noted in animals with pleural effusion secondary to a diaphragmatic hernia. Thorough palpation of the mammary chain for masses or irregularities is warranted. Rectal palpation for masses and observation of the quality of the stool may provide diagnostic clues. Fever may be found with pleural effusions due to inflammatory lesions, infection, or neoplasia.

DEFINITIVE DIAGNOSIS OF PLEURAL EFFUSION

Pleural effusion can be confirmed radiographically, ultrasonographically, or via thoracocentesis (Fig. 52–1). Positioning for thoracic radiographs can be stressful and should be done with caution in animals with respiratory distress. Stabilization with thoracocentesis should be performed prior to thoracic radiographs in animals with respiratory compromise. Removing the fluid prior to radiography will help stabilize the dog or cat as well as optimize the chance to recognize any underlying lung or cardiac pathology that may be causing the effusion.

Equipment for thoracocentesis includes a 20-cc syringe, three-way stopcock, IV extension tubing, and an 18- or 20-gauge needle (1 to 1.5 inches long). The three-way stopcock should be connected to the tip of the syringe. The intravenous extension tubing is then connected to the stopcock, and the needle is attached to the distal end of the extension tubing. The location for thoracocentesis should be the seventh or eight intercostal space at the level of the costochondral junction. The area should be clipped and aseptically prepared prior to the procedure. The animal should be in sternal recumbency. The procedure is generally well tolerated, and sedation or local anesthesia is rarely needed. At least two people are required, with one individual aspirating the syringe while the other advancing the needle. The needle should be inserted just cranial to the rib to avoid the nerves and vessels that run along the caudal aspect. As the needle is advanced, gentle negative pressure should be applied to the syringe. Needle advancement should be stopped when fluid appears in the extension tubing. This will minimize the chance of causing damage to the underlying lung tissue. Ideally, as much fluid as possible should be removed if the pleural effusion is causing respiratory compromise. There should be quick and significant relief of the respiratory distress once the fluid is removed. If respiratory distress is still present, more fluid remains or there is another cause of the respiratory distress. Both sides of the chest should be aspirated if all the fluid cannot be obtained and respiratory compromise is still present. If pleural fluid cannot be ob-

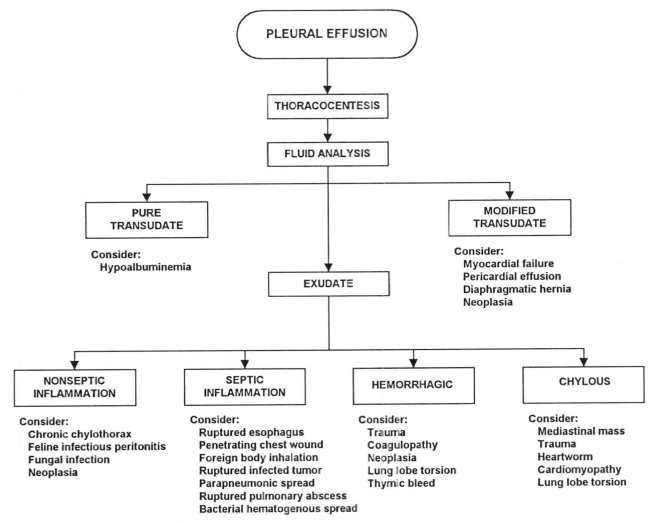

Figure 52–1. Algorithm for differential diagnosis of pleural effusion.

tained from multiple sites despite strong evidence of its presence, the fluid may be loculated, the needle may be obstructed, the needle may not be long enough to enter the pleural space, or the dog or cat may have chronic pleuritis with fibrous adhesions and "pseudo-effusion." Ultrasound-guided thoracocentesis may be required in some instances. Thoracic ultrasound may also provide information as to the underlying cause, and pleural fluid facilitates the ultrasonic visualization of normal intrathoracic structures, masses, diaphragmatic hernia, or lung lobe torsion. Complications associated with thoracocentesis are uncommon and include damage to underlying lung tissue, hemorrhage, pneumothorax, infection, and reexpansion pulmonary edema.

Fifty to one hundred milliliters of pleural fluid must be present in dogs before pleural effusion can be recognized radiographically. The radiographic signs of pleural effusion include pleural fissure lines, rounding of the lung borders, separation of the lung borders from the thoracic wall, loss of the cardiac silhouette, and widening of the mediastinum. It should also be recognized that a diaphragmatic hernia cannot be ruled out if the shadow of the diaphragm cannot be visualized without interruption.

FLUID EVALUATION

Analysis of the pleural fluid often provides the most important diagnostic clue diagnosing the cause of pleural effusion. Fluid samples obtained by thoracocentesis should be placed in a tube containing an anticoagulant such as EDTA for cell counts and a clot tube for biochemical analysis such as triglyceride or cholesterol concentrations. Samples for aerobic and anaerobic culture should be saved for submission in the event that cytologic assessment indicates a septic process.

Classifying the fluid as a transudate, modified transudate, or exudate is helpful in delineating the underlying pleural fluid balance derangement. Transudates are relatively acellular (<1500 nucleated cells/µL), clear, and have a low total protein content (<3.0 g/dL). Transudates are usually a result of a decrease in intravascular oncotic pressure owing to hypoalbuminemia (usually <1.0 g/dL). Modified transudates have a total protein content around 3.0 g/dL or slightly higher and are moderately cellular (1500 to 5000 nucleated cells/µL). Modified transudates are most commonly due to long-standing transudates or to an increase in lymphatic or venous hydrostatic pressure (e.g., right-sided heart failure). Exudates are defined by an increased total protein content (usually much greater than 3.0 g/dL) and a high total nucleated cell count (>5000/µL). These fluids are turbid as a result of the increased nucleated cell concentration. Exudates usually are caused by increased vascular permeability. Many disease processes are dynamic, and effusion characteristics can alter as the disease progresses.

The gross physical characteristics of the fluid can provide information for the diagnosis of the underlying cause. White turbid fluid suggests that the fluid is chyle, whereas a bloody effusion indicates hemorrhage. Foamy or viscous effusions are often high in protein content, and dark brown or foul-smelling fluid indicates that a bacterial infection is present.

Cytologic evaluation is essential in determining the underlying cause of the pleural effusion. A direct smear of the fluid may be prepared similar to a blood smear and stained with Diff-Quik stain (Harleco). Transudates and modified transudates may be centrifuged, the majority of the supernatant removed, and the pellet resuspended in the remaining

supernatant. A smear of this mixture can then be made and will enhance assessment of cells, debris, and organisms present. Presence of inflammation and infection should be determined. Inflammation can be further characterized as acute, chronic active, or chronic. Finally, the smear should be scanned for evidence of malignancy.

Acute inflammation is recognized when nearly all of the white blood cells are neutrophils, while chronic active inflammation is characterized by a mixed population of white blood cells composed of 50 to 70 per cent neutrophils with the remainder being macrophages and mesothelial cells. Greater than 50 per cent of the inflammatory cells are macrophages and reactive mesothelial cells in chronic inflammation. Septic inflammation is characterized by degenerative changes within the neutrophils including nuclear hypersegmentation, nuclear pyknosis, karyolysis, karyorrhexis, and cytoplasmic changes such as basophilia and vacuolization. Identification of organisms such as bacteria provides a more definitive diagnosis of a septic process but is not always made cytologically despite true infection.

SPECIFIC EFFUSIONS

Low intravascular oncotic pressure due to hypoalbuminemia is the most common cause of pleural effusions that are pure transudates. Categorization of a pleural effusion as a pure transudate warrants measurement of blood albumin concentration and investigation for the cause of the hypoalbuminemia if this is confirmed.

Modified transudates may be due to a long-standing pure transudate or to an increase in hydrostatic pressure of veins or lymphatics. Myocardial failure, pericardial effusion, neoplasia, diaphragmatic hernia, and lung lobe torsions are potential causes of modified transudates.

Hemorrhagic effusions are red, and even a small amount of blood in the fluid can impart an extremely bloody appearance. A packed cell volume should be determined on the fluid and compared with the packed cell volume of a simultaneously collected peripheral blood sample. Nearly equivalent packed cell volumes suggest a pure and active hemorrhage as the cause of the pleural effusion, whereas lower effusion packed cell volume indicates that other components are contributing to the formation of the pleural effusion. Common causes of hemorrhagic pleural effusions include trauma, coagulopathies, neoplasia, lung lobe torsion, and spontaneous thymic hemorrhage in young dogs. Packed cell volumes lower in fluid than blood also help prove that the fluid is not being directly drained from a blood vessel, as well as noting that pleural effusions rarely clot.

Chylous effusions are opaque white but may be less so if the animal has fasted. These effusions may also have a pink or "tomato soup" appearance if blood is present. Chylomicrons present in the effusion form a cream layer at the top of the supernatant if the fluid sample is refrigerated and left to stand. Cytologically, the predominant cell type is the mature lymphocyte, although nondegenerate neutrophils may be present as well. A pleural fluid cholesterol:triglyceride ratio of less than 1 is suggestive of a chylous effusion, but a definitive diagnosis is provided by finding a higher concentration of triglycerides in the fluid compared with blood. Causes of chylous effusions include mediastinal masses, trauma, heartworm infection, cardiomyopathy, and lung lobe torsion. Many are considered idiopathic because an underlying cause cannot be determined.

Feline infectious peritonitis virus, long-standing chylothorax, fungal infections, and some malignancies may cause nonseptic inflammation. Nonseptic, eosinophilic effusions may be caused by parasitic infections, granulomatosis, chronic eosinophilic disorders, and hypereosinophilic syndrome.

Septic inflammatory effusions are caused by bacterial contamination of the pleural space. This contamination may occur as a result of ruptured esophagus, penetrating chest wound, hematogenous spread of bacteria, foreign body inhalation, ruptured necrotic and infected tumors, ruptured pulmonary abscess, and parapneumonic spread.

Pleural effusions associated with malignancies may be modified transudates, exudates, or hemorrhagic depending upon the predominant effect that the tumor has on pleural fluid balance such as lymphatic obstruction, blood vessel erosion, or increased membrane and capillary permeability. Adenocarcinoma, mesothelioma, lymphosarcoma, and thymoma are often associated with pleural effusion.

OTHER DIAGNOSTIC MEASURES

Thoracic radiography and pleural fluid analysis do not always fully characterize the underlying disease or the overall health of the animal. Complete assessment of the dog or cat with pleural effusion often requires a constellation of diagnostic tools including complete blood count, serum chemistry profile, urinalysis, special positioning for thoracic radiographs (e.g., standing lateral), abdominal radiography, thoracic and abdominal ultrasound, infectious disease titers, and blood coagulation profiles. Initial thoracic radiograph results and fluid analysis provide the clinician with information that will help determine the remaining diagnostic evaluation.

THERAPY FOR PLEURAL EFFUSION

Treatment of the underlying cause is the definitive mode of therapy, since pleural effusion is a secondary process. Pleural drainage through thoracocentesis or chest tubes will help minimize the effects of the pleural effusion while the underlying disease process is treated.

PROGNOSIS

Most diseases associated with pleural effusion are quite serious. In many instances, the underlying disease may be treated or controlled but not cured. Exceptions include diaphragmatic hernia, lung lobe torsion, traumatic hemorrhagic pleural effusions, hemorrhagic pleural effusions associated with some acquired coagulopathies, and pleural effusions associated with systemic inflammation.

CHAPTER 53

CARDIOPULMONARY ARREST AND RESUSCITATION

Mary Anna Labato

PREDISPOSITION FOR CARDIOPULMONARY ARREST

Cardiopulmonary arrest is defined as a sudden and often unexpected cessation of ventilation and effective circulation. Cardiopulmonary resuscitation is a common procedure in veterinary practice, although there is variation in basic cardiac life support technique. Although some clinicians report encouraging resuscitation rates, low hospital discharge rates still indicate that the reality of poor success rates with CPR be considered carefully before starting.

SIGNS OF CARDIOPULMONARY ARREST

A trained staff and well-equipped hospital are important components of successful resuscitation. Teamwork is essential because one-person CPR is ineffective. Recent work suggests that a minimum of three people are necessary for efficient CPR. The presence of a properly stocked resuscitation box, whose contents are checked weekly, is also of crucial importance (Table 53–1). Ideally, "practice drills" should take place at 12-week intervals.

There is no typical presentation of incipient cardiopulmonary arrest in the veterinary patient. Decreases in heart rate, cyanosis, slow or delayed respirations, dyspnea, or disorientation warrants evaluating the animal's pulse, and respiratory rate. Capillary refill time is a poor indicator of the circulatory status. Hypothermia (rectal temperature <100°F [37.8°C]) was noted in 80 per cent of cats and 34 per cent of dogs prior to the onset of arrest in one study and may be a good indicator of circulatory failure and impending arrest.

TABLE 53–1. EMERGENCY CART SUPPLIES

Drugs
Atropine
Bretylium tosylate
Calcium chloride
Dexamethasone sodium phosphate
Diltiazem
Epinephrine
Furosemide
Lidocaine
Magnesium chloride
Naloxone
Sodium bicarbonate
Saline flushes

Supplies
Ambu bag
Various size endotracheal tubes
Laryngoscopes
Hypodermic needles, various sizes
Assorted intravenous catheters
Intravenous administration sets
2-inch roll of gauze
$2 \times 2''$, $4 \times 4''$ gauze sponges
$\frac{1}{2}$-, 1-, 2-inch tape
Syringes, various sizes
Polyethylene urinary catheters
Suture material
T-connectors
Stopcocks
Cut-down tray with loaded scalpel
Suction tips

CARDIOPULMONARY RESUSCITATION
(Fig. 53–1)

Step 1: Basic Life Support

Basic life support is the technique of providing temporary pulmonary and circulatory support to an animal with respiratory compromise or cardiovascular collapse. It is usually performed by the manual administration of artificial respiration and cardiac compression so that adequate oxygenation of the heart and brain can be maintained. Primary respiratory arrest will usually allow the heart to continue to pump oxygenated blood for several minutes. Early intervention for animals in which respirations have ceased can prevent cardiac arrest. This is a primary indication for the commencement of basic life support. When there is a primary cardiac arrest, oxygen is not circulated, and oxygen stored within vital organs is depleted in seconds. The ABCs of life support include establishing an airway (A), breathing (B), and supporting circulation (C).

Airway. An *Airway* must be established, then *Breathe* for the animal, and maintain *Circulation* by use of cardiac compression. Once these basic life support measures have been instituted, advanced and prolonged life support measures must be addressed. It is important to note the time in order to allow realistic duration of treatment. Advanced life support measures include the following: the definitive diagnosis of the cardiac abnormality; defibrillation, if necessary; administration of emergency drugs; and, finally, gauging the animal's response to resuscitative efforts and providing intensive care monitoring in the post-arrest animal.

Breathing. Initially assess the breathlessness of the animal. Watch for the chest to rise and fall, listen for air escaping during exhalation, and feel for air flow. The assessment phase should last no longer than a few seconds. Once breathlessness has been recognized, breathe for the animal.

Ventilations can be administered using an Ambu bag attached to an oxygen source. Anesthetic machines are satisfactory alternatives once the anesthetic residues have been flushed out of the rebreathing circuit. Room air (21 per cent oxygen) may also be administered using an Ambu bag. If there is no other source, mouth-to-tube breathing should be initiated; this will provide 16 to 17 per cent oxygen.

An acupuncture technique may be utilized to reestablish spontaneous ventilation if other efforts prove futile. The Jen Chung acupuncture site (GV-26) may be used. This technique is performed by inserting a 25-gauge needle into the base of the nasal philtrum, midline level with the lower edge of the nares, down to the periosteum. The needle is then twirled or pecked up and down. One should not wait for an unconscious animal to breathe in response to acupuncture during CPR. This technique should be reserved for animals with spontaneous circulation that have not initiated ventilations. Additionally, if ventilations are stimulated by this technique, one must be certain that there is a sustained ventilatory effort.

Two initial breaths of 1 to 1.5 seconds' duration are recommended for dogs and cats. The recommended rates of artificial ventilation vary from 12 to 35 breaths per minute (the author and her colleagues suggest 25 to 35). Recent recommendations suggest breathing techniques that provide for moderate hyperventilation to offset the developing metabolic acidosis associated with cardiopulmonary arrest.

The use of simultaneous ventilation and chest compression cardiopulmonary resuscitation has been shown to be most effective. Using this technique, airway pressures of 80 to 100 mmHg are generated. This also increases the ventilatory rate.

Circulation. Determine the pulselessness of the animal. If no pulse is palpated, the diagnosis of cardiac arrest is confirmed. Cardiac compression in cats and small dogs less than 15 pounds (7 kg) is best accomplished in lateral recumbency. The compression is applied over the heart and the chest wall compressed 25 to 30 percent of its dimension. Cardiac compression in dogs over 15 pounds (7 kg) is performed with the patient in dorsal recumbency. This position will maximize the increase in intrathoracic pressure due to the larger ventrodorsal dimension of the thorax. Chest compression is applied over the distal third of the sternebrae. The best body position for the animal during cardiopulmonary resuscitation may be dictated by stability.

Chest compressions should be delivered at a rate of 80 to 120 compressions per minute, with the higher rates being used for small dogs and cats. Approximately 50 per cent of the compression cycle should be spent in actual compression and 50 per cent in release.

Step 2: Closed Chest Compression Versus Open Chest Compression

The effectiveness of closed chest cardiopulmonary resuscitation depends on the transmission of high-pressure forces to generate movement of blood. Conditions that may lessen the generation or transmission of these pressures, such as rib fractures, or predispose to inadequate ventilation/perfusion, such as pleural effusion or hemorrhage, pneumothorax, or cardiac tamponade, may serve as an indication for open chest cardiac massage.

Open chest cardiac massage results in improvement in systolic, diastolic, and mean arterial pressures; in coronary artery perfusion pressure; and in carotid artery blood flow. Direct massage of the heart may provide near-normal perfusion of the brain and heart when performed correctly; how-

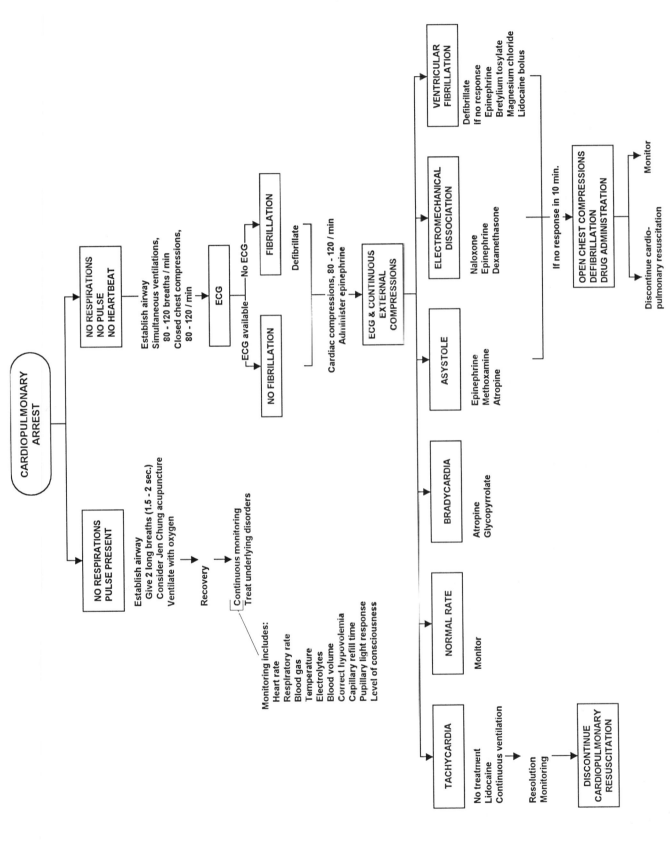

Figure 53-1. Algorithm for management of cardiopulmonary arrest.

ever, its invasiveness often lessens the rescuer's willingness to use the technique.

Step 3: Electrocardiography of Cardiopulmonary Arrest

It is important not to delay the initiation of cardiopulmonary resuscitation to obtain an electrocardiogram. However, the identification of the cardiac rhythm is important for proper antiarrhythmic treatment and supportive care. Cardiac arrhythmias commonly associated with cardiopulmonary arrest include sinus bradycardia, sinus tachycardia, electromechanical dissociation, ventricular asystole, ventricular fibrillation, and ventricular tachycardia.

Ventricular Asystole. Ventricular asystole always indicates cardiac arrest and carries a poor prognosis. The treatment of choice for ventricular asystole is epinephrine 0.1 mg/lb (0.2 mg/kg) intravenously and continued cardiopulmonary resuscitation methods. When ventricular asystole results from high vagal tone, atropine 0.02 mg/lb (0.04 mg/kg) intravenously should be administered. If all else fails, a thump to the chest, the so-called precordial thump, may initiate a ventricular rhythm in some animals.

Electromechanical Dissociation. Electromechanical dissociation (EMD) has been found to be the most common dysrhythmia occurring in dogs and cats in cardiac arrest. The prognosis of successful resuscitation of animals with EMD is poor. When EMD results from hypovolemia, cardiac tamponade, tension pneumothorax, or severe pleural effusion, the chance for successful resuscitation is better than when due to severe metabolic disease.

Recommendations for treatment include epinephrine 0.1 mg/lb (0.2 mg/kg) intravenously and high doses of dexamethasone sodium phosphate—2 mg/lb (4 mg/kg) intravenously. Naloxone may be beneficial in the treatment of EMD. It has been hypothesized that endogenous opiates lead to myocardial depression. The suspected mechanism of action is that naloxone, an opiate antagonist, may make the myocardium more catecholamine-responsive.

Step 4: Drug Therapy

Sometimes basic life support measures are all that is required to reinstitute pulmonary and cardiac function. However, the administration of additional drugs may prove to be necessary (Table 53–2).

Methoxamine is a pure alpha-agonist that increases diastolic pressure without contributing to myocardial hypoxia and cardiac arrhythmias. Its pressor effects decrease blood flow to the kidneys, intestines, skin, and skeletal muscle. In dogs with asphyxia-induced EMD, methoxamine administration resulted in quick resuscitation versus a slower response in dogs receiving either atropine or epinephrine. Methoxamine has been advocated in EMD for increasing aortic diastolic pressure, maintaining the ratio of endocardial to epicardial blood flow, and protecting against dysrhythmias.

Diltiazem has both a membrane-stabilizing effect and a bradycardia effect. Diltiazem has been demonstrated to improve resuscitation from experimentally induced ventricular fibrillation when administered before or early during CPR. This response may have important clinical implications in the treatment of animals undergoing cardiac arrest and CPR.

TABLE 53–2. COMMONLY USED DRUGS IN CARDIOPULMONARY RESUSCITATION

DRUG	DOSAGE AND ROUTE	ACTION	INDICATIONS
Amiodarone	10–15 mg/kg IV	Class 3 antiarrhythmic	Ventricular fibrillation
Atropine sulfate	0.04 mg/kg IV	Parasympatholytic	Sinus bradycardia Ventricular asystole AV block
Bretylium tosylate	5–10 mg bolus IV 1–2 mg/min CRI	Class 3 antiarrhythmic	Ventricular fibrillation
Calcium chloride	0.1 mg/kg IV	Positive inotrope	Hypocalcemia Hyperkalemia Calcium channel blocker toxicity
Dexamethasone sodium phosphate	4 mg/kg IV	Anti-inflammatory glucocorticosteroid	Cerebral edema EMD
Diltiazem	0.05–2.0 mg/kg IV 1–10 μg/kg/min	Calcium channel blocker	Ventricular fibrillation
Epinephrine	1:1000 0.2 mg/kg IV	Alpha- and beta-agonist	Ventricular asystole EMD Ventricular fibrillation
Furosemide	0.5–2.2 mg/kg IV	Loop diuretic	Pulmonary edema Cerebral edema
Glycopyrrolate	0.005–0.010 mg/kg IV	Parasympatholytic	Sinus bradycardia Ventricular asystole AV block SA block
Lidocaine hydrochloride	1.0–2.2 mg/kg IV	Antiarrhythmic	Ventricular tachycardia Ventricular fibrillation
Magnesium chloride	5–10 mL/patient IV	Cofactor	Ventricular fibrillation
Mannitol	2.2 g/kg IV	Osmotic diuretic	Cerebral edema Free radical scavenger
Methoxamine	2.2–10 mg/kg IV	Alpha-agonist	Ventricular asystole Ventricular fibrillation EMD
Naloxone	0.01–0.04 mg/kg IV	Opiate antagonist	EMD
Sodium bicarbonate	1 mEq/kg IV	Alkalinizing agent	Metabolic acidosis

EMD = electromechanical dissociation; IV = intravenous; CRI = continuous rate infusion.

Diltiazem (0.05 to 2.0 mg/kg intravenously; or 1 to 10 μg/kg/min) has shown an excellent response in the treatment of supraventricular arrhythmias.

Bretylium tosylate is a class 3 antiarrhythmic that inhibits release of norepinephrine from adrenergic nerves. It increases the action potential duration and prolongs the refractory period of myocardial cells without directly decreasing conduction velocity or automaticity. Bretylium has been used to treat ventricular fibrillation but does not have consistent effects on the amount of current required for defibrillation. It does not appear to measurably increase defibrillation threshold.

Magnesium chloride has been used as an intravenous bolus and continuous-rate infusion to control refractory ventricular tachycardia and ventricular fibrillation. The mechanism of action is not completely understood but is thought to be related to the involvement of Mg as a cofactor in the Na^+/K^+-ATPase pump. Hypomagnesemia may lead to Purkinje fiber excitability and subsequent arrhythmias. MgCl is currently used at a dose of 5 to 10 mL/patient IV of a 200-mg/mL solution. Alternative dosing is 15 mg/kg bolus, or 10 to 25 mg/kg/hr.

Amiodarone may be useful in refractory ventricular fibrillation. It has been used in humans with ventricular fibrillation when there is no response to lidocaine or electrical defibrillation.

Fluid therapy in cardiopulmonary resuscitation should be determined by the animal's pre-arrest status. Selection and dosing of intravenous fluids should not be arbitrary. Fluid therapy should be used in hypovolemic animals. There is an increase in capillary permeability during cardiopulmonary arrest, predisposing the animal to the development of pulmonary edema.

Step 5: Defibrillation

The treatment of choice for ventricular fibrillation is immediate defibrillation. The most important factor for determining ease and success of defibrillation is the time delay between onset of fibrillation and the administration of the electrical countershock. Ventricular fibrillation lasting longer than 5 minutes is usually difficult to convert. In fact, early defibrillation is so important that blind defibrillation, if no ECG monitor is available, has been recommended.

For external defibrillation, the initial setting should be 1 J/lb (2 J/kg) for animals under 15 pounds (7 kg), 2.2 J/lb (5 J/kg) for those 17.6 to 88 pounds (8 to 40 kg), and 2.2 to 4.5 J/lb (5 to 10 J/kg) for dogs heavier than 88 pounds (40 kg). With open chest resuscitation, if the electrodes are applied directly to the heart, the electrical settings should start at 0.1 J/lb (0.2 J/kg). If initial shocks are unsuccessful, the energy level should be doubled and two countershocks delivered consecutively.

POST-RESUSCITATION THERAPY

Constant monitoring of the animal's condition during and immediately after cardiopulmonary resuscitation allows prompt recognition of potentially treatable sequelae. There should be frequent assessment of the animal's level of consciousness, body movements, pupillary light reflexes, mucous membrane color, respiratory rate, heart rate, and rhythm. Acute changes or a progressive deterioration may indicate a change in outcome.

CONCLUSIONS AND ETHICAL CONSIDERATIONS

Recent studies have shown that hospital discharge rates for animals with cardiopulmonary arrest are low and consistent with those reported from studies in human beings. There are much higher rates for successful resuscitation and survival in otherwise healthy animals that have anesthetic- or drug-related arrests, and in hypovolemic animals with primary pulmonary arrest.

Cardiopulmonary resuscitation should not be undertaken when the animal is in the terminal stages of an incurable disease or when there is no reasonable chance to regain central nervous system function. Owners should be advised to choose, in advance, if resuscitative methods should be initiated if the situation arises. As our resuscitative techniques improve, we must justify to the owners that attempts at cardiopulmonary resuscitation are ethical and in the best interest of the animal. One approach suggested in human medicine is to regard cardiopulmonary resuscitation as an experimental procedure. In animals with progressive and chronic disease, the factors that contribute to arrest generally remain regardless of whether circulation and ventilation are artificially maintained. In these animals, cardiopulmonary resuscitation contributes little toward long-term survival. It may have contributed emotional trauma to the owners and resulted in substantial costs. Veterinarians must be cognizant of these facts.

CHAPTER 54

SNEEZING AND NASAL DISCHARGE

Brendan C. McKiernan

Sneezing and nasal discharge are the primary signs of sinus, nasal, and/or nasopharyngeal disorders in the dog and cat. If one of these problems persists, sneezing may decrease over time, but nasal discharge usually increases in severity and may change in character.

DEFINITIONS AND GENERAL PATHOPHYSIOLOGY

Sneezing. Sneezing is an involuntary airway protective reflex, which, like coughing, is initiated following stimulation of subepithelial receptors. Multiple direct causes of sneezing have been reported, including congenital (cleft palate, cilial defects), inflammatory (allergic, parasitic), and infectious (viral, bacterial, fungal); mechanical and chemical stimuli (foreign bodies, environmental dusts); and simple trauma.

Reverse Sneezing. This well-recognized condition in veterinary medicine is associated with violent, *paroxysmal inspiratory efforts* that function to move secretions and other debris from the nasopharynx into the oropharynx where they can be swallowed.

Nasal Discharge. Initially, owners may not appreciate that nasal discharge exists, owing to an animal's tendency to clear secretions by licking. Later, as the volume of secretion increases, the character changes, or as secretions accumulate on the nostril/facial hair, the discharge may become more apparent to the owner and the frequency of sneezing increases. Nasal secretions arise from a variety of sources, including the epithelial mucous cells, submucosal glands, and well-developed anterior nasal glands. *Nasal discharge* may be characterized as serous, mucoid, mucopurulent, purulent, blood-tinged to overtly bloody (epistaxis), or containing food particles. Blood may occur subsequent to focal irritation/inflammation or erosion, secondary to mucosal capillary trauma during violent sneezing episodes, or as part of a systemic disease such as a coagulopathy or thrombocytopenia. Nasal discharge may also be associated with extranasal diseases (e.g., pneumonia). Additional discharge characteristics that may help to localize the problem are presented in Table 54–1.

INTERPRETATION OF HISTORICAL FINDINGS

In addition to sneezing and nasal discharge, owners may recognize other signs that may assist in localizing the problem and/or prioritizing a list of differential diagnoses (Fig. 54–1).

Signalment. *Age:* Young animals are suspect for congenital diseases (e.g., cleft palate, ciliary dyskinesia, nasal polyps in cats); tumors and chronic dental disease are typically encountered in middle-aged to older animals. *Breed:* Few breed-associated nasal diseases are reported in veterinary medicine, but hyperplastic rhinitis has been associated with Irish wolfhounds; research-bred beagle dogs have an increased incidence of rhinitis secondary to IgA immunodeficiency; and brachycephalic animals have a variety of upper airway problems.

Animal Husbandry. Various management factors may be associated with specific diseases, including the animal's *use* (foreign body is most common in hunting dogs), the *environment* to which the animal is exposed (air pollutants, dusty cat litter), home or *travel* history (fungal diseases are common in specific regions), and *exposure* history (congregations of animals—boarding; shows—increase the risk of infectious disease transmission).

TABLE 54–1. CHARACTERISTICS THAT ASSIST IN THE INITIAL LOCALIZATION, INTERPRETATION, AND DIFFERENTIAL DIAGNOSIS OF NASAL DISCHARGE IN CATS AND DOGS

Features
  Evidence of dried discharge; unilateral vs. bilateral discharge
  Depigmentation of the alar cartilage
  Character—serous, mucoid, mucopurulent, purulent, blood-tinged, epistaxis, food content
  Epistaxis—may be secondary to
    Nasal disease (trauma, tumor, fungal, foreign body)
    Oral disease (tooth, tumor)
    Systemic disease (thrombocytopenia, coagulopathy)

Discharge (unilateral when it initially began) may be associated with
  Dental disease in the upper arcade
  Nasal polyps (C)
  Nasal foreign body
  Nasal tumor
  Fungi—*Cryptococcus* (C), *Aspergillus* (D), *Penicillium* (D), *Rhinosporidium* (D), *Sporothrix* (D)
  Parasites—*Pneuminosoides* (D), *Cuterebra* (D,C), *Linguatula* (C), *Capillaria* (D,C)

Discharge (bilateral when it initially began) may be associated with
  Infection—viral, bacterial, *Chlamydia* (C)
  Immunoglobulin deficiency (IgA)
  Hyperplastic rhinitis (Irish wolfhound)
  Cilial dyskinesia
  Allergy
  Lymphoplasmacytic rhinitis
  Environmental agents—dusts, smoke
  Extranasal disease—pneumonia, esophageal stricture, megaesophagus, cricopharyngeal disease
  Nasopharyngeal foreign body
  Parasites—*Pneuminosoides* (D), *Cuterebra* (D,C), *Linguatula* (C), *Capillaria* (D,C)
  Trauma

C = cat; D = dog.

194

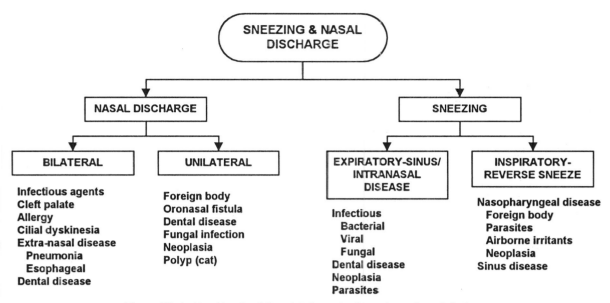

Figure 54–1. Algorithm for differential diagnosis of sneezing and nasal discharge.

Medical History. The medical history may provide considerable information regarding the current problem. Past skull *trauma* or *surgery* has been associated with nasal aspergillosis and bone sequestration. Previous *dental problems* should remind the clinician that this common cause of rhinitis should be carefully considered. The *vaccination* history and *response to previous medical treatments* are helpful in prioritizing a list of differential diagnoses.

Sneezing. If the owner can determine whether the sneezing episode is *inspiratory* or *expiratory* in nature, reverse sneezing can be differentiated from primary conditions affecting the anterior nasal cavity and sinuses. The *onset* and *duration* of the problem may be important; sneezing often lessens with chronicity (although nasal discharge usually persists), whereas an acute onset of violent sneezing suggests that a foreign body should be considered.

Nasal Discharge. The type of discharge (serous, mucoid, purulent, bloody, or food materials), onset, duration, and response to therapy should be ascertained. It is also helpful to determine whether the process began as a unilateral or bilateral process (see Table 54–1). Sinus and nasopharyngeal processes may not show any nasal (anterior) discharge; rather, secretions in these cases often are moved caudally into the oropharynx and swallowed.

Abnormal Sounds. *Wheezing* or *whistling* sounds are produced by air flowing through a narrowed lumen and commonly are reported in animals with dried secretions at the nostrils or a stenotic air passageway (e.g., stenotic nares, nasopharyngeal web, mass). *Stertor* (snoring or noisy inspiratory sounds) may be encountered secondary to anatomic disorders (e.g., elongated soft palate in brachycephalic dogs) or in animals with secretions in the nasopharynx. *Stridor* refers to an inspiratory wheeze (usually high pitched) and is associated most frequently with narrowing or obstruction of the upper airway (cervical trachea or larynx).

Bony Involvement. Animals suffering from diseases associated with periosteal involvement (tumor, fungal infection) may demonstrate *pain* when petted or touched. *Gross swelling* or *facial distortion* is most often due to tumor growth.

Tissue Growth. In addition to gross facial distortion, tissue growth within the nasal cavity may be detected in the oral cavity (depression of the hard or soft palate) or at the external nares. Biopsies of tissue growing out the external nares may be obtained without anesthesia; common differentials for tissue visible at the nares include fungal granulomas (*Cryptococcus, Sporothrix, Rhinosporidium* spp.) and various nasal tumors.

Pawing at Face. Intranasal foreign bodies, nasal parasites, and occasionally severe dental disease may be associated with an animal pawing at its face.

INTERPRETATION OF PHYSICAL EXAMINATION FINDINGS

Nasal Discharge. Evidence of discharge is usually found upon careful examination of the nares and adjacent hair or the hair on the front legs. Chronic nasal discharge (particularly fungal rhinitis in the dog) has been associated with depigmentation of the epithelium of the alar fold (Fig. 54–2).

Air Flow. Nasal discharge and/or the process responsible for causing the discharge typically results in a decrease in air flow at the nostrils. Techniques used to *see, hear,* or *feel* that there is a difference in *air flow* between the left and right nostrils include (1) visually comparing the area (size) of condensation on a cool glass slide or steel table during exhalation through each nostril, and (2) listening to or feeling the air flow from each nostril while the opposite one is occluded. A calm, healthy animal, while *at rest*, should be able to breathe comfortably through one nostril while the other is shut off; no difference in sound, air flow, or visible condensation should be detected between nostrils.

Bony Changes. The nasal and sinus regions, as well as the oral cavity, should be palpated and examined for any evidence of *distortion* or *swelling*. Cats with nasal cryptococcosis frequently have a swelling over the bridge of the nose. In large dogs, *percussion* may be used to determine that there is sinus filling. *Pain* may also be noted during percussion or palpation and is thought to be secondary to periosteal involvement.

Oral Examination. A careful examination of the oral cavity is mandatory in rhinitis cases. Attention should be

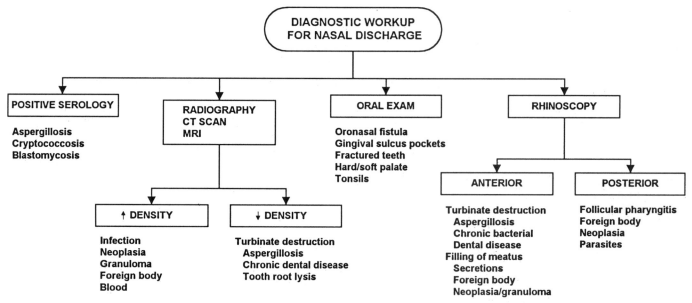

Figure 54–2. Algorithm for diagnostic work-up for nasal discharge.

given to the *hard palate* (defect/clefts, swellings, erosions, trauma secondary to malocclusion); *soft palate* (mucosal erosions, ventral depression from nasopharyngeal masses); *tonsils, teeth,* and *periodontia* (gingival hyperemia, deep periodontal pockets/root abscesses, fractures, defects in enamel, oronasal fistulas, and abnormal occlusion); and the *oral mucosa* in general (the palate, tongue, and cheeks for erosions/ulcers [e.g., feline calicivirus] and petechiae).

Regional Lymph Nodes. Chronic inflammation, infection, or tumor may result in involvement of the tonsils and/or regional (submandibular, retropharyngeal) lymph nodes.

DIAGNOSTIC PLAN

Reverse sneezing localizes the site of the irritation to the nasopharynx. A calm, healthy animal, while *at rest*, should be able to breathe comfortably through one nostril while the other is shut off. If there is a noticeable differences in the sound produced, the air flow detected, or the animal's ability to comfortably breathe through either nostril, the clinician should suspect involvement in that side of the nasal cavity. Lack of appetite, dropping food when eating, ptyalism, gross periodontal disease, and/or overt tooth sensitivity may suggest dental disease (see Table 54–1).

Clinical Pathologic Testing. Although valuable in the overall assessment of the patient, clinical pathologic testing rarely establishes a specific cause for sneezing and nasal discharge. *General anesthesia* is required for positioning during skull radiography as well as for rhinoscopy; a CBC, chemistry profile, and a urinalysis are recommended as part of the database in these animals prior to anesthesia. Systemic disorders may occasionally be a cause of nasal discharge, and specific laboratory tests (platelet count, coagulation profile) may be of benefit in these instances.

Serologic Testing. Serologic testing has been used as an aid in diagnosing nasal fungal conditions including infections due to *Aspergillus* and *Penicillium* spp. as well as *Cryptococcus neoformans*. A positive serology is supportive of a fungal disease but should be interpreted in light of other diagnostic tests and not as being absolutely diagnostic.

Likewise, a negative result does not necessarily rule out a fungal etiology.

Nasal Bacterial and Fungal Cultures. Results of culture must be interpreted cautiously because they may only reflect airway colonization and not actually be the cause of a given disease process. Bacteria are rarely the primary cause of nasal disease; secondary bacterial infections are common. *Aspergillus* and *Penicillium* have been cultured from the nose of both healthy and diseased animals.

Cytologic Evaluation. Secretions and/or biopsies obtained from the nasal cavity may be evaluated cytologically, although it is uncommon for cytology to be of assistance in establishing an etiologic diagnosis. Exceptions to this statement are selected nasal conditions in which the type of cells and/or organisms seen confirm the diagnosis, such as allergic rhinitis, neoplasia, and certain nasal fungal diseases. Final confirmation of nasal tumors should always be based on histopathologic analysis.

Skull Radiography. General anesthesia is necessary for optimal patient positioning and detailed visualization of anatomic structures. Table 54–2 lists various radiographic views and the anatomic regions that are best evaluated using those positions. Loss of structural symmetry, changes in nasal cavity density (increased or decreased), bony abnormalities (loss of turbinates, nasal septum erosion, periosteal reaction, tooth root lysis), and the presence of foreign bodies are some of the more typical radiographic findings encountered. *Computed tomography (CT)* and *magnetic resonance imaging (MRI)* have been used to provide additional information regarding the nasal passages, extent of bony lesions (e.g., the cribriform plate), and brain involvement. In several hospitals, CT and MRI have completely replaced radiographs in the evaluation of dogs and cats with nasal disease because these studies provide more information for the same expense (see Chapter 123).

Rhinoscopy. *After* obtaining skull radiographs, CT, or MRI, a visual assessment of the nasal cavity (anterior rhinoscopy) and nasopharynx (posterior rhinoscopy) should be performed. Abnormal rhinoscopic findings, along with their interpretations, are outlined in Table 54–3. For *anterior rhinoscopy,* a simple otoscope, a rigid arthroscope or pediat-

TABLE 54–2. RADIOGRAPHIC EXAMINATIONS FOR SNEEZING AND NASAL DISCHARGE IN THE DOG AND CAT

RADIOGRAPHIC POSITION	AREA EVALUATED	ADVANTAGES AND DISADVANTAGES
Lateral	Nasal bones	Periosteal reaction may be seen
	Frontal sinuses	Inability to localize diseased side (e.g., right vs. left)
	Nasopharynx	Can assess for extent of caudal tumor growth; presence of polyps and foreign bodies in nasopharynx
	Teeth	Inability to localize diseased side (due to overlying structures)
VD or DV		Poor nasal detail due to overlying structures (mandible, tongue, lower dental arcade)
Open mouth DV	Nasal cavity, turbinates	Good turbinate detail, views maxillary sinus; localizes diseased side
Intraoral (nonscreen film)	Nasal cavity, turbinates	Provides best detail of turbinates and maxillary sinus; good detail of upper teeth, localize disease to an affected side
Lateral oblique	Maxillary dental arcade	Provides good detail of upper arcade
Large dental film (DV or lateral)	Maxillary dental arcade	Provides best detail for tooth roots on the upper arcade, excellent for maxilla of cats and small dogs
Rostrocaudal ("frog eye")	Frontal sinuses	Localizes disease to affected side; evaluates frontal sinus for filling and/or bony defects

ric cystoscope, or small-diameter flexible endoscope may be used. For *posterior rhinoscopy*, a dental mirror may provide some visualization of the nasopharynx, although the best assessment is made by retroflexing a small flexible endoscope over the soft palate.

Nasal Flushing/Biopsy Techniques. Saline may be forcefully injected through the nasal cavity in order to wash out material for evaluation. More traumatic flushing (e.g., using a rigid plastic catheter) may result in a greater yield of cells, and often small pieces of tissue for histopathology. A variety of nasal biopsy techniques have been described. Plastic catheters cut to a sharply angled tip may be inserted into suspect tissue while suction is applied with a syringe. Tissue samples are typically left within the lumen of the catheter with this technique. *Endoscopic cup forceps* may be used during rhinoscopy to obtain a "pinch biopsy" under direct visualization or passed blindly once a tissue mass is localized (*caution:* never insert the catheter past the level of the medial canthus). Nasal and sinus trephination or actual surgical rhinotomy must be considered if other biopsy techniques have not provided diagnostic samples.

TABLE 54–3. RHINOSCOPICALLY DETECTED ABNORMALITIES OF THE NOSE AND NASOPHARYNX

Anterior rhinoscopy (nasal cavity)
Mucosa—color, friability, vascularity, edema
Secretions—amount, location, character
Plaques/inspissated secretions (e.g., fungal)
Loss of normal turbinates—destructive rhinitis (secondary to chronic fungal or bacterial infections)
Septum—deviation, perforation
Obstruction of meatus
  By tissue (tumor or granuloma)
  By foreign body
  By secretions
Parasites
Maxillary/frontal sinuses—entry implies turbinates loss

Posterior rhinoscopy (nasopharynx and choanae)
Soft palate—length, thickness, focal disease
Secretions—amount, location, character
Foreign body—nasopharynx or caudal nasal cavity
Follicular pharyngitis (lymphoid hyperplasia)
Choanae—mass protruding, foreign body
Eustachian tube openings (drainage)
Tissue masses, polyps
Mucosal proliferation, friability

Oral Examination. A complete oral examination, performed while the animal is still under anesthesia, includes evaluation of the hard and soft palate, tonsils, and the gums and teeth. A careful dental examination including *periodontal probing* is a mandatory part of all nasal work-ups.

TREATMENT GOALS

The overall goals of treatment of nasal, sinus, and nasopharyngeal diseases are, briefly, (1) to normalize nasal function and thereby improve air flow, smell, and clearance of secretions; (2) to decrease pain and excessive sneezing; and (3) to minimize secretion production. Antibiotic therapy may decrease the amount of purulent nasal discharge, but the underlying cause (e.g., foreign body, tooth root abscess) must be treated. Nasal fungal diseases require antifungal therapy (see Chapter 123). Surgery may be indicated for feline nasal polyps, and deeply embedded nasal foreign bodies that could not be removed endoscopically. Nasal tumors respond better to radiation therapy than to surgery or chemotherapy.

OUTCOME

Sneezing and nasal discharge are signs of irritation to the nasal epithelium. Unilateral discharge in an older animal should be carefully evaluated to rule out neoplasia. Animals presenting with a history of bloody nasal discharge, as well as those with acute, paroxysmal sneezing, should be fully evaluated (including radiography and rhinoscopy), especially in areas where foreign bodies ("foxtails") are commonly encountered. Systemic disorders (pneumonia, thrombocytopenia) may result in nasal discharge. Reverse sneezing, although often alarming to owners, is rarely a significant health concern for the animal but is an important condition to recognize because it alerts the clinician to possible nasopharyngeal disorders. Chronic nasal discharge may be associated with sufficient inflammation to result in "destructive rhinitis" (endoscopically, the gross loss of turbinates); it is commonly encountered in chronic bacterial rhinitis (secondary to foreign bodies, feline viral rhinitis, and tooth root abscess) as well as canine aspergillosis. Destructive rhinitis results in some degree of persisting nasal discharge regardless of treatment.

CHAPTER 55
ANEMIA

Kenita S. Rogers

Red blood cells (RBCs) carry oxygen to the tissues. The clinical consequences of anemia, or diminished red cell mass, are related primarily to insufficient oxygen delivery to vital organs. With few exceptions, anemia is a reflection of an underlying disease process rather than being a primary disease. Therefore, except in an emergency, most attention is directed to diagnosing and correcting the cause rather than specifically treating the anemia. Understanding normal bone marrow function and the systemic abnormalities that affect this function is fundamental to accurately characterizing the cause of anemia and determining the adequacy of the bone marrow response. Anemia is termed *regenerative* if there is ample evidence that the bone marrow is responding appropriately to a low packed cell volume (PCV). If the marrow does not appear to be responding adequately, the anemia is termed *nonregenerative*.

Regenerative anemia usually results from excessive loss of RBCs caused by hemorrhage or hemolysis. The response to this type of anemia is enhanced erythropoiesis with increased numbers of young red cells (reticulocytes) noted in the circulation. Thus, a simple measure of bone marrow activity in the dog and cat is a reticulocyte count (Table 55–1). However, it must be remembered that the bone marrow needs adequate time to respond to blood loss: 2 to 3 days in cats and 4 to 5 days in dogs after an acute episode of hemorrhage or hemolysis. Chronic external blood loss may have a different sequela: a regenerative response to the anemia initially, but then a progressive deficiency in iron stores. When adequate quantities of this important hemoglobin constituent are not available for erythropoiesis, the anemia will become nonregenerative, and the red cells will eventually appear microcytic.

Nonregenerative anemia is characterized by hypoproliferation or ineffective proliferation of erythroid elements of the bone marrow and is most often secondary to another disease process. Treatment of the underlying disease generally leads to resolution of this typically mild to moderate anemia. Less frequently, nonregenerative anemia is due to primary bone marrow disease, which may be progressive, severe, and associated with alterations in other bone marrow elements, potentially resulting in concurrent thrombocytopenia and leukopenia.

Understanding the differences in pathophysiology and clinical signs associated with acute versus chronic anemia is important. Although acute blood loss implies loss of a substantial quantity of blood in a sudden episode, the source of the bleeding may not be immediately obvious. If the loss is both acute and severe, it may result in hypovolemic shock, because both RBCs and plasma are lost simultaneously. RBC parameters are often unchanged during the 12 hours immediately following the blood loss, but the animal gradually begins to reestablish the intravascular volume by equilibrating with extravascular fluids. Normocytic, normochromic anemia becomes apparent with the resultant hemodilution but appears nonresponsive, with a low reticulocyte count. When the marrow has had adequate time to respond, the anemia becomes regenerative.

Owing to the slow onset of anemia with chronic, progressive, moderate blood loss, the body has sufficient time to initiate compensatory physiologic mechanisms. These mechanisms include increased RBC 2,3-diphosphoglycerate, which lowers the oxygen-hemoglobin affinity and enhances tissue delivery of oxygen. Additional responses include changes in tissue perfusion with preferential shunting of blood to the most vital organs, increased cardiac output with a persistent tachycardia, and increased erythropoietin levels to stimulate RBC production. This anemia remains responsive unless iron stores are depleted by chronic external loss (such as intestinal bleeding). As iron stores diminish, the anemia becomes progressively less responsive. Chronic, recurring internal hemorrhage, such as abdominal hemorrhage due to hemangiosarcoma, does not cause iron deficiency.

TABLE 55–1. GATHERING DIAGNOSTIC INFORMATION FROM THE COMPLETE BLOOD COUNT

I. Description of red blood cell (RBC) morphology (see Table 55–2)

II. Reticulocyte assessment
   A. Absolute count: Reticulocytes/μL = (% reticulocytes $\times$ RBC/μL) $\div$ 100.
   Canine normal = 0–60,000/μL; feline normal = 0–50,000/μL.
   B. Corrected reticulocyte count: % reticulocytes $\times$ patient packed cell volume (PCV)/normal PCV.
   Normal: canine PCV = 45; feline PCV = 35.
   Canine normal = < 1%; feline normal = < 0.5%.
   C. In feline blood, distinguish between punctate and aggregated reticulocytes; only the latter are considered useful in calculations.

III. RBC indices
   A. Indices can be a valuable aid for classifying anemias but are limited to counts from automated analyzers calibrated for the species of interest, owing to inaccuracies encountered in manual counts.
   B. Mean cell volume (MCV): (PCV $\times$ 10) $\div$ RBC (millions) = MCV (femtoliters).
   C. Mean cell hemoglobin (Hb) concentration (MCHC): (Hb $\times$ 100) $\div$ PCV = MCHC (g/dL).

IV. Red cell distribution width
   A. Available from some laboratories.
   B. More sensitive measure of cell volume than MCV.
   C. Quantifies degree of anisocytosis in the erythrocyte population.

V. Plasma protein
   A. Often decreased with acute hemorrhage.
   B. May be increased with hemolytic disease.

VI. Platelet count or estimate
   A. May be decreased owing to acute hemorrhage.
   B. May help indicate a cause for ongoing hemorrhage.
   C. Can substantiate concurrent bone marrow disease.
   D. Thrombocytosis can be associated with iron-deficiency anemia, splenectomy, and chronic inflammatory disorders.

SIGNIFICANCE OF HISTORICAL FINDINGS

Data as basic as the signalment may provide important clues to the etiology of anemia. Congenital coagulation defects have an increased incidence in certain breeds. Basenjis, beagles, English springer spaniels, and cocker spaniels have congenital enzymopathies that may result in profound hemolytic anemia. Immune-mediated hemolytic anemia is diagnosed most commonly in middle-aged female dogs, particularly poodles, cocker spaniels, and terriers. Cats are susceptible to feline leukemia virus and feline immunodeficiency virus, which can cause anemia by a variety of mechanisms.

The pet's environmental history should relate potential exposure to internal and external parasites that can independently cause external blood loss and transmit systemic diseases such as *Ehrlichia canis* and *Haemobartonella felis* that can result in anemia. The animal's vaccination status and exposure to infectious diseases can provide important information. Leptospirosis can be associated with a hemolytic anemia, whereas infectious canine hepatitis can result in disseminated intravascular coagulation (DIC) and bleeding. The myeloid series is most profoundly affected by feline panleukopenia, but anemia can be a sequela of infection. Recent vaccination with modified live viruses can lead to a transient thrombocytopenia, but perhaps more importantly, it has been associated with precipitation of immune-mediated hemolytic anemia in some dogs.

Recent exposure to drugs or toxins should alert the clinician to the possibility of a causal relationship, and a history of recent systemic disease or surgery could be important. After a splenectomy, abnormalities on the complete blood count (CBC) are expected, and the animal is more susceptible to developing a protozoal hemolytic anemia. Chronic renal disease can result in a nonregenerative anemia (in part owing to erythropoietin deficiency), and severe intestinal parasitism can produce blood-loss anemia and iron deficiency. Neoplasia can lead to anemia by a number of mechanisms, including blood loss, iron deficiency, marrow infiltration, anemia of chronic disease, and immune-mediated phenomena.

The owner's perception of performance status can relate signs compatible with anemia, including exercise intolerance, lethargy, and weakness. Nonspecific clinical signs may be present that point to systemic illness as a cause for the anemia, including weight loss, anorexia, fever, and lymphadenopathy. There may have been evidence of bleeding such as epistaxis, melena, hematuria, and bruising. The owner may have noted respiratory difficulty related to severe anemia, hemorrhage, or pleural effusion, or an enlarging abdomen related to organomegaly or hemorrhage. The mucous membranes may have been noted to be pale, discolored, or icteric.

SIGNIFICANCE OF PHYSICAL EXAMINATION FINDINGS

Clinical signs of anemia result from reduced oxygen-carrying capacity of the blood and resultant physiologic adjustments. The most readily recognized abnormality on the physical examination of an anemic animal is pallor of nonpigmented areas of the body, including the skin, lips, tongue, nail beds, buccal cavity, and other mucous membranes. The degree of pallor is only a rough guide to the severity of the anemia and can be particularly deceptive in cats. Muffled heart sounds or abdominal distention may indicate bleeding into the pericardial, pleural, and peritoneal spaces. Evidence of overt hemorrhage could include hematemesis, melena, hematuria, epistaxis, hemarthrosis, or subcutaneous hemorrhage. Signs of oxygen deficiency such as dyspnea and tachypnea may be present at rest in animals with severe anemia, but slight exertion may be necessary to produce such signs in those with moderate anemia. Tachycardia and poor tolerance of handling and stress may be apparent, particularly in cats. Additionally, a soft systolic murmur may develop in animals with severe or acute anemia owing to increased turbulence of blood flow. The severity of the symptoms of oxygen deficiency are more often related to the rapidity of onset rather than the degree of anemia, because chronic development of anemia allows time for adaptive changes by the cardiovascular and respiratory systems.

Evidence of systemic illness that could account for the anemia may be present. Fever may indicate underlying infectious, inflammatory, or neoplastic disease. Organomegaly may be associated with infiltrative diseases as well as extravascular hemolysis. Regional and generalized lymphadenopathy and ocular changes such as hemorrhage or exudates should be noted. Icterus may be associated with acute hemolysis and primary or secondary hepatobiliary disease. Methemoglobin, which is incapable of carrying oxygen, is formed from hemoglobin when iron is oxidized from its ferrous to its ferric form. Methemoglobinemia and brown mucous membranes can be seen with acetaminophen intoxication in cats.

HELPFUL DIAGNOSTIC TESTS

The most important laboratory data to collect in an anemic dog or cat are a CBC with an assessment of RBC morphology, calculation of red cell indices, and reticulocyte count (see Table 55–1). There are several common changes in RBC morphology that can have specific diagnostic value in anemic animals (Table 55–2).

When immune-mediated hemolytic anemia (IMHA) is suspected, particularly in a dog, a Coombs' test or direct antibody test (DAT) is often performed. Approximately two thirds of canine patients with IMHA are DAT-positive, although there does not appear to be a correlation between the strength of the reaction and the severity of clinical disease. Most standard canine reagents are pooled antisera directed against canine IgG, IgM, and complement. Unfortunately, the test may be negative despite clinical evidence of IMHA, owing to the presence of few antibody molecules on the RBCs, use of incorrect species-specific reagents, drug-induced antibody, or incorrect laboratory techniques. Spherocytes, commonly noted with IMHA, can also be detected by the osmotic fragility test. This test detects a population of osmotically fragile spherocytes as the erythrocytes are exposed to a graded series of hypotonic saline solutions.

Erythrocyte number and size and hemoglobin concentration are not good indicators of iron adequacy. Serum iron can be affected by several pathophysiologic processes. It is usually decreased with iron deficiency and acute and chronic inflammatory reactions and increased with hemolytic anemia, refractory anemias, and iron overload. A reliable indicator of body iron stores in many species is serum ferritin, which is low in animals with iron deficiency and increased in those with acute inflammatory processes because it is an acute-phase reactant. The total iron-binding capacity increases during iron deficiency in most species, but variable results make interpretation of this test difficult in the dog.

TABLE 55–2. RBC MORPHOLOGY CHANGES WITH DIAGNOSTIC VALUE

MORPHOLOGY CHANGES	MECHANISM	DISEASE PROCESSES	OTHER INFORMATION
Spherocyte	Excessive loss of surface membrane by partial phagocytosis	IMHA, post-transfusion, occasionally with Heinz body anemias	Increased osmotic fragility; difficult to identify in cats
Autoagglutination	IgM on RBC surface	IgM-mediated IMHA	Differentiate from rouleaux by mixing with a drop of saline; nonagglutinating cells will disperse
Polychromasia	Color variation among RBCs on Wright-stained blood smears	Part of regenerative response to anemia	Usually correlates with reticulocytes in circulation
Anisocytosis	Different RBC sizes on a blood smear	A variety of conditions, including a regenerative response and iron deficiency	Must assess whether cell population is larger or smaller than normal
Nucleated RBCs	Early release from bone marrow or not removed by RE system	Responsive anemia, altered bone marrow release, diminished splenic clearance, lead toxicity, vascular neoplasia, hypoxemia	Must have reticulocytosis to be part of a regenerative response
Heinz bodies	Aggregates of precipitated oxidatively denatured hemoglobin	Administration or ingestion of oxidant: acetaminophen, onions, antibiotics, benzocaine, others	Small number normally found in cats; cats more likely to develop owing to hemoglobin structure
Schistocytes	Irregular RBC fragment resulting from mechanical trauma	DIC, vascular neoplasia, caval syndrome, splenic torsion	Consider causes of microangiopathic hemolysis
Hemoparasites	Parasites identified on RBC membrane	Haemobartonellosis, babesiosis, cytauxzoonosis	May increase after splenectomy; assess FeLV status in cats; can have concurrent infections

RBC = red blood cell; IMHA = immune-mediated hemolytic anemia; IgM = immunoglobulin M; RE = reticuloendothelial; DIC = disseminated intravascular coagulation; FeLV = feline leukemia virus.

Bone marrow examination is indicated in a dog or cat that has unexplained nonregenerative anemia. A CBC and reticulocyte count should always be performed within 24 hours before bone marrow collection, however, because this test is not usually indicated with a regenerative process. Bone marrow aspirates provide cytologic specimens for evaluation of cellularity, myeloid-to-erythroid ratios, orderly maturation, and evidence of specific diseases such as neoplasia. Bone marrow biopsies are indicated with hypocellular cytologic specimens and may provide evidence of processes such as myelofibrosis, marrow necrosis, and neoplasia.

The categories of disease processes that can result in regenerative and nonregenerative anemia are found in Figure 55–1. Table 55–3 outlines specific diagnostic tests that may be helpful in differentiating individual disease processes in each of these categories.

DIFFERENTIAL DIAGNOSIS

REGENERATIVE ANEMIAS

The two categories of anemia that characteristically lead to a regenerative response are excessive blood loss and hemolysis (see Fig. 55–1). Animals with an acute 30 to 40 per cent loss of blood volume typically exhibit hypovolemic shock, whereas loss of 50 per cent or greater usually results in death if immediate treatment is not instituted. Clinical signs of shock are often apparent before the PCV is lowered. The presence of microcytic, hypochromic anemia is consistent with chronic rather than acute external hemorrhage. If hemorrhage has been into a body cavity, it can be easily detected by centesis, but this procedure does not indicate the exact source of the bleeding. In addition, lack of clotting of the blood withdrawn from a body cavity does not distinguish coagulopathies from other causes of hemorrhage, because blood within the pleural and peritoneal spaces becomes defibrinated within 45 to 60 minutes.

Hemolytic disease can be divided into intravascular and extravascular sites of hemolysis. Intravascular hemolysis usually represents a more severe disease process and is due to destruction of RBCs within the vascular space. Intravascular hemolysis leads to the formation of numerous vasoactive and chemotactic substances that can be harmful to the physiologic status of the animal and lead to DIC. Extravascular hemolysis is usually caused by phagocytosis of RBCs by macrophages within the reticuloendothelial system, particularly the spleen and liver. With intravascular or extravascular hemolysis, hemoglobin is degraded, with bilirubin being one of the by-products. If more bilirubin is formed than can be conjugated by the liver and excreted, hyperbilirubinemia (icterus) and bilirubinuria result. Premature loss of RBCs by immune-mediated destruction is one of the most common causes of severe anemia in the dog. A nonregenerative form with the immune-mediated process directed at erythroid precursor cells in the bone marrow has been recognized. This form may exhibit spherocytosis or be DAT-positive, but the bone marrow shows maturation arrest at some stage of erythroid progression. It must be recognized that a normal regenerative process can be dampened by the presence of other concurrent diseases such as chronic renal disease or an inflammatory state.

NONREGENERATIVE ANEMIAS

The causes of nonregenerative anemia can be discussed in six categories (see Fig. 55–1).

Primary Failure of Erythropiesis. Primary failure of erythropoiesis is an uncommon, selective, severe erythroid hypoplasia of the bone marrow. The etiology may be immune-mediated, and some cases are DAT- or antinuclear antibody–positive. It is most commonly acquired and may be associated with a number of disease conditions. The criteria for diagnosis include documenting a severe, chronic, normocytic, normochromic nonregenerative anemia, with a cellular bone marrow that retains active granulopoiesis and thrombopoiesis.

Secondary Failure of Erythropoiesis. Secondary fail-

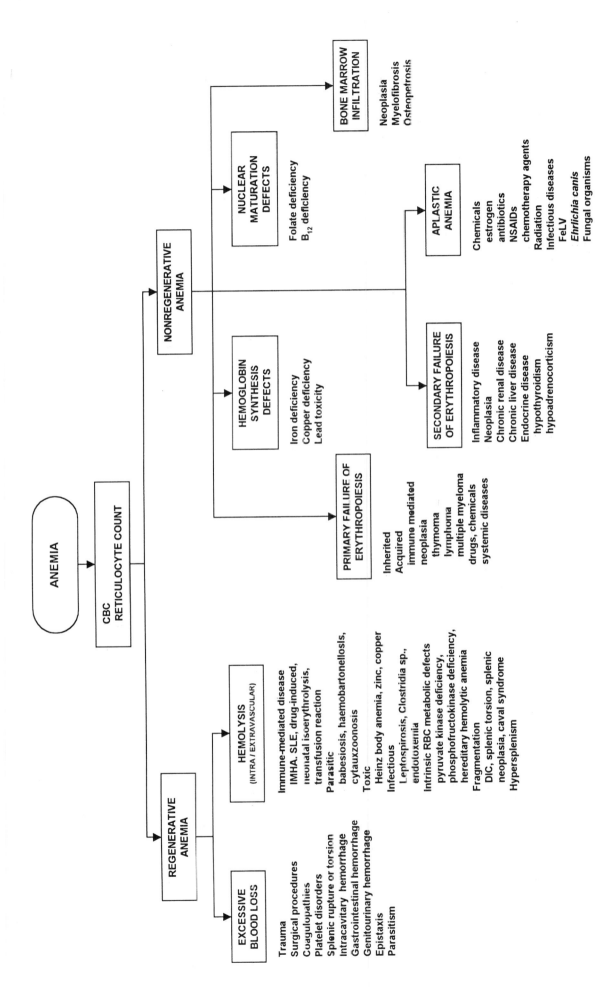

Figure 55–1. Algorithm for differential diagnosis of anemia.

TABLE 55–3. SPECIFIC DIAGNOSTIC TESTS FOR ANIMALS WITH ANEMIA

I. Excessive blood loss
   A. Identification of external and internal parasites
   B. Fecal flotation
   C. Occult fecal blood
   D. Platelet count or estimate
   E. Coagulation testing
   F. Urinalysis
   G. Total protein
   H. Body cavity imaging (radiography, ultrasonography, computed tomography [CT], magnetic resonance imaging [MRI])
   I. Evaluation of fluids in body cavities
   J. Endoscopy

II. Hemolysis (intra/extravascular)
   A. Red blood cell (RBC) morphology changes (see Table 55–2)
   B. Immune testing: direct antibody test; antinuclear antibodies if systemic lupus erythematosus is suspected
   C. Coagulation testing
   D. Biochemical panel
   E. Urinalysis
   F. Osmotic fragility
   G. Abdominal radiography/ultrasonography
   H. Heartworm testing

III. Primary failure of erythropoiesis
   A. Bone marrow aspirate/biopsy
   B. Biochemical panel
   C. Immune testing
   D. Thoracic radiography

IV. Secondary failure of erythropoiesis
   A. Biochemical panel
   B. Urinalysis
   C. Thyroid hormone assay
   D. Adrenocorticotropic hormone stimulation or dexamethasone suppression test
   E. Kidney or liver biopsy
   F. Assessment of iron metabolism: serum iron, serum ferritin, total iron-binding capacity
   G. Imaging

V. Hemoglobin synthesis defects
   A. Assessment of iron metabolism
   B. Bone marrow aspirate/biopsy
   C. Serum lead levels

VI. Nuclear maturation defects
   A. Serum folate levels
   B. Serum B_{12} levels
   C. Endoscopy
   D. Bone marrow aspirate/biopsy

VII. Bone marrow infiltration
   A. Bone marrow aspirate/biopsy
   B. Assessment of neoplastic infiltration of other organs

VIII. Aplastic anemia
   A. Bone marrow aspirate/biopsy
   B. Assessment for systemic disease

IX. Tests for evaluation of systemic diseases associated with anemia
   A. Rickettsial titers: canine ehrlichiosis, Rocky Mountain spotted fever
   B. Feline leukemia virus and feline immunodeficiency virus tests
   C. Lymph node aspiration/biopsy
   D. Hepatic or splenic aspirate/biopsy
   E. Radiography of the thorax and abdomen
   F. Ultrasonography
   G. Nuclear scintigraphy
   H. CT or MRI

ure of erythropoiesis encompasses many of the most common causes of nonregenerative anemia. Examples include inflammatory disease, neoplasia, chronic renal and liver disease, and certain endocrine disorders. Bone marrow examination is normal or shows mild erythroid hypoplasia. Anemia of inflammatory disease (AID) is characterized by altered iron metabolism and must be differentiated from iron deficiency, because serum iron levels are often low in either condition. In AID, there is suppression of erythropoiesis owing to relative iron unavailability. Total body stores of iron are adequate, but much of it is sequestered in the reticuloendothelial system, particularly in the liver and bone marrow. There may be a mild to moderate decrease in RBC life span. Anemia is the most common hematologic complication in animals with cancer and is frequently accompanied by AID. Other causes for anemia in cancer patients include blood loss, microangiopathic hemolysis, immune-mediated hemolysis, pure red cell aplasia, chemotherapy-induced erythroid suppression, and hypersplenism. The anemia associated with chronic renal disease is primarily due to ineffective erythropoiesis attributable to decreased production of erythropoietin by diseased kidneys, although blood loss and decreased RBC life span also contribute. With chronic liver disease, mechanisms leading to anemia include AID, blood loss, and microangiopathic disease. Certain endocrine disorders, particularly hypothyroidism and hypoadrenocorticism, may be associated with anemia. Thyroxine may have a direct effect on erythroid colony formation in vitro, and the anemia may be a physiologic adaptation to decreased oxygen demand. Anemia caused by bleeding into the intestinal tract and due to "chronic disease" may be masked by hemoconcentration in some animals with hypoadrenocorticism.

Nuclear Maturation Defects. Nuclear maturation defects are primarily associated with deficiencies of folate and vitamin B_{12}, which are required for biosynthesis of purines and pyrimidines. Macrocytic, normochromic anemia results from a defect in DNA synthesis, as defective nuclear maturation leads to a decreased number of cellular divisions and the appearance of large nucleated erythroid cells (megaloblasts) and mature non-nucleated cells (macrocytes) in peripheral blood. The bone marrow is characterized by erythroid hyperplasia with maturation arrest at the rubricyte stage. Mild thrombocytopenia and leukopenia may occur, because nuclear maturation affects all developing cells in the bone marrow.

Hemoglobin Synthesis Defects. Hemoglobin synthesis defects are associated primarily with iron deficiency but can also be seen with copper deficiency and lead intoxication. Iron deficiency occurs gradually, so hematologic changes depend on the extent of iron depletion. Microcytic, hypochromic anemia characterizes the blood picture of advanced iron deficiency and results from decreased hemoglobin production in individual cells. Hemoglobin functions as a signal for termination of cell division, and cells with limited ability to produce hemoglobin undergo additional divisions, resulting in microcytic erythrocytes. Young animals with rapid growth rates and low dietary sources of iron are most susceptible to iron deficiency. In adult animals, iron deficiency usually results from excessive iron loss rather than inadequate intake. Iron loss can usually be equated with blood loss, and this loss must be protracted to lead to a deficient state.

Aplastic Anemia. Aplastic anemia is characterized by an acellular or hypocellular marrow that results in pancytopenia. Bone marrow failure can be due to marrow necrosis or inflammation, an alteration in the marrow microenvironment, or a defect in the proliferative capacity of the pluripotential stem cell. Aplastic anemia in veterinary patients is usually due to chemicals such as estrogen, certain antibiotics, chemotherapy drugs, or infectious agents such as feline leukemia virus and *Ehrlichia canis*. Neutropenia and thrombocytopenia often occur before anemia, as RBCs have the longest life span in circulation.

Marrow Infiltration. Marrow infiltration can be associated with neoplasia (myelophthisis), myelofibrosis, or osteopetrosis. Myelophthisic disease can act by "crowding out" normal hematopoietic cells, altering the marrow microenvironment, competing for nutritional factors, and producing tumor-related factors that suppress normal hematopoiesis. Myelofibrosis may be a primary pathologic process or a sequela of damaged marrow that leads to hypoplasia of marrow elements and eventual replacement by collagen. Osteopetrosis is an inherited disorder characterized by a generalized increase in bone density and failure to develop normal marrow cavities.

CHAPTER 56

POLYCYTHEMIA

Andreas H. Hasler and Urs Giger

Polycythemia is defined as an abnormally increased packed cell volume (PCV), red blood cell count (RBC), and hemoglobin concentration (Hb). It is important to recognize that normal upper values of erythrocyte parameters for dogs are different from those for cats. Upper limits for dogs versus cats are PCV 55 versus 45 per cent, RBC 8.5 versus $10 \times 10^6/\mu L$, and Hb 18 versus 14 g/dL. Furthermore, certain breeds, such as greyhounds and dachshunds, generally have higher values than most other breeds of dogs.

PATHOPHYSIOLOGY

Polycythemia can be either relative or absolute. Relative polycythemia is defined as an increased PCV with a normal total RBC mass, resulting from a decrease in plasma volume. External loss of body fluids, shifting of body fluids from the vascular space into the interstitial space, or inadequate fluid intake can result in relative polycythemia. Thus, relative polycythemia occurs when plasma volume decreases to a greater extent than red cell volume. Depending on the amount of concomitant protein loss or shift, total plasma protein will be low, normal, or high. Splenic contraction can lead to an increase in circulating red cells but not in the total number of red cells and hence to relative polycythemia in dogs but not in cats.

In contrast, absolute polycythemia is caused by an increased total RBC mass. Although it is rarely clinically necessary, the total red cell mass can be calculated based on the degree of dilution of a labeled erythrocyte sample during circulation. Absolute polycythemia is divided according to its pathophysiology into primary and secondary polycythemia (Fig. 56–1). Secondary polycythemia is further classified as physiologically appropriate or inappropriate.

Under normal circumstances, the red cell mass is tightly regulated by a classic endocrine feedback system. Erythropoietin (EPO) plays the key role in the regulation of red cell mass and erythrocyte production. Renal hypoxia, but not the number or mass of circulating red cells, stimulates the renal production of EPO. The oxygen sensor in the kidney is believed to be one of the heme proteins. When the oxygen tension is sufficiently low, the heme protein is in its deoxy conformation and triggers the synthesis of EPO. The cellular site of production in the kidney has been localized in interstitial renal cells in the inner cortex lying in immediate proximity to the proximal tubules. The number of cells that are recruited parallels the degree of hypoxia. As a consequence of hypoxia, EPO is released, and its plasma level increases. EPO acts in the bone marrow both as a growth factor and as a differentiating factor. In its presence, colony-forming unit-erythroid (CFU-E) grows and matures, and globin synthesis is activated. The resulting increase in circulating red cells enhances the oxygen carrying capacity and, as a consequence, improves renal oxygenation. Hence, renal EPO production decreases, and the regulatory loop is complete.

This physiologic mechanism allows both the primary and secondary forms of absolute polycythemia to occur. In primary polycythemia there is an autonomous, i.e., EPO-independent, production of red cells; in secondary polycythemia the red cell production is EPO-dependent.

In veterinary medicine, the term primary polycythemia is used synonymously with polycythemia vera. To our knowledge, no attempts have been made to characterize different forms of primary polycythemia in dogs and cats. Conversely, in human medicine, polycythemia vera is a well-defined disease and is separated from other forms of the condition. Familial polycythemia, for example, involves mutations of the EPO receptor. Polycythemia vera, considered a myeloproliferative disease, has not been associated with changes

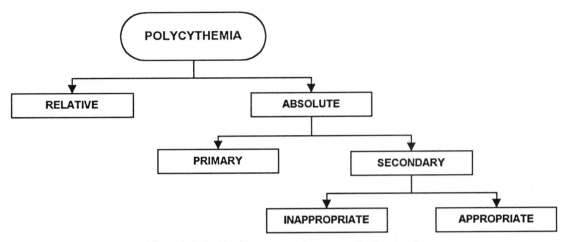

Figure 56–1. Algorithm categorizing causes of polycythemia.

in the EPO receptor. Other receptors (such as insulin-like growth factor-1 and Bcl-x) have recently been incriminated.

Secondary appropriate polycythemia is a consequence of persistent hypoxia. The most common cause is living at high altitudes. The most common disorders causing appropriate polycythemia are congenital heart defects with right-to-left shunting of blood. The mixing of venous and arterial blood causes systemic hypoxemia and activation of EPO production. Decreased oxygen partial pressure, abnormal ventilation, or ventilation-perfusion mismatch can lead to polycythemia. We are aware of one cat with eosinophilic bronchitis that developed polycythemia, but it is our opinion that polycythemia is a rare consequence of respiratory disease.

Hemoglobin function abnormalities that cause polycythemia are extremely rare in dogs and cats. One cat with methemoglobinemia caused by methemoglobin-reductase deficiency was noted to have moderate polycythemia (PCV 55 per cent). Alterations of hemoglobin structure or decreases in 2,3-diphosphoglycerol that lead to polycythemia have yet to be documented in cats or dogs but have been described in people.

Secondary inappropriate polycythemia refers to rare renal or other diseases leading to elevated serum EPO levels without systemic hypoxia. Malignancies may produce EPO as a paraneoplastic syndrome. Definitive proof that neoplastic tissue produces EPO—by detecting EPO-mRNA in tumor cells—has not been described in veterinary medicine. Renal disease such as renal neoplasia, amyloidosis, infection, and inflammation may cause local hypoxia and hence trigger EPO synthesis.

Regardless of the cause, the consequence of increased red cell mass cell mass is an increase in blood viscosity. Hematocrit is the major determinant of blood viscosity. The rise in blood viscosity becomes more pronounced when the hematocrit rises above 50 to 60 per cent (for dogs). As a consequence, workload increases, and cardiac hypertrophy may occur. Depending on the degree of viscosity and vascular hindrance, microcirculation decreases, blood flow becomes sluggish, and local hypoxia occurs. Most likely the neurologic complications seen in polycythemic animals, such as seizures, blindness, or ataxia, are caused by impaired microcirculation in the brain. Thrombosis of cortical arteries associated with seizures and polycythemia has been reported.

PRESENTING COMPLAINT AND PHYSICAL FINDINGS

The signs of relative polycythemia are generally obvious and depend on the severity of dehydration and the underlying disease process. Tacky mucous membranes and prolonged capillary refill time are noticed and skin turgor is decreased when dehydration persists for more than a few hours.

Animals with absolute primary polycythemia have signs secondary to hyperviscosity. More than half of polycythemic cats and dogs have neurologic complications such as seizures, ataxia, blindness, tremors, or behavior changes. Other complaints, such as polyuria-polydipsia, vomiting, diarrhea, or epistaxis, are much less common. Animals with secondary polycythemia can have signs referable to hyperviscosity or to the underlying disease or both. Neurologic complaints are less frequent than in primary polycythemia. The mucous membranes are typically hyperemic, although there may be cyanosis in cases of secondary polycythemia resulting from cardiopulmonary disease or methemoglobinemia.

DIAGNOSTIC PLAN

The type of polycythemia must be determined, because the appropriate treatment is dependent on the cause. All proposed diagnostic tests are used to identify a secondary cause of the polycythemia, and primary polycythemia is diagnosed by excluding other causes.

MINIMAL DATABASE

A complete minimal database with complete blood count (CBC), chemistry panel, and urinalysis is recommended for the diagnostic evaluation of a polycythemic animal and as a baseline to assess therapeutic success. It usually enables the clinician to distinguish relative from absolute polycythemia and to determine the degree of polycythemia. Total red cell mass determination is not necessary to distinguish relative from absolute polycythemia in clinical practice. An absolute reticulocyte count ($>40,000/\mu L$) is an inexpensive way to appreciate the increased erythropoietic activity despite an increased hematocrit.

DIAGNOSTIC TESTING (Fig. 56–2)

Assessment of systemic hypoxia is a crucial step in the differentiation of appropriate versus inappropriate or primary polycythemia. Signs of cyanosis may be obvious but could be restricted to caudal body parts, as seen with reversed patent ductus arteriosus (rPDA). We recommend stabilizing

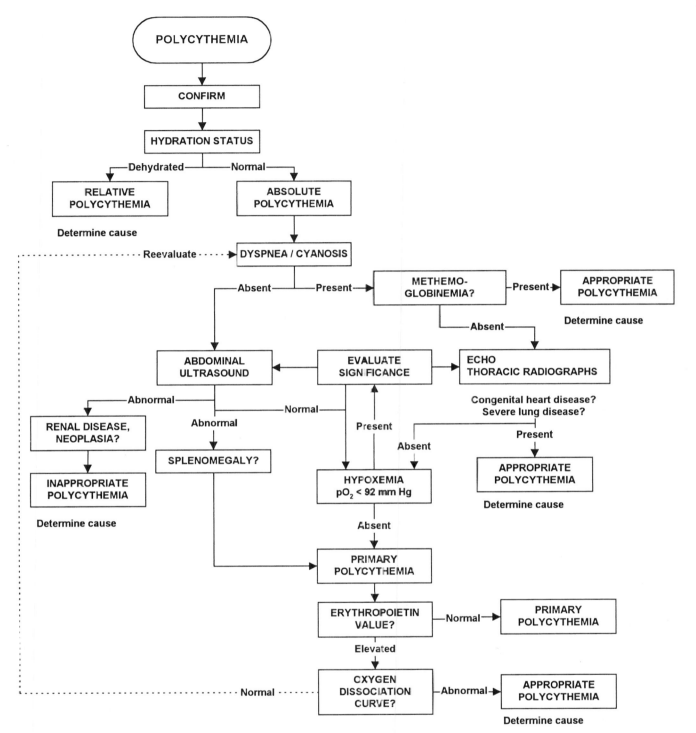

Figure 56–2. Algorithm for differential diagnosis and treatment of polycythemia.

(phlebotomizing) the animal before getting an arterial blood gas, because the high viscosity can make it difficult to obtain a proper sample and reading. Normal values (i.e., oxygen partial pressure >92 mmHg) are expected in all but appropriate polycythemia (except hemoglobinopathy, where P_{O_2} is normal). In cases of mildly reduced P_{O_2} values (about 85 to 92 mmHg), the clinician must judge whether the cause is a sampling error or a true abnormality. If blood gas determination is not available, pulse oximetry can be used to assess oxygen saturation and estimate oxygen partial pressure. A low saturation (<80 per cent) with a reliable recording suggests hypoxia.

Abdominal ultrasonography and radiographs are used in an attempt to detect neoplasia or renal disease. Mild changes such as hyperechoic kidneys may also be found in animals with primary polycythemia. Furthermore, splenomegaly is detected in about 10 per cent of dogs and 25 per cent of cats with primary polycythemia. Thoracic radiographs are directed toward identifying pulmonary and cardiac abnormalities. Most animals with primary polycythemia have unremarkable imaging studies, although mild bronchointerstitial changes or enlarged ventricles resulting from hyperviscosity have been reported.

Because there are no characteristic erythroid markers for primary polycythemia, bone marrow examination is not helpful in differentiating primary from secondary polycythemia. Polycythemic animals have erythroid hyperplasia with a low myeloid-to-erythroid (M:E) ratio. Hence, this procedure is generally not recommended. Erythroid precursors in primary polycythemia grow in EPO-free medium or are hypersensitive to EPO, whereas erythropoiesis in secondary polycythemia is EPO-dependent. Therefore, evaluating the growth behavior of bone marrow cells from animals with suspected primary polycythemia may be most useful. Because use of this method is restricted to established research laboratories, it has been reported only once in a polycythemic cat.

Erythropoietin concentrations are presently measured by immunologic methods, although no species-specific immunologic assays are currently available for dogs and cats. However, at least two human assays have been validated for animals. An increased serum EPO value is diagnostic for secondary polycythemia, and EPO concentrations may be as high as 50-fold above control. In our experience, however, in about half of the cases of secondary polycythemia, values are in the normal range, despite the fact that secondary polycythemia is EPO-dependent. Hence, a low to normal EPO value does not exclude secondary polycythemia. In primary polycythemia, values are in the low or normal range. If clinical evaluation led to a diagnosis of primary polycythemia but a high serum EPO concentration is found repeatedly, further clinical evaluation is recommended to detect the cause.

TREATMENT AND PROGNOSIS

Relative polycythemia is corrected by administering adequate intravenous fluids and addressing the underlying cause. Initial treatment of severe absolute polycythemia is limited to phlebotomy. Serial phlebotomies of 10 to 20 mL/kg blood are recommended rather than a single phlebotomy to reach the target hematocrit of about 55 percent in dogs and 50 percent in cats. Phlebotomy regimens alone may be sufficient to control primary polycythemia, and intervals may increase with time as iron deficiency develops. If intervals continue to be short or phlebotomies are difficult, chemotherapy with hydroxyurea can be initiated. The initial dose is 30 to 50 mg/kg by mouth once a day for 1 week, then titrated to effect, considering myelosuppression and gastrointestinal side effects. For primary polycythemia, a PCV in the normal range is desirable. Combination of hydroxyurea and phlebotomy is an alternative to single-mode therapy. The prognosis for primary polycythemia is guarded, but survival for more than 6 years has been achieved in treated animals.

Treatment of secondary polycythemia also needs to be directed against the underlying disease. In inappropriate polycythemia caused by neoplasia, removal of the tumor has resolved the polycythemia. In cases in which no curative treatment is possible, such as with rPDA, palliative phlebotomies and eventually hydroxyurea can improve quality of life. In animals with cyanotic cardiopulmonary disease, the target hematocrit is in the high-normal range to provide higher oxygen-carrying capacity, and careful fluid replacement at the time of phlebotomy is recommended to prevent hypovolemic crisis. Survival of more than 4 years has been reported in cases of rPDA.

CHAPTER 57

CYANOSIS

Rebecca L. Stepien

DEFINITIONS AND PATHOPHYSIOLOGY

Cyanosis is defined as a bluish discoloration of skin or mucous membranes due to excessive amounts of desaturated (or reduced) hemoglobin (Hb) in the capillary blood. It is clinically recognized as tissue coloration ranging from deep red-purple to dusky blue. Cyanosis may be central or peripheral. *Central cyanosis* is a result of systemic arterial Hb desaturation and affects all tissues; *peripheral cyanosis* is due to localized increases in desaturated Hb and affects cutaneous tissues or, in the case of thrombosis or tourniquet application, regional tissues supplied by the affected vessel. Central cyanosis may also be detected in the peripheral tissues; all animals with peripheral cyanosis should be examined for signs of central cyanosis.

Detection of cyanosis is possible when absolute concentration of reduced Hb (RHb) in *capillary* blood reaches approximately 5 g/100 mL. This is the level most frequently quoted in the literature, but numerous studies have confirmed that *arterial* RHb need only reach approximately 3 to 3.5 g/100 mL to cause detectable cyanosis. The amount of RHb depends on Hb concentration and per cent saturation of Hb in arterial blood (SaO_2), a value that is related to arterial oxygen tension (PaO_2). When breathing room air, the alveolar oxygen tension (PO_2) is approximately 100 mmHg and SaO_2 is approximately 97 per cent, resulting in a PaO_2 of approximately 95 mmHg. In the normal animal with a packed cell volume (PCV) of 45 per cent, total Hb concentration is approximately 15 g/100 mL, and arterial RHb is 3 per cent, or about 0.45 g/100 mL, well below the arterial RHb necessary to appear cyanotic. When decreased inspired oxygen concentration results in decreased SaO_2, arterial RHb increases; cyanosis becomes clinically evident when arterial RHb exceeds the 3 to 3.5 g/100 mL threshold. An animal with a normal PCV must have an SaO_2 between 73 and 78 per cent (PaO_2 = 39–44 mmHg) in order to have clinically detectable cyanosis. Thus, detection of central cyanosis in an animal without cyanotic heart disease is an acute emergency, indicating severe arterial hypoxemia.

Adequate intensity of light appears to be more important than the source for detection of cyanosis. Pigmented mucous membranes may limit evaluation of oral mucous membrane color in some dog breeds, but vaginal or preputial mucous membrane color may be evaluated. Cyanosis may be difficult to detect in anemic animals; an animal with a PCV of 18 per cent (total Hb 6 g/100 mL) must have a PaO_2 of less than 30 mmHg before cyanosis is detectable (i.e., cyanosis is detectable only after death). Conversely, polycythemia may result in a PCV of 60 per cent or more; these animals may appear cyanotic when their oxygen saturation drops below about 87 per cent (PaO_2 = 55 mmHg). In general, the lower the total Hb concentration, the more SaO_2 may fall before the detection of cyanosis. Higher total Hb concentrations result in earlier detection of cyanosis, before SaO_2 has decreased markedly.

Peripheral cyanosis results from desaturation of Hb in the arterial blood supply (i.e., as a result of central cyanosis) or excessive desaturation of Hb in peripheral tissues due to an imbalance in oxygen supply relative to the metabolic needs of the tissues served. Imbalances may occur when metabolic needs of local tissues are increased but flow is limited (e.g., exercise in an animal with congestive heart failure) or when cutaneous capillary blood flow is sluggish (e.g., peripheral vasoconstriction or venous stasis). Sluggish blood flow through the tissue capillaries increases the amount of time oxygenated erythrocytes are in contact with tissues, allowing increased oxygen extraction at the tissue level. More Hb is desaturated, resulting in detectable cyanosis and reduced venous oxygen tension (PvO_2).

CAUSES OF CYANOSIS

Peripheral cyanosis occurs when there is inadequate oxygenation of peripheral capillary blood. This may be a reflection of central cyanosis or result from decreased local capillary perfusion due to a variety of causes (Table 57–1). Causes of decreased peripheral perfusion include local or regional thrombosis (e.g., aortic saddle thrombus) or decreased cardiac output as a result of cardiac disease, arrhythmias, or severe hypovolemia (e.g., shock). With the exception of severe heart failure associated with pulmonary edema, these clinical diagnoses are not usually associated with central cyanosis, and PaO_2 is normal.

Central cyanosis describes a situation in which increased arterial RHb is systemic (i.e., arterial hypoxemia is present). Central cyanosis may result from a number of causes (see Table 57–1). In young animals, congenital heart disease that results in right-to-left shunting is the most likely cause of cyanosis. Severe pulmonary disease may result in cyanosis at any age. Congenital abnormalities in Hb are rare in companion animals, but methemoglobinemia due to toxicity may lead to chocolate colored blood, resulting in a cyanotic appearance in affected animals. Methemoglobin is a normal product of Hb oxidation and is maintained at low concentrations (approximately 1 per cent of total Hb) by erythrocyte

TABLE 57-1. CAUSES OF CENTRAL AND PERIPHERAL CYANOSIS

Central Cyanosis

Cardiac (right-to-left shunting)
  Intracardiac
    Tetralogy of Fallot
    Atrial or ventricular septal defect with pulmonic stenosis or pulmonary hypertension
  Extracardiac
    Reversed patent ductus arteriosus* (patent ductus arteriosus with pulmonary hypertension)
Pulmonary
  Hypoventilation (mechanical or functional limitation of breathing)
    Pleural effusion, pneumothorax
    Respiratory muscle failure (due to fatigue, myopathy, or neurologic abnormalities)
    Central neurologic abnormalities (e.g., sedative or anesthetic overdose, primary neurologic disease)
  Obstruction
    Laryngeal paralysis
    Mass lesion of large airways (larynx, trachea, primary bronchi)
    Large airway foreign body
  Inadequate oxygen in inspired gas (e.g., anesthetic accident)
  Ventilation-perfusion mismatch
    Pulmonary thromboembolism
    Severe pulmonary infiltration
      Edema
      Inflammation
      Neoplasia
      Acute respiratory distress syndrome (ARDS)
      Chronic obstructive pulmonary disease (COPD) or pulmonary fibrosis
  Abnormal hemoglobin (e.g., methemoglobinemia)

Peripheral Cyanosis

Inadequate oxygenation of circulating hemoglobin (i.e., central cyanosis)
Alterations in capillary blood flow
  Decreased arterial supply
    Peripheral vasoconstriction (e.g., hypothermia)
    Arterial thromboembolism
    Low cardiac output
  Obstruction of venous drainage (e.g., tourniquet, venous thrombosis, severe right-sided heart failure)

* Associated with differential cyanosis unless the animal is markedly polycythemic.

methemoglobin reductase within the circulating red blood cells. The percentage of methemoglobin may increase due to ingestion of or exposure to oxidants or if erythrocyte methemoglobin reductase deficiency is present. Common oxidants associated with production of methemoglobin include nitrates, nitrites, acetaminophen, methylene blue, phenazopyridine, Cetacaine, and topical benzocaine. Clinical recognition of color changes in arterial blood is possible if methemoglobin content exceeds 10 per cent of total Hb, but it may be difficult to detect in dark venous blood samples.

Causes of central cyanosis responsive to oxygen supplementation include hypoventilation, obstructive diseases of the major airways, and ventilation-perfusion mismatch, often related to severe pulmonary parenchymal disease. These causes may be differentiated with a variety of clinical tests, including response to administration of 100 per cent oxygen.

EVALUATION OF THE CYANOTIC ANIMAL

Clinical differentiation of cyanosis is based on history, physical examination findings, and diagnostic testing. Because cyanosis is a clinical sign rather than a disease, diagnostic tests are directed toward both definition of arterial oxygen status (e.g., blood gas analysis, pulse oximetry, PCV determination, response to 100 per cent oxygen) and identification of any underlying cause (e.g., radiography, echocardiography).

HISTORY

Some causes of cyanosis (e.g., sedative overdose resulting in hypoventilation) are easily ascertained based on review of the clinical history. Other causes, such as cyanotic congenital heart disease, typically are diagnosed in a specific subset of the population (e.g., animals younger than 3 years old). Acquired causes of peripheral or central cyanosis may have a supportive clinical history (e.g., history of chronic heart disease) but are primarily differentiated based on clinical examination and diagnostic findings.

PHYSICAL EXAMINATION

The character of cyanosis may be used to differentiate peripheral from central disease. Peripheral cyanosis involves cutaneous tissues, but mucous membrane and tongue color remains normal unless central cyanosis is coexistent (Fig. 57–1). Central cyanosis is detected by identification of cyanotic mucous membranes and tongue. A special case of central cyanosis is the differential cyanosis noted in cases of reversed patent ductus arteriosus. In these cases, the cranial mucous membranes are pink, but caudal mucous membranes are cyanotic. Causes of regionally isolated peripheral cyanosis that are usually readily detected by physical examination include generalized hypothermia (diagnosed based on history and detection of low core body temperature), mechanical

venous obstructions (e.g., rubber band or tourniquet), and arterial thromboembolism (detected based on typical findings of pain, pulselessness, paresis, pallor, and palpable coolness of affected area). The causes of central cyanosis are often associated with abnormal physical findings reflecting the etiology (Fig. 57–2).

DIAGNOSTIC TESTING

Much of the information necessary to narrow the list of differential diagnoses for central cyanosis is obtained by manipulation of oxygen supplementation with analysis of arterial blood gas (ABG) values and pulse oximetry results (Table 57–2; see Figs. 57–1 and 57–2).

ABG analysis is the gold standard for evaluation of cyanosis. Although venous samples can contribute helpful information toward a diagnosis, arterial samples provide definitive evidence of baseline abnormalities and response to oxygen. For maximal diagnostic value, oxygenated ABG values must be obtained while the animal is receiving *100 per cent oxygen*.

Pulse oximetry is a readily available resource the for evaluation of cyanosis in many clinics. The probe is applied to the axillary or inguinal fold, a lip, or the tongue (in an anesthetized animal). If a satisfactory signal can be recorded, there is reasonably good correlation between pulse oximetry estimates and invasive measures of SaO_2 in dogs. Given a normal PCV, pulse oximetry values can be used to reflect PaO_2 (Table 57–3). Pulse oximetry has important limitations for continual monitoring but can be useful in the evaluation of baseline oxygenation and response to oxygen supplementation when ABG analysis is not available.

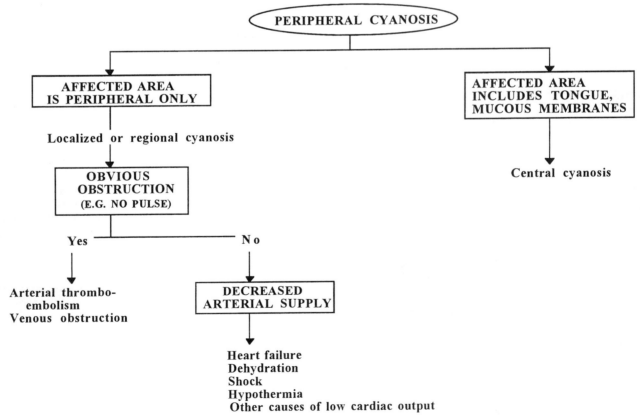

Figure 57–1. Algorithm for the differential diagnosis of peripheral cyanosis. All tentative diagnoses should be confirmed with appropriate specific diagnostic testing.

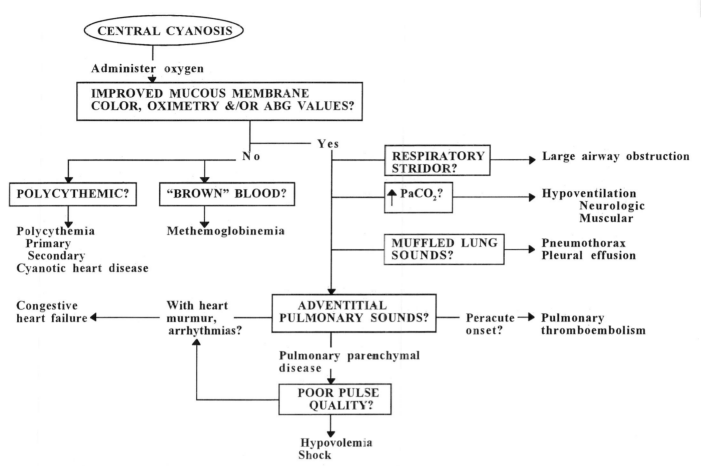

Figure 57–2. Algorithm for the differential diagnosis of central cyanosis. All tentative diagnoses should be confirmed with appropriate specific diagnostic testing. PaCO$_2$ = arterial CO$_2$ tension; ABG = arterial blood gas.

THERAPY

Therapy of cyanosis is dependent on understanding the cause of the condition. Peripheral cyanosis, although often indicative of serious disease conditions, is not usually life-threatening, and therapy is directed toward resolution of the underlying disease. Successful therapy of the underlying condition usually results in resolution of peripheral cyanosis.

Central cyanosis is treated as an emergency until the cause can be ascertained, and reduced oxygen supply is assumed until disproved. Presence of a patent airway is confirmed or one is established, and oxygen is administered immediately using an oxygen mask, nasal insufflation, an oxygen cage, or intubation. Life-threatening pleural effusions (e.g., pyo-

thorax, pneumothorax) may be removed via thoracocentesis. A combination of examination, therapeutic manipulations with oxygen, and other diagnostic tests may be used to delineate the cause of the cyanosis.

Congenital heart disease resulting in right-to-left shunting may be palliated surgically; supplemental oxygen is not helpful, because the amount of desaturated (venous) blood added to the arterial blood is fixed. In most cases, animals with cyanotic heart disease are relatively comfortable at rest, and emergency intervention is not necessary. Therapy of methemoglobinemia involves elimination of the cause and attempts to limit tissue injury. Methemoglobin cannot bind oxygen, so oxygen supplementation is not useful, but once the oxidant has been eliminated, erythrocytes can convert a

TABLE 57–2. BLOOD GAS MEASUREMENTS, OXYGEN SATURATIONS, AND RESPONSE TO OXYGEN SUPPLEMENTATION IN VARIOUS CYANOTIC DISORDERS

PROBLEM	Sao$_2$ (ROOM AIR)*	Pao$_2$ (ROOM AIR)*	Paco$_2$*	Pao$_2$ RESPONSE TO 100% O$_2$
Peripheral cyanosis	Normal†	Normal†	Normal†	(−)
Right-to-left intracardiac shunt	↓↓	↓↓	Normal	(−)
Pulmonary parenchymal disease	↓↓	↓↓	↑	↑
Hypoventilation	↓	↓	↑↑↑	↑
Systemic hypoperfusion	↓	↓	Normal / ↑	↑
Ventilation-perfusion mismatch	↓	↓	Normal / ↓	↑
Methemoglobinemia	↓	Normal	Normal	(−)

* Normal Sao$_2$ (room air) = ∼ 97%; normal Pao$_2$ (room air) = ∼ 100 mmHg; normal Paco$_2$ (room air) = ∼40 mmHg.
† Unless drawn from affected area.

large portion of the methemoglobin back to Hb within about 24 hours. Methylene blue and N-acetylcysteine have been recommended for acute therapy of methemoglobinemia.

Neurologic or musculoskeletal causes of hypoventilation may be temporary (e.g., sedative overdose, respiratory muscle fatigue) or permanent (e.g., neoplasia involving or compressing respiratory centers). Respiratory support, including oxygen supplementation with or without mechanical ventilation, may be used to support the animal until the drug effects subside or can be reversed (e.g., narcotic sedative reversal) or until the underlying problem can be definitively treated.

Obstruction of major airways should be relieved immediately, either by removing the obstruction (e.g., large airway foreign body) or by bypassing the obstruction (e.g., intubation past the obstruction or tracheostomy below the level of obstruction). Therapy of pulmonary thromboembolism is controversial and may involve administration of fluids, anticoagulants, and/or plasma, but supplemental oxygen is recommended as supportive therapy. Definitive resolution of pulmonary parenchymal diseases results in resolution of the cyanosis, but supplemental oxygen may be helpful in the short term to maximize Hb saturation. Use of mechanical ventilation is helpful in cases of severe, prolonged dyspnea

TABLE 57–3. ARTERIAL OXYGEN TENSION AT VARIOUS ARTERIAL OXYGEN SATURATIONS (ASSUMING NORMAL HEMOGLOBIN CONCENTRATIONS)

ARTERIAL OXYGEN SATURATION (%) (SaO_2)	ARTERIAL OXYGEN TENSION (mmHg) (PaO_2)
98	98
97	95
95	80
93	70
90	60
85	50
75	40

with respiratory muscle fatigue. Obstructive pulmonary disease and pulmonary fibrosis are chronic conditions, making oxygen supplementation impractical. In these cases, animals may benefit from exercise restriction, weight loss, and management of complications. In all cases in which oxygen is administered, repeated evaluation of mucous membrane color and measurements of oxygen saturation and blood gas values are used to judge efficacy of therapy.

CHAPTER 58

JAUNDICE

Jan Rothuizen

Jaundice or icterus is the accumulation of bilirubin in plasma and tissues to such an extent that the yellow pigment causes a visible yellow discoloration of the sclera, the skin, and the mucous membranes. Bilirubin levels are below 0.4 mg/dL in healthy dogs and cats, and icterus usually becomes distinct when the level exceeds 2 mg/dL. Hence only severe hyperbilirubinemia is clinically apparent.

PHYSIOLOGY

Bilirubin is the normal product of all hemoproteins and is derived from the degradation of the heme moiety. Hemoglobin is the most important source of bilirubin, but bilirubin is also produced from other hemoproteins. The liver is the primary source of these hemoproteins, which include catalases, peroxidases, and cytochromes. Erythrocytes contain the bulk of the hemoproteins and account for 70 per cent of the bilirubin production. Despite their small mass, the hepatic hemoproteins contribute about 30 per cent of bilirubin production because their turnover is much higher. In dogs the corresponding lifetimes are 98 days for erythrocytes versus 0.5 to 3 days for hepatic hemoproteins. The values are presumably similar in cats.

Heme is enzymatically cleaved by heme oxygenase to form biliverdin, which is reduced to bilirubin by biliverdin reductase. Because heme oxygenase is rate limiting, pathologic conditions may lead to accumulation of yellow but never of green pigment in dogs and cats. Heme oxygenase and biliverdin reductase are equally distributed in the liver and in the spleen. Hepatic clearance of plasma bilirubin is quite inefficient; thus most of the bilirubin produced appears in the systemic circulation instead of being immediately cleared from the portal blood by the liver. The relative inefficiency of bilirubin clearance implies that hepatic conjugation and biliary excretion rather than hepatic perfusion determine the concentration in plasma. Therefore, jaundice is not seen in animals with severely impaired hepatic perfusion, as in congenital portosystemic shunts. In contrast, ammonia is almost completely cleared by the liver in a single passage, and ammonia levels in blood are therefore almost exclusively determined by hepatic perfusion.

Bilirubin is hydrophobic and can be transported in blood only when bound to albumin. Excretion into bile (or urine) requires conjugation, which makes it hydrophilic and thus water-soluble. A bilirubin molecule can bind two conjugating moieties, and in most species conjugated bilirubin is diglucuronide. Dogs also exploit other sugars such as glucose and xylose, and they make monoconjugates as well as diconjugates. The diconjugates consist of different combinations of the possible conjugating groups. Upon conjugation, bilirubin is excreted into the bile. Conjugated bilirubin is not absorbed from the intestinal tract, but deconjugation by bacterial enzymes can result in some enterohepatic circulation of bilirubin when there is small intestinal bacterial overgrowth.

In the colon, conjugated bilirubin is further processed by bacterial enzymes to form the colorless urobilinogens, which in the oxidized form give the brown color to feces. Little urobilinogen is absorbed, and less than 1 per cent escapes clearance by the liver to be excreted by the kidneys. Attempts have been made to use the measurement of urobilinogen in urine as an indicator of hepatobiliary excretion of bilirubin. The absence of urobilinogen in the urine was presumed to indicate severe impairment of the bile flow, as could occur in extrahepatic cholestasis. There are, however, so many factors influencing the minute amount of urobilinogen in the urine that its measurement has proved to be meaningless clinically.

In dogs, unlike in other species, the kidneys have an active role in bilirubin metabolism. Male dog renal tubular cells, especially, have all the enzymes necessary to produce bilirubin from heme and to conjugate it, after which it may be excreted in the urine. As a consequence, dog urine may normally contain detectable amounts of bilirubin. Moreover, when there is hemolysis, the kidneys excrete more bilirubin, even in the absence of hyperbilirubinemia. The presence of bilirubin in the urine, which in other species is a clear sign of conjugated hyperbilirubinemia and liver disease, is not necessarily related to hepatobiliary dysfunction in male dogs.

Bilirubin is a highly effective antioxidant, binding oxygen radicals to form biliverdin, which is converted into bilirubin again in the liver and spleen. However, unconjugated bilirubin is toxic to the brain. Human infants may have high unconjugated bilirubin levels in the first week after birth because conjugating enzymes are not yet fully functional. At this age, bilirubin passes the blood-brain barrier easily and may cause irreversible brain damage. Such "kernicterus" also occurs rarely in kittens, but not in puppies.

DIFFERENTIAL DIAGNOSIS (Fig. 58–1)

Pathologic bilirubin concentrations and jaundice may occur in conditions associated with increased bilirubin production, decreased clearance, inadequate conjugation, or impaired biliary excretion. When bile flow or biliary excretion of conjugated bilirubin is impaired, the accumulating pigment is conjugated; in all other cases it is unconjugated. Increased production alone does not result in jaundice, because the normally functioning liver has a huge reserve capacity and can handle large amounts of bilirubin.

HEMOLYSIS

The main mechanism of increased bilirubin production is hemolysis. In dogs with severe (e.g., autoimmune) hemolysis, the erythrocyte lifetime is reduced to 10 days or less, and bilirubin production is increased five- to 10-fold. Unexpectedly, in such dogs the conjugated fraction of plasma bilirubin is higher. Analysis of the factors influencing bilirubin concentration has shown that severe hemolysis is accompanied by reduced bile flow and, as a result, cholestasis. Conjugated pigment is the main determinant of hyperbilirubinemia. In dogs with hemolytic jaundice, there is hepatic centrilobular necrosis, which causes the cholestasis. Because the centrilobular zone is the last part of the liver lobule to receive blood, a suddenly reduced oxygen supply due to anemia may induce irreversible damage to these cells. When anemia develops gradually, the hepatocytes develop a much more efficient uptake of oxygen, so that even severe anemia has little effect. Hemolytic jaundice therefore occurs only in acute, severe hemolysis and is the result of secondary cholestasis rather than increased bilirubin production. The degree of cholestasis is comparable to that in primary liver disease. Only in extremely early stages of severe hemolysis or when hemolysis is moderate is there no visible jaundice, but there may be slight hyperbilirubinemia owing to the increased production of unconjugated bilirubin.

LIVER AND BILIARY DISEASES

Jaundice also occurs in many different liver and biliary diseases, including extrahepatic bile duct obstruction, different forms of hepatitis, cirrhosis, and malignancies. Jaundice in these diseases is the result of derangement of various steps in the metabolism of bilirubin. Cholestasis, a decreased bile flow, is the most prominent feature in these conditions. Cholestasis may be intrahepatic, predominantly at the level of bile canaliculi, or extrahepatic due to obstruction of the

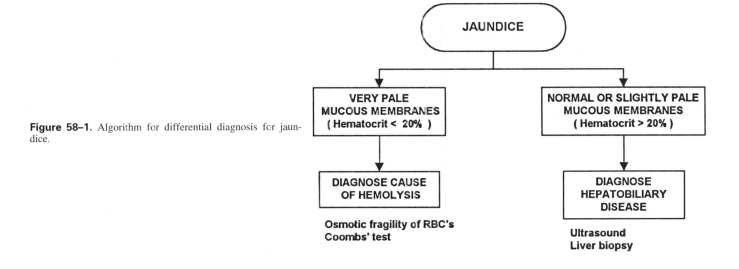

Figure 58–1. Algorithm for differential diagnosis for jaundice.

common bile duct. Both intra- and extrahepatic cholestasis results in decreased bile flow in the canaliculi, accumulation of bile constituents such as conjugated bilirubin in the hepatocytes, and regurgitation of these materials into Disse's space via the sinusoidal membrane of hepatocytes and the intercellular space between them. This results in increased concentrations of conjugated bilirubin, bile salts, and enzymes such as AP and γGT in plasma. The increased bilirubin content in hepatocytes also hampers the conjugation and the clearance of bilirubin. Cholestasis therefore leads to accumulation of not only conjugated but also unconjugated bilirubin in the plasma. Apart from the direct effects of cholestasis, the conjugating and clearing capacities of the liver are also reduced by a decrease in funcional liver mass, depending on the severity of hepatic damage. Another factor influencing bilirubin metabolism in hepatobiliary diseases is hemolysis. In icteric dogs with such diseases, erythrocyte life span is often 20 to 60 days (normally 98 days), and bilirubin production from erythrocytes is two to five times greater. Factors responsible for hemolysis secondary to hepatobiliary diseases may be decreased stability of the erythrocyte membranes, caused by increased bile salt concentrations, and hypersplenism with prolonged trapping of erythrocytes when there is portal hypertension. The production of bilirubin from hepatic hemoproteins is quite variable in liver diseases. It remains normal in most cases but may be highly increased by unexplained mechanisms. For the previously stated reasons, plasma bilirubin in liver disease or in extrahepatic cholestasis is both conjugated and unconjugated.

DIAGNOSTIC TESTING

It is not possible to differentiate hemolytic jaundice from hepatobiliary icterus by measuring conjugated and unconjugated bilirubin, because in all cases the conjugated form prevails (50 to 90 per cent), but unconjugated bilirubin is increased as well. The conjugation pattern of bilirubin changes when there is cholestasis. Cholestasis is a component of all diseases associated with jaundice. Normally, dogs use different conjugating groups to conjugate bilirubin, and they make mono- as well as diconjugates. Most other mammals use glucuronide and make only diglucuronide. However, in cholestatic disease in all species, both mono- and diconjugates are formed using sugars and sulfate. This results in a mixture of different bilirubin conjugates with a wide range of polarities, which has implications for the generally used techniques of measuring bilirubin. The colorimetric measurement is based on cleavage of the tetrapyrrole structure of bilirubin and coupling of the two dipyrrole products to an azo dye. The velocity of the color reaction depends on the polarity of the original molecules. Bilirubin diglucuronide reacts quickly ("direct bilirubin"), and unconjugated bilirubin reacts only after addition of a reaction accelerator ("indirect bilirubin"). In healthy animals, plasma contains only indirect bilirubin, but when there is cholestasis, direct bilirubin prevails. Measurement of direct and indirect bilirubin has been used as a basis to explain the underlying process. However, owing to the variable mixture of conjugates with different polarities in cholestatic diseases, the difference between conjugated and unconjugated bilirubin is not well defined, and the results of measurements are highly arbitrary. This, together with the absence of a pathophysiologic basis for differentiating between various hepatobiliary diseases and hemolytic disease using the ratio of conjugated to unconjugated bilirubin, makes the clinical application of such measurements useless.

Normally, bilirubin is reversibly bound to albumin in the plasma, permitting an easy exchange with tissues and clearance by the liver. In cholestatic plasma, conjugated bilirubin slowly undergoes irreversible, covalent binding to albumin. The reaction also occurs in vitro when plasma or serum is stored at room temperature. The fraction of conjugated bilirubin captured in "biliprotein" depends on the duration of the hyperbilirubinemia. In chronic cases it may account for over 80 per cent of the conjugated bilirubin. Biliprotein is detected by conventional bilirubin measurements. In contrast to loosely bound bilirubins, biliprotein is not cleared from the plasma by the liver, and it remains in the circulation with the half-life of albumin. Thus persistence of hyperbilirubinemia or jaundice does not necessarily indicate persistence of the underlying disease.

Jaundice is a clear indication of hepatobiliary disease with cholestasis, which is either primary or secondary to hypoxia as a result of acute hemolysis. However, jaundice is present in only a minority of animals with such diseases. Cats tend to have jaundice more frequently than dogs, but in either species it occurs in only 10 to 30 per cent of the cases of hepatobiliary disease. Although specific, jaundice is an insensitive indicator of hepatobiliary diseases. Determining direct and indirect bilirubin in plasma is useless, because differences are not related to the causes of icterus and because biliprotein can make the results artifactitious. Far better for the detection or evaluation of hepatobiliary diseases are plasma bile acids, because they are sensitive and specific. The presence of visible jaundice is direct evidence of hepatobiliary disease, indicating the need for diagnostic evaluation of the underlying disease. When there is severe, acute anemia, diagnostic efforts should be directed to the cause of hemolysis; when there is no more than moderate anemia, the liver disease should be evaluated by ultrasonography and histologic examination of a liver biopsy.

CHAPTER 59

BLEEDING DISORDERS:
Epistaxis and Hemoptysis

Orla Mahony

DEFINITIONS

Epistaxis refers to actual hemorrhage from the nasal cavity. *Hemoptysis,* by strict definition, refers to spitting up of blood or blood-stained sputum. However, the term is used for the coughing up of blood, grossly bloody sputum, or even blood-tinged sputum.

PATHOPHYSIOLOGY

Epistaxis. Local processes cause epistaxis through direct damage to blood vessels from trauma, the erosive nature of infectious, inflammatory, or neoplastic disease; weakening of vascular malformations; or violent sneezing. Coagulopathies commonly cause epistaxis through defects of platelet number or platelet function or, rarely, from decreased concentrations of coagulation factors. Polycythemia causes an expanded blood volume, venous engorgement, and impaired blood flow, which may occasionally cause epistaxis from hypoxia, thrombosis, and rupture of small vessels. Sustained primary or secondary hypertension can result in weakening and eventual rupture of small arteries and arterioles.

Hemoptysis. The pathologic mechanisms responsible for hemoptysis include pulmonary hypertension (dirofilariasis, congestive heart failure, pulmonary thromboembolism), loss of vascular integrity (trauma, inflammation, neoplasia), cavitary pulmonary lesions (infectious, neoplastic, congenital, traumatic), and mucosal necrosis with rupture of underlying blood vessels (bronchiectasis).

EPISTAXIS

HISTORICAL FINDINGS

The history should include the following.
Signalment. Young, pure-bred animals are more likely to have hereditary coagulopathies; young to middle-aged animals are more prone to infections; middle-aged animals more commonly acquire immune-mediated diseases; and older animals are more likely to develop neoplastic disease.

Surgical History. Hereditary coagulopathies are unlikely if the animal has had no bleeding complications following surgery in the past. A possible exception would be an animal with von Willebrand's disease and an acquired secondary problem such as aspirin administration or hypothyroidism.

Current Medications. Drugs can cause quantitative and qualitative platelet abnormalities through bone marrow suppression (cytotoxic drugs, phenylbutazone, estrogen), immune-mediated destruction (sulfonamides, arsenicals), and acquired platelet dysfunction (aspirin, other nonsteroidal anti-inflammatory drugs, and the penicillin derivatives). However, the drugs causing platelet dysfunction rarely cause excessive bleeding unless there is an underlying coagulopathy.

Vaccination History. Modified live virus vaccines can cause immune-mediated thrombocytopenia within 3 to 4 weeks of vaccine administration.

Environment. Palatine injury can be caused by chewing on wood or catching sticks. Animals may also consume vitamin K antagonists.

History of Trauma. Attempts should be made to rule out trauma, particularly for a single, self-limited episode of epistaxis. If hemorrhage persists or recurs after trauma, an underlying coagulopathy may be present.

Travel History. In certain geographic areas, rickettsial, fungal, and parasitic diseases are common.

Nature and Chronicity of the Problem. It is important to differentiate epistaxis from hemoptysis, as they are sometimes confused. Careful questioning and a thorough physical examination should localize the source of hemorrhage. Acute epistaxis following trauma is likely to be self-limited. If epistaxis is preceded by or associated with a serous or mucopurulent nasal discharge, a local process within the nasal cavity is likely. Stertorous breathing is indicative of a local problem. Coagulopathy is likely if a discharge is only hemorrhagic, especially if it is bilateral and recurrent.

History of Bleeding From Other Sites. Hematuria or melena may point to a bleeding disorder. However, melena can result from nasal bleeding and swallowing of that blood. Hematemesis can be due to vomiting swallowed blood.

Pawing at the Face or Paroxysmal Sneezing. This commonly occurs following recent inhalation of a foreign body.

Breed or Family History of Bleeding Problems. Either history may point to a coagulopathy.

PHYSICAL FINDINGS

The integument and mucous membranes should be examined for evidence of petechiae, ecchymoses, or bruises, which are suggestive of a coagulopathy. The animal's face should be examined for evidence of visual or palpable asymmetry. Facial distortion is most often caused by neoplasia, but infectious or inflammatory processes should also be considered. Evidence of pain on palpation of the face, protrusion of the eye, or epiphora suggests a local process. A thorough examination is essential to rule out palatine defects, dental disease, or masses that communicate with the nasal cavity. Patency of the nostrils is assessed by holding a glass slide in front of each nostril and examining the slide for condensation. A fundic examination can reveal retinal lesions caused by rickettsial or fungal diseases, coagulopathies, neoplasms, or hypertension.

DIFFERENTIAL DIAGNOSIS

The differential diagnosis can be divided into systemic and local problems (Table 59–1). However, it is important to remember that even when a local problem is diagnosed, the animal may have an underlying coagulopathy that is exacerbating the problem.

Systemic Processes

Bleeding disorders are important causes of epistaxis. Defects of primary hemostasis (platelet plug formation) are much more common causes of epistaxis than are defects of secondary hemostasis (coagulation cascade). The former is associated with mucosal and cutaneous hemorrhage clini-

cally, whereas the latter is generally associated with hemorrhage into body cavities and joint spaces.

Disorders of primary hemostasis include quantitative and qualitative platelet defects (see Chapter 180). Thrombocytopenias can be subdivided into diseases causing increased destruction, increased consumption, or decreased production of platelets. Many of these diseases are also associated with platelet function abnormalities. Increased destruction of platelets can be caused by immune-mediated processes, some drugs, or infection. Increased consumption of platelets occurs in disseminated intravascular coagulation (DIC), vasculitis, or sepsis. Decreased production of platelets occurs with bone marrow disorders such as malignancy and aplasia. Aplastic anemia is usually idiopathic but is sometimes caused by drugs or infections. In the absence of other abnormalities, thrombocytopenia is unlikely to result in bleeding until the count is less than 50,000 to 75,000/μL. In idiopathic thrombocytopenic purpura, platelet counts often drop below 10,000/μL before bleeding occurs. This is because increased production of young active platelets protects against bleed-

---

TABLE 59–1. CAUSES OF EPISTAXIS

SYSTEMIC PROCESSES

Quantitative Platelet Abnormalities

Increased destruction
  Idiopathic thrombocytopenic purpura—idiopathic or secondary to
    modified live virus vaccines or drugs (e.g., sulfonamides,
    methimazole)
  Infections (e.g., ehrlichiosis)
Increased consumption
  Disseminated intravascular coagulation
  Vasculitis or sepsis (e.g., Rocky Mountain spotted fever)
Decreased production
  Hematopoietic malignancy
  Aplasia
  Drugs (e.g., estrogen [endogenous or exogenous], phenylbutazone,
    chemotherapy)
  Infections (e.g., ehrlichiosis, feline leukemia virus, feline
    immunodeficiency virus)
  Osteosclerosis
  Idiopathic

Coagulation Factor Abnormalities

Vitamin K–responsive coagulopathies
Hereditary coagulopathies
Paraproteinemias

Qualitative Platelet Abnormalities

  Hereditary (e.g., von Willebrand's disease, basset hound thrombopathia)
  Ehrlichiosis
  Drugs (e.g., aspirin, nonsteroidal anti-inflammatories, anesthetics
    antibiotics, heparin)
  Uremia
  Paraproteinemias (e.g., multiple myeloma, Waldenstrom's
    macroglobulinemia, lymphocytic leukemia)

Polycythemia

  Polycythemia vera
  Polycythemia secondary to renal or adrenal tumors
  Cardiopulmonary disease

Hypertension

  Primary
  Secondary to renal, endocrine, neurogenic disorders

LOCAL PROCESSES

Neoplasia

  Nasal adenocarcinoma
  Fibrosarcoma
  Chondrosarcoma
  Osteosarcoma
  Lymphoma
  Squamous cell carcinoma
  Transmissible venereal tumor
  Benign polyp

Inflammation

  Lymphoplasmacytic rhinitis

Infection

  Fungal
    Aspergillus
    Penicillium
    Cryptococcus
    Rhinosporidium
    Phaeohyphomycosis
  Parasitic
    Linguatula
    Leishmania
    Cuterebra
  Bacterial
    Bordetella
    Pasteurella
  Viral
    Feline viral rhinotracheitis
    Feline calicivirus

Other

  Foreign body
  Trauma
  Vascular malformation

ing. Qualitative disorders include congenital thrombocytopathias, such as von Willebrand's disease, and acquired disorders secondary to uremia, canine ehrlichiosis, paraproteinemias, or drugs such as aspirin. Polycythemia occasionally causes epistaxis. Absolute polycythemia, characterized by an expanded red cell mass, may occur in polycythemia vera or be seen secondary to diseases with appropriate or inappropriate erythropoietin elevations. Hypertension has recently been recognized as a cause of epistaxis in cats and dogs.

Local Processes

Epistaxis secondary to neoplastic, infectious, and inflammatory processes is usually preceded by a chronic mucopurulent discharge (see Chapter 123). Trauma to the nasal cavity can cause mild to severe epistaxis, which is usually self-limited although it occasionally requires packing of the nasal cavity to control the hemorrhage.

Neoplasia. Malignant nasal tumors, especially adenocarcinomas that originate within the ethmoidal turbinates, are much more common in dogs than in cats. Benign anterior nasal cavity fibrous polyps are occasionally seen in cats and dogs. Cats may get nasopharyngeal polyps.

Fungal Rhinitis. *Aspergillus fumigatus* is the most common fungus isolated in dogs, whereas *Cryptococcus neoformans* is most common in cats.

Parasitic Rhinitis. *Linguatula serrata*, named after its tonguelike appearance, is an arthropod that parasitizes the nasal cavity of dogs. It sometimes causes a severe rhinitis with coughing, sneezing, and epistaxis. Leishmaniasis is a protozoal disease that causes epistaxis in 10 per cent of infected dogs and is thought to be the result of ulceration within the nasal cavity. *Capillaria aerophila*, a nematode, and *Cuterebra*, a botfly larva, can also parasitize the nasal cavity and cause epistaxis.

Bacterial Rhinitis. Bacteria usually require predisposing inflammation or damage in order to become established, with the exception of *Bordetella bronchiseptica* and *Pasteurella multocida*, which may be primary pathogens in the dog.

Viral Rhinitis. Viruses rarely cause a blood-tinged nasal discharge. Feline rhinotracheitis virus and feline calicivirus represent important causes in the cat. Multiple viruses have been shown to cause rhinitis in dogs, including distemper virus, adenovirus, reovirus, and a parainfluenza virus.

Inflammatory Rhinitis. Lymphoplasmacytic rhinitis is an immune-mediated, corticosteroid-responsive disease of unknown etiology, usually causing a mucopurulent discharge. However, hemorrhagic discharges also occur.

Foreign Body Rhinitis. The majority of foreign bodies are inhaled. Others enter through the palate of the mouth or behind the soft palate, and some are intentionally pushed into the nasal cavity either unwittingly or maliciously.

DIAGNOSTIC PLAN

The specific diagnostic approach is dependent on the history, physical examination, and initial laboratory findings (Fig. 59–1). An important factor is whether the animal has a coagulopathy. The minimal database must include a complete blood count (CBC) with platelet count, a chemistry profile, and urinalysis.

Complete Blood Count. The CBC provides data regarding the presence of anemia, polycythemia, thrombocytopenia, leukocytosis, or leukopenia. If there is no history of

trauma or a mucopurulent discharge, the platelet count is quite important. Examination of a well-made blood smear permits estimation of the platelet number, with less than four platelets per high-power field indicative of severe thrombocytopenia. The feathered edge should be examined for clumps of platelets.

Chemistry Profile. Hypoalbuminemia may occur in acute ehrlichiosis, Rocky Mountain spotted fever, and severe hemorrhage. Hyperglobulinemia is usually present in ehrlichiosis and may occur with inflammation, chronic antigenic stimulation, and neoplasia. Serum chemistries also help rule out systemic diseases that may cause coagulopathies, such as uremia or liver disease. However, these diseases usually have other clinical signs in addition to epistaxis.

Urinalysis. Because the bladder has a mucosal surface, hematuria can occur with platelet problems. Proteinuria can occur with hyperglobulinemias or immune-mediated diseases.

Hemostatic Studies. If bleeding persists or recurs and the animal is anemic, a reticulocyte count is indicated to characterize the anemia as regenerative or nonregenerative and to help determine whether the marrow is normal. An activated clotting time is a useful screening test that evaluates abnormalities of the intrinsic coagulation system. It may also be prolonged if the platelet count is less than 10,000/μL. A coagulation profile (prothrombin time, partial thromboplastin time, fibrinogen, and fibrin degradation products) evaluates the intrinsic and extrinsic coagulation pathways (see Chapter 181). If the platelet count is over 100,000/μL, platelet function can be evaluated with buccal mucosal bleeding time. New tests are being developed to measure antiplatelet antibody. Older tests, such as platelet factor 3 release, lack specificity and have variable sensitivity. A bone marrow aspirate and/or biopsy is indicated if thrombocytopenia, nonregenerative anemia, leukopenia, paraproteinemia, or abnormal circulating cells are present.

Serology. Serologic testing is helpful in the diagnosis of canine ehrlichiosis, Rocky Mountain spotted fever, feline leukemia virus, and feline immunodeficiency virus.

Electrophoresis. Electrophoresis is used to distinguish between monoclonal and polyclonal gammopathies. Monoclonal gammopathies in dogs have been reported to be idiopathic as well as associated with myeloma, macroglobinemia, ehrlichiosis, lymphocytic leukemia, plasma cell leukemia, and cutaneous amyloidosis.

Parasitology. *Linguatula serrata* and *Capillaria aerophila* ova are found in nasal swabs or fecal flotations.

Rhinoscopy/Imaging. With a cuffed endotracheal tube in place, general anesthesia is required for thorough evaluation of the nasal cavity and oral cavities once coagulation has been assessed to be normal. Plain radiographs and computed tomography help determine the nature and the extent of the disease process. Rhinoscopy may allow visualization of foreign bodies, tumors, necrotic tissue, and fungal plaques, and may be used to obtain biopsies and remove some foreign bodies or small polyps. However, foreign bodies may be buried in granulation tissue, necessitating a rhinotomy for removal. The use of a flexible endoscope allows visualization of the caudal nasal conchae and in some cases, the frontal sinus. A diagnosis of aspergillosis may be missed if the frontal sinus is not evaluated. However, rhinoscopy has its limitations, with fresh hemorrhage and blood clots often obscuring the view. A dental mirror can also be used to visualize the nasopharynx.

Nasal Flushing. Through an endoscope or a red rubber catheter introduced into the nose or retroflexed over the soft

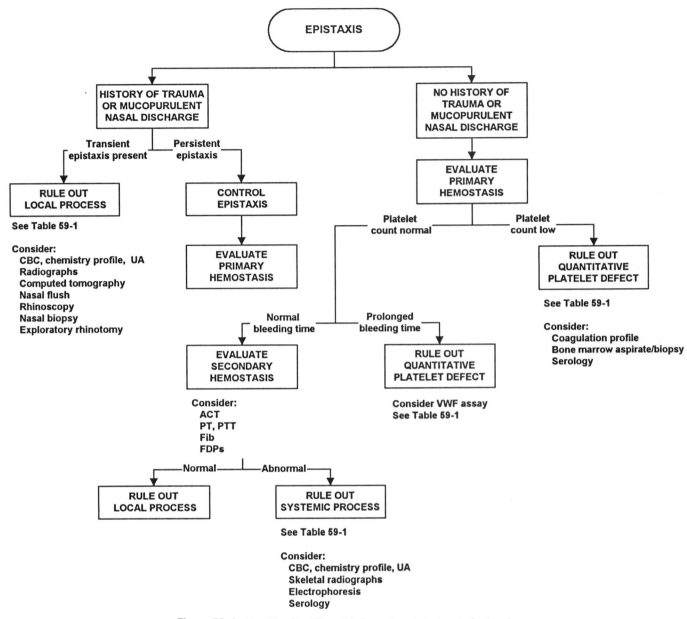

Figure 59–1. Algorithm for differential diagnosis and treatment of epistaxis.

palate, nasal flushing can be used to dislodge foreign bodies, or the fluid can be collected and submitted for cytologic evaluation.

Nasal Biopsy. If the coagulation profile is normal and a local process is suspected, a biopsy may be required to reach a definitive diagnosis. An endoscopically guided biopsy can be performed, or a blind biopsy may be performed with Jackson cup biopsy forceps. The forceps must not be inserted beyond the level of the medial canthus of the eye. Radiographs may be used as a guide to suspected lesions. Biopsies can result in life-threatening hemorrhage, for which one should be prepared.

Blood Pressure. Indirect blood pressure measurement can be obtained by means of Doppler and oscillometric techniques.

GOALS OF TREATMENT

The goal of treatment is to control epistaxis until a definitive diagnosis is made and then to treat the underlying disease. Moderate epistaxis is usually controlled with cage rest. Sedatives (e.g., butorphanol or oxymorphone, with or without diazepam) may be required to calm a distressed dog or cat. Drugs such as phenothiazines, which cause hypotension, should be avoided, especially if there is severe blood loss. Rarely, epistaxis requires further intervention such as intravenous fluids and/or a blood transfusion. Fresh whole blood provides red cells, platelets, and coagulation factors. Packed red cells are sufficient in most cases. In cases of idiopathic thrombocytopenic purpura, it is generally impossible to supply enough platelets to be useful in stopping the bleeding.

Persistent epistaxis may necessitate general anesthesia and ligation of the external carotid artery on the affected side or packing of the external nares and posterior nasal pharynx with gauze soaked in dilute epinephrine (1:100,000). A cuffed endotracheal tube ensures that no blood is aspirated.

Animals with severe epistaxis secondary to trauma must be observed carefully for any evidence of airway obstruction. If the animal is obtunded, blood clots can be removed from

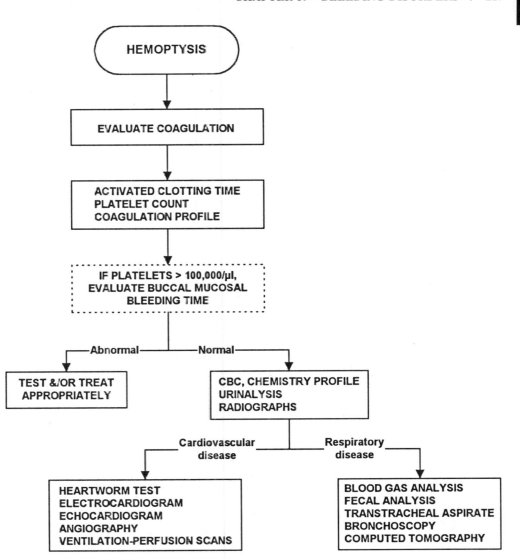

Figure 59–2. Algorithm for management of hemoptysis.

the pharynx if necessary. If a dog or cat is unable to ventilate adequately, a tracheostomy tube should be placed. The nasal obstruction will resolve over a couple of days.

HEMOPTYSIS

HISTORICAL FINDINGS

It is important to distinguish hemoptysis from hematemesis and bleeding from the gums and nasopharynx. Pertinent information includes known heart and lung disease, current medications, heartworm status, toxin exposure, and travel history.

TABLE 59–2. CAUSES OF HEMOPTYSIS

Dirofilariasis
Acute pulmonary edema
Cavitary pulmonary lesions
Neoplasia, trauma, infection, congenital causes
Severe pulmonary contusions
Coagulopathies
Tracheal or bronchial foreign bodies
Complication of diagnostic procedures
Other parasites (e.g., *Paragonimus, Filarioides, Angiostrongylus*)
Bacterial bronchopneumonia

PHYSICAL FINDINGS

A thorough physical examination should help localize the problem to a particular system. An abbreviated, nonstressful examination is required for a severely dyspneic animal. Appropriate therapeutic measures should be undertaken whenever necessary. Special attention should be paid to the respiratory and cardiac systems. A good oral examination should be performed to identify any bleeding lesions. Evaluation for a coagulopathy is the same as that described for epistaxis.

DIFFERENTIAL DIAGNOSIS (Table 59–2)

Hemoptysis is seldom seen in small animals, because they rarely expectorate after coughing. If hemoptysis is seen, it suggests either serious disease of the lower respiratory tract or a bleeding disorder. Heartworm disease can cause hemoptysis in both dogs and cats. Thromboembolic and parenchymal disease resulting in hemoptysis most frequently develops following the death of adult worms, especially after adulticide treatment. Exercise is usually the inciting factor. Hemoptysis has also been seen in the heartworm caval syndrome. Pulmonary thromboembolism caused by Cushing's disease, immune-mediated hemolytic anemia, or indwelling catheters is rarely associated with hemoptysis. Acute pulmonary edema sometimes results in expectoration of frothy pink sputum. Primary lung tumors (e.g., bronchoalveolar carcinoma) have been associated with hemoptysis. Metastatic lung tumors are less likely to cause hemoptysis, because their distribution tends to be interstitial rather than connecting with airways. Examples of infectious cavitary lesions include lung abscesses and parasitic cysts (paragonimiasis). Hemoptysis with severe traumatic pulmonary contusions is an ominous sign. Hemorrhage into the pulmonary parenchyma secondary to coagulopathies is rare but can result in hemoptysis. Iatrogenic hemoptysis can occur secondary to diagnostic procedures such as transtracheal aspirate, percutaneous fine-needle aspiration biopsy, and transbronchial biopsy. Animals should be closely monitored after these procedures.

DIAGNOSTIC PLAN

The minimal database includes a CBC with platelet count, chemistry profile, urinalysis, and thoracic radiographs (Fig. 59–2). Thoracic radiography is essential, provided the animal is able to withstand the stress of the procedure. Radiographs help localize the problem to either the respiratory or the cardiovascular system. The radiographs should be evaluated for fractured ribs, pulmonary contusions, cardiac enlargement, pruning of the pulmonary arteries (pulmonary thromboembolism), pleural effusions, pulmonary edema, pulmonary cavitary lesions, and foreign bodies. Occasionally, radiographs are normal in spite of severe pulmonary disease, such as contusions immediately following trauma and thromboembolism. Evaluation of hemostasis is an important component of the initial evaluation and is carried out in a manner similar to that described for epistaxis.

Depending on the initial findings, further tests could include blood gas analysis, occult heartworm antigen and microfilaria tests, cardiac evaluation, fecal analysis for parasites, transtracheal aspirates for culture and cytology, lung biopsies, and exploratory thoracotomy. Bronchoscopy can be used to visualize the tracheobronchial tree and to collect specimens, as well as for the removal of foreign bodies. It may even be possible to determine the origin of the hemorrhage. Computed tomography has been shown to be useful in human patients with hemoptysis who have negative radiographic and bronchoscopic findings.

GOALS OF TREATMENT

Initial stabilization of the acutely dyspneic animal includes cage rest, minimal stress, oxygen, maintenance of a patent airway, and the use of appropriate drugs, depending on the nature of the problem. Hemoptysis may be life-threatening—not from exsanguination, but from asphyxiation—and therefore requires intubation, suctioning, and ventilation.

CHAPTER 60

PETECHIAE AND ECCHYMOSES

Mary Beth Callan

Superficial bleeding into the skin or mucous membranes is referred to as purpura. Purpura can be categorized as petechiae or ecchymoses. Petechiae are small pinpoint hemorrhages (< 3 mm) resulting from extravasation of blood from capillaries, whereas ecchymoses are larger areas of hemorrhage resulting from leakage of blood from small arterioles and venules. Petechiae and ecchymoses are observed in primary hemostatic defects, i.e., platelet-vessel abnormalities. They represent a mild form of surface bleeding without external blood loss but may be associated with more serious hemorrhage. Both are commonly seen in dogs but rarely in cats.

PATHOPHYSIOLOGY

The vasculature is lined by a layer of endothelial cells that are linked by continuous and well-organized tight junctions varying in width from 0 to 4 nm. This provides a selectively impermeable membrane that prevents the passive transfer of blood into the extravascular space. The subendothelial matrix and additional layers of the vessels (media and adventitia) also act as barriers against extravasation of blood. Vascular integrity is influenced by many factors, one of which is platelets. Ultrastructural and functional changes develop in the vascular endothelium of thrombocytopenic animals, and these abnormalities are promptly reversed by a rise in the platelet count. However, the molecular basis for the observed changes remains unclear.

Thrombocytopenia (reduced platelet numbers), either as a sole hemostatic defect or as part of a combined hemostatic disorder, is the most common cause of petechiae and ecchymoses in dogs and cats. However, thrombopathias and vascular disorders may also cause capillary bleeding.

THROMBOCYTOPENIA

Thrombocytopenia may be a result of decreased platelet production by the bone marrow or increased platelet destruction, consumption, or sequestration (Table 60–1). Frequently more than one mechanism is involved. For example, bone marrow suppression, consumption of platelets secondary to vasculitis, splenic sequestration, increased destruction of platelets by both immune-mediated and non-immune-mediated mechanisms, and virus-associated myelodysplasia and myeloproliferative disorders may contribute to thrombocytopenia in dogs and cats with infectious diseases. Thrombocytopenia was recently reported in dogs with anticoagulant rodenticide poisoning, but the bleeding observed, mainly bleeding into body cavities, is typical of a coagulopathy.

The most common cause of petechiae and ecchymoses in the dog is increased platelet destruction associated with immune-mediated thrombocytopenia (IMT), a disorder in which antibody bound to the surface of the platelet results in premature removal by the reticuloendothelial system. The bone marrow typically has normal to increased numbers of megakaryocytes. However, antibodies may also be directed against the megakaryocytes, resulting in decreased platelet production. Dogs suspected of having IMT should also be evaluated for anemia due to immune-mediated destruction of red cells, proteinuria due to immune-mediated damage to glomeruli, polyarthritis due to immune-mediated inflammatory disease, and vasculitis. If any of these complications exist, systemic lupus erythematosus should be suspected. IMT occurs rarely in cats, but thrombocytopenia may be seen with infectious diseases (especially viral infections), neoplasia, and drug reactions.

Increased sequestration of platelets resulting in thrombocytopenia has been observed in dogs with splenomegaly, hepatomegaly, and endotoxemia, as well as in experimental hypothermia in dogs. However, petechiae and ecchymoses are not typically observed as a result of sequestration of platelets.

TABLE 60–1. CAUSES OF PETECHIAE AND ECCHYMOSES IN DOGS (D) AND CATS (C)

Thrombocytopenia

Decreased platelet production
  Drug
    Albendazole (D)
    Azathioprine (D,C)
    Chemotherapeutic agents (D,C)
    Chloramphenicol (D,C)
    Estrogen (D)
    Griseofulvin (C)
    Meclofenamic acid (D)
    Phenobarbital (D)
    Phenylbutazone (D)
    Trimethoprim-sulfadiazine (D)
  Infection
    Ehrlichia sp.
    Feline leukemia virus
    Feline immunodeficiency virus
    Disseminated histoplasmosis
  Myelophthisis
  Myelofibrosis
  Immune-mediated disorder
    (antimegakaryocytic)
Increased platelet destruction
  Immune-mediated
      thrombocytopenia (IMT)
    Primary
      Idiopathic thrombocytopenic
        purpura (ITP)
      Systemic lupus
        erythematosus (SLE)
    Secondary IMT
      Infection
      Neoplasia
      Vaccine
      Drug
        Sulfonamides (D)
        Cephalosporins (D)
        Gold salts (D)
        Methimazole (C)
        Propylthiouracil (C)
        Dextrans (D)
    Ehrlichia sp.
Increased platelet consumption
  Disseminated intravascular
    coagulation
  Vasculitis
    Infection
      Rickettsia rickettsii
      Leptospira sp
      Ehrlichia sp.
      Feline infectious peritonitis
        virus

  Neoplasia
  Inflammation
  Immune-mediated disorder
  Drug reaction

Thrombopathia

Inherited
  Chédiak-Higashi syndrome of
    Persian cat
  Thrombasthenia of otterhound
  Delta-storage pool disease of
    American cocker spaniel
  Other thrombopathias
    Basset hound
    Spitz
    Grey collies with cyclic
      hematopoiesis
    Domestic shorthair cat
Acquired
  Drug
    Aspirin
    Cephalothin
    Acepromazine
  Systemic disease
    Uremia
    Liver disease
  Hematologic disorders
    IMT
    Myelo-/lymphoproliferative
      disorders
    Dysproteinemia (e.g.,
      multiple myeloma)

Vascular Disorders

Vasculitis (see increased platelet
  consumption)
Hyperadrenocorticism
Dysproteinemia

THROMBOPATHIA

Thrombopathias may be classified as acquired or inherited defects (see Table 60–1). Except for a few hereditary thrombopathias and acquired platelet dysfunctions associated with other hemostatic defects, clinical bleeding is mild and not spontaneous. Platelet function, as assessed by the bleeding-time test and various in vitro tests, may be affected by a large number of drugs and by various systemic and hematologic disorders. Whereas drugs of nearly every classification have been associated with acquired platelet dysfunction in humans, Table 60–1 lists only drugs that have caused thrombopathia in dogs and cats. Platelet dysfunction induced by aspirin, cephalothin, and acepromazine has been documented in vitro, but the in vivo effects of these drugs are less clear. Nevertheless, it is prudent to avoid the use of such drugs in dogs with bleeding disorders. Inherited disorders of platelet function have been identified in several breeds of dogs and in a few cats. Mucosal surface bleeding is a common feature of these disorders, and fatal hemorrhage has been observed in some.

Von Willebrand's disease (vWD), the most common canine inherited bleeding disorder, results from a reduction in the amount of functional plasma von Willebrand factor, leading to impaired platelet-vessel adhesion. vWD rarely causes petechiae, although ecchymoses may be observed in some dogs with vWD following surgical procedures. As with other primary hemostatic defects, typical signs of vWD include bleeding from mucosal surfaces (e.g., epistaxis, melena, hematuria) and excessive bleeding following surgery or trauma.

VASCULAR DISORDERS

In the absence of a quantitative or qualitative platelet abnormality, the presence of purpura suggests a vascular disorder. Vasculitis, secondary to infectious, inflammatory, immune-mediated, or neoplastic diseases or drug reactions, is the most common cause of vascular purpura (see Table 60–1). Some dogs with Cushing's disease also are prone to develop ecchymoses following minor trauma (e.g., cystocentesis), possibly as a result of increased protein catabolism leading to dermal and connective tissue atrophy and thus altered dermal vascular support.

HISTORY AND PHYSICAL EXAMINATION

In a dog or cat presenting with petechiae and/or ecchymoses, the history may provide important clues as to the etiology of the disorder. Given the many possible effects of various drugs on primary hemostasis (bone marrow suppression, IMT, platelet dysfunction, and vasculitis), a complete medication history is imperative. Likewise, recent vaccinations, tick exposure, and previous or concurrent medical problems are relevant. A history of previous episodes of mucosal surface bleeding or purpura in an otherwise healthy animal, or a family history of similar bleeding, may be suggestive of an inherited thrombopathia.

Given that thrombocytopenia, thrombopathia, and vascular disorders may be associated with an underlying disease, a complete physical examination is essential. Peripheral lymphadenopathy, hepatomegaly, and/or splenomegaly may indicate an underlying infectious, inflammatory, or neoplastic disease. Petechiae are most readily seen on mucous membranes of the gingiva, prepuce, and vulva, as well as on sparsely haired skin of the ventral abdomen and pinnae. Following phlebotomy, ecchymoses are commonly observed around the venipuncture site.

DIAGNOSTIC APPROACH (Fig. 60–1)

Because thrombocytopenia is the most common cause of petechiae and ecchymoses, the initial laboratory evaluation should always include a platelet count. Although platelet count determinations are performed quickly and accurately by electronic particle counters in the dog, a blood smear should also be evaluated. However, cell counting instruments with a threshold function to separate platelets and red blood cells (RBCs) by volume may not be accurate in the cat (there is considerable overlap between erythrocyte and platelet volumes), resulting in spuriously low platelet counts. In addition, feline platelets tend to clump. A manual platelet count is recommended for all cats and for dogs in which the automated platelet count is low. In an emergency situation, evaluation of a blood smear to obtain an estimate of platelet number is sufficient; 10 to 20 platelets per oil immersion field is deemed adequate. Platelet counts are often less than 10,000/μL in dogs with IMT. In addition to providing an estimate of platelet number, evaluation of a blood smear may reveal evidence of RBC regeneration (polychromasia, anisocytosis, and macrocytosis), blood parasites, RBC agglutination, spherocytosis, or RBC fragments.

If the dog or cat is thrombocytopenic, evaluation of the complete blood cell count (CBC) to determine whether other cytopenias are present will aid in the formulation of a list of differential diagnoses and a focused diagnostic plan. Pancytopenia is most suggestive of bone marrow disease, whereas concurrent anemia and thrombocytopenia may be the result of blood loss anemia due to thrombocytopenia, immune-mediated destruction of both RBCs and platelets, or bone marrow disease.

A bone marrow aspirate or biopsy is indicated in dogs and cats with pancytopenia, nonregenerative anemia and thrombocytopenia, persistent thrombocytopenia despite therapy, or atypical cells noted in the peripheral blood. A bone marrow aspirate is not necessary in all dogs with IMT but should be considered when the platelet count has not increased within 5 to 7 days of initiating immune-suppressive therapy. Despite severe thrombocytopenia, excessive bleeding is rarely a complication of bone marrow aspiration or biopsy.

The buccal mucosal bleeding time (BMBT) evaluates only primary hemostasis or the platelet-vessel interaction. A BMBT is indicated in animals with petechiae and ecchymoses that are not thrombocytopenic. The BMBT is performed using a spring-loaded device that is standardized to produce uniform incisions. Simplate devices (Organon Technika Corp., Durham, NC) are available with one or two blades and produce incisions approximately 5 mm long and 1 mm deep (do not use blades with only 0.5 mm depth). Single-blade devices are recommended for cats and small dogs. To perform a BMBT, the animal is placed in lateral recumbency, and the upper lip is everted to expose the buccal mucosa and secured with gauze tied tightly enough around the muzzle to impair venous return, resulting in slight congestion of the mucous membranes. The device is placed against the mucosa horizontal to the lip, the blade is released, and timing begins. Filter paper or a gauze square is positioned 2 to 3 mm below the incision to blot shed blood from the mucosa, being careful not to touch the incision. Normal BMBT in the dog is less than 4 minutes and in the cat is less than 2 minutes. A prolongation of the BMBT in an animal with a normal platelet count suggests thrombopathia, vWD, or a vascular disorder. Because vWD is much more common in the dog than intrinsic platelet function defects or vascular disorders, measurement of plasma von Willebrand factor concentration is recommended before platelet function testing, particularly in dogs being evaluated for development of ecchymoses following surgery rather than spontaneous formation of petechiae.

The clot retraction assay may crudely suggest a platelet dysfunction in practice, but platelet aggregation and secretion studies are needed to define such defects.

The cuticle bleeding time assesses both primary and secondary hemostasis and thus cannot differentiate between a thrombopathia and a coagulopathy. In addition, clipping the nail too short is painful, and it is difficult to standardize this bleeding-time test, potentially providing misleading results. Therefore, the BMBT is preferred to the cuticle bleeding time in the evaluation of animals with suspected disorders of primary hemostasis.

An activated clotting time (ACT), which assesses the intrinsic and common pathways of the coagulation cascade and thus provides similar information to the activated partial thromboplastin time (aPTT), is useful in ruling out a concurrent coagulopathy. Normal ACT in the dog is 60 to 110 seconds and in the cat is 50 to 75 seconds. In animals with severe thrombocytopenia ($< 10,000/μL$), the ACT may be slightly prolonged by approximately 10 seconds because of decreased availability of platelet phospholipid to support coagulation.

TREATMENT

Medical management of dogs or cats with petechiae and ecchymoses varies widely. Treatment is aimed at the underlying disorder (e.g., rickettsial infections, neoplasia, immune-mediated diseases). Most thrombocytopenic dogs should be initially treated with doxycycline and prednisone. Discontinuation of medications (e.g., methimazole) may be all that is necessary to resolve the primary hemostatic disorder.

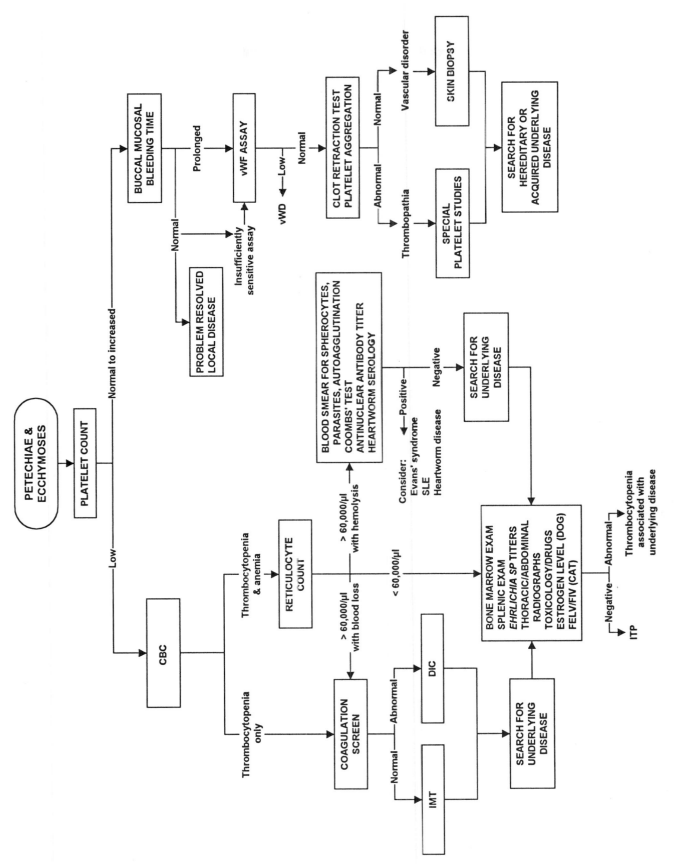

Figure 60–1. Algorithm for diagnostic approach to petechiae and ecchymoses.

Dogs and cats presenting with petechiae and ecchymoses as the sole form of bleeding rarely require blood transfusion support. However, if there is concurrent mucosal surface bleeding, particularly into the gastrointestinal tract, leading to anemia, transfusion of packed RBCs may be indicated to provide additional oxygen-carrying support. Platelet transfusions in the form of fresh whole blood, platelet-rich plasma, or platelet concentrate are indicated in life-threatening or uncontrolled bleeding. A small amount of bleeding into the brain, myocardium, lungs, or oropharynx could have devastating consequences without resulting in anemia. Platelet transfusions are generally not recommended in animals with IMT (unless there is uncontrolled or life-threatening bleeding) because the transfused platelets will immediately be covered with antibodies and therefore have a short life span (minutes to hours).

CHAPTER 61

HYPONATREMIA AND HYPOKALEMIA

Yonatan Peres

HYPONATREMIA

Hyponatremia is defined as a serum concentration of sodium below reference limits (usually <140 mEq/L). Serum sodium concentrations reflect the relative amount of sodium to water in extracellular fluid. Therefore, hyponatremia should be regarded as a disorder of water balance rather than sodium balance.

CAUSES (Table 61–1)

Hyponatremia is usually associated with hypo-osmolality, because sodium is the major determinant of plasma osmolality. The animal may be hypovolemic (dehydrated), normovolemic, or hypervolemic (overhydrated). Hyponatremia can also be documented in dogs or cats that are hyperosmolar or euosmolar (pseudohyponatremia).

Hypo-osmolar Hyponatremia

Hypovolemia

Solute loss can lead to volume depletion and decreased effective circulating plasma volume. Solute loss is most commonly a result of vomiting or diarrhea. Other causes of solute loss include third space losses; cutaneous losses; or renal loss owing to renal failure, use of diuretics, or hypoadrenocorticism. In most cases, solute and fluid losses do not significantly decrease serum sodium concentrations. Hyponatremia and hypo-osmolality occur if losses are replaced with hypotonic fluid, such as water, or if the ability of the kidneys to excrete free water is impaired.

Nonrenal Loss. Gastrointestinal disease, third space losses, and fluid loss via cutaneous lesions may result in dehydration and volume depletion. In order to maintain plasma volume, in spite of the hypo-osmolality, antidiuretic hormone (ADH) release is stimulated. The ADH inhibits free water excretion via the kidney. The result is hypo-osmolar hyponatremia. In severe volume depletion, the delivery of solute to the distal tubule is compromised, which further limits loss of water.

Renal Loss. In dogs or cats with renal disease, decreases in glomevular filtration rate, as well as solute losses owing to vomiting or diarrhea, can cause hypo-osmolar hyponatremia. Hyponatremia may also occur with diuretic therapy through similar mechanisms. In hypoadrenocorticism, aldosterone deficiency causes renal and gastrointestinal sodium loss as

---

TABLE 61–1. CAUSES OF HYPONATREMIA

Hypo-osmolar Hyponatremia

Hypovolemia
  Gastrointestinal loss
  Third space loss
  Cutaneous loss (e.g., burns)
  Hypoadrenocorticism
  Renal disease, failure
  Diuresis
Normovolemia
  SIADH
  Primary polydipsia
  Severe hypothyroidism
Hypervolemia
  Congestive heart failure
  Liver disease
  Renal disease
  Nephrotic syndrome

Hyperosmolar Hyponatremia

Diabetes mellitus
Mannitol infusion

Euosmolar Hyponatremia (Pseudohyponatremia)

Hyperproteinemia
Lipemia

well as dehydration. Usually the hyponatremia is accompanied by hyperkalemia.

Hypervolemia

Inadequate tissue perfusion can lead to decreased effective circulating plasma volume. Hypervolemic states with concurrent inadequate tissue perfusion can be caused by congestive heart failure, liver disease, nephrotic syndrome, or oliguric renal failure. Factors that contribute to volume depletion in these states include decreased cardiac output, decreased oncotic pressure owing to hypoalbuminemia, decreased renal perfusion, arteriovenous shunting, splanchnic venous pooling, portal hypertension, and ascites. These factors stimulate ADH release and activate the renin-angiotensin-aldosterone system. Sodium is retained, and solute delivery to the distal renal tubule is decreased. Sodium retention and impaired water excretion result. In spite of an increase in total body sodium content, hyponatremia may develop.

Normovolemia

Increased concentrations of endogenous ADH and primary polydipsia can cause hyponatremia. The syndrome of inappropriate ADH secretion (SIADH) is rare in small animals but has been reported in dogs with dirofilariasis and hypothalamic neoplasia. The syndrome is characterized by excess ADH unrelated to any osmotic or volume stimuli. Retention of ingested water inhibits aldosterone secretion, leads to loss of sodium in the urine, and limits expansion of the plasma volume. Cyclophosphamide, vincristine, barbiturates, and chlorpropamide may stimulate ADH release or potentiate its action. Administration of exogenous ADH may also result in water retention and hyponatremia.

Primary (psychogenic) polydipsia is a behavioral abnormality. Extremely excessive water intake may impair the ability of the kidney to excrete free water, resulting in hyponatremia.

Hyperosmolar Hyponatremia

Hyperosmolar hyponatremia can occur secondary to severe hyperglycemia in diabetes mellitus or the administration of hypertonic solutions such as mannitol. Shifting of water from the intracellular fluid (ICF) to the extracellular fluid (ECF) results in dilutional hyponatremia.

Euosmolar Hyponatremia (Pseudohyponatremia)

Pseudohyponatremia is secondary to severe hyperlipidemia or hyperproteinemia. The sodium concentration in the aqueous phase of the plasma and the osmolality are unchanged.

CLINICAL SIGNS

Major clinical signs in hyponatremic dogs or cats are usually those of the underlying condition. The clinical signs of hyponatremia depend on the degree and rate of decrease. Mild hyponatremia may not cause clinical signs. Clinical signs are not usually observed until the serum sodium concentration falls below 125 mEq/L, when weakness, depression, confusion, nausea, vomiting, seizures, and coma may be observed. Acute decreases are more likely to be associated with severe signs than are slow, chronic decreases. Shifting of water from ECF to ICF results in cellular swelling and cerebral edema.

DIAGNOSIS

The clinical approach to the diagnosis and treatment of hyponatremia is shown in Figure 61–1. The initial diagnosis of the underlying cause should be based on history and physical examination findings. Hydration status is important. Hyperosmolar and euosmolar hyponatremia can be ruled in or out by measuring the levels of protein, lipids, and glucose. Further diagnostic tests may be needed to determine the underlying cause. The measurement of serum osmolality is often quite helpful in determining which intravenous fluids to use in therapy. Serum osmolality can be measured directly, using an osmometer, or calculated using the following formula:

$$2 \left([Na] + [K]\right) + \frac{glucose}{18} + \frac{blood\ urea\ nitrogen}{2.8}$$

TREATMENT

Effort should be made to determine and correct the underlying cause. The initial treatment for a dehydrated or volume-depleted animal is fluid replacement with isotonic sodium chloride solution. Overhydrated animals may be treated with diuretics, as needed. Hyponatremia in dogs or cats with normal effective circulating volume, in cases of SIADH or primary polydipsia, can be controlled by restricting water intake and correcting the underlying cause.

Dogs or cats with severe hyponatremia, associated with neurologic signs, may be treated with hypertonic saline (3 per cent NaCl). The rate at which hyponatremia should be corrected is controversial. The following formula is used to calculate the amount of sodium required to return the sodium concentration to normal:

$$Na\ deficit\ (mEq/L) = 0.6 \times body\ weight\ (kg) \times (140\text{-}Na)\ (mEq/L)$$

HYPOKALEMIA

Hypokalemia is defined as a serum potassium concentration below reference limits for the laboratory used (usually <3.5 mEq/L). Potassium balance is normally maintained by matching input from the diet to output through the urinary and gastrointestinal tracts. Serum potassium balance, in acute changes, is maintained by translocation of potassium from the intracellular space to the extracellular fluid. In general, hypokalemia caused by a shift of potassium from ECF to ICF is associated with metabolic acidosis.

CAUSES

Hypokalemia can result from anorexia, vomiting, diarrhea, or renal losses. Hypokalemia can also result from translocation of this electrolyte from ECF to ICF. Causes of hypokalemia are listed in Table 61–2.

External Balance

Decreased Intake. Hypokalemia is usually not caused solely by decreased dietary intake. Hypokalemia usually

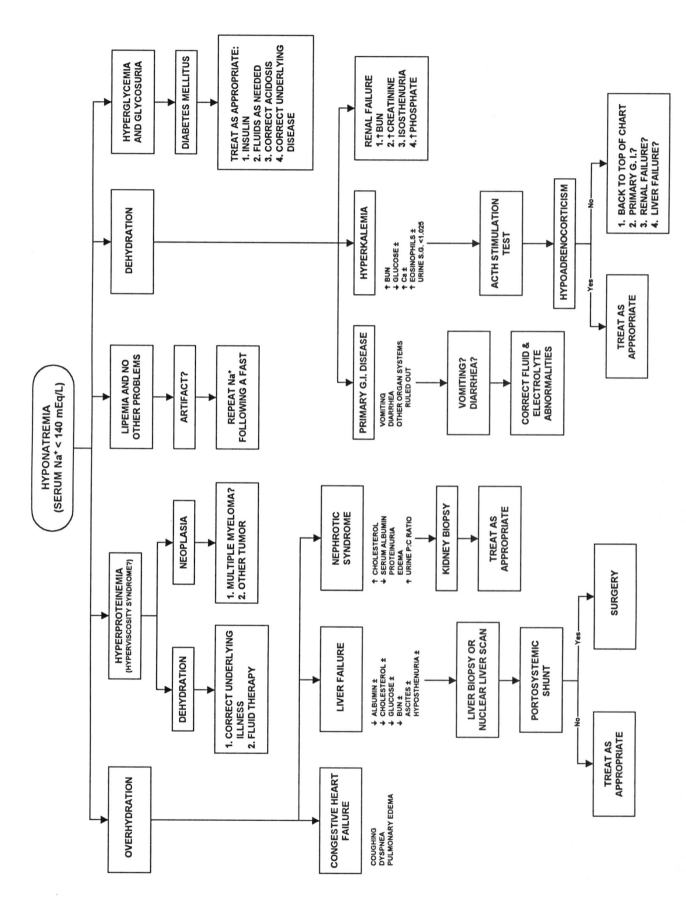

Figure 61–1. Algorithm for differential diagnosis and management of hyponatremia.

TABLE 61–2. CAUSES OF HYPOKALEMIA

Decreased Intake

  Anorexia (unlikely alone)
  Administration of intravenous fluids that contain little or no potassium

Increased Loss

  Renal
    Chronic renal failure
    Hypokalemic nephropathy in cats
    Renal tubular acidosis
    Postobstructive diuresis
    Polyuric phase of acute renal failure
    Dialysis
    Hyperaldosteronism (primary; secondary due to liver insufficiency,
      congestive heart failure, nephrotic syndrome)
    Hyperadrenocorticism
    Diuretics
    Renal glycosuria
    Hyperglycemia
    Fanconi's syndrome
    Drugs
  Gastrointestinal
    Vomiting, diarrhea
    Enemas
    Hyperthyroidism
  Translocation
    Alkalemia (e.g., bicarbonate therapy)
    Insulin therapy
    Catecholamines
    Hypokalemic periodic paralysis
    Hypothermia
    Diabetic ketoacidosis
    Hypomagnesemia
  Pseudohypokalemia
    Hyperlipidemia
    Hyperproteinemia
    Hyperglycemia
    Azotemia

results from a combination of prolonged anorexia, vomiting, diarrhea, and urinary losses. Anorexic hospitalized dogs or cats receiving intravenous fluids low in potassium (0.9 per cent NaCl, 5 per cent dextrose, lactated Ringer's) may become hypokalemic. Appropriate supplementation of intravenous fluids is imperative.

Gastrointestinal Loss. The most common cause of hypokalemia is loss due to vomiting, usually associated with metabolic alkalosis, or diarrhea, associated with metabolic acidosis. Further losses of sodium and chloride due to volume depletion enhance urinary losses of potassium and hydrogen. Repeated enemas may also cause potassium depletion.

Renal Loss. Hypokalemia due to chronic renal failure is more common in cats than in dogs. Renal tubular acidosis (RTA) is much less common. Type I (distal) RTA is associated with an increase in aldosterone secretion, leading to urinary loss. In type II (proximal) RTA, urinary loss is a result of large doses of sodium bicarbonate, administered to correct acidosis.

Cats fed on diets that are low in potassium and that contain urinary acidifiers may develop hypokalemic nephropathy. This syndrome is characterized by chronic tubulointerstitial nephritis. Hypokalemia is common in cats with postobstructive diuresis. This is most likely to be severe during the first 24 to 72 hours following relief of urinary obstruction. Hypokalemia may also be recognized in dogs or cats in the polyuric phase of acute renal failure.

Primary hyperaldosteronism is rare in dogs but has been reported in a few dogs with aldosterone-secreting adrenal tumors. Hypomagnesemia can enhance secretion of aldosterone, resulting in hypokalemia. Dogs with hyperadrenocorticism rarely have severe hypokalemia due to excess glucocorticoids and mineralocorticoids. However, low-normal or mildly decreased serum potassium concentrations are common. Administration of loop or thiazide diuretics increases flow rate in the distal tubules, and, secondary to volume depletion, aldosterone secretion is increased. As a result, hypokalemia may occur, although it is usually mild.

Hyperglycemia and glucosuria in diabetes mellitus induce osmotic diuresis with enhanced renal loss of potassium. These potassium losses can become severe and life-threatening, especially in ketoacidosis, with its associated anorexia, vomiting, and diarrhea.

Renal loss of potassium has been described in a disease in basenji dogs, similar to Fanconi's syndrome, and in dogs with renal glycosuria. Administration of various drugs may cause hypokalemia. Penicillin derivatives may increase potassium secretion in the distal tubules. Amphotericin B may cause hypokalemia owing to increasing permeability of cell membranes. Peritoneal dialysis can cause hypokalemia if potassium-free dialysate is used for extended periods.

Internal Balance

Hypokalemia may occur as a result of translocation of potassium from ECF to ICF. In alkalemia, potassium ions enter the cells in exchange for hydrogen ions. Insulin release or administration drives glucose and potassium into the cells, potentially resulting in hypokalemia if the dog or cat is anorexic or has vomiting and diarrhea. Catecholamines in stress can cause hypokalemia. Hypothermia may be another cause of hypokalemia, due to potassium shift into cells. A syndrome similar to hypokalemic periodic paralysis in humans has been reported in young Burmese cats. This syndrome is thought to be due to episodes of sudden translocation of potassium from ECF to ICF.

Pseudohypokalemia

The measurement of potassium by flame photometry and ion-selective potentiometry is reliable. Pseudohypokalemia may be secondary to severe hyperlipidemia, hyperproteinemia, hyperglycemia, or azotemia, if a laboratory uses dry reagent methods (less common with flame photometry). The concentration of potassium in the aqueous phase of the plasma remains unchanged. These considerations are irrelevant when direct potentiometry methods are used.

CLINICAL SIGNS

Most dogs and cats with mild hypokalemia have no clinical signs. However, as serum potassium concentrations decrease below 3 mEq/L, signs become obvious and include generalized muscular weakness, impaired gastrointestinal motility with ileus and constipation, decreased myocardial contractility and cardiac arrhythmias, and polyuria-polydipsia. Young Burmese cats (4 to 12 months old) with hypokalemic periodic paralysis have recurrent episodes of limb muscle weakness and neck ventroflection. Chronic depletion of potassium results in growth retardation, weight loss, and poor haircoat.

DIAGNOSIS

The clinical approach to the diagnosis and treatment of hypokalemia is shown in the Figure 61–2. The initial diagno-

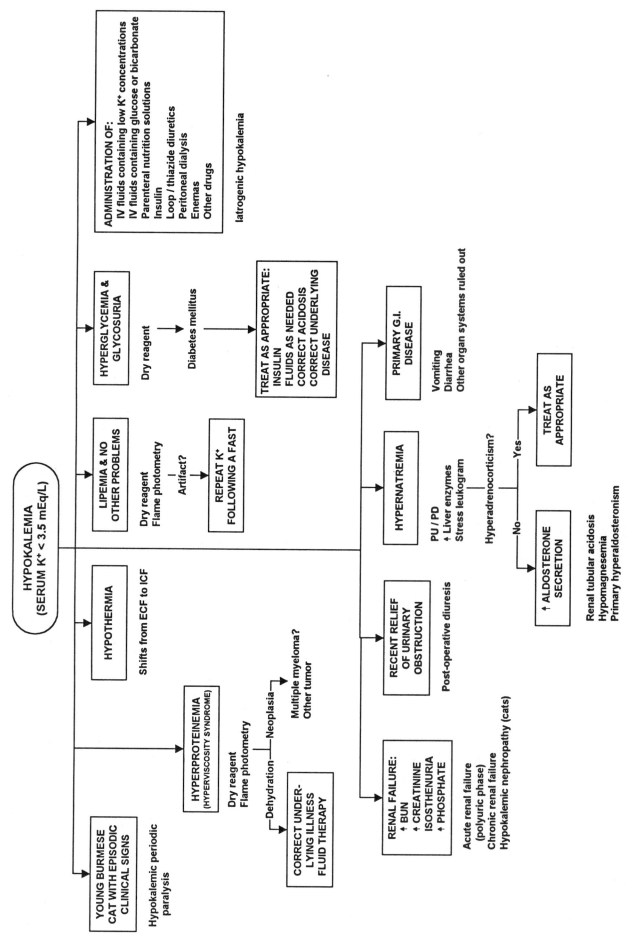

Figure 61-2. Algorithm for differential diagnosis and management of hypokalemia.

sis of the underlying cause is based on the history and physical examination findings. Pseudohypokalemia, if using flame photometry or dry reagent methods, may be ruled out by measuring levels of protein, lipids, glucose, and blood urea nitrogen.

Determination of the fractional excretion of potassium (FEk) may help differentiate renal from nonrenal sources of potassium loss. FEk can be calculated using the following formula:

$$\frac{Uk/Sk \ (mEq/L)}{Ucr/Scr} \times 100,$$

where Uk is the urine concentration of potassium, Sk is the serum concentration of potassium, Ucr is the urine concentration of creatinine, and Scr is the serum concentration of creatinine. FEk values up to 6 per cent are considered normal in potassium-depleted animals with normal renal function. FEk values above 6 per cent may indicate inappropriate renal loss.

Hypokalemia prolongs the ventricular action potential and delays the ventricular repolarization of the myocardium. Electrocardiogram abnormalities include prolonged Q-T interval, decreased amplitude of T wave, depression of S-T segment, appearance of U waves, and premature contractions.

TREATMENT

Treatment consists of determination and correction of the underlying disease, together with potassium supplementation. The treatment of choice is intravenous administration of potassium chloride (KCl). The rate of infusion should not exceed 0.5 mEq/kg/hour, to avoid potential adverse cardiac effects. The concentration of potassium in the infused fluid should not exceed 60 mEq/L, to avoid pain and sclerosis of the veins. Oral supplementation should be initiated as soon as possible. The preparation of choice is potassium gluconate. The oral dose for dogs is 2 to 44 mEq/day, depending on body size, and 2 to 4 mEq/day for cats.

CHAPTER 62

HYPERKALEMIA AND HYPERNATREMIA

Michael Schaer

HYPERKALEMIA

Hyperkalemia is defined as a serum potassium concentration exceeding approximately 5.5 mEq/L. Concentrations in excess of 7.5 mEq/L are particularly dangerous, especially with respect to cardiac function, because this degree of hyperkalemia causes neuromuscular cell membrane depolarization, with impairment of excitation and conduction. Because severe hyperkalemia is life-threatening, clinicians must remain vigilant to successfully treat the condition.

CAUSES

Hyperkalemia has three main causes: increased intake, decreased excretion, and increased transfer from the intracellular to the extracellular space. Some causes are listed in Table 62–1. In the dog and cat, hyperkalemia is most commonly associated with acute oliguric renal failure, urinary outflow obstruction, and adrenocortical insufficiency. Pseudohyperkalemia, such as occurs in the Akita dog, should be recognized to avoid needless diagnostic effort and treatment expense. Although metabolic acidosis is commonly associated with a compartmental shift of potassium from the intracellular to the extracellular space, this tendency is usually restricted to conditions in which inorganic ion accumulations associated with metabolic acidosis are the main cause. Respiratory acidosis produces little or no effect.

EFFECTS ON THE ANIMAL

Physical Examination Findings

The most important signs associated with hyperkalemia are muscular weakness and myocardial abnormalities, which may not be evident until the serum potassium level exceeds 7 mEq/L. The skeletal muscle weakness is typically diffuse. In contrast to the detrimental effects of hypernatremia on the central nervous system, hyperkalemia's effect concentrates mainly on the peripheral neuromuscular tissues. Hyperkalemic dogs and cats may have bradycardia and palpably weak pulses. Cardiac arrest can occur in the advanced stages of hyperkalemia.

Electrocardiographic Changes

Life-threatening hyperkalemia, owing to its effect on the myocardium when serum levels exceed 7.5 mEq/L, initially increases myocardial excitability but subsequently depresses

TABLE 62–1. CAUSES OF HYPERKALEMIA

Pseudohyperkalemia

Hemolyzed blood sample associated with poor collection technique*,†
Thrombocytosis* (as seen in Cushing's disease)
Extreme leukocytosis

Redistribution of Potassium

Metabolic acidosis*
Hypertonic solutions
Hyperkalemic periodic paralysis (very rare)
Drugs
    Prostaglandin inhibitors
    Beta-blocking agents
    Succinylcholine

Potassium Loading

Endogenous
    Hemolysis (rare in the dog and cat)
    Rhabdomyolysis (rare without renal failure)
Exogenous
    Potassium salts* (when infused K^+ exceeds a rate of 0.5–1.0 mEq/kg
        body weight/hour)

Reduced Potassium Excretion

Acute renal failure* (oliguric, anuric)
    Urinary outflow obstruction*
    Urinary bladder rupture*
Hypoadrenocorticism*
Primary hypoaldosteronism
Effective circulating volume depletion (any illness causing marked
    hypovolemia)
Drugs
    Potassium-sparing diuretics
    Converting enzyme inhibitors
    Nonsteroidal anti-inflammatory agents

Other

Hyperkalemia associated with pleural effusion
Hyperkalemia associated with trichuriasis

*Common cause in the dog and cat.
†Red blood cells in the Akita dog contain higher-than-usual amounts of potassium.

both excitability and conduction velocity secondary to persistent depolarization and inactivation of the sodium channels within the cell membranes. Typical progressive electrocardiographic alterations include peaking or depression of the T wave, decreased R-wave and P-wave amplitudes, increased duration of the P wave, prolongation of the PR interval, eventual disappearance of the P wave, widening of the QRS complex, and sine wave–type QRS complexes. When the serum potassium concentration exceeds 8 to 9 mEq/L, the impaired conduction can result in heart blocks, idioventricular complexes, ventricular escape beats, and eventually ventricular fibrillation or asystole.

DIAGNOSIS

An attempt to identify hyperkalemia in any dog or cat should be prompted by the clinical presentation (Fig. 62–1). In any animal showing signs of mental depression, generalized muscular weakness, and dehydration in the setting of oliguria, anuria, urinary outflow obstruction, or gastrointestinal signs of vomiting, diarrhea, and anorexia, hyperkalemia should be suspected. These latter signs are also compatible with adrenocortical insufficiency (see Chapter 155).

Although laboratory quantitation is ideal for the diagnosis of hyperkalemia, many clinical situations do not allow for immediate access to serum electrolyte assessment. Therefore, clinicians must have an index of suspicion for the presence of hyperkalemia in the appropriate clinical settings. Alternatively, clinicians should obtain a lead II electrocardiogram (ECG) in an attempt to identify characteristic changes in any ill animal when immediate serum or plasma electrolyte analysis is not available. Not every hyperkalemic dog and cat has characteristic ECG alterations, but their occurrence is common, helping to establish a tentative diagnosis and to justify emergency treatment.

TREATMENT GOALS

Treatment should be aimed at correcting the underlying disorder as well as immediately reversing any myocardial abnormalities observed on the ECG. If the ECG is normal, treatment with intravenous isotonic saline solution is sufficient if the animal's urine output is normal or increased. In more urgent situations characterized by marked ECG abnormalities, additional treatment measures (Table 62–2) may be necessary to decrease the serum potassium concentration or to counteract its adverse effects. Ideally, 20 to 40 minutes of aggressive intravenous saline administration should precede ancillary measures directed at hyperkalemia. The prognosis for hyperkalemia is good if the appropriate treatment measures are instituted in a timely manner and the underlying cause is reversible.

HYPERNATREMIA

Hypernatremia is defined as a serum sodium concentration exceeding 155 mEq/L. Because serum sodium concentrations vary inversely with the amount of total body water, it is anticipated that hypernatremia will occur most often when hypotonic fluid losses are combined with a disturbance in water intake. It is less frequently associated with excessive sodium intake.

CAUSES

Hypernatremia can develop with deficient, normal, or excessive amounts of total body sodium. Hypernatremia can be further categorized as hypovolemic, isovolemic, or hypervolemic (Table 62–3). Animals suffering from a deficiency of sodium and a relatively greater loss of water may have hypernatremia despite low total body amounts of sodium. In dogs and cats, extrarenal loss of hypotonic fluid occurs most frequently as a result of diarrhea. Hypotonic losses can also follow osmotic diuresis due to diabetes mellitus, or the administration of mannitol, or urea. The hypotonic losses that accompany uremia may explain the hypernatremia that follows relief of urinary obstruction in tomcats being treated with intravenous isotonic saline. Because glucose enhances osmotic movement of water from the intracellular to the extracellular fluid compartment, some hyperglycemic dogs or cats have a normal or low serum sodium concentration in spite of serum hypertonicity.

Loss of free water without loss of electrolytes such as sodium, as seen in dogs or cats with diabetes insipidus (DI), does not result in severe plasma volume contraction unless intake of water is restricted. Water-deprived animals with DI may rapidly undergo cellular hypertonicity because of water transfer from the intracellular to the extracellular space. It is because of this intercompartmental transfer of water that dogs and cats often retain adequate skin turgor despite detrimental amounts of fluid volume loss. Eventually, however,

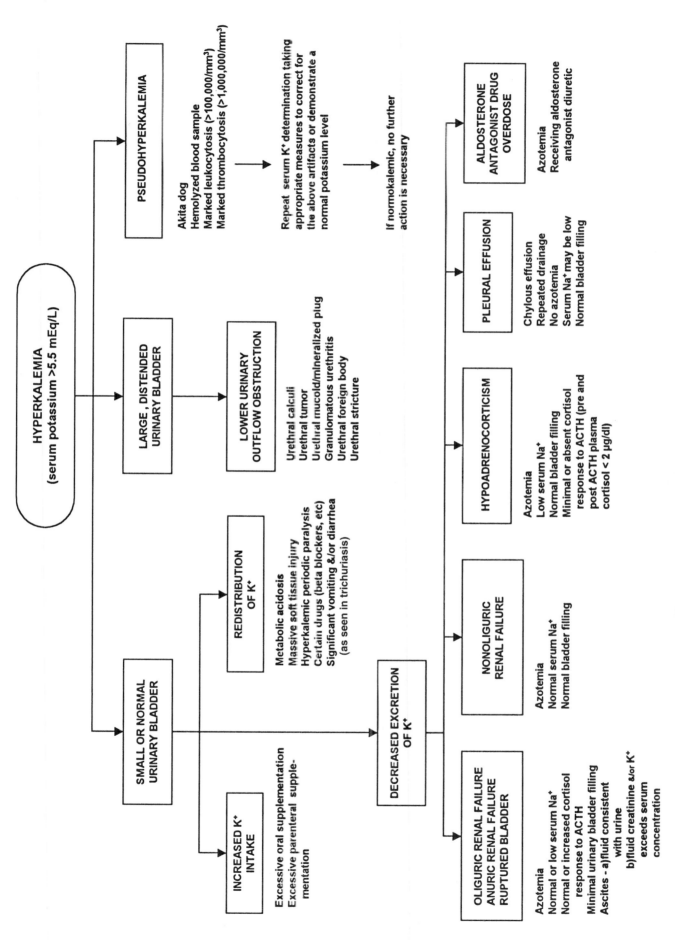

Figure 62–1. Algorithm for differential diagnosis and management of hyperkalemia.

TABLE 62–2. PRINCIPLES OF TREATING HYPERKALEMIA

OBJECTIVE	METHOD
Enhancing potassium excretion	Relieve any urinary tract obstruction Intravenous isotonic saline Cation exchange resin Peritoneal or hemodialysis
Intercompartmental transfer	Intravenous sodium bicarbonate Intravenous insulin and glucose combination Intravenous glucose alone
Counteract myocardial cell membrane toxicity	Intravenous 10 per cent calcium gluconate

continued diuresis in the absence of water intake leads to severe hypernatremia, plasma volume contraction, hypotension, renal ischemia, and renal shutdown.

Essential hypernatremia, a failure of the hypothalamic osmoreceptors to respond appropriately to an increase in serum osmolality, is rare in dogs and cats. There is usually an adequate antidiuretic hormone response to hypovolemia. These dogs and cats are neither polydipsic nor polyuric; characteristically, they are adipsic.

EFFECTS ON THE ANIMAL

The main physiologic effect of hypernatremia is the formation of a hypertonic extracellular fluid environment. As plasma hypertonicity progresses, water moves from the intracellular to the extracellular compartment, resulting in cellular dehydration. These adverse effects are particularly evident in the brain. Hypovolemia eventually occurs when hypotonic fluid losses exceed water intake.

TABLE 62–3. CAUSES OF HYPERNATREMIA

HYPERNATREMIA ASSOCIATED WITH WATER LOSS	HYPERNATREMIA ASSOCIATED WITH SALT GAIN
Pure Water Loss—Isovolemia	*Water Loss With High Urine Sodium—Hypervolemia*

Normal total body Na+ and normal ECF volume
  Pituitary diabetes insipidus
  Nephrogenic diabetes insipidus
  Heatstroke
  Fever
  Inadequate access to water (CNS disease, infirmity)
  Burns
  Essential hypernatremia
	Increased total body Na+ and increased ECF volume
	  Increased salt intake
	  Dietary
	  Sea water
	  Saline emetics
	  IV hypertonic fluids
	  IV sodium bicarbonate
	  Hyperaldosteronism
	  Hyperadrenocorticism

Hypotonic Water Loss—Hypovolemia	

Decreased total body Na+ and decreased ECF volume
  Diarrhea
  Vomiting
  Oral hyperalimentation
  Osmotic diuresis
    Acute renal failure
    Chronic renal failure
    Diabetes mellitus
    Diuretic use
    IV solute administration (mannitol, glucose, urea)	

ECF = extracellular fluid; CNS = central nervous system; IV = intravenous.
Modified from Hardy RM: Hypernatremia. Vet Clin North Am 19:231–239, 1989.

In the brain, movement of water out of cells and down the osmotic gradient created by the rise in the effective plasma osmolality leads to decreased volume and rupture of cerebral veins, resulting in focal intracerebral and subarachnoid hemorrhages. These changes are dramatic with acute-onset hypernatremia. Venous sinus thrombosis also can occur. The resulting neurologic dysfunction may be irreversible. The clinical signs include restlessness, irritability, lethargy, muscular twitching, spasticity, seizures, coma, and death.

When the onset of hypertonicity is gradual, the brain counteracts osmotic dysequilibrium and shrinkage by forming and accumulating substances known as idiogenic osmols, or osmolytes. These idiogenic osmols are assumed to attempt to restore or maintain cell volume. This compensatory mechanism is of limited benefit if hypertonicity is not corrected, but it explains why some animals with chronic hypernatremia can be asymptomatic.

Hypernatremic dogs and cats with low total body sodium and hypotonic fluid loss exhibit signs of hypovolemia: weakness, lethargy, tachycardia, palpably weak pulses, prolonged capillary refill time, and decreased skin turgor. With extreme hypovolemia, renal ischemia may occur, causing acute tubular necrosis and renal failure.

Hypernatremia caused by sodium loading is uncommon, and it causes extracellular fluid overload as well as cellular dehydration. This overload on the cardiovascular system can cause peripheral edema and, eventually, pulmonary edema due to congestive heart failure. Neurologic signs similar to those already described can also occur. There are no characteristic ECG abnormalities associated with hypernatremia.

DIAGNOSIS

Hypernatremia is typically a serendipitous finding in the assessment of an ill dog or cat (Fig. 62–2). The presence or absence of normal skin turgor varies with the cause. Those conditions of hypotonic fluid loss and decreased total body sodium exhibit decreased skin turgor and hypovolemia. These dogs and cats have normal renal capacity to conserve water and sodium, allowing them to form hypertonic urine with a low sodium concentration.

Water-deprived dogs and cats with DI retain normal skin turgor until the advanced stages of water depletion. By this phase, severe renal ischemia has already occurred. Characteristically, these animals have hyperosmolar plasma and hypoosmolar urine, and eventually they become azotemic, acidotic, and anuric. Never deprive these animals of water overnight without monitoring.

Dogs and cats with essential hypernatremia usually have gradual-onset hypernatremia and normal skin turgor. Neurologic signs might not occur until serum sodium concentrations exceed 175 mEq/L. Azotemia is not typical, but hypertonic plasma and retention of the ability to concentrate urine should be expected. Those animals whose hypernatremia is due to excess sodium intake can also concentrate their urine, which typically contains large quantities of sodium.

Hypernatremia is diagnosed by laboratory sodium quantitation. The serum chloride is invariably elevated as well, because it is sodium's obligate extracellular anion. Serum hyperosmolality (normal, 290 to 310 mOsm/L) can be calculated using the formula:

$$2\left([Na] + [K]\right) + \frac{glucose}{18} + \frac{BUN}{2.8}$$

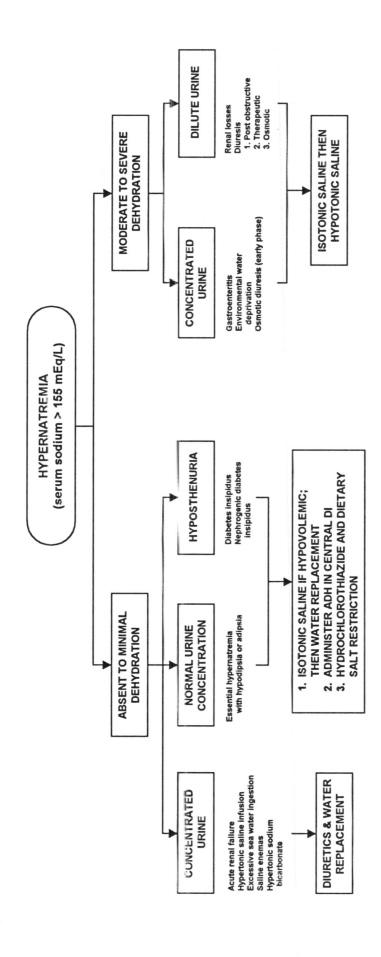

Figure 62–2. Algorithm for differential diagnosis and management of hypernatremia.

HYPERNATREMIA
(serum sodium > 155 mEq/L)

ABSENT TO MINIMAL DEHYDRATION

MODERATE TO SEVERE DEHYDRATION

CONCENTRATED URINE

Acute renal failure
Hypertonic saline infusion
Excessive sea water ingestion
Saline enemas
Hypertonic sodium bicarbonate

DIURETICS & WATER REPLACEMENT

NORMAL URINE CONCENTRATION

Essential hypernatremia with hypodipsia or adipsia

HYPOSTHENURIA

Diabetes insipidus
Nephrogenic diabetes insipidus

1. ISOTONIC SALINE IF HYPOVOLEMIC; THEN WATER REPLACEMENT
2. ADMINISTER ADH IN CENTRAL DI
3. HYDROCHLOROTHIAZIDE AND DIETARY SALT RESTRICTION

CONCENTRATED URINE

Gastroenteritis
Environmental water deprivation
Osmotic diuresis (early phase)

DILUTE URINE

Renal losses
Diuresis
1. Post obstructive
2. Therapeutic
3. Osmotic

ISOTONIC SALINE THEN HYPOTONIC SALINE

where Na+ and K+ are measured in mEq/L. Alternatively, it can be measured by the freezing point depression technique using an osmometer.

TREATMENT GOALS

Readers are referred to Chapter 148 for details on treatment. When a dog or cat has decreases in total body sodium as evidenced by hypovolemia, isotonic sodium chloride solution should be administered until hemodynamic stability is restored. Once this is accomplished, intravenous fluids can be changed as required by the individual. Acute-onset symptomatic hypernatremia can be treated with intravenous fluids. The goal is a decline of serum sodium approximating 1 mEq/L per hour. Chronic hypernatremia, however, must be treated slowly, so that the rate of decline of serum sodium does not exceed 0.5 mEq/L per hour (12 mEq/day). Rapid lowering may lead to severe neurologic consequences. Seizure control can be accomplished by administering diazepam, phenobarbital, or pentobarbital. The comatose dog or cat requires meticulous care, with special attention to the skin, urinary bladder, and airway. Urine output should be closely monitored. Anuria is an ominous sign, and restoration of urine production may require dialysis.

Hypernatremia caused by excessive sodium intake should be treated with furosemide to promote sodium excretion. Cautious administration of 5 per cent dextrose solution should also be used in the absence of dehydration and hypovolemia. Dogs and cats with essential hypernatremia require extra water added to their food to compensate for their adipsia. This is done by feeding a balanced canned food ration mixed with the animal's daily water requirements. Food and water requirements should be provided in divided portions over each 24-hour period.

The prognosis for acute hypernatremia is guarded owing to its adverse effects on the brain. Timely, appropriate treatment, along with a reversible underlying disease process, can result in an improved prognosis.

CHAPTER 63

ABNORMALITIES OF MAGNESIUM, CALCIUM, AND CHLORIDE

Lisa K. Kurosky

MAGNESIUM

Over the past decade, the role of magnesium in homeostasis and disease has received increasing attention. In people, magnesium has been implicated as an important factor in the development of atherosclerosis, hypertension, arrhythmias resulting in sudden cardiac death, thrombosis causing ischemic heart disease, and diabetes mellitus due to insulin resistance. The role of magnesium is being evaluated in critical care patients and sports medicine. In veterinary medicine, a syndrome of hypomagnesemic tetany (grass tetany) has long been recognized in cattle.

Physiology. Magnesium is the most abundant intracellular divalent cation. It is an important cofactor for various enzymes, including those of oxidative phosphorylation, and can influence the activity of adenyl cyclase. Magnesium helps maintain normal cardiac electrical physiology as it modulates several types of calcium channels and potassium currents within cardiac cells. Approximately 1 per cent of total body magnesium exists in a diffusible form in the extracellular fluid. Serum magnesium ranges between 1.8 and 2.5 mg/dL in both humans and dogs (normals not established for cats). The remaining 99 per cent of body magnesium resides intracellularly (30 per cent) and within bone (69 per cent). Magnesium in the intracellular space, in plasma, and bound to organic compounds, primarily adenosine triphosphate (ATP), is in equilibrium. Absorption of magnesium from the jejunum and ileum is enhanced by vitamin D. It is excreted via the kidneys.

Hypomagnesemia. Clinical consequences of hypomagnesemia in humans may include anorexia, nausea, vomiting, lethargy, and weakness. In severe depletion, paresthesia, muscular cramps, irritability, and mental confusion may occur. About 50 per cent of hypomagnesemic human patients develop hypokalemia (mechanism unknown). Attempts to correct the hypokalemia are unsuccessful without correction of the magnesium deficiency. With a decrease in serum magnesium below 1.2 mg/dL, hypocalcemia may also occur. This is caused by inhibition of parathyroid hormone (PTH) release and an impaired response to PTH in bone. Hypomagnesemic hypocalcemia may be severe enough to cause clinical signs of tetany. Such patients require correction of the magnesium deficiency in order to resolve the hypocalcemia. Hypomagnesemia also causes electrocardiogram (ECG) and rhythm changes similar to those seen with hypokalemia. ECG changes include S-T segment depression, flattening of T waves, Q-T prolongation, and arrhythmias.

Determination of magnesium deficiency may be made by direct measurement of serum magnesium. If the value is below normal, a definitive diagnosis of hypomagnesemia can be made. However, as is the case with serum potassium determinations, serum values do not always accurately reflect total body stores. A normal serum magnesium level may be found concurrently with depletion of total body magnesium. A method for the determination of magnesium depletion established for human patients is measurement of the percentage magnesium retained following administration of an oral or intravenous loading dose.

Causes of hypomagnesemia include inadequate intake; primary gastrointestinal disorders (specific absorptive defects, malabsorption syndromes, prolonged diarrhea); pancreatitis (Mg^{++} and Ca^{++} saponification of fat); endocrine disorders, including hypo- and hyperparathyroidism; hyperthyroidism; hyperaldosteronism; and diabetic ketoacidosis. One common cause for hypomagnesemia is polyuria from any cause, including diuretic administration. This is noteworthy, because cardiac patients on diuretic therapy are at risk for hypomagnesemia.

Treatment of hypomagnesemia includes treatment of the underlying disorder. Humans with life-threatening cardiac arrhythmias, myocardial infarctions, or hypocalcemia associated with hypomagnesemia are given intravenous magnesium sulfate. Oral administration with magnesium oxide or other magnesium salts is used for chronic supplementation. In affected patients receiving diuretic therapy, spironolactone or triamterene may be substituted for loop diuretics to minimize magnesium loss.

Because of its effects on the electrophysiology of cardiac tissue, magnesium has emerged in human medicine as a treatment for cardiac arrhythmias, specifically for torsades de pointes and other ventricular arrhythmias. Magnesium was recently recommended by the American Heart Association as the third drug of choice in resuscitation of human patients with pulseless ventricular tachycardias or ventricular fibrillation. Magnesium, administered intravenously or orally, prolongs sinoatrial node recovery time, prolongs the atrioventricular node relative and effective refractory periods, and decreases conduction velocity in the ventricular myocardium. Magnesium takes on additional significance in cardiovascular medicine, as it decreases platelet aggregation, reduces synthesis of thromboxane A_2, and acts as a cofactor for two enzymes essential in lipid metabolism, lecithin-cholesterol acyltransferase and lipoprotein lipase. Magnesium also has vasodilatory effects.

Hypermagnesemia. Symptomatic hypermagnesemia is uncommon, but signs include sedation, hypoventilation, muscle weakness, hypotension, bradycardia, and vasodilatation. At extreme concentrations, coma and respiratory paralysis occur. Causes of hypermagnesemia include severe rhabdomyolysis and overadministration of magnesium in patients with insufficient renal function. Normal renal function almost precludes the possibility of overdose. Treatment includes administration of intravenous saline and furosemide to promote excretion.

CALCIUM

Physiology. Calcium normally exists in plasma within the narrow reference range of 9.0 to 11.5 mg/dL. About 40 per cent of total plasma calcium is present in a nondiffusible, protein-bound form; 10 per cent in a diffusible, nonionized form; and about 50 per cent in a diffusible, ionized state. Ionized calcium is the physiologically active component. Regulation of plasma calcium concentration is achieved by interactions of PTH, active vitamin D, and, to a small extent, calcitonin.

Hypocalcemia. Clinical signs of hypocalcemia in small animal patients are variable and typically occur with serum calcium concentrations below 6.5 mg/dL. Nonspecific signs include weakness, listlessness, inappetence, vomiting, and diarrhea. Nervous system signs of irritability, trembling, muscle twitching or cramping, facial rubbing, lameness, seizures, and tetany are common. Clinical signs may wax and wane, potentially making clinical diagnosis difficult.

Causes of hypocalcemia include primary or iatrogenic hypoparathyroidism, hypomagnesemia, chronic renal failure (rare), acute renal failure secondary to ethylene glycol toxicity, acute pancreatitis, puerperal tetany, malnutrition, malabsorption syndromes, and phosphate enemas. Other causes include vitamin D deficiency, administration of citrated blood products, trauma (rare), and medullary carcinoma of the thyroid (rare). Because 40 per cent of calcium exists in plasma bound to proteins (primarily albumin), hypoalbuminemia may result in an apparent hypocalcemia. Therefore, interpretation of calcium in the presence of hypoalbuminemia first requires correction by the formula:

Corrected total Ca (mg/dL) = measured total Ca (mg/dL)
 − albumin (g/dL) + 3.5

Treatment of hypocalcemic tetany requires slow intravenous administration of calcium given to effect, with dosing guidelines of 5 to 15 mg/kg. Calcium gluconate (10 per cent solution) is most commonly used, as it will not cause irritation if extravasation from a vein occurs. ECG monitoring is advised during treatment, and administration should be slowed or discontinued if bradycardia, premature ventricular complexes, or shortening of the Q-T interval is observed. Short-term patient management after tetany can be achieved by subcutaneous administration every 6 to 8 hours of the same intravenous dose used to initially control signs mixed with an equal volume of saline. Long-term maintenance of persistent hypocalcemia requires oral administration of vitamin D and calcium (see Chapter 149).

Hypercalcemia. Clinical signs of hypercalcemia may include listlessness, depression, weakness, anorexia, vomiting, constipation, polyuria, polydipsia, obtundation, and even coma. Causes of hypercalcemia include primary hyperparathyroidism, hypercalcemia of malignancy, neoplastic bony metastases, vitamin D toxicity, hypoadrenocorticism, chronic or acute renal failure, septic bone disease, disseminated mycosis, disuse osteoporosis, hemoconcentration, and hypothermia. Neoplasms documented to cause hypercalcemia as a paraneoplastic syndrome include hematologic cancers such as lymphosarcoma, myeloproliferative diseases, lymphocytic leukemia, and myeloma; solid tumors with bony metastases—primarily carcinomas (nasal, pancreatic, pulmonary); and solid tumors without bony metastases such as apocrine gland adenocarcinoma of the anal sac, squamous cell carcinoma, thyroid adenocarcinoma, pulmonary carcinoma, pancreatic adenocarcinoma, and fibrosarcoma (Fig. 63–1).

Treatment of hypercalcemia involves treatment of the primary underlying disease. Intravenous fluid therapy with 0.9 per cent sodium chloride and furosemide administration are

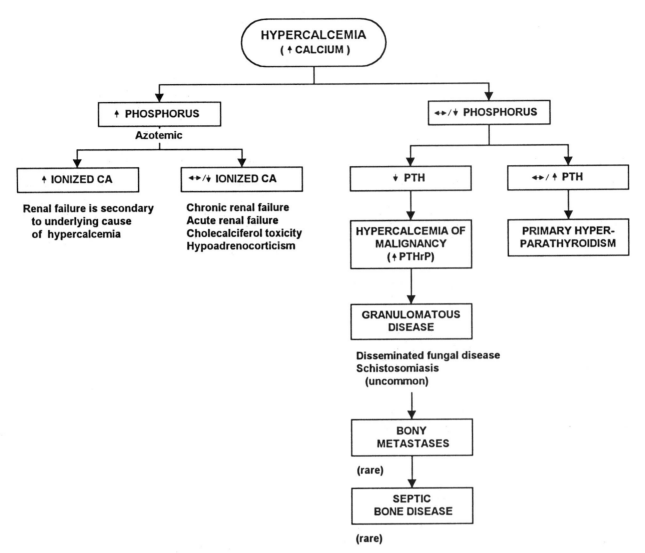

Figure 63–1. Algorithm for differential diagnosis of hypercalcemia.

beneficial in reducing hypercalcemia in the immediate short term.

CHLORIDE

Physiology. Chloride is an abundant anion in the extracellular fluid compartment. Chloride generally moves passively across electrical gradients following shifts in sodium. It is a strong anion and plays an important role, with other strong ions, in regulation of acid-base balance. A difference in net Cl^- excretion relative to net Na^+ excretion effects a change in acid-base status. Chloride also is used in the calculation of anion gap (AG), where AG = ([Na^+] + [K^+]) − ([Cl^-] + [HCO_3^-]). The loop of Henle and distal renal tubules are responsible for passive and active chloride excretion.

Hypochloremia. Shifts in plasma levels of chloride frequently follow shifts in sodium concentration. Examples of clinical conditions leading to hyponatremia with concurrent hypochloremia include those in which the extracellular fluid (ECF) volume is expanded (with a decreased effective circulating volume), such as congestive heart failure, hepatic cirrhosis, and nephrotic syndrome; those conditions with near normal ECF volume (and decreased effective circulating arterial volume), such as hypothyroidism and adrenal insufficiency; and conditions that are euvolemic, such as the syndrome of inappropriate antidiuretic hormone secretion. Clinical situations in which the Cl^- concentration changes *without* a concurrent change in Na^+ concentration result in acid-base disturbances. Hypochloremic metabolic alkalosis occurs with specific loss of chloride ions, such as with gastric vomiting or administration of diuretics that cause Cl^- wasting (e.g., furosemide).

Hyperchloremia. An increase in plasma chloride concentration in conjunction with hypernatremia occurs with renal water loss. Clinical examples include osmotic diuresis, as in diabetes mellitus, or nonosmotic renal water loss, as in central or nephrogenic diabetes insipidus. The acid-base disturbance of hyperchloremic metabolic acidosis arises with alkali loss from the gastrointestinal tract (diarrhea) or kidneys (renal tubular acidosis [RTA]). Both proximal and distal RTA result in hyperchloremic metabolic acidosis (mechanism unknown in distal RTA). Also, early chronic renal failure can result in hyperchloremic metabolic acidosis.

SECTION II

DIETARY CONSIDERATIONS OF SYSTEMIC PROBLEMS

CHAPTER 64

NUTRITION OF HEALTHY DOGS AND CATS IN VARIOUS STAGES OF ADULT LIFE

James G. Morris and Quinton R. Rogers

Although both dogs and cats are classified as carnivores, their nutrient requirements are not identical. The metabolism and nutritional needs of dogs approach those of omnivores, whereas the metabolism of cats is consistent with that of a strict meat-eating mammal.[1–3]

FOOD INTAKE AND PALATABILITY

The diet of feral cats is based largely on small mammals, birds, lizards, and insects. When domesticated cats are fed free choice, they eat 10 to 20 meals per day (12 mice per day provide the energy requirement of a normal cat) about equally divided between the light and the dark period. There are significant breed differences in the feeding behavior of dogs: beagles have feeding patterns similar to cats, whereas basenjis and poodles eat only during the light period. The number of meals can vary widely from 5 to 20. Adult dogs adapt to one meal a day, and cats at maintenance can adapt to a similar regimen. During gestation and lactation, however, performance is enhanced by feeding several times a day or by feeding free choice. During the latter part of gestation and lactation, bitches should be offered food at least twice a day and preferably fed free choice. Both cats and dogs prefer meat-based canned products rather than dry expanded diets, in part owing to the higher moisture content of canned products and in part because blood and fluids contain positive palatability factors. Texture is important; cats and dogs both prefer soft moist foods to dry powdery foods. Dogs respond positively to protein, peptides, certain free amino acids, sugar, and mononucleotides, together with certain electrolytes. The response of cats is neutral to protein and sugar, positive to peptides and certain free amino acids, and negative to mononucleotides. Good-quality animal fats enhance palatability for both cats and dogs. Medium chain triglycerides are strongly aversive to cats but not to dogs. Both dogs and cats respond positively to fresh meat extracts, whereas cats but not dogs generally show strong negative palatability to oxidized or rancid fats and breakdown products of trinucleotides or mononucleotides. In summary, cats are more sensitive to adulteration, oxidation, and rancidity in foods than are dogs. Uncooked or cooked meat extracts (broth) are the most palatable natural ingredients to use to enhance the palatability of unpalatable foods for both dogs and cats.

Food intake of cats and dogs fed diets of low or high palatability is quite well controlled. The level at which the animal controls its weight is complex and depends on factors such as genetics (breed and strain), life stage, physical activity, whether neutered, food availability, and food palatability. Both dogs and cats maintain their weight and stay healthy if their diet is complete and balanced, even if the diet has poor palatability. Highly palatable high-fat diets increase the risk for obesity. Nevertheless, dogs and cats control their food intake, albeit at a higher level of body weight, even when fed highly palatable high-fat diets. It is always easier to prevent obesity by selecting or manipulating the aforementioned factors before obesity occurs rather than to try to limit food intake to effect weight loss. In herbivores and omnivores, food intake is depressed and strong avoidance of a particular diet is exhibited when animals are fed diets with various nutrient deficiencies or excesses (e.g., deficiencies of thiamine, sodium, phosphate, protein, specific essential amino acids). In most species, including cats and dogs, emetics (e.g., lithium chloride or apomorphine) induce an aversion to the taste of the food just previously eaten. This behavior is called a learned taste aversion. In cats there appears to be a neural disassociation between the neural response to the nutrient deficiency and feeding behavior. For those deficiencies and excesses that have been examined (protein deficiency and excess, individual essential amino acid deficiency and excess, sodium deficiency), no learned taste aversions have been demonstrated, despite the fact that food intake may have been depressed.[3, 4] Thus palatability may override nutrient metabolic effects in cats, whereas nutrient metabolic effects (caused by nutrient deficiencies and excesses) override palatability effects in herbivores and omnivores (Fig. 64–1). It is notable that even though cats do not appear to develop learned aversions to simple nutrient deficiencies or excesses, it has been shown that cats do avoid diets that cause hyperammonemia[5] or metabolic acidosis.[6]

GENERAL FEEDING RECOMMENDATIONS

Practitioners should advise clients to choose a commercial diet that has passed an Association of American Feed Control Officials (AAFCO) animal protocol test for the particular life stage of the cat or dog. This ensures that the diet has undergone an animal feeding test. An AAFCO nutrient profile label means only that a diet meets a calculated nutrient profile. In most cases it is safest to feed a diet that has passed an AAFCO all-stages protocol. The exception would be if a particular dog or cat has a medical problem; then a specific therapeutic diet should be fed. In selecting an appropriate therapeutic diet, one should always select a diet that has been tested for the intended purpose. If no particular diet has been tested clinically for the particular medical

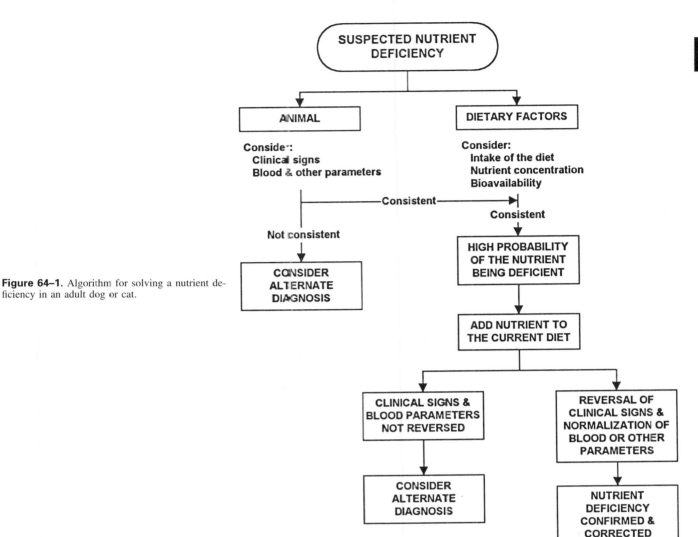

Figure 64–1. Algorithm for solving a nutrient deficiency in an adult dog or cat.

condition, a clinical nutritionist should be consulted for advice, or to formulate a balanced homemade diet that is appropriate. It is prudent to check whether a commercial diet (regular or therapeutic) has been properly tested in animals for the intended purpose. There is no reason not to feed a diet that has large built-in safety factors in nutritional requirements, but likewise there is no reason to pay for extra nutrients if they have not been shown to be of extra benefit to the cat or dog. When a diet is complete, balanced, and tested and has been shown to be fully adequate in animals, there is no reason to feed a diet containing even more of one or more essential nutrients. Nevertheless, there is a paucity of information on specific nutrient requirements in adult life stages, including maintenance. There has been considerable research on the nutrient requirements for dogs and cats for growth, because it is the easiest life stage for which to determine requirements. Therefore, requirements for growth have been used to formulate requirements during pregnancy. Additional information from epidemiologic evidence and from other species has been used to formulate requirements for maintenance.

MEETING ENERGY NEEDS

About 80 per cent of the food eaten by mature cats and dogs is used to provide their energy needs. The requirements

for protein, minerals, and vitamins can be met in the remaining dry matter. Therefore, meeting energy needs is the first consideration in feeding cats and dogs. Energy unlike individual amino acids, vitamins, and minerals, is not supplied by any single nutrient but is provided by the oxidation of substrates, primarily fats, carbohydrates, and proteins. The energy needs of dogs or cats may be supplied by diets with varying ratios of these three nutrients. The only avenue an animal has for disposal of excess energy is by oxidation to produce adenosine triphosphate or to store the excess energy in the form of adipose tissue. Mature dogs and cats that are in energy balance convert all the available or metabolizable energy (ME) from food into heat. To calculate the amount of food required by dogs or cats, the ME value of the food should be known.

The energy requirements of mature, nonpregnant cats and dogs are not constant but decrease on a unit-body-weight basis with age, which is related to the reduction in general activity with age. As indicated, many individual cats and dogs adjust their energy intake from food to balance their energy needs. However, in some adults, this balance is not maintained, leading either to body weight loss, resulting in catabolism of body energy stores, or to obesity and body weight gain owing to excessive energy intake.

The maintenance energy requirements of adult cats and dogs may be estimated from formulas relating ME requirements to body weight. Because mature dogs have about a 50-fold range in body weight, and because ME requirements per unit of body weight decrease with body weight, formulas generally include some power function of body weight (e.g., body weight raised to $\frac{3}{4}$ power). A common linear formula used for dogs is $ME = 30 W + 70$, and an exponent formula is $ME = 132 W^{3/4}$, where W is body weight in kilograms and ME is kilocalories per day. The first equation approximates the relationship for small dogs such as beagles but overpredicts energy requirements for large breeds. As the body-weight range of adult cats is much less than that of adult dogs, a power function is not used with cats. The formula $ME = 80 W$ has been used for active cats and $ME = 70 W$ for inactive cats.

Although these formulas are useful starting points, they are not absolute requirements, because there is considerable individual animal variation. It has been shown that there is a large variation in the prediction interval of maintenance energy requirement.[7, 8] However, when enteral or parenteral nutritional support is necessary, a requirement estimate must be made. Similarly, when a weight reduction program is undertaken, an estimate of maintenance energy requirements is desirable. All adult cats and dogs that are voluntarily consuming food should be fed relative to their body condition and not by a formula. If an adult dog or cat is fed free choice and becomes obese, either the amount of food offered or the energy density (available caloric density) of the food should be reduced. When an adult cat or dog is not maintaining body weight, either more food or a more palatable food should be fed to increase intake, and/or a diet of a higher caloric density should be fed.

Pregnancy causes a demand for energy greater than normal adult maintenance requirements. Different responses to pregnancy occur in the ingestive behavior of bitches versus queens, even though the length of gestation is similar. Queens increase food intake soon after conception and have an almost linear increase in body energy stores with duration of gestation. In contrast, bitches normally do not increase food and energy intake until the latter stages of pregnancy. Queens and bitches in normal body condition may be given food free choice during pregnancy to allow for the increase in body tissue that will be mobilized during lactation and by fetal energy demands. Whereas the latter stages of pregnancy increase energy requirements by about a third, lactation places a huge demand on the bitch and queen and can result in energy intakes three to four times above maintenance. Depending on the number of kittens or pups, queens or bitches sustain a loss of body weight during lactation. This tissue loss should be largely the tissue gained during the prepartum period, and with a good diet, the weaning body weight of the mother should not be less than the body weight at conception.

PROTEINS AND AMINO ACIDS

Proteins are added to diets to provide essential amino acids and nitrogen. Nitrogen requirements are usually expressed as the crude protein requirement, because crude protein is defined as the quantity of nitrogen times 6.25. Nitrogen is used for the biosynthesis of dispensable amino acids, heme, purines, pyrimidines, and so forth. Both essential and dispensable amino acids are necessary at the cellular level for protein synthesis. Several amino acids are precursors for hormones and neurotransmitters. If the amino acid

and crude protein requirements are known for each life stage, the clinical nutritionist can formulate a diet using amino acid composition tables for particular proteins and ensure that both essential amino acid and nitrogen requirements are met. However, a weakness of diet formulation using nutrient composition tables is that the bioavailabilities of amino acids and nitrogen from food sources are usually not known, or the effect of processing on the particular food (or food combinations) is not known. The most accurate way to tell if the diet is adequate in protein is to evaluate plasma amino acid concentrations during the absorptive state after feeding a particular diet. Amino acid patterns can be used not only to verify that essential amino acid requirements have been met but also to diagnose various nutritional problems (e.g., protein-energy malnutrition, essential amino acid deficiency) and metabolic problems (e.g., liver or kidney disease).

Carnivores have no problem meeting their protein or amino acid requirements if they eat other animals, because the body composition of various animals is quite similar and is high in good-quality protein. Nutritional problems arise only if a client attempts to feed a carnivore a vegetarian diet or a diet that has poor-quality ingredients (e.g., by-products that are high in collagen, such as skin and bone) or products that have been excessively processed. Quality control of ingredients in pet foods is a problem in the pet food industry, because large quantities of animal by-products do not always have a constant composition; thus these by-products may have variable digestibilities and bioavailabilities for nitrogen and amino acids. Specific amino acid deficiencies or excesses can cause a variety of problems, such as cataracts, dermatitis, hair loss and/or reddening of black hair, irritability, neurologic deficits, hyperammonemia, fatty liver, low glutathione, and emesis. After reviewing the literature and using our experience in feeding dogs and cats, we have developed an estimate of dietary nutrient allowances (Table 64–1). These allowances include an approximate 25 to 50 per cent in excess the minimal requirement to allow variation in bioavailability. Our estimate of minimal requirement is undoubtedly high for several of the amino acids, because so many data are missing, especially for the adult life stages. Nevertheless, these values may be used as guidelines until more refined data are available. It is possible, using diet composition tables, that these recommendations may be too low owing to poor-quality ingredients with low digestibility coefficients. Most cat and dog foods are formulated to meet or exceed these recommendations. Major pet food companies have competent nutritionists who take digestibility and bioavailability values into account in formulating diets, and most of the major diets have been tested. Therefore, veterinarians should be confident in recommending any pet food that has passed the AAFCO feeding protocol for the life stage in question. The bottom line is simple for adult dogs and cats, feed a commercial diet for the appropriate life stage from a reputable company. The only other safe course is consultation with a small animal nutritionist to attempt to evaluate a diet or to formulate a homemade diet. The latter is not recommended, because of the difficulty in predicting bioavailability of ingredient nutrients and the difficulty in getting good compliance in making and feeding such a diet.

MINERALS AND VITAMINS

Adult cats and dogs require the same minerals and vitamins that are essential to growing kittens and puppies. Al-

TABLE 64–1. SUGGESTED NUTRIENT ALLOWANCES* FOR ADULT DOGS AND CATS AT MAINTENANCE (NUTRIENT PER 1000 KCAL OF DIETARY METABOLIZABLE ENERGY)

NUTRIENT	UNIT	ADULT DOG	ADULT CAT
Protein†	g	37.5	75.0
Arginine	g	1.43	3.13
Histidine	g	0.54	0.90
Isoleucine	g	1.05	1.75
Leucine	g	1.80	3.75
Lysine	g	2.25	3.00
Methionine + cysteine	g	1.50	2.75
Methionine	g	0.75	1.50
Phenylalanine + tyrosine	g	2.10	2.50
Phenylalanine	g	1.05	1.25
Threonine	g	1.20	2.00
Tryptophan	g	0.35	0.50
Valine	g	1.28	1.75
Calcium	g	1.6	1.2
Phosphorus	g	1.2	1.2
Potassium	g	1.2	1.25
Sodium	g	0.40	0.40
Chloride	g	0.20	0.20
Magnesium	g	0.11	0.08
Iron	mg	20	20
Copper	mg	0.8	1.1
Manganese	mg	1.4	1.1
Zinc	mg	9.7	11
Iodine	mg	0.16	0.07
Selenium	mg	0.03	0.02
Vitamin A (retinol)	mg	0.3	0.21
Vitamin D (cholecalciferol)	μg	2.75	2.6
Vitamin E (alpha-tocopherol)	mg	6.1	7.0
Vitamin K	μg	—	21
Thiamine	mg	0.3	1.1
Riboflavin	mg	0.7	0.9
Pyridoxine	mg	0.3	0.9
Niacin	mg	3.0	10.0
Pantothenic acid	mg	2.7	1.0
Folic acid	mg	0.54	0.17
Vitamin B$_{12}$	μg	7.0	4.0
Biotin	μg	—	15
Choline	mg	340	500

*Note: These values are not minimal nutrient requirements, but nutrient allowances. Requirements have been increased to accommodate variation in digestibility and bioavailability of nutrients in natural foods and individual animal variation.

†For a protein of good quality. The requirement for protein and amino acids needs to be increased for proteins of lower quality or lower digestibility.

though the requirements for growing kittens and puppies are fairly well defined, those for adults are not known with the same precision. The dietary concentration for growth satisfies adult requirements, even though the food intake of adults on a unit-body-weight basis is less than that during growth. The function and clinical role of vitamins have recently been reviewed.[9]

MINERALS

Mineral requirements for adult cats and dogs for maintenance expressed per 1000 kcal dietary ME are given in Table 64–1. These requirements are based on published values[10, 11] with updated information. Expression on an equivalent energy basis shows that the requirements of adult cats and dogs are similar. The requirements given in Table 64–1 are for minerals with a high bioavailability, such as from mixtures of the salts of these minerals or from bone. Applying these values to practical diets requires bioavailability values to be taken into account. Although these have not been determined in cats and dogs, values originating in other

simple-stomached species give useful approximations. The bioavailability of calcium, phosphorus, and magnesium from plant sources is considerably less than that from mineral salts or bone and should be discounted by 50 per cent. In contrast, sodium, potassium, and chloride are readily exchangeable, and no adjustments is necessary in regard to their source.

Bioavailability of trace elements, especially as they pertain to cats and dogs, is not known, but observations indicate that the availability of zinc and copper in diets containing high proportions of plant products is compromised. Zinc deficiency is not uncommon in dogs fed some of the lower-quality dry diets containing a high proportion of plant products. Clinical signs of copper deficiency have been reported in newborn kittens from queens given diets containing copper oxide as a supplementary source of copper. Reproductive performance of the queens was also reduced. The requirements for many of the major minerals (e.g., calcium, potassium, and sodium) increase greatly in lactation. However, as food intake is also increased about fourfold, the percentage in the diet need not change.

Diagnosis of mineral deficiencies should be based on specific clinical signs, blood or plasma concentrations for the species, and reversal of clinical signs following supplementation with the specific mineral while the cat or dog is maintained on the same diet.

VITAMINS

Vitamin requirements of adult cats and dogs expressed on the basis of 1000 kcal of metabolizable energy are given in Table 64–1. The values are based on published data[10, 11] that have been modified when newer information is available. For the fat-soluble vitamins A, D, and E, the requirements are similar for adult cats and dogs. Cats, unlike dogs, are unable to utilize beta-carotene as a precursor for retinol, so they depend on preformed vitamin A in the diet. The values for vitamin A and D are in excess of minimal requirements, and further supplementation in normal animals is unwarranted. Neither cats nor dogs are capable of synthesizing vitamin D from ultraviolet light.[12] Although vitamins A and D are regarded as the most toxic of all the vitamins when given in excess, adult cats can tolerate large excesses (50 times requirement) of these two vitamins with no discernible deleterious effects. In normal cats and dogs, in contrast to most other animals, large concentrations of retinyl esters occur in plasma. Requirements for vitamin E are a function of the total polyunsaturated fatty acids (PUFAs) in the diet. As cats frequently consume diets high in PUFAs, the requirement to prevent steatitis in cats is higher than that for dogs that are subjected to lower dietary inputs of PUFAs. Both cats and dogs require an exogenous source of vitamin K, but intestinal synthesis appears to be adequate to supply this need in dogs. When cats are fed some high-fish diets, they have a prolongation of clotting time and require supplemental vitamin K.

In contrast to the fat-soluble vitamins, the requirements for the water-soluble vitamins for cats versus dogs are different. Cats have a higher requirement than dogs for thiamine (vitamin B₁) and are exposed to dietary ingredients that often contain both thiaminases (e.g., fish) and to canned diets that have sustained extensive processing, causing loss of thiamine. As thiamine stores are rapidly exhausted, thiamine deficiency can readily occur in cats given deficient diets. Cats, unlike dogs, are unable to use tryptophan as a precursor for niacin synthesis, so niacin is an absolute essential dietary nutrient for cats. Niacin is normally obtained from foods by hydrolysis of NAD and NADP (nicotinamide adenosyl dinucleotide and phosphodinucleotide) in the gut. Meats contain high levels of these nucleotides and thus are a principal source of this vitamin.

The published vitamin requirements[10, 11] for growing kittens and puppies appear to satisfy the requirements of mature cats and dogs. However, in applying these values, it is necessary to take into consideration the bioavailability of the vitamin and its stability in the product. The bioavailability of the fat-soluble vitamins is high in the absence of most fat malabsorption syndromes, whereas the bioavailability of most of the B vitamins in natural products is variable and can be quite low.

TAURINE

Taurine, a beta-sulfur amino acid, occurs in all animal cells and is virtually the sole conjugate of the bile acids in cats and dogs. Taurine is synthesized de novo by dogs and cats from the sulfur amino acids cysteine and methionine. Although cat diets contain a higher level of sulfur amino acids than do dog diets, the rate of taurine synthesis by cats is low, and cats given a low-taurine diet are readily depleted of this amino acid. This very low rate of taurine synthesis in cats is a consequence of low activities of two enzymes in the pathway of synthesis. Taurine depletion is associated with a wide range of clinical conditions, including feline central retinal degeneration, reversible dilated cardiomyopathy, reproductive failure in queens, and developmental defects and growth retardation in kittens. The amount of dietary taurine required for cats to maintain adequate blood concentrations varies twofold with the type of diet. For expanded (dry) diets, 1250 mg taurine/kg dry matter is adequate. Canned diets, which promote higher intestinal degradation of taurine exposed in the enterohepatic circulation, require 2500 mg/kg dry matter to maintain blood concentrations in the normal range.

ESSENTIAL FATTY ACIDS

Natural diets for dogs and cats should contain a source of PUFAs that these animals cannot synthesize de novo. They are the essential fatty acids (EFAs). Dogs require two EFAs in the diet: linoleic acid C18:2 n-6, and linolenic acid C18:3n-3. The letter followed by the number (e.g., n-6 or n-3) refers to the location of the first double bond in the fatty acid from the methyl or omega end of the fatty acid. Animals cannot insert double bonds further than nine carbons from the carboxyl end of a fatty acid. Besides linoleic and linolenic acids, cats require arachidonic acid in the diet. In cats, the activity of the $\Delta 6$-desaturase enzyme is extremely low, so they are unable to desaturate the elongation product of linoleic acid to produce arachidonic acid. Fatty acids function as precursors of eicosanoids, which include prostaglandin, leukotrienes, and thromboxanes. These extremely active biologic compounds have both paracrine and endocrine activity. As a group, the eicosanoids of the n-6 series tend to be involved in a more pro-inflammatory role, whereas those of the n-3 have an anti-inflammatory or only a mildly inflammatory role.

Of the three fatty acids, the quantitative requirement of cats and dogs is greatest for linoleic acid. A deficiency of linoleic acid results in hyperkeratosis of skin, fatty degeneration of the liver, and degeneration of the testis. In addition, there is increased water loss through the skin. Cats and dogs require about 1 to 2 per cent of their calories as linoleic acid to prevent clinical signs of deficiency, though higher levels of total fat have been associated with better coat condition. The n-3 fatty acids are high in marine animal fats and linseed oil.

Clinical signs of arachidonate deficiency in cats are associated with eicosanoid dysfunction and include defective reproduction and changes in blood platelet aggregation. Cats' requirement for arachidonic acid is on the order of 200 mg/kg dry matter. Arachidonate in the diet comes from animal tissue membranes. Recently a fungal source of arachidonate has become commercially available, so it is possible to circumvent an obligate source of animal fat in cat diets.

OTHER NUTRIENTS AND NUTRACEUTICALS

Choline is often included among the "essential" vitamins because it supplies labile methyl groups. Methionine and betaine can also supply methyl groups. A lack of total methyl groups in the diet leads to fatty liver because of an inability to mobilize hepatic fat.

Ascorbate, or vitamin C, is synthesized de novo by dogs and cats from glucose, and there is no substantiated evidence except in liver disease (only anecdotal reports) that dogs or cats benefit from the addition of ascorbate to the diet. In contrast, some breeds of dogs have a limited capacity to synthesize adequate carnitine and benefit from its supplementation. Synthetic antioxidants are frequently added to human and animal diets to prevent lipid peroxidation during storage. There is substantial evidence that the consumption of lipid peroxides is contraindicated. Whether these synthetic antioxidants are deleterious when used at the recommended concentrations in the diet is debatable. Natural antioxidants such as alpha-tocopherol, though less effective than the synthetic antioxidants, can also be used. A number of human foods such as onions and chocolate cause adverse effects in cats and dogs, respectively; thus some human foods should not be fed to cats and dogs indiscriminately. Food fadism in human nutrition has resulted in malnutrition, toxicities, and deficiencies.[7] These same practices occur in dog and cat nutrition and should be avoided.

REFERENCES

1. MacDonald ML, Rogers QR, Morris JG: Nutrition of the domestic cat, a mammalian carnivore. Nutr Rev 4:521, 1984.
2. Morris JG, Rogers QR: Comparative aspects of nutrition and metabolism of dogs and cats. In Burger IH, Rivers JPW (eds): Nutrition of the Dog and Cat. New York, Cambridge University Press, 1989, pp 35–66.
3. Rogers QR, Morris JG: Nutritional peculiarities of the cat. In Leibetseder J (ed): Proceeding of XVI WSAVA World Congress. Vienna, 1991, pp 261–266.
4. Yu SF, Rogers QR, Morris JG: Absence of a salt (NaCl) preference or appetite in sodium replete or depleted kittens. Appetite 29:1, 1997.
5. Morris JG, Rogers QR: Ammonia intoxication in the near-adult cat as a result of dietary deficiency of arginine. Science 199:431, 1978.
6. Cook NE, Rogers QR, Morris JG: Acid-base balance affects dietary choice in cats. Appetite 26:175, 1996.
7. Herbert V, Barrett S: Twenty-one ways to spot a quack. Nutrition Forum Newsletter, Sept 1986, pp 65–68.

8. Heusner AA: Body mass, maintenance and basal metabolism in dogs. J Nutr 121:88, 1991.
9. Rucker RB, Morris JG: The vitamins. *In* Kaneko JJ, Harvey JW, Bruss ML (eds): Biochemistry of Domestic Animals, 5th ed. San Diego, Academic Press, 1997, pp 702–739.
10. National Research Council: Nutrient Requirements of Dogs. Washington, DC, National Academy Press, 1985.
11. National Research Council: Nutrient Requirements of Cats. Washington, DC, National Academy Press, 1986.
12. Morris JG: Ineffective synthesis of vitamin D in kittens exposed to sun and ultraviolet light is reversed by an inhibitor of 7-dehydrocholesterol-Δ7-reductase. *In* Norman AW, Bouillon R, Thomasset M (eds): Vitamin D Chemistry, Biology and Clinical Applications of the Steroid Hormone. Riverside, University of California, 1997, pp 721–722.

NUT

CHAPTER 65

NEONATAL AND PEDIATRIC NUTRITION

Johnny D. Hoskins

The nutritional requirements, feeding, and care of puppies and kittens from birth to early adulthood are substantially different during their different stages of growth. Proper nutrition consists of supplying all necessary nutrients in adequate amounts and in proper proportions. Growth is a critical time in a puppy's or kitten's life that involves the interaction of heredity, hormonal regulation, health issues, and proper nutrition. Puppies and kittens will fail to grow to the size determined by their hereditary factors unless they consume appropriate food of adequate quality. If poor-quality commercially prepared diets, homemade diets of single food items, or indiscriminate mixtures of single food items are fed to the animals during their growth period, nutrition-related problems can occur. Supplementation of poor or questionable diets with specific nutrients such as calcium, phosphorus, vitamin A, vitamin D, or organ tissues can create dietary imbalances that may lead to a number of nutritional problems, especially during the growth period.

FEEDING THE PUPPY

Mothers should be fed to attain proper body condition throughout gestation and lactation. Normal maintenance levels of food should be fed through breeding and for the first 6 weeks of gestation. Food intake should then be increased gradually until the mother is consuming approximately 25 per cent more than maintenance at the end of gestation. Energy needs for the lactation peak, which occurs during the third to fourth week of lactation, may be two to three times maintenance needs.

Healthy puppies, during the first 2 to 3 weeks of life, should only eat and sleep. Nursing should be vigorous and active, with each puppy receiving sufficient milk from its mother. If the mother is healthy and well nourished, the puppy's nutritional needs for its first 3 to 4 weeks of life should be provided completely by her. Indications that the puppy is not receiving sufficient milk are constant crying, extreme inactivity, and/or failure to achieve weight gains in accordance with the general guidelines that a puppy should gain 1 to 2 g/day/lb (2 to 4 g/day/kg) of anticipated adult weight, or at least 10 per cent gain per day.[1] For example, if the adult dog is expected to weigh 30 pounds, as a puppy it should gain 30 to 60 g/day during its first 5 months of life.

The transition from mother's milk to solid food should be a gradual process beginning at about 3 weeks of age (4 weeks of age for toy breeds); however, if necessary, supplemental feeding may be started as soon as the puppy fails to show sufficient weight gain. During the changeover to solid food, the puppy can be offered a thick, gruel-like mixture of good-quality puppy food designed for growth and water (one part dry food blended with three parts water, or two parts canned food blended with one part water). To get the puppy eating, the gruel is placed in a shallow food dish, and the puppy is encouraged to lap the gruel by touching its lips to the food, or the feeder can put a finger in the gruel and then into the puppy's mouth. It can also be force fed using a commercial dosing syringe. Once the puppy is eating the gruel well, the amount of water in the gruel is gradually reduced until it is omitted.

By 6 weeks of age, the puppy should be getting at least 25 per cent of its requirements from the weaning diet. The puppy may be permanently separated from the mother as soon as it learns to eat readily and drink satisfactorily. Most puppies are completely weaned at 7 to 8 weeks of age, depending somewhat on the dog's size and breed. Early weaning and separation from littermates before 6 weeks of age can cause malnutrition or numerous behavioral problems later in life. Because of this, complete weaning should not be attempted until puppies are at least 6 weeks old and close human contact has been established.

The primary challenges of feeding a growing puppy are providing adequate energy and essential nutrients and avoiding a rapid growth rate. An appropriate growth food provides adequate nutrients and energy in a volume that can be easily consumed by the puppy. Supplementation with meat, table scraps, or other items is not recommended, because it is likely to create a finicky eater, nutritional deficiencies or excesses, or both. Because the puppy's eating habits are still in the developmental stage, it is important that a good-quality growth-formulated puppy food be fed daily at regular intervals and that fresh water in a clean bowl be available at all times.

Feeding the weaned puppy should always be directed to attaining the moderate growth rate for the breed.[1] Instead of making food available to the puppy at all times (free-choice feeding), time-limited meal feeding is recommended. At each feeding, give the puppy 15 to 20 minutes to eat all that it wants and then remove the remaining food. From the time of weaning to 4 to 6 months of age (9 months for giant breeds), puppies are best fed at least three times a day at regular intervals. Thereafter, puppies should be fed twice a day, on a regular schedule.

FEEDING LARGE AND GIANT BREEDS

Some large and giant breeds of dogs (those over 30 kg body weight at maturity) have the genetic capacity to grow rapidly and will do so if provided with a food that meets or exceeds their nutrient and energy needs. However, a rapid growth rate is not compatible with normal skeletal growth and may result in certain types of developmental bone disease.

Several studies have shown that diet and feeding management have an important influence on the development of osteochondrosis and hypertrophic osteodystrophy in large and giant breeds of dogs.[2, 3] Puppies fed a diet with a reduced fat content for a lower caloric intake and medium levels of calcium and phosphorus (0.8 and 0.67 per cent as fed, respectively) grew at a satisfactory rate. After 4 months of age, puppies were larger and had appropriate skeletal development.

Beginning at weaning and continuing until they reach maturity, large and giant breeds of dogs should be fed for a moderate growth rate. This can be accomplished by limiting food intake or, even better, by feeding a growth-formulated puppy food for large and giant breeds. If osteochondrosis or hypertrophic osteodystrophy occurs, nutritional management should be aimed at reducing caloric intake by decreasing the amount of food that is fed or feeding a growth-formulated puppy food for large and giant breeds.

FEEDING THE KITTEN

Love, care, and attention are important factors in raising a well-adjusted kitten, but a proper diet is the most important factor in the kitten's physical development. If the mother is healthy and well nourished, the nutritional needs of the kittens for the first 4 weeks of life should be filled completely by her. During this time, healthy kittens should nurse vigorously and actively. Each kitten should receive sufficient milk from its mother. Kittens not receiving sufficient milk cry constantly, are restless or extremely inactive, and/or fail to achieve the expected weight gain of 10 to 15 g/day.[1]

Kittens should be encouraged to begin eating solid food at 4 weeks of age. At this time, the kitten can be offered a thick, gruel-like mixture of good-quality kitten food designed for growth and milk or water (one part dry food blended with three parts milk, or two parts canned food blended with one part milk). The gruel is fed to kittens from a shallow bowl or force fed by using a commercial dosing syringe. The feeder can encourage the kitten to eat the gruel by smearing some of the gruel on the kitten's lips, being

careful not to get any in the nose, or placing a finger in the gruel and then into the kitten's mouth. This usually encourages the kitten to eat from a bowl at an early age. Once the kitten is eating the gruel well, the amount of milk or water in the gruel is gradually reduced until the kitten is consuming only solid food. The kitten may be permanently separated from the mother as soon as it learns to eat readily and drink satisfactorily. Most kittens are completely weaned at 6 to 8 weeks of age. Early weaning and separation from littermates before 6 weeks of age can result in behavioral problems such as slowness to learn and suspicious, cautious, and aggressive actions.[4]

The food that is given to the weaned kitten should be one specifically formulated for growth. Feeding between 3 and 3.5 ounces of dry food per day or 8 to 10 ounces of canned food per day usually meets the growth requirements of most kittens. Any supplementation with meat, table scraps, or other items is not recommended, because it can create dietary imbalances, finicky eaters, or nutritional deficiencies or excesses. Because the kitten's eating habits are still in the formative stage after weaning, it is important that easily digested, high-quality, calorically dense food be provided daily and that fresh water in a clean bowl be available at all times. Cow's or goat's milk is often fed to kittens after weaning and is a good food, provided that it does not cause diarrhea. However, milk should never be given in place of fresh water.

Kittens should be fed all the food they will consume. Excessive caloric intake and excessively rapid growth rate are seldom problems in growing kittens. Most kittens are nonvoracious, noninhibited eaters, and when food is always available, they nibble at it frequently. Kittens fed unlimited amounts of food (free-choice feeding), regardless of the form of food (dry or canned), eat every few hours. Free-choice feeding, or at least three-times-a-day feeding, is preferred during growth.

At 12 weeks of age, the kitten's energy needs are three times greater than those of an adult cat, or more than 200 kcal/kg of body weight. As kittens mature past 6 months of age, their growth rate slows and their food needs decrease. Their energy needs are still greater than those of adult cats, or approximately 90 kcal/kg of body weight.

Male kittens tend to grow more rapidly and for a longer time than female kittens. A female kitten's growth rate slows down at 7 months, but she continues to grow through the ninth month. A male kitten's growth slows at 9 months, but he continues to grow through the twelfth month.

REARING NURSING PUPPIES AND KITTENS

Successful rearing of orphaned puppies and kittens requires providing them with a suitable environment; the correct quantity and quality of nutrients for different stages of growth; a regular schedule of feeding, sleeping, grooming, and exercise; and the stimulus that provokes micturition and defecation.

Newborn puppies and kittens are unable to effectively control their body temperature.[5] They gradually change, during their first 4 weeks of life, from being largely poikilothermic to being homeothermic. That is, for the first week of life, their body temperature is directly related to the environmental temperature, and a steady ambient temperature of 30 to 32°C (86 to 90°F) is needed. Over the next 3 weeks, the ambient temperature can be gradually lowered to

24°C (75°F). Humidity should be maintained at 55 to 60 per cent. It is equally important that sudden changes of environmental conditions be avoided and that disturbances be minimized outside of socialization, exercise, and hygiene activities.

Feeding orphaned puppies and kittens that still require mother's milk can be rewarding. The most obvious alternative to a mother rearing her own young is for another nursing mother to act as a foster mother. Although this is a more satisfactory arrangement than trying to hand rear orphaned puppies and kittens, the chances of having access to a foster mother at the right stage of lactation and with sufficient resources to rear a litter are poor.

If a foster mother is not available, it is necessary to hand feed the puppies or kittens a replacement food that is a prototype of nutritive substance formulated to meet the optimal requirements of the puppy or kitten. Mother's milk is the ideal food. Various modifications of homemade and commercially prepared formulas simulating mother's milk have been used with good success.[5–7] Several homemade or commercial formulas for rearing puppies and kittens are identified in Table 65–1. Commercially prepared formulas are preferred, because they more closely compare with mother's milk. These formulas generally provide 1 to 1.24 kcal of metabolizable energy per milliliter of formula. The caloric needs for most nursing-age puppies and kittens is 22 to 26 kcal per 100 g of body weight. Therefore, the average puppy or kitten should daily receive approximately 13 mL of formula per 100 g of body weight during the first week of life, 17 mL of formula per 100 g of body weight during the second week, 20 mL of formula per 100 g of body weight during the third week, and 22 mL of formula per 100

TABLE 65–1. MILK-REPLACEMENT FORMULA FOR ORPHANED PUPPIES AND KITTENS

Commercial Prepared Formula for Puppies or Kittens

Begin Milk Replacer for Puppies (Performer Brand, St. Joseph, MO)
Begin Milk Replacer for Kittens (Performer Brand, St. Joseph, MO)
Esbilac Powder for Puppies (Pet-Ag Inc., Elgin, IL)
Esbilac Liquid for Puppies (Pet-Ag Inc., Elgin, IL)
GME Powder for Puppies (a goat-milk formula; Pet-Ag Inc., Elgin, IL)
Kittylac Powder for Kittens (Lander Corp., Post Falls, ID)
KMR Liquid for Kittens (Pet-Ag Inc., Elgin, IL)
KMR Powder for Kittens (Pet-Ag Inc., Elgin, IL)
Multi-Milk for Multi-Animals (milk replacer for animals with lactose intolerance; Pet-Ag Inc., Elgin, IL)
Nurturall Liquid for Puppies (Veterinary Products Laboratories, Phoenix, AZ)
Nurturall Powder for Puppies (Veterinary Products Laboratories, Phoenix, AZ)
Nurturall Liquid for Kittens (Veterinary Products Laboratories, Phoenix, AZ)
Nurturall Powder for Kittens (Veterinary Products Laboratories, Phoenix, AZ)
Veta-Lac Powder for Puppies (Vet-A-Mix, Shenandoah, IA)
Veta-Lac Powder for Kittens (Vet-A-Mix, Shenandoah, IA)

Homemade Prepared Formula for Puppies

120 mL cow's or goat's milk
120 mL water
2 to 4 egg yolks
1 to 2 tsp vegetable oil
1000 mg calcium carbonate

Homemade Prepared Formula for Kittens

90 mL condensed milk
90 mL water
120 mL plain yogurt (not low-fat)
3 large or 4 small egg yolks

g of body weight during the fourth week. These amounts of formula should be given in equal portions three or four times daily. For the first 3 weeks of life, the formula should be warmed before each feeding to about 100°F (37.8°C) or near the animal's body temperature.

After each feeding, the abdomen should be enlarged but not overdistended. When a formula is used, less than the prescribed amount should be given per feeding for the first day's feedings. The amount is then gradually increased to the recommended feeding amount by the second or third day. The amount of formula is increased accordingly as the puppy or kitten gains weight and a favorable response to feeding occurs. Puppies should gain 1 to 2 g/day/lb (2 to 4 g/day/kg) of anticipated adult weight for the first 5 months of their lives. At birth, the kitten should weight 80 to 140 g (most weigh around 100 to 120 g) and should gain 50 to 100 g weekly.[1]

When preparing the formula, follow the manufacturer's directions for its proper preparation, and keep all feeding equipment scrupulously clean. A good way of handling prepared formula is to prepare only a 48-hour supply at a time and divide this into portions required for each feeding. Store prepared formula in the refrigerator at 4°C.

The easiest and safest way of feeding prepared formula to nursing-age puppies and kittens is by nipple bottle, dosing syringe, or tube.[1] Nipple bottles made especially for feeding orphaned puppies or kittens or bottles equipped with preemie infant nipples are preferred. When feeding with a nipple bottle, hold the bottle so that the puppy or kitten does not ingest air. The hole in the nipple should be such that when the bottle is inverted, milk slowly oozes from the nipple. It may be necessary to enlarge the nipple hole with a hot needle to get milk to ooze from the bottle when inverted. When feeding, squeeze a drop of milk onto the tip of the nipple and then insert the nipple into the puppy's or kitten's mouth. Never squeeze milk out of the bottle while the nipple is in the animal's mouth; doing so may result in laryngotracheal aspiration of the milk into the lungs. In addition, prepared formula should never be fed to a puppy or kitten that is chilled or that does not have a strong sucking reflex. Only when the sucking reflex is present should bottle feeding be attempted.

Tube feeding is the fastest way to feed orphaned puppies or kittens. Most owners can do it easily with a little training. The following may be used: a number 5 French infant feeding tube for puppies or kittens weighing less than 300 g; a number 8 to 10 French infant feeding tube for puppies or kittens weighing over 300 g; or an appropriately sized, soft, male urethral catheter. Once a week, mark the feeding tube clearly to indicate the depth of insertion to ensure gastric delivery; that is, the distance from the last rib to the tip of the nose can be measured and marked off on the feeding tube as a guide. Never feed into the distal esophagus. When feeding, fill a syringe with warm prepared formula and fit it to the feeding tube, being sure to expel any air in the tube or syringe. Open the animal's mouth slightly, and with the animal's head held in the normal nursing position, gently pass the feeding tube to the marked area. If an obstruction is felt or coughing occurs before reaching the mark, the tube is in the trachea. If this does not happen, slowly administer the prepared formula over a 2-minute period to allow sufficient time for slow filling of the stomach. Regurgitation of formula rarely occurs, but if it does, withdraw the feeding tube and interrupt feeding until the next scheduled meal.

A vital aspect of tending orphaned puppies and kittens is

to simulate, after feeding, the mother's tongue action on the anogenital area, which provokes reflex micturition and defecation. Application of this stimulus has to be taken over by the person tending the puppies or kittens. The necessary result can be achieved by swabbing the anogenital area with moistened cotton or dry, soft tissue paper to manually stimulate the reflex elimination. It is sometimes possible to effect the same response simply by running a forefinger along the abdominal wall. This stimulation should be provided after each bottle or tube feeding. After 3 weeks of age, puppies and kittens are usually able to relieve themselves without simulated stimulation.

Most puppies and kittens benefit from gentle handling before feeding to allow for some exercise and to promote muscular and circulatory development. In addition, at least once a week the orphaned puppy or kitten should be washed gently with a soft moistened cloth for general cleansing of the skin, simulating the cleansing licks of the mother's tongue.

As mentioned before, the orphaned puppy or kitten should be encouraged to begin eating solid food at 3 or 4 weeks of age, respectively. Once it is eating satisfactorily from a bowl, the amount of prepared formula is gradually reduced until only the puppy or kitten food designed for growth is being fed, at least three times a day.

MALNUTRITION OF THE PUPPY AND KITTEN

Malnutrition occurs when nutritional requirements are not being met. Malnutrition is especially common during the time puppies and kittens depend entirely on the mother for their nutritional needs. Nursing puppies and kittens have similar nutritional requirements, and survival for each depends on the mother's ability to care for them; their ability to digest, absorb, and utilize nutrients; and the gradually increasing plane of nutrition provided.

Several factors can contribute to malnutrition in the nursing puppy or kitten.[5, 6] The puppy or kitten may ingest insufficient milk because the mother dies or disowns her young, because the mother cannot adequately care for a large litter, or because of partial or complete lactation failure by the mother owing to illness, mastitis, metritis, or underdeveloped mammae. In addition, the puppy or kitten may be born prematurely or underdeveloped; it may be so weak and sick that it cannot suckle normally, or it may have congenital defects that preclude adequate milk intake. Failure to provide an appropriate growth-formulated diet at 3 to 4 weeks of age and older can result in nutrient intake inadequate to meet the needs of growth.

Immediate recognition of a malnourished puppy or kitten is usually based on its smaller, lighter appearance, its feeble attempts to feed, or its inability to attain adequate weight gain for its age. High-pitched, constant crying or inactivity accompanied by a weak sucking reflex are advanced indications that the nursing puppy or kitten is receiving insufficient milk. Reduced body tone and muscle strength may be evident on handling. Coexisting congenital defects that are not immediately life-threatening may be detected on physical examination.

The treatment of malnutrition in the nursing puppy and kitten generally requires that proper nourishment be provided.[6] Complications that are frequently encountered during the management of malnutrition are diarrhea, dehydration, hypoglycemia, and hypothermia.[8] If diarrhea occurs while feeding adequate amounts of properly prepared milk-replacement formula, immediately reduce the amount of solid intake by half. This can be done by diluting the formula 1 to 1 with water or, preferably, with a mixture of equal parts of multiple-electrolyte solution and 5 per cent dextrose and water solution. As the condition of feces improves, the amount of solids can be gradually increased to the recommended level.

Hypoglycemia and dehydration occur quickly when a malnourished puppy or kitten is not fed adequately. To help alleviate dehydration and mild hypoglycemia, administer an equal mixture of warm multiple-electrolyte solution and 5 per cent dextrose and water solution parenterally until the puppy or kitten responds. No type of milk-replacement formula should be given to a weak and severely chilled puppy or kitten that displays a diminished sucking reflex or a rectal temperature below 35°C (95°F).

It is important to maintain the rectal body temperature above 35°C (95°F). Warming of the puppy or kitten should be done slowly over 1 to 3 hours, depending on the degree of chilling. Until the rectal temperature is about 100°F, only warmed fluid solutions, as mentioned previously, should be given. Once the rectal temperature is 100°F, warmed milk-replacement formula may be substituted for the fluid solution.

REFERENCES

1. Lewis LD, et al: Small Animal Clinical Nutrition III. Topeka, KS, Mark Morris Associates, 1987.
2. Brawner WR, et al: Body composition of growing Great Dane puppies fed diets varying in calcium and phosphorus concentration evaluated by dual energy x-ray absorptiometry. ACVR 12:1, 1996.
3. Goodman SA, et al: Orthopedic observations in Great Dane puppies fed diets varying in calcium and phosphorus content: A preliminary report. Proceedings of the 24th annual Veterinary Orthopedic Society, San Francisco, 1997, p 51.
4. Beaver BV: Behavior development and behavioral disorders. In Hoskins JD (ed): Veterinary Pediatrics: Dogs and Cats From Birth to Six Months. Philadelphia, WB Saunders, 1995, p 23.
5. Bjorck G: Care and feeding of the puppy in the postnatal and weaning period. In Bjorck G (ed): Nutrition and Behavior in Dogs and Cats. New York, Pergamon Press, 1982, p 25.
6. Baines FM: Milk substitutes and the hand rearing of orphan puppies and kittens. J Small Anim Pract 22:555, 1981.
7. Remillard RL, et al: Comparison of kittens fed queen's milk with those fed milker replacers. Am J Vet Res 54:901, 1993.
8. Mosier JE: Causes and treatment of neonatal deaths. In Kirk RW (ed): Current Veterinary Therapy VI. Philadelphia, WB Saunders, 1977, p 44.

CHAPTER 66

DEVELOPMENTAL ORTHOPEDIC DISEASE OF DOGS

Daniel C. Richardson and Steven C. Zicker

Developmental orthopedic disease (DOD) is a diverse group of musculoskeletal disorders that occur in growing animals (most commonly fast-growing large and giant breed dogs) and in some cases may have a nutrition-related etiology. The prevalence of musculoskeletal problems in dogs of all breeds younger than 1 year of age is about 22 per cent, with 20 per cent of these cases having a possible nutrition-related etiology.[1] Osteochondrosis and canine hip dysplasia (CHD) account for the overwhelming majority of nutrition-related problems.[1]

CHD is the most frequently encountered orthopedic disease with heritability and a potential nutrition-related etiology in veterinary medicine.[2] CHD is an abnormal development or growth of the hip joint manifested by varying degrees of laxity of surrounding soft tissues, instability, and malformation of the femoral head and acetabulum with osteoarthrosis. The actual number of cases is estimated to be in the millions worldwide.[3]

Osteochondrosis is widespread among young, rapidly growing, warm-blooded domesticated species and humans. Generally, osteochondrosis is a disruption in endochondral ossification that results in a focal lesion. Osteochondrosis occurs in the physis and/or epiphysis of growth cartilage and may be considered a generalized or systemic disease.

When osteochondrosis affects physeal cartilage, it may cause growth abnormalities in long bones, such as angular limb deformities. Osteochondrosis of articular epiphyseal cartilage commonly occurs in the shoulder (proximal humerus), stifle (distal femur), hock (talus), and elbow (distal humerus). Acute inflammatory joint disease (or degenerative joint disease) may ensue subsequent to development of osteochondrosis when the cartilage surface is disrupted and subchondral bone is exposed to synovial fluid (osteochondritis dissecans). Inflammatory mediators and cartilage fragments are released into the joint, which perpetuates the cycle of degenerative joint disease. Other disease processes such as spondylolisthesis, intra-articular fracture, complete or partial epiphysiolysis, and deformed joint surfaces have been associated with osteochondrosis, but their etiology is still undetermined.

LABORATORY INFORMATION

Uncomplicated cases of DOD rarely produce alterations in complete blood counts, serum biochemistries, or urinalyses.[4] On occasion, serum concentrations of calcium and phosphorus may be elevated or decreased during the genesis of DOD. However, absence of calcium or phosphorus perturbations does not negate a diagnosis of DOD.[4] Increased bone remodeling may result in increased activity of alkaline phosphatase (ALP) in serum. This parameter is already high in young, growing animals and may not be a very sensitive indicator of ongoing metabolic bone disease. Other enzymatic activities in serum are not useful indicators for the diagnosis of DOD. Biochemical markers of human metabolic bone disease such as type I collagen propeptides, tartrate-resistant acid phosphatase, and osteocalcin may prove useful in the future for veterinary diagnostics.[5] Analysis of urine for markers of bone turnover such as hydroxylysine glycosides, free pyridinolines, or pyridinoline cross-links of collagen may prove useful in the future.

RISK FACTORS

Despite improved nutrient content and balance of foods, the frequency of canine DOD has not decreased markedly. Genesis of DOD is presumed to be a multifactorial process that appears to have significant input from management (environmental), genetic, and nutritional interactions in young, growing animals. Specific factors that are currently thought to increase risk in young dogs include large and giant breed dogs (genetic), ad libitum feeding (management), foods with high energy (fat) density (nutrition), and excessive calcium intake from food or treats (nutrition).

ETIOPATHOGENESIS

A number of mechanisms are possible when considering the genesis of DOD, but no one specific etiology is considered ultimately responsible for all observed clinical manifestations. Historically, feeding dogs and cats imbalanced foods, especially those deficient in calcium, phosphorus, or vitamin D_3, was the main risk factor for skeletal diseases such as secondary hyperparathyroidism.[6] Today, dietary deficiencies are rare in young, growing dogs, because most are fed commercial foods formulated to have internal safety margins for specific nutrients.[7] Two theories are currently popular for the pathogenesis of some types of DOD: (1) excessive energy intake, which results in rapid growth and biomechanical "triggering" of skeletal lesions, and (2) excessive calcium intake, which results in hypercalcitoninism and interferes with normal endochondral ossification and bone remodeling.

ENERGY, GROWTH, AND BIOMECHANICAL STRESS

The risk of DOD appears to be increased in large and giant breed dogs fed well-balanced, highly palatable, energy-dense foods,[6, 8–10] presumably because of their genetic propensity for rapid growth.[6, 11] The musculoskeletal system changes constantly throughout life, with the most rapid changes occurring in the first few months of life (Fig. 66–1). The skeletal system apparently is most susceptible to physical, nutritional, and metabolic insults during the first 12 months of life, for several possible reasons.

First, overfeeding of energy in young large and giant breed dogs affects growth velocity directly through nutrient supply and indirectly through growth hormone, insulin-like growth factor 1 (IGF-1), triiodothyronine (T_3), thyroxine (T_4), and insulin.[12–14] Dysregulation of these endocrine factors, whether attributable to nutrition, feeding management, or genetics, during this critical period of skeletal growth may produce an environment in which DOD develops.

Second, histologic examinations reveal that articular cartilage is not as well supported by solid bone plates in rapidly growing dogs compared with smaller breeds or littermates that were fed restricted amounts after weaning.[6] The epiphyseal spongiosa of giant breed dogs is inherently less dense and therefore inferred to be less strong than the spongiosa in small breeds, a tendency that may be exaggerated by overnutrition. Ad libitum feeding may lead to a mismatch between bone growth and body growth, resulting in a lower ratio of long bone diaphyseal shaft cross-sectional area to body weight and in the formation of a less dense epiphyseal spongiosa.

The result of this bone growth–body growth mismatch is biomechanical stress, which has been suggested as an etiology for DOD. It is unknown, and somewhat contested, whether small focal cartilaginous lesions occur first and are then exacerbated by biomechanical stress[6, 15] or whether biomechanical stress induces cartilaginous lesions.[8, 16] In either case, immature skeletons may be damaged by increased static (weight load) and dynamic (muscle pull) forces, which are of special importance in large and giant breed dogs. Taken together, dysregulation of nutrient supply, bone formation, and endocrine regulation may interfere with skeletal maturation, thus increasing the risk for DOD in young animals.

EXCESS CALCIUM AND HYPERCALCITONINISM

A contrasting theory involves increased rates of DOD observed in dogs with high calcium intakes.[4, 17–19] Dogs raised on food with a high calcium content or a high calcium plus phosphorus content exhibited disturbed endochondral ossification,[16, 20] retained cartilaginous cores in the distal radius and ulna,[19] and delayed skeletal maturation and growth of bone length.[19] Calcium intake, therefore, seems to be a significant determining factor in DOD. The effect may occur either directly or indirectly, possibly by calcium competing with other minerals or stimulating calciotropic hormones.[21]

The total concentration of calcium in serum is determined by the interplay of homeostatic mechanisms involving influx (gastrointestinal absorption), efflux (gastrointestinal and renal loss), and the less labile bone pool. The concentration of ionized calcium is the most important determinant of calciotropic homeostatic regulation. Sudden increases in concentrations of ionized calcium stimulate release of calcitonin from the thyroid gland, whereas decreases in concentrations of ionized calcium stimulate release of parathyroid hormone (PTH) from the parathyroid gland. Calcitonin released into blood results in decreased concentrations of calcium and phosphorus, possibly through increased osteoblastic and decreased osteoclastic activity (decreased skeletal remodeling).[22, 23]

Dogs ingesting excessive amounts of calcium for prolonged periods exhibited hyperplastic C-cells (calcitonin-producing cells) in their thyroid glands.[20, 21] These same dogs had clinical and radiographic evidence of DOD compared with controls.[8, 16] Accordingly, hypercalcitoninism may be a contributing factor to DOD in dogs.[8, 16]

KEY NUTRITIONAL FACTORS

Nutrients must be provided in appropriate amounts and balances for optimal bone development. Excesses of specific nutrients, such as calcium and energy, together with rapid growth appear to predispose to disorders such as osteochondrosis and CHD.[8, 11] However, severe excesses, deficits, or imbalances of any nutrient may affect bone development.

ENERGY AND FAT

Energy intake, which is dependent on a variety of physiologic factors, is the main nutritional factor that determines growth intensity, as long as other nutrients are supplied in adequate and balanced amounts. Determination of appropriate energy requirements for growing dogs is difficult, because minimal comparative data from well-controlled studies are available. Energy intake reaches a maximum, in relation to body weight, in the second to fourth months of life (< 45 per cent adult body weight) (see Fig. 66–1). General recommendations for the amount of energy to feed are presented later in this chapter.

Large breed dogs (German shepherd, rottweiler, Labrador retriever, and golden retriever) fed high-energy-density (3.98 kcal/g metabolizable energy [ME]: 23.9 per cent fat dry matter [DM]), medium-energy-density (3.5 kcal/g ME: 10.8 per cent fat DM), and low-energy-density (3.16 kcal/g ME: 8.0 per cent fat DM) foods ad libitum actually grew slower and had less fat deposition when consuming the low-energy-density food.[24] This indicates that growing dogs may receive better satiety signals from low-energy-density foods than from high-energy-density foods and thus avoid overconsumption of energy. However, a certain amount of fat (Association of American Feed Control Officials [AAFCO] mini-

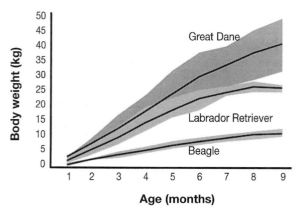

Figure 66–1. Growth curves (weight vs. age) for Great Danes, Labrador retrievers, and beagles. (From Richardson DC, Zentek J, Hazewinkel HAW, et al: Developmental Bone Disease of Dogs, SACN IV. Topeka, KS, Mark Morris Institute, 1997.)

mum recommendation for growth = 8.0 per cent) in the food is important for fat-soluble vitamin absorption and palatability. Concentrations of essential nutrients may need to be adjusted in order to meet nutritional requirements when the energy density of foods is altered.

Because increased rate of growth is a risk factor in fast-growing large and giant breed dogs, it follows that increased fat content, or increased metabolizable energy per gram of dry matter of foods, must be considered a risk factor. As the fat content of foods increases, the energy density also necessarily increases, unless fiber is substituted for other metabolizable nutrients. In general, it is best to keep the energy content of a growth food for large breed puppies below 3.8 kcal/g, which approximates 12 per cent fat on a dry-matter basis.

CALCIUM

The amount of true calcium absorption in dogs ranges from 25 to 90 per cent, depending on the amount of intake and the age of the animal.[4, 25] Calcium is absorbed through three modalities: active absorption, facilitated diffusion, and passive diffusion. Passive diffusion is especially important in young animals. Active absorption is most important in the proximal gastrointestinal tract. Passive and facilitated absorption, however, are important in the distal gastrointestinal tract, mainly because of prolonged transit time and increased calcium concentration through that section. Vitamin D_3 metabolites, especially 1,25-dihydroxyvitamin D_3, are the most important hormonal regulators of gastrointestinal calcium absorption.[26] Regulation of renal calcium excretion is also subject to regulation, mainly by PTH.

The absolute level of calcium in the food, rather than an imbalance in the calcium-phosphorus ratio, influences skeletal development.[16, 25] Young giant breed dogs ingesting foods containing excess calcium (3.3 per cent dry-matter basis) with either normal phosphorus (0.9 per cent dry-matter basis) or high phosphorus (3 per cent dry-matter basis, to maintain a normal calcium-phosphorus ratio) had a significantly increased prevalence of DOD.[25] These puppies apparently were unable to protect themselves from the negative effects of chronic calcium excess.[16] Because the previously discussed studies demonstrate the safety and adequacy of 1.1 per cent calcium (dry-matter basis) and the AAFCO suggested recommended allowance is 1.0 per cent (dry-matter basis), calcium levels for growth foods should range from 0.9 to 1.5 per cent for at-risk puppies, with no supplementation.[27]

DIGESTIBILITY

Although not a nutrient, this nutritional factor becomes important in certain physiologic states, such as growth. During the growth period, the ability to ingest and absorb adequate amounts of various nutrients is dependent on food intake capacity and the quality of ingredients. It is especially important to consider quality of ingredients when trying to limit energy intake in at-risk dogs. The goal of energy restriction is not to provide low-quality foods that are poorly digestible but to provide high-quality foods in a low-energy-density product that will promote appropriate growth. It is important to assess digestibility and recommend foods with above-average digestibility for growth. Above-average digestibility can be considered more than 5 per cent above the average values defined by AAFCO.[28]

OTHER MINERALS

Phosphorus. The level of phosphorous recommended must be considered in conjunction with calcium recommendations. Excessive as well as inadequate phosphorus intake may affect calcium homeostasis and thus bone development. Excessive phosphorus intake, together with inadequate calcium intake, may result in nutritional secondary hyperparathyroidism. The calcium-to-phosphorus ratio should be maintained at 1.1:1 to 2:1. When calcium intake is set at 0.9 to 1.5 per cent of the food, as recommended previously for large breeds at risk for DOD, the phosphorus content of the food should be 0.8 to 1.4 per cent of the dry matter.[29]

Copper. Copper plays an important role in the metabolism of collagen and elastin; however, the overall prevalence of primary (dietary) copper deficiency should not be overestimated.[30] Dietary copper levels less than 1 mg/kg dry matter resulted in severe growth deformities, fractures, wide "knotty" epiphyses, and especially severe hyperextension of the limb axis in growing dogs.[31] In young beagles, clinical signs of copper deficiency were less severe than those previously described, but hyperextension of the forelegs was also found as a characteristic feature.[32]

Most common ingredients are rich in copper; however, some homemade, unsupplemented foods (made of rice, dairy products, fat, starch) may contain low or suboptimal concentrations of copper. Under certain circumstances, this may contribute to the development of skeletal disease, even if copper levels are higher than in deficient experimental foods. A suboptimal copper supply could evoke negative effects, especially if combined with a high growth intensity or additional dietary imbalances. The recommendation for copper in growth foods is 7.3 ppm,[28] but to achieve a safety margin for at-risk dogs, a level of 10 ppm is encouraged. Most commercial foods for growth deliver copper in a range from 10 to 20 ppm to ensure that this minimum recommendation is met.

Zinc. Inadequate zinc supply, especially in growing animals, may lead to severe clinical signs within days, resulting in growth depression, skin defects, impaired immune function, and growth disorders of the skeleton. These disorders may be linked to the role of zinc as a cofactor in multiple enzymes, including those important for connective tissue metabolism. A low activity of alkaline phosphatase (< 300 IU/L) is a good indicator of low zinc status in young dogs.[33] Experimental zinc deficiency in beagles led to a significant decrease of zinc concentrations in the skeleton,[33] especially in metaphyseal bone, which represents newly formed tissue. It is not known to what extent marginal zinc intake, because of either subnormal dietary zinc concentrations or high concentrations of interacting substances (e.g., phytic acid, calcium, copper, low-digestible carbohydrates), contributes to DOD. There are no reports demonstrating detrimental effects of excess zinc on skeletal development in dogs; however, excess zinc may be presumed to be toxic at higher levels, as observed in other species.

Foods for growing dogs should contain a safety margin of zinc to compensate for negative interactions exerted by other dietary ingredients, especially if the originally balanced food is "improved" by dog owners who add large amounts of calcium carbonate or other calcium salts. It is recommended that foods contain zinc in the 120- to 130-ppm range. Most commercial foods for growth contain 200 to 300 ppm to ensure that this minimum recommendation is met.

Iodine. Iodine is essential for function of the thyroid gland.[34] Both thyroid hormones, particularly triiodothyronine, influence normal degeneration of growth cartilage, penetration of capillaries, and mineralization of newly formed bone. Thyroid hormones also stimulate formation and resorption of bone, which results in remodeling of the skeleton.[35] Congenitally hypothyroid Boxers had shortened limb bones and severe disturbances of the ossification and mineralization process, which were alleviated by L-thyroxine supplementation.[36] Stunted limb development, hyperplasia of the thyroid gland, edema, and loss of hair typically occur in young pups born to bitches that were iodine deficient during pregnancy. Most commercial foods meet the recommended iodine level of 1.5 ppm.[28]

Manganese. Manganese acts as a coenzyme in glycosyl transferases in the metabolism of the ground substance in cartilage. Experimental dietary deficiency leads to disproportionate, shortened, and thickened long bones in different species; defective development of the skull; and formation of otoliths in the inner ear during gestation.[37] Currently, no reports on naturally occurring manganese deficiency in dogs exist. Compared with most other species, the dietary requirements of dogs appear to be lower (1.4 mg/1000 kcal ME).[38] Most commercial foods meet or exceed the recommended level of 5 mg/kg dry-matter basis.[28]

PROTEIN

Protein is required for a variety of structural and functional molecules in order to achieve proper growth. The minimal adequate level of dietary protein depends on digestibility, amino acid composition, proper ratios among the essential amino acids, energy density of the food, and dietary protein's availability from protein sources. The dietary protein requirements of healthy growing dogs decrease as they approach adulthood.[27]

Protein excess has not been demonstrated to negatively affect health or skeletal development during growth in Great Danes when compared with isoenergetically fed controls.[39] Protein deficiency may affect the general health of developing puppies, decrease plasma growth hormone levels, and reduce skeletal growth.[38] A growth food with average energy density should contain 25 to 30 per cent protein (dry-matter basis) of high biologic value.[29]

VITAMINS

Vitamin D. Metabolites of vitamin D_3 act in concert with other hormones to regulate calcium metabolism and therefore skeletal development in dogs. Vitamin D_3 metabolites aid in absorption of calcium and phosphorus from the gut as well as influence bone cell activity.[40] Vitamin D_3 has been suggested as a requirement in foods for dogs because endogenous synthesis may be limited.[41]

Clinical cases of vitamin D_3 deficiency (rickets) are extremely rare in animals eating commercial foods.[7] Diagnosis of vitamin D_3 deficiency can be made by measuring circulating levels of vitamin D_3 metabolites. Increased growth plate width is not associated with low-calcium, high-phosphorus foods but is a strong indicator of rickets.[40]

In growing dogs, supplementation with excess vitamin D can markedly disturb normal skeletal development.[27, 40] Excess vitamin D may cause hypercalcemia, hyperphosphatemia, anorexia, polydipsia, polyuria, vomiting, muscle weakness, generalized soft tissue mineralization, and lameness. Minimal recommendations for foods are 500 IU vita-

min D/kg dry matter (143 IU/1000 kcal ME).[7, 28, 29] Commercial pet foods contain from two to 10 times the minimal amount recommended by AAFCO.[28] Because commercial foods contain added vitamin D_3, and in light of potentially limited endogenous synthesis, measurement of vitamin D_3 in serum may reflect dietary changes rather than specific disease states.

Vitamin A. Vitamin A is an essential factor involved in bone metabolism, especially osteoclastic activity.[42] Deficiency or excess may lead to severe metabolic bone disease in growing dogs.[38] Hypervitaminosis A may result in anorexia, decreased weight gain, hyperesthesia, narrowing of long bone epiphyseal cartilage, ankylosis, new bone formation without osteolysis, and thin bone cortices. Hypovitaminosis A results in a variety of clinical signs, including anorexia, weight loss, ataxia, xerophthalmia, metaplasia of bronchiolar epithelium, conjunctivitis, and increased susceptibility to infection.

Concentration of vitamin A in dog foods is recommended at 5000 IU/kg dry matter (1429 IU/1000 kcal ME).[28, 38] Most commercial dog foods are supplemented well above the minimal requirement for vitamin A.

Vitamin C. The relationship between vitamin C and developmental disorders of the skeletal system in dogs is unproved, and supplementation is not recommended.[43] There are no dietary requirements for vitamin C in dogs.[29]

FEEDING PLAN

PREVENTION FOR AT-RISK DOGS

1. Determine if the dog is at risk for DOD (all large and giant breeds).
2. If at risk, control nutrients of concern by diet composition and feeding method.
3. Do not add vitamin or mineral supplements to balanced foods, particularly calcium, phosphorus, vitamin D, and vitamin A. If a nutritionally adequate growth food is being fed, supplementation is contraindicated.
4. Take a body condition score (BCS) every 2 weeks. Dogs should have a BCS of 2 to 3 (Table 66–1).

FOOD SELECTION

The food should consist of a commercial or well-balanced homemade food specific for the unique nutrient requirements of fast-growing large and giant breed puppies. Recommended nutrient intake in fast-growing large and giant breed dogs is similar to that in other breeds, except for more stringent restrictions regarding fat, energy, and calcium intake. Several commercial foods are available that have been formulated for fast-growing large and giant breed puppies. However, even foods specifically formulated for large breeds have considerable differences in key nutrients that are considered risk factors for skeletal disease in large breed puppies.

In general, dry foods are more economical and less energy dense than canned foods. Considering that most DOD occurs in large and giant breed dogs, dry food is usually selected. However, canned foods may be fed as long as special attention is paid to key nutritional factors.

Foods for growth should have passed an AAFCO feeding trial specific for that life stage. However, AAFCO trials do not ensure adequacy or safety for every breed. In dogs at risk for DOD, special attention should be focused on energy density and calcium content of the food, as well as feeding method.

DETERMINATION OF A FEEDING METHOD

Both the nutrient profile of a food and how it is fed may help control nutrition-related risk factors for DOD. The aim of feeding programs for large breed growing puppies is to achieve moderate energy restriction. This energy restriction may be as high as 10 to 25 per cent of ad libitum intake if high-energy-density foods are currently fed ad libitum.[8, 9, 44] This recommendation does not mean that one should starve a dog or feed it a weight-control food formulated for obese adult dogs. If healthy growing dogs eat to satisfy their satiety needs, foods formulated for weight control may result in insufficient mineral, protein, or vitamin intake. Rather, correct dietary allowances must be supplied to puppies in order to satisfy physiologic needs for optimal skeletal growth in conjunction with moderate energy restriction.[28] Slow growth during the first year does not have a deleterious effect on final adult skeletal size.

There are three basic methods of feeding growing dogs: free choice (ad libitum), time limited, or food limited. In any feeding regimen, an initial estimate of the amount to be fed is required, whether it is the manufacturer's feeding guide or a calculated amount. In general, free-choice feeding is contraindicated in at-risk dogs until they have reached skeletal maturity (about 12 months of age, or at least 80 to 90 per cent of adult weight). If time-limited feeding is used, 10-minute, 5-minute, or even shorter feeding periods (three times per day for the first month after weaning, then twice per day) may be required to achieve the desired decreased food intake in some puppies.

TABLE 66–1. BODY CONDITION SCORING SYSTEM FOR DOGS

SCORE	DESCRIPTION
1 Very thin	Ribs: Easily palpable with no fat cover Tail base: Prominent raised bony structures with no subcutaneous tissue Abdomen: Severe abdominal tuck, accentuated hourglass shape
2 Underweight	Ribs: Easily palpable with minimal fat cover Tail base: Raised bony structures with little subcutaneous tissue Abdomen: Abdominal tuck, marked hourglass shape
3 Ideal	Ribs: Palpable with slight fat cover Tail base: Smooth contour or some thickening, bony structures palpable under thin layer of subcutaneous fat Abdomen: Abdominal tuck, well-proportioned lumbar "waist"
4 Overweight	Ribs: Difficult to palpate, moderate fat cover Tail base: Smooth contour or some thickening, bony structures remain palpable Abdomen: Little or no abdominal tuck or waist, back slightly broadened
5 Obese	Ribs: Very difficult to palpate, thick fat cover Tail base: Appears thickened, difficult to palpate bony structures Abdomen: Pendulous ventral bulge, no waist, back markedly broadened; trough may form when epaxial areas bulge dorsally

From Proceedings of a Symposium on Health and Nutrition of Geriatric Cats and Dogs, Orlando, FL, 1996.

TABLE 66–2. NUTRITIONAL RECOMMENDATIONS FOR DOGS AT RISK FOR DEVELOPMENTAL ORTHOPEDIC DISEASE

KEY NUTRITIONAL FACTOR	ALLOWANCE/RECOMMENDATION
Feeding method	Calculated food dose
Energy	Weaning to 4 months = 3 × RER 4–12 months = 2 × RER
Body condition score	Adjust food dose as needed to achieve a body condition score between 2 and 3
Energy density of food	3.2–3.8 kcal/g (13.4–15.9 kJ/g)
Fat	Limit to approximately < 12% of dry matter
Calcium	0.9–1.5% of dry matter
Protein	25–30% of dry matter
Supplements	None recommended, especially if fed commercial foods recommended for large breed dogs
Digestibility	Above average

RER = resting energy requirement.
From Richardson DC, Zentek J, Hazewinkel HAW, et al: Developmental Bone Disease of Dogs, SACN IV. Topeka, KS, Mark Morris Institute, 1997.

The method of choice for feeding at-risk puppies is limiting food intake by calculating a food dose to maintain optimal growth rate and body condition. Food-limited feeding requires feeding a measured amount of food based on calculated energy requirement, or as recommended by the manufacturer, divided into two or three meals per day. Energy requirement is most easily calculated by using resting energy requirement (RER) as a base. RER can be calculated using either of the following equations:

$$RER \text{ (kcal/day)} = 70 \, (BW_{kg})^{0.75} \text{ or } (30 \times BW_{kg}) + 70$$

As a starting point, use 3 × RER for the first 4 months of life and 2 × RER from 4 months of age to 80 per cent of expected mature weight (about 10 to 12 months for most breeds). Once the daily caloric requirement has been calculated (kcal/day, kJ/day), divide this number by the energy density of the food (kcal or kJ/cup or kcal or kJ/can) to determine the number of cups or cans to feed per day. Most large and giant breed dogs continue to increase body weight and muscle mass after 12 months, but the growth rate is reduced, and most if not all growth plates are closed. At 12 months they can be fed as adults (1.6 × RER for neutered dogs and 1.8 × RER for intact dogs). Remember, calculations and manufacturers' recommendations are only starting points and should be followed by BCS.

CONCLUSION

Regular clinical evaluation of growing puppies and adjustment of food offered are crucial. Rapidly growing large and giant breed dogs have a very steep growth curve, and their intake requirements can change dramatically over short periods. These puppies should be weighed and evaluated (BCS) and their daily feeding amounts adjusted at least once every 2 weeks (Fig. 66–2).

Skeletal disease can be influenced during growth by feeding technique and nutrient profile. However, nutritional management alone will not completely control DOD. Dietary deficiencies are of minimal concern with today's commercial foods specifically prepared for young, growing dogs. The major potential for harm is in overnutrition from excess

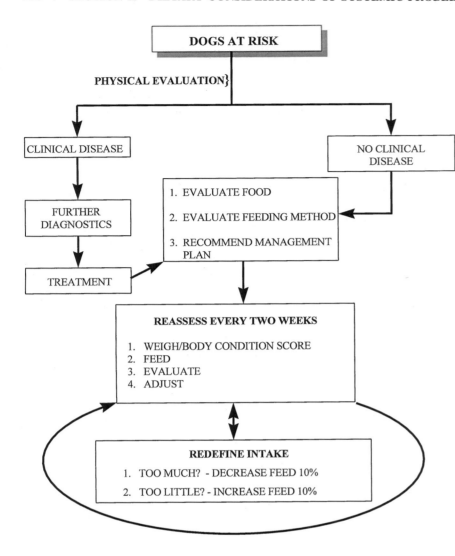

Figure 66–2. Paradigm for working up dogs at risk for developmental orthopedic disease. (From Richardson DC, Zentek J, Hazewinkel HAW, et al: Developmental Bone Disease of Dogs, SACN IV. Topeka, KS, Mark Morris Institute, 1997.)

consumption and oversupplementation of foods with excessive energy and calcium (Table 66–2).

REFERENCES

1. Breuer GJ: Unpublished data, Purdue University.
2. Johnson JA, Austin C, Breuer GJ: Incidence of canine appendicular musculoskeletal disorders in 16 veterinary teaching hospitals from 1980–1989. JVCOT 7:56, 1994.
3. Brinker WO, Piermattei DL, Flo GL: Physical examination for lameness. In Handbook of Small Animal Orthopedics and Fracture Treatment, 2nd ed. Philadelphia, WB Saunders, 1990, pp 267–277.
4. Nap RC, Hazewinkel HAW: Growth and skeletal development in the dog in relation to nutrition; a review. Vet Q 16:50, 1994.
5. Robey PG, Termine JD: Biochemical markers of metabolic bone disease. In Avioli LV, Krane SM (eds): Metabolic Bone Disease and Clinically Related Disorders, 2nd ed. Philadelphia, WB Saunders, 1990, pp 244–263.
6. Daemmrich K: Relationship between nutrition and bone growth in large and giant dogs. J Nutr 121:S114, 1991.
7. Kallfelz FA, Dzanis DA: Overnutrition: An epidemic problem in pet animal practice. Vet Clin North Am Small Anim Pract 19:433, 1989.
8. Hedhammar A, Wu F, Krook L, et al: Overnutrition and skeletal disease. An experimental study in growing Great Dane dogs. Cornell Veterinarian 64 (Suppl. 5):1, 1974.
9. Kealy RD, Olsson SE, Monti KL, et al: Effects of limited food consumption on the incidence of hip dysplasia in growing dogs. JAVMA 210:857, 1992.
10. Richardson DC: The role of nutrition in canine hip dysplasia. Vet Clin North Am Small Anim Pract 22:529, 1992.
11. Meyer H, Zentek J: Energy requirements of growing Great Danes. J Nutr 121:S35, 1991.
12. Eigenmann JE, DeBruijne JJ, Froesch ER: Insulin-like-growth-factor I and growth hormone in canine starvation. Acta Endocrinol (Kbh) 108:161, 1985.
13. Danforth E, Burger AG: The impact of nutrition on thyroid hormone physiology and action. Annu Rev Nutr 9:201, 1989.
14. Nap RC, Hazewinkel HAW, Voorhout G, et al: The influence of the dietary protein content on growth in giant breed dogs. JVCOT 6:1, 1993.
15. Carlson CS, Meuten DJ, Richardson DC: Ischemic necrosis of cartilage in spontaneous and experimental lesions of osteochondrosis. J Orthop Res 9:317, 1991.
16. Hazewinkel HAW, Goedgebuure SA, Poulos PW, et al: Influences of chronic calcium excess on the skeletal development of growing Great Danes. J Am Anim Hosp Assoc 21:377, 1985.
17. Slater MR, Scarlett JM, Donoghue S, et al: Diet and exercise as potential risk factors for osteochondritis dissecans in dogs. Am J Vet Res 53:2119, 1992.
18. Dobenecker B, Kienzle E, Matis U: Mal- and overnutrition in puppies with or without clinical disorders of skeletal development (abstract). Proc Eur Soc Vet Comp Nutr, Munich, 25, 1997.
19. Voorhout A, Hazewinkel HAW: A radiographic study on the development of the antebrachium in Great Dane pups on different calcium intakes. Vet Radiol 28:152, 1987.
20. Goedegebuure SA, Hazewinkel HAW: Morphological findings in young dogs chronically fed a diet containing excess calcium. Vet Pathol 23:594, 1986.
21. Nunez EA, Hedhammar A, Wu FM, et al: Ultrastructure of the thyroid C cells and the parathyroid cells in growing dogs on a high calcium diet. Lab Invest 31:96, 1974.
22. Martin TJ, Moseley JM: Calcitonin. In Avioli LV, Krane SM (eds): Metabolic Bone Disease and Clinically Related Disorders. Philadelphia, WB Saunders, 1990, pp 131–154.
23. Weisbrode SE, Capen CC: The ultrastructural effects of parathyroid-hormone, calcitonin, and vitamin D on bone. In Bonucci E, Motta PM (eds): Ultrastructure of Skeletal Tissues. Bone and Cartilage in Health and Disease. Netherlands, Kluwer Academic Publishing, Dordrecht, 1990, pp 253–269.
24. Toll PW, Richardson DC: Unpublished data, Hill's Pet Nutrition, Inc., Science and Tech Center, Topeka, KS.
25. Hazewinkel HAW, Vandenbrom WE, Van't Klooster AT, et al: Calcium metabolism in Great Dane dogs fed diets with various calcium and phosphorous levels. J Nutr 121:S99, 1991.
26. Birge SJ, Avioli LV: Pathophysiology of calcium and phosphate disorders. In

Avioli LV, Krane SM (eds): Metabolic Bone Disease and Clinically Related Disorders. Philadelphia, WB Saunders, 1990, pp 196–221.

27. Richardson DC, Toll PW: Relationship of nutrition to developmental skeletal disease in young dogs. Vet Clin Nutr 4:6, 1997.
28. Association of American Feed Control Officials: Official publication 1997.
29. Dzanis DA: The AAFCO dog and cat nutrient profiles. In Bonagura JD (ed): Current Veterinary Therapy XII. Philadelphia, WB Saunders, 1995, pp 1418–1421.
30. Harris ED, Rayton JK, Balthrop JE, et al: Copper and the synthesis of elastin and collagen. In Ciba Foundation Symposium 79, Biological Roles of Copper. Amsterdam, Excerpta Medica, 1980, pp 163–182.
31. Baxter JH, Van Wyk JJ: A bone disorder associated with copper deficiency. I. Gross morphological, roentgenological, and chemical observations. Bull Johns Hopkins Hosp 93:1, 1953.
32. Zentek J, Daemmrich K, Meyer H: Untersuchungen zum Cu-Mangel beim wachsenden Hund. J Vet Med A 38:561, 1991.
33. Zentek J: Unpublished data, University of Hannover, Hannover, Germany.
34. Belshaw BE, Cooper TB, Becker DV: The iodine requirement and influence of iodine intake on iodine metabolism and thyroid function in the adult beagle. Endocrinology 96:1280, 1975.
35. High WB, Capen CC, Black HE: Effect of thyroxine on cortical bone remodeling in adult dogs. A histomorphometric study. Am J Pathol 102:438, 1981.

36. Saunders HM, Jezyk P: The radiographic appearance of canine congenital hypothyroidism: Skeletal changes with delayed treatment. Vet Radiol 32:171, 1991.
37. Hurley LS, Keen CL: Manganese. In Mertz W (ed): Trace Elements in Human and Animal Nutrition. Orlando, FL, Academic Press, 1986, pp 185–223.
38. National Research Council: Nutrient Requirements of Dogs. Rev. ed. Washington, DC, National Academy of Sciences, 1985.
39. Nap RC, Mol JA, Hazewinkel HAW: Age-related plasma concentrations of growth hormone (GH) and insulin-like growth factor 1 (IGF-1) in Great Dane pups fed different dietary levels of protein. Domest Anim Endocrinol 10:237, 1993.
40. Hazewinkel HAW: Nutrition in orthopedics. In Bojrab MJ (ed): Disease Mechanisms in Small Animal Surgery, 2nd ed. Philadelphia, Lea & Febiger, 1993, pp 1119–1128.
41. How KL, Hazewinkel AW, Mol JA: Dietary vitamin D dependence of cat and dog due to inadequate cutaneous synthesis of vitamin D. Gen Comp Endocrinol 96:12, 1994.
42. Hayes KC: On the pathophysiology of vitamin A deficiency. Nutr Rev 29:3, 1971.
43. Richardson DC: Developmental orthopedics: Nutritional influences in the dog. In Ettinger SJ, Feldman EC (eds): Textbook of Veterinary Internal Medicine, 4th ed. Philadelphia, WB Saunders, 1995, pp 252–257.
44. Lavelle RB: The effects of overfeeding of a balanced complete commercial diet to a group of growing Great Danes. In Burger IH, Rivers JW (eds): Nutrition of the Dog and Cat. Cambridge, Cambridge University Press, 1989, pp 303–315.

NUT

CHAPTER 67

ADVERSE REACTIONS TO FOODS: Allergies Versus Intolerance

Philip Roudebush and W. Grant Guilford

An adverse reaction to food is a clinically abnormal response to an ingested food or food additive. In general, the pathogenic mechanisms that lead to an adverse food reaction include ingestion of the inciting agent followed by interaction of the agent with a biologic amplification system that leads to inflammation and clinical signs.

In view of the number of diverse foods that are routinely ingested by the dog and cat, it is not surprising that adverse reactions develop to dietary substances. The fact that food-related reactions appear relatively infrequently is testimony to the effectiveness of the intestinal mucosal barrier and oral tolerance. Adverse reactions to food have been blamed for a variety of clinical syndromes in the dog and cat, usually involving the skin and gastrointestinal tract.

TERMINOLOGY

Adverse reactions to food comprise a variety of subclassifications based on pathomechanisms.[1, 2] The terminology is often confusing, but the following terms and definitions are those recommended by the American Academy of Allergy and Immunology (Fig. 67–1).[1, 2] Food allergy (food hypersensitivity) is an adverse reaction to a food or food additive with a proven immunologic basis. Food anaphylaxis is an acute food allergy with systemic consequences such as respiratory distress, vascular collapse, and urticaria. Food intolerance is a nonimmunologic, abnormal physiologic response to a food or food additive. Food intolerance can be further classified as food idiosyncrasy, food poisoning, and pharmacologic reactions to food. Food idiosyncrasy is an abnormal response that resembles food allergy but does not involve immune mechanisms. A direct nonimmunologic action on the host of food or a toxin in food is termed food poisoning. Adverse reactions due to a druglike or pharmacologic effect of a food substance on the host are termed pharmacologic reactions to food. Adverse reactions resulting from such behaviors as gluttony, pica, or ingestion of indigestible materials are called dietary indiscretion. Traditionally, the terms food hypersensitivity and food allergy have been used to describe all adverse reactions to food in dogs and cats, including reactions that were truly food intolerance. The newer terminology is used throughout this chapter and should be used to describe adverse food reactions in veterinary patients.

FOOD ALLERGENS

The specific food allergens that cause problems in animals have been poorly documented. In general, the major food

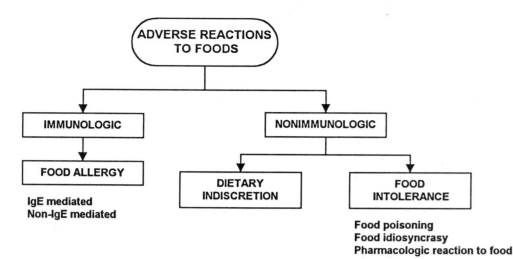

Figure 67–1. Algorithm for adverse reactions to foods.

allergens that have been identified in people are water-soluble glycoproteins that have molecular weights ranging from 10,000 to 60,000 daltons and are stable to treatment with heat, acid, and proteases.[3] Other physiochemical properties that account for their unique allergenicity are poorly understood.

A survey of veterinarians in North America incriminated food preservatives and dyes, wheat, beef, chicken egg, corn, poultry, soy, and dairy products as common causes of dermatologic signs of food allergy in dogs.[4] It is interesting to compare these clinical perceptions with documented case studies in the literature. Ten different studies, representing 253 dogs, described cutaneous lesions associated with adverse reactions to specific foods or ingredients.[5] In these studies, adverse reactions to beef, dairy products, and wheat accounted for two thirds of all the reported cases. Adverse reactions to chicken, chicken egg, lamb, soy, or pork accounted for approximately one fifth of the reported canine cases.

Food allergens incriminated in North American cats with dermatologic disease include fish, beef, chicken or other poultry, dairy products, preservatives, and dyes.[4] Eight different studies, representing 45 cats, described cutaneous lesions associated with adverse reactions to specific foods or ingredients.[5] In these studies, adverse reactions to beef, dairy products, and fish accounted for more than 80 per cent of all the reported feline cases.

Human allergy reference books often contain phylogenetic tables of animal and vegetable foods, so food-allergic persons can avoid other closely related foods.[3, 6] In clinical practice, human patients often report cross-reactivity among various fish and crustaceans but less cross-reactivity within vegetable food groups. Results of oral food challenges in children demonstrate that clinically important cross-reactivity to legumes (peanut, soybean, green bean, lima bean, pea, lentil) is very rare. Wheat, rye, and barley cross-react in allergic people, but oat allergens appear to cross-react only weakly. Cross-reactivity among milk proteins from cows, goats, and sheep has been noted. Children allergic to chicken egg have also been shown to cross-react with egg proteins of other birds. Certain allergens are apparently common to both foods and pollens. Common allergens have been reported in melon, banana, and ragweed pollen; celery and mugwort pollen; and apple and birch pollen. Cross-reactivity among food allergens has not been well investigated in pet animals.

FOOD INTOLERANCE

Nonimmunologic, abnormal physiologic reactions to food include food intolerance and dietary indiscretion (see Fig. 67–1). Like the terms food allergy and food hypersensitivity, the term food intolerance has been applied inappropriately to any and all adverse reactions to food. Food intolerance mimics food allergy, except that it can occur on the first exposure to a food or food additive, because nonimmunologic mechanisms are involved. The incidence of food intolerance versus food hypersensitivity or food allergy in veterinary patients is unknown.

REACTIONS TO FOOD ADDITIVES

Idiosyncratic adverse reactions to food additives often occur in people. Food additives frequently incriminated in human adverse reactions include sulfites, monosodium glutamate, tartrazine and other azo or nonazo dyes, benzoates, parabens, and spices. Few of the adverse reactions to food additives appear to involve an immunologic mechanism, although IgE-mediated reactions may occur. Confirmed reactions to food additives are best described as food intolerances or food idiosyncrasies, because clinical signs resulting from their ingestion are thought to be nonimmunologically mediated.[7] Examples are reactions to azo dyes, nonazo dyes, and antioxidants that can directly cause histamine release from leukocytes of clinically normal people.[8]

Although food additives are frequently incriminated in adverse reactions in dogs and cats, few data confirm this perception. Propylene glycol has been documented to cause hematologic abnormalities in cats and subsequently has been eliminated from cat foods sold in the United States and some other countries.[9]

Some veterinary dermatologists have incriminated food colorants and other food additives as causes of erythema multiforme and other "druglike" skin eruptions.[10, 11] Erythema multiforme is a cutaneous reaction pattern of multifactorial etiology seen uncommonly in dogs and rarely in cats. Lesions include erythematous macules and papules that spread to produce annular target and arciform lesions. The oral and nasal mucosa, pinnae, axillae, and groin areas are commonly involved. Most documented cases of erythema multiforme in dogs and cats are associated with drug hypersensitivity; neoplasia and infection are less common causes.

Food additives have been suspected in some cases, but their role has been poorly documented.[10, 11] Further studies are needed to document the occurrence of adverse reactions to pet food additives and the responsible pathomechanisms.

REACTIONS TO VASOACTIVE AMINES IN FOOD

Another cause of food intolerance is pharmacologic reactions to substances found in food. Vasoactive or biogenic amines such as histamine cause clinical signs in people when present in excessive levels in food.[12, 13] Scombroid fish such as tuna, mackerel, skipjack, and bonito that spoil before consumption are a frequent cause of histamine toxicosis in people.[12, 13] Clinical signs usually include diarrhea, flushing, sweating, nausea, vomiting, urticaria, facial swelling, and erythroderma.

The role of histamine and other vasoactive amines in food intolerance in animals is unknown. Adverse reactions to ingested scombroid fish have been observed in cats and dogs.[14] Recent surveys to detect histamine in pet foods found the highest levels of histamine in canned fish-based cat foods or those cat foods containing fish solubles.[14, 15] Vasoactive amines such as cadaverine may also exacerbate adverse reactions to spoiled fish by inhibiting histamine metabolism. Tyramine, spermine, spermidine, phenethylamine, putrescine, and cadaverine are other vasoactive amines found in pet foods.[16] Vasoactive or biogenic amines may not be present in levels high enough to cause clinical signs but could lower the threshold levels for allergens in individual dogs and cats. Idiosyncratic intolerances to small quantities of histamine have been reported to occur in people and animals.[14]

CARBOHYDRATE INTOLERANCE

Adult hypolactasia, infantile lactase deficiency, congenital lactose intolerance, and congenital glucose-galactose malabsorption are disorders of carbohydrate intolerance in people.[17] Fewer conditions are associated with recognized carbohydrate intolerance in dogs and cats. However, neonatal death following episodes of diarrhea are common, and the same spectrum of metabolic disorders resulting in carbohydrate intolerance in people may occur in dogs and cats.

The diarrhea, bloating, and abdominal discomfort that occur when animals with lactose intolerance ingest milk are relatively common metabolic adverse reactions in dogs and cats. Puppies and kittens normally have adequate levels of intestinal lactase to permit digestion of lactose in the mother's milk. In many subjects, brush border disaccharidase activity decreases after weaning to a fraction of the activity found in young animals. Osmotic diarrhea often occurs when excessive levels of lactose are consumed. Puppies, kittens, or adult animals may develop diarrhea when given cow's or goat's milk, because these milk sources contain more lactose than either bitch's or queen's milk.

Intolerance to disaccharides commonly occurs secondary to enteritis or rapid food changes. Loss of intestinal brush border disaccharidase activity contributes to the diarrhea associated with enteritis. Inadequate intestinal disaccharidase activity is also one of the factors responsible for diarrhea subsequent to rapid food changes. Several days are required for intestinal disaccharidase enzyme activity to adapt to changes in food carbohydrate sources.

CLINICAL FEATURES IN DOGS AND CATS

DERMATOLOGIC RESPONSES IN DOGS

NUT

Reports of adverse food reactions in dogs with cutaneous disease did not document a gender predisposition, and ages ranged from 4 months to 14 years.[18, 19] Up to one third of canine cases, however, may occur in dogs younger than 1 year old.[18, 19] Because many adverse food reactions occur in young dogs, the index of suspicion for food allergy may rise above that for atopic disease when pruritic dermatoses occur in dogs younger than 6 months old.[19] Most investigators have not found a breed predilection, whereas others have found that cocker spaniels, springer spaniels, Labrador retrievers, collies, miniature schnauzers, Chinese Shar Peis, West Highland white terriers, wheaten terriers, Boxers, dachshunds, Dalmatians, Lhasa apsos, German shepherds, and golden retrievers are at increased risk.[19]

Adverse food reactions in dogs typically occur as nonseasonal pruritic dermatitis, occasionally accompanied by gastrointestinal (GI) signs. The pruritus varies in severity. Lesion distribution is often indistinguishable from that seen with atopy: feet, face, axillae, perineal region, inguinal region, rump, and ears are often affected.[18, 19] One fourth of dogs with adverse food reactions have lesions only in the region of the ears.[20] This finding suggests that adverse food reactions should always be suspected in dogs with pruritic, bilateral otitis externa, even if accompanied by secondary bacterial or *Malassezia* infections.

Adverse food reactions in dogs produce no set of pathognomonic cutaneous signs. A variety of primary and secondary skin lesions occur, including papules, erythroderma, excoriations, hyperpigmentation, epidermal collarettes, pododermatitis, seborrhea sicca, and otitis externa. Adverse food reactions often mimic other common canine skin disorders, including pyoderma, pruritic seborrheic dermatoses, folliculitis, and ectoparasitism.[18, 19] Twenty to 30 per cent or more of dogs with suspected adverse food reactions may have concurrent allergic disease, such as flea-allergic dermatitis or atopy.[20] Some dogs present with only recurrent bacterial pyoderma, with or without pruritus, and all clinical signs resolve with antibiotic therapy.

Food anaphylaxis is an acute reaction to food or food additives with systemic consequences. The most common clinical manifestation in dogs occurs in localized form, referred to as angioedema or facioconjunctival edema.[19] Angioedema is typically manifested by large edematous swellings of the lips, face, eyelids, ears, conjunctiva, and/or tongue, with or without pruritus.[19] Angioedema is evoked by the same types of substances that induce systemic anaphylaxis. Most veterinary practitioners attribute angioedema solely to insect envenomation (biting or stinging insects), but a number of other common causes include food, drugs, vaccines, infections, atopy, and blood transfusions.[19] Urticarial reactions (hives) are characterized by localized or generalized wheals, which may or may not be pruritic. They usually occur within minutes of allergen exposure and generally subside after one to two hours.

One author (PR) has seen angioedema of the tongue, palate, and throat repeatedly in the same dogs after indiscreet ingestion of mushrooms, domestic flowers, or other plants. This presentation resembles the oral allergy syndrome in people, which is a form of contact urticaria confined almost exclusively to the oropharynx.[3] Symptoms in people include rapid onset of pruritus and angioedema of the lips, tongue, palate, and throat. Symptoms usually resolve rapidly. This syndrome in people is most commonly associated with the ingestion of various fresh fruits and vegetables.

DERMATOLOGIC RESPONSES IN CATS

Gender predisposition has not been documented in adverse food reactions in cats, and ages have ranged from 6 months to 12 years.[18, 19] Siamese or Siamese cross cats may be at increased risk, because they have accounted for nearly one third of cases.

Dermatologic signs include several different clinical reaction patterns, such as severe, generalized pruritus without lesions; miliary dermatitis; pruritus with self-trauma centered around the head, neck, and ears; traumatic alopecia; moist dermatitis; and scaling dermatoses (Fig. 67–2).[18, 19] In one study, angioedema, urticaria, or conjunctivitis occurred in one third of cats with adverse food reactions.[21] Adverse reactions to food may also cause self-inflicted alopecia (psychogenic alopecia, neurodermatitis), eosinophilic plaques, and indolent ulcers of the lips in some cats.[18, 19] Concurrent flea-allergy dermatitis or atopy may occur in up to 30 per cent of cats with suspected adverse food reactions.[21]

Moderate to marked peripheral lymphadomegaly is found in up to one third of cats with dermatologic manifestations of food allergy.[19] Absolute peripheral eosinophilia occurs in 20 to 50 per cent of feline cases.[19]

GI RESPONSES IN DOGS AND CATS

Gender predilections have not been established for GI disease resulting from adverse reactions to foods.[2] Similarly, there are no well-documented breed predispositions to GI

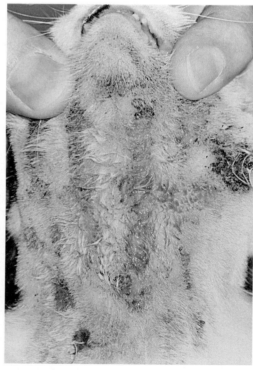

Figure 67–2. Domestic shorthair feline with severe pruritus and self-trauma around the face, head, and neck due to atopy and an adverse reaction to food. Neck excoriations are shown here. The cat reacted positively by intradermal skin testing to a small number of inhalant allergens and partially responded to a commercial lamb and rice diet.

food allergy, but Chinese Shar Pei and German shepherd dogs are commonly affected.[2] Furthermore, gluten-sensitive enteropathy has been well-documented in Irish setter dogs.[2] A wide age range is affected, including dogs and cats as young as weaning age.

Every level of the GI tract can be damaged by food allergies. In dogs, cats, and people, clinical signs usually relate to gastric and small bowel dysfunction, but colitis can also occur.[2,22] Vomiting and diarrhea are prominent features. The diarrhea can be profuse and watery, mucoid, or hemorrhagic. Intermittent abdominal pain is occasionally seen. Concurrent cutaneous signs may be seen. GI disturbances occur in 10 to 15 per cent of dogs and cats with cutaneous manifestations of food sensitivity.[18,19] In experimentally induced food hypersensitivity, the most common clinical signs are diarrhea, an increase in the number of bowel movements, and occasional vomiting. One veterinary dermatologist observed that pruritic dogs with more than three bowel movements per day are more likely to have an adverse reaction to food as part of the reason for their dermatoses.[18]

There are at least five subacute to chronic GI conditions thought to involve food allergy in people: food protein–induced enterocolitis, food-induced colitis syndrome, food-induced malabsorption syndrome, gluten-sensitive enteropathy, and allergic eosinophilic gastroenteritis.[23] All these conditions can occur in dogs and cats. The role of food allergy in canine and feline inflammatory bowel disease (IBD) is unknown. Hypersensitivity to food is probably involved in the pathogenesis of this syndrome; at least some affected animals could be more appropriately diagnosed as suffering from food protein–induced enterocolitis. Dogs with IBD have been tested for the presence of fecal and serum antibodies against a variety of food and parasitic antigens, but the search has been unrewarding.

Currently, 10 per cent of dogs with IBD diagnosed by one of the authors (WGG) have positive gastroscopic food sensitivity tests (GFSTs) to food antigens. Positive GFST results to foods used in the treatment of the disease are often detected during follow-up endoscopic studies. This finding strongly implies that food allergy is involved in the perpetuation of IBD but that it may not be the primary cause. That is, inflammation of the mucosa predisposes animals to the development of acquired food allergies. Therefore, a change in food antigens may temporarily reduce the immune-mediated mucosal inflammatory response. The longevity of this amelioration is questionable, however, because the so-called hypoallergenic foods commonly used in veterinary medicine contain intact proteins that are hypoallergenic primarily by virtue of their novelty to the host's immune system. The duration of protein novelty to the gut-associated lymphoid tissue (GALT) is likely to be very limited if the antigen is fed to an animal with a highly porous mucosal barrier. The subclassification of IBD in which hypersensitivity to food antigens is most likely to play a causal role is eosinophilic enterocolitis.

Irritable bowel syndrome is a disease of dogs characterized by chronic recurrent abdominal pain and large bowel diarrhea. Feeding changes often alleviate the signs of irritable bowel disease, implying that food sensitivity plays a role in this syndrome. In the experience of one of the authors (WGG), avoiding gas-producing foods (e.g., homemade vegetable-based foods) or foods with a high fat content is particularly advantageous in the management of dogs with irritable bowel syndrome. In affected dogs, the adverse reactions to these nutrients are most likely due to a food intolerance rather than a food allergy.

DIAGNOSIS

Dietary elimination trials are the main diagnostic method used in dogs and cats with suspected adverse food reactions. At the present time, intradermal skin testing, radioallergosorbent tests (RASTs), and enzyme-linked immunosorbent assays (ELISAs) for food hypersensitivity are considered unreliable in animals with dermatologic disease.[3, 24, 25]

The ideal elimination food should (1) include a reduced number of novel, highly digestible protein sources; (2) avoid protein excesses; (3) avoid additives and vasoactive amines; and (4) be nutritionally adequate for the animal's life stage and condition. The ideal elimination food should provide preferably one or two different types of protein to which the animal has not been previously exposed. This recommendation often includes a commercial or homemade food with one animal protein source and one vegetable protein source. Excess protein levels should be avoided to reduce the amount of potential allergens to which the animal is exposed. A higher protein level may be necessary to counteract protein losses from the GI tract or impaired absorption in animals with hypoproteinemia and weight loss associated with severe GI disease.

Protein digestibility is also an important factor when assessing an elimination food. Complete digestion of food protein results in free amino acids and small peptides that are poor antigens.[26] Thus, an incompletely digested food protein has the potential to incite an allergic response because of residual antigenic proteins and large polypeptides. Protein digestibility has been documented for some commercial pet foods marketed as hypoallergenic or elimination foods.[27] A protein digestibility exceeding 90 per cent is recommended for such foods.

Although specific pet food additives have not been documented to cause adverse food reactions, food additives generally should be avoided in elimination foods. The ideal elimination food should avoid ingredients such as fish that are known to contain higher levels of vasoactive amines than do other pet food ingredients.[14, 15]

Finally, although elimination trials are performed only for several weeks to months, the food used in the trial should be nutritionally complete and balanced for the intended species, age, and lifestyle of the animal. Elimination trials are often performed with young animals in which nutritionally inadequate foods are more likely to result in nutritional disease.

HOMEMADE ELIMINATION FOODS

Homemade foods are often recommended as the initial test food for dogs and cats with suspected food allergy.[4] Homemade test foods usually include a single protein source or a combination of a single protein source and a single carbohydrate source. Ingredients recommended for homemade feline foods include lamb baby food, lamb, rice, and rabbit. Ingredients recommended for homemade canine foods include lamb, rice, potato, fish, rabbit, venison, and tofu.

Many homemade foods fail to meet nutritional requirements because they are made from a minimum of ingredients.[4] In general, homemade foods lack a source of calcium, essential fatty acids, certain vitamins, and other micronutrients and contain excessive levels of protein, which are contraindicated in food allergy cases. Feeding nutritionally inadequate homemade foods for more than three weeks may result in nutritional disease, especially in young animals.

COMMERCIAL ELIMINATION FOODS

A variety of foods with limited and different protein sources are manufactured by several companies. These commercial products are attractive because they are convenient, often contain novel protein sources, and are nutritionally complete and balanced for either dogs or cats. Protein digestibility varies markedly among these products.[27] Further, few of these commercial foods have been adequately tested in dogs and cats with known adverse food reactions; only a few commercial foods have undergone the scrutiny of clinical trials using animals with dermatologic or GI disease. In published clinical trials, two thirds to three fourths of animals with suspected adverse food reactions showed significant improvement in clinical signs when fed commercial foods.[5]

PERFORMING ELIMINATION TRIALS IN ANIMALS WITH DERMATOLOGIC DISEASE

Before an elimination trial is initiated, the client should feed the dog or cat its usual food for 7 to 14 days (Fig. 67–3). During this time, the client should record the type and amount of food ingested; any other ingested food items such as table scraps, treats, and snacks; and the occurrence and character of adverse reactions. The animal is then fed a controlled elimination food for 4 to 12 weeks. No other substances should be ingested, including treats, flavored vitamin supplements, chewable heartworm preventive tablets, fatty acid supplements, and chew toys. During the elimination trial, the client should document daily the type and amount of food ingested and the occurrence and character of adverse reactions. A daily food diary helps document progression of clinical signs during the elimination trial and whether a strict elimination trial was performed in the home environment. The diary often reveals different findings from those offered to the clinician by the client during the recheck examination.

A tentative diagnosis of an adverse food reaction in dermatologic patients is made if the level of pruritus markedly decreases. This improvement may be gradual and may take 4 to 12 weeks to become evident.

A diagnosis of an adverse food reaction is confirmed if clinical signs reappear 10 to 14 days after the animal's former food and other ingested substances are offered as a challenge. Provocation involves introducing single ingredients until as many positive reactions as possible can be documented. Clients and veterinarians are often reluctant to pursue challenge and provocation once clinical signs have improved or been eliminated. Provocation may also be difficult to perform in many dogs and cats because commercial pet foods contain large numbers of ingredients, and feeding the same ingredients often cannot be duplicated in challenge studies. As an example, use of chicken meat in a provocative food challenge may not duplicate the types or levels of antigens found in poultry by-product meal.

Elimination trials are often difficult to interpret because of concurrent allergic skin disease. In several studies, at least 20 to 30 per cent of dogs and cats with adverse food reactions had concurrent allergies. These animals may respond only partially to an elimination trial. Flea-allergy dermatitis and atopy are the most common canine and feline allergies and should be eliminated through other diagnostic testing.

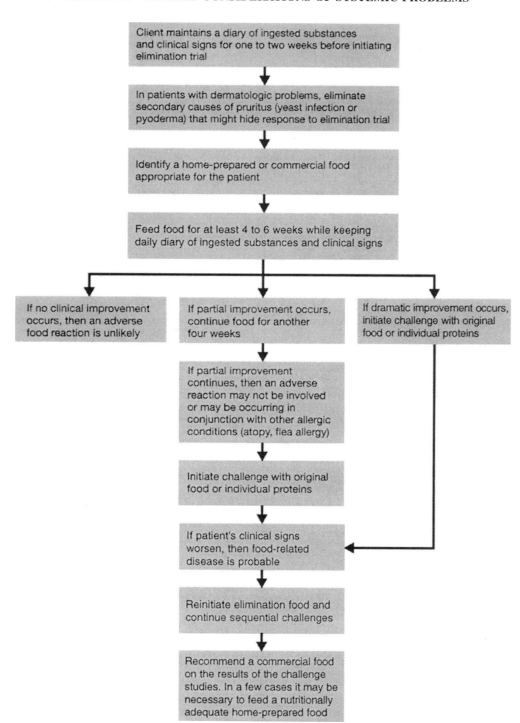

Figure 67–3. Protocol for elimination-challenge trials for the diagnosis of adverse reactions to food. (From Hand MS, Thatcher CD, Remillard RL [eds]: Small Animal Clinical Nutrition, 4th ed. Topeka, KS, Mark Morris Institute, 1999.)

PERFORMING ELIMINATION TRIALS IN ANIMALS WITH GI DISEASE

Elimination-challenge trial designs for animals with GI food disease are similar to those for animals with dermatologic problems (see Fig. 67–3). However, shorter elimination periods are usually satisfactory (two to four weeks). In chronic relapsing conditions, the elimination period chosen must be greater than the usual symptom-free period to allow reliable assessment of how food sensitivity contributes to the animal's signs.

As with skin disease, the degree of clinical improvement during the elimination trial will be 100 per cent only if food sensitivity is the sole cause of the animal's problems. For instance, resolution of allergies acquired as a *result* of GI disease will not eliminate the clinical signs caused by the primary GI disease process. Recrudescence of GI signs after challenge of a food-sensitive animal with the responsible allergen usually occurs within the first three days but may take as long as seven days, particularly if the responsible allergen was removed from the food for longer than one month.

TREATMENT

For most food allergies, avoiding the offending foods is the most effective treatment. How selective or meticulous an avoidance diet must be depends on the individual animal's sensitivity. Some dogs and cats may suffer adverse reactions to even trace quantities of an offending food, while others may have a higher tolerance level. Concurrent allergies influence the threshold level of clinical signs in some animals. Symptomatic therapy in pruritic animals can also include corticosteroids and antihistamines. Corticosteroids along with dietary change are often used in cats with IBD. One third of human beings on strict avoidance diets for one to two years have tolerated the reintroduction of food allergens into their diets. This suggests that strict avoidance in animals with food allergy may allow some of these dogs and cats to tolerate exposure to certain food allergens later in life.

Both homemade and commercial foods can be used for long-term maintenance of animals with suspected food allergy. It is important that any homemade recipe for long-term maintenance ensure a nutritionally adequate ration. An attempt should always be made to find an acceptable commercial food, which will raise owner compliance with the dietary change and ensure a nutritionally adequate ration.

REFERENCES

1. Anderson JA: The establishment of common language concerning adverse reactions to foods and food additives. J Allergy Clin Immunol 78:140, 1986.
2. Guilford WG: Adverse reactions to food. In Guilford WG, Center SA, Strombeck DR, Williams DA, Meyer DJ (eds): Small Animal Gastroenterology, 3rd ed. Philadelphia. WB Saunders, 1996, pp 436–450.
3. Sampson HA: Adverse reactions to foods. In Middleton E, Reed CE, Ellis EF, et al(eds): Allergy: Principles and Practice. St Louis, Mosby-Year Book, 1993, pp 1661–1636.
4. Roudebush P, Cowell CS: Results of a hypoallergenic diet survey of veterinarians in North America with a nutritional evaluation of homemade diet prescriptions. Vet Dermatol 3:23, 1992.
5. Roudebush P, Guilford WG, Shanley KJ: Adverse reactions to food. In Hand MS, Thatcher CD, Remillard RL, et al (eds): Small Animal Clinical Nutrition, 4th ed. Topeka, KS, Mark Morris Institute, 1999.
6. Sampson HA: Eczema and food hypersensitivity. In Metcalfe DD, Sampson HA, Simon RA (eds): Food Allergy: Adverse Reactions to Foods and Food Additives. Boston. Blackwell Scientific, 1991, pp 114–128.
7. Hannuksela M, Haahtela T: Hypersensitivity reactions to food additives. Allergy 42:561, 1987.
8. Murdoch RD, et al: Effects of food additives on leukocyte histamine release in normal and urticaria subjects. J R Coll Physicians Lond 21:251, 1987.
9. Hickman MA, et al: Effect of diet on Heinz body formation in kittens. Am J Vet Res 50:475, 1990.
10. Affolter VK, Shaw SE: Cutaneous drug eruptions. In Ihrke PJ, Mason IS, White SD (eds): Advances in Veterinary Dermatology, vol 2. New York, Pergamon Press, 1993, p 450.
11. Mason KW: Personal communication, Queensland, Australia.
12. Taylor SL: Histamine food poisoning: Toxicology and clinical aspects. CRC Crit Rev Toxicol 17:91, 1986.
13. Morrow JD, et al: Evidence that histamine is the causative toxin of scombroid-fish poisoning. N Engl J Med 324:716, 1991.
14. Guilford WG, et al: The histamine content of commercial pet foods. N Z Vet J 42:201, 1994.
15. Guraya HS, Koehler PE: Histamine in cat foods: Survey and comparison of methodologies. Vet Hum Toxicol 33:124, 1991.
16. Roudebush P: Unpublished data.
17. Halliwell REW: Comparative aspects of food intolerance. Vet Med 87:893, 1992.
18. MacDonald JM: Food allergy. In Griffin CE, Kwochka KW, MacDonald JM (eds): Current Veterinary Dermatology. St Louis, Mosby-Year Book, 1993, pp 121–132.
19. Scott DW, Miller WH, Griffin CE: Small Animal Dermatology, 5th ed. Philadelphia, WB Saunders, 1995.
20. Rosser EJ: Diagnosis of food allergy in dogs. JAVMA 203:259, 1993.
21. Rosser EJ: Food allergy in the cat: A prospective study of 13 cats. In Ihrke PJ, Mason IS, White SD (eds): Advances in Veterinary Dermatology, vol 2. New York, Pergamon Press, 1993, pp 33–39.
22. Nelson RW, et al: Nutritional management of idiopathic chronic colitis in the dog. J Vet Intern Med 2:133, 1988.
23. Proujansky R, et al: Gastrointestinal syndromes associated with food sensitivity. Adv Pediatr 35:219, 1988.
24. Jeffers JG, et al: Diagnostic testing of dogs for food hypersensitivity. JAVMA 189:245, 1991.
25. Kunkle G, Horner S: Validity of skin testing for diagnosis of food allergy in dogs. JAVMA 200:677, 1992.
26. Yunginger JW: Food antigens. In Metcalfe DD, Sampson HA, Simon RA (eds): Food Allergy: Adverse Reactions to Foods and Food Additives. Boston, Blackwell Scientific, 1991, pp 36–51.
27. Roudebush P, et al: Protein characteristics of commercial canine and feline hypoallergenic diets. Vet Dermatol 5:69, 1995.

CHAPTER 68

NUTRITIONAL MANAGEMENT OF GASTROINTESTINAL, HEPATIC, AND ENDOCRINE DISEASES

Kathryn E. Michel

Dietary therapy has a requisite role in the management of most gastrointestinal (GI) disorders. Depending on the underlying disease, dietary modification may be a specific, and at times the primary, therapeutic intervention, or it may simply be an aspect of supportive care. The presence of food in the GI tract provides a variety of trophic signals, including direct provision of nutrients to the enterocytes, increased mesenteric blood flow, and stimulation of the release of digestive enzymes and enterohormones, all of which can influence intestinal cell proliferation and differentiation. Conversely, dietary factors may cause a variety of adverse reactions, including immunologic and inflammatory responses, osmotic diarrhea, and altered GI transit time. Nutritional therapy involves general considerations, such as diet digestibility and feeding schedules, as well as manipulation of the type and quantities of specific nutrients.

BOWEL REST

In many instances, withholding food and water temporarily constitutes the sole treatment for animals with acute GI disturbances. The animal receives supportive care, with particular attention paid to maintaining normal hydration and electrolyte status.

For an animal whose nutritional status was normal at the outset of its illness, fasting for several days should have no impact on clinical outcome, as long as dehydration is avoided. There are other GI diseases, however, that might entail longer periods of fasting, such as pancreatitis or parvovirus enteritis. Two issues must be considered for these animals. First is whether the animal's nutritional status will deteriorate to the point where it will affect clinical outcome during the period of fasting. Second is the effect that lack of enteral intake will have on the GI tract itself, and whether recovery of function could actually be impeded.

It is possible to nourish an animal parenterally when enteral feeding is unfeasible or contraindicated. Parenteral nutritional support can maintain an animal's nutritional status, but it will not prevent gut mucosal atrophy and diminished absorptive capacity.[1]

How important it is to restore the presence of enteral nutrients and how much of an impact this has on clinical recovery are currently unknown and under active investigation. The conventions for the management of acute diarrhea in humans have changed over the past two decades. Continued feeding, generally with milk or cereal-based rehydration formulas, minimizes malnutrition, possibly supports GI structure and function, and does not appear to exacerbate or prolong the diarrhea.[2] It has been pointed out, however, that most studies have involved humans with secretory diarrhea, whereas the type of diarrhea most common in dogs and cats is osmotic.[3]

DIET DIGESTIBILITY

Once the clinical signs of GI upset begin to resolve, first water and then food are reintroduced. Typically what is offered is a "bland" diet. For veterinary patients, this is often boiled ground beef or chicken and white rice, or one of the growing number of prescription diets. Probably the most important aspect of the bland diet is a high degree of digestibility. Typically, pet foods have a dry-matter digestibility in the range of 80 to 85 per cent, although some products are closer to 90 per cent. Prescription diets designed specifically for GI disease are usually in the range of 88 to 91 per cent. Intake of fiber, lactose, and other nondigestible carbohydrates should be minimal.

High digestibility facilitates absorption in the proximal small bowel. This should lessen the potential for the development of osmotic diarrhea. By promoting complete absorption, it should limit the availability of nutrients to enteric microorganisms, thus decreasing ammonia production and the gaseous by-products of fermentation.

MEAL SIZE, FREQUENCY, AND CONSISTENCY

On reintroduction of feeding, small meals should be offered three or more times a day. Small frequent feedings may limit the duration of gastric acid secretion and also result in less gastric distention, which could lessen the potential for nausea. The maximal gastric capacity is estimated to be 90 mL/kg for adult dogs and 45 to 60 mL/kg for adult cats.[4] Limiting meal portions to 20 to 30 per cent of thecretic capacity is a reasonable starting point. Blending a diet with water to a more liquid consistency should enhance the rate at which it is emptied from the stomach. It may also improve the palatability of the food for some animals, especially if the food is warmed to slightly below body temperature.

The animal's resting energy requirement $(RER = 30WT_{KG} + 70)$ should be estimated and used as a minimal goal for caloric intake. Because the animal has already experienced some caloric restriction, it is important that the clinician have some notion of animal's requirements and of the caloric density of the food being offered. This way, a rational "food dosage" can be arrived at, and the all too common practice of writing food orders such as "feed a little bit four times a day" can be avoided.

There are two additional considerations when reintroducing food to animals that have been fasted for acute gastroenteritis. First is the potential for the development of a learned food aversion. The animal may associate a particular food with nausea, vomiting, or other forms of GI upset. Therefore, forms of coaxed or forced feeding, where food is placed near or in the animal's mouth, may have the opposite effect of that intended. For an animal that is still feeling unwell, offering a variety of foods may only increase the number of foods that the animal will refuse. In such cases, it may be best to continue the fast until the animal shows spontaneous interest in food. The use of antiemetic drugs and tube feeding for nutritional support may be necessary in some cases.

A second consideration is the potential development of a dietary hypersensitivity to proteins fed during acute gastroenteritis, when gut mucosal permeability may be abnormally increased.[5] This hypothesis requires further investigation but argues in favor of feeding these animals a diet containing an uncommon protein source until convalescence is achieved, to reduce the likelihood of developing an allergy to more common food ingredients.

PROTEIN AND AMINO ACIDS

First and foremost, a diet must contain adequate protein and an appropriate amino acid profile to meet the requirements of the species consuming it. Protein turnover is increased in illness and injury, and although information on the specific needs of dogs and cats with different GI disorders is lacking, it is safe to say that their requirements likely exceed those established for maintenance. The increased requirements of illness are compounded in cases in which enteric protein losses are above normal.

Protein source is also important. Some animals may have true food allergies, and in all but a few cases, the antigenic component of the food is a protein. Even though dietary hypersensitivity has not been proved to be the etiology of inflammatory bowel disease, animals often show improvement when placed on a controlled diet containing a novel protein source.[6]

It is recognized that gut mucosal atrophy can occur despite using an enteral route of feeding when animals are given purified diets containing amino acids instead of intact protein.[7] One explanation for these findings may be that the purified diets are lacking in the dispensable amino acid glutamine. Glutamine is abundant in most dietary proteins and serves as the principal respiratory fuel for the enterocyte. Addition of glutamine to amino acid–based diets improves mucosal structure and barrier function, but not to the extent seen in animals consuming diets with intact protein.[8] There

is evidence that some proteins are more potent secretagogues for GI hormones than others.[7, 9] Part of the trophic effect of intact protein on the gut may be secondary to the stimulation of hormone secretion, in addition to serving as a source of glutamine.

FAT

Restriction of dietary fat intake is advocated in the management of a variety of GI diseases. Although fat is one of the most digestible components of the diet, fat malassimilation is not uncommon. Fatty acids reaching the colon are hydroxylated by bacteria and can have toxic effects on the mucosa, resulting in diarrhea.

In circumstances of fat malabsorption, such as lymphangiectasia, medium-chain triglycerides (MCTs) can be used to replace some of the long-chain triglycerides in the diet as a calorie source. MCTs contain fatty acids that are 8 to 12 carbons in length and provide approximately 8 kcal/g. MCTs are less dependent on micelle formation for digestion and absorption than are long-chain triglycerides and are absorbed directly into the portal circulation. Chronic consumption of a diet containing MCTs has been associated with fatty liver in cats, so supplementation with MCTs should be used with caution in this species.[10] Also, because dogs and cats often find MCTs unpalatable, their usefulness as a caloric supplement may be limited.

Because fat is a potent stimulus for pancreatic secretion, low-fat diets are generally prescribed for animals recovering from acute pancreatitis. Although conclusive evidence is lacking, chronic high-fat intake may be involved in the pathogenesis of canine pancreatitis. Therefore, dietary fat restriction may help prevent recurrence of this disease.

There have been some preliminary investigations of essential fatty acids as a means of mediating inflammatory bowel disease in human patients. So far, benefits of fish oil supplementation have been modest at best, but further investigation is warranted.

FIBER

Fiber is a generic term, and although there are disorders of the GI tract that can be considered "fiber-responsive" diseases, it is imperative to recognize which type of fiber is appropriate in each case. Fiber includes both carbohydrates and noncarbohydrates (e.g., lignin) of plant origin that cannot be digested by mammalian enzymes. Fibers can be classified according to their function in the cell wall, solubility in aqueous solutions, or fermentability. The latter two classifications are important when considering the role of fiber in the management of GI diseases.

Soluble fibers tend to gel in water. This property may delay gastric emptying and inhibit absorption in the small intestine. Insoluble fibers, in contrast, do not gel and generally have little effect on gastric emptying or nutrient absorption. They increase fecal bulk and appear to normalize intestinal transit time. These qualities are beneficial for treating animals with constipation.

Soluble fibers are usually more fermentable than insoluble fibers, although this is not always the case. Fiber is fermented to short-chain fatty acids (SCFAs) in the colon. One of the SCFAs, butyrate, is the principal metabolic fuel of the colonocyte. SCFAs have been shown to have a trophic effect on the colonic mucosa and have been used in a therapeutic enema for human patients with ulcerative colitis. There have been some preliminary investigations of the use of fiber for the treatment of large bowel diarrhea in dogs. Both soluble and insoluble fiber types have been reported to be effective. However, most clinical trials have been nonblinded and without a control group. In a recent controlled and blinded prospective clinical trial, results were inconclusive.[11] Further investigation of the role of fiber in the management of large bowel disease is definitely required. However, at this time, empiric use of fiber supplementation or prescription diets containing moderate amounts of fiber in animals with idiopathic large bowel disease is warranted.

NUTRITIONAL MANAGEMENT OF HEPATIC DISEASE

There are some disorders of the liver for which nutritional management has a specific therapeutic objective. For the most part, however, the role of nutrition in the treatment of animals with hepatic dysfunction is supportive.

Given the central function of the liver in the digestion, metabolism, and storage of nutrients, maintaining metabolic homeostasis and adequate nutritional status when hepatic function is impaired can be challenging. Nutritional management in the face of liver disease involves balancing two objectives: providing sufficient nutrients to maintain the host, and promoting hepatocellular regeneration without overwhelming the remaining metabolic capacity of the organ, which might lead to the accumulation of toxic metabolites.

GENERAL CONSIDERATIONS

Particular attention should be paid to ensuring that the animal has adequate caloric intake. This not only promotes hepatic repair and recovery of function but also minimizes catabolism of endogenous tissues. Depending on the animal's activity level, calories equal to RER may be sufficient, particularly for hospitalized patients. Caloric intake should be adjusted to maintain current weight. Placing an animal in a positive energy balance to promote weight gain should be done cautiously, and only when the animal is clinically stable and convalescent. Feeding numerous small meals throughout the day improves total intake for many animals and minimizes the clinical signs associated with aberrations of protein and carbohydrate metabolism, which are usually most pronounced during periods of fasting.

PROTEIN

Although the pathogenesis of hepatic encephalopathy (HE) remains obscure, a number of theories involve derangement of protein metabolism. Hyperammonemia secondary to impaired ureagenesis occurs in animals with severe liver dysfunction or portosystemic shunts (PSS). Ammonia is generated principally from the metabolism of amino acids, particularly when dietary protein exceeds requirements, and by the activity of enteric microorganisms.

In theory, a diet for an animal with signs of HE should contain enough protein to meet but not exceed nutritional requirements. Clinically, there is no simple or precise way to evaluate an animal's protein needs. One investigation found that the protein requirement of dogs with PSS was no different from that of normal dogs.[12] In practice, animals with liver disease should be fed as much protein as they will tolerate.

If an animal develops signs of HE, the protein content of the diet being consumed at that time should be evaluated by calculating the percentage of calories coming from protein. The minimal protein intake for adult maintenance is 18 per cent of calories for dogs and 26 per cent for cats, according to the Association of American Feed Control Officials guidelines; however, many commercial pet foods contain protein far in excess of these amounts.[13] By way of comparison, canine protein-restricted prescription renal-failure diets contain around 12 per cent protein calories, and the comparable feline diets contain around 20 per cent. Therefore, the degree of protein restriction for an animal exhibiting signs of HE should be based on its current intake and what it will tolerate once nondietary management, such as the use of lactulose and neomycin, is instituted. Proteins with high biologic value can be fed in smaller quantities than proteins with limited amounts of one or more of the essential amino acids. In addition, the diet should be highly digestible and fed in small portions to promote complete absorption in the small intestine.

Abnormal plasma amino acid concentrations have been noted in dogs with PSS or chronic hepatitis. Plasma concentrations of the branched chain amino acids (BCAAs) leucine, isoleucine, and valine are decreased, reflecting catabolism by peripheral tissues, whereas concentrations of the aromatic amino acids (AAAs) tyrosine, phenylalanine, and tryptophan are increased, secondary to reduced hepatic metabolism. It has been proposed that these alterations in plasma amino acid concentrations may lead to altered neurotransmitter synthesis in the brain. BCAA-enriched diets have been formulated with the objective of normalizing amino acid concentrations in the plasma and the central nervous system. To date, however, these formulas have not shown clinical efficacy in human patients, and in one investigation of dogs with PSS, dogs consuming a diet enriched with BCAAs showed more neurologic dysfunction than those consuming a diet enriched with AAAs.[12]

Source of dietary protein is another consideration in the management of hepatic disease. Dogs with experimentally created PSS and human patients with cirrhosis have fewer signs of HE when fed milk or vegetable diets as opposed to meat diets.[14, 15] It may be that meat contains heme and other nitrogenous substances that exacerbate HE. In addition, the fiber in vegetable diets and the lactose in milk diets may decrease intestinal transit time and increase elimination of fecal nitrogen. It should be noted that cats have higher protein requirements than other species and that vegetable protein sources do not provide the essential amino acid taurine.

CARBOHYDRATES AND FATS

Derangement of carbohydrate metabolism has been reported in dogs with chronic hepatitis or PSS and in cats with idiopathic hepatic lipidosis (IHL). Clinically evident fasting hypoglycemia occurs presumably because of the inability of the diseased liver to store sufficient glycogen or because of impaired gluconeogenesis. Animals may also show abnormal glucose tolerance.[16] This may become a limiting factor in an animal's ability to meet its caloric requirements with dietary carbohydrate.

Although liver dysfunction may lead to decreased secretion of bile salts, moderate dietary fat consumption is usually well tolerated. In cases in which steatorrhea is evident, MCTs can be used to replace some of the long-chain triglycerides as a source of energy in the diet, as they can be digested and absorbed without micelle formation. It should be noted, however, that cholesterol and the fat-soluble vitamins are dependent on micelle formation for absorption. Therefore, lack of bile salt secretion in cases of cirrhosis or chronic cholestatic disease could lead to deficiencies of these nutrients.

COPPER

Hepatic copper accumulation occurs in certain breeds of dogs, including the Bedlington terrier and the West Highland white terrier, as an inherited defect of the copper-binding protein metallothionein. Copper accumulation and hepatocellular injury are progressive with age, so dietary restriction of copper intake is effective only in affected dogs that are identified while still young. Currently there are no manufactured diets available that are both copper-restricted and suitable for growth or long-term management of dogs with hepatic disease. Because the nutritional requirements for growth are more stringent, preparation of copper-restricted homemade diets for immature dogs should be done with great care and caution.

Zinc supplementation reduces absorption of dietary copper. Zinc induces the synthesis of the protein metallothionein in the intestinal mucosa. This protein binds copper strongly and prevents its absorption systemically. When the enterocyte is sloughed, the copper is excreted in the feces.

NUTRITIONAL MANAGEMENT OF ENDOCRINE DISEASES

With the exception of diabetes mellitus, the role of diet in the management of endocrine disorders of dogs and cats is largely uninvestigated.

DIABETES MELLITUS

With few exceptions, dietary management of diabetes mellitus in dogs and cats is done in conjunction with insulin replacement therapy. The objectives of dietary management are to establish and maintain an optimal body weight, to integrate feeding and insulin injection schedules, and to optimize glycemic control through diet composition. Beyond these general goals, it is important to recognize that there is no single diet or dietary regimen that is appropriate for all or even the majority of cases. Each animal must be evaluated based on its presenting body condition, insulin replacement therapy, and presence or absence of coexisting diseases. Once a regimen is in place, it is critical to adhere to it as closely as possible, as alterations will affect the efficacy of insulin replacement therapy.

Body Condition

Obese dogs and cats can show insulin resistance that resolves with weight loss.[16, 17] Some diabetic cats have spontaneous resolution of their condition once excess weight has been lost. Many diabetic animals first present in some form of medical crisis. Often they have excess body fat but also a severe degree of muscle wasting. It is important that these animals be stabilized before any kind of calorie restriction for weight reduction is instituted. Many diabetic animals are underweight at presentation, and in those cases, stabilized animals should be fed a modest increase in calories to promote repletion.

Meal Timing and Diet Composition

The timing of meals is necessarily linked to the insulin dosage schedule. Ideally, the feeding timetable and the diet composition should promote slow, steady absorption of nutrients from the GI tract at times of peak insulin activity. Complex carbohydrates are absorbed in this fashion and should provide 50 to 60 per cent of the calories in diets for canine diabetics. Soft, moist pet foods should be avoided, because they contain a high proportion of simple sugars. Cats have evolved eating relatively little dietary carbohydrate. They can tolerate it, but it is not clear whether substitution of fat calories with carbohydrate calories would be of any advantage in the management of diabetic cats.

Diets high in soluble fiber have been used to improve glycemic control in human diabetics. One investigation of dogs with alloxan-induced diabetes mellitus found that diets containing either insoluble or soluble fiber improved glycemic control compared with a low-fiber diet.[18] These findings may be applicable to dogs with naturally occurring diabetes mellitus; however, confirmation of this awaits clinical trials. The use of high-fiber diets to improve glycemic control in feline diabetics likewise requires investigation.

High-fiber diets may be less palatable to some animals and can cause increased stool volume. More importantly, most of the high-fiber diets currently on the market were designed for weight reduction and would be contraindicated for debilitated animals. Therefore, even if the clinical benefits of high-fiber diets for the management of canine and feline diabetics become more clearly defined, these diets must be used judiciously.

REFERENCES

1. Mukau L, Talamini MA, Sitzmann JV: Elemental diets may accelerate recovery from total parenteral nutrition-induced gut atrophy. JPEN 18:75, 1994.
2. Isolauri E, Juntunen M, Wiren S, et al: Intestinal permeability changes in acute gastroenteritis: Effects of clinical factors and nutritional management. J Pediatr Gastroenterol Nutr 8:466, 1989.
3. Guilford WG: Nutritional management of GI diseases. In Guilford WG, Center SA, Strombeck DR, et al (eds): Strombeck's Small Animal Gastroenterology, 3rd ed. Davis, Stonegate Publishing, 1996, pp 889–910.
4. Lewis LD, Morris ML, Hand NS: Small Animal Clinical Nutrition, 3rd ed. Topeka, KS, Mark Morris Associates, 1987.
5. Gryboski JD: Gastrointestinal aspects of cow's milk protein intolerance and allergy. Immunol Allergy Clin North Am 11:733, 1991.
6. Nelson RW, Stockey LJ, Kazacos E: Nutritional management of idiopathic chronic colitis in the dog. J Vet Intern Med 2:133, 1988.
7. Zaloga GP, Ward KA, Prielipp RC: Effect of enteral diets on whole body and gut growth in unstressed rats. JPEN 15:42, 1991.
8. Fox AD, Kripke SC, DePaula J, et al: Effect of glutamine-supplemented enteral diet on methotrexate-induced enterocolitis. JPEN 12:325, 1988.
9. Marks SL, Reader R, Backus R, et al: Dietary soy protein helps maintain intestinal mucosal integrity in cats with methotrexate-induced enteritis (abstract). Vet Clin Nutr 3:30, 1996.
10. MacDonald ML, Anderson BC, Rogers QR, et al: Essential fatty acid requirements of cats: Pathology of essential fatty acid deficiency. Am J Vet Res 45:1310, 1984.
11. Leib MS, Saunders GK, Willard MD, et al: Fiber-responsive large bowel diarrhea. Proc 15th ACVIM Forum, Orlando, FL, 1997, pp 319–321.
12. Laflamme DP, Allen SW, Huber TL: Apparent dietary protein requirements of dogs with portosystemic shunt. Am J Vet Res 54:719, 1993.

13. American Association of Feed Control Officials: Official publication, 1993.
14. Schaeffer MC, Rogers QR, Buffington CA, et al: Long-term biochemical and physiological effects of surgically placed portacaval shunts in dogs. Am J Vet Res 47:346, 1986.
15. Weber FL Jr, Minco D, Fresard KM, et al: Effects of vegetable diets on nitrogen metabolism in cirrhotic subjects. Gastroenterology 89:538, 1985.
16. Biourge V, Nelson RW, Feldman EC, et al: Effect of weight gain and subsequent weight loss on glucose tolerance and insulin response in healthy cats. J Vet Intern Med 11:86, 1997.
17. Wolfsheimer KJ, Kombert M, Jeansonne L: The effects of caloric restrictions on IV glucose tolerance tests in obese and non-obese beagle dogs (abstract). J Vet Intern Med 7:113, 1993.
18. Nelson RW, Ihle SL, Lewis LD, et al: Effects of dietary fiber supplementation on glycemic control in dogs with alloxan-induced diabetes mellitus. Am J Vet Res 52:2060, 1991.

CHAPTER 69

DIETARY MODIFICATIONS IN CARDIAC DISEASE

Stephen J. Ettinger

Dietary modification is a traditional method of managing cardiac disease associated with congestive heart failure (CHF) and systemic hypertension. Low-sodium diets are recommended by most veterinarians for the management of dogs with degenerative valvular disease and clinical signs of CHF. Dietary modification was identified as the most common tool used by practicing veterinarians for the clinical management of heart disease.[1] It continues to be so, even with the introduction of other effective therapeutic products. This fact does not support the sole use of dietary management in treating heart failure. The benefit of combined methodology should be considered as the total approach to treating CHF. Understanding the pathophysiology of heart failure allows a scientific approach to nutritional management. The practitioner should not be too hasty to use just one approach to cardiac disease that best benefits from a combination of treatment strategies.

In light of the discussion that follows, this author believes that it is prudent to make the following recommendations regarding restricted salt therapy:

- *If there is no to minimal cardiac pathology and no signs of quantifiable cardiac pathophysiology, normal dietary measures are suggested.*
- *If there is no to minimal pathology and no signs of quantifiable cardiac pathophysiology in an older animal with evidence (blood and/or urine) of chronic renal insufficiency, feed a diet designed for senior pets with moderate salt and protein restriction.*
- *If diminished cardiac function is present as detected by elevated neuroendocrine levels, radiography, echocardiography, or invasive measures, dietary salt restriction should be instituted using a moderate to marked reduction based on symptoms, severity of ventricular dysfunction, and other therapeutic interventions being administered.*

OBJECTIVES OF DIETARY MODIFICATION

The primary goal of the cardiovascular system is to maintain the supply of oxygen and nutrients to the body tissues.

Another priority is maintenance of venous pressures. In heart failure, the body sacrifices the maintenance of venous pressures to maintain tissue nourishment, and thus life. Increased venous pressures are partially responsible for the clinical signs of CHF. The compensatory responses of the body attempting to nourish tissue are the result of a combination of neurohumoral mechanisms, including the sympathetic nervous system, vasopressin, and the renin-angiotensin-aldosterone pathway.[2] Compensatory changes maintain tissue nutrient levels in the short term, but ultimately these result in sodium and water retention, increased extracellular fluid volume, and increased venous pressures, resulting in fluid accumulation with the subsequent clinical signs of right- and/or left-sided heart failure. The objective of dietary modification is to reduce the magnitude of these compensatory changes and the resulting clinical signs.

Controversy exists about when to start therapeutic interventions, including dietary ones, in the treatment of heart disease. There is agreement that cardiac dysfunction—something that can be quantitatively identified—requires drug and dietary therapy. In dogs and cats, cardiac dysfunction is associated with elevated neuroendocrine (NE) levels. In normal animals, volume contraction induced by diuretic therapy (or possibly severely salt-restricted diets) has been shown to turn on the NE system, increasing plasma renin activity and aldosterone levels. Premature therapeutic interventions, unless of proven benefit, are not generally recommended, because they may aggravate the vicious circle of self-perpetuating heart failure.

IMPORTANT DIETARY CONSIDERATIONS

Reduce Sodium Intake to Prevent Fluid Accumulation. Excess dietary sodium is readily excreted in the urine by normal dogs and cats. In the course of cardiac disease, the dog begins to lose the ability to excrete excess sodium. This probably represents a neurohumoral renal response. This reduced rate of salt excretion progresses as heart failure worsens. The dietary level of sodium that can be tolerated without the appearance of clinical signs depends on the type and severity of the cardiac lesions, neurohumoral mechanisms, and state of congestion present. These are highly individual. The application of dietary sodium restriction as a clinical tool is divided into three levels: mild or reduced salt, 7 to 13 mg/lb; moderate restriction, 5 to 7 mg/lb; and severe restriction, 2 to 6 mg/lb.

The use of sodium-restricted diets may or may not be beneficial for geriatric dogs or small-breed dogs with heart murmurs but no clinical signs of heart failure. Normal geriatric dogs without clinical signs of heart disease do not appear to have distinctive abnormalities in NE levels (plasma renin activity [PRA] or aldosterone [ALDO]). The development of clinical signs of heart failure in humans and dogs is generally associated with increasing NE levels. Normal geriatric dogs fed low-salt diets developed a mild increase in both PRA and ALDO, whereas the same dogs fed low-salt diets and given high-dose loop diuretic therapy (furosemide) significantly increased their NE levels.[8] Thus the question of the benefit of early low-salt diet (or diuretic therapy) in the therapeutic management of heart disease—not heart failure—is reinvented. There is near universal agreement as to its benefit once the pet has entered the congestive failure state.

Dogs in phase II/IV heart disease (i.e., mild signs, especially with physical exertion) often can be effectively maintained with minimal clinical signs on only a moderately restricted-sodium diet (senior-type diet). Avoiding loop diuretics at this time appears to be a good general recommendation. Markedly restricted-sodium diets are required for all dogs exhibiting clinical signs of CHF, (i.e., phase III/IV and IV/IV heart disease). Therapeutic management of heart failure by other modalities is presented in Chapter 111. This chapter limits its discussion to dietary modifications.

Table 69–1 presents the sodium levels of the best-selling dog and cat foods in the United States. Popular canned dog and cat foods have the highest average sodium content, with levels averaging up to 16 times the adult canine requirement[3] and 5 times the adult feline requirement.[7] Popular dry dog foods and premium canned and dry dog foods have lower sodium levels but still 6 to 7 times the adult requirement.[3] Premium canned and dry cat foods average 1.5 to 2 times the adult feline requirement.[7] Table 69–2 identifies levels of selected nutrients in commercial foods used in animals with cardiovascular disease. Salt is an inexpensive ingredient that enhances palatability. Increased salt levels are an inexpensive way of enhancing the acceptance of potentially less expensive ingredients.

Reduced salt intake can be achieved with several premium foods and with most of those sampled in the dietary foods category. Moderate sodium restriction can be achieved with most foods designed for geriatric dogs and all those except one in the dietary foods category. Severe sodium restriction can be achieved only with diets specifically designed for the management of cardiac disease. Even those diets designed for animals with cardiac disease contain sodium levels above the maintenance requirement for normal adult dogs or cats.[3, 7] Hyponatremia should be of no practical consideration for dogs or cats eating restricted-sodium diets to prevent salt and water retention. This may not be true if potent diuretics such as thiazide or loop diuretic agents are being administered. No therapeutic diuretic agent is able to overcome the effect of significant salt loading. Diuretic therapy is not a substitute for reduced dietary sodium intake. Further, diuretic side effects, including electrolyte disorders and blood volume contraction stimulating the NE system, are disadvantageous.

Dilutional hyponatremia is the consequence of excessive fluid accumulation in the body. The effective circulating blood volume in the body is inadequate owing to systolic pump failure, and the total body fluid level is increased. Sodium levels in the blood may appear to be decreased when in reality there is an excessive level of total body sodium. Recognition of dilutional hyponatremia from the history and the blood chemistry panel alerts the clinician to the need to eliminate more pure water and not to attempt to increase salt levels.

Prevent or Correct Hypoproteinemia. Hypoproteinemia is of little concern if any of the foods in Tables 69–1 and 69–2 are being fed, because they contain two to four times the protein requirement for normal adult dogs. Protein excess is of far greater concern, owing to the common presence of reduced renal function in older dogs afflicted with congestive heart disease. Dogs and cats with acute or chronic CHF may have reduced total protein levels due to hemodilution.

Maintain Total Body Potassium Balance. Dietary potassium is an important consideration owing to the common use of diuretic agents that increase urinary excretion of potassium and magnesium. All severely restricted-sodium dietary foods in Table 69–1 designed for animals with cardiac disease contain levels of potassium exceeding 0.7 per cent of the dry matter. Thus, the foods likely to be fed to dogs receiving high dosages of these diuretics already contain levels of potassium that substantially exceed 0.32 per cent of dry matter, a level shown to be adequate for puppy growth.[6] Of perhaps more concern are recent reports of hyperkalemia in dogs being given certain angiotensin-converting enzyme (ACE) inhibitors.[5] With the widespread use of these drugs in managing canine cardiac disease, additional potassium supplementation of restricted-sodium dietary foods appears to be contraindicated. Recently, a large multicenter study was completed using enalapril and traditional cardiac therapy and dietary measures in dogs with CHF due to mitral valvular insufficiency or congestive cardiomyopathy. There was no significant change in serum potassium levels at any time during therapy in either the placebo control group or those given the ACE inhibitor enalapril.[9, 10] Renal insufficiency in animals with CHF treated with drug and/or dietary therapy continues to be a concern. Renal failure is a frequent sequela of long-term successfully managed heart failure. Using an ACE inhibitor such as benazepril may be helpful, since this group of drugs is not renally excreted.

Hypokalemia and hypomagnesemia are also to be avoided, because these electrolyte disorders can aggravate arrhythmogenesis, decrease myocardial contractility, and induce profound muscle weakness and may potentiate or induce drug-related toxicities (digoxin, diuretics, antiarrhythmics).

Provide Taurine and Carnitine. Deficient levels of available dietary taurine have been linked to the production of certain forms of dilated cardiomyopathy in cats. Cats synthesize taurine from cysteine and methionine, but only in a limited manner. Taurine is believed to be important in myocyte calcium binding and modulation of contractility. Cats fed a taurine-deficient diet may develop dilated cardiomyopathy (see Chapter 117). All feline foods that meet AAFCO guidelines should contain added taurine unless the food has been shown to maintain normal taurine blood levels owing to the taurine content of the ingredients.[7] Cats with taurine-deficient cardiomyopathy should be treated with a

TABLE 69–1. SODIUM CONTENT OF SELECTED COMMERCIAL DIETS* (% DRY MATTER)

Popular Dry Dog Foods

Alpo Beef Dinner	0.36
Field Trial Chunks	0.48
Friskies Com 'N Get It	0.55
Gaines Cycle-2 Adult	0.14
Gaines Cycle-4 Senior	0.12
Gaines Gravy Train	0.40
Kal Kan Pedigree Meal Time	0.68
Purina Dog Chow	0.42
Purina Hi-Pro	0.38
Purina O.N.E. Adult	0.50

Premium Dry Dog Foods

Hill's Science Diet Canine Maintenance	0.27
Hill's Science Diet Canine Senior	0.18
Iams Chunks	0.54
Iams Eukanuba Adult	0.55
Iams Less Active	0.34
Iams Senior Formula	0.25
Iams Lamb & Rice	0.60
Neura Chicken Formula	0.21
Nutro Max	0.48
Purina Pro Plan Adult	0.47

Dietary Dry Dog Foods

Hill's Healthblend Geriatric	0.17
Hill's Prescription Diet k/d	0.23
Hill's Prescription Diet h/d	0.08
Kal Kan Waltham Low Protein	0.29
Neura Formula 200 Heart	0.11
Neura Formula 300 Kidney	0.17
Provisions CNM NF-Formula	0.23

Popular Dry Cat Foods

Alpo Gourmet Dinner	0.44
Friskies Chef's Blend	0.43
Friskies Ocean Fish Flavor	0.59
Kal Kan Whiskas Original Recipe	0.56
Kozy Kitten Gulf Fish & Shrimp Flavor	0.35
9-Lives Real Tuna & Egg Flavor	0.32
Purina Alley Cat	0.42
Purina Cat Chow	0.36
Purina Meow Mix	0.46

Premium Dry Cat Foods

Hill's Science Diet Feline Maintenance	0.32
Hi-Tor Felo Diet	0.44
Iams Adult	0.29
Neura Cat Diet	0.45
Nutro Max Cat	0.44
Purina Pro Plan Adult	0.31

Dietary Dry Cat Foods

Hill's Healthblend Adult	0.28
Hill's Prescription Diet Feline c/d	0.37
Hill's Prescription Diet Feline k/d	0.25
Provisions CNM Feline UF-Formula	0.38
Iams Less Active	0.30

Popular Canned Dog Foods

Alpo Beef Chunks Dinner	0.64
Friskies Mighty Dog Beef	1.02
Gaines Cycle-2 Adult	0.60
Kal Kan Grand Gourmet with Chunky Beef	1.19
Kal Kan Pedigree with Chunky Beef	1.38
Kal Kan Pedigree Select Dinner	1.40
Quaker Oats Ken L Ration Original	1.61
Quaker Oats King Kuts with Real Beef	1.01
Recipe Chunky Beef Stew	0.53
Skippy Chunky Beef Dinner	0.96

Premium Canned Dog Foods

Hill's Science Diet Canine Maintenance	0.29
Hill's Science Diet Senior	0.26
Iams Beef Formula	0.33
Iams Lamb & Rice Formula	0.44
Nature's Recipe Maintenance Lamb & Rice	0.50
Neura Chicken Dog Food	0.19
Neura Lamb & Rice	0.41
Nutro Natural Choice Lamb & Rice	0.39

Dietary Canned Dog Foods

Hill's Healthblend geriatric	0.17
Hill's Prescription Diet k/d	0.22
Hill's Prescription Diet h/d	0.08
Kal Kan Waltham Low Sodium	0.10
Kal Kan Waltham Low Protein	0.33
Neura H Diet	0.11
Provisions CNM CV-Formula	0.12
Provisions CNM NT-Formula	0.23

Popular Canned Cat Foods

Alpo Beef & Liver Banquet	0.77
Alpo Tuna Treat	0.90
Amore Simmered Beef & Chicken Entree	1.08
Friskies Mixed Grill	0.61
Friskies Ocean Whitefish & Tuna Dinner	0.19
Friskies Fancy Feast Chopped Grill Feast	0.84
Kal Kan Whiskas Choice Cuts in Sauce with Beef	1.60
Kal Kan Whiskas Mealtime	0.77
Kal Kan Sheba with Beef in Aspic	1.06
Kozy Kitten Fish Dinner	0.61
9-Lives Seafood Platter	1.10
Puss 'N Boots Supreme Salmon Flavor	1.18
Purina Premium Turkey & Giblets	1.20
Purina Premium Tuna	0.54

Premium Canned Cat Foods

Hill's Science Diet Feline Maintenance	0.34
Iams Chicken Formula	0.57
Iams Ocean Fish Formula	0.36

Dietary Canned Cat Foods

Hill's Healthblend Adult	0.24
Hill's Prescription Diet Feline c/d	0.34
Hill's Prescription Diet Feline h/d	0.24
Kal Kan Waltham Low Protein	0.36
Provisions CNM CV-Formula	0.22
Provisions CNM UR-Formula	0.46

*The foods are classified by location of purchase. Popular foods are purchased primarily in supermarkets. Premium foods are purchased primarily in pet shops, large-format pet retailers, or veterinary clinics. Dietary foods are purchased primarily in veterinary clinics.

taurine-rich diet as well as oral supplementation of 250 to 500 mg oral taurine divided daily.

Recent studies relate taurine-deficiency dilated cardiomyopathy to American cocker spaniels and golden retriever dogs. When the dogs were provided with supplemental oral taurine, there was evidence of echocardiographic and clinical improvement (see Chapter 116). Taurine supplementation of commercial canine low-sodium diets is now usually provided, and oral taurine supplementation should be considered in those dogs with lowered serum taurine levels.

L-Carnitine concentrates in cardiac and skeletal muscle cells and is considered to be an important component of the

TABLE 69–2. LEVELS OF SELECTED NUTRIENTS IN COMMERCIAL FOODS USED IN ANIMALS WITH CARDIOVASCULAR DISEASE*

	PROTEIN	FAT	SODIUM	CHLORIDE	POTASSIUM	MAGNESIUM	PHOSPHORUS
Canned Canine Products							
Hill's Prescription Diet Canine h/d	17.3	28.8	0.10	0.35	0.83	0.13	0.47
Hill's Prescription Diet Canine k/d	14.8	27.3	0.21	0.25	0.30	0.13	0.11
Hill's HealthBlend Canine Geriatric	17.4	14.0	0.15	0.59	0.63	0.09	0.41
Hill's Prescription Diet Canine w/d	16.2	12.1	0.26	0.78	0.60	0.08	0.42
Purina CNM Canine CV-Formula	17.8	31.9	0.12	1.27	1.21	0.06	0.40
Purina CNM Canine NF-Formula	16.15	27.4	0.24	0.43	0.72	0.08	0.30
Select Care Canine Modified Formula	16.8	21.8	0.24	na	0.96	0.07	0.35
Waltham Low Sodium	26.3	38.0	0.10	na	1.50	0.10	0.67
Leo Specific Cardil CHW	17.7	21.3	0.11	na	1.31	0.07	0.57
Dry Canine Products							
Hill's Prescription Diet Canine h/d	17.2	20.9	0.07	0.35	0.72	0.11	0.62
Hill's Prescription Diet Canine k/d	14.6	19.5	0.21	0.38	0.32	0.06	0.29
Hill's HealthBlend Canine Geriatric	17.7	10.0	0.15	0.52	0.60	0.10	0.51
Hill's Prescription Diet Canine w/d	16.7	6.9	0.21	0.50	0.60	0.12	0.51
Purina CNM Canine NF-Formula	15.9	15.7	0.22	0.57	0.86	0.07	0.29
Select Care Canine Modified Formula	14.4	19.7	0.28	na	0.88	0.09	0.34
MediCal Cardio	18.6	17.2	0.17	na	1.04	0.10	0.60
Canned Feline Products							
Hill's Prescription Diet Feline h/d	43.6	27.0	0.24	0.75	0.90	0.06	0.73
Hill's Prescription Diet Feline k/d	29.3	41.1	0.26	0.27	1.00	0.04	0.57
Hill's HealthBlend Feline Adult	41.1	22.3	0.24	0.70	0.79	0.06	0.65
Hill's HealthBlend Feline Geriatric	40.9	20.5	0.33	0.67	0.88	0.10	0.61
Purina CNM Feline CV-Formula	42.5	26.8	0.20	1.09	1.33	0.07	0.92
Select Care Feline Modified Formula	35.0	53.0	0.23	na	1.07	0.06	0.49
Leo Specific FHW	44.3	26.7	0.14	na	1.31	0.11	0.71
Dry Feline Products							
Hill's Prescription Diet Feline k/d	28.1	27.4	0.28	0.50	0.89	0.05	0.57
Hill's HealthBlend Feline Adult	32.7	20.2	0.23	0.62	0.65	0.07	0.70
Hill's HealthBlend Feline Geriatirc	33.2	18.6	0.33	0.89	0.79	0.07	0.68
Purina CNM Feline NF-Formula	28.8	11.8	0.18	0.60	0.82	0.09	0.38
Select Care Feline Modified Formula	28.3	22.1	0.27	na	0.92	0.07	0.52

*This list represents products with the largest market share for which manufacturers' published values are available; expressed as % dry matter.
na = information not published by manufacturer.
Modified from *Small Animal Clinical Nutrition IV*, 4th ed, 1999, Table 17–9. Topeka, KS, Mark Morris Institute.

enzymes that transport long-chain fatty acids from the cytosol of cells into the mitochondria. Then the fatty acids are oxidized to generate energy. This is considered important in the heart, where fatty acids are an energy source sustaining contraction and relaxation. Additionally, carnitine serves as a mitochondrial detoxifying agent by scavenging toxic metabolites and transporting them out of the mitochondria as carnitine esters.[11, 12] It is synthesized in the liver from the amino acids methionine and lysine.

A subset of dogs, primarily but not limited to Boxers and American cocker spaniels, has been identified with carnitine-deficient dilated cardiomyopathy (see Chapter 116). Some of these dogs have lowered serum carnitine levels, a specific but insensitive marker for this disease (below 12 to 40 μmol/L). Right ventricular endomyocardial biopsy determination provides greater information on such a deficiency (normal, 6.7 to 11 nmol/mg). Investigators are uncertain whether the dilated cardiomyopathy is the cause or the effect of the carnitine deficiency. Supplementation with oral L-carnitine (22–44 mg/lb three times a day) is recommended, but this is expensive and should not be considered a universal recommendation.[11, 12]

Control Caloric Intake and Body Weight

Cardiac Cachexia. Cachexia is defined as unintentional weight loss of greater than 10 per cent, particularly involving lean tissue wasting. Cachexia occurs with many disease states, including heart failure, when there is negative nitrogen and energy balance owing to inadequate food intake, excessive energy loss, or altered metabolism.[12]

Cardiac cachexia has been related to the accumulation of cytokines in the body, such as tumor necrosis factor-α (TNF-α; cachectin) and interleukin-1. Cytokines suppress specific genes that encode for lipogenic enzymes (lipoprotein lipase), thus promoting the breakdown of adipose tissue and skeletal muscle.

TNF-α is a proinflammatory cytokine with negative inotropic effects. Levels are elevated in human patients with heart failure. While most of the biologic effects of TNF-α are beneficial, through inflammation or cell growth, there are definite adverse effects in the heart failure patients.[13] TNF-α promotes LV dysfuntion, pulmonary edema, cardiomyopathy, LV remodeling, and abnormal myocardial metabolism. Myocardial depression is through a direct effect on calcium handling and/or through nitric oxide production.[13]

Cachexia is further aggravated by increased workload on the part of the muscles of respiration (dyspnea and tachypnea), by anorexia induced by drug therapy and extravascular fluid accumulation, and by concomitant organ disease such as renal insufficiency. Decreased renal blood flow results in prostaglandin release, which further stimulates release of TNF-α from circulating monocytes. Such starvation or cachexia catabolizes structural proteins, including cardiac muscle, which further impairs cardiac function.

Food intake should be at a level that will maintain normal

body weight for the animal. Cardiac cachexia develops progressively in most animals with chronic cardiac disease, ultimately resulting in significant weight loss and weakness. This occurs despite what appears to be adequate caloric intake. Fish oils high in omega-3 fatty acids have been implicated in the improvement of cytokine production. Supplementing the diet with such products may be helpful in counteracting some of the effects of cachexia, but studies proving these points in pets are lacking.

It is not unusual for a dog or cat to lose up to 25 per cent of initial body weight, if one discounts fluid accumulations, while being treated for CHF. Throughout dietary therapy in animals with heart failure, the appropriate goal is to maintain nutrient intake and avoid caloric and vitamin deficiencies. This is particularly important when owners prepare their own homemade diets. Stimulation of the appetite through any and all mechanisms is very important. Reevaluation of drug dosages is critical as significant weight loss occurs. Food preparation in a manner that stimulates the desire to eat can be beneficial. Psychologically, owners are more concerned about starvation and weight loss than about heart failure. Excessive concern on the veterinarian's part about the need for a low-salt diet when anorexia and cachexia are present may be regarded as cold and uncaring by the owner. Use caution and common sense at this critical point.

Obesity. Obesity can be as significant a problem in older dogs with heart failure as is being underweight. Obesity is associated with blood volume expansion and increased cardiac output, increased plasma and extracellular volume, increased neurohumoral activation, reduced urinary sodium and water excretion, increased heart rate, systolic and diastolic dysfunction, exercise intolerance, and blood pressure irregularities. Blood pressure changes are due to the presence of increased ALDO, insulin, and NE levels.

Weight may be difficult to regulate because most salt-restricted diets are high in fat. Excessive weight increases the stress of cardiac function and exacerbates clinical heart failure. The best way to manage and control weight excess in an animal with cardiac disease is to reduce the total intake of the sodium-restricted dietary food. Commercial reducing diets contain sodium levels above that appropriate for managing heart failure. Caution is advised while managing animals with heart failure, because progressive weight loss may continue to the point of cachexia.

SOURCES OF SODIUM INTAKE OTHER THAN DIET

Treats. As shown in Table 69–3, the sodium content of manufactured treats is highly variable. Some are similar to premium foods, and others are extremely high in sodium. If owners feel that they must give treats to their pets, these should be limited to pieces of the sodium-restricted diet, fruits, vegetables, or low-sodium treats. Other safe treats include homemade (or bakery made) no-salt (not sugar-free) cookies, plain melba toast with or without salt-free margarine or jams, Passover-type matzoh, small slices of cooked chicken or beef, and unsalted popcorn or peanuts. Most manufactured foods such as processed meats, cheeses, cookies, pretzels, and snack foods are contraindicated owing to their high sodium content. Rawhide bones contain 0.2 per cent sodium and are safe in limited quantities.

Fresh Water. Animals with cardiac disease should always have access to fresh water. A significant source of sodium intake occurs when the water has been softened by

TABLE 69–3. SODIUM CONTENT OF SELECTED COMMERCIAL TREATS (% DRY MATTER)

LOWER-SODIUM TREATS (<0.5%)		HIGH-SODIUM TREATS (>0.5%)	
Canine Treats			
Alpo Stew Biscuits	0.31	Alpo Jerky Strips	1.03
Fiber Formula Biscuits	0.08	Alpo Liv-a Snaps	0.57
Hill's Science Diet Adult Treats	0.25	Champion Valley Farms Recipe Dog Treats	2.30
Hill's Science Diet Senior Treats	0.17	Purina Beggin' Strips	1.20
Iams Lamb & Rice Biscuits	0.12	Purina Hearty Chews	2.08
Iams Less Active Biscuits	0.12	Quaker Oats 100% Natural	0.52
Iams Original Biscuits	0.15	Quaker Oats Snausages	1.13
OM Formula Biscuits	0.21	Star Kist Jerky Treats	3.40
Purina Cheese Dawgs	0.42	Star Kist Meaty Bone	0.80
Purina Short Ribz	0.37		
Feline Treats			
Quaker Oats Puss 'N Boots Pounce	0.30	Martha White Bonkers (Liver)	0.99
Star Kist 9-Lives Finicky Bits	0.50	Purina Whisker Lickin's	1.03

an ion exchange softener that uses salt. When the water in the house is softened by this method, the pet's water should be obtained from an exterior water faucet, which usually supplies unsoftened water. If the entire water supply of the house is softened, distilled or nonsoftened water should be given, especially during the period of active diuresis. Distilled water or water with less than 150 ppm sodium is generally considered acceptable.

DIETARY USE OF SODIUM

The only known need for increased salt intake in the normal dog or cat is during reproduction. Because sodium and chloride can become limited during gestation and lactation, sodium-restricted diets should not be fed during this time. Once a dog or cat reaches adulthood (with the exception of during gestation and lactation), a diet containing no more than 0.4 per cent sodium in the dry matter is adequate and avoids the potential adverse effects of the long-term consumption of high-sodium diets. There are few reasons to feed dogs and cats high-salt diets except to increase water intake and urine volume as a part of a therapeutic protocol for the dissolution of struvite urolithiasis. Other unusual requirements for salt supplementation in the diet might include hypoadrenocorticism, high-dose diuretic administration, hypoaldosteronism, essential hyponatremia, psychogenic polydipsia, and SIADH (the syndrome of inappropriate antidiuretic hormone secretion). Many foods are simply salted to enhance palatability, perhaps in an effort to disguise the quality of the food ingredients.

PRACTICAL CONSIDERATIONS

Classification of Prepared Pet Foods by Sodium Content. To be able to effectively use dietary sodium restriction in clinical cases, it is necessary to know the relative sodium content of different classes of foods. The therapeutic objective is to reduce the sodium intake by feeding a palatable diet with a lower sodium content. Table 69–4 classifies prepared pet foods according to sodium con-

TABLE 69–4. CLASSIFICATION OF PREPARED PET FOODS BY SODIUM CONTENT

	AVERAGE SODIUM CONTENT (% DRY MATTER)
High (>0.5% DM)	
Popular canine and feline canned	0.9–1.0
Reduced-salt diets (0.35–0.5% DM)	
Popular canine and feline dry	0.40–0.44
Premium canine and feline canned and dry	0.35–0.42
Moderate salt restriction (0.1–0.35% DM)	
Canine geriatric/senior	0.12–0.17
Dietary-canine and feline renal	0.23–0.33
Dietary-feline cardiac	0.23
Severe salt restriction (<0.1% DM)	
Dietary-canine cardiac	0.08–0.12
Minimum Adult Requirement	
Canine	0.06
Feline	0.20

DM = dry matter.

tent and eliminates the need to know the content of each specific brand of dog and cat food.

Changing the Diet to a Salt-Restricted Product. Changing the diet can be a problem with some pets. Often, preconceived ideas by owners make it a difficult sell for veterinarians. Many pets, especially dogs, readily accept a change to a restricted-sodium diet by the third day. A complete switch from a high-sodium popular canned food or a homemade diet to a severely restricted-sodium prepared food should not be attempted all at once. Dietary sodium restriction should be initiated by selecting a lower-sodium diet from Table 69–1. Dietary foods designed for renal failure are excellent alternatives, as they are moderately restricted in sodium and usually quite palatable. The combined use of drug therapy, especially potent diuretics, and lowered-salt diets can be too restrictive. Volume depletion results, further stimulating the production of NE, ALDO, and PRA. In such cases, using moderately restricted-sodium renal diets is an excellent option for the management of animals with heart failure. Another alternative is to change to a senior diet, which often reduces sodium intake by 70 to 80 per cent. After a few weeks, the change to a severely restricted-sodium diet can often be accomplished, if needed, to control clinical signs.

Homemade Diets. Some owners choose not to feed prepared foods to their pets or refuse to believe that their pets will consume a commercially prepared food. Although it is useful to stress the positive benefits of commercial diets, it is wrong to believe that every client will accept such a change. Identify the client and work within the parameters he or she sets. Foolishly believing that the animal is actually receiving a low-salt diet when the owner is "flavoring" the product with salted home-cooked items is a disservice to the pet and the client. In such instances, the owner should be provided with a specific recipe for a sodium-restricted diet. Recipes and guidelines for preparing homemade low-salt diets for dogs and cats are contained in Tables 69–5 and 69–6. In general, equal quantities of fresh fish, beef, or poultry; vegetables; and cereals (rice or potatoes) plus two calcium carbonate tablets (Tums; Titralac) provide a well-balanced diet low in sodium. It is nearly impossible under such conditions to guarantee a nutritionally complete product designed for weight control that contains proper levels of protein and salt. The owner must be advised that a home-made diet restricted in both salt and calories is a less than ideal alternative and that such a diet may not meet all nutritional needs. Avoiding calorie and vitamin excess or deficiency is a concern. Ensuring adequate intake of vitamins is important but difficult, because most commercial vitamin supplements contain salt. A high-calorie, low-salt vitamin-mineral substitute (Nutrical) may be helpful in preventing this problem when added to the recipe in Table 69–5. Some clients even find Nutrical useful as an expedient for administering tablet medications.

Anorexic pets brought home after a bout with heart failure may be a challenge to the veterinarian and the owner. Finding a diet acceptable to the pet may be difficult, making drug administration even more frustrating. Junior meat-type baby foods without vegetables or additives, such as lamb, veal, and chicken, are low in sodium (35 to 50 mg/4-oz jar) and often prove useful in these situations. Never allow a dog or cat on high-dose diuretics to starve, as this will seriously aggravate hyponatremia, hypochloremia, and renal dysfunction. Similarly, never withhold or restrict access to water in dogs or cats with heart disease, whether or not they are on drug or diet therapy.

Veterinary Instructions. In initiating any clinical regi-

TABLE 69–5. GENERAL RULES TO OBSERVE IN PREPARING A LOW-SODIUM DIET

1. Use NO salts in food or in cooking.
2. Milk products are generally HIGH in sodium.
3. Canned, frozen, and prepared foods are usually HIGH in sodium.
4. Fresh meats are generally LOW in sodium.
5. All shellfish and prepared fish are HIGH in sodium.
6. DO NOT feed these foods, since they are HIGH in sodium:
   a. Cereals—All breads and prepared cereals are high in sodium except puffed rice, macaroni, rice, oatmeal, and potatoes.
   b. Snacks—milk, ice cream, puddings, gelatin dessert, salted crackers, baking soda or baking powder products.
   c. High-sodium-content meats and fish—luncheon meats, frankfurters, dried beef, sausage, sweetbreads, brains, kidney. Also clams, crabs, scallops, lobster, fish fillets. Cured meats such as ham, bacon, smoked pork, and corned beef. Canned or frozen items, unless marked "SALT FREE."
   d. Cheese and milk—all except unsalted cottage cheese or low-sodium cheddar.
   e. Fats—salted butter or margarine. Fat from salted meats.
   f. Vegetables—fresh artichokes, beets, celery, kale, spinach, chard, and turnips. All canned types, unless salt-free.
   g. Seasoning—all mixed salts.
   h. Condiments—catsup, chili sauce, soy sauce, mustard, horseradish, steak sauce, and prepared dressings.
   i. Miscellaneous—all salted nuts, potato chips, pretzels, olives, relish, pickles, molasses, brown sugar, peanut butter, candy, pudding, and glazed fruits.
   j. Special foods—baby foods, broths, and organ meats should be strictly avoided, since salt is a common ingredient in these food preparations.

Recipes for Low-Sodium Diets

Low-Sodium Diet for Dogs	*Low-Sodium Diet for Cats*
½ lb lean ground beef	1 lb regular ground beef
2 cups cooked rice without salt	¼ lb liver
1 tbs vegetable oil	1 cup cooked rice without salt
2 Tums tablets, crushed	1 tsp vegetable oil
	1 tsp calcium carbonate or
Braise meat, retaining fat.	10 Tums tablets, crushed
Add other ingredients and mix.	
Yield: 1.1 lb (480 g)	Braise meat and liver, retaining fat.
Sodium content: 0.05% in dry matter	Add other ingredients and mix.
	Yield: 1.7 lb (750 g)
	Sodium content: 0.16% in dry matter

Modified from Ettinger SJ, Suter PF: Canine Cardiology. Philadelphia, WB Saunders, 1970.

TABLE 69–6. SODIUM AND CALORIE CONTENT OF FOODS

FOOD	AMOUNT	SODIUM (mg)	CALORIES
Bread, cereals, and potatoes			
Recommended			
Potato	1 (small)	1	70
Polished rice	½ cup	1–10	360
Macaroni	1 cup	1–10	465
Puffed wheat	1 oz	1–10	100
Spaghetti	1 cup	1–10	355
Not recommended			
Bread	1 slice	200	60
Pretzels	1	275	58
Potato chips	1 oz	300	170
Cheese pizza	1 slice	650	245
Margarine and oil			
Recommended			
Unsalted margarine	1 tsp	0–1	50
Vegetable shortening	1 tbs	0–1	120
Not recommended			
Mayonnaise	1 tbs	60–90	110
Margarine (stick)	1 tbs	105	102
Dairy products			
Not recommended			
Milk (regular)	1 cup	122	160
Milk (skim)	1 cup	122	90
Cream cheese	1½ oz	100–120	160
Cottage cheese	3 oz	200–300	90
American cheese	1 oz	400	105
Butter			
Salted	1 tbs	90	100
Unsalted	1 tbs	0	100
Cheddar cheese	1 oz	176	100
Parmesan cheese	1 oz	112	45
Meats, poultry, fish			
Recommended			
Beef (fresh)	3½ oz	50	200
Pork (fresh)	3½ oz	62	275
Lamb (fresh)	3½ oz	84	175
Veal	3½ oz	67	300
Chicken (no skin)			
Light meat	3½ oz	64	180
Dark meat	3½ oz	86	180
Turkey (no skin)			
Light meat	3½ oz	82	230
Dark meat	3½ oz	98	230
Not recommended			
Egg	1	70	80
Bacon	2 slices	385	95
Ham (processed)	3 oz	940	225
Frankfurter	1	560	310
Cheeseburger	1	750	610
Vegetables (fresh or dietetic canned)			
Asparagus	½ cup	<5	20
Green beans	½ cup	<5	15
Peas	½ cup	<5	55
Green pepper	¼ cup	<5	10
Tomato	1	<5	30
Lettuce	¼ head	<5	15
Corn	½ cup	<5	70
Cucumber	½ cup	<5	<20
Celery	1 cup	104	35
Fresh fruits			
Most are low in sodium and are permitted			
Desserts			
Recommended			
Sherbet	½ cup	15–25	120
Not recommended			
Gelatins	½ cup	60–85	50–80
Ice cream	½ cup	60–85	200
Puddings	½ cup	100–200	175

Modified from Ettinger SJ, Suter PF: Canine Cardiology. Philadelphia, WB Saunders, 1970.

men, instructions to the owner are important. It is just as necessary to emphasize the importance of dietary modifications as the dosage and frequency of administration of drugs. Negative statements such as "Your pet may not like this food, but give it a try" almost assures that the owner will not be successful in changing the pet's diet. The alternative of "If you wish to enhance the quality of life while treating heart disease, your pet must eat a low-salt diet. I recommend. . ." greatly enhances the probability that the change will be accomplished. An additional point that the owner will appreciate is the ability to reduce drug (diuretic) therapy when sodium intake is lowered. Further, discuss the benefits of gradual dietary change versus total emergence into the new diet overnight.

Owners may find that commercial preparations appear unpalatable to their pets because of the unfamiliar method of preparation. Warming, chopping, or even pan frying such foods often changes the presentation to one that is more familiar to both the pet and the owner. Supplementing such food with unsalted condiments (e.g., garlic or onion powder, honey, maple syrup, oregano, parsley) is likely to make the product more familiar or tasty. Salt substitutes may be of use to those pets familiar with high levels of salt in their usual diet. Caution needs to be exercised because of their high potassium content. Salt substitutes should never be used in diets supplemented with potassium, particularly when potassium-sparing therapeutic agents are being administered.

LOW-SALT DIETS IN HYPERTENSIVE CARDIAC DISEASE

Recognition of the importance of systemic hypertension in both dogs and cats has brought a newly recognized demand for reduced-salt diets. Essential hypertension in humans is often treated successfully with dietary measures alone. Such is not the case with cats or dogs, as pets usually suffer from a secondary cause of hypertension rather than essential hypertension.

Alterations of the blood pressure in dogs and cats are controlled by regulating the kidneys' ability to excrete sodium and water. The control of systemic blood pressure requires sophisticated balancing of the central and peripheral nervous systems, the peripheral vasculature, the kidneys, and systemic neurohumoral factors.

Systemic hypertension in small animals is associated with heart rate variations due to such diseases as hyperthyroidism, anemia, polycythemia, hyperviscosity syndrome, and pheochromocytoma. Renal failure, hyperaldosteronism, and hyperadrenocorticism all increase salt and water retention and induce hypertension. Activation of the renin-angiotensin-aldosterone axis in cardiac disease promotes peripheral vasoconstriction (hypertension), salt and water retention, and elevation of catecholamine levels. Virtually all chronic renal diseases have the potential to induce systemic hypertension as well.

It is beyond the scope of this chapter to discuss the therapeutic measures required for each of the previously mentioned systemic diseases. Nevertheless, universal dietary measures are available for ameliorating the clinical effects of the induced hypertensive state. Gradual introduction of "renal diets" is the recommended approach for animals with hypertensive disease. Moderately restricted-salt diets are beneficial, because renal disease is frequently associated with hypertension. The concomitant use of ACE inhibitors, beta-blocking agents, calcium channel blocking agents, and/or diuretics may be indicated (see Chapter 50).

Acknowledgment

Dr. Ettinger wishes to acknowledge the assistance of Dr. Mark L. Morris, Jr., in preparing this chapter for the previous edition. Changes and new recommendations in this edition are those of Dr. Ettinger.

REFERENCES

1. Goodwin JK, Hamlin RL: Preference of veterinarians for drugs used to treat heart disease in dogs and cats—a 20 year follow-up study. J Vet Intern Med 7:118, 1993.
2. Knight DH: Pathophysiology of heart failure. In Ettinger SJ (ed): Textbook of Veterinary Internal Medicine, 3rd ed. Philadelphia, WB Saunders, 1989, pp 899–910.
3. AAFCO Nutrient Profiles for Dogs. Official Publication, AAFCO, 1993, p 93.
4. Nutrient Requirements of Dogs. Washington, DC, National Academy of Sciences, 1985, p 17.
5. Roudebush P, et al: The effect of combined therapy with captopril, furosemide, and a sodium restricted diet on serum electrolyte concentrations and renal functions in normal dogs and dogs with congestive heart failure. J Vet Intern Med 8:337, 1994.
6. Lewis LD, et al: Recipes for homemade diets. In Small Animal Clinical Nutrition III. Topeka, KS, Mark Morris Associates, 1987, p A3-1.
7. AAFCO Nutrient Profiles for Cat Foods. Feline Nutrition Experts Subcommittee Report, Washington, DC, 1991.
8. Roudebush P, Allen TA: Effect of dietary sodium and furosemide on hematologic, biochemical and endocrine parameters in normal geriatric dogs (abstract). Proceedings of the 14th annual ACVIM Forum, San Antonio, TX, 1996, 753.
9. COVE multicenter study group: Controlled clinical evaluation of enalapril in dogs with heart failure. J Vet Intern Med 9:243, 1995.
10. Ettinger SJ, et al: Relationships of enalapril with other CHF treatment modalities. Proceedings of the 12th annual ACVIM Forum, San Francisco, 1994, p 251.
11. Sanderson S, et al: Heart disease management—indicators for non-drug therapies. Vet Forum December: 14:36, 1996.
12. Roudebush P, et al: Dietary modifications in cardiovascular disease. In Hand MS, Thatcher CD, Remillard R, Roudebush P (eds): Small Animal Clinical Nutrition IV. Topeka, KS, Mark Morris Institute, 1999.
13. Bristow MR: Tumor necrosis factor–α and cardiomyopathy. Circulation 97:1340, 1998.

CHAPTER 70

DIETARY CONSIDERATIONS FOR URINARY DISEASES

Scott A. Brown, Joseph W. Bartges, Delmar R. Finco, and Jeanne A. Barsanti

Many urinary diseases are important in the clinical practice of veterinary medicine. Unfortunately, our understanding of dietary considerations for dogs and cats with diseases of the urogenital systems is limited to cases of chronic renal failure, protein-losing nephropathies, renal disease with systemic hypertension, and urolithiasis. The possible role of diet in the pathogenesis of idiopathic feline lower urinary tract disease is considered in Chapter 175. Here we address considerations related to the nutritional management of urinary tract disorders in dogs and cats and provide information on currently available commercial diets that may be used in the management of these disorders.

CHRONIC RENAL DISEASE AND DIET

Renal disease is a frequent cause of illness and death in dogs and cats, affecting approximately 1 per cent of all dogs.[1] The prevalence increases with advancing age, with chronic renal failure reaching a peak prevalence of 1 in 10 dogs and 1 in 3 cats over 15 years of age.[2] Renal failure sufficient to cause uremia is associated with a high mortality rate and considerable financial outlay for therapy (e.g., intensive fluid therapy, renal transplantation, and/or dialysis). For animals with chronic renal failure, the goals of dietary management are to maximize the quality and quantity of life by ensuring adequate intake of energy, limiting the extent of uremia, and slowing the rate of progression of renal disease.

INTERACTION OF DIET AND RENAL DISEASE

Maintaining Homeostasis

The kidney is an organ of homeostasis, maintaining or controlling extracellular fluid and blood volume, systemic arterial pressure, red blood cell production, nitrogenous waste excretion, and the balance of a variety of electrolytes and minerals. When renal disease is severe enough to produce an alteration of renal function, many important abnormalities occur as a result of failure of renal homeostatic mechanisms (see Chapters 167–170). If these derangements in body homeostasis are severe enough to produce clinical signs, the condition is referred to as uremia. An important principle of dietary therapy is that the extent of the abnormalities produced by the disruption of homeostasis in an animal with renal disease can be modified by dietary intake. For example, ingestion of a diet with low phosphorus content may lessen hyperphosphatemia, hyperparathyroidism, and renal osteodystrophy. Other clinical problems affected by dietary intake include hypokalemia, acidosis, systemic hypertension, and general clinical signs of uremia (e.g., vomiting and lethargy).

Progressive Nephropathy

A second principle of dietary therapy for animals with chronic renal disease is that the kidney is susceptible to further injury, and the extent of this injury may be modified by adjustments in dietary intake. Studies in dogs and cats indicate that dietary changes, such as phosphorus restriction or alteration of fatty acid composition, may alter the rate of progression of renal disease from early injury to end-stage uremia.[3–13]

Potassium

Hypokalemia is often observed in dogs and cats with renal failure, particularly those with marked polyuria or renal tubular disorders. Although cause and effect have not been clearly established, it is hypothesized that renal failure leads to kaliuresis and hypokalemia, which reduce renal function. This decline in renal function further enhances kaliuresis, setting up a vicious cycle. Thus, it is important to ensure adequate potassium intake for cats (and dogs) with renal failure. To achieve this goal, the diet can be supplemented with potassium salts (see Chapter 169), if needed, to maintain eukalemia. Because acidosis or dietary acidification enhances kaliuresis, care should be taken in assessing and maintaining the acid-base balance in animals with renal disease (see later).

Preventing Acidosis

Diets with animal-source protein are generally acidifying; additional acidification is frequently used in feline diets in an attempt to reduce the prevalence of lower urinary tract disease. When rats with chronic renal failure develop metabolic acidosis, enhanced renal ammoniagenesis activates the alternate complement cascade, leading to tubulointerstitial injury,[14] particularly in acute renal injury. Metabolic acidosis also contributes to uremia and muscle wasting. Although cats do not appear to respond to metabolic acidosis with an increase in renal ammoniagenesis, dietary acidification should be avoided in cats with renal disease, and until further information is available, dietary alkalinization should be used in all dogs and cats with renal disease and metabolic acidosis. Metabolic acidosis in animals with renal failure can be ameliorated by dietary alkalinization, restriction of dietary protein intake, or change from an animal-source to a vegetable-source protein (e.g., soy protein but not corn gluten). Dietary alkalinization (e.g., calcium carbonate, potassium citrate, or sodium bicarbonate) effectively controls acidosis without the need for other dietary manipulations (see Chapter 169). Consequently, this alternative offers the simplest solution, and calcium, potassium, or sodium salts should be used. The goal of this therapy is to achieve a normal value for plasma bicarbonate or total carbon dioxide content.

Protein

Many studies have examined the relationship between dietary protein intake and progression of experimental or spontaneous renal disease in dogs.[3–13] Although a thorough review of available data is beyond the scope of this chapter, it is apparent that these studies do not support the use of low-protein diets to slow the progression of renal failure in dogs. There are few studies of the progressive nature of renal disease in cats. One such study indicates that cats with induced renal disease have fewer glomerular lesions if fed a diet restricted in protein and energy.[12] However, the use of a reduced-protein diet was associated with weight loss in cats with experimentally induced renal disease.[12] Because studies

in rodents have shown that energy malnutrition is more effective than protein restriction in delaying the progression of renal disease, it is important to separate the effects of protein and energy restriction before firm recommendations can be made for dietary protein intake in cats with early renal failure. A recent study found that dietary protein restriction did not slow progression in cats with induced renal insufficiency.[10]

In animals with clinical signs attributable to biochemical disturbances from renal dysfunction, modification of dietary intake may ameliorate clinical signs. In uremic animals, restriction of dietary protein intake has routinely been recommended to reduce the generation of a variety of toxins derived from protein metabolism. Dietary protein restriction may limit the genesis of nitrogenous wastes and thus lessen the extent of uremic complications of chronic renal failure, such as lethargy and vomiting. Efforts to restrict dietary intake of protein should be undertaken only if adequate intake of calories can be maintained. One clinical trial supports the use of dietary protein restriction for this purpose.[15] Although there are no strict guidelines to follow for the restriction of dietary protein intake to ameliorate uremia, there is a general principle that dietary protein restriction should be considered whenever blood urea nitrogen concentration exceeds 80 mg/dL; the more severe the renal dysfunction, the greater the degree of protein restriction required to ameliorate uremia.

On the basis of current evidence, a moderate-protein diet (15 to 25 per cent protein content on a dry weight basis supplying approximately 1.2 to 2.0 g protein/lb body weight/day [2.5 to 4 g/kg/day]) is appropriate for dogs with moderate azotemia (blood urea nitrogen <75 mg/dL) that do not exhibit signs of uremia. However, there is no apparent advantage of diets within this range. Diets higher in protein may be tolerated by dogs with renal disease that exhibit little or no azotemia. Further restriction of protein intake (9 to 15 per cent protein content on a dry weight basis supplying approximately 0.6 to 1.2 g protein/lb body weight/day [1.3 to 2.5 g/kg/day]) is warranted only if uremia is present or blood urea nitrogen exceeds 80 mg/dL. Dietary protein restriction in cats with azotemic renal failure should be attempted much more cautiously and typically employs a diet containing 28 to 32 per cent protein (dry weight basis) that supplies 1.7 to 2.0 g protein/lb body weight/day (3.8 to 4.4 g/kg/day). The rationale for dietary protein restriction in cats is controversial, and it should be attempted only in azotemic or uremic cats.

Phosphorus

Studies have documented a relationship between dietary phosphorus intake and mortality in dogs[3, 7] and cats[16] with induced chronic renal failure. Although the exact mechanism of phosphorus nephrotoxicity remains to be established, dietary restriction of phosphorus intake has been associated with a preservation of renal function, a lessening of tubulointerstitial lesions, and a reduction in the extent of hyperphosphatemia, hyperparathyroidism, and hyperlipidemia. The most appropriate goal for dietary phosphorus restriction is unknown, but effectiveness can be monitored through the measurement of plasma concentrations of phosphorus and/or parathyroid hormone or determination of the fractional excretion of phosphate (see Chapters 167 and 169). The most readily monitored goal is the establishment of normophosphatemia.

Dietary phosphorus restriction should be in proportion to

the degree of renal dysfunction. In general, diets comprising less than 0.5 per cent phosphorus on a dry weight basis should be used initially. It is likely that further reductions in phosphorus intake will be necessary to achieve normophosphatemia in some affected animals. A variety of factors besides dietary restriction of phosphorus intake can lower intestinal absorption of phosphorus. Diets with a high phytin (plant source) content, an elevated calcium-to-phosphorus ratio, and a high ratio of organic to inorganic phosphorus reduce intestinal absorption of ingested phosphorus. A dietary calcium-phosphorus imbalance (ratio <1.0) should be avoided at any level of phosphorus intake and at any value for renal function in dogs and cats. Theoretically, dietary restriction of phosphorus leading to an increase in the calcium-phosphorus ratio would be beneficial by increasing relative calcium-phosphorus binding in the gut. However, hypercalcemia could result in an animal fed a diet with an excessively high calcium-phosphorus ratio. Because intestinal phosphorus binders reduce absorption of ingested phosphorus, they should be added in animals remaining hyperphosphatemic despite dietary phosphate restriction. These agents should be given with meals and dosed to effect (see Chapter 169). Calcium- or aluminum-containing agents are acceptable. Calcium-containing phosphorus binding agents may induce hypercalcemia and should not be used in animals with hypercalcemia or in conjunction with vitamin D therapy (e.g., calcitriol).

In some animals, the therapy outlined earlier leads to normophosphatemia, but manifestations attributable to renal secondary hyperparathyroidism, such as renal osteodystrophy, remain. In those cases, the oral administration of calcitriol (initial dose of 1 to 3 ng/lb/day) may be used as adjunct therapy (see Chapters 167 and 169). Frequent dose adjustments of calcitriol, based on plasma concentrations of parathyroid hormone and calcium, may be required. Calcitriol therapy does not lower plasma parathyroid hormone concentrations in all animals.

Dietary Fatty Acid Composition

Two recent studies documented that dietary supplementation with polyunsaturated fatty acids (PUFAs) can alter renal hemodynamics and prevent or delay progressive renal injury in dogs with induced chronic renal failure.[8, 9] Compared with safflower oil (omega-6 PUFA) supplementation, the addition of menhaden fish oil (omega-3 PUFA) to the diet lowered intraglomerular pressure and preserved renal structure and function.[8] This dietary modification should be considered as a means of delaying progression in dogs with azotemic chronic renal failure, although it remains controversial.[9]

Sodium

Systemic hypertension is frequently present in dogs and cats with chronic renal failure.[17, 18] High systemic arterial pressures may produce hypertensive injury within the kidney, though this remains to be established. It has not been clearly established that moderate dietary sodium restriction will lower systemic arterial pressure in dogs and cats with spontaneous renal disease. In animals with renal failure in which measurement of blood pressure establishes the presence of marked systemic hypertension (systolic arterial blood pressure >200 mm Hg), dietary sodium restriction is an appropriate therapeutic maneuver, although of unknown effectiveness.

Although there is no clear evidence that sodium bicarbon-

ate is associated with elevations of blood pressure, dietary sodium supplementation should be used cautiously in animals with renal failure. Potassium or calcium salts (see Chapters 168 and 169) are usually recommended for dietary alkalinization in animals with renal failure. In cats, potassium salts have the added advantage of supplying additional dietary potassium. Alkalinizing calcium salts (e.g., calcium carbonate or calcium acetate) may result in hypercalcemia, and serial measurements of the plasma calcium concentration should be made at intervals during therapy.

Dietary sodium restriction, when attempted, should be moderate, with a goal of approximately 7 to 18 mg/lb/day (15 to 40 mg/kg/day). Special diets for animals with renal failure (Table 70–1) all have a moderately low sodium content. (Commercially available diets for normal cats and dogs contain approximately 0.5 to 1.5 per cent sodium on a dry weight basis and typically provide 35 to 70 mg sodium/lb/day [75 to 150 mg/kg/day].) Because homeostatic mechanisms for sodium balance may be less effective in animals with renal dysfunction, changes in sodium intake (oral or parenteral) should be accomplished gradually, over 7 to 14 days. Excessive or rapid sodium restriction may produce extracellular volume depletion, dehydration, and systemic hypotension. Ideally, the effectiveness of dietary sodium restriction should be assessed by blood pressure measurements. Minimally, physical examination and serum creatinine measurements should be performed 1 to 2 weeks after adjusting dietary sodium intake.

DIETARY CONSIDERATIONS FOR STAGES OF RENAL FAILURE

For the purposes of dietary management of renal failure, animals with chronic renal failure can be divided into several stages (see Table 70–1) on the basis of laboratory and clinical findings: nonazotemic (normal blood urea nitrogen and serum creatinine concentrations), azotemic (elevated blood urea nitrogen and serum creatinine concentrations in the absence of clinical signs), uremic (elevated blood urea

TABLE 70–1. SUMMARY OF DIETARY RECOMMENDATIONS BENEFICIAL IN THE TREATMENT OF URINARY DISEASES IN DOGS AND CATS

CLINICAL PROBLEM	DIETARY RECOMMENDATION
Nonazotemic renal failure	None
Azotemic renal failure	Nonacidifying, reduced phosphorus, potassium supplemented (especially cats), and omega-3 polyunsaturated fatty acid enriched (dogs)
Uremic renal failure	Nonacidifying, reduced phosphorus, reduced protein, potassium supplemented (especially cats), and omega-3 polyunsaturated fatty acid enriched (dogs)
Protein-losing nephropathy	Reduced protein (if azotemic or uremic, see appropriate category above for additional recommendations)
Systemic hypertension	Reduced sodium
Calcium oxalate urolithiasis	Alkalinizing, reduced protein, and reduced sodium or increased fiber
Cystine urolithiasis	Alkalinizing, reduced protein, and reduced sodium
Struvite urolithiasis	Acidifying, diuresis inducing, reduced magnesium, reduced phosphorus, reduced protein
Urate urolithiasis	Alkalinizing, reduced protein

TABLE 70–2. POTENTIAL INDICATIONS FOR SELECTED COMMERCIAL DIETARY PREPARATIONS FORMULATED FOR THE TREATMENT OF URINARY TRACT DISEASES IN DOGS

CLINICAL PROBLEM	DIET
Nonazotemic renal failure	No special dietary modifications indicated
Azotemic renal failure	Kidney Formula Early Stage* Low Protein† Medium Protein† Modified Formula‡ NF-Formula§ Prescription Diet k/d‖
Uremic renal failure	Kidney Formula Advanced Stage* Low Protein† Medium Protein† Modified Formula‡ NF-Formula§ Prescription Diet k/d‖ Prescription Diet u/d‖
Protein-losing nephropathy	Kidney Formula Early Stage* Kidney Formula Advanced Stage* Low Protein† Medium Protein† Modified Formula‡ Prescription Diet k/d‖ Prescription Diet u/d‖
Systemic hypertension	CV-Formula§ Prescription Diet h/d‖
Calcium oxalate urolithiasis	*Prevention* NF-Formula§ Control Formula‡ HiFiber Formula‡ Prescription Diet k/d‖ Low Protein† Medium Protein† Mature Formula‡ Modified Formula‡ Prescription Diet k/d‖ Prescription Diet u/d‖ Prescription Diet w/d‖
Cystine urolithiasis	*Dissolution and Prevention* Prescription Diet u/d‖
Struvite urolithiasis	*Dissolution* Prescription Diet s/d‖ *Prevention* Prescription Diet c/d‖
Urate urolithiasis	*Dissolution and Prevention* Prescription Diet k/d‖ Prescription Diet u/d‖

*Eukanuba Veterinary Diets, Iams Co., Lewisburg, OH.
†Veterinary Diets, Waltham, Leicestershire, UK.
‡Select Care Diets, Vet's Choice, Santa Monica, CA.
§CNM Diets, Ralston Purina Co., St. Louis, MO.
‖Prescription Diets, Hill's Pet Nutrition, Inc., Topeka, KS.

nitrogen and serum creatinine concentrations plus clinical signs such as vomiting, lethargy, or inappetence), and proteinuric (elevated urine protein-to-creatinine ratio in the absence of urinary tract inflammation, plus hypoalbuminemia).

NONAZOTEMIC RENAL FAILURE

Currently, there is no evidence to support the use of special modified diets in dogs or cats with nonazotemic renal disease unless they are proteinuric.

AZOTEMIC RENAL FAILURE

In animals with azotemic renal failure in which the blood urea nitrogen concentration is less than 80 mg/dL, the goals of therapy are to limit the extent of complications of uremia and to delay further progression of renal disease. To accomplish the first goal, the diet should be nonacidifying and potassium-supplemented. To delay progression, the diet should be reduced in phosphorus content; for dogs, benefit may be observed from dietary supplementation with omega-3 PUFAs.

UREMIC RENAL FAILURE

In animals with clinical signs attributable to biochemical disturbances from renal dysfunction and/or a blood urea nitrogen concentration greater than 80 mg/dL, modification of dietary protein intake may help other measures in ameliorating clinical signs. Metabolic acidosis, hypokalemia, and hyperphosphatemia all may contribute to uremic complications such as lethargy, depression, and weakness.

PROTEINURIC RENAL FAILURE

In animals with an elevated urine protein-to-creatinine ratio in the absence of urinary tract inflammation and concurrent hypoalbuminemia, dietary protein restriction is indicated. The use of a restricted-protein diet generally limits

TABLE 70–3. POTENTIAL INDICATIONS FOR SELECTED COMMERCIAL DIETARY PREPARATIONS FORMULATED FOR THE TREATMENT OF URINARY TRACT DISEASES IN CATS

CLINICAL PROBLEM	DIET
Nonazotemic renal failure	No special dietary modifications indicated
Azotemic or uremic renal failure or protein-losing nephropathy	Low Protein† Mature Formula‡ Modified Formula‡ NF-Formula§ Prescription Diet k/d‖
Systemic hypertension	CV-Formula§ Prescription Diet h/d‖
Calcium oxalate urolithiasis	*Prevention* Control Formula‡ Mature Formula‡ Modified Formula‡ Weight Formula‡ Low Protein† NF-Formula§ Prescription Diet k/d‖ Prescription Diet w/d‖ Urinary Formula Moderate pH/O*
Cystine urolithiasis	*Prevention* Prescription Diet u/d‖
Struvite urolithiasis	*Dissolution* Prescription Diet s/d‖ *Prevention* Prescription Diet c/d‖ Control Formula‡ Control pHormula† UR-Formula§ Urinary Formula Low pH/S*
Urate urolithiasis	*Dissolution and Prevention* Prescription Diet k/d‖

*Eukanuba Veterinary Diets, Iams Co., Lewisburg, OH.
†Veterinary Diets, Waltham, Leicestershire, UK.
‡Select Care Diets, Vet's Choice, Santa Monica, CA.
§CNM Diets, Ralston Purina Co., St. Louis, MO.
‖Prescription Diets, Hill's Pet Nutrition, Inc., Topeka, KS.

both glomerular albumin loss and hepatic generation of albumin. In individual animals, the net effect of these opposing effects varies. The efficacy of any change in dietary protein intake should be judged on the basis of sequential determinations of the urine protein-to-creatinine ratio and serum albumin concentration at 2- to 4-week intervals (less frequently after stability has been documented). In proteinuric animals with azotemia or uremia, other dietary recommendations (see Table 70–1) should be applied.

COMMERCIALLY AVAILABLE DIETS

RENAL DISEASE

Unfortunately, little is known about the minimal dietary needs of animals with renal failure, and it is generally assumed that they are similar to those of normal animals. This is not necessarily valid. For example, the U.S. National Research Council's recommended minimal daily intake of phosphorus is 89 mg/kg body weight/day.[9] However, dogs with induced chronic renal failure fed less than 89 mg/kg/day were hyperphosphatemic, suggesting that the optimal daily requirements of phosphorus for dogs with renal failure are substantially below this recommended minimal value.[3, 7] Since minimal daily requirements for nutrient intake have not been established for animals with renal failure, careful attention to plasma biochemistries, body condition, daily food intake, and the animal's behavior is required in the medical management of animals with chronic renal failure.

A variety of special diets is available for the treatment of animals with renal failure (Tables 70–2 and 70–3). Some pets find special diets unpalatable, particularly if they are uremic. If a pet ingests less than its daily energy needs, malnutrition will result. To obtain required energy, body protein stores are broken down, liberating nitrogenous wastes. Because special diets for animals with renal failure are generally restricted in protein and sodium content, hypoproteinemia and extracellular fluid volume depletion may ensue. One can prevent this state of imbalance and secondary azotemia by modifying the offered diet or by seeking a diet that the animal will ingest. Such modifications include warming the diet or supplementing it with a small amount of a substance to enhance palatability (e.g., 1 to 2 tablespoons of turkey fat). The latter modification alters the nutrient content of ingested food and should be done sparingly.

Although a number of recipes are available for homemade diets for pets with chronic renal failure,[20] educating the owner and ensuring compliance are difficult. Consequently, a commercially available preparation is likely to be more practical when dietary modification is instituted.

Choosing an appropriate commercial diet for an animal with renal disease can be difficult. Pet food companies are not required to demonstrate efficacy for claims they may make, and they can (and occasionally do) alter the content and nutrient profiles of foods without notice. The "guaranteed analyses" provided on pet food labels are not intended to approximate the actual nutrient content of the food but rather to guarantee that it contains either more or less than the stated amount. These guaranteed minimal or maximal values may differ from actual nutrient content by 50 per cent or more and do not provide reliable information for making decisions about the dietary intake of dogs and cats with renal failure. Although some nutrient profiles are based on calculations, reliable nutrient profiles can be derived only from chemical analyses of average lots. The Association of American Feed Control Officials (AAFCO) Pet Food Committee has issued recommended minimal and maximal values for nutrient profiles for dog foods, but these recommendations for normal dogs may not apply to animals with renal disease. Consequently, the veterinarian is left with considerable uncertainty about what food to use. In this setting, individualized management with careful monitoring is required. Serial measurements of serum concentrations of creatinine, blood urea nitrogen, phosphate, calcium, bicarbonate, protein, and albumin and a complete blood count and urinalysis should be performed 1 month after a diet change and repeated every 3 months throughout the life of an animal with renal failure. This allows the veterinarian to identify abnormalities and institute appropriate therapy (see Chapters 167–170).

TABLE 70–4. APPROXIMATE NUTRIENT INTAKE* PER KILOGRAM BODY WEIGHT FOR A DOG CONSUMING SELECTED DIETS FORMULATED FOR THE TREATMENT OF CHRONIC RENAL FAILURE

DIET	FORM	PROTEIN (g/kg)	PHOSPHORUS (mg/kg)	SODIUM (mg/kg)	POTASSIUM (mg/kg)
Kidney Formula Early Stage†	Dry	3.00	63.4	76.1	101.5
Kidney Formula Advanced Stage†	Dry	2.04	33.6	67.3	78.9
Low Protein‡	Dry	2.24	52.8	35.2	105.6
	Canned	2.47	71.1	82.3	119.8
Medium Protein‡	Dry	2.85	62.5	27.8	95.5
	Canned	3.26	71.4	89.3	116.1
Modified Formula§	Dry	2.08	51.6	40.6	128.1
	Canned	2.34	48.8	29.3	112.3
NF-Formula‖	Dry	2.26	40.7	31.3	122.2
	Canned	2.21	39.8	31.0	97.4
Prescription Diet k/d#	Dry	2.03	43.8	28.6	45.2
	Canned	1.97	25.0	29.6	39.4
Prescription Diet u/d#	Dry	1.18	25.0	30.1	78.0
	Canned	1.40	18.8	30.6	48.1

*These values are based solely on nutrient content information provided by pet food manufacturers; they have not been independently verified by the authors. Nutrient intake is for a 20-kg dog consuming 1250 kcal daily. Factors such as digestibility, palatability, biologic value of protein, availability of phosphorus for absorption, effect on acid-base status, fatty acid profile, and interlot variability are likely to vary substantially among diets.
†Eukanuba Veterinary Diets, Iams Co., Lewisburg, OH.
‡Veterinary Diets, Waltham, Leicestershire, UK.
§Select Care Diets, Vet's Choice, Santa Monica, CA.
‖CNM Diets, Ralston Purina Co., St. Louis, MO.
#Prescription Diets, Hill's Pet Nutrition, Inc., Topeka, KS.

TABLE 70–5. APPROXIMATE NUTRIENT INTAKE* PER KILOGRAM BODY WEIGHT FOR A CAT CONSUMING SELECTED DIETS FORMULATED FOR THE TREATMENT OF CHRONIC RENAL FAILURE

DIET	FORM	PROTEIN (g/kg)	PHOSPHORUS (mg/kg)	SODIUM (mg/kg)	POTASSIUM (mg/kg)
Low Protein†	Dry	3.80	70	28	124
	Canned	4.26	66	71	132
Mature Formula‡	Dry	5.35	118	69	167
	Canned	5.69	75	44	94
Modified Formula‡	Dry	4.82	91	47	153
	Canned	4.37	61	28	85
NF-Formula§	Dry	5.06	68	32	144
	Canned	4.21	70	23	131
Prescription Diet k/d‖	Dry	4.25	92	43	131
	Canned	3.93	77	34	134

*These values are based solely on nutrient content information provided by pet food manufacturers; they have not been independently verified by the authors. Nutrient intake is for a 4-kg cat consuming 280 kcal daily. Factors such as digestibility, palatability, biologic value of protein, availability of phosphorus for absorption, effect on acid-base status, fatty acid profile, and interlot variability are likely to vary substantially among diets.
†Veterinary Diets, Waltham, Leicestershire, UK.
‡Select Care Diets, Vet's Choice, Santa Monica, CA.
§CNM Diets, Ralston Purina Co., St. Louis, MO.
‖Prescription Diets, Hill's Pet Nutrition, Inc., Topeka, KS.

If uremia, hyperphosphatemia, hypokalemia, and/or systemic hypertension are present in an animal consuming a commercially available preparation, changing intake to a diet with a different nutrient profile should be considered. Nutrient content expressed as a percentage of dry matter or as a percentage as fed can be misleading. Nutrient information on commercially available preparations based on actual intake per kilogram of body weight for a 44-pound dog (assumes 1250 kcal of metabolizable energy/day[19]) and for an 8.8-pound cat (assumes 280 kcal of metabolizable energy/day[21]) demonstrates that although several of the commercially available preparations are similar, there are some apparent differences in protein, phosphorus, sodium, and potassium content (Tables 70–4 and 70–5). These differences can be used to make choices among various preparations for the management of individual animals with renal failure, but they should be interpreted with caution. This information represents approximations based on current formulations of these diets provided on typical analyses by the manufacturers. These data have not been independently tested by the authors, nor is information currently available on the variability of nutrient contents among lots for these various commercial preparations. Finally, these diets have not been tested by comparative feeding trials. Factors such as digestibility, palatability, biologic value of protein, availability of phosphorus for absorption, effect on acid-base status, and fatty acid profiles are likely to vary among diets. However, until comparative studies are done, there are no objective criteria for evaluating diets with similar nutrient profiles, again emphasizing the need for individualized nutritional management of affected pets.

UROLITHIASIS

A variety of commercial preparations is available for the management of urolithiasis. For a further discussion of general dietary recommendations (see Table 70–1) and alternative commercial preparations (see Tables 70–2 and 70–3), the reader is referred to Chapters 175 and 176.

REFERENCES

1. MacDougall DG, et al: Canine chronic renal disease: Prevalence and types of glomerulonephritis in the dog. Kidney Int 29:1144, 1986.
2. Polzin D, et al: Medical management of feline chronic renal failure. *In* Kirk RW (ed): Current Veterinary Therapy XI. Philadelphia, WB Saunders, 1992, p 848.
3. Brown SA, et al: Beneficial effects of dietary mineral restriction in dogs with marked reduction of functional renal mass. J Am Soc Nephrol 1:1169, 1991.
4. Brown SA, et al: Single-nephron adaptations to partial renal ablation in the dog. Am J Physiol 258:F495, 1990.
5. Brown SA, Brown CA: Single-nephron adaptations to partial renal ablation in cats. Am J Physiol 269:R1002, 1995.
6. Brown SA, et al: Dietary protein intake and the glomerular adaptations to partial nephrectomy in dogs. J Nutr 121:S125, 1991.
7. Finco DR, et al: Effects of phosphorus/calcium-restricted and phosphorus/calcium-replete 32% protein diets in dogs with chronic renal failure. Am J Vet Res 53:157, 1992.
8. Brown SA, et al: Beneficial effects of chronic administration of dietary omega-3 polyunsaturated fatty acids in dogs with renal insufficiency. J Lab Clin Med 131:447, 1998.
9. Bauer J, et al: Dietary omega-6 fatty acid supplementation improves ultrafiltration in spontaneous canine chronic renal failure. J Vet Int Med 11:126, 1997.
10. Finco DR, et al: Protein and calorie effects on progression of induced chronic renal failure in cats. Am J Vet Res 59:575, 1998.
11. Polzin DJ, et al: Influence of reduced protein diets on morbidity, mortality, and renal function in dogs with induced chronic renal failure. Am J Vet Res 45:506, 1983.
12. Adams L, et al: Influence of dietary protein/calorie intake on renal morphology and function in cats with 5/6 nephrectomy. Lab Invest 70:347, 1994.
13. Robertson JL, et al: Long-term renal responses to high dietary protein in dogs with 75% nephrectomy. Kidney Int 29:511, 1986.
14. Nath KA, Hostetter MK, Hostetter TH: Pathophysiology of chronic tubulo-interstitial disease in rat. J Clin Invest 76:667, 1985.
15. Grandjean D, et al: Interet d'une alimentation hypoproteique et hypophosphoree dans l'evolution post seuil critique d'une insuffisance renale chronique chez le chien. Rec Med Vet 166:865, 1990.
16. Ross LA, Finco DR, Crowell WA: Effect of dietary phosphorus restriction on the kidneys of cats with reduced renal mass. Am J Vet Res 43:1023, 1982.
17. Cowgill LD: Systemic hypertension. *In* Kirk RW (ed): Current Veterinary Therapy IX. Philadelphia, WB Saunders, 1986, p 360.
18. Littman MP: Spontaneous systemic hypertension in 24 cats. J Vet Intern Med 8:79, 1994.
19. National Research Council: Nutrient Requirements of Domestic Animals: Dogs. Washington, DC, National Academy Press, 1985.
20. Lewis LD, Morris ML, Hand MS: Small Animal Clinical Nutrition, 3rd ed. Topeka, Mark Morris Associates, 1987.
21. National Research Council: Nutrient Requirements of Domestic Animals: Cats. Washington, DC, National Academy Press, 1986.

CHAPTER 71

ENTERAL AND PARENTERAL NUTRITIONAL SUPPORT

Stanley L. Marks

The goal of nutritional support is to provide a formula of fuels and nutrients in proportions that can be used by the animal with maximal efficiency. Choosing the proper access technique and nutrition formulation requires knowledge, skill, and time. Many techniques for obtaining enteral access are available, and the approach used depends on several issues, including anticipated duration of enteral support, aspiration risk, condition of the gastrointestinal tract, the animal's temperament, and its degree of malnutrition.

RATIONALE FOR ENTERAL NUTRITIONAL SUPPORT

Enteral feeding is indicated for dogs and cats that cannot ingest adequate amounts of calories but have sufficient gastrointestinal function to allow digestion and absorption of feeding solutions delivered via an enteral feeding device. The rationale for prescribing enteral rather than parenteral nutrition (PN) is superior maintenance of intestinal structure and function. The most important stimulus for mucosal cell proliferation is the direct presence of nutrients in the intestinal lumen.[1] Other advantages of enteral nutrition are safety of administration and relatively low cost. The average daily cost of PN for maintaining caloric requirements of a dog or cat can be 5 to 10 times that of enteral feeding.

PATIENT SELECTION FOR NUTRITIONAL SUPPORT

Objective methods of assessing nutritional status, such as body composition measurement (anthropometry, impedance measurements, dual energy X-ray absorptiometry), are still in their infancy in veterinary medicine. Thus, subjective assessment of each animal's nutritional status is recommended. This technique is based on easily collected historical information (changes in oral intake, degree of weight loss, presence of vomiting or diarrhea) and changes found on physical examination (muscle wasting, body condition, presence of edema or ascites). Measurements of the animal's serum albumin concentration and total lymphocyte count are insensitive determinants of nutritional status because of the number of disease processes that influence these parameters. Nutritional support should be considered for animals demonstrating recent weight loss exceeding 10 per cent of optimal body weight or for those whose oral intake has been or will be interrupted for more than 5 days. Animals with nutrient losses from chronic diarrhea and vomiting, renal disease, or burns should also be considered for nutritional support.

ENTERAL FEEDING ACCESS DEVICES

The best feeding tubes for prolonged use are made of polyurethane or silicone. For short-term feeding (<10 days), polyvinylchloride (PVC) tubes are appropriate. Silicone is softer and more flexible than other tube materials and has a greater tendency to stretch and collapse. Polyurethane is stronger than silicone, allowing for thinner walls and a larger internal diameter, despite the same French size.[2] The French unit measures the outer lumen diameter of a tube (each French unit is equal to 0.33 mm).

NASOESOPHAGEAL TUBES

Nasoesophageal tubes are a simple and efficient choice for feeding an animal in need of short-term (<10 days) nutritional support. This includes most anorectic hospitalized animals that have a normal nasal cavity, pharynx, esophagus, and stomach.[3-5] Nasoesophageal tube feeding is contraindicated in animals that are vomiting or comatose or lack a gag reflex. PVC (Infant Feeding Tube, Argyle Division of Sherwood Medical, St. Louis, MO) or red rubber tubes (Sovereign Feeding Tube, Monoject Division of Sherwood Medical, St. Louis, MO) are the least expensive tubes for dogs and cats, although the PVC tubes may harden within 2 weeks of insertion and cause irritation or ulceration of the pharynx or esophagus.[6] Tubes made of polyurethane (Travasorb Feeding Tube, Travenol Laboratories, Deerfield, IL, or Peditube, Biosearch Medical Products, Somerville, NJ) are more expensive; however, they are less irritating and more resistant to gastric acid, allowing prolonged usage. An 8 French × 42 inch tube (preferably with a stylet) is suitable for dogs weighing more than 15 kg. A 5 or 6 French × 36 inch tube is recommended for dogs weighing less than 15 kg and for cats.

The end of the tube should terminate in the distal esophagus rather than the stomach to decrease the likelihood of reflux esophagitis. Desensitization of the nasal cavity with four or five drops of 0.5 per cent proparacaine hydrochloride is recommended. The tube tip should be lubricated and passed into the ventral nasal meatus by positioning the animal's head in a normal angle of articulation (Fig. 71–1A). In the dog, the tube is directed in a ventromedial direction while pushing the external nares dorsally.[7] This maneuver opens the ventral meatus and guides the tube into the oropharynx. A tape tab should be secured to the skin on the dorsal midline between the eyes, and the tube should be secured as close to the nostril as possible with either suture material or glue (Superglue, Loctite Corp., Cleveland, OH) (see Figs. 71–1B and C). An Elizabethan collar is usually required to prevent inadvertent tube removal.

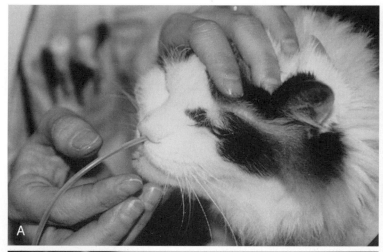

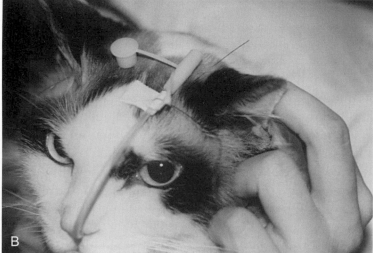

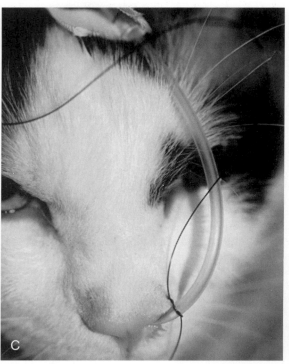

Figure 71–1. *A,* The tip of the nasoesophageal tube has been lubricated and passed into the ventral meatus by positioning the animal's head in a normal angle of articulation. *B,* The nasoesophageal tube can be secured to the skin on the dorsal midline between the eyes with tape "butterflies." *C,* A second tape tab should be secured as close to the nostril as possible, with either suture material or glue.

After placement, the tube position should be checked by injecting 5 to 10 mL of air while auscultating the cranial abdomen for borborygmus, or by infusing 3 to 5 mL of sterile saline or water through the tube and observing for a cough response. Confirmation of correct tube placement can also be obtained by a lateral survey thoracic radiograph and observing the position of the radiopaque tube in the esophagus.

The most common complications associated with the use of nasoesophageal tubes include epistaxis, dacryocystitis, rhinitis, tracheal intubation causing pneumonia, and vomiting.[5]

PHARYNGOSTOMY TUBES

The increasing availability of endoscopic equipment and the superior benefits of percutaneous gastrostomy tube placement have resulted in pharyngostomy tubes becoming virtually obsolete. Nevertheless, placement modifications have resulted in a dramatic reduction in complications associated with the interference of epiglottic movement and partial laryngeal obstruction.[8] The correct placement of a pharyngostomy tube is dorsal and caudal to the stylohyoid and epihyoid bones.[8] The indications for pharyngostomy tube placement are similar to those for nasoesophageal tube placement; however, the procedure requires general anesthesia.

Complications of pharyngostomy tube placement include airway obstruction, aspiration of food, vomiting or reflux,

epiglottic entrapment, laryngeal obstruction, recurrent laryngeal nerve injury, tube displacement, chewing of the tube, esophagitis, and infection of the wound site.[4, 8]

ESOPHAGOSTOMY TUBES

Three techniques for esophagostomy tube placement have been described.[9, 10] The first method is a percutaneous (needle) technique that involves use of an intravenous jugular vein catheter inside a 14-gauge needle.[9] A curved Carmalt forceps is inserted into the esophagus, and the tip is turned outward as a directional guide for the needle catheter. The needle is inserted through the skin and into the esophagus between the parted blades of the forceps. The premeasured catheter is fed through the needle and into the thoracic esophagus, whereupon the needle is removed. The second technique involves placing a small-bore feeding tube (5 to 12 French) in the esophagus via a surgical cutdown.[9]

An alternative esophagostomy tube technique using an Eld Gastrostomy Tube Applicator (Jorgensen Laboratories, Loveland, CO) was recently described by Devitt and Seim.[10] This technique was well tolerated in all animals and was not associated with major complications. The time required for healing of the esophagostomy site following tube removal was less than 2 weeks. In all placement methods, the tube is fixed in place with a friction suture or a tape "butterfly."

The ostomy site is allowed to heal by granulation and epithelialization when the esophagostomy tube is removed.[9]

GASTROSTOMY TUBES

Gastrostomy tube feeding is indicated for long-term (weeks to months) nutritional support of anorectic or dysphagic animals.[11, 12] Gastrostomy feeding tubes are of comparatively large diameter (18 to 24 French), allowing the economic use of blended pet foods and the direct administration of medications. Gastrostomy tube feeding is contraindicated in animals with persistent vomiting, decreased consciousness, or gastrointestinal obstruction. Caution should be exercised in animals with megaesophagus and conditions in which the stomach cannot be apposed to the body wall (severe ascites, adhesions, space-occupying lesions).[13]

Gastrostomy tubes can be placed percutaneously or during laparotomy. Placement is usually accomplished via a percutaneous endoscopic gastrostomy (PEG) technique,[11, 12] or a blind percutaneous gastrostomy (BPG) technique.[14–16] Preadapted gastrostomy kits from Mill Rose Labs (Mentor, OH) or Cook Veterinary Products (Bloomington, IN) are marketed for veterinary use and are economical (less than $30 each). We do not recommend cutting the small nipple on the mushroom tip to enhance the flow of food through the tube. Removing the tip of the mushroom compromises the integrity of the mushroom and hinders percutaneous removal of the tube.

Percutaneous Endoscopic Gastrostomy Technique

Endoscopic and blind placement of gastrostomy tubes requires brief anesthesia. The animal should be placed in right lateral recumbency so that the stomach tube can be placed through the greater curvature of the stomach and the left body wall. Preparation for both percutaneous procedures is identical and involves a surgical prep of the skin caudal to the left costal arch. The endoscope should be introduced into the stomach, which is then inflated. The left body wall is transilluminated with the endoscope to ensure that the spleen is not positioned between the stomach and body wall. An appropriate site for tube insertion should be determined by endoscopically monitoring digital palpation of the gastric wall. A small incision is made in the skin with a scalpel blade, and an intravenous catheter is stabbed through the body wall into the lumen of the stomach (Fig. 71–2A). The stylet is removed, and nylon or polyester suture is threaded through the catheter into the lumen of the stomach. The suture material is grasped with the endoscopic biopsy forceps, and the endoscope and forceps are carefully withdrawn through the esophagus and out the mouth (see Fig. 71–2B). The suture material is secured to the feeding tube (see Fig. 71–2C), and gentle traction is applied to the suture material at its point of exit from the abdominal wall (see Fig. 71–2D). The feeding tube is pulled out through the body wall, allowing the mushroom end to draw the stomach wall against the body wall (see Fig. 71–2E). The feeding tube is anchored in this position by the external bumper placed over the catheter at the skin surface. The endoscope is then reinserted into the stomach to verify the correct placement of the mushroom against the gastric mucosa. A stockinette jacket is fitted to protect the tube after it has been clamped and capped (see Fig. 71–2F).

Complications related to PEG tubes include those associated with placement of the tube (splenic laceration, gastric hemorrhage, and pneumoperitoneum) and delayed complications such as vomiting, aspiration pneumonia, tube extraction, tube migration, peritonitis, and stoma infection.[11, 12] Splenic laceration can be minimized by insufflating and transilluminating the stomach before placement of the needle or catheter into the abdominal wall.

Blind Percutaneous Gastrostomy Technique

An alternative technique for nonendoscopic and nonsurgical gastrostomy tube placement has been described.[14–16] The gastrostomy tube placement device can be prepared with a length of vinyl or stainless steel tubing (diameter 1.2 to 2.5 cm) purchased from a hardware store, or an Eld Gastrostomy Tube Applicator (Jorgensen Laboratories, Loveland, CO) or gastrostomy tube introduction set (Cook Veterinary Products, Bloomington, IN) can be used. The reported complication rate of BPG is similar to that of PEG; however, the risk of penetrating the spleen, stomach, or omentum is greater when the stomach is not insufflated with air before positioning the tube against the lateral abdominal wall.[17] Contraindications to using the blind technique include severe obesity that precludes accurate palpation of the tube against the abdominal wall and esophageal disease.

Surgical Tube Gastrostomy Technique

Surgical placement of gastrostomy tubes has been superseded by the percutaneous techniques because of their ease and speed of placement, lower cost, and decreased morbidity. A surgical approach may be indicated in obese animals, in those with esophageal obstruction, or when a laparotomy is planned for reasons other than tube placement.

Gastrostomy Tube Removal

For percutaneously placed tubes, it is recommended that the tube be left in place for a minimum of 7 to 10 days. Animals receiving immune-suppressive therapy or those that are severely debilitated may require longer than 10 days for a peritoneal seal to form. The tube should be removed only when oral food intake is sufficient to meet caloric requirements. One of two methods of tube removal can be applied. The tube can be cut at the body wall and the mushroom tip pushed into the stomach to be passed in the feces. This method is safe in medium to large size dogs, because the mushroom and internal bumper should be easily passed in the stool. Alternatively, a stylet can be inserted into the tube to flatten the mushroom tip while exerting firm traction on the tube. This method is recommended for cats and small dogs, because the mushroom can cause intestinal obstruction. The gastrocutaneous tract should seal with minimal or no leakage within 24 hours.

Gastrostomy Tube Replacement

Premature removal of a gastrostomy tube (within 10 days of placement; before establishment of the gastrocutaneous tract) requires a PEG procedure to evaluate the gastric mucosa and verify correct positioning of the replacement gastrostomy tube. If the tube is inadvertently removed once the gastrocutaneous tract is well healed, the original catheter can be replaced with a balloon-type catheter (Flexiflo Gastrostomy Tube, Ross Laboratories, Columbus, OH)[18] or a low-

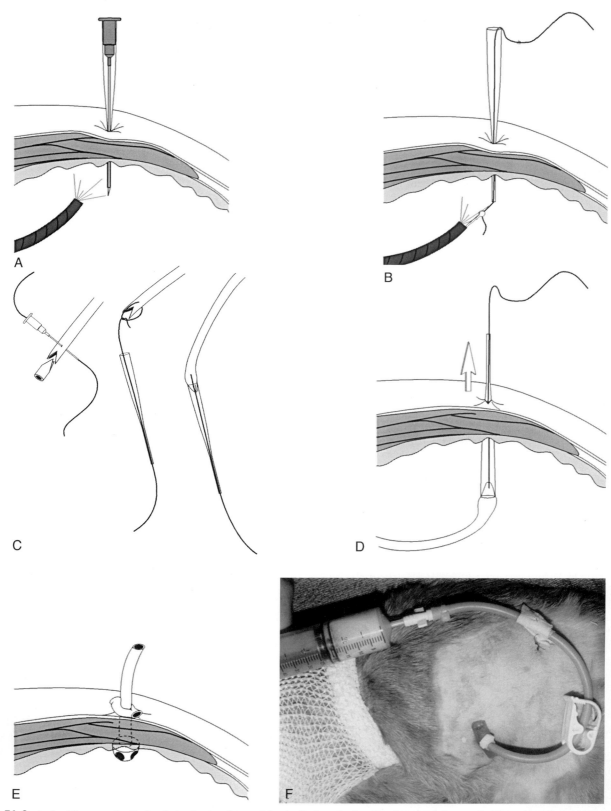

Figure 71–2. *A,* An 18-gauge sheathed catheter is placed transabdominally into the insufflated stomach lumen. *B,* The catheter stylet is removed, and nylon suture is advanced through the needle until it can be grasped with endoscopic retrieval forceps. The nylon suture is pulled out through the mouth as the endoscope is withdrawn. *C,* The end of the catheter opposite the mushroom tip is modified by removing a V-shaped wedge. Nylon suture is securely attached to the catheter just under the trimmed portion via a hypodermic needle. The suture is tied in a square knot, and the gastrostomy tube is drawn snugly into the flared end of the catheter. *D,* The lubricated catheter is drawn down the esophagus and into the stomach as the assistant applies traction on the suture exiting the body wall. *E,* The catheter is advanced until the mushroom tip rests gently against the gastric mucosa. Endoscopy should be repeated to confirm the correct position of the gastrostomy tube tip. An external flange is fitted down the tube against the skin to prevent the tube from slipping into the stomach. *F,* Gastrostomy feeding tube in place, with the clamp in the open position. The stockinette jacket is pulled over the gastrostomy tube once feeding is completed.

profile gastrostomy device (LPGD) (Fig. 71–3). Neither catheter requires an endoscopic procedure for placement.

ENTEROSTOMY TUBES

Enterostomy tubes are indicated for animals unable to tolerate intragastric feeding despite having normal distal small-intestine and colon function.[19, 20] Specific indications for feeding via jejunostomy tube include gastric outlet obstruction, gastroparesis, recurrent or potential aspiration, proximal small-bowel obstruction, and partial gastrectomy.[19, 20] Jejunal tube feeding minimizes the stimulation of pancreatic secretion and is an excellent way to provide nutrition to animals with severe pancreatitis.[21] The surgical (open) jejunostomy technique is a quick and easy method developed by Delany that uses a 5 French PVC tube (Infant Feeding Tube, Argyle Division of Sherwood Medical, St. Louis, MO) introduced into the bowel lumen through a hypodermic needle.[22]

Percutaneous Endoscopic Jejunostomy Technique

Percutaneous endoscopic jejunostomy (PEJ) techniques have been used extensively in humans.[23] Two basic techniques for PEJ have been described. The most common method involves the placement of a transpyloric (postpyloric) feeding tube through a previously placed PEG using endoscopic guidance.[23] Although the procedure is simple to perform, results of studies evaluating the long-term efficacy of transpyloric PEJ have been disappointing.[24] Efforts to develop a gastrojejunal feeding tube for the dog have had limited success.[25] Preliminary investigations indicate that percutaneous duodenostomy is a safe and feasible technique.[26] A direct PEJ was described in humans that avoids the complications associated with transpyloric PEJ.[27] The technique is virtually identical to the PEG technique, with the exception that the endoscope is used to transilluminate the abdominal wall adjacent to a loop of small bowel. The external sutures are cut, and the catheter is slowly withdrawn upon completion of enteral feeding. Complications of enterostomy tube placement include catheter dislodgment and subsequent peritonitis, focal cellulitis around the stoma site, abdominal cramping, diarrhea, and vomiting.[20]

CALCULATION OF NUTRITIONAL REQUIREMENTS

Nutritional support provides substrates for gluconeogenesis and protein synthesis. It also provides the energy needed

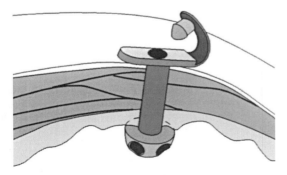

Figure 71–3. Low-profile gastrostomy device with mushroom tip that serves as an internal stabilizer. The tip must be stretched with an obturator tube to facilitate placement. A feeding adaptor attaches a syringe directly into the feeding port.

TABLE 71–1. ENTERAL FEEDING WORKSHEET FOR DOGS AND CATS

1. Calculate resting energy requirement (RER)
   Body weight 2 to 45 kg: RER (kcal) = 30 Wt_{kg} + 70
   Body weight <2 or >45 kg: RER = 70($Wt_{kg}^{0.75}$)
   Body weight = _____ kg
   RER = _____ kcal

2. Calculate illness energy requirement (IER)
   Illness factor = 1.2 to 1.5 for dogs
   Illness factor = 1.1 to 1.2 for cats
   IER = RER × illness factor
   IER = _____ kcal

3. Calculate amount of diet to feed
   Daily volume to feed: IER ÷ energy density (kcal/mL)
   Daily volume = _____ mL

4. Evaluate responses and modify as needed

Weight changes often reflect fluid dynamics in the early period following injury.
Calculate daily caloric intake and compare with goal.
Caloric requirement may need to be increased or decreased, depending on the animal's metabolic rate and response to nutritional support.

From Marks SL: The principles and practical application of enteral nutrition. Vet Clin North Am Small Anim Pract 28:677–708, 1998.

to meet the demands of host defense, wound repair, cell division, and growth. An estimate of an animal's nutrient requirements (Table 71–1) is needed to determine the minimal amount of food necessary to sustain critical physiologic processes. The resting energy requirement (RER) is the animal's energy requirement at rest in a thermoneutral environment and in a postabsorptive state. A linear formula can be applied to determine the RER of dogs and cats weighing at least 2 kg. Alternatively, one can use an allometric formula that can be applied to dogs and cats of all weights.

$$\text{Linear formula: RER (kcal/day)} = (30 \times BW_{kg}) + 70$$
$$\text{Allometric formula: RER (kcal/day)} = 70\,(BW_{kg}^{0.75})$$

Accurate, direct measurements of energy expenditure in sick dogs and cats are not available. Use of "fudge factors" extrapolated from the human literature to calculate the energy requirements of critically ill animals is discouraged. The term "illness energy requirement" (IER) is used to determine caloric requirements of critically ill animals and can be determined from these formulas:

$$\text{Canine IER (kcal/day)} = 1.2 \text{ to } 1.5 \times \text{RER}$$
$$\text{Feline IER (kcal/day)} = 1.1 \text{ to } 1.2 \times \text{RER}$$

Close observation of changes in body weight, physical examination findings, and ongoing losses help determine whether to increase or decrease an animal's IER.

DIET SELECTION

The type of formula selected depends on the route of feeding, the functional status of the gastrointestinal tract, and the nutrient requirements. Other factors such as cost, availability, and ease of use may also be important. Animals fed via nasoesophageal or jejunostomy feeding tubes are limited to receiving liquid enteral formulas that have a caloric density of approximately 1 kcal/mL. When selecting a liquid formula for feeding, one should pay particular attention to the amount of protein in the formula, the type of protein (intact proteins, peptides, and amino acids), and the quality of the protein. Most liquid formulas for people (Table 71–2) contain less than 20 per cent protein calories, preclud-

TABLE 71–2. MACRONUTRIENT COMPOSITION OF SELECTED HUMAN LIQUID ENTERAL FORMULATIONS

PRODUCT	PROTEIN TYPE	PROTEIN SOURCE	CALORIC DENSITY (kcal/mL)	NUTRIENTS (% of total kcal)			FORMULA CHARACTERISTICS
				Protein	Fat	Carbohydrate	
Vitaneed (Sherwood Medical)	Intact	Pureed beef, sodium and calcium caseinates	1.0	16	36	48	Isotonic, fiber 8 g/L, taurine free
Osmolite HN (Ross)	Intact	Soy protein isolate, sodium and calcium caseinates	1.06	16.7	30	53.3	Isotonic, lactose free, fiber free, taurine 114 mg/L
Jevity (Ross)	Intact	Sodium and calcium caseinates	1.06	16.7	30	53.3	Isotonic, lactose free, fiber 14.4 g/L, taurine 114 mg/L
Impact (Sandoz Nutrition)	Intact	Sodium and calcium caseinates, L-arginine	1.0	22	25	53	Isotonic, high protein, lactose free, fiber free, taurine free
Traumacal (Mead Johnson)	Intact	Sodium and calcium caseinates	1.5	22	40	38	Hyperosmolar (490 mOsm/kg), high protein, lactose free, fiber free, taurine free
Immun-Aid (McGaw)	Intact	Lactalbumin, L-arginine, L-glutamine, BCAA, nucleic acid	1.0	32	20	48	Hyperosmolar (460 mOsm/kg), high protein, lactose free, fiber free, taurine 200 mg/L
Travasorb HN (Clintec Nutrition)	Hydrolyzed	Hydrolyzed lactalbumin	1.0	18	12	70	Hyperosmolar (560 mOsm/kg), lactose free, fiber free, taurine free
Perative (Ross)	Hydrolyzed	Partially hydrolyzed sodium caseinate, lactalbumin hydrolysate	1.3	20.5	25	54.5	Hyperosmolar (425 mOsm/kg), lactose free, fiber free, taurine 130 mg/mL
Peptamen (Clintec Nutrition)	Hydrolyzed	Hydrolyzed whey protein	1.0	16	33	51	Isosmolar, lactose free, fiber free, taurine 80 mg/mL
Vital HN (Ross)	Hydrolyzed	Partially hydrolyzed whey, meat and soy, L-amino acids	1.0	16.7	9.4	74	Hyperosmolar (500 mOsm/kg), lactose free, fiber free, low fat, taurine free
Vivonex TEN (Norwich Eaton)	Amino acids	Crystalline amino acids	1.0	15.0	3	82	Hyperosmolar (630 mOsm/kg), lactose free, fiber free, low fat, taurine free

BCAA = branched chain amino acid.
From Marks SL: The principles and practical application of enteral nutrition. Vet Clin North Am Small Anim Pract 28:677–708, 1998.

ing their use for the long-term (>3 weeks) feeding of cats. The lower-protein formulas should be supplemented with protein modules such as Promod (Ross Laboratories, Columbus OH), Casec (Mead-Johnson, Evansville, IN), or Promagic (Animal Nutrition Laboratories, Burlington, NJ) at 15 to 30 g casein or whey powder added to each 8-fluid-ounce container. Almost all human liquid enteral formulas lack taurine, an essential amino acid in cats, necessitating its supplementation (250 mg taurine per 8-fluid-ounce container).

Polymeric solutions contain macronutrients in the form of isolates of intact protein (casein, lactalbumin, whey, egg white), triglycerides, and carbohydrate polymers. The osmolality varies between 300 and 450 mOsm/kg in solutions with a caloric density of 1 kcal/mL; however, the osmolality may reach 650 mOsm/kg in solutions with a greater caloric density. Monomeric solutions contain protein as peptides or amino acids, fat as long-chain triglycerides (LCTs) or a mixture of LCTs and medium-chain triglycerides (MCTs), and carbohydrates as partially hydrolyzed starch maltodextrins and glucose oligosaccharides. These solutions require less digestion than regular foods or polymeric solutions; however, the partially digested macronutrients contribute to the higher osmolality, which is between 400 and 700 mOsm/kg.

Commercial blenderized pet food diets are excellent for pharyngostomy, esophagostomy, or gastrostomy tubes. There are also a number of complete and balanced veterinary enteral formulations (Table 71–3) that contain adequate amounts of protein, taurine, and micronutrients. Feeding

should be delayed for 24 hours after placing a gastrostomy tube, to allow return of gastric motility and formation of a fibrin seal. Diet can be administered as bolus feedings or continuous infusion when feeding via gastrostomy tube. Improved weight gain and decreased gastroesophageal reflux have been reported in humans given continuous feedings,[28] although similar studies are lacking in the veterinary literature. Delayed gastric emptying and vomiting can be managed by decreasing the feedings or treating with metoclopramide (1 to 2 mg/kg intravenously every 24 hours as a continuous infusion). Jejunal feeding can be started within 6 hours of tube placement if peristalsis is present. Continuous feeding must be used with jejunostomy feeding to avoid abdominal cramping and diarrhea associated with bolus feeding. The initial flow rate of 1 mL/kg per hour should be increased gradually over 48 hours until the total daily volume can be given over a 12- to 18-hour period.[9]

With bolus feeding, the required daily volume of food should be divided into four to six feedings. Animals are usually fed approximately 25 per cent of their caloric requirement on the first day of feeding, with a 25 per cent increase in calories (volume) per day. Most animals are able to reach their complete energy requirement by the fourth or fifth day of feeding. The food should be warmed to room temperature and fed slowly through the tube to prevent vomiting. Flushing of the tube with 15 to 20 mL of lukewarm water helps prevent clogging. Before each feeding, aspirate the tube with an empty syringe to check for residual food left in the stomach from the previous feeding. If more than half of the last feeding is removed from the stomach,

TABLE 71–3. MACRONUTRIENT COMPOSITION OF SELECTED VETERINARY ENTERAL FORMULATIONS

PRODUCT	PROTEIN TYPE	CALORIC DENSITY (kcal/mL)	NUTRIENTS (% of total kcal)			FORMULA CHARACTERISTICS
			Protein	Fat	Carbohydrate	
Prescription diet a/d gel (Hill's)	Intact	1.3	34	53	13	Isosmolar, lactose free, fiber 1.3% DM, adequate taurine
Iams' Eukanuba Recovery Formula (Iams')	Intact	2.1	29	5	66	Isosmolar, lactose free, fiber 1.6% DM, adequate taurine
Canine CliniCare (Abbott)	Intact	1.0	20	55	25	Isosmolar, lactose free, fiber free, taurine 88 mg/mL
Feline Clinicare (Abbott)	Intact	1.0	30	45	25	Isosmolar, lactose free, fiber free, adequate taurine
Feline Clinicare RF (Abbott)	Intact	1.0	22	57	21	Isosmolar, lactose free, fiber free, adequate taurine

DM = dry matter.
From Marks SL: The principles and practical application of enteral nutrition. Vet Clin North Am Small Anim Pract 28:677–708, 1998.

skip the feeding and recheck residual volume at the next feeding.

RATIONALE FOR PARENTERAL NUTRITIONAL SUPPORT

The functional capacity of the gastrointestinal tract is a key determinant in the selection of enteral versus parenteral nutrition. Dogs or cats with an inability to absorb nutrients via the gastrointestinal tract, e.g., those with massive small-bowel resection, diseases of the small intestine, intractable vomiting or diarrhea, moderate to severe acute pancreatitis, and severe malnutrition with a nonfunctional gastrointestinal tract, are likely to benefit the most from PN support.[29] Parenteral nutrition can be delivered by either central or peripheral access. Total parenteral nutrition (TPN) is the provision of all essential nutrients intravenously, usually via the cranial vena cava. Peripheral parenteral nutrition (PPN) is often used as a temporary maneuver to provide short-term (<5 days) nutritional support in dogs and cats unable to tolerate full enteral nutrition or when central venous catheterization is contraindicated. The major limitation in using PPN is the high incidence of thrombophlebitis.[30] Consequently, a PN solution administered by peripheral vein must be relatively dilute (<900 mOsm/L), thus providing fewer calories and less protein per volume.

PARENTERAL NUTRITION COMPONENTS

The three basic components of PN solutions are amino acids, lipids, and dextrose. Crystalline amino acid solutions, available in concentrations of 3 to 15 per cent, maintain nitrogen balance and replete lean tissue in cachectic animals. The standard amino acid solutions (Travasol, Clintec Nutrition, Deerfield, IL) contain all the essential and dispensable amino acids for dogs and cats, with the exception of taurine. Modified parenteral amino acid solutions have been developed for specific disease states such as renal failure and hepatic encephalopathy. These formulations are expensive, and their superiority as the sole source of nitrogen over standard solutions has not been demonstrated in prospective clinical trials. The use of amino acid solutions that contain electrolytes added by the manufacturer (Travasol 8.5%, Clintec Nutrition, Deerfield, IL, or Aminosyn 8.5%, Abbott Laboratories, North Chicago, IL) is recommended and is ade-

quate for the majority of dogs and cats not experiencing severe ongoing losses or deficiencies.

Lipid emulsions provide an intravenous source of fat calories and essential fatty acids. Cats cannot convert linoleic acid to arachidonic acid, and they should receive supplementation with an animal fat source if TPN is administered for longer than 2 weeks. Lipid emulsions are available as 10 per cent (1.1 kcal/mL) or 20 per cent (2.0 kcal/mL) solutions with osmolarities that range from 270 to 340 mOsm/L, respectively. Lipid emulsions contain soybean oil (Intralipid, Clintec Nutrition, Deerfield, IL) or a combination of soybean and safflower oil triglycerides (Liposyn II, Abbott Laboratories, North Chicago, IL), egg-yolk phospholipids as an emulsifying agent, and glycerin to achieve isotonicity with plasma. Sodium hydroxide is added to these products to adjust the pH to 6.0 to 7.9.

Carbohydrate in the form of dextrose is a vital source of fuel and has important nitrogen-sparing effects. Providing calories as glucose stimulates insulin secretion, reduces muscle protein catabolism, and inhibits hepatic glucose output, thereby eliminating the need for skeletal muscle protein to provide amino acid precursors for gluconeogenesis. Dextrose is the least expensive intravenous energy source and is available in concentrations ranging from 5 to 70 per cent. The dextrose in intravenous solutions is hydrated, so that each gram of dextrose monohydrate provides 3.4 kcal.

Standard parenteral maintenance doses of all vitamins should be provided as an additive to the TPN solution. Multivitamin preparations for TPN provide all fat- and water-soluble vitamins with the exception of vitamin K, which may be given subcutaneously once weekly. No formal recommendations are currently available for supplementation of trace minerals to dogs and cats receiving PN.

PARENTERAL NUTRITION COMPOUNDING

The preparation and administration of PN solutions create problems owing to stability and compatibility. Factors that enhance precipitation include high molar concentrations, increases in solution pH, decreases in amino acid concentration, use of calcium as the chloride salt, increases in temperature, contact with intravenous fat emulsions, and the order of calcium and phosphate addition.[31] Total nutrient admixtures (TNAs) facilitate the combination of dextrose, amino acid, fat emulsion, electrolytes, and multivitamins in one container. These components are aseptically mixed in one bag

TABLE 71–4. SAMPLE CALCULATION FOR DESIGNING A TOTAL PARENTERAL NUTRITION BASE FORMULA FOR THE DOG

Four-year-old male beagle (10 kg) with complaints of anorexia, profuse vomiting, and severe weight loss of 6 weeks duration.

1. Calculate resting energy requirement (RER) (see Table 71–1)
   RER = 394 kcal/day
2. Calculate illness energy requirements (IER) (see Table 71–1)
   IER = 394 × 1.3 = 512 kcal/day
3. Calculate protein requirement
   Adult canine: 4–6 g/100 kcal energy
   Adult feline: 6–9 g/100 kcal energy
   Protein requirement for this dog = 4 g/100 kcal × 512 kcal
   Protein requirement = 4 × 5.12 = ± 20 g/day
4. Calculate volumes of nutrient solutions required
   8.5% amino acid solution contains = 85 mg protein/mL
   To supply 20 g of protein, need 235 mL of 8.5% amino acids
   In dogs, give calculated IER as nonprotein calories; i.e., use lipid emulsion and dextrose in a 1:1 ratio to meet *total* energy requirements. In cats, the protein calories are calculated (4 kcal/g of protein) and subtracted from the IER. The remaining calories are provided as a 50:50 mixture of lipid and dextrose.
   50% dextrose = 1.7 kcal/mL
   To supply 50% of IER (256 kcal), need 151 mL of 50% dextrose
   20% lipid emulsion = 2.0 kcal/mL
   To supply 50% of IER (256 kcal), need 128 mL of 20% lipid emulsion
5. Add multivitamin and supplemental electrolytes as warranted
6. Total volume of total parenteral nutrition solution = 514 mL/day
   Administer at 21 mL/hour after 24-hour gradual acclimation

(up to 3 L) and provide a total nutrient supply for 24 to 48 hours. The advantages of the TNA system include decreased nursing time involved in intravenous setup and tubing changes, decreased risk of contamination, and time saved in the pharmacy during preparation. Amino acid solutions should be added to the lipid emulsion before the dextrose solution is added. This prevents deterioration of the emulsion and oiling out, which can occur when dextrose (pH approximately 4.0) is added directly to the lipid emulsion.[32] Although compounding under a laminar flow hood is desirable, asepsis can be maintained in a clean, low-traffic area such as a surgery suite.

PARENTERAL NUTRITION ADMINISTRATION

Cannulation of a large-bore, high-flow central vein, such as the cranial vena cava, permits infusion of hyperosmolar (usually >1600 mOsm/L) nutrient solutions that would not be tolerated by smaller, low-flow peripheral veins. A percutaneously placed multi-lumen polyurethane catheter (Arrow International Inc., Reading, PA) is recommended. Dressings and tubing connecting the parenteral solutions with the catheter should be changed every 48 to 72 hours. A 0.22-μm filter is inserted between the intravenous tubing and the catheter when lipid-free PN is used and should be changed with the tubing. A 1.2-μm filter should be used when a TNA containing a lipid emulsion is infused. Caloric requirements should be calculated as previously described. Unlike cats, dogs may be given the calculated IER as nonprotein calories,[33] with approximately 50 per cent of the calories provided as lipid, and the remainder as dextrose (Table 71–4). Standard TPN formulas are suitable to facilitate PN administration in most dogs and cats (Table 71–5).

MONITORING

A complete blood count and serum biochemical profile should be performed before initiation of PN support. Body weight, fluid intake, and fluid output should be measured daily, whereas serum electrolytes, phosphorus, and glucose concentrations can be determined every 48 hours until stable and then rechecked weekly. Serum triglyceride concentrations should be evaluated early in the course of PN to document adequate triglyceride clearance. Triglyceride concentrations greater than 400 mg/dL necessitate either reduction of the rate of infusion or complete discontinuation of lipid supplementation. Providing 30 to 40 per cent of total calories as lipid does not stimulate the pancreas and can attenuate any hyperglycemia associated with pancreatitis.[21]

COMPLICATIONS

A total of 473 complications were recorded in 209 dogs receiving TPN over an 84-month period at our teaching hospital.[34] Metabolic complications were the most commonly encountered problems during TPN administration (70 per cent of complications), with transient hyperglycemia being most common. Other less common metabolic complications included hyperbilirubinemia, increased alkaline phosphatase activity, and hyperlipemia. Mechanical problems constituted 25 per cent of the complications observed and included inadvertent catheter removal or occlusion, disconnection or breakage of the line, and venous thrombosis. Mechanical complications can be reduced with meticulous catheter care and close monitoring. Catheter- or solution-related sepsis was a relatively infrequent complication (5 per cent) because of scrupulous catheter care and insertion techniques.

TABLE 71–5. STANDARD FORMULAS FOR TOTAL PARENTERAL NUTRITION

	CRITICALLY ILL FORMULA: DOGS	CRITICALLY ILL FORMULA (RENAL/HEPATIC FAILURE): DOGS	CRITICALLY ILL FORMULA: CATS	CRITICALLY ILL FORMULA (RENAL/HEPATIC FAILURE): CATS
50% dextrose	300 mL	300 mL	150 mL	300 mL
20% Intralipid	250 mL	250 mL	125 mL	250 mL
8.5% Travasol	500 mL	250 mL	500 mL	500 mL
Multivitamin B	2 mL	2 mL	2 mL	2 mL
KPO_4	12 mEq	17 mEq	1 mEq	12 mEq
Protein yield	4.2 g protein/100 kcal	2.1 g protein/100 kcal	6.3 g protein/100 kcal	3.6 g protein/100 kcal
Potassium yield	40 mEq potassium/L	40 mEq potassium/L	40 mEq potassium/L	40 mEq potassium/L
Caloric density	1.0 kcal/mL*	1.3 kcal/mL*	0.9 kcal/mL†	1.1 kcal/mL†

*Calculated without amino acids.
†Calculated with amino acids.

REFERENCES

1. Johnson LR: Regulation of gastrointestinal growth. *in* Johnson LR (ed): Physiology of the Gastrointestinal Tract, 2nd ed. New York, Raven Press, 1987, p 301.
2. Geraghty ME: Tube feeding equipment update. Dietitians in Nutrition (support newsletter), July/August 1989, p 1.
3. Abood SK, Buffington CA: Enteral feeding of dogs and cats: 51 cases (1989–1991). JAVMA 201:619, 1992.
4. Armstrong PJ, et al: Enteral nutrition by tube. Vet Clin North Am Small Anim Pract 20:237, 1990.
5. Crowe DT: Clinical use of an indwelling nasogastric tube for enteral nutrition and fluid therapy in the dog and cat. J Am Anim Hosp Assoc 22:675, 1986.
6. Hayhurst ER, Wyman M: Morbidity associated with prolonged use of polyvinyl feeding tubes. Am J Dis Child 129:72, 1975.
7. Abood SK, Buffington CA: Improved nasogastric intubation technique for administration of nutritional support in dogs. JAVMA 199:577, 1991.
8. Crowe DT, Downs MO: Pharyngostomy complications in dogs and cats and recommended technical modifications: Experimental and clinical investigations. J Am Anim Hosp Assoc 22:493, 1986.
9. Crowe DT: Nutritional support for the hospitalized patient: An introduction to tube feeding. Compend Contin Educ Pract Vet 12:1711, 1990.
10. Devitt CM, Seim HB: Clinical evaluation of tube esophagostomy in small animals. J Am Anim Hosp Assoc 33:55, 1997.
11. Armstrong PJ, Hardie EM: Percutaneous endoscopic gastrostomy. A retrospective study of 54 clinical cases in dogs and cats. J Vet Intern Med 4:202, 1990.
12. Bright RM, Burrows CF: Percutaneous endoscopic tube gastrostomy in dogs. Am J Vet Res 49:629, 1988.
13. Gauderer MWL, et al: Gastrostomy without laparotomy: A percutaneous endoscopic technique. J Pediatr Surg 15:872, 1980.
14. Fulton RB, Dennis JS: Blind percutaneous placement of a gastrostomy tube for nutritional support in dogs and cats. JAVMA 201:697, 1992.
15. Marks SL, et al: Blind percutaneous gastrostomy: A new technique. ACVIM Abstracts. J Vet Intern Med 8:150, 1994.
16. Mauterer JV, et al: New technique and management guidelines for percutaneous nonendoscopic tube gastrostomy. JAVMA 205:574, 1994.
17. Clary EM, et al: Nonendoscopic antegrade percutaneous gastrostomy: The effect of preplacement gastric insufflation on tube position and intra-abdominal anatomy. J Vet Intern Med 10:15, 1996.
18. Kadakia S, et al: Comparison of Foley catheter as a replacement gastrostomy tube with commercial replacement gastrostomy tube: A prospective randomized trial. Gastrointest Endosc 40:188, 1994.
19. Crowe DT: Enteral nutrition for critically ill or injured patients—part I. Compend Contin Educ Pract Vet 8:603, 1986.
20. Orton EC: Enteral hyperalimentation administered via needle catheter jejunostoma as an adjunct to cranial abdominal surgery in dogs and cats. JAVMA 188:1406, 1986.
21. Stabile BE, et al: Intravenous mixed amino acids and fats do not stimulate exocrine pancreatic secretion. Am J Physiol 246:G274, 1984.
22. Delany HM, et al: Jejunostomy by needle catheter technique. Surgery 73:786, 1973.
23. Bumpers HL, et al: A simple technique for insertion of PEJ via PEG. Surg Endosc 8:121, 1994.
24. Disario JA, et al: Poor results with percutaneous endoscopic jejunostomy. Gastrointest Endosc 36:257, 1990.
25. Hardie EM, Armstrong J: Development of a gastro-jejunal tube for the dog. J Nutr 121:S154, 1991.
26. McCrackin MA, et al: Endoscopic placement of a percutaneous gastroduodenostomy feeding tube in dogs. JAVMA 203:792, 1993.
27. Pritchard TJ, Bloom AD: A technique of direct percutaneous jejunostomy tube placement. Surg Gynecol Obstet 178:173, 1994.
28. Coben RM, et al: Gastroesophageal reflux during gastrostomy feedings. Gastroenterology 106:13, 1994.
29. American Society for Parenteral and Enteral Nutrition Board of Directors: Guidelines for use of total parenteral nutrition in the hospitalized adult patient. J Parenter Enter Nutr 10:41, 1986.
30. Stokes MA, Hill GL: Peripheral parenteral nutrition: A preliminary report on its efficacy and safety. J Parenter Enter Nutr 17:145, 1993.
31. Niemiec PW, Vanderveen TW: Compatibility considerations in parenteral nutrient solutions. Am J Hosp Pharm 41:893, 1984.
32. Black CD, Popovich NG: A study of intravenous emulsion compatibility: Effects of dextrose, amino acids, and selected electrolytes. Drug Intell Clin Pharm 15:184, 1981.
33. Lippert AC, et al: Total parenteral nutrition in clinically normal cats. JAVMA 194:669, 1989.
34. Reuter JD, et al: Use of total parenteral nutrition in dogs: 209 cases (1988–1995). J Vet Emerg Crit Care, 8:201, 1998.

CHAPTER 72

HYPERLIPIDEMIAS

John E. Bauer

Hyperlipidemia refers to the presence of excess lipid in the bloodstream. Because lipids are transported primarily by lipoproteins, the term hyperlipoproteinemia is sometimes used interchangeably. However, in a strict sense, the term hyperlipoproteinemia should be used only if steps have been taken to determine whether lipoprotein elevations exist. In some cases, hyperlipidemia is grossly apparent by virtue of a turbid or milky serum or plasma. When turbidity is present the sample is described as hyperlipemic, and this is seen only when serum triglyceride (TG) concentrations are markedly elevated. By contrast, elevations of serum cholesterol concentrations alone do not impart turbidity to the specimen, although it can be described as hyperlipidemic. Thus a hyperlipidemic specimen is not always hyperlipemic. A normal-appearing sample may be hyperlipidemic, but this can be determined only after laboratory analysis of its TG or cholesterol concentration. It should be noted that marked cholesterol elevations can impart a slight haziness to the sample. However, only TG elevations cause hyperlipemia.

Primary hyperlipidemias occur in dogs and cats and are often familial or hereditary. Secondary disorders of lipid metabolism have also been described in these species. In dogs, fasting hyperlipemias can be associated with pancreatitis, ocular abnormalities, and cutaneous xanthomas. They may be secondary to diabetes mellitus, renal disease, hypothyroidism, cholestasis, hypoadrenocorticism, and ultra-high-fat diets or the result of some metabolic effect on lipid metabolism.[1, 2] Cats may be similarly affected.

Most hyperlipidemias seen in dogs and cats are secondary to another disease or acquired by diet. Regarding incidence, one study in the United Kingdom reported that fasting hypertriglyceridemia occurred in 53 of 362 dogs (14.3 per cent) presented to the University of Glasgow Veterinary School.[3] Similar figures in other countries have not yet been obtained. In view of this finding, evaluation of a hyperlipidemic animal and the differential diagnoses of primary abnormalities require familiarity with lipid metabolic phenomena, awareness of hereditary lipid problems, an appreciation for the pathophysiology of possible lipid derangements, and knowledge of those conditions that cause secondary hyperlipidemias. Evaluation also requires a basic understanding of species differences in lipoprotein characteristics and metabolism and familiarity with laboratory procedures used in their evaluation.

ROLE OF PLASMA LIPOPROTEINS IN LIPID TRANSPORT

Transport of water-insoluble lipids in the aqueous environment of the circulatory system requires the presence of specific protein-lipid complexes. In the circulation, non-esterified fatty acids are complexed with albumin, albeit only briefly, as they are readily taken up by tissues for metabolism. Thus normal concentrations of these "free" fatty acids usually do not exceed 1.0 mmol/L. The other lipids, namely triglycerides, phospholipids, and free and esterified cholesterol, are transported as lipoprotein complexes associated with specific proteins known as apolipoproteins (apoproteins). Molecular complexes of these materials consist of an amphoteric shell of proteins, free cholesterol, and phospholipids surrounding a hydrophobic core of TG and cholesteryl esters (CEs), most frequently in a spheric particle. The apoproteins and phospholipids have distinct solubilization effects on the fat-soluble TG and CE. In addition, the apoproteins have structural and functional attributes that serve to help direct lipoprotein metabolism via receptor- and non-receptor-mediated phenomena and enzymatic and exchange reactions. In these ways, the apoproteins serve as regulators of lipid metabolism.

FRACTIONATION AND CLASSIFICATION OF SERUM LIPOPROTEINS

Plasma lipoproteins differ in size, density, electrical charge, lipid and apopeptide composition, and metabolic function. As such, they are characterized by their hydrated densities (ultracentrifugal behavior), electrophoretic mobilities (agarose or polyacrylamide gels), chromatographic separation (gel filtration, ion exchange, affinity), or chemical precipitation (heparin-MnCl$_2$). The lipoproteins of dogs and cats can be compared with those of humans, but it should be remembered that distinct species differences exist.

In humans, four main classes of lipoproteins are recognized. These same four fractions are also observed in dogs and cats and consist of chylomicrons, very low-density lipoproteins (VLDL), low-density lipoproteins (LDL), and high-density lipoproteins (HDL) (Table 72–1). An intermediate-density lipoprotein (IDL), with hydrated density between VLDL and LDL, also exists. Within the LDL and HDL categories, lipoprotein subclasses are also recognized and are usually referred to as HDL$_1$, HDL$_2$, and so forth. A full description of these subclasses can be found elsewhere.[4]

METABOLISM OF EXOGENOUS (DIETARY) LIPID

Chylomicrons are the largest of the lipoproteins and are involved in the transport of dietary lipid (primarily TG) from the small intestine after absorption (see Table 72–1; Figs. 72–1 and 72–2). Absorption is facilitated by pancreatic lipase within the intestinal lumen causing the release of fatty acids and mono- and diglycerides. It should be noted that once they are within the enterocytes, the glycerides are reesterified with the fatty acids to produce triglycerides, which are then packaged along with free and esterified cholesterol, phospholipids, and the apo-B$_{48}$ protein to form chylomicrons. These particles are then secreted into the lacteals and enter the general circulation at the thoracic duct. These postprandial particles are especially enriched in exogenous triglyceride. In the circulation, the chylomicrons acquire the apo-C and apo-E peptides from HDL, thereby providing the determinants of their metabolic fates. One of the apo-C peptides (apo-C-II) functions as a cofactor for lipoprotein lipase (LPL). This reaction releases fatty acids and glycerol from chylomicrons as they travel through capillary beds of adipose and muscle tissues for subsequent metabolism. Because TGs are in the core of the particle, further hydrolysis results in a reduction in the size of the chylomicron. The build-up of excess surface materials such as apo-C and phospholipids occurs in this fashion until the point at which these components are transferred back to HDL (see Fig. 72–1). Such particles are termed chylomicron remnants, and these can be rapidly removed from the circulation by virtue of hepatic receptor binding of the remaining apo-E peptide (see Fig. 72–2).[5]

METABOLISM OF ENDOGENOUS (SYNTHESIZED) LIPID

Besides chylomicrons, all other lipoprotein classes are involved in the transport and metabolism of endogenously synthesized lipids (see Table 72–1 and Fig. 72–1). VLDLs are the primary carriers of TG in the fasting state. They are synthesized mainly in the liver, although some intestinal contribution has been observed.[6] Endogenously synthesized TGs are combined with cholesterol, CEs, phospholipids, and the apo-B$_{100}$ peptide. Dogs are one of a few species that have also been observed to secrete apo-B$_{48}$-containing VLDL.[7] Although reasons for this are unclear, the presence of this apopeptide may explain the low concentrations of apo-B-containing lipoproteins in dogs due to rapid recognition and hepatic receptor binding of these particles, resulting in their rapid clearance.[7, 8] Their metabolic fate is similar to that of the chylomicrons in that once VLDLs are secreted into the circulation, they also acquire apo-C and apo-E peptides, resulting in similar fatty acid delivery via tissue perfusion of capillary beds, remnant production, and uptake.

Although VLDL remnants may be removed by hepatic mechanisms, in some cases, circulating VLDLs undergo further transformation to LDL. This process appears to be dependent not only on LPL but also on a similar endothelial lipase found in the liver. As further delipidation occurs, the VLDL is again reduced in size to form LDLs, which contain primarily CE and apo-B$_{100}$. These LDLs can also bind specific receptors (apo-B, E-receptors) that are known to have a wide tissue distribution. In this way, the ubiquitous delivery of cholesterol for steroid hormone production, cell membrane synthesis, and hepatic metabolism takes place.[9]

The HDLs are relatively abundant in dogs and cats. They serve as both donors and acceptors of apo-C, apo-E, and various lipids from other lipoproteins in the circulation. In addition, they are involved in the return of cholesterol back to the liver for excretion or redistribution (see Table 72–1; Fig. 72–3). Synthesized primarily in the liver, discoid-shaped HDLs are secreted as a phospholipid bilayer containing cholesterol and its protein determinant, apo-AI. In the circu-

TABLE 72–1. PHYSICAL CHARACTERISTICS OF CANINE AND FELINE LIPOPROTEINS COMPARED WITH HUMANS

LIPOPROTEIN/FUNCTION	SIZE (nm)	HYDRATED DENSITY (g/ml)	MOBILITY (ELECTROPHORESIS)	MAJOR APO-PROTEINS
Chylomicrons—dietary lipid transport				
Dog, cat, human	75–1200	<0.960	Origin	B_{48}
VLDL—hepatic TG/cholesterol transport				
Dog, cat	30–80	0.093–1.006	Pre-beta	B_{100}, B_{48}, E, C
Human	30–80	0.093–1.006	Pre-beta	B_{100}, E, C
LDL—cholesterol transport				
Dog	18–25	1.019–1.087	Beta	B_{100}, B_{48}
Cat	18–25	1.030–1.043	Beta	B_{100}
Human	18–25	1.019–1.063	Beta	B_{100}
HDL$_1$ (HDL$_c$)—reverse cholesterol transport				
Dog	10–35	1.025–1.100	Alpha$_2$	E, A, C
HDL$_2$—reverse cholesterol transport				
Dog	9–12	1.063–1.100	Alpha$_1$	E, A, C
Cat	9–12	1.063–1.100	Alpha$_1$	E, A-I, C
Human	9–12	1.063–1.125	Alpha	A-I, A-II, E, C
HDL$_3$—reverse cholesterol transport				
Dog, cat	5–9	1.100–1.210	Alpha$_1$	A, C
Human	5–9	1.125–1.185	Alpha	A-I, A-II, E, C

VLDL = very low-density lipoprotein; TG = triglyceride; LDL = low-density lipoprotein; HDL = high-density lipoprotein.

lation, apo-AI functions as a cofactor for the lecithin-cholesterol acyltransferase (LCAT) reaction. This reaction is significant in that it is the first metabolic step in a process known as reverse cholesterol transport. Briefly, HDL-phospholipid donates one of its fatty acids to cholesterol during this reaction taking place on the HDL surface. The resultant hydrophobic CE thus formed enters the particle's core, causing spheric HDL to form (see Fig. 72–1). This HDL is referred to as HDL$_3$.

In humans, a further lipid exchange process takes place between HDL and the apo-B-containing lipoproteins (i.e., chylomicrons, VLDL, LDL). This exchange is mediated by the cholesteryl ester transfer protein (CETP) and results in transfer of TG from the apo-B lipoprotein for CE in HDL (see Fig. 72–3). As the resultant CE-rich apo-B-containing lipoproteins are taken up by hepatic receptor–mediated events, reverse cholesterol transfer is completed. This cholesterol can be secreted in bile. The HDLs remaining in the circulation are relatively glyceride-rich and are known as HDL$_2$. Hepatic lipase helps remove this glyceride-associated

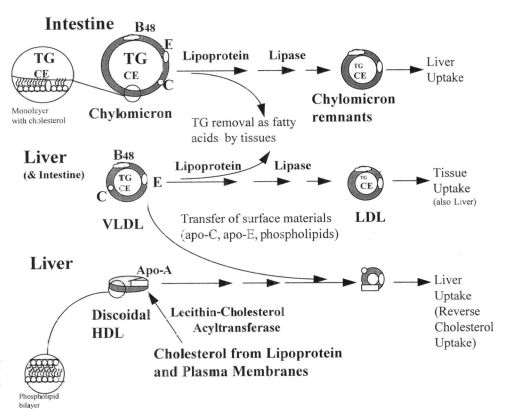

Figure 72–1. Summary of lipoprotein metabolism. Dietary fat is digested in the small intestine and incorporated into chylomicrons containing apo-B$_{48}$. The chylomicrons are transported via the lymphatics to the circulation. The particles then acquire apolipoproteins (apo-E and apo-C) from high-density lipoproteins (HDLs) and lose their triglyceride (TG) via lipoprotein lipase (LPL)–mediated lipolysis and fatty acid uptake by tissues. Remnant particles formed are removed by receptor- and non-receptor-mediated pathways in the liver. The very low-density lipoproteins (VLDLs) are assembled in the liver, secreted into the circulation, and acquire apo-E and apo-C peptides. They are similarly metabolized via LPL, leaving TG-depleted remnant particles, which ultimately form TG-poor, cholesterol-rich low-density lipoprotein (LDL). The LDL and associated cholesterol can be taken up by hepatic and other cells by receptor-mediated events. Discoidal HDLs are synthesized in the liver and acted on by lecithin-cholesterol acyltransferase (LCAT) using tissue or cellular cholesterol and lipoprotein phospholipid to form cholesteryl esters (CEs), resulting in a spheric HDL particle. These particles subsequently transfer their cholesterol to the liver. B$_{48}$ = apo-B$_{48}$; C = apo-C; E = apo-E.

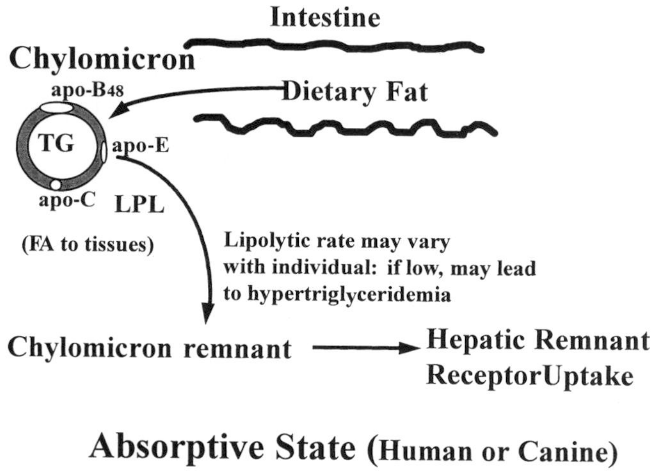

Intestine

Chylomicron

apo-B48 — **Dietary Fat**

TG) apo-E

apo-C LPL

(FA to tissues)

Lipolytic rate may vary
with individual: if low, may lead
to hypertriglyceridemia

Chylomicron remnant ⟶ **Hepatic Remnant ReceptorUptake**

Absorptive State (Human or Canine)

Figure 72–2. Chylomicron formation and metabolism in the absorptive state after eating. Lipoprotein lipase (LPL) mediates the transfer of fatty acids (FA) to tissues and the formation of triglyceride (TG)-poor remnants. The remnants are subsequently taken up by hepatic mechanisms. Hyperchylomicronemia may occur if intestinal synthesis is high or if lipolysis is reduced. Individual variability may occur.

fatty acid, and in the process, HDL_3 is again formed. In this way, the HDL particle is prepared for reutilization in further reverse cholesterol transport events.

By contrast, in dogs and cats, alternative pathways of reverse cholesterol transport must exist, because neither species appears to have any appreciable CETP activity in circulation.[10, 11] In dogs, HDLs become enriched in CE and apo-E, forming unique particles known as HDL_1 (see Fig. 72–3). Although similar to HDL_3, HDL_1 is lighter than typical HDL with a hydrated density similar to human LDL.[12] Their electrophoretic mobility is slower ($alpha_2$ vs. $alpha_1$; see later) when compared with HDL_2 and HDL_3 fractions. It is this HDL_1 fraction that is elevated whenever hypercholesterolemia occurs in dogs.

PRACTICAL DIAGNOSTIC METHODS

TURBIDITY

Inspection of the extent of serum lactescence or turbidity often provides a useful clue to TG concentration. Normal, straw-colored serum usually indicates TG less than 200 mg/dL. Hazy serum contains approximately 300 mg/dL, and opaqueness is seen with TG greater than 600 mg/dL. When turbidity similar to that of skim milk is observed, TG concentration is approximately 1000 mg/dL; when it is similar to whole milk, concentrations of 2500 to 4000 mg/dL may be found. Specific determinations of serum TG are useful especially when follow-up samples are available and to evaluate lipid-lowering regimens.

REFRIGERATION TEST

The refrigeration test may be useful in the absence of other more specific techniques. By simply allowing the serum to remain undisturbed in a refrigerator overnight, the sample can be inspected for the existence of "cream" layer. Under this condition, chylomicrons will float, resulting in a positive test. If the underlying serum is clear, a pure hyperchylomicronemia is indicated. Reasons for this condi-

tion include either a non-fasted animal at the time of sample collection or the possibility of a primary hyperchylomicronemia. If the underlying serum remains turbid with or without a "cream" layer, other lipoproteins are also present in excess. This finding is referred to as a "mixed" hyperlipoproteinemia in the absence of other, more specific characterizations by ultracentrifugation, electrophoresis, or precipitation techniques.

INTERFERENCE WITH LABORATORY LIPID MEASUREMENTS

Hyperlipemia interferes with serum direct bilirubin determination, resulting in moderate elevations. It may also decrease serum cholesterol, chloride, amylase, and lipase measurements and directly interfere with plasma protein and hemoglobin assays. When chylomicrons are present in excess, they displace water in a defined volume of serum, thereby falsely decreasing other serum components, especially electrolytes, by dilution. Other interferences that may affect cholesterol determinations include hyperbilirubinemia, which yields lower cholesterol concentrations. Conversely, hypercholesterolemia may also lower TG concentrations.

DIAGNOSTIC APPROACH TO HYPERLIPIDEMIA AND HYPERLIPOPROTEINEMIA

The possibility that a non-fasted serum sample was submitted for analysis should always be considered. For most animals, an 8- to 10-hour fast is sufficient for general screening purposes. Animals that are hyperlipidemic after a 12-hour fast, however, may have a lipid abnormality that warrants further investigation.

Both serum total cholesterol and TG determinations are helpful in initially evaluating lipid abnormalities. Preliminary work using previously frozen samples indicates that dogs (n = 9) and cats (n = 2) appear to have high glycerol blanks determined as free glycerol.[13] Although this is of interest in relation to the assessment of normal laboratory values, it remains to be determined whether this effect is due to freeze-thaw or autohydrolysis under storage conditions.

Lipoprotein electrophoresis, though nonspecific, is helpful when pre- and posttreatment samples are available. It is easily performed but usually requires access to scanning densitometry for quantification. Precipitation techniques may become more applicable in future studies as more laboratories become familiar with these methods.[14] Ultracentrifugation is usually not indicated, except in investigative work, and requires additional laboratory skills and equipment to perform reliably. In conjunction with complete blood counts, serum biochemical profiles, T_3, T_4, amylase, lipase, and so forth, secondary hyperlipidemias can be ruled out and a diagnosis made.

It should be noted that major differences exist between dog or cat plasma lipoproteins and human lipoproteins in the circulation. In dogs and cats, HDL predominates, whereas LDL is the major lipoprotein in humans. These differences can be most readily appreciated through densitometric evaluation of lipoproteins stained for their lipid content after agarose gel electrophoresis (Fig. 72–4). It is of interest that HDL-predominant animals such as dogs and cats, as a group, are more resistant to LDL cholesterol elevations and associated atherogenesis than are the LDL-

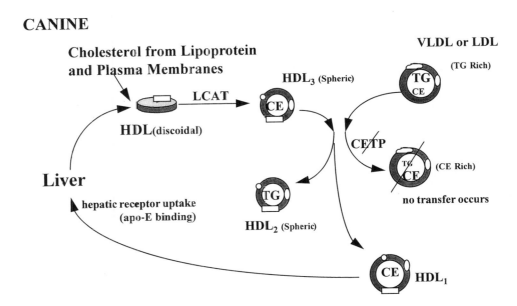

Figure 72–3. Comparative differences of high-density lipoprotein (HDL) metabolism in humans and canines. Discoidal HDL acquires tissue or cellular cholesterol facilitated by lecithin-cholesterol acyltransferase (LCAT), becoming spheric HDL₃. In humans: Cholesteryl ester transfer protein (CETP) transfers cholesteryl ester (CE) from HDL to either very low-density lipoprotein (VLDL) or low-density lipoprotein (LDL) in exchange for triglyceride (TG), generating CE-rich VLDL or LDL and relatively TG-rich HDL₂. The HDL₂ is acted on by hepatic lipase, again resulting in HDL₃, or is taken up by receptor mechanisms. In canines: No transfer of HDL-CE to VLDL or LDL occurs. Instead, HDL₁ (HDL_c) is taken up by hepatic receptor mechanisms. The lack of CETP in dogs may protect LDL from becoming cholesterol enriched, thereby helping to protect CETP-deficient species from potential atherogenic LDL.[1]

predominant species such as humans. Reasons for this intriguing difference are not completely understood but are of considerable interest in comparative medicine.

Owing to the extensive literature on and the health significance of human lipoproteins, most commercial laboratories offering either precipitation or electrophoretic techniques generally analyze and interpret dog and cat serum specimens based on human patterns. However, as noted earlier, the distribution of serum lipids and lipoproteins of canine and feline species is unlike those of humans, and caution should be exercised when interpreting lab values in this fashion. Precipitation techniques used for human lipoprotein fractionation do not universally quantify canine HDL and LDL types.[15] A precipitation technique has been published for canine plasma lipoprotein quantitation but has not been widely adapted for routine use in veterinary clinical pathology settings.[14] For these reasons, the author's laboratory prefers to use agarose gel electrophoresis to assess relative lipoprotein distributions. Overall, it may not be as quantitative as carefully modified and validated precipitation techniques. Nonetheless, most human clinical pathology laboratories can perform lipoprotein electrophoresis. With practice, using laboratory normal values, such results can be readily interpreted. Normal values from the author's laboratory have been published previously.[8]

CANINE LIPOPROTEINS

Dogs exhibit TG-rich postprandial chylomicrons after ingesting dietary fat. These particles do not migrate on electrophoresis and remain at the point of application of the sample. There are four additional lipoprotein classes, three of which are similar to the VLDL, LDL, and HDL fractions of humans.[16] Canine VLDLs contain TG-rich particles ranging in size from 30 to 80 nm in diameter. When isolated and concentrated, these VLDLs have a pre-beta mobility on electrophoresis. However, VLDLs are observed only rarely in a typical, normal canine serum sample after electrophoresis. This fraction often co-migrates with other beta lipoproteins and is hidden within the beta band (see Fig. 72–4). Although a pre-beta band can occasionally be seen, some commercial and human hospital labs often identify the alpha₂ band as pre-beta. The reason for this error is because human

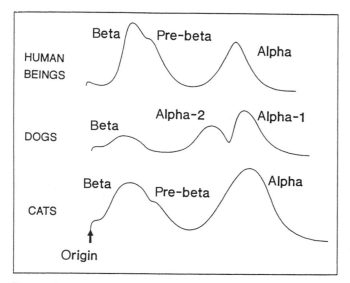

Figure 72–4. Densitometric tracings of serum lipoprotein distributions after agarose gel electrophoresis and lipid staining. Species differences are as indicated. (From Bauer JE: Diet-induced alteration of lipoprotein metabolism. JAVMA 201:1691, 1992.)

serum lipoprotein electrophoresis results in only a single alpha band, whereas canine serum yields both alpha₁ and alpha₂ bands.

Human serum contains beta, pre-beta, and alpha bands on electrophoresis and contains a preponderance of beta lipoproteins. Normal dog serum most consistently shows beta, alpha₂, and alpha₁ bands, with a preponderance of alpha₁ lipoproteins. In hypothyroid cholesterol-fed dogs and other hypercholesterolemic states, the alpha₂ lipoprotein becomes cholesterol-enriched.[1, 16–18] This lipoprotein is also known as HDL_1 or HDL_c. Its hydrated density is similar to human LDL. By contrast, in humans, elevations of LDL cholesterol are usually found when serum total cholesterol concentration is elevated. Also, the alpha₁-lipoproteins contain most of the cholesterol in normal dogs and are the major carrier of it; in humans, LDL serves in this capacity. When canine alpha₁-lipoproteins become cholesterol enriched owing to some metabolic alteration, it may be possible for them to become transformed into an alpha₂ migrating lipoprotein, with the resultant elevation of this latter fraction observed when electrophoresis is performed.[19]

A combination of laboratory methods may be necessary to specifically evaluate a given canine lipoprotein class for investigative study. Techniques such as precipitation, electrophoresis, and density ultracentrifugation have been used. Immunologic methods also may hold promise but have not been investigated to any appreciable extent to date. An awareness of the limitations of existing techniques should help prevent erroneous interpretations of clinical data in individual cases.

Using ultracentrifugal techniques, additional differences between dogs and humans are seen. But because most hospital laboratories do not offer this technique as a clinical test, these differences should not confuse the practice setting. However, for the sake of completeness, within the typical density range of human LDL, two classes of canine lipoproteins have been found: an LDL-type, 20 nm in diameter, which has beta mobility; and an HDL-type, 10 to 30 nm in diameter. This latter lipoprotein has an alpha₂ mobility[16] and has been termed HDL_c or HDL_1. It may have a human HDL

counterpart, but further studies are needed to substantiate this possibility.

FELINE LIPOPROTEINS

Although the centrifugal conditions established for the isolation of human plasma lipoproteins do not appear to be suitable for dogs, they do appear to be directly applicable to feline species.[7, 16, 20] Feline lipoproteins have been fractionated into four distinct classes by density gradient ultracentrifugation (VLDL + IDL, LDL, HDL_2, and HDL_3) and are similar to human plasma. Chylomicrons and three additional broad migrating fractions are seen on agarose electrophoresis. Unlike humans, however, cats have five to six times more HDL than LDL. The combined VLDL plus IDL fraction isolated at a density of less than 1.019 g/mL has pre-beta mobility on agarose, supporting the concept that the pre-beta band seen is feline VLDL. This particle is more TG-rich than human VLDL. In the 1.019 to 1.063 g/mL density range, particles similar to human LDL are found. Although these lipoproteins are somewhat smaller with more negative charge than human LDL, they show beta migration on agarose. Two distinct subfractions of feline HDL have been isolated. These particles have a hydrated density of 1.063 to 1.21 g/mL and similar size and electrophoretic mobility as human HDL.[20] Thus, human and feline electrophoretic terminologies coincide, and interpretations from human and hospital laboratories should be directly applicable. Comparisons using ultracentrifugal and precipitation methods are presently ongoing in a number of laboratories, but validation and widespread use of precipitation techniques have not been performed to date.

DISEASES ASSOCIATED WITH HYPERLIPIDEMIAS

PRIMARY IDIOPATHIC HYPERLIPIDEMIAS

Primary idiopathic hyperlipidemia appears most consistently in miniature schnauzers and beagles. It appears to be familial in these two breeds, although other breeds are also affected. The problem is poorly understood and metabolically complex. Animals are often seen with abdominal pain or seizures. Pancreatitis may also be present, and an etiologic link with hypertriglyceridemia may exist (see Pancreatitis later). High serum TG content may thus be a risk factor for pancreatitis, as in human beings. Because pancreatitis may lead to diabetes mellitus, hyperlipidemic dogs also may be at risk for that disorder. Indeed, many dogs appear to have combinations of some or all of these conditions when hyperlipidemia is first diagnosed. Spontaneous resolution and recurrence are also features of this syndrome, which makes evaluation of treatment modalities frustrating.

Other metabolic features observed include insulin resistance, fasting hyperinsulinemia, glucose intolerance, and hypertension.[21] Laboratory findings include hypertriglyceridemia with or without hypercholesterolemia and elevations of beta-migrating lipoproteins on electrophoresis. Increases in chylomicron and alpha₂ migrating lipoproteins may also be seen, the latter usually in association with cholesterol elevations. In recent years, an association between seizures and hypertriglyceridemia has been anecdotally reported in dogs. These dogs are usually being treated concurrently with barbiturates to control seizure activity. Dogs are initially evaluated and treated for seizures, with high serum TG concentrations subsequently seen.

The severity of serum TG elevations is variable and may be related to the wide variability of TG clearance in plasma (even after 12 hours of withholding of food) in affected dogs.[21] Moderately high TG content in serum samples (i.e., high concentration but no lactescence) from dogs in which food has been withheld may be of less concern; however, when this is first observed, a decrease in fat intake and monthly reevaluation are advised.

Proposed Pathogenesis

Metabolic mechanisms of this disorder remain speculative but include delayed VLDL clearance or increased production. Delayed clearance may be due to a familial deficiency of LPL activity.[1, 3, 21] Located on the capillary endothelial surface of peripheral tissues, this enzyme is responsible for the hydrolysis of chylomicron and VLDL-TG.[22] Such deficiencies have been reported in humans.[22] Congenital LPL deficiency has been reported in a mixed breed puppy[23] and implicated in hypertriglyceridemia in two Brittany spaniels.[24] It is also recognized as the cause of a primary hyperchylomicronemia in cats.[25, 26] An additional possibility relating to delayed lipoprotein clearance, although more speculative, is the existence of a hepatic receptor defect involved in the uptake or internalization of chylomicron and other TG-rich lipoprotein remnants. Lack of such a receptor activity would explain, in part, the variability of the fasting hypertriglyceridemias seen in individual animals. In addition, to the extent that such a receptor may be up- or down-regulated by various hormonal or dietary means, an explanation for the spontaneous but sometimes temporary resolution of serum TG elevations would be possible.

Treatment

Dietary modifications, lipid-lowering drugs, or marine-life oil supplements are generally advocated as potentially beneficial in cases of idiopathic hypertriglyceridemia. Cases of pure hyperchylomicronemias (i.e., no VLDL-TG elevation) appear to respond to dietary fat restriction more readily than do mixed hypertriglyceridemias (i.e., both chylomicron and VLDL fractions are elevated).[18] In the former cases, the refrigeration test should result in a significant chylomicron layer with a clear serum layer below. Hypercholesterolemias are not typically seen in cases of pure hyperchylomicronemia. Decreasing dietary fat is the therapy of choice and may help minimize long chylomicron residence times in the circulation because their intestinal production is reduced.

Numerous low-fat diets are commercially available for dogs. Formulas with and without fiber exist, and readers are advised to become familiar with the range of products available by examining label information of representative product categories. Low-fat diets may not always be efficacious, especially when elevations of VLDL-TG exist, because these lipids are endogenously produced. However, if the low-fat diet selected is complete and balanced and palatable to the animal, it will do no harm and may be used in combination with other lipid-lowering agents. Some endogenous TG elevations have been successfully lowered by administration of menhaden fish-oil capsules (1 g/4.55 kg body weight) daily, combined with dietary fat restriction. The n-3 fatty acid content of fish oils has been shown to lower TG concentrations in human beings and in animal studies.[27] The partial efficacy in dogs suggests that overproduction of VLDL may be at least partially responsible for the hypertriglyceridemia observed. In one case, a dog with seizures and a high serum TG content was treated with a low-fat diet and dietary fish-oil supplement regimen, which controlled the high serum TG content for up to 1 year. However, rebound hypertriglyceridemia was noticed thereafter, and the condition remained refractory to treatment with higher oil doses and other lipid-decreasing agents such as gemfibrozil and niacin. Gemfibrozil (Lopid, Parke-Davis) at a fixed dose of 200 mg/day has been used in an effort to stimulate LPL activity and reduce VLDL-TG secretion.[27] Use of 100 mg of niacin daily reportedly reduced serum TG content in four dogs with idiopathic hypertriglyceridemia for several months without problems. In one case in the author's experience, niacin treatment resulted in erythema and pruritus of the dog's muzzle reported by the owner when either 100 mg/day or 25 mg/day doses were used within 1 to 2 days time. Skin flushing and erythema have also been reported in human beings as an adverse effect of high niacin doses.

Whether similar rebound hypertriglyceridemia is a consistent feature, independent of the type of lipid-decreasing agent used, is unknown. This rebound has not been reported with the use of fish-oil treatment for high serum TG concentrations in human beings or in studies using experimental animals. The preceding treatment recommendations, however, should be used with care until the safety and efficacy of lipid-decreasing agents in dogs are more firmly established.

SECONDARY HYPERLIPIDEMIAS

Pancreatitis

Hypertriglyceridemia is often present in dogs with pancreatitis, although hyperlipemic plasma is not always noted. Moderate hypercholesterolemia may also be present.[28] In some cases, alpha$_2$ migrating lipoproteins are elevated, with electrophoretic changes manifesting themselves within 48 to 72 hours of inflammation. In many cases, hyperlipemia is due to mixed hypertriglyceridemias, with both chylomicrons and VLDL being elevated. Lipoprotein electrophoresis yields variable results, with elevations of both the origin and the beta regions. Because LPL activity is stimulated by circulating insulin, it has been hypothesized that pancreatic inflammation compromises the ability of the pancreas to make sufficient insulin to maintain normal LPL activity.[28]

There is evidence that in some cases, hyperlipidemia may have been the cause of pancreatitis.[2, 28] In humans, hyperchylomicronemia is a recognized risk factor for pancreatitis.[29] It has been speculated that increased chylomicrons may lead to circulatory stasis, resulting in local ischemia of the pancreas and lipase leakage. Pancreatic lipase from cells damaged in this fashion may then partially hydrolyze chylomicron TG, yielding further tissue damage from free fatty acid release and concomitant inflammation.[29] Although not all dogs with hyperlipemia necessarily develop pancreatitis, modifying the diet in an attempt to reduce serum TG concentrations and advising owners of potential risks are recommended.

Diabetes Mellitus

Both dogs and cats with diabetes frequently exhibit marked hypertriglyceridemia and moderate hypercholesterolemia. Elevated cholesterol concentrations with normal TG have also been reported.[30] Untreated dogs with ketoacidosis often have beta-migrating lipoproteins. In some cases, hyper-chylomicronemia and increased alpha$_2$ and/or pre-beta lipo-protein elevations may also occur.[28] In insulin-deficient dogs, the elevations of beta and/or pre-beta lipoproteins may be caused in part by insulin lack, because this hormone is necessary for the normal production and activity of LPL. Increased VLDL synthesis (beta and/or pre-beta fractions) may also exist owing to lipid mobilization and reassembly of these TG-rich particles. Hyperlipidemias often improve with successful treatment of the diabetic animal.

In cats, long-term progestogen (megestrol acetate) therapy may result in diabetes mellitus and hyperlipidemia. With-drawal of the drug usually resolves this problem, although some cats may require permanent insulin replacement ther-apy.[31]

Hypothyroidism

Mild to marked hypercholesterolemia is common in hypo-thyroid dogs. Animals with serum cholesterol concentrations in excess of 750 mg/dL should be tested for serum T$_3$ and T$_4$ concentrations. Elevated beta and alpha$_2$ lipoprotein fractions are observed electrophoretically. Increased serum TG and associated beta and pre-beta fractions may also occur, especially when serum cholesterol concentrations are in excess of 750 mg/dL. This latter observation may be due to increased de novo hepatic synthesis of beta lipoproteins in an effort to metabolize excess cholesterol overall.

Lipoprotein alterations have been experimentally induced by fat and cholesterol feeding of hypothyroid fox hounds and random-bred mongrel dogs.[19] Under this condition, hy-percholesterolemia and atherosclerosis occurred. Cholesterol concentrations in excess of 750 mg/dL were usually required for as long as 2 years, however, for atherosclerosis develop-ment. In addition, the topographic distribution and severity of atherosclerotic lesions appeared to be altered by the type of dietary fat fed. For example, when the dietary fat was unsaturated (cottonseed oil), the disease involved the entire aorta, with only moderate involvement of peripheral arter-ies.[19] When the dietary fat source was saturated (beef tallow or tallow plus lard), the abdominal aorta and coronary and peripheral arteries became severely diseased. Lipid meta-bolic alterations seen when hypothyroid dogs were fed diets containing 16 per cent hydrogenated coconut oil (saturated plus medium-chain triglycerides) and 5 per cent cholesterol (dry weight basis) included elevations of serum total choles-terol concentrations and alpha$_2$ lipoproteins. In clinical cases of hypothyroidism, lipid abnormalities usually resolve with treatment of the primary condition.[30] Nonetheless, dietary fat type and amount and dietary cholesterol may be important factors to consider in cases characterized by very high serum cholesterol concentrations. Consequently, serum cholesterol determinations should be performed when following these cases.

Coronary artery disease is uncommon in dogs and cats. However, in view of the previously described experimental studies in dogs, it may be important to bear in mind the possibility of subclinical atherosclerosis and stroke due to embolic phenomena when excessively high serum choles-terol concentrations are found. Thus, extremely high choles-terol values in dogs should be pursued diagnostically. In the author's opinion, most marked cholesterol elevations are likely to be due to hypothyroidism, which can be ruled in or out and dealt with as appropriate. Euthyroid dogs with serum cholesterol values greater than 750 mg/dL for a protracted period may need to be treated with cholesterol-lowering

drugs such as the HMG-CoA reductase inhibitors with or without cholestyramine. Target goals in this setting should be to reduce the hypercholesterolemia below 750 mg/dL. It should be noted that primary hypercholesterolemia was reported in Briard dogs in the United Kingdom. However, serum values did not exceed 350 mg/dL.[32]

Cholestasis

Liver disorders, including cholestasis, are frequently ac-companied by alterations of serum and tissue lipids. Abnor-mal lipoprotein distributions, including the occurrence of lipoprotein X, with a hydrated density similar to human LDL, may occur. Surgical ligation of common bile ducts has provided an effective way to study lipoprotein alterations due to cholestasis.[17] Although elevations of serum total cho-lesterol concentrations may not be of sufficient magnitude to yield diagnostic or prognostic information, characteriza-tion of lipoprotein changes via ultracentrifugation and/or electrophoresis may be helpful. Whether an elevation of the alpha$_2$ lipoprotein band occurs in cholestasis cases is pres-ently unknown. Proper interpretation of serum lipoprotein electrophoresis in future clinical cases may help address this question.

Hypoadrenocorticism

Dogs with hypoadrenocorticism may show mild hyperlip-idemias, as do humans. Early studies have characterized these changes as being due to increased pre-beta lipoproteins and LDL cholesterol.[30] Alterations, however, tend to be mild (TG <500 mg/dL) and may be due to some degree of peripheral insulin resistance as a result of excess corticoste-roid concentrations.[31]

Nephrotic Syndrome

In humans, attention has been paid to the possible relation-ship between hypercholesterolemia and renal disease. This alteration may be due, in part, to increased hepatic choles-terol synthesis. In dogs, hypercholesterolemia has been re-ported with nephrotic syndrome, but this finding has been inconsistent.[28] It should be noted that in studies of dietary management of spontaneously occurring canine renal dis-eases, both normal and affected dogs became mildly hyper-cholesterolemic (350 to 450 mg/dL) with alpha$_2$ lipoprotein elevations when fed commercially prepared protein- and phosphorus-restricted diets.[33] These diets are typically rec-ommended for renal disease management and contain higher total dietary fat than many maintenance-type dog foods. Hypercholesterolemia under these conditions rarely exceeds 450 mg/dL and may not pose any appreciable canine health risk. Nonetheless, a detailed dietary history should be ob-tained when such diets are fed in an effort to evaluate the cholesterol response in animals with nephrotic syndrome or other types of renal failure, because the diet itself may be the source of moderate hypercholesterolemia and hyperlipo-proteinemia.

High-Fat Diets

A final example of altered canine plasma lipoprotein dis-tribution and metabolism can be seen when very high-fat diets are fed. Dogs maintained on diets containing 55 per cent (on an as-is basis) fat primarily from beef tallow exhibit marked alterations in lipoprotein cholesterol distribution compared with a typical maintenance diet (about 16 per cent fat, as is). Indeed, elevations in various LDL and/or HDL (possibly alpha$_2$) fractions and a shift of all lipoprotein fractions to lower-density forms occur.[34] Recent studies using diets containing approximately 67 per cent calories as fat have confirmed these findings and extended them to include measured increases in both free and esterified cholesterol, along with elevations of the alpha$_2$ and, to a lesser extent, the alpha$_1$ fractions. LCAT activities were also increased, indicating heightened reverse cholesterol transport with high dietary fat. The cholesterol content of these latter diets was not high at approximately 0.1 g/100 kcal of diet.[35]

PRIMARY HYPERCHOLESTEROLEMIA OF BRIARD DOGS

Fasting hypercholesterolemia in 78 Briard dogs that was not secondary to some primary metabolic derangement was reported in the United Kingdom.[32] Follow-up studies on 15 of these animals demonstrated that, apart from hypercholesterolemia, the dogs were otherwise normal, including their serum TG concentrations. Elevations of alpha$_2$ lipoproteins were seen on electrophoresis. Thus an abnormal accumulation of this fraction, presumably HDL$_1$, appeared to be the primary metabolic derangement. Although reasons for this alteration are unclear, it should be noted that the cholesterol elevations did not exceed approximately 350 mg/dL. As such, these animals may not be at risk for arterial or associated disease. However, it remains to be established whether this abnormality may play a role in retinal pigment epithelial dystrophy, which has been associated with this breed.

OCULAR MANIFESTATIONS OF HYPERLIPOPROTEINEMIA

Ocular manifestations of altered lipid metabolism have been observed for numerous years but not systematically studied biochemically. Nonetheless, a review of these findings summarized many of the most salient features of these ocular changes.[36] Such changes include lipemia of ocular blood vessels, corneal opacities, lipemic aqueous, and lipid infiltration of the globe. This latter change is most readily seen in the peripheral cornea and uveal tract. Lipid manifestations appear more commonly in dogs than in cats and depend on the type and amount of lipoprotein abnormality involved. Both primary and secondary hyperlipidemias may show ocular signs and have been reviewed.[36]

FELINE DYSLIPOPROTEINEMIAS

Feline disorders in which plasma lipoprotein alterations occur include those secondary to diabetes mellitus and the nephrotic syndrome, or they may be drug induced (megestrol acetate diabetes mellitus). Lipoprotein changes appear to be generally similar to those seen secondarily in dogs, although unrecognized differences likely exist.

Primary disorders are also recognized. Most notable is an inherited hyperchylomicronemia that has been studied in New Zealand[26] and documented in the United States[25] and the United Kingdom.[32] This syndrome is characterized as a persistent fasting hypertriglyceridemia similar to human type I hyperlipoproteinemia in which LPL activities are low or absent. In cats, it has been demonstrated that post-heparin plasma LPL activities are also decreased, although LPL mass is unaffected. In addition to chylomicron elevation and hypertriglyceridemia, lipemia retinalis, xanthomas, peripheral neuropathies, and granulomas may be seen. Moderate elevations of serum total cholesterol may also occur. Studies by Peritz et al found that a point mutation has occurred that prevents the LPL enzyme from binding its normal physiologic capillary endothelial surface.[37] A more recent study investigated severe hyperchylomicronemia in two litters of suckling kittens that was accompanied by anemia. It was determined that defective LPL activity rather than a deficiency of the apo-CII activating cofactor of LPL or LPL inhibitor was responsible and that it appeared to be inherited in an autosomal recessive manner.[38] It is unclear to what extent anemia may be related to this disorder, although one study also noted a severe anemia associated with LPL deficiency in kittens.[25] In this latter case, the anemia was explained by severe flea infestations in these young animals.

Other primary lipid abnormalities are also likely in cats. Preliminary data on a disorder of feline lipoprotein metabolism have been reported.[39] In that case, a 1.5-year-old castrated Siamese cat was presented with hypercholesterolemia and numerous xanthomas, including radiologic evidence of thoracic granulomas. Plasma lipoprotein distributions on agarose gels revealed elevations of a beta band consistent with increased LDL cholesterol. This alteration appears to be similar to human familial type IIa hyperlipoproteinemia, a form of primary hypercholesterolemia. The extent to which diet may be able to control this disorder is presently unknown, although dietary and other management has been used successfully in human patients.

REFERENCES

1. Rogers WA, et al: Lipids and lipoproteins in normal dogs and in dogs with secondary hyperlipoproteinemia. JAVMA 166:1092, 1975.
2. Rogers WA: Lipemia in the dog. Vet Clin North Am Small Anim Pract 7:637, 1977.
3. Watson TDG, Barrie J: Lipoprotein metabolism and hyperlipidaemia in the dog and cat: A review. J Small Anim Pract 34:479, 1993.
4. Gotto AM Jr, et al: Introduction to the plasma lipoproteins. Methods Enzymol 128:3, 1986.
5. Hui D, et al: Isolation and characterization of the apolipoprotein E receptor from canine and human liver. J Biol Chem 261:4256, 1986.
6. Brindley DN: Metabolism of triacylglycerols. In Vance DE, Vance J (eds): Biochemistry of Lipids, Lipoproteins and Membranes. Amsterdam, Elsevier, 1992, p 184.
7. Bauer JE: Comparative lipid and lipoprotein metabolism. Vet Clin Pathol 25:49, 1996.
8. Bauer JE: Diet-induced alteration of lipoprotein metabolism. JAVMA 201:1691, 1992.
9. Brown MS, Goldstein JL: How LDL receptors influence cholesterol and atherosclerosis. Sci Am 251:58, 1984.
10. Ha YC, Barter PJ: Differences in plasma cholesteryl ester transfer activity in sixteen vertebrate species. Comp Biochem Physiol 71B:265, 1982.
11. Watson TDG, et al: Development of methods for analyzing plasma lipoprotein concentrations and associated enzyme activities and their use to measure the effects of pregnancy and lactation in cats. Am J Vet Res 56:289, 1995.
12. Koo C, et al: Obligatory role of cholesterol and apolipoprotein E in the formation of large cholesterol-enriched and receptor-active high density lipoproteins. J Biol Chem 260:11934, 1985.
13. Bauer JE, Puppione DL: Unpublished observations.
14. Barrie J, et al: Quantitative analysis of canine plasma lipoproteins. J Small Anim Pract 34:226, 1993.
15. Rhodes DC, et al: Evaluation of methods for the determination of HDL-cholesterol in normal dogs and dogs with hypercholesterolemia by polyanion precipitation and density gradient ultracentrifugation (abstract). Proceedings, 42nd annual meeting, ACVP, Orlando, FL, 1991, p 18.
16. Mahley RW, Weisgraber KH: Canine lipoproteins and atherosclerosis. 1. Isolation and characterization of plasma lipoproteins from control dogs. Circ Res 35:713, 1974.
17. Bauer JE, et al: Lipoprotein cholesterol distribution in experimentally produced canine cholestasis. In Burger IF, Rivers JPW (eds): Nutrition of the Dog and Cat. Cambridge, Cambridge University Press, 1989, p 308.

18. Rogers WA, et al: Idiopathic hyperlipoproteinemia in dogs. JAVMA 166:1087, 1975.
19. Mahley RW, et al: Canine lipoproteins and atherosclerosis. 1. Characterization of the plasma lipoproteins associated with atherogenic and non-atherogenic hyperlipidemia. Circ Res 35:722, 1974.
20. Demacker PNM, et al: A study of the lipid transport system in the cat, *Feline domesticus.* Atherosclerosis 66:113, 1987.
21. Whitney MS, et al: Ultracentrifugal and electrophoretic characterization of the plasma lipoproteins of miniature schnauzer dogs with idiopathic hyperlipoproteinemia. J Vet Intern Med 7:253, 1993.
22. Grundy SM: Hypertriglyceridemia: Mechanisms, clinical significance, and treatment. Med Clin North Am 66:519, 1982.
23. Baum D, et al: Congenital lipoprotein lipase deficiency and hyperlipemia in the young puppy. Proc Soc Exp Biol Med 131:183, 1969.
24. Hubert B, et al: Hypertriglyceridemia in two related dogs. Companion Anim Pract 1:33, 1987.
25. Bauer JE, Verlander JW: Congenital lipoprotein lipase deficiency in hyperlipemic kitten siblings. Vet Clin Pathol 13:7, 1984.
26. Jones BR, et al: Occurrence of idiopathic familial hyperchylomicronemia in a cat. Vet Rec 12:543, 1983.
27. Bauer JE: Evaluation and dietary considerations in idiopathic hyperlipidemia in dogs. JAVMA 206:1684, 1995.
28. Whitney MS: Evaluation of hyperlipidemia in dogs and cats. Semin Vet Intern Med Surg (Small Anim) 292, 1992.
29. Greenberger NJ: Pancreatitis and hyperlipemia. N Engl J Med 289:586, 1973.
30. Armstrong PJ, Ford RB: Hyperlipidemia. *In* Kirk RW (ed): Current Veterinary Therapy X (Small Animal Practice). Philadelphia, WB Saunders, 1989, p 1046.
31. Johnson RK: Canine hyperlipidemia *In* Ettinger SJ (ed): Textbook of Veterinary Internal Medicine, vol 1, 3rd ed. Philadelphia, WB Saunders, 1989, p 198.
32. Watson P, et al: Hypercholesterolemia in Briards in the United Kingdom (abstract). Proceedings of the 10th ACVIM Forum, San Diego, CA, 1992, p 814.
33. Malchik KL, et al: Lipoprotein metabolism and LCAT activities of dogs with chronic renal failure (abstract). Proceedings of the 14th ACVIM Forum, San Antonio, TX, 1996, p 777.
34. Bauer JE: Single spin density gradient systems and micropreparative ultracentrifugation. *In* Perkins EG (ed): Analyses of Fats, Lipids and Lipoproteins. Champaign, American Oil Chemists' Society, 1991, p 555.
35. McAlister KG, et al: Canine plasma lipoproteins and LCAT activities in dietary oil supplemented dogs. Vet Clin Nutr 3:50, 1996.
36. Crispin SM: Ocular manifestations of hyperlipoproteinemia. J Small Anim Pract 34:500, 1993.
37. Peritz LN, et al: Characterization of a lipoprotein class III type defect in hypertriglyceridemia. Clin Invest Med 13:259, 1990.
38. Watson TDG, et al: Inherited hyperchylomicronemia in the cat: Lipoprotein lipase function and gene structure. J Small Anim Pract 33:207, 1992.
39. Bauer JE: Alterations of lipoprotein metabolism. Proceedings of the 9th ACVIM Forum, New Orleans, LA, 1991, p 511.

SECTION III

THERAPEUTIC CONSIDERATIONS IN MEDICINE

CHAPTER 73

PRINCIPLES OF DRUG THERAPY

Dawn Merton Boothe

DOSE-RESPONSE RELATIONSHIP

The most common adverse drug reactions are type A or "augmented" reactions. The magnitude of a pharmacologic response to a drug is proportionately related to (log of) drug concentration at the tissue site, which in turn reflects the plasma drug concentration (PDC).[1-3] Type A reactions are dose- or duration-dependent and generally are caused by PDCs that either exceed the maximum or drop below the minimum effective therapeutic range. They tend to be manifested as an exaggerated but normal pharmacologic response or as therapeutic failure. Failure to modify a dose appropriately is probably one of the more common, albeit unrecognized, causes of type A adverse reactions. Doses that are anecdotal rather than based on scientific, controlled studies are a frequent cause of type A adverse drug reactions. However, even drug therapy and doses based on scientific data may fail, because the animals studied tend to be healthy and small in number. However, if the clinician is sufficiently familiar with the drug and its kinetics in a given species, type A reactions are largely predictable and thus potentially avoidable.

DETERMINANTS OF DRUG DISPOSITION

DRUG MOVEMENT

Following administration of a fixed dose of a drug, several drug movements act in concert to determine PDC (Fig. 73–1): absorption, distribution, metabolism, and excretion. These drug movements are dynamic (see Fig. 73–1), occurring simultaneously, and their net effect determines PDC and tissue drug concentrations at any time during the dosing interval.[1-3]

Plasma Drug Concentration–Versus–Time Curve

Drug movements can be described mathematically by plotting PDC against time on semilogarithmic paper following administration of a known dose (Fig. 73–2). The PDC versus time curve is linearized if it follows first-order kinetics: a constant fraction rather than a constant amount of drug is moved per unit of time (see Fig. 73–2).[1-3] Each component of the curve might reflect a different drug movement and can be described by the respective slope of the line that constitutes the movement. To distinguish the rate of each movement, each slope is separated from the remainder of the curve by computer-generated programs that "strip" and "best fit" each component using linear regression. An equation comprised of the slope and a y intercept for each component describes the curve (see Fig. 73–2) and can be used to predict PDC at any time following administration of a dose. The equation also provides information needed to establish a dosing regimen.[1-3]

Mechanisms of Drug Movement

Each drug movement is affected by a number of physiologic factors, the most important being the rate and extent

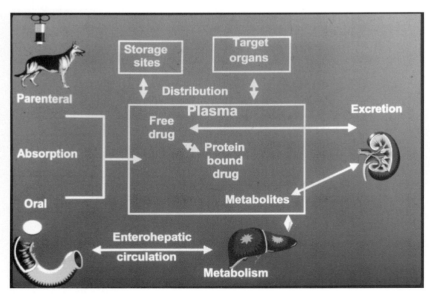

Figure 73–1. The determinants of plasma drug concentration act in concert following administration of a fixed dosing regimen, absorbed usually from the gastrointestinal tract; distribution of drug not bound to plasma proteins (free drug) from the systemic circulation into tissues and back; and elimination of the drug or its metabolites by (generally hepatic) metabolism and renal biliary secretion.

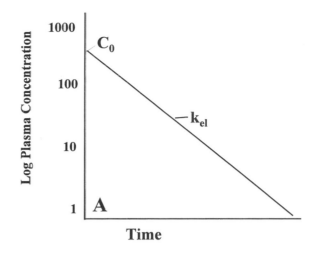

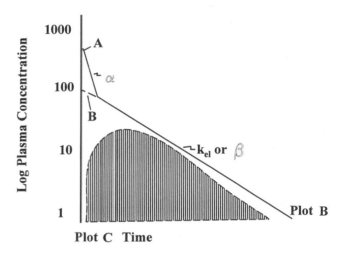

Figure 73–2. Plasma drug concentration (PDC)–versus–time curves. Following intravenous administration, a drug that fits a one-compartment open model (plot A) will plot as a straight line on semilogarithmic paper. There is no distribution phase, and the volume of distribution is based on PDC extrapolated *(dotted line)* back to time zero (C_0). Following intravenous administration, a drug characterized by distribution into peripheral tissues generally results in two or more components or phases (plot B). The first, more rapid phase reflects both distribution into tissues and elimination. Once distribution equilibrium has been reached, PDC declines owing to elimination only (second or terminal phase of this curve). The phases of PDC can be separated by stripping, most effectively accomplished by linear regression. The first (stripped) component of the curve usually represents distribution, and the slope (α) is the distribution rate constant. The volume of distribution (Vd) for such a drug is based on PDC (plot B) after distribution is complete, usually determined by extrapolating *(dotted line)* the terminal or elimination phase of the PDC-versus-time curve. The slope of the second phase of the curve is the elimination rate constant (β or k_{el}), and it is from this component that elimination half-life is determined (see Fig. 73–3 inset). Following oral administration (plot C), absorption is manifested as the upswing of the PDC, which generally follows first-order input (a constant fraction is absorbed per unit of time). Distribution and elimination of the absorbed drug are also occurring at the same time. The absorption rate constant (k_a) can be derived or stripped from the upswing of the curve, but only after the elimination component of the curve is stripped. Generally, the distribution phase of non-intravenous doses is masked by the absorptive phase. Bioavailability (F) of the oral drug is determined from the area under the curve ratios measured from the extravascular dose *(dotted line)* to the intravenous dose.

of passive diffusion.[1-3] Lipid solubility, molecular weight, and drug pK_a reflect the chemical structure of the drug and are important determinants of passive diffusion. The concentration gradient of nonionized drug across the site of drug movement is one of the most important determinants of passive drug diffusion. The easiest way to increase passive drug movement is simply by increasing the concentration of drug at the site by increasing the dose. However, a drug must be dissolved and should be un-ionized in order to passively diffuse. Ionized drugs not only cannot traverse lipid membranes but may be "trapped" in the environment. A drug is generally ionized when surrounded by an environmental pH greater than its pK_a if a weak acid, or less than its pK_a if a weak base. For example, as weak bases, orally administered aminoglycosides (pK_a 9 to 10) are ionized and trapped in the acidic environment of the gastrointestinal tract and thus are not absorbed. However, as weak acids, the beta-lactam antibiotics are predominantly un-ionized and well absorbed. Other host determinants of passive diffusion include thickness of the membrane to be traversed (e.g., edematous versus normal tissues), surface area (e.g., small intestine vs. stomach), and temperature.[1-3]

Absorption

The rate and extent of gastrointestinal drug absorption depend on a number of host factors, most of which affect passive diffusion.[1-3] These include gastrointestinal pH, which favors absorption of weak acids; surface area, which favors absorption in the small intestine compared with the stomach; motility, which mixes the drug, thus increasing the concentration of diffusible drug at the site of movement; permeability and thickness of the mucosal epithelium; and, for selected (few) drugs, intestinal blood flow, which maintains the concentration gradient across the mucosal epithelium.

The percentage of an administered dose that reaches systemic circulation is referred to as bioavailability (F).[1-3] Bioavailability is determined by measuring the area under a PDC-versus-time curve (AUC) following non-intravenous administration and comparing this number (dividing it) with the AUC measured following intravenous administration of the same dose (see Fig. 73–2). If the AUCs for both curves are equal, bioavailability is 100 per cent (F = 1). Bioavailability is used to predict drug efficacy following administration of the same drug by different routes or formulations. Factors that determine absorption of a drug also determine its bioavailability. In addition, bioavailability of an orally administered drug is decreased if the drug is metabolized by intestinal epithelial cells, microbes, or the liver. An orally administered drug is exposed to hepatocytes via the portal circulation before entering the systemic circulation. Drugs characterized by a high hepatic extraction ratio (>70 per cent) are almost completely removed from the blood by hepatocytes during the first passage of blood through the liver (first-pass metabolism or "flow-limited" drugs).[1-3] As a result, following oral administration, the drug may not reach the systemic circulation in concentrations sufficiently high to cause a pharmacologic response. Either such drugs are administered parenterally or the oral dose is sufficiently high to compensate for first-pass metabolism. The negative effects of first-pass metabolism on pharmacologic response may be reduced if the drug metabolites are also pharmacologically active (e.g., propranolol and diazepam). Novel routes of drug administration have been designed to overcome the detrimental effects of first-pass metabolism of some drugs. For example, transdermal patches allow for continuous delivery of opioid analgesics (e.g., fentanyl). Rectal administration of diazepam not only largely circumvents first-pass metabolism but also is a viable option in animals for whom an intravenous route is not possible.

Distribution

Once a drug reaches the systemic circulation, it must be distributed from the central (blood) compartment to peripheral tissues (including the site of drug action) and back into the central compartment, from which it is eliminated. The major factors that determine drug distribution to and from tissues include the lipid solubility of the drug and its ability to penetrate cell membranes, the concentration of drug unbound to plasma or tissue proteins, and regional (organ) blood flow.

The amount of tissue to which a drug is distributed, often estimated by the volume of distribution (Vd) of the drug, directly influences—and for many drugs, determines—PDC following administration of a fixed dose.[1-3] The volume is theoretic, in that it is calculated from the peak PDC that occurs after a distribution steady state has occurred. The volume is that to which the drug must be distributed (or the volume that would dilute the drug) if the drug were present throughout the body at the same concentration as that measured in the plasma. The Vd is measured by administering a known amount (dose) of drug intravenously (to assure that all drug reaches the systemic circulation, that is, F = 100 per cent. The maximum PDC is determined after (distribution) equilibrium has been reached but before elimination has begun. The maximum concentration in such instances is referred to as C_o. The Vd of a drug can then be calculated:

$$Vd = dose/C_o$$

Because the dose is generally in milligrams per kilogram and C_o is generally in milligrams per milliliter (the same as grams per liter), Vd is generally reported as liters per kilogram. The PDC achieved following administration of a fixed dose varies inversely with Vd. Thus, if Vd increases, the dose also must increase if the same drug concentration is to be maintained. Volume of distribution differs among and within species. A newborn or pediatric patient generally has a Vd that is up to 30 per cent greater than that of a young adult, and the PDC can, subsequently, be 30 per cent less.[4] Geriatric patients often have a contracted Vd, and a dose decrease might be indicated.[5, 6] Diseases associated with fluid retention (ascites, edema), obesity, or intensive fluid therapy often cause Vd to increase, whereas dehydration or weight loss causes Vd to decrease. The impact of changes in Vd differs with the chemistry of the drug. Lipid-soluble drugs generally distribute to all body compartments, and as long as drugs are dosed on a mg/kg basis, dosing regimens should be modified based on the weight. However, if the drug is distributed to extracellular fluid, changes in Vd induced by physiologic (e.g., obesity) or pathologic (e.g., ascites or fluid retention) states suggest a need for changing the dose or, in the case of fluid accumulation, the dose should be determined using estimated lean body weight.

Drug binding to proteins affects several determinants of drug movement, but particularly distribution. Weakly acidic drugs tend to bind to albumin, and weakly basic drugs tend to bind to alpha$_1$ glycoproteins.[1-3, 7] Many drugs are also bound to tissue proteins. Although plasma protein binding renders a drug more water-soluble and facilitates its movement in circulation, protein-bound drugs cannot be distributed from plasma into tissues, or from tissues back to plasma. In addition, a "bound drug" is not pharmacologically active, cannot be filtered into the glomerulus (although it can be renally excreted), and, in many cases, is more slowly metabolized by the liver. Drugs that are highly protein-bound (>80 per cent) may be more likely to be involved in adverse reactions early in the dosing regimen, because displacement of only a small proportion of drug from the protein (owing to competition with other protein-bound drugs or hypoalbuminemia) can increase the total amount of free, active drug. For example, displacement of only 1 per cent of a drug that is 99 per cent protein-bound such that it becomes 98 per cent bound (e.g., nonsteroidal anti-inflammatories) can double the concentration of pharmacologically active drug.[8]

Because drugs that are highly protein-bound remain in the systemic circulation bound to the protein, their volume of distribution tends to be small (<0.1 L/kg), reflecting the plasma central compartment. Drugs that distribute to extracellular fluid (ECF) or intracellular fluid (ICF, i.e., total body water [TBW]) take longer to reach equilibrium compared with drugs that are limited to plasma (e.g., highly protein-bound). Water-soluble drugs tend to be distributed to ECF and thus are often characterized by a Vd of 0.1 to 0.3 L/kg. Lipid-soluble drugs may cross cell membranes and thus distribute to ECF plus ICF (i.e., TBW); such drugs have a larger volume of distribution (>0.6 L/kg). Drugs that are bound to tissues may take even longer to reach distribution equilibrium, and the PDC-versus-time curves may be made up of three or more components. The Vd of such drugs (e.g., digoxin in cardiac tissue and aminoglycosides in renal tubular cells) can be large (>2 L/kg). Although Vd is a useful parameter with which to predict the magnitude of distribution of a drug (and thus to determine dose), it is important to remember that it is only theoretic and does not confirm to which tissue or compartment (ECF, ICF, TBW, or binding to tissues) the drug has distributed. The ability of a drug to penetrate cell membranes is an important consideration when therapeutic success is dependent on reaching intracellular sites. Selected tissues are recognized to be particularly difficult to reach with drugs. These include the brain, prostate, eye, and others. Lipid-soluble drugs with a large Vd are more likely to reach these tissues than are water-soluble drugs.

The rate at which a drug is distributed to tissues can be scientifically represented by the slope of the initial component or phase of the PDC-versus-time line (see Fig. 73–2). The distribution half-life, generally derived from the first component of a fitted curve (often referred to as α), is the time necessary for 50 per cent of distribution to be completed and offers a means for estimating the time that must elapse before drug distribution to tissues is complete. Clinically, this parameter becomes important, because maximum concentration (C_{max}) will not be achieved in tissues until distribution has reached an equilibrium. If PDCs are being monitored in an animal, blood samples for peak drug concentrations should not be collected until distribution has reached an equilibrium. For many drugs, both absorption and distribution are complete within one to two hours after administration. If a drug is given orally, intramuscularly, or subcutaneously, the graphic representation of distribution may be "hidden" in the absorptive phase of drug movement.

Metabolism

The rate at which a drug is eliminated from the body is the final determinant of PDC. Most drugs are eliminated by hepatic metabolism and/or renal excretion. Lipid-soluble drugs require conversion to a water-soluble form before they can be eliminated by the kidneys.[1-3] Such drugs usually are subject to hepatic metabolism, which can occur in two phases. Phase I metabolism chemically changes the drug so that it is (usually) more water-soluble and more susceptible to phase II metabolism. Reactions include oxidation, hydrolysis, or reduction. Phase I metabolites are usually inactive (e.g., phenobarbital) but can be equally active, more active (e.g., a pro-drug such as enalapril), or less active (e.g., diazepam) or more toxic (e.g., acetaminophen) compared with the parent compound. Phase II metabolism, also known as conjugation, occurs when a large water-soluble molecule is chemically added to either the parent drug or a phase I metabolite. Glucuronidation is the most common phase II reaction. Addition of glutathione to a reactive metabolite is an important mechanism by which reactive metabolites can be scavenged before tissue damage occurs. Sulfonation and acetylation are less common phase II reactions. With rare exceptions, phase II metabolites (including those that are toxic) are inactive. Acetylation occasionally results in formation of active metabolites (e.g., procainamide). Most drug metabolites are eliminated in the urine, but some may be eliminated in the bile.

Factors that can affect hepatic drug metabolism include the amount and activity of drug-metabolizing enzymes and, if the drug is characterized by a high extraction ratio (>70 per cent), hepatic blood flow. Changes in protein binding of highly bound drugs can also affect the rate of hepatic metabolism of drugs characterized by a low (<70 per cent) extraction ratio. The rate of elimination of such drugs is inversely proportional to their degree of protein binding. The greater the protein binding, the slower the rate of metabolism. Drugs that are highly protein-bound that become displaced may initially cause an adverse reaction. However, the hepatic clearance of the unbound drug increases as the drug becomes unbound, thus tending to offset the effect of drug displacement from protein. Diseases, drug interactions, and species differences can have a profound impact on drug metabolism and thus duration of drug elimination. For example, drugs that induce drug-metabolizing enzymes (phenobarbital, rifampin) increase the clearance of other drugs metabolized by the liver and can cause therapeutic failure with those other drugs. Inducing drugs may increase the risk of hepatotoxicity caused by reactive drug metabolites. Inhibitors (e.g., chloramphenicol, cimetidine, ketoconazole) prolong the half-lives of other drugs and may result in drug toxicity. Inhibitors can be used therapeutically, as is exemplified by the use of cimetidine to decrease the toxicity of acetaminophen.

Excretion

Renal excretion is the most important route of drug elimination for both parent drugs and their metabolites. The elimination of water-soluble drugs (e.g., aminoglycosides and beta-lactams) is particularly dependent on renal excretion. Host factors that determine renal excretion include glomerular blood flow, active tubular secretion, and tubular resorption. Each of the determinants of renal excretion can be influenced by renal blood flow. The kidney is also capable of metabolizing some drugs (e.g., imipenem), although this capacity is only occasionally of clinical importance.

Glomerular filtration is a passive process. Drugs enter the glomerulus by bulk flow, being excluded if too large (>60,000 molecular weight) or if bound to large molecules such as albumin. In contrast, active transport of drugs in the proximal tubules is efficient and rapid but is susceptible to competition among drugs. Separate transport proteins exist for acidic, basic, and neutral drugs. Probenecid has been used clinically to compete with and thus inhibit the renal excretion of expensive beta-lactam antibiotics (e.g., imipenem), thus prolonging therapeutic PDC. Resorption of drugs from renal tubules into peritubular capillaries slows renal excretion. The extent to which a drug is reabsorbed depends on its lipid solubility and its ionization.[1-3] Weakly acidic drugs are more likely to be resorbed in acidic urine but will be trapped and excreted in alkaline urine. Urinary pH can be therapeutically altered so that the renal excretion rate of a drug can be modified. Note that for antimicrobial drugs that are renally excreted (e.g., amoxicillin), minimum inhibitory concentrations (MICs) referring to PDC are inappropriate guides to antimicrobial therapy of urinary bladder (but not renal) infections, because drug concentrations achievable in the urine are much higher than those in the plasma. A drug can be concentrated in the urine more than 300-fold compared with plasma concentrations, thus achieving concentrations that far surpass those on which plasma MICs are based.

In contrast to renal excretion, biliary excretion is slow and less important. Characteristics that determine biliary excretion of drugs include chemical structure, polarity, and, importantly, molecular weight (generally >600). Drugs excreted in the bile are in greater contact with the intestine and its flora compared with other drugs and are thus more likely to cause adverse reactions in the gastrointestinal tract. In addition, drugs excreted by this route may undergo enterohepatic circulation. When excreted into the bile in the conjugated form, drugs cannot be reabsorbed from the intestine because of the large molecule weight. However, bacterial degradation can result in free, unconjugated drug that can then be reabsorbed into the systemic circulation. Enterohepatic circulation prolongs drug half-life. Doxycycline, clindamycin, and naproxen (in dogs) are examples of drugs that undergo enterohepatic circulation.

Elimination

The combined effects of renal and biliary excretion, as well as other routes of elimination not discussed (e.g., pulmonary, sweat), irreversibly remove drug from the body. The rate of drug elimination (slope, i.e, k_{el}; also β or γ, depending on the number of linear components that make up the PDC-vs.-time curve) describes the fraction of drug in the body irreversibly eliminated per unit of time (time^{-1}) (see Fig. 73–2). This rate is represented by the slope of the terminal (last) component of a PDC-versus-time curve (the initial components, if present, generally represent both distribution and elimination).

Because k_{el} is a slope, it can be calculated from only two points on the PDC-versus-time curve, such as might be obtained from a peak and trough sample collected as part of therapeutic drug monitoring.[6-8] The k_{el} is simply the rise over the run, or $C_1 - C_2/t_2 - t_1$, where C = concentration of sample 1 or 2, respectively, and t = the time that samples 1 and 2 were collected (see Fig. 73–2). Because the PDC is plotted logarithmically, the actual equation becomes:

$$\ln \frac{(C_1 / C_2)}{t_2 - t_1}$$

For example, if gentamicin samples collected at 2 hours and 12 hours following an intravenous dose were 10.5 and 2 μg/mL, the k_{el} for gentamicin in this animal would be 0.17 hours^{-1}. The elimination half-life of a drug is the time necessary for half the drug to be eliminated from the body. It is derived from k_{el} ($t_{1/2} = 0.693/k_{el}$) (see Fig. 73–2) and is one of the most useful parameters for determining an appropriate dosing interval. It also can be derived directly from the plot of drug concentration (semilog)–versus–time curve. In the earlier example, the half-life of gentamicin in this animal would be 4.2 hours. At one drug elimination half-life, 50 per cent of the dose has been eliminated; by five drug half-lives, over 97 per cent of the drug has been eliminated. Thus, approximately 21 hours must elapse before most of the drug would be eliminated from this dog. For most cases of drug intoxication, elapse of one to two elimination half-lives is generally sufficient for PDC to drop below the toxic range. However, this is not always true and depends in part on how much drug initially was ingested and what constitutes a toxic concentration.

Clearance is a parameter often used to assess the elimination capacity and thus the physical well-being of an organ. Plasma clearance is the volume of plasma irreversibly cleared of the drug per unit of time and represents the sum total of organ clearance.[1-3] Note that clearance differs from elimination because it is a volume, not a rate per unit of time. If the drug is cleared exclusively by one organ (e.g., renal clearance of aminoglycosides or hepatic clearance of caffeine), then plasma clearance also represents clearance of the specific organ and can be used to evaluate the function of the organ. The volume of blood cleared per unit of time by an organ is independent of PDC. The same volume of blood will be irreversibly cleared of drug by an organ regardless of how much drug is in the blood.

Although half-life is a clinically useful estimate of how long a drug stays in the body, it is a "hybrid" parameter, in that it is determined by both distribution and clearance. Obviously, the more rapidly a drug is cleared by an organ, the shorter the drug half-life. However, if a drug is distributed to a large tissue volume, the organs of clearance cannot access the drug, and the rate of elimination decreases. Thus, drug elimination half-life changes directly and proportionately with the Vd of a drug, but inversely (and proportionately) with the clearance of the drug. The clinical significance of these relationships can be demonstrated with a dog or cat that has become dehydrated as a result of uncompensated chronic renal disease. As tissue volume contracts with dehydration, the Vd decreases. Although PDC (and the risk of drug toxicity) increases, more drug is in each milliliter of blood, and thus more drug is eliminated per unit of time, even though clearance does not increase. If all else remains normal, drug half-life decreases. In an animal that is not dehydrated but suffers from significantly compromised renal function (and the drug is eliminated by the kidney), clearance decreases (a smaller volume of drug goes through the organs of clearance). If no other change occurs, drug elimination half-life would increase. In an animal with both volume

contraction and compromised renal function (the more common situation), the effects of the changes in clearance and Vd balance each other, and drug half-life may not change, even though renal function may be impaired and body fluid compartments have changed.

FIXED DOSING REGIMENS

DOSE

A fixed dosing regimen comprises a dose and an interval (or frequency). The dose necessary to achieve a specified target PDC (e.g., C_{max}) depends on the volume of tissue that will dilute the dose administered, estimated by Vd.

$$\text{Dose} = [C_{max}][Vd]$$

The dose of drug must be increased or decreased proportionately with changes in Vd in order to achieve the same target PDC. The Vd of a drug is the sole determinant of PDC for drugs that do not accumulate.[1-3] For drugs that do accumulate, the initial dose of the drug must also take into account the magnitude of accumulation, which in turn depends on the elimination half-life of the drug in relation to the dosing interval.

INTERVAL

The frequency of dosing or the dosing interval is determined by the time (T_{max}) it takes for maximum PDC (C_{max}) to drop to a point below which the desired response no longer occurs, C_{min} (Fig. 73–3). Thus, T_{max} depends on the amount of fluctuation in PDC (the therapeutic range) desired or acceptable during the dosing interval and the elimination rate constant (k_{el}). If C_{min} for a drug is close to half of C_{max}, then approximately one drug half-life (i.e., $T_{max} = t_{1/2}$) can elapse before the next dose must be administered. The longer the elimination half-life of a drug, the longer the interval (or T_{max}) can be between doses.[1-3]

Frequently, in order to effect a pharmacologic response or to maintain owner compliance, clinicians are tempted to modify the recommended dosing interval. Yet decreasing a dosing interval is of no benefit for drugs whose half-lives are long. For example, an 8-hour dosing interval for phenobarbital (drug half-life 50 to 100 hours) offers no advantage over a 12-hour interval, because very little drug will be eliminated during the 12-hour period between doses. An exception is made if induction of drug-metabolizing enzymes by phenobarbital has decreased the drug half-life to less than 24 hours. For drugs with short half-lives (e.g., many antibiotics), prolonging the dosing interval from every 8 hours to every 12 hours may be accompanied by a dramatic decrease in PDC, quite possibly below C_{min}. For example, if the half-life is two hours, a four-hour increase in the dosing interval will result in a 75 per cent decrease in PDC, because two additional half-lives will elapse. Note, however, that some drugs are effective even if the PDC is essentially nondetectable. Examples include antimicrobials that exhibit a postantibiotic effect (e.g., aminoglycosides), drugs that accumulate in tissues (e.g., omeprazole), drugs such as diazepam whose metabolites are active (some with drug half-lives longer than the parent compound), and drugs that inactivate chemicals or destroy receptors that must be resynthesized before the physiologic effect resolves (e.g., antiprostaglandins). These drugs need not be given every half-life (often two hours or less) in order to remain effective.

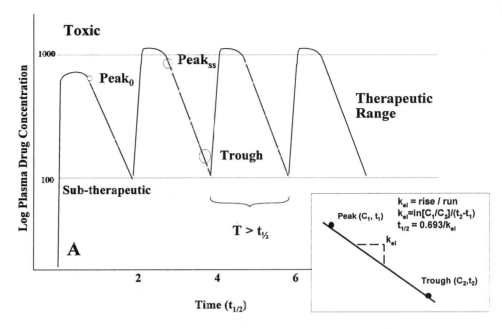

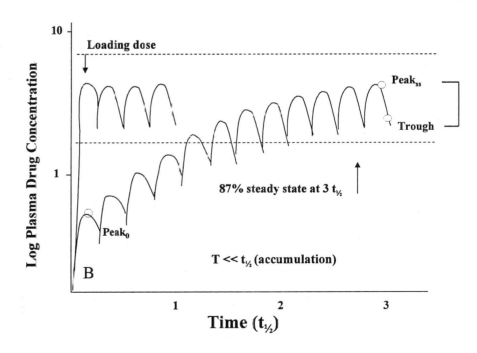

Figure 73–3. Plasma drug concentration (PDC)–versus–time curves following multiple extravascular dosing. The therapeutic range of a drug is defined by a peak or maximum concentration (C_{max}) above which toxicity is more likely, and a trough or minimum concentration (C_{min}) below which therapeutic failure is more likely. The relationship between dosing interval T and drug half-life ($t_{1/2}$) determines the amount of fluctuations in PDC during a dosing interval and the amount that a drug will accumulate. A drug whose dosing interval is longer than its half-life *(A)* accumulates little to not at all, because most of the drug will be eliminated during a dosing interval. In contrast, a drug administered at an interval shorter than its half-life *(B)* will accumulate, because most of the drug is still in the body by the next dose. Drug half-life can be determined from peak (C_{max}) and trough (C_{min}) (inset, *A*).

Drug half-lives can be as short as two minutes or less (e.g., epinephrine and dobutamine) or as long as several weeks (e.g., potassium bromide). Drugs with half-lives that are too short for convenient dosing either are given as constant intravenous infusions (e.g., lidocaine) or may be prepared as slow-release preparations (e.g., benzathine penicillin). Although the elimination half-life of the drug does not vary for these slow-release preparations compared with other preparations of the drug, the absorption of the drug is much slower. The intent, although not always successful, is to maintain constant therapeutic concentrations by assuring continuous addition of drug into plasma. Note, however, that absorption may be so slow that therapeutic concentrations are never reached. Many oral drugs are prepared as slow- or continuous-release preparations (e.g., quinidine, theophylline). However, these preparations have been formulated for humans, and the release kinetics may vary substantially in animals. Use of these preparations should be reserved for drugs that have been studied in animals. Alternatively, therapeutic drug monitoring for some drugs can be used to assure that drug concentrations fall within the therapeutic range.

ACCUMULATION

For drugs with very long half-lives, dosing intervals are correspondingly prolonged. However, a dosing interval that is too long may also be inconvenient. In addition, for many drugs, the therapeutic range is very narrow, and fluctuation of PDC during the dosing interval must be minimized. In both situations, the recommended dosing interval is often shorter than the elimination half-life. With each subsequent dose of drug administered at an interval (T) that is much shorter than the drug half-life, the majority of the previous dose may still be in the body, and the drug begins to accumulate with multiple doses (see Fig. 73–3). Eventually, a steady state is reached, such that the amount of drug administered with each dose equals the amount eliminated during the dosing interval. As with drug elimination, approximately five drug half-lives must elapse following a fixed dosing regimen before steady state is reached. Steady state is a relevant issue only for drugs that accumulate, that is, drugs that are administered at a dosing interval that is shorter than the drug elimination half-life (e.g., phenobarbital, potassium bromide, digoxin, selected antimicrobials). The amount that a drug will accumulate as steady-state PDCs are reached depends on the relationship between the drug elimination half-life and the dosing interval. The greater the difference between the two (the larger the half-life is compared to the interval), the more the accumulation.[1–3] The relationship between elimination half-life and dosing interval also determines the amount that the PDC may fluctuate during a dosing interval. For drugs administered at an interval equal to the elimination half-life, PDC will fluctuate twofold between doses. The relationship between drug half-life and dosing interval provides a basis for collecting samples when using therapeutic drug monitoring to guide therapy. For example, a single sample is sufficient for drugs with long half-lives (e.g., bromide), because little drug is eliminated between each interval. For drugs with short half-lives (e.g., clorazepate or digoxin in some animals), both a peak (generally two to four hours) and a trough (just before the next dose) are indicated.

Drugs that accumulate present problems that are not encountered with other drugs. Maximal therapeutic efficacy will not be realized until steady-state concentrations have been reached, which may be an unacceptable time for some animals (e.g., epileptics receiving potassium bromide). In such situations, a loading dose can be administered. This single dose, based on Vd of a drug and target concentrations (usually between C_{max} and C_{min}), is intended to achieve therapeutic concentrations with the first dose (assuming 100 per cent bioavailability). The daily maintenance dose is begun after loading has occurred. A disadvantage that may preclude administration of a loading dose is that the body is not allowed to gradually adapt to the drug. Note that the maintenance dose may not maintain the PDC reached by loading. In such cases, PDC may gradually decrease below C_{min} or increase above C_{max}, and the change may not be evident until a new steady state has been reached five drug half-lives later.

THERAPEUTIC RANGE

Fixed dosing regimens comprise a route, a dose (e.g., mg/kg), and an interval (e.g., every eight hours) that are designed to generate and maintain PDC in the therapeutic range throughout most of the dosing interval.[1–3] The therapeutic range is defined by the minimal effective PDC (trough or C_{min}), below which therapeutic failure is likely to occur, and a maximal effective PDC (peak or C_{max}), above which a type A adverse reaction is more likely (see Fig. 73–3). Although a therapeutic range can be helpful for targeting drug therapy, it can also be misleading. A common misconception is that once a therapeutic range has been reached (as might be documented by therapeutic drug monitoring), if the desired response has not occurred, drug therapy has failed. However, a therapeutic range generally reflects concentrations between which a large proportion (e.g., 95 per cent) of the population will respond. Where in the therapeutic range a particular animal will respond is not predictable. Indeed, a small percentage of animals will respond outside of the therapeutic range (high or low end), and some animals will show clinical signs of toxicity below the maximal therapeutic range.

Although dosing regimens are designed to achieve a targeted PDC, the determinants of PDC are susceptible to changes by a number of factors. Factors to be taken into account when modifying recommended doses in an animal include physiologic factors such as species and age; pathologic factors (or disease), particularly cardiac, renal, or hepatic; and pharmacologic factors (e.g., drug interactions) resulting from administration of the drug alone or in combination with other drugs.[7] Each of the factors can alter any drug movement and profoundly alter an animal's response to a drug. However, the discerning clinician can make modifications in a dosing regimen that are designed for a particular animal if he or she has sufficient knowledge about the animal's physiologic status and the pharmacology of each drug the animal is receiving. Professional flexible labels, a recent change for drugs approved for use in animals, are intended to facilitate selection of a proper dosing regimen by providing information pertinent to the drug, its disposition in the target species, adverse effects, and drug interactions. Professional flexible labels offer a range of doses and/or intervals, thus allowing clinicians flexibility (without fear of extralabel use) when administering drugs.

REFERENCES

1. Ritschel WA: Handbook of Basic Pharmacokinetics Including Clinical Applications. Hamilton IL, Drug Intelligence Publications, 1992.

2. Rowland M, Tozer TN: Clinical Pharmacokinetics: Concepts and Applications. Philadelphia, Lea & Febiger, 1989.
3. Baggott JD: Principles of Drug Disposition in Domestic Animals: The Basis of Veterinary Clinical Pharmacology. Philadelphia, WB Saunders, 1977, pp 73–112.
4. Boothe DM, Tannert K: Special considerations for drug and fluid therapy in the pediatric patient. Compend Contin Educ Pract Vet 14:313, 1991.
5. Aucoin DP: Drug therapy in the geriatric animal: The effect of aging on drug disposition. Vet Clin North Am Small Anim Pract 19:41, 1989.
6. Ritschel WA: Gerontokinetics: The Pharmacokinetics of Drugs in the Elderly. Calcwell, NJ, Telford Press, 1988, pp 1–16.
7. Belpaire FM, DeRick A, Dello C, et al: Alpha 1–acid glycoprotein and serum binding of drugs in healthy and diseased dogs. J Vet Pharmacol Ther 10:43, 1987.
8. Pond SM: Pharmacokinetic drug interactions. In Benet LZ, Massoud N, Gambertoglio JG (eds): Pharmacokinetic Basis for Drug Treatment. New York, Raven Press, 1985, pp 195–220.

RX

CHAPTER 74

ANTIMICROBIAL DRUGS

Mark G. Papich

Antimicrobial drug treatment is the most common therapy in veterinary medicine. This chapter will review some of the important aspects of antimicrobial treatment and provide guidelines for treating infections in small animals. When treating bacterial infections, evaluate the location of the infection and determine if there are barriers to drug penetration or whether there are local factors such as tissue pH or cellular debris that may affect antimicrobial drug activity. Next, one should consider the most likely pathogen causing infection, based upon culture results, cytologic examination, or historical data. In some instances, antimicrobial susceptibility testing will be necessary to determine drug activity against the pathogen. The pharmacokinetics of the drug and the pharmacokinetic-pharmacodynamic relationships should be known to maximize the antibacterial effect with the proper dosing regimen. Finally, the effect of antimicrobial drugs on the patient's health and physiologic status must be known. If the administered antimicrobial drug will affect the patient's health, these risks must be understood.

TISSUE PENETRATION OF ANTIBIOTICS

Because there is no barrier to impede diffusion of antibiotics from the vascular compartment to extracellular fluid of most tissues (exceptions listed below), antibiotic drug concentrations in the serum or plasma represent the drug concentration in the extracellular space (interstitial fluid).[1] Pores in the endothelium of capillaries are large enough to allow drug molecules to pass through unless the drug is highly protein bound in the blood. But there are few antibiotics of clinical significance used in small animals for which plasma protein binding is high enough to affect clinical efficacy of drugs.

PERFUSION-LIMITED DRUG DIFFUSION

Diffusion of most antibiotics in tissues is *perfusion limited* rather than *permeability limited*. This implies that, if adequate drug concentrations can be achieved in plasma, it is unlikely that a barrier will prevent drug diffusion to the site of infection as long as the tissue has an adequate blood supply. There is little evidence that differences in efficacy among antibiotic drugs can be attributed to differences in drug's lipid solubility when perfusion-limited perfusion applies.

PERMEABILITY-LIMITED DRUG DIFFUSION

Drug diffusion is *permeability limited* when a lipid membrane (such as tight junctions on capillaries) presents a barrier to drug diffusion. These tissues include certain sequestered sites such as the central nervous system and eye, the epithelial lining fluid of the lung, and glandular tissues such as the prostate and mammary gland. To treat infections in tissues for which permeability-limited diffusion applies, a drug must be sufficiently lipid-soluble to diffuse through the lipid barrier.

Characteristics of Tissues Affected by Permeability-Limited Diffusion

Central Nervous System. The central nervous system generally restricts poorly lipid-soluble and polar antibiotics. Most cephalosporins (except those classified as third generation), penicillins, and aminoglycosides do not attain adequate concentrations in the central nervous system when administered systemically. Antibiotics with better penetrating ability include metronidazole, trimethoprim, and some third-generation cephalosporins such as cefotaxime. When other drugs are administered, high doses must be given in order to attain effective antibacterial concentrations.

Eye. Following systemic administration, lipid-soluble drugs such as chloramphenicol and tetracycline can attain therapeutic intraocular concentrations (or concentrations in the tears or conjunctival fluid). If less lipophilic drugs (e.g., penicillin) are administered systemically, they may not attain adequate antibacterial concentrations in the eye.

Respiratory Tract. Antibiotic drugs distribute into the parenchyma of lung tissue to achieve therapeutic drug concentrations because there are no major barriers to diffusion as long as there are not consolidated lung lobes. Antibiotics administered to animals with pneumonia will achieve concentrations in the extracellular fluid of the lungs that are at least equal to the plasma concentrations. However, some drugs may not diffuse well into bronchial secretions because of the presence of a blood-bronchus barrier. In these cases, there may not be sufficient drug concentrations in the epithelial lining fluid of the respiratory tract to treat infections associated with bronchitis.[2] Drugs with poor lipid solubility such as penicillins and aminoglycosides have low concentrations in bronchial secretions after systemic administration, but this barrier may be diminished when it is inflamed. Drug concentrations may be higher in the bronchial mucosa because this tissue concentration represents the extracellular fluid.

Prostate. Antibiotic penetration into the prostate is limited because of a barrier between prostatic glandular cells and the serum or plasma. Most drugs in the plasma do not penetrate this gland. Drugs that are weak acids (penicillins and cephalosporins) may diffuse into the prostate in small concentrations but easily diffuse back to the plasma owing to the acidic nature of the prostatic fluid, but drugs that are weak bases (trimethoprim, macrolides) diffuse into the prostate and become trapped in the fluid because they become protonated in the more acidic prostatic fluid.[3] Drugs that are amphoteric, such as the fluoroquinolones, diffuse easily into the prostate. Enrofloxacin has been shown to reach concentrations in prostatic fluid and tissues that exceed plasma concentrations.[4] Chloramphenicol and tetracycline concentrations in prostate fluid of dogs are low after systemic administration.[3]

INTRACELLULAR INFECTIONS

Only lipid-soluble drugs are able to reach high concentrations in cells, unless they are internalized via an active process such as pinocytosis. Intracellular organisms such as *Brucella, Chlamydia, Rickettsia, Bartonella,* and *Mycobacteria* are examples of obligate intracellular pathogens. Staphylococci, a facultative intracellular organism, may, in some cases, become resistant to treatment because of intracellular survival. The concentration of drugs in cells often is expressed as the cellular to extracellular concentration ratio (C:E ratio). Examples of drugs that accumulate in leukocytes and other cells (that is, they have C:E ratios greater than 1) are fluoroquinolones (enrofloxacin, ciprofloxacin, difloxacin or orbifloxacin), lincosamides (clindamycin, lincomycin), macrolides (erythromycin, clarithromycin), and the azalides (azithromycin).[5] Beta-lactam antibiotics and aminoglycosides do not reach effective concentrations within cells.

TISSUE-DIRECTED ANTIBIOTIC THERAPY

As stated in the section above, because some drugs exhibit high intracellular concentrations in leukocytes (high C:E ratios), this has been proposed as a mechanism to deliver antibiotic to infected sites. This phenomenon has been called *tissue-directed antibiotic therapy,*[6] and this approach may be effective for treating infection in inflamed tissues. Presumably, leukocytes loaded with antibiotic (e.g., azithromycin, clindamycin, fluoroquinolones) could deliver drug directly to infected tissue guided by chemotactic stimuli. For this strategy to be effective, active drug must be released from leukocytes at the site of infection. For a drug sequestered in lysosomes, such as clindamycin, drug activity may

be low, but when phagocytes accumulate in infected tissues, active drug is released to produce an antibacterial effect.[7]

LOCAL FACTORS THAT AFFECT ANTIBIOTIC EFFECTIVENESS

Although drugs may demonstrate in vitro antibacterial activity, this is no guarantee that it will be effective in vivo. Tissue components may inactivate or interfere with drug activity to decrease effectiveness. Pus and necrotic debris may bind and inactivate vancomycin or aminoglycoside antibiotics (gentamicin, amikacin), causing them to be ineffective. Foreign material in a wound (such as surgical implants) can protect bacteria from antibiotics and phagocytosis by forming a biofilm (glycocalix) at the site of infection.

An acidic environment of infected tissue or acidic urine may decrease the effectiveness of clindamycin, erythromycin, fluoroquinolones (e.g., enrofloxacin, orbifloxacin), and aminoglycosides. Penicillins and tetracyclines are not affected as much by a change in the pH of the tissue, but their activity is diminished by the presence of hemoglobin (such as in a blood clot). An anaerobic environment decreases the effectiveness of aminoglycosides, whereas metronidazole has no activity against aerobic bacteria. Effective drug concentrations may not be attained in tissues that are poorly vascularized (e.g., extremities during shock, sequestered bone fragments, and endocardial valves) because an adequate blood flow is necessary to deliver an antibiotic to the site of infection.

STRATEGIES FOR SELECTING AN APPROPRIATE ANTIBIOTIC

IDENTIFY THE BACTERIA

Initial, empiric antibiotic selection can be based on a presumptive identification. A Gram stain of exudate or tissue fluids will differentiate gram-positive versus gram-negative and cocci versus bacilli. A simple cytologic examination from infected tissue, with the microscope slide stained with Wright's stain, also can show the presence of bacteria and identify the organism as a coccus or bacillus. Antibacterial therapy can be initiated from a presumptive diagnosis on the basis of these initial tests and clinical examination.[8] More specific therapy should be based on a culture and interpretation of susceptibility tests.

EMPIRIC DRUG SELECTION

If identification and antibacterial susceptibility of bacteria causing an infection are not immediately possible, initial therapy may be empiric. Prescribing empirically is possible when there are many resources that provide guidelines on the susceptibility of bacteria.[9] If one suspects the bacteria to be streptococci (but not *Enterococcus*), beta-streptococci, *Bacillus, Actinomyces,* or *Pasteurella,* successful therapy can be achieved by administering a penicillin such as ampicillin, or amoxicillin, a tetracycline, or trimethoprim-sulfonamide.

The most common *Staphylococcus* causing infections in small animals is *Staphylococcus intermedius.* Susceptibility can be expected to first-generation cephalosporins (for example, cephalexin, cefadroxil, or cefazolin), amoxicillin-clavulanate (Clavamox, Pfizer), a beta-lactamase–resistant penicillin such as oxacillin, or one of the fluoroquinolones (for example, enrofloxacin or orbifloxacin). All of these drugs have been effective in clinical practice.

Bacteria that are likely to be resistant to many commonly used antibiotics are *Pseudomonas aeruginosa,* Enterobacteriaceae (*E. coli, Klebsiella, Enterobacter*), *Proteus* spp. (indole-positive), and enterococci. In these cases, a susceptibility test is advised because resistance can be unpredictable. Therapy to treat infections caused by gram-negative enteric bacteria can be initiated with a fluoroquinolone (enrofloxacin, ciprofloxacin, orbifloxacin), a cephalosporin, amoxicillin-clavulanate, or an aminoglycoside (for example, gentamicin or amikacin).

If the bacterium is an anaerobe, such as *Clostridium, Actinomyces, Fusobacterium,* or *Bacteroides* (except beta-lactamase–producing strains of the *Bacteroides fragilis* group), administer penicillin G, amoxicillin-clavulanate, metronidazole, clindamycin, or a second-generation cephalosporin (for example, cefoxitin or cefotetan). The activity of first-generation cephalosporins and trimethoprim-sulfonamide combinations may be unpredictable for anaerobic infections.[10]

BACTERIAL SUSCEPTIBILITY TESTING

Agar-Disk Diffusion Test

The most familiar test for measuring bacterial susceptibility to antimicrobials has been the agar-disk diffusion test (ADD), also known as the Kirby-Bauer test. Details for performing this test are described in the book by Lorian.[9] This test measures the inhibition of bacterial growth against a concentration of antimicrobial that diffuses from an impregnated paper disk placed on the agar. The zone size can be directly correlated with the minimum inhibitory concentration (MIC). The larger the zone size, the lower the MIC, and vice versa. The ADD test is a valuable qualitative method for determining susceptibility. To perform this test according to the guidelines established by the National Committee for Clinical Laboratory Standards (NCCLS), the inoculation variables must be well controlled and the test should be performed according to strict procedural guidelines.[9] The precise depth of the agar, incubation time (usually 18 to 24 hours), and selection and preparation of the agar are important. The agar should be free of PABA, which interferes with the susceptibility test for sulfonamides, and free of thymidine, which interferes with the test for trimethoprim. Since each antibiotic diffuses at different rates throughout the agar, one must use published standards for interpreting the sensitivity.

MIC Determination

A test that directly measures the minimum inhibitory concentration (MIC) is more quantitative than the ADD test. Results of studies involving human patients show that an MIC determination of susceptibility correlates better with clinical success than an ADD test. The interpretation of the MIC test relies on knowing the breakpoints for each drug. An example of breakpoints for bacteria is shown in Table 74–1. Since susceptibility is reported as a specific drug concentration, pharmacokinetic data can be used to relate dosages to drug concentrations desired. Knowing the MIC can also be helpful for treating infections in the lower urinary tract. For these infections, the MIC can be related to the drug levels achieved in urine.[11]

TABLE 74–1. INTERPRETATION OF SERUM/PLASMA CONCENTRATIONS FOR BACTERIA

ANTIMICROBIAL	SUSCEPTIBLE* (µg/mL)	RESISTANT (µg/mL)
Amikacin	≤16	≥64
Ampicillin	≤8**	≥16
Ampicillin/clavulanic acid	≤4/2**	≥8/4
Cefazolin	≤8	≥32
Cefotaxime	≤8	≥64
Cephalothin	≤8	≥32
Cefoxitin	≤8	≥32
Ciprofloxacin	≤2	≥4
Clindamycin	≤0.5	≥4
Erythromycin	≤0.5	≥8
Gentamicin	≤4**	≥16
Imipenem	≤4	≥16
Oxacillin	≤2**	≥4
Rifampin	≤1	≥4
Tetracycline	≤4	≥16
Ticarcillin	≤64**	≥128
Trimethoprim/sulfa	≤2/38	≥4/76
Vancomycin	≤4	≥32

*Values between the susceptible and resistant range are interpreted as "intermediate."

**There are exceptions for interpreting some pathogens; consult NCCLS, or Lorian[9] (1996) for details.

From National Committee for Clinical Laboratory Standards (NCCLS) Guidelines M7-A3, 1995.

Guidelines for Interpretation of MIC. In Table 74–1, the MICs that define susceptible and resistant breakpoints are listed. The following rules are helpful for interpretation: If the MIC is below the susceptible breakpoint, the organism is sensitive and a cure can be expected using standard doses. Occasionally, even when the breakpoint is below the "susceptible" range, the organism is resistant in vivo. For example, a cephalosporin will not be effective for treating methicillin-oxacillin–resistant staphylococci even though the in vitro MIC may be in the susceptible range. If the MIC is above the resistant breakpoint, the organism is resistant and drug therapy with that drug is not recommended. MIC values between resistant and sensitive categories are in an "intermediate" zone. (This also has been called "moderately susceptible.") If the MIC is intermediate, the organism should ordinarily be considered resistant, but successful therapy can be achieved when the drug concentrates at high levels as it does when treating a lower urinary tract infection, or when topical therapy is used. In extreme cases, high doses have been used to achieve drug levels above the intermediate range, but this should not be considered unless the safety of the drug at high doses is known.

Limitation of Bacterial Sensitivity Testing

There are important limitations to consider when assessing the clinical relevance of in vitro antibacterial susceptibility tests. Sensitivity tests assume equal plasma and tissue concentrations and will overestimate the antimicrobial activity in the central nervous system, prostatic fluid, and mammary gland. Sensitivity tests will underestimate activity of topical treatments, local infusions, and antibacterials that concentrate in the urine. Susceptibility also may underestimate activity at drug concentrations below the MIC (sub-MIC effects). Sensitivity tests do not detect potentially synergistic antibiotic combinations (except for trimethoprim-sulfonamides and amoxicillin-clavulanate). An example of a synergism is the combination of a beta-lactam antibiotic and an aminoglycoside. Bacteria may be resistant to either drug alone, but sensitive when administered in combination. Finally, sensitivity tests cannot consider the local factors that may affect antimicrobial activity such as pus, necrotic tissue, low oxygen tension, and poor blood perfusion. For example, an aminoglycoside may not be effective in vivo if the infection is in necrotic tissue or an abscess, despite an in vitro test that indicates susceptibility.

RELATIONSHIP OF MIC TO CLINICAL OUTCOME

PHARMACOKINETIC-PHARMACODYNAMIC RELATIONSHIPS

The MIC is determined by in vitro tests and is defined as the lowest concentration that inhibits visible bacterial growth. This is considered a *pharmacodynamic* measurement. Studies in laboratory animals and clinical patients have defined the relationship of the MIC to clinical outcome.[12–15] This relationship has been correlated to certain variables such as the peak plasma concentration (C_{MAX}), the area of the plasma concentration versus time curve (AUC), and the length of time that the plasma concentration is above the MIC during a 24-hour interval. These parameters are *pharmacokinetic* measurements and are depicted graphically in Figure 74–1. Together, these measurements provide the basis for pharmacokinetic/pharmacodynamic markers to predict clinical outcome:[14] the ratio of the maximum plasma concentration (C_{MAX}, or peak) to the MIC, the time above MIC (measured in hours during a 24-hour interval), and the ratio of the total area under the plasma concentration versus time curve (AUC) for 24 hours to the MIC (AUC:MIC ratio).

Bacteriostatic Drugs

Drugs considered bacteriostatic include tetracyclines, macrolides (erythromycin), and clindamycin. For these drugs, drug concentrations should be maintained at the site of infection above the MIC throughout the dosing interval. Time above MIC is the most important marker.

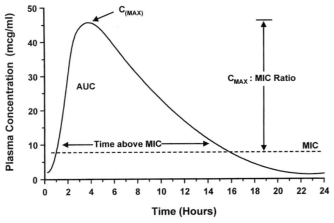

Figure 74–1. The pharmacokinetic variables from an antibiotic drug plasma concentration versus time profile and their relationship to the pharmacodynamic parameter of MIC. Pharmacokinetic and pharmacodynamic variables for antibiotics can be used as markers for clinical outcome. The variables of minimum inhibitory concentration (MIC), maximum (peak) plasma concentration (C_{MAX}), and area under the curve for the plasma concentration versus time profile (AUC) have been used to derive the time above MIC, C_{MAX}:MIC ratio, and AUC:MIC ratio.

Bactericidal Drugs

Time-Dependent Drugs. Beta-lactam antibiotics such as penicillins, potentiated-aminopenicillins, and cephalosporins are slowly bactericidal, and the concentration of beta-lactam antibiotics should be kept above the MIC throughout most of the dosing interval. Therefore, time above MIC is the best pharmacokinetic/pharmacodynamic marker. There is a threshold of four to five times the MIC, above which increased bacterial killing is not observed. A more effective treatment is expected with these drugs when they are administered at more frequent intervals, to maximize time >MIC, rather than by increasing the dose. Since the MICs of beta-lactam antibiotics are lower for gram-positive bacteria, and antibacterial effects occur at concentrations below the MIC, longer dose intervals may be possible for infections caused by gram-positive as compared with gram-negative bacteria.

Dosage regimens for the beta-lactam antibiotics should consider these pharmacokinetic-pharmacodynamic relationships. For treating a gram-negative infection, especially a serious one, administer penicillin derivatives and cephalosporins three to six times per day. Some of the third-generation cephalosporins have long half-lives, and less frequent regimens have been used for some of these drugs. For treating a gram-positive infection, such as a skin infection caused by *Staphylococcus*, twice-daily therapy with beta-lactams at moderate doses is sufficient. Twice-daily regimens have been shown as effective as three-times-daily regimens for treating bacterial pyoderma.[16]

Concentration-Dependent Drugs. Aminoglycoside antibiotics such as gentamicin or amikacin are most bactericidal when the peak plasma concentrations above the MIC are high. The C_{MAX}:MIC ratio is the most important pharmacokinetic/pharmacodynamic marker. After attaining this peak, plasma concentrations can fall below the MIC for 8 to 12 hours and still achieve a cure. Currently used dosage regimens for these drugs are designed to produce a peak of 8 to 10 × the MIC (C_{MAX}:MIC ratio of 8 to 10), with administration of only once daily. This regimen is at least as effective, and perhaps less nephrotoxic, than lower doses administered more frequently.[17] Our clinical regimens in small animals now employ this strategy. Gentamicin can be administered safely and effectively at a dose of 6 mg/kg once daily, IV. The corresponding dose for amikacin is 10 mg/kg, IV.

For the fluoroquinolone antimicrobials, either the peak concentration (C_{MAX}:MIC ratio) or the area under the plasma concentration curve (AUC:MIC ratio) predict antibacterial success.[14] Published work in experimental animals[18] and clinical studies in people[19] suggest that the C_{MAX}:MIC ratio should be above 8 to 10, or the AUC:MIC ratio should be above 125. In addition to better cure rates, high C_{MAX}:MIC ratios have been associated with a lower incidence of development of resistance.[14]

To achieve this goal, low doses of fluoroquinolones can be administered to treat highly susceptible organisms, for example, those with an MIC value of 0.06 μg/mL or less for ciprofloxacin or enrofloxacin. Susceptible bacteria of the Enterobacteriaceae are expected to have MIC values in this range. For bacteria that are more resistant, a correspondingly higher dose will be needed. For example, to achieve the necessary peak concentration for a *Staphylococcus* or *Pseudomonas aeruginosa* with a MIC of 0.5 μg/mL, a dose of 5 to 7.5 mg/kg/day for orbifloxacin and 10 to 20 mg/kg/day for enrofloxacin should be used. When the MIC values are high (for example, ≥1.0 μg/mL), the effectiveness of fluoroquinolones is doubtful because even at doses at the high end of the accepted range, a sufficient AUC:MIC ratio will be difficult to achieve.

TREATMENT OF SPECIFIC INFECTIONS

Treatment of common infections is listed in the following section. Listed here are empiric treatments based on the usual susceptibility pattern and clinical experience. Information on the pharmacology of specific drugs mentioned can be found in many pharmacology textbooks, and drug doses are listed in current veterinary textbooks.[20] For refractory infections resistant to the drugs listed in this section, consult a specific reference on treating resistant infections.[21]

SKIN AND SOFT TISSUE INFECTIONS

Bacteria

The most important skin pathogen in dogs is *Staphylococcus intermedius*. Other bacteria identified usually are opportunistic. For example, when deep skin infections occur, *Pseudomonas aeruginosa* or bacteria of the Enterobacteriaceae (*Escherichia coli* and *Proteus*) have been identified. Occasionally, other gram-positive cocci cause infection, including enterococci. Anaerobic bacteria, including *Actinomyces,* have been isolated from deep infections. Bacteria causing skin infection in cats induced by a bite wound can be *Pasteurella*, streptococci, or other inhabitants of the oral cavity, including anaerobes.

Antibiotic Considerations

Since most skin and soft tissue infections are extracellular, the most important feature of drug delivery is to ensure that there is sufficient antibiotic drug concentrations in the extracellular fluid.[1] As was discussed earlier, adequate concentrations in plasma usually ensure effective concentrations in these tissues. Recall that in some situations, even when there are sufficient drug concentrations, drug activity can be diminished. For example, the components of pus may bind and inactivate certain drugs and a necrotic environment with cellular debris may inhibit activity of aminoglycosides and trimethoprim-sulfonamides. This issue may be important when treating an infection associated with an abscess or when treating otitis externa.

Drug Selection

Staphylococcus. Surveys have shown that the incidence of resistance (in vitro) for *Staphylococcus intermedius* is lowest for first-generation cephalosporins (e.g., cefadroxil, cephalexin), beta-lactamase–resistant penicillins (e.g., oxacillin, cloxacillin, dicloxacillin), beta-lactamase inhibitor combinations (e.g., amoxicillin-clavulanate; Clavamox), and fluoroquinolones (enrofloxacin, orbifloxacin). These drugs have been effective for treatment of skin infections. Other drugs that have been used successfully include erythromycin, lincomycin, clindamycin, and trimethoprim-sulfonamide or ormetoprim-sulfonamide combinations.

The incidence of staphylococcal resistance to erythromycin, clindamycin, lincomycin, chloramphenicol, and trimethoprim-sulfonamides is variable. Clinical studies support the assumption that naive bacteria are usually sensitive to these drugs, but after treatment, resistance can be acquired, especially in cases of recurrent pyoderma.[22–24]

Pseudomonas. Occasionally, especially in deep or chronic infections, *Pseudomonas aeruginosa* is the cause of infection. *Pseudomonas aeruginosa* has inherent resistance to many drugs because it lacks high-permeability porin proteins by which antibiotics gain access to bacteria. A wild strain of *Pseudomonas aeruginosa* has inherent resistance to most common drugs but should be susceptible to amikacin, gentamicin, or tobramycin; extended-spectrum penicillins (ticarcillin, piperacillin); some selected third-generation cephalosporins (e.g., ceftazidime); carbapenems (meropenem or imipenem); and perhaps a fluoroquinolone (ciprofloxacin, difloxacin, enrofloxacin, or orbifloxacin).

Pasteurella. Skin and soft tissues may be infected with *Pasteurella*, if caused from a bite wound. Susceptibility of this bacteria is predictable. Usually, it is sensitive to most antibiotics, including ampicillin/amoxicillin, cephalosporins, fluoroquinolones, and potentiated sulfonamides.

Other Gram-Negative Bacilli. If the infecting organism is *Enterobacter, Klebsiella, E. coli,* or *Proteus* (indole-positive), resistance to many antibiotics is possible and a susceptibility test may be advised. A first-generation cephalosporin or trimethoprim-sulfonamide may be active against enteric gram-negative bacteria of this group, but resistance is common. For initial therapy, we usually expect the gram-negative enteric bacteria to be susceptible to fluoroquinolones and aminoglycosides. Fluoroquinolones are an effective choice, if oral therapy is to be considered.

Enterococci. Enterococci are gram-positive cocci that have emerged as important causes of infections, especially those that are nosocomial. The most common species identified are *Enterococcus faecalis* and *E. faecium*. Wild-strain enterococci may be sensitive to penicillin G, ampicillin, or amoxicillin, but susceptibility to the cephalosporins and fluoroquinolones is unpredictable. These strains are usually resistant to trimethoprim-sulfonamide combinations, clindamycin, and erythromycin. If the *Enterococcus* isolated is sensitive to penicillins, administer amoxicillin or ampicillin at the high end of the dose range (because of higher breakpoint). Whenever possible, combine an aminoglycoside with a beta-lactam antibiotic for treatment of serious infections. Each drug alone is poorly bactericidal against enterococci. Often, the only drug effective against enterococci is vancomycin. Vancomycin should be given only as an intravenous infusion administered over 30 to 60 minutes to avoid toxicity. Guidelines for administration are available in other references.[25]

Anaerobic Bacteria. Anaerobic bacteria isolated from dogs and cats include bacteria of the *Bacteroides fragilis* group, *Peptostreptococcus*, *Fusobacterium*, and *Porphyromonas*.[26] Infections of the head, neck, and mouth may be caused by the genera *Prevotella* and *Porphyromonas*. Ordinarily, most anaerobes are highly susceptible to penicillins (including ampicillin), amoxicillin–clavulanic acid, clindamycin, chloramphenicol, and metronidazole. Bacteria of the *Bacteroides fragilis* group can be an exception and can cause resistant infections, especially in the abdomen.[21] The inducible beta-lactamase from *B. fragilis* is a cephalosporinase (not inhibited by clavulanate). Fluoroquinolones and aminoglycosides are not effective, and trimethoprim-sulfonamides, although active on a susceptibility test, may not be effective clinically.[10]

Urinary Tract Infections

Bacteria

The most common bacteria in dogs and cats causing infection of the urinary tract are *Proteus mirabilis, Staphylo-*

coccus spp., and gram-negative bacilli such as *Pseudomonas*, *E. coli*, *Klebsiella*, and *Enterobacter*.[11] Occasionally enterococci also cause infection in dogs and cats.

Antibiotic Considerations and Drug Selection

For treatment, consider the antibiotics that are excreted via the kidneys and concentrate in the urine. These drugs include any of the penicillins and cephalosporins, tetracyclines (except doxycycline), fluoroquinolones, aminoglycosides, and trimethoprim-sulfonamides. These drugs are concentrated 10- to 100-fold in the urine compared with the plasma.[11] Therefore, attaining drug concentrations in urine for susceptible bacteria is rarely a problem, which is a reason for high success rates for many drugs. Dose rates administered usually can be at the lower end of a dose range because of the extent of concentration of drug in the urine. Selection of drugs based on empiric activity can be made on the same basis as was listed for soft tissue infections.

If the patient is an intact male, infection of the prostate gland is possible. Drug penetration into the prostate gland was discussed in an earlier section. In these cases, a drug that can diffuse into the prostate such as a fluoroquinolone or trimethoprim should be administered.

TREATMENT OF INFECTIONS IN BONES AND JOINTS

Bacteria

Staphylococci, *E. coli*, *Pseudomonas*, *Proteus*, and anaerobes have been causes of joint and bone infections in small animals. Often these may be mixed infections. As reviewed by Lew and Waldvogel,[27] *Staphylococcus* can be particularly troublesome because it adheres to bone by expressing receptors for components of bone matrix. It also may be internalized by cultured osteoblasts and survive intracellularly.

Treatment Considerations

Aggressive treatment is necessary because the consequences of treatment failure are often loss of a limb or long-term morbidity. Drug selection should be made on the basis of a reliable susceptibility test taken from a culture deep within the wound. Drug safety also is an important consideration, since treatment is required for a long duration, usually a minimum of 6 weeks. Bone and joints do not present a barrier for drug diffusion; therefore, one drug group is not preferred over another because of superiority of better penetration. However, the presence of pus, necrotic tissue, devitalized bone, or foreign body may delay antibiotic diffusion. Surgery to remove or decrease this material is recommended.

Antibiotic Choices. Beta-lactam antibiotics that can be administered orally for long periods and that are active against staphylococci are rational initial choices. Drugs used for this purpose include first-generation cephalosporins (cefadroxil, cephalexin) and amoxicillin-clavulanate. Other drugs administered to small animals that are effective are the fluoroquinolones (enrofloxacin, orbifloxacin, or difloxacin) and clindamycin. For resistant infections caused by *Pseudomonas*, *E. coli*, or *Enterobacter*, susceptibility to the fluoroquinolones should be examined because they can be effective oral drugs. In some instances, parenteral therapy with an aminoglycoside or parenteral beta-lactam (third-generation cephalosporin, or carbapenem) may be necessary.[21]

ANTIMICROBIAL ADMINISTRATION FOR SURGICAL PROPHYLAXIS

In order to reduce the risk of postsurgical complications caused by infection, prophylactic antibiotics have been administered. To be effective, the antibacterial must be present in tissues at the time of bacterial contamination, which requires optimum timing of drug administration.

Patient Factors

One must consider the duration and extent of bacterial contamination that is likely. If it is a clean surgery (that is, a surgery that will not encounter a contaminated site), prophylactic antibiotics may not be necessary.[28] If the surgery will involve a contaminated site, or if the patient is at a high risk for developing a postoperative infection, administration of prophylactic antibiotics is encouraged. Factors that will increase the risk of postoperative infection are the presence of poorly perfused or devitalized tissue, presence of foreign material (such as orthopedic fixation devices), and entry into a contaminated organ (such as large intestine).

Duration of surgery has a strong influence on the risk of postoperative infection. Studies in both human and veterinary medicine have demonstrated that the risk of postoperative infection increases with the duration of surgery. For example, in animals the risk of postoperative infection is twice as high for patients that undergo a 90-minute procedure compared with a 60-minute procedure.[28]

Antimicrobial Spectrum

The antimicrobial choice will depend on the type and location of the surgery. A good surgeon should be familiar with the normal flora, the opportunistic bacteria, and the most likely pathogens at the surgical site. For example, coliforms and anaerobes are common organisms associated with bowel surgery; for soft tissue surgery, staphylococci are common. It is not necessary to eradicate every potential pathogen, but it is important to have good activity against the most likely opportunistic bacteria.

Drug Considerations: Choice, Timing, and Route

The drug *must* be administered preoperatively if prophylactic antimicrobial use is to be effective. Since there is a lag of at least 30 minutes between peak plasma concentration and peak tissue concentration, in most hospitals, the drug is administered 20 to 30 minutes prior to the actual surgery. Delaying the administration of antibiotics until after surgery may not be any more effective than administration of a placebo. In most cases, redosing should be done 90 minutes to 2 hours after the surgery begins. The practice of continuing antibiotic administration after surgery is not necessary, unless there is evidence of infection.[29]

The route of administration should usually be intravenous. Slow or incomplete absorption of antibiotics from intramuscular or subcutaneous sites is likely following injection of slow-release drugs (e.g., procaine penicillin, oxytetracycline), and they are poor choices. For prophylaxis of bowel surgery, oral treatment with neomycin or metronidazole prior to surgery is accepted.

The drugs most often administered prophylactically for surgery are the first-generation cephalosporins (e.g., cefazolin). Administration of cefazolin every 90 to 120 minutes has been shown to maintain adequate drug concentrations in anesthetized animals when administered during surgery.[30] If the surgery will involve a site in which anaerobic bacteria can be encountered, antibiotics with activity against anaerobes are administered. In these cases, the second-generation cephalosporins cefoxitin or cefotetan, metronidazole, or clindamycin have been used.

REFERENCES

1. Nix DE, Goodwin SD, Peloquin CA, et al: Antibiotic tissue penetration and its relevance: Impact of tissue penetration on infection response. Antimicrob Agents Chemother 35:1953, 1991.
2. Baldwin DR, Andrews JM, Honeybourne D: Bronchoalveolar distribution of cefuroxime axetil and in-vitro efficacy of observed concentrations against respiratory pathogens. J Antimicrob Chemother 30:377, 1992.
3. Meares EM: Prostatitis: Review of pharmacokinetics and therapy. Rev Infect Dis 4:475, 1982.
4. Dorfman M, Barsanti J, Budsberg SC: Enrofloxacin concentrations in dogs with normal prostate and dogs with chronic bacterial prostatitis. Am J Vet Res 56:386, 1995.
5. Pascual A: Uptake and intracellular activity of antimicrobial agents in phagocytic cells. Rev Med Microbiol 6:228, 1995.
6. Schentag JJ, Ballow CH: Tissue-directed pharmacokinetics. Am J Med 91(Suppl 3A):3A–5S, 1991.
7. Yancey RJ, Sanchez MS, Ford CW: Activity of antibiotics against Staphylococcus aureus within polymorphonuclear neutrophils. Eur J Clin Microbiol Infect Dis 10:107, 1991.
8. Hirsh DC, Ruehl WW: A rational approach to the selection of an antimicrobial agent. J Am Vet Med Assoc 10:1058, 1984.
9. Lorian V: Antibiotics in Laboratory Medicine, 4th ed. Media, PA, Williams & Wilkins, 1996.
10. Dow SW: Management of anaerobic infections. Vet Clin North Am Small Anim Pract 18:1167, 1988.
11. Ling GV: Therapeutic strategies involving antimicrobial treatment of the canine urinary tract. J Am Vet Med Assoc 185:1162, 1984.
12. Vogelman B, et al: Correlation of antimicrobial pharmacokinetic parameters with therapeutic efficacy in an animal model. J Infect Dis 158:831, 1988.
13. Nicolau DP, Quintiliani R, Nightingale CH: Antibiotic kinetics and dynamics for the clinician. Med Clin North Am 79:477, 1995.
14. Hyatt JM, McKinnon PS, Zimmer GS, Schentag JJ: The importance of pharmacokinetic/pharmacodynamic surrogate markers to outcome. Clin Pharmacokinet 28:143, 1995.
15. Drusano GL: Role of pharmacokinetics in the outcome of infections. Antimicrob Agents Chemother 32:289, 1988.
16. Frank LA, Kunkle GA: Comparison of the efficacy of cefadroxil and generic and proprietary cephalexin in the treatment of pyoderma in dogs. J Am Vet Med Assoc 203:530, 1993.
17. Freeman CD, Nicolau DP, Belliveau PP, Nightingale CH: Once-daily dosing of aminoglycosides: Review and recommendations for clinical practice. J Antimicrob Chemother 39:677, 1997.
18. Meinen JB, McClure JT, Rosin E: Pharmacokinetics of enrofloxacin in clinically normal dogs and mice and drug pharmacodynamics in neutropenic mice with Escherichia coli and staphylococcal infections. Am J Vet Res 56:1219, 1995.
19. Forrest A, Nix DE, Ballow CH, et al: Pharmacodynamics of intravenous ciprofloxacin in seriously ill patients. Antimicrob Agents Chemother 37:1073, 1993.
20. Papich MG: Doses for selected drugs (Appendix). In Bonagura JD (ed): Current Veterinary Therapy XII. Philadelphia, WB Saunders, 1995.
21. Papich MG: Bacterial resistance. In Bonagura JD (ed): Current Veterinary Therapy XIII. Philadelphia, WB Saunders, 1999, in press.
22. Lloyd DH, Lamport AI, Feeney C: Sensitivity of antibiotics amongst cutaneous and mucosal isolates of canine pathogenic staphylococci in the UK, 1980–1996. Vet Derm 7:171, 1996.
23. Medleau L, Long RE, Brown J, et al: Frequency and antimicrobial susceptibility of staphylococcus species isolated from canine pyoderma. Am J Vet Res 47:229, 1986.
24. Noble WC, Kent LE: Antibiotic resistance in Staphylococcus intermedius isolated from cases of pyoderma in the dog. Vet Derm 3:71, 1992.
25. Papich MG: Antibacterial drug therapy: Focus on new drugs. Vet Clin North Am Small Animal Pract 28:215–231, 1998.
26. Jang SS, Breher JE, Dabaco LA, Hirsh DC: Organisms isolated from dogs and cats with anaerobic infections and susceptibility to selected antimicrobial agents. J Am Vet Med Assoc 210:1610, 1997.
27. Lew DP, Waldvogel FA: Osteomyelitis. N Engl J Med 336:999, 1997.
28. Brown DC, Conzemius MG, Shofer F, et al: Epidemiologic evaluation of postoperative wound infections in dogs and cats. J Am Vet Med Assoc 210:1302, 1997.
29. Kaiser AB: Antimicrobial prophylaxis in surgery. N Engl J Med 315:1129, 1986.
30. Marcellin-Little DJ, Papich MG, Richardson DC, DeYoung DJ: Pharmacokinetic model for cefazolin distribution during total hip arthroplasty in dogs. Am J Vet Res 57:720, 1996.

CHAPTER 75

GLUCOCORTICOID THERAPY

John M. MacDonald

Glucocorticoids represent a variety of compounds used in veterinary medicine for a wide range of organ-system diseases. They are one of the most used medications and also one of the most abused therapies. While glucocorticoid therapy is often an essential part of the treatment plan in most inflammatory and autoimmune disorders, an understanding of how steroids work and a basis for rational therapeutic choices are often missing.

Glucocorticoids are used predominantly for their anti-inflammatory and immunosuppressive effects, although they are incorporated in the treatment of some neoplastic diseases for their tumoricidal activity.[1–6]

Glucocorticoids are naturally produced by the zona reticularis and zona fasciculata of the adrenal cortex and are necessary for their life-sustaining activity. Cortisol (hydro-cortisone) is the predominant natural glucocorticoid in the dog and cat and is one of the unique hormones that are regulated by response to their own levels, unlike others, such as insulin, that respond to glucose levels (Fig. 75–1). In general, glucocorticoid synthesis and release are dependent on the release of the anterior pituitary hormone adrenocorticotrophin (ACTH). ACTH, in turn, is controlled by corticotropin-releasing hormone (CRH) produced by the hypothalamus. A direct negative feedback mechanism establishes control of the amounts of CRH and ACTH produced and thereby the amount of adrenal glucocorticoid production and release.[2–6] In humans, this seems to follow a diurnal rhythm, although this has not been observed in the dog, where multiple episodes of cyclic changes may occur.[7] Nevertheless, it is important to remember that exogenous glucocorti-

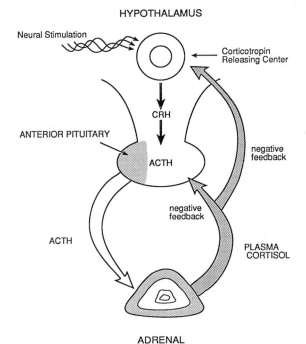

Figure 75–1. Regulation of adrenocortical function. Neural stimulation affects the corticotropin-releasing center, resulting in the production and release of corticotropin-releasing factor (CRF). CRF in turn increases the production and release of adrenocorticotropic hormone (ACTH) from the anterior pituitary. ACTH stimulates the production and release of cortisol in the adrenal cortex. The increased plasma cortisol results in negative feedback on the corticotropin-releasing center and the anterior pituitary, resulting in decreased CRF and ACTH.

coid administration will impact this regulatory mechanism with variation in individual tolerance. Iatrogenic adrenocortical insufficiency can result if therapeutic principles are not adhered to and is not always dose-dependent or relative to duration of therapy.

WHAT ARE GLUCOCORTICOIDS?

Glucocorticoids are hormones like other adrenocortical compounds and are derived from exogenous cholesterol. All adrenal glucocorticoids contain a steroid nucleus consisting of 17 carbon atoms that is replicated in many synthetic formulations particularly to enhance glucocorticoid activity and diminish the mineralocorticoid activity (Fig. 75–2). Incorporation of fluoride within the steroid structure increases the steroid potency. Other molecular manipulations are performed to alter potency and duration of activity. In addition to the actual structure of the glucocorticoid, the base of the steroid compound will affect the duration of activity. Sodium phosphate and succinate have a less prolonged activity, whereas acetonide and acetate have the longest. Bioavailability of all glucocorticoids requires separation of the active chemical from the steroid ester. Solubility factors of succinate, phosphate, or sulfate make their actions more rapid, while the acetate, diacetate, or acetonide compounds are less soluble and provide more sustained effect by the slow release of the glucocorticoid from the base. This has been used to an advantage in cases of intra-articular or intralesional injections, but has also been the source of adverse effects when repeated doses have been used inappropriately in cases requiring long-term maintenance therapy. Injectable, long-acting glucocorticoids often contain acetate or acetonide bases for the steroid to decrease the solubility.

GLUCOCORTICOID TRANSPORTATION AND STEROID RECEPTORS

Transportation of glucocorticoids is predominantly through binding proteins. Greater than 90 per cent of cortisol is bound to plasma protein with corticosteroid-binding globulin (CBG or transcortin) being the predominant one with less binding to albumin. The protein-bound glucocorticoid represents the reservoir with only the unbound or free steroid capable of tissue association. This relationship represents changes in the equilibrium between these two states. The glucocorticoid enters the cell predominantly by passive mechanisms. The affinity of a glucocorticoid and the amount of carrier protein present (CBG or albumin) determine the amount of bound and unbound glucocorticoid.[2–6, 8] Glucocorticoids bind to albumin less preferentially and after the CBG binding has reached the maximal capacity.

STEROID RECEPTORS

The predominance of steroid receptors is somewhat variable depending on the types of tissue or cell. Some tissues are more "steroid-sensitive" than others, although most body tissues are affected to some degree by glucocorticoids and contain receptors. Glucocorticoid receptors are located in the cytosol and vary in number by both cell type and with some species variation. The cat has fewer by as much as 50 per cent compared with other species.[9] The structure of the glucocorticoid receptor consists of three parts: the carboxy-terminal where the glucocorticoid binds, a DNA-binding domain in the middle of the receptor where nuclear binding takes place, and finally the amino terminal domain, also known as the immunogenic domain of unknown activity.[4]

RECEPTOR ACTIVITY

Receptor binding to active glucocorticoid is proportional to some intrinsic factors. For example, dexamethasone seems to bind tighter than cortisol and other glucocorticoids. The affinity, however, does not seem to parallel the glucocorticoid activity on a dose administration basis. Binding of the steroid occurs by active conformation of the receptor, which is in equilibrium with an inactive form (Fig. 75–3). Certain antagonists may bind predominantly on the inactive form, which prevents further conformational changes to occur and hence interfere with glucocorticoid binding. Glucocorticoid binding to the inactive receptor stabilizes the receptor in a high-affinity state, which then becomes activated involving a change in the receptor activity. This activation is thought to be a phosphorylation and the activation is a consequence of dephosphorylation, and the conversion of the inactive receptor to the active one capable of binding hormone occurs by rephosphorylation. The activated receptor carries a different charge and enters the nucleus where it is now able to bind to specific DNA sites. In addition, accessory proteins may be involved in binding the receptor to the DNA (see Fig. 75–3). The glucocorticoid receptor complex in the nucleus regulates transcription of a very small percentage (<1 per cent) of a subset of expressed genes in that cell. Sites of glucocorticoid-receptor complex have action in the nucleus of specific DNA sequences termed glucocorticoid regulatory element (GRE). Interaction of the GRE with glucocorticoid-receptor complex affects the transcription at a nearby promoter. The GRE acts as a hormone-responsive enhancer element; in other words, it can affect the efficiency by which the promoter initiates transcription. GRE can act either on one side or the other from the promoter and at a considerable distance from the promoter. DNA flanking the GRE may also influence the GRE function. The interaction of the receptor-glucocorticoid complex with the GRE probably af-

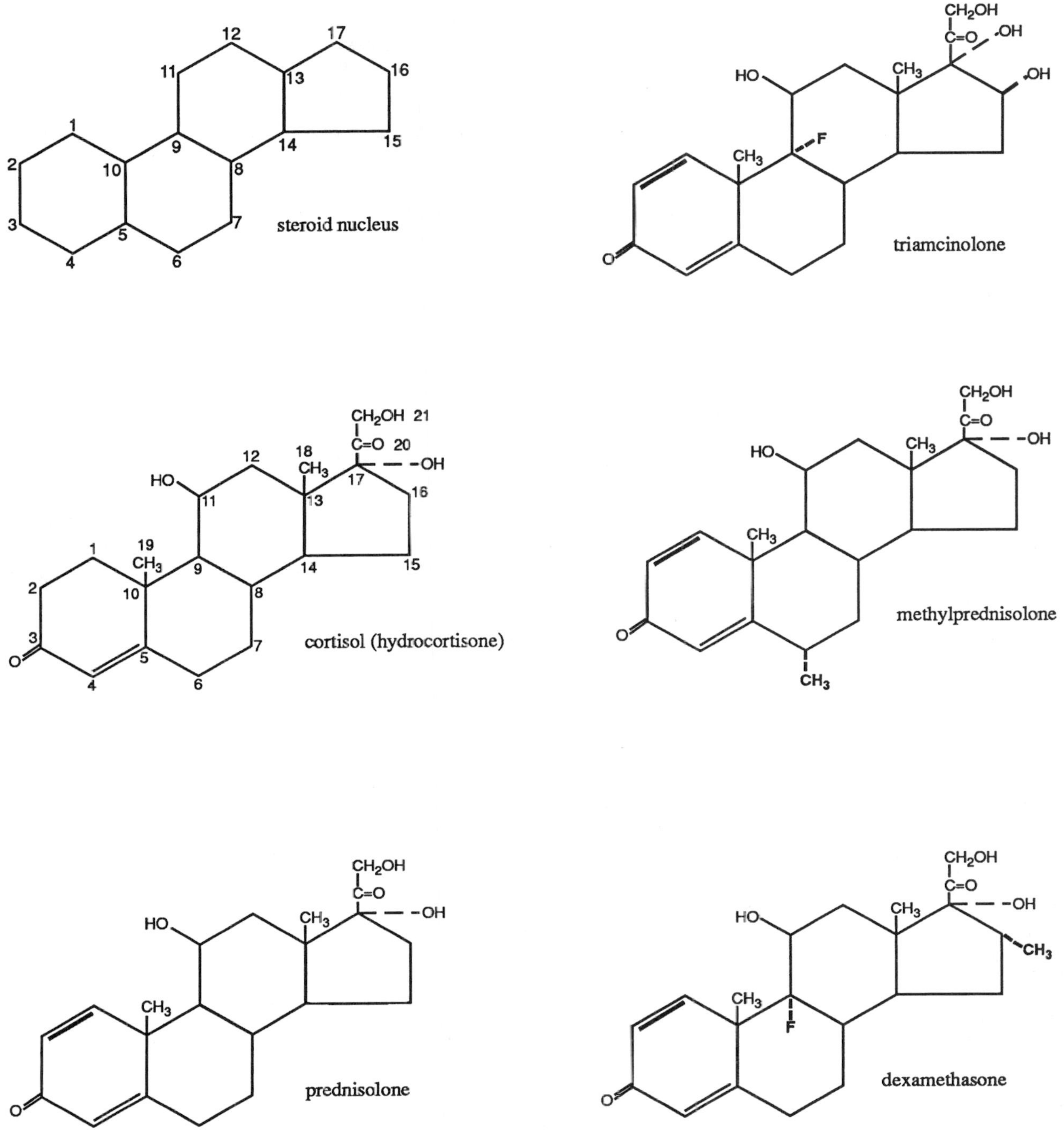

RX

Figure 75–2. Glucocorticoid structure. All glucocorticoids contain a steroid nucleus. Modifications in this structure result in the formation of specific glucocorticoids, often with major alteration in activity. A large number of synthetic glucocorticoids have been produced. Some of the variations among the steroids depicted are indicated in bold.

fects chromatin structure with subsequent effects on transcription initiation, although the primary way in which this occurs is not totally known.[2, 4]

The hormone-receptor complex translocated to the nucleus crucially influences the activity of the gene in triggering a transcription process, thus inducing specific messenger RNA to produce a specific effector protein that may be unique, or it may alter the rate of production of proteins routinely synthesized. This process may stimulate the synthesis of inhibitory proteins and hence produce a catabolic effect. Glucocorticoids also appear to have a permissive effect for actions of many other types of hormones by inducing enzymes subsequently activating cyclic adenosine monophos-

phate (cAMP). After DNA binding, the receptor is recycled with the glucocorticoid released and receptor in the inactive form available for reactivation. Antagonists may bind to the receptor in the inactive form, which would prevent further activity. Other proteins may interact with the receptor, changing their activity and limiting their glucocorticoid effectiveness (see Fig. 75–3).

Responsiveness of glucocorticoids can be extensively regulated and involves modifying some steps following the binding of the steroid to the receptor. Change of responsiveness may also be caused by effects of other hormones or factors on the expression of the glucocorticoid-regulated gene or on the capability of glucocorticoids to regulate that

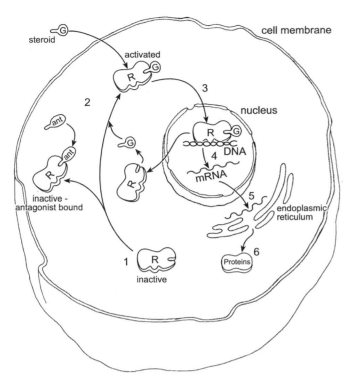

Figure 75–3. Glucocorticoid receptor activity. Free glucocorticoids (G) passively diffuse across the cell membrane into the cell. (1) Glucocorticoid receptors (R) are present in the cell in an inactive state and may bind with either a glucocorticoid (G) or an antagonist (ant). (2) The receptor becomes activated when a glucocorticoid binds to it. (3) The activated receptor migrates to the nucleus, where it contacts specific areas of DNA. (4) Transcription of messenger RNA (mRNA) occurs, which results in protein production from the endoplasmic reticulum (5–6). The glucocorticoid receptor will release the glucocorticoid in the cytoplasm, leaving the receptor in an inactive form that is free to bind with either antagonist or glucocorticoid.

gene. Also glucocorticoids and other factors regulate receptor levels or receptor activity affecting responsiveness. The determinant of response to steroid therapy depends on several other factors, including the systemic disposition of the compounds. This includes the protein-binding characteristics of that particular glucocorticoid with transcortin or albumin. In addition, certain drugs are administered in an active form that must be converted to an active metabolite. Prednisone is the inactive form of prednisolone, and cortisone is converted to hydrocortisone. Finally, there is a lag time for the physiologic effect itself to take place.[2, 4, 6]

ANTI-INFLAMMATORY EFFECTS OF GLUCOCORTICOIDS

The anti-inflammatory action of glucocorticoids is believed to be mediated by anti-inflammatory protein(s) synthesized in target cells under the influence of the glucocorticoid. Part of this mode of action of anti-inflammatory protein is that of reduced production of proinflammatory metabolites, especially those derived from arachidonic acid. Prostaglandins I_2 and E_2 plus leukotrienes C_4, D_4, E_4, and B_4 may be responsible for the end-inflammatory response modified by decreased metabolism of arachidonic acid. In general, glucocorticoids induce an antiphospholipase effect by using second-messenger proteins called lipocortins. These proteins inhibit cellular phospholipase A, thus reducing the release of arachidonic acid and all subsequent proinflammatory mediators (prostaglandins, prostacycline, thromboxane, and leu-

kotrienes). Lipocortins regulate cellular metabolism of phospholipases as well. Many cells release arachidonic acid when stimulated by neurotransmitters and certain drugs. Lipocortins are present even in cells not treated with glucocorticoids and are naturally enzymatically digested by proteases. They promote the maturation as well of suppressor T cells and inhibit the proliferation response to T cells by mitogens. Beta-lipocortins have a dose-dependent inhibitory effect on the acute phase of cytotoxic T cells. They also inhibit antibody-dependent cytotoxicity by natural killer cells. Further, they protect cells from complement-mediated lysis.[10–12]

The anti-inflammatory action of glucocorticoids is related to the mediation by anti-inflammatory protein(s) synthesized in target cells under their influence. They affect a wide range of inflammatory cells and mediators of inflammation. The effect of glucocorticoids on neutrophils produces an absolute leukocytosis with a neutrophilia that is not related to the original neutrophil count. This is accomplished by increasing release of cells from the marginated granulocyte pool to the circulation. In addition, the neutrophils' half-life is prolonged as a consequence of glucocorticoid influence. There is also a decreased egress of neutrophils from circulation to sites of inflammation. Endothelial adherence of leukocytes is blocked by glucocorticoids, although studies show cortisone has minimal effect on the vascular stasis or extravascular migration of leukocytes once they have entered the tissue. Glucocorticoids also affect neutrophil metabolism. Cortisol decreases neutrophil cell glycolysis and aerobic production of lactic acid but does not effect the oxygen utilization. Some evidence suggests that neutrophil lysosomes are not stabilized by glucocorticoids similar to other cell lysosomes. Mediator release from human neutrophils can be inhibited by glucocorticoids.[2, 13, 14]

There have been conflicting reports on the effect of glucocorticoids on the ability of neutrophils to ingest and kill bacteria. It is, however, well established that glucocorticoids compromise host defense mechanisms and depress resistance to infection. Glucocorticoids have demonstrated inhibition of metabolic processes that are important to the intracellular killing of microorganisms.[2, 12, 13]

Glucocorticoids influence lymphocytes by shifting the traffic of circulating cells. Lymphopenia usually occurs shortly after glucocorticoid exposure within 4 to 6 hours, and there appears to be a differential sensitivity of lymphocyte subsets. T lymphocytes are more sensitive than B cells. Further, helper or inducer lymphocytes (CD4) are more sensitive than the cytotoxic suppressor cells (CD8). In general, the absent number of any subset either is unchanged or decreased in number. The bone marrow has been postulated as the site of extravascular redistribution, although this has not been unequivocally determined in humans. Further, the mechanism of steroid-induced redistribution of lymphocytes is not clearly delineated. Although the direct influence of the lymphocyte distribution pattern is often gone 24 hours after pulse therapy, some of the immunomodulating effects of the drug may have long-term activity.[2, 12]

The response of T lymphocytes to phytomitogens is affected by glucocorticoids. Glucocorticoids suppress T-cell proliferation, whereas B-cell proliferation is not as sensitive. Proliferation response to antigens is particularly important with reference to immunosuppressive effects. Steroid influence on natural killer lymphocytes has a variable activity that tends to suppress this action. Steroids also inhibit the production of interleukin-2, which results in inhibition of lymphocyte proliferation and cytotoxic function. In addition, glucocorticoids cause suppression of B-cell growth factors (BCGF) affecting the proliferation of this cell type.

Cell lysis is more prominent in certain subsets but predominantly affects those in nonperipheral blood compartments and lymphocytes that have been activated. The immunoglobulin production of B lymphocytes is variable. IgG and IgA have greater suppressive effect from glucocorticoids than IgM. Early B-cell activity is inhibited by glucocorticoids and suppression of immunoglobulin synthesis. Immunoglobulin production, however, is not the most important aspect of anti-inflammatory or immunosuppressive activity of glucocorticoids. As well as having a direct effect upon lymphocytes, glucocorticoids also induce immunomodulation by their effects on production of soluble factors as well as modulation of accessory cell function.[2, 12, 14]

Glucocorticoids induce eosinopenia, which is most likely a consequence of change in distribution to various tissues. Supportive evidence for a lytic or toxic effect on eosinophils has not been determined unequivocally. Supporting evidence, however, suggests that the reticuloendothelial system is important for the redistribution of the eosinophils. Glucocorticoids increase eosinophil migration to lymph nodes and thymus. In addition, eosinophils have a higher phagocytosis by macrophages under this influence. The spleen may also concentrate eosinophils, but it is not necessary for eosinopenia to occur. There is no evidence that the lungs serve as a reservoir for eosinophils, and there is little evidence that eosinophilopoiesis is affected by glucocorticoids. Bone marrow release of eosinophils may be prevented, but eosinophilopoiesis is not inhibited from in vivo studies.[2, 13] This anti-inflammatory effect of glucocorticoids on eosinophils is beneficial for the treatment of many diseases where hypersensitivity or parasitism results in an eosinophilic inflammatory response. It also appears that eosinophil adherence can be transiently reduced by glucocorticoids as well as inhibition of eosinophil chemotaxis. Eosinophils also exhibit capacity for antibody-dependent cell-mediated cytotoxicity (ADCC). This is an important immunologic mechanism in host defense against parasites. Inhibition of ADCC occurs at nonphysiologic concentrations of glucocorticoids.[2, 5, 13, 14]

Mononuclear cells are key to many bodily functions:

1. They serve as antigen-presenting accessory cells during the induction of cell-mediated and humoral immune responses.
2. They also function as "professional" phagocytes against bacteria, fungi, viruses, etc.
3. In combination with antibody, they may have tumor cell–killing capacity.
4. They are also essential for the role of clearing senescent cells, particularly erythrocytes and bone remodeling, wound healing, and lung surfactant turnover.

Glucocorticoid receptors for macrophages are similar to other tissues, although they appear to have more receptors than lymphocytes or neutrophils, either as a consequence of their larger size or as a difference in a phenotypic change. Glucocorticoid effects on mononuclear cells and macrophages result in a transient monocytopenia, although there is no evidence for decreased chemotactic activity. There is evidence of inhibition of maturation of monocytes to active macrophages. Glucocorticoids inhibit the production, distribution, and certain functions of mononuclear phagocytes. Some of the effects may be a consequence of production of lipocortins by macrophages that play a central role by decreasing arachidonic acid production as well as other immunosuppressive effects. Glucocorticoids also inhibit production of tumor necrosis factor (TNF), which affects a wide variety of inflammatory processes. The major anti-inflammatory effect of glucocorticoids is related also to decreased accumulation of mononuclear phagocytes at the inflammatory foci. This may be a consequence of decreased chemotactic factors by other cells, including T-lymphocytes outside the mononuclear cell population. Antienzymic effects of glucocorticoids may also be a factor. Inhibition of cytokines such as IL-1, IFN-gamma, and TNF/cachectin are caused by glucocorticoids.[2, 14, 15]

Glucocorticoids reduce the number of circulating basophils most likely through reduced production. Glucocorticoid effect on mast cells has been substantiated showing reduction of the number of mucosal mast cells, although the subtype of mast cell found in connective tissue is less sensitive. The reduction of mast cells most likely is a consequence of inhibition of IL-3 or mast cell growth factor, although there may be a direct glucocorticoid effect on mast cells that occurs. Migration of basophils is significantly reduced by glucocorticoids. There is little evidence that steroids directly inhibit production and release of inflammatory mediators by mast cells, and may represent decreased number of mast cells thereby achieving the minimized effect of degranulation. The application of glucocorticoids topically resulting in decreased response to antigen may involve the decreased number of mast cells or the decreased access of antigen to mast cells in the tissue.[2, 13, 15]

GENERAL EFFECTS OF GLUCOCORTICOIDS

Physiologic levels of glucocorticoids are necessary for the maintenance of nearly all body systems and are recognized for altering deleterious effects of stress. The extent of the effect of the glucocorticoid is dependent on its potency and dose in addition to individual response.

The catabolic effects of glucocorticoids are responsible for muscle weakness and atrophy. Osteoporosis may also be observed and interference with growth hormone release and decrease in fibrocartilage growth. Carbohydrate, protein, and lipid metabolism is influenced by glucocorticoids. Increased gluconeogenesis and a diabetogenic effect are observed with elevations of blood glucose seen clinically. Mobilization of amino acids from peripheral tissue and breakdown of triglycerides in adipose tissue are consequences of glucocorticoid influence. Free fatty acids and amino acids are subsequently available for conversion to hepatic glycogen.[3, 5, 6, 14, 16]

Glucocorticoids affect water and electrolyte balance predominantly by increasing glomerular filtration rate and inhibiting the action of antidiuretic hormone (ADH) on renal tubules. Glucocorticoids also have increased ADH inactivation. Retention of sodium, excretion of potassium, and diuresis are expectations of glucocorticoid influence but will vary with regard to the specific steroid used and the individual's responsiveness. There is an expansion of extracellular fluid volume as a result of glucocorticoid therapy.[3, 16]

Adrenal steroid hormones influence the physiologic actions of adrenergic agents. Catecholamine stimulation of both hepatic glucose production and muscle uptake of glucose is enhanced by steroid hormones. Positive ionotropism, positive chronotropism, and increased arrhythmogenicity are enhanced by glucocorticoids through effect on adrenergic receptors.[17]

CONCEPTS OF GLUCOCORTICOID USE

Glucocorticoids are most commonly used for antipruritic, anti-inflammatory, or immunosuppressant effects. There are many factors that should be considered in determining the gluococorticoid to be used. They include the route of administration and the regimen of therapy (how much, how often, and for how long?).[5, 14, 18–21] Considerations for glucocorticoid treatment require responding to an inventory of questions:

(1) What is the condition to be treated, and how serious is the disorder? Variation of life-threatening disease states to minor cutaneous irritations is observed in veterinary practice, and consideration of the risk:benefit ratio should be evaluated when selecting the mode of therapy. (2) How long will the glucocorticoid treatment be used? Short-acting parenterally administered drugs would be appropriate for short durations of treatment, or repositol glucocorticoid may be indicated for a pruritic condition whose underlying cause is resolvable in a short time. An animal with atopic or autoimmune disease will require protracted therapy and would be a candidate for alternate-day therapy with an oral short-acting glucocorticoid. (3) Which glucocorticoid preparation best fits the needs for the specific situation? This again is contingent upon the disease treated, the anticipated duration of therapy, and the individual tolerance of specific glucocorticoids. (4) What is the anticipated effective steroid dose? This will vary, depending on drug potency and indication of administration (shock, immunosuppression, antipruritic). This may have a major impact on increasing adverse effects in diseases requiring high-dose therapy. (5) Is the patient predisposed to known hazards of steroid therapy, or is there a known intolerance? Animals with diabetes mellitus, hepatopathies, pancreatitis, coexisting infections/parasitism, or renal failure may pose concern for the use of glucocorticoids. Sensitivity to polydipsia and polyuria may appear to be more of a nuisance, but to the pet owner it may represent a major intolerance. Many allergic dogs have a propensity to develop secondary infections (staphylococcal pyoderma, cutaneous *Malassezia,* and dermatophytosis) when treated with glucocorticoids. A thorough medical history should be determined, particularly in older patients or those with suspected systemic disease. (6) Have other methods of treatment been considered or utilized to minimize the glucocorticoid dosage and side effects? This is particularly important in animals requiring prolonged therapy as in the pruritic patient or in cases such as autoimmune disease where a high dose of glucocorticoid is used. Antihistamines, essential fatty acid therapy, and topical antipruritics should always be considered first in the pruritic patient and incorporated with steroid treatment. Use of immunosuppressants such as azathioprine, chlorambucil, or gold salts may be considered in treating the autoimmune patient. (7) Is the use of an alternate-day regimen indicated? In general, any animal requiring glucocorticoid treatment for longer than 3 to 4 weeks should be placed on an alternate-day regimen requiring the use of short-acting, low-potency glucocorticoids by oral administration. Prednisolone, prednisone, and methylprednisolone are suitable for this purpose, although oral triamcinolone has also been used in this type of regimen.

DRUG SELECTION

There continue to be certain myths regarding potency variations among glucocorticoids and their effectiveness for attaining an anti-inflammatory response. Variation in drug potency represents a difference in the properties of the chemical in receptor binding and duration of activity on the receptor with respect to a specific tissue. The receptor does not respond differently with each glucocorticoid but essentially the same. The potency difference between prednisolone and dexamethasone, for example, means it takes far less of the dexamethasone to attain an equipotent effect of the prednisolone (Table 75–1).

Choosing a more potent glucocorticoid when presented with a clinical case solely to cause a greater therapeutic impact on the disease is an unacceptable practice. The first objective of glucocorticoid therapy is to use the least potent drug at the lowest possible dosage. A single rule cannot be set for selecting a specific steroid for therapy. Experience based on specific diseases with given patients can be useful. In some cases, steroids may lose effectiveness as a consequence of tachyphylaxis and the selection of a different drug at equipotent dosage may result in control once again.[5, 14, 19] Aside from steroid tachyphylaxis, the more common cause of decreased steroid effectiveness in pruritic dermatitis is concurrence of coexisting or complicating disease(s) such as infection, parasitism, or excess allergen exposure.

Prednisone, prednisolone, and methylprednisolone are the most often used glucocorticoids. These are short-acting glucocorticoids with minimal mineralocorticoid activity and low-potency anti-inflammatory effect (see Table 75–1). Prednisone is converted to prednisolone in the liver, but essentially the drugs may be dosed the same. More potent drugs

TABLE 75–1. RELATIVE POTENCY OF GLUCOCORTICOIDS

DRUGS	ANTI-INFLAMMATORY POTENCY	MINERALO-CORTICOID POTENCY	EQUIVALENT DOSE (mg)	HALF-LIFE (hr) PLASMA	HALF-LIFE (hr) TISSUE
Short-Acting					
Cortisone	0.8		25		
Hydrocortisone	1.0	2	20	1	8–12
Intermediate-Acting					
Prednisone	4.0	1	5	1	12–36
Prednisolone	4.0	1	5	1	12–36
Methylprednisolone	5.0	0	4	1.5	12–36
Long-Acting					
Triamcinolone	40.0	0	1.3	5	12–36
Flumethasone	15.0	0	0.5	35–54	35–54
Dexamethasone	40.0	0	0.5	3.5	35–54
Betamethasone	50.0	0	0.4	35–54	35–54

such as betamethasone and dexamethasone are reserved for specific and infrequently observed indications. Triamcinolone is an intermediate-acting drug with comparable potency to methylprednisolone. It has been considered a longer-acting drug as a result of its persistent pharmacologic activity. One should consider not only the response of the disease to the steroid treatment, but also the tolerance or intolerance of the patient.

ROUTE OF ADMINISTRATION

The oral route is most commonly chosen and is preferred because it is most easily regulated and dosage change can be accomplished more regularly. Since many of the drugs used are short or intermediate acting, there is minimal residual effect in the event of intolerance. Most oral forms are tablets containing the free steroid alcohol resulting in rapid absorption with rather short half-lives. One should be reminded that biologic activity may persist long after the plasma half-life has been surpassed because of the mechanism by which glucocorticoids work. The oral route is also preferred because it is simple to use and relatively inexpensive and is the only safe and therapeutically effective way to provide chronic glucocorticoid therapy, especially in dogs. Liquid suspension formulations of prednisolone and prednisolone are available for administration to smaller dogs.

PARENTERAL GLUCOCORTICOID ADMINISTRATION

Parenteral administration of glucocorticoids should be reserved for those selective cases where the duration of disease is relatively short (4 weeks or less), the treatment is performed under life-threatening conditions (shock, cerebral/spinal cord edema, septic shock, etc.), or limitations of oral therapy exist (pet personality, comatose or semicomatose state, vomiting, etc.). Injectable steroids are most commonly administered by intramuscular or subcutaneous injection, although intravenous or intralesional injections are performed (Table 75–2). Although most injectable steroids are not approved for subcutaneous administration, it is a common practice to avoid the discomfort of an intramuscular injection. Obese patients should, on the other hand, be administered an intramuscular injection to minimize the sequestration of the steroid in fat tissue.[14] Another concern for subcutaneous administration is local atrophy, although focal alopecia, pigmentary changes, and epidermal and dermal atrophy are more common.[14]

Glucocorticoids that contain either sodium succinate or

sodium phosphate formulations can be administered either intramuscularly or intravenously. Prednisolone sodium succinate is often administered by intravenous injection for the treatment of traumatic or hypovolemic shock or acute neurologic trauma. The relative rapid bioavailability of the glucocorticoid in this preparation makes it ideal for these circumstances. The acetate- and acetonide-formulated steroids produce an insoluble compound that results in greater duration of therapy by a more sustained release. Methylprednisolone acetate is an example of a repositol glucocorticoid with long duration of activity despite the comparative shorter-acting methylprednisolone properties. Repositol drugs such as these are not intended for chronic (>3 to 4 weeks) treatment of cases, with the exception of the cat. Triamcinolone acetonide is another example of extending the duration of activity by combining the steroid with an ester resulting in poor solubility and longer duration of action. The latter is often used for intra-articular or intralesional injections. Both methylprednisolone acetate and triamcinolone acetonide are inappropriately overused in pruritic dermatologic disease. These drugs are acceptable for short-duration problems such as a dog with scabies receiving scabicidal therapy or a flea allergy case receiving insecticidal therapy. In both cases, the primary disease is being treated and the steroid injection is required only once or twice.

TOPICAL ADMINISTRATION

Topical glucocorticoids are used in dermatologic therapy in a variety of formulations and active steroid compounds. Applied topically, they will still be systemically absorbed and have been associated with deleterious effects. They are available in creams, lotions, foams, gels, solution, shampoos, rinses, and ointments. Topical glucocorticoids are frequently incorporated in otic medications and contribute a desirable anti-inflammatory effect in most cases. They are usually combined with antimicrobial agents. Topical glucocorticoids may be used as adjunctive therapy to systemic nonsteroidal antipruritic treatment or alternate-day oral glucocorticoid treatment. Glucocorticoids commonly used include hydrocortisone, prednisone, dexamethasone, betamethasone, triamcinolone acetonide, and fluocinolone acetonide. More details on this specific modality of treatment may be found elsewhere.[5, 14, 21–24]

ORAL GLUCOCORTICOID THERAPY

Anti-inflammatory Steroid Therapy. The most common use of glucocorticoids is for the anti-inflammatory effect in treating skin disease, although the drugs and regimens are applicable to treating other organ-system diseases. Oral prednisone and prednisolone are most commonly employed and at interchangeable dosages. Conversion of prednisone to prednisolone is not a practical concern in typical cases.[14, 21] The first phase of treatment (induction) is implemented when the steroid therapy is first initiated. The oral glucocorticoid is administered on a daily basis for 7 to 14 days before converting to the maintenance phase (Table 75–3). The anti-inflammatory dosage for prednisone or prednisolone is 0.5 mg/lb (1.1 mg/kg) every 24 hours for the dog, and 1.1 to 2.2 mg/lb (2.2 to 4.4 mg/kg) for the cat. Some prefer to divide the dosage to twice daily, but experience using both alternatives appears to have little clinical difference. In general, cats require about twice the dosage of dogs for both

TABLE 75–2. INJECTABLE GLUCOCORTICOIDS FOR ANTIPRURITIC THERAPY IN DOGS AND CATS

DRUG	DOSAGE	SPECIES
Prednisone or prednisolone	0.5 mg/kg q24h	Dog/cat
Triamcinolone	0.1–0.2 mg/kg	Dog/cat
Methylprednisolone acetate	2–40 mg/animal	Dog
	10–20 mg/animal	Cat
Flumethasone	0.06–0.25 mg/animal	Dog
	0.03–0.125 mg/animal	Cat
Dexamethasone	0.25–1.0 mg/animal	Dog
	0.125–0.5 mg/animal	Cat
Betamethasone	0.2–0.4 mg/kg	Dog

Modified from Scott DW, Miller WH, Griffin CE: Dermatologic therapy In Small Animal Dermatology. Philadelphia, WB Saunders, 1995, p 242.

TABLE 75–3. ORAL GLUCOCORTICOID ANTIPRURITIC/ANTI-INFLAMMATORY THERAPY FOR THE DOG

DRUG	DOSAGE
Prednisone or prednisolone	0.5–1.0 mg/kg daily for induction, then every other day for maintenance
Methylprednisolone	1.0–2.0 mg/5 kg daily for induction, then 0.5–1.0 mg/5 kg every other day for maintenance
Triamcinolone	0.1–0.2 mg/kg daily for induction, then 0.025–0.05 mg/kg every 72 hours

induction and maintenance therapy. It is proposed that cats require more glucocorticoid because they have 50 per cent fewer glucocorticoid receptors in steroid-sensitive cells.[9]

Methylprednisolone is another short-acting, low-potency glucocorticoid suitable for long-term therapy. The addition of the methyl group to the existing prednisolone structure enhances the potency (see Fig. 75–2) but also has more sparing effect of the polydipsia or polyuria. The dosage is variable at 0.1 to 0.4 mg/lb (0.25 to 0.8 mg/kg) for the dog but usually requires doubling the dose for cats.

Triamcinolone is used less commonly for oral anti-inflammatory therapy but is an alternate drug. The initial dose for the dog is 0.1 to 0.15 mg/lb/day (0.2 to 0.3 mg/kg/day) and then tapered to a dose of 0.02 to 0.5 mg/lb (0.05 to 0.1 mg/kg) every other day. The dosage for cats is 0.25 to 0.5 mg/lb/day (0.5 to 1.0 mg/kg/day). As with other oral glucocorticoids, the maintenance alternate-day regimen may be preceded by an induction phase where the drug is administered once daily or divided twice daily.

Cats have a higher tolerance for glucocorticoids, and therefore drugs that would not be acceptable for longer-term therapy in the dog may safely be employed in the cat. Dexamethasone is a long-acting, potent glucocorticoid with limited application in treatment of most inflammatory diseases, particularly those with long-term management. The use of oral dexamethasone in the cat, however, has the advantage of less frequent administration on a maintenance regimen (twice weekly), and because the cat has greater glucocorticoid tolerance, there is less concern for side effects. The dosage is 0.05 mg/kg (0.25 mg tablet/cat) orally for 7 to 10 days for induction and then on a maintenance regimen of twice weekly (Table 75–4).

It is reported by some veterinarians that oral glucocorticoids are not effective in controlling the disease compared with injectable steroids. This impression may be the result of coexisting problems as often seen in dermatologic cases such as infection (bacterial pyoderma, dermatophytosis, or cutaneous *Malassezia*) in addition to allergic dermatoses (flea allergy, canine atopy, or food allergy). Removing the infectious or parasitic components or administering proper and equivalent oral steroid dosage would likely result in the

TABLE 75–4. ORAL GLUCOCORTICOID ANTIPRURITIC/ANTI-INFLAMMATORY THERAPY FOR THE CAT

DRUG	DOSAGE
Prednisone or prednisolone	2.2–4.4 mg/kg once daily for 7–14 days then 0.5–2.2 mg/kg every other day
Triamcinolone	0.5–1.0 mg/kg daily for 7–14 days, then 2–3 times/week for maintenance
Dexamethasone	0.1 mg/kg once daily for 7 days, then twice weekly

control of the pruritus in these cases. Another approach often used in practice is the sequential administration of glucocorticoids with an initial injection of steroid followed by a regimen of oral therapy. This technique is used to induce a more immediate steroid effect by the injection and maintain a protracted steroid effect from the oral therapy. The mind set that injectables work faster is *not* supported by the absorption rates of oral versus intramuscular therapy or the mechanism by which glucocorticoids work. There is **no** indication for routine use of this technique. Use of properly dosed oral therapy will attain pharmacologic levels of the drug in the same time as the injectable and will eliminate another therapeutic step.

One of the most common errors in steroid therapy is not attaining proper dosage. Comparing equipotency of drugs is important to determine a desirable dose. Variation in both treatment response and tolerance of steroids should be considered. In lieu of selecting a higher than recommended dosage of a steroid or resorting to an injectable form, it is prudent to first reevaluate the problem and possibly try a different low-potency steroid. Oftentimes the glucocorticoid is underdosed for the body weight of the animal, although individual variation of response is also observed. Steroid tachyphylaxis also accounts for decreased drug efficiency.

Immunosuppressive Glucocorticoid Therapy. Immunosuppression therapy may be accomplished using the same drugs used for anti-inflammatory treatment but at a higher dosage. Prednisone is most commonly used, but prednisolone may be used interchangeably. The dosage for dogs is 1 to 3 mg/lb (2.2 to 6.6 mg/kg) every 24 hours or divided twice daily for induction. Since this dosage is double that of the anti-inflammatory dose, dividing the treatment to twice daily may reduce gastritis, although it will not affect other gastrointestinal adverse effects (ulceration and hemorrhage). The immunosuppressive dosage of prednisone or prednisolone for cats is 2 to 5 mg/lb/day (4 to 10 mg/kg/day). Induction is used initially by daily therapy until remission of clinical signs is observed. This usually requires 3 to 4 weeks or longer in most cases. Conversion to an alternate-day regimen should be done gradually.

MAINTENANCE GLUCOCORTICOID THERAPY

Maintenance glucocorticoid therapy includes any treatment that exceeds 3 to 4 weeks in duration. This often includes hypersensitivity conditions (canine atopy, flea allergy dermatitis, contact allergy, allergic pulmonary disease), inflammatory neuropathies, and gastroenteritis. Anticipation of the progression of the disease by its characteristics or the medical history of the individual patient is used to project the duration of therapy.

ALTERNATE-DAY GLUCOCORTICOID THERAPY

The only safe and efficacious maintenance regimen for glucocorticoid therapy is alternate-day oral administration. Glucocorticoids are limited to those having short duration of activity, minimal or no mineralocorticoid activity, and low potency. Prednisone, prednisolone, and methylprednisolone have the qualities ideal for this treatment. Triamcinolone has been used on an every-3-day treatment regimen in the dog and cat for maintenance, although every-other-day regimens have been used by clinicians for protracted times without recognition of deleterious effects by evaluating blood parameters (complete blood cell counts and serum chemistries) or monitoring the patient for outward signs of hyperglucocorticoidism.

The purpose of alternate-day steroid therapy is to minimize side effects while maintaining pharmacologic activity. The hypothesis is that the anti-inflammatory glucocorticoid activity persists longer than the side effects. The intermittent treatment of the glucocorticoid produces a cyclic pattern somewhat similar to physiologic changes allowing some time without the adverse influence of the steroid. Because full expression of the disease may occur only when the inflammatory activity reaches a certain level for a protracted time, readministration of the glucocorticoid prior to attaining that threshold of inflammation is sufficient to curtail development of symptoms. An interval of therapy at 12, 24, or even 36 hours is accompanied by adrenocortical suppression, and an interval of 72 hours usually does not provide effective control of the disease. Therefore, the optimal interval is every 48 hours, although certain clinical diseases may be controlled with medication every 72 hours.[5, 14, 18, 20–22]

Alternate-day steroid therapy should be expected to be nearly as effective as daily therapy without the risks of adrenocortical suppression or marked signs of hyperglucocorticoidism. Conversion from daily therapy to alternate-day therapy is somewhat contingent on the type of disease being treated. Conversion of daily therapy of glucocorticoids using an anti-inflammatory or antipruritic dosage may be done simply by administering the daily treatment (either a once a day or divided twice a day dose) as a single treatment every 48 hours. The time of the treatment is not critical in veterinary medicine because there is not a well-defined diurnal steroid cycle observed in the species veterinarians most often treat. Owner convenience is more of a factor, as well as anticipated side effects such as polyuria/polydipsia on the day of treatment.

The conversion from continuous (daily) immunosuppressive glucocorticoid therapy to an alternate-day treatment regimen is best done gradually. There is less tendency for exacerbations when conversion is not made abruptly. There are several methods described for this process and probably others that individuals find preferable for their purposes. This is an area where there is a lot of variation and no hard-and-fast rules about the protocol. Animals with autoimmune skin diseases may not achieve complete disease resolution through this therapy even when combined with other chemotherapeutic pharmaceuticals. A level of acceptance by the pet owner of residual symptoms may be necessary. The clinician should be cautious in regard to the treatment being worse than the disease, particularly if the problem is not a life-threatening process. The following represent methods of converting to an alternate-day regimen when using immunosuppressive therapy. Tailoring of the treatment to each individual patient, however, is mandatory to attain that delicate balance between disease control and adversities of the therapy.

1. If a divided daily dose is used, the first objective is to decrease the frequency so that the total dose is administered only once daily. The dosage of the once-daily treatment is then increased gradually, but only for the administration on the alternate day. This is done while continuing the next-day dose as previous so that the first day of the 2-day cycle will have the increased dose and the second day will maintain the conventional dose. Next, the second-day dose will be eliminated gradually by decreasing the amount. Finally, the alternate-day treatment will be tapered to reach the optimal dosage. A change in dosage should not be attempted more frequently than every 10 to 14 days (five to seven treatments).

2. Another approach less complicated than the former is to double the daily dose on the first day of each 2-day cycle and then gradually taper the dose on the second day, remembering to make adjustments gradually and not more frequently than every five to seven treatments. This is continued until the alternate-day dose has been eliminated. The dose then used on the alternate-day regimen is gradually adjusted until the level of disease control has been optimized with the lowest possible dosage of glucocorticoid.

There is no evidence that one of the conversion plans is better than the other. Modifying the treatment to the individual patient is of major importance. If the simplified plan does not work and exacerbation is observed during the conversion, it may indicate that (1) the conversion to alternate-day therapy was premature, (2) adjunctive therapy may be necessary to attain maximal control of the problem (e.g., azathioprine, chlorambucil, chrysotherapy), (3) a more gradual transition is necessary for that given case (do not rush the process). This may require returning to a daily regimen for a period of time before attempting conversion again. Conversion to an alternate-day regimen should not be initiated hastily and is best accomplished using gradual conversion after an induction period sufficient to resolve clinical symptoms. This is particularly important in most autoimmune diseases.

Immunosuppressive glucocorticoid therapy even in combination with other immunosuppressants may result in exacerbations requiring treatment modification. Typically the dosage of glucocorticoid is increased or the animal is returned to an induction (daily) regimen of glucocorticoid at a standard dosage. Another option for either recurrent or refractory cases or simply to initiate induction is the use of a pulse therapeutic regimen with methylprednisolone sodium succinate; 0.05 mg/lb (0.11 mg/kg) is added to a sterile solution of 5 per cent dextrose in water and administered via indwelling intravenous catheter over 1 hour and repeated for 3 consecutive days. Cimetidine has been administered at 2 mg/lb (4 mg/kg) every 8 hours by mouth during the administration of steroid.[25] Maintenance therapy may be initiated 24 hours after the third day of pulse therapy. The additional treatment with other immunosuppressant drugs would be indicated if relapses are observed with glucocorticoid therapy alone.

The maintenance alternate-day glucocorticoid therapeutic dosage for immunosuppressive effect is usually between 0.5 and 1.0 mg/lb (1.0 to 2.0 mg/kg) but may be higher in certain cases. Initiation of other adjunctive therapy should be included if optimal control cannot be attained with this regimen.

SPECIFIC USES OF GLUCOCORTICOIDS

Glucocorticoids used for shock or cerebrospinal trauma often include different glucocorticoids and dosages than conventional anti-inflammatory or immunosuppression therapy.[5, 18, 20, 26] Although there may be some variation in the reports of efficacy based upon experimental data, it is usually an accepted treatment regimen to include glucocorticoid treatment in certain CNS disease. Methylprednisolone has been beneficial in cats with induced spinal cord trauma at 7 to 14 mg/lb (15 to 30 mg/kg) administered intravenously. The equipotent dose of dexamethasone is 1.2 to 2.2 mg/lb (2.5

to 5 mg/kg). A follow-up treatment in 3 to 4 hours with methylprednisolone is often recommended. Conversion to a short duration of maintenance therapy may be indicated with oral therapy.[26]

Glucocorticoids are also advocated in the treatment of shock. Controversy exists with regard to septic or hemorrhagic shock. Large doses are usually administered for shock and should be administered as early in the condition as possible.[5] Methylprednisolone should be used at 7 to 14 mg/lb (15 to 30 mg/kg) body weight and dexamethasone is 2 to 4 mg/lb (4 to 8 mg/kg).

Adrenocortical insufficiency requires glucocorticoid replacement whether the disease is primary (Addison's) or secondary (e.g., exogenous glucocorticoid therapy or Lysodren). Low-potency, short-acting glucocorticoids should be used at a dosage sufficient to provide for the glucocorticoid requirement. This has been estimated as 0.1 mg/lb/day (0.2 mg/kg/day) of hydrocortisone.[14] This dosage may be used on a daily basis with restoration of the hypothalamic-pituitary-adrenal axis. The use of more potent glucocorticoids such as prednisone or prednisolone is not necessary unless there is an active inflammatory disease requiring therapy. Using these drugs on an alternate-day regimen will not hasten the recovery from iatrogenic Cushing's or the coexisting adrenocortical insufficiency. Evaluation of the adrenal reserve by performing an ACTH stimulation test is necessary to determine when supplementation can safely be discontinued. Hydrocortisone should be withheld 24 to 48 hours before performing the test so as not to interfere with test results (the assay will measure the exogenous hydrocortisone). Prednisone and prednisolone will also cross-react with many radioimmunoassays. Prednisolone often cross-reacts more, but since prednisone is converted to prednisolone, either may produce erroneous results unless a short lapse of treatment precedes the test (24 to 48 hours). Evaluation of the adrenal activity in the case of iatrogenic Cushing's is usually not indicated until 4 to 6 weeks of replacement therapy has been used. Alternate-day therapy may be less desirable in the case of adrenocortical insufficiency because there is more time when the drug is at a minimal level, although in animal species this is much less a concern than in humans.

GLUCOCORTICOID TREATMENT CONTRAINDICATIONS AND SIDE EFFECTS

The side effects of glucocorticoids have all been well documented.[17–32] There appear to be three categories of veterinarians who administer steroids. The first is the group who throw caution to the wind and use glucocorticoids without regard to therapeutic principles or concern for conservative therapy. They represent the "live on the edge" types who truly take advantage of the steroid tolerance of animal species despite the ill effects induced. The second group are those who have exaggerated concern for the adverse effects of steroids and consequently undertreat cases with less than desirable control of the problem. The last group have judicious use of glucocorticoids and institute therapy for specific conditions according to therapeutic guidelines and treatment principles. There is no doubt that the greatest use and misuse of glucocorticoid therapy is related to the treatment of dermatologic diseases. The adverse effects of glucocorticoid therapy, however, are often related to much deeper structures than the skin.

Glucocorticoids have more potential for adverse effects in humans than in animal species. Cats have been well recognized for their extreme tolerance of glucocorticoids. Because glucocorticoids have a mechanism of action that affects protein, lipid, and carbohydrate metabolism, it is inevitable that abnormal physiologic function is induced. Suppression of host defense mechanisms, change in fluid balance, and modification of endocrine function are likewise affected to an extent proportional to the drug used, dosage, interval of therapy, duration of treatment, and individual variation in tolerance. Adverse effects are not predictable and definitely do not require protracted or excessive steroid therapy. Common side effects include polyuria, polydipsia, polyphagia, and excessive panting. Personality changes (usually for the worse) are not often discussed with pet owners but may be a major side effect of steroids. Aggressive behavioral change concomitant with steroid therapy is likely related, and alternative treatment should be sought. Many older dogs, particularly females, develop urinary incontinence, which is not a side effect well tolerated by the pet owner. Weakness and decreased activity are side effects aggravated by the weight gain from the polyphagia. Dietary counseling should always be included when discussing steroid therapy with pet owners. A common relationship observed in treating the pruritic dog is the tendency for chronic relapsing bacterial pyoderma. There is a direct correlation between the amount of steroid usage and antibiotic usage in these cases. Some of the adverse effects may go unnoticed, including lower urinary tract infection and gastrointestinal disease. Although there may be specific cases where glucocorticoids are used in the presence of an infection, the combination is not routinely recommended.[33] Gastric ulcers result from acute or chronic high-dose (immunosuppressant) glucocorticoid therapy and may not be prevented by treatment with H_2 blockers.

The development of adult-onset demodicosis is almost always related to hyperglucocorticoidism, either spontaneously occurring hyperadrenocorticism or an exogenous source of steroid. Fungal infections are likewise seen as complications. Either dermatophytosis or cutaneous *Malassezia* is most frequently represented as a cutaneous manifestation. Endocrine changes with steroid therapy are often occult without prominent outward signs. Aside from adrenocorticoid suppression, the diabetogenic effect may lead to overt diabetes mellitus. Thyroid hormone synthesis may be suppressed and increase in parathyroid hormone levels observed.

Wound healing is altered with glucocorticoid therapy, which effects many stages of the normal event. Muscle atrophy and osteoporosis are a consequence of catabolic effect of glucocorticoids with changes in protein metabolism and inhibitions of fibroblast activity. Bone healing, particularly in older animals, is impaired by glucocorticoids.[34] Glucocorticoids used in accident victims with fractures should include short-acting drugs and avoidance of protracted therapy.

WITHDRAWAL OF STEROIDS

Glucocorticoid withdrawal in humans is often associated with anorexia, myalgia, nausea, emesis, lethargy, headaches, fever, weight loss, postural hypotension, desquamatia, and arthralgia. Many of these symptoms occur when the patient's cortisol levels are normal and there is no impairment of the hypothalamic-pituitary-adrenal (HPA) axis responsiveness. Since the symptoms may be reproduced by prostaglandin (PGE_2 and PGI_2) administration, it has been postulated that steroid withdrawal syndrome may be the result of sudden increase in prostaglandin production following withdrawal.[27]

Steroid withdrawal is not as great a concern in veterinary medicine, although gradual tapering of the dose may allow a better transition to the natural physiologic state of the animal. The only real concern for steroid withdrawal is the case of adrenocortical insufficiency (iatrogenic Cushing's), although the dog and cat rarely demonstrate problems when there is minimal adrenal reserve and no supplementation is used. The paradox of this condition must be emphasized where the clinical features are the result of hyperglucocorticoidism while the adrenal glands are atrophied with loss of adrenal reserve, leaving the animal vulnerable to the effects of stress with no reserve for steroid response. Supplementation with hydrocortisone 0.1 mg/lb/day (0.2 mg/kg/day) orally will provide maintenance glucocorticoid while allowing restoration of the HPA axis. The gradual withdrawal of alternate-day glucocorticoid administration with prednisone or prednisolone may also be used. Evaluation by ACTH stimulation testing is necessary to determine recovery of the insufficiency to normal response. Although the ACTH stimulation test is a measure of adrenocortical response, it is also an effective measure of the entire HPA axis. The hypothalmus and pituitary return to normal before the adrenal cortex; therefore, a normal ACTH stimulation test implies normal hypothalamic and pituitary activity.

Feedback mechanisms of glucocorticoids are two types, referred to as fast and delayed. Fast feedback is detectable within minutes of steroid therapy, and its effect is dependent upon a rising level of glucocorticoid. Delayed feedback is further divided into two components: intermediate feedback and slow feedback. Intermediate feedback occurs within 2 to 10 hours post exposure. Slow feedback occurs as a consequence of classic steroid mechanism of action on transcription by decreasing mRNA encoded for proopiomelanocortin, the precursor of ACTH.[27] Decreased ACTH results in decreased adrenocortical stimulation and may lead to atrophy.

REFERENCES

1. Claman HN: Glucocorticoids and autoimmune disease. In Schleimer RP, Claman HN, Oronsky A (eds): Anti-inflammatory Steroid Action, Basic and Clinical Aspects. New York, Academic Press, 1989, p 409.
2. Cohn LA: The influence of corticosteroids on host defense mechanisms. J Vet Int Med 5(2):95, 1991.
3. Dluhy RG, Newmark SR, Lauler DP, et al: Pharmacology and chemistry of adrenal glucocorticoids. In Azarnoff DL (ed): Steroid Therapy. Philadelphia, WB Saunders, 1975, p 14.
4. LaPointe MC, Baxter JD: Molecular biology of glucocorticoid hormone action. In Schleimer RP, Claman HN, Oronsky A (eds): Anti-inflammatory Steroid Action, Basic and Clinical Aspects. New York, Academic Press, 1989, p 3.
5. McDonald RK, Langston VC: Use of corticosteroids and nonsteroidal anti-inflammatory agents. In Ettinger SJ, Feldman EC (eds): Textbook of Veterinary Internal Medicine, 4th ed. Philadelphia, WB Saunders, 1995, p 284.
6. Munck A, Guyre PM: Glucocorticoid physiology and homeostasis in relation to anti-inflammatory actions. In Schleimer RP, Claman HN, Oronsky A (eds): Anti-inflammatory Steroid Action, Basic and Clinical Aspects. New York, Academic Press, 1989, p 30.
7. Kemppainen RJ, Sartin JL: Evidence of episodic but not circadian activity in plasma concentrations of adrenocorticotropin, cortisol, and thyroxine in dogs. J Endocrinol 103:219, 1984.
8. Corticosteroids in veterinary medicine. Technical bulletin of The Upjohn Company Animal Health Division, Kalamazoo, Michigan.
9. van den Broek AHM, Stafford WL: Epidermal and hepatic glucocorticoid receptors in cats and dogs. Res Vet Sci 52:312, 1992.
10. Flower RJ: Glucocorticoids and the inhibition of phospholipase A. In Schleimer RP, Claman HN, Oronsky A (eds): Anti-inflammatory Steroid Action, Basic and Clinical Aspects. New York, Academic Press, 1989, p 409.
11. Hirata, F: The role of lipocortins in cellular function as a second messenger of glucocorticoids. In Schleimer RP, Claman HN, Oronsky A (eds): Anti-inflammatory Steroid Action, Basic and Clinical Aspects. New York, Academic Press, 1989, p 67.
12. Cupps TR: Effects of glucocorticoids on lymphocyte function. In Schleimer RP, Claman HN, Oronsky A (eds): Anti-inflammatory Steroid Action, Basic and Clinical Aspects. New York, Academic Press, 1989, p 132.
13. Butterfield JH, Gleich GJ: Anti-inflammatory effects of glucocorticoids on eosinophils and neutrophils. In Schleimer RP, Claman HN, Oronsky A (eds): Anti-inflammatory Steroid Action, Basic and Clinical Aspects. New York, Academic Press, 1989, p 13.
14. Scott DW, Miller WH, Griffin CE: Dermatologic therapy—hormonal agents. In Small Animal Dermatology, p 240. Philadelphia, WB Saunders, 1995.
15. Munck A, Guyre PM: Glucocorticoid actions on monocytes and macrophages. In Schleimer RP, Claman HN, Oronsky A (eds): Anti-inflammatory Steroid Action, Basic and Clinical Aspects. New York, Academic Press, 1989, p 199.
16. Szefler SJ: General pharmacology of glucocorticoids. In Schleimer RP, Claman HN, Oronsky A (eds): Anti-inflammatory Steroid Action, Basic and Clinical Aspects. New York, Academic Press, 1989, p 354.
17. Davies AO: Steroid hormone induced regulation of adrenergic receptors. In Schleimer RP, Claman HN, Oronsky A (eds): Anti-inflammatory Steroid Action, Basic and Clinical Aspects. New York, Academic Press, 1989, p 156.
18. Boothe DM: Controlling inflammation with nonsteroidal anti-inflammatory drugs. Vet Med Sept:875, 1989.
19. Calvert CA, Cornelius LM: The pharmacodynamic differences among glucocorticoid preparations. Vet Med 85:860, 1990.
20. Kemppainen RJ: Principles of glucocorticoid therapy in nonendocrine disease. In Kirk RW (ed): Current Veterinary Therapy IX. Philadelphia, WB Saunders, 1986. p 954.
21. Scott D: Rational use of glucocorticoids in dermatology. In Bonagura J, Kirk RW (eds): Kirk's Current Veterinary Therapy XII. Philadelphia WB Saunders, 1995, p 573.
22. Maibach HI, Stoughton RB: Topical corticosteroids. In Azarnoff DL (ed): Steroid Therapy. Philadelphia, WB Saunders, 1975, p 174.
23. Robertson DB, Maibach HI: Topical glucocorticoids. In Schleimer RP, Claman HN, Oronsky A (eds): Anti-inflammatory Steroid Action, Basic and Clinical Aspects. New York, Academic Press, 1989, p 494.
24. Rosenthal AS, Kirkpatrick CH: Glucocorticoids and allergic reactions. In Azarnoff DL (eds): Steroid Therapy. Philadelphia, WB Saunders, 1975, p 238.
25. White SD, Stewart LJ, Bernstein M: Corticosteroid (methylprednisolone sodium succinate) pulse therapy in five dogs with autoimmune skin disease. JAVMA 191(9):1121, 1987.
26. Hoerlein BF, et al: Evaluation of naloxone, crocetin, thyrotropin-releasing hormone, methyl-prednisolone, partial myelotomy, and hemilaminectomy in the treatment of acute spinal cord trauma. JAAHA 21:67, 1985.
27. Axelrod, L: Side effects of glucocorticoid therapy. In Schleimer RP, Claman HN, Oronsky A (eds): Anti-inflammatory Steroid Action, Basic and Clinical Aspects. New York, Academic Press, 1989, p 377.
28. Calvert CA, Cornelius LM: Corticosteroid hormones: Endogenous regulation and the effects of exogenous administration. Vet Med 85:810, 1990.
29. Hoening M, Moore GE: Duration of pituitary and adrenocortical suppression after long-term administration of anti-inflammatory doses of prednisone in dogs. JAVMA 53(5):720, 1992.
30. Ihrke PJ, et al: Urinary tract infection associated with long-term corticosteroid administration in dogs with chronic skin diseases. JAVMA 186:43, 1985.
31. Murtaugh RJ, et al: Use of synthetic prostaglandin E (misoprostol) for prevention of aspirin-induced gastroduodenal ulceration in arthritic dogs. JAVMA 202(2) 251, 1993.
32. Romatowski J: Topics in drug therapy (iatrogenic adrenocortical insufficiency in dogs). JAVMA 196(7):1144, 1990.
33. Ford RB: Concurrent use of corticosteroids and antimicrobial drugs in the treatment of infectious disease in small animals. JAVMA 195:1142, 1984.
34. Calvert CA, Cornelius LM: Avoiding the undesirable effects of glucocorticoid hormone therapy. Vet Med 1990 85:846, 1990.

RX

CHAPTER 76

OVER-THE-COUNTER PHARMACEUTICALS

Etienne Côté

Using human nonprescription (over-the-counter, or OTC) drugs in veterinary medical therapy is an attractive option because these drugs are usually inexpensive and widely available. Veterinarians deal with OTC drugs either when they advocate their use for medical treatment or when they manage OTC drug intoxications.

A dizzying variety of brand names and products exists on the OTC pharmaceuticals market. Many drugs have similar names but quite different components. Therefore, the veterinarian needs to specify the active ingredients of the drug in question to avoid confusion. For example, many products containing acetylsalicylic acid (ASA) can safely be used for treating dogs and cats, yet varieties of these same products are available in nearly identical packaging and are labeled "aspirin-free," "pain-relief," "cold," "flu," or "sinus." These versions often contain acetaminophen as the active ingredient instead of ASA and are thus potentially toxic. A brand name alone (e.g., Anacin, Benadryl) is inadequate and could be disastrously misleading. Furthermore, manufacturers may change the contents of a product while keeping the same name. The active ingredient in Kaopectate was formerly kaolin-pectin; now, the active ingredient is attapulgite, but the name of the product remains the same. Again, it is best to avoid confusion by stressing active ingredient rather than brand name. When the veterinarian advocates the use of a product, confusion can be minimized by giving the client the names of the desired active ingredients and the names of active ingredients to avoid, in writing, and urging the client to seek pharmacist confirmation when selecting the product.

Human drugs approved for OTC sale in the United States must be proved to be safe and efficacious in humans, but not in animals. The absorption characteristics of OTC human preparations, particularly time-release or enteric-coated formulations, are optimal for the human gastrointestinal (GI) tract but not for that of dogs or cats. Clinical trials assessing the effectiveness of any human OTC-formulated drug against placebo in the veterinary setting are rare. Therefore, when a prescription veterinary drug is available, it may often be safer and more reliable to prescribe it rather than to advocate a human OTC equivalent.

None of the drugs described in this chapter has Food and Drug Administration approval for use in dogs or cats in the United States. Advocating the use of these drugs in an extralabel manner signifies that the veterinarian and client understand the risk inherent in using medications not specifically designed for use in animals.

ANALGESICS

Aspirin, plain (e.g., Norwich, St. Joseph, Bayer, Anacin, ASA) or buffered (e.g., Bufferin, Ascriptin, Ecotrin), is a common treatment for musculoskeletal pain in dogs and cats. Although the recommended dose in dogs is 5 to 12 mg/lb (10 to 25 mg/kg) by mouth two to three times a day, dogs may require 10 to 39 mg/lb (23 to 86 mg/kg) twice a day to control osteoarthritis. Substantial overlap between therapeutic and toxic doses exists; in dogs, doses of 12 mg/lb (25 mg/kg) three times a day for 14 days systematically produced adverse GI effects, and doses of 45 to 50 mg/lb (100 to 110 mg/kg) once a day for 1 to 4 weeks were lethal. Concurrent treatment with misoprostol reduces GI toxicity, but treatment with the H_2-receptor blocking drug cimetidine does not. Parenteral administration of the salicylates also produces GI toxicity; administering aspirin in pulverized form and/or with a full meal may reduce topical irritation in the stomach, but not all adverse GI effects can be eliminated this way. One regular aspirin tablet, plain or buffered, typically contains 325 mg ASA; "baby" or "low-dose" tablets, 81 mg; and "extra-strength" tablets, 500 mg or more.

Aspirin is indicated for anticoagulation in dogs and cats at a dose much lower than the anti-inflammatory dose. Few adverse side effects can be expected at these doses, but effectiveness in animals in a hypercoagulable state is questionable.

Acetaminophen (Excedrin, Feverall, Liquiprin, Midol, Panadol, Pamprin, Percogesic, Tempra, Tylenol, Bromo-Seltzer, paracetamol, and many others, including most "aspirin-free" formulations) is an analgesic drug used in dogs. It is contraindicated in cats because it can induce methemoglobinemia and hemolytic anemia. Hematologic and hepatic adverse effects occur in dogs ingesting large doses (usually >45 mg/lb [100 mg/kg], but as little as approximately 9 mg/lb [20 mg/kg] in one case). Acetylcysteine is an antidote.

Newer OTC nonsteroidal anti-inflammatory drugs are not currently recommended for veterinary use. Naproxen (e.g., Aleve, Naprosyn) and ibuprofen (e.g., Advil, Motrin, Nuprin) are associated with severe GI ulcerations and perforations in dogs. Ketoprofen (e.g., Actron, Orudis) may eventually be approved for use in dogs and cats in the United States, given its common use in veterinary medicine in other countries. The current OTC human formulation, like other enteric-coated preparations, may have variable absorption characteristics in small animals.

ANTIDIARRHEALS

Adsorbents such as kaolin-pectin and attapulgite (e.g., Kaopectate, Donnagel) are considered generally harmless but of questionable clinical efficacy. Bismuth subsalicylate (e.g., Pepto-Bismol, 8.6 mg salicylate/mL; Pepto-Bismol Maximum Strength, 15.7 mg salicylate/mL; Pepto-Bismol Caplets, 99 mg salicylate/caplet) has been shown to have a beneficial effect on the morbidity of acute diarrhea in humans. The liquid is given at a dose of 0.125 mL/lb (0.25 mL/kg) by mouth every 4 to 6 hours in dogs and cats; up to 0.9 mL/lb (2 mL/kg) every 6 to 8 hours has been advocated for dogs only. Cats are more sensitive to salicylates than dogs and should probably not receive frequent or high doses of bismuth subsalicylate, because some of the salicylate is absorbed systemically.

Loperamide (e.g., Imodium A-D) is an effective opiate antidiarrheal medication. The recommended dose for dogs, 0.04 mg/lb (0.08 mg/kg) by mouth three to four times a day may be difficult to achieve in smaller animals, given the concentration of active ingredient in the OTC product (2 mg/tablet; 0.2 mg/mL oral liquid), and caution is warranted. Intoxication, manifesting with central nervous system (CNS) signs and vomiting, has been reported in dogs (especially collies) and cats. Naloxone is an antidote.

ANTIEMETICS

The efficacy of OTC human antiemetics in small animal medicine remains unproved. Drugs such as dimenhydrinate (e.g., Dramamine), meclizine (e.g., Bonine, Dramamine II), and cyclizine (e.g., Marezine) are sometimes given for the prophylaxis of motion sickness in dogs and cats. Toxicity appears unlikely, but CNS signs could occur at very high doses (45 mg/lb [100 mg/kg] in a human case).

CHRONIC RENAL FAILURE DRUGS

Phosphate binders such as aluminum hydroxide (e.g., Amphojel, 64 mg Al(OH)$_3$/mL) AlternaGEL, 120 mg Al(OH)$_3$/mL) are used in the treatment of hyperphosphatemia. Exact titration of the dose depends on serum phosphorus levels. Constipation and loss of appetite are possible side effects. Another phosphate binder is calcium carbonate (e.g., Titralac, Tums).

COUGH SYRUPS

Most OTC cough syrups contain one or more of the following six active ingredients: acetaminophen, phenylpropanolamine, pseudoephedrine, guaifenesin, chlorpheniramine (or brompheniramine), and dextromethorphan. Acetaminophen and phenylpropanolamine are described elsewhere in this chapter. Pseudoephedrine is rarely indicated in veterinary medicine, and toxicity (excitement, tachycardia) is common. Guaifenesin is considered to be of minimal therapeutic value in the treatment of coughs. Antihistamines are considered minimally useful in nonallergic causes of cough. Dextromethorphan has successfully been used (though empirically) in the treatment of coughing in dogs. It is an effective cough suppressant and therefore is contraindicated when cough is beneficial, such as in the expectoration of pus in cases of pneumonia. Most cough syrups contain multiple active ingredients, and currently only a few, such as Vicks Formula 44 (not 44D, 44E), contain only dextromethorphan (2 mg/mL). Unwanted and potentially dangerous active ingredients are present in many preparations. For instance, NyQuil liquid contains dextromethorphan as a cough suppressant, but it also contains pseudoephedrine and over 300 mg acetaminophen/5 mL teaspoon.

DERMATOLOGIC DRUGS

Several antihistamines are used in veterinary dermatology. Chlorpheniramine (e.g., Chlor-Trimeton) effectively controls 70 per cent of seasonally pruritic cats and is of some value for the same problem in dogs. Clemastine fumarate (e.g., Tavist-1) and diphenhydramine (e.g., Benadryl Allergy) also control pruritus in some dogs.

Topical antibacterials such as neomycin (e.g., Neosporin) and triple antibiotic combinations (e.g., Mycitracin) are probably minimally effective but also minimally harmful. Antifungals such as clotrimazole (e.g., Lotrimin, Cruex) and miconazole (e.g., Micatin) are effective against several types of fungi, including *Malassezia* yeasts, dermatophytes, and saprophytes such as *Aspergillus* spp. The reader is referred to additional sources for exact protocols for the use of these drugs.

Zinc oxide creams (e.g., Desitin) are frequently applied to burned or irritated skin. The usefulness of zinc oxide in treating such conditions, and as a sunscreen, must be weighed against the potential for toxicity, which manifests as vomiting and lethargy after animals lick the product off the skin.

Benzocaine is present in many OTC dermatologic "soothing" preparations (e.g., Lanacaine, Solarcaine). It can cause hemolytic anemia in cats and dogs who ingest it and should be used cautiously, if at all, in these species.

EMETICS

For those situations in which emesis is to be induced, oral administration of syrup of ipecac is effective and safe. Only one additional dose is recommended if vomiting has not occurred within 15 minutes. Orally administered hydrogen peroxide also effectively induces emesis in dogs and cats. Both of these products are available as generics. Large doses of table salt, though sometimes emetic, are not recommended because of the serious consequences of hypernatremia if vomiting does not occur.

GASTRIC ACID–REDUCING DRUGS

The phosphate binders described earlier are also antacids. They are rarely used in canine and feline medicine because of the frequent dosing needed to maintain a high gastric pH. The H$_2$-receptor blocking drugs cimetidine (e.g., Tagamet HB 200), ranitidine (e.g., Zantac), famotidine (e.g., Pepcid AC), and nizatidine (Axid AR) all decrease gastric acid secretion. Some (ranitidine, nizatidine) have GI prokinetic activity. Famotidine and nizatidine do not affect hepatic p450 enzymes. The H$_2$-blockers have a wide margin of safety.

LAXATIVES AND ENEMAS

Although no clinical veterinary trials have compared OTC laxatives to one another or to placebo, a variety of OTC preparations is available to effectively manage constipation. Stimulant laxatives such as bisacodyl (e.g., Dulcolax) increase myenteric nervous activity and peristalsis. They are advocated for short-term use only. Emollient laxatives such as docusate (Colace, Surfak) soften the stool and are said to be more effective in acute rather than chronic constipation. Constipation prevention may be achieved using soluble fiber such as psyllium mucilloid (Metamucil), with the exact dose titrated to result in soft, formed feces. Phenolphthalein (e.g., Ex-Lax) is not superior to other laxatives and is associated with diarrhea and colic.

Phosphate enemas (e.g., Fleet) are contraindicated in cats, and possibly small dogs, because of the severe hyperphosphatemia they induce. Pediatric emollient enemas (e.g., docusate sodium) have been used successfully and safely.

OPHTHALMIC DRUGS

Irrigating solutions (e.g., Dacriose, Collyrium for Fresh Eyes) are used for clearing debris and pus from the eyes on a short- to long-term basis. Artificial tears (e.g., Adsorbotear, Tears Naturale II) are used for tear replacement; solutions containing polyvinyl alcohol may be irritating, however. Ophthalmic decongestants (e.g., Visine, OcuClear) are of essentially no therapeutic worth; they obscure the diagnosis and may cause chronic conjunctivitis.

URINARY INCONTINENCE DRUGS

Phenylpropanolamine (e.g., Dexatrim, Acutrim; 75 mg/tablet) is a recognized treatment for urinary incontinence caused by lower urinary sphincter incompetence (e.g., estrogen-responsive incontinence and others). Because a single tablet contains 75 mg, dosing (0.7 mg/lb [1.5 mg/kg]) must be done carefully to avoid side effects such as restlessness, CNS stimulation, and cardiovascular effects. Phenylpropanolamine is also present in combination with various other antihistamines, analgesics, and cough suppressants in mixtures used for treating the common cold.

Over-the-counter drugs may be useful in specific therapeutic situations in which convenience, lack of an effective veterinary equivalent, or cost play an important role in drug selection. These advantages need to be weighed against the drawbacks of drug formulations meant for humans, frequent lack of proven efficacy, absence of veterinary labeling for most of these products, and the potential for selection of the wrong product by the client.

REFERENCES

1. Adams HR (ed): Veterinary Pharmacology and Therapeutics, 7th ed. Ames, Iowa State Press, 1995.
2. Côté E: Over-the-counter human medications in small animal practice. Part 1. Gastrointestinal, urinary, and ophthalmic drugs. Comp Cont Ed Pract Vet 20(5):603–617, 1998.
3. Côté E: Over-the-counter human medications in small animal practice. Part 2. Analgesic, respiratory, and dermatologic drugs. Comp Cont Ed Pract Vet 20(7):791–808, 1998.
4. Covington TR (ed): American Pharmaceutical Association Handbook of Nonprescription Medications. Washington, DC, American Pharmaceutical Association, 1996.
5. Guilford WG, Center SA, Strombeck D, et al (eds): Strombeck's Small Animal Gastroenterology, 3rd ed. Philadelphia, WB Saunders, 1996.
6. Papich MG: Toxicoses from over-the-counter human drugs. Vet Clin North Am Small Anim Pract 20:431, 1990.
7. Physicians' Desk Reference for Nonprescription Drugs, 18th ed. Montvale, NJ, Medical Economics, 1997.
8. Polzin DJ, Osborne CA, Bartges JW, et al: Chronic renal failure. In Ettinger SJ, Feldman EC (eds): Textbook of Veterinary Internal Medicine, 4th ed. Philadelphia, WB Saunders, 1995, pp 1734–1760.
9. Scott DW, Miller WH, Griffin C (eds): Small Animal Dermatology, 2nd ed. Philadelphia, WB Saunders, 1995.
10. Slatter DH: Fundamentals of Veterinary Ophthalmology, 2nd ed. Philadelphia, WB Saunders, 1990.

CHAPTER 77

ADVERSE DRUG REACTIONS

Jill Maddison

An adverse drug reaction (ADR) is any response to a drug that is noxious and unintended and that occurs at doses used for prophylaxis, diagnosis, or therapy.[1] Lack of apparent efficacy has been classified as an ADR by some, but therapeutic failure may be excluded as an ADR. Many factors contribute to therapeutic failure (including incorrect diagnosis), and it is possible that a drug may be ineffective under certain conditions or may be administered in such a manner that effective concentrations at the site of action were not achieved.

ADRs frequently reported in dogs and cats involve vaccines, antimicrobial drugs, nonsteroidal anti-inflammatory drugs, ectoparasiticides, anthelmintics, and anesthetic agents. These are probably the most common therapeutic or prophylactic agents used. Thus the higher incidence of ADRs related to these agents probably reflects usage pattern rather than increased ADR potential.

CLASSIFICATION OF ADVERSE DRUG REACTIONS

Type A ADRs are expected but exaggerated pharmacologic or toxic responses to a drug. This may be an exaggeration of the intended response to the drug, a secondary response affecting an organ other than the target organ but predictable based on the pharmacology of the drug, or a toxic response.[2]

Most ADRs of this type are attributable to differences in drug disposition that cause higher plasma drug concentrations as a result of, for example, organ failure, reduced protein binding attributable to displacement by another drug, or inappropriate dosage of a non-lipid-soluble drug in an obese dog. These reactions are usually dose-dependent and avoidable if sufficient drug and patient information is available.

Type B reactions are unexpected or aberrant responses that are unrelated to the drug's pharmacologic effect. They are not dose-dependent and are unpredictable and idiosyncratic. Type B ADRs include allergic reactions, direct toxic effects on organs that are associated with actions unrelated to any desired therapeutic effect (the mechanisms for which may be complex and obscure), and aberrant responses in different species.

INCIDENCE OF ADVERSE DRUG REACTIONS

The incidence of ADRs in veterinary medicine is unknown. In human medicine it has been estimated that 3 to 5 per cent of all hospitalized patients are admitted because of an ADR.[3] Some studies give a wide variety of estimates that 1.5 to 35 per cent of patients develop an ADR while hospitalized.[4] There are few studies in the veterinary literature that estimate incidence. In one study, 130 of 39,451 cases (0.33 per cent) seen at the University of California–Davis Veterinary Teaching Hospital in 1975–1976 were suspected drug reactions, and of these, 66 had evidence linking the drug to the reaction.[5] However, this does not give an estimate of the incidence of ADRs in animals treated with drugs, because data were not available on the number that had been administered drugs. It has been estimated that 1 per cent of the veterinary hospital population treated with drugs experience ADRs, but there are divergent opinions among clinicians about the frequency and importance of ADRs.[1] One author concluded that how often ADRs occur depends on how intensively one searches, on what one means by an ADR, and on the group of patients in whom one looks.[4]

DIFFICULTIES IN DIAGNOSING ADRs

Appropriate diagnosis of an ADR is heavily dependent on the expertise of the attending clinician and the quality of the information available. Even experienced clinicians have difficulty determining causality, and experts have been shown to agree less than 50 per cent of the time when assigning causality to an ADR.[3] The clinical signs of an ADR are almost always nonspecific and rarely if ever pathognomonic. In human medicine the most common symptoms of ADRs (e.g., nausea or vomiting, diarrhea, abdominal pain, rash, pruritus, drowsiness, headache) are also reported in 80 per cent of healthy patients on no medication.[4] Placebo administration causes an increase in the percentage of patients with symptoms and the number of symptoms per patient.[4] Although a true placebo effect presumably does not exist in animals, veterinarians must rely on the observations of owners, who may be subject to various conscious or subconscious factors that influence interpretation of their pets' behavior.

Other factors that contribute to difficulties in determining whether a true ADR has occurred include multiple medications, underlying pathology, and the assumption that it is the active principal of a medication that is responsible for the

ADR. Many reactions are due to excipients, and some may be due to in vitro degradation products.[6]

Even though all new drugs are extensively evaluated before release onto the market, evaluation before registration cannot assure safety. Premarketing clinical trials are usually too small and conducted for too short a period to detect rare or delayed ADRs. In addition, it is difficult to include in trials all groups of animals, including different breeds, the aged, the young, diseased animals, and others that may have a high risk of developing an ADR. Hence, postmarketing surveillance of ADRs is important in ensuring drug safety and detecting unusual and uncommon ADRs.

POSTMARKETING DRUG SURVEILLANCE

Postmarketing surveillance occurs in various forms—phase IV clinical trials, spontaneous reporting schemes, intensive monitoring within hospitals (uncommon in veterinary medicine), analysis of health registers (more relevant to human medicine), and prospective studies. ADR reports rarely indicate the need to remove the drug from the market, but such reports may indicate the need for changes in dose rate; additional labeling or clarification of labeling; additional warnings, precautions, and contraindications; and formulation changes.[7]

Phase IV clinical trials may be conducted by the manufacturer after marketing approval, are based on usual clinical use of the drug, and usually do not include control groups.[8] However, it has been demonstrated in human medicine that despite the relatively large size of the cohorts monitored in phase IV studies, spontaneous reporting methods are more likely to detect previously unsuspected ADRs.[8]

Spontaneous ADR reporting schemes can involve reporting of suspected ADRs by practitioners and animal owners through a variety of means—case reports in the literature, reports submitted to an ADR reporting center (which may or may not involve regulatory authorities, depending on the country), and reports made directly to the manufacturer. In various countries, manufacturers are now required to report ADRs to appropriate regulatory authorities. Spontaneous reporting schemes are relatively cheap and potentially include all patients taking the drug. However, underreporting is a serious disadvantage—it is estimated that only about 5 to 25 per cent of all ADRs are eventually reported.[3]

The ADR reporting rate is low within the medical profession and almost certainly even lower within the veterinary profession. Even in countries where ADR reporting is mandatory, the reporting rate by medical practitioners remains low.[9] An analysis of the attitudes of medical practitioners in South Africa to ADR reporting revealed that there were differences in reporting rates among groups within the profession (a larger number of medical specialists reported ADRs compared with general practitioners, and surgical specialists did not report any ADRs during the study).[9] The major reasons identified for failure to report ADRs were the belief of medical practitioners that unusual or serious reactions were infrequent and that common or trivial ADRs did not warrant reporting, apathy, and being too busy to do the paperwork. Fear of personal consequences (criticism and medicolegal action) was not deemed to be an important impediment to reporting. The authors concluded somewhat pessimistically that "the prognosis is poor [for improved ADR reporting] and it appears that, like all else which passes between doctors and their patients, ADRs will continue to remain largely outside the reach of an external agency."

Similar studies have not been done within the veterinary profession, but there is no reason to assume that veterinarians' attitudes about ADR reporting are radically better than those of their medical colleagues.

IDENTIFICATION OF ADVERSE DRUG REACTIONS

Any drug has the potential to affect an individual patient adversely. The justification for using a drug is the favorable ratio of anticipated benefits to potential risks. In life-threatening situations, use of a drug with a narrow therapeutic ratio may be warranted, whereas use of a drug with a narrow therapeutic ratio is not justifiable to treat trivial problems.

Accurate identification of an ADR is often difficult, and it may go undetected if the clinical signs induced are indistinguishable from those of common disease syndromes. A clinician should always be alert to the possibility that the clinical abnormalities an animal presents with or develops during the course of an illness are due to the treatment rather than to the disease process itself.

The following questions should be considered when attempting to ascertain whether an ADR has occurred:

1. *Is there a plausible temporal relationship between administration of drugs and effect?* However, note that ADRs for some drugs can take months to years to develop (e.g., those given to treat neoplasia).

2. *Is there an improvement in the clinical syndrome when the drug is discontinued?*

3. *Does the ADR recur if the animal is reexposed to the drug?* This last criterion is often difficult to fulfill because of understandable owner reluctance to subject the animal to further discomfort and because of the possibility that a recurrence of the ADR (particularly with an allergic basis) may be life-threatening.

FACTORS THAT INFLUENCE TYPE A ADRs

It is important to understand the factors that modify the effects of drugs and their dosages in order to anticipate when an animal may be at increased risk of a type A ADR. Many factors modify the effects of drugs in the individual. Some factors result in qualitative differences in the effects of the drug and may preclude its safe use in that animal. Other factors may produce a quantitative change in the usual effects of the drug that can be offset by appropriate adjustment in dose. Factors that may be important in modifying the effects of a drug in an individual include the following.

SPECIES

In veterinary medicine we have to deal with animals of different species, different ages, and different weights (even within the same species). Therefore it is particularly important that we are aware of species-specific peculiarities in drug metabolism, the effect of body size on dosing recommendations, and, most importantly, that drug doses cannot necessarily be extrapolated between cats and dogs, even if they are of similar weights. Species differences in drug disposition may occur owing to differences in absorption (differences in the anatomy of the gastrointestinal tract), metabolism, protein binding, and many other factors.

Cats have a slow rate of biotransformation for many drugs that depend on glucuronyl transferases for glucuronide conjugation in the liver. They have a substantially reduced ability to conjugate drugs such as acetaminophen and aspirin with glucuronic acid. As a result, hepatic clearance of aspirin in cats is prolonged, resulting in a half-life of 37.5 hours, compared with 8.5 hours in dogs. However, the drug can be used safely provided the dosage interval is appropriately extended. In contrast, acetaminophen is extremely toxic to cats and cannot be used under any circumstances, because alternative metabolic pathways to glucuronidation produce toxic metabolites. Other drugs that are metabolized more slowly in cats include dipyrone, chloramphenicol, and hexachlorophene.

Some sulfate conjugation pathways are well developed in cats, which may represent an alternative pathway for drugs that are normally conjugated with glucuronides in other species. Cats also have unusual receptor site sensitivity for many drugs; for example, high doses of morphine result in excitement rather than sedation.

Cat erythrocytes are more susceptible to oxidative changes. The grooming habits of cats facilitate ingestion of substances on their fur; thus they can receive unpredictably larger doses of aerosols or dusts. It is believed that this is the major route by which cats develop lead toxicity. Cats are more susceptible to aminoglycoside neurotoxicity than are other species. The differences between factors that influence drug disposition in dogs and cats have been reviewed extensively.[2]

Dogs do not have the ability to acetylate drugs. When this pathway is responsible for drug inactivation (e.g., sulfonamides), the drug will have a longer duration of action than in other species.

BODY SIZE AND PERCENTAGE FAT

Metabolic rate (and therefore ability to metabolize a drug) is more closely related to body surface area than body weight. Smaller animals within a species require a higher dose per kilogram than do larger animals. This is particularly relevant to dogs, where body size within the species covers such a large range. When there is a narrow therapeutic range for the drug, this factor can become very important. The dose of a drug with a narrow therapeutic ratio (e.g., digoxin, cytotoxic drugs) is usually calculated based on body surface area rather than body weight. There can be a large difference in the calculated dose for dogs of extreme size (small or large) when weight rather than body surface area is used. For drugs with a wide margin of safety, such accurate dosage is not particularly important. However, for drugs with a narrow margin of safety, failure to calculate the dose appropriately can result in toxicity or reduced therapeutic efficacy.

Another consideration when adjusting dosages for body size is the fat component of the body weight. Drug dosages are usually expressed per weight within a particular species. One should attempt to estimate the appropriate lean body weight and use this to calculate an appropriate dosage for non-lipid-soluble drugs even if using body surface area. Drugs that have a narrow margin of safety and are not lipid-soluble include digoxin and the aminoglycoside antibiotics.

AGE

Neonates have a reduced capability for drug biotransformation and have underdeveloped hepatic and renal excretory mechanisms. This accounts for the increased sensitivity to and prolonged recovery from barbiturate anesthetics that may be observed in dogs and cats younger than 4 months. Other factors that influence drug disposition in young animals include increased gastrointestinal permeability, differences in body water and protein binding (greater percentage of body water, less extensive protein binding), and increased blood-brain barrier permeability.

Because older animals may have reduced hepatic or renal function, less body water, and reduced lean body mass, they often require lower doses of drugs compared with younger animals. It is important to be aware that the aging process varies greatly between individuals. Patient-specific physiologic and functional characteristics are probably more important than age per se in predicting ADRs.

Sex

During pregnancy or lactation, caution should be observed in administration of drugs that might affect the fetus or neonate. Drugs that should be avoided or used with caution in pregnant animals include corticosteroids, cytotoxic drugs,

griseofulvin, ketoconazole, prostaglandins, salicylates, sex hormones, tetracyclines, and live vaccines. Drugs that may adversely affect lactation, causing agalactia, include atropine, bromocriptine, and furosemide. Adverse drug reactions occur more commonly in female humans, but it is not known if this phenomenon occurs in domestic animals.

Pathology

Dosage recommendations are usually based on pharmacokinetic data obtained from healthy animals under controlled conditions, even though many drugs will be given to diseased animals. Drug metabolism and excretion may be adversely affected by pathology of various organs, particularly the liver and kidney. Adjustment in dosage may be required, depending on the site of metabolism and route of elimination of the particular drug.

Hepatic disease can alter the bioavailability and disposition of a drug, as well as influence the pharmacologic effects of the drug (Table 77–1). The enhanced effects of drugs in patients with liver disease are primarily due to decreased drug metabolism. Fortunately, glucuronidation, a common

TABLE 77–1. DRUGS THAT SHOULD BE AVOIDED OR USED WITH CAUTION IN ANIMALS WITH HEPATIC OR RENAL DISEASE

DRUG CLASS	USE WITH CAUTION IN HEPATIC DISEASE	USE WITH CAUTION IN RENAL DISEASE
Antimicrobials	Chloramphenicol Chlortetracyclines* Erythromycin estolate* Flucytosine Griseofulvin Ketoconazole Lincosamides Macrolides Metronidazole Sulfonamide-trimethoprim*† Sulfonamides Tetracyclines	Aminoglycosides*† Amphotericin*† Fluoroquinolones Lincomycin Nafcillin Nalidixic acid Nitrofurantoin Polymyxins† Sulfonamide-trimethoprim Sulfonamides Tetracyclines (except doxycycline)
Anesthetics (general, local, sedatives, anticonvulsants)	Anticonvulsants Barbiturates*† Chlorpromazine Diazepam† Halogenated anesthetics Ketamine Lignocaine Propofol	Acepromazine Chlorpromazine Ketamine Methoxyflurane*† Procainamide
Cardiac drugs	Beta blockers Lignocaine Quinidine	Angiotensin-converting enzyme inhibitors*† Cardiac glycosides Procainamide
Diuretics		Spironolactone Thiazides
Anti-inflammatories/analgesics	Butorphanol Corticosteroids Meclofenamic acid Phenylbutazone Polysulfated glycosaminoglycan	Nonsteroidal anti-inflammatories*† Pethidine Polysulfated glycosaminoglycan
Cytotoxic drugs	Doxorubicin	Cisplatin*† Doxorubicin*† Fluorouracil Methotrexate*†
Miscellaneous	Doxapram Heparin Suxamethonium	Allopurinol Doxapram Gallamine Piperazine

*Avoid.
†Toxic.

method by which lipid-soluble drugs are metabolized in dogs, appears to be relatively unaffected by hepatic disease.[10] The effect of hepatic disease on bioavailability and disposition of drugs is difficult to predict. In general, when administering drugs that are extensively metabolized by the liver to animals with liver disease, the dosage interval should be prolonged.

The degree to which impaired renal function affects drug elimination is determined by the fraction of the dose that is excreted unchanged by the kidneys. Some drugs are nephrotoxic (e.g., aminoglycosides, amphotericin). The potential for nephrotoxicity is increased in animals with preexisting renal disease and those that are dehydrated owing to water or sodium loss or diuretic (especially furosemide) usage.

Drug absorption and distribution may also be adversely affected by cardiac insufficiency. Regional blood flow is altered in cardiovascular disease, resulting in the brain and heart receiving more blood and the kidneys, skeletal muscles, and splanchnic organs receiving less. Infiltrative gut disease alters the absorption of orally administered drugs. Dehydration or acidosis may alter the biotransformation or distribution of a drug. For example, a dehydrated animal does not absorb drugs or fluids well from subcutaneous sites.

Drug Interactions

A drug interaction can occur if one member of a class of drugs alters the intensity of the pharmacologic effects of another drug given concurrently. The net result of a drug interaction may be enhancement of the effects of one or the other drug (hence increasing the risk of an ADR occurring), development of totally new effects not seen when either drug is used alone, inhibition of the effect of one drug by another, or no change in the net result despite the kinetics or metabolism of one or both drugs being substantially altered.

Drug interactions may be classified as *pharmacokinetic*—defined as an alteration in the absorption, distribution, or disposition of one drug by another—which is the most common type of drug interaction, or as *pharmacodynamic,* in which one drug affects the action of the other drug. Drug interactions can involve direct chemical or physical interaction, interaction in gastrointestinal absorption, competition between drugs for protein binding sites, interaction at receptor sites, interaction owing to accelerated metabolism, inhibition of metabolism, alteration of renal excretion, and alteration of pH or electrolyte concentrations.

TYPE B ADVERSE DRUG REACTIONS (HYPERSENSITIVITY)

Type B ADRs are unrelated to dose, hard to predict, and difficult to avoid. The major example of an idiosyncratic or type B ADR is an allergic or hypersensitivity reaction. Drug hypersensitivity reactions are more common in patients with a prior history of allergic reactions to the drug or in atopic patients, but they can occur in any individual.

Penicillin-induced hypersensitivity is the most well characterized drug-induced hypersensitivity in small animals. Other drugs that have been reported to cause allergic reactions include sulfonamides, doxorubicin, penicillamine, dipyrone, and quinidine.[11] In human medicine, allergic drug reactions account for approximately 5 to 10 per cent of ADRs.[12]

Any component of a drug preparation may induce a hypersensitivity reaction, and microbiologic contamination may also stimulate such a reaction. Drug hypersensitivity should be considered in the differential diagnosis of any apparent immune-mediated disease (e.g., polyarthropathy, hemolytic anemia, vesicular or ulcerative dermatitis).

Allergic drug reactions may occur as a result of a number of different immunologic mechanisms, including immediate hypersensitivity (type I), cytotoxic hypersensitivity (type II), immune complex formation (type III), and delayed hypersensitivity (type IV). However, the pathophysiology of many drug reactions eludes precise characterization, and some immune reactions are a result of a combination of mechanisms.[12]

Relatively few drugs are responsible for inducing allergic drug reactions, as most drugs are not capable of forming covalent bonds with proteins, a requisite step to render a molecule immunogenic. The drug–drug metabolite–protein complex must have multiple antigenic combining sites to stimulate a drug-specific immune response and to elicit an allergic reaction.[12] For those drugs that are capable of inducing an immunologic response, it is generally the metabolites of the drug that are chemically reactive and easily form covalent bonds with macromolecules.[11]

For example, the principal reactive product of penicillin appears to be the penicilloyl moiety resulting from the cleavage of the lactam ring. Hydroxylamine metabolites, formed from oxidation of the para-amino group of sulfonamide drugs and capable of covalently binding to protein, are believed to be involved in allergic reactions to this class of drug. Doberman pinschers appear to be at increased risk of sulfonamide hypersensitivity. This has been postulated to be at least partially related to a decreased ability to detoxify hydroxylamine metabolites.[13]

Cross-reactivity to other apparently unrelated drugs can occur if the particular portion of the drug molecule that is acting as the hapten also occurs in pharmacologically disparate groups of drugs. For example, the sulfamyl group is present in sulfonamide antimicrobial drugs, furosemide, thiazide diuretics, and the sulfonylurea group of oral hypoglycemic agents (e.g., glipizide). Thus an animal that has a reaction to a sulfonamide may also react to these seemingly unrelated drugs.

Drug hypersensitivity may manifest in different ways. Acute anaphylaxis is associated with IgE and mast cell degranulation. It is characterized by one or all of the following clinical signs: hypotension, bronchospasm, angioedema, urticaria, erythema, pruritus, pharyngeal and/or laryngeal edema, vomiting, and colic. The main shock or target organ for anaphylactic reactions varies between species; hepatic veins are the main target in dogs, and the bronchi, bronchioles, and pulmonary vein are the main target in cats.[11]

A systemic allergic reaction associated with drug use may be related to deposition of immune complexes in tissues and activation of complement. Clinical signs include lymphadenopathy, neuropathy, vasculitis, nephritis, arthritis, urticaria, and fever. Various hematologic perturbations may occur related to drug-induced antibody production, resulting in hemolytic anemia, thrombocytopenia, and, rarely, agranulocytosis. Cutaneous reactions may also occur related to development of immune complex deposition or delayed hypersensitivity.

Prior exposure to the drug is not essential, as hypersensitivity may develop over the course of drug administration. In humans, five to seven days is required for drug hypersensitivity to develop in a patient previously unexposed to the drug.

Allergic drug reactions should be managed by withdrawing the drug and treating with corticosteroids if needed. Adrenaline and fluid therapy may be needed for acute anaphylactic reactions.

PSEUDOALLERGIC DRUG REACTIONS

Drug reactions may occur that resemble drug allergies but do not have an immunologic basis. These reactions are often termed anaphylactoid reactions and do not require prior exposure to the drug. They occur most frequently when a drug is given rapidly intravenously. Anaphylactoid reactions may be caused by nonspecific release of mediators of hypersensitivity or by the direct effects of the drug on tissues.[11]

Acute cardiovascular collapse can be induced by intravenous administration of chloramphenicol, aminoglycosides, tetracyclines, and propylene glycol. Intravenous precipitation of water-insoluble drugs can also cause acute collapse. Direct release of hypersensitivity mediators can occur, particularly with administration of iodinated contrast media, some intravenous anesthetics and opiates (e.g., morphine), polymyxin, and thiamine. Administration of drugs in hypotonic solutions or some organic vehicles can cause erythrocyte lysis and therefore acute hemolytic reactions that are not immunologically mediated. Non-immunologically-mediated drug fevers have also been reported—most frequently after the administration of penicillins and cephalosporins in dogs and tetracyclines in cats. In humans, aspirin and other nonsteroidal anti-inflammatory drugs can induce anaphylactoid reactions through interference with arachidonic acid metabolism.

REFERENCES

1. Hoskins JD, Hubbert WT, et al: A questionnaire for the clinical assessment of veterinary adverse drug reactions. Cornell Vet 72:3, 1982.
2. Boothe DM: Drug therapy in cats: Mechanisms and avoidance of adverse drug reactions. JAVMA 196:1297, 1990.
3. Bukowski JA, Wartenberg D: Comparison of adverse drug reaction reporting in veterinary and human medicine. JAVMA 209:40, 1996.
4. Kramer MS: Difficulties in assessing the adverse effects of drugs. Br J Clin Pharmacol 11:105S, 1981.
5. Ndiritu CG, Enos LR: Adverse reactions to drugs in a veterinary hospital. JAVMA 171:335, 1977.
6. Edwards IR: Adverse drug reaction monitoring: The practicalities. Med Tox 2:405, 1987.
7. Knobloch CP: Adverse reaction reporting program. JAVMA 176:29, 1980.
8. Ross AC, Knapp DE, Anello C, et al: Discovery of adverse drug reactions. JAMA 249:2226, 1983.
9. Robins AH, Weir M, Biersteker EM: Attitudes to adverse drug reactions and their reporting among medical practitioners. S Afr Med J 72:131, 1987.
10. Debuf Y: The Veterinary Formulary, 2nd ed. London, Pharmaceutical Press, 1994, pp 60–64.
11. Davis LE: Hypersensitivity reactions induced by antimicrobial drugs. JAVMA 185:1131, 1984.
12. Anderson JA, Adkinson F: Allergic reactions to drugs and biologic agents. JAMA 258:2891, 1987.
13. Cribb AE: Idiosyncratic reactions to sulfonamides in dogs. JAVMA 195:1612, 1989.

CHAPTER 78

FLUID AND ELECTROLYTE THERAPY

Rebecca Kirby and Elke Rudloff

All creatures depend upon body fluids for survival. Oxygen is bound to intravascular hemoglobin in the lungs for transport to the peripheral tissues and cells. This *oxygen delivery* is dependent upon the functions of the cardiovascular system and an adequate fluid volume to carry the oxygen to the tissues. The fluid at the tissue level (interstitial) is responsible for delivering nutrients to the cells, support of the tissue structures, and uptake and transport of waste products for elimination. Water and electrolytes are used in all normal cell functions and are made available by capillary exchange.

The goal of fluid resuscitation and maintenance is to restore perfusion and hydration while preventing volume overload and its complications of pulmonary, peripheral, and brain edema. Fluid deficits in the intravascular space cause poor perfusion and inadequate tissue oxygenation. Fluid deficits in the extravascular space cause dehydration. Criteria for proper fluid selection begin with deciding where the fluid deficit is located. Capillary dynamics and the composition of the fluids administered determine how the administered fluid is distributed.

FLUID COMPARTMENT AND CAPILLARY DYNAMICS

Sixty per cent of body kilogram weight is water. Of this water, 66.6 per cent is intracellular and 33.3 per cent is extracellular. Of the body water that is extracellular, 25 per cent is intravascular and 75 per cent is interstitial water. Transcellular fluid is composed of cerebrospinal fluid, gastrointestinal fluid, lymph, bile, glandular and respiratory secretions, and synovial fluid. Because these fluids are produced by the action of specific cells and not transudates from the plasma, they are not considered when assessing extracellular fluid volumes.[1]

The intracellular compartment is contained within a cell membrane. Most of the cell membranes are permeable to water but not to most charged particles (ions). The extravascular space between the tissue compartments and cells is the interstitial compartment. The arteries, veins, and capillaries contain the fluid of the intravascular compartment.

Within the intravascular compartment, the capillaries are the site of normal fluid exchange between the intravascular and interstitial spaces. The capillary "membrane" is composed of endothelial cells and a basement membrane (Fig. 78–1). Lipid-soluble molecules such as oxygen and carbon dioxide are freely permeable and rapidly cross through the endothelial cells to the area of lower concentration. Nonlipid soluble particles, including water, must diffuse through tight endothelial intercellular clefts. The size of the solute determines whether or not that particle can move freely across this capillary "membrane."

The interstitium is composed of collagen fiber bundles, proteoglycan filaments, and lymphatics. The collagen extends a long distance, providing most of the tensile strength of the tissues. Proteoglycan filaments form a fine reticular network that contains most of the interstitial fluid. The fluid moves molecule by molecule using kinetic motion. For the short distances, this diffusion occurs rapidly and also moves electrolytes, nutrients, cellular excreta, oxygen, carbon dioxide, proteins, and other substances. Occasionally small rivulets of "free" fluid and small free fluid vesicles are present. This fluid flows freely, usually along the surfaces of collagen fibers or surfaces of cells.[2] The amount of free fluid in normal tissues is slight—less than 1 per cent.

The lymphatics are scavengers that remove excess fluid, protein molecules, debris, and other matter from the tissue spaces.[2] The interstitial fluid enters terminal lymphatic capillaries and is propelled to the systemic circulation by movement of the surrounding tissues. The lymphatics of most normal tissues can pump a slight intermittent negative pressure that gives an average negativity in the loose interstitial tissues.

The need for filtering and exchanging interstitial fluid is critical for cellular metabolism and survival. Starling's law (Fig. 78–2) defines the forces that affect the volume of fluid that is distributed between the intravascular and interstitial compartments. As the blood passes throughout the length of the capillary, the hydrostatic pressure gradient causes a continuous, dynamic movement of water and solutes into the interstitium (Fig. 78–3). Approximately 90 per cent of the volume of fluid that leaves the arterial capillary is taken up at the venular end of the capillary. Though the hydrostatic pressure gradient is not that different, uptake occurs as a result of the increased permeability and number of venular capillaries compared with the arterial end. The remaining 10 per cent of filtered fluid volume is deposited into the lymphatics, along with waste products and proteins, to maintain volume equilibrium.

The filtration of water and solutes from the capillary into the interstitium allows delivery of water, nutrients, oxygen, and electrolytes to the cells for metabolism. The nutrients and oxygen are extracted from this fluid filtered at the arterial end of the capillary, and waste products are then deposited into this same fluid. This waste-containing fluid then diffuses through the interstitium and back into the venular capillary circulation. Once in the circulation, the waste products are transported to organs such as the liver, lung, and kidneys for degradation and excretion. In addition, proteins and other solutes are transported in the interstitial fluid and deposited into the lymphatics as needed, with the lymphatics emptying into the venous circulation. The number and capacity of the lymphatics varies from tissue to tissue, and when their ability is overwhelmed, interstitial edema occurs.

The dynamics of the various fluid compartments changes during critical illness and shock. Separation of capillary endothelial junctions during reperfusion of hypoxic tissue and active transcellular-vesicular transport of proteins result in leakage of albumin and fluids out of the intravascular space.[3, 4] Intracellular and interstitial water content increases following hemorrhagic shock as a result of electrogenic pump depression.[5–7] The resultant hypovolemia and edema

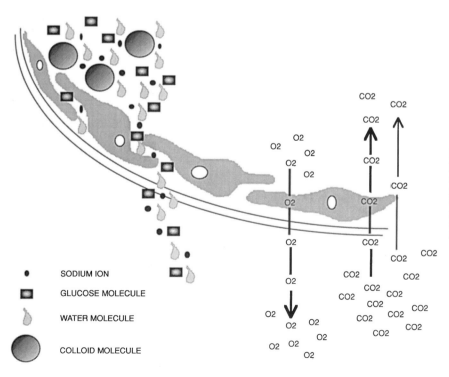

SODIUM ION

GLUCOSE MOLECULE

WATER MOLECULE

COLLOID MOLECULE

Figure 78–1. A capillary is illustrated in cross-section. Lipid-soluble molecules such as oxygen and carbon dioxide diffuse through the endothelial cell membranes, passing freely between the interstitial and intravascular space. Nonlipid-soluble particles, to include water, must pass through intercellular clefts, between endothelial cells. Molecules that are too large to pass through the membrane cleft will be retained within the capillary.

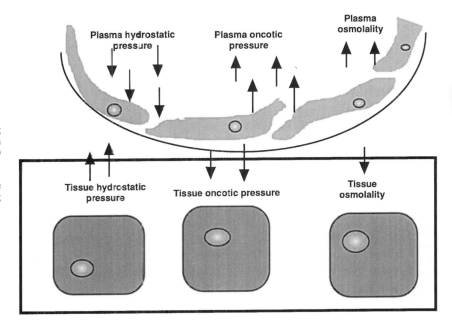

Figure 78–2. Starling's principle. The forces affecting fluid movement between the capillary and interstitium are defined by Starling's equation: v = [kf(P$_c$ − P$_f$) − sigma(π_c − π_{if})] − Q lymph. v = volume; kf = filtration coefficient; P = hydrostatic pressure; c = capillary; if = interstitial fluid; sigma = membrane pore size; π = COP; Q = lymph flow returning interstitial fluid and albumin back to circulation.

affect oxygen transport and diffusion to the cell, adding insult to the already dysfunctional cell membrane.[8]

There are many disease processes that result in increased permeability of the capillaries and postcapillary venules of the body. Vascular leakage of albumin as a result of inflammatory mediator action during the systemic inflammatory response syndrome (SIRS) occurs at the postcapillary venules with diameters of 10–50 μm.[9] These endothelial cells contract and pull away from each other, resulting in large interendothelial gaps.[10, 11] Albumin (69,000 daltons) will flux across the capillary membrane into the interstitium at and remote from the injured site as a result of cytokine action.[12–14] Hypoalbuminemia associated with SIRS implies that the capillary pore size is at least 69,000 daltons in diameter when there is adequate liver function and no evidence of significant renal or intestinal albumin loss.

FLUID CHARACTERISTICS

The number, charge, and size of the particles in water, together with capillary dynamics, determine the movement of that fluid throughout the different fluid compartments. Whenever a membrane between two fluid compartments is permeable to water but not to some of the dissolved solutes, and the concentration of the solutes is greater on one side of the membrane than the other, water passes through the membrane toward the side with the greater concentration of solutes. This is called *osmosis.* The amount of pressure required on the opposite side of the membrane to oppose this movement of water molecules is *osmotic pressure.* The osmotic pressure is determined by the number of particles, not the mass. Osmolality expresses osmotic pressure as milliosmoles per kilogram of water, and osmolarity indicates

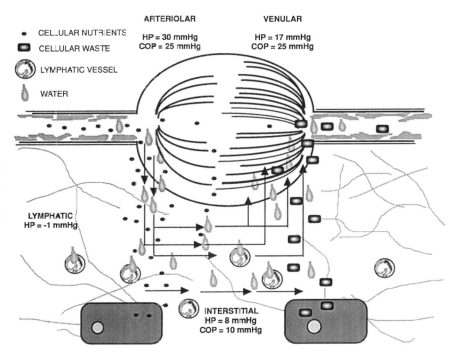

Figure 78–3. The arteriolar (left) side of the capillary presents a hydrostatic pressure of 30 mmHg. Starling's forces favor the movement of fluid into the interstitium. This fluid carries oxygen and nutrients for the cells. The fluid diffuses across the interstitium, depositing these products in exchange for waste products and carbon dioxide. Fluid that is not taken back into the venular side of the capillary is removed by the lymphatics.

osmoles per liter solution. There must be an equal number of cations and anions present on either side of the membrane to ensure electrochemical neutrality between the intravascular and interstitial compartments.

Approximately four fifths of the total osmolality of the interstitial fluid and plasma is caused by sodium and chloride ions, where almost half of the intracellular osmolality is caused by potassium ions. This makes sodium the most osmotically significant ion in the intravascular and extravascular fluid. The ability of fluid to move water across the cellular membrane depends upon the osmolality of that fluid compared with the intracellular osmolality and is called *tonicity*.

The proteins are the only dissolved substances in the plasma and interstitial fluid that do not diffuse readily through the capillary membrane. This maintains the protein concentration in the plasma approximately three times that of the interstitial fluid. It is the proteins that are responsible for the osmotic pressure at the capillary membrane. To distinguish this osmotic pressure at the capillary membrane from that exerted at the cell membrane, the term *colloid osmotic pressure* or *colloid oncotic pressure (COP)* is used. The Gibbs-Donnan effect (Fig. 78–4) causes the colloid osmotic pressure to be about 50 per cent greater than that caused by the proteins alone.

FLUID SELECTION

There are two major catagories of administered fluids: crystalloids and colloids. A *crystalloid* is a water-based solution with small molecules that are permeable to the capillary membrane. The sodium and glucose concentrations of these fluids determine the osmolality and tonicity of the fluid and the distribution between the fluid compartments. The most commonly administered crystalloids and their specific characteristics are listed in Table 78–1.

A *colloid* fluid is a water-based solution with both small molecules that are permeable to the capillary membrane as well as large molecules that cannot cross the capillary membrane. Natural colloids consist of plasma proteins from donor animals and are administered as fresh-frozen plasma, frozen plasma, whole blood, albumin concentrate, and oxyhemoglobin. Synthetic colloids are man-made large molecules dissolved in normal saline. It is the sodium of the saline that determines the osmolarity of the solution, and it is the size of the synthetic molecule that determines the distribution of the solution. Natural and synthetic colloids and their specific characteristics are listed in Table 78–1.

CRYSTALLOIDS

Starling's forces favor the movement of intravascular crystalloids from the capillary into the interstitial space. For example, only approximately 20 per cent of lactated Ringer's solution administered intravenously remains in the intravascular space with 80 per cent moving into the interstitium after 1 hour.[15] Crystalloids are therefore considered primarily as interstitial volume replacement and maintenance fluids.

The critical role that interstitial fluid plays in cells' metabolism and survival makes crystalloid administration an important part of every resuscitation and maintenance fluid therapy plan. The specific crystalloid to administer is selected primarily by the tonicity of the fluid.

ISOTONIC CRYSTALLOIDS

In most clinical situations, resuscitation with crystalloids is best accomplished utilizing an isotonic, balanced electrolyte solution, such as lactated Ringer's, Plasma-Lyte A, or Normosol-R. These solutions provide electrolytes and buffers in concentrations typical of normal plasma and are called *replacement* fluids. If there are ongoing losses of plasma water after resuscitation, such as vomiting or diarrhea, the replacement fluids are utilized to continuously replace these deficits. Isotonic saline is also a replacement fluid but is not "balanced," since it contains only sodium, chloride, and water. There are specific clinical situations that will direct the clinician to utilize isotonic saline instead of the other balanced solutions or to select a specific balanced

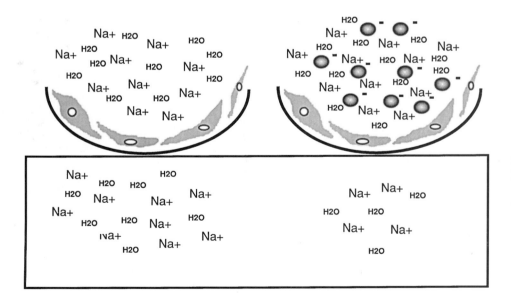

Figure 78–4. Gibbs-Donnan effect. Effect of nondiffusible protein anions (illustrated by larger gray circles) on the distribution of diffusible ions (Na^+ = sodium) across the membrane. Water (H_2O) is retained within the capillary.

● ⁻ **Albumin molecule**

TABLE 78–1. CHARACTERISTICS AND CONTENTS OF COMMONLY USED CRYSTALLOIDS AND COLLOIDS

NAME	FLUID COMPARTMENT	OSMOLARITY (mOsm/L)	pH	Na$^+$ (mEq/L)	Cl$^-$ (mEq/L)	K$^+$ (mEq/L)	Mg^{2+} (mEq/L)	Ca^{2+} (mEq/L)	DEXTROSE (g/L)	BUFFER
Crystalloid										
REPLACEMENT										
0.9% Saline	Extracellular	308 (isotonic)	5.0	154	154	0	0	0	0	None
Lactated Ringer's	Extracellular	275 (isotonic)	6.5	130	109	4	0	3	0	Lactate
Plasmalyte-A pH 7.4	Extracellular	294 (isotonic)	7.4	140	98	5	3	0	0	Acetate, gluconate
Normosol-R	Extracellular	295 (isotonic)	5.5–7	140	98	5	3	0	0	Acetate, gluconate
7.0% saline	Extracellular	2396 (hypertonic)		1197	1197	0	0	0	0	None
5% dextrose in water	Intracellular	252 (hypotonic)	4.0	0	0	0	0	0	50	None
MAINTENANCE										
2.5% dextrose in 1/2-strength lactated Ringer's	Extracellular	264 (isotonic)	4.5–7.5	65.5	55	2	0	1.5	25	Lactate
ProcalAmine	Extracellular	735 (hypertonic)	6–7	35	41	24	5	0	30	Acetate, phosphate
3% FreAmine III	Extracellular	405 (hypertonic)	6–7	35	41	24	5	0	0	Acetate, phosphate
Normosol-M and 5% dextrose	Extracellular	363 (hypertonic)		40	40	13	3	0	50	Acetate
Colloid										
NATURAL										
Whole blood	Extracellular	300 (isotonic)	variable	140	100	4	0	0	0–4	None
Frozen plasma	Extracellular	300 (isotonic)	variable	140	110	4	0	0	0–4	None
SYNTHETIC										
6% Hetastarch	Extracellular	310 (isotonic)	5.5	154	154	0	0	0	0	None
10% Pentastarch	Extracellular	326 (isotonic)	5.0	154	154	0	0	0	0	None
Dextran 40	Extracellular	311 (isotonic)	3.5–7.0	154	154	0	0	0	0	None
Dextran 70	Extracellular	310 (isotonic)	3–7	154	154	0	0	0	0	None
Oxypolygelatin	Extracellular	200 (hypotonic)	7.4	155	100	0	0	1	0	None

solution (Table 78–2). This decision is based on the electrolyte (Na$^+$, K$^+$, Mg^{2+}, Ca^{2+}) concentrations, osmolarity, and pH of the fluid to be administered compared with the needs of the patient.

HYPOTONIC CRYSTALLOIDS

These solutions have water in excess of solutes. The administration of 5 per cent dextrose in water (D5W) is essentially the same as administering free water. The glucose is rapidly metabolized, and the free water moves into the interstitial and intracellular compartments. The use of D5W should be restricted to slow infusion to replace calculated free water deficits, slow administration of constant-rate infusion drugs, or in combination with replacement fluids to create a maintenance composition fluid, resulting in 2.5 per cent dextrose in half-strength replacement fluid. It is not to be used as a resuscitation fluid.

Other hypotonic solutions include half-strength saline or half-strength lactated Ringer's. These are utilized when sodium administration should be minimized. Administration must be slow to allow redistribution and uptake of free water into the interstitial and intracellular spaces.

HYPERTONIC CRYSTALLOIDS

Crystalloid solutions are made hypertonic by the addition of sodium or glucose. Hypertonic crystalloids include 3.0

per cent, 7.0 per cent, and 7.5 per cent saline, and 5 per cent glucose added to balanced electrolyte solutions or maintenance solutions. The hypertonicity draws water into the intravascular space after administration. If there is ongoing loss of plasma water, or if there is already interstitial dehydration, these fluids should be avoided.

The use of hypertonic saline in resuscitation leads to rapid intravascular volume expansion after administration of a small volume of this crystalloid. However, this increase is transient, as the diffused water dilutes the intravascular hypertonic sodium solution. This diluted solution then redistributes back into the interstitial spaces, often taking additional sodium. Cellular dehydration is a sequela, which in some resuscitative situations may be advantageous (brain in cerebral edema; myocardium in shock) but in general is not beneficial. Often hypertonic saline is combined with colloids to retain more of the water and sodium within the intravascular space.

COLLOIDS

Whole blood, plasma products, and concentrated albumin contain natural colloids in the form of proteins, primarily albumin. Oxypolygelatin, dextran 40 and 70, and hydroxyethyl starches (hetastarch and pentastarch) are synthetically derived colloids. Whether a colloid is natural or synthetic in origin, it is the difference in their macromolecular structure and weight that dictates the oncotic effect, method of excre-

TABLE 78–2. CLINICAL SITUATIONS THAT WARRANT SELECTION OF A SPECIFIC CRYSTALLOID IN THE FLUID THERAPY PLAN

DISEASE	CRYSTALLOID	REASON	COMMENTS
Acidosis	Lactated Ringer's Plasmalyte-A Normosol-R	Buffered solutions	Lactate requires degradation to bicarbonate by the liver. Consider choosing other crystalloids Do not administer blood products in the same IV line as lactated Ringer's to prevent calcium precipitation with the anticoagulant
Alkalosis	0.9% sodium chloride	There can be a loss of chloride with hydrogen Lower pH	May require potassium supplementation
Heart failure	Isotonic 1/2-strength isotonic crystalloids, e.g., as lactated Ringer's	Least amount of sodium that may cause exacerbation of fluid overload by increasing intravascular volume	Do not administer blood products in the same IV line as lactated Ringer's to prevent calcium precipitation with the anticoagulant
Hypercalcemia	0.9% sodium chloride	Contains no calcium Relatively higher sodium level will induce greater diuretic effect	May require potassium supplementation
Hypernatremia	Lactated Ringer's	Least amount of sodium compared with other replacement isotonic crystalloids	Do not administer blood products in the same IV line as lactated Ringer's to prevent calcium precipitation with the anticoagulant
Hypoadrenocorticism	0.9% sodium chloride	Contains no potassium Highest amount of sodium augmenting sodium replacement	
Liver failure—end stage	Plasmalyte-A Normosol-R	Avoid lactate buffers Least amount of sodium in the face of portal hypertension	
Renal failure—hypernatremic end stage	Plasmalyte-A Normosol-R 1/2-strength lactated Ringer's	Avoid higher sodium level while decreased glomerular filtration prevents adequate filtering	Do not administer blood products in the same IV line as lactated Ringer's to prevent calcium precipitation with the anticoagulant
Renal failure—oliguric/anuric	0.9% sodium chloride	Avoid contributing to potassium retention	Monitor sodium levels closely
Shock resuscitation—hypovolemic	Lactated Ringer's Plasmalyte-A Normosol-R	Buffered solutions Replace intravascular volume	Lactate requires degradation to bicarbonate by the liver. Consider choosing other crystalloids Do not administer blood products in the same IV line as lactated Ringer's to prevent calcium precipitation with the anticoagulant

tion, and half-life of the solution. Colloids are primarily intravascular volume replacing fluids.

The number average molecular weight of a colloid is the arithmetic mean of the molecular weights of the polymers in solution, and is the weight that produces the most physiologic effect. Weight-average molecular weight is the weight as determined by light scattering and is the sum of the number of molecules at each number average molecular weight divided by the total number of all molecules in solution. This weight is generally larger when larger polymers exist and indicates the potential of molecular longevity in plasma. In general, the greater the number of small molecules that exist per unit volume, the greater the initial oncotic effect and plasma volume expansion. Colloids listed in order of greatest plasma volume expansion are: 25 per cent albumin, oxypolygelatin, dextran 40, pentastarch, dextran 70 hetastarch, 5 per cent albumin, whole blood, plasma.

The degree of molar substitution, the size of the molecule, and the enzymatic processes required for breakdown deter-

mine the half-life of the molecule in the body. Synthetic colloids are eliminated by several processes.[16] Rapid renal elimination of polymeric material whose size is well below the glomerular threshold (<70,000 daltons) occurs 1 to 3 hours after injection. Larger molecules are degraded into smaller pieces and voided. A decrease in glomerular filtration rate will affect synthetic colloid elimination, increasing the half-life of circulating colloid molecules.[16] Extravasated polymeric material, lost from the bloodstream but not voided in the urine, accounts for 20 to 30 per cent of the total dose of macromolecules (>70,000 daltons) administered IV. Both natural and synthetic colloids can be found extravasated into the interstitial space, reaching the maximum within the first 24 hours.

The third process of elimination is via the gastrointestinal system and is of little consequence. Commercially available synthetic colloids listed in order of longest half-life are: hetastarch, dextran 70, pentastarch, dextran 40, oxypolygelatin.

Much of the basic pharmacology of colloids is similar between natural and synthetic colloid groups. However, there are significant differences between groups and within each group (see Table 78–1). These differences are what makes each colloid unique, and are the basis for making an appropriate colloid selection for a specific animal patient. Often a combination of colloids is the best therapeutic approach.

NATURAL COLLOIDS

Whole blood, plasma, and concentrated albumin are natural colloids, with the largest number of oncotic molecules being albumin. Albumin has an average molecular weight of 69,000 daltons and provides 75 per cent of the oncotic pressure in normal vessels. The rest of the colloid oncotic pressure (COP) is attributed to fibrinogen (average molecular weight of 320,000 daltons) and globulins (average molecular weight of 140,000 daltons).[17]

Natural colloids are obtained by volunteer donation and processed according to the product desired.[18] Canine and feline blood products are available (see Chapter 79).

Concentrated human albumin solutions are available for rapid low-volume resuscitation. In humans, concentrated 5 per cent albumin is used during hypovolemic resuscitation, and 25 per cent albumin has been administered to the edematous patient requiring volume resuscitation. Unfortunately, concentrated canine and feline albumin is not readily available.

Natural colloids contain more than just oncotic proteins. Fresh whole blood contains red blood cells, coagulation factors, platelets, albumin, fibrinogen, globulins, white blood cells, and antithrombin. Fresh-frozen plasma contains coagulation factors, albumin (3.5 to 5 per cent concentration), fibrinogen, globulins, and antithrombin, while frozen plasma contains these substances with virtually no concentration of factors V and VIII.

Fresh-frozen or frozen plasma transfusion may be appropriate for animals that acutely lose albumin from the vasculature as a result of an increase in capillary membrane pore size. When the serum albumin level is less than 2.0 g/dL, the authors will administer plasma products in an effort to support the body's requirement of albumin as a buffer and carrier molecule.[19–22]

Dogs and cats receiving whole blood or a combination packed red blood cell–colloid transfusion should be blood-typed and cross-matched, time permitting.

Patients receiving plasma transfusions do not require cross-matching. Plasma should be defrosted in a warm water bath to patient temperature and administered via an 18-micron micropore filter.

Potential concerns with administering natural colloids include a risk of a transfusion reaction, expense, and availability. Time is a factor when treating the acutely hemorrhaging patient. Waiting for blood-typing and a cross-match of whole blood products, or waiting for blood product warming prior to administration, is not always feasible. Although minimized with proper screening of blood donors, transmission of blood-borne illnesses is also a possibility with natural colloid infusion. Serum calcium should be monitored during multiple transfusions. Administration of large volumes of blood products can also cause a dilutional coagulopathy.

SYNTHETIC COLLOIDS

Synthetic colloids were developed to provide timely and convenient fluid resuscitation while avoiding the problems encountered with rapid natural colloid infusions. They provide an increase in COP beyond what is attainable with natural colloids and can be used in conjunction with whole blood or plasma. They are not, however, to be considered a substitute for blood products when albumin, red blood cells, antithrombin, or coagulation proteins are needed.

Oxypolygelatin, dextrans, and hydroxyethyl starches (HES) are synthetic colloids, each with pharmacology, specific qualities, and potential side effects that make them unique. The specific characteristics of the synthetic colloids are listed in Tables 78–1 and 78–3. Indications for use are presented in Table 78–4, and doses and rate of administration are in Table 78–5. Selection of a specific synthetic colloid is based upon these individual characteristics, and questions to consider when making this selection are outlined in Table 78–6.

OXYPOLYGELATIN

The standard gelatin products are either modified fluid, urea-linked, or oxypolygelatin. Oxypolygelatin differs from the other two in the way it is cross-linked. It is produced from cattle–bone marrow gelatin, prepared by gradual controlled heating and oxidation with hydrogen peroxide. Excretion of oxypolygelatin is primarily by glomerular filtration

TABLE 78–3. COMPARISON OF COLLOIDS

	5% ALBUMIN	25% ALBUMIN	OXYPOLY-GELATIN	DEXTRAN 40	DEXTRAN 70	PENTASTARCH	HETASTARCH
Weight-average molecular weight (daltons)	69,000	69,000	30,000	40,000	70,000	280,000	450,000
Number-average molecular weight (daltons)	69,000	69,000	22,000–24,000	25,000	39,000	39,000	70,000
Molecular weight range (daltons)	—	—	5600–100,000	10,000–80,000	15,000–160,000	10,000–1 mil	10,000–3.4 mil
Solvent	—	—	Electrolyte solution	0.9% saline or 5% dextrose	0.9% saline or 5% dextrose	0.9% saline	0.9% saline
Maximum water binding (mL H_2O/g colloid)	18	18	39	37	29	30	20
Concentration (%)	5	25	5.6	10	6	10	6
Half-life (hrs)	14–16 days	14–16 days	2–4	2.5	25	2.5	25
Plasma % (hrs)	—	—	12	18	29	7	38
Extravascular % (24 hrs)	—	—	—	22	33	33	39
Overall survival in blood	—	—	168 hrs	44 hrs	4–6 weeks	96 hours	17–26 weeks
Colloid oncotic pressure (mmHg)	20	100	45–47	40	—	25	30

TABLE 78–4. INDICATIONS FOR USE OF SPECIFIC COLLOIDS

Natural Colloids

Fresh whole blood:	Rapid volume resuscitation acute hemorrhage; anemia with hypoalbuminemia; significant bleeding from coagulopathy/thrombocytopenia
Stored whole blood	As above except bleeding thrombocytopenia, factor V or VIII deficiency
Autotransfused blood*	Rapid intravascular volume resuscitation for life-threatening hemorrhage when no transfusion available
Plasma:	Coagulopathies (fresh-frozen for factor V or VII deficiency); disseminated intravascular coagulation; low antithrombin; acute hypoalbuminemia

Synthetic Colloids

Oxypolygelatin	Acute, short-term intravascular volume resuscitation from hypovolemic shock
Dextran 40	Rapid short-term intravascular volume resuscitation from hypovolemic shock; rapid improvement of microcirculatory flow; prophylaxis deep vein thrombosis/pulmonary emboli
Dextran 70	Rapid intravascular volume resuscitation from hypovolemic, traumatic, or hemorrhagic shock
Hydroxyethyl starch	Rapid intravascular volume resuscitation from all forms of shock; SIRS with increased capillary permeability/albumin leakage; small-volume resuscitation

*Purvis, D: Autotransfusion in the emergency patient. Vet Clin North Am Small Anim Pract 24:1291, 1995.

and secretion into the feces.[23] A small percentage will appear in expired air. Breakdown into smaller peptides and amino acids occurs via proteolytic enzyme degradation. The rate of metabolism depends only on the molecular weight size distribution of macromolecules present in blood after the first phase of elimination is completed.

Oxypolygelatin administration results in intravascular volume 2.0 times the amount administered owing to osmosis of an equal amount of water from the interstitium. Simultaneous administration of crystalloids for interstitial volume replacement is recommended. Because of its rapid and dramatic volume-expanding capabilities, postinfusion vascular volumes should be closely monitored to avoid volume overload. An osmotic diuresis occurs through the excretion of the small gelatin molecules.[24] Oxypolygelatin has not been associated with renal failure.[23] There are no direct effects on coagulation proteins or platelets.

Antibodies to raw unmodified gelatin can be found in animals without prior administration of the gelatin products. By adjusting the cross-linking, oxypolygelatin has relatively less risk for inducing these reactions than the other gelatins. However, a clinically relevant risk of allergic reaction remains with oxypolygelatin, mediated by histamine and complement activation.[23, 25] The reported incidence of anaphylactic reactions for all species of gelatins is higher than for either dextran or HES.

A dilutional coagulopathy has been reported,[24] similar to dextran 40, and the clotting time was significantly increased after equal volume oxypolygelatin infusion.[26] Because gelatins have been reported to initiate tetany by lowering serum calcium, the oxypolygelatin product for veterinary use is supplemented with calcium. The manufacturer of oxypolygelatin recommends using it with extreme caution in animals with coagulation disorders, hypoproteinemia, cardiac and pulmonary insufficiency, and renal diseases. Gelatins may cause depression of serum fibronectin levels, but the clinical significance is unknown.[27]

DEXTRAN

Dextrans are polysaccharides composed of linear glucose residues.[28] They are produced by the enzyme dextran sucrase during growth of various strains of bacterium *Leuconostoc* in media containing sucrose. Different molecular weight dextrans can be produced by acid hydrolysis of the parent macromolecule. High-molecular-weight dextrans (250,000 and 500,000) have been investigated in horses and in rodents, respectively.[29, 30] Dextrans are carried in sodium chloride or 5 per cent dextrose solutions, are isotonic, and can be stored at room temperature.

Survival of dextrans in plasma is determined by the molecular weight. Large polymers are retained in blood until they are metabolized to a size able to penetrate the endothelial cell barrier. The smallest dextran molecules are rapidly

TABLE 78–5. DOSAGE AND RATE OF ADMINISTRATION OF SPECIFIC COLLOIDS

Natural Colloids

Whole blood:	Dog: 20 mL/kg or until PCV can support tissue oxygenation (generally 25–30%) Cat: 10 mL/kg or until PCV can support tissue oxygenation (generally 25–30%)

Whole blood is administered as quickly as possible in acute life-threatening hemorrhagic shock to sustain an MAP of 80 mmHg, or over a 4–6 hour period when hemodynamically stable. For dogs and cats in distributive shock due to SIRS, once the PCV is above 25%, the initial infusion of blood can be followed by a CRI of hetastarch

Plasma:	Dog: 250 mL/10–20 kg over 4–6 hours or until the plasma albumin >2.0 g/dL Cat: 10 mL/kg over 4–6 hours or until the plasma albumin >2.0 g/dL

From our experience, as many as 6–10 units of frozen plasma may be required to raise the plasma albumin level to 2.0 g/dL in large-sized dogs with SIRS. For dogs and cats in distributive shock due to SIRS, once the plasma albumin is above 2.0 g/dL, the initial infusion of plasma can be followed by a CRI of hetastarch

Synthetic Colloids

Oxypolygelatin:	5 mL/kg over 15 minutes, titrate to effect Do not exceed 15 mL/kg total dose

If further volume is required for volume resuscitation, another synthetic colloid can be administered. For dogs and cats in distributive shock due to SIRS, the initial resuscitation can be followed by a CRI of hetastarch

Dextran:	Dogs: 10–40 mL/kg/day IV bolus to effect Cats: 5 mL/kg increments given over 5–10 minutes, repeated to effect, up to 40 mL/kg

For dogs and cats in distributive shock due to SIRS, the initial bolus of dextran can be followed by a CRI of hetastarch

Hydroxyethyl starch:	Dogs: 10–40 mL/kg/day IV bolus to effect Cats: 5 mL/kg increments given over 5–10 minutes, repeated to effect, up to 40 mL/kg

For dogs and cats in hypovolemic cardiogenic shock, with pulmonary contusions, or with head injury: 5 mL/kg increment boluses are administered to effect, using the smallest volume possible to maintain an MAP of at least 80 mmHg

For dogs and cats in distributive shock due to SIRS, the initial bolus of colloid is followed by CRI of hetastarch to maintain an MAP of at least 80 mmHg and a COP >14 mmHg:

> Dogs: 10–20 mL/kg/day
> Cats: 10–40 mL/kg/day in the cat (2–8 mL/cat/hour)

TABLE 78–6. QUESTIONS TO IDENTIFY CHARACTERISTICS OF SPECIFIC COLLOIDS

1. Rate of administration?
Dogs: Rapid IV bolus (within 5 min): dex, heta, penta
                Slow IV bolus (total within 15–30 min): all colloids
Cats: Slow IV to effect (total within 15–30 min): all colloids

2. Small volume resuscitation needed:
Traumatic or hypovolemic shock: dex, heta, penta, gel
Cardiogenic shock: heta, penta

3. Duration and strength of effect desired?
Strongest colloid effect wanted for 2–4 hours: dex-40, gel
Moderate colloid effect wanted for 2–4 hours: penta, dex-70
Moderate colloid effect needed for >24 hours: heta

4. Anticipated capillary integrity?
Losing electrolytes and water: heta, penta, dex-70, plasma
Losing electrolytes, water and albumin: heta, penta, +/− plasma

5. Systemic inflammatory response syndrome anticipated?
Heta, penta

6. Ongoing hemorrhage occurring?
Traumatic loss: Whole blood with dex, heta, penta, gel
                 PRBC with plasma, heta, dex, gel
DIC: Plasma (with heparin) and heta combination
Coagulopathy: Whole blood alone or with heta, penta, dex, gel
                 Plasma alone or with heta, penta, dex, gel

7. Rheologic effect desired?
Improved microvascular flow: heta, dex, gel, penta
Decrease red blood cell or platelet aggregation or adhesion: dex-40

dex = dextran; heta = hetastarch; penta = pentastarch; gel = oxypolygelatin; PRBC = packed red blood cells.

filtered by the kidneys and induce a mild diuresis. Because of their linear structure, many molecules easily enter through the capillary membranes into the interstitial space and eventually return to the bloodstream via the lymphatics. Larger molecules are briefly stored in hepatocytes, renal tubular cells, and reticuloendothelial system without producing toxicity.[27] Dextran is broken down completely to CO_2 and H_2O by dextranase present in spleen, liver, lung, kidney, brain, and muscle at a rate approaching 70 mg/kg every 24 hours.[31, 32] The plasma half-life of dextran 40 is 2.5 hours, and for dextran 70 is 25 hours.

The reported degree of dextran-induced volume expansion varies based on the type and concentration of solution used and the experimental setting. A 500-mL bolus of 6 per cent dextran 40 produces a 750-mL expansion in intravascular volume at 1 hour and a 1050-mL expansion at 2 hours.[33] In normal dogs, dextran 70 increased the plasma volume 1.38 times (138 per cent) the volume infused.[34]

Dextran is not an anticoagulant but has antithrombotic effects that are due to hemodilution of blood, temporary change in the function of factor VIIIR:Ag, and decreasing platelet aggregability and thrombus stability, especially at a lower molecular weight.[35, 36] Dextran copolymerizes with the fibrin monomer, destabilizing clot formation.[37] Thrombi formed in blood of human patients given dextran are significantly more lysable than thrombi obtained from untreated controls.[38] The small molecules in dextran 40 provide a coating of the red cells and platelets, and an inhibition of thrombus formation that may prevent thrombosis.

Blood glucose levels may be elevated during dextran metabolism into its glucose residues. This may be a response to rapid degradation of the glucose polymers, or a catecholamine response to shock. Bilirubin values can be falsely increased for unknown reasons. Dextran 70 may cause a change in the total solids value that does not reflect actual protein content. Clinical significance of these changes is not known.[39] Dextran 70 may interfere with blood cross-match as a result of red blood cell cross-linking.[40–42]

Dextran 40 has been associated with acute renal failure,[43] anaphylaxis, and bleeding diathesis. As tubular water is reabsorbed by the kidney, the filtered dextran may precipitate and irreversibly obstruct the tubules. Renal problems are more likely to occur when there is underlying renal disease or preexisting dehydration. Dextran 70 has rarely been associated with acute renal failure.[27]

There are naturally occurring antibodies to dextran in the general human population. Dextran is found in sugar and other foods. Moderate to life-threatening dextran-induced anaphylactic reactions in man can be classified as immune complex–mediated (type III) anaphylaxis.[44] Mild reactions appear to have a different mechanism. Clinical and experimental experience with dextran 70 in the dog finds moderate to life-threatening reactions rare.

Hemostatic changes in healthy experimental dogs given dextran 70 include an increase in the buccal mucosal bleeding time and partial thromboplastin time (PTT), and a decrease in von Willebrand factor antigen and factor VIII coagulant activity, without clinical bleeding.[39] Fibrinogen concentration decreases in excess of that which can be explained by dilution in dogs.

HYDROXYETHYL STARCH

Hydroxyethyl starch (HES) is the parent name of a polymeric molecule made from a waxy species of either maize or sorghum, and is composed primarily of amylopectin (98 per cent). It is a highly branched polysaccharide closely resembling glycogen, formed by the reaction between ethylene oxide and amylopectin in the presence of an alkaline catalyst.[28] The molecular weight and molar substitution can be adjusted by acid hydrolysis of the parent amylopectin molecule.

Two species of HES are currently commercially available for fluid resuscitation and maintenance: 6 per cent hetastarch and 10 per cent pentastarch.[28, 40, 45–47] The disappearance of HES molecules from the body depends on their rate of absorption by tissues (liver, spleen, kidney, and heart), gradual return to the circulation, uptake by the reticuloendothelial system, enzymatic degradation to smaller particles by amylase, and clearance through the urine and bile. Blood alpha-amylase–mediated hydrolysis reduces the molecular weight to less than 72,000 daltons. The metabolism of HES retained in tissue probably occurs by the action of cytoplasmic lysosomes.[48] Resident macrophages do not contain enzymes for biodegradation of HES molecules, prolonging elimination. HES molecules are stored transiently in the renal tubular epithelium, causing morphologic changes but no alteration in renal function.[42] A rise in serum amylase is to be expected without alteration in pancreatic function.

The degree of substitution rather than molecular weight is the major determinant of how long the different types of HES survive in the blood. Pentastarch is more rapidly degraded and excreted than hetastarch owing to a lower molar substitution. When hetastarch is infused at 25 mL/kg in normal dogs, the initial increase in plasma volume is 1.37 times the volume infused.[34] Administration of a 500-mL infusion of pentastarch results in a 700-mL increase in plasma volume within 30 minutes of infusion.[49] The intravascular persistence of hetastarch is significantly greater than that of dextran 70, with 38 per cent of hetastarch remaining compared with 19 per cent of dextran 24 hours after infusion.[27] Administration of hetastarch by constant-rate infusion (CRI) may provide a constant supply of larger molecular weight particles, perhaps maintaining and augmenting plasma COP in the animal with albumin loss.

Pentastarch is being used in humans as an adjunct for leukapheresis and is also used in Europe and Canada as a hemodiluting and volume-expanding agent.[50, 51] Pentastarch has been investigated for inducing hypervolemia in hemodilution treatment of acute stroke victims,[52] as well as for volume expansion in human cardiac patients undergoing surgery,[53, 54] septic patients,[55] and for burn resuscitation.[56]

HES has been shown to reverse changes in microvascular permeability caused by oxygen free radicals during reperfusion injury.[57–59] It also decreases plasma concentration of soluble adhesion molecules, decreasing leukocyte-endothelial adhesion and improving microcirculation.[60] Whether this is an effect of improved microvascular perfusion or an independent characteristic of its molecular architecture has yet to be determined. Hetastarch has been investigated as a carrier for deferoxamine (an iron chelator) in ischemia-reperfusion studies.[61, 62]

Hetastarch favors retention of intravascular fluid and prevents washout of interstitial proteins.[63–65] In hypooncotic situations, hetastarch infusion has a great advantage over the other colloids because the larger molecules remain intravascular, limiting pulmonary fluid flux.[66] Lung lymph flow in the animal chronically protein depleted receiving lactated Ringer's was dramatically increased in comparison with those receiving hetastarch. This is attributed to hetastarch's ability to increase plasma oncotic pressure.

The incidence of anaphylaxis with hetastarch infusion has been reported in humans as 0.0005 to 0.085 per cent.[67, 68] Reactions can be divided into mild (skin reactions and/or mild elevation in temperature), moderate (tachycardia, hypotension, nausea, or disturbance in respiration), and life-threatening. Hetastarch is nontoxic and nonallergenic in doses up to 100 mL/kg in dogs.[69] Hetastarch has been shown to cause complement activation.[70] In the authors' experience, a large number of cats have a moderate reaction, displaying nausea and occasionally vomiting when hetastarch is infused rapidly. However, when the drug was given slowly (over 15 to 30 minutes) to the cat, this side effect is eliminated.

There are conflicting reports of HES-induced coagulopathies. It appears that the molecular weight range plays a role, as well as the amount administered.[28, 71–73] Studies of the effects of hetastarch on platelets have yielded contradictory results after one-time administration.[74] Induced thrombocyte aggregation was inhibited after perioperative administration of high-molecular-weight starch, and a platelet concentration decrease proportional to the dilutional effect has been reported.[75, 76] There are a few published letters concerning a hetastarch-related decrease in von Willebrand factor concentrations.[77, 78]

Dilutional effects on coagulation factors and proteins are produced in response to the volume expansion of the plasma. Bleeding time and volume of blood lost were most significant in dogs receiving more than the recommended dose.

There is a notable increase in activated partial thromboplastin time (aPTT) in patients receiving hetastarch, attributable to precipitation of factor VIII by hetastarch.[78–81] This effect is reportedly less than that of dextran. The authors have administered hetastarch to over 700 dogs and 250 cats over an 8-year period. Activated clotting times (ACT) in these animals were prolonged without clinical evidence of hemorrhage. It is the authors' impression that the ACTs may increase to 180 seconds in the dog (normal ACT = 90 to 120 seconds) and 120 seconds in the cat (normal ACT = 75 to 90), attributable to the direct and dilutional effects of hetastarch, without concern for clinical hemorrhage. However, when hetastarch has been administered during resuscitation to dogs with massive trauma in quantities that exceed 20 mL/kg/day, there has been an occasional increase in incisional bleeding. This may be due to an increase in microcirculatory flow and blood pressure, as well as dilutional and direct effects of the hetastarch on coagulation.

In another experimental model of canine hemorrhage, bleeding from incisions was three to four times longer than saline controls in those receiving 20 to 30 mL/kg of hetastarch.[82] Results of coagulation profiles were not significantly different from other experimental studies and were attributed to hemodilution. Hetastarch was associated with the least bleeding from the incisions in comparison with the dextrans at equal volume.

Pentastarch has similar effects on coagulation parameters as hetastarch; however, no significant changes are noted for urokinase-activated clot lysis and bleeding times with pentastarch.[83] In addition, effects on factor VIII moieties are a result of hemodilution alone with pentastarch.

STROMA-FREE HEMOGLOBIN

It has been proposed that hemoglobin solution might be a temporary substitute for red blood cells.[84] Hemoglobin has the ability to bind oxygen, with 1 g of hemoglobin chemically binding 1.3 mL of oxygen. Hemoglobin can become fully saturated for oxygen at ambient oxygen pressures, and the oxygen is normally unloaded at the capillary in oxygen pressures of approximately 40 mmHg.

The hemoglobin solution is made stroma-free to avoid complications of nephrotoxicity. The molecule is modified by the addition of pyridoxal phosphate, giving the molecule a higher ability for oxygen saturation. Also, the molecule is polymerized to normalize the oxygen capacity while maintaining the COP within normal (20 to 25 mmHg).

Preliminary studies are favorable for using stroma-free hemoglobin in the dog as a temporary substitute for red blood cells. Long-term studies are necessary to determine the safety and efficacy at various doses and rates of administration.

THE FLUID THERAPY PLAN

The fluid therapy plan is based on the characteristics of the specific fluids and the distribution of those fluids within the body. Determining ongoing fluid requirements can be challenging because of vascular leakage, vasodilatation, excessive vasoconstriction, inadequate cardiac function, alterations in fluid composition, and/or ongoing fluid loses. Fluid therapy must be adequate to replace the deficits and meet the ongoing requirements of the animal. Decisions must often be made quickly, ordering the ideal fluid(s) at the right rate, in sufficient amounts, and given by the most efficient route.

Tolerance for error is less in the critical patient than in the usual hospitalized patient. Normal kidney and cardiovascular systems can correct most fluid therapy miscalculations, but in the critically ill animal, these organs may be compromised. Often the clinician must determine the best approach for restoring organ function on an hour-to-hour basis, using end-point resuscitation techniques. It must be determined whether the animal needs a resuscitation and maintenance fluid plan or only maintenance.

RESUSCITATION

Resuscitation fluid therapy is the administration of fluids to rapidly replace a fluid deficit that is causing or has the potential to cause life-threatening organ compromise. When the fluid deficit is in the intravascular space, this is manifested primarily as a *perfusion* problem. When the fluid deficit is in the interstitial or intracellular space, the physical signs reflect a *hydration* problem.

Perfusion

Fluid deficit in the intravascular space causes *poor perfusion* and inadequate tissue oxygenation. This volume deficit results in a lower vessel wall tension and a decrease in the tonic stimulation of the baroreceptors. There is blunting of vagal stimulation of the sinus node and increased sympathetic stimulation. Poor perfusion is manifested by tachycardia and vasoconstriction in the dog and, most commonly, by a normal or slower than normal heart rate in the cat. The earliest stages of hypovolemic shock in the dog cause hyperemic mucous membranes and bounding pulses. This is not typically seen in the cat. Later stages in the dog and cat are manifested by poor pulse quality, prolonged capillary refill time, grey mucous membrane coloration, and low rectal temperatures. Enough fluids must be rapidly administered to remain in the intravascular space, increase the vessel wall tension, and obliterate the need for the baroreceptor compensatory response. Microvascular flow must be rapidly restored for return of tissue oxygenation and cellular energy production.

Resuscitation of perfusion deficits associated with hypovolemia requires rapid intravascular volume expansion by intravenous or intraosseous routes of administration. Crystalloids can be used alone for this purpose; however, perfusion end-points may be more difficult to reach and maintain without complications of edema. Standard recommended crystalloid resuscitation volumes to administer for shock are equivalent to replacing one blood volume per hour (dog: 90 mL/kg/hour; cat: 40 to 60 mL/kg/hour). This must be titrated to effect.

When large quantities of crystalloids are rapidly administered intravenously, there is an immediate increase in hydrostatic pressure and extravasation of large quantities into the interstitial spaces. Many animals can handle the extra interstitial volume for a short period. In normal tissues, the lymphatics will return the excess fluid to the vascular space to be excreted by the kidneys. However, there are two major organs that fail when the quantity of interstitial fluid surpasses the capacity of the lymphatics: the brain and lungs. Extreme care must be given when replacing perfusion deficits with crystalloids alone in animals with pathology in either of these organs, or if there is significant impairment of renal function.

The use of colloids during fluid resuscitation requires less volume than with crystalloids alone, there is less tendency toward fluid overload, and resuscitation times are shorter.[85–87] Plasma COP can be maintained near normal (20 to 25 mmHg) with synthetic colloids, favoring intravascular fluid retention.

When colloids are to be administered, it must be decided whether natural colloids, e.g., plasma or whole blood, a synthetic colloid, or a combination of both is to be used (Fig. 78–5). When the animal requires red blood cells, clotting factors, antithrombin III, or albumin, blood products are necessary. However, because the COP of transfused plasma and whole blood is the same as that of the patient's blood or plasma (unless the animal is hypoproteinemic), the blood products cannot be expected to raise the COP. The blood volume will be increased by an amount equal to the amount infused. The addition of synthetic colloids may be required for this effect and will result in an increase in intravascular volume greater than the volume infused.

A colloid should be administered that is larger than the pore size of the capillaries. When there is increased capillary permeability and loss of albumin through the capillary membrane, hetastarch or pentastarch is the colloid of choice. Persisting in giving crystalloids alone will raise the intravascular hydrostatic pressure, further dilute the COP, and accelerate fluid flow across the membrane into the interstitial fluid compartment.

Resuscitation and maintenance fluid therapy for shock and systemic inflammatory response syndrome (SIRS) disease conditions (such as sepsis, pancreatitis, heat stroke) with increased capillary permeability are often best accomplished with a synthetic colloid combined with a crystalloid, and with natural colloids as indicated. The amount of crystalloid administered with colloids must be reduced by 40 to 60 per cent of what would be administered if crystalloids were used alone. This is to prevent a dramatic increase in intravascular hydrostatic pressure and decrease in intravascular COP, causing interstitial edema. Techniques for resuscitation with colloids include rapid intravascular volume resuscitation for dogs and small volume resuscitation.

Rapid Intravascular Volume Resuscitation for Dogs. Unless there is closed cavity hemorrhage, pulmonary contusions, cardiac dysfunction, or head trauma, dogs experiencing shock due to hypovolemia or maldistribution of blood flow benefit from rapid intravascular volume resuscitation techniques. The 10 to 20 mL/kg daily dose of dextran, hetastarch, or stroma-free hemoglobin is administered as quickly as possible by IV bolus.

Whole blood products can be administered by rapid intravenous volume resuscitation techniques in catastrophic hemorrhagic situations, with input at least matching ongoing loss. Rapid intravascular volume resuscitation techniques with synthetic colloids are not recommended in the cat.

Small Volume Intravascular Resuscitation. Oxypolygelatin requires a slower administration over 15 minutes, as recommended by the manufacturer, and is best administered by a small volume intravascular resuscitation technique. Crystalloid fluids are titrated to replace interstitial fluid deficits. Additional colloids can be administered using small volume intravascular resuscitation techniques if perfusion has not improved to the desired end-point after the initial bolus. Hypovolemic dogs with closed cavity hemorrhage, head trauma or pulmonary contusions, cardiogenic shock, and oliguric renal failure, and all hypotensive cats will benefit from careful resuscitation using small volume intravascular resuscitation techniques. The synthetic colloid is administered at 5 mL/kg increments, over 5 to 10 minutes. The perfusion parameters are reassessed and the 5 mL/kg bolus repeated as needed until the end-point of resuscitation is reached. The goal is to administer the smallest volume of colloid possible to successfully resuscitate the intravascular compartment. This minimizes extravasation of fluids into the brain or lungs, titrates the preload to the heart, and reduces the probability of disturbing clot formation.[88–90] Animals

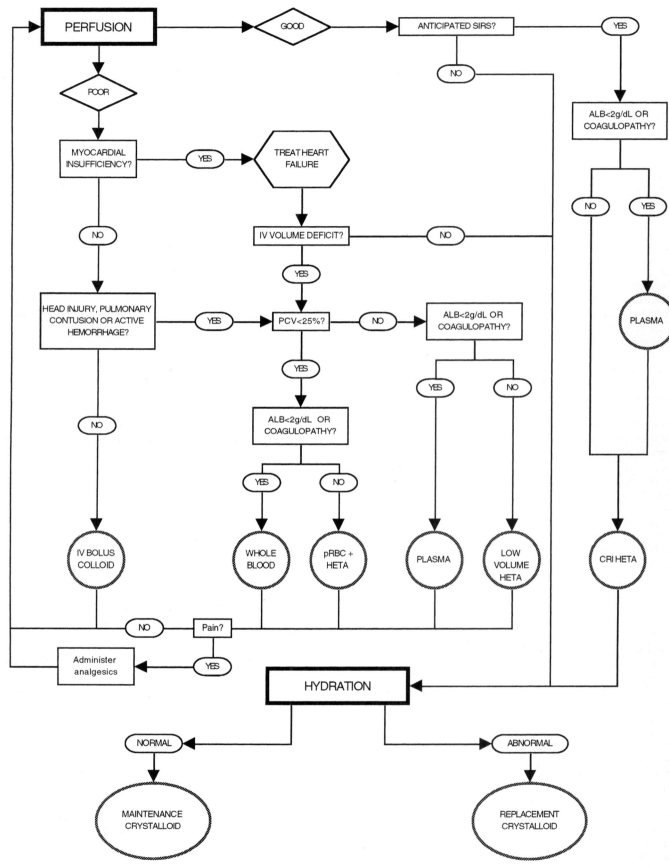

Figure 78–5. Algorithm for selection of colloid for resuscitation of poor perfusion.

requiring resuscitation by techniques described above will be prepared for maintenance colloid infusion immediately post-resuscitation.

When hypovolemia plays a significant role in the decompensation from cardiogenic shock, careful small volume resuscitation with a colloid can replace intravascular volume while minimizing crystalloid extravasation into the lungs.[91] However, the mainstay of therapy is directed toward controlling arrhythmias, augmenting contractility as necessary, and manipulating preload and afterload.[92]

Hydration

Fluid deficit in the extravascular space (interstitial and intracellular) causes *dehydration*. This results in tenting of the skin, dry mucous membranes, sunken eyes, and dullness to the cornea. Severe dehydration can lead to impaired perfusion as a result of fluid moving from the intravascular space to the dehydrated interstitium. To replenish the extravascular spaces, crystalloid fluids that are the same tonicity as normal plasma are administered. Over 75 to 80 per cent of the isotonic crystalloid administered intravenously will be in the extravascular space within 1 hour in a normal animal.

The amount of crystalloids to administer is determined by using physical parameters to estimate the per cent of dehydration. The formula

Per cent dehydration $\times$ kg body weight = fluid deficit (liters)

is used to arrive at a total volume. These fluids are administered by intravenous or intraosseous routes when used for resuscitating hydration. Though subcutaneous routes can be used, the disbursement of fluids throughout the body will often be too slow for effective resuscitation. A balanced isotonic fluid is most often used initially; however, some clinical situations warrant selection of a specific balanced electrolyte solution or isotonic saline as the fluid of choice (see Table 78–2).

The rate of administration will depend upon the urgency of interstitial resuscitation and the rate at which the fluids were lost. Acute loss warrants acute replacement over 1 to 4 hours. Chronic losses or dysfunction of the lungs, heart, or brain directs a slower resuscitation rate, over 4 to 12 hours, as long as perfusion is adequate. The total amount administered and the rate of administration will be determined by monitoring for specific end-points.

End-point Resuscitation

Formulas have been proposed for calculating the quantities of fluids to be delivered for successful resuscitation. However, these formulas have not proven to be consistently accurate, owing to individual variations such as vascular permeability; differences in cardiac, pulmonary, and renal function; and ongoing losses. Successful resuscitation therapy depends upon administering quantities of fluids sufficient to reach specified end-points (Table 78–7). This process is termed *end-point resuscitation*.

The goal of volume resuscitation in shock or SIRS diseases is to provide adequate resuscitation while preventing volume overload and its complications of pulmonary, peripheral, and brain edema. The clinician must determine prior to resuscitation what end-point values for monitored parameters will indicate successful resuscitation. Physical, hemodynamic, and blood chemistry parameters are the mainstay of monitoring end-points. Further investigations may lead to monitoring gastric mucosal pH and serum lactate for end-point determination. The inciting cause of the fluid deficit and vital organ function will dictate the end-points selected and end-point resuscitation techniques employed.

Supranormal End-point Resuscitation. Below a critical level of oxygen delivery to the tissue, tissue extraction cannot increase in proportion to the reduced delivery, and oxygen consumption begins to fall. Cellular hypoxia and decreased energy production result. Clinical studies in critically ill humans have found a higher mortality rate in those that are unable to increase their oxygen extraction rate in response to decreases in oxygen transport. The highest surviving group had their oxygen consumption dependent upon oxygen transport.[93] For hypovolemic and SIRS shock, resuscitation of perfusion to supranormal values to increase oxygen delivery is recommended (see Table 78–7).[94] Restoration of physical perfusion parameters (lowering of heart rate, stronger pulses, normal capillary refill time, pink mucous membranes) is used in conjunction with hemodynamic parameters.

Hypotensive End-point Resuscitation. Traumatic shock with closed cavity hemorrhage warrants hypotensive resuscitation. The animal is resuscitated to end-points of improved physical perfusion parameters, but blood pressures remain in the low-normal range rather than utilizing supranormal values. This is to avoid dislodging clots that may be providing life-saving hemostasis.

Isovolemic Hemodilution. Isovolemic hemodilution can be employed to conserve blood, reduce risks associated with transfusion, and improve microcirculatory blood flow.[95] It has been used in humans during cardiac surgery, for Jehovah's Witnesses, in patients difficult to cross-match, and in renal transplant patients who must avoid homologous blood to prevent alloimmunization.

Normally total body oxygen delivery exceeds oxygen uptake by the tissues. This provides a large oxygen reserve. When oxygen delivery is decreased as a result of hemodilution, there is a corresponding increase in oxygen extraction. Maintenance of normal tissue oxygenation during limited hemodilution is attributed to increased tissue perfusion. Although the number of red cells per unit volume is reduced, they are delivered more rapidly, and possibly more uniformly to the capillary beds. It has been demonstrated that there are disproportionately large increases in coronary blood flow during hemodilution compared with other regional vascular beds. This is due to both decreased viscosity and direct vasodilatation of coronary vascular beds.[96]

During deliberate hemodilution, blood is extracted and preserved for reinfusion at a later time. The blood loss is matched by a cell-free infusion, keeping the blood volume constant.[95] The estimated blood to withdraw to achieve the target hematocrit is:

$$BL = BV \times (H_o - H_f)/H_o$$

where BL = blood loss; BV = blood volume; H_o = initial hematocrit; H_f = final hematocrit; hemoglobin concentration may be substituted for hematocrit.

Studies in dogs and humans have shown that colloid hemodilution resulted in better compensatory changes than did hemodilution with lactated Ringer's solution in terms of oxygen transport and changes in lung water.[97] The end-point of volume infusion is not only the target hematocrit but also physiologically stable end-points such as mean arterial pressure and cardiac output.

TABLE 78–7. FLUID SELECTION, DOSE, AND RATE BASED ON PATHOLOGY

STATUS	FLUID TYPE	DOSE/RATE	END POINT	COMMENTS
Compensatory shock Red MM, CRT < 1 sec Rapid heart rate Normal to increased MAP Normal to decreased CVP	Isotonic, replacement crystalloid Or isotonic, replacement crystalloid with synthetic colloid	Dog: 90 mL/kg/hr IV, IO Cat: 40–60 mL/kg/hr IV, IO Dog: 35–55 mL/kg/hr IV, IO Cat: 24–36 mL/kg/hr IV, IO with HES/DEX: 20mL/kg IV, IO bolus or OXY: 15 mL/kg in 5 mL/kg increment boluses IV	Pink MM, 1–2 sec CRT Normal heart rate MAP ≥ 80 mmHg CVP > 6 & < 8 cm H_2O COP ≧ 14 mm Hg ALB > 2.0 g/dL	Follow with rehydration and maintenance fluid administration
Early decompensatory shock Pale MM, CRT > 2 sec Rapid heart rate Normal to decreased MAP Decreased CVP	Isotonic, replacement crystalloid Or isotonic, replacement crystalloid with synthetic colloid	Dog: 90 mL/kg/hr IV, IO Cat: 40–60 mL/kg/hr IV, IO Dog: 35–55 mL/kg/hr IV, IO Cat: 24–36 mL/kg/hr IV, IO with HES/DEX: 20 mL/kg IV, IO bolus or OXY: 15 mL/kg in 5 mL/kg increment boluses IV	Pink MM, 1–2 sec CRT Normal heart rate MAP ≥ 80 mmHg CVP > 6 & < 8 cmH₂O COP ≧ 14 mmHg ALB > 2.0 g/dL	If it is difficult maintaining resuscitation, place on a CRI of hetastarch Dog: 0.8–1.2 mL/kg/hr Cat: 2–8 mL/cat/hr Follow with rehydration and maintenance fluid administration
	Or hypertonic saline with synthetic colloid	7% saline: Dog: 4–8 mL/kg IV, IO and HES/DEX: 20 mL/kg bolus IV, IO Cat: 1–4 mL/kg IV, IO and HES/DEX: 20 mL/kg bolus IV, IO		Administer hypertonic saline with extreme caution in dehydrated animal, or if brain or pulmonary hemorrhage is suspected
Late decompensatory shock Pale to grey MM, CRT > 2 sec Normal to slow heart rate Decreased MAP Normal/increased/decreased CVP Organ failure	Isotonic, replacement crystalloid with synthetic colloid	Dog: 35–55 mL/kg/hr IV, IO Cat: 24–36 mL/kg/hr IV, IO with HES/DEX: 20 mL/kg IV, IO or OXY: 15 mL/kg in 5 mL/kg increment boluses IV	Pink MM, 1–2 sec CRT Normal heart rate MAP ≥ 80 mmHg CVP > 6 & < 8 cm H_2O COP ≧ 14 mmHg ALB > 2.0 g/dL	If it is difficult maintaining resuscitation, place on a CRI of betastarch Dog: 0.8–1.2 mL/kg/hr Cat: 2–8 mL/cat/hr May require additional cardiovascular support with positive inotropes or blood pressure support
	Or hypertonic saline with synthetic colloid	7% saline: Dog: 4–8 mL/kg IV, IO and HES/DEX: 20 mL/kg bolus IV, IO Cat: 1–4 mL/kg IV, IO and HES/DEX: 20 mL/kg bolus IV, IO		Administer hypertonic saline with extreme caution in dehydrated animal, or if brain or pulmonary hemorrhage is suspected Follow with rehydration and maintenance fluid administration
Acute hemorrhage (PCV < 20%)	Whole blood or packed red blood cells mixed with isotonic saline, plasma, HES or DEX	As quickly as possible to reach end-point IV, IO	PCV > 25% MAP > 80 mmHg ALB > 2.0 g/dL	May require active hemostasis May require additional synthetic colloid dose for intravascular resuscitation Follow with rehydration and maintenance fluid administration

Condition	Fluid	Dose / Rate	End-point	Comments
Chronic hemorrhage or hemolysis (PCV < 15%)	Packed red blood cells mixed with isotonic saline	Over 4–6 hours IV, IO to reach end-point	PCV > 25%	Follow with rehydration and maintenance fluid administration
Pulmonary hemorrhage, head hemorrhage, cardiac insufficiency	Hetastarch With isotonic, replacement crystalloid	5 mL/kg increment boluses until end-point reached Dog: 35–55 mL/kg/hr IV, IO Cat: 24–36 mL/kg/hr IV, IO	MAP = 80 mmHg COP ≥ 14 mmHg ALB > 2.0 g/dL	If it is difficult maintaining resuscitation, place on a CRI of hetastarch Dog: 0.8–1.2 mL/kg/hr Cat: 2–8 mL/cat/hr Follow with rehydration and maintenance fluid administration
Low plasma albumin (< 2.0 g/dL) **Coagulopathy** (Prolonged PT/aPTT) **Low antithrombin** (< 90%)	Plasma	10–20 mL/kg or until end-point is reached over 4–6 hours IV, IO	Normal coagulation protein activity ALB > 2.0 g/dL	Follow with rehydration and maintenance fluid administration
Systemic inflammatory response syndrome	Hetastarch	Dog: 0.8–1.2 mL/kg/hr IV, IO Cat: 2–8 mL/cat/hr IV, IO	COP ≥ 14 mmHg ALB > 2.0 g/dL	Must have intravascular volume replaced Adjust maintenance fluid rates accordingly Monitor closely for fluid overload
Interstitial dehydration Decreased skin turgor Sunken eyes Dry MM Loss of eye moisture	Isotonic, replacement crystalloid	Fluid deficit (L) = % dehydration × BW (kg) IV over 1–4 hours if acute dehydration IV over 12–24 hours if chronic dehydration SQ if normovolemic not to exceed 20 mL/kg over several injection sites	Rehydration	Must have intravascular volume replaced Must receive maintenance fluids during rehydration May require adjustment based on ongoing fluid losses
Free water loss (high plasma sodium)	5% dextrose in water	H_2O deficit (L) = 0.6 × BW (kg) × (New Na − 140/140) IV, IO IV over 12–24 hours if acute dehydration IV or oral over 24–48 hours if chronic dehydration	Plasma sodium in the normal range	Must have intravascular and interstitial volume replaced Must receive maintenance fluids during rehydration
Maintenance	Isotonic, maintenance crystalloid	60 mL/kg/day IV, IO, PO, SQ		Must have intravascular and interstitial volume replaced

MM = mucous membrane color; CRT = capillary refill time; MAP = mean arterial blood pressure; CVP = central venous pressure; PCV = packed cell volume; ALB = albumin; PT = prothrombin time; aPTT = activated partial thromboplastin time; COP = colloid oncotic pressure; IV = intravenous; IO = intraosseous; PO = per os; SQ = subcutaneous; HES = hetastarch; DEX = dextran; OXY = oxyglobin.

Maintenance

Often, the fluid combination chosen for initial stabilization is not the same as what is required for maintenance. Once the interstitial fluid deficit has been replaced and replacement of plasma water is no longer required, the interstitial fluid volume must be maintained. Water is used in cellular metabolism and is lost by way of the kidneys, respiration, and evaporation. Potassium is secreted by the kidney in large quantities. The need for free water by the cells directs the sodium concentration in *maintenance* fluids to be approximately 50 per cent of the plasma concentration. The need to replace lost potassium requires potassium concentrations in maintenance fluids up to three times replacement fluid concentrations. These solutions are made isotonic by the addition of a 2.5 per cent concentration of glucose. However, once these isotonic maintenance fluids are distributed into the interstitium, the glucose is quickly metabolized and there is additional free water to use in metabolic processes. The use of replacement fluids for maintenance therapy requires active excretion of sodium by the kidney to provide the needed free water and supplementation of the replacement fluids with potassium.

Normal maintenance fluid rates account for insensible, obligatory (urinary and fecal), and metabolic losses of water and electrolytes. The standard fluid maintenance requirements are estimated at 40 to 60 mL/kg/day. Ongoing losses through diuresis, vomiting, diarrhea, or extravasation of fluid into third-body spaces such as the peritoneum, pleural cavity, or uterus are estimated and added to the total daily fluid volume, and oral intake volumes are subtracted. The maintenance fluid therapy plan will need reassessment throughout the day and adjustments made according to ongoing losses, metabolic requirements, oral intake of water and food, and renal and cardiac function.

It has been suggested that current methods for assessing fluid needs may overestimate the patient's actual requirements since sick patients are inappetent and inactive.[1] Water requirements have been based on formulas for maintenance energy requirements: $140 \times$ (kg body weight)$^{0.73}$ but it is felt that this might overestimate the needs.[98] The use of calorimetry for measuring actual energy requirements has been proposed as a means of determining actual needs. Frequently perfusion parameters must also be supported, and medullary washout from aggressive resuscitation fluid administration can make the ongoing fluid requirement higher than what is required for energy needs alone. Most patients respond well to the standard fluid replacement regimen because excessive fluid and electrolytes are readily excreted by the kidney.

Crystalloids will be the mainstay of maintenance fluid therapy, with the selection made to suit the specific needs of the animal. The maintenance fluids can also provide electrolytes, colloidal oncotic pressure, proteins, coagulation factors, glucose, and nutrients depending upon the fluids selected and how they are supplemented. Increased capillary permeability and hypoproteinemic states can require ongoing maintenance of COP. This can be accomplished by a CRI of large-molecular-weight colloid, such as hetastarch, combined with a maintenance crystalloid (see Tables 78–5 and 78–7). The crystalloid volume infused should be reduced by 40 to 60 per cent from standard calculations to avoid intravascular volume overload.

Albumin, coagulation factors, and antithrombin III can be maintained by infusion of fresh-frozen or frozen plasma. Red blood cells can be replaced and maintained by infusing packed red cells diluted in saline or whole blood. Nutrients can be provided in the form of amino acids (FreAmine, ProcalAmine, Travenol 8% amino acids), lipids (Intralipid), and glucose according to the fluid chosen for maintenance. The composition and volumes of these nutritional supplements are based on metabolic requirements.

Alterations in sodium, potassium, calcium, magnesium, and phosphorous can cause life-threatening complications when unrecognized or uncorrected. Significant electrolyte imbalances can necessitate selection of a specific crystalloid (see Table 78–2) or supplementation of the crystalloid to obtain and maintain electrolyte homeostasis.

ELECTROLYTE IMBALANCES

Electrolyte abnormalities are an important factor in the survival of critical patients. Sodium, potassium, magnesium, calcium, and/or phosphorus disequilibrium cause serious alterations in cellular function and lead to life-threatening complications.

SODIUM DISORDERS

Blood sodium concentration reflects the ratio of sodium to water in the extracellular fluid and accounts for most of the osmotically active particles in the serum. Figure 78–6 represents algorithms for the management of sodium disorders.

Hypernatremia

Rapid volume replacement can cause serious complications. Acute elevation of extracellular sodium concentration leads to intracellular dehydration. High sodium concentration occurs in the CSF and interferes with the sodium-potassium pump. Sodium is trapped within the CSF, and profound neurologic signs (depression, weakness, confusion, seizures, coma, and finally death) can occur as a result of dehydration of neurons.

When sodium elevation is chronic, the nervous system is initially protected by production of intracellular idiogenic osmoles that counterbalance the hyperosmolarity of the serum. This protective mechanism can be overwhelmed, and, in time, neurologic abnormalities become apparent.

Rapid volume replacement with a low sodium containing fluid causes a disequilibrium between the serum and CSF sodium concentration. Water moves from the vasculature into the CSF. In the acute patient, this causes extracellular volume overload, and in the chronic patient causes intracellular hypervolemia. Either mechanism can elevate intracranial pressure and cause neurologic compromise.

Severe dehydration and poor perfusion should be anticipated with hypernatremia. Volume is rapidly replaced utilizing sodium-containing cyrstalloids or colloids to restore perfusion using hypotensive resuscitation techniques. Hydration deficits should be replaced slowly over 12 to 24 hours using lactated Ringer's, normal saline, or half-strength saline once adequate perfusion has been restored.

Once rehydrated, the sodium is remeasured and the new sodium value is utilized to determine the remaining ECF water deficit through the following formula:

$$(\text{New Na} - 140/140) \times \text{kg body wt} \times 0.6 = \text{water deficit in liters}$$

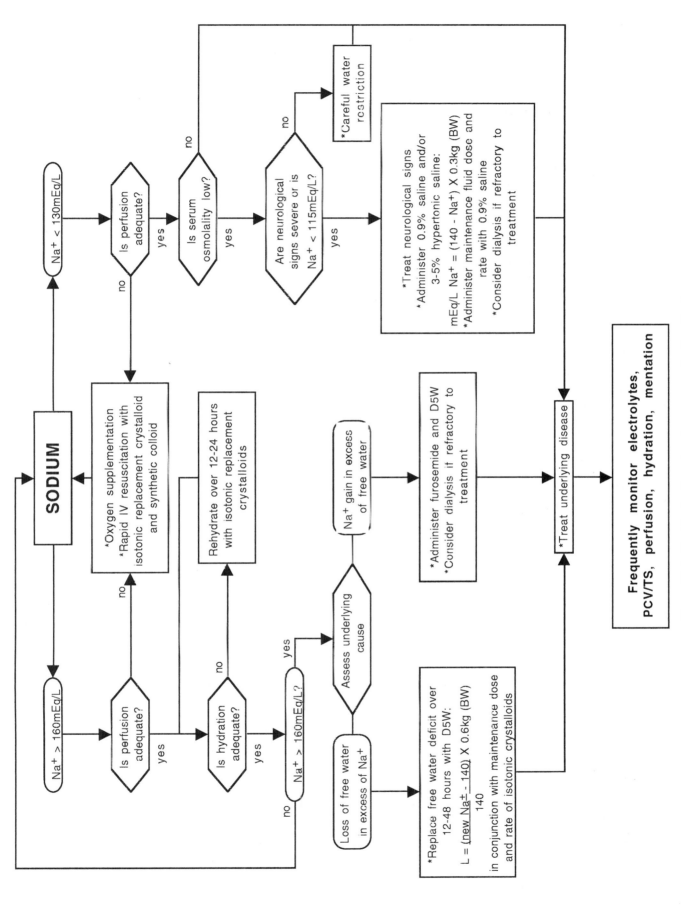

Figure 78–6. Algorithm for diagnosis and management of sodium disorders.

This volume is replaced by 5 per cent dextrose in water over 12 to 24 hours. Maintenance fluid requirements are provided utilizing a balanced electrolyte solution and potassium supplementation as needed.

Hyponatremia

Serum osmolarity aids in identifying the origin of hyponatremia. Hypoosmolar serum (osmolarity <280 mOsm/L) suggests total body water in excess of sodium. This can be due to excessive water intake, inappropriate reabsorption of water in proportion to sodium, or failure to reabsorb sodium by the kidney. Severe signs include stupor, coma, seizures, and dementia.

It is important to assess hydration and replace volume deficits with isotonic saline. Hyponatremia less than 115 mEq/L in a patient with severe neurologic alterations may require sodium supplementation. Hypertonic saline (3 per cent or 5 per cent) can be used during maintenance therapy and the sodium deficit calculated using the following formula:

$$(140 - \text{measured Na}) \times \text{kg body wt} \times 0.3 = \text{mEq/L Na deficit}$$

This should be replenished slowly over 12 to 24 hours. Rapid replacement has resulted in central pontine myelinolysis.

Mild signs most commonly manifest as generalized weakness and mental depression. Hypovolemia is best managed with normal saline volume replacement. When excessive water intake or renal retention results in normovolemia or hypervolemia, water restriction is effective therapy.

Severe neurologic signs are associated with normal or excessive intravascular fluid volume that necessitates furosemide therapy to promote renal water excretion. Sodium can be supplemented as described above. Hypokalemia may result, requiring potassium supplementation. When water excess is not responsive to diuretic therapy, peritoneal dialysis may be effective.

Hyponatremia associated with normal serum osmolarity (pseudohyponatremia) is due to other serum substances that provide a dilutional factor. Hyperlipemia, hyperglycemia, and hyperproteinemia can each attract water into the intravascular space and dilute sodium. The underlying disease is identified and treated.

Hyperosmolar hyponatremia occurs when there are substances in the blood such as glucose, urea nitrogen, and toxins that elevate serum osmolarity, attract water, and dilute serum sodium concentration. Disorders to consider include diabetes mellitus, toxins such as ethylene glycol, and renal failure. It is important to diagnose and manage the underlying disorder.

POTASSIUM DISORDERS

Potassium is the principal intracellular electrolyte. Serum potassium values may not accurately reflect the total body potassium stores, and many factors affect serum concentration. Blood pH affects the distribution of potassium between the plasma and the cell, with acidosis promoting extracellular movement of potassium and alkalosis causing potassium to enter the cell. When there is massive cell injury such as crush injuries, burns, or heat stroke, large amounts of intracellular potassium can be released to the plasma. Disorders altering renal regulation and urine output will affect serum potassium concentrations because potassium content is regulated by the kidney. Figure 78–7 represents algorithms for the management of potassium disorders.

Hyperkalemia

Hyperkalemia should be suspected in any small animal patient with renal compromise, urinary obstruction, bradycardia, arrhythmias, poor perfusion, massive tissue destruction, or severe generalized weakness. Inadequate tissue perfusion warrants immediate ECG assessment. Hyperkalemia affects electrical conduction within the myocardium, prolonging repolarization and eventually depolarization. Electrocardiographic changes consistent with hyperkalemia include bradycardia, tall-spike T waves, prolongation of the P-R interval, flattening of the P wave, widening of the QRS complex, and eventually sine wave formation.

When poor perfusion is due to volume deficiency, low-potassium fluids should be rapidly infused. When inadequate perfusion is due to hyperkalemia and its effects on the myocardium, therapy to shift potassium into the intracellular space is required until the underlying disease can be identified and treated. Regular insulin (0.2 units/kg body weight IV) followed by dextrose (2 g/unit of insulin administered IV and supplement fluids with 2.5 per cent dextrose) will decrease serum potassium within 5 minutes and lasts between 20 to 45 minutes. Or, glucose (0.1 to 1.5 mg/kg body weight IV) may offset the myocardial effects of hyperkalemia.

Other alternatives are to administer sodium bicarbonate or calcium gluconate. Sodium bicarbonate (0.2 to 0.5 mEq/kg IV slowly or diluted in fluids) changes serum pH and drives potassium into the cell. However, sodium bicarbonate has other side effects and should be used cautiously in critical patients. Calcium gluconate (10 per cent solution at 0.5 to 1.5 mL/kg body weight IV) may offset the myocardial effects of hyperkalemia.

The mainstay of therapy for hyperkalemia is fluid diuresis and, when indicated, furosemide therapy to promote kaliuresis. Should oliguric or anuric renal failure be the inciting cause and diuresis is not possible, dialysis is required.

An arterial blood gas is taken to determine the effects of acidosis on potassium concentration. Acidosis will cause a 0.6 mEq/L rise in serum potassium for each 0.1 decrease in pH. When hyperkalemia persists in the face of severe metabolic acidosis (pH < 7.1), conservative bicarbonate therapy should be considered.

When severe hyperkalemia is refractory to therapy or mineralocorticoids, consider potassium exchange resin or peritoneal dialysis.

Hypokalemia

Clinical signs are generalized muscle weakness, flaccid paralysis, ileus, impaired ventilation, and arrhythmias. An arterial blood gas is performed and the serum potassium corrected for alkalosis. Should hypokalemia persist, potassium supplementation can be required.

Hypokalemia becomes a life-threatening problem when serum values of less than 2.5 mEq/L are associated with ECG changes (T-wave depression, prolonged QT interval, U waves, and ST-segment depression have been described), severe weakness, or ventilatory compromise. Potassium should be administered with IV fluids in a peripheral vein and infused at a rate less than 0.5 mEq/kg/hr. Extreme caution must be taken when renal insufficiency is present.

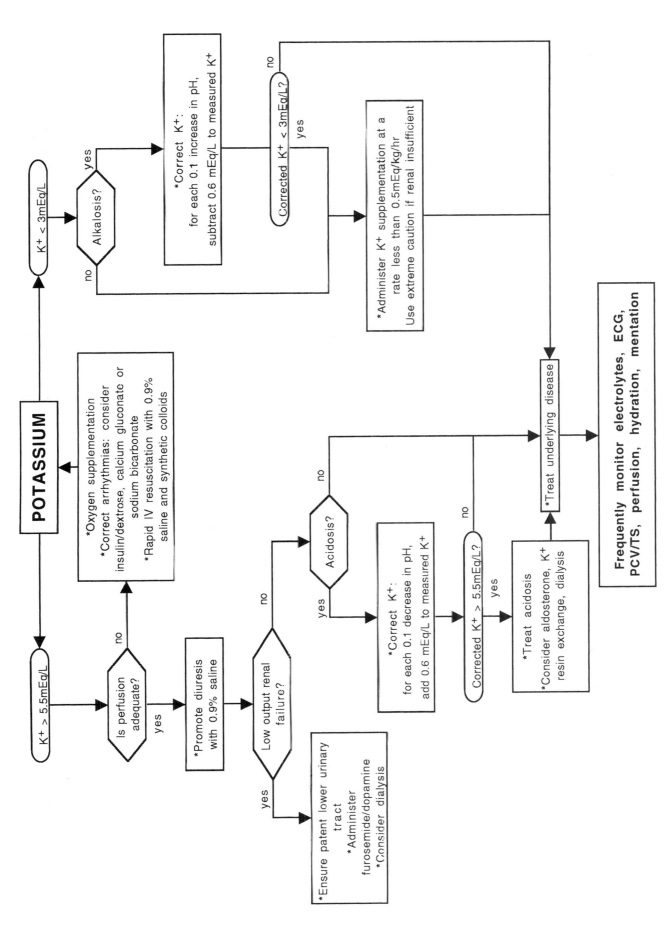

POTASSIUM

K⁺ < 3mEq/L

Alkalosis?

yes → *Correct K⁺:
for each 0.1 increase in pH,
subtract 0.6 mEq/L to measured K⁺

no

Corrected K⁺ < 3mEq/L?

yes / no

*Administer K⁺ supplementation at a
rate less than 0.5mEq/kg/hr
Use extreme caution if renal insufficient

*Oxygen supplementation
*Correct arrhythmias: consider
insulin/dextrose, calcium gluconate or
sodium bicarbonate
*Rapid IV resuscitation with 0.9%
saline and synthetic colloids

K⁺ > 5.5mEq/L

Is perfusion adequate?

no
yes

*Promote diuresis
with 0.9% saline

Low output renal failure?

no → Acidosis?

yes

yes → *Correct K⁺:
for each 0.1 decrease in pH,
add 0.6 mEq/L to measured K⁺

no

Corrected K⁺ > 5.5mEq/L?

yes / no

*Treat acidosis
*Consider aldosterone, K⁺
resin exchange, dialysis

*Ensure patent lower urinary
tract
*Administer
furosemide/dopamine
*Consider dialysis

*Treat underlying disease

**Frequently monitor electrolytes, ECG,
PCV/TS, perfusion, hydration, mentation**

Figure 78–7. Algorithm for diagnosis and management of potassium disorders.

RX

343

When potassium supplementation is not urgent, a slower infusion given according to the following guidelines is desirable.

SERUM POTASSIUM	POTASSIUM ADDED TO 250 ML FLUIDS
<2.0 mEq/L	20 mEq/250 mL
2.0–2.5 mEq/L	15 mEq/250 mL
2.5–3.0 mEq/L	10 mEq/250 mL
3.0–3.5 mEq/L	7 mEq/250 mL

CALCIUM DISORDERS

Calcium is present in the blood bound to albumin for transport, or in an ionized physiologically active form. When total calcium is measured, an estimate of the calcium related to the albumin can be made by adding or subtracting 0.8 mg/dL for each g/dL of albumin above or below normal. Figure 78–8 represents algorithms for the management of calcium disorders.

Hypercalcemia

Clinical signs of polyuria and polydipsia, unexplained shock, heart failure, oliguria, abdominal pain, constipation, vomiting, restlessness, altered mentation, and tachypnea are suggestive of hypercalcemia. Initial assessment of the hypercalcemic patient should concentrate upon peripheral perfusion and glomerular filtration. Capillary refill time, pulse rate, rhythm and intensity, body temperature, and blood pressure are assessed by physical examination and myocardial conduction investigated by ECG. Shock is to be treated by rapid IV infusion of normal saline, and arrhythmias are treated according to ECG diagnosis. When poor cardiac function is attributed to hypercalcemia, resulting in failure and potentially death, calcium channel blockers can be utilized. Ionized serum calcium can be rapidly lowered by administering sodium bicarbonate or sodium phosphate. This does, however, result in precipitation of calcium into the soft tissues with major organ compromise. Avoid this therapeutic measure when possible.

It has been demonstrated experimentally in the dog that serum calcium levels greater than 16 mg/dL are associated with vasomotor spasms of the afferent glomerular arteriole.[99] This results in poor glomerular and tubular perfusion and renal failure. Serum creatinine and urine output are monitored as a reflection of glomerular blood flow and filtration rate. Volume deficits are quickly restored with IV isotonic saline. Calciuresis is promoted by using furosemide (1 mg/kg/hr administered by CRI). Dopamine (2 to 3 µg/kg/min CRI) is given to offset the preglomerular arteriolar spasms.

Fluid diuresis is promoted by matching the volume of saline infusion with the volume of urine produced unless oliguric renal failure or congestive heart failure is present. Hypokalemia, hypomagnesemia, and hypophosphatemia can result and should be corrected by adding the appropriate supplement to the IV fluids. When phosphate supplementation is required, it is important to maintain the calcium phosphorous product below 55 to avoid soft tissue calcification. Urine output; central venous pressure; packed cell volume; total solids; serum calcium, phosphorus, potassium, and magnesium; EKG; and blood pressure should be monitored.

When little response is noted from the general therapy, more specific modalities can be used. These include glucocorticoids to decrease intestinal calcium absorption and promote calciuresis and calcitonin or mithramycin to promote calcium deposition in bone. Mithramycin has potential side effects of blood dyscrasia and is reserved for patients with nonresponsive hypercalcemia associated with cancer. When these methods fail or when severe renal insufficiency is present, peritoneal dialysis or hemodialysis using a calcium-free dialysate can be effective. The definitive therapy is directed toward the underlying disease.

Hypocalcemia

Hypocalcemia should be suspected in any patient showing severe generalized weakness, seizures, tremors, tonic-clonic muscle activity, facial pawing and scratching, or hyperexcitability. When severe generalized weakness, tetany, or seizures are detected in a suspected hypocalcemic patient, a blood sample should be obtained for serum calcium and 10 per cent calcium gluconate (0.5 to 1.5 mL/kg IV slowly) administered.

Frequently hypocalcemia will be chronic in origin and not associated with acute life-threatening problems. Calcium gluconate can then be given orally or slowly in the IV fluids.

Definitive therapy is aimed at the underlying disease. CBC and complete biochemical profile to include BUN, creatinine, serum sodium, potassium, calcium, magnesium, albumin, amylase, lipase, and alkaline phosphatase should be requested. Alkalosis can cause hypocalcemia and/or acute hypocalcemia can cause hypoventilation, warranting arterial blood gas analysis.

PHOSPHORUS DISORDERS

Phosphorus is an important intracellular ion necessary for the generation of adenosine triphosphate (ATP), the principal intracellular energy source. It is absorbed through the small intestines and excreted by the kidney. High concentrations are found in bone. Acidosis causes phosphorus to shift from the cell into the plasma, and alkalosis results in movement from the plasma into the cell. Disorders in serum phosphorus can present life-threatening complications and should be assessed in relation to serum concentration of potassium, sodium, magnesium, and calcium.

Hyperphosphatemia

Hyperphosphatemia occurs when the serum phosphorous is greater than 7 mg/dL. These are no specific clinical signs to suggest hyperphosphatemia, but historical or clinical findings can reveal acute renal failure, chronic renal failure, urinary obstruction, hypoparathyroidism, massive cell lysis, phosphate enemas, ischemic bowel, or ingestion of phosphate or vitamin D. Hypocalcemia occurs when the calcium-phosphorus product is greater than 55 owing to soft tissue deposition of calcium phosphate.

Therapy involves reducing gut phosphate absorption by administering phosphate-binding antacids such as aluminum hydroxide gel. Volume expansion with isotonic saline will promote phosphate excretion by the kidneys when renal function is normal. When renal failure is present, dialysis may be required.

Hypophosphatemia

Hypophosphatemia occurs when the serum phosphorus is less than 1.5 mg/dL. Acute hypophosphatemia rarely causes

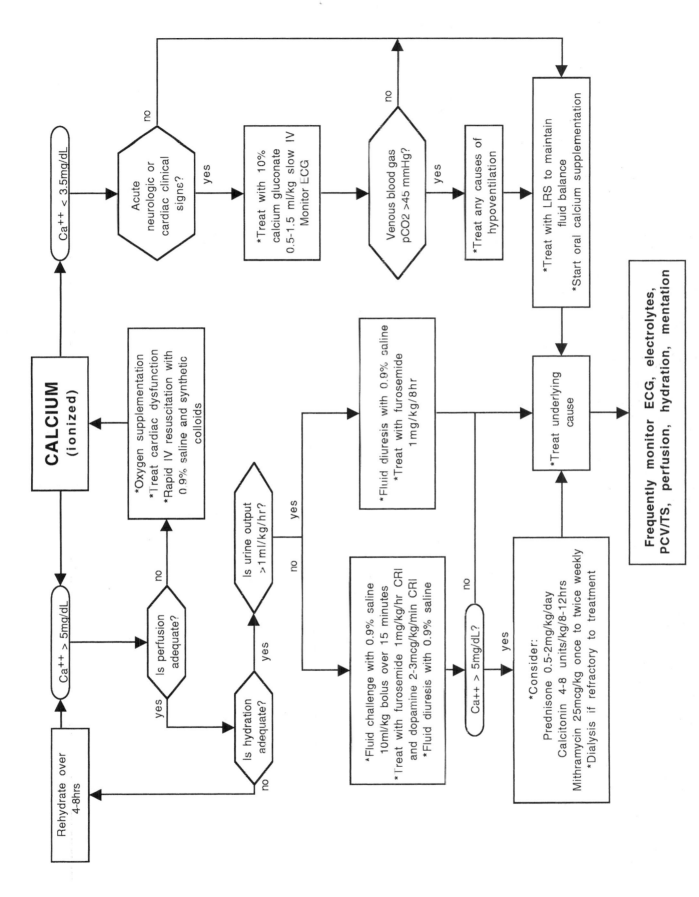

Figure 78–8. Algorithm for diagnosis and management of calcium disorders.

immediate problems, but prolonged deficiency results in total body phosphorus and ATP energy store depletion. It occurs when a severe catabolic state is rapidly changed to an anabolic state, such as in diabetic ketoacidosis, burns, or severe emaciation.

Severe hypophosphatemia (<1.0 mg/dL) has effects related to energy depletion. Red blood cell lysis, impaired white blood cell phagocytic and bactericidal capabilities, platelet dysfunction, muscle disease, cardiomyopathy, and central nervous system signs have been reported. Severe respiratory alkalosis can cause a transient hypophosphatemia but will generally correct when the pH has normalized.

Mild asymptomatic hypophosphatemia can be treated by oral supplementation utilizing skim milk or hyperalimentation fluids. Diarrhea is a common complication. Parenteral administration is indicated for severely affected patients and can be accomplished by administration of sodium or potassium phosphate (3.0 mmol/mL) at a dosage of 0.01 to 0.03 mmol of phosphate/kg/hr for 3 to 6 hours in a calcium-free fluid. Serum phosphorus is then reevaluated. Hypocalcemia, hypernatremia, hypotension, hyperkalemia, and metastatic calcification are complications.

MAGNESIUM DISORDERS

Magnesium functions as a cofactor in many enzymatic reactions involved in the hydrolysis or transfer of phosphate groups. It participates in activating amino acids and synthesizing protein, in stabilizing nucleic acid, in muscle contractility, and in neuronal transmission.

Magnesium is important for maintenance of intracellular potassium and is second only to potassium in intracellular cation concentration. Serum and tissue magnesium levels do not correlate well, but serum measurement is the most clinically useful method of magnesium evaluation. Approximately two thirds of the serum magnesium is ionized, while the remainder is bound to albumin.

Hypermagnesemia

Hypermagnesemia is diagnosed when serum magnesium concentrations are greater than 2.0 mmol/L or 4.9 mg/dL. Clinical signs include peripheral vasodilatation, hypotension, nausea, vomiting, drowsiness, depressed deep tendon reflexes, respiratory depression, skeletal muscle paralysis, cardiac arrhythmias, coma, and death. In humans, the prevalence of hypermagnesemia in hospitalized patients is 9.3 per cent.[100]

Therapy involves discontinuing magnesium administration and/or treating the underlying renal insufficiency. When renal function is normal, isotonic saline volume replacement and diuresis with furosemide are of benefit. Intravenous infusion of calcium will temporarily neutralize the neuromuscular effects of hypermagnesemia. However, severe hypermagnesemia can be treated by dialysis with a magnesium-free dialysate.

Hypomagnesemia

Hypomagnesemia is diagnosed when serum concentrations are less than 0.5 mmol/L or 1.2 mg/dL. Magnesium depletion is associated with a shift of magnesium from the extracellular to intracellular space and is not due to increased renal excretion. Low magnesium and low calcium occur simultaneously in many patients. In a study in people, hypomagnesemia was diagnosed in 11 per cent of the hospitalized population and 23 per cent of the patients with hypocalcemia.[100, 101]

Clinical signs of tetany, tremors, hyperexcitability, tachycardia, ventricular arrhythmias, seizures, and cardiac arrhythmias have been described in humans, though many patients are asymptomatic. Oral replacement is preferred with chronic problems. Parenteral supplementation is reserved for critical patients with evidence of myoneural or cardiac dysfunction. Magnesium sulfate can be given IM or magnesium chloride IV very slowly. The extracellular deficit can be estimated by the following formula, to be infused over 48 hours: (desired Mg − measured Mg) × kg body weight × 0.2 − mg deficit. Hypocalcemia associated with hypomagnesemia responds quickly to magnesium supplementation.

REFERENCES

1. Kohn CW, DiBartola SP: Composition and distribution of body fluids in dogs and cats. In Dibartola SP (ed): Fluid Therapy in Small Animal Practice. Philadelphia, WB Saunders, 1992, p 29.
2. Guyton AC, Hall JE: The microcirculation and the lymphatic system: Capillary fluid exchange, interstitial fluid, and lymph flow. In Guyton AC, Hall JE (eds): The Textbook of Medical Physiology. Philadelphia, WB Saunders, 1996, pp 183–197.
3. Rackow EC, Fein AL, Siegel J: The relationship of colloid osmotic pressure gradient to pulmonary edema and mortality in critically ill patients. Chest 82:4, 1982.
4. Persson NH, et al: The hamster cheek pouch: An experimental model to study post ischemic macromolecular permeability. Int J Microcirc Clin Exp 4:257, 1985.
5. Granger DN, et al: Effect of local arterial hypotension on cat intestinal capillary permeability. Gastroenterology 79:474, 1980.
6. Slonim M, Stahl WM: Sodium and water content of connective tissue versus cellular tissue following hemorrhage. Surg Forum 19:53, 1968.
7. Shires GT, et al: Alterations in cellular membrane function during hemorrhagic shock in primates. Ann Surg 176:288, 1972.
8. Fulton RL: Adsorption of sodium and water by collagen during hemorrhagic shock. Ann Surg 172:861, 1970.
9. Zikria BA, Subbarao C, Oz MC, et al: Macromolecules reduce abnormal microvascular permeability in rat limb ischemia-reperfusion injury. Crit Care Med 17:1306, 1989.
10. Majno G, Palade GE: Studies on inflammation. 1. The effect of histamine and serotonin on vascular permeability: An electron microscopic study. J Biophys Biochem Cytol 11:571, 1961.
11. Joris I, et al: The mechanism of vascular leakage induced by leukotriene E₄. Endothelial contraction. Am J Pathol 126:19, 1987.
12. Horan KL, et al: Evidence that prolonged histamine suffusions produce transient increases in vascular permeability subsequent to the formation of venular macromolecular leakage sites. Proof of the Majno-Palade hypothesis. Am J Pathol 123:570, 1986.
13. Davidson I, et al: Hemodilution and recovery from experimental intestinal shock in rats: A comparison of the efficacy of three colloids and one electrolyte solution. Crit Care Med 9:42, 1981.
14. Hoye RC, et al: Fluid volume and albumin kinetics occurring with major surgery. JAMA 222:1255, 1972.
15. Zornow MH, Prough DS: Fluid management in patients with traumatic brain injury. New Horizons 3(3):495, 1995.
16. Klotz U, Kroemer H: Clinical pharmacokinetic considerations in the use of plasma expanders. Clin Pharm 12:123, 1987.
17. Kaminski MV, Haase TJ: Albumin and colloid osmotic pressure implications for fluid resuscitation. Crit Care Clin 8(2):311, 1992.
18. Cotter SM: Clinical transfusion medicine. Comp Trans Med 36:188, 1991.
19. Kirby R: Colloids: Those magic fluids. IVECCS VI Proceedings 1994, p 648.
20. Doweiko JP, Nompleggi DJ: Role of albumin in human physiology and pathophysiology. J Paren Enteral Nutr 15:207, 1991.
21. Jusko WJ, Gretch M: Plasma and tissue protein binding of drugs in pharmacokinetics. Drug Metab Rev 5:43, 1976.
22. Karp WB, et al: Binding properties of glycosylated albumin and acetaldehyde albumin. Alcohol Clin Exp Res 9:429, 1985.
23. Lundsgaard-Hansen P, Tschirren B: Modified fluid gelatin as a plasma substitute. In Blood Substitutes and Plasma Expanders. New York, Alan R. Liss, 1978, pp 227–257.
24. Frawly JP, et al: Plasma retention and urinary excretion of dextran and modified fluid gelatin in combat casualties. Surgery 37:784, 1955.
25. Watson J: Mechanisms of hypersensitivity to intravenous agents. Vet Res Commun 7:195, 1983.
26. Lutz H: Animal experiments on the effect of colloidal plasma substitutes in hemorrhagic shock in the dog. Bibl Haemat. New York, Basel, S. Karger, 1969, pp 232–247.
27. Griffel MI, Kaufman BS: Pharmacology of colloids and crystalloids. Crit Care Clin 8(2):235, 1992.

28. Mishler JM: Synthetic plasma volume expanders: Their pharmacology, safety and clinical efficacy. Clin Hematol 13:75, 1984.

29. Moore RM, et al: Effect of high-molecular-weight dextran macromolecules on low-flow ischemia and reperfusion of the large colon in horses. AJVR 57:1067, 1996.

30. Huch K, et al: Hyperoncotic dextran and systemic aprotinin in necrotizing rodent pancreatitis. Scand J Gastroenterol 30:812, 1995.

31. Ammon R: Das Vorkommen von Dextranase im Menschlichen Gewebe. Enzymologia 25:245, 1963.

32. Gray I: Metabolism of plasma expanders studied with carbon-14–labeled dextran. Am J Physiol 174:462, 1953.

33. Hauser CJ, et al: Oxygen transport responses to colloids and crystalloids in critically ill surgical patients. Surg Gynecol Obstet 150:811, 1980.

34. Thompson WL, et al: Intravascular persistence, tissue storage, and excretion of hydroxyethyl starch. Surg Gynecol Obstet 131:965, 1970.

35. Bergqvist D: Dextrans and haemostasis, a review. Acta Chir Scand 31:320, 1982.

36. Aberg M, et al: Effect of dextran and induced thrombocytopenia on the lysability of ex vivo thrombi in dogs. Acta Chir Scand 143:91, 1977.

37. Aberg M, et al: Effect of dextran on factor VIII and platelet function. Ann Surg 189:243, 1979.

38. Gruber U, Messmer K: Colloids for blood volume support. Prog Surg 15:49, 1977.

39. Concannon KT, et al: Hemostatic defects associated with two infusion rates of dextran 70 in dogs. AJVR 53:1369, 1992.

40. Rampling MW: Red cell agglutination and yield stress. In Lowe GDO (ed): Clinical Blood Rheology. Boca Raton, FL, CRC Press, 1988, pp 45–64.

41. Janes AW, et al: Serial infusion effects of hydroxyethyl starch on ESR, blood typing and crossmatching and serum amylase levels. Vox Sang 32:131, 1977.

42. Ibister JP, Fischer MD: Adverse effects of plasma volume expancers. Anaesth Intens Care 8:145, 1980.

43. Matheson NA, Diomi P: Renal failure after administration of dextran 40. Surg Gynecol Obstet 131:661, 1970.

44. Hedin H, and Richter W: Pathomechanisms of dextran-induced anaphylactoid/anaphylactic reactions in man. Int Arch Allergy Appl Immunol 68:122, 1982.

45. Webb AR, et al: A comparison of the effects of artificial plasma substitutes, albumin and saline solutions on in vitro apparent blood viscosity. Clin Hemorheol 10:287, 1990.

46. Webb AR, et al: Advantages of a narrow-range, medium molecular weight hydroxyethyl starch for volume maintenance in a porcine model of fecal peritonitis. Crit Care Med 19:409, 1991.

47. Webb AR, et al: In vitro colloid osmotic pressure of commonly used plasma substitutes: A study of the diffusibility of colloid molecules. Intensive Care Med 15:116, 1989.

48. Hulse JD, Yacobi A: Hetastarch: An overview of the colloid and its metabolism. Drug Intell Clin Pharm 17:334, 1983.

49. Khosropour R, et al: Comparison of the effect of pre- and intra-operative administration of medium molecular weight hydroxyethyl starch (HES200/0.5) and dextran 40(60) in vascular surgery. Anaesthetist 29:616, 1980.

50. Kortilla K, Grohn P, Gordin A, et al: Effect of hydroxyethyl starch and dextran on plasma volume and blood hemostasis and coagulation. J Clin Pharmacol 24:273, 1984.

51. Köhler H, Zschiedrich H, Clasen R, et al: Blutvolumen, kollodosmotischer Druck und Nieren Funktion von Probanden nach Infusion mittelmolekularer 10% Hydroxyäthylstärke 200/0.5 und 10% Dextran 40. (The effects of hydroxyethyl starch 200/0.5 and 10% dextran 40 on blood volume, colloid osmotic pressure and renal function in human volunteers.) Anesthesist 31:61, 1982.

52. Rainey TG, Read CA: Pharmacology of colloids and crystalloids. In Chernow B (ed): The Pharmacologic Approach to the Critically Ill Patient. Baltimore, Williams & Wilkins, 1994, pp 272–290.

53. London M, et al: A randomized clinical trial of 10% pentastarch (low molecular weight hydroxyethyl starch) versus 5% albumin for plasma volume expansion after cardiac operations. J Cardiovasc Surg 97:785, 1989.

54. Mastroianni L, et al: Hemodynamic effects of pentastarch versus albumin in post open-heart surgery patients. Clin Pharmacol Ther 43:168, 1988.

55. Rackow EC, et al: Effects of pentastarch and albumin infusion on cardiorespiratory function and coagulation in patients with severe sepsis and systemic hypoperfusion. Crit Care Med 17:394, 1989.

56. Waxman K, et al: Hemodynamic and oxygen transport effects of pentastarch in burn resuscitation. Ann Surg 209:341, 1988.

57. Oz MC, et al: Hydroxyethyl starch macromolecules protect against increases in microvascular permeability following ischemia-reperfusion injury. Surg Forum 40:48, 1989.

58. Zikria BA, et al: Macromolecules reduce abnormal microvascular permeability in rat limb ischemia-reperfusion injury. Crit Care Med 17:1306, 1989.

59. Zimmerman BJ, Granger DN: Role of xanthine oxidase–derived oxidants and granulocytes in ischemia/reperfusion. In Schlag G, Redl H, Siegel JH (eds): Shock, Sepsis, and Organ Failure: First Wiggers Bernard Conference. New York, Springer-Verlag, 1990, pp 382–403.

60. Boldt J, et al: Influence of different volume therapies and pentoxifylline infusion on circulating soluble adhesion molecules in critically ill patients. Crit Care Med 24:385, 1996.

61. Lewis D, et al: Effect of intravenous administration of hydroxyethyl-starch-deferoxamine on oxygen-derived free radical generation in cancellous bone specimens obtained from dogs. Am J Vet Res 11:1613, 1994.

62. Hallaway PE, et al: Modulation of deferoxamine toxicity in clearance by covalent attachment of biocompatible polymers. Proc Natl Acad Sci USA 1989:10108, 1989.

63. Rackow EC, et al: Fluid resuscitation in circulatory shock: A comparison of the cardiorespiratory effects of albumin, hetastarch and saline solutions in patients with hypovolemic and septic shock. Crit Care Med 111:839, 1983.

64. Demling RH, et al: Acute versus sustained hypoproteinemia and post traumatic pulmonary edema. Surgery 92:79, 1982.

65. Kramer GC, et al: Effects of hypoproteinemia and increased vascular pressure on lung balance in sheep. J Appl Physiol 55:1514, 1983.

66. Harms BA, et al: Pulmonary transvascular fluid filtration response to hypoproteinemia and Hespan infusion. J Surg Res 48:408, 1990.

67. Nearman HS, Herman ML: Toxic effects of colloids in the intensive care unit. Crit Care Clin 7:713, 1991.

68. Ring J, Messmer K: Incidence and severity of anaphylactoid reactions to colloid volume substitutes. Lancet 1:467, 1977.

69. Ballinger WF II, et al: Effect of hydroxyethyl starch upon survival of dogs subjected to hemorrhagic shock. Surg Gynecol Obstet 122:33, 1966.

70. Porter SS, Goldberg RJ: Intraoperative allergic reactions to hydroxyethyl starch: A report of two cases. Can Anaesth Soc J 33:394, 1986.

71. Strauss RG: Review of the effects of hydroxyethyl starch on the blood coagulation system. Transfusion 21:299, 1981.

72. Macintyre E, et al: The haemostatic effects of hydroxyethyl starch used as a volume expander. Int Care Med 11:300, 1985.

73. Howard J, et al: Studies of dextrans of various molecular sizes. Ann Surg 143:369, 1956.

74. Haass A, et al: Hemodilution in cerebral circulatory disturbances: Indications, implementation, additional drug treatment and alternatives. In Koscielny J, Kiesswetter H, Jung F, Haass A (eds): Haemodilution. Berlin, Springer-Verlag, 1992, pp 52–114.

75. Boldt J, et al: Influence of different intravascular volume therapies on platelet function in patients undergoing cardiopulmonary bypass. Anesth Analg 76:1185, 1993.

76. Scherer R, et al: Effects of hypertonic saline hydroxyethyl starch solution on collagen-induced platelet aggregation and ATP secretion. Infusionsther Transfus Med 21:310, 1994.

77. Stump DC, et al: Effects of hydroxyethyl starch on blood coagulation, particularly factor VIII. Transfusion 25:349, 1985.

78. Strauss RG, et al: Effects of hydroxyethyl starch on fibrinogen, fibrin clot formation and fibrinolysis. Transfusion 25:230, 1985.

79. Trumble ER, et al: Coagulopathy with the use of hetastarch in the treatment of vasospasms. J Neurosurg 82:44, 1995.

80. Alexander B: Effects of plasma expanders on coagulation and hemostasis: Dextran, hydroxyethyl starch, and other macromolecules revisited. Prog Clin Biol Res 19:293, 1978.

81. Alexander B, et al: Coagulation, hemostasis, and plasma expanders: A quarter century enigma. Fed Proc 34:1429, 1975.

82. Karlson KE, et al: Increased blood loss associated with administration of certain plasma expanders: Dextran 75, dextran 40, and hydroxyethyl starch. Surgery 62:670, 1967.

83. Strauss RG, et al: Pentastarch may cause fewer side effects on coagulation than hetastarch. Transfusion 28:257, 1988.

84. Gould SA, et al: Aritificial blood: Current status of hemoglobin solutions. Crit Care Clin 8(2):294, 1992.

85. Haupt MT, Rackow EC: Colloid osmotic pressure and fluid resuscitation with hetastarch, albumin and saline solutions. Crit Care Med 10:159, 1982.

86. Demling RH, Manohar M, Will JA: Response of the pulmonary microcirculation to fluid loading after hemorrhagic shock and resuscitation. Surgery 87:552, 1980.

87. Shoemaker WC, Schluchter M, Hopkins JA, et al: Fluid therapy in emergency resuscitation: Clinical evaluation of colloid and crystalloid regimens. Crit Care Med 9:367, 1981.

88. Bickell WH, et al: Immediate versus delayed fluid resuscitation for hypotensive patients with penetrating torso injuries. N Engl J Med 331:1105, 1994.

89. Martin RR, et al: Prospective evaluation of preoperative fluid resuscitation in hypotensive patients with penetrating truncal injury: A preliminary report. J Trauma 33:354, 1992.

90. Kowalenko T, et al: Improved outcome with hypotensive resuscitation of uncontrolled hemorrhagic shock in a swine model. J Trauma 33:349, 1992.

91. Klein LW: Cardiovascular therapeutics. In Parrillo JE (ed): Current Therapy in Critical Care Medicine, 3rd ed. St. Louis, CV Mosby, 1977, pp 72–78.

92. Fox PR: Canine and Feline Cardiology. New York, Churchill Livingstone, 1988.

93. Gutierrez G, Pohil R: Oxygen consumption is clearly related to O_2 supply in critically ill patients. Crit Care Med 1:45, 1986.

94. Shoemaker WC, et al: Hemodynamic and oxygen transport monitoring to titrate therapy in septic shock. New Horizons 1:145, 1993.

95. Mathru M, Rooney M: Hemodilution. Probl Crit Care 5(3):400, 1991.

96. Race C, et al: Regional blood flow during dextran-induced normovolemic hemodilution in the dog. J Thorac Cardiovasc Surg 53:578, 1967.

97. Karanko MS, et al: Restoration of volume by crystalloid versus colloid after coronary artery bypass: Hemodynamics, lung water, oxygenation, and outcome. Crit Care Med 15:559, 1987.

98. Haskins SC: Fluid and electrolyte therapy. Compend Cont Ed Pract Vet 6:244, 1984.

99. Chomdej B, et al: Renal hemodynamic and autoregulatory responses to acute hypercalcemia. Am J Phys 232(6):F490, 1977.

100. Wong ET, et al: A high prevalence of hypomagnesemia and hypermagnesemia in hospitalized patients. Am J Clin Path 73:348, 1980.

101. Whang R, et al: Predictors of clinical hypomagnesemia: Hyokalemia, hypophosphatemia, hyponatremia, and hypocalcemia. Arch Intern Med 144:1794, 1984.

CHAPTER 79

BLOOD BANKING AND TRANSFUSION MEDICINE

Ann E. Hohenhaus

Most veterinarians agree that transfusion of blood and components is a lifesaving therapy, yet transfusion does not cure any disease. It replaces a deficiency of blood cells or plasma coagulation factors until the animal resumes production of these substances. As with other medical therapy, the potential risks of transfusion should be weighed against the expected benefits, and every effort should be made to provide a safe transfusion by adequate donor screening, aseptic collection and storage of blood, blood typing and cross-matching before transfusion, and careful monitoring during transfusion. Adherence to these recommendations will aid the veterinarian in providing safe and efficacious transfusions.

BLOOD COLLECTION

The simplest method of obtaining blood for transfusion is to purchase the blood from a commercial blood bank (Table 79–1). According to one study, most veterinarians use their own dogs or employees' dogs or maintain a blood donor on the premises as the source of blood for transfusion.[1] Selec-

TABLE 79–1. VETERINARY BLOOD BANKS (USA)

Animal Blood Bank
PO Box 1118
Dixon, CA 95620
800-243-5759

"Buddies for Life"
Canine Blood Bank
1940 S. Telegraph Rd.
Bloomfield Hills, MI 48302-0245
248-334-6877

Eastern Veterinary Blood Bank
2138-B Generals Highway
Annapolis, MD 21401
800-949-3822

Hemopet
938 Stanford St.
Santa Monica, CA 90403
310-828-4804

Midwest Animal Blood Services
120 East Main St.
Stockbridge, MI 49285
517-851-8244

Penn Animal Blood Bank
Veterinary Hospital of University of Pennsylvania
3850 Spruce St.
Philadelphia, PA 19104
215-573-PABB

tion of appropriate donors is essential to providing safe and efficacious transfusions.

BLOOD DONOR SELECTION

Determination of the suitability of a dog or cat as a blood donor should include a thorough physical examination. Animals with signs of illness or poor condition should be excluded. Blood donors should be vaccinated against infectious diseases and treated with heartworm preventatives. Before each donation, a hemoglobin level or hematocrit should be obtained to prevent blood collection from an anemic donor. Additional tests of the potential donor include evaluation of coagulation parameters, investigation of the animal's infectious disease status, and blood type.

Canine. The ideal blood donor dog should weigh more than 27 kg, because dogs of this size are able to donate 450 mL of whole blood in one donation at 3-week intervals for 2 years.[2] Dogs chosen as blood donors must have a docile temperament and a lean neck to facilitate venipuncture for collection of blood. Because von Willebrand's disease is prevalent in dogs, a von Willebrand's factor level should be obtained from each donor so that the level will be known when the plasma is needed for treatment of von Willebrand's disease. Dogs with low levels of this clotting factor would not be ideal plasma donors.

Feline. The ideal blood donor cat should weigh more than 5 kg and, like the blood donor dog, have a docile temperament. The author avoids choosing brachycephalic cats, such as the Persian and Himalayan, as blood donors, because phlebotomy seems to be more difficult to perform. Using these breeds of cats may be unavoidable when type B blood is needed, owing to the high prevalence of blood type B in these particular breeds (Table 79–2).

INFECTIOUS DISEASE SCREENING OF BLOOD DONORS

Canine. The approach to screening dogs for infectious diseases varies depending on the geographic region of the dog's residence. The most common disease tested for is heartworm disease. Both *Babesia canis* and *Haemobartonella canis* have been transmitted to a dog by blood transfusion.[3, 4] All donor dogs should have negative titers against *B. canis*. It is especially important to evaluate *B. canis* titers in greyhounds because of the high seroprevalence in that population.[5] *Ehrlichia sp.* and *Trypanosoma cruzi* are blood-borne organisms that can be transmitted via blood transfusion and should be screened for before using dogs as blood donors. Borreliosis has not been documented as a

TABLE 79–2. BLOOD TYPE FREQUENCY OF CATS IN THE UNITED STATES

BREED	TYPE A (%)	TYPE B (%)
Abyssinian	86	14
Birman	84	16
British shorthair	60	40
Burmese	100	0
Cornish rex	66	34
Devon rex	59	41
Domestic shorthair (by region)		
Northeast	99.7	0.3
North Central	99.6	0.4
Southeast	98.5	1.5
Southwest	97.5	2.5
West Coast	95.3	4.7
Himalayan	93	7
Japanese bobtail	84	16
Maine coon	98	2
Norwegian forest cat	93	7
Persian	86	14
Scottish fold	82	18
Siamese	100	0
Somali	83	17
Sphinx	81	19
Tonkinese	100	0

From Oakley DA, Giger U: Just their type: Feline transfusions and blood donors. Vet Tech 18:747, 1997.

transfusion-transmitted disease in humans; dogs believed to have Lyme disease should be excluded as donors, however.

Feline. Two viruses likely to cause severe posttransfusion infection are feline leukemia virus (FeLV) and feline immunodeficiency virus (FIV). To prevent donor cats from acquiring retroviral infections, they should reside indoors. Before their initial donation, all donor cats should have at least three negative FeLV and FIV tests at 1-month intervals. Both tests should be repeated on an annual basis and whenever the donor is sick. Eliminating cats with subclinical feline infectious peritonitis from the donor pool is more problematic because of the lack of a sensitive and specific test for the disease. *Bartonella henselae* is an emerging feline infectious disease that has been transmitted to cats via infected blood.[6] All donor cats should be cultured for *B. henselae* and, if positive, should not be used as blood donors. Fleas are believed to be the vector for *B. henselae*; consequently, flea control is essential in donor cats. *Haemobartonella felis* is another blood-borne parasite that should be screened for before donation.

COLLECTION PROCESS

A detailed description of the collection of blood from donors is beyond the scope of this chapter. An excellent description of the process has been published.[7]

Blood must be collected by aseptic methods. Whenever possible, the items used for phlebotomy should be sterile, single-use, and disposable. Improper aseptic methods can result in bacterial contamination of blood.[8] Hair overlying the venipuncture site should be clipped and the skin prepared using a surgical scrub technique. The optimal solutions for skin disinfection have not been identified in veterinary transfusion medicine, but in human blood donors, a 70 per cent isopropyl alcohol scrub followed by a 2 per cent tincture of iodine scrub resulted in better skin surface disinfection than alcohol followed by chlorhexidine or green soap.[9] Once

scrubbed, the venipuncture site should not be palpated before venipuncture.

Canine. Most dogs do not require sedation for blood donation. If sedation is required, the author prefers butorphanol (0.1 mg/kg IV 10 to 15 minutes before donation). It is most convenient to collect dog blood in commercially available bags containing anticoagulant. Attached to these bags are needles, facilitating the collection of blood directly into the bags. Either jugular veins or femoral arteries can be used to collect blood; the choice is based on individual preference. Blood can flow into the collection bag by gravity flow or by a vacuum device, which has not been associated with excessive hemolysis.[10]

Feline. Most cats require sedation for blood donation. The author prefers a combination of ketamine and diazepam (10 mg and 0.5 mg IV per cat, respectively). Protocols using midazolam and isoflurane have been suggested.[7] Without modification, commercially available blood collection systems cannot be used to collect feline blood, because the bags are designed to collect 450 mL of whole blood. Most of the anticoagulant may be moved from the primary bag of a standard double blood bag into the plasma collection bag, and then the blood can be collected in the primary bag.[11] A vacuum collection system, as is often used for dogs, can also be used.[12] The simplest system requires large (35- to 60-mL) syringes to which anticoagulant is added; the blood is drawn into the syringe through a 19-g butterfly catheter placed in the jugular vein.[7] Technically, only the first collection method is a "closed" system, making it appropriate for storage of blood for longer than 24 hours.[13]

PROCESSING OF DONOR BLOOD

All bags of blood and components should be labeled with the donor identification code, the donor's blood type, the component contained in the bag, the date collected, and the date of expiration. The species of animal the blood was collected from must be clearly recorded on the bag to prevent an inadvertent cross-species transfusion.

A sample of donor blood should be maintained in the blood bank in the tubing attached to the blood bag or in stoppered tubes. These samples may be used to perform a crossmatch, double-check a blood type, or examine a blood smear without the need to open the bag of blood itself.

The typical veterinary hospital does not have a centrifuge of adequate size to manufacture blood components; consequently, the reader is referred elsewhere if additional information on that topic is needed.[7, 13, 14] A human hospital blood bank may centrifuge and process the whole blood collected by the veterinarian into components.

BLOOD COMPONENTS: STORAGE, DESCRIPTION, AND INDICATIONS

STORAGE OF BLOOD AND COMPONENTS

Blood and components should be stored in a blood bank refrigerator or freezer equipped with thermometers and alarms to prevent accidental warming of the stored products; however, this is not practical in the typical veterinary hospital. Consequently, the refrigerator and freezer chosen for storage should be the least frequently opened ones available to maintain as consistent a temperature as possible. The refrigerator should be maintained at 1 to 6°C. Coagulation factors in plasma or its derivative, cryoprecipitate, are best preserved at temperatures of −18°C or less, which are not achievable in a household freezer. The shelf life of coagulation factors in plasma has been based on storage at these temperatures and has not been evaluated in a household freezer. A shelf life of 3 months has been recommended for plasma frozen in a household freezer.[15] A platelet concentrate may be stored at room temperature (20 to 24°C) with gentle agitation for up to 5 days if it was collected in a closed system.[16] Otherwise, platelets should be transfused as soon as possible after collection. Neutrophils do not have any appreciable shelf life and should be transfused as soon as they are obtained.

PREPARATION OF COMPONENTS

The three goals for the preparation of components from whole blood are (1) to maximize the utilization of a limited resource, blood; (2) to optimally preserve the constituents of blood, red blood cells, by refrigeration and plasma by freezing; and (3) to minimize bacterial contamination and proliferation. These goals are accomplished by the collection of whole blood, using aseptic technique, in commercially available sterile primary collections bag containing anticoagulant with attached satellite bags (Fig. 79–1). Collection and storage of blood in bags allow separation of blood into components, and plastic bags minimize mechanical trauma to the red blood cells, require less storage space, and are not breakable, as are vacuum bottles. Storage of blood in plastic bags also preserves red blood cell function better than storage in vacuum bottles, as indicated by the smaller changes in 2, 3, diphosphoglycerate (DPG) and pH during storage in plastic bags.[17] After centrifugation, the red blood cells and plasma are separated using the tubing interconnecting the satellite bags, designed to maintain sterility. If the tubing or bags are opened to the environment, the blood or component should be used within 24 hours or discarded, because sterility cannot be ensured. Storage of blood as components allows animals needing only the elements of plasma to receive a plasma transfusion, and those needing an increase in oxygen-carrying capacity to receive only red blood cells, thus maximizing the usage of a single donation. Separate

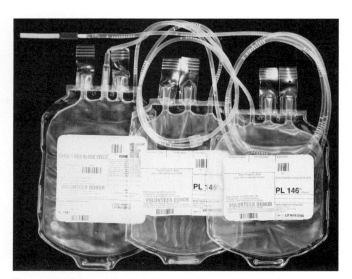

Figure 79–1. A standard triple-pack collection system consisting of a primary bag on the far left containing CPDA-1 anticoagulant and two satellite bags for production of components.

TABLE 79–3. ANTICOAGULANTS AND PRESERVATIVES FOR BLOOD

CANINE BLOOD		
	Ratio with Blood	*Storage Time at 0–6°C*
Anticoagulant		
Heparin	625 U/50 mL blood	For immediate transfusion
3.8% sodium citrate	1 mL/9 mL blood	For immediate transfusion
Anticoagulant-preservative		
CPDA-1	1 mL/7 mL blood	20 days
ACD-B	1 mL/7 mL blood	21 days
Additive solutions	100 mL/250 mL packed red blood cells	37–42 days

FELINE BLOOD		
	Ratio with Blood	*Storage Time at 0–6°C*
Anticoagulant		
Heparin	625 U/50 mL blood	For immediate transfusion
3.8% sodium citrate	1 mL/9 mL blood	For immediate transfusion
Anticoagulant-preservative		
ACD-B	1 mL/7 mL blood	30 days
Additive solutions		Not evaluated

storage of plasma also permits its long-term storage, despite the relatively short shelf life of red blood cells.

ANTICOAGULANTS AND PRESERVATIVES

Anticoagulants are solutions that prevent coagulation of blood so that it can be transfused. Anticoagulants include heparin and 3.8 per cent sodium citrate (Table 79–3). These solutions have no preservative function, and blood collected in these solutions should be transfused within 8 hours of collection.[13]

The use of several different preservative solutions has been described in veterinary blood banking. All preservative solutions contain citrate as the anticoagulant, but the preservative composition varies, resulting in different shelf lives for red blood cells stored in the different media (see Table 79–3). Preservative solutions both prevent coagulation of blood and provide nutrients for metabolism and stabilization of red blood cells during storage.

Acid citrate dextrose (ACD) solution is an early preservative solution developed during World War II. Two forms of the preservative are available: solution A and solution B. Storage time for canine blood in ACD-B is 3 weeks; for feline blood, it is 4 weeks.[18, 19]

Citrate phosphate dextrose adenine (CPDA-1) is available in commercially prepared blood collection systems. It is commonly used to produce canine blood components and to store canine packed red blood cells; it has a shelf life of 20 days.[20] The posttransfusion viability of feline red blood cells stored in CPDA-1 has not been fully evaluated but may be as long as 35 days.[21]

Additive solutions are the newest development in citrate-based preservatives for red blood cell storage. Several different solutions are available in multibag systems designed for the collection of 450 mL of whole blood that is processed into plasma and packed red blood cells. Once the plasma is removed, the additive solution is added from its bag to the packed red blood cells to provide additional nutrients for prolonged storage. Nutricel (Miles Pharmaceutical Division, West Haven, CT) and Adsol (Fenwal Laboratories, Baxter Health Care Corp., Deerfield, IL) have been evaluated for the storage of canine red blood cells but not for the storage of feline packed red blood cells.[22, 23]

WHOLE BLOOD

Blood collected from the donor, plus the anticoagulant, is termed whole blood. Most veterinary practices use whole blood for transfusion, which, when transfused within 8 hours of collection, provides both oxygen-carrying capacity and coagulation factors.[1] Whole blood stored longer only increases oxygen-carrying capacity. The use of whole blood would be most appropriate in an anemic animal with a simultaneous coagulation factor deficiency. If whole blood is used as a source of coagulation factors in an animal that is not yet anemic, there is a risk of iatrogenic polycythemia. The dosage of whole blood is 13 to 22 mL/kg.

PACKED RED BLOOD CELLS

After whole blood is centrifuged to separate the red blood cells from plasma, the plasma is expressed into a satellite bag, and the remaining red blood cells and a small amount of plasma are designated packed red blood cells. Although no standard unit size has been defined in veterinary medicine, 1 unit of packed red blood cells can be considered the volume of cells produced from 1 unit of whole blood. In the dog, approximately 200 mL of packed red blood cells, with a hematocrit of 80 per cent, is obtained when a commercial collection system is used. The primary indication for the transfusion of red blood cells is to restore or maintain an adequate supply of oxygen to meet tissue demands. Packed red blood cells are indicated for the treatment of anemia due to blood loss, hemolysis, or bone marrow dysfunction.[24, 25] The hematocrit or hemoglobin concentration does not adequately assess the need for red blood cell transfusion; consequently, a value for hematocrit or hemoglobin alone cannot serve as a guide for transfusion. The animal's cardiovascular status, anticipated blood loss, chronicity of anemia, and ability of the bone marrow to respond to the anemia should all play a role in the decision to transfuse. Blood transfusions should not be used to make an animal "feel better," to promote healing, or as a volume expander.[26]

FRESH FROZEN PLASMA

Fresh frozen plasma is frozen within 8 hours of collection to maintain activity of the labile clotting factors (factors VIII and V). To manufacture plasma, whole blood is centrifuged, and the supernatant plasma is expressed into a satellite bag. The resulting plasma contains electrolytes, albumin, globulins, coagulation factors, and other proteins. Typically, plasma is used as a source of coagulation factors (Fig. 79–2). Therapeutic indications for the use of fresh frozen plasma are coagulation factor deficiencies such as rodenticide intoxication, vitamin K–dependent coagulopathy of Devon rex cats, and hemophilia B (factor IX deficiency).[27–29] Canine von Willebrand's disease and hemophilia A (factor VIII:C deficiency) can be treated with fresh frozen plasma, but

treatment with cryoprecipitate minimizes the risk of volume overload.[30] Plasma therapy has been recommended for human patients with disseminated intravascular coagulation associated with active hemorrhage or requiring an invasive procedure.[31] For any of these disorders, an initial dosage of fresh frozen plasma of 6 to 10 mL/kg should be given and the clinical status of the animal reevaluated for continued hemorrhage. Reevaluation of the coagulation profile is useful when making the decision to continue plasma therapy. Ongoing hemorrhage or persistent abnormalities of the coagulation profile indicate the need for additional transfusions. The choice of plasma as a source of albumin requires that a large volume of plasma be available, because approximately 45 mL/kg is needed to raise the albumin 1 g/dL.

CRYOPRECIPITATE

Cold insoluble globulin or cryoprecipitate is a subfraction of plasma prepared by thawing fresh frozen plasma at 1 to 6°C. During the thawing process, a thick white precipitate forms and is separated from the remaining plasma via centrifugation.

Factors VIII:C (antihemophiliac factor) and XIII, von Willebrand's factor, and fibrinogen are contained in cryoprecipitate; therefore, cryoprecipitate is used to treat hemophilia A, von Willebrand's disease, and fibrinogen deficiency. The advantages of this product over fresh frozen plasma for the treatment of these disorders are the much smaller volume of cryoprecipitate required and possibly improved hemostasis in von Willebrand's disease.[30] One unit of cryoprecipitate is suspended in 10 to 15 mL of plasma. The initial dosage of cryoprecipitate is 1 unit per 10 kg body weight.

PLATELET TRANSFUSION

Platelet transfusions are rarely reported in veterinary medicine, except in unusual circumstances such as bone marrow transplantation, Chédiak-Higashi disease, and the treatment of immune-mediated thrombocytopenia with vincristine-loaded platelets.[32–34] The infrequent use of platelet transfusions is due to two factors: First, platelets are time-consuming to harvest from whole blood and should be used immediately unless stored at room temperature under constant agitation.[16, 32] Second, one of the more common causes of thrombocytopenia that would result in a platelet count low enough to result in hemorrhage and require platelet transfusion is immune-mediated thrombocytopenia. In that case, transfused platelets would likely be destroyed as rapidly as the animal's own platelets. One unit of platelets is the amount of platelets derived from 1 unit of whole blood. Platelets are transfused at 1 unit per 10 kg of body weight.

NEUTROPHIL TRANSFUSION

Transfusions of neutrophils can be performed in dogs with neutropenia, but to achieve the recommended dose of neutrophils (1.5×10^8 neutrophil/kg), a cell separator is required.[35] Whole blood for the production of neutrophils must be stored at 20 to 24°C before transfusion, and the neutrophil transfusion must be given within hours of collection, or the cells become dysfunctional. Consequently, neutrophil transfusions are impractical in routine transfusion medicine.

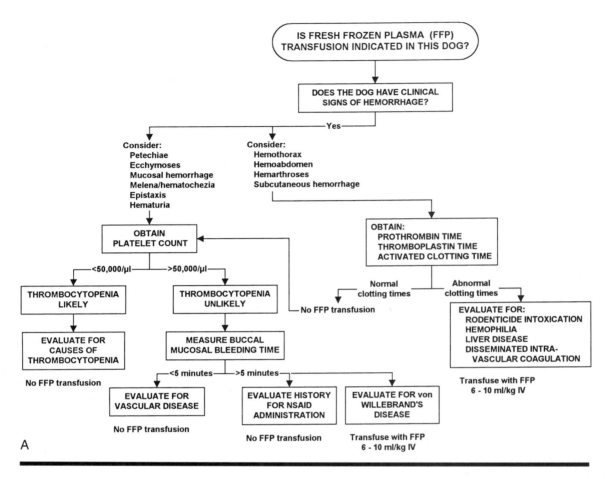

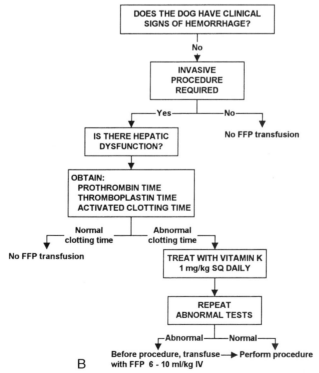

Figure 79–2. Algorithms for use of fresh frozen plasma transfusions with *(A)* and without *(B)* clinical signs of hemorrhage.

HUMAN IMMUNOGLOBULIN

Although it is not a product produced from canine plasma, human immunoglobulin G (IgG) has been recommended as an adjunct to immunosuppressive therapy in dogs with immune-mediated hemolytic anemia, at a dosage of 0.5 to 1 g/kg body weight infused over 6 to 8 hours.[36, 37] Prepared from pooled human plasma by cold ethanol fractionation, the IgG is stored in the refrigerator as a lyophilized powder until reconstitution immediately before administration. It is believed that the immunoglobulins have an immunosuppressive effect by inducing Fc receptor blockade or alteration of the reticuloendothelial cell system function, but the actual mechanism is unknown. Only one dose of IgG per dog has been given because of the risk of a severe immunologic reaction in a dog receiving a human protein. The major negative aspect of IgG therapy is the cost of the product, which is $300 to treat a 10-kg dog.

IMPORTANCE OF BLOOD GROUPS IN DOGS AND CATS

CANINE DEA SYSTEM

More than 13 canine blood groups have been described, but typing sera are available for only 6 of these types: DEA (dog erythrocyte antigen) 1.1, 1.2, 3, 4, 5, 7. Blood typing of dogs is typically performed at a reference laboratory, but a simple card typing system is now available to determine dogs' DEA 1.1 status (dmsLaboratories, 2 Darts Mills Road, Flemington, NJ 08822; telephone 800–567–4367). Naturally occurring alloantibodies against blood groups are not believed to play a role in acute hemolytic transfusion reactions. The DEA 1 blood group has multiple alleles, including DEA 1.1, 1.2, 1.3, and a null type; of these, DEA 1.1 is believed to be the most antigenic. If a donor is positive for DEA 1.1, the transfusion can sensitize the DEA 1.1–negative recipient, resulting in a transfusion reaction if a second DEA 1.1–positive transfusion is given.[38] Dogs positive for DEA 1.1 should be excluded as donors. It has been suggested that donor dogs positive for DEA 1.2 will sensitize recipients that are negative for that type, but reports of transfusion reactions in dogs transfused with DEA 1.2–positive cells are currently lacking in the literature.[39] DEA 7 is believed to be structurally related to a common bacterial antigen, and a naturally occurring antibody against DEA 7 has been described in 20 to 50 per cent of DEA 7–negative dogs. Some believe that the presence of this antibody results in premature removal after transfusion of DEA 7–positive cells.[40] Thus, a recommendation has been made to choose donors that are negative for DEA 7.

Because 98 per cent of dogs have red blood cells positive for DEA 4, dogs positive for this antigen and negative for all others have been termed "universal donors."[39]

FELINE AB SYSTEM

Only one blood group system has been identified in the cat. This blood group system has three blood types: A, B, AB. Blood types vary among breeds of cats and among geographic locations. Most American cats are type A, and type AB is extremely rare (<1 per cent of all cats; see Table 79–2). Type AB is found only in breeds of cats with type B in their populations.[41] All cats with blood type B have natural alloantibodies against type A cells, and all type A cats have alloantibodies against type B cells. The anti-B antibodies are generally weak, but both types of antibodies result in shortened red blood cell survival following incompatible transfusions.[42] An acute hemolytic transfusion reaction occurs when type A blood is given to a type B cat. Kittens of type A that are born to a type B queen and allowed to nurse during the first 24 hours of life consume antibodies in the colostrum and are at risk for neonatal isoerythrolysis.[43]

Blood types in cats can be determined by a reference laboratory, and now a simple card system is available for use in veterinary hospitals (Fig. 79–3). It requires only a few drops of blood, and results are available within a minute (dmsLaboratories, 2 Darts Mills Road, Flemington, NJ 08822; telephone 800–567–4367). If blood typing is not available, crossmatching blood of the recipient to a type A donor will infer the type of the recipient. An incompatible major crossmatch implies a type B cat, and a compatible major crossmatch implies a type A cat.

PRETRANSFUSION TESTING

CROSSMATCHING

A crossmatch determines the compatibility of the transfusion being considered and does not predict future compatibility or prevent sensitization of the recipient to this transfusion. Because each transfusion can induce the production of new antibodies that could result in incompatibility, the crossmatch should be repeated if more than 4 days elapse between transfusions. Several crossmatch procedures have been described.[44, 45] The variations among the procedures are minor; some methods incorporate multiple temperatures (4°C, 37°C, and 42°C) for incubation, and others add an additional

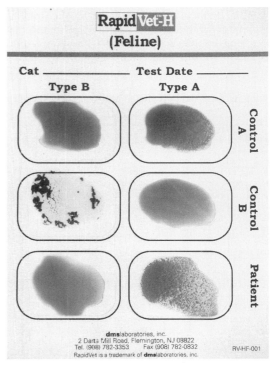

Figure 79–3. A feline blood typing card showing a typical reaction for the type A and type B controls and a type A patient. The agglutination reaction is easily interpreted. (Courtesy of dmsLaboratories, Inc., Flemington, NJ.)

step at the end using species-specific Coombs' reagent to increase test sensitivity. The protocol used at the Animal Medical Center can be found in Table 79–4.

CROSSMATCH INTERPRETATION

Incompatibility in the crossmatch is indicated by hemolysis or agglutination. A grading scale for the degree of agglutination is often used in human transfusion medicine.[13]

    0   = no agglutination
    1 + = many small agglutinates admixed with free cells
    2 + = large agglutinates mixed with smaller clumps
    3 + = many large agglutinates
    4 + = single agglutinate, no free cells

Units of blood that are incompatible should not be used unless all available units are incompatible based on the crossmatch results. If that occurs, the least reactive unit should be transfused. When the recipient control shows hemolysis or agglutination, as often occurs in hemolytic anemia, the crossmatch cannot be interpreted.

CLINICAL CONSIDERATIONS IN TRANSFUSION PRACTICES

ADMINISTRATION OF BLOOD AND COMPONENTS

Every unit of blood or plasma should be closely inspected before administration. A brown discoloration of blood is indicative of bacterial contamination.[8] The label on each unit should be checked to ensure that blood from the proper species of animal is being administered. The results of blood typing and crossmatching in the medical record should be compared with the donor identification code and blood type on the unit to ensure that the correct unit has been released from the blood bank. This prevents the most common cause of acute hemolytic transfusion reaction in human medicine from occurring in veterinary patients—the administration of a unit of blood not intended for the patient.[46]

TABLE 79–4. ANIMAL MEDICAL CENTER CROSSMATCH PROTOCOL

1. Obtain EDTA anticoagulated blood from the recipient and the potential donor or from the crossmatch tubing segments from the units of blood being considered for transfusion.
2. Centrifuge both donor and recipient blood for 5 minutes at $1000 \times g$.
3. Using pipettes, save plasma in separate labeled tubes.
4. Wash the red blood cells by adding phosphate-buffered saline to the red cells to fill the tube. Resuspend red cells in the saline by tapping the bottom of the tube with a finger.
5. Centrifuge red cells and saline for 5 minutes at $1000 \times g$. Pipette off saline and discard.
6. Repeat steps 4 and 5 twice.
7. After the third washing of red cells in saline, resuspend red cells to a 3 to 5 per cent solution. It will appear bright cherry red in color.
8. For each potential donor, mix 2 drops of recipient plasma and 1 drop of donor red cell suspension for the major crossmatch. Mix gently.
9. For each potential donor, mix 2 drops of donor plasma and 1 drop of recipient red cell suspension for the minor crossmatch. Mix gently.
10. For the recipient control, mix 2 drops of recipient plasma and 1 drop of recipient red cell suspension. Mix gently.
11. Incubate the tubes at room temperature for 15 minutes.
12. Centrifuge for 15 seconds at $1000 \times g$.
13. Observe the plasma for hemolysis.
14. Resuspend the centrifuged cells by shaking gently.
15. Observe the red blood cell pellet for agglutination.

The American Association of Blood Banks recommends that no medications or fluid be added to blood or blood products except for 0.9 per cent sodium chloride.[13] This regulation is designed to prevent hemolysis of red blood cells from exposure to hypotonic solutions such as 5 per cent dextrose in water or coagulation of blood by calcium-containing fluids such as lactated Ringer's solution. Sodium chloride is usually added to packed red blood cells to reduce their viscosity and speed transfusion.

Blood warming is not necessary in most transfusions, even though red blood cells are refrigerated; plasma must be thawed before administration.[47] An adult animal receiving 1 unit of blood or components can use body heat to warm the unit. Neonates or animals receiving massive (greater than 1 blood volume) transfusions are at risk for transfusion-induced hypothermia, and blood should be at least room temperature before administration. Blood that is warmed is at greater risk for bacterial overgrowth or hemolysis due to overheating. Red blood cells that have been warmed to 37°C deteriorate rapidly and if not used should be discarded.

Fresh frozen plasma must be thawed before administration. When frozen, the plastic bags become very brittle; consequently, plasma bags are frozen in cardboard boxes to protect them from cracking when handled. Plasma from the freezer should not be handled until the plastic warms and becomes supple. Then, if immediate transfusion is necessary, thawing can be facilitated by placing the plasma in a plastic bag and thawing in a 37°C water bath. Plasma can be thawed in a microwave oven, but the author has found this method unsatisfactory.[48]

All blood and components should be administered through an administration set with an integral filter designed to remove clots and debris formed during collection and storage. Typically, a 170-micron filter is used; however, for small-volume transfusions given from a syringe, the use of an 18-micron filter attached to the syringe has been recommended.[49]

Intravenous administration is the most common route for blood and components. In cases of vascular collapse or in very small puppies and kittens, blood can be successfully administered via an intraosseous catheter. Over 90 per cent of red blood cells administered this way are found in the circulation within 5 minutes.[50]

The administration rate for blood products varies with the clinical condition and the product administered. Whatever the administration rate chosen, the blood should be delivered at a rate fast enough to complete the transfusion within 4 hours. This reduces the potential for bacterial overgrowth. In a normovolemic, anemic animal, an initial rate of 0.25 mL/kg should be tried for the first 30 minutes; if no reaction is observed, the rate can be increased.[15] Dogs and cats with hemorrhagic shock should be transfused as rapidly as possible. Plasma may be administered more rapidly (4 to 6 mL/minute) than red blood cell–containing products.[51] Infusion devices such as pumps may be used to control the delivery rate of blood products only if the devices have been approved for use with blood products. The IVAC 530 pump has been determined to be efficacious with both fresh and stored canine blood.[52]

ADVERSE EFFECTS OF BLOOD TRANSFUSION

Acute hemolytic transfusion reactions are mediated by the immune system and occur either because of naturally occurring, preformed alloantibodies against red blood cell antigens, such as an A-B mismatch transfusion in the cat, or because of antibodies induced by a previous transfusion, as has been reported in the dog.[38] The presence of antibodies against red blood cell antigens rapidly induces hemolysis of red blood cells, resulting in hemoglobinemia, hemoglobinuria, icterus, and fever. The Coombs' test may become positive. The clinical signs of an acute hemolytic transfusion reaction are slightly different in the cat and dog. In the dog, restlessness, salivation, incontinence, dyspnea, hypotension, collapse, convulsions, and vomiting occur. Acute death is uncommon.[53] In cats, acute death has been reported to occur in type B cats given type A blood.[54] The first sign of a transfusion reaction in a cat is extension of limbs and apnea, followed by increases in respiratory and heart rates. Shock, consisting of hypotension, and heart block can also occur. Acute oliguric or anuric renal failure has not been reported in veterinary patients.[38, 53–55]

Febrile nonhemolytic transfusion reactions have been reported in both dogs and cats.[25, 56] A transfusion-associated fever is defined as a 1°F body temperature rise over the pretransfusion temperature. In humans, the presence of recipient antibodies against donor leukocytes is responsible for these reactions. The cause in veterinary patients has not been investigated.

Urticaria is the result of recipient antibody against donor plasma proteins and has been described as the most common adverse event associated with plasma transfusion.[57] It has also been reported as a complication of whole blood transfusion.[25] Typically, facial swelling is most severe.

Contamination of blood by microorganisms has long been known to be a potential complication of blood transfusion. The use of sterile collection systems has reduced the risk of contamination but has not eliminated it. Contaminated blood can cause sepsis or shock, if the organism produces an endotoxin, and this should be suspected if there is a transfusion-associated fever or discolored blood.[3, 8]

Posttransfusion purpura is a recently reported complication of transfusion in a dog.[58] Thrombocytopenia and petechiation occurred 5 to 8 days following a transfusion in a dog that had received a previous transfusion for hemophilia. An immune mechanism for platelet destruction was suspected, because the platelets collected during a thrombocytopenic episode were positive for platelet-bound IgG.

Circulatory overload can occur in animals with compromised cardiac or pulmonary systems or chronically anemic animals that are transfused too rapidly. Clinical signs include coughing, cyanosis, and dyspnea. Thoracic radiography can be used to confirm vascular congestion or overt edema.

Metabolic complications of transfusion include hypocalcemia and hyperkalemia. Neither has been reported in veterinary medicine but could occur in animals receiving massive transfusions. Hypocalcemia results not from the administration of blood but from the administration of citrate in the anticoagulant. Clinical signs include a long Q-T interval with a normal heart rate or, with severe hypocalcemia, acute death.[59] Hyperkalemia also results from massive transfusion of stored blood. As red blood cells are stored, potassium leaks out of the cell into the plasma. In transfusion recipients with compromised renal function, this can result in potassium intoxication.

MANAGEMENT OF TRANSFUSION REACTIONS

If a transfusion reaction is suspected, the transfusion should be stopped immediately and an investigation as to the cause undertaken. The intravenous line should be kept open with an infusion of crystalloid solution. An acute hemolytic transfusion reaction, a febrile nonhemolytic reaction, circulatory overload, and microbial contamination all have some similar clinical features. To differentiate among them, the following procedures should be followed:

1. Check blood bag labels and information in the medical record to determine whether the animal transfused was the intended recipient and that the correct unit of blood was given.

2. Obtain blood and urine from the recipient to document hemoglobinemia and hemoglobinuria. Perform a Coombs' test on the posttransfusion sample. Positive results indicate incompatible transfused cells. A negative test, in the face of hemolysis, suggests that the hemolysis is caused by physical damage to red blood cells, such as thermal damage or mechanical trauma.

3. Repeat blood type and crossmatch to determine whether a pretransfusion error was made.

4. Perform a Gram stain and a culture on the donor unit, especially if the unit is discolored. Bacteria are not always visible in contaminated units.[8]

5. Auscultate the heart and lungs, and obtain thoracic radiographs to evaluate for circulatory overload. Measure blood pressure or central venous pressure; both increase with circulatory overload.

6. Measurements of serum potassium and calcium should be obtained. If rapid assessment of electrolytes is not possible, an electrocardiogram may reveal prolonged Q-T intervals with hypocalcemia and decreased height of P waves, loss of P waves, or widening of the QRS complex with large T waves with hyperkalemia.

If these tests do not indicate an acute hemolytic transfusion reaction or bacterial contamination, the transfusion may be restarted. If a febrile, nonhemolytic reaction is diagnosed, antipyretics may be given if the animal is uncomfortable. Urticaria is treated with antihistamines and a slower rate of transfusion. Animals with circulatory overload should receive diuretics and supplemental oxygen and be transfused at a rate less than 4 mL/kg/hour.[60] Either calcium chloride or calcium gluconate can be given to correct hypocalcemia.[61] A combination of insulin-dextrose and 0.9 per cent saline should be administered to correct hyperkalemia. Posttransfusion purpura is a delayed complication of transfusion, so no immediate therapy is possible. Whether or not immunosuppression with corticosteroids ameliorates the process is unknown.

Transfusion recipients that have received an incompatible unit or a contaminated unit require aggressive medical therapy. Fluids should be administered intravenously with continuous blood pressure monitoring to control hypotension and maintain adequate urine output. If fluid therapy does not maintain blood pressure, pressors are indicated. Empiric antibiotic therapy should be given based on the results of the Gram stain. If no bacteria are seen but contamination is suspected, a broad-spectrum approach should be taken. Because disseminated intravascular coagulation may result from an incompatible transfusion or sepsis, a coagulation profile should be evaluated.

REFERENCES

1. Howard A, Callan B, Sweeny M, et al: Transfusion practices and costs in dogs. JAVMA 210:1697, 1992.
2. Potkay S, Zinn RD: Effects of collection interval, body weight, and season on the hemograms of canine blood donors. Lab Anim Care 19:197, 1969.

3. Freeman MJ, Kirby BM, Panciera DL, et al: Hypotensive shock syndrome associated with acute *Babesia canis* infection in a dog. JAVMA 204:94, 1994.

4. Lester SJ, Hume JB, Phipps B: *Haemobartonella canis* infection following splenectomy and transfusion. Can Vet J 36:444, 1995.

5. Taboada J, Harvey JW, Levy MG, et al: Seroprevalence of babesiosis in greyhounds in Florida. JAVMA 200:47, 1992.

6. Kordick DL, Breitschwerdt EB: Relapsing bacteremia after blood transmission of *Bartonella henselae* to cats. Am J Vet Res 58:492, 1997.

7. Schneider A: Blood components: Collection, processing and storage. Vet Clin North Am Small Anim Pract 25:1245, 1995.

8. Hohenhaus AE, Drusin LM, Garvey MS: *Serratia marcescens* contamination of feline whole blood in a hospital blood bank. JAVMA 210:794, 1997.

9. Goldman M, Roy G, Frechette N, et al: Evaluation of donor skin disinfection methods. Transfusion 37:309, 1997.

10. Eibert M, Lewis DC: Post transfusion viability of stored canine red blood cells after vacuum facilitated collection. J Vet Intern Med 11:143, 1997.

11. Price LS: A method for collecting and storing feline whole blood. Vet Tech 7:561, 1991.

12. Kaufman PM: Management of the feline blood donor. *In* Hohenhaus A (ed): Problems in Veterinary Medicine, Transfusion Medicine. Philadelphia, JB Lippincott, 1992, p 555.

13. Walker R (ed): Technical Manual, 11th ed. Bethesda, MD, American Association of Blood Banks, 1993.

14. Mooney SC: Preparation of blood components. *In* Hohenhaus A (ed): Problems in Veterinary Medicine, Transfusion Medicine. Philadelphia, JB Lippincott, 1992, p 594.

15. Turnwald GH, Pichler ME: Blood transfusion in dogs and cats. Part II. Administration, adverse effects and component therapy. Comp Cont Ed 7:115, 1985.

16. Allyson K, Abrams-Ogg ACG, Johnstone IB: Room temperature storage and cryopreservation of canine platelet concentrates. Am J Vet Res 58:1338, 1997.

17. Eisenbrandt DL, Smith JE: Evaluation of preservatives and containers for storage of canine blood. JAVMA 163:988, 1973.

18. Eisenbrandt DL, Smith JE: Use of biochemical measures to estimate viability of red blood cells in canine blood stored in acid citrate dextrose solution. JAVMA 163:984, 1973.

19. Marion RS, Smith JE: Posttransfusion viability of feline erythrocytes stored in acid citrate dextrose solution. JAVMA 183:1459, 1983.

20. Price GS, Armstrong PJ, McLeod DA, et al: Evaluation of citrate phosphate dextrose adenine as a storage medium for packed canine erythrocytes. J Vet Intern Med 2:126, 1988.

21. Buchler J, Cotter SM: Storage of feline and canine whole blood in CPDA-1 and determination of the posttransfusion viability. J Vet Intern Med 8:172, 1994.

22. Wardrop KJ, Tucker RL, Munai K: Evaluation of canine red blood cells stored in a saline, adenine and glucose solution for 35 days. J Vet Intern Med 11:5, 1997.

23. Wardrop KJ, Owen TJ, Meyers KM: Evaluation of an additive solution for preservation of canine red blood cells. J Vet Intern Med 8:253, 1994.

24. Kerl ME, Hohenhaus AE: Packed red blood cell transfusions in dogs: 131 cases (1989). JAVMA 202:1495, 1993.

25. Callan MB, Oakley DA, Shofer FS, et al: Canine red blood cell transfusion practice. J Am Anim Hosp Assoc 32:303, 1996.

26. Audet AM, Goodnough LT: Practice strategies for elective red blood cell transfusion. Ann Intern Med 116:403, 1992.

27. Mount ME, Feldman BF, Buffington T: Vitamin K and its therapeutic importance. JAVMA 180:1354, 1982.

28. Littlewood JD, Shaw SC, Coombes LM: Vitamin K dependent coagulopathy in a British Devon rex cat. J Small Anim Pract 36:115, 1995.

29. Feldman DG, Brooks MB, Dodds WJ: Hemophilia B (factor IX deficiency) in a family of German shepherd dogs. JAVMA 206:1901, 1995.

30. Meyers KM, Wardrop KJ, Meinkoth J: Canine von Willebrand's disease; pathobiology, diagnosis and short-term treatment. Comp Cont Ed 14:13, 1992.

31. Feinstein DI: Treatment of disseminated intravascular coagulation. Semin Thromb Hemost 14:351, 1988.

32. Abrams-Ogg ACG, Kruth SA, Carter RF, et al: Preparation and transfusion of canine platelet concentrates. Am J Vet Res 54:635, 1993.

33. Cowles BE, Meyers KM, Wardrop KJ, et al: Prolonged bleeding time of Chediak-Higashi cats corrected by platelet transfusion. Thromb Haemost 67:708, 1992.

34. Helfand SC, Jain NC, Paul M: Vincristine-loaded platelet therapy for idiopathic thrombocytopenia in a dog. JAVMA 185:224, 1984.

35. Epstein RB, Waxman FJ, Bennett BT, et al: *Pseudomonas* septicemia in neutropenic dogs. I. Treatment with granulocyte transfusions. Transfusion 14:51, 1974.

36. Scott-Moncrieff JCR, Regan WJ, Glickman LT, et al: Treatment of nonregenerative anemia with human gamma-globulin in dogs. JAVMA 206:1895, 1995.

37. Scott-Moncrieff JCR, Regan WJ, Snyder PQ, et al: Intravenous administration of human immune globulin in dogs with immune mediated hemolytic anemia. JAVMA 210:1623, 1997.

38. Giger U, Gelens CJ, Callan MB, et al: An acute hemolytic transfusion reaction caused by dog erythrocyte antigen 1.1 incompatibility in a previously sensitized dog. JAVMA 206:1358, 1995.

39. Hale AS: Canine blood groups and their importance in veterinary transfusion medicine. Vet Clin North Am Small Anim Pract 25:1323, 1995.

40. Smith CA: Transfusion medicine: The challenge of practical use. JAVMA 198:474, 1991.

41. Griot-Wenk ME, Callan MB, Chisholm-Chait A, et al: Blood type AB in the feline AB blood group system. Am J Vet Res 57:1438, 1996.

42. Giger U, Bucheler J: Transfusion of type-A and type-B blood to cats. JAVMA 198:411, 1991.

43. Casal ML, Jezyk PF, Giger U: Transfer of colostral antibodies from queens to their kittens. Am J Vet Res 57:1653, 1996.

44. Giger U: Feline transfusion medicine. *In* Hohenhaus A (ed): Problems in Veterinary Medicine, Transfusion Medicine. Philadelphia, JB Lippincott, 1992, p 600.

45. Bucheler J, Cotter SM: Outpatient blood donor program. *In* Hohenhaus A (ed): Problems in Veterinary Medicine, Transfusion Medicine. Philadelphia, JB Lippincott, 1992, p 572.

46. Szama K: Reports of 355 transfusion associated deaths: 1976–1985. Transfusion 30:583, 1990.

47. Iserson KV, Huestis DW: Blood warming: Current applications and techniques. Transfusion 31:558, 1991.

48. Hurst TS, Turrentine MA, Johnson GS: Evaluation of microwave-thawed canine plasma for transfusion. JAVMA 190:863, 1987.

49. Kaufman PM: Supplies for blood transfusions in dogs and cats. *In* Hohenhaus A (ed): Problems in Veterinary Medicine, Transfusion Medicine. Philadelphia, JB Lippincott, 1992, p 582.

50. Clark CH, Woodley CH: The absorption of red blood cells after parenteral injection at various sites. Am J Vet Res 10:1062, 1959.

51. Killingsworth C: Use of blood and blood components for feline and canine patients. JAVMA 185:1452, 1984.

52. Stiles J, Raffe MR: Hemolysis of canine fresh and stored blood associated with peristaltic pump infusion. Vet Emerg Crit Care 1:50, 1991.

53. Yuile CL, VanZandt TF, Ervin DM, et al: Hemolytic reactions produced in dogs by transfusion of incompatible dog blood and plasma. Blood 4:1232, 1948.

54. Auer L, Bell K: Blood transfusion reactions in the cat. JAVMA 170:729, 1982.

55. Giger U, Akol KG: Acute hemolytic transfusion reaction in an Abyssinian cat with blood type B. J Vet Intern Med 4:315, 1990.

56. Henson MS, Kristensen AT, Armstrong PJ, et al: Feline blood component therapy: Retrospective study of 246 transfusions. J Vet Intern Med 8:169, 1994.

57. Wardrop KJ: Canine plasma therapy. Vet Forum 14:36, 1997.

58. Wardrop KJ, Lewis D, Marks S, et al: Posttransfusion purpura in a dog with hemophilia A. J Vet Intern Med 11:261, 1997.

59. Killen DA, Grogan EL, Gower RE, et al: Response of canine plasma-ionized calcium and magnesium to the rapid infusion of acid-citrate-dextrose (ACD) solution. Surgery 70:736, 1971.

60. Green CE: Blood transfusion therapy: An updated overview. Proceedings of the American Animal Hospital Association, 49th Annual Meeting, 187, 1982.

61. Cote CJ, Drop LJ, Daniels AL, et al: Calcium chloride versus calcium gluconate: Comparison of ionization and cardiovascular effects in children and dogs. Anesthesiology 66:465, 1987.

CHAPTER 80

TOXICOLOGY

Steven S. Nicholson

Specific therapy, including antidotes, when available, is provided for each toxicant discussed. Emergency detoxification procedures such as induction of emesis, gastric lavage, use of activated charcoal or a cathartic, and bathing to remove toxicants from the skin and hair are noted when they are indicated.

INSECTICIDES, MOLLUSCACIDES, REPELLENTS

AMITRAZ

Exposure to excessive levels of amitraz via application to the skin for *Demodex* control and ingestion of tick collars has resulted in poisoning. Amitraz is an alpha-adrenergic agonist and a weak monoamine oxidase inhibitor. Signs of poisoning include hypotension, mydriasis, hypothermia, bradycardia, hypoperistalsis, ataxia, sedation, vasoconstriction, vomiting, and diarrhea (Fig. 80–1). Hypoglycemia caused by insulin release occurs and may be supportive of a diagnosis of amitraz poisoning.[1] Atropine may aggravate some signs (e.g., further inhibit peristalsis) and may cause hypertension.[1] Treatment with yohimbine at 0.45 mg/lb or 0.1 mg/kg intravenously (IV) effectively reverses the signs of amitraz poisoning.

BORIC ACID, BORATES

Boric acid is not a corrosive agent but is cytotoxic to cells. The toxic dose is greater than 1 g/kg. It is rapidly absorbed and eliminated in the urine. Dogs poisoned by oral ingestion develop vomiting, depression, and occasionally diarrhea. Seizures, renal tubular nephrosis, and, rarely, hepatotoxicity are seen.

DEET

The insect repellent diethyltoluamide has an oral median lethal dose (LD_{50}) of 1 to 2 g/kg in rats. At toxic levels it induces seizures, hypotension, and bradycardia. A commercial flea and tick product containing 9 per cent fenvalerate and deet was associated with clinical illness in dogs and cats. Too frequent application was the primary problem. Vomiting, anorexia, tremors, excitation, hypersalivation, and seizures occurred. Decontamination and supportive care are generally adequate for mild cases.

METALDEHYDE

Metaldehyde products are used as snail and slug poison and generally contain a carbonate insecticide as well. The pesticides are mixed with bran as flakes or pellets. Ingestion of 2 ounces of a 3 per cent bait (1800 mg metaldehyde) by a 22-pound dog will induce signs within an hour. Vomiting may occur owing to stomach irritation. Hypersalivation, abdominal pain, tremors, hyperesthesia, nystagmus (especially in cats), and incoordination are seen. Significant elevation of body temperature is common. Opisthotonos and continuous tonic convulsions similar to those of strychnine poisoning, but not induced by light or noise, develop. Severe acidosis develops in poisoned animals. Tests for metaldehyde or acetaldehyde in the stomach contents or suspect bait are offered by some laboratories. Detoxification procedures include control of seizures with diazepam, correction of acidosis with sodium lactate in fluids, and provision of supportive care.

NAPHTHALENE

A commercial mothball, naphthalene at a dosage of more than 400 mg/kg is said to be toxic to dogs. Cats are more susceptible. Signs and lesions of poisoning include vomiting, hepatic damage, lethargy, Heinz body anemia, hemoglobinuria, and nephrosis secondary to intravascular hemolysis.[2] Ascorbic acid 20 mg/kg is the treatment for methemoglobinemia, and fluids with bicarbonate reduce precipitation of hemoglobin in the kidneys.

NICOTINE

Nicotine sulfate is still sold as an insecticide. Nicotine in cigarettes, gum, and skin patches may poison animals. Signs of poisoning are largely the result of stimulation of sympathetic and parasympathetic ganglia and include hyperexcitability, muscle fasciculations, hypersalivation, vomiting, and dyspnea, soon progressing to paresis and paralysis. Toxicosis is confirmed by analysis of stomach contents, urine, and skin. Treatment includes atropine if parasympathetic signs are severe. General detoxification and supportive procedures are required.

ORGANOCHLORINE INSECTICIDES

Few of these compounds remain in use today. Parts per billion–level residues may be present in the blood and fat of animals exposed to traces of insecticides in soil and food products. Endosulfan remains in use for gardens and agricultural application. Endosulfan, with an oral LD_{50} of 65 mg/kg, has been used maliciously to kill neighborhood dogs. Endosulfan is highly toxic to cats, with an oral LD_{50} of 2 mg/kg. Convulsions and muscle twitching involving the eyelids, ears, and limbs are common. Signs may persist for several days. Excitement or handling may cause the signs to

357

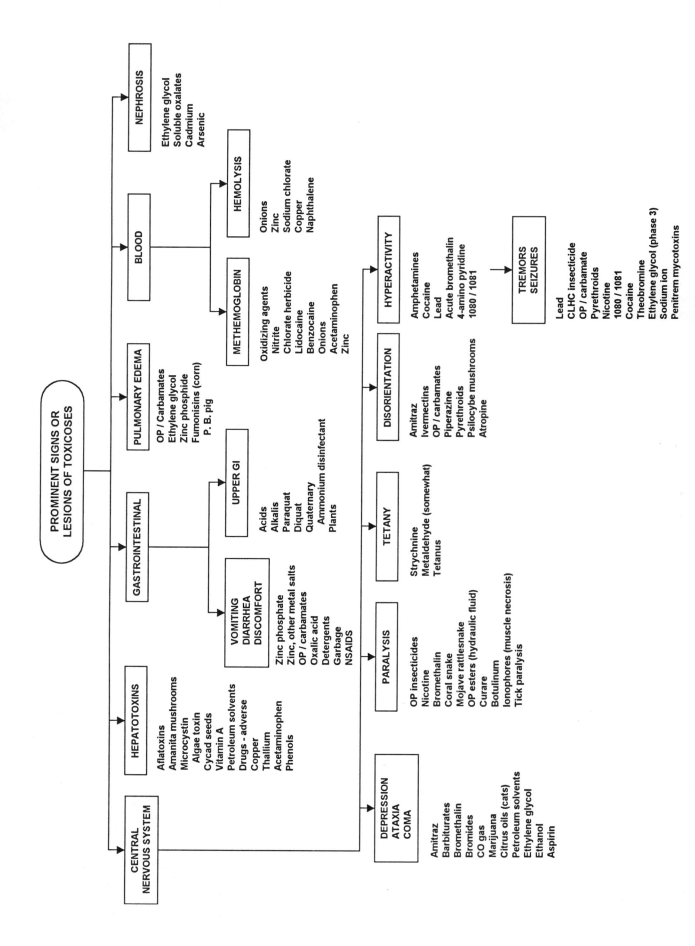

Figure 80–1. Algorithm for prominent signs or lesions of toxicoses.

reappear or increase. Animals may appear normal between episodes of neuromuscular activity. Serum, vomitus, liver, fat, and brain may be chemically analyzed. Enterohepatic circulation may prolong the period of elimination, requiring pulse dosing with activated charcoal orally at 1.0 g/kg (0.5 g/lb) at four- to six-hour intervals even in dermal exposures.

ORGANOPHOSPHORUS AND CARBAMATE INSECTICIDES

These are anticholinesterase insecticides. Onset of signs generally occurs within minutes to an hour of exposure to a toxic dose. With dermal contact from dips or sprays, there may be a longer period to onset of poisoning. Salivation, lacrimation, urination, and defecation (SLUD) occur in acutely poisoned animals. Muscle fasciculations are prominent, and the pupils are constricted unless the animal is in shock. Convulsions may be continuous in severe cases and lead to respiratory failure. Depression, weakness, and paralysis may develop. Bronchoconstriction and pulmonary congestion and edema contribute to respiratory distress. Laboratory findings of red blood cell cholinesterase activity reduced by 25 per cent or more (based on the normal range for that laboratory) confirm exposure. Marked reduction of red cell cholinesterase activity may be noted in poisoned animals that are not exhibiting clinical signs. Cats normally have much lower red cell cholinesterase activity than dogs, making interpretation difficult. The carbamate-cholinesterase bond is quickly reversed, which limits the value of this procedure. Retina and brain cholinesterase determinations are available at some laboratories. Stomach contents, liver, urine, hair, skin, and fat can be used for chemical analysis, depending on the type of exposure and the compound in question. Favorable response to atropine supports the diagnosis. Severely poisoned, cyanotic animals may require additional oxygen before atropinization to avoid possible ventricular fibrillation. Atropine is administered (0.1 to 0.2 mg/lb or 0.2 to 0.4 mg/kg) slowly IV over five minutes. Additional atropine may be necessary to achieve the desired response. A favorable response is seen within three to five minutes and includes drying of mucous membranes of the mouth and relief of bronchospasm. Repeated administration of atropine, as needed to control signs, can be given at a lower dosage IV or subcutaneously (SC).

Carbamate poisoning usually responds promptly to atropine therapy and removal of the pesticide. Severe toxicosis induced by ingestion of a massive dose of a highly toxic agricultural product is an exception. Organophosphorus poisoned animals may recover slowly owing to profound cholinesterase depression. Slow absorption and elimination of the pesticide and/or retention in fat with delayed elimination, as in chlorpyrifos toxicosis in the cat, also slows recovery. Maintaining activated carbon in the gastrointestinal tract, 0.5 g/kg four times a day, may bind pesticide that is recycling in saliva and bile. Diphenhydramine has antinicotinic activity and may be useful in dogs and cats.[2] Signs of depression that may be caused by diphenhydramine should be considered. Pralidoxime chloride (2-PAM, Protopam Chloride), a cholinesterase reactivator, can be administered in addition to atropine as a 10 per cent solution at 5 mg/lb (10 mg/kg) for cats and 20 mg/lb (40 mg/kg) for dogs slowly IV or with fluids over 30 minutes. The intramuscular (IM) route can be used for subsequent treatments. Response to cholinesterase reactivators decreases with time after organophosphorus exposure; therefore, treatment should begin within 24 to 48

hours. There seems to be a benefit to its use in animals poisoned several days earlier when slowly eliminated compounds such as fenthion and chlorpyrifos are involved.

PYRETHRIN AND PYRETHROID INSECTICIDES

Pyrethroids are synthetic insecticides that are chemically similar to pyrethrins and have a similar mode of action. They are rapidly metabolized by liver and plasma esterases. Synergists in insecticidal products slow metabolism of pyrethroids by altering the effectiveness of mixed-function oxidase enzymes. Pyrethroids are rapidly metabolized by mammals into inactive acid and alcohol components. Pyrethrins are neurotoxic, with the development and severity of clinical signs being proportional to the nervous tissue concentration. Cats appear to be more susceptible to pyrethroid poisoning than dogs. Onset of signs may be delayed in dermal exposures for several hours to a day or two. Signs include tremors, increased salivation, ataxia, vomiting, depression, hyperexcitability or hyperactivity, seizures, and dyspnea.[3] Death may occur but is not common. Signs generally abate and the animal returns to normal within 72 hours. Control seizures or hyperactivity with diazepam or barbiturates, and employ detoxification procedures as indicated. Recovery within 72 hours is expected in most cases.

ROTENONE

Cats are more commonly affected than dogs by rotenone. Vomiting occurs and may eliminate a portion of ingested rotenone. Gastric irritation, lethargy, stupor, and respiratory depression are seen.[2] Tremors and seizures have been reported. Removal of rotenone from the skin and administration of activated charcoal and sorbitol orally should be effective.

RODENTICIDES

ANTICOAGULANTS

The second-generation anticoagulant indanediones (diphacinone) and 4-hydroxycoumarins bind to plasma proteins and are slowly released, requiring vitamin K_1 therapy for two to four weeks. Brodifacoum is most commonly used and most toxic. The acute LD_{50} dose for dogs is as low as 0.25 mg/kg body weight. Four grams of 0.005 per cent brodifacoum bait per kilogram body weight is the approximate toxic dose for a dog. That is about 1 ounce of bait per 16 pounds of dog. Secondary or relay poisoning can occur. Cats are more resistant to toxicity. Coumarins and indanediones depress the hepatic vitamin K–dependent synthesis of prothrombin. Peak plasma levels are reached in 12 hours, and prolongation of the prothrombin time begins when clotting factors present at the time of anticoagulant ingestion are consumed, usually within 24 to 36 hours after ingestion, reaching a maximum within 36 to 72 hours. Prolongation of the prothrombin time may precede prolongation of the partial thromboplastin time. PIVKA (proteins induced by vitamin K absence or antagonism) testing detects noncarboxylated vitamin K–dependent factors. Lethargy, respiratory distress, dyspnea, and ventral hematomas were prominent initial signs in 15 dogs and cats in two reports.[4, 5] Epistaxis, hematuria, and melena are additional signs. Bleeding into the joints, brain, and spinal cord can occur. Anticoagulants cross the placental barrier and may affect fetuses. Laboratory testing exists for some anticoagulants in plasma or serum and liver. The need for lifesaving measures such as blood or plasma transfusions, treatment of shock, oxygen therapy, and drugs for pulmonary edema must be considered. Vitamin K_1 should be administered orally at 1 to 2.5 mg/lb (2 to 5 mg/kg), followed by a fatty meal such as moist dog food to enhance absorption. Oral dosing is effective and rapid and avoids the potential for hemorrhage at the injection site.[6] A loading dose of vitamin K_1 at 2.5 mg/lb (5 mg/kg) SC in multiple sites using a small-gauge needle can be given if oral dosing is thought inappropriate. Follow this in 12 hours with 0.75 to 1.25 mg/lb (1.5 to 2.5 mg/kg) orally, and continue oral dosing twice a day for 21 to 30 days. Prothrombin time should be checked two to three days after cessation of therapy.[7] Activated coagulation time is easily performed in a clinic setting and is often satisfactory to monitor response to treatment.[1]

CHOLECALCIFEROL

Cholecalciferol (vitamin D_3) poisoning results in hypercalcemia (>12.5 mg/dL), which, if not successfully treated, leads to calcification of soft tissues and nephrosis. Signs and lesions attributed to cardiac, pulmonary, renal, gastrointestinal, and nervous system effects may be seen.[8] Five grams of bait per kilogram body weight is a toxic dose. Polyuria and polydipsia (PU/PD) and hypercalcemia occur within 24 hours after ingestion. Anorexia, depression, lethargy, constipation, vomiting, hematemesis, and a bloody stool may develop three to five days after ingestion. Therapy is aimed at returning serum calcium to below 12.5 mg/dL by promoting calcium elimination through calciuresis and reducing absorption from the intestine (prednisolone) and bone (calcitonin). Treatment consists of normal saline (0.9 per cent sodium chloride) and furosemide (initial bolus 2.5 mg/lb or 5 mg/kg repeated three times a day, or first dose followed by a constant-rate infusion of 2.5 mg/lb or 5 mg/kg per hour) and prednisolone 0.5 to 1 mg/lb (1 to 2 mg/kg) twice a day. Salmon calcitonin can be used at 4 to 6 IU SC every two to three hours until serum calcium stabilizes at less than 12.5 mg/dL. The dosage can be increased to 5 to 10 IU/lb (10 to 20 IU/kg) if the initial dosage is not effective.[6] Furosemide and prednisolone treatment may be necessary for two to four weeks. A low-calcium diet should be fed.

BROMETHALIN

Bromethalin rodenticide toxicity results in cerebral edema, and an increase in cerebrospinal fluid pressure places pressure on nerve axons, causing decreased nerve impulse conduction, paralysis, and death. Lesions produced in dogs from a fatal single oral dose of 6.25 mg/kg include diffuse white matter spongiosis, mild microgliosis, and optic nerve vacuolization.[9] The minimal toxic dose for dogs is 1.67 mg/kg; the minimal lethal dose is 1.25 mg/lb or 2.5 mg/kg (25 g of bait/kg body weight). The minimal toxic dose for cats is less, 0.3 g of bait/kg, and the minimal lethal dose is 1.1 g of bait/kg body weight. Clinical signs are varied and dose-dependent. A large dose causes a convulsant syndrome, generally within 24 hours, characterized by tremors, hyperthermia, extreme hyperexcitability, and focal motor and generalized seizures. A lower dose induces signs in one to five

days, including hind limb ataxia and/or paresis and/or central nervous system depression. Lesions are said to be minimal with mild edema and spongy degeneration in the white matter of the brain, spinal cord, and optic nerve. Tests that detect bromethalin or the metabolite desmethyl bromethalin in tissues may be offered by some labs but may have limited clinical value in chronic cases.[9] In addition to oral dosing with activated charcoal three times daily, suggested therapy includes dexamethasone 1 mg/lb (2 mg/kg) every six hours or prednisolone 1 to 3 mg/lb (2 to 6 mg/kg) orally daily and mannitol solution 250 mg/lb (500 mg/kg) IV every six hours to relieve cerebral edema.

STRYCHNINE AND SODIUM FLUOROACETATE

These extremely toxic rodenticides have presented veterinarians with emergency situations for many years. Use of 1080/1081 is restricted to licensed pest-control operators for limited use and is seldom, if ever, used in the United States. Baits containing 0.5 per cent strychnine are available for gopher control. Strychnine is thought to be a competitive inhibitor of the inhibitory neurotransmitter glycine. This results in uninhibited stimulation of motor neurons, affecting all striated muscle. The lethal dose is in the range of 0.25 to 2 mg/kg for most animals. The 0.5 per cent product contains 5 mg strychnine per gram of bait, an amount toxic to a 10- to 12-pound dog. Nervousness and apprehension precede tetanic seizures, which develop 15 minutes to 2 hours following ingestion. Tetanic seizures are triggered by noise, bright light, and touch. Death is the result of respiratory paralysis and may come with the first seizure or after exhaustive bouts of seizures. Sodium fluoroacetate poisons the tricarboxylic acid cycle, causing citrate accumulation and hyperactive behavior; death ensues within an hour. Strychnine alkaloid can be identified in stomach contents, liver, and urine. Compound 1080/1081 tissue levels can be detected by capillary gas chromatography–mass spectrometry, but few laboratories offer the service. Pentobarbital (15 mg/lb or 30 mg/kg) given IV to effect is useful for controlling the tetanic seizures. Light anesthesia, adequate to control seizures, is maintained until strychnine is eliminated in the urine (approximately 42 hours). Gastric lavage followed by installation of activated charcoal is recommended. Acidification of the urine by IV or oral ammonium chloride may enhance urinary excretion. The prognosis for 1080/1081 poisoning is grave, as there is no effective, readily available antidote.

ZINC PHOSPHIDE

Zinc phosphide is a rodenticide that has replaced strychnine in several products. It is stable for long periods in a dry environment. Secondary poisoning can occur. Stomach acid releases phosphine gas from zinc phosphide. A lethal dose for a 30-pound dog with a full stomach would be delivered in 2 tablespoons or 30 g of bait containing 2 per cent zinc phosphide. On an empty stomach, the lethal dose is greater than 300 mg/kg.[6] Phosphine is responsible for the acute effects, which include severe gastrointestinal inflammation, abdominal distention, pulmonary congestion and edema, and cardiovascular insufficiency. Signs develop within 15 minutes to several hours after ingestion and may include vomiting, running fits, convulsions, abdominal discomfort, labored respiration, and depression. Catarrhal to hemorrhagic gastroenteritis can occur. A rotten fish or garlic-like odor is characteristic of acute cases at necropsy. Submit promptly frozen stomach contents and bait for zinc phosphide/phosphine determination. Treatment includes control of seizures, acidosis, and shock. Gastric lavage and supportive care follow.

AUTOMOTIVE PRODUCTS

ETHYLENE GLYCOL

Synonyms for ethylene glycol include 1,2-dihydroxymethane, 1,2-ethanediol, ethylene alcohol, ethylene dihydrate, glycol, monoethylene glycol, and MEG. The minimal lethal dose of the undiluted product for a cat is 0.7 mL/lb (1.5 mL/kg). That dose is delivered by 1 tablespoonful (15 mL) of 50:50 radiator fluid. The minimal lethal dose for a dog is 3.3 mL/lb (6.6 mL/kg), or approximately 4.5 ounces for a 20-pound dog. The initial metabolism of ethylene glycol is to glycoaldehyde. Early signs of intoxication become apparent within an hour and are similar to those seen following consumption of ethanol. Peak absorption and highest blood level develop within one to three hours after ingestion. Detectable levels of ethylene glycol persist up to 48 hours in serum and urine. Drunken behavior may be seen, with vomiting, ataxia, knuckling, and depression during this first phase of toxicosis. Signs may progress to coma and death during the first few hours. In most cases, after four to six hours the animal appears to be normal. Glycolic acid then causes severe metabolic acidosis in the second phase of clinical toxicosis, which develops 12 to 24 hours after ethylene glycol ingestion.[10] Urinary concentration of glycolate correlates with clinical signs and mortality. Further metabolism of glycolic acid produces formic acid, oxalic acid, and oxalate. These acids add to the anion gap metabolic acidosis. Oxalate combines with calcium to form calcium oxalate crystals in renal tubules, urine, and blood vessels of the brain and other tissues. Glycolate and oxalate are thought to produce the tubular damage. The third phase of poisoning is associated with renal failure and becomes apparent 24 to 96 hours after ingestion.

Ethylene glycol colorimetric spot test kits for urine and serum are available to practitioners to support a diagnosis of ethylene glycol toxicosis during the first 24 hours after exposure. Propylene glycol may cause a positive spot test.[10] Anion gaps greater than 40 to 50 mEq/L are considered typical of ethylene glycol toxicosis.[11] Serum osmolality is increased as well. Calcium oxalate crystals may be seen in urine by five hours after ingestion in dogs and three hours in cats. The birefringent crystals appear in the monohydrate and dihydrate forms when viewed under polarized light—the former as sheaf, dumbbell, six-sided, elongated, or prism-shaped forms, and the latter as the classic Maltese cross. Serum osmolality increases as the ethylene glycol serum level increases; 100 mg/dL accounts for a 16 mOsm/kg increase.[12] Calculation of the osmolar gap can provide the initial clue or strong support for suspected ethylene glycol ingestion. The osmolar gap remains markedly wide for the first six hours and then gradually decreases until the normal reference range is reached in 24 hours. In the third phase, hypocalcemia, elevated blood urea nitrogen, and creatinine accompany depression, anorexia, gastroenteritis, encephalopathy, coma, and death. Presence of crystals in renal biopsy material or crystals viewed via cytologic examination of renal cortex scrapings at necropsy are very supportive if not diagnostic.

Therapy can be successful if started within six to eight hours of ingestion and before renal damage is indicated by azotemia. Emesis can be induced safely if the animal is alert and the gag reflex is functional. Activated carbon and sodium sulfate should be given by stomach tube during the first three hours after ingestion. Dehydration and acidosis must be corrected and fluid therapy maintained to promote excretion of the toxicants. The potential for overhydration in the face of renal shutdown must be considered. Peritoneal dialysis may be a lifesaving procedure when oliguria is present.

Ethanol and 4-methylpyrazole (fomepizole, Antizol-Vet) inhibit ethylene glycol metabolism. If treatment is begun within eight hours in dogs not already azotemic, the prognosis should be fair to guarded. It is not recommended for use in cats. Fomepizole (Antizol-Vet) therapy of ethylene glycol toxicosis is safe and effective and does not cause the side effects seen with ethanol.[13] Administer an initial loading dose of 10 mg/lb (20 mg/kg) IV as soon as practical upon suspicion of ethylene glycol poisoning. Following the initial loading dose, doses of 6.8, 6.8, and 2.5 mg/lb should be administered at 12, 24, and 36 hours, respectively. Ethanol therapy for dogs includes 2.5 mL/lb (5.5 mL/kg) in saline IV, plus 4 mL/lb (8 mL/kg) of 5 per cent sodium bicarbonate intraperitoneally (IP), each given every four hours for five treatments, then every six hours for four treatments. For cats, 20 per cent ethanol is administered at 2.5 mL/lb (5 mL/kg) in saline IV and 5 per cent bicarbonate at 3 mL/lb (6 mL/kg) IV every six hours for five treatments, then every eight hours for four treatments.

PROPYLENE GLYCOL

Colorimetric ethylene glycol spot tests on serum or urine may be positive in the presence of propylene glycol. Propylene glycol is metabolized to lactic and pyruvic acid, and the toxicity from oral or intravenous drug forms is low. The acute oral LD_{50} in dogs is 9 mL/kg.[10] The toxic syndrome induced by propylene glycol is similar to the acute phase of ethylene glycol intoxication. Treatment largely depends on symptomatic and supportive care, as use of ethanol or 4-methylpyrazole is generally not recommended.[10] Activated charcoal–saline cathartic could be administered.

METHANOL

Windshield wiper fluids may contain methanol as an antifreeze agent, and a warning is generally stated on the product label. Ethanol is the recommended treatment (see earlier).

METALS

LEAD

Absorption of lead is greater in young animals, and low dietary calcium may increase absorption.[14] Lead may cross the blood-brain barrier in greater amounts in young animals. Lead shot embedded in tissue is poorly absorbed unless it is in or near joints, where contact with the relatively acidic synovial fluid may increase absorption. Gastrointestinal and neurologic signs such as anorexia, vomiting, abdominal pain, diarrhea, and constipation precede the onset of central nervous system disturbance by several days. Megaesophagus is a less common finding. Hysteria characterized by increased irritability, whining or barking, continuous running, and snapping may occur in young dogs. Opisthotonos, clonic-tonic activity, apparent blindness, dullness, or unusual behavior may be noticed by the owner. Cats display anorexia, lethargy, and seizures.[15, 16] A large number of nucleated red blood cells (5 to 40/100 white blood cells), accompanied by a packed cell volume of not less than 30 per cent, supports a suspicion of lead toxicosis. Torso radiographs may reveal lead paint chips or other materials, but they must be differentiated from bone chips, zinc, or other metals and rocks. Whole blood is the preferred sample for confirmatory diagnosis in the living animal. The lead is associated with the red blood cells. Lead concentration of 35 μg/dL (0.35 ppm) or higher is highly supportive of lead poisoning. A level of 40 μg/dL (0.40 ppm) in the presence of compatible signs is considered diagnostic. A lead level of 10 μg/dL (0.10 ppm) to 35 μg/dL (0.35 ppm) suggests a higher than normal lead burden.[16, 17] If blood lead levels are not conclusive, the urinary calcium EDTA postchelation test, comparing urine lead before and 24 hours after a dose of the antidote, is useful. An increase in urine lead of greater than 10 times is seen in lead poisoning. Kidney and liver lead levels of 4 ppm and above indicate abnormal lead accumulation, and greater than 8 ppm is associated with fatal cases.

Removal of lead from the digestive tract with a magnesium or sodium sulfate cathartic may be indicated. Surgical removal of an object might be necessary. Thiamine, 1 mg/lb or 2 mg/kg of body weight SC or IM every 12 hours is beneficial in alleviating signs. Chelation therapy using commercial calcium EDTA diluted to 1 per cent (10 mg/mL) in isotonic saline or 5 per cent dextrose is recommended. Specific treatment involves administration of calcium EDTA at a dosage of 35 to 55 mg/lb (75 to 110 mg/kg), diluted to a 1 or 2 per cent solution in 5 per cent dextrose in water (IP, SC, or slowly IV), divided every 12 hours.[18] Treat for two days, rest for two days, and treat for two additional days if indicated. Severe cases can be treated for five days. Diarrhea, renal tubular necrosis, and depletion of zinc and magnesium can occur with excessive use of calcium EDTA. It is important that hydration be maintained to promote renal function and urinary excretion of the chelated lead. D-penicillamine 50 mg/lb (110 mg/kg) daily, divided every six to eight hours and given orally 30 minutes before feeding for one to two weeks, is effective when signs are minimal. It can be used following a course of calcium EDTA therapy or as chelation treatment in animals that are exhibiting less severe cases of lead poisoning. D-Penicillamine often causes anorexia, vomiting, and depression, which may be alleviated by premedication with 1 to 2 mg/lb (2 to 4 mg/kg) dimenhydrinate (Dramamine). An alternative plan is to reduce the dose of penicillamine to 15 to 25 mg/lb/day (33 to 55 mg/kg/day). D-Penicillamine can be dissolved in fruit juice to facilitate treatment at home. Succimer (Chemet) in 100-mg capsules is an oral chelating agent that is effective and reasonably safe for the treatment of lead intoxication in dogs at the label dosage for humans. Blood lead levels tend to fluctuate and to rebound following treatment, not returning to a normal range for weeks. It is imperative that the animal not be returned home to a hazardous situation where lead exposure would continue.

THALLIUM

The sale of thallium pesticides has been prohibited since 1972 in the United States, but they may still be in use in many countries. A case of thallium toxicosis in a dog was reported in 1992.[19] Gastroenteritis and hepatic, renal, and cardiac effects are seen. Alopecia and conjunctivitis accompany chronic cases. Urine is the best sample to examine for levels.

MERCURY

Mercury poisoning is seldom reported in the pet practice setting. In acute exposure to ingested mercuric salts, oral administration of milk and eggs to bind mercury to protein may be beneficial. Succimer (Chemet) has been used successfully as an oral chelating drug in a limited number of human cases.

ZINC

Sources of zinc in reported cases of poisoning in dogs and birds have included pennies minted since 1983 (96 per cent zinc), zinc nuts on collapsible transport cages, galvanized drip points on metal fences, toy chains, and zinc oxide ointment. Zinc leaches from galvanized containers into food or water that is acidic. Hemolytic anemia is a consistent finding in dogs. Signs of depression, abdominal discomfort, vomiting, diarrhea, and anorexia may precede the appearance of red urine and icterus. Clinical pathology often includes azotemia, elevated pancreatic and hepatic enzymes, and evidence of anemia. Abdominal survey radiographs may provide the first evidence of a retained metal object. Serum zinc levels are elevated well above the normal range of 0.7 to 1.2 mg/L in dogs, confirming exposure. Special blood tubes (metal-free) should be used. Liver zinc concentrations (normal = 30 to 70 ppm) may be greater than 200 ppm. Treatment involves supportive measures and removal of the metal object by endoscopy or gastrotomy. Blood transfusion may be indicated. Fluid therapy can correct fluid loss and electrolyte imbalances associated with vomiting and improve renal function. Chelation therapy for zinc toxicosis with calcium EDTA, similar to treatment of lead poisoning, should be administered.

IRON

Iron salts in the form of ferrous sulfate tablets have fatally poisoned children. Gastroenteritis (sometimes hemorrhagic), nausea, and vomiting may be accompanied by shock and lethargy in moderate to severe poisoning. Deferoxamine mesylate (Desferal) is the antidote for human iron intoxication.

COPPER

Hepatic copper accumulation (in lysosomes) and chronic poisoning caused by the autosomal recessive disorder of Bedlington terriers and the similar condition reported in West Highland white terriers account for most copper toxicoses in small pet animals. Doberman pinschers may also accumulate high liver copper levels. On a dry-weight basis, copper levels above 1000 ppm have been used for confirmation in dogs.[20] Acute copper poisoning is rare. D-Penicillamine is a treatment.

ARSENIC

Products containing 1 to 2 per cent arsenic trioxide in a sweet liquid are marketed as ant bait. Herbicides are readily available containing 4 to 48 per cent MSMA (an arsenical) for use as an edger. Severe diarrhea, dehydration, shock, metabolic acidosis, and anuria develop. Hepatic necrosis and renal tubular necrosis are additional findings. Serum, urine, and kidney are the biologic specimens to submit for toxicologic analysis. Intensive fluid and electrolyte therapy is needed. Oral activated charcoal is considered beneficial. If the source of exposure is from licking contaminated hair and feet, thorough washing is essential. Dimercaprol (British antilewisite, or BAL) is an antidote for inorganic arsenic, and D-penicillamime (see Lead) is useful.

HERBICIDES

PARAQUAT AND DIQUAT

Paraquat is pneumotoxic, and both paraquat and diquat are corrosive. They cause gastroenteritis and hepatic and renal damage. Pulmonary edema develops in one to three days, followed by progression of pulmonary changes to fibrosis and death. Reducing absorption from the gastrointestinal tract is best achieved by gastric lavage with a slurry of Fuller's earth (up to 30 per cent). Oxygen therapy is contraindicated. Contact the manufacturer for further information.

CHLORPHENOXY COMPOUNDS

The acute, oral LD_{50} of 2,4-D for dogs is approximately 50 mg/lb of body weight (100 mg/kg). It is rapidly excreted in urine. Treated lawns should be allowed to dry before returning animals to them. Myotonia is a prominent sign in 2,4-D poisoned dogs.

GLYPHOSATE

Glyphosate herbicides are available as Round-up, Sting, and Rodeo (among many). Some dogs and cats exposed to freshly treated weeds and grass have had transient signs of irritation to the eyes and skin.

REFERENCES

1. Murphy MJ: Clinical update toxin exposures in dogs and cats: Pesticides and biotoxins. JAVMA 205:414, 1994.
2. Osweiler GD: Insecticides and molluscacides. In Osweiler GD (ed): Toxicology, 1st ed. Philadelphia, Williams & Wilkins, 1996, pp 231–245.
3. Valentine WM, et al: Pyrethrin and pyrethroid insecticides. Vet Clin North Am Small Anim Pract 20:375, 1990.
4. DuVall MD, et al: Case studies on second generation anticoagulant rodenticide toxicities in nontarget species. J Vet Diagn Invest 1:66, 1989.
5. Schulman A, et al: Diphacininone induced coagulopathy in the dog. JAVMA 188:402, 1986.
6. Osweiler GD: Rodenticides. In Osweiler GD (ed): Toxicology. Philadelphia, Williams & Wilkins, 1996, pp 275–295.
7. Woody BJ, et al: Coagulopathic effects and therapy of brodifacoum toxicosis in dogs. J Vet Intern Med 6:23, 1992.
8. Moreau R, Squires RA: Hypercalcemia. Compendium Small Anim 14:1077, 1992.
9. Dorman DC, et al: Diagnosis of bromethalin toxicosis in the dog. J Vet Diagn Invest 2:123, 1990.
10. Owens JG, Dorman DC: Common household hazards for small animals. Vet Med 92:140, 1997.
11. Osweiler GD: Common household products. In Osweiler GD (ed): Toxicology. Philadelphia, Williams & Wilkins, 1996, pp 317–330.
12. Mount ME: Toxicology. In Ettinger SL (ed): Textbook of Veterinary Internal Medicine, 2nd ed. Philadelphia, WB Saunders, 1989, pp 456–483.
13. Connally HE, Thrall MA, Forney SD: Safety and efficacy of 4-methylpyrazole for treatment of suspected and confirmed ethylene glycol intoxication in dogs: 107 cases (1983–1995). JAVMA 209:1880, 1996.
14. Osweiler GD: Metals and minerals. In Osweiler GD (ed): Toxicology. Philadelphia, Williams & Wilkins. 1996, pp 179–211.
15. Miller S, Baulk TJ: Lead toxicosis in a group of cats. J Vet Diagn Invest 4:362, 1992.
16. Van Alstine WG, Wickliffw LW, Everson RJ, et al: Acute lead toxicosis in a household of cats. J Vet Diagn Invest 5:496, 1993.
17. Berny PJ, Cote LM, Buck WB: Low blood lead concentration associated with various biomarkers in household pets. Am J Vet Res 55:55, 1994.
18. Murphy MJ: Toxin exposures in dogs and cats: Drugs and household products. JAVMA 205:557, 1994.
19. Waters CB, et al: Acute thallium toxicity in a dog. JAVMA 201:883, 1992.
20. Brewer MD, Dick RD, Schall W: Use of zinc acetate to treat copper toxicosis in dogs. JAVMA 201:564, 1992.

CHAPTER 81

COMMON PLANT TOXICITIES

Lynn Hovda

Worldwide, plants are involved in 10 to 15 per cent of all companion animal poison exposures. Dogs account for 70 per cent, cats for 25 per cent, and other animals for the remaining 5 per cent.[1] Exposures involving dogs are evenly split between interior and exterior plants, whereas cat exposures mainly involve plants found within the home. Youth, confinement, and boredom are the most common reasons for plant ingestion, although some pets may inadvertently be poisoned by well-meaning owners.

Recognition of exposure is often frustrating. Many pet owners report known exposures, but some are not witnessed, making the diagnosis difficult. Knowledge of indigenous toxic plants and several reliable sources of plant identification aid in the formulation of a treatment plan.

Treatment is frequently symptomatic and supportive, as few antidotes are available. The specific plant; quantity and parts ingested; time of ingestion; and species, breed, and weight of the animal all need to be considered before treatment is begun. If an unknown plant toxicity is presumed, unless contraindicated, the stomach contents should be evacuated with induced emesis or gastric lavage, followed by activated charcoal with a cathartic. Close examination of the stomach contents for berries, seeds, and plant pieces may confirm ingestion, assist in plant identification, and guide therapy.

PLANTS AFFECTING PRIMARILY THE GASTROINTESTINAL SYSTEM

Oxalate-containing plants (family Araceae) are the most frequently reported exposures.[1, 2] Common household plants containing insoluble crystals include dumbcane (*Dieffenbachia* spp.), philodendron (*Philodendron* spp.), peace lily (*Spathiphylum* spp.), and devil's ivy (*Epiprenum aureum*). Crystals are usually concentrated in a raphide structure within the stalk. Disruption of the raphides by chewing on the stalk releases oxalate crystals and unidentified enzymes. Clinically, three scenarios can occur:

1. Stomatitis/glossitis. Irritation to the mucous membranes of the mouth and throat causes immediate pain, local swelling, and profuse salivation. These may be accompanied by head shaking, loss of vocalization, and airway compromise. Treatment is primarily symptomatic. The mouth should be examined thoroughly and remaining plant pieces removed. Cool fluids, ice chips, and analgesics increase comfort until the signs resolve.

2. Ocular. Eye exposures, although rare in animals, cause intense burning pain and swelling. Left untreated, conjunctivitis, abrasions, and corneal ulcers may develop. Treatment includes a 10- to 15-minute eye irrigation, followed by a thorough ocular examination. Ophthalmic medications should be used as needed.

3. Systemic. Systemic effects occur primarily in cats exposed to *Philodendron* spp. The signs are referable to the renal and central nervous systems (hyperexcitability, tetany, seizures). Treatment is symptomatic and supportive.

Rhubarb (*Rheum* spp.) contains soluble oxalate crystals. The stalk is edible and causes no systemic effects. When the leaves are ingested, soluble oxalates can be absorbed and bind with calcium. Although symptoms are primarily related to the gastrointestinal tract, systemic hypocalcemia sometimes results. Oral calcium hydroxide is used to bind oxalates in the gastrointestinal tract. If systemic signs are noted, intravenous calcium should be administered.

Christmas plants receiving bad publicity include the holly (*Ilex* spp.)[3] and poinsettia (*Euphorbia pulcherrima*).[4] There are well over 300 species of holly in the United States alone. The toxin remains unidentified but may be ilicin (ilexanthin and ilex acids), a saponin causing gastrointestinal effects. Treatment is symptomatic and includes demulcents and antacids. Poinsettias produce only mild toxicity. The unidentified toxin in the latex sap rarely causes more than mucous membrane irritation or contact dermatitis. Mistletoe (*Phoradendron flavescens*) has the potential for more serious effects.[5] The toxin is a phytotoxin or toxalbumin. Severe gastroenteritis with prolonged emesis may occur 18 to 24 hours after ingestion of leaves or berries. Treatment is symptomatic and supportive.

English ivy (*Hedera helix*), a common houseplant and ground cover, contains hederagenin, a saponin.[3, 5] Ingestion of leaves and berries may cause profuse salivation, abdominal pain, emesis, and diarrhea. Treatment is primarily symptomatic and supportive.

Several varieties of poisonous plants grow from bulbs, roots, or corms. Included are amaryllis, jonquil, and daffodil (family Amaryllidaceae); tulip (family Liliaceae); and iris (family Iridaceae). The toxic principles are unknown, but ingestion of the bulbs, roots, or corms has been associated with a mild to moderate gastroenteritis. All parts of the Easter lily (*Lilium longiflorum*)[6] and daylily (*Hemerocallis* spp.)[5] have been associated with nephrotoxicity in cats. The toxic principle is unknown. Ingestion causes gastrointestinal distress, depression, and anorexia, followed in 2 to 4 days by acute renal failure. Early intervention is necessary for survival. Treatment includes aggressive gastrointestinal decontamination and fluid diuresis for a minimum of 24 hours.

Solanine-containing plants are members of the Solanaceae family. Included are the tomato (*Solanum lycopersicon*), potato (*S. tuberosum*), eggplant (*S. melongena*), bittersweet (*S. dulcamara*), deadly or black nightshade (*S. nigrum*), and Jerusalem cherry (*S. pseudocapsicum*). The primary toxin is solanine. Some plants produce tropane belladonna (deadly nightshade) or solanocapsine (Jersulaem cherry). Solanine is poorly absorbed orally, and most members of this family act only as gastrointestinal irritants. Systemic absorption occurs when there is substantial mucosal damage. Systemically, solanine causes central nervous system (CNS) depression and cardiac arrhythmias. Deadly nightshade may cause a mixed picture, depending on which toxin is prevalant. Solanine usually predominates, but sometimes anticholinergic signs occur, and physostigmine is indicated.[7] Solanocapsine affects cardiac muscle, causing decreased heart rate and conductive changes. Treatment is symptomatic.

Life-threatening mushroom ingestions include amanitin poisoning (*Amanita virosa, Amanita phalloides, Conocybe filaris*), orellanine poisoning (*Cortinarius orellanus, Cortinarius rainierensis*), and monomethylhydrazine poisoning (*Gyromita esculenta*).[8] Of these, amanitin poisoning is the most widely reported in dogs.[8, 9] *Amanita phalloides* are found in wooded areas throughout the United States and Canada. Signs usually do not develop for 6 to 24 hours after ingestion. Typically, signs include a 24- to 36-hour gastrointestinal phase, followed by a 24-hour remission phase, and then a late hepatic phase characterized by jaundice, coma, and death. Survivors of the hepatic phase may ultimately die from renal tubular necrosis. Diagnosis is difficult. Liver enzymes are markedly elevated early in the process, and blood urea nitrogen and creatinine increase later. Occasionally, spores are found in gastrointestinal contents or feces. A few commercial laboratories are able to perform amatoxin tests on urine. If a sample mushroom is available, the Meixner blue test is a useful qualitative test for amatoxins. Early treatment includes gastric lavage and activated charcoal with a cathartic. Charcoal hemoperfusion may be helpful but is rarely performed on animals. Experimentally, high-dose penicillin, silymarin, prednisone, thioctic acid, cimetidine, and cytochrome c have been used with some success. Liver transplant is the proven therapy.

Abrus precatorius, the jequirity bean, has been used for centuries in Latin American necklaces and jewelry. It has long been illegal to import this jewelry to the United States. The toxin is abrin, a toxalbumin similar to botulinum, cholera, and diphtheria. The toxin must be released from its hard shell to be active. Dogs are poisoned by chewing on the shell and ingesting the contents. Signs of toxicity include abdominal pain, vomiting, diarrhea, seizures, and cerebral edema. There is no antidote; treatment is symptomatic and supportive. The castor bean plant *(Ricinus communis)* is a similar plant widely used as an ornamental shrub throughout the United States. The toxin is ricin. Signs and treatment are identical to those of abrin poisoning.

PLANTS AFFECTING PRIMARILY THE CARDIOVASCULAR SYSTEM

Plants with cardiac glycoside activity include the common oleander *(Nerium oleander)*, yellow oleander *(Thevetia peruviana)*, foxglove *(Digitalis purpurea)*, and lily of the valley *(Convalleria majalis)*.[3] Five different types of cardiac glycosides have been identified in the common oleander. The seeds, stems, and roots are toxic. Yellow oleander contains the cardiac glycosides thevetin A, thevetin B, and peruvoside. All parts of the plant contain cardiac glycosides, with seeds having the highest concentration. Although the lethal quantity of oleander is small, spontaneous vomiting and an extremely bitter taste help limit the number of deaths. The sap has been associated with contact dermatitis and blistering of the nose and footpads. Convallatoxin, convallarin, and convallamarin are toxins in lily of the valley.[10] Signs associated with all these plants are generally related to the gastrointestinal tract and cardiovascular system. Vomiting and abdominal pain begin several hours before any deterioration in myocardial function. Marked bradycardia with first-, second-, or third-degree atrioventricular block, ventricular arrhythmias, and asytole can occur. Hyperkalemia is usually prominent, although a few reports of hypokalemia exist.[3, 11] Oleander and foxglove cardiac glycosides, but not those of lily of the valley, cross-react to a certain extent with most digoxin assays. The correlation between serum levels and degree of toxicity is poor for oleander. Correction of potassium abnormalities, antiarrhythmic drugs, temporary pacemakers, and large doses of antidigitalis antibody fragments (Fab) (1.5 vials/kg body weight) have all been used in poisonings from cardiac glycoside–containing plants.[10, 11]

Azaleas *(Rhododendron* spp.) are associated with severe toxicity and death. The precise mechanism is unknown, but it appears that grayanotoxins act by binding to closed sodium channels.[12] Slower opening and increased sodium permeability cause a decreased resting membrane potential in Purkinje's fibers. Clinical signs include severe weakness, hypotension, dyspnea, and respiratory failure. Gastrointestinal signs unrelated to grayanotoxins include salivation, vocalization, vomiting, and diarrhea.[12, 13] Sodium channel blocking antiarrhythmic drugs such as quinidine and procainamide have been suggested.[13]

PLANTS AFFECTING PRIMARILY THE NEUROLOGIC SYSTEM

The Japanese yew *(Taxus cuspidata)* is a common ornamental shrub found in the northern United States and Canada. Taxine is the toxin. All parts of the plant, except the aril, are toxic. Death may be sudden. Vomiting, diarrhea, weakness, trembling, bradycardia, and convulsions occur in less toxic cases.[14] Treatment includes early emesis or gastric lavage, activated charcoal with a cathartic, and supportive care.

Animals ingest tobacco *(Nicotiana tabacum)* from cigarettes, chewing tobacco, cigars, or pipe tobacco.[3] Nicotine is a rapidly acting toxin that stimulates and then depresses the autonomic ganglia.[3, 5] Centrally mediated emesis often occurs before significant absorption, and no further signs develop. Animals with severe poisoning show signs of CNS involvement and cardiac abnormalities. Death is from paralysis of the muscles of respiration. Treatment should be aimed first at assisting respiration and then at removing residual tobacco from the gastrointestinal tract.

Many plants are associated with hallucinogenic effects. Poisoning may be accidental or intentional. Diagnosis is often difficult, as many owners are reluctant to cooperate. Sporadically reported in dogs are poisonings from psilocybins, or "magic mushrooms."[8, 15] Muscle weakness, ataxia, abnormal mentation, vocalization, and temperature changes occur 20 to 30 minutes after ingestion.[15] Marijuana *(Cannabis sativa)* poisoning has also been reported in dogs.[16] Dogs generally become glassy eyed, ataxic, and hyperactive or comatose. Other less common hallucinogenic plants are jimsonweed *(Datura stramonium)*, thorn apple *(Datura metaloidyl)*, blue morning glory *(Ipomoea violace)*, nutmeg *(Myristica fragrans)*, and peyote (family Cactaceae). Signs vary from plant to plant, but in general, all cause changes in the CNS. Treatment is supportive, and signs generally resolve in 24 to 48 hours.

Nettle toxicity (family Urticaceae) is seen primarily in hunting or field dogs. Some species of nettles contain hairs that break off when an animal rubs against them, allowing injection of the contents into the animal. The toxic agents are histamine, acetylcholine, serotonin, and formic acid. Clinical signs are variable and depend on which toxin predominates. Muscle weakness is the most common sign but may be accompanied by salivation, vomiting, pawing at the mouth, tremors, dyspnea, and a slow, irregular heartbeat. Atropine in large doses, antihistamines, and sedation are useful. Generally, animals respond to treatment in 24 hours or less.

REFERENCES

1. Hornfeldt CS: Poisoning in animals. Mod Vet Pract 68:25, 1987.
2. Hornfeldt CS: Plant toxicity in small animals: Oxalate-containing plants. Vet Pract Staff 1:3, 1993.
3. Fowler ME: Poisonous plants affecting the gastroenteric system. *In* Plant Poisoning in Small Companion Animals. St. Louis, Ralston Purina Company, 1980, 7–19.
4. Hornfeldt CS: Confusion over toxicity of poinsettia. JAVMA 194:1004, 1989.
5. Osweiler GD: Plant-related toxicosis: *In* Osweiler GD: Toxicology. Philadelphia, Williams & Wilkins, 1996, pp 361–409.
6. Hall JO: Nephrotoxicity of Easter lily *(Lilium longiflorum)* when ingested by the cat. J Vet Intern Med 3:121, 1992.
7. Hornfeldt CS: Solanine poisoning in small animals. Vet Pract Staff 6:1, 1994.
8. Wilson RB, Holladay JA: Mushroom poisoning. Comp Cont Ed 9:791, 1987.
9. Kallet A, Sousa C, Spangler W: Mushroom *(Amanita phalloides)* toxicity in dogs. Cal Vet 42:9, 1988.
10. Moxley RA, Schneider NR, Steinegger DH, et al: Apparent toxicosis associated with lily-of-the-valley *(Convallaria majalis)* ingestion in a dog. JAVMA 195:485, 1989.
11. Clark RF, Selden BS, Curry SC: Digoxin specific FAB fragments in the treatment of oleander toxicity in a canine model. Ann Emerg Med 20:1073, 1991.
12. Frape D, Ward A: Suspected rhododendron poisoning in dogs. Vet Rec 132:515, 1993.
13. Rose A, Pitchford W, Monin T, et al: Acute weakness and death in a cat. Vet Hum Toxicol 30:334, 1988.
14. Evans KL, Cook JR: Japanese yew poisoning in a dog. J Am Anim Hosp Assoc, 27:300, 1991.
15. Kirwan AP: "Magic mushroom" poisoning in a dog. Vet Rec 126:149, 1990.
16. Schwartz RH, Riddile M: Marijuana intoxication in pets. JAVMA 187:206, 1985.

CHAPTER 82

ACUPUNCTURE IN SMALL ANIMAL PRACTICE

Luc A.A. Janssens

A CRITICAL VIEW ON MEDICAL TREATMENTS

The word *acupuncture* is probably familiar to every veterinarian and veterinary student in Europe and the Americas. That was quite different 25 years ago, when acupuncture was a mystical term for most non-Asian people apart from a small group of "alternative" Western individuals.

If we look at the Western population today, there are two groups of people who unconditionally believe in the efficacy of acupuncture: (1) academics, neuroscientists, and researchers involved in neurophysiology and pain research; and (2) credulous people—those who believe in the superiority of alternative healing methods (homeopathy, herbal medicine, acupuncture, etc.). A large-scale inquiry by consumer organizations in some West European countries revealed that more than 50 per cent of the population believes in the efficiency of alternative medical treatments. It must also be said that important organizations such as the World Health Organization (WHO) and the National Institutes of Health (NIH) have officially recognized acupuncture as an effective treatment for several diseases. Still, the group of nonbelievers, with the opinion that acupuncture is a placebo based on suggestion or a form of hypnosis, is in many Western countries much larger than the one of believers.

It is as incorrect to believe uncritically in a type of medicine with no scientific foundation (e.g., precious stone therapy) as it is to disbelieve in the efficacy of alternative therapies (such as acupuncture) with overwhelming—but unprecedented—scientific data that construct its foundation.

TRADITIONAL CHINESE ACUPUNCTURE—A CRITICAL REVIEW

Acupuncture is an ancient Chinese art of healing that consists of diagnosing and treating disease.[1,2] The diagnostic aspects consist basically of pressure point diagnosis and pulse diagnosis. The treatment aspects consist of "activation" of acupuncture points (AP) that are thought to be localized on one of 12 meridians (Mer). Each Mer contains a certain number of AP. The minimum number is 9; the maximum is 67. Traditionally, the total number of AP is 365 (one for each day).

Pressure point diagnosis is performed by minute palpation of the body surface with emphasis on exploring the AP areas, the anatomic location of which should be memorized. Sensitive or painful points under palpation pressure suggest an energy disturbance. Recognized focal painful points or areas in Western medicine include right trapezius muscle pain in gallbladder disease, McBurney's point in appendicitis, left arm pain in myocardial hypoxia, the experimental

pain zones of Head (in humans), as well as the Clavier of Roger in the horse.[3] These sensitive areas are anatomically standardized, are often localized far away from the locus of disease, and become sensitive when internal organs are inflamed or experimentally irritated. There are *viscerocutaneous reflexes* on the basis of this phenomenon.[3] These reflexes start with intestinal irritation. The neurogenic pathway runs from here through the afferent visceral sympathetic to the dorsal root ganglion and dorsal horn and communicates with the efferent sympathetic neuron in the lateral horn. From there, an efferent signal runs through the ventral root into the sympathetic ganglion and to the segmental periphery (skin, muscle, blood vessels). This causes referred skin sensitivity, vasoconstriction, contraction of the erector pili muscles, muscle hypertonicity, and sweating in the referred area.[3] Kothbauer[4] searched experimentally for these reflexes in the cow by injecting iodine solutions at different points of the urogenital tract while he searched for sensitive areas or points on the animal's back with the help of an electric measuring device. Before the iodine injections, no painful areas or points were detectable on the skin. Injection, however, produced reproducible sensitive areas in which very focal points were identified that were extremely painful under pressure and electrical current and that developed a decreased local skin resistance. These points are considered to be AP. They can then be used diagnostically because a specific sensitive point under palpation refers to a specific internal origin. This reflex has also been examined experimentally in different animal species. In these, destruction of the sympathetic chain, but not the spinal cord or vagus, destroyed the reflex.

Also, *a cutaneovisceral reflex* exists. Stimulation of the skin in rats, rabbits, amphibians, and fish[3] induced gastrointestinal changes in vascularity and motility that were again abolished only when the sympathetic trunk was destroyed. These two reflexes reflect the basics explaining the working mechanism of acupuncture therapy (AT).

Acupuncture pulse diagnosis is the second diagnostic tool. It is not comparable with our Western method of pulse palpation. It is a much more elaborate and sophisticated method. It has been explained in much detail for human use in old and recent Chinese texts, but only in one ancient equine text. The method consists of sensing the arterial pulse with three different fingers on the left and right wrist (Fig. 82–1). The pulse is felt with minor finger pressure (superficial pulse) and deep pressure (deep pulse). As thus, 12 different pulses are perceived. Each of these correlates with a different Mer and gives information about its condition or "energy" status. It seems to take several years of practice to study the subtlety of pulse diagnostics, and no apparatus exists yet to record the many variables in each pulse described by experts. This makes the system subjective, non-

RX

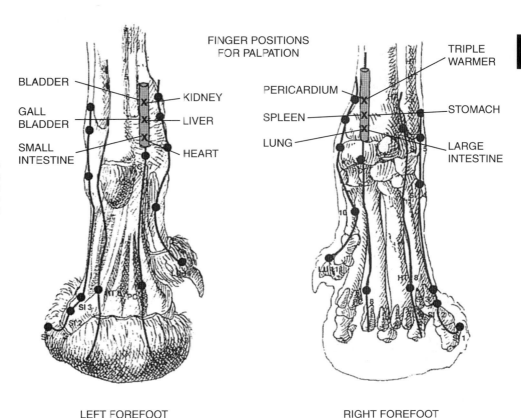

Figure 82–1. Pulse diagnosis in the dog. The left and right ulnar artery is palpated with three fingers at the same time. The pulse is felt with minor (superficial pulse) or hard pressure (deep pulse) to observe 12 pulses (3 × 2 × 2), each correlating with a meridian.

reproducible, and non-recordable. Although it might be a valuable and subtle diagnostic method for humans, if applied by well-trained experts, it is impractical for veterinary use. Yet pulse diagnosis is the core of classic acupuncture because it determines the "energy" disturbances in each Mer. Only after that examination will one logically determine, by the use of certain reasoning patterns, which AP on which Mer to stimulate.

There are 12 different symmetric meridians (also called channels or vessels) in the body, each with a different name (Fig. 82–2). Each name relates to a hypothetical "organ system" (e.g., lung, heart, kidney). Some of these systems have, however, no meaning to us (e.g., triple heater). Some names have questionable translations (e.g., large intestine might also mean long intestine and thus small intestine). However, the fact that most Mer have anatomic names does not mean that they "represent" this organ or that all AP on this Mer have an influence on that organ.

The Chinese were aware of the blood flow and intestinal motility (food flow) a few thousand years ago. Since their nature philosophy was one of consistent change and thus flow from one state into another (such as the seasons, for example), they saw the body as a system with many channels (tendons, blood vessels, nerves, etc.) through which the body's energy and fluids were circulating. The Mer were thought to be one among the many types of channel systems in which this "energy" flows, from one channel into the next, orderly, directed, and at a certain speed with a maximal energy state of an organ/Mer system at a certain hour of the day. The total energy flow circle takes 24 hours. There is no

scientific evidence of any such circle, but this flow description is probably the first mention of biorhythms.

It is unclear how the Chinese detected AP, but probably most were defined by palpation of sensitive spots and recognition of spontaneous painful spots. AP can now be searched for with modern methods. Indeed, the skin impedance (resistance) of an AP is much lower (7 to 70 kOhm) than of surrounding skin (300 to 2000 kOhm) in humans and in the dog.[5] The surface of this low-resistance spot is about 1 mm². A lower skin resistance means better electric conductivity, which explains why many AP are motor points. A motor point is the skin point where the lowest electrical current still causes muscle contraction of the underlying muscle. Still[5] examined the canine skin over reported Mer for low-resistance points and found that these are stable in location if searched for over time. About 80 per cent of the points correspond with known anatomic AP.[6] There is no difference in localization depending on sex, breed, weight, body condition, temperament, time of day, or year. The number of low-resistance points found on Mer tracts was always higher (115 to 226 per cent) than the defined number on accepted anatomic charts. Measurements outside of Mer also revealed the existence of low-resistance points. Discovering so many low-resistance points nowadays correlates with the historical evolution of acupuncture. Indeed, the number of AP gradually increased from 365 to about 1000 in recent times. It is puzzling to see that so many low-resistance points exist on and next to Mer. Can all these be used as effective treatment points too? And why was the course of the Mer designed to run through certain AP and not through other nearby (nowa-

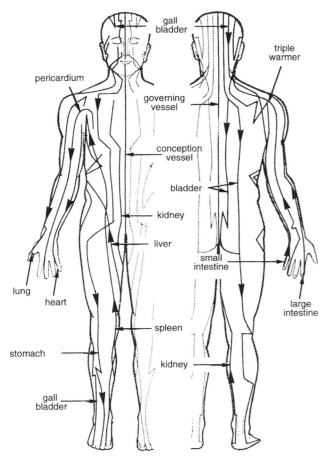

Figure 82–2. Schematic representation of the 12 symmetric and 2 midline meridians (channels, vessels) in humans. There are three meridians on the outer side of each arm and leg, three on the inner side of each arm and leg, three on the chest, and three on the back. The arrows indicate the directions of the so-called energy flow.

days non-meridian) points? These questions will be resolved later.

Some work was performed on the anatomic variability of AP in different dogs using impedance meters. There was variability at some points, while others were very stable. The fact that some anatomic variability exists and that treatments are based on stimulation of chart-based anatomic AP signifies that often vicinity points and not the "real" AP are stimulated. This seems not to affect clinical results.

Another phenomenon of AP is that in internal disease, specific AP will display a decrease in electrical resistance that reverses increase after recovery from disease. This is the case not only for AP on the body, but even more so for AP on the ear lobes. The latter represent and connect to internal organs. They were discovered in the 1960s and can be used for diagnostic as well as therapeutic reasons. Skin resistance is determined by extracellular ion concentrations and thus by sweat production and local blood flow. The latter is defined by the local cutaneosympathetic tone. Histologic research of AP has identified many local neurovascular (ateriovenous) bundles under the point. These bundles have a high incidence of arteriovenous shunts that are always richly innervated by the sympathetic nervous system. This finding helps to explain lower local skin resistance of AP than that of surrounding skin and also that it is variable and under the influence of the viscerocutaneous sympathetic reflex.

Although there is convincing evidence of the existence of

AP, there is no scientific evidence that Mer are physiologically measurable entities.[7] We assume that they are imaginary lines connecting AP. Their origin is probably based on the sometimes radiating sensation humans experience when an AP is stimulated (called T' chi, Chi of Qi sensation). The sensation is, however, anatomically vague. The fact that they are imaginary allows for arbitrariness when decisions have been made on which of three anatomically close and sensitive points have to be incorporated into one Mer, which to make a non-meridian point, and which to assign to another Mer. These decisions have been made historically, and a general consensus of acceptance of the system exists now. This explains why consecutive points may have totally different clinical indications.[2]

In traditional (Taoist) Chinese medical philosophy (TCM), there are three fundamental statements (axioms) that are at its origin. The first axiom is that all living creatures possess life energy, called Qi, which flows through the body in Mer in a 24-hour circle. If the circulation is disturbed, disease originates. This disturbance can be observed by pulse diagnosis. The second axiom is that all phenomena can be divided in two opposite categories: yin or yang. Six of the twelve Mer are yin, the other six yang; the six hollow organs are yang, the six solid yin. In a healthy body, there is an equilibrium between yin and yang. If the balance is disturbed (e.g., too much yang in one organ), disease originates. The third axiom is that all phenomena can be classified in one out of five element categories: earth-metal-water-wood and fire (Fig. 82–3). These elements have an influence on each other. This influence can be constructive (X forms Y, e.g., wood creates fire) or destructive (e.g., metal destroys wood). A pentagon schematically represents these interactions.

Treatment of disease consists of a specific sort of activation (stimulation or sedation) of a specific AP on a specific Mer. To decide on which AP to use, one has to understand the previously described interactions. One of the most important is that stimulation of one Mer will automatically stimulate the next one, draw energy from the former one, and sedate the second next one. This allows one to stimulate a Mer by using AP not on the Mer itself but, for example, on the former one. To find out which specific AP to activate on the Mer that has to be stimulated, the system had to be made more complex because not any arbitrary AP on that Mer will do the job. Therefore, one AP on each Mer (localized distal from knee or elbow) represents one of the five element categories. There is, however, no consistency in the follow-up of these element points, and some AP are skipped without logical explanation. This is a first inconsistency. A

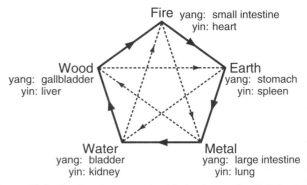

Figure 82–3. The five element cycle with the constructive (full lines) and destructive (dotted lines) interactions. Each of the five elements is allotted two organs, one hollow (yang) and one solid. The two organs of one element are said to be coupled.

second inconsistency exists in the Mer follow-up in the energy and five element cycles. The energy cycle runs in the reverse direction from the constructive pentagon cycle and thus might be considered a mirror flow. But in the latter there are some unexplainable jumps. Two Mer are skipped (liver and gallbladder), and the flow then returns from where it came from. A third inconsistency originates when trying to fit 12 meridian/organs into a pentagonal system. Indeed, two organs are left over. As an exception, these are attributed to the element fire, which thus contains 4 Mer. These three exceptions are just a few examples of the many that can be discovered after careful analysis of the TCM reasoning system.

Once one has defined which AP on which Mer to activate, there are two methods to activate each AP. Activation, also called tonification, is produced by manipulating (rotating, twirling, lifting, and thrusting) the needle, while sedation is caused by inserting a needle without further manipulation. For a long time, and sometimes even now, two different types of needles were used for each purpose: tonification was performed with golden needles, sedation with silver needles (again the yin/yang idea), and golden needles were often heated. There is no scientific proof, however, that the material of the needle has any influence on treatment efficiency. Important seems to be that the correct AP is stimulated with a stimulus strong enough to effectively activate the afferent nerve endings of importance for acupuncture. This can be done by needles, massage, electricity, laser, etc.

TCM theories have been elaborately expanded over the centuries, and many more interactions, many more meridians, and many more AP have been added to the original system. The reasoning and theories were relatively clear and simple in the beginning but grew to an elaborate, overcomplex system that tried spasmodically to fit exceptions or new observations into the framework of the existing theories. It did so by introduction of new connections and new laws or by accepting exceptions and keeping them out of the theory framework. Clearly this system uses post-factum reasoning. For a new phenomenon, a new theory was constructed and integrated more or less in the existing system. This way of theorizing does not allow to extract new knowledge or predict facts except by coincidence. TCM lacks globalization and unity even in its early form.

TCM is phenomenally complex and can be admired for its inventiveness. The reasonings can be used in practice to perform acupuncture therapy (AT), but in the absence of pulse diagnosis, the treatment will lack fine tuning and accuracy. Pulse diagnosis, however, is hardly ever used by Western doctors and veterinarians who apply acupuncture as a therapy. Instead, traditionally oriented practitioners will use symptom classifications that attribute disease to an element and an energy state (e.g., tachycardia is excess of heart energy, is thus fire element yin excess). They will start the classic reasoning based from there and not from palpation of the pulse.

There is another way to decide which AP to use for a certain disease. This is consulting human formula books (cookbook acupuncture). In these, a certain formula (a prescription of certain AP) is mentioned for a certain disease. These formulas are the result of many centuries of clinical acupuncture experience. One author[8] computerized these formulas from a massive amount of books that were valued on importance. The result is a disease-oriented appreciation list of AP. We recommend the use of this list for small animal applications and restrict ourselves to the top 3 to 5 AP for those conditions on which no specific veterinary publications

exist. Up to now, there has been no clinical or statistical proof that the use of TCM theories is superior to cookbook acupuncture. It is tempting to expect a complex system to be better, but there is no proof for it. As Dr. Felix Mann described in his last book on acupuncture[3] after studying TCM for 20 years, after learning Chinese language and reading all texts in their original writing: "After . . . I mastered the subject . . . I seriously examined the validity of all I had learned, only to discover that most of it was fantasy . . . and that most of the laws of acupuncture are laws about non-existent entities."

A SHORT FLIGHT OVER THE WORKING MECHANISM OF ACUPUNCTURE

Classic theories are incapable of explaining the working mechanism of acupuncture in a physiologic way. So how must we think about acupuncture? Is it a form of hypnosis; a complex placebo therapy; a method of stress analgesia; or other?

Acupuncture is not hypnosis, since it does not use suggestion and repetitive stimulation and since no immobility is obtained. Hypnosis can cause analgesia in 10 per cent of its patients, while acupuncture analgesia (AA) has proved to be successful in 70 to 90 per cent in treated patients.

Acupuncture is not a placebo, since double-blind studies including placebo treatments have proved acupuncture to be far more successful than placebo treatments, which generally obtain a 20 to 30 per cent success ratio.[9]

Acupuncture is not stress analgesia. Stress analgesia can be induced by a very short stimulus period, while a 15- to 20-minute induction-stimulation period is needed to produce AA and stress analgesia is not naloxone-reversible while AA is.

Is acupuncture a stimulation method that works by means of humoral and neurologic pathways? Humoral pathways of acupuncture certainly exist because cross-over tests with dogs and rats both with linked blood circulation and transfer of cerebrospinal fluid produced analgesia in the recipient animals that did not receive acupuncture treatment while the donor animals did. The substances involved here are mainly endorphins, since naloxone treatment of the recipient animals abolished analgesia.[10] However, humoral factors are not involved in acupuncture stimulus propagation because avascularization of a limb in which acupuncture stimulation is applied still results in normal acupuncture effects.

Neurogenic pathways are without a doubt the most important factors in the working mechanism of acupuncture. Local anesthesia of the skin around the AP did not abolish acupuncture-induced oral analgesia in monkeys, while deep local anaesthesia did. Local anesthesia or section of the innervating nerve of the periostal and musculoskeletal structures beneath the AP did abolish acupuncture effects. When AP are used in the lower limbs (legs), no acupuncture effects occur after epidural anesthesia or somatic and sympathetic denervation.

Acupuncture stimuli are captured by somatic and sympathetic free nerve endings in deep tissues. From here, afferent impulses run mostly through A delta fibers, to arrive in an interactive gatelike system in the dorsal horn of the spinal cord grey matter. There connections run to segmental and intersegmental sympathetic neurons or segmental interneurons, ascending and descending spinal segments, and the brain.

AA mechanisms have been studied the most in detail.

Most of these pathways were unraveled by focal transection or administration of chemical agonists or antagonists of different neuropeptides in experimental animals. We know now that acupuncture is effective through interactions with segmental (mostly ipsilateral) spinal cord pain pathways and with activation of the enkephalin-endorphin and serotonin production and release.

The endorphins produced under AA are multiple, but dynorphin seems to be important in the spinal cord and beta-endorphin in the brain.[10] This type of analgesia is naloxone-reversible and produced by low-frequency (2 to 8 Hz) stimulation of the needles (manual twirling, mechanical twirling, or low-frequency electric stimulation). Twenty to thirty per cent of patients do not respond to AA. Many can turn into responders by preloading them with D-phenylalanine or L-tryptophan. Both block carboxypeptidase a catabolic enzyme for endorphins. Serotonin, on the other hand, is produced in the brain's nucleus raphe magnus, preferentially by high-frequency stimulation (about 200 Hz) of the AP. This centrally produced serotonin flows through a spinal descending pathway in the lateral white matter adjacent to the dorsal horn and blocks or attenuates incoming pain signals at the spinal level. There are several other important substances involved in AA (e.g., cholecystokinin [CCK], norepinephrine, GABA).[11]

The therapeutic effects of acupuncture have revealed that the autonomic nervous system plays a pivotal role. For example, stimulation of AP stomach 36 causes parasympathetic phenomena that are counteracted by atropine administration. AP governing vessel 26 stimulation causes respiratory and cardiac activation that is counteracted by propranolol (beta-blocker) and to a lesser extent by phentolamine (alpha-blocker). Acupuncture is capable of releasing endorphins, serotonin, and epinephrine. Endorphins have a negative influence on intestinal motility, and serotonin and norepinephrine are important modifiers of mood and appetite. The link between trigger points (TP) and AP (70 per cent of TP are AP) and the vast amount of TP research and understanding[12] explain the working mechanisms of acupuncture in muscle and joint disease.

APPLICATIONS OF ACUPUNCTURE IN SMALL ANIMAL PRACTICE (Figs. 82–4 and 82–5)

Acupuncture can be used during surgical procedures for analgesic purposes or as a form of therapy.

AA can be used in practice as one part of the cocktail of anesthetic methods or as a sole procedure. We found it to be time-elaborate, requires a lot of technical assistance, is unpredictable, and suffers from several inconveniences such as muscle tension, patient movement, patient reaction, vagal reactions, and incomplete analgesia in certain regions. As thus, it cannot compete with modern anesthetic techniques, but it may still be of value in animals with a high anesthetic risk if sophisticated methods are not available.

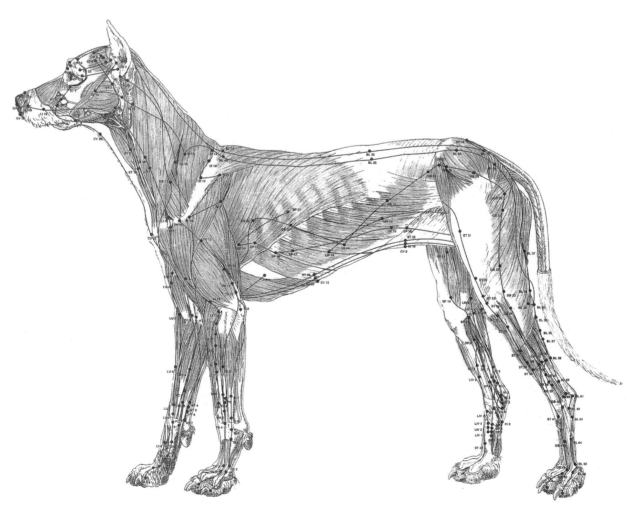

Figure 82–4. A lateral body view on the anatomy of acupuncture points in the dog.

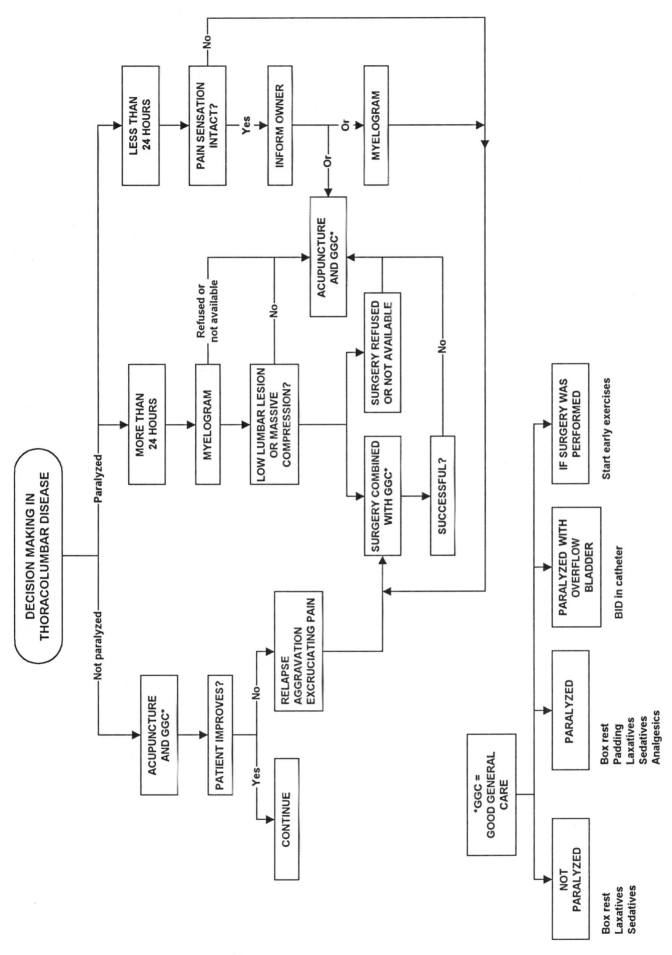

Figure 82–5. Algorithm for decision making regarding use of acupuncture in animals with thoracolumbar disease.

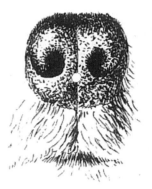

Figure 82–6. The representation of point governing vessel 26 on the plane of the nose in the dog. This point can be used for activation of respiratory and cardiac functions and in respiratory and cardiac arrest.

Most frequently acupuncture will be used as a therapy and most often for neurologic and musculoskeletal problems. Acupuncture can be of benefit for other conditions such as respiratory and cardiac arrest under anesthesia, after trauma, or due to heart failure.[13, 14] If a 25- to 28-gauge hypodermic needle is placed in the midline of the nasal plane (Fig. 82–6) between the nostrils about 1 to 5 cm deep and vigorous twirling and pecking is applied for 10 to 600 seconds, there is a strong activation of the respiratory and cardiovascular system. Several methods of stimulation of this point have been compared for effectiveness. Manual needle stimulation and heat (80°C) were most effective. Still applied the method in pentobarbital-overdosed dogs and cats and tried to revitalize them. The method was highly successful in dogs and produced more favorable results (88 per cent) than IV epinephrine injection (75 per cent) or needling of a very nearby non-AP (40 per cent). In cats, stimulation of the point yielded comparable results to doxapram injection (res. 76 and 69 per cent) but better results than seen with stimulation of a nearby non-AP.[15] Patients with respiratory arrest react more rapidly and favorably than those with cardiac arrest. Experimental work in cats with hemorrhagic shock showed that the group that received stimulation of this point had a much higher survival rate than the group of nontreated cats.

Acupuncture is effective in a high percentage of chronic arthropathies in humans and in animals with arthritis. In general, a 60 to 70 per cent success rate can be expected in dogs. Some joints, such as the shoulder, hip, and knee, seem to be better acupuncture candidates than carpi, tarsi, and elbows, but this observation is preliminary and may change when more effective treatment protocols are discovered.[16] In deciding on when to use acupuncture as a treatment modality for chronic conditions, one should identify whether the arthritic joint is stable or not. If not (hip dysplasia in young dogs with a positive Ortolani sign and clinical subluxation; recent rupture of an anterior cruciate ligament with a positive drawer movement or a dog with vascular necrosis of the femoral head and progressive crumbling of the cartilage), acupuncture is of limited and short-lasting benefit because its analgesic and anti-inflammatory actions will automatically be deleted by new joint trauma induced by abnormal biochemical movement. These joints require surgical stabilization. If a joint is stable, shows arthritis, and causes symptoms, two treatment options exist: surgery (e.g., total hip replacement) or conservative treatment. The latter may consist of weight reduction, restricted and controlled movement, and drug therapy. If these treatment options are refused or if there are drug side effects or unfavorable clinical results,

acupuncture is an alternative. The advantage of acupuncture is that it does not produce side effects apart from a 1- to 2-day clinical aggravation in most animals after the first treatments. Different treatment protocols have been used by different authors, but mostly one or two treatments a week are administered for 3 to 10 weeks. Thereafter, animals often function well for long periods of time (months to years) and most will need one or two periodic booster treatments. (This type of treatment schedule is quite comparable with polysulfated glycosaminoglycan injection therapy.) It is not fully understood why acupuncture is effective in arthritis, but many pathophysiologic processes that occur in chronic osteoarthritis are also unknown. One aspect of acupuncture in the treatment of musculoskeletal problems has been understood: namely that AT is largely TP therapy. Indeed, more then 70 per cent of human TP correspond with acupuncture points and many canine TP correspond with AP.[12, 17] TP are hard, palpable nodular structures that occur in muscles and fascia often after even minimal strain or trauma. They are much more prevalent in older than younger individuals. Although most TP disappear spontaneously, some tend to persist for many years. When acute, TP cause active local pain (e.g., sore back). When chronic (passive), they are silent causing muscle shortening, stiffness, and weakness without atrophy. Many TP cause referred pain, often at a distance from their origin. When squeezed or compressed, they are painful (healthy muscle is not painful under compression) and then trigger the referred pain. These painful points have since long been described in acupuncture texts as Ashi points and were always added to the classic treatment protocol. Chronic TP can become active and thus spontaneously painful under certain conditions such as exercise, stress, fever, viral infections, and fatigue. Although TP have become quite well known to practitioners, they are unknown to most small animal practitioners. Research has revealed that the basic pathology of a TP is a muscle end-plate disease. Neuromuscular end-plates of TP show that acetylcholine levels are 100 times as high as in normal end-plates. This hyperactivity allows us to see TP actively on EMG recordings. In these, typical seashell noise is heard and rapid, low-voltage activity is recorded. This activity disappears once the TP is abolished. Sympathetic activity seems to play a pivotal role in TP because general and local sympathetic blockade abolished TP temporarily. The main treatment for TP, however, is TP stimulation. This is achieved by dry needling or injection. There is no advantage to injection of any fluid (water, physiologic, vitamin B, local anesthetics); moreover, injection techniques cause more afterpain. When needling TP, it is pivotal to obtain (see and feel) the twitch response. This is a rapid contraction of a small number of muscle fibers when the TP is hit. Since one TP consists often of many small TP in the same vicinity, dry needling must consist of hitting all TP and thus several twitches will be evoked. Treatment is considered finished when no new twitches can be produced. Since these treatments are often painful, it is often necessary to sedate the animal, especially when many TP have to be treated. As in acupuncture treatments, once-a-week therapies are mostly performed and often three to five treatments are sufficient. TP therapy can improve the quality of functioning, the speed of recovery, and the angles and range of motion of arthritic joints. TP become objectively smaller or disappear after therapy. TP may also exist in muscles without concurrent joint disease. We found the left triceps muscle to be quite susceptible to TP development. Treatment of this TP yielded very favorable results, with 80 per cent of the chronically lame animals becoming free of lameness in a mean of 3 weeks.[17] We encourage practitioners to search for TP in lame dogs that show no arthritic or neurologic abnormalities.

Acupuncture assists in dogs with disk protrusions or herniations. Cervical, thoracolumbar, and lumbosacral disk disease (CDD, TLDD) have all been treated successfully. A variety of treatment protocols exist with veterinary acupuncturists. Different choices of the type and number of AP, stimulation methods (injections, dry needling, electrostimulation, etc.), duration, and interval are used. There is agreement, however, that success rates are comparable. If this is true, we think the simplest method may be the best.

Two authors have reported detailed studies of large groups of dogs with TLDD or CDD.[18–21] In both cases, distant and local AP were used and clinical results were comparable. Most protocols treat the animals once a week, but there is evidence that more frequent treatments (two or three a week) lead to faster recovery in acute nonparalyzed TLDD cases.[18] The simplest method for TLDD treatment consisted of dry needling of one AP on the hindleg between the tibia plateau and the head of the fibula and several local paravertebral tense and painful (Ashi or TP) back AP. There seems to be no benefit in stimulating the latter points with injection therapy in regard to plain needling in back pain patients. In all acutely (<24 hours) presented patients, and independent from whether they will undergo surgery or not, we now advocate to administer one bolus of sodium prednisolone succinate at 30 mg/kg IV as a free radical scavenger. About 90 to 95 per cent of nonparalyzed animals (pain only or grade 1, pain plus paresis or grade 2) were cured with this technique in 2 to 3 weeks. Approximately 80 per cent of paralyzed dogs with intact pain sensation (grade 3) were cured in about 6 weeks, and 25 per cent of those paralyzed with absence of pain sensation (grade 4) recovered in 3 to 6 months. We have proved that treating these animals with normal-dose and long-term corticosteroids before or during the onset of AT prolongs recovery significantly.[12] The success of AT for nonparalyzed patients is greater than for other treatments both surgical and conservative. Results for grade 3 patients are comparable with rapid decompression and better than conservative treatments, and success percentages in grade 4 patients are half that for rapid surgical decompression. Therefore, we recommend acupuncture as the first treatment option in grades 1 and 2. If dogs do not respond favorably to AT, if the condition aggravates neurologically, if there is excruciating pain, if there are frequent relapses, or if it is the owner's wish, surgery should be performed (see Fig. 82–5). In grade 3 dogs, we leave the decision of surgery versus AT to the owner if the animal is presented within 24 hours after the onset of symptoms. The advantage of surgery here is that recovery is faster and that there is a smaller risk for aggravation to grade 4. If the animal is presented for treatment more than 24 hours after the onset of paralysis, surgery may not be of use unless the lesion is in the low lumbar region or of a very confirmed and very compressive nature. In that case, the pathology is more of compressive than kinetic origin and there is still some logic in retarded decompression. If dogs are presented in grade 4 within 24 hours, we advocate rapid decompression. If refused, nonavailable, or if the patient is presented later, we propose AT. AT is always accompanied by good general care (GGC), which consists of cage or playpen rest for 4 weeks (the healing-sealing period of the dorsal anulus); sedatives (diazepam or acepromazine, 4 weeks); and stool softeners (4 weeks) to prevent straining during defecation. These animals are indeed almost always constipated, and

augmented abdominal pressure leads to elevated pressures in the disk and in the vertebral canal. This creates extra pain and a higher risk for new extrusions. When the dog is paralyzed, the cage should be padded and analgesics administered. When bladder paralysis is present (overflow bladder), the bladder should be emptied twice a day. This can be done by catheterization or the Credé maneuver, and urine should be checked weekly for infection. Physical exercises are started after the 4-week period in all animals that were not operated upon. When permanent or long-standing paralysis is present, dogs are given a two-wheel cart to walk in, a low-bulk diet, rectal stimulation–induced defecation after feeding, and perineal rubbing to induce urination.

In CDD patients, acupuncture results are less favorable than in TLDD.[21] About 80 per cent of neck pain patients and two thirds of neck pain plus paresis patients are cured within 2 to 4 weeks. Treatment schedules are mostly once a week, but in severe acute cases more regular treatments are beneficial. It is extremely important in CDD patients to treat all the TP in the neck region efficiently. We do not recommend to treat tetraparetic animals with AT, and although we have treated dogs in this group successfully, we find the recovery too long-standing, the complication rate too high, and the pain too excessive. GGC consists in CDD animals of cage rest, sedatives, laxatives, and strong analgesics or non-steroidal anti-inflammatory drugs (NSAIDs) or low-dosage corticosteroids. Since pain in CDD dogs may be excruciating, long-lasting, exhausting, and nonresponsive to medication, we strongly suggest an ethical solution and advocate ventral slot surgery if animals are not responding to AT in 21 days, if pain is excessive, or if there are frequent relapses. Dogs that suffer pain after surgery are routinely treated with AT with emphasis on TP. In disk patients that were treated successfully, relapses occur as with all conservative treatments. These were, in our series, about 25 per cent in TLDD over a 5-year period, and 33 per cent over a 3-year period in CDD.

Acupuncture has been used successfully in many other clinical conditions in companion animals. Describing these is beyond the scope of this chapter. The interested reader may obtain detailed information in the references of this chapter.

Acknowledgments

I am grateful to Roger Belderbosch from the Service of Science Philosophy of the University of Ghent, Belgium, who was extremely helpful in critical analysis of the Taoist medical reasoning. Lambert Leijssens is thanked for preparing the figures. Marsha Feldman and Steve Ettinger are thanked for their valuable help with the algorithm, linguistics, and content.

REFERENCES

1. Mann F: Basic principles of acupuncture. In Mann F (ed): The Ancient Chinese Art of Healing. London, W Heinemann Medical Books, 1971, p 3.
2. Anon: Basics of Acupuncture. In Academy of Traditional Chinese Medicine (ed): An Outline of Chinese Acupuncture. Peking, Foreign Language Press, 1975, p 12.
3. Mann F: Dermatomes, myotomes, sclerotomes. In Mann F (ed): Scientific Aspects of Acupuncture. London, W Heinemann Medical Books, 1977, p 50.
4. Kothbauer O: Die provokation einer hyperalgetische Zone die Haut und eines Schmertzpunkt durch die Reizung eines Uterushornes beim Rind. Wiener Tierarztlicher Monatschau 56:803, 1973.
5. Still J: Relationships between electrically active skin points and o points in the dog. Am J Acupuncture 16:55, 1988.
6. Janssens LAA, Still J: Acupuncture Points and Meridians in the Dog, 2nd ed. Brussels, Van Wilderode Print, IVAS Distribution, 1997.

RX

7. Bensoussan A: The nature of meridians. *In* Bensoussan A (ed): The Vital Meridian. Melbourne, Churchill Livingstone, 1991, p 51.

8. Rogers PAM: Choice of AP points for particular conditions. *In* Postgraduate Committee in Veterinary Science (ed): Acupuncture in Animals. Sydney, Postgraduate Committee in Veterinary Science Publications, 1991, p 223.

9. Pomeranz B: Relation of stress induced analgesia to acupuncture analgesia. N Y Acad Sci 467:444, 1986.

10. Peets JM, Pomeranz B: Acupuncture-like transcutaneous electrical nerve stimulation analgesia is influenced by spinal cord endorphins but not by serotonin. *In* Bonagura W (ed): Advances in Pain Research and Therapy. New York, Raven Press, 1985, p 519.

11. Han JS, Terenius L: Acupuncture analgesia. Ann Rev Pharmacol Toxicol 22:193, 1982.

12. Travell JG, Simons DG: General issues. *In* Travell JG, Simons DG (eds): Myofascial Pain and Dysfunction: The Trigger Point Manual. Baltimore, Williams & Wilkins, 1992, p 1.

13. Janssens L, et al: Respiratory and cardiac arrest under general anaesthesia: Treatment by acupuncture of the nasal philtrum. Vet Rec 105:273, 1977.

14. Lee DC et al: Some effects of acupuncture at jen soun on cardiovascular dynamics in dogs. Can J Comp Med 41:446, 1977.

15. Still J: Comparision between stimulation of respiration through treatment by acupuncture or by noradrenalin in dogs suffering from respiratory arrest due to use of barbiturates. Ann Med Vet 132:57, 1988.

16. Janssens LAA: Observations on acupuncture therapy in chronic osteoarthritis in dogs: A review of sixty-one cases. J Small Anim Pract 27:825, 1986.

17. Janssens LAA: Trigger points in 48 dogs with myofascial pain syndromes. Vet Surg 20:274, 1991.

18. Still J: Analgesic effects of acupuncture in thoracolumbar disc disease in dogs. J Small Anim Pract 30:298, 1989.

19. Janssens LAA, De Prins EM: Treatment of thoracolumbar disk disease in dogs by means of acupuncture: A comparison of two techniques. JAAHA 25:169, 1989.

20. Still J: Acupuncture treatment of type-III and type-IV thoracolumbar disc disease. Mod Vet Pract 7:35, 1987.

21. Janssens LAA: The treatment of canine cervical disc disease by means of acupuncture: A review of 32 cases. J Small Anim Pract 26:203, 1985.

CHAPTER 83

COMPLEMENTARY/ ALTERNATIVE CANCER THERAPY—FACT OR FICTION?

Gregory K. Ogilvie and Narda G. Robinson

In 1993 David Eisenberg, physician and member of Harvard University's Center for Alternative Medicine Research, published a landmark study in the *New England Journal of Medicine*.[1] He showed that one third of all Americans routinely use alternative and complementary therapies, especially as a supplement to conventional health care methods. Interestingly, Americans visit alternative practitioners more often than mainstream physicians, at a cost of $14 billion a year.[1] An additional $4 billion is spent annually on alternative products such as vitamins and herbs. This same trend is occurring in veterinary health care, especially in the treatment of cancer, where traditional treatment options are limited and often toxic. Veterinary specialists often view unconventional treatment options with suspicion. Many are not aware of the potential for complementary treatments to support or directly treat animals with cancer. Many cultures and health care systems have been employing complementary therapy for thousands of years with apparent success. Because these treatment modalities have been entrenched for generations as the standard of care, few practitioners from these cultures see the logic of instituting Western-style studies to document efficacy. For these reasons and many others, few traditional data exist documenting the effectiveness of complementary therapeutics.

The objectives of this chapter are to introduce and define some complementary therapeutics that have been used to treat cancer and other diseases in animals and humans. Specific attention is directed toward defining what is known about the efficacy of these modalities for the support of the cancer patient, as well as in the prevention and treatment of cancer. Because complementary veterinary medicine in the United States is in its infancy, several examples using human cancer patients are discussed. The reader is encouraged to seek additional information in the references provided.

ACUPUNCTURE

Acupuncture involves the stimulation of specific anatomic points on the body for therapeutic purposes with needles, heat, pressure, friction, suction, or impulses of electromagnetic energy. This ancient healing art is generally well accepted and widely used by human and veterinary health care professionals to treat a wide variety of ailments. Acupuncture is used to normalize or correct the flow of *qi* (pro-

Supported in part by grants from the National Cancer Institute (#2 CA 29582). The content is solely the responsibility of the authors and does not necessarily represent the official views of the National Cancer Institute. The editors neither recommend nor dismiss the alternative methods discussed. They are presented to the reader in the hope that open discussion allows for individual choices.

nounced "chee," which refers to the body's vivifying force) to restore health. Sound scientific data have shown that stimulation of specific points on the body alters the chemical neurotransmitters in the body. Well-designed studies show efficacy for the treatment of osteoarthritis, chemotherapy-induced nausea, asthma, back pain, and headaches, to name a few. Since 1960, there have been at least 3425 articles published on the efficacy of medical acupuncture.[2] The most common disorders treated were organic in nature and pain problems. Ailments directly related to cancer therapy constituted 3 per cent of all organic lesions reported. Cancer-induced pain represented 1 per cent of the cases.[2] Although the number of disorders directly related to cancer was minimal, there are many important lessons in the other reports that can be used to support cancer patients. For example, the most dramatic reports have involved the use of acupuncture in surgical analgesia.[2] In 1973, up to 25 per cent of all surgeries in mainland China were performed using acupuncture analgesia, with efficacy reported in up to 90 per cent of the cases.[2, 3] Acupuncture anesthesia is not widely used in the United States in human or veterinary surgery. This modality continues to be used in China, especially for surgeries of the head, neck, pelvis, skin, and muscle.[3–5] This modality obviously has a potential benefit for veterinary cancer patients, where surgery is the mainstay of therapy.[4, 5]

Two uncontrolled studies of acupuncture to treat large case series of human cancer patients in 1985 and 1990 were conducted and published.[6, 7] The results suggested that this treatment modality can be used to relieve pain. Few well-designed studies exist demonstrating the efficacy of acupuncture for the treatment of pain in veterinary cancer patients.

Several studies were completed between 1986 and 1993 that showed that acupuncture was effective for the treatment of postoperative and chemotherapy-induced nausea and vomiting in people. This would be of obvious benefit for the veterinary cancer patient. Five of nine similarly constructed studies evaluating acupuncture to treat postoperative nausea found this method superior to controls.[8–10] One report found that acupuncture was superior to conventional medication for nausea and restlessness.[11] Another study showed that if saline or glucose were injected at antiemetic points, this approach was more effective than standard antiemetic medications.[12]

One investigator demonstrated that acupuncture could be used effectively to prevent chemotherapy-induced nausea and vomiting in large numbers of human patients.[12] In another study, acupuncture combined with antiemetics was shown to be more effective than antiemetics alone to treat chemotherapy-induced vomiting.[13]

Acupuncture can be an effective palliative therapy for controlling pain related directly to a malignant process or cancer therapy (Table 83–1). Improving quality of life by reducing nausea and vomiting is another important beneficial effect of acupuncture.

CHIROPRACTIC SCIENCE

Chiropractic science is a healing method that concerns itself with the relationship between structure and function.[1, 23, 24] The structure of the spine and function of the nervous system are the primary areas of interest of many practitioners. Healing occurs by manual procedures and interventions, not by surgical or chemotherapeutic treatments. Chiropractic care involves integration of the disciplines of radiology, sports medicine, neurology, osteopathy, and ortho-

TABLE 83–1. WHEN ACUPUNCTURE MAY BE OF BENEFIT TO CANCER PATIENTS

CANCER-RELATED AILMENT	EVIDENCE OF EFFECTS OF ACUPUNCTURE
Immune hypofunction	Natural killer cell cytotoxicity enhanced[14]; increases the percentage of peripheral blood T lymphocytes[15]
Postoperative ileus	Acupuncture group had restoration of gastrointestinal motility in less than half the time required by the control group[16]
Chemotherapy- and opioid-induced nausea	Acupuncture shows consistent results in reducing emetic effects of chemotherapy and opioids[8, 11, 12, 13, 17]
Preoperative anxiety	Patients receiving acupuncture experienced less palmar sweating prior to anesthesia[17]

Malignant pain
  Postradiation fibrosis
  Muscle spasms
  Vascular problems
  Hyperesthesia and dysesthesia
  Resistant bone pain
	82% of 183 selected patients experienced improvement following acupuncture[18]

Poorly healing wounds	Acupuncture treatment with electrical stimulation and laser facilitates wound healing[19]
Phantom limb pain of amputees	62% of patients had marked improvement, and 23% had moderate improvement[20]
Radiation-induced xerostomia	68% of patients receiving classic acupuncture, and 50% of patients receiving superficial acupuncture, had increased salivary flow rates[21]
Cancer-related breathlessness	70% reported marked symptomatic benefit, with significant improvements in breathlessness, relaxation, and anxiety[7, 22]

pedics. Research within the profession is still in its infancy. Many of the early data were lost because of the lack of an appropriate scientific forum in which to publish data. Although good data exist concerning the efficacy of this treatment discipline, there are few data involving cancer patients. Areas of efficacy include back and other orthopedic pain and somatovisceral disorders such as hypertension. Chiropractic care for the veterinary cancer patient revolves around improving function and reducing pain, especially in areas of orthopedic or neurologic disorders.

MASSAGE THERAPY

Massage therapy is the manipulation of soft body parts to a state of normalcy.[1, 23–26] This modality incorporates the use of fixed or movable pressure and holding or causing the body to move. This ancient healing art affects the musculoskeletal, circulatory-lymphatic, and nervous systems. Healing by touch in massage therapy involves *vis medicatrix naurae* (helping the body heal itself). Techniques include Swedish massage, deep-tissue massage, neuromuscular massage, and manual lymphatic massage. Various adaptations of these techniques in human medicine are being used in veterinary medicine, although few data exist documenting efficacy in animals. In the last 50 years, over 100 clinical trials have been published in the English language, including those in *Archives of Surgery* and the *British Medical Journal*. These trials have shown efficacy in acute and chronic pain, acute and chronic inflammation, chronic lymphedema, nausea, muscle spasm, various soft tissue dysfunctions, grand mal epileptic seizures, anxiety, and depression.[24] Massage has also been shown to stimulate the body's ability to control pain naturally by producing endorphins.[25] Some suggest that massage therapy is contraindicated in cancer patients because increased blood flow may result in increased metastases. Applications of massage therapy for the veterinary cancer patient revolve around relieving pain and discomfort and maintaining function.

BIOFIELD THERAPY

Biofield therapeutics is the ancient art of laying on of hands. The earliest record of this healing method dates between 2500 and 5000 years ago. The first complete record is in Huang Ti Nei Ching Su Wen (the Yellow Emperor's Classic of Internal Medicine).[1, 23, 24] Healing appears to come from two sources. The first is a source other than the practitioner, such as God, the cosmos, or another supernatural entity. The second source is the practitioner, who modifies or amplifies the patient's biofield. During this type of healing, the practitioner places his or her hands on or near the patient's body to improve general health or to improve a disease condition. Treatments take from 30 minutes to several hours. Numerous treatments may be required. Practitioners note that a biofield emanates for a distance beyond the physical body and that the strength, distance, and color of the field depend on the health and emotional state of the individual. Three forms of biofield therapeutics are used[1, 23, 24]: healing touch (Reiki), therapeutic touch, and SHEN therapy. Reiki originated in Japan in the 1800s, and its theoretic basis involves providing spiritual energy with innate intelligence, channeled through the practitioner. In Reiki, the spiritual body is healed and is then expected to heal the physical body. In SHEN therapy, healing is reported to occur through a biofield conforming to the natural laws of physics with a discernible flux pattern throughout the body. Therapeutic touch involves a practitioner who restores the correct vibrational component to the patient's universal, unitary field. It has been estimated that approximately 18 million sessions are held on human patients annually. Only a fraction of this number is performed on veterinary patients. In an overall report, Benor reported an analysis of 151 healing studies.[24] Sixty-one were controlled. Fifty-six per cent showed significant results, including decreased anxiety of hospitalized patients (four studies), improved hemoglobin in hospitalized human patients (four studies), increased speed and completeness of healing of full-thickness wounds (one study), and improved tension headaches (one study). A number of rodent or tissue culture studies were completed, including one showing the efficacy of treating cancer cells.[18]

AYURVEDA

Ayurveda is an ancient natural system of healing from India that provides an integrated approach for the prevention and treatment of a wide variety of illnesses.[1, 23, 24] Ayurvedic theory states that all disease begins with an imbalance or stress in the individual's consciousness. Although the yoga posturing used in ayurveda is not applicable to veterinary patients, herbal and other treatments used in this discipline may be helpful (see Herbal and Botanical Medicine). Laboratory and clinical studies on ayurvedic herbal preparations and other therapies have shown them to be effective for the treatment of a number of diseases by free-radical scavenging effects, immune system modulation, and hormonal effects. Human health practitioners have reported efficacy for the treatment of a wide variety of cancers, including breast cancer, in people.[26] The National Cancer Institute (NCI) has included ayurvedic compounds on the list of substances that may have cancer prevention properties. Several NCI-funded studies have begun to evaluate two ayurvedic compounds, maharadis amrit kaash 4 and 5 (MAK-4 and MAK-5). MAK-4 and MAK-5 have been shown to significantly inhibit the growth of cancer cells in people and rats.[27] Other applications are listed in Table 83–2.

HOMEOPATHIC MEDICINE

Homeopathic medicine is practiced worldwide, especially in Europe, Latin America, and Asia.[1, 23, 24] Despite the relatively modest number of veterinary or human homeopathic practitioners in the United States, homeopathic remedies are a multimillion-dollar industry. These homeopathic remedies are made of naturally occurring substances from plants, animals, and minerals. These substances are recognized (but not approved or dismissed) by the Food and Drug Administration. The remedies are diluted to as low as 10^{-30} to $10^{-20,000}$. Critics of homeopathy suggest that such extreme dilutions of compounds preclude any probability for efficacy. Scientists who have not rejected the potential benefits of homeopathy suggest that the efficacy can be explained by quantum physics, whereby the electromagnetic energy of these remedies may interact with the body for beneficial purposes. A phenomenon known as the "memory of water" is used to explain how extreme dilutions can result in retained efficacy. In this theory, the structure of water and alcohol solution is altered during the procedure of making the remedies so that the structure of the molecule is retained even after none of the actual substance remains.

The British Medical Journal published a meta-analysis on 96 published reports of 107 controlled trials.[28] Trials were scored using a predefined system, and 22 were designated as well-designed clinical trials involving homeopathy. Fifteen of 22 showed positive results. These rarely included any cancer patients. The types of human patients that were improved included those with allergic diseases and arthritis. Homeopathy may be of benefit in supporting a cancer patient, but few data exist to suggest that it can be used to directly treat or prevent a malignant process.

The issue of vaccine-associated sarcomas in cats has led many homeopathic practitioners to suggest that homeopathic remedies should be used instead of traditional vaccines. This may have great appeal, but efficacy data are very limited in veterinary patients.

NATUROPATHIC MEDICINE

Naturopathic medicine is a health care profession that is 100 years old.[1, 23, 24] This American care system began around the turn of the century. Naturopathic medicine incorporates botanical medicine, clinical nutrition, homeopathy, acupuncture, traditional oriental medicine, hydrotherapy, and naturopathic manipulative therapy. Many nontraditional veterinary practitioners formally or informally use this type of therapy. Medical research is based on the empiric documentation of treatments with case history observations, medical records, and summaries of practitioners' experiences. Limited data

TABLE 83–2. AYURVEDIC HERBS REPORTED TO HAVE ANTICANCER OR SUPPORTIVE BENEFIT FOR CANCER PATIENTS

AYURVEDIC HERB	BOTANY	INDICATIONS FOR THE CANCER PATIENT
Ashwaganda (*Withania somnifera*)	Solanaceae: nightshades: datura, mandragora, hyoscyamus niger, Lyopersicon esculentrum, Nicotiana glauca, Atropina belladona	Tumor inhibitory effect in mice; anti-inflammatory
Forskolli (*Coleus forskohli*)	Libiatae (Lamiaceae)	Inhibits pulmonary metastases of implantable tumors in mice
Phyllanthus (*Phyllanthus amarius*): Bhumy amalaki	Epuphorbaciae	Inhibits growth of P-388 lymphocytic leukemia in vitro
Turmeric (*Curcuma longa*) (also haridra)	Zingiberacea	Preventative for mammary tumor development in vivo; anti-inflammatory, analgesic

Adapted from Silver RJ. Ayurvedic Veterinary Medicine. *In* Schoen AM, Wynn SG (eds): Complementary and Alternative Veterinary Medicine. St. Louis, Mosby, 1998, pp 456–459.

exist in a controlled trial format documenting the efficacy of this treatment modality in cancer patients.

PHARMACOLOGIC AND BIOLOGIC TREATMENT

Pharmacologic and biologic treatments use a wide variety of drugs and vaccines that have not been accepted by mainstream medicine and surgery. Some of the more common agents being used are[1, 23, 24]:

- *Antineoplastons*—peptide fractions originally derived from blood and urine. They are used to treat a wide variety of malignancies in people. This controversial treatment is being evaluated in a study funded by the National Institutes of Health. Early studies showed efficacy in a number of tumors.[29, 30]
- *Cartilage products*, especially those from sharks and cattle. Cartilage has been shown to have antiangiogenic properties. In addition, it has tissue inhibitors of metalloproteinases (TIMPs) that inhibit tumor metastasis. Shark cartilage has become very popular because of reports out of Mexico and Cuba suggesting that this product is an effective cancer treatment in people. These original studies were soundly criticized because of faulty study design, lack of controls, and failure to confirm that patients had malignancies. Current studies are being performed in several human cancer centers, but final reports have not been published. One report suggested a reduction in prostate cancer in men.[31] Despite the lack of documentation of efficacy, 50,000 Americans use cartilage products costing $7000 a year per person. One report published in the *Proceedings of the Veterinary Cancer Society* (1995) failed to confirm the efficacy of shark cartilage for the treatment of cancer in veterinary patients.[32]
- *Ethylenediaminetetraacetic acid (EDTA) chelation therapy* has been used to treat a number of conditions, but the mechanism for treating cancer has not been clearly stated. It is interesting that metalloproteinases, especially those of gelatinase capability, are indeed inhibited by EDTA. Metalloproteinases 2 and 9 are critical for tumor growth and invasion. This is the explanation for the potential value of this type of therapy.
- *Immunoaugmentive therapy* is an experimental form of cancer therapy consisting of daily injections of blood products. Work done in dogs with osteosarcoma suggests that specific immunoaugmentive therapy improves disease-free intervals and survival.[33, 34] Similarly, dogs that have limb-sparing surgery for osteosarcoma and get infected allografts have a significantly longer disease-free interval than those that do not have infected allografts. This may occur because of enhancement of factors that augment the immune system. Other studies suggest the efficacy of administering derivatives of aloe vera.[35]
- *714-X* is a nitrogen-producing compound that is injected into the lymphatic system to treat a number of malignancies.[8]
- *Coley's toxin* is derived from *Streptococcus pyogenes* and *Serratia marcescens* and has been touted as a treatment for cancer.[18]
- *MTH-68* is a vaccine from the Newcastle disease virus of chickens that may interfere with oncornaviruses.
- *Iscador* is a lipid extract of mistletoe plants that has been used to treat many tumors.

HERBAL AND BOTANICAL MEDICINE

Eighty per cent of the world population, or approximately 4 billion people, use herbal and botanical medicine.[1, 23, 24] Almost every native medicine around the world uses herbal treatments. Despite this widespread use, acceptance differs throughout the world. In the United States, herbal remedies are considered to be without efficacy by many in regulatory bodies. Many drugs we use routinely today are derived from plants (Table 83–3). European governments, especially the German and French, have formally approved herbs for therapeutic purposes. Indeed, some of the best studies on the efficacy of these herbs have been done in Europe. In China, herbs and other plant derivatives have been used to treat cancer. Agents used in China include sesquiterpenes, diterpenes, triterpenes, quinones, podophyllotoxins, taxol, alkaloids, and others.[36] Many of these have been adapted for Western-style cancer therapy. The number of herbs and other plant-based materials used therapeutically is staggering and beyond the scope of this chapter. As an example of the potential benefit of these agents, in 1981, the U.S. Department of Agriculture, in conjunction with the NCI, concluded a 25-year study of plants with anticancer properties. The work includes 365 folk medicinal species and identifies more than 1000 pharmacologically active phytochemicals.[37]

NUTRITIONAL THERAPY

Nutritional therapy revolves around the notion that nutrients can be used to support and treat people and animals

TABLE 83–3. DRUGS DERIVED FROM HERBS OR BOTANICALS THAT HAVE PROVEN OR POTENTIAL BENEFITS TO CANCER PATIENTS

DRUG	PLANT SOURCE	USE
Proven Drugs		
Aspirin	*Filipendula ulmaria*	Analgesic, anti-inflammatory, reduces platelet aggregation to inhibit metastases, reduces colon cancer
Codeine	*Papaver somniferum*	Analgesic and antitussive
Paclitaxel	*Taxus brevifolia*	Anticancer agent
Vincristine, vinblastine	*Catharanthus roseus*	Anticancer agent (lymphoma)
Reported Potential		
3-(3,3-di-methylallyl)-5(3-acetyl-2,4-dugtdrixt-5-methyl-6-methoxybenzyl)-phloracetophenone	*Mollotus japonicus*	In vitro and in vivo anticancer effects vs. human carcinoma (Hep-2), lung (PC-13), and mouse B16 melanoma, P-388 and L51788Y leukemia
Diterpene acids: pseudolaric acid-A and -B	*Pseudolarix kaempferi*	In vitro and in vivo anticancer effects vs. P-388, HL-60TB, melanoma cell line SK-MEL-5, and ovarian cancer A2780
Indarubin	*Danggui luiwei Wan*	Human leukemia clinical trials in China
Arnica	*Arnica montana L.*	Cancer therapy, immunostimulant, anti-inflammatory
Barberry bark	*Berberis vulgaris*	Anticancer, antiseptic, antidiarrheal
Blessed thistle	*Cnicus benidictus*	Antibiotic, anti-inflammatory, antileukemic, antitumor, bacteriocidal, antiemetic
Bogbean, buckbean	*Menyanthes trifoliata*	Inhibits melanoma growth in athymic mice
Colchicum	*Colchicum autumnale*	Anticancer, especially for leukemias; anti-inflammatory
Dandelion	*Taraxacum officale Wigg.*	Anti-inflammatory, anticancer compound
Echinacea, coneflower	*Echinacea angustifolia, Echinacea purpufea*	Antibacterial, antiviral, immunostimulant, induces release of tumor necrosis factor, reported to reduce side effects of radiation therapy, anticancer
Evening primrose oil	*Oenothera biennis*	Anticancer
Fenugreek	*Trigonela foenumgraecum*	Cervical cancer in China
Ginger	*Zingiber officinale*	Analgesic, anticancer, anti-inflammatory
Pau d'Arco	*Tabebuia impetiginosa*	Anticancer, antifungal
Red clover	*Trifolium pratense*	Antitumor, sedative
Tea	*Camillia sinensis*	Anticancer, antioxidant

From Lin J-H, Rogers PAM, Yamada H: Chinese herbal medicine: Pharmacological basis. *In* Schoen AM, Wynn SG (eds): Complementary and Alternative Veterinary Medicine. St. Louis, Mosby, 1998, pp 379–404.

with cancer and a wide variety of other diseases, as well as to prevent such diseases (Table 83–4).[1, 23, 24] Indeed, nutrients have been used as a therapeutic tool for as long as records have been kept. A large quantity of data exists documenting the beneficial and adverse effects of nutrients. Animals and humans have evolved considerably from their original Paleolithic diets. The increased use of energy-dense foods rich in animal fats, partially hydrogenated vegetable oils, and refined carbohydrates and the lack of whole grains, fruits, and vegetables may cause significant health problems. Improving the diet of animals could have beneficial consequences. Similarly, the use of specific nutrients as therapeutic tools is attaining greater prominence. Veterinary food companies have pioneered the use of diets to treat a wide variety of diseases, including obesity, renal disease, heart disease, and renal calculi. Recent research suggests that specific diets can be of benefit to both veterinary and human cancer patients.

Dietary therapy has taken several approaches. Some advocate increasing supplementation of specific nutrients to prevent or treat diseases such as cancer. Therapies suggested but not proved to be of benefit in cancer patients include N-3 fatty acids, betacarotene, or vitamin C. Others suggest a massive supplementation of certain nutrients, and still others suggest revision of the entire dietary profile for optimization of health. An example of the latter would be a vegan diet.

Orthomolecular medicine is a discipline that promotes the improvement of health and the treatment of disease by using the optimal amount of substances normally present in the body. To prevent overt deficiencies and diseases, advocates suggest increasing the intake of such nutrients. This has been linked to positive responses in the treatment of AIDS,

bronchial asthma, cardiovascular disease, strokes, and cancer.[1, 23, 24]

A great deal of information has been gained by the study of lifestyle diets. For example, Asian and Mediterranean diets have been shown for different reasons to reduce cardiovascular disease and cancer. This has led to research in veterinary medicine in which eicosanoids of the N-3 series (eicosapentaenoic acid and docosahexaenoic acid) are being used to treat dogs with lymphoma and hemangiosarcoma. Omega-3 (N-3) fatty acids have also been shown to inhibit tumorigenesis and cancer spread in animal models, and they form the basis for treatment of cancer in humans.[39] As a general rule, N-3 fatty acids (eicosapentaenoic acid, docosahexaenoic acid) have an inhibiting effect on tumor growth. Metastases are enhanced by the N-6 fatty acids (linoleic acid, gamma-linolenic acid). In vivo studies have shown that eicosapentaenoic acid has selective tumoricidal action without harming normal cells.[38–40] Studies are under way to determine if this phenomenon can reduce morbidity in dogs receiving external beam radiation therapy.

CONCLUSION

Caution needs to be employed when assessing the efficacy of complementary therapies. These modalities may be helpful in treating the veterinary cancer patient. Well-controlled studies are essential to document efficacy and toxicity. The biggest concern is that unproven therapies may be used instead of known treatments. The owner should be informed of all the benefits and risks of traditional and nontraditional therapies alike.

TABLE 83–4. CHEMOPREVENTIVE AGENTS

AGENT	TUMOR TYPE
Single Agents	
Retinoids (vitamin A, tretinoin, isotretinoin, fenretinide)	Many
Betacarotene	Many
Tamoxifen	Breast cancer
Calcium	Colon cancer
Finasteride	Prostate
dl-alpha tocopherol	Many
Selenium	Skin, esophagus
Ascorbic acid	Esophagus, stomach, colon, cervix
N-acetylcysteine	Oral/GI, lung, breast, colon, bladder
NSAIDs (aspirin, sulindac, piroxicam, ibuprofen)	Colon, bladder, skin, breast, UADT, esophagus, cervix
DFMO	Oral/GI, lung, skin, breast, bladder, colon
Dithiolthiones (oltipraz)	Oral/GI, lung, skin, breast, colon, bladder
Glycyrrhetinic acid	Colon, skin, breast
Carbenoxolone	Colon, breast
DHEA analogs (fluasterone)	Oral/GI, lung, skin, colon, breast
Curcumin	Oral/GI, lung, skin, colon, breast
Protease inhibitors	Oral/GI, lung, colon
Polyphenols (ellagic acid)	Skin, colon, bladder, esophagus, breast
Organosulfur compounds (*N*-allyl-*l*-cysteine)	Skin, cervix, colon, esophagus, lung
Fumaric acid	Lung, breast, liver
Phenhexyl isothiocyanate	Breast, lung
Combinations	
Vitamin A/betacarotene	Lung, oral/GI
Vitamin A/*N*-acetylcysteine	Lung, oral/GI
dl-alpha tocopherol/betacarotene	Lung, oral/GI
DFMO/piroxicam	Colon
Fenretinide/tamoxifen	Breast
Fenretinide/oltipraz	Lung, bladder
Fenretinide/betacarotene	Lung
Fenretinide/DFMO	Bladder

GI-gastrointestinal; NSAIDS = nonsteroidal anti-inflammatory drugs; UADT = upper abdominal digestive tract; DFMO = difluoromethylornithine; DHEA = dehydroepiandrosterone.

From Ogilvie GK: Nutritional approaches to cancer therapy. *In* Schoen AM, Wynn SG (eds): Complementary and Alternative Veterinary Medicine. St. Louis, Mosby, 1998, p 94.

REFERENCES

1. Eisenberg DM, Kessler RC, Foster C, et al: Unconventional medicine in the United States. Prevalence costs and patterns of use. N Engl J Med 328:246, 1993.
2. Helms JM: Acupuncture Energetics: A Clinical Approach for Physicians. Berkeley, CA, Medical Acupuncture Publishers, 1995, pp 42–57.
3. Diamond EG: Acupuncture analgesia: Western medicine and Chinese traditional medicine. JAMA 218:1558, 1971.
4. Report of the medical delegation to the People's Republic of China, June 15–July 6, 1973. Washington, DC, National Academy of Sciences, Institute of Medicine, 1973.
5. Lee MHM: Acupuncture analgesia in dentistry. A clinical investigation. N Y State Dent J 39:288, 1973.
6. Filshie J, Redman D: Acupuncture and malignant pain problems. Eur J Surg Oncol 11:389, 1985.
7. Filshie J: Acupuncture for malignant pain. Acupuncture in Medicine. 8:38, 1990.
8. Dundee JW: Reduction in the emetic effects of opioid preanesthetic medication by acupuncture. BMJ 22:583, 1986.
9. Dundee JW: Traditional Chinese acupuncture: A potentially useful antiemetic. BMJ 293:583, 1986.
10. Ghally RG: Antiemetic studies with traditional Chinese acupuncture: A comparison of manual needling with electrical stimulation and commonly used antiemetics. Anesthesiology 42:1108, 1987.
11. Ghally RG: Acupuncture also reduces the emetic effects of pethidine. Br J Anaesth 59:135, 1987.
12. Yang LC: Comparison of P6 acupoint injection with 50% glucose in water and intravenous droperidol for the prevention of vomiting after gynecological laparoscopy. Acta Anaesthesiol Scand 37:192, 1993.
13. Dundee JW: Acupuncture prophylaxis of chemotherapy-induced sickness. J R Soc Med 82:268, 1989.
14. Sato T, Yu Y, Guo SY, et al: Acupuncture stimulation enhances splenic natural killer cell cytotoxicity in rats. Jpn J Physiol 46:131, 1996.
15. Jianguo Y, Rongxing Z, Mingsheng Z, Qimei G: Effect of acupuncture on peripheral T lymphocytes and their subgroups in patients with malignant tumors. Int J Clin Acupun 4:53, 1993.
16. Xunshi W, Zhaolin Z, Chenrang S, et al: Clinical study on the use of second metacarpal holographic acupoints for re-establishing gastrointestinal motility in patients following abdominal surgery. Am J Acupun 22:353, 1994.
17. Aglietti L: A pilot study of metaclopramide, dexamethasone, diphenhydramine and acupuncture in women treated with cisplatin. Cancer Chemother Pharmacol 26:239, 1990.
18. Lewis GBH: An alternative approach to premedication: Comparing diazepam with auriculotherapy and a relaxation method. Am J Acupun 15:205, 1987.
19. Muxeneder R: Die konservative Behandlung chronischer Hautveränderungen des Pferdes durch Laserpunktur. Der praktische Tierarzt 69:12, 1988.
20. Liaw M, Wong AM, Cheng P: Therapeutic trial of acupuncture in phantom limb pain of amputees. Am J Acupun 22:205, 1994.
21. Blom M, Dawidson I, Fernberg J-O, et al: Acupuncture treatment of patients with radiation-induced xerostomia. Eur J Cancer B Oral Oncol 32B:182, 1996.
22. Filshie J, Penn K, Ashley S, Davis CL: Acupuncture for the relief of cancer-related breathlessness. Palliat Med 10:145, 1996.
23. Alternative Medicine: Expanding Medical Horizons, A Report to the National Institutes of Health on Alternative Medical Systems and Practices in the United States. 1994.
24. Bennor DJ: Healing research. Helix Verlab 1:1, 1992.
25. Kaarda B, Tosteinbo O: Increase of plasma beta endorphins in connective tissue message. Gen Pharmacol 20:487, 1989.
26. Sharma HM, Dwvedi C, Satter HA, et al: Antineoplastic properties of maharishi 4 against DMBA-induced mammary tumors in rats. J Pharm Biochem Behav 35:767, 1990.
27. Arnold JT, Korytynski EA, Wilkinson BP, et al: Chemopreventative activity of maharishi amrit kalash and related agents in rat tracheal epithelial and human tumor cells. J Proc Am Assoc Cancer Res 32:128, 1991.
28. Kleijnen J, Knipschild P, Reir GT: Clinical trials of homeopathy. BMJ 302:316, 1991.
29. Bertelli A, Mathe G: Antineoplastons (1). Drugs Exp Clin Res 12 (Suppl 1), 1985.
30. Bartelli A, Mathe G: Antineoplastons (2). Drugs Exp Clin Res 13 (Suppl 1), 1987.
31. Simone C: Presentation at a hearing on alternative medicine before a subcommittee of the Committee on Appropriations, US Senate, 103rd Congress, June 24, 1993.
32. Meyer JA, Dueland RT, et al: Canine osteogenic sarcoma treated by amputation and MER. Cancer 49:1613, 1982.
33. MacEwen EG, Kurzman ID, Rosenthal RC, et al: Therapy for osteosarcoma in dogs with intravenous injection of liposome-encapsulated muramyl tripeptide. J Natl Cancer Inst 81:935, 1989.
34. Harris C, Pierce K, King G, et al: Efficacy of acemannan in treatment of canine and feline spontaneous neoplasms. Mol Biother 3:207, 1991.
35. Lin J-H, Rogers PAM, Yamada H: Chinese herbal medicine: Pharmacological basis. *In* Schoen AM, Wynn SG (eds): Complementary and Alternative Veterinary Medicine. St. Louis, Mosby, 1998, pp 379–404.
36. Lien EJ, Li WY: Structure Activity Relationship Analysis of Chinese Anticancer Drugs and Related Plants. Taiwan, Oriental Healing Arts Institute, 1985, pp 1–140.
37. Duke JA, Ayensu ES: Handbook of Medicinal Herbs. Boca Raton, FL, CRC Press, 1985.
38. Begin ME, Ellis G, Das UN, et al: Differential killing of human carcinoma cells supplemented with N-3 and N-6 polyunsaturated fatty acids. J Natl Cancer Inst 77:2053, 1986.
39. Begin ME, Das UN, Ellis G, et al: Selective killing of human cancer cells by polyunsaturated fatty acids. Prostaglandins Leukot Med 19:177, 1985.
40. Mengeaud V, Nano JL, Fournel S, Rampal P: Effects of eicosapentaenoic acid, gamma-linolenic acid and prostaglandin E₁ on three human colon carcinoma cell lines. Prostaglandins Leukot Essent Fatty Acids 47:313, 1992.

RX

SECTION IV

INFECTIOUS DISEASE

CHAPTER 84

FREQUENTLY ASKED QUESTIONS ABOUT ZOONOSES

Michael G. Groves, Kathleen S. Harrington, and Joseph Taboada

Veterinarians often are consulted by the public, and occasionally by physicians and other veterinarians, for information regarding zoonoses (diseases that are transmitted to humans from animals). When a person is diagnosed with an illness that is somewhat out of the ordinary, many times relatives are worried that the family pet was the source of the trouble. Usually, however, the diseases in question are not zoonoses. There are physicians who, perhaps seeking "zero risk," advise patients to dispose of pets to prevent or alleviate a zoonotic illness. Pregnant women have been advised to get rid of their cats to prevent their contracting toxoplasmosis; HIV-positive people may be told they that should not have animals at all. Although this advice may be well intended, it is often ill informed. Too often, what is missing is some reasonable approximation of the true risk of disease transmission balanced against the benefits of pet ownership. Of the true zoonoses, a few diseases account for most of the questions: cat scratch disease, larva migrans, rabies, and toxoplasmosis. (See Table 84–1 for less common zoonotic infections and Table 84–2 for some diseases that are not acquired from animals.)

CAT SCRATCH DISEASE

Cat scratch disease (CSD) is caused by *Bartonella henselae*, a gram-negative bacterium. As the name suggests, it is carried by cats and is usually associated with cat-inflicted trauma, e.g., a scratch (in most cases) or a bite. Some 22,000 people reportedly have this disease each year, but its incidence is probably much higher because most cases are asymptomatic. Clinical CSD in humans typically is characterized by swollen, painful lymph nodes, usually those immediately proximal to the site of inoculation; low-grade fever, muscle aches, and general malaise are common. In more than 90 per cent of cases the disease is mild and self-limited, and symptoms resolve without treatment within a few weeks to a few months. More severe disease that requires hospitalization does occur. Rarely, *B. henselae* infection may cause a more serious syndrome called bacillary angiomatosis. This form of the disease affects mainly immunocompromised individuals, particularly AIDS patients. Bacillary angiomatosis causes angioproliferative lesions on the skin and in various organs. When it affects the liver and spleen, it is referred to as bacillary peliosis. Bacillary angiomatosis can be life-threatening. Early diagnosis and prompt treatment with antibiotics are important.

How Common Is *B. henselae* Infection in Cats?

Prevalence of antibodies to *B. henselae* in cats varies widely in different geographic regions, with highest rates occurring in warm, humid areas. In the southeastern United States more than 50 per cent of cats are seropositive, whereas in the Rocky Mountains and Great Plains less than 4 per cent have antibodies to *B. henselae*.[1]

What Are the Signs of *B. henselae* Infection in Cats?

B. henselae infection in cats produces a prolonged and often intense bacteremia, but most animals develop few, if any, clinical signs. Occasionally, cats may show a transient lymphadenopathy and low-grade fever when the infection is first acquired, but there seem to be no lasting ill effects associated with infection, despite the long duration of bacteremia.

How Can One Tell if a Cat Is Infected?

Antibodies to *B. henselae* can be detected by an indirect fluorescent antibody test. When bacteremia is present, the organism can sometimes be cultured directly from the cat's blood.

What Groups of Cats Are Most Likely to Be Infected?

Kittens appear to have the highest prevalence of bacteremia, and epidemiologically, kittens, especially if they have fleas, are most commonly associated with disease transmission. Also, feral cats are more likely to be infected than are pet cats.

How Long Does the Bacteremia Last?

This has not yet been determined, but various studies have shown detectable bacteremia for as long as a year or more.[2, 3] There is evidence that levels of bacteremia wax and wane, so the organism may not always be present at a culturable level.[4]

If *B. henselae* Is Only in the Cat's Blood, How Can It Be Transmitted by a Scratch or Bite?

There are at least two plausible theories about this. One is that the bacteria get into the mouth from the blood, e.g., from teething or gum irritations, and contaminate the saliva.

TABLE 84–1. OTHER ZOONOTIC INFECTIONS

DISEASE/AGENT	TYPE OF ORGANISM	ASSOCIATED SMALL ANIMALS	MODE OF TRANS-MISSION	SITE OF INFECTIVE AGENT IN HOST	TYPE OF DISEASE IN HUMANS	FREQUENCY OF OCCURRENCE IN HUMANS IN USA	SEVERITY OF TYPICAL DISEASE	GROUPS AT RISK
Babesiosis (*Babesia microti*)	Parasite (protozoan)	Rodents	Tick bite	Blood	Nonspecific, febrile	Very rare	Severe, sometimes fatal	Asplenic, immuno-compromised, elderly
Brucellosis (*Brucella canis*)	Bacterium (gram-negative rod)	Dogs	Direct contact, laboratory accident	Aborted fetuses, blood, placenta, tissues, urine, vaginal discharge	Febrile	Very rare	Moderate, recurrent or chronic	Animal handlers, kennel workers, laboratory personnel, veterinarians
Campylobacteriosis (*Campylobacter* spp.)	Bacterium (gram-negative rod)	Cats, dogs, birds	Fecal-oral	Feces	Diarrhea, enterocolitis	Uncommon in direct transmission; common foodborne	Mild to severe	Children, immuno-compromised
Capnocytophaga canimorsus infection	Bacterium (gram-negative rod)	Dogs, cats	Bite or scratch	Oral cavity, saliva	Septicemia	Very rare	Severe to fatal	Asplenic, immuno compromised
Cryptococcosis (*Cryptococcus neoformans*)	Fungus (yeast)	Birds (present in droppings, esp. from pigeons; also environment)	Inhalation	Feces	Deep mycosis, meningitis	Common in at-risk group	Severe	HIV+, AIDS
Cryptosporidiosis (*Cryptosporidium parvum*)	Parasite (protozoan)	Dogs, cats	Fecal-oral	Feces	Diarrhea	Uncommon	Asymptomatic to moderate; severe to fatal in HIV+	Children, HIV+, AIDS
Dermatophytoses (*Microsporum canis*)	Fungus (derma-tomycete)	Dogs, cats	Direct contact	Hair, dander	Cutaneous lesions	Common	Mild	Any exposed
Dipylidiasis (*Dipylidium caninum*)	Parasite (cestode)	Dogs	Fecal-oral	Feces	Gastrointestinal	Rare	Asymptomatic to mild	Children
Dirofilariasis (*Dirofilaria immitis*)	Parasite (nematode)	Dogs	Mosquito bite	Blood	Pulmonary	Very rare	Severe	
Echinococcosis (*Echinococcus granulosus*)	Parasite (cestode)	Dogs	Fecal-oral	Feces	Visceral lesions	Uncommon	Severe	Children
Ehrlichiosis, human granulocytic (unnamed *Ehrlichia* sp.)	Bacterium	Dogs (?)	Tick bite	Blood	Nonspecific, febrile	Very rare	Mild to severe; sometimes fatal	Most cases in adult males
Ehrlichiosis, human monocytic (*Ehrlichia chaffeensis*)	Bacterium	Dogs (?), rodents	Tick bite	Blood	Nonspecific, febrile	Rare	Mild to severe; sometimes fatal	Most cases in adult males

Table continued on following page

TABLE 84–1. OTHER ZOONOTIC INFECTIONS *Continued*

DISEASE/AGENT	TYPE OF ORGANISM	ASSOCIATED SMALL ANIMALS	MODE OF TRANSMISSION	SITE OF INFECTIVE AGENT IN HOST	TYPE OF DISEASE IN HUMANS	FREQUENCY OF OCCURRENCE IN HUMANS IN USA	SEVERITY OF TYPICAL DISEASE	GROUPS AT RISK
Fish-fancier's finger, fish-tank granuloma—see *Mycobacterium marinum* infection								
Hantavirus infection								
Hemorrhagic fever with renal syndrome	Virus	Rodents	Inhalation, contaminated food or water, bites	Saliva, urine, blood	Febrile, renal	Does not occur	Mild to severe; sometimes fatal	Anyone exposed to wild rodents
Hantavirus pulmonary syndrome	Same as above	Same as above	Same as above	Same as above	Pulmonary	Very rare	Severe to fatal	
Heartworm—see Dirofilariasis								
Herpesvirus simiae (cercopithecine herpesvirus, B-virus)	Virus	Monkeys, esp. macaques	Bites, mucous membrane exposure	Saliva, secretions from lesions	Meningoencephalitis	Very rare	Usually fatal	Animal handlers, laboratory researchers, veterinarians, zoo personnel
Leptospirosis (*Leptospira* spp.)	Bacterium (spirochete)	Dogs, rodents	Direct contact, contaminated food or water, mucous membrane exposure	Urine	Nonspecific and highly variable febrile	Rare	Asymptomatic to severe; sometimes fatal	Gardeners, people exposed to water from ponds or streams
Lyme disease (*Borrelia burgdorferi*)	Bacterium (spirochete)	Ticks (dogs may bring ticks in proximity to humans)	Tick bite	Saliva	Skin lesions, arthritis, systemic and neurologic symptoms	Common	Moderate to severe	Most cases in children and young adults
Lymphocytic choriomeningitis	Virus (arenavirus)	Rodents	Fecal-oral, inhalation, ingestion of contaminated food or water, direct contact	Urine	Influenzalike; meningitis possible	Common	Mild to moderate; rarely severe	Laboratory personnel working with rodents, anyone exposed to wild rodents
Mycobacterium marinum infection	Bacterium (acid-fast)	Fish, shellfish, etc. (organism naturally occurs in marine and fresh waters)	Wounds from fish or other aquatic animals; open skin in contact with contaminated water	Surface	Cutaneous granulomatous lesions	Rare	Mild to severe	Fishermen, aquarium owners or workers
Pasteurellosis (*Pasteurella multocida*)	Bacterium (gram-negative rod)	Cats, dogs	Bite, scratch	Oral cavity, saliva	Cellulitis, febrile	Uncommon	Mild to severe	Any exposed
Plague (*Yersinia pestis*)	Bacterium (gram-negative rod)	Rodents (rarely cats or dogs that have been in contact with rodents)	Flea bite; rarely inhalation from cat or dog with pulmonary infection	Blood	Lymphadenitis; septicemia, pulmonary	Very rare	Severe; sometimes fatal	Any exposed to wild rodents in endemic areas, e.g., campers/hikers in western U.S.
Psittacosis (*Chlamydia psittaci*)	Bacterium	Birds (esp. psittacines)	Inhalation	Respiratory secretions	Fever, pneumonia	Rare	Mild to moderate, sometimes severe	Bird owners, pet shop workers, veterinarians, zoo personnel; disease worse in elderly

Disease	Organism	Reservoir/Host	Transmission	Source	Clinical features	Frequency	Severity	Population at risk
Q fever (*Coxiella burnetii*)	Bacterium	Dogs, cats	Inhalation, direct contact	Aborted fetuses, placenta, vaginal secretions	Acute febrile; endocarditis may appear many years later	Very rare	Asymptomatic to severe; sometimes fatal	Laboratory workers, veterinarians, animal handlers; disease worse in elderly
Rat-bite fevers								
Spirillosis (sodoku) (*Spirillum minus*)	Bacterium (spirochete)	Rodents	Bites	Oral cavity, saliva	Febrile	Very rare	Mild to severe; rarely fatal	People living in proximity to rodents, laboratory or animal care personnel who work with rodents
Streptobacillosis (*Streptobacillus moniliformis*)	Bacterium (gram-negative rod)	Rodents	Bites, ingestion of contaminated food or water	Oral cavity, saliva, urine	Fever, rash, arthritis; relapses common	Very rare	Mild to severe; sometimes fatal	People living in proximity to rodents, laboratory or animal care personnel who work with rodents
Ringworm—see Dermatophytoses								
Rocky Mountain spotted fever (*Rickettsia rickettsii*)	Bacterium	Ticks (dogs may bring ticks in proximity to humans)	Tick bite	Saliva	Fever, rash	Rare	Severe; sometimes fatal	Most cases in children and young adults
Salmonellosis, reptile-associated	Bacterium (gram-negative rod)	Reptiles	Fecal-oral	Feces, oral and nasal secretions	Diarrhea, gastroenteritis	Rare	Mild to severe	Children, pregnant women, immuno-compromised
Sporotrichosis (*Sporothrix schenckii*)	Fungus	Armadillos, cats (organism naturally occurs in plants and soil)	Puncture wounds, scratches	Cutaneous and subcutaneous lesions	Ulcerative lymphangitis affecting subcutaneous tissues	Rare	Moderate to severe	Gardeners, armadillo hunters
Tularema (*Francisella tularensis*)	Bacterium (gram-negative rod)	Ticks, rabbits	Tick bite, direct contact with tissues or body fluids of infected animals, ingestion of infected meat, inhalation; rarely bite of infected cat	Blood, viscera, body fluids	Ulceroglandular, febrile	Rare	Mild to severe; sometimes fatal	Most cases in young adults and children
Typhus, flea-borne (murine or endemic typhus) (*Rickettsia typhi*)	Bacterium	Rodents, wildlife, cats	Flea bite	Blood	Febrile	Rare	Mild to moderate	Most cases in children and young adults
Typhus, sylvatic (*Rickettsia prowazekii*)	Bacterium	Flying squirrels	Inhalation (?); louse is vector in squirrels	Blood, feces (?)	Febrile	Very rare	Mild to moderate	Most cases in U.S. among rural dwellers

TABLE 84–2. SOME DISEASES NOT ACQUIRED FROM ANIMALS

AIDS (HIV infection)
Botulism
Cholera
Coccidioidomycosis
Cytomegalovirus
Diphtheria
Hand, foot, and mouth disease (coxsackievirus)
Hepatitis
Histoplasmosis
Legionellosis
Parvovirus (human parvovirus infection; parvovirus B19; erythema infectiosum)
Pinworms
Shigellosis
Streptococcosis (group A)

From there the organism could be transmitted to a human by a bite, or it could be transferred to claws when the cat grooms itself, and then transmitted by a scratch. Another possibility is flea-mediated transmission. Flea bites may well be the means of cat-to-cat transmission of *B. henselae*. Experimental studies have shown that the cat flea readily acquires *B. henselae* from infected cats and can transmit the infection to uninfected animals.[5] This is not likely to be the primary means of transmission to humans, however. Because viable bacteria are excreted in flea feces,[6] transmission of the organism could easily occur if contaminated "flea dirt" comes into contact with a person's open wound, whether a cat scratch or bite or a non-cat-inflicted cut or abrasion.

What Can Be Done to Eliminate the Bacteremia?

There is no known effective means of clearing the cat of *B. henselae* infection. Efforts to completely and permanently eliminate the organism by using antibiotic therapy have met with only limited success.[3] Thus treatment of cats is not considered a reliable strategy for preventing CSD in humans.

Is Declawing an Effective Means of Preventing Human Infection?

No. Although most cases of clinical CSD in humans can be traced to a cat scratch, a significant number are associated with bites, with wounds not inflicted by cats, or with no known site of inoculation.

Should a Person Who Contracts CSD Get Rid of His or Her Cat?

Although having CSD is not a pleasant experience, permanent sequelae are almost nonexistent. People rarely become reinfected, and more than one case in a household is unusual. Rather than deprive oneself of the pleasures of cat ownership, a better approach is to take some commonsense precautions to minimize the chances of becoming infected.

What Can Be Done to Prevent Human Infection With CSD?

Start with aggressive flea control, involving both pets and the environment. Prevent cat scratches or bites by discouraging aggressive behavior. Do not tease kittens into rough play, and do not allow children to annoy cats or kittens. Immediately wash any bite or scratch thoroughly with soap and warm water and cover the wound to keep it clean. Do not allow cats to lick broken skin.[7]

If the offending animal is a kitten, clients should be advised that risk of transmission diminishes greatly as the cat matures. This may be due to at least two factors: levels of bacteremia wane with age, and older cats tend to be more sedate and less likely to scratch.

Should Those Who Are HIV-Positive Even Consider Getting Cats? Or if They Already Have Cats, Should They Get Rid of Them?

HIV-positive individuals and AIDS patients should be able to have cats if they follow the prevention guidelines given earlier. CSD is not a common disease; there are more than 57 million pet cats in the United States and more than one third of all households have at least one cat, yet only 22,000 cases of CSD are reported each year. Bacillary angiomatosis is rare. To be on the safe side, it might be prudent for someone who is HIV-positive to avoid acquiring a kitten or getting a cat from an animal shelter, because kittens and strays tend to have a higher rate of seroprevalence. A combination of serologic testing and blood culture can be used as a screening tool. Although it should be noted that negative results on both tests do not necessarily guarantee that the cat is free from infection, the probability of the cat truly being disease-free is increased. An older, flea-free cat that is kept indoors has less chance of carrying *B. henselae*. The benefits of a companion animal for some people may outweigh any risks of pet ownership, provided steps are taken to keep the risk at a minimum.[8] However, anyone who is seriously immunocompromised should tell his or her physician about any animals in the household to increase the chances of early recognition of zoonoses.

LARVA MIGRANS: TOXOCARIASIS, BAYLISASCARIASIS, AND ANCYLOSTOMIASIS

Larva migrans is a broad term for the conditions that can result when humans become infected with ascarids or hookworms of dogs, cats, or wild animals. Because humans are not the normal hosts, the parasites do not complete their life cycle in the intestines; instead, the larval forms migrate through various organs and tissues, hence the name.

Toxocariasis. Toxocariasis is caused by *Toxocara* spp., *T. canis* being the species most often implicated.[9] When only a few larvae are present, as is usually the case, infection is likely to be asymptomatic or subclinical.[10] Heavier infestations may cause visceral larva migrans (VLM) or ocular larva migrans (OLM). Toxocaral VLM is usually a relatively mild disease, characterized by enlargement of the liver, pulmonary symptoms, and chronic abdominal pain.[9, 10] Fatalities have occurred but are rare; they are mostly associated with larvae invading the central nervous system or heart.[10] OLM occurs when larvae enter the eye; this condition may result in permanent blindness.[9] Toxocariasis, in one form or another, is probably the most common zoonotic disease associated with pet animals that occurs in the United States.[11]

Baylisascariasis. Baylisascariasis is caused by *Baylisascaris procyonis*, a large ascarid of raccoons. Like toxocariasis, most baylisascariasis cases are subclinical and associated with light infections. *Baylisascaris* can cause VLM and OLM but is more pathogenic than *Toxocara* spp. and is more likely to produce neural larva migrans (NLM) when large numbers of larvae are present. Symptoms of NLM may range from lethargy, hemiparesis, and torticollis to coma and death. Baylisascariasis is being diagnosed more frequently in people.[12]

Ancylostomiasis. Hookworms (*Ancylostoma* spp.) have the potential to cause cutaneous larva migrans, an acute dermatitis with intense itching that spreads as the larvae migrate intracutaneously. In some patients, the larvae penetrate to deeper tissues; *A. caninum* sometimes reaches the small intestine, where it can cause eosinophilic enteritis. Ancylostomiasis usually is a self-limited condition, but symptoms may persist weeks or months before natural resolution.[9]

How Do People Contract Toxocariasis or Baylisascariasis?

These two diseases are contracted by ingestion of infective eggs or viable larvae. Soil contaminated by feces of infected animals is the source of infective eggs. When soil is consumed (e.g., geophagia or on unwashed vegetables), eggs can be transferred to the mouth. Raw liver (chicken, beef, or sheep) can be a source of infective larvae.

How Likely Is Soil to Be Contaminated?

Any place that dogs, cats, or wild animals may defecate should be considered potentially contaminated. In the United States and United Kingdom, up to 30 per cent of soil samples from public parks were found to contain toxocaral eggs.[10]

How Long Do Infective Eggs Persist in Contaminated Soil?

Infective eggs may survive in soil for as long as several months. Although they are sensitive to desiccation, where soil is somewhat moist, the eggs can persist for prolonged periods.[10]

Who Is Most at Risk of Developing Severe Disease due to Toxocariasis or Baylisascariasis?

Most severe infections occur in toddler-age children with pica (usually geophagia) who have contact with puppies.[13] As many as 30 per cent of children between 1 and 6 years of age may be affected by pica, and when it involves eating soil, the risk increases tremendously.[10] In addition, many children are less than attentive to personal hygiene, such as washing hands before eating. When they have been playing with puppies or kittens, or outside in the soil or in sandboxes, their hands may well be contaminated with infective eggs.

How Do People Contract Ancylostomiasis?

Ancylostomiasis is the result of hookworm larvae penetrating the skin. People whose bare skin contacts damp, sandy soil contaminated with feces of infected dogs or cats are at risk. This can include children, gardeners, utility workers, and people on beaches.

What Can Veterinarians Do to Prevent the Various Types of Larva Migrans?

Pet owners should be educated about the intestinal parasites of dogs and cats, their potential public health hazard, and appropriate anthelmintic treatment to minimize risk. "Veterinarians are in an optimal position to provide pet owners with this service because of their unique training, frequent contact with the high proportion of pet owners who use veterinary services, and their rapport with clients." This statement is from *How to Prevent Transmission of Intestinal Roundworms From Pets to People*, a set of guidelines for veterinarians to help them help their clients avoid larva migrans. This pamphlet was prepared by the Centers for Disease Control and Prevention (CDC) in association with veterinary public health and parasitology groups and can be obtained from the CDC or downloaded from its web site.[14]

Early deworming can help prevent the massive environmental contamination that infected puppies and kittens can cause. The optimal treatment schedule for puppies is deworming at 2, 4, 6, and 8 weeks of age in areas where both ascarids and hookworms are prevalent; if only ascarids are likely to be present, treatment may commence at 3 weeks of age. Kittens should be started on anthelmintic treatments at 6 weeks of age, with repeat treatments at 8 and 10 weeks. Nursing bitches and queens should be treated concurrently.[14]

Is There Anything Parents Can Do to Help Prevent These Conditions?

Parents can help prevent their children from becoming infected by covering sandboxes when they are not in use to keep cats from using them as litterboxes. They also should teach children not to put dirty objects in their mouths and to always wash their hands after handling animals or playing in the soil and before eating.[9] Keeping raccoons as pets increases the risk of human baylisascariasis. Infected animals may shed millions of *Baylisascaris* eggs daily in their feces, and having raccoons in the domestic environment makes human contact with contaminated areas more likely.[12]

RABIES

Rabies is an acute viral encephalomyelitis that is almost always fatal in any animal or human. It is transmitted only when the virus enters the body through breaks in the skin or via contact with mucous membranes. When a person is exposed to rabies, postexposure prophylaxis (PEP) should be initiated immediately. If there is no true exposure to the virus, such treatment is not necessary.

What Constitutes an Exposure to Rabies?

According to information provided by the CDC,[15] there are two possible routes of exposure to rabies: bite and nonbite. Any penetration of the skin by teeth of a rabid animal constitutes a bite exposure. Nonbite exposures include scratches, abrasions, open wounds, or mucous membranes that come in contact with saliva or other potentially infectious material, e.g., brain or spinal cord tissue, from a rabid animal.

What Does Not Constitute an Exposure to Rabies?

In the absence of a bite or other exposure described earlier, the act of petting or touching a rabid animal is *not* an exposure to rabies and does not require PEP. Likewise, contact with blood, urine, or feces of an infected animal is not an exposure; rabies virus is found only in saliva and nervous tissue.[15]

What Animals Are Most Likely to Be Rabid?

In the United States, rabies is mostly a problem in wildlife. The only cases that occur now in domestic animals are caused by spillover from wildlife epizootics. In 1996, there were 7124 cases of wildlife rabies reported in the United States and Puerto Rico, as compared with 574 cases in domestic animals.[16] Along the eastern seaboard, raccoons are the species most often affected. In the central states and in California, skunks present the most danger. Various fox species cause problems in western New York and Canada (red foxes), Alaska (arctic and red foxes), and Arizona and Texas (grey foxes). Rabid bats of several different species are found throughout North America, but the prevalence of rabies in any given species is not known. Among domestic animals in the United States, cats account for the highest number of cases, followed by cattle and dogs (266, 131, and 111 cases, respectively, in 1996). Most of the reports of cat rabies are from states in which raccoon rabies is epizootic.[16] Dogs are the most significant reservoir in Africa, much of Asia, and parts of Central and South America. In Europe, foxes account for most confirmed cases.

Does Rabies Occur in Squirrels or Other Rodents?

Rabies can occur in any mammalian species but is rarely reported in rodents, perhaps because the small size of most species makes surviving a bite from a rabid animal unlikely. Questions often arise about squirrels, which may nip people who feed them in parks and in other peridomestic situations. Between 1971 and 1994, there were 24 reports of rabid squirrels in the United States.[17] However, neither squirrels nor any other rodents have ever been implicated in the transmission of rabies to humans in this country. Perhaps of more importance is the increasing number of reports of rabid woodchucks or groundhogs (*Marmota monax*). Between 1985 and 1994, more than 300 of these large rodents were found to be infected with the rabies strain associated with raccoons in the eastern United States, and there are reports of rabid woodchucks attacking and biting humans.[17]

In any bite situation, it is important to distinguish between a provoked bite and an unprovoked bite, in which an animal attacks without warning. A provoked bite is one that occurs as a result of some preceding interaction between the human and the animal, including feeding or petting. Provoked bites are not considered abnormal behavior. In contrast, an unprovoked bite is one that occurs without prior interaction, such as when an animal suddenly attacks and bites or scratches someone without apparent cause. In such cases, rabies should be suspected, regardless of species.

Which Animals Are Most Likely to Transmit Rabies to Humans?

In the United States, most cases of indigenously acquired human rabies are caused by viral strains carried by various species of bats. Between 1980 and 1997, 21 of the 36 cases of human rabies in the United States were associated with bat-related virus variants.[18] In the rest of the world, dogs are responsible for most human deaths. (Most of the non-bat-associated cases in the United States occurred in returning travelers who had been exposed to rabid dogs in other countries.)

What Are the Recommendations Regarding Human Exposure to Bats?

Anyone who has had bite, scratch, or mucous membrane exposure to a bat should undergo PEP, unless the bat can be tested and is found negative for rabies. However, data on bat-associated human rabies cases in the United States suggest that "seemingly insignificant physical contact with bats may result in viral transmission, even without a clear history of animal bite."[19] Therefore, when the bat is unavailable for testing, PEP is also recommended in the absence of an obvious bite, scratch, or mucous membrane exposure when there is even a possibility that such contact may have occurred. Situations in which administration of PEP is indicated include a sleeping person awakening to find a bat in the room or an adult seeing a bat in the same room with a previously unattended child or mentally disabled or intoxicated person. Bats should never be handled by untrained persons and should never be kept as pets.

What Should Be Done if a Dead or Moribund Bat Is Found in the House?

Because up to 50 per cent of dead or grounded bats may test positive for rabies,[20] precautions should be taken when approaching such an animal. Do not touch even a dead bat with bare hands. Wear gloves or use a disposable object, such as a piece of cardboard, to scoop the bat into a box or plastic bag; seal the container. Submit the specimen for rabies testing as soon as possible. Refrigerate the specimen if it cannot be submitted immediately.

What Should Be Done if a Cat or Dog Is Found With a Bat?

When a bat is found in proximity to a pet, it is prudent to assume that exposure may have occurred and immediately submit the bat for testing (follow the procedure in the previous paragraph). If rabies is confirmed, or if the bat escapes or is otherwise not available for testing, take appropriate action as outlined in the most current version of the National Association of Public Health Veterinarians' annual publication "Compendium of Animal Rabies Control." The 1997 version states: "Unvaccinated dogs and cats exposed to a rabid animal should be euthanized immediately. If the owner is unwilling to have this done, the animal should be placed in strict isolation for 6 months and vaccinated 1 month before being released. Animals with expired vaccinations need to be evaluated on a case-by-case basis. Dogs and cats that are currently vaccinated should be revaccinated immediately, kept under the owner's control, and observed for 45 days."[21]

TOXOPLASMOSIS

Toxoplasmosis is a systemic disease caused by *Toxoplasma gondii*, a coccidian parasite that has the domestic cat as its definitive host. Primary *Toxoplasma* infections in immunocompetent adults and children are often asymptomatic or cause only a mild flulike illness. After the initial parasitemia subsides owing to the body's immune response, the organism may encyst in various tissues. In healthy people this is not a problem, but HIV-positive and other immunocompromised individuals are at risk of developing life-threatening cerebral toxoplasmosis when the decline in the immune system allows reactivation of viable tissue cysts. If a pregnant woman contracts a primary infection, the parasite can cross the placenta and infect the fetus. When this happens, abortion or premature birth may occur; babies that survive may be permanently neurogically impaired.

Are Cats the Main Source of Human Infection?

Indirectly, yes. Cats are the definitive host of this parasite, i.e., they are the only animals in which the parasite can complete its life cycle, and therefore the only animals that excrete infective oocysts. However, it is thought that most people contract toxoplasmosis through consuming undercooked meat or food that has been cross-contaminated from raw meat, rather than directly from infected cats.[22]

What Meats Are Most Likely to Be Infected With *Toxoplasma* Cysts?

In the United States, fresh pork probably is the main source of human infection. Meat from sheep and from game animals such as deer, bear, moose, and pronghorn also may contain viable infective cysts, as may chicken. The prevalence of *T. gondii* cysts in cattle is not known, but beef is not thought to represent an important source of infection for humans.[22]

How Do Food Animals Become Infected?

A cat with active toxoplasmosis sheds oocysts in its feces; if sporulated oocysts are ingested by another animal, infection will result. Food animals often consume cat feces while grazing. Omnivores, such as swine, may contract the infection via ingestion of contaminated meat, rodents, or birds. In animals other than cats, *T. gondii* encysts in muscle tissue after the initial acute infection subsides; these cysts remain viable in meat from infected animals.

How Likely Is It That a Person Changing a Litterbox Will Become Infected With Toxoplasmosis?

Not likely at all, provided some common sense and good hygiene are practiced. It takes a day or more at ambient temperature for oocysts in feces to sporulate and become infective.[23] Therefore, daily removal and proper disposal of feces from the litterbox will prevent the development of the infective stage, even if the cat is shedding oocysts. Of course, one should always wash one's hands thoroughly with soap and water after handling used litter.

Does an Infected Cat Always Shed Oocysts?

An infected cat typically sheds oocysts for about three weeks following primary infection. Although recurrent shedding is known to occur, it is rare, and repeated exposures to the organism usually do not cause further shedding of oocysts.[23]

Can a Person Get Toxoplasmosis From Handling an Infected Cat?

Cats that are actively shedding oocysts seldom have diarrhea, and normal, firm cat feces do not significantly contaminate the fur. What fecal contamination there is generally does not remain on a cat's fur long enough for sporulation to occur; most cats are so fastidious that they clean themselves thoroughly immediately after defecation.[22]

Is It Safe for a Pregnant Woman to Have a Pet Cat?

Yes. Her chances of contracting toxoplasmosis from eating undercooked meat are higher than those of contracting it from her cat. But unless she knows that she is immune to toxoplasmosis (via serologic testing to detect antibodies from an earlier infection), common sense suggests erring on the side of caution to prevent a primary infection. A pregnant woman should avoid any contact with cat feces by having someone else change litterboxes, if at all possible. If she

must change them herself, she should wear gloves and change the boxes daily, as mentioned earlier. She also should thoroughly wash her hands after handling a cat or anything potentially contaminated with cat feces.

What Else Can a Pregnant Woman Do to Avoid Toxoplasmosis?

A pregnant woman who is not immune or does not know whether she is immune to toxoplasmosis should avoid contact with soil (because of the possibility of contamination with cat feces) and raw meat. She should wear gloves while gardening and wash vegetables thoroughly. If she must handle raw meat, she should be scrupulous about cleanliness (hands, kitchen utensils, surfaces) during and after preparation to avoid transfer of viable cysts from the food to her mouth. Likewise, she should avoid eating undercooked meats. *Toxoplasma* cysts are killed by thorough cooking (155°F or above) or by freezing (-20°F or below) for at least a day.

Are HIV-Positive Individuals at Special Risk of Contracting Toxoplasmosis From Their Pet Cats?

Most HIV-positive people who develop toxoplasmosis do so as a result of reactivation of latent tissue infection as their immune system declines. No correlation has been shown between cat ownership and presence of *Toxoplasma* antibodies in HIV-infected adults.[23, 24]

How Can People Prevent Their Cats From Becoming Infected With *T. gondii*?

Pet cats should be fed only commercial cat food or other cooked foods. They should not be given raw meat or poultry, viscera, or bones. Pet cats should be kept indoors to prevent hunting and scavenging.[22]

REFERENCES

1. Jameson P, et al: Prevalence of *Bartonella henselae* antibodies in pet cats throughout regions of North America. J Infect Dis 172:1145, 1995.
2. Kordick DL, et al: Prolonged *Bartonella* bacteremia in cats associated with cat-scratch disease patients. J Clin Microbiol 33:3245, 1995.
3. Regnery RL, et al: Experimentally induced *Bartonella henselae* infections followed by challenge exposure and antimicrobial therapy in cats. Am J Vet Res 57:1714, 1996.
4. Kordick DL, Breitschwerdt EB: Blood transmission of *Bartonella henselae* in cats (abstract). Programs and abstracts of the 95th general meeting of the American Society for Microbiology, Washington, DC, 1995.
5. Chomel BB, et al: Experimental transmission of *Bartonella henselae* by the cat flea. J Clin Microbiol 34:1952, 1996.
6. Higgins JA, et al: Acquisition of the cat scratch disease agent *Bartonella henselae* by cat fleas (Siphonaptera: Pulicidae). J Med Entomol 33:490, 1996.
7. Harrington KS, Groves MG: Cat scratch disease. *In* Farris R, et al (eds): Health Hazards in Veterinary Practice, 3rd ed. Schaumburg, IL, American Veterinary Medical Association, 1995, p 23.
8. Angulo FJ, et al: Caring for pets of immunocompromised persons. JAVMA 205:1711, 1994.
9. Benenson AS: Toxocariasis. *In* Benenson AS (ed): Control of Communicable Diseases Manual, 16th ed. Washington, DC, American Public Health Association, 1995, p 465.
10. Schantz PM: Toxocariasis. *In* Farris R, et al (eds): Health Hazards in Veterinary Practice, 3rd ed. Schaumburg, IL, American Veterinary Medical Association, 1995, p 70.
11. Schantz PM: Of worms, dogs, and human hosts: Continuing challenges for veterinarians in prevention of human disease. JAVMA 204:1023, 1994.
12. Kazakos KR: Baylisascariasis. *In* Farris R, et al (eds): Health Hazards in Veterinary Practice, 3rd ed. Schaumburg, IL, American Veterinary Medical Association, 1995, p 13.
13. Glickman LT, Magnaval J-F: Zoonotic roundworm infections. Infect Dis Clin Am 7:717, 1993.
14. http://www.cdc.gov/ncidod/diseases/roundwrm/roundwrm.htm

15. Centers for Disease Control: Rabies prevention—United States, 1991: Recommendations of the Immunization Practices Advisory Committee (ACIP). MMWR 40 (RR–3), 1991.
16. Krebs JW, et al: Rabies surveillance in the United States during 1996. JAVMA 211:1525, 1997.
17. Childs JE, et al: Surveillance and spatiotemporal associations of rabies in rodents and lagomorphs in the United States, 1985–1994. J Wildl Dis 33:20, 1997.
18. Centers for Disease Control and Prevention: Human rabies—Texas and New Jersey, 1997. MMWR 47:1, 1998.
19. Centers for Disease Control and Prevention: Human rabies—Montana and Washington, 1997. MMWR 46:770, 1997.
20. Anonymous: Of bats, rabies, and men: Epidemiology report. Alabama Department of Public Health, December 1994, p 3.
21. Jenkins SR, et al: Compendium of animal rabies control, 1997. JAVMA 210:33, 1997.
22. Dubey JP: Toxoplasmosis. JAVMA 205:1593, 1994.
23. Acha PN, Szyfres B: Toxoplasmosis. In Acha PN, Szyfres B (eds): Zoonoses and Communicable Diseases Common to Man and Animals, 2nd ed. Washington, DC, Pan American Health Organization, 1987, p 628.
24. Glaser CA, Angulo FJ, Rooney JA: Animal-associated opportunistic infections among persons infected with the human immunodeficiency virus. Clin Infect Dis 18:14, 1994.

CHAPTER 85

BACTERIAL DISEASES

Craig E. Greene

SALMONELLOSIS

Salmonella are ubiquitous gram-negative bacilli that can reside in the intestinal tract of a wide variety of mammals, birds, reptiles, and even insects. Under certain circumstances they can cause systemic disease. Species of *Salmonella* that are recognized to be of major pathogenic significance in veterinary microbiology include *S. choleraesuis, S. arizonae, S. enteritidis,* and *S. typhimurium. S. enteritidis* has been further divided into more than 1700 bioserotypes, each with a distinguishing name; usually the bioserotype name is substituted for that of the species. The majority of serotypes show little or no specific host adaptation and have been isolated from vertebrates, invertebrates, and the environment. Serotypes or individual isolates vary widely in their ability to produce disease. The species most commonly isolated from dogs and cats is *S. typhimurium.*

The most common source of infection, which occurs through the gastrointestinal route, is contact with contaminated food, water, or fomites. Salmonellae can survive for relatively long periods outside the host. Finding *Salmonella* in the environment usually indicates direct or indirect fecal contamination. Dogs and cats may acquire their infections by drinking contaminated water or foodstuffs or preying on infected animals. Uncooked or unprocessed meat or animal by-products in the diet have most often been incriminated.[1] However, salmonellae can contaminate and then replicate in processed foods during storage.

The frequency of fecal isolation from clinically healthy or hospitalized dogs is reported to be 1 to 36 per cent; from normal cats it is 0 to 14 per cent. The actual prevalence varies, based on the age, diet, and exposure of the animal to puppies and kittens younger than 1 year of age. Stress caused by hospitalization, anesthesia, surgical and medical or immune-suppressive therapy, concurrent diseases, and overcrowding has been correlated with an increased risk of salmonellosis in dogs and cats.[2, 3] By virtue of altering normal intestinal microflora, antibiotic therapy reduces host resistance to salmonellosis. Salmonellae attach preferentially to the tips of mucosal villi in the intestine, which they invade and in which they multiply. Localization and persistence of the organisms in the intestinal epithelium and lymph nodes account for shedding, which usually occurs for 3 to 6 weeks on an intermittent basis. Endotoxemia or bacteremia may occur in some animals as a result of intestinal colonization and proliferation.

Clinical findings in salmonellosis vary according to the number of infecting organisms, the immune status of the host, and complicating factors or concomitant diseases. The syndromes can be artifically divided into gastroenteritis, bacteremia and endotoxemia, organ localization, and persistence of an asymptomatic carrier state. Clinical signs associated with *Salmonella* gastroenteritis are variable, and most occur a few days following stress or hospitalization. Fever, malaise, and anorexia are noted initially, followed by vomiting, abdominal pain, and diarrhea.[4] Weight loss and dehydration become evident within several days of illness. Shock or central nervous system (CNS) signs may develop in severely affected bacteremic or endotoxemic animals. Pneumonic signs can also be associated with bacterial embolization. Metastatic infection may occur in other tissues following clinical or subclinical bacteremia, with the clinical signs referable to the organ of localization. Abortion, stillbirth, and birth of weak puppies or kittens may result from in utero infection.

Diagnosis is based on clinical suspicion. Hematologic and biochemical findings are nonspecific, being typical of infectious diarrhea or septicemia. Isolation of *Salmonella* organisms is the most definitive means of confirming infection. However, because of the carrier state, mere isolation from the gastrointestinal tract or its secretions does not indicate that the organisms are causing clinical disease. Selective media improve the isolation rate from enteric specimens.[5, 6] Serologic testing is also inconclusive. Therefore, finding organisms in samples of normally sterile body fluids or tissues allows for the most definitive diagnosis of systemic salmonellosis. Samples for culture taken at surgery or necropsy should include liver, spleen, lung, mesenteric lymph nodes, and intestinal tract.

Gross lesions are found at necropsy in animals that develop severe clinical illness. A diffuse mucoid to hemorrhagic enteritis is usually confined to the distal small bowel, cecum, and colon. Histologic lesions are of a hemorrhagic ulcerative enteritis. Lesions, usually of a suppurative nature, may be found in the lungs, liver, and brain of animals that die from bacterial dissemination.

Appropriate therapy for canine and feline salmonellosis varies according to the type and severity of clinical illness. Acute *Salmonella* gastroenteritis, without systemic signs, is best treated with parenteral polyionic isotonic fluids to replace losses from vomitus and diarrhea. Antibiotics usually effective against *Salmonella* include chloramphenicol and trimethoprim-sulfonamides (Table 85–1). In vivo resistance may be encountered. Aminoglycosides may be considered when bacterial resistance is anticipated, but the risk of renal toxicity often precludes their use. Variable resistance to erythromycin, ampicillin, cephapirin, or nitrofurans occurs. Fluoroquinolones, such as enrofloxacin, have been shown to be effective in treating *Salmonella* enteritis or bacteremia in people and animals. Because *Salmonella* gastroenteritis is usually self-limited, routine antimicrobial treatment may not be indicated, because when only single-agent therapy is used, there may not be elimination of the convalescent excretion period. Another inherent problem with routine antibiotic administration for *Salmonella* gastroenteritis is that an increased prevalence of transferable resistance has been demonstrated among *Salmonella* isolates from dogs, cats, and humans.[2] With severe endotoxemia, antisera commercially available for this purpose could be considered.

Prevention of salmonellosis following an outbreak involves hygiene and strict isolation of infected animals, followed by routine disinfection of cage areas they have contacted. Salmonellosis is a zoonosis, and care should be taken to avoid human contact.

CAMPYLOBACTERIOSIS AND HELICOBACTERIOSIS

Campylobacter are gram-negative, slender, curved or spiral-shaped rods that colonize the intestinal tract of animals.

C. jejuni is the organism routinely associated with diarrheal disease in animals and people. A catalase-negative species, *C. upsalensis,* has been isolated from asymptomatic and diarrheic dogs, as well as asymptomatic cats.[7] Like salmonellae, the isolation rate of *C. jejuni* varies according to the age and environmental background of the animal. Stray or group-housed animals have the highest fecal rates. *C. jejuni* has been isolated from approximately 20 to 30 per cent of diarrheic cats and dogs, respectively, compared with less than 10 per cent isolation from normal cats and dogs. Puppies and kittens appear more likely to acquire *C. jejuni* and to have clinical disease. The fecal-oral route is the primary means of organism spread, usually via contaminated food or water supplies. Meat, especially poultry, and unpasteurized milk have been commonly incriminated.

The severity of campylobacteriosis is dependent on prior exposure, number and virulence of organisms ingested, development of protective antibody, and presence of other enteric pathogens. Environmental, physiologic, or surgical stress or concurrent enteric infections may exacerbate disease severity. Dogs and cats appear to be better adapted than people to *Campylobacter,* and most animals are asymptomatic carriers.[8] When clinical illness develops, it is usually in animals younger than 6 months of age. Also, animals may be more susceptible to clinical disease when they are stressed. *Campylobacter*-associated diarrhea has a wide clinical spectrum ranging from loose feces to watery diarrhea to bloody mucoid diarrhea. Severe signs are not common. Fever, anorexia, and vomiting are also rare. The condition usually lasts 1 to 3 weeks. Biliary and systemic infection with *Campylobacter* has been described,[9] but this may have actually been a *Helicobacter.* Fecal contamination from puppies and kittens can serve as sources of *Campylobacter* infection in people, although contact with undercooked poultry is most common. Disease in humans is often severe, and the diarrhea may be accompanied by vomiting, fever, and abdominal discomfort.

Presumptive clinical diagnosis should be based on microscopy of fresh fecal samples under dim or other contrasting illumination, looking for the rapid motion and characteristic shape of *C. jejuni.* Gram's stains show slender gull-wing-

TABLE 85–1. DRUGS FOR BACTERIAL DISEASES

GENERIC	DOSAGE (mg/lb)	ROUTE	FREQUENCY (hours)	DISEASE INDICATION
Chloramphenicol	12.5–25	PO, IV, SC	8	Salmonellosis, campylobacteriosis, helicobacteriosis, actinomycosis, streptococcosis
Trimethoprim-sulfonamide	7.5–15	PO	12	Salmonellosis, brucellosis, nocardiosis
Gentamicin	1.0	IM, SC	12–24*	Salmonellosis, brucellosis, nocardiosis, rhodococcosis, leptospirosis carrier
Enrofloxacin	2.5–5	PO	12	Salmonellosis, campylobacteriosis, opportunistic mycobacteriosis, bartonellosis
Erythromycin	4–7.5	PO	8–12	Campylobacteriosis, streptococcosis, borreliosis
Tetracycline	2.2	PO	8	L-form infections, opportunistic mycobacteriosis, borreliosis, brucellosis
Dapsone	0.5	PO	6–8	Lepromatous mycobacterial infection
Clofazimine	4	PO	24	Lepromatous and opportunistic mycobacterial infections
Rifampin	15	PO	24	Mycobacterial infections
Minocycline	5	PO	12	Brucellosis,† borreliosis
Penicillin	10–30 × 10³ units	IM, IV	8–12	Actinomycosis, streptococcosis, leptospirosis, tetanus, botulism, feline abscesses
Ampicillin/amoxicillin	10–15	PO, IV	8–12	Helicobacteriosis, streptococcosis, borreliosis, feline abscesses
Doxycycline	5	PO	12	Borreliosis, opportunistic mycobacterial infections, brucellosis,† leptospirosis carrier, bartonellosis
Metronidazole	5	PO	8	Tetanus, botulism, feline abscesses

PO = oral; IM = intramuscular; SC = subcutaneous; IV = intravenous.
*Watch for nephrotoxicity; higher dosages are only for life-threatening infections.
†Doses of 6.25 mg/lb PO every 12 hours for 4 weeks are used for treating brucellosis in conjunction with gentamicin for 2 weeks.

shaped rods. For culture, the organism can survive a few days in feces or as long as a week under refrigeration. Cultures should be performed on specific *Campylobacter* isolation media in an oxygen-reduced atmosphere at 42°C. Strain differences can be recognized, and many of the isolates frequently found in diarrheic and normal laboratory beagles and cats have had serotypes frequently encountered in humans.[10]

Gross and microscopic lesions most frequent in neonates are of an acute to chronic ileocecocolitis. Microscopically, the colon and cecum have decreased epithelial cell height, brush borders, and a number of goblet cells. Hyperplasia of epithelial glands results in a thickened mucosa, and inflammatory infiltrates may be noted. Using silver stains, *Campylobacter*-like organisms may be demonstrated attached to, but not within, colonic epithelium.

Efficacy of antibiotic therapy for *Campylobacter*-associated diarrhea in the dog and cat is not known; however, antibiotics should be used to minimize exposure to humans and other pets. Erythromycin is the drug of choice for *Campylobacter*-induced diarrhea in humans and presumably in animals (see Table 85–1); however, vomiting is a common side effect. Feces should be cultured from 1 to 4 weeks after treatment to confirm efficacy. Chloramphenicol has been used with variable efficacy in dogs and cats. Although the fluoroquinolones are highly effective in treating people, their use in dogs and cats should be reserved for resistant cases because of the public health risk of inducing the development of antimicrobial resistance in animal bacteria. Furthermore, because clinical campylobacteriosis is often observed in young animals, the use of fluoroquinolones is contraindicated because of toxicity to developing cartilage.

Helicobacter are gram-negative, microaerophilic bacteria with similar morphology to *Campylobacter*. A number of species have been isolated from the gastrointestinal tract of dogs and cats, and many may have been previously confused with *Campylobacter*. Some species live in the acid conditions of the gastric mucosa, where they may proliferate and cause chronic gastritis and peptic ulcer disease. *H. pylori* is the species that infects people and has been isolated from the stomach of cats in one instance.[11] Other *Helicobacter* such as *H. felis, H. bizzozeronii,* and other as yet unnamed gastric *Helicobacter*-like organisms colonize various mammalian hosts and have been linked to gastritis in dogs and cats. They are transmitted orally to other animals and through close contact between animals, or nosocomial spread through fomites can occur. These organisms can proliferate in the stomach of clinically healthy animals and produce gastric inflammation and lymphoid proliferation, which may result in clinical illness. Because their presence is not always associated with clinical disease, commensurate pathologic changes should always accompany culture-positive or histologic detection of *Helicobacter*. Clinical signs may include vomiting, weight loss, and diarrhea.

Helicobacter that inhabit the stomach of dogs and cats are fastidious and difficult to cultivate in the laboratory, requiring specialized conditions and often being overgrown by contaminants unless selective media are used. Properly equipped laboratories should be notified in advance, and transport broth should be used for sending specimens. In routine clinical practice, histologic examination is the usual means of diagnosis. A clinically useful test in people is the carbon-labeled urea breath test. Therapy for gastric helicobacteriosis involves the combination of at least two antimicrobials such as metronidazole and amoxicillin (see Table 85–1) plus antacids (see Chapter 136).

In addition to gastric helicobacters, a number of species have been isolated from the intestinal tract of normal and diarrheic animals. The significance of these organisms in causing inflammatory bowel disease is uncertain. In addition, some species colonize the liver of animals, possibly causing hepatic inflammation. A novel organism, *H. canis,* was found in the liver of a young dog with acute multifocal necrotizing hepatitis.[12] The host range and zoonotic potential of these helicobacters need further investigation.

TYZZER'S DISEASE

Tyzzer's disease, caused by *Clostridium piliforme,* a spore-forming, gram-negative bacterium, affects a wide range of animals, including dogs and cats.[13] *C. piliforme* is a commensal of the intestinal tract of laboratory rodents and is found on fecal cultures of normal and diseased animals. Clinical illness is rodents is precipitated by various stresses. Immunosuppressed dogs and cats presumably acquire infection by contact with or ingestion of rodent feces containing bacterial spores. Most cats with this disease have been laboratory-reared and exposed to rodents. Following local proliferation in the intestine, organisms spread by the portal circulation to the liver and produce multifocal hepatic necrosis.

Clinical signs include a rapid onset of lethargy, depression, anorexia, abdominal discomfort, hepatomegaly, and abdominal distention. These signs are followed by hypothermia, a moribund attitude, and death within 24 to 48 hours. Profuse diarrhea is rare, and scant amounts of pasty feces are more characteristic. Icterus has been apparent in some animals, especially cats.

Because of the rapidly fatal nature of this disease, diagnosis is usually made by gross examination of specimens collected at necropsy. Multiple whitish-gray to hemorrhagic foci, 1 to 2 mm in diameter, are found on the capsule and cut surface of the liver and on other viscera. The intestinal mucosa may be thickened and congested in the region of the terminal ileum and proximal colon. Foamy, dark brown feces are usually present in the lumen, and mesenteric lymph nodes are generally enlarged.

Histologic findings usually include multifocal periportal hepatic necrosis and necrotic ileitis or colitis. There are typically numerous intracellular filamentous organisms in hepatocytes at the margins of necrotic lesions and in the intestinal epithelial cells. Spore forms have also been observed. Because *C. piliforme* cannot be isolated on artificial medium that lacks living cells, specimens for culture must be inoculated into mice or cell culture. Treatment has not been successful.

L-FORM INFECTIONS

Cell-wall-deficient or L-form bacteria have been isolated from cats with a syndrome of fever and persistently draining, spreading cellulitis and synovitis. It often involves the extremities. The usual source of infection is contamination of penetrating wounds. Abscesses develop at the point of inoculation, and lesions spread, drain, dehisce, and do not permanently heal. Bacteremic spread of infection may result in polyarthritis or distant abscess formation. The exudates from draining lesions contain predominantly macrophages and neutrophils, with a few lymphocytes. Diagnosis is difficult because these organisms are hard to demonstrate by light microscopy or by culture. Infection can be transmitted to cats experimentally by subcutaneous inoculation with cell-free material from tissues or exudates of affected cats. Electron microscopic evaluation of tissues may show the characteristically pleomorphic, cell-wall-deficient organisms in phagocytes. Tetracycline is the treatment of choice (see Table 85–1).

MYCOBACTERIOSIS

Mycobacterium is a genus comprising morphologically similar, aerobic, environmentally resistant, non-spore-forming acid-fast bacteria. They have a wide host affinity and pathogenic potential. Because of their structural properties and ability to survive intracellularly, they produce granulomatous inflammations. Mycobacterial infections can be divided into three forms—tuberculous, lepromatous, and opportunistic—based on the types of organisms that cause the disease.

The tuberculous mycobacteria, *M. tuberculosis, M. bovis,* and *M. avium,* produce indistinguishable nodular granulomas in their hosts. *M. tuberculosis*-complex includes *M. microti,* a rodent pathogen, and *M. africanum,* a human pathogen in Africa. *M. bovis* is closely related to *M. tuberculosis* var. *bovis,* an unclassified species that infects cats in Great Britain.[14] The *M. avium-intracellulare* complex (MAC) includes a large number of closely related saprophytic organisms that produce tuberculous granulomas in their hosts. Dogs and cats are susceptible to infections by *M. tuberculosis* and *M. bovis* but are more resistant to infection by MAC. Because *M. tuberculosis* is primarily a human pathogen, canine and feline infections are considered an inverse zoonosis. The overall prevalence of human and animal *M. tuberculosis* infections had been decreasing in recent years, but a surge in reported drug-resistant cases in people has occurred in densely populated urban areas, in economically disadvantaged regions, and in people with acquired immunodeficiency syndrome (AIDS).[15] Although herbivores and wildlife prey are the primary hosts of *M. bovis* infections,[16] cats and dogs can potentially become disseminators when the organism localizes in the intestinal or respiratory tracts. Cats usually excrete the organism via feces and dogs via respiratory secretions. Cats and dogs may acquire intestinal infections from ingestion of contaminated unpasteurized milk, uncooked meat, or offal from infected cattle. *M. tuberculosis* var. *bovis* infections are probably acquired by cats from ingestion of infected rodents.

Owing to innate resistance, infections with MAC tubercle bacilli are less common in dogs and cats compared with other hosts. Poultry is the usual source of infection, and feces of infected birds contain large numbers of bacilli. Infection is acquired by eating infected meat or via contact with contaminated soil or fomites.

Tubercle bacilli induce granuloma formation at the site of inoculation, usually the respiratory tract, gastrointestinal tract, or local lymph nodes. Host immunity is an important determinant of infection dissemination. In cases of host immunoincompetence, the tuberculous mycobacteria may disseminate throughout the body by direct extension or by mechanical means. A higher prevalence of *M. avium* infection has been observed in breeds such as the basset hound and the Siamese cat.[17, 18]

The nontuberculous forms of mycobacterial infection include feline leprosy caused by *M. lepraemurium,* the same acid-fast, difficult-to-culture organism responsible for murine leprosy and the atypical mycobacterioses. *M. lepraemurium*

and its resultant disease appear to occur more frequently in areas of the world with cold, wet climates. Transmission is thought to occur from bites or contact with infected rats. The atypical forms of mycobacteriosis are caused by numerous saprophytic mycobacterial species called opportunistic, or anonymous, mycobacteria. These atypical mycobacteria are ubiquitous in nature, and although they are not highly pathogenic, they can produce pyogranulomatous lesions following penetrating trauma to the skin or soft tissues. Of the identified species causing infection in cats and dogs, *M. fortuitum, M. chelonei, M. smegmatis,* and *M. phlei* are most common.[19–21] Cats seem more susceptible and exhibit a higher infection rate than do dogs.

Tubercular mycobacterial infections in dogs and cats are often asymptomatic or insidious. When clinical signs occur in dogs and cats, they reflect the site of granuloma formation. Bronchopneumonia, pulmonary nodule formation, and hilar lymphadenopathy are most commonly seen in dogs, causing fever, weight loss, anorexia, and harsh, nonproductive coughing. Dogs and cats may develop dysphagia, retching, hypersalivation, and tonsillar enlargement as the result of oropharyngeal lesions. Cats, which develop primary intestinal localization more commonly than dogs, may have weight loss, anemia, vomiting, and diarrhea as signs of intestinal malabsorption. Mesenteric lymph nodes may be palpably enlarged. Abdominal effusion is present in some cases. With dissemination, the clinical signs reflect the organ system of involvement. With MAC infections, dissemination of infection may be the first sign of clinical illness, with generalized lymphadenomegaly, anorexia, weight loss, and fever. Masses or enlargement of parenchymal organs may be detected. With feline leprosy, lesions are usually soft, fleshy, focal nodules in the skin and subcutis of the head and extremities. The lesions develop rapidly and are usually freely movable and nonpainful. They may be haired or superficially ulcerated, and regional lymph nodes may be enlarged.

Opportunistic mycobacteriosis in cats most commonly occurs with multiple fistulous draining tracts associated with purulent drainage into the caudal abdominal, inguinal, and lumbar subcutaneous tissues. Draining nodules may also occur. Signs of systemic illness, such as fever and anorexia, are rare. Dogs with atypical mycobacteriosis usually have a history of fight wounds or trauma followed by granulomatous proliferation of cutaneous tissues with serous or seropurulent drainage. Clinical laboratory findings in tuberculosis are frequently nonspecific, although hyperglobulinemia may be apparent. Radiographically visible masses and tracheobronchial lymphadenopathy may be apparent in the thoracic cavity. Abdominal palpation, radiography, or ultrasonography may reveal enlargement of parenchymatous organs such as the liver and spleen or solitary abdominal masses. Fluid may be present in the abdominal cavity, and calcified mesenteric lymph nodes may be noted. Osteoproliferative lesions may also be found in the axial or appendicular skeleton.

Intradermal (ID) skin testing in dogs with tuberculin has been reported to be inconsistent and unreliable. However, use of the medial side of the pinna may yield more consistent results.[22] Cats do not react strongly to ID-administered tuberculin. Culture is the definitive means of identifying the specific mycobacterial agent. These pathogens are slow growing, requiring special media and several weeks to establish visible colonies. Granulomatous lesions consist of areas of focal necrosis surrounded by infiltrations of plasma cells and macrophages and an outer connective tissue capsule. Calcification of granulomas may occur. Definitive diagnoses can be made by demonstrating intracellular acid-fast organisms within a lesion via biopsy and histologic examination of lesions or with direct smears of exudates or fluids. Tuberculous bacilli that are observed in cells are not usually numerous unless MAC is responsible. In contrast, the diagnosis of lepromatous infections in cats is made by finding large numbers of acid-fast bacilli on histologic or cytologic samples. Culture results are routinely negative. Confirming opportunistic mycobacteriosis is not always easy, because a diligent search for organisms in impression smears from exudates or tissue biopsy is usually required. Tissue biopsies generally reveal extensive granulomatous to pyogranulomatous inflammation of the dermis and panniculitis. Bacterial culture and identification of the organism are helpful for definitive diagnosis and long-term management; however, the time for bacterial isolation is long, necessitating treatment on the basis of cytologic and histologic findings. Polymerase chain reaction has facilitated diagnosis of human infections.[23]

Treatment of human tuberculosis involves several drug regimens, depending on whether the patient has been exposed and whether subclinical or active disease has been demonstrated. Similar guidelines might apply to affected pets, but the zoonotic aspect of a pet harboring *M. tuberculosis* must be considered. Long-term (6 months to 1 year) single-drug (isoniazid) regimens are used prophylactically when exposure with concurrent immunosuppression increases the likelihood of producing active disease. Combination chemotherapy using several agents is employed in treating active disease for a minimum of 6 to 9 months. An isoniazid-ethambutol-rifampin combination is used to treat people, but this is often hepatotoxic for dogs and cats. In most cases, active tuberculosis in dogs and cats is not treated and the animals are euthanized. Treatment of animals with *M. bovis* or *M. tuberculosis* var. *bovis* is also with combination therapy such as rifampin, fluoroquinolones, and clarithromycin. *M. avium* may temporarily respond to drugs used to treat both opportunistic or tuberculous mycobacterial infections. In most cases, there is minimal response to any drugs used, and the inevitable dissemination of the organism proves fatal. In a few dogs and cats, therapy with a combination of drugs including clofazimine has been successful in eliminating or suppressing active infection.[24, 25]

Surgical removal of lepromatous granulomas is the desired treatment. When surgery is not feasible or when removal is incomplete, cats have been treated with dapsone, rifampin, or clofazimine. Opportunistic mycobacteria are usually resistant to antituberculous drugs but respond variably to more conventional antibiotics such as aminoglycosides, tetracyclines, quinolones, and clofazimine (see Table 85–1).

BRUCELLOSIS

Brucella canis is a small gram-negative bacterium that naturally infects Canidae, causing an insidious bacteremia and reproductive disturbances. *B. canis* is most commonly transmitted venereally, penetrating the mucous membranes and entering the lymphoreticular system. Infection is transmitted during breeding or following abortion. Low numbers of organisms are seen in semen and urine. The highest number of organisms is found in aborted material. After contacting the mucous membranes, bacteria enter phagocytic cells and are transported to lymphatic and genital tract tissues, where they persist intracellularly. *B. canis* may also spread to nonreproductive tissues, such as intervertebral disks, eyes, and kidneys.

Despite generalized systemic infection with *B. canis,* adult dogs are rarely seriously ill. The organism has relatively low virulence. Fever is uncommon, and lymph node enlargement may be noted. The primary problems in intact male dogs are epididymitis, scrotal enlargement, and scrotal dermatitis. Bitches in late gestation (40 to 60 days) usually abort dead pups but show no other clinical signs. Pups are usually partially autolyzed. Conception failures also occur. In utero death with fetal resorption or abortion and ingestion of fetuses are usually interpreted as signs of infertility. Some pups are stillborn or weak. Nonreproductive abnormalities may include spinal hyperesthesia, paresis, or paralysis. Recurrent anterior uveitis has been detected in some infected dogs.

Hematologic and biochemical values are either unaltered or nonspecific in canine brucellosis. Hyperglobulinemia with concomitant hypoalbuminemia has been the most consistent finding in chronically infected dogs. Semen abnormalities include immature sperm, deformed acrosomes, swollen midpieces, detached tails, and head-to-head agglutination. Neutrophilic and mononuclear inflammation accompanies these changes.

Serologic testing is the most frequently used diagnostic method for detecting canine brucellosis. But with all antibody tests, they can be subject to errors in interpretation from cross-reactivity with other organisms. False-negative results can occur during the first 4 weeks after infection. Low or intermediate titers may be noted in early or prior infection. The rapid slide agglutination test (RSAT) is preferred as an in-office screening procedure because it is inexpensive, rapid, and sensitive and detects antibodies early (D-Tec CB, Synbiotics, San Diego, CA). There is a high correlation between a negative test and lack of infection. The tube agglutination test (TAT) is used by some laboratories following a positive RSAT to obtain confirmation and quantitative titers. Unfortunately, it suffers from the same nonspecific results and has not been well standardized among laboratories. Generally, with the TAT, titers of 200 or greater are highly presumptive of active infection, because they often correlate with positive blood culture. Titers of 100 are considered suspicious, and those less than 50 are considered negative. An agar gel diffusion test (AGID) has been developed as a sensitive procedure for the serodiagnosis of canine brucellosis. Two antigens, from either cell wall or cytoplasm, have been used in this test. With cytoplasmic antigens the test is more specific in detecting infection in dogs when other tests are equivocal or negative.[26] This test, performed by certain commercial laboratories, should be used as a confirmatory serologic procedure. Enzyme-linked immunosorbent assay (ELISA) and fluorescent antibody (FA) methods have been developed, but these have not been well standardized or widely evaluated.[27] Culture, if positive, is the only definitive way to resolve serologic differences. Blood is the best source for isolating the organism. False-negative results may occur in chronically infected dogs with intermittent bacteremia. Culture of the organism from urine or semen is unreliable. The organism may be found with culture of tissues at necropsy. Macroscopic changes in adults or surviving pups are usually confined to lymphadenopathy and splenomegaly. Histologic changes are those of diffuse lymphoreticular hyperplasia. A necrotizing vasculitis occurs in reproductive tissues, including the prostate, scrotum, sheath, and vulva.

Therapy of *B. canis* is difficult because of the intracellular persistence of the organism. Relapses are common once antimicrobial therapy is discontinued. For these reasons, repetitive courses are often indicated. Infected male dogs rarely, if ever, recover. They may become sterile. Infected female dogs have recovered in some instances and have been returned to breeding programs with extreme caution. It is recommended that pets be neutered. There is a public health risk of infecting people via canine genital secretions. Various antimicrobial agents have been considered for treatment.[28] Combination therapy offers the best chance for eliminating infection, usually with tetracyclines and aminoglycosides (see Table 85–1). Aminoglycosides such as gentamicin are given for the first and fourth weeks, with doxycycline or minocycline being given at high dosages for 4 weeks. Less efficacy has been seen with the substitution of tetracycline or chloramphenicol, but such regimens are less expensive and therefore more practical. The organism is also sensitive in vitro to ampicillin, trimethoprim-sulfonamides, and fluoroquinolones. However, dogs may respond poorly or not at all to these drugs when they are used alone or for a single course of therapy. Infected animals may have to be treated with two or more courses of antimicrobial therapy. Sequential serologic titers at 3- to 6-month intervals are used to monitor treatment efficacy. Cases of human infection caused by B. canis have been most common following contact with aborting bitches. Human infections with this species can be effectively treated with tetracyclines.

ACTINOMYCOSIS AND NOCARDIOSIS

Actinomycetales are branching, filamentous, gram-positive bacteria including the microaerophilic genus *Actinomyces* and the aerobic genus *Nocardia*. *Actinomyces* are commensal organisms found in the oral cavities of animals and people. Infection follows bite or puncture wounds or tissue trauma, which creates favorable environments for growth. Contamination of wounds may occur when they are licked by the affected host. *Nocardia* are acid-fast-staining, soil saprophytes that enter the body through contamination of wounds or by respiratory inhalation. Host immunocompetence is important in determining the entry and spread of both infections.

Actinomycosis has primarily been seen in large sporting breeds of dogs and in cats, producing localized pyogranulomatous infections.[29] Lesions include localized abscesses, chronic draining fistulas, bony infections, or infections of body cavities. Drainage from lesions is serosanguineous and often contains small yellow granules. Clinical signs are referable to the area of involvement and may be referable to localized swellings or accumulation of fluid in body cavities. Paraspinal or appendicular osteomyelitis causes signs of fever, reluctance to move, swelling of the extremities, or persistently draining fistulas. Paresis or paralysis develops in those animals with paraspinal lesions. Radiographic lesions seen in the bone are those of both lysis and periosteal proliferation.

Nocardia may cause clinical syndromes in dogs and cats that are similar to those of actinomycosis; however, in addition to localized pyogranulomas and body cavity effusions, a disseminated form that begins in the respiratory tract has been seen primarily in young dogs.[30, 31] Hematologic and biochemical findings in both infections are nonspecific and typical of any pyogenic inflammatory process. A leukocytosis with a left shift is typical. Cytologic examination of lesion exudate is most helpful and sometimes more specific if granules are present. When examined by microscopy, these gram-stained squash preparations consist of colonies

of gram-positive branching, filamentous rods and cocci. Acid-fast staining of the organisms helps to incriminate many *Nocardia*. Definitive diagnosis can be obtained only through culture of *Nocardia*, which grow aerobically or with carbon dioxide enrichment. For *Actinomyces*, samples should be obtained anaerobically in capped vials, and the laboratory should be alerted so that special growth conditions can be performed. Lesions compatible with these diseases should be biopsied and examined histologically; although they cannot be distinguished, the presence of the organisms can at least be established. Nocardial organisms may have to be visualized using Gram's or acid-fast stain.

Treatment for both diseases involves surgical drainage and debridement of affected areas, except in those cases in which infection is disseminated. Treatment for weeks to months with antibiotics is essential. Antimicrobial therapy is instituted based on the finding of the exudates. Antibiotic therapy is usually initiated before cultural identification of the organism. The majority of infections containing gram-positive branching, filamentous bacteria are mixed anaerobic infections with *Actinomyces*. They are sensitive to many antibacterials such as penicillins, chloramphenicol, or clindamycin (see Table 85–1). Although effective against the organism, penicillin has difficulty penetrating pyogranulomatous lesions. Therefore, high doses and long courses of treatment are recommended. In contrast, antimicrobial therapy for *Nocardia* infections includes trimethoprim-sulfonamides as the first choice, followed by aminoglycosides or tetracyclines (see Table 85–1). Combination therapy may be needed if resistance is noted. Treatment is usually for a 6-week period unless early and dramatic resolution is noted. Therapy should not be discontinued until several weeks after all signs are gone, because relapse is frequent. Foreign bodies (especially "foxtails") should be suspected, and surgical drainage should be considered, if lesions recur after therapy is stopped.

STREPTOCOCCOSIS

Streptococci are gram-positive, nonmotile, facultatively anaerobic cocci that cause localized to widespread pyogenic infections. Most are commensals of the skin and mucous membranes with a few pathogenic variants. Those species that produce beta-hemolysis or clearing around colonies on blood agar tend to be more pathogenic. Organisms in the nonhemolytic group are found on mucous membranes and skin of clinically healthy animals and are considered contaminants. Streptococci are usually classified into groups based on the antigenic reaction of their cell wall carbohydrates.

Group A streptococci are primarily commensal and pathogenic species in people. Two species, S. pyogenes and S. pneumoniae, are mainly involved. The latter species has been isolated in only one cat.[32] Reports of infection with S. pyogenes are more frequent in dogs and cats. Group A streptococcal infections are acquired by dogs and cats from direct or close contact with humans.[33] Some humans are carriers and show no signs of illness. Prevalence rates for group A streptococci are higher in young children. Domestic pets that contract the infection show no clinical illness or tonsillar enlargement. Dogs and cats are only transiently infected, unlike their human counterparts. Isolates of group A streptococci from dogs have shown the greatest susceptibility to penicillin, erythromycin, and chloramphenicol (see Table 85–1).

Group B streptococci have been reported to cause endometritis, with birth of pups that develop bacteremia, pyelone-phritis, and necrotizing pneumonia. Group G streptococci have been more commonly isolated than group B as causes of neonatal sepsis. Similarly, peritonitis with septicemia, parturient endometritis, and placentitis have been described in cats. Therapy is similar to that for group A streptococcal infections.

Group C infections have been described only in dogs, although both dogs and cats have these organisms as commensal flora. Acute hemorrhagic and purulent pneumonia has been described in dogs. Weakness, coughing, dyspnea, fever, hematemesis, and red urine have been the predominant clinical signs, which may or may not precede acute death. Group C isolates have been made from less severe infections in dogs, and septicemia and pneumonia have been described in captive coyotes.[34]

Group G streptococci are the predominant resident micro-floral isolates that cause the majority of streptococcal infections in cats and dogs.[35, 36] In neonatal animals, the source of streptococci is the vagina of the queen or bitch, and subsequent umbilical infections may result in bacteremic spread. Cervical lymphadenitis results in surviving juveniles, and spread to joints is possible. Other group G infections that affect cats are often opportunistic and follow wounds, trauma, surgical procedures, viral infections, or immune-suppressive conditions. These suppurative infections can result in septicemia and embolic lesions, most often in the lung and heart. As with other streptococci, those in group G are sensitive to penicillin and its derivatives. Appropriate surgical drainage hastens response to antimicrobial therapy. For prevention of infection in newborns, dipping the umbilical cord in 2 per cent tincture of iodine and treatment of all kittens at birth with ampicillin, amoxicillin, or procaine and benzathine penicillin combined have been successful.

Toxic shock and necrotizing fasciitis are syndromes of toxigenic streptococcal infections in people, and similar syndromes have been observed in dogs and cats.[37, 38] This has also been termed flesh-eating bacterial infection. Most cases follow wound infections or respiratory or urinary infections. Ulcerative and purulent skin lesions associated with lymphadenomegaly may initially appear, followed by rapidly advancing cellulitis and associated discomfort. Animals may develop signs of septic shock. Streptococcal organisms may be identified in exudates or aspirates of affected tissues. Surgical debridement with systemic antimicrobial therapy is required. Penicillin G and aminopenicillins are the preferred antibiotics for treatment of affected dogs and cats.

RHODOCOCCOSIS

Rhodococcus equi (previously *Corynebacterium equi*) is a soil-borne, pleomorphic, gram-positive bacillus that has been associated primarily with suppurative infections in domestic livestock. *R. equi* has been isolated from lesions in dogs, but abscesses in cats have been most commonly reported. Affected animals are typically from an environment with exposure to domestic herbivores. The organism usually gains access to the body from penetrating wounds. Pyogranulomatous lesions develop at the site of inoculation, with localized swelling and ulceration. Diagnosis is made by culture, and treatment involves surgical drainage and antimicrobial therapy. Although amputation may seem excessive for extremity lesions, infection commonly recurs even with such radical measures. Lincomycin and gentamicin have been the most effective choices for antimicrobial therapy (see Table 85–1).

BORRELIOSIS

Lyme borreliosis is one of a larger group of tick-borne spirochetoses that affect people and animals worldwide. These diseases can be divided into the Lyme disease group transmitted by ixodid ticks and the relapsing fever group transmitted by soft ticks. The Lyme disease group has been recognized more recently. It is caused by *Borrelia burgdorferi sensu lato,* which is divided into at least four species affecting people and dogs worldwide.[39–41] Other species have been isolated from ticks and wildlife in various countries. *B. burgdorferi sensu stricto* predominates in affected people in the United States, and *B. garinii* and *B. afzelii* predominate in Europe. *B japonica* has been isolated from ticks on people and dogs in Japan. The presence of disease and its clinical features are dependent on the isolate that is responsible for infection in a given geographic region. Genetic variability of isolates also occurs within each continent. The natural disease in cats is poorly documented, although cats can be infected experimentally.

The primary established vectors causing Lyme borrelioses worldwide are various species of the *Ixodes ricinus* complex. As a model species in North America, *I. scapularis* is a three-host tick with a 2-year life cycle. Infected nymphs overwinter, and in the spring they transmit infection to reservoir hosts, which in turn infect feeding larvae. Larvae and nymphs feed primarily on rodents and small mammals, whereas adult ticks feed on deer or larger mammals. People and pets are usually infected by nymphs or adult ticks. Other ticks and insect vectors have been found to harbor *B. burgdorferi sensu lato* but do not seem to maintain the infection or be important in transmission.

The pathogenesis of the clinical syndrome is produced primarily by the host reaction to the organism, which has the ability to survive for extended periods in tissue. Following tick attachment, organisms enter hosts and spread into connective tissue, joints, and other tissues. After several weeks of infection, organisms are present in extremely small quantities in host tissues. The host inflammatory response to their presence causes disease manifestations.[42]

Cats have been found to be seropositive for this infection, and experimental infection has been produced,[43] but naturally acquired disease has not been documented. In experimentally infected dogs, clinical illness begins 60 to 90 days after inoculation.[44] Clinical signs include fever, inappetence, lethargy, lymphadenopathy, and episodic shifting limb lameness related to polyarthritis. The dermatologic lesion of expanding erythema around the site of a tick bite has not been well documented in affected dogs. Protein-losing glomerulopathy progressing to renal failure has also been observed.[45] Neurologic manifestations caused by meningitis or encephalitis have not been well documented in either experimental or natural canine infections.

No specific hematologic or biochemical changes have been associated with Lyme disease. Dogs with renal localization of infection may have azotemia, proteinuria with variable hematuria, pyuria, and tubular casts. Synovial fluid analysis findings are typical for a suppurative polyarthritis, with leukocyte counts ranging from 2000 to 100,000 nucleated cells/μL. Spirochetes have rarely been isolated from joint fluid. Serotesting has been the mainstay for diagnosis of this disease. Screening titers using whole bacteria as antigen have some cross-reactivity with other spirochetes, and subclinical infections occur in endemic areas. Both these features contribute to seroreactivity observed in uninfected dogs. Immunoglobulin M (IgM) titers usually increase within the first weeks of infection in experimentally infected dogs; however, in naturally infected dogs and people, the IgM titers can persist. Interlaboratory variation means that absolute titers cannot be equated.[46] Antibody titers of clinically ill and asymptomatic dogs often overlap in endemic areas, making titer information difficult to interpret. Purified-protein antigen assays or immunoblotting has been used in an attempt to identify nonspecific reactions, but they do not distinguish active disease from past infections. Identification or isolation of *B. burgdorferi* from tissues or body fluids is definitive but extremely difficult and requires Barbour-Stoenner-Kelly II media. Tissue or fluid samples can be evaluated microscopically for the presence of pathogenic spirochetes using immunofluorescence and specific monoclonal antibodies or with polymerase chain reaction (PCR) in research laboratories.[47, 48]

Antibiotics that are most effective for treating borreliosis are tetracyclines, ampicillin or amoxicillin, some third-generation cephalosporins, or erythromycin and its derivatives.[49] Doxycycline is usually the drug of choice for treatment of dogs with acute infection (see Table 85–1). The other drugs are usually reserved for refractory or chronic infections. Research suggests that the organism is difficult to eliminate from animals with established infection, and relapses occur despite seemingly adequate treatment regimens. Aspirin or other nonsteroidal anti-inflammatory drugs or glucocorticoids may be helpful for pain relief during episodes of recurrent synovitis. Only anti-inflammatory doses of glucocorticoids should be used in the face of spirochetemia. Infected dogs serve as a sentinel for human infection but in themselves probably pose a minimal health risk. Greater danger might be associated with dogs bringing ticks into close proximity of people. Vaccines are available in the United States that are protective in challenge exposure studies.[50] There are two whole-cell and one genetic recombinant vaccine. To be effective, vaccines must be given before exposure to infected ticks. Vaccination may induce serum antibody titers, which may make subsequent titer interpretations difficult, and is not generally recommended in nonendemic areas. Immunoblotting must be used to distinguish vaccine-induced from natural exposure titers. Tick control using residual insecticides or growth regulators is important in endemic areas.

LEPTOSPIROSIS

Leptospirosis, a disease of worldwide significance in many animals, is caused by infection with antigenically distinct serovars of the motile spirochetal bacterium *Leptospira interrogans sensu lato*. Domestic and wild animals serve as potential reservoirs of infection for humans and other animal hosts. *L. grippotyphosa, L. pomona*, and *L. bratislava* are the most common serovars isolated from or serologically detected among infected dogs. *L. icterohaemorrhagiae* and *L. canicola* are now less frequent, presumably because of vaccination. Clinical reports of leptospirosis in cats are rare. Leptospires can be transmitted directly between animals by close contact as the organism penetrates the mucosa. Shedding by infected animals is usually via the urine. Indirect transmission, which is more frequent, occurs through exposure of susceptible animals to a contaminated environment, especially one with stagnant or slow-moving warm water.

Leptospires multiply rapidly upon entering the blood vascular space and produce damage to many organs in suscepti-

ble hosts. Inflammation caused by initial replication of the spirochete causes damage to the kidneys and liver. Recovery from infection is dependent on increased specific antibody production. Renal colonization occurs in most infected animals because the organism can persist in renal tubular epithelial cells. Coagulation dysfunction in severe acute infection may occur as a result of disseminated intravascular coagulation. Clinical signs in canine leptospirosis depend on age and immunity of the host, environmental factors affecting the organisms, and virulence of the infecting serovar. Peracute leptospiral infections cause massive leptospiremia, shock, and death. Less severe infections cause fever, anorexia, vomiting, dehydration, increased thirst, and reluctance to move. Progressive deterioration in renal function results in oliguria or anuria. Icterus occurs in some dogs. A majority of leptospiral infections in dogs are chronic or subclinical, but the animals may have acute renal failure. Serologic and microbiologic evaluation for leptospirosis should be performed on dogs with fever of unknown origin or unexplained renal dysfunction. Clinical signs are usually mild or inapparent in feline leptospirosis, despite the presence of leptospiremia and leptospiruria and histologic evidence of renal and hepatic inflammation.

Hematologic findings in typical cases of canine leptospirosis include leukocytosis and thrombocytopenia.[51, 52] Serum urea nitrogen and creatinine concentration increases occur in dogs with varying severity of renal failure. Electrolyte alterations usually parallel the degree of renal and gastrointestinal dysfunction. Liver damage is demonstrated by high serum hepatic transaminase activity and bilirubinuria.

The microscopic agglutination test is the standard serologic method for diagnosing leptospirosis. Demonstration of a fourfold rise in a titer is often required for serologic confirmation of disease. Because titers are often negative in the first week of illness, a second and sometimes a third serum sample should be obtained within 2- to 4-week intervals. Proper timing and technique are essential for the recovery of leptospires; they are fastidious, and sampling should precede institution of antimicrobial therapy. Urine is the best fluid for dark-field examination and culture purposes. Fluorescent antibody and PCR techniques have been adapted to identify leptospiral serovars in tissues and body fluids.[53] At necropsy of dogs dying acutely, lesions can include icterus, petechiation on the surfaces of many organs, and diffuse swelling of the lungs, liver, and kidneys. Renal function abnormalities in chronically infected animals do not always correlate with the severity of histologic changes.

Supportive therapy for animals with leptospirosis depends on the severity of infection and the presence of renal or hepatic dysfunction and other complicating factors. Fluids must be given to overcome shock and dehydration, and chemical diuresis with osmotic agents (10 per cent glucose at 2.5 mL/lb) or tubular diuretics (furosemide) is needed for oliguric animals. Antibiotics immediately inhibit multiplication of the organism and rapidly reduce fatal complications of infection such as hepatic and renal failure. Penicillin is the antibiotic of choice for terminating leptospiremia, as it is effective and is not contraindicated in renal failure. Following recovery, doxycycline or aminoglycosides should be given to eradicate the carrier state (see Table 85–1).

Prevention of leptospirosis involves elimination of the carrier state. Control of shedding by wild animal reservoirs is impossible. For this reason, vaccination of dogs is essential. Bivalent inactivated bacterins that contain two main serovars, *L. canicola* and *L. icterohaemorrhagiae*, are available for dogs. Immunization has been effective in reducing the prevalence and severity of canine leptospirosis, but it does not prevent the carrier state, nor does it protect against infection with other serovars. Because highest titers are produced by multiple injections, annual vaccinations should be given to dogs in endemic areas, and all dogs should receive at least three injections in their primary vaccination series. From a public health standpoint, contaminated urine is highly infectious for people and for susceptible animal species; therefore, contact on mucous membranes or skin abrasions should be avoided.

TETANUS

Tetanus is caused by the action of a potent neurotoxin formed in the body by *Clostridium tetani*, a motile, gram-positive, nonencapsulated, anaerobic, spore-forming bacillus. Resistant spores of the organism can be found in the environment, especially in rich soil, and it enters the body when wounds become contaminated. Dogs and cats are relatively resistant to the effects of the toxin compared with other species. Toxin enters the axons of the nearest motor nerves at the neuromuscular end plate and migrates by retrograde transport within motor axons to the neuronal cell body within the spinal cord or brain stem. Toxin can spread within the CNS in this fashion or be taken in the bloodstream from the area of the wound to nerves at distant sites. Thus the disease can present as a localized progressive illness or as a more generalized syndrome. Tetanus toxin has been shown to block inhibitory transmission to motor neurons. It has additional actions on the neuromuscular junction and autonomic ganglia, which can cause additional visceral and motor neuron disturbances.

Clinical signs of tetanus usually occur within 5 days to 3 weeks of injury. Because dogs and cats have innate resistance to the disease, their injuries are often substantial enough to warrant notice. Localized tetanus is manifest by increased stiffness of a muscle or an entire limb, first noted in close proximity to the wound site.[54] The stiffness usually spreads gradually from there and may involve the entire nervous system. An animal with tetanus holds its ears erect and has its ears and facial muscles drawn back (risus sardonicus), with protrusion of the third eyelid. Other signs include trismus (lockjaw), increased salivation, altered heart and respiratory rates, laryngeal spasm, and dysphagia. Regurgitation and gastroesophageal reflux may result from esophageal hiatal hernia.[55] Mild stimulation may precipitate periodic generalized tonic contraction of all muscles with opisthotonos or may precipitate grand mal convulsions. Death results from inability to breathe properly.

The history of a recent wound and the clinical signs are the primary means of making a diagnosis of tetanus. Isolation of *C. tetani* from wounds can be a difficult procedure and is unrewarding in most cases.

Therapy for severely affected animals is costly and labor intensive. Mildly diseased animals recover from their neurologic dysfunction with wound management alone. Antitoxin is administered intravenously at a rate of 5 to 50 IU/lb, although precautions must be taken to reduce anaphylaxis. Pretesting the animal for hypersensitivity can be done by ID injection. Antihistamines can be preadministered if allergic complications are anticipated. Glucocorticoids and epinephrine may be needed if a reaction develops. Local and parenteral antibiotic therapy should be instituted in an attempt to kill any vegetative *C. tetani* organisms present in the wound. Penicillin G is the drug of choice and is usually given intravenously or intramuscularly in high dosages. Other drugs that should be effective are tetracycline and metronidazole (see Table 85–1). Sedation may be needed for an excitable animal, and phenothiazines appear to be highly effective, even though they are contraindicated in most seizure disorders. Supportive measures are imperative in the successful management of an animal with tetanus. Fluids are needed for hydration, and tracheostomy may be required if laryngeal spasm is severe. Esophagostomy or gastrostomy tubes may be needed if trismus prevents eating. In mildly affected animals, normal function usually returns within 3 weeks after treatment is instituted. The prognosis for severely affected animals is extremely guarded, and many die as a result of complications associated with cardiovascular dysfunction or uncontrollable muscle spasms.

BOTULISM

Clostridium botulinum is a gram-positive, anaerobic, spore-forming soil saprophyte that produces a neurotoxin that causes neuromuscular paralysis. Most cases of botulism in animals are caused by ingestion of the preformed toxin in food. Natural cases in dogs have been attributed to eating carrion or raw meat. The disease in cats is similar to that in dogs, although there are no reports of naturally occurring disease. Once ingested, the toxin is absorbed from the stomach and upper small bowel into lymphatics. The toxin circulates to the neuromuscular junction of cholinergic nerves, where it exerts its effects. Botulinal toxin prevents the presynaptic release of acetylcholine. The blockage of acetylcholine release results in generalized lower motor neuron disease and parasympathetic dysfunction.

Clinical signs are of a symmetric, ascending weakness from the rear to the forelimbs that can result in quadriplegia. Limb reflexes are depressed, and cranial nerve motor responses are affected, causing mydriasis, decreased jaw tone, decreased gag reflexes, and excess salivation. Megaesophagus may be present. Pain perception is intact, and muscle atrophy and hyperesthesia do not develop. Death may result from respiratory paralysis. The duration of illness in dogs that recovered ranged from 1 to 3 weeks.

Hematologic and biochemical parameters are unaffected. Electromyography shows conduction defects primarily in the neuromuscular junction and less in the peripheral nerve. Confirmatory diagnosis of botulism is based on the finding of the toxin in serum, feces, vomitus, or samples of the food that was ingested.

Supportive treatment is most important, because spontaneous recovery occurs in moderately affected animals if respiratory and urinary tract infections can be avoided. Affected animals should be padded when recumbent and assisted to eat and drink. For specific treatment, antitoxin is relatively unavailable, and its use is controversial. Despite ingestion of preformed toxin, penicillin or metronidazole has been recommended to reduce any potential intestinal population of clostridia (see Table 85–1). Botulinal toxin is destroyed by heating for 100°C for 10 minutes. Preventing access to carrion and thorough cooking of any food fed to dogs can reduce the prevalence of the disease.

FELINE ABSCESSES

Percutaneous abscesses are the most common bacterial infection of feline skin. Because abscesses usually result from bites and scratches, the most common organisms found within them are resident oral microflora, and anaerobes predominate. *Pasteurella multocida* is the most common aerobic organism isolated. Clinical signs of abscess formation in cats reflect the site and severity of infection. Abscesses are usually located around the cat's legs, face, back, and base of the tail. Some cats develop mild swellings with few other signs of illness, whereas others have fever, anorexia, depression, hyperesthesia, and regional lymphadenopathy. Drainage of creamy, purulent material occurs spontaneously or following surgical lancing, and systemic signs often abate once the abscess ruptures. In complicated cases, the abscess can migrate in tissues or infection can disseminate hematogenously, causing signs typical to the organ system involved. A mature neutrophilia is characteristic of a walled-off or mature abscess, whereas diffuse cellulitis or septicemia is manifest by a lower white blood cell count with a degenerative left shift.

Small localized abscesses may drain spontaneously by the time the cat is presented for examination, in which case only clipping and cleansing of the area are required. Deeper or more extensive abscesses require surgical drainage. Antibiotics alone are ineffective in penetrating walled-off abscesses, which require surgical drainage. Penicillin derivatives are the antibiotics of choice for treating abscesses because they are bactericidal and have marked activity against the more frequently encountered organisms. Penicillin V, amoxicillin, or ampicillin may be dispensed in oral forms to be administered by the client. Drugs such as metronidazole can be used if foul-smelling or discolored discharges suggest a predominance of anaerobic infection (see Table 85–1). Castration is recommended as a preventive measure because it reduces the fighting and roaming behavior of male cats.

BARTONELLOSIS

Bartonella are arthropod-transmitted gram-negative bacteria that cause disease in people and animals. Their human health significance has been established for many years, but infection in dogs and cats has only recently been elucidated. Trench fever from World War II was caused by *B. quintana*, a louse-borne organism that is now also known to cause bacillary angiomatosis (BA), endocarditis, and lymphadenomegaly in people. *B. henselae* and *B. clarridgeiae* are the cause of cat scratch disease and are presumed to be flea transmitted.[56] *B. henselae* has been associated with bacteremia, meningitis, BA, and endocarditis in people. Both these *Bartonella* species infect cats, but their significance in causing clinical illness in their reservoir host is uncertain. Experimental infections have been associated with clinical signs, but naturally infected cats have few signs. *B. vinsonii* subsp. *berkhoffii*, which is transmitted by *Rhipicephalus sanguineus*, has been isolated from the blood of healthy and diseased dogs.[57, 58] Affected dogs have shown signs of endocarditis, including shifting leg lameness, fever, and heart murmurs.

Diagnosis of bartonellosis is based on cultivation of the organism from blood. The bacteria are associated with the erythrocytes, and whole blood must be used. Efficacy of treatment of bacteremia in cats has not been clearly established. There is some suppression of the level of bacteremia with doxycycline or enrofloxacin (see Table 85–1), but it may rebound within several weeks after therapy is discontinued.[59] Treatment for 2 to 4 weeks is recommended, and follow-up cultures should be taken to confirm its effectiveness. Because fleas appear to be important in the acquisition

and transmission of infection between cats, control measures should be instituted. Although scratch or bite injuries have been related to human infections, fleas may be involved in transmitting infection to people through their bites or by contaminating the animal's haircoat or local environment with excreta.

REFERENCES

1. Chengappa MM, Staats J, Oberst RD, et al: Prevalence of *Salmonella* in raw meat used in diets of racing greyhounds. J Vet Diagn Invest 5:372, 1993.
2. Wall PG, Davis S, Threlfall EJ, et al: Chronic carriage of multidrug resistant *Salmonella typhimurium* in a cat. J Small Anim Pract 36:279, 1995.
3. Weber A, Wachowitz R, Weigl U, et al: Occurence of *Salmonella* in fecal samples of dogs and cats in northern Bavaria from 1975 to 1994. Berl Munch Tierarztl Wochenschr 108:401, 1995.
4. Dow SW, Jones RL, Henik RA, et al: Clinical features of salmonellosis in cats: Six cases (1981–1986). JAVMA 194:1464, 1989.
5. Dusch H, Altwegg M: Evaluation of five new plating media for isolation of *Salmonella* species. J Clin Microbiol 33:802, 1995.
6. Sugiyama Y, Sugiyama F, Yagami K: Isolation of *Salmonella* from impounded dogs introduced in a laboratory. Exp Anim 42:119, 1993.
7. Stanley J, Jones C, Burnens A, et al: Distinct genotypes of human and canine isolates of *Campylobacter upsalensis* determined by 16S rRNA gene typing and plasmid profiling. J Clin Microbiol 32:1788, 1994.
8. Burnens AP, Angeloz-Wick B, Nicolet J: Comparison of *Campylobacter* carriage rates in diarrheic and healthy pet animals. Zentralbl Veterinarmed 39:175, 1992.
9. Oswald GP, Twedt DC, Steyn P: *Campylobacter jejuni* bacteremia and acute cholecystitis in two dogs. J Am Anim Hosp Assoc 30:165, 1994.
10. Fox JG, Taylor NS, Penner JL, et al: Investigation of zoonotic acquired *Campylobacter jejuni* enteritis with serotyping and restriction endonuclease DNA analysis. J Clin Microbiol 27:2423, 1989.
11. Handt LK, Fox JG, Dewhirst FE, et al: *Helicobacter pylori* isolated from the domestic cat: Public health implications. Infect Immun 62:2367, 1994.
12. Fox JG, Drolet R, Higgins R, et al: *Helicobacter canis* isolated from a dog liver with multifocal necrotizing hepatitis. J Clin Microbiol 34:2479, 1996.
13. Duncan AJ, Carman RJ, Olsen GJ, et al: Assignment of the agent of Tyzzers disease to *Clostridium* piliforme comb-nov on the basis of 16S ribosomal-RNA sequence analysis. Int J Syst Bacteriol 43:314, 1993.
14. Gunn-Moore DA, Jenkins JA, Lucke VM: Feline tuberculosis: A literature review and discussion of 19 cases caused by an unusual mycobacterial variant. Vet Rec 138:53, 1996.
15. Frieden TR, Sterling T, Pablos-Mendez A, et al: The emergence of drug-resistant tuberculosis in New York City. N Engl J Med 328:521, 1993.
16. de Lisle GW, Collins DM, Loveday AS, et al: A report of tuberculosis in cats in New Zealand and the examination of strains of *Mycobacterium bovis* by DNA restriction endonuclease analysis. N Z Vet J 38:10, 1990.
17. Jordan HL, Cohn LA, Armstrong DJ: Disseminated *Mycobacterium avium* complex infection in three Siamese cats. JAVMA 204:90, 1994.
18. Clercx C, Coignoul F, Jakovljevic S, et al: Tuberculosis in dogs: A case report and review of the literature. J Am Anim Hosp Assoc 28:207, 1992.
19. Fox LE, Kunkle GA, Homer BL, et al: Disseminated subcutaneous *Mycobacterium fortuitum* infection in a dog. JAVMA 206:53, 1995.
20. Grooters AM, Couto CG, Andrews JM, et al: Systemic *Mycobacterium smegmatis* infection in a dog. JAVMA 206:200, 1995.
21. Malik R, Hunt GB, Goldsmid SE, et al: Diagnosis and treatment of pyogranulomatous panniculitis due to *Mycobacterium smegmatis* in cats. J Small Anim Pract 35:524, 1994.
22. Greene CE: Tuberculous mycobacterial infections. *In* Greene CE (ed): Infectious Diseases of the Dog and Cat. Philadelphia, WB Saunders, 1990, pp 558–566.
23. Kocagoz T, Yilmaz E, Ozkara S, et al: Detection of *Mycobacterium tuberculosis* in sputum samples by polymerase chain reaction using a simplified procedure. J Clin Microbiol 31:1435, 1993.
24. Kaufman AC, Greene CE, Rakich P, et al: Treatment of localized *Mycobacterium avium* complex infection in a cat with clofazimine and doxycycline. JAVMA 207:457, 1995.
25. Miller MA, Greene CE, Brix AE: Disseminated *Mycobacterium avium-intracellulare* infection in a miniature schnauzer. J Am Anim Hosp Assoc 31:213, 1995.
26. Carmichael LE, Joubert JC, Jones L: Characterization of *Brucella canis* protein antigens and polypeptide antibody responses of infected dogs. Vet Microbiol 19:373, 1989.
27. Mateu de Antonio EM, Martin M, Soler M: Use of indirect enzyme-linked immunosorbent assay with hot saline solution extracts of a variant (M−) strain of *Brucella canis* for diagnosis of brucellosis in dogs. Am J Vet Res 54:1043, 1993.
28. Mateu de Antonio EM, Martin M: In vitro efficacy of several antimicrobial combinations against *Brucella canis* and *Brucella melitensis* strains isolated from dogs. Vet Microbiol 45:1, 1995.
29. Donohue DE, Brightman AH: Cervicofacial *Actinomyces viscosus* infection in a Brazilian fila: A case report and literature review. J Am Anim Hosp Assoc 31:501, 1995.

30. Marino DJ, Jaggy A: Nocardiosis: A literature review with selected case reports in two dogs. J Vet Intern Med 7:4, 1993.
31. Kirpenstein J, Fingland RB: Cutaneous actinomycosis and nocardiosis in dogs: 48 cases (1980–1990). JAVMA 201:917, 1992.
32. Stallings B, Ling GV, Lagenaur LA, et al: Septicemia and septic arthritis caused by *Streptococcus pneumoniae* in a cat: Possible transmission from a child. JAVMA 191:703, 1987.
33. Wilson KS, Maroney SA, Gander RM: The family pet as an unlikely source of group A beta-hemolytic streptococcal infection in humans. Pediatr Infect Dis J 14:372, 1995.
34. Gates NL, Green JS: Epizootic streptococcal pneumonia in captive coyotes. J Wildl Dis 15:497, 1979.
35. Iglauer F, Kunstyr I, Moerstedt R, et al: *Streptococcus canis* arthritis in a cat breeding colony. J Exp Anim Sci 34:59, 1991.
36. Bjurstrom L: Aerobic bacteria occurring in the vagina of bitches with reproductive disorders. Acta Vet Scand 34:29, 1993.
37. White S: Further evidence of streptococcal toxic shock syndrome in pets. JAVMA 209:1994, 1996.
38. Prescott JF, Mathews K, Gyles CL, et al: Canine streptococcal toxic shock syndrome in Ontario: An emerging disease? Can Vet J 36:486, 1995.
39. Baranton G, Postic D, Saint GI, et al: Delineation of *Borrelia burgdorferi sensu stricto, Borrelia garinii* sp nov., and group VS461 associated with Lyme borreliosis. Int J Syst Bacteriol 42:378, 1992.
40. Filipuzzi-Jenny E, Blot M, Schmid-Berger N, et al: Genetic diversity among *Borrelia burgdorferi* isolates: More than three genospecies? Res Microbiol 144:295, 1993.
41. Canica MM, Nato F, du Merle L, et al: Monoclonal antibodies for identification of *Borrelia afzelii* sp nov. associated with late cutaneous manifestations of Lyme borreliosis. Scand J Infect Dis 25:441, 1993.
42. Persing DH, Rutledge BJ, Rys PN, et al: Target imbalance: Disparity of *Borrelia burgdorferi* genetic material in synovial fluid from Lyme arthritis patients. J Infect Dis 169:668, 1994.
43. Gibson MD, Young CR, Tawfik OM, et al: *Borrelia burgdorferi* infection of cats. JAVMA 202:1786, 1993.
44. Appel MJG, Allan S, Jacobson RH, et al: Experimental Lyme disease in dogs produces arthritis and persistent infection. J Infect Dis 167:651, 1993.
45. Dembach DM, Smith CA, Lewis RM, et al: Morphologic, immunohistochemical, and ultrastructural characterization of a distinctive renal lesion in dogs puta-

46. Greene RT, Hirsch D, Rottman PL, et al: Interlaboratory comparison of titers of antibody to *Borrelia burgdorferi* and evaluation of a commercial assay using canine sera. J Clin Microbiol 29:16, 1991.
47. Nocton JJ, Dressler F, Rutledge BJ, et al: Detection of *Borrelia burgdorferi* DNA by polymerase chain reaction in synovial fluid from patients with Lyme arthritis. N Engl J Med 330:229, 1994.
48. Salinas-Metendez JA, Tamez-Gonzalez R, Welsh-Lozano O, et al: Detection of *Borrelia burgdorferi* DNA in human skin biopsies and dog synovial fluid by the polymerase chain reaction. Rev Latinoam Microbiol 37:7, 1995.
49. Johnson RC, Kodner CB, Jurkovich PJ, et al: Comparative in vitro and in vivo susceptibilities of the Lyme disease spirochete *Borrelia burgdorferi* to cefuroxime and other antimicrobial agents. Antimicrob Agents Chemother 34:2133, 1990.
50. Chu HJ, Chaavez LG, Blumer BM, et al: Immunogenicity and efficacy study of a commercial *Borrelia burgdorferi* bacterin. JAVMA 201:403, 1992.
51. Brown CA, Roberts AW, Miller MA, et al: *Leptospira interrogans* serovar grippotyphosa infection in dogs. JAVMA 209:1265, 1996.
52. Rentko VT, Clark N, Ross LA, et al: Canine leptospirosis: A retrospective study of 17 cases. J Vet Intern Med 6:235, 1992.
53. Merien F, Amouriaux P, Perolat P, et al: Polymerase chain reaction for detection of *Leptospira* spp. in clinical samples. J Clin Microbiol 30:2219, 1992.
54. Malik R, Church DB, Maddison JE, et al: Three cases of localized tetanus. J Small Anim Pract 30:469, 1989.
55. Van Ham L, Van Bree H: Conservative treatment of tetanus associated with hiatus hernia and gastroesophageal reflux. J Small Anim Pract 33:289, 1992.
56. Chomel BB, Kasten RW, Floyd-Hawkins K, et al: Experimental transmission of *Bartonella henselae* by the cat flea. J Clin Microbiol 34:1952, 1996.
57. Kordick DL, Swaminathan B, Greene CE, et al: *Bartonella vinsonii* subsp. *berkhoffii* subsp. nov., isolated from dogs; *Bartonella vinsonii* subsp. *vinsonii*; and emended description of *Bartonella vinsonii*. Int J Syst Bacteriol 46:704, 1996.
58. Pappalardo BL, Correa MT, York CC, et al: Epidemiologic evaluation of the risk factors associated with exposure and seroreactivity to *Bartonella vinsonii* in dogs. Am J Vet Res 58:467, 1997.
59. Greene CE, McDermott M, Jameson PH, et al: *Bartonella henselae* infection in cats: Evaluation during primary infection, treatment, and rechallenge infection. J Clin Microbiol 34:1682, 1996.

tively associated with *Borrelia burgdorferi* infection: 49 cases (1987–1992). Vet Pathol 34:85, 1997.

CHAPTER 86

THE RICKETTSIOSES

Edward B. Breitschwerdt

Rickettsiae are arthropod-transmitted, small, obligate intracellular, gram-negative, pleomorphic coccobacilli bacterial organisms in the order Rickettsiales. The family Rickettsiaceae continues to be redefined by new molecular classification techniques. The families Bartonellaceae and Anaplasmataceae are no longer included in the order Rickettsiales. The family Rickettsiaceae includes three tribes: Rickettsiae, Ehrlichieae, and Wolbachieae. Organisms within the tribe Wolbachieae are arthropod pathogens or symbiotes and are not known to be pathogenic for vertebrates. Within the genera *Rickettsia* and *Ehrlichia* there are numerous species that are pathogenic for animals and humans. Rickettsial pathogens are found throughout the world; can be transmitted by ticks, fleas, or chiggers; and can induce disease ranging in severity from subclinical to life-threatening.

SPOTTED FEVER GROUP RICKETTSIAE

The spotted fever group (SFG) rickettsiae have been described from all continents. The group includes nine species—*Rickettsia rickettsii* (the type species), *R. africae, R. akari, R. australis, R. conorii, R. montana, R. parkeri, R. rhipicephali,* and *R. sibirica*—although many other SFG rickettsiae have been described. SFG rickettsiae are transmitted by *Dermacentor, Rhipicephalus, Haemaphysalis,* and *Amblyomma* species of ticks. Rickettsia-induced endothelial cell damage results in vasculitis, altered vascular permeability, edema, and necrosis.[1] As the most pathogenic of the SFG rickettsiae, *R. rickettsii* is considered in detail.

ROCKY MOUNTAIN SPOTTED FEVER

Rocky Mountain spotted fever (RMSF) is a tick-transmitted rickettsial disease of dogs, people, and other vertebrate species. The causative agent is *R. rickettsii*. Although canine susceptibility to *R. rickettsii* was established in 1933, information related to the naturally occurring disease first appeared in the literature in 1979. RMSF is a relatively common cause of canine illness, and untreated disease can be fatal.[2, 3] The majority of human and presumably canine cases of RMSF occur in the southeastern United States, with cases reported from throughout the United States, western Canada, Mexico, and South America. Distribution of the disease is related to the distribution of the vector ticks *Dermacentor variabilis*, the American dog tick found in the eastern United States, and *Dermacentor andersoni*, the wood tick, which is the principal vector in the western United States. Although not considered vectors in North America, *Rhipicephalus sanguineus* and *Amblyomma cajennense* are capable of transmitting *R. rickettsii* in Central and South America. In ticks, *R. rickettsii* is transmitted both transovarially and transstadially. Within the tick population in a given region, few ticks contain potentially infective *R. rickettsii*. However, there are geographic foci that contain large numbers of infective ticks, most likely related to transovarial transmission of *R. rickettsii* and to restricted territorial movement of small mammals that also serve as hosts. Because of the process called reactivation, attachment of a tick to the host for 5 to 20 hours is required before rickettsial transmission can take place. For this reason, routine "tick checks" are recommended in endemic areas to prevent transmission of *R. rickettsii*.

The tick transmits *R. rickettsii* through the saliva during feeding. A necrotic lesion (eschar) can occur at the site of tick attachment. The rickettsiae enter the circulatory system and replicate in endothelial cells of small blood vessels and capillaries. Similar to other SFG rickettsiae, *R. rickettsii* cause direct damage to endothelial cells. This causes vascular inflammation, then necrosis, and finally increased vascular permeability. This process results in extravasation of fluid and blood cells into the extravascular fluid space and contributes to edema, hemorrhage, hypotension, and shock. Central nervous system edema may contribute to the development of neurologic signs, rapid clinical deterioration, and death. Myocardial inflammation can induce conduction abnormalities such as heart block or potentially life-threatening arrhythmias. Pulmonary edema, radiographically depicted as a moderate pulmonary interstitial pattern with mild alveolar infiltration, may cause tachypnea, dyspnea, or coughing in some dogs. Ocular abnormalities, including subconjunctival hemorrhage, retinal petechiae, focal areas of retinal edema, and perivascular inflammatory cell infiltrates, reflect varying degrees of damage.[4, 5] Gangrene affecting the distal extremities, scrotum, mammary glands, nose, or lips is associated with severe vascular obstruction and can induce substantial tissue loss, necessitating reconstructive surgery.[6] In severe cases, decreased renal perfusion can predispose to acute renal failure. Because of difficulties associated with confirming the diagnosis of acute fulminant RMSF with currently available diagnostic tests, the extent to which *R. rickettsii* causes fatal disease in dogs in the southeastern United States is unknown.

Experimentally, a dose-related influence on the severity of *R. rickettsii*–induced vascular injury has been demonstrated in dogs. Following experimental infection with *R. rickettsii*, the severity of illness varies from mild to fatal, depending on the concentration of rickettsial inoculum. Therefore, veterinarians should anticipate a spectrum of illness following naturally occurring infection in endemic regions. Similarly, infection with less pathogenic SFG rickettsiae may result in subclinical or mild disease manifestations.

Clinical abnormalities associated with RMSF include fever, anorexia, depression, mucopurulent ocular discharge, scleral injection, tachypnea, coughing, vomiting, diarrhea, muscle pain, neutrophilic polyarthritis, and a diverse group of neurologic signs including hyperesthesia, ataxia, vestibular signs, stupor, seizures, and coma. In some dogs weight loss is severe, considering the short duration of illness. Poorly localizing joint, muscle, and/or neurologic pain suggestive of polyarthritis, polymyositis, or meningitis may represent the only or most prominent clinical finding. Retinal hemorrhages are a consistent finding but may be absent early in the course of the disease.[1, 5] Epistaxis, melena, hematuria, and petechial to ecchymotic hemorrhages occur in some dogs but may not develop unless diagnosis and treatment are delayed for five or more days after the onset of clinical signs. Scrotal edema, hyperemia, hemorrhage, and epididymal pain are frequently observed in male dogs. Signs associated with cardiovascular collapse, oliguric renal failure, or brain death can develop in the terminal stages of the disease.

R. rickettsii causes a diverse spectrum of clinical, hematologic, biochemical, and pathologic abnormalities that mimic many other infectious and noninfectious diseases. Differential diagnostic considerations might include canine distemper, bacterial discospondylitis, pneumonia, acute renal failure, pancreatitis, colitis, meningitis, vestibulitis, encephalitis, or immune-mediated polyarthritis. RMSF is clinically indistinguishable from acute ehrlichiosis, thereby necessitating diagnostic testing for differentiation.[2] Unlike ehrlichiosis, in which chronic infection can persist for years, the total duration of illness following *R. rickettsii* infection is generally short (two weeks or less). Because protective immunity develops rapidly following infection, canine RMSF is an acute disease that generally occurs during the spring and summer (April to October) months in the southeastern United States. In nearly all respects, canine RMSF is identical to human RMSF.

Diagnosis

Seasonal occurrence, history of tick infestation, fever, and combinations of the previously described clinical findings should suggest the possibility of RMSF. Owing to marked variation in clinical presentation, confirmation of the diagnosis of RMSF is important for the clinician to gain familiarity with the disease. In addition, confirmation of RMSF in household pets warrants owner education as to the enhanced risk associated with tick exposure in that environment. Thrombocytopenia, generally mild in degree, is the most consistent hematologic finding. Leukopenia generally occurs during the early stages of infection (first 24 to 48 hours), followed by progressive leukocytosis, which increases in proportion to the severity of vascular injury. Toxic granulation of neutrophils, metamyelocytes, eosinopenia, lymphopenia, and monocytosis may accompany the more typical changes in platelet and neutrophil number. A mild anemia may occur. Severe anemia, leukopenia, and thrombocytopenia can accompany fulminant canine RMSF.

Biochemical abnormalities reflect the effects of generalized vascular damage and vary with the severity and duration of infection. Hypoproteinemia, hypoalbuminemia, azotemia, hyponatremia, hypocalcemia, and increased liver enzymes (serum alkaline phosphatase, alanine aminotransferase) may occur in dogs with RMSF. Bilirubinuria and, rarely, bilirubinemia occur in dogs with RMSF. Synovial or cerebrospinal fluid analysis usually reveals a mild increase in protein and cells, which, in the early disease process, are composed of a high percentage of neutrophils and, later, mononuclear cells.

Confirmation of a diagnosis requires either direct immunofluorescent testing for *R. rickettsii* antigen in tissue biopsy or necropsy specimens, serologic testing, polymerase chain reaction (PCR) amplification of rickettsial DNA, or rickettsial culture, which requires a biosafety level 3 laboratory and specialized technical expertise. With the indirect fluorescent antibody test, documentation of a fourfold or greater increase in antibody titer between acute and convalescent sera confirms a diagnosis of RMSF.[4] To facilitate the accurate interpretation of serologic results, it is important to obtain the acute-phase sample as early in the disease course as possible and the convalescent sample two to three weeks thereafter. If acute-phase serum is obtained several days after the onset of clinical signs, a high antibody titer will be obtained. Although early initiation of antirickettsial antibiotic therapy will slightly decrease the intensity of the humoral immune response to *R. rickettsii* antigen, experimental studies indicate that collection of appropriately timed serum samples should still facilitate an accurate diagnosis of RMSF in dogs.[7]

Frequent or constant tick exposure can result in serum antibodies to nonpathogenic SFG rickettsiae, most notably *R. rhipicephali* and *R. montana*, that cross-react with *R. rickettsii*. This can complicate the interpretation of a single serologic result derived from dogs with suspected RMSF. Because the possibility of exposure to ticks containing nonpathogenic SFG rickettsiae is much greater than the possibility of exposure to *R. rickettsii*, many dogs tested for RMSF in the summer have low-positive ($\geq$ 1:64) titers to *R. rickettsii* as a result of exposure to closely related rickettsiae. This observation emphasizes the need for evaluation of both acute and convalescent serum samples or use of PCR to confirm a diagnosis of RMSF.

Direct immunofluorescent testing provides the opportunity for rapid diagnosis by demonstrating *R. rickettsii* in skin biopsies.[8] Organisms are generally more readily demonstrated in human patients in areas of hemorrhage, although organisms may be more readily identifiable in clinically unaffected skin from dogs.[8] Prior initiation of antibiotic therapy can cause a false-negative test result.

Treatment

Tetracycline (22 mg/kg three times a day for 14 days) or doxycycline (5 mg/kg twice a day for 14 days) is effective treatment of SFG rickettsiae or *Ehrlichia* species infestation. Chloramphenicol or enrofloxacin is equally effective for treating RMSF.[7] Following initiation of treatment, a rapid clinical response occurs in dogs without severe vascular damage or neurologic sequelae. Defervescence should be anticipated within 24 hours after the initiation of antibiotics. Delay in diagnosis or the use of antibiotics such as penicillin, cephalosporin derivatives, or aminoglycosides that lack antirickettsial spectrums may result in increased morbidity or mortality. Owing to severe vascular damage, fluid therapy should be used with caution. Prednisolone administered at anti-inflammatory or immune-suppressive dosages in conjunction with doxycycline does not potentiate the severity of *R. rickettsii* infection in experimentally infected dogs.[9]

Prevention

Three years following experimental infection with *R. rickettsii*, challenge inoculation of dogs failed to induce a clinical or serologic response, suggesting that immunity following natural infection is probably lifelong. It is possible that undiagnosed mild or asymptomatic *R. rickettsii* infections, or repeated exposure to nonpathogenic SFG rickettsiae, contribute to the prevention of severe RMSF in dogs with heavy tick exposure in endemic regions. Minimizing tick exposure and routine removal of ticks from dogs represent the most effective means of prevention. Following infection with *R. rickettsii*, the duration of rickettsemia is brief, approximately 5 to 14 days.[9] Therefore, infected dogs do not play an important reservoir role and pose a minimal zoonotic threat to humans.

Care should be exercised in removing ticks, so as not to contaminate one's hands with infective hemolymph from ticks. Although the risk of inadvertent transmission is small, contact with rickettsemic blood during intravenous catheter placement, blood collection procedures, or laboratory sample analysis should be avoided. Zoonotic warning labels are recommended for blood samples obtained from dogs in which a differential diagnosis of RMSF is being considered.

TYPHUS GROUP RICKETTSIAE

The typhus group (TG) rickettsiae include *R. typhi, R. prowazekii, R. canada,* and *R. felis. R. typhi,* transmitted by the rat flea, causes endemic typhus. *R. prowazekii,* transmitted by the human body louse or flying squirrel fleas in the United States, causes epidemic typhus. In general, little is known about the pathogenic potential of TG rickettsiae in domestic animals. Experimentally, disease manifestations were not observed in dogs infected with *R. prowazekii* or *R. canada.*[10] However, seroepidemiologic evidence suggests that dogs and humans in the eastern United States may be infected with a TG rickettsia.

Since 1990, three novel organisms, *Bartonella henselae, Bartonella clarridigiae,* and *Rickettsia felis,* have been identified as zoonotic flea-transmitted pathogens. Vector competence has been demonstrated experimentally for cat-to-cat transmission of *B. henselae* and *R. felis* by fleas. The extent to which cats and other animals such as opossums serve as a reservoir for *R. felis* is currently being studied. The pathogenicity of these three organisms in cats has not been established. *R. felis* was only recently recognized as a cause of febrile illness in a human patient from Texas.[11]

THE EHRLICHIAE

The genus *Ehrlichia* consists of three genogroups: the *E. canis* genogroup, which includes *E. canis, E. chaffeensis, E. ewingii, E. muris,* and *Cowdria ruminantium*; the *E. phagocytophila* genogroup, which includes *E. phagocytophila, E. equi, E. platys,* and the agent of human granulocytic ehrlichiosis (HGE); and the *E. sennetsu* genogroup, which consists of *E. sennetsu, E. risticii,* and *Neorickettsia helminthoeca.* Historically, *Ehrlichia* species were believed to infect a very narrow host range. Evolving evidence indicates that several *Ehrlichia* species can infect multiple host species.

CANINE MONOCYTIC EHRLICHIOSIS

Canine monocytic ehrlichiosis, caused by *E. canis* or *E. chaffeensis,* is generally characterized by a reduction in cellular blood elements. *E. canis* was first recognized in Algeria in 1935 and first reported in the United States in 1963. *E. chaffeensis* was first reported in naturally infected dogs in 1996[12] and has subsequently been shown to cause severe disease manifestations that are clinically and serologically indistinguishable from *E. canis* infection.[13] Ehrlichiosis has been reported from most tropical and subtropical regions throughout the world.

The distribution of ehrlichiosis is related to the distribution of the vector tick, *Rhipicephalus sanguineus*, the brown dog tick. The distribution vector and relative pathogenic importance of *E. chaffeensis* in dogs await further study. Although ehrlichiosis is diagnosed most frequently in dogs living in the southeastern and southwestern United States, the disease has been reported from nearly every state. Because of chronic, subclinical infection,[14] a dog can be transported from an endemic to a nonendemic region and subsequently develop disease manifestations years after initial infection.

E. canis is a small pleomorphic rickettsial organism that infects circulating mononuclear cells. Morulae, which are intracellular inclusions composed of clusters of rickettsial organisms, are occasionally observed in blood smears during the early stage of infection but rarely in association with chronic infection. Early reports suggested infection of nonhuman primates, and a recent report describes the isolation of an organism genetically related to *E. canis* from a veterinarian in Venezuela.[15] *E. chaffeensis*, a closely related rickettsial organism that serologically cross-reacts with *E. canis*, causes ehrlichiosis in people.[16]

E. canis infections have been reported in dogs with concurrent infection with *Babesia canis* or *Hematozoon canis* (both tick-transmitted protozoa) or with *Bartonella vinsonii*, suggesting simultaneous transmission of organisms from vector ticks. Concurrent infection with organisms such as phaeohyphomycosis or cryptococcus may represent coincidental infections or potentially secondary opportunistic infections associated with chronic ehrlichiosis.

Canine infection probably occurs when salivary secretions from the tick contaminate the attachment site during ingestion of a blood meal. *E. canis* infection can also be introduced in susceptible dogs by blood transfusion. This has been accomplished with blood obtained from dogs chronically infected with *E. canis* for up to five years. This fact has obvious implications for canine blood donors in endemic regions. Ticks are thought to represent the primary reservoir for the disease, and adult *R. sanguineus* are capable of transmitting *E. canis* for at least 155 days following detachment from the host. Ticks can acquire *E. canis* only if engorgement occurs during the acute phase of the disease in dogs.

Following experimental infection, *E. canis* causes acute, subclinical, and chronic disease phases. After an incubation period of 8 to 20 days, the infected dog enters into the acute phase of ehrlichiosis, which lasts two to four weeks. During this time, the organism multiplies within circulating mononuclear cells and the mononuclear phagocytic tissues of the liver, spleen, and lymph nodes. This causes lymphadenomegaly and lymphoreticular hyperplasia of the liver and spleen. Infected cells are transported via blood to other body organs, especially the lungs, kidneys, and meninges. Infected cells adhere to the vascular endothelium, inducing a vasculitis and subendothelial tissue infection. Platelet consumption, sequestration, and destruction all appear to contribute to thrombocytopenia during the acute phase. Leukocyte counts are variable, and anemia, related to suppression of erythrocyte production and accelerated erythrocyte destruction, develops progressively during the acute phase.

The subclinical phase of infection occurs six to nine weeks after inoculation and is characterized by the variable persistence of thrombocytopenia, leukopenia, and anemia in the absence of clinical signs. Experimentally, dogs with

adequate immunocompetence are reported to eliminate the parasite and do not develop the chronic phase of the disease. Dogs that are unable to mount an effective immune response to the organism are chronically infected.[17] Hyperglobulinemia, not related to the humoral immune response to *E. canis*, is typically associated with chronic disease.[18, 19] The mechanism responsible for bone marrow suppression in chronic ehrlichiosis is not yet understood.

Clinical signs during the acute phase of disease vary from depression, anorexia, and fever to severe loss of stamina, weight loss, ocular and nasal discharges, dyspnea, lymphadenopathy, and edema of the limbs or scrotum. Acute-phase clinical signs are transient and usually resolve in one to two weeks without treatment. Thrombocytopenia and leukopenia generally occur 10 to 20 days following infection. Despite moderate to severe thrombocytopenia, hemorrhages are rarely observed. A variety of central nervous system signs, including hyperesthesia, muscle twitching, and cranial nerve deficits, may occur owing to inflammation or bleeding into the meninges. Clinical findings in the acute phase of ehrlichiosis can be identical to those in canine RMSF.

Clinical signs associated with the chronic phase of the disease are mild to absent in some dogs and severe in other dogs. For example, it is not unusual in endemic areas to detect hematologic abnormalities due to chronic *E. canis* infection in healthy dogs being evaluated for heartworm adulticide therapy. Undetected thrombocytopenia in these dogs might potentiate the severity of pulmonary hemorrhage associated with thromboembolism.

Bleeding tendencies, pallor due to anemia, severe weight loss, debilitation, abdominal tenderness, anterior uveitis, retinal hemorrhages, and neurologic signs consistent with meningoencephalitis typify dogs that develop disease manifestations during chronic infection. Due to immunosuppression, secondary bacterial infections may be documented. Numerous patterns of hemorrhage may occur in dogs with ehrlichiosis. Epistaxis, once considered a hallmark of the disease, is reported infrequently in more recent case studies.

In addition to clinical signs that may be suggestive of ehrlichiosis, severe laboratory abnormalities can contribute to the index of suspicion for the disease. Hematologic abnormalities including pancytopenia, aplastic anemia, neutropenia, or thrombocytopenia would be consistent with *E. canis* infection. Thrombocytopenia is the most consistent hematologic abnormality in both the acute and chronic stages of ehrlichiosis. However, following experimental infection, platelet numbers are frequently in the low laboratory reference range. Pancytopenia is documented in less than 25 per cent of dogs in retrospective clinical studies. Profound lymphocytosis, accompanied by atypical or reactive lymphocytes, has been associated with ehrlichiosis. Because *E. canis* causes defective platelet function, bleeding can be detected in dogs with normal, increased, or mildly suppressed platelet counts. Finding morulae in peripheral blood smears or buffy coat smears is diagnostic for monocytic ehrlichiosis; however, morulae are generally found only during the first two weeks following infection, and usually in very low numbers.

Anemia, if present, varies in severity among affected dogs. Positive Coombs' tests suggest that immune damage, due to circulating erythrocyte antibodies, can contribute to an acute hemolytic crisis in some dogs with ehrlichiosis. In this situation, a regenerative anemia may be encountered; however, a nonregenerative anemia is most frequently documented in chronically infected dogs. Although highly variable, bone marrow examination usually reveals a hypocellular marrow with varying degrees of suppression of the erythroid, myeloid, and megakaryocytic series. Hyperplasia of the bone marrow, especially megakaryocytic hyperplasia, occurs during the acute phase of the disease. Although encountered in other chronic inflammatory diseases, plasmacytosis is a frequently reported bone marrow finding in ehrlichiosis.

Serum proteins are increased above expected values in approximately 50 to 75 per cent of *E. canis* seropositive dogs.[18, 19] Hyperglobulinemia is characterized by increased beta and/or gamma globulins. Serum protein electrophoresis may reveal a polyclonal or monoclonal gammopathy.[19] A monoclonal gammopathy, in association with severe bone marrow plasmacytosis, could be easily misdiagnosed as a plasma cell myeloma; when found in association with lymphocytosis, it may be misdiagnosed as lymphocytic leukemia. Hypoalbuminemia occurs in association with protein-losing nephropathy or a reciprocal decrease in albumin associated with hyperglobulinemia. Experimentally, a transient, reversible protein-losing nephropathy associated with ultrastructural glomerular damage occurs two to five weeks after inoculation.[20] In the chronic disease phase, *E. canis* can induce a severe protein-losing nephropathy most likely related to immune complex glomerulonephritis. Less frequently encountered serum laboratory abnormalities include azotemia and increased serum alanine aminotransferase, alkaline phosphatase, and total bilirubin.

Diagnosis of monocytic ehrlichiosis requires visualization of morulae, detection of *E. canis* antibodies, or PCR amplification of *E. canis* or *E. chaffeensis* DNA. The indirect fluorescent antibody (IFA) technique or the dot enzyme-linked immunosorbent assay (ELISA) is available for detection of *Ehrlichia* species antibodies. Because they are derived from the same genogroup, *E. canis, E. chaffeensis*, and *E. ewingii* produce cross-reacting antibodies. Although interlaboratory variation in serologic results occurs owing to interpretation error, the IFA test for *E. canis* is highly sensitive. Serologic cross-reaction has not been reported in association with *R. rickettsii, B. canis, E. platys*, or *E. equi*. A positive titer is considered indicative of infection, because most experimentally infected dogs become seronegative within six to nine months after effective treatment, whereas untreated dogs remain seropositive. Infection with *E. canis* does not infer protective immunity; therefore, subsequent exposure to infected ticks after treatment results in disease recurrence, generally of decreased severity. Following antirickettsial antibiotic treatment, some dogs become asymptomatic but maintain high *E. canis* antibody titers for years.[21] Clinically, these dogs are assumed to have eliminated the rickettsia if hyperglobulinemia resolves progressively following treatment or if *E. canis* DNA cannot be amplified from EDTA blood samples. Infrequently, a dog maintains a high antibody titer, and a hematologic abnormality such as thrombocytopenia persists, for years following antirickettsial therapy. Although it is unclear whether these dogs are chronically infected with *E. canis* or infected with other pathogens, or whether the persistent hematologic abnormalities are mediated through altered immunoregulation induced by the organism, there is little evidence to support antimicrobial rickettsial resistance leading to persistent infection.

Tetracycline (22 mg/kg three times a day for 14 days) or doxycycline (5 mg/kg twice a day for 21 days) is currently recommended for treatment of monocytic ehrlichiosis. Chloramphenicol and enrofloxacin may be effective, but controlled therapeutic studies are unavailable. Although imidocarb dipropionate has gained clinical acceptance in some endemic regions for treating severe, chronic, or presumed refractory cases of ehrlichiosis, lack of efficacy has been demonstrated in treating some dogs with ehrlichiosis. Clinical improvement may be observed with penicillin or sulfonamides, but the response is variable, and infection generally persists.

The prognosis for canine ehrlichiosis is generally good. Dramatic clinical improvement usually occurs within 24 to 48 hours after initiation of tetracycline in dogs with acute-phase or mild chronic-phase disease. Rapid clinical improvement is frequently noted in chronically infected dogs; however, up to a year may be necessary for complete hematologic recovery. Continuous or long-term administration of antibiotics, such as tetracycline, has apparently contributed to delayed hematologic recovery in dogs with obvious clinical improvement. Hemorrhage or concurrent infection may contribute to death of chronically infected dogs, despite the initiation of tetracycline therapy. The duration of antirickettsial drug treatment for chronically affected dogs or those with severe pancytopenia or aplastic anemia remains controversial. Supportive therapy, including fluids, blood transfusion, vitamins, and anabolic steroids, is required in some dogs. Long-term tetracycline prophylaxis (6.6 mg/kg once daily) and repositol oxytetracycline (200 mg intramuscularly twice weekly) has been used in military working dogs to prevent *E. canis* infection in highly endemic regions. This approach may be appropriate for recurrent infections in kennels if tick-control measures are of limited effectiveness. Because of extensive dog transport and chronic asymptomatic *E. canis* infection, there is always the potential for establishment of new endemic foci in previously naive regions. Tick control is very important but may not always be effective in preventing the disease. No vaccine is currently available.

CANINE GRANULOCYTIC EHRLICHIOSIS

Historically, neutrophilic morulae, when found on blood smears from dogs, were thought to represent a less pathogenic strain of *E. canis*. More recently, neutrophilic rickettsiae have been isolated or characterized using molecular probes. Unfortunately, conclusions regarding the identity of granulocytic organisms in many clinical reports have not been possible until recently. In the United States, neutrophilic morulae appear to represent infection with at least two species of *Ehrlichia, E. equi* or *E. ewingii*.[22, 23] In endemic regions, *Ixodes scapularis, Ixodes pacificus*, or *Ixodes ricinus* (Europe) transmit members of the *Ehrlichia phagocytophilia* genogroup to cats, dogs, sheep, horses, and human beings. California, Minnesota, Wisconsin, and several New England states report a high prevalence of infection, generally in dogs, horses, and human beings. Neutrophilic ehrlichiosis, presumably caused by *E. ewingii*, has been most frequently described in dogs in Missouri, Oklahoma, Tennessee, North Carolina, and Virginia.[24, 25] Because the disease occurs in spring and early summer, tick transmission is suspected, but a definitive vector has not been confirmed. Dogs can be co-infected with monocytic and granulocytic *Ehrlichia* species.

Clinical signs include lameness involving one or more limbs, muscular stiffness, a stilted gait, reluctance to rise, an arched back posture, and joint swelling and pain. Polyarthritis, characterized by a predominantly neutrophilic inflammatory response and generally accompanied by fever, is the most frequently reported abnormality associated with granulocytic ehrlichiosis. Hematologic abnormalities, similar to those observed with *E. canis* infection, include anemia, neutropenia, thrombocytopenia, lymphocytosis, monocytosis, and eosinophilia.

Granulocytic *Ehrlichia* morulae have been observed frequently in neutrophils from dogs receiving glucocorticoid or cancer chemotherapeutic drugs. Although the importance of this clinical observation is unclear, it may suggest that chronically infected dogs develop ehrlichiemia if immunosuppressed or that immunosuppression potentiates morulae development during an acute infection. Because of serologic cross-reactivity, dogs infected with *E. ewingii* but not *E. equi* develop a humoral antibody response to *E. canis* antigen. PCR amplification with *Ehrlichia* species-specific primers can facilitate determination of the infecting species.

Therapeutically, tetracycline hydrochloride or doxycycline elicits rapid improvement in clinical status. Experimental transmission of a granulocytic *Ehrlichia* derived from a dog from Missouri suggests that dogs can attain an immunologic cure without antimicrobial therapy following asymptomatic infection.[26]

CANINE CYCLIC THROMBOCYTOPENIA

Canine cyclic thrombocytopenia is caused by *Ehrlichia platys*, a rickettsial organism that replicates only in platelets. The mode of *E. platys* transmission is presumed to be by tick vector, but experimentally, *Rhipicephalus sanguineus*, the vector for *E. canis*, did not transmit *E. platys* infection.[27] In the United States, *E. platys* is generally considered to be minimally pathogenic and is usually recognized as an incidental observation during blood smear examination. The distribution of *E. platys* infection in the United States has not been established, but most reports have originated from the South and Southeast, with occasional reports from the north and north-central portions of the country.[28] With the exception of a single case report of uveitis, naturally occurring and experimental infections have not been associated with clinical signs. *E. platys* causes cyclic rickettsemia and thrombocytopenia at approximately 10- to 14-day intervals.[29, 30] At its nadir, thrombocytopenia can be severe (20,000 to 50,000 platelets/μL), and platelets are hypoaggregatable. A mild normocytic, normochromic nonregenerative anemia, associated with anemia of inflammation, leukopenia, hypoalbuminemia, and hyperglobulinemia, has been reported in association with experimental *E. platys* infection.[29] On Giemsa-stained blood smears, *E. platys* appears as single or, less frequently, multiple basophilic inclusions within platelets. The duration of rickettsemia in untreated dogs has not been clearly established.

Diagnosis of *E. platys* requires visualization of rickettsiae in platelets or detection of serum antibodies by indirect immunofluorescence or PCR amplification. Owing to antigenic divergence, *E. platys* does not cross-react serologically with *E. canis, E. ewingii, E. risticii,* or *E. equi.* Antibodies appear in the serum two to three weeks following experimental infection and are usually detectable during the initial thrombocytopenic episode. In a study of thrombocytopenic and healthy kennel dogs in Louisiana, seroprevalence to *E. platys* was 40.7 per cent in the thrombocytopenic group and 54.2 per cent in healthy kennel dogs.[31] *E. platys* morulae were detected in only one of the thrombocytopenic dogs. These results suggest that exposure to *E. platys* in southern states is extensive and that premunition probably develops following several cycles of thrombocytopenia. Co-infection with *E. canis* and *E. platys* is common, and it has been theorized that *E. platys* infection might intensify the clinical course of monocytic ehrlichiosis.

Treatment with oral tetracycline (22 mg/kg every 8 hours for 14 days), or presumably doxycycline (5 mg/kg every 12 hours for 14 days), should eliminate the organism. Because experimental studies have not identified abnormal clinical signs associated with *E. platys* infection, caution should be exercised in ascribing clinical illness to *E. platys*, and other infectious and noninfectious causes of thrombocytopenia should be pursued diagnostically.

EHRLICHIA RISTICII

In 1994, Kakoma et al. reported serologic evidence of over 100 cases of atypical canine ehrlichiosis with three fatalities.[32] These dogs were not seroreactive to *E. canis* antigen by IFA, but they were reactive to *E. risticii* antigen, at generally low antibody titers. *E. risticii* is the cause of Potomac horse fever. Serum samples in this study were derived from California, Texas, Arizona, Illinois, Washington, Florida, and Michigan. Isolates obtained from three dogs were morphologically and genetically (based on partial 16S rRNA gene sequence) indistinguishable from *E. risticii.* Successful experimental transmission of a dog isolate was not reported. Clinical abnormalities were described for six dogs and included lethargy, vague signs of abdominal discomfort with intermittent vomiting, persistent bleeding or petechial hemorrhages, polyarthritis, dependent edema, and posterior paralysis. Hematologic abnormalities were variably present and included anemia, thrombocytopenia, prolongation of prothrombin time, and hypercalcemia. Therapy with tetracycline also appears to be variably efficacious for treatment of this infection, with substantial improvement in some dogs and a complete lack of response in other dogs. The authors propose that, pending additional research, the canine isolate be referred to as *E. risticii* subsp. *atypicalis.* The definitive pathophysiologic characterization of this rickettsia as a cause of disease in dogs awaits additional study.

FELINE EHRLICHIOSIS

Ehrlichia-like inclusion bodies have been observed in monocytes, lymphocytes, or granulocytes from cats living in Kenya, France, Sweden, and the midwestern and western United States. Antibody reactivity to *E. canis* or *E. risticii* antigens has also been reported.[33, 34] Although the precise clinical significance of these observations awaits the results of future studies, it seems probable that cats can be infected by one or more rickettsiae of the genus *Ehrlichia.* Experimentally, inoculation of *E. equi* in cats has resulted in asymptomatic infection or mild fever and depression and the development of neutrophilic and eosinophilic morulae. Because *E. equi* induces morulae in polymorphonuclear cells rather than mononuclear cells, it is likely that there is a feline monocytic *Ehrlichia* that causes disease in cats.

Anorexia; loss of body condition; fever; splenomegaly; lymphadenopathy; normocytic, normochromic anemia; radiographic evidence of interstitial lung disease; and mononuclear intracytoplasmic inclusions typical of the genus *Ehrlichia* were described in three cats from Kenya. Neutropenia and hyperglobulinemia were each reported in one cat. These cats were infested with *Haemaphysalis leachi* ticks. Resolution of disease signs was reported following treatment with either tetracycline hydrochloride or imidocarb dipropionate.

Intracytoplasmic inclusions resembling *Ehrlichia* morulae have been observed during cytologic evaluation of a lymph node aspirate from a cyclically febrile, anorexic cat from Colorado.[33] Laboratory abnormalities included a normocytic, normochromic, nonregenerative anemia; hyperglobulinemia; and pyogranulomatous lymphadenitis. Serum IgG antibodies to *E. canis* antigen were detected, and the cat responded rapidly to doxycycline despite a previous lack of response to several nonrickettsiostatic antibiotics. Serologic evidence of ehrlichiosis was detected in 12 sick cats with clinical and laboratory abnormalities including fever, malaise, weight loss, anorexia, lymphadenopathy, nonseptic suppurative polyarthritis, anemia, thrombocytopenia, neutropenia, and polyclonal or monoclonal gammopathy. Each of these cats responded favorably to doxycycline. Antibody reactivity (IFA and Western immunoblot) to *E. risticii* antigens was described in five cats from California.[34] Hematologic abnormalities included leukopenia, anemia, and thrombocytopenia. Attempts to isolate, transmit, or detect *E. risticii* by PCR were unsuccessful. Additional studies are needed to isolate and genetically characterize feline *Ehrlichia* organisms and to clarify the pathogenic importance of *Ehrlichia* species in cats.

SALMON-POISONING DISEASE

Salmon-poisoning disease is caused by two rickettsiae, *Neorickettsia helmintheca* and the Elokomin fluke fever agent.[35] The Elokomin fluke fever agent, potentially another strain of *N. helmintheca*, causes less mortality in dogs than typically encountered with salmon-poisoning disease. Both organisms can be transmitted during ingestion of fish containing trematode *(Nanophyetus salmincola)* metacercariae. *N. helmintheca* can be found in all stages of the trematode life cycle, from egg to adult fluke. Salmon-poisoning disease is limited geographically by the distribution of the trematode's first intermediate host, a small snail, *Auxodrome silicula*, to the coastal areas of Washington, Oregon, and California.

Following ingestion of metacercariae-infected fish, adult flukes develop in the dog's intestine in approximately six days, after which rickettsiae are inoculated, presumably into villus epithelial and intestinal lymphoid cells. Subsequently, rickettsemia develops and organisms are disseminated, potentially by circulating monocytes, to many organ systems. Following ingestion of parasitized fish, the incubation period before the development of clinical signs is usually about seven days but can be as long as a month. Clinical signs associated with *N. helmintheca* infection appear to be limited to domestic and wild Canidae. Experimentally, the rickettsiae can be transmitted by parenteral injection of blood, spleen, or lymph suspensions from infected dogs.

Salmon-poisoning disease is characterized by a sudden onset of fever greater than 40°C, depression, and anorexia. Vomiting and diarrhea, accompanied by weight loss, contribute to dehydration and hypokalemia. Serous nasal and mucopurulent ocular discharge occurs in some dogs. Terminally, weight loss may be severe, and diarrhea may consist primarily of blood. There is progressive lymph node enlargement and splenomegaly. In untreated dogs, death usually occurs 7 to 10 days after the onset of clinical signs.

The diagnosis of salmon-poisoning disease can be implied by finding operculated trematode eggs in dog feces. Eggs can be detected by direct fecal smears or by the sugar flotation technique. Identification of characteristic intracytoplasmic rickettsial inclusion bodies on a Giemsa-stained lymph node aspirate, particularly in mononuclear phagocytic cells, can be used to confirm the disease. Similar to the treatment of other rickettsial diseases, tetracycline is the drug of choice.

HEMOBARTONELLOSIS

Haemobartonella are hemotropic organisms that have been differentiated on the basis of their host range. They include *H. muris*, infecting rats; *H. felis*, infecting cats; and *H. canis*, infecting dogs. Based on 16S rRNA gene sequence, *Haemobartonella* species are closely related to mycoplasma species and may be reclassified in the family Mycoplasmataceae.[36]

Experimentally, *H. felis* can be transmitted by intravenous, intraperitoneal, and oral inoculation of infected blood. It is probable that transmission occurs by bloodsucking arthropods and potentially by cat-bite wounds. Although the mode of transmission is unclear, newborn kittens from female cats with clinical disease can be infected.

Feline hemobartonellosis is characterized by acute or chronic anemia, pallor, weight loss, anorexia, and occasionally splenomegaly or icterus. Because of the epicellular location of the organism, immune-mediated erythrocyte destruction is associated with antierythrocytic antibodies; reticuloendothelial cell erythrophagocytosis, particularly in the spleen; increased erythrocyte fragility; and a shortened erythrocyte half-life. For reasons that remain unclear, the severity and rate of decline of anemia in cats with hemobartonellosis are variable. Many infected cats become Coombs' test–positive, indicating the presence of infection-induced antierythrocyte antibodies. Without therapy, approximately one third of cats with acute hemobartonellosis die as a result of severe anemia. Cats that recover without treatment develop recurrent episodes of rickettsemia and remain chronically infected for months to years, if not indefinitely. Chronically infected carrier cats appear clinically normal but may have mild regenerative anemia. Experimentally, the severity of rickettsemia can vary dramatically within a 24-hour period, and intervals of several weeks can exist between episodes of rickettsemia. Clinically, this observation emphasizes that failure to visualize *H. felis* organisms on a blood smear does not eliminate the possibility that hemobartonellosis is responsible for anemia.

Risk factors for hemobartonellosis include anemia, positive status for feline leukemia virus (FeLV), lack of vaccinations, history of cat-bite abscesses, age younger than 4 years, or outdoor roaming status.[37] Interestingly, sex, multicat households, and the presence of fleas were not significant risk factors. *H. felis* organisms were found on 3.6 per cent of the blood smears from healthy cats and on 7.5 per cent from ill cats.[37] Owing to the difficulty in detecting small numbers of organisms during blood-smear examination, and because of the episodic nature of *H. felis* rickettsemia, the prevalence of *H. felis* in both healthy and sick cat populations is probably underestimated in most survey studies.[38] Immune suppression associated with FeLV infection, splenectomy, or corticosteroid therapy potentiates visualization of rickettsia on blood smears and may influence disease susceptibility and severity.

Experimentally, *Haemobartonella canis* can be transmitted by *Rhipicephalus sanguineus*. Similar to *H. felis*, *H. canis* can be transmitted iatrogenically by blood transfusion. It is generally accepted that *H. canis* is an incidental finding during blood-smear examination, that the rickettsia is of minimal pathogenic significance, and that concurrent infectious or noninfectious disease should be sought in a rickett-semic dog. In contrast to these considerations, selected reports support a more serious pathogenic role for *H. canis*. Similar to cats, immune suppression in dogs potentiates rickettsemia and, in the case of splenectomy, increases the severity of anemia.

The diagnosis of hemobartonellosis in dogs and cats requires detection of the organism on Wright-Giemsa–stained thin smears of peripheral blood or PCR amplification. Hematologic and biochemical changes are nonspecific and of limited diagnostic value. Tetracycline appears to be the treatment of choice. Concurrent immune-suppressive drug therapy with glucocorticoid or other agents is frequently necessary to stop immunologically mediated erythrocyte destruction. Chlorpromazine (2 mg/kg orally for 8 days) and metronidazole (40 mg/kg orally for 21 days) has been recommended for resistant French strains of *H. felis*[39] and infrequently for treatment of refractory feline hemobartonellosis in the author's experience. Drowsiness associated with chlorpromazine is an anticipated side effect.

COXIELLA BURNETII

Coxiella burnetii causes Q fever in people and is an occupational hazard for personnel in the livestock industry, meat processing plants, and laboratories performing investigations in which sheep or other animals might be unknowingly infected with the rickettsia.[40] Because humans become infected by inhalation of aerosols containing *C. burnetii*, acute outbreaks of fever, pneumonic illness, hepatitis, or, rarely, endocarditis can occur. Chronic *C. burnetii* infection is being recognized as an emerging zoonosis that may contribute to a chronic fatigue–like syndrome. Contact with animals is a major risk factor for human infection. Although cattle, sheep, and goats are the main reservoirs for *C. burnetii* in humans, recent reports indicate that exposure to infected dogs and cats poses an as yet ill-defined risk for human infection.[41, 42] The organism can be found in urine, feces, milk, and reproductive tissues of animals. Because the placentas of chronically infected animals contain large numbers of *C. burnetii*, infectious aerosols are created during parturition. Epidemiologically, exposure to newborn kittens, and particularly stillborn kittens, is a significant risk factor for Q fever in people in Nova Scotia, Canada. Q fever occurs worldwide and has been reported from at least 51 countries and 31 states. Many tick species, including *R. sanguineus*, are naturally infected with *C. burnetii*.

The extent to which *C. burnetii* causes illness in cats or dogs remains unclear. Experimentally, fever, lethargy, inappetence, and *C. burnetii* rickettsemia of at least one month's duration developed following subcutaneous inoculation. Clinical signs were not observed in cats infected by oral feeding or by contact urine and/or aerosol exposure; however, half of these cats became rickettsemic and seroconverted to *C. burnetii*. Detection of agglutinating serum antibodies to *C. burnetii* in 53 per cent of 1040 dogs in California indicates that canine exposure is extensive in that state, which has the highest Q fever incidence in the United States. Because of the human health hazard associated with aerosol infection, veterinarians should exercise caution when managing periparturient problems, particularly in regions known to be endemic for Q fever.

REFERENCES

1. Davidson MG, Breitschwerdt EB, Walker DH, et al: Vascular permeability and hemostatic mechanisms during *Rickettsia rickettsii* infection in dogs. Am J Vet Res 51:165, 1990.

2. Greene CE, Burgdorfer W, Cavagnolo R, et al: Rocky Mountain spotted fever in dogs and its differentiation from canine ehrlichiosis. JAVMA 186:465, 1985.

3. Breitschwerdt EB, Meuten DM, Walker DH, et al: Rocky Mountain spotted fever: A kennel epizootic. Am J Vet Res 46:2124, 1985.

4. Breitschwerdt EB, Levy M, Davidson MG, et al: Kinetics of IgM and IgG responses to experimental and naturally occurring *Rickettsia rickettsii* infection in dogs. Am J Vet Res 51:1312, 1990.

5. Davidson M, Breitschwerdt EB, Nasisse M, et al: Ocular manifestations of Rocky Mountain spotted fever in dogs. JAVMA 194:777, 1989.

6. Weiser I, Greene CE: Dermal necrosis associated with Rocky Mountain spotted fever. JAVMA 195:1756, 1989.

7. Breitschwerdt EB, Davidson MG, Aucoin DP, et al: Efficacy of chloramphenicol, enrofloxacin and tetracycline for treatment of experimental Rocky Mountain spotted fever in dogs. Antimicrob Agents Chemother 35:2375, 1991.

8. Davidson MG, Breitschwerdt EB, Walker DH, et al: Identification of rickettsiae in cutaneous biopsies from dogs with experimental Rocky Mountain spotted fever. J Vet Intern Med 3:8, 1989.

9. Breitschwerdt EB, Davidson MG, Hegarty BC, et al: Prednisolone at anti-inflammatory or immunosuppressive dosages in conjunction with doxycycline does not potentiate the severity of *Rickettsia rickettsii* infection in dogs. Antimicrob Agents Chemother 48:141, 1997.

10. Breitschwerdt EB, Hegarty BC, Davidson MG, et al: Evaluation of the pathogenic potential of *Rickettsia canada* and *Rickettsia prowazekii* organisms in dogs. JAVMA 207:58, 1995.

11. Schriefer ME, Sacci JB, Dumler JS, et al: Identification of a novel rickettsial infection in a patient diagnosed with murine typhus. J Clin Microbiol 32:949, 1994.

12. Dawson JE, Biggie KL, Warner CK, et al: Polymerase chain reaction evidence of *Ehrlichia chaffeensis*, an etiologic agent of human ehrlichiosis, in dogs from southeast Virginia. Am J Vet Res 57:1175, 1996.

13. Breitschwerdt EB, Hegarty BC, Hancock SI: Sequential evaluation of dogs naturally infected with *Ehrlichia canis*, *Ehrlichia ewingii* or *Ehrlichia chaffeensis*. In press.

14. Waner T, Harrus H, Bark H, et al: Characterization of the subclinical phase of canine ehrlichiosis in experimentally infected beagle dogs. Vet Parasitol 69:307, 1997.

15. Perez M, Rikihisa Y, Wen B: *Ehrlichia canis*–like agent isolated from a man in Venezuela: Antigenic and genetic characterization. J Clin Microbiol 34:2133, 1996.

16. Anderson BE, Dawson JE, Jones DC, et al: *Ehrlichia chaffeensis*, a new species associated with human ehrlichiosis. J Clin Microbiol 29:2838, 1991.

17. Codner EC, Roberts RE, Ainsworth G: Atypical findings in 16 cases of canine ehrlichiosis. JAVMA 186:166, 1985.

18. Kuehn NF, Gaunt SD: Clinical and hematologic findings in canine ehrlichiosis. JAVMA 186:355, 1985.

19. Breitschwerdt EB, Woody BJ, Zerbe CA, et al: Monoclonal gammopathy associated with naturally occurring canine ehrlichiosis. J Vet Intern Med 1:2, 1987.

20. Codner EC, Maslin WR: Investigation of renal protein loss in dogs with acute experimentally induced *Ehrlichia canis* infection. Am J Vet Res 53:294, 1992.

21. Bartsch RC, Greene RT: Post-therapy antibody titers in dogs with ehrlichiosis: Follow-up study on 68 patients treated primarily with tetracycline and/or doxycycline. J Vet Intern Med 10:271, 1996.

22. Greig B, Asanovich KM, Armstrong PJ, et al: Geographic, clinical, serologic, and molecular evidence of granulocytic ehrlichiosis, a likely zoonotic disease, in Minnesota and Wisconsin dogs. J Clin Microbiol 34:44, 1996.

23. Anderson BE, CE Greene, DC Jones, et al: *Ehrlichia ewingii* sp. nov., the etiologic agent of canine granulocytic ehrlichiosis. Int J Syst Bacteriol 42:299, 1992.

24. Stockham SL, Schmidt DA, Curtis KS, et al: Evaluation of granulocytic ehrlichiosis in dogs of Missouri, including serologic status to *Ehrlichia canis*, *Ehrlichia equi*, and *Borrelia burgdorferi*. Am J Vet Res 53:63, 1992.

25. Goldman EE, Breitschwerdt EB, Grindem CB, et al: Granulocytic ehrlichiosis in dogs from North Carolina and Virginia. J Vet Intern Med 12:61, 1998.

26. Stockham SL, Tyler JW, Schmidt DA, et al: Experimental transmission of granulocytic ehrlichial organisms in dogs. Vet Clin Pathol 19:99, 1990.

27. Simpson TM, Gaunt SD, Hair JA, et al: Evaluation of *Rhipicephalus sanguineus* as a potential biologic vector of *Ehrlichia platys*. Am J Vet Res 52:1537, 1991.

28. Wilson J: *Ehrlichia platys* in a Michigan dog. J Am Anim Hosp Assoc 28:381, 1992.

29. Gaunt SD, Baker DC, Babin SS: Platelet aggregation studies in dogs with acute *Ehrlichia platys* infection. Am J Vet Res 51:290, 1990.

30. Mathew JS, Ewing SA, Murphy GL, et al: Characterization of a new isolate of *Ehrlichia platys* (order Rickettsiales) using electron microsurgery and polymerase chain reaction. Vet Parasitol 68:1, 1997.

31. Hoskins JD, Breitschwerdt EB, Gaunt SD, et al: Antibodies to *Ehrlichia canis*, *Ehrlichia platys*, and spotted fever group rickettsiae in Louisiana dogs. J Vet Intern Med 2:55, 1988.

32. Kakoma I, Hansen RD, Anderson BE, et al: Cultural, molecular and immunological characterization of the etiologic agent for atypical canine ehrlichiosis. J Clin Microbiol 32:170–175, 1994.

33. Bouloy T, Lappin MR, Holland CJ, et al: Clinical ehrlichiosis in a cat. JAVMA 204:1475, 1994.

34. Peavy GM, Holland CJ, Dutta SK, et al: Suspected ehrlichial infection in five cats from a household. JAVMA 210:231, 1997.

35. Rikihisa Y, Stills H, Zimmerman G: Isolation and continuous culture of *Neorickettsia helminthoeca* in a macrophage cell line. J Clin Microbiol 29:1928, 1991.

36. Rikihisa Y, Kawahara M, Wen B, et al: Western immunoblot analysis of *Haemo-*

INF

bartonella muris and comparison of 16S rRNA gene sequences of *H. muris, H. felis* and *Eperythrozoon suis.* J Clin Microbiol 35:823, 1997.

37. Grindem CB, Corbett WT, Tompkins MT: Risk factors for *Haemobartonella felis* infection in cats. JAVMA 196:96, 1990.

38. Van Steenhouse JL, Taboada J, Millard JR: Feline hemobartonellosis. Compendium for Continuing Education 15:535, 1993.

39. Gretillat S: Feline hemobartonellosis. Fel Pract 14:22, 1984.

40. Marrie TJ, Stein A, Janigan D, et al: Route of infection determines the clinical manifestations of acute Q fever. J Infect Dis 173:484, 1996.

41. Marrie TJ, Langille D, Papukna V, et al: Truckin' pneumonia—an outbreak of Q fever in a truck repair plant probably due to aerosols from clothing contaminated by contact with new born kittens. Epidemiol Infect 102:119, 1989.

42. Laughlin T, Waag D, Williams J, et al: Q fever: From deer to dog to man (letter). Lancet 337:676, 1991.

CHAPTER 87

PROTOZOAL AND MISCELLANEOUS INFECTIONS

Michael R. Lappin

There are multiple pathogenic protozoans that can infect dogs and cats. The group can be divided into amoebae, ciliates, coccidians, flagellates, Microspora, and Piroplasmia. Protozoans generally cause gastrointestinal tract disease (enteric protozoans), polysystemic disease, or, in the case of *Toxoplasma gondii*, both enteric and polysystemic disease.

ENTERIC PROTOZOAL DISEASES

Etiologies. The most common protozoal agents infecting the gastrointestinal tract of dogs and cats are *Giardia, Cryptosporidium parvum, Cystoisospora* spp., *Sarcocystis* spp., *Besnoitia* spp., *Hammondia* spp., *Toxoplasma gondii, Entamoeba histolytica, Balantidium coli,* and *Pentatrichomonas hominis. Giardia* and *P. hominis* are flagellates; *Cystoisospora* spp., *Sarcocystis* spp., *Besnoitia* spp., *Hammondia* spp., *T. gondii,* and *C. parvum* are coccidians[1, 2]; *B. coli* is a ciliate; and *E. histolytica* is an amoeba. *Cystoisospora* spp., *Sarcocystis* spp., *Besnoitia* spp., *Hammondia* spp., and *T. gondii* complete the intestinal cycle in only one species. Some isolates of *C. parvum, Giardia, E. histolytica, B. coli,* and *P. hominis* replicate in multiple warm-blooded vertebrates and so can potentially be zoonotic.

Epidemiology. Fecal-oral transmission occurs with all the enteric protozoans (Table 87–1). The coccidians produce oocysts. *Cryptosporidium parvum* oocysts are immediately infectious when passed by the host; *T. gondii* (1 to 5 days) and *Cystoisospora* spp. (8 hours) must sporulate outside the host to be infectious. Both trophozoites and cysts of *Giardia, B. coli,* and *P. hominis* are potentially infectious; however, transmission occurs most frequently after ingestion of cysts, because trophozoites are generally killed by gastric secretions. Ingestion of the organism in the tissues of transport hosts can also result in infection by *Cystoisospora* spp., *Besnoitia* spp., *Hammondia* spp., and *T. gondii.* Carnivorism can result in infection by *C. parvum, Giardia, E. histolytica,*

B. coli, and *P. hominis* if the organisms were present in the intestines of the prey species. Infections can be self-limited for each of the agents, but with the exception of *T. gondii,* fecal shedding periods are variable. Following tissue cyst ingestion, infected cats rarely shed oocysts of *T. gondii* for more than two weeks.

The enteric protozoans have worldwide distribution. Because they are maintained in nature primarily by fecal-oral transmission, more cases are associated with crowded and unsanitary environments. In general, *Giardia, T. gondii, Cystoisospora,* and *C. parvum* infections are common in dogs and cats of the United States; *E. histolytica, B. coli,* and *P. hominis* infections are rare. Antibodies against *T. gondii* (40 per cent)[3] and *C. parvum* (8.3 per cent)[4] are commonly detected in serum from client-owned cats, suggesting that exposure is common. Prevalence of the agents varies by region in coprologic studies.

Pathogenesis. Pathogenic mechanisms have not been ascertained for each of the enteric protozoans. *Cystoisospora* spp. and *T. gondii* replicate in intestinal cells and may result in clinical illness from cell destruction. Tissue invasion also can occur with *E. histolytica.*[5, 6] *Giardia* and *C. parvum* are found on the surface of enterocytes, so pathogenesis is unlikely to be secondary to direct cell damage. Some of the pathogenic mechanisms proposed for enteric pathogens include production of toxins, disruption of normal flora, induction of inflammatory bowel disease, inhibition of normal enterocyte enzymatic function, blunting of microvilli, and induction of motility disorders. *Cystoisospora* spp. generally result in clinical disease only in puppies or kittens, and *Sarcocystis* spp., *Besnoitia* spp., and *Hammondia* spp. are almost never pathogenic in dogs or cats; all other enteric protozoans can cause disease regardless of age. Clinical disease is more common, and duration of organism shedding into the environment may be prolonged, in dogs and cats with an immunodeficiency condition.

TABLE 87–1. ENTERIC PROTOZOAL INFECTIONS OF THE DOG AND CAT

ORGANISM	FORM IN FECES	SIZE (μ)
Balantidium coli	Trophozoite	60×35
	Cyst	40×60
Besnoitia spp.		
Feline		
B. besnoiti	Oocyst	15×13
B. wallacei	Oocyst	17×12
B. darlingi	Oocyst	12×12
Cryptosporidium spp.	Oocyst	$3–6$
Cystoisospora spp.		
Feline		
C. felis	Oocyst	30×40
C. rivolta	Oocyst	20×25
Canine		
C. canis	Oocyst	30×38
C. ohioensis	Oocyst	19×23
C. neorivolta	Oocyst	11×13
C. burrowsi	Oocyst	17×20
Entamoeba histolytica	Trophozoite	$10–30$
	Cyst	$5–20$
Giardia	Trophozoite	$15 \times 10 \times 3$
	Cyst	10×8
Hammondia spp.		
Feline		
H. hammondi	Oocyst	12×11
Canine		
H. heydorni	Oocyst	11×12
Pentatrichomonas hominis	Trophozoite	$5–20 \times 3–14$
Sarcocystis spp.		
Feline		
S. hirsuta	Oocyst	12×8
S. tenella	Oocyst	12×8
S. porcifelis	Oocyst	13×8
S. muris	Oocyst	10×8
S. leporum	Oocyst	13×10
Canine		
S. cruzi	Oocyst	16×11
S. capracams	Oocyst	—
S. ovicanis	Oocyst	15×10
S. mischeriana	Oocyst	13×10
S. bertrami	Oocyst	15×10
S. fryeri	Oocyst	12×8
S. hemionilatrantis	Oocyst	14×9
S. idiciukeicabus	Oocyst	11×15
Toxoplasma gondii	Oocyst	10×12

Adapted from Lappin MR: Protozoal diseases. *In* Morgan RV (ed): Handbook of Small Animal Practice, 3rd ed. Philadelphia, WB Saunders, 1997, p 1172.

Clinical Findings. Owner observations regarding dogs or cats with enteric protozoal infections usually include vomiting, inappetence, or diarrhea; fever is uncommon. *Giardia*, *C. parvum*, and *T. gondii* infections are commonly associated with small-bowel diarrhea; *E. histolytica*, *B. coli*, and *P. hominis* infections are most commonly associated with large-bowel diarrhea. *Cystoisospora* spp. infections can cause clinical signs of large- or small-bowel diarrhea. Physical examination findings in dogs or cats with enteric protozoal infections are nonspecific but can include abdominal discomfort, increased gas or fluid in the intestinal tract, or thickened intestinal loops.

Diagnosis. All dogs and cats with large-, small-, or mixed-bowel diarrhea should be assessed for enteric protozoal infections. Diagnosis of gastrointestinal protozoal infection is based primarily on documentation of oocysts, trophozoites, or cysts on direct fecal examination or fecal flotation.[7] A direct smear of diarrheic stool can be used to examine for trophozoites of *E. histolytica*, *B. coli*, *P. hominis*, or *Giardia*. More frequently, a small quantity of feces is mixed with a drop of 0.9 per cent sodium chloride on a clean microscope

slide and examined at $100\times$ after placing a coverslip. When a motile organism is noted, structural features are assessed by examining at $400\times$. Application of a stain such as Lugol's solution, methylene blue, or acid methyl green to the wet mount at the edge of the coverslip will aid in visualizing internal structures of protozoa.[7] Trophozoites are rarely found in formed stools. Duodenal aspiration for cytologic examination for *Giardia* trophozoites is effective for the diagnosis of giardiasis in the dog. However, this technique is not effective in the cat because the organism lives in the distal small intestine.

Protozoal cysts or oocysts are best demonstrated following fecal concentration; Sheather's sugar centrifugation and zinc sulfate centrifugation are two techniques commonly used in clinical practice.[7] These solutions are inexpensive and generally effective. Sugar solution is hypertonic and distorts *Giardia* cysts; the cytoplasm is pulled to one slide and appears as a half or quarter moon. Zinc sulfate is considered by some to be the flotation solution of choice for *Giardia* cysts.

Owing to their small size and limited number in feces, *C. parvum* oocysts are often not seen when concentrated feces are examined at $100\times$. Sugar solution flotation may be the optimal procedure. Acid-fast staining or fluorescein-labeled monoclonal antibody staining of a fecal smear aids in the diagnosis of cryptosporidiosis in dogs and cats. Oocysts stain pink with acid-fast stain. A fluorescein-labeled monoclonal antibody system is also available for identification of *Giardia* cysts.

Antigens of *Giardia* and *C. parvum* can be detected in feces by enzyme-linked immunosorbent assay. Results of these assays should be interpreted with results from fecal examination techniques. Polymerase chain reaction for demonstration of some enteric protozoans in feces is being studied.

The presence of enteric protozoans in diarrheic stool does not prove that disease was caused by the organism. Some enteric protozoans, especially *Giardia*, *C. parvum*, and *Cystoisospora* spp., live chronically in the intestinal tract of normal animals; other conditions causing gastrointestinal tract disease can induce shedding. Thus, animals with enteric protozoal infections that do not improve with therapy should be evaluated for underlying causes of disease. *Giardia*, *C. parvum*, *Cystoisospora* spp., and *Sarcocystis* spp. are commonly found in animals with normal stools, so yearly fecal examinations are indicated in all dogs and cats.

Treatment. Withholding food for 24 to 48 hours is indicated in dogs and cats with acute vomiting or diarrhea. Highly digestible, bland diets are used most frequently if vomiting and small-bowel diarrhea are the primary manifestations of disease. High-fiber diets are used if large-bowel diarrhea is occurring. Feeding a high-fiber diet may also aid in the treatment of giardiasis, owing to inhibition of trophozoite attachment to duodenal epithelial cells.

Entamoeba histolytica, *Giardia*, *B. coli*, and *P. hominis* generally respond to metronidazole (Table 87–2). Central nervous system (CNS) toxicity occasionally occurs with this drug[8]; it is unlikely with appropriate doses. Fenbendazole and albendazole are commonly prescribed alternative anti-*Giardia* drugs.[9, 10] However, activity of these drugs against the other enteric protozoans is unknown. Because dogs or cats with giardiasis could also be infected with these other potentially zoonotic enteric protozoans, metronidazole is a logical primary drug. Metronidazole also helps correct the anaerobic bacterial overgrowth that commonly accompanies giardiasis. If inflammatory changes exist, metronidazole may

TABLE 87–2. DRUGS USED IN THE MANAGEMENT OF PROTOZOAL DISEASES

ORGANISM/GENERIC DRUG NAME	COMMON CANINE DOSAGE	COMMON FELINE DOSAGE
Babesia spp.*		
Clindamycin	12.5 mg/kg, q12h, for 2 weeks, PO	NA
Imidocarb dipropionate	2–7 mg/kg, q7–14days, IM, SC	NA
Phenamidine isethionate	15 mg/kg, q24h, daily for 2 days, SC	NA
Balantidium coli		
Metronidazole	25 mg/kg, q12h, for 8 days, PO	25 mg/kg, q12h, for 8 days, PO
Cryptosporidium parvum		
Paromomycin	As for cats	165 mg/kg, q12h, for 5 days, PO
Tylosin	As for cats	10–15 mg/kg, q8–12h, for 21 days, PO
Cystoisospora spp.		
Trimethoprim-sulfonamide	15–30 mg/kg, q12h, for 5 days, PO	15 mg/kg, q12h, for 5 days, PO
Sulfadimethoxine	50–60 mg/kg, daily, for 5–20 days, PO	50–60 mg/kg, daily, for 5–20 days, PO
Furazolidone	8–20 mg/kg, q12–24h, for 5 days, PO	8–20 mg/kg, q12–24h, for 5 days, PO
Amprolium	300–400 mg, daily, for 5 days	60–100 mg, daily, for 5 days
Cytauxzoon felis		
Buparvaquone	NA	10 mg/kg, q24h, IM, SC
Imidocarb	NA	5 mg/kg, q14days, IM
Parvaquone	NA	10–30 mg/kg, q24h, IM, SC
Tetracycline	NA	5–10 mg/kg, q12–24h, IM, IV
Encephalitozoon†	NA	NA
Entamoeba histolytica		
Metronidazole	25 mg/kg, q12h, for 8 days, PO	25 mg/kg, q12h, for 8 days, PO
Giardia		
Metronidazole	25 mg/kg, q12h, for 8 days, PO	25 mg/kg, q12h, for 8 days, PO
Albendazole	25 mg/kg, q12h, for 2–5 days, PO	Unknown
Fenbendazole	25 mg/kg, q12h, for 3–7 days, PO	Unknown
Ipronidazole	126 mg/L water, for 7 days, PO	Unknown
Furazolidone	4 mg/kg, q12h, for 7 days, PO	4 mg/kg, q12h, for 7 days, PO
Hepatozoon canis‡		
Trimethoprim-sulfadiazine	15 mg/kg, q12h, for 2–4 weeks, PO	NA
Pyrimethamine	0.25 mg/kg, q24h, for 2–4 weeks, PO	NA
Clindamycin	10 mg/kg, q8h, for 2–4 weeks, PO	NA
Leishmania		
Allopurinol	15 mg/kg, q12h, for months	NA
Amphotericin B (liposomal)	3–3.3 mg/kg, 3 times weekly, for 3–5 treatments, IV	NA
Meglumine antimonate	100 mg/kg, q24h, IV, IM, SC	NA
Sodium stibogluconate	30–50 mg/kg q24h, IV, SC	NA
Neospora§		
Trimethoprim-sulfonamide	15 mg/kg, q12h, for 4 weeks, PO	NA
Pyrimethamine	1 mg/kg, q24h, for 4 weeks, PO	NA
Clindamycin	10 mg/kg, q12h, for 4 weeks, PO	NA
Pentatrichomonas hominis		
Metronidazole	25 mg/kg, q12h, for 8 days, PO	25 mg/kg, q12h, for 8 days, PO
Pneumocystis carinii		
Pentamidine isethionate	4 mg/kg, q24h, for 2 weeks, IM	Unknown
Trimethoprim-sulfonamide	15 mg/kg, q6–12h, for 2 weeks, PO	15 mg/kg, q12h, for 4 weeks, PO
Toxoplasma gondii		
Clindamycin hydrochloride	12.5 mg/kg, q12h, for 28 days, PO, IM	12.5 mg/kg, q12h, for 28 days, PO, IM
Pyrimethamine	0.25–0.5 mg/kg, q24h, for 28 days, PO	Usually not used owing to toxicity
Trimethoprim-sulfonamide	15 mg/kg, q12h, for 28 days, PO	15 mg/kg, q12h, for 28 days, PO
Doxycycline	5–10 mg/kg, q12h, for 4 weeks, PO	5–10 mg/kg, q12h, for 4 weeks, PO
Trypanosoma cruzi		
Nifurtimox	2–7 mg/kg, q6h, for 3–5 months, PO	NA

IM = intramuscular, IV = intravenous, SC = subcutaneous, PO = oral, NA = not applicable.
Babesia gibsoni is most likely to respond to phenamidine.
†No treatment has been reported for encephalitozoonosis in small animals.
‡It has been recommended to use pyrimethamine, clindamycin, and trimethoprim-sulfonamide concurrently.
§It has been recommended to use either pyrimethamine or clindamycin concurrently with trimethoprim-sulfonamide.

also be beneficial because of inhibition of lymphocyte function. Tinidazole administered orally at 44 mg/kg every 24 hours for 3 days, ipronidazole administered orally at 126 mg/L of water ad libitum for 7 days, and furazolidone (see Table 87–2) are other potential anti-*Giardia* drugs. Paromomycin is an effective treatment of cryptosporidiosis in dogs and cats (see Table 87–2).[11] Sequential administration of clindamycin 12 mg/kg orally twice a day followed by tylosin 11 mg/kg orally three times a day for 21 days may be a useful treatment regimen.[12]

The *T. gondii* oocyst shedding period can be shortened by administration of clindamycin 12.5 to 25 mg/kg orally twice a day for 7 to 14 days. Alternatively, the combination of sulfonamides and pyrimethamine, monensin, or toltrazuril can be used.[3] The most commonly prescribed drugs (see Table 87–2) to treat *Cystoisospora* spp. infections of dogs and cats are trimethoprim-sulfonamide, sulfadimethoxine, furazolidone, amprolium, or amprolium-sulfadimethoxine (150 mg amprolium and 25 mg/kg sulfadimethoxine orally once a day for 14 days). Quinacrine, spiramycin, toltrazuril, and roxithromycin have been used on a limited basis.

Zoonotic Potential and Prevention. *Cryptosporidium*

parvum, T. gondii, Giardia, E. histolytica, B. coli, and *P. hominis* are potentially zoonotic. Although not all isolates of *Giardia* are zoonotic, it is impossible to determine whether an individual strain is infectious to people. Clinical cryptosporidiosis is characterized by small-bowel diarrhea and is generally self-limited in immunocompetent humans, but fatal infection can occur in humans with AIDS. Annually, from 5 to 10 per cent of humans with AIDS will be infected by *C. parvum.*[13] Some isolates of *C. parvum* infect multiple species; others have a limited host range. Oocysts are rarely found in dog and cat feces in North America, but antibodies are commonly detected in serum from cats, suggesting that exposure is common.[4] Person-to-person contact with oocysts by fecal-oral contamination and the ingestion of contaminated water are the most likely routes of exposure to *C. parvum. C. parvum* infection in people following exposure to infected calves is well documented. Cryptosporidiosis has been detected in humans and small animals in the same environment.

Toxoplasma gondii is one of the most significant small animal zoonoses. Primary infections, but not subsequent infections, of mothers during gestation can lead to severe clinical toxoplasmosis in the fetus. Stillbirth, CNS disease, and ocular disease are common clinical manifestations. The fetus is unlikely to be infected during a first-trimester exposure, but if infection occurs, it generally results in severe disease. Second- and third-trimester fetal infections have less severe consequences. Immunocompetent individuals can have self-limited fever, malaise, and lymphadenopathy after primary infection; subsequent infections are usually subclinical. In people with AIDS, toxoplasmosis is the most common opportunistic CNS infection. Most are thought to have encephalitis from activation of bradyzoites in tissue cysts after decline of CD4+ lymphocyte counts.

Cats shed *T. gondii* oocysts only for days to several weeks following primary inoculation. Most cats are fastidious and do not allow feces to remain on their skin for one to five days to allow oocyst shedding; the organism was not isolated from the fur of cats shedding millions of oocysts seven days previously.[14] Administration of clinical doses of glucocorticoids or co-infection with feline immunodeficiency virus (FIV) or feline leukemia virus (FeLV) does not induce oocyst shedding in chronically infected cats.[3] Veterinary health care providers and people with AIDS who own cats are not at increased risk for toxoplasmosis. These findings suggest that touching individual cats is an unusual way to contract toxoplasmosis. However, four of nine seropositive cats challenged with *T. gondii* six years after primary inoculation shed oocysts, so gut immunity is not permanent.[14] To prevent contact with oocysts, people should avoid feeding cats undercooked meats, not allow cats to hunt, clean the litter box daily with scalding water or use a litter box liner, incinerate or flush the feces, wear gloves when working with soil, wash hands thoroughly with soap and hot water following gardening, wash fresh vegetables well before ingestion, keep children's sandboxes covered, boil water for drinking that has been obtained from the general environment, control potential transport hosts, and treat oocyst-shedding cats with anti-*Toxoplasma* drugs.[3]

Many people are infected by ingestion of *T. gondii* in tissues. Meats (particularly pork, lamb, and goat) should be cooked to medium-well to inactivate tissue cysts. Gloves should be worn when handling raw meats (including field dressing) for cooking, or hands should be cleansed thoroughly afterward. Freezing meat inactivates many but not all tissue cysts.

Because humans are unlikely to be infected with *T. gondii* from contact with individual cats, serologic testing of healthy cats for toxoplasmosis is not required.[15] There also is no serologic assay that accurately predicts when a cat shed *T. gondii* oocysts in the past, and most cats that are shedding oocysts are seronegative. Most seropositive cats have completed the oocyst-shedding period and are unlikely to repeat shedding; most seronegative cats would shed the organism if infected. If an owner is concerned about toxoplasmosis, he or she should see a physician for testing. It is advisable for women to know their *T. gondii* serologic status before pregnancy.

Dogs do not complete the enteroepithelial phase of *T. gondii.* Like all other warm-blooded vertebrates, dogs are infected by the ingestion of sporulated oocysts or tissue cysts. Toxoplasmosis in dogs can be prevented by not allowing dogs to be coprophagic and by feeding only cooked meat and meat by-products.

Trophozoites of enteric protozoans are susceptible to most disinfectants and rapidly die outside the host. Cysts and oocysts are resistance to most disinfectants. Cleanliness is the best method for avoiding contamination of the environment. Steam cleaning ruptures and inactivates most oocysts. Transport and paratenic hosts should be controlled in the environment. A vaccine against *Giardia lamblia* is currently being evaluated.[16]

POLYSYSTEMIC PROTOZOAL DISEASES

The primary protozoans that induce polysystemic disease in dogs and cats are *Acanthamoeba* spp., *Hepatozoon canis, Neospora caninum, Toxoplasma gondii, Leishmania* spp., *Trypanosoma cruzi, Cytauxzoon felis, Babesia* spp., and *Pneumocystis carinii.*

COCCIDIANS

Toxoplasmosis

Etiology and Epidemiology. *Toxoplasma gondii* is a coccidian with worldwide distribution; the seroprevalence of infection is approximately 40 per cent in cats and humans and approximately 20 per cent in dogs in the United States.[3] The oocysts in feces at the completion of the intestinal phase in cats are unsporulated and are not infectious; infectious sporozoites develop in oocysts after one to five days of exposure to oxygen, appropriate environmental temperature, and humidity. Once sporulated, oocysts are infectious for most warm-blooded vertebrates and can survive in the environment for months to years. Tachyzoites and bradyzoites are the two tissue stages of *T. gondii* found in the tissues of infected cats, dogs, and other intermediate hosts.[3] Tachyzoites are the rapidly dividing, dissemination stage; they replicate intracellularly until infected cells are destroyed or the immune system attenuates replication. Bradyzoites are the slowly dividing, persistent stage; they form in extraintestinal tissues (particularly CNS, muscles, and visceral organs) of immunocompetent individuals. It is likely that bradyzoites persist in tissues for the life of the host. Infection with *T. gondii* occurs following ingestion of any of the three life stages or transplacentally when the host has its primary infection during gestation. Ingesting *T. gondii* bradyzoites during carnivorous feeding most commonly infects cats. Because dogs are more likely than cats to be coprophagic, ingestion of sporulated oocysts is a likely means of infection.

Clinical Features. During the one- to two-week intestinal cycle that occurs after primary exposure, approximately 10 to 20 per cent of experimentally inoculated cats develop self-limited small-bowel diarrhea. This is presumed to be due to enteroepithelial replication of the organism. Inflammatory bowel disease may be an uncommon manifestation of the intestinal cycle in cats.[17]

In cats, fatal extraintestinal toxoplasmosis can develop from overwhelming intracellular replication of tachyzoites following primary infection of kittens or immune-suppressed adult cats; the course of illness is acute.[18, 19] Hepatic, pulmonary, CNS, and pancreatic tissues are commonly involved. Disseminated toxoplasmosis in cats results in depression, anorexia, fever followed by hypothermia, peritoneal effusion, icterus, dyspnea, and death. Acquired immunodeficiency can allow bradyzoites in tissue cysts to revert to tachyzoites and disseminate. This occurs in some people with AIDS, cats infected with FeLV, FIV, and feline infectious peritonitis virus, or those immune-suppressed with drugs.

Chronic clinical syndromes occur in some cats from extraintestinal infection.[20, 21] *T. gondii* infection apparently can cause anterior or posterior uveitis, fever, muscle hyperesthesia, weight loss, anorexia, seizures, ataxia, icterus, diarrhea, and pancreatitis. The pathogenesis of chronic, sublethal toxoplasmosis may be due to immune complex formation and deposition in tissues with delayed hypersensitivity reactions. *Toxoplasma* cannot be cleared from the body by drugs, so recurrence of subfatal disease is common.

Dogs with generalized toxoplasmosis usually have respiratory, gastrointestinal, or neuromuscular infection resulting in fever, vomiting, diarrhea, dyspnea, and icterus.[3] Dogs with myositis have weakness, stiff gait, or muscle wasting; rapid progression to tetraparesis and paralysis with lower motor neuron dysfunction can occur. Many dogs with suspected neuromuscular or CNS toxoplasmosis probably had neosporosis (see the following section). Ataxia, seizures, tremors, cranial nerve deficits, paresis, and paralysis are the most common manifestations of CNS toxoplasmosis. Ventricular arrhythmias from myocardial infection occur in some infected dogs. Ocular manifestations, including retinitis, anterior uveitis, iridocyclitis, and optic neuritis, occur in some dogs with toxoplasmosis but are less common than in the cat.

Diagnosis. There are no pathognomonic clinicopathologic or radiographic abnormalities in dogs or cats with clinical toxoplasmosis. Abnormalities consistent with feline toxoplasmosis are nonregenerative anemia, neutrophilic leukocytosis, lymphocytosis, monocytosis, neutropenia, eosinophilia, proteinuria, and bilirubinuria, as well as increases in serum protein, bilirubin, creatinine kinase, alanine aminotransferase, alkaline phosphatase, and lipase.[3] Diffuse interstitial or alveolar patterns and pleural effusion are the most common radiographic abnormalities. Cerebrospinal fluid (CSF) protein concentrations and cell counts (small mononuclear cells and/or neutrophils) are often abnormally increased with CNS toxoplasmosis.

The antemortem definitive diagnosis of feline or canine toxoplasmosis can be made if the organism is demonstrated; however, this is uncommon, particularly if the disease is chronic. Bradyzoites or tachyzoites are rarely detected in tissues, effusions, bronchoalveolar lavage fluids, aqueous humor, or CSF. Detection of $10 \times 12\ \mu$ oocysts in feces from cats with diarrhea suggests toxoplasmosis but is not definitive, because *Besnoitia darlingi* and *Hammondia hammondi* infections of cats produce morphologically similar oocysts.

Toxoplasma gondii–specific antibodies can be detected in the serum of normal cats and dogs, as well as in those with clinical signs of disease, so it is impossible to make an antemortem diagnosis of clinical toxoplasmosis based on these tests alone.[22] Of the serum tests, IgM correlates the best with clinical toxoplasmosis. The antemortem diagnosis of clinical toxoplasmosis can be tentatively based on the combination of

- Demonstration of antibodies in serum, which documents exposure to *T. gondii*.
- Demonstration of an IgM titer greater than 1:64 or a fourfold or greater increase in IgG titer, which suggests recent or active infection.
- Clinical signs of disease referable to toxoplasmosis.
- Exclusion of other common causes of the clinical syndrome.
- Positive response to appropriate treatment.

Some cats and dogs with clinical toxoplasmosis will have reached their maximal IgG titer or will have undergone antibody class shift from IgM to IgG by the time serologic evaluation is performed. Thus, the failure to document an increasing IgG titer or a positive IgM titer does not exclude the diagnosis of clinical toxoplasmosis. Because some healthy cats and dogs have extremely high serum antibody titers and some clinically ill cats and dogs have low serum antibody titers, the magnitude of titer is relatively unimportant in the clinical diagnosis of toxoplasmosis. Because the organism cannot be cleared from the body, most cats and dogs will be antibody-positive for life, so there is little use in repeating serum antibody titers after clinical disease has resolved.

The combination of aqueous humor or CSF *T. gondii*–specific antibody detection and organism detection by polymerase chain reaction (PCR)[22] is the most accurate way to diagnose ocular or CNS toxoplasmosis in cats (Diagnostic Laboratory, College of Veterinary Medicine and Biomedical Sciences, Colorado State University, Fort Collins, CO 80523). Although limited numbers of CSF or aqueous humor samples from dogs have been evaluated this way, trends are similar to those from cats (MR Lappin, unpublished data). *Toxoplasma gondii*–specific IgA, IgG, and the organism (by PCR) can be detected in aqueous humor and CSF of both normal and clinically ill cats. *Toxoplasma gondii*–specific IgM has been detected only in the aqueous humor or CSF of clinically ill cats and may be the best indicator of clinical disease.

Therapy. Supportive care is given as needed. Clindamycin hydrochloride or trimethoprim-sulfonamide combination administered for four weeks can be utilized (see Table 87–2). Pyrimethamine combined with sulfa drugs is effective for the treatment of human toxoplasmosis but is toxic in cats. Other anti-*Toxoplasma* drugs include doxycycline, minocycline, azithromycin, and clarithromycin.[3] Cats and dogs with uveitis should be treated with anti-*Toxoplasma* drugs in combination with topical, oral, or parenteral corticosteroids to avoid secondary damage to the eye induced by inflammation. Glaucoma and lens luxations are common in cats. Chorioretinitis may respond to clindamycin hydrochloride alone.

Excluding ocular, CNS, and neuromuscular disease, signs of toxoplasmosis usually resolve within the first two to three days of clindamycin or trimethoprim-sulfonamide administration. Ocular, CNS, and neuromuscular toxoplasmosis responds more slowly. If fever or muscle hyperesthesia is not resolving after three days of treatment, other causes should be considered. Recurrence of clinical signs may be more common if treatment duration is less than four weeks. There is currently no drug that can totally clear the body of the organism, so recurrences are common. The prognosis is poor for cats and dogs with disseminated toxoplasmosis owing to organism replication, particularly if immunodeficiency exists. Dogs with neuromuscular disease also have a poor prognosis.

Zoonotic Potential and Prevention. See the section on enteric protozoal pathogens for a complete discussion.

Neosporosis

Etiology and Epidemiology. *Neospora caninum* is a tissue coccidian that is antigenically distinct from *T. gondii*.[3, 23] *N. caninum* and *T. gondii* have a similar morphologic appearance; it is likely that many dogs once thought to have clinical toxoplasmosis had neosporosis. Tachyzoites and bradyzoites in tissue have been identified. It is proposed but not proved that the sexual cycle (oocyst production) of *N. caninum* is completed in a carnivore. The only proven route of transmission in dogs is transplacental. Repeated transplacental infection of puppies from infected bitches can occur during subsequent pregnancies.[24] Neuromuscular disease in dogs and abortion in cattle are the most common naturally occurring manifestations of neosporosis. Kittens experimentally inoculated with *N. caninum* develop encephalomyelitis and myositis; naturally infected cats have not been reported.[3] Although canine neosporosis has been reported from many countries, the prevalence of disease is largely undetermined.

Clinical Features. In puppies with congenitally transmitted neosporosis, ascending paralysis with rigid contracture and atrophy of the hind limbs is the most common clinical manifestation of the disease.[3] Disease is due to intracellular replication of *N. caninum* tachyzoites and resultant scar tissue formation. Ruptured tissue cysts in CNS structures are associated with mononuclear cell infiltrates, which suggests an immune-mediated component to the pathogenesis of disease. Polymyositis and multifocal CNS disease can occur alone or in combination and can result in neonatal death. Clinical signs can be evident soon after birth or may be delayed for several weeks. Several other clinical manifestations of neosporosis, including myocarditis, dysphagia, ulcerative dermatitis, pneumonia, and hepatitis, have been recognized in dogs as old as 15 years.[3, 25] It is unknown whether clinical disease in older dogs is due to acute primary infection or exacerbation of chronic infection. Administration of glucocorticoids may activate bradyzoites in tissue cysts, resulting in clinical illness. Untreated neosporosis is usually fatal.

Diagnosis. The laboratory and radiographic abnormalities induced by neosporosis are nonspecific. Myositis commonly results in increased serum activities of creatine kinase and aspartate aminotransferase. CSF abnormalities include increased protein concentration (20 to 50 mg/dL) and a mild, mixed inflammatory cell pleocytosis (10 to 50 cells/dL) consisting of monocytes, lymphocytes, neutrophils, and, rarely, eosinophils. *N. caninum* tachyzoites are rarely identified on cytologic examination of CSF, imprints of dermatologic lesions, and bronchoalveolar lavage but cannot be distinguished from those of *T. gondii* under the light microscope. Tissue cysts of the two organisms can be differentiated; *N. caninum* tissue cysts have a wall greater than 1 μ; *T. gondii* tissue cysts have a wall less than 1 μ. The organism can also be differentiated from *T. gondii* by electron microscopy, immunohistochemistry, and PCR.[3]

To make a presumptive diagnosis of neosporosis, combine appropriate clinical signs of disease, positive serology or presence of antibodies in CSF, and exclusion of other causes of the clinical syndromes, in particular *T. gondii*. Immunoglobulin G antibody titers of 1:200 or greater have been detected in all dogs with clinical neosporosis; there is minimal serologic cross-reactivity with *T. gondii* at titers of 1:50 or greater.[3] Serology is commercially available.

Therapy. Surviving dogs to date have been treated with trimethoprim-sulfadiazine combined with pyrimethamine; sequential treatment with clindamycin hydrochloride, trimethoprim-sulfadiazine, and pyrimethamine; or clindamycin alone.[3, 25] Administration of trimethoprim-sulfadiazine with pyrimethamine or clindamycin (see Table 87–2) for four weeks is currently recommended for the treatment of canine neosporosis. Treatment of clinically affected dogs should be initiated before the development of extensor rigidity, if possible. It is possible to arrest the progress of disease in some dogs, but scar formation and dysfunction are unlikely to resolve.

Zoonotic Potential and Prevention. *Neospora caninum* is not known to be zoonotic, but until the definitive host is identified, final recommendations concerning prevention cannot be made. Bitches that whelp clinically affected puppies should not be bred. Glucocorticoids should not be administered to seropositive animals, because a potential exists for activation of infection.

Hepatozoonosis

Etiology and Epidemiology. *Hepatozoon canis* infects dogs and cats in Africa, southern Europe, Asia, and the United States and maintains its life cycle in *Rhipicephalus sanguineus*.[26–29] Hepatozoonosis in the United States is most common in the Texas Gulf coast, Louisiana, Alabama, Georgia, and Oklahoma. It has been proposed that the American form of hepatozoonosis is a separate species (*H. americanum*) transmitted by *Amblyomma maculatum*.[26] Sexual reproduction of *H. canis* occurs in *R. sanguineus*; the organism is transmitted when the vertebrate host ingests ticks containing oocysts that release sporozoites. Sporozoites infect mononuclear phagocytes and endothelial cells of the spleen, liver, muscle, lungs, and bone marrow and ultimately form cysts containing macromeronts and micromeronts. Pyogranulomatous inflammation results and causes the clinical disease. Replication of the organism in muscles around bones results in marked periosteal reaction. Gamonts can be found in circulating neutrophils and monocytes and are the source of new tick infections. Vertical transmission also has been documented in dogs.[30]

Clinical Findings. Most infected dogs remain clinically normal; disease is most common in young or immunocompromised dogs.[26–29] Most dogs with hepatozoonosis live in rural, wooded areas and are diagnosed from April to October, when ticks are most active. Fever, weight loss, and hyperesthesia over the paraspinal regions are the most common findings. Pale mucous membranes from anemia, bloody diarrhea, anorexia, depression, and oculonasal discharge occur in many dogs. Clinical signs can be intermittent and recurrent. Although cats can develop hepatozoonosis, most have concurrent diseases, so it is unclear whether the organism is a primary pathogen in cats.

Diagnosis. Definitive diagnosis is based on identification of gamonts in neutrophils or monocytes in Giemsa or Leishman's stained blood smears or by demonstration of the organism in muscle biopsy sections.[26–29] A presumptive diagnosis can be made based on combining appropriate geographic location or travel history, presence of extreme neutrophilic leukocytosis (20,000 to 200,000 cells/μL) with a left shift, and periosteal reaction, which can occur around any bone other than the skull. Eosinophilia, regenerative anemia, hypoalbuminemia, hypoglycemia, proteinuria, and increased alkaline phosphatase and creatine kinase activities are detected in some dogs.

Therapy. It is unclear whether drug administration speeds resolution of disease. The combination of trimethoprim-sulfadiazine, pyrimethamine, and clindamycin (see Table 87–2) may be successful.[26, 29] Diminazene, imidocarb, toltrazuril, and primaquine have been used in some infected dogs but are not routinely available in the United States. Administration of toltrazuril failed to prevent relapse in 18 of 21 treated dogs.[27] Administration of nonsteroidal anti-inflammatory agents may be the most successful aspect of therapy in most cases. The periosteal reaction may never resolve radiographically.

Zoonotic Potential and Prevention. There is no evidence for zoonotic transfer of *H. canis* from infected dogs to people. Tick control is the best form of prevention. Glucocorticoid administration should be avoided, as it may exacerbate clinical disease.

PIROPLASMIA

Babesiosis

Etiology and Epidemiology. *Babesia* spp. parasitize red blood cells, leading to progressive anemia. *Babesia* spp. have worldwide distribution; infections of dogs with *B. canis* and *B. gibsoni* have been documented primarily in the southern United States.[31] None of the *Babesia* spp. that infect cats, *B. cati* (India), *B. felis* (South Africa and Sudan), *B. herpailuri* (South America and Africa), and *B. pantherae* (Kenya), is found in the United States. *Rhipicephalus sanguineus*, *Dermacentor* spp., *Haemaphysalis leachi*, and *Hyalomma plumbeum* can transmit *B. canis*. *Haemaphysalis bispinosa* and *R. sanguineus* can transmit *B. gibsoni*. *Babesia* spp. can also be transmitted by blood transfusion. Severity of disease depends on the strain of *Babesia* and the host immune status; the strains infecting dogs in the United States are of lower pathogenicity than those in other countries.[32] The organism can be maintained in the body chronically in a quiescent state. Administration of glucocorticoids or splenectomy may activate chronic disease.

Clinical Findings. There are subclinical, peracute, acute, chronic, and atypical infections in dogs. The incubation period of *Babesia* spp. infections varies from 10 days to 3 weeks. Red blood cells are destroyed by intracellular organism replication or immune-mediated reactions against the parasite or altered self-antigens. Anemia and fever leading to pale mucous membranes, tachycardia, tachypnea, depression, anorexia, and weakness are common with peracute and acute disease. Hypoxia from rapidly developing hemolytic anemia can result in metabolic acidosis and renal disease. Icterus, petechiation, and hepatosplenomegaly are present in some dogs, depending on the stage of infection and the presence of disseminated intravascular coagulation. Chronically infected dogs are usually subclinically affected but may have weight loss and anorexia. Ascites, gastrointestinal signs, CNS disease, edema, and clinical evidence of cardiopulmonary disease occur in some dogs with atypical infection.

Diagnosis. Regenerative anemia, hyperbilirubinemia, bilirubinuria, hemoglobinuria, thrombocytopenia, metabolic acidosis, azotemia, polyclonal gammopathy, and renal casts are common in dogs with peracute or acute babesiosis.[31] *Babesia* spp. can occasionally be demonstrated in red blood cells using Wright's or Giemsa stains on thin blood smears, but parasitemia is variable. *Babesia canis* is typically found as paired, piriform bodies measuring 2.4 × 5.0 μ. *B. gibsoni* is typically found as single, annular bodies measuring 1.0 × 3.2 μ.

A presumptive diagnosis of babesiosis can be based on historical findings, physical examination findings, test results, and positive serology. Indirect fluorescent antibody titers for *B. canis* and *B. gibsoni* greater than 1:80 are positive. Recent or active infection can be confirmed by demonstration of increasing titers over two to three weeks. False-negative serologic test results can occur in peracute cases or in dogs with concurrent immune suppression. Because clinically normal dogs can be seropositive, setology alone should not be used to make a definitive diagnosis.

Therapy. Blood transfusion, sodium bicarbonate therapy for acidosis, and fluid therapy should be administered as indicated when treating peracute or acute babesiosis. Phenamidine isethionate is effective for *B. canis* and *B. gibsoni* infections; imidocarb dipropionate and diminazene aceturate are effective for *B. canis*. Because these drugs are not yet available in the United States, dogs with suspected babesiosis should be treated with clindamycin hydrochloride or metronidazole.[31, 32] Doxycycline was effective prophylactically at lessening clinical illness in dogs experimentally inoculated with *B. canis*.[33] The organism may not be cleared from the body following treatment. Relapses may occur.

Zoonotic Potential and Prevention. *Babesia* spp. infecting dogs and cats do not appear to cause human disease. Tick control is the primary means of prevention. Administration of immune-suppressive drugs and splenectomy should be avoided in previously infected dogs. Blood donors should be serologically screened for *B. canis* and *B. gibsoni* infection and not used if seropositive.

Cytauxzoonosis

Etiology and Epidemiology. *Cytauxzoon felis* is a generally fatal disease of domestic cats in the southern and southeastern United States.[26] Because bobcats are usually subclinically affected, they may be the natural host of the organism. *C. felis* is experimentally transmitted from infected bobcats to domestic cats by *Dermacentor variabilis*; clinical illness occurs after an incubation period of 5 to 20 days.[34] Schizonts and macroschizonts form in mononuclear phagocytes, which line the lumen of veins throughout the body, obstructing blood flow through tissues (tissue phase). The erythrocyte phase develops when merozoites released from the infected macrophages infect erythrocytes; hemolytic anemia is a sequela.

Clinical Findings. Fever, anorexia, dyspnea, depression, collapse, icterus, pale mucous membranes, and death are the most common clinical findings.[26, 34–36] Although most cases of cytauxzoonosis are in cats allowed to go outdoors, ticks are generally not identified on affected cats. The course of disease is generally one week or less.

Diagnosis. Regenerative anemia, neutrophilic leukocytosis or leukopenia, thrombocytopenia or thrombocytosis, hemoglobinemia, hemoglobinuria, bilirubinemia, and bilirubinuria are the most common laboratory abnormalities.[26, 34–36] An antemortem diagnosis can be made if the ring-shaped erythrocytic phase can be detected on thin blood smears or infected macrophages can be detected in bone marrow, spleen, liver, or lymph node aspirates stained with Wright's or Giemsa stains. Serologic testing can also be used to confirm exposure.[35]

Therapy. Fluid therapy and blood transfusion should be administered as indicated. Parvaquone, buparvaquone, thiacetarsamide, and tetracycline therapy have been attempted, but only six of approximately 500 reported cases have survived.[26, 34, 36] Diminazene aceturate and imidocarb dipropionate may be more effective (see Table 87–2).[34]

Zoonotic Potential and Prevention. *Cytauxzoon felis* is not known to infect people. Tick control should be maintained, and cats in endemic areas should be housed indoors.

FLAGELLATES

Leishmaniasis

Etiology and Epidemiology. Old World leishmaniasis in people is induced by *L. tropica* complex (cutaneous) and *L. donovani* complex (visceral). Cutaneous (*L. mexicana* complex and *L. braziliensis* complex), mucocutaneous (*L. braziliensis* complex), and visceral (*L. donovani* complex) forms of New World leishmaniasis occur in people. Rodents and dogs are primary reservoirs of *Leishmania* spp. People and cats are probably incidental hosts; sand flies are the vectors. Canine leishmaniasis has been reviewed.[37–39] Flagellated promastigotes develop in the sand fly and are injected into the vertebrate host when the sand fly feeds. Promastigotes are engulfed by macrophages and disseminate through the body. Cutaneous lesions containing amastigotes (nonflagellate) develop after an incubation period of one month to seven years; sand flies are infected during feeding. Polyclonal (and occasionally monoclonal) gammopathies proliferation of macrophages, histiocytes, and lymphocytes in lymphoreticular organs; and immune complex formation resulting in glomerulonephritis and polyarthritis are common manifestations of immune reactions against the intracellular organism.

Clinical Findings. If poor cell-mediated immune responses occur, dogs generally develop visceral leishmaniasis.[37–39] Weight loss with normal to increased appetite, polyuria, polydipsia, muscle wasting, depression, vomiting, diarrhea, cough, epistaxis, sneezing, and melena are common presenting complaints. Splenomegaly, lymphadenopathy, skin disease, fever, rhinitis, dermatitis, increased lung sounds, icterus, swollen painful joints, and uveitis are commonly identified on physical examination. Cutaneous lesions characterized by hyperkeratosis, scaling, thickening, mucocutaneous ulcers, and intradermal nodules on the muzzle, pinnae, ears, and footpads are detected in approximately 90 per cent of infected dogs. Cats are usually subclinically infected. One cat had cutaneous nodules on the ear pinna.[40]

Diagnosis. Hyperglobulinemia, hypoalbuminemia, proteinuria, increased liver enzyme activities, thrombocytopenia, azotemia, lymphopenia, and leukocytosis with left shift are common clinicopathologic abnormalities associated with leishmaniasis in dogs.[37–39] The hyperglobulinemia is usually a polyclonal gammopathy, but an IgG monoclonal gammopathy was reported in a dog. Neutrophilic polyarthritis occurs in some dogs as a manifestation of a type III hypersensitivity reaction or joint infection.[41] Demonstration of amastigotes (2.5 to 5.0 μ × 1.5 to 2.0 μ) in lymph node aspirates, bone marrow aspirates, or skin imprints stained with Wright's or Giemsa stain gives a definitive diagnosis. The organism can also be identified by histopathologic or immunoperoxidase evaluation of skin or organ biopsy, culture, inoculation of hamsters, or PCR.[42] Antibodies against *Leishmania* can be detected in serum; IgG titers develop 14 to 28 days after infection and decline 45 to 80 days after treatment. Because dogs are unlikely to naturally eliminate infection, a true-positive test indicates infection.

Treatment. Meglumine antimonate, sodium stibogluconate, liposomal amphotericin B, and allopurinol are the most commonly prescribed treatments. Because meglumine and stibogluconate are not routinely available in the United States, liposomal amphotericin B[43] or allopurinol[44] are the drugs of choice (see Table 87–2). The prognosis is variable; most cases are recurrent. Dogs with renal insufficiency have a poor prognosis. Antibody titers can be used to assess efficacy of therapy.

Zoonotic Potential and Prevention. Dogs act as a reservoir host for *Leishmania* spp., allowing for infection of sand flies. Direct contact with amastigotes in draining lesions is unlikely to result in human infection. Avoidance of infected sand flies is the only means of prevention; use of deltamethrin-impregnated collars lessened sand fly exposure of dogs in France.[45] Breeding places of sand flies should be controlled, and animals should be housed at night when sand flies feed.

American Trypanosomiasis

Etiology and Epidemiology. *Trypanosoma cruzi* causes American trypanosomiasis. Infected reservoir mammals (dogs, cats, raccoons, opossums, armadillos) and vectors (reduviid bugs, kissing bugs) are found in the United States, but infection is rare when compared with South America.[46, 47] When infected kissing bugs defecate during feeding, epimastigotes (flagellated vector form) enter the vertebrate host, are engulfed by macrophages and myocytes, and transform into amastigotes (nonflagellated intracellular form). Trypomastigotes (flagellated stage found free in blood) form as the amastigotes divide by binary fission until the host cell ruptures. Ingesting trypomastigotes during a blood meal then infects the vector. Transmission to mammalian hosts can also occur by ingestion of the vector, blood transfusion, ingestion of infected tissues or milk, or transplacentally. Acute disease occurs during peak parasitemia that occurs two to three weeks after infection.

Clinical Findings. Myocardial cells are damaged by parasite replication or immune-mediated reactions. Myocarditis or heart failure results in exercise intolerance or weakness. Generalized lymphadenopathy, pale mucous membranes, tachycardia, pulse deficits, hepatomegaly, anorexia, diarrhea, neurologic signs, and abdominal distention can occur. Chronic dilatative cardiomyopathy develops in some dogs that survive acute infection.

Diagnosis. Clinicopathologic, thoracic radiographic, abdominal radiographic, and echocardiographic findings are consistent with cardiac disease and failure but are not specific for trypanosomiasis. The primary electrocardiogram findings are ventricular premature contractions, heart block, and T-wave inversion. Demonstration of trypomastigotes (1 flagellum, 15 to 20 μ long) in thick blood films, buffy coat smears, lymph node aspirates, or abdominal effusions stained with Giemsa or Wright's stain can be used to make a definitive diagnosis. Histopathologic evaluation of cardiac tissue may reveal amastigotes (1.5 to 4.0 μ). Trypomastigotes can also be cultured from blood or grown by bioassay in mice. Because exposure to *T. cruzi* is rare in dogs living in the United States, the combination of appropriate clinical findings and positive serum antibody titers can be used to make a strong presumptive diagnosis.

Therapy. Drugs effective for trypanosomiasis are not available in the United States; nifurtimox 2 to 7 mg/kg orally four times a day for three to five months has been prescribed most frequently in other countries. Glucocorticoid therapy may improve survival of acutely infected dogs with myocarditis. Therapy for arrhythmias or heart failure should be instituted as needed.

Zoonotic Potential and Prevention. Infected dogs can serve as a reservoir of *T. cruzi* for vectors, and blood from infected dogs can be infectious to humans. Vector control is the primary means of prevention. Dogs should be kept from other reservoir hosts such as opossums and should not be fed raw meat. Potential blood donors from endemic areas should be serologically screened.

AMOEBA

Acanthamoeba spp.

Acanthamoeba castellani and *A. culbertsoni* are free-living amoebae rarely associated with disease in dogs.[48–50] Several cases have been reported in greyhounds. Young dogs seem to be affected most often. Clinical signs resemble canine distemper virus infection and consist primarily of oculonasal discharge, fever, anorexia, lethargy, dyspnea, and CNS disease. There are no pathognomonic laboratory or radiographic abnormalities, but leukopenia is common. The organism can be demonstrated histologically or in culture; antemortem diagnosis is not usually made. There is no known effective treatment. There is no known zoonotic risk.

MICROSPORA

Encephalitozoon cuniculi

Dogs and cats can develop clinical illness following exposure to *Encephalitozoon cuniculi*.[51–53] Schizonts and sporonts are found intracellularly in many cell types, including renal tubular epithelial cells, endothelial cells, tissue macrophages, and hepatocytes. Spores are the extracellular stage of the organism that is passed in urine. Infection is probably from oronasal exposure to spores passed in urine. In utero infection can also occur; infected puppies are weak, have stunted growth, and develop renal failure and CNS disease. Muscle spasms, depression, paralysis, and death have been reported in naturally infected cats. There are no pathognomonic laboratory abnormalities, but azotemia, increased activities of hepatic enzymes, and increased CSF cell counts (neutrophils) and protein concentrations commonly occur. Diagnosis is based on demonstration of spores in urine sediment stained with Gram or Ziehl-Neelsen stains. Serologic testing is available but is not specific for *E. cuniculi*. Although no drug has been shown to be effective for treatment of *E. cuniculi* in infected dogs or cats, fumagillin and albendazole were effective in vitro.[54] The zoonotic risk is considered minimally important, but a 10-year-old girl in a home with two infected puppies seroconverted to *E. cuniculi*.[53] Sanitation is the best form of control.

MISCELLANEOUS INFECTIOUS AGENTS

PNEUMOCYTOSIS

Pneumocystis carinii is a saprophytic organism with worldwide distribution that occasionally causes respiratory

disease in the immunocompromised mammalian host.[55–58] The organism is transmitted by direct contact with respiratory secretions and causes disease by replicating in the alveoli; this induces infiltrates of lymphocytes, plasma cells, and macrophages, which interferes with gaseous exchange. It is a rare disease, with most dogs and all cats to date subclinically infected.

Dry cough, dyspnea, and progressive weight loss are common clinical findings. Laboratory abnormalities are nonspecific. Thoracic radiographic abnormalities include mixed alveolar or interstitial lung pattern and cor pulmonale. Diagnosis is based on cytologic demonstration of the organism in transthoracic aspirates, transtracheal wash specimens, or lung biopsies. Trimethoprim-sulfonamide or pentamidine and supportive care as for any pneumonia are potentially effective treatments. Because the organism is saprophytic, there is little to no zoonotic potential.

PROTOTHECOSIS

Prototheca zopfii and *P. wickerhamii* are the two species in this genus of green algae incriminated as pathogens; prototothecosis is a disseminated disease in the dog (*P. zopfii*) and a cutaneous disease in the cat (*P. wickerhamii*).[59–61] The organism is found in sewage and animal wastes and is transmitted by ingestion of contaminated food, water, or soil. Disease generally occurs only in individuals with decreased cell-mediated immune responses. There may be strain differences in virulence and genetic predispositions.

The disseminated disease is most common in collies that present for evaluation of weight loss, large-bowel diarrhea, CNS disease, or uveitis. The cutanueous disease occurs in dogs and cats and appears as draining ulcers and crusts of the trunk, extremities, and mucous membranes in dogs and as firm cutaneous nodules on the limbs, feet, and head of cats. CSF abnormalities include pleocytosis with either lymphocytes or granulocytes as the predominant cell type and increased total protein. Diagnosis is confirmed by cytologic, histologic, or culture documentation of the organism in CSF, rectal scrapings, or rectal biopsies. Cutaneous lesions should be excised if possible. Liposomal amphotericin B, ketoconazole, itraconazole, and fluconazole may be effective treatments (see Chapter 93 for a discussion of these drugs). CNS and ocular manifestations have a poor prognosis; fluconazole may be the drug of choice for disease of these systems. There is minimal zoonotic risk.

REFERENCES

1. Dubey JP: A review of *Sarcocystis* of domestic animals and of other coccidia of cats and dogs. JAVMA 169:1061, 1976.
2. Kirkpatrick CE, Dubey JP: Enteric coccidial infections. *Isospora, Sarcocystis, Cryptosporidium, Besnoitia,* and *Hammondia*. Vet Clin North Am Small Anim Pract 17:1405, 1987.
3. Dubey JP, Greene CE, Lappin MR: Toxoplasmosis and neosporosis. *In* Greene CE (ed): Infectious Diseases of the Dog and Cat, 2nd ed. Philadelphia, WB Saunders, 1998, pp 493–509.
4. McReynolds, Lappin MR, Thrall MA, et al: Regional seroprevalence of *Cryptosporidium* spp. IgG antibodies of cats in the United States. Vet Parasitol, in press, 1998.
5. Ajuwape ATP, Nottidge HO: Amoebiasis in a four-month old puppy: A case report. Trop Vet 11:69, 1993.
6. Shimada A, Muraki Y, Awakura T, et al: Necrotic colitis associated with *Entamoeba histolytica* in a cat. J Comp Pathol 106:195, 1992.
7. Lappin MR, Calpin J: Laboratory diagnosis of protozoal infections. *In* Greene CE (ed): Infectious Diseases of the Dog and Cat, 2nd ed. Philadelphia, WB Saunders, 1998, pp 437–441.
8. Dow SW, LeCouteur RA, Poss ML, et al: Central nervous system toxicosis associated with metronidazole treatment of dogs: Five cases (1984–1987). JAVMA 195:365, 1989.

9. Barr SC, Bowman DD, Heller RL, et al: Efficacy of albendazole against giardiasis in dogs. Am J Vet Res 54:926, 1993.

10. Barr SC, Bowman DD, Heller RL, et al: Efficacy of fenbendazole against giardiasis in dogs. Am J Vet Res 55:988, 1994.

11. Barr SC, Guilford WG, Jamrosz GF, et al: Paromomycin for the treatment of *Cryptosporidium* infection in dogs and cats. Proceedings of the 12th American College of Veterinary Internal Medicine Forum, San Francisco, May 1994, p 1008.

12. Lappin MR, Dowers K, Edsell D, et al: Cryptosporidiosis and inflammatory bowel disease in a cat. Feline Pract 25:10, 1997.

13. Juranek DD: Cryptosporidiosis: Sources of infection and guidelines for prevention. Clin Infect Dis 21:S57, 1995.

14. Dubey JP: Duration of immunity to shedding *Toxoplasma gondii* oocysts by cats. J Parasitol 81:410, 1995.

15. Angulo FJ, Glaser CA, Juranek DD, et al: Caring for pets of immunocompromised persons. JAVMA 205:1711, 1994.

16. Olson ME, Morck DW, Ceri Ceri H: The efficacy of a *Giardia lamblia* vaccine in kittens. Can J Vet Res 60:249, 1996.

17. Peterson JL, Willard MD, Lees GE, et al: Toxoplasmosis in two cats with inflammatory intestinal disease. JAVMA 199:473, 1991.

18. Dubey JP, Carpenter JL: Histologically confirmed clinical toxoplasmosis in cats: 100 cases (1952–1990). JAVMA 203:1556, 1993.

19. Dubey JP, Lappin MR, Thulliez P: Diagnosis of induced toxoplasmosis in neonatal cats. JAVMA 207:179, 1995.

20. Lappin MR, Greene CE, Winston S, et al: Clinical feline toxoplasmosis: Serologic diagnosis and therapeutic management of 15 cases. J Vet Intern Med 3:139, 1989.

21. Lappin MR, Roberts SM, Davidson MG, et al: Enzyme-linked immunosorbent assays for the detection of *Toxoplasma gondii*–specific antibodies and antigens in the aqueous humor of cats. JAVMA 201:1010, 1992.

22. Lappin MR: Feline toxoplasmosis: Interpretation of diagnostic test results. Semin Vet Med Surg 11:154, 1996.

23. Dubey JP, Carpenter JL, Speer CA, et al: Newly recognized fatal protozoan disease of dogs. JAVMA 192:1269, 1989.

24. Dubey JP, Koestner A, Piper RC: Repeated transplacental transmission of *Neospora caninum* in dogs. JAVMA 197:857, 1990.

25. Ruehlmann D, Podell M, Oglesbee M, et al: Canine neosporosis: A case report and literature review. J Am Anim Hosp Assoc 31:174, 1995.

26. Macintire DK: Emerging tick-borne diseases. Comp Cont Ed Pract Vet 19:S66, 1997.

27. Macintire DK, Vincent Johnson N, Dillon AR, et al: Hepatozoonosis in dogs: 22 cases. JAVMA 210:916, 1997.

28. Panciera RJ, Gatto NT, Crystal MA, et al: Canine hepatozoonosis in Oklahoma. J Am Anim Hosp Assoc 33:221, 1997.

29. Vincent-Johnson N, Macintire DK, Baneth G: Canine hepatozoonosis: Pathophysiology, diagnosis, and treatment. Comp Cont Ed Pract Vet 19:51, 1997.

30. Murata T, Inoue M, Tateyama S, et al: Vertical transmission of *Hepatozoon canis* in dogs. J Vet Med Sci 55:867, 1993.

31. Taboada J: Canine babesiosis. *In* Bonagura JD (ed): Current Veterinary Therapy XII. Philadelphia, WB Saunders, 1995, pp 315–319.

32. Breitschwerdt EB: Babesiosis: Clinical experiences. Comp Cont Ed Pract Vet 19:S54, 1997.

33. Vercammen F, De Deken R, Maes L: Prophylactic treatment of experimental canine babesiosis (*Babesia canis*) with doxycycline. Vet Parasitol 66:251, 1996.

34. Kier AB, Greene CE: Cytauxzoonosis. *In* Greene CE (ed): Infectious Diseases of the Dog and Cat, 2nd ed. Philadelphia, WB Saunders, 1998, pp 470–473.

35. Hoover JP, Walker DB, Hedges JD: Cytauxzoonosis in cats: Eight cases (1985–1992). JAVMA 205:455, 1994.

36. Walker DB, Cowell RL: Survival of a domestic cat with naturally acquired cytauzoonosis. JAVMA 206:1363, 1995.

37. Bravo L, Frank LA, Brenneman KA: Canine leishmaniasis in the United States. Comp Cont Ed Pract Vet 15:699, 1993.

38. Kontos UJ, Koutinas AF: Old World canine leishmaniasis. Comp Cont Ed Pract Vet 15:949, 1993.

39. Slappendel RJ: Canine leishmaniasis: A review based on 95 cases in the Netherlands. Vet Q 10:1, 1988.

40. Craig TM, Barton CL, Mercer SH, et al: Dermal leishmaniasis in a Texas cat. Am J Trop Med Hyg 35:1100, 1986.

41. Spreng D: Leishmanial polyarthritis in two dogs. J Small Anim Pract 34:559, 1993.

42. Ashford DA, Bozza M, Freire M, et al: Comparison of the polymerase chain reaction and serology for the detection of canine visceral leishmaniasis. Am J Trop Med Hyg 53:251, 1995.

43. Oliva G, Gradoni L, Ciaramella P, et al: Activity of liposomal amphotericin B (AmBisome) in dogs naturally infected with *Leishmania infantum*. J Antimicrob Chemother 36:1013, 1995.

44. Lester SJ, Kenyon JE: Use of allopurinol to treat visceral leishmaniasis in a dog. JAVMA 209:615, 1996.

45. Killick Kendrick R, Killick Kendrick M, Focheux C, et al: Protection of dogs from bites of phlebotomine sandflies by deltamethrin collars for control of canine leishmaniasis. Med Vet Entomol 11:105, 1997.

46. Meurs KM, Miller MW, Helman RG: Canine Chagas' myocarditis. *In* Bonagura JD (ed): Current Veterinary Therapy XII. Philadelphia, WB Saunders, 1995, pp 850–854.

47. Barr SC, Van Beek O, Carlisle-Nowak MS, et al: *Trypanosoma cruzi* infection in Walker hounds from Virginia. Am J Vet Res 56:1037, 1995.

48. Bauer RW, Harrison LR, Watson CW, et al: Isolation of *Acanthamoeba* sp. from a greyhound with pneumonia and granulomatous encephalitis. J Vet Diagn Invest 5:386, 1993.

49. Harrison LR, Bauer RW: Acanthamebiasis. *In* Greene CE (ed): Infectious Diseases of the Dog and Cat. Philadelphia, WB Saunders, 1990, pp 815–817.

50. Pearce JR, Fowel HS, Chandler FW, et al: Amebic meningoencephalitis caused by *Acanthamoeba castellani* in a dog. JAVMA 187:951, 1985.

51. Szabo JR, Pang V, Shadduck JA: Encephalitozoonosis. *In* Greene CE (ed): Infectious Diseases of the Dog and Cat. Philadelphia, WB Saunders, 1990, pp 786–791.

52. Cole JR, Sangster LT, Sulzer CR, et al: Infections with *Encephalitozoon cuniculi* and *Leptospira interrogans*, serovars, *grippotyphosa*, and *ballum* in a kennel of foxhounds. JAVMA 180:435, 1982.

53. Mcinnes EF, Stewart CG: The pathology of subclinical infection of *Encephalitozoon cuniculi* in canine dams producing pups with overt encephalitozoonosis. J S Afr Vet Assoc 62:51, 1991.

54. Beauvais B, Sarfati C, Challier S, et al: In vitro model to assess effect of antimicrobial agents on *Encephalitizoon cuniculi*. Antimicrob Agents Chemother 38:2440, 1994.

55. Lobetti RG, Leisewitz AL, Spencer JA: *Pneumocytis carinii* in the miniature dachshund: Case report and literature review. J Small Anim Pract 37:280, 1996.

56. Botha WS, VanRensburg IBJ: Pneumocytosis: A chronic respiratory distress syndrome in the dog. J S Afr Vet Assoc 50:173, 1979.

57. Hagler DN, Kim CK, Walzer PD: Feline leukemia virus and *Pneumocystis carinii* infection. J Parasitol 73:1284, 1987.

58. McCully RM, Lloyd J, Kuys D, Schneider DJ: Canine *Pneumocystis* pneumonia. J S Afr Vet Assoc 50:207, 1979.

59. Wolf AM: Opportunistic fungal and algal infections. *In* Bonagura JD (ed): Current Veterinary Therapy XII. Philadelphia, WB Saunders, 1995, pp 324–327.

60. Finnie JW, Coloe PJ: Cutaneous protothecosis in a cat. Aust Vet J 57:307, 1981.

61. Gaunt SD, McGrath RK, Cox HU: Disseminated protothecosis in a dog. JAVMA 185:906, 1984.

CHAPTER 88

CANINE VIRAL DISEASES

Johnny D. Hoskins

CANINE DISTEMPER

Canine distemper virus (CDV) causes a highly contagious disease of dogs and all animals in the Canidae family (dingo, fox, coyote, wolf, jackal), the Mustelidae family (ferret, mink, skunk, badger, marten, weasel, otter), and the Procyonidae family (raccoon, panda, kinkajou, coati).[1]

Etiology. Canine distemper (CD) is caused by *Morbillivirus,* a large RNA virus that is closely related to measles and rinderpest viruses. CDV is a relatively labile virus, with infectivity being destroyed by heat, drying, detergents, lipid solvents, and disinfectants.

Epidemiology. CDV is transmitted by aerosol droplets from all body excretions of infected animals, and infection spreads rapidly among susceptible young dogs. Some CDV strains are mildly virulent and cause inapparent infections. Others cause acute CD with a high incidence of encephalitis and high mortality.[2] Some CDV strains are more viscerotropic and cause a debilitating disease with high mortality and a low incidence of encephalitis. Secondary bacterial infections from the immune-suppressive effects of CDV are usually responsible for the clinical signs associated with acute CD. These secondary infections also contribute to the mortality rate of CD. Occurrence of toxoplasmosis, neosporosis, coccidiosis, viral enteritis, cryptosporidiosis, and giardiasis may be enhanced by the immune-suppressive effects of concurrent CDV infection.

Clinical Signs. After CDV exposure, a transient fever and leukopenia occur without overt signs of disease. Coughing, diarrhea, vomiting, anorexia, dehydration, and weight loss with debilitation commonly follow. Mucopurulent oculonasal discharges and pneumonia may occur from secondary bacterial infections. A skin rash progressing to pustules may occur on the abdomen. Multifocal chorioretinitis with grey to pink irregular areas of degeneration in peripheral and midperipheral nontapetal fundus and optic neuritis can be observed in acute CD. Retinal atrophy and scar formation may be observed in dogs that have recovered from CD infection or those with chronic CD. Scar formation is characterized by areas of hyperreflectivity of light. Irregularities in dental surfaces may be present owing to hypoplasia of enamel. Metaphyseal osteopathy may be present as a result of effects of the CDV. CDV RNA has been detected in metaphyseal bone cells and could be responsible for the metaphyseal osteopathy.[3–5]

Myoclonus, chewing gum seizures, ataxia, incoordination, circling, hyperesthesia, muscle rigidity, vocalization as if in pain, fear responses, and blindness are the common neurologic signs of acute CD. Neurologic signs may also have a delayed onset, weeks or months after recovery from inapparent infections or after recovery from acute CD. Dogs with late-onset neurologic signs usually have immunity to CDV. Dogs that survive may have residual neurologic deficits of myoclonus or visual and olfactory dysfunction.

CDV has also been associated with chronic encephalitis in older dogs. The clinical signs include incoordination, weakness in pelvic limbs, menace deficits, visual impairment, head tilt, nystagmus, facial paralysis, and head tremors without myoclonus. As the encephalitis progresses, affected dogs become mentally depressed, develop compulsive circling or head pressing, and show temperament changes.

Diagnosis. The diagnosis of CD is usually based on history and clinical signs.[6] A definitive diagnosis can be made by detection of CDV in epithelial cells by fluorescent antibody (FA) test or by virus isolation. Serologic testing may or may not be helpful in diagnosing acute CD, because dogs with acute disease usually fail to respond immunologically. Dogs that recover from acute CD have lower titers of antibody than dogs with inapparent infections or with vaccine-induced immunity.

The FA test is done on epithelial cells collected from the conjunctiva or other mucous membranes or on smears of blood or buffy coat cells, because CDV infects lymphocytes, thrombocytes, and sometimes immature erythrocytes. Interpretation of the FA test is based on detection of CDV antigen only within intact cells. The FA test is good at detecting cells positive for CDV during the first few days of acute CD. The FA test is negative in cases of delayed-onset or chronic CD encephalitis, because dogs with these disorders usually have neutralizing antibody that has eliminated the virus or that blocks the FA reaction. Viral antigen persists longer in macrophages and epithelial cells in the lower respiratory tract and in epithelial cells of footpads in dogs that have recovered from acute CD. A negative FA test for CDV does not rule out CD. A positive test for CDV indicates that CDV antigen was detected in the cells observed, and the results should be interpreted in conjunction with the history and clinical signs. Attenuated CDV vaccines are not disseminated from lymphoid tissue to epithelial cells, and therefore are not detected by the FA test. Systemic immunity prevents dissemination of the virus and limits replication and immune response, which maintains immunity in adult dogs with frequent exposure to CDV.

Treatment and Prevention. There are no antiviral drugs for the treatment of CD. Broad-spectrum antibiotics are used to control secondary bacterial infections, and fluids, electrolytes, and nutritional supplements are indicated for supportive therapy. The prognosis is guarded for most cases of acute CD, especially if neurologic signs are present and progressing, but control of secondary infections and supportive therapy improve the chances for recovery and quality of life.

The available attenuated and recombinant CDV vaccines induce effective immunity to CD.[7] A single dose of attenuated vaccine or multiple doses of recombinant vaccine usually immunize dogs that are free of antibody and are susceptible to CD. The age at which puppies become susceptible to CD is proportional to the titer of antibody of their mother and varies according to the colostral transfer of antibody to the puppies. Because of the variable age at which puppies become immunizable to CD, a series of vaccinations are given to puppies according to schedules that are practical but that maximize the probability of inducing immunity (Table 88–1).

INFECTIOUS CANINE HEPATITIS

Infectious canine hepatitis (ICH) is a multisystemic viral disease that affects primarily the liver of dogs and foxes.

Etiology. ICH is caused by canine adenovirus type 1 (CAV-1), a DNA virus. CAV-1 is moderately resistant and survives in the environment for days to months, depending on the temperature and humidity. CAV-1 is moderately resistant to disinfectants, but quaternary ammonium compounds inactivate its infectivity within 10 minutes.

Epidemiology. After oronasal exposure, CAV-1 localizes in the tonsils and regional lymph nodes, where primary replication occurs with subsequent viremia. Clinical signs caused by CAV-1 infection are due to cellular damage as a result of direct effects of viral replication. Damage to endothelial cells may lead to hemorrhagic diathesis. During acute ICH, CAV-1 is present in all body excretions. Contamination of the environment by CAV-1 occurs from shedding of virus in feces and urine.

Clinical Signs. Clinical signs of ICH occur in young seronegative dogs. The incubation period is four to seven days. Transient or biphasic fever, depression, and lethargy are early signs. Later signs include reluctance to move, abdominal tenderness, pale mucous membranes, and anorexia. Tonsillitis, pharyngitis, and cervical lymphadenopathy are common findings. Dogs with uncomplicated ICH usually recover after an illness lasting three to five days. Corneal opacity may occur during convalescence. In more severe cases, hemorrhagic diathesis with petechial and ec-

chymotic hemorrhages may occur. Bleeding times are prolonged, and coagulation abnormalities typical of disseminated intravascular coagulation (DIC) occur. Neurologic signs related to vascular damage may occur. Abdominal distention may result from serosanguineous ascites. Hepatomegaly occurs, and in some cases the liver can be palpated. The prognosis is guarded in dogs with multisystemic involvement.

Diagnosis. With the onset of clinical signs, moderate to severe leukopenia, neutropenia, lymphopenia, and thrombocytopenia are present. Serum alanine transaminase activity may be increased. Demonstration of rising antibody titer in paired serum samples confirms the diagnosis of ICH. Intranuclear inclusion bodies may be detected in hepatic parenchymal cells.

Treatment and Prevention. Most infected dogs recover with supportive therapy. Prevention is provided by immunization with vaccines containing attenuated CAV-1 or CAV-2. Most vaccines marketed in the United States contain attenuated CAV-2 in combination with other canine viruses. Vaccines containing attenuated CAV-2 are essentially free of postvaccinal reactions or complications. Vaccination schedules for immunization of puppies against CAV-1 are the same as those for immunization against CD (see Table 88–1).

INFECTIOUS TRACHEOBRONCHITIS

Any contagious respiratory disease of dogs that is manifested by coughing and not caused by CD is referred to as infectious tracheobronchitis or kennel cough.

Etiology. Incriminated viruses include CAV-2, canine parainfluenza (CPI), CAV-1, canine reovirus-1, canine reovirus-2, canine reovirus-3, and canine herpesvirus. CAV-2 and CPI, the more common viral causes of kennel cough, may damage the respiratory epithelium to such an extent that invasion by various bacteria and/or mycoplasmas results in severe airway disease.[8] CAV-2 is moderately resistant and can survive for months in the environment. CPI virus is relatively labile and does not survive long in the environment. Quaternary ammonium disinfectants are effective against both CAV-2 and CPI virus.

Epidemiology. CAV-2 and CPI virus are transmitted by aerosol droplets. Both viruses cause localized infections of the respiratory tract without dissemination to other organs and are shed in respiratory secretions. Most CAV-2 and CPI virus infections are mild or inapparent.

Clinical Signs. The primary sign of CAV-2 or CPI virus infection is paroxysmal coughing of varying frequency and intensity. Fever and decreased appetite are variable. Coughing results from irritation at the tracheal-bronchiolar level of the respiratory tract. Dogs usually recover three to seven days after the onset of clinical signs. Experimentally, it is difficult to reproduce respiratory disease with CPI virus alone. Experimental infection with CAV-2 reveals an inverse relationship between magnitude of the febrile response and duration of clinical signs. Dogs that developed a rectal temperature greater than 104.5°F recovered more quickly than those that had a low-grade fever.

Diagnosis. A diagnosis of kennel cough is based on history and clinical signs. Definitive viral diagnosis depends on isolation and identification of the virus or demonstration of a rising titer of antibody to a specific virus in paired serum samples.

Treatment and Prevention. There are no antiviral drugs for the treatment of CAV-2 or CPI virus infection.

TABLE 88–1. SUMMARY OF SUGGESTED VACCINATION PROTOCOL FOR IMMUNIZATION OF DOGS AGAINST VIRAL INFECTIONS

AGE	DISEASE
6 weeks	Canine distemper
	Infectious canine hepatitis
	Parvovirus
	Coronavirus
	Parainfluenza
9 weeks	Canine distemper
	Infectious canine hepatitis
	Parvovirus
	Coronavirus
	Parainfluenza
12 weeks	Canine distemper
	Infectious canine hepatitis
	Parvovirus
	Coronavirus
	Parainfluenza
	Rabies
15–16 weeks	Immunity check*
Yearly†	Canine distemper
	Infectious canine hepatitis
	Parvovirus
	Coronavirus
	Parainfluenza
	Rabies‡

*Immunity check means determining serum antibody titer for canine parvovirus, especially in rottweilers and Doberman pinschers.

†Instead of using an annual vaccination schedule, a biennial vaccination schedule is preferred.

‡Rabies vaccinations are given annually or triennially, depending on the vaccine used and local statutes.

Most dogs recover naturally without complications. Broad-spectrum antibiotics are indicated when there is secondary bacterial infection. Attenuated CAV-2 and CPI virus vaccines are available and are given in combination with other canine viruses according to the schedule used for CD vaccine (see Table 88–1). Attenuated CPI virus is also available in combination with attenuated *Bordetella bronchiseptica* for intranasal administration. When kennel cough becomes a serious problem in a kennel, intranasal vaccines are recommended for use in puppies as young as 2 to 4 weeks of age.

CANINE PARVOVIRUS

Natural canine parvovirus (CP) infection may occur in domestic dogs, bush dogs, coyotes, crab-eating foxes, maned wolves, and raccoon dogs, and it is probable that most if not all Canidae are susceptible.[9] Experimentally, CP infections can be produced in ferrets and minks; however, the infection is generally self-limited. The newer viral strains may infect cats under experimental and natural conditions.[10]

Etiology. Canine parvovirus type 2 (CPV-2) is the primary cause of systemic and intestinal infections in domestic dogs younger than 6 months old. During the past 20 years, CPV-2 has undergone genetic alterations in the dog, developing new virus strains. In 1980 the original CPV-2 strain evolved into type 2a (CPV-2a), and in 1984 another variant designated type 2b (CPV-2b) appeared. These CPV-2 alterations were genetic adaptations, enabling the virus to replicate and spread more effectively. In the United States, CPV-2b has largely replaced previously isolated strains, whereas in the Far East and Europe, both CPV-2a and CPV-2b predominate.

CPV-2 is extremely stable and resistant to adverse environmental influences. CPV-2 can persist on inanimate objects, such as clothing, food pans, and cage floors, for longer than five months. Most detergents and disinfectants fail to inactivate CPV-2 strains; one exception is sodium hypochlorite (common household bleach).

Epidemiology. In domestic dogs, CPV-2 infection does not necessarily result in apparent disease; many naturally infected dogs never develop overt clinical signs. When it occurs, clinical illness is most severe in young, rapidly growing puppies that harbor intestinal parasites, protozoa, and certain enteric bacteria such as *Clostridium perfringens*, *Campylobacter* spp., and *Salmonella* spp.

Most CP results from exposure to contaminated feces. In addition, people, instruments (equipment in veterinary clinics or kennels), insects, and rodents can serve as vectors. Dogs may carry the virus on their haircoat for as long as contaminated feces are attached to the hairshafts. With newer CPV-2 strains, the incubation period can be as brief as four to six days. Acute CP can be seen in dogs of any breed, age, or sex. Nevertheless, puppies between 6 weeks and 6 months of age and rottweilers, Doberman pinschers, Labrador retrievers, American pit bull terriers, German shepherds, Staffordshire terriers, and Alaskan sled dogs seem to have an increased risk.

CPV-2 spreads rapidly among dogs via oronasal exposure to contaminated feces. Virus replication begins in lymphoid tissue of the oropharynx, mesenteric lymph nodes, and thymus and is disseminated to the intestinal crypts of the small intestine via viremia. Marked plasma viremia is observed one to five days after infection. Subsequent to the viremia, CPV-2 localizes predominantly in the epithelium lining the tongue, oral cavity, esophagus, small intestine, and lymphoid tissue, such as thymus and lymph nodes. Virus may also be isolated from the lungs, spleen, liver, kidneys, and myocardium. Secondary bacterial infection from gram-negative and anaerobic microflora causes complications related to intestinal damage, bacteremia and endotoxemia, and DIC. Active CPV-2 excretion begins on the third or fourth day after exposure, generally before signs appear. CPV-2 is shed extensively in the feces for 7 to 10 days.

Clinical Signs. CP is associated with disease in two distinct organ systems: the gastrointestinal tract, which is common, and the myocardium, which is rare. Marked variations exist in the clinical response of dogs to intestinal CPV-2 infection, ranging from inapparent to an acute fatal disease. Inapparent, or subclinical, infection occurs in most dogs. The severity depends on the animal's age, stress level, breed, and immune status. The most severe infections are usually seen in puppies younger than 12 weeks old, because they lack protective immunity and have an increased number of growing, dividing cells. CP may progress rapidly, especially the newer CPV-2 strains.[11] Vomiting is often severe and is followed by diarrhea, anorexia, and rapid onset of dehydration. Yellow-grey feces can be streaked or darkened by blood. Elevated rectal temperature (40 to 41°C [104 to 105.8°F]) and leukopenia may be present. Death can occur as early as two days after the onset of illness and is often associated with gram-negative sepsis or DIC.

CPV-2 myocarditis can develop from infection in utero or in puppies younger than 8 weeks old. Usually all puppies in a litter are affected. Puppies with CPV-2 myocarditis are often found dead or succumb within 24 hours after the appearance of signs, which include dyspnea, crying, and retching. Signs of cardiac dysfunction may be preceded by the enteric form of CP or may occur suddenly without apparent previous illness. The spectrum of myocardial disease in individuals is wide and may include any of the following: acute diarrhea and death without cardiac signs; diarrhea and apparent recovery followed by death weeks or months later as a result of heart failure; or a sudden onset of heart failure, which occurs in apparently normal puppies at 6 weeks to 6 months of age. Myocarditis occasionally occurs in puppies born to isolated, unvaccinated mothers.

Diagnosis. The sudden onset of a foul-smelling bloody diarrhea in a young (<2 years) dog is often considered indicative of CPV-2 infection. However, all signs characteristic of CP are seldom present at any one time. The degree of leukopenia is usually proportional to the severity of illness and the disease stage.

Fecal enzyme-linked immunosorbent assay (ELISA) antigen tests are available for in-hospital testing for acute CP.[12] These user-friendly tests are relatively sensitive and specific for detecting acute CP. However, the period of fecal antigen shed is brief and somewhat cyclic; it corresponds to five to seven days of clinical illness. CPV-2 antigen is seldom detectable after 10 to 12 days in a natural infection. In addition, direct fecal sampling from the rectum of suspected dogs is more sensitive for detecting CPV-2 antigen than is sampling from expelled feces alone. Positive ELISA results confirm CP or may be induced by the attenuated CPV-2 vaccines (vaccine virus can yield a false-positive result in dogs 5 to 12 days after vaccination); negative results do not eliminate the possibility of CP.

CPV-2 can be easily isolated from small-intestinal tissue or feces using tissue culture systems if performed early. Later in the disease course, virions are coated by antibodies and cleared. Immunochemical methods can also be used to detect virus in tissue culture or tissue. Polymerase chain reaction (PCR) testing has been used as a specific and sensitive means of detecting CPV-2 in feces of infected dogs. This method can also differentiate between field and vaccine CPV-2 strains.[13]

Inhibition of hemagglutination by CPV-2 antisera can be used to demonstrate antibody. A high hemagglutination inhibition titer in a single serum sample collected after the dog has been clinically ill for three or more days is diagnostic for CP. Rising titers can be demonstrated by the comparison of acute and 10- to 14-day convalescent serum samples using either canine or feline parvovirus in hemagglutination inhibition and virus neutralization tests. Vaccination interferes with interpretation, but field CP generally produces a higher titer than vaccination does.

Serum ELISAs that permit distinction between IgG and IgM levels are available at a few diagnostic laboratories. Increased serum IgM concentrations can be noted within the first week of CP and by recent vaccination with the attenuated CPV-2 vaccines. Thereafter, serum IgG concentrations are increased with either CP or through vaccination. Consequently, serum ELISA tests have limited value in distinguishing recent CP from attenuated CPV-2 vaccination.

Treatment. The goals of symptomatic treatment for CP are restoring fluid and electrolyte balance and resting the gastrointestinal tract. Fluid therapy is probably the most important aspect of clinical management and should be continued as long as vomiting and/or diarrhea persist. The dog's serum electrolytes must be evaluated at least once, and in the ill puppy two or three times daily. The electrolyte status of the dog aids in selecting appropriate fluid therapy—saline if the dog is hyponatremic, lactated Ringer's if the serum sodium concentration is normal, potassium supplementation dictated by the serum concentration, and so forth. Further complicating fluid balance requirements is the frequency of anemia due to severe gastrointestinal bleeding and hypoproteinemia (especially hypoalbuminemia) due to severe gastrointestinal losses. These complications must be recognized, monitored, and treated continuously. An anemic puppy may require blood transfusions. A "toxic" and hypoalbuminemic puppy benefits the most from plasma or blood. A stable but hypoproteinemic puppy may benefit from colloid in addition to crystalloid therapy. These treatments are critical, together with nursing care and antibiotics. There is no set antibiotic protocol for puppies with CP, but their need is unquestioned because of tremendous sloughing of gastrointestinal mucosa associated with the disease and loss of this barrier to infection.

Antiemetic drugs do little for the primary treatment of CP and are indicated only for persistent vomiting. Metoclopramide hydrochloride has proved useful in most dogs with persistent vomiting. Prochlorperazine or chlorpromazine may be used in dogs that do not respond to metoclopramide. Using drugs to alter gut motility is seldom recommended in treating CP. Narcotic analgesics that act as antidiarrheal agents (e.g., diphenoxylate hydrochloride, loperamide hydrochloride) are preferred when motility modifiers are needed.

Within the first 24 hours of clinical CP, recommended adjunctive therapy includes transfusing specific hyperimmune plasma (8 to 10 mL/kg intravenously once), administering recombinant human granulocyte colony-stimulating factor (5 µg/kg subcutaneously daily until neutrophil numbers exceed 1500/µL), or giving antiendotoxin sera (dose according to manufacturer's guidelines). All three of these adjuncts reportedly decrease mortality and hospitalization time.[14] Recombinant human granulocyte colony-stimulating factor has been advocated for use in treating severe neutro-

penias induced during CP. However, supplementing CPV-2-neutropenic puppies with this factor did not change any aspect of their clinical outcome.[15]

In dogs with CP, food should be withheld until 24 to 48 hours after vomiting ceases and diarrhea is reduced. Small amounts of water should be offered over the next 24 hours. If vomiting of water does not occur, small portions of a highly digestible, low-fiber, moderately low-fat diet (e.g., cooked rice or cereal supplemented in a 4:1 ratio with low-fat cottage cheese, boiled lean ground beef, chicken, or commercial baby food) can be given three to six times a day. Commercial low-residue diets formulated for gastrointestinal disease may also be used. If commercial diets are used, the dog should initially be given one third the amount needed to meet normal maintenance energy needs. Over the next several days, the amount of food should be gradually increased to meet the dog's regular needs.

After gastrointestinal signs abate, a broad-spectrum dewormer and treatment for *Giardia* infection such as fenbendazole (50 mg/kg orally once a day for seven days) should be given.[9] Puppies that survive the first three to four days of CP and that have an increasing total white blood cell count usually recover rapidly, generally within one week in uncomplicated cases. Severely ill dogs that develop sepsis or other complications may require prolonged hospitalization.

Prevention. A puppy that recovers from CP is immune to reinfection for at least 20 months and possibly for life. Upon reexposure to the various CPV-2 strains, protected puppies do not have an increased serologic titer, show overt signs of illness, or shed virus in the feces. There is a good correlation between serum antibody titer, determined by either hemagglutination inhibition or virus neutralization testing, and resistance to infection. Serum antibody titers remain high for a prolonged period after CP, even if reexposure does not occur. If serum antibody titers become low, a localized infection is possible, but viremia and generalized illness are unlikely to occur.

Attenuated and inactivated CPV-2 vaccines are available. These vaccines produce varying levels of protective immunity and are safe for use either alone or in combination with other canine virus components. Transient lymphopenia occurs four to six days after the administration of some attenuated CPV-2 vaccines. Most attenuated CPV vaccine strains replicate in the intestinal tract and are briefly shed in the feces. The events after administration of attenuated CPV-2 vaccines parallel those that result from field CP. On day 2 after vaccine administration, viremia and systemic distribution occur, with shedding from the gastrointestinal tract on days 3 through 10. One difference between vaccine-induced and field infections is that lower quantities of virus are shed after vaccination. Humoral immune responses to attenuated CPV-2 vaccines are similar to those observed with field CP. Serum antibody is usually detectable three days after vaccination, with concentrations rising rapidly to those observed after field infection. Even if reexposure does not occur, protective antibody titers may persist for at least two years, and dogs exposed during this time should not become infected.

To solve the previous problems of maternal antibody interference and lack of sufficient seroconversion to most attenuated and inactivated CP vaccines, CPV-2 vaccines that contain highly immunogenic, attenuated CPV-2 strains produced at a high titer and low passage are preferred. Vaccine studies have demonstrated that a CPV-2 vaccine from a highly immunogenic strain produced at a high titer will actively immunize puppies with low to moderate levels of maternal immunity to CPV-2.[16] With such vaccines, puppies are more likely to develop protective antibody titers. Puppies of unknown immune status should be vaccinated with a high-titer attenuated CPV-2 vaccine at 6, 9, and 12 weeks old and be revaccinated annually. A check for serum antibody titer or an additional vaccination could be done at 15 to 16 weeks old, especially in those breeds at high risk for CP. Additional CPV-2 vaccines do not have to be given through 20 to 22 weeks of age. CPV-2 vaccine is given in combination with vaccines for other canine viruses (see Table 88–1).

CANINE CORONAVIRUS

Canine coronavirus (CCV) is a cause of acute gastroenteritis in most Canidae.

Etiology. CCV, an enveloped RNA virus, is a member of the Coronaviridae. Several CCV strains have been isolated from outbreaks of diarrheal disease in dogs. CCV is fairly resistant and can remain infectious for long periods during winter months. CCV can be inactivated by most commercial detergents and disinfectants.

Epidemiology. The true importance of CCV as a cause of infectious enteritis in dogs is not known. Available information suggests that CCV has been present indefinitely in the dog population and is an infrequent cause of infectious enteritis. When present, CCV spreads rapidly through groups of susceptible dogs.[17] Neonatal puppies are more severely affected than are puppies of weaning age and adult dogs. CCV is shed in the feces of infected dogs for two weeks or longer, and fecal contamination of the environment is the primary source for its transmission.

Clinical Signs. It is difficult to differentiate CCV from other causes of infectious enteritis. The clinical signs can vary, and dogs of any breed, age, and sex are affected. Infected dogs usually have a sudden onset of diarrhea preceded sometimes by vomiting.[18] The feces are orange, malodorous, and infrequently contain blood. Loss of appetite and lethargy are common signs. Fever is not constant, and leukopenia is not a recognized feature. In severe cases, diarrhea can become watery, and dehydration and electrolyte imbalances can follow. Most affected dogs recover naturally after 8 to 10 days. When secondary complicating factors are present, the clinical course of CCV can be prolonged.

Diagnosis. It is difficult to make a definitive diagnosis of CCV-induced disease. The detection of CCV in fresh feces can be done by electron microscopy. Viral isolation is difficult, as CCV does not grow well on tissue or cell culture systems. A serum virus neutralization and ELISA tests for CCV have been developed. Positive CCV serum titers of affected dogs may help in differentiating CCV enteritis from other viral infections.

Treatment and Prevention. Management of CCV should emphasize supportive treatment to maintain fluid and electrolyte balance as described for CP. Although rarely indicated, broad-spectrum antibiotics can be used to treat secondary bacterial infections. Good nursing care is certainly essential. Inactivated and attenuated CCV vaccines are available.[19] They provide incomplete protection against infection owing to the localized, superficial CCV infection in the intestinal tract of dogs. It is difficult to assess the role of CCV vaccines in protection against enteritis, because CCV infections are usually inapparent or cause only mild signs.

CANINE HERPESVIRUS

Canine herpesvirus (CHV), an enveloped DNA virus, primarily causes severe illness and death in puppies younger than 3 weeks old. Newborn puppies usually become infected with CHV during passage through an infected birth canal or by contact with infectious vaginal or nasal secretions of the mother or littermates. Transplacental transmission may also occur. The incubation period varies from three to six days in puppies younger than 3 weeks old. Affected puppies cease nursing; cry persistently; become weakened, depressed, and hypothermic; and often pass soft, yellow-green feces. Petechial hemorrhages often occur in mucous membranes. Death usually occurs in 24 to 72 hours after onset of clinical signs. Older puppies (three to five weeks old) show mild respiratory signs with subsequent recovery. Puppies that recover usually have latent CHV infections, and some may develop neurologic signs such as ataxia and blindness. Multifocal petechial and ecchymotic hemorrhages in kidneys, liver, lungs, lymph nodes, and the gastrointestinal tract are typical findings at necropsy. Intranuclear inclusion bodies may be present surrounding foci of necrosis and hemorrhage.

Treatment of affected puppies is usually supportive. Serum antibody can be detected in puppies known to have recovered from CHV infection. Mothers may lose a litter of puppies to CHV and raise healthy litters subsequently. Spread of CHV infection can be controlled by not breeding dogs known to have been infected.

RABIES

Rabies is an acute viral encephalitis characterized by altered behavior, aggressiveness, progressive paralysis, and death in warm-blooded animals.

Etiology. Rabies virus is a labile RNA virus that does not persist in the environment. Sunlight, warm temperatures, drying, and common disinfectants destroy its infectivity. Although there is only one antigenic type, antigenic differences have been identified with the use of monoclonal antibodies.

Epidemiology. All warm-blooded animals are susceptible to rabies virus, with skunks, wild canids, raccoons, bats, and cattle being the most susceptible. Dogs, cats, horses, sheep, goats, nonhuman primates, and humans are intermediate in susceptibility. Wild animals are the primary rabies reservoirs, but domestic animals are the principal source for transmission of rabies to humans. When rabies in dogs and cats is controlled, the occurrence of rabies in humans is reduced. Vaccination of at least 70 per cent of the dog and cat population controls dog and cat rabies and provides an effective barrier for humans.

Infection occurs by contact of infected saliva from a rabid animal with nerve endings or damaged nerve fibers as a result of a bite. Contamination of a fresh wound with saliva containing rabies virus, or rabies virus making contact with the conjunctiva or olfactory mucosa, can also result in rabies transmission.

The incubation period from the time of exposure to the onset of clinical rabies is usually three to eight weeks, but it can vary from one week to more than one year. The location of the bite, type of exposure, and amount of virus present at exposure are the important factors that affect the incubation period. Bites that occur on the face, head, and neck result in shorter incubation periods. After rabies virus inoculation, it migrates centripetally in peripheral nerve fibers to the central nervous system and eventually affects the neurons. After the virus reaches the brain and multiplies in neurons, it migrates centrifugally in nerve fibers from the central nervous system to the salivary glands, allowing for shedding of virus in the saliva and further transmission.

Clinical Signs. The stages of rabies are prodromal, furious, and paralytic. The prodromal stage is characterized by change in behavior and temperament, such as restlessness, snapping at imaginary objects, or vocalization at the slightest provocation. The prodromal stage usually lasts for two to three days and is followed by the furious stage. Dogs may show prominent excitability to external stimuli or may be easily excited and attempt to bite or ingest anything, including solid objects such as wood, metal, and fences. Self-mutilation may occur. Viral-induced damage to motor neurons may cause seizures or ascending paralysis and ataxia of the back legs. Paralysis of muscles of deglutition is responsible for drooling of saliva and inability to swallow. Change in tone of vocalization, dysphagia, protrusion of third eyelids, pupil dilatation, or pupil constriction may occur. The paralytic stage may last for two to four days and is followed by death due to respiratory arrest.

Diagnosis. Rabies should be suspected on the basis of history and clinical signs. Confirmation of the diagnosis usually depends on postmortem examination for rabies virus in the brain or brain stem. Fluorescent antibody and immunoperoxidase techniques have been applied to biopsies of skin at the nape of the neck or sensory vibrissae from the maxillary area for antemortem diagnosis of rabies. Monoclonal antibody techniques may also be used to distinguish the source of rabies virus, differentiating between vaccine and field rabies virus.

Treatment and Prevention. Treatment is not recommended for dogs with rabies because of the risk of human exposure. Dogs that have clinical signs consistent with rabies should be placed in strict isolation to prevent possible exposure of other animals or humans, or they should be euthanized and the brain examined for rabies virus.

Rabies is preventable by immunization of dogs and cats and by control or immunization of stray animals. Excellent inactivated rabies vaccines are available for use in dogs, cats, and ferrets and, in some instances, for use in horses, cattle, and sheep. These vaccines are safe and effective, with many of them providing immunity for three years. A list of licensed animal rabies vaccines is revised annually as part of a "Compendium of Animal Rabies Control" that is published in the *Journal of the American Veterinary Medical Association*.[20] It is recommended that dogs and cats be vaccinated at 3 months of age, again one year later, and either annually or triennially thereafter, depending on the rabies vaccine used. Three-year vaccines are recommended even in areas where state or local laws require annual vaccination for rabies. There are no inactivated rabies vaccines approved for use in wild or exotic animals.

PSEUDORABIES

Pseudorabies, primarily a disease in swine, affects the central nervous system of dogs and cats. Pseudorabies in dogs occurs only in areas where pseudorabies virus is endemic in the swine population. Naturally acquired infections occur following ingestion of the herpesvirus. Infected dogs typically show sudden onset of change in behavior, seizures, and intense pruritus of the head and limbs. The disease progresses rapidly, and death usually occurs within 48 hours after onset of signs. Intense pruritus may result in self-mutilation. Paresis and paralysis may occur shortly before death. The diagnosis of pseudorabies should be suspected based on the history and clinical signs. Definitive diagnosis is dependent on histopathologic examination of the brain or by virus isolation.

REFERENCES

1. Appel MJ, Summers BA: Pathogenicity of morbilliviruses for terrestrial carnivores. Vet Microbiol 44:187, 1995.
2. Mitchell WJ, et al: Viral expression in experimental canine distemper demyelinating encephalitis. J Comp Pathol 104:77, 1991.
3. Mee AP, et al: Canine distemper virus transcripts detected in the bone cells of dogs with metaphyseal osteopathy. Bone 14:59, 1993.
4. Baumgärtner W, et al: Metaphyseal bone lesions in young dogs with systemic canine distemper virus infection. Vet Microbiol 44:201, 1995.
5. Khan SA, et al: Paget's disease of bone and unvaccinated dogs. Bone 19:47, 1996.
6. Blixenkrone-Moller M, et al: Studies on manifestations of canine distemper virus infection in an urban dog population. Vet Microbiol 37:163, 1993.
7. Chappuis G: Control of canine distemper. Vet Microbiol 44:351, 1995.
8. Bemis DA: *Bordetella* and *Mycoplasma* respiratory infection in dogs. Vet Clin North Am Small Anim Pract 22:1173, 1992.
9. Hoskins JD: Update on canine parvoviral enteritis. Vet Med 92:694, 1997.
10. Mochizuki M, et al: Isolation of canine parvovirus from a cat manifesting clinical signs of feline panleukopenia. J Clin Microbiol 34:2101, 1996.
11. Harrington DP, et al: A retrospective study of canine parvovirus gastroenteritis: 89 cases. J Vet Intern Med 10:157, 1996.
12. Hoskins JD, et al: Evaluation of a fecal antigen ELISA test for the diagnosis of canine parvovirus. J Vet Intern Med 10:159, 1996.
13. Uwatoko K, et al: Rapid method utilizing the polymerase chain reaction for detection of canine parvovirus in feces of diarrheic dogs. Vet Microbiol 43:315, 1995.
14. Dimmit R: Clinical experience with cross-protective anti-endotoxin antiserum in dogs with parvoviral enteritis. Canine Pract 16:23, 1991.
15. Rewerts JM, et al: Effect of rhG-CSF administration on the clinical outcome of neutropenic parvovirus-infected puppies. J Vet Intern Med 10:178, 1996.
16. Larson LJ, Schultz RD: High-titer canine parvovirus vaccine: Serologic response and challenge-of-immunity study. Vet Med 90:210, 1996.
17. Tennant BJ, et al: Studies on the epizootiology of canine coronavirus. Vet Rec 132:7, 1993.
18. Tennant BJ, et al: Canine coronavirus infection in the dog following oronasal inoculation. Res Vet Sci 51:11, 1991.
19. Pardo C, Mackowiak M: Efficacy of a new canine origin, modified live virus vaccine against canine coronavirus. Athens, GA, Rhone Merieux, 1995.
20. Compendium of animal rabies control, 1997. JAVMA 210:33, 1997.

INF

CHAPTER 89

FeLV AND NON-NEOPLASTIC FeLV-RELATED DISEASE

Julie K. Levy

VIROLOGY

Household clusters of lymphosarcoma and lymphocytic leukemia cases have been observed among young cats for many years, but it was not until the discovery of retrovirus particles in a leukemic cat in 1964 that an infectious etiology was considered likely.[1] Over the next few years, the agent, named feline leukemia virus (FeLV), was isolated and shown to be capable of transmitting lymphocytic neoplasia among cats. An indirect fluorescent antibody test to detect antigenemia, developed in 1973, made the clinical screening of privately owned cats possible.[2] The mass testing that followed revealed that the virus was present at low rates throughout the world's domestic cat population, that it appeared to be spread both vertically (from queen to fetus or nursing kitten) and horizontally (from cat to cat), and that infection was associated with a variety of illnesses in addition to neoplasia, including anemia and immunodeficiency.

FeLV is a retrovirus, which means that its genetic material is transmitted from host to host as RNA. In infected cells, DNA copies of the virus are transcribed, and it is these copies that are inserted randomly into the host DNA. Once this provirus is integrated, cell divisions result in daughter cells that also contain the viral DNA. The virus encodes three major protein groups: gag (group-specific antigens), pol (reverse transcriptase), and env (envelope). One of the gag proteins, p27, is abundant in the plasma of infected cats and in the cytoplasm of individual infected cells, which is why most clinically available enzyme-linked immunosorbent assay (ELISA) or immunofluorescent antibody (IFA) tests are designed to detect this protein. The envelope protein gp70 defines the virus subgroup and appears to be important for inducing immunity.[3]

FeLV isolates occur in three subgroups (A, B, and C), which vary in their clinical pathogenesis. Subgroup A is the most common isolate and is the primary subgroup passed horizontally among cats in nature. Following infection with subgroup A, viral recombinations may occur with the feline endogenous retrovirus, leading to the emergence of subgroup B, which is associated with immune suppression and malignancy. Subgroup C is rare in nature and arises from mutations of the subgroup A strains. Thus, all FeLV-infected cats carry subgroup A; fewer are co-infected with subgroup B or C. In experimental infections with defined strains of virus, a group AB strain (Rickard) causes lymphosarcoma in nearly 100 per cent of kittens by one year after infection, whereas subgroup C isolates are more likely to produce fatal anemia.[3]

EPIDEMIOLOGY

FeLV infection exists in domestic cats worldwide. Interestingly, the infection rate of free-roaming cats is similar throughout the world, ranging from 1 to 8 per cent of healthy cats. Infection rates of up to 21 per cent have been reported from large surveys of clinically ill cats.[4] Certain diseases were originally associated with high rates of FeLV infection when testing first became available, such as lymphosarcoma and myelogenous leukemia (75 per cent) and feline infectious peritonitis (FIP; 32 per cent). In recent years, FeLV-negative cases of these diseases have become more common as the overall prevalence of FeLV has decreased.[5]

Susceptibility to FeLV infection is highest in young kittens. Experimental infections with some laboratory strains of virus can be difficult to achieve in kittens older than 16 weeks of age.[6] This also appears to be true in nature, as the prevalence of anti-FeLV antibody increases steadily over time, indicating an increasing rate of exposure to the virus throughout life. In one survey in Scotland, only 6 per cent of kittens younger than 5 months old had antibodies. This percentage increased to 55 per cent at 1 to 2 years of age and to 74 per cent by 3 years. In the United States, antibody prevalence (virus exposure) was related to the degree of exposure to other cats and to the time spent outdoors. Cats in Boston and Detroit, where many cats are allowed to roam outside, had 63 and 47 per cent antibody rates, respectively, whereas only 5 per cent of New York City cats, primarily confined to high-rise apartments, had any antibodies.[3] Despite the evidence for increased risk of exposure to FeLV throughout life, the cumulative rate of infection is opposite that of antibody production. Of 8642 cases of FeLV reported by North American veterinary teaching hospitals since 1973, the highest rate of infection was reported in cats younger than 2 years of age.[7] Although FeLV was reported in cats of all ages, the rate declined steadily as cats aged. Taken together with the antibody serosurveys, this suggests that exposure to FeLV accumulates with age but that susceptibility to infection simultaneously decreases. This age-related resistance is not absolute, however, as evidenced by the increased rate of infection observed among adult cats brought into households with endemic FeLV and by natural exposure studies of vaccine efficacy in which a high proportion of unvaccinated adult controls became infected when they were housed with other infected cats.

There is evidence that the overall rate of FeLV infection is decreasing.[5, 7] This is particularly true in catteries that produce purebred animals. The availability of routine testing in these closed facilities made it possible to remove all infected animals. Likewise, the current practice of testing cats at animal shelters and testing new pets has contributed to the decline of this virus. The first vaccine was introduced in 1985, but the observed decline in overall infection rate began before this. At least one model of FeLV infection dynamics estimates that the rate of FeLV vaccination is still too low to contribute to a general decrease in the prevalence of FeLV.[8]

FeLV infection is slightly more common among male cats than females. Unlike feline immunodeficiency virus (FIV), which is spread among cats primarily by biting during fights, FeLV is also efficiently passed both vertically and horizontally from infected queens to kittens and among communal cats with prolonged close contact. FeLV is shed in high levels in the saliva, urine, and other secretions, so sharing food and water dishes, mutual grooming, and using common litter areas all contribute to the equal spread of the virus to males and females. The wandering and fighting behavior of unneutered males is an additional risk factor for infection among this group.

Infected cats can pass the virus to their offspring in utero or to newborn kittens through milk. Reproductive failure, in the form of fetal resorption, abortion, and neonatal death, is common in this situation, although up to 20 per cent of vertically infected kittens may survive the neonatal period to become persistently infected adults. The distinction between vertical transmission from queen to kitten and horizontal transmission among a family group is a somewhat arbitrary one from a clinical perspective. It is common, however, to observe that newborn kittens from persistently or latently infected queens may test negative at birth, only to seroconvert one by one over the following weeks to months. Thus, if the queen or any one of her litter is infected, the entire family should be treated as suspect and isolated from other uninfected cats until they are retested.

DIAGNOSIS

Routine screening for FeLV infection became available when Hardy developed the IFA in 1973. When the ELISA was developed several years later, clinicians gained the ability to perform rapid and reliable in-house testing. These two tests have remained the mainstay of clinical FeLV testing.[9] Both tests detect the FeLV core protein p27, which is produced abundantly in most infected cats. The ELISA is performed on serum, plasma, and whole blood samples. In some studies, higher rates of false-positives were recorded when whole blood samples were used, particularly when the samples were hemolyzed. False-positive results were also a problem in some test systems that used murine-derived reagents in cats that had naturally occurring anti-mouse antibodies. User error contributes to false-positive results in ELISA testing as well. This is most likely to occur in the washing steps of kits using a micro-well or wand format. The use of membrane-based tests offers the advantage of eliminating separate washing steps and including both positive and negative controls for each test sample. Some test systems have been developed for tear or saliva samples in place of blood.[10] In general, these tests are not as accurate, and because the consequences of both false-positive and false-negative test results can be disastrous for individual cats or for multiple-cat populations, they are not recommended for routine screening.

The IFA detects p27 antigen within the cytoplasm of infected blood cells. Because it requires special processing and fluorescent microscopy, the IFA must be performed by a qualified reference laboratory. Generally, two or more quality blood or bone marrow smears are air-dried and mailed, unfixed, to the laboratory. Because the antigen is present at highest concentrations in neutrophils and platelets, false-negatives may result when these two cell lines are deficient. False-positive results may occur when smears are too thick, when background fluorescence is high, and when the test is prepared and interpreted by inexperienced personnel. Both the ELISA and the IFA are extremely sensitive and specific when performed correctly, but quality-control variability among facilities has been reported to affect the reliability of test results. Thus, careful attention should be paid to the performance of FeLV screening tests in clinics and in the selection of reference labs. ELISA tests detect viral antigens circulating freely in the blood, whereas the IFA identifies infected leukocytes and platelets. Because FeLV generally replicates in lymphoid tissue and other sites before reaching the bone marrow, the ELISA may detect infection a few weeks earlier than the IFA. Some cats are apparently able to clear the infection at this stage and may revert to ELISA-negative status within a few weeks to months. IFA-positive tests indicate that the bone marrow is infected with FeLV. In this case, most cats will be persistently infected for life.[11] In general, the ELISA is considered to be slightly more sensitive, and the IFA is slightly more specific. With either test, however, the reliability (predictive value) of the test is dependent on the rate of infection within different populations of cats. For example, FeLV is present in most cats with thymic lymphoma, so a positive test is likely to be accurate in this situation. In a lower-risk population, such as a closed cattery known to be free of FeLV, a positive test should be viewed with more suspicion, and additional confirmatory tests should be performed.[12]

Recently, the polymerase chain reaction (PCR) test has been adapted to clinical use for the diagnosis of FeLV infection. This test differs from earlier screening tests in that it detects viral nucleic acid sequences (RNA or DNA) instead of protein antigens. It is sensitive because the process involves amplification of FeLV sequences many times in order to enhance detection. The PCR must be performed by well-equipped and well-trained laboratories, because minor alterations in sample handling can destroy the delicate nucleic acid material or introduce minute amounts of cross-contamination, leading to either false-negative or false-positive results. With this in mind, however, the PCR has also greatly enhanced the ability to detect FeLV infection in blood, solid tissues, tissue cultures, and fixed specimens. Commercial FeLV PCR tests detect proviral DNA, that is, virus sequences that have been integrated into the host genome. The detection of viral DNA does not necessarily mean that a cat is persistently infected or that it is shedding infectious virus. FeLV provirus has been detected in both transiently and latently infected cats, as well as in apparently uninfected cats that reside with FeLV-infected cats. PCR may be useful in helping to determine the true status of cats with discordant results from other testing techniques.

Because no test is accurate 100 per cent of the time, and because various testing modalities target somewhat different specimens and disease stages, it is possible to have test results that disagree. The challenge for the clinician is to determine which test result most likely reflects the true status of the cat. For example, it is possible for infected cats to be antigenemic (viral proteins circulating in the blood) but to have negative virus blood cultures if the infection is sequestered in another tissue compartment such as the bone marrow or lymphoid system. In one study of cats that were positive by ELISA but negative by culture, viral DNA was detected by PCR in samples from 7 of 39 cats, indicating that the cats were, most likely, truly infected with FeLV. The sensitivity of the PCR was increased to detect DNA in 13 of the 39 cats if a second round of amplification with nested (internal) primers was performed.[13]

The combination of routine screening with one or two confirmatory tests will accurately determine the FeLV infection status of most cats. Some animals, however, will have repeatedly discordant test results or occult infections. Rarely, some cats that test negative for viremia have been shown to secrete infectious virus in body fluids such as milk and urine. It is particularly difficult to know the true status of cats that have been exposed to FeLV and have apparently cleared the virus. Surveys conducted before the development of FeLV vaccines indicate that many, if not most, free-roaming cats acquire anti-FeLV antibodies, indicating at least transient exposure and infection with the virus.[14] Although almost all these antibody-positive cats are seronegative for viral antigens, it is not possible to know whether they are truly clear of infection, resistant to further exposure, or latently infected.

The American Association of Feline Practitioners (AAFP) has developed recommendations for testing cats for FeLV.[15] Based on the premise that "FeLV is transmitted contagiously among cats and is associated with the illness and death of more cats than any other pathologic condition," the AAFP recommends testing all existing household cats and any new kittens and cats before they are introduced into the household. Identifying infected cats before other cats are exposed provides an opportunity to prevent the spread of the disease. In addition, it is preferable to identify infected cats before they are adopted or before a strong pet-owner bond develops. The AAFP further recommends retesting cats that become ill with clinical signs consistent with FeLV infection and before vaccination for FeLV. The ELISA is the association's preferred screening test, with the IFA being the most appropriate confirmatory test. Because false-positive test results may occur with whole blood samples, the AAFP recommends confirmation of positive tests with serum or plasma. The use of saliva or tears is not recommended. The FeLV test detects viral antigens and not antibody, so maternal immunity has no effect on the test results. Therefore, cats may be tested at any age. Because cats may be in the early stage of infection at the time of the first test, it is recommended that a follow-up test be performed at least 90 days after the initial test or after a potential exposure to FeLV.

PATHOGENESIS

Horizontal transmission of FeLV among susceptible cats occurs most commonly via the oronasal route and by bite wounds. Although a majority of cats within a population may demonstrate evidence of exposure to FeLV by the presence of anti-FeLV antibodies, only a portion of exposed cats will become persistently viremic. There are several reasons for this low rate of persistent infection, including the rapid inactivation of the virus outside of the host, the large viral dose required for successful infection, and the natural resistance of many cats. Thus, cats are most likely to become infected in situations in which they have extended, close contact with actively shedding cats. True "outbreaks" of FeLV infection are unlikely to occur.

Following mucosal or percutaneous inoculation of FeLV, the virus replicates in local lymphoid tissues. From there, infected cells carry the virus to other target tissues, such as thymus, spleen, and lymph nodes. At this stage of acute viral replication, fever, malaise, diarrhea, and leukopenia are common. In addition, generalized lymphadenopathy may be so marked as to be mistaken for lymphoma. Regardless of the often dramatic clinical presentation, this stage of infection is generally transient, and most affected cats survive with supportive care.[16]

Later, the virus infects the salivary gland and the mucosal glandular epithelium. These sites of infection may secrete most of the infectious virus that is responsible for horizontal transmission. About the same time, bone marrow cells become involved, producing infected leukocytes and platelets that circulate in the blood. Early in infection, circulating viral antigens may be detected in the circulation before the bone marrow is infected. This results in discordant test results (ELISA positive, IFA negative) and explains the slightly higher sensitivity of the ELISA tests. During this stage of infection, before the bone marrow is affected, most cats mount an immune response capable of eliminating the viremia within weeks.[16] Although viremia (circulating virus) is not detected in these cats, it is believed that the virus is still present in a latent form. Latent infections can reactivate spontaneously or in response to concurrent immune suppression.[17] As time passes, however, latent infections become more difficult to reactivate, even with the administration of high doses of corticosteroids. By one year after infection, reactivation of the virus is considered unlikely. If viremia persists more than 16 weeks, or if the bone marrow is infected, as indicated by a positive IFA test, chances are high that the cat will remain persistently infected, viremic, and infectious to other cats for the remainder of its life.

The ability of FeLV to become part of the host's own DNA is one of the most important factors in the lifelong presence of the virus following persistent infection. In essence, every infected cell would have to be recognized and destroyed to "cure" the infection. Once the pool of hematologic and immune stem cells becomes infected, true elimination of the virus becomes unlikely.

The exact mechanisms for the varied clinical responses of infected cats are poorly understood. It is clear that the clinical course is determined by a combination of viral and host factors. Some of these differences can be traced to properties of the virus itself. Subgroup A, which is the form that is passed horizontally among cats, is the least pathogenic type. Subgroups B and C arise de novo in cats infected first with subgroup A and are believed to be responsible for most of the clinical syndromes associated with FeLV. Subgroup B induces immune suppression and malignant transformation. Subgroup C causes severe nonregenerative anemia.

Perhaps the most significant host factor that determines the clinical outcome of cats infected with FeLV is the age of the cat at the time of infection.[6] Neonatal kittens develop marked thymic atrophy following infection, resulting in severe immune suppression, wasting, and early death. As cats mature, they acquire a progressive resistance to infection. When older cats do become infected, they tend to have milder signs and a more protracted period of apparent good health, although they remain infectious to other cats.

Cats infected with FeLV have 62 times the risk of developing lymphoma compared with uninfected cats. Persistently infected cats, which have the longest duration of host-virus interaction, have 50 times the incidence of lymphoma compared with FeLV-recovered cats. FeLV does not contain oncogenes, so malignant transformation is not a direct consequence of viral infection. Instead, it is believed that lymphomas arise when viral replication, budding, and reinsertion into the genome of new cells result in random rearrangement of viral pieces and host DNA (insertional mutagenesis).[18] When these chance insertions alter the relationship of genes to cell cycle control mechanisms, rapidly replicating clones result.

Bone marrow suppression, resulting in nonregenerative anemia, leukopenia, or thrombocytopenia, results from both primary infection of hematopoietic stem cells and infection of stromal cells that constitute the supporting environment for hematopoietic cells. One form of FeLV-induced anemia is associated with red blood cell (RBC) macrocytosis. This is believed to represent a virus-induced defect in the cell division that accompanies RBC maturation. Much more common is pure red cell aplasia, a severe nonregenerative anemia associated with marked depletion and maturation arrest of erythroid precursors in the bone marrow. In this case, serum erythropoietin levels are markedly increased, indicating that the anemia is not due to a deficiency of erythropoietin. In addition to primary viral anemia, infected cats may have decreased hematocrits for a number of secondary reasons.[3, 19, 20]

Regenerative anemia in FeLV-infected cats, indicated by increased reticulocytes and, in some cases, nucleated RBCs, occurs most commonly in the presence of hemobartonellosis, autoimmune hemolytic anemia, or hemorrhage. The myeloproliferative disease erythremic myelosis causes a peculiar FeLV-related anemia characterized by extremely high numbers of nucleated RBCs (sometimes exceeding 500 nRBCs/100 white blood cells) and an extremely low hematocrit. Although the anemia may appear to be regenerative because of the high number of nucleated RBCs, the absence of reticulocytes indicates that it is, in fact, a nonregenerative anemia. Erythremic myelosis is resistant to chemotherapy and is virtually always fatal, although affected cats may have extended survival if supported with blood transfusions.

Nonregenerative anemia may be a nonspecific response to chronic disease in cats, or it may be due to bone marrow infiltration by lymphoma, leukemia, or infectious agents such as systemic mycoses. Other cell lines may also be affected by the virus. FeLV and myeloproliferative disease accounted for 44 per cent of cats with thrombocytopenia in one report. Neutropenia is also common in FeLV-infected cats, especially in the early and late stages of infection. There is also a "panleukopenia-like syndrome" of FeLV that mimics feline parvoviral infection with severe leukopenia and enteritis.[21] Cyclic neutropenia has been reported to be associated with FeLV infection in a few cats. The cycles are regular, ranging from 8 to 14 days. In one such cat, platelet count and reticulocyte count also cycled. Various cytopenias may wax and wane in FeLV-infected cats, seemingly responding to a variety of therapeutic interventions, but these syndromes are just as likely to resolve spontaneously. Some persistent cytopenias are associated with myelodysplasia and may eventually evolve into a terminal myelodysplastic syndrome or leukemia.[3, 19, 20]

Diseases associated with immune suppression account for a large portion of the morbidity and mortality of FeLV-infected cats.[20–22] Exactly how the virus damages the immune system is poorly understood, as is why different animals have such varying degrees of immune suppression in response to the same virus. Once again, viral strain, inoculum route and dose, and age of the host are all factors in the severity of subsequent immune suppression, as are other unknown host resistance factors. Cats may develop thymic atrophy or depletion of lymph node paracortical zones following infection. Neutropenia and lymphopenia are common findings. In some cats, lymphopenia may be characterized by preferential loss of CD4+ helper T cells, resulting in an inverted CD4+:CD8+ ratio more typical of FIV infection.[23]

More commonly, there are substantial losses of both helper cells and cytotoxic-suppressor (CD8+) cells. Many immune function tests of naturally infected cats have been reported to be abnormal, including poor response to T-cell mitogens, prolonged allograft rejection, reduced immunoglobulin production, depressed neutrophil function, and complement depletion. Interleukin-2 (IL-2) and interleukin-4 (IL-4) are decreased in some infected cats. Studies disagree on whether interferon gamma (IFN-γ) is deficient or increased. FeLV does not appear to suppress interleukin-1 (IL-1) production from infected macrophages. Several studies support the finding of increased tumor necrosis factor-alpha (TNFα) in both the serum of infected cats and infected cells in culture. Although each cytokine plays a vital role in the generation of a healthy immune response, the excess production of certain cytokines, such as TNFα, can also cause illness.

There are many reports of FeLV-infected cats having concurrent bacterial, viral, protozoal, and fungal infections, but few studies exist that prove that these cats have a higher rate of infection than FeLV-negative cats or that they have a less favorable response to therapy. Thus, although FeLV is well known to suppress immune function, it should not be assumed that all concurrent infections are a result of FeLV infection. Secondary infections most commonly associated with FeLV include FIP, upper respiratory infections, and hemobartonellosis.

In addition to immune suppression, FeLV-infected cats are subject to a variety of immune-mediated diseases. Hemolytic anemia, glomerular nephritis, and the syndromes of fever and wasting are often due to an overactive or dysregulated immune response to the virus. The loss of T suppressor cell activity and the formation of antigen-antibody complexes may contribute to these syndromes.[3]

Clinical evaluation of the immune status of FeLV-infected cats is hampered by the lack of well-characterized immune function tests. Thus, clinicians remain largely dependent on complete blood count (CBC) and clinical presentation for diagnosing immune dysfunction. Most serious clinical disease syndromes occur in cats that have been persistently infected for six months or more. Although the virus was named after the contagious malignancy that first drew attention to it, most infected cats are brought to veterinarians for chronic anemias or immune suppression. Of 8642 FeLV-infected cats examined at North American veterinary schools, various co-infections (FIP, upper respiratory infection, FIV, hemobartonellosis, stomatitis) were the most frequent finding (15 per cent), followed by anemia (11 per cent), lymphoma (6 per cent), leukopenia or thrombocytopenia (5 per cent), and leukemia or myeloproliferative disease (4 per cent).[7] From a clinical standpoint, it is important to realize that many of these syndromes are treatable and that not all disease that occurs in FeLV-infected cats is actually due to the virus. When infected cats do succumb from direct viral effects, it is usually the result of severe anemia or neoplasia.

PREVENTION AND CONTROL

TEST AND REMOVAL FOR CLOSED POPULATIONS

When FeLV was first described in the mid-1960s, the highest rates of infection were found in large multicat households and catteries. In contrast, free-roaming cats had lower rates of infection, and cats housed singly indoors were rarely infected. Convenient and reliable testing for FeLV became available in the mid-1970s. Very quickly, cat breeders implemented test and removal programs, which proved to be extremely reliable for eliminating the virus from catteries. The most dramatic example of this was a mandatory test and removal program imposed on all members of a cat breeding society in the Netherlands in 1974.[24] When testing was first implemented, the prevalence of FeLV in purebred catteries was 11 per cent. Following the removal program, the rate was reduced to less than 2 per cent within four years, and no infected cats have been reported since 1984. Cat fanciers in other countries responded similarly, although on a more voluntary basis, so that FeLV is now considered an anomaly in well-run catteries. Suppliers of cats for research and many stray cat shelters also implemented mass testing programs, thus further reducing the rate of FeLV infection within certain cat communities.

INDIRECT CONTACT

The elimination of FeLV from closed catteries is facilitated by the fragility of the virus outside of the host's body. The virus begins losing viability immediately on dry surfaces and is completely inactivated within two to three hours.[25] Thus, environmental contamination from cats that are removed following detection is easily inactivated by routine disinfection (quaternary ammonium, dilute bleach). Likewise, indirect exposure between cats at shows or veterinary clinics is not a risk for transmission, as long as the cats are not allowed direct contact. There is no need to house FeLV-infected cats in special isolation rooms so long as cats are housed in separate cages. Veterinarians and handlers, however, should take precautions to avoid inadvertent transmission of the virus through body fluids such as blood, urine, and saliva. Clinical practices that risk nosocomial transmission include serial surgeries performed with the same instruments; reuse of inadequately sterilized syringes and of saliva-contaminated endotracheal tubes and anesthetic circuits; unscreened or latently infected blood donors; and fluid bags shared between animals. The same universal precautions employed in human health facilities to prevent the spread of HIV and hepatitis viruses should be incorporated into veterinary practices to prevent the transmission of FeLV and other infectious agents.

VACCINATION

The simplest protection from infection is to keep susceptible cats confined indoors. For cats that are allowed to wander outdoors, vaccination against FeLV may offer some level of protection. Development of a safe and effective vaccine against FeLV presented special challenges that other diseases did not. Because of the ability of retroviruses to integrate into the host genome and to cause disease years later, even in apparently recovered cats, there is reluctance to pursue the use of a live virus preparation. Thus, most vaccine development research focused on the use of whole killed virus preparations or subunit vaccines. The first anti-FeLV vaccine was licensed in 1985. Since that time, the original vaccine has undergone modification, and several other products have appeared on the market. The relative efficacy of the various vaccines is the subject of much controversy. Many of the published vaccine efficacy trials were performed or funded by the manufacturers, raising questions about the independence of the studies. Furthermore, the testing protocols varied widely among studies, making meaningful comparisons difficult.[26, 27] Because of natural resistance to FeLV infection, investigators often used artificial immune suppression (corticosteroids) and administration of large viral dosages to increase the challenge virulence in FeLV vaccine efficacy studies. This makes it difficult to know what the actual effect of the vaccine in a natural exposure environment would be. The results of efficacy trials of vaccines currently available in the United States are summarized in Figure 89–1.

There is an epidemiologic association between vaccination against FeLV (and rabies) and the development of sarcomas at the site of injection.[28] Although the rate of tumor formation is controversial (estimated at 1 to 3/10,000 vaccines administered), the tumors are particularly aggressive and often recur after resection. The mechanism of malignant transformation is not known, but it is possible that adjuvants used in inactivated vaccines may be involved. The recognition of these tumors and other problems associated with widespread annual vaccination has led the AAFP to develop revised vaccination recommendations for cats.[29] The AAFP questions the automatic annual revaccination of cats for numerous infectious diseases, regardless of risk. Instead, it recommends tailoring vaccine protocols for each feline patient. In terms of FeLV vaccinations, the AAFP recommends immunizing only those cats with potential risk of exposure to the virus: cats allowed outdoors and cats residing in households with infected cats or with cats of unknown FeLV infection status. Furthermore, it is recommended that all cats be tested for the presence of FeLV before immunization, because FeLV vaccination of infected cats is not believed to be of benefit (although it is probably of no harm either). Prevaccination screening also avoids the situation in which an unscreened but infected vaccinated cat later develops FeLV-related disease, leading an owner or veterinarian to have concerns about vaccine failure. The AAFP further recommends administering any vaccine with FeLV antigen in the lower left leg. This is to aid in the treatment of subsequent sarcomas (by amputation), as well as to help identify the offending product. It is important to keep detailed medical records of vaccine administration (including date, injection site and route, product, and lot number). The use of peel-off vaccine labels that are placed in the permanent medical record is helpful in this regard. It is also important to report adverse vaccine reactions to the manufacturer and to the U.S. Department of Agriculture.

THERAPY FOR FeLV-RELATED DISEASES

Despite the fact that persistent FeLV infection is associated with a decreased life expectancy, many owners elect to provide treatment for the myriad clinical syndromes that accompany infection. It is important for both the owner and the veterinarian to realize that FeLV-positive cats are subject to the same diseases that befall negative cats, and that an illness may not be related to the FeLV infection at all. Each cat must be evaluated as an individual and be carefully assessed for treatable disease. For the most part, secondary diseases in FeLV-infected cats are treated the same as in uninfected cats. Some secondary infectious conditions in FeLV-infected cats may require more intensive and prolonged therapy than in uninfected cats.

If secondary or unrelated diseases have been ruled out, a search is commenced to identify an FeLV-related syndrome. Neoplastic conditions are generally diagnosed by biopsy.

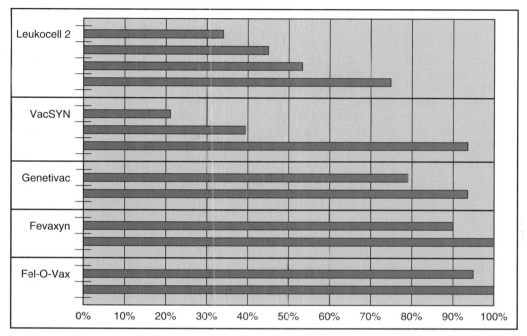

Figure 89–1. Comparison of FeLV vaccine efficacy. Studies were included if group size was at least 10 cats and if at least 50 per cent of unvaccinated controls became persistently viremic following challenge.

$$PF = \text{persistent viremia; } PF\,(\%) = \frac{\%\text{ controls with persistent viremia} - \%\text{ vaccinates with persistent viremia}}{\%\text{ controls with persistent viremia}}$$

(Based on data in Sparkes AH: Feline leukemia virus A review of immunity and vaccination. J Small Anim Pract 38:187, 1997.)

In the case of hematologic abnormalities, a bone marrow examination is frequently indicated to rule out neoplastic or infectious infiltrates. If no other cause can be identified, the abnormality may be attributed to direct viral effects.

If cytopenias are severe, or if treatable underlying etiologies are not discovered, therapy may be attempted with hematologic growth factors.[30] Erythropoietin (Epogen, Amgen; 35 to 100 IU/kg subcutaneously every other day to correct anemia, then weekly to sustain packed cell volume [PCV]) has been of benefit to some cats with FeLV-associated anemia, although many do not respond. Reasons for resistance to erythropoietin include iron deficiency, concurrent infection, FeLV infection of bone marrow stromal cells, and the development of antierythropoietin antibodies. In some nonresponsive cats, repeated blood transfusions may be the only treatment possible.

Granulocyte-colony stimulating factor (Neupogen, Amgen; 5 μg/kg subcutaneously twice a day) was designed to prevent the neutropenia associated with aggressive human chemotherapy protocols. In cats, it has been used successfully to treat neutropenia due to drug toxicity, infectious diseases, FeLV-associated cyclic neutropenia, and idiopathic causes. Long-term use of the drug is limited by cost and the development of neutralizing antibodies against the human product within a few weeks but it is often effective for acute or life-threatening neutropenia. There is no growth factor currently available to stimulate platelet production, and recovery from thrombocytopenia depends on identifying and correcting the underlying cause.

THERAPY FOR FeLV-INFECTED CATS

The evaluation of anti-FeLV therapies is hampered by the lack of well-controlled clinical trials in which new treatments are compared against standard care or placebo. Host

factors such as the age of the cat at the time of infection, genetic variables, immune function, and concurrent diseases are as important as viral strain, dose, and route of infection in determining the clinical outcome of infection. The marked natural variation in disease expression among infected cats makes it risky to predict which cats will have rapid progression of disease and which will be long-term survivors.

In addition to host and viral factors that impact infected cats, the attitudes and motivations of both owners and treating veterinarians have a profound effect on clinical outcome. Many healthy cats are found to be infected on routine screening examinations. These cats may be routinely euthanized because of the risk of transmitting infection to other cats or because of the perceived inevitability of disease development. Likewise, owners and veterinarians of infected cats may have a negative attitude about pursing diagnosis and treatment of illness in these cats, even though the current illness may be unrelated to the viral infection and may respond well to specific therapy.

Most reports in the veterinary literature describe naturally infected cats treated with a variety of specific therapies in combination with routine supportive care. These studies generally do not include controls but may compare results to historic reports. Unfortunately, historic controls include cats that were euthanized routinely after testing positive or that did not undergo thorough diagnosis and treatment. Despite the difficulty and expense of conducting well-designed clinical trials with large numbers of naturally infected cats, a few have been done and represent the greatest contribution to this field.

IMMUNE MODULATOR THERAPY

Immune modulators are proposed to benefit retrovirus-infected cats by restoring compromised immune function, thereby allowing the cat to decrease its viral burden and recover from associated clinical syndromes. These agents are proposed to stimulate early events in the immune cascade, which may lead to a systemic response against viral infection and secondary diseases.[31] Based on in vitro results in other species, most of the immune modulators are proposed to stimulate release of cytokines such as TNFα, IL-1, and IFN-γ. It is not known whether these agents cause the same effect in vivo or whether cat cells react in the same way as do those of other species. Immune function is notoriously difficult to measure, and there is marked interspecies variation in normal immune responses. Thus, it is risky to assume that findings in one species will be identical or even beneficial in another. Even if the proposed cytokines are stimulated in cats, it is not clear that this would be beneficial or even safe. Studies in cats with both natural and experimental FeLV infection suggest that these cats already have increased serum levels of TNFα and IL-6, both of which are produced by activated macrophages and are known to produce weight loss and fever in cats with infections or cancer.

Acemannan (Carrisyn, Carrington Laboratories) is a complex carbohydrate (mannan) polymer derived from the aloe vera plant. In murine tissue cultures, acemannan induces macrophages to produce TNFα and IL-1. In one noncontrolled open-label trial, 50 cats with natural FeLV infection were treated with acemannan (2 mg/kg intraperitoneally every week for six weeks).[32] Whether concurrent supportive care was permitted was not described. At the end of the 12-week study period, 9 cats had been excluded from evaluation. Of the remaining 41 cats, 29 (71 per cent) were known to be alive. All cats remained ELISA-positive for FeLV antigen, and there was no significant change in clinical or hematologic scores from baseline.[32] Although there was no control group in this study, the authors reported that previously, 10 of 11 FeLV-infected cats had been euthanized or died within 64 days of diagnosis at their clinic. However, they also acknowledged that their clinic considered euthanasia to be an appropriate response to a diagnosis of FeLV infection and that it was impossible to know what the survival rate would have been if the cats had been treated and allowed to live. Because the study did not include a control group, and because clinical and laboratory evaluations failed to document improvement from pretreatment evaluations, it is difficult to determine whether the use of acemannan improved the outcome of infection in treated cats. The reported survival times have been achieved by others without the use of immune modulators, so it is possible that the cats were responding to supportive care or would have survived with no medical care at all.

Propionibacterium acnes (ImmunoRegulin, ImmunoVet) is a killed bacterial product that has been shown to enhance interferon, T-cell, and natural killer cell (NK) activity in mice. No prospective studies have been reported on the use of this product in retrovirus-infected cats, but veterinarians have described their clinical experience in published roundtable discussions and in anecdotal reports. In one discussion, a practitioner reported treating 76 clinically ill cats with natural FeLV infection with ImmunoRegulin (0.25 to 0.5 mL intravenously twice weekly, then every other week for 16 weeks) and supportive care, including prednisone, antibiotics, and vitamins.[33] Although no specific clinical and laboratory evaluations were discussed, the practitioner reported that 55 of the cats (72 per cent) became seronegative for FeLV antigens and survived for an unspecified period of time.[33] In another discussion, a veterinarian reported treating 700 cats with natural FeLV infection with ImmunoRegulin

(0.5 mL intravenously every three days, then every week for six or more weeks) in conjunction with antibiotics, fluids, and other supportive care. He estimated that 50 per cent of the cats improved, although seroconversion to negative was rare.[34]

Staphylococcus protein A (SPA, Sigma) is a bacterial polypeptide product purified from the cell wall of *Staphylococcus aureus* Cowan I. It has the ability to bind the Fc portion of IgG and also stimulates T-cell, NK, and IFN-γ activities. A variety of SPA sources and treatments have been used in FeLV-infected cats. Interest was first generated when plasma from FeLV-infected lymphosarcoma-bearing cats was passed over SPA or *S. aureus* columns to remove circulating immune complexes and then returned to the cats. More than 100 cats were treated in this manner, generally undergoing twice-weekly treatments for 10 to 20 weeks. In some studies, a high rate of tumor remission and conversion to FeLV-negative status was observed; in others, responses were less dramatic and were short-lived.[35] Subsequently, it was determined that SPA and other products may have leached from the filters and columns used for immunosorption and been returned to the cats as contaminants in the treated plasma. The possibility that these products exerted a positive immunomodulatory effect caused investigators to treat cats with small doses of SPA. In such a study of kittens with experimental FeLV infection, treatment (20 μg/2.75 kg intraperitoneally twice weekly for eight weeks) neither reversed viremia nor improved humoral immune function.[36] Again, the lack of placebo-treated controls in any of these reports makes it difficult to determine the true effect of SPA therapy.

Interferon alfa is only one of many interferons that have shown promise as direct antiviral agents (at high doses) and as immune modulators (at low doses). Interferons have a wide range of effects on immune function, including enhancing T-cell, macrophage, and NK activity and inducing release of other cytokines. There have been anecdotal reports of beneficial responses in cats with FeLV infection treated with low doses (0.5 to 30 U orally every day) of various forms of IFN-α. The most positive responses are reported with human IFN in contrast to bovine or feline products. The mechanism by which oral IFN-α acts is unknown, but the product is not believed to be present in the blood or oral cavity in concentrations high enough to exert a direct antiviral effect. It is possible that IFN-α binds to mucosal receptors, triggering an immunologic cascade with advantageous systemic effects. In a small, unpublished study, IFN-α failed to improve hematologic or lymphocyte subset abnormalities in cats with chronic FeLV infection. In another study designed to test the ability of natural human IFN-α to prevent the development of experimental FeLV-related disease, cats were treated (0.5 or 5 U orally every 24 hours for seven days on alternate weeks for one month) beginning at the time of virus challenge.[37] Although 12 of 13 cats became infected, cats treated with the lower dose survived longer (mean 500 days) than cats treated with the higher dose (mean 313 days) or with placebo (72 days). Possible explanations for the unusually short survival time of the placebo-treated cats were not discussed.[37] In a review of more than 100 FeLV-infected cats treated with various protocols for low-dose IFN in combination with antibiotics, blood transfusions, fluids, and other supportive care, it was recommended to treat cats with 15 to 30 U orally every day for seven days on alternate weeks (recombinant human IFN-α; Roferon, Hoffman LaRoche).[38] If natural human (Cantell) IFN-α was used, decreasing the dose to 0.5 U was recommended. Roferon is supplied in 3-million-U vials. The protocol for diluting the drug for oral use is to mix 3 million U in 1 L sterile saline; freeze in 1- or 10-mL aliquots; as needed, thaw aliquots and mix into the working solution by further diluting into 100 mL (1-mL aliquot) or 1000 mL (10-mL aliquot). The final working concentration of 30 U/mL is considered an appropriate cat dose. This working solution may be stored in the refrigerator for several months. Recombinant human IFN-α (rh-IFN-α) is also available from Schering Plough (Intron A).

PIND-ORF (Baypamun, Bayer) is derived from inactivated *Parapoxvirus ovis* and is proposed to induce nonspecific or "para" immunity. This preparation caused a sensation when veterinary practitioners in Germany reported that they were able to cure 80 to 100 per cent of FeLV-infected cats, even those in moribund condition.[39–41] Following their reports of eliminating viral infection and disease in hundreds of FeLV-infected cats, Baypamun (1 mL subcutaneously one to three times a week for 4 to 30 weeks) quickly became the most commonly used treatment for FeLV infection in Europe. In the only double-blind, placebo-controlled clinical trials of an immune modulator reported to date, 150 cats with natural FeLV infection were randomized to receive Baypamun (1 mL subcutaneously twice the first week, then once a week for six weeks) or placebo.[42, 43] Neither the owners nor the investigators were aware of the treatment group. There were no significant differences in clinical score, hematology score, lymphocyte subsets, FeLV p27 concentration, pterin concentration, reversion to negative status, or survival between the groups. In fact, although the difference was not statistically significant, 33 per cent of the treated cats survived, compared with 60 per cent of the placebo group. Overall, between 7 and 12 per cent of the cats in both groups became negative for FeLV p27 antigen. This study demonstrates the marked differences that can be observed in uncontrolled or retrospective case studies compared with randomized, controlled clinical trials. The ability of clinicians to select the most effective treatments for their retrovirus-infected patients is severely hampered by the lack of controlled trials reported in the veterinary literature.

SPECIFIC ANTIVIRAL AGENTS

In contrast to immune modulators, which are designed to combat viral infection by enhancing immune function, antiviral agents directly inhibit virus infection and replication. Experimental work with antiviral therapeutics is generally conducted in three stages. Antiviral drugs are usually first tested for their ability to suppress viral infection in vitro. Drugs that prove promising in tissue culture are often next tested for their ability to prevent infection in a viral challenge study. This is because it is easier to prevent retroviral infection than to cure it once it is established. Although prevention is not a clinically relevant application of antiviral therapy, this stage of experimentation further narrows the field of candidate drugs. Finally, cats with well-characterized chronic retroviral infections are treated with promising drugs, and various outcomes such as survival, clinical disease, viral burden, and immune function are measured and compared with a control group. Unfortunately, few therapies have received such rigorous investigation.

AZT/zidovudine (Retrovir, Glaxo-Wellcome) is the most widely used antiviral agent for both human and feline retroviral infection. It is a nucleoside analog inhibitor of the viral enzyme reverse transcriptase, preventing conversion of viral RNA into DNA, which would then enter the host genome. AZT is so effective that it is often used as the gold standard against which new candidate drugs are compared. The drug has been shown to prevent persistent FeLV infection if treatment is begun around the time of viral inoculation.[44, 45] In one study, AZT alone prevented FeLV antigenemia, but not latent infection, when started at the time of FeLV challenge. Adding rh-IFN-α (1.6 million U/kg subcutaneously every day for 7 days, then 1.6×10^5 U/kg subcutaneously every day for 35 days) to AZT (10 to 20 mg/kg orally three times a day for 49 days) prevented the development of latent infection as well. The PCV should be monitored periodically in AZT-treated cats, as anemia is a common side effect. If the PCV drops below 20 per cent, treatment may be stopped for a few days and then reinstituted when the PCV is normal again.

Only one controlled clinical trial has been reported in which cats with natural FeLV infections were treated with antiviral drugs.[46] In this study, 32 FeLV-infected cats, all with chronic oral inflammation (stomatitis), were treated with AZT (5 mg/kg subcutaneously twice a day), PMEA (2.5 mg/kg subcutaneously twice a day), or placebo for three weeks in a double-blind design. No other treatments were permitted. AZT- or PMEA-treated cats had improved stomatitis scores and decreased FeLV p27 antigenemia compared with placebo-treated cats. Both treatment groups experienced a mild decrease in mean hematocrit, and some cats in the PMEA group had to discontinue treatment owing to severe anemia. The authors concluded that PMEA at the dose used was too toxic for clinical use in cats. The importance of this study is the clear advantage of AZT treatment for clinical and immunologic recovery compared with placebo. The dose of 5 mg/kg twice a day, which is lower than previously recommended, offers the advantages of reduced hematologic toxicity and lower cost.

Interferon alfa (Intron A, Schering Plough; Roferon, Hoffman LaRoche) has potent antiviral activity, preventing final virion assembly and budding. When administered to cats with chronic (> 12 weeks) experimental FeLV infection, rh-IFN-α (10,000 to 1 million U/kg subcutaneously every day) effectively reduced FeLV p27 antigenemia. The effect was most rapid and complete in the high-dose treatment group. However, neutralizing antibodies developed against the human protein and appeared earliest in the high-dose group. Thus, the authors concluded that the intermediate dose of 100,000 U/kg provided the most beneficial balance of efficacy and duration of action, which lasted approximately 50 days. Interestingly, the addition of AZT to the rh-IFN-α treatment did not enhance the antiviral effect in this study of chronically infected cats, as it did in the study of FeLV prophylaxis.[47] Even a transient suppression of virus load may benefit FeLV-infected cats, because the immune system may achieve some level of reconstitution during this time of suppressed viral activity. A recombinant feline IFN product (1000 to 1 million U/kg) available in Japan failed to prevent infection during FeLV challenge. Furthermore, continued treatment of the chronically infected cats failed to reduce FeLV p27 antigenemia or to prevent lymphoma formation.

OTHER ANTIVIRAL THERAPIES

The nucleoside analog DDC is effective for preventing infection of lymphoid cells in vitro, although bone marrow cells appear to be more difficult to protect. In cats, however, tolerable doses were ineffective in preventing infection with

FeLV.[48] Other antiviral therapies, including passive transfer of specific antibodies and activated leukocytes, IL-2, vaccination of infected cats, and bone marrow transplantation, have been attempted in FeLV-infected cats, but none of these therapies was predictably effective.

REFERENCES

1. Jarrett WFH, et al: Leukemia in the cat. A virus-like particle associated with leukemia (lymphosarcoma). Nature 202:567, 1964.
2. Hardy WD, et al: Detection of the feline leukemia virus and other mammalian oncornaviruses by immunofluorescence. *In* Dutcher RM, Chieco-Bianchi L (eds): Unifying Concepts of Leukemia. Basel, Karger, 1973, p 778.
3. Pedersen NC: Feline leukemia virus infection. *In* Feline Infectious Diseases. Santa Barbara, American Veterinary Publications, 1988, p 83.
4. Conner TP, et al: Report of the National FeLV/FIV Awareness Project. JAVMA 199:1348, 1991.
5. Cotter SM: Changing epidemiology of FeLV. Proceedings of the 15th Annual ACVIM Forum, Lake Buena Vista, FL, 1997, p 518.
6. Hoover EA, et al: Feline leukemia virus infection: Age-related variation in response of cats to experimental infection. J Natl Cancer Inst 57:365, 1976.
7. Veterinary Medical Data Base, College of Veterinary Medicine, Purdue University.
8. Romatowski J, Lubkin SR: Use of an epidemiologic model to evaluate feline leukemia virus control measures. Feline Pract 25:4, 1997.
9. Hardy WD, Zuckerman EE: Ten-year study comparing enzyme-linked immunosorbent assay with the immunofluorescent antibody test for detection of feline leukemia virus in cats. JAVMA 199:1365, 1991.
10. Hawkins EC: Saliva and tear tests for feline leukemia virus. JAVMA 199:1382, 1991.
11. Hardy WD: The feline leukemia virus. J Am Anim Hosp Assoc 17:951, 1981.
12. Romatowski J: Interpreting feline leukemia test results. JAVMA 195:928, 1989.
13. Miyazawa T, Jarrett O: Feline leukaemia virus proviral DNA detected by polymerase chain reaction in antigenaemic but non-viraemic ('discordant') cats. Arch Virol 142:323, 1997.
14. Rogerson P, et al: Epidemiologic studies on feline leukaemia virus infection: I. A serological survey in urban cats. Int J Cancer 15:781, 1975.
15. American Association of Feline Practitioners: Recommendations for Feline Leukemia Virus Testing, 1995.
16. Rojko JL, Kociba GJ: Pathogenesis of infection by the feline leukemia virus. JAVMA 199:1305, 1991.
17. Rojko JL, et al: Reactivation of latent feline leukemia virus infection. Nature 298:385, 1982.
18. Athas GB, et al: Genetic determinants of feline leukemia virus–induced multicentric lymphomas. Virology 214:431, 1995.
19. Reinacher M: Diseases associated with spontaneous feline leukemia virus (FeLV) infection in cats. Vet Immunol Immunopathol 21:85, 1989.
20. Ogilvie GK, et al: Clinical and immunologic aspects of FeLV-induced immunosuppression. Vet Microbiol 17:287, 1988.
21. Pardi D, et al: Selective impairment of humoral immunity in feline leukemia virus–induced immunodeficiency. Vet Immunol Immunopathol 28:183, 1991.
22. Diehl LJ, Hoover EA: Early and progressive helper T-cell dysfunction in feline leukemia virus–induced immunodeficiency. J Acquir Immune Defic Syndr 5:1188, 1992.
23. Quackenbush SL, et al: Lymphocyte subset alterations and viral determinants of immunodeficiency disease induction by the feline leukemia virus FeLV-FAIDS. J Virol 64:5465, 1990.
24. Weijer K, et al: Control of feline leukemia virus infection by a removal programme. Vet Rec 119:555, 1986.
25. Francis DP, et al: Feline leukemia virus: Survival under home and laboratory conditions. J Clin Microbiol 9:154, 1979.
26. Loar AS: Feline leukemia virus: Immunization and prevention. Vet Clin North Am 23:193, 1993.
27. Sparkes AH: Feline leukaemia virus: A review of immunity and vaccination. J Small Anim Pract 38:187, 1997.
28. Kass PH, et al: Epidemiologic evidence for a causal relation between vaccination and fibrosarcoma tumorigenesis in cats. JAVMA 203:396, 1993.
29. American Association of Feline Practitioners: Feline Vaccination Guidelines, 1997.
30. Ogilvie GK: Hematopoietic growth factors: Frontiers for cure. Vet Clin North Am 25:1441, 1995.
31. Tizard I: Use of immunomodulators as an aid to clinical management of feline leukemia virus–infected cats. JAVMA 199:1482, 1991.
32. Sheets MA, et al: Studies of the effect of acemannan on retrovirus infections: Clinical stabilization of feline leukemia virus–infected cats. Mol Biother 3:41, 1991.
33. Round-table discussion: Immune modulation can be an alternative for practice problems. Vet Forum 9:43, 1993.
34. Lies M: Volume of opinion warrants merit. Vet Forum 6:42, 1990.
35. Weiss RC: Immunotherapy for feline leukemia, using staphylococcal protein A or heterologous interferons: Immunopharmacologic actions and potential use. JAVMA 192:681, 1988.
36. Lafrado LJ, et al: Biological effects of staphylococcal protein A immunotherapy in cats with induced feline leukemia virus infection. Am J Vet Res 51:482, 1990.
37. Cummins KM, et al: Oral use of human alpha interferon in cats. J Biol Response Mod 7:513, 1988.
38. Weiss RC, et al: Low-dose orally administered alpha interferon treatment for feline leukemia virus infection. JAVMA 199:1477, 1991.
39. Hörber D, et al: [Beneficial effects of para-immunization of leukaemia-positive cats with "Baypamun HK."] Tierarztl Umschau 47:556, 1992.
40. Hörber D, Mayr B: [Paramunization of FeLV-positive cats with PIND-AVI.] Tierarztl Prax 19:311, 1991.
41. Guller K, Bigler B: [The treatment of FeLV-positive cats with Baypamun.] Kleintierpraxis 40:379, 1995.
42. Block A: [Double-blind placebo-controlled study of the efficacy of an inducer of para-immunity in cats naturally infected with feline leukemia virus.] Tierarztliche Fakultat, 1996 (thesis).
43. Hartmann K, et al: Treatment of feline leukemia virus–infected cats with paramunity inducer. In press.
44. Mathes LE, et al: Pre- and postexposure chemoprophylaxis: Evidence that 3'-azido-3'-dideoxythymidine inhibits feline leukemia virus disease by a drug-induced vaccine response. Antimicrob Agents Chemother 36:2715, 1992.
45. Mathes LE, et al: Evidence that high-dose zidovudine at time of retrovirus exposure reduces antiviral efficacy. Antimicrob Agents Chemother 40:2183, 1996.
46. Hartmann K, et al: Use of two virustatica (AZT, PMEA) in the treatment of FIV and of FeLV seropositive cats with clinical symptoms. Vet Immunol Immunopathol 35:167, 1992.
47. Zeidner NS, et al: Alpha interferon (2b) in combination with zidovudine for the treatment of presymptomatic feline leukemia virus–induced immunodeficiency syndrome. Antimicrob Agents Chemother 34:1749, 1990.
48. Polas PJ, et al: In vitro and in vivo evidence that the antiviral activity of 2',3'-dideoxycytidine is target cell dependent in a feline retrovirus animal model. Antimicrob Agents Chemother 34:1414, 1990.

CHAPTER 90

FIV AND FIV-RELATED DISEASE

Margaret C. Barr and Tom R. Phillips

The retrovirus family, the Retroviridae, is a large group of viruses that share certain physical, biochemical, and genetic characteristics. The Retroviridae are divided into three subfamilies: the Spumavirinae, the Oncornavirinae, and the Lentivirinae. Cats are susceptible to infection with viruses from each of these subfamilies. Feline immunodeficiency virus (FIV) belongs to the lentivirus subfamily of retroviruses.[1] Lentiviruses infect a broad range of mammals and include human (HIV), simian, and bovine immunodeficiency viruses; equine infectious anemia virus; and maedi-visna virus of sheep. The immunodefiency disease resulting from FIV infection in domestic cats is quite similar to human acquired immunodeficiency syndrome (AIDS) and thus provides a useful animal model for HIV infection and AIDS.

The FIV virion has characteristic lentivirus morphology and size. An envelope with short membrane peplomers or spikes surrounds an electron-dense wedge-shaped core, consisting of two identical single strands of RNA surrounded by viral core proteins (Fig. 90–1). Each virion also carries an enzyme called reverse transcriptase. Retroviruses use reverse transcriptase to produce a double-stranded DNA copy of the virion RNA (the flow of information from RNA to DNA is "backwards," hence the name *retro*virus). This DNA copy, called a provirus, integrates into the host cell chromosomal DNA and thus can replicate along with the infected cell. The genomic organization of the FIV provirus is similar to that of other lentiviruses, with long terminal repeat (LTR) regions flanking three large open reading frames (ORFs) and at least four small ORFs. The larger ORFs represent the *gag*, *pol*, and *env* genes that encode the major structural and enzymatic proteins of FIV, and the smaller ORFs encode proteins involved in the regulation of viral replication.[1]

EPIZOOTIOLOGY AND TRANSMISSION OF FIV

FIV infection is found throughout the world in domestic cats and has been well established in some populations for more than 25 years. The prevalence of FIV infection in the United States is estimated to be 1.5 to 3 per cent in healthy cats and 7 to 15 per cent in cats with signs of clinical illness or at high risk for exposure.[2] In contrast, about 29 per cent of Japanese cats are infected with FIV, with 44 per cent of ill cats testing positive.[3] The high prevalence of FIV infection in these cats may result from the relatively high density of free-roaming cats in Japan.

Male cats are almost three times as likely to be infected with FIV as female cats. Free-roaming cats have a greater risk of infection than cats housed strictly indoors, while very few pure breed cats housed in catteries are infected with FIV. The prevalence of FIV infection increases with age, with a mean age of about 5 years at the time of diagnosis.[2, 3] The higher prevalence of infection in male cats can be attributed to their greater territorial aggression and disproportionate number of bite wounds. Likewise, free-roaming cats have a much greater chance of aggressive contact with other cats than do indoor cats, and older cats have had more opportunity for such contact to occur.

FIV is efficiently transmitted through bite wounds because virus is shed in the saliva of infected cats. Initial attempts to demonstrate transmission of FIV through casual or sexual contact among cats were unsuccessful; however, viral RNA and proviral DNA have been detected in samples from some FIV-seronegative cats housed in contact with FIV-infected cats.[4] In addition, FIV has been transmitted to female cats by artificial insemination using semen from FIV-infected male cats.[5] The significance of these findings is unknown, and additional study will be required to determine the actual risk of FIV transmission through casual or sexual contact.

Placental or colostral transmission for FIV from a queen to her offspring is probably infrequent. Experimental in utero and postnatal transmissions are most efficient when the queen's initial exposure to FIV occurs during gestation or lactation.[6] Thus, fetuses or kittens exposed to FIV prior to antibody development in the queen appear to be at highest risk of infection. This suggests that strong humoral and cellular immune responses and/or low levels of viremia present in many queens with established FIV infections may prevent perinatal infections of kittens. However, some strains of FIV have a much higher propensity for maternal transmission. Queens infected with these strains have high viral loads

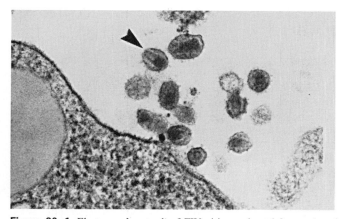

Figure 90–1. Electron micrograph of FIV virions released from cultured lymphocytes demonstrating typical lentivirus morphology (arrowhead). Note the cone-shaped electron-dense core of mature particles. Magnification × 68,000. (Courtesy of Edward Dougherty.)

and low numbers of CD4$^+$ T lymphocytes, which may account for differences in transmission.[7]

IMMUNITY AND PATHOGENESIS

IMMUNE RESPONSE TO FIV

When cats are experimentally infected with FIV, neutralizing antibodies appear 3 to 4 weeks after infection; however, virus can be isolated from infected cats in spite of high neutralizing antibody titers. Antibodies to the envelope glycoprotein and the major core proteins develop first, with antibodies to the transmembrane protein and the *pol* gene products generally appearing 4 to 8 weeks after infection. Antibody levels peak after several weeks and remain high for months to years following infection. Although most cats develop high antibody levels within a few weeks after FIV infection, some cats have delayed or weak responses and some lose antibodies during the terminal stages of disease.[2, 4]

Cellular immune responses also develop early in infection. Virus-specific cytotoxic T cells probably play an important role in controlling FIV replication and decreasing viremia, especially during asymptomatic infection.[8] CD8$^+$ T cells from some chronically infected cats exhibit antiviral activity in FIV-infected lymphocyte cultures. This CD8$^+$-associated suppression may result from a direct cytotoxic effect on infected cells, the influence of soluble factors (cytokines) released from certain CD8$^+$ cell subtypes, or a combination of these activities.[9]

IMMUNOPATHOGENESIS OF FIV INFECTION

The underlying immunopathology of FIV infection is similar to that seen in HIV-infected humans.[10] Unlike HIV infection of human lymphocytes, which is restricted to CD4$^+$ lineages, FIV lytically infects both feline CD4$^+$ (helper) and feline CD8$^+$ (cytotoxic) T lymphocytes. In spite of this ability to infect both CD4$^+$ and CD8$^+$ subsets of T cells in vitro, FIV selectively and progressively decreases feline CD4$^+$ cells in vivo. In cats with short-term experimental infections, the CD4$^+$:CD8$^+$ ratio is decreased slightly as a result of an increase in CD8$^+$ cells. The inversion of the CD4$^+$:CD8$^+$ ratio becomes significant in cats infected for longer than 18 months. Cats with experimental FIV infections of more than 25 months have an absolute decrease of CD4$^+$ T lymphocytes, with little or no change in absolute numbers of CD8$^+$ cells.[2, 4, 10]

Proliferative responses of peripheral blood mononuclear cells (PBMCs, which include lymphocytes) from experimentally and naturally FIV-infected cats are decreased compared with the responses of PBMCs from uninfected control cats. After long-term FIV infection, cats may have a decreased ability to respond to T-dependent antigens, but immunologic responses to T-independent antigens are not impaired.[4, 10] Naive T cells exhibit reduced proliferation in response to foreign antigens as early as 5 weeks after infection, whereas memory T-cell responses are impaired later in infection.[11] Cytokine production by infected cells is also abnormal, with elevated levels of tumor necrosis factor–alpha (TNF-α), interleukin-1 (IL-1), and IL-6 corresponding to decreased proliferative responses of PBMCs.[10]

In addition to lymphocyte infection and perturbation of their function, FIV also infects macrophages, megakaryocytes, and mononuclear bone marrow cells.[12, 13] Macrophages are thought to be a major reservoir of HIV in infected humans, and they probably play a similar role in FIV-infected cats. In laboratory cultures, macrophages in an early stage of activation support transient productive FIV replication, while more highly differentiated macrophages do not release virus.[12]

NEUROPATHOGENESIS OF FIV INFECTION

FIV has been isolated from cerebrospinal fluid, cerebral cortex, caudate nucleus, midbrain, cerebellum, and rostral and caudal brain stem.[14] The virus infects the brain early, with virus-induced central nervous system (CNS) lesions sometimes developing within 2 months of infection.[15] Cats infected with FIV demonstrate a variety of CNS disturbances, including delayed pupillary response, anisocoria, delayed auditory and visual evoked potentials, delayed righting reflex, increased sensory and spinal conduction velocities, and disturbed sleep patterns.[14, 16–18] Pathologic findings include the presence of perivascular infiltrates of mononuclear cells, diffuse gliosis, glial nodules, and white matter pallor.[14, 15] These lesions are usually located in the caudate nucleus, midbrain, and rostral brain stem.

Brain cells infected by FIV include microglia and astrocytes. The virus does not infect neurons; however, neuronal death has been associated with FIV infections.[19, 20] The mechanism of neuronal damage is unclear. It may result from the effects of FIV on the neuron supportive functions of astrocytes, toxic products released from infected microglia, or cytokines produced in response to the viral infection. Astrocytes are by far the most common cell type of the brain and are important in maintaining CNS neuronal microenvironment. One of the most important functions of astrocytes is to regulate the level of extracellular glutamate, a major excitatory neurotransmitter that accumulates as a consequence of neuronal activity. Excessive extracellular glutamate often results in neuronal toxicity and death. Infection of astrocytes with FIV can significantly inhibit the glutamate-scavenging ability of feline astrocytes, potentially resulting in neuronal damage.[20] Also, HIV-1–infected microglia cultures produce the neurotoxic compounds TNF-α, IL-1, quinolinate, eicosanoids, and Ntox. It is probable that microglia infected with FIV produce similar neurotoxins, although the relevance of these products in FIV-induced CNS pathogenesis is unknown.

CLINICAL PRESENTATION OF FIV-RELATED DISEASES

Suppression of immune function by FIV infection in domestic cats results in a plethora of clinical signs.[3, 4] Diseases associated with FIV infection cannot be distinguished clinically from feline leukemia virus (FeLV)–associated immunodeficiencies (see Table 90–1 and Chapter 89). FIV infection in domestic cats resembles HIV infection in humans, with stages similar to the acute (first), asymptomatic carrier (AC, second), persistent generalized lymphadenopathy (PGL, third), AIDS-related complex (ARC, fourth), and AIDS (fifth) stages of HIV infection.[4, 21]

The acute phase begins about 4 weeks after FIV infection and persists as long as 4 months. Some cats have lymphadenopathy, neutropenia, fever, and diarrhea. Others have no clinical signs during acute infection. The AC stage, during which clinical evidence of disease is absent, may last several

TABLE 90–1. DISEASES ASSOCIATED WITH FIV AND FeLV INFECTIONS

Immunosuppression with opportunistic infections
Gingivitis/stomatitis (FIV > FeLV)
Myeloproliferative disease/erythroleukemia (FeLV >> FIV)
Lymphosarcoma/lymphoid leukemias (FeLV >> FIV)
Diarrhea/panleukopenia-like syndrome
Weight loss/cachexia
Chronic fever
Glomerulonephritis
Anterior uveitis/pars planitis/glaucoma (FIV >> FeLV)
Behavioral changes/dementia/peripheral neuropathies
Hypergammaglobulinemia (FIV > FeLV)
Hemolytic anemias/aplastic anemias (FeLV >> FIV)
Lymphopenia/neutropenia
Thrombocytopenia (FeLV >> FIV)
Abortion/fetal resorptions/thymic atrophy (FeLV >> FIV)
Chronic progressive polyarthritis

months to years. A short period (2 to 4 months or less) of PGL follows the AC stage. The ARC and AIDS stages of disease are not clearly defined for FIV infection, but cats with ARC often have chronic respiratory, gastrointestinal, and skin disorders, accompanied by lymphadenopathy. The development of opportunistic infections, severe emaciation, and lymphoid depletion signals a progression to AIDS.[4, 21]

Many FIV-positive cats have histories of recurrent illnesses with periods of relative health between episodes. In one study of naturally FIV-infected cats, the rate of progression was variable, with death occurring in about 18 per cent of infected cats within the first 2 years of observation (4.5 to 6 years after the estimated time of infection). An additional 18 per cent of infected cats developed increasingly severe disease, but more than 50 per cent of the infected cats remained clinically asymptomatic during the same time period.[21] The average life expectancy of cats once they enter the ARC or AIDS stage of disease is less than 1 year.[4]

The lymphadenopathy observed during FIV infection is associated with follicular hyperplasia and massive paracortical infiltration with plasmacytes. In some lymph nodes, a mixture of follicular hyperplasia and follicular depletion or involution may be observed (Fig. 90–2). In the terminal stage of disease, lymphoid depletion is the predominant finding.[4]

Among the most common clinical findings in FIV-infected cats are gingivitis, stomatitis, and periodontitis. The oral lesions in 25 to 50 per cent of positive cats may be ulcerative

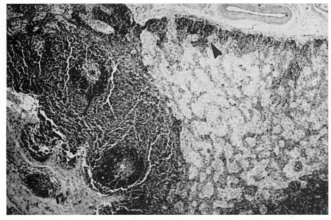

Figure 90–2. Micrograph of the corticomedullary junction of a mesenteric lymph node of an FIV-infected cat. An area of follicular hyperplasia (*) is juxtaposed with an area of lymphoid depletion (arrowhead).

and/or proliferative.[2] Both ulcerative and proliferative lesions consist of lymphocytic and plasmacytic infiltrates that may extend to the draining lymph nodes and spleen of affected cats.[4]

Chronic, nonresponsive, or recurrent infections of the external ear and skin are commonly seen. Skin lesions and abscesses are often caused by *Staphylococcus* or other bacterial infections. Abscesses from cat bites and other trauma may heal slowly in spite of aggressive treatment. Cases of generalized notoedric and demodectic mange, parasitic diseases that are uncommon in otherwise healthy cats, have been reported in FIV-positive cats.[3] The dermatophytosis may be particularly aggressive and difficult to treat. Severe neutropenias have been induced in several FIV-infected cats treated for dermatophytosis with griseofulvin.[22] The neutropenia is reversible if the drug is withdrawn early enough, but secondary infections associated with the condition can be life-threatening.

Chronic upper respiratory tract disease occurs in about 30 per cent of FIV-positive cats, and persistent diarrhea occurs in 10 to 20 per cent of infected cats.[3] Feline herpesvirus and calicivirus infections may be partially responsible for upper respiratory disease including rhinitis, conjunctivitis, and keratitis. Intestinal lesions similar to those seen with feline parvovirus infection have been observed in several cats with diarrhea. The etiology of the enteritis may be bacterial, fungal, or parasitic; however, some of the pathology may be FIV induced.[4]

Clinically ill cats are more likely than asymptomatic FIV-infected cats to have hematologic abnormalities, especially cytopenias.[22] Anemia, lymphopenia, neutropenia, and hypergammaglobulinemia are the most frequent abnormalities, while thrombocytopenia is found in less than 10 per cent of FIV-infected cats. Neutrophilia and lymphocytosis have been observed in some cats with secondary infections or neoplasia.[3, 2] Cats infected with FIV may be more susceptible to *Haemobartonella felis*–induced anemia and related disease. Bone marrow abnormalities in some FIV-infected cats include increased cellularity as a result of lymphocytes, plasma cells, or eosinophils; myeloproliferative disease; dysmorphic syndromes; and neoplasia.[22]

Ophthalmic diseases associated with FIV infection include anterior uveitis, pars planitis, and glaucoma.[23] The anterior uveitis is characterized by aqueous flare, iridial hyperemia, hypotony of the ocular globe, miosis or anisocoria, posterior synechia, and anterior subcapsular cataracts. Pars planitis is recognized as punctate white infiltrates in the anterior vitreous ("snow"). In most cats, pars planitis is clinically inapparent although extreme cases may result in lens luxation or retinal detachment. Glaucoma usually develops secondary to intraocular inflammation or neoplasia. Findings on examination include increased intraocular pressure (>25 mmHg), optic disk cupping, buphthalmia, lens luxation, and loss of vision.[23] The underlying cause of ocular disease in FIV infection is unclear. Potential causes include one or more of the following mechanisms: (1) direct damage to the uveal or vascular epithelium by the virus, (2) immune-mediated or autoimmune disease, or (3) opportunistic infections, such as cytomegalovirus and *Toxoplasma gondii* infections.[23] FIV-positive cats are frequently coinfected with *Toxoplasma*, and reactivation of latent toxoplasmosis is suspected to occur in these cats when they become immunosuppressed.[24]

Although FIV is primarily known for causing immunodeficiency disease, it is important to recognize that FIV infection can also affect the CNS. Because CNS signs may or may not be accompanied by other clinical abnormalities,

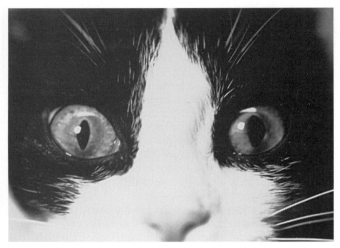

Figure 90–3. Anisocoria in an FIV-infected cat. The response to light is delayed and incomplete in one eye, resulting in pupil inequality. This condition has been seen in experimental infections with certain strains of FIV.

FIV should be included in the differential diagnosis for any cat presented with unexplained alterations of CNS function. Infected cats may demonstrate behavioral alterations such as becoming more aggressive or fearful, or exhibiting compulsive behavior patterns. Posterior paresis may be observed as ataxia or the inability to successfully negotiate small jumps.[17] Anisocoria is also associated with FIV infection (Fig. 90–3).[14] These problems have been seen within the first year of FIV infection. However, these early CNS signs are frequently transient in nature and may resolve after a few weeks or months. This reversal of clinical signs may reflect the adaptive ability of the feline brain or resolution of transient lesions.

Lentiviruses are not considered to be directly oncogenic. Because older cats are most likely to both be infected with FIV and develop nonretrovirus-related tumors, it is difficult to determine just what role FIV has in the neoplastic process. Lymphomas associated with FIV infection frequently are extranodal in origin (Fig. 90–4) and may be of B, T, or non-T, non-B cell lineage.[25] Statistically, FIV-infected cats are five times more likely to develop leukemia/lymphoma than uninfected cats. This relative risk increases to 62 times normal for FeLV-infected cats and to 77 times normal for cats with dual FeLV/FIV infections. In addition to leukemia/lymphoma, neoplastic diseases that have been reported in FIV-positive cats include fibrosarcoma, mastocytoma, squamous cell carcinoma, and myeloproliferative disease.[4]

Coinfection of cats with FIV and FeLV occurs under natural conditions. Preexisting FeLV infection acts as a potentiator for FIV-related disease in experimentally infected cats.[26] Specific pathogen–free cats generally exhibit only

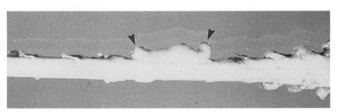

Figure 90–4. Extradural lymphosarcoma in an FIV-infected cat. The lesion was located at the level of thoracic vertebra 3 and was responsible for progressive hindlimb paresis in the cat (arrowheads).

mild, transient signs (low-grade fever, neutropenia, lymphadenopathy) after experimental inoculation with FIV. In contrast, when cats persistently (but asymptomatically) infected with FeLV are infected with FIV, many develop severe disease characterized by leukopenia, anorexia and weight loss, diarrhea, fever, dehydration, depression, and neurologic disease. Cats with naturally acquired dual infections have severe disease and thus have a poorer prognosis than cats infected with either virus alone.[3, 27]

PREVENTION AND DIAGNOSIS OF FIV INFECTION

CONTROL OF FIV TRANSMISSION AND INFECTION

Prevention of exposure to FIV-infected cats is the only available method to control the spread of the virus. Because casual contact between cats and contact with fomites are inefficient methods of transmission, preventing exposure to FIV is relatively straightforward. Cats should not be allowed to roam free or to interact with feral or free-roaming cats. All new cats should be screened for FIV infection prior to entering an FIV-negative multiple-cat household or cattery. If possible, a 6- to 8-week quarantine period should be enforced to allow time for recently infected cats to develop detectable levels of antibody.

Commercial vaccines for protection against FIV infection or disease are not available. Experimental inactivated virus or fixed infected cell vaccines provide protection against challenge with homologous strains of FIV but are not always effective against heterologous strains. Recombinant and peptide-based FIV vaccines have been less successful in early trials.[28–30]

DIAGNOSTIC TESTS FOR FIV

Infections with FIV and FeLV can be differentiated only by appropriate laboratory tests. In most circumstances, concurrent testing for both viruses is indicated. Cats with signs of immunosuppression or entering multiple-cat facilities should be tested for both FIV and FeLV.

The diagnosis of FIV infection usually depends on the detection of FIV-specific antibodies in serum, plasma, or whole blood. Commercial ELISA tests are available for use in veterinary clinics and diagnostic laboratories; some laboratories also offer IFA or immunoblot (Western blot) assays for FIV antibodies.[31] In general, FIV ELISAs have similar sensitivities to the IFA and immunoblot procedures; however, false-positives (decreased specificities) with ELISAs may result from operator error (especially inadequate washing) or nonspecific reactivity with cell culture components. Positive ELISA tests for FIV antibody should be confirmed by IFA or immunoblot, especially when the cat is asymptomatic or at low risk for infection, or when euthanasia of an FIV-positive cat is considered. It is also important to recognize that the presence of maternally derived FIV antibody in kittens less than 4 to 5 months of age causes positive test results with any of the antibody assays, whether or not the kitten is infected with FIV.[31]

Causes of false-negative FIV tests include insufficient levels of antibody in the sample tested (early infection or poor immune response), inadequate sensitivity of the assay, and operator error (incorrect sample preparation or interpretation of results). False-negative tests in some ELISA formats appear to result from a prozonal effect in samples with high levels of antibodies.[31] Indeterminant or equivocal FIV test results are obtained when antibody levels are near the limit of detection in an assay. High levels of background (nonspecific) reactivity also may result in indeterminant tests. Cats with indeterminant tests or discordant results should be retested in 6 to 8 weeks; most cats will have a clearly positive or negative result on retesting. In addition, FIV antibody–positive kittens should be retested at 8 to 12 months of age to allow time for maternal antibodies to disappear and active seroconversion to occur.[31]

Circulating blood levels of free virus, viral antigen, and cell-associated virus are too low to be detected consistently in most FIV-infected cats.[4] Virus isolation and detection of FIV DNA or RNA by polymerase chain reaction (PCR) may be useful in diagnosis of FIV infection in cats with negative or indeterminant antibody tests. Virus isolation and PCR are not available as commercial assays but are performed in some research facilities.

TREATMENT OF FIV INFECTION AND ASSOCIATED DISEASES

ANTIVIRAL THERAPEUTIC AGENTS

Safe and consistently effective antiviral agents are not available for use in FIV-infected cats. Two primary approaches to antiretroviral therapy have been used in cats: (1) reverse transcriptase inhibitors have been administered to suppress viral replication, and (2) immunomodulatory drugs have been given to potentiate the cat's immune response against the retrovirus. The reverse transcriptase inhibitor 3'-azido-2',3'-dideoxythymidine (AZT) acts by blocking the incorporation of nucleosides into the DNA copy of the virus during the initial phase of replication. General clinical improvement of FIV-associated stomatitis, gingivitis, and diarrhea has been observed following AZT treatment.[4] If AZT or other reverse transcriptase inhibitors are used, treated cats should be monitered closely for the development of anemia, cytopenias, and hepatotoxicities. Dosages should be adjusted as needed.

Immunomodulatory drugs may be useful in alleviating clinical signs associated with retroviral infections. Low-dose, orally administered human recombinant alpha interferon (HuIFN-α) has been successful in increasing survival rates and improving clinical status of retrovirus-infected cats. Oral HuIFN-α treatment is thought to act by stimulating the release of soluble cytokines, such as IL-1, from oropharyngeal macrophages and lymphocytes; these cytokines then circulate systemically and modulate immune function. Additional immunomodulatory drugs that have shown some promise in the treatment of feline retroviral diseases include *Propionibacterium acnes*, acemannan, and staphylococcal protein A (SPA). All of these drugs induce the release of endogenous interferons and IL-1.[2, 4]

Perhaps the best strategy for antiretroviral therapy is combining two or more of the drugs mentioned above. Until more extensive field trials of these agents have been performed, no single treatment can be recommended. Table 90–2 outlines treatment regimens for AZT and some of the immunomodulatory drugs.

TREATMENT OF FIV-RELATED DISEASES

Management of secondary and opportunistic infections is a primary consideration in the treatment of cats immunosuppressed by FIV. Accurate diagnosis of a secondary infection is required before adequate chemotherapy can be instituted. Toxoplasmosis, haemobartonellosis, and cryptococcosis are frequently associated with feline retroviral infections; suggested chemotherapies are outlined in Table 90–2. Additional supportive therapy, such as parenteral fluids and nutritional supplements, may be required. Management of weight loss and cachexia associated with FIV infection is also critical. Inactivated vaccines should be used for protection against respiratory and enteric viruses. The ability of some FIV-infected cats to respond appropriately to vaccination is questionable; the immune response of immunocompromised cats to vaccines, especially rabies virus vaccines, requires additional evaluation.[4]

Retrovirus-related gingivitis tends to be refractory to treatment. Antibacterial or antimycotic drugs are effective if the primary lesions are caused by overgrowth of bacteria or fungi, but prolonged therapy or increased dosages may be required. Metronidazole or clindamycin is useful for treating anaerobic bacterial infections. Judicious but aggressive use of corticosteroids or gold salts may be helpful in controlling immune-mediated inflammation. These immunosuppressive agents should be restricted or avoided in cats with overt signs of opportunistic bacterial or fungal infections.

Treatment of anterior uveitis consists of application of topical corticosteroids, but long-term response to therapy may be incomplete or poor. Pars planitis will often regress spontaneously and may recur; response to topical and systemic corticosteroid therapy is variable. Standard therapeutic protocols for glaucoma treatment may be used.[23]

Currently, there are no specific therapeutic approaches that target FIV-associated CNS disease. Supportive therapy, immunomodulators, and antiviral agents may be useful. It is important to emphasize that CNS signs often naturally but transiently improve.

TABLE 90–2. DRUG APPENDIX

GENERIC	TRADE	DOSAGE	ROUTE	FREQUENCY	DESCRIPTION
AZT (3'-azido-2',3'-dideoxythimidine)	Retrovir	5 mg/kg	SQ	q12h for 3 weeks	Antiretroviral drug (monitor for anemia)
Interferon-alpha (recombinant human IFN)	Roferon	30 IU/cat	PO	Daily—7 days on; 7 days off	Immune function modulator
Propionibacterium acnes	Immunoregulin	0.5 mL/cat	IV	Once or twice weekly	Immune function modulator
Acemannan	Carrisyn	100 mg/cat or 2 mg/kg	PO or SQ, IV	Daily or weekly	Immune function modulator
Metronidazole	Flagyl	7 to 15 mg/kg	PO	q8h to q12h	Antimicrobial—anaerobes
Oxytetracycline	Terramycin	15 mg/kg or 7.5 mg/kg	PO or IM, IV	q8h or q12h	Antimicrobial—*Haemobartonella*
Clindamycin	Antirobe	11 mg/kg	PO	q12h	Antimicrobial—*Toxoplasma*
Itraconazole	Sporanox	5 mg/kg long term	PO	q12h	Antifungal—*Cryptococcus*

Surgical removal of isolated tumors may be useful, but care must be taken to ensure proper healing of incisions. Established chemotherapy protocols can be utilized for treatment of lymphoproliferative diseases. Combined therapy with nonspecific immunopotentiators such as *Staphylococcus* protein A or *Propionibacterium acnes*, or interferons may also be used to control FIV-related tumors.

PUBLIC HEALTH SIGNIFICANCE

FIV infection in domestic cats poses little or no public health hazard. Like other lentiviruses, FIV appears to be species-specific. Initial isolation of FIV requires growth of the virus in primary feline PBMCs, thymic cultures, or spleen cells, although the cell tropism may broaden for some strains of FIV that have been adapted to or selected for growth in a feline kidney cell line. Additionally, FIV antibodies have not been detected in any samples from veterinarians, cat owners, or researchers exposed to FIV by bite wounds, needle punctures, or close contact with FIV-positive cats.[4] However, cats with retrovirus-induced immunosuppression may serve as a reservoir for diseases such as active toxoplasmosis and cryptosporidiosis and thus may present a health risk to individuals with immune dysfunction.

REFERENCES

1. Miyazawa T, et al: The genome of feline immunodeficiency virus. Arch Virol 134:221, 1994.
2. Barr MC, et al: Feline viral diseases. *In* Ettinger SJ, Feldman EC (eds): Textbook of Veterinary Internal Medicine, 4th ed. Philadelphia, WB Saunders, 1994, pp 409–439.
3. Ishida T, et al: Feline immunodeficiency virus infection in cats of Japan. JAVMA 194:221, 1989.
4. Sparger EE: Current thoughts on feline immunodeficiency virus infection. Vet Clin North Am Small Anim Pract 23:173, 1993.
5. Jordan HL, et al: Transmission of feline immunodeficiency virus in domestic cats via artificial insemination. J Virol 70:8224, 1996.
6. Wasmoen T, et al: Transmission of feline immunodeficiency virus from infected queens to kittens. Vet Immunol Immunopathol 35:83, 1992.
7. O'Neil LL, et al: Frequent perinatal transmission of feline immunodeficiency virus by chronically infected cats. J Virol 70:2894, 1996.
8. Beatty JA, et al: A longitudinal study of feline immunodeficiency virus–specific cytotoxic T lymphocytes in experimentally infected cats, using antigen-specific induction. J Virol 70:6199, 1996.
9. Jeng CR, et al: Evidence for CD8+ antiviral activity in cats infected with feline immunodeficiency virus. J Virol 70:2474, 1996.
10. Willett BJ, et al: FIV infection of the domestic cat: An animal model for AIDS. Immunol Today 18:182, 1997.
11. Bishop SA, et al: An early defect in primary and secondary T cell responses in asymptomatic cats during acute feline immunodeficiency virus (FIV) infection. Clin Exp Immunol 90:491, 1992.
12. Brunner D, Pedersen NC: Infection of peritoneal macrophages in vitro and in vivo with feline immunodeficiency virus. J Virol 63:5483, 1989.
13. Beebe AM, et al: Detection of feline immunodeficiency virus infection in bone marrow of cats. Vet Immunol Immunopathol 35:37, 1992.
14. Phillips TR, et al: Neurological abnormalities associated with feline immunodeficiency virus infection. J Gen Virol 979, 1994.
15. Hurtrel M, et al: Comparison of early and late feline immunodeficiency virus encephalopathies. AIDS 6:399, 1992.
16. Henriksen SJ, et al: Feline immunodeficiency virus as a model for study of lentivirus infection of the central nervous system. Curr Top Microbiol Immunol 202:167, 1995.
17. Phillips TR, et al: Neurologic dysfunctions caused by a molecular clone of feline immunodeficiency virus, FIV-PPR. J Neurovirol 2:388, 1996.
18. Podell M, et al: AIDS-associated encephalopathy with experimental feline immunodeficiency virus infection. J Acquir Immune Defic Syndr 6:758, 1993.
19. Meeker RB, et al: Cortical cell loss in asymptomatic cats experimentally infected with feline immunodeficiency virus. AIDS Res Hum Retroviruses 13:1131, 1997.
20. Zenger E, et al: Cellular mechanisms of feline immunodeficiency virus (FIV)–induced neuropathogenesis. Front Biosci 2:D527, 1997.
21. Ishida T, et al: Long-term clinical observations on feline immunodeficiency virus infected asymptomatic carriers. Vet Immunol Immunopathol 35:15, 1992.
22. Shelton GH, et al: Hematologic abnormalities in cats seropositive for feline immunodeficiency virus. JAVMA 199:1353, 1991.
23. English RV, et al: Intraocular disease associated with feline immunodeficiency virus infection in cats. JAVMA 196:1116, 1990.
24. Lappin MR, et al: Effect of primary phase feline immunodeficiency virus infection on cats with chronic toxoplasmosis. Vet Immunol Immunopathol 35:121, 1992.
25. Endo Y, et al: Molecular characteristics of malignant lymphoma in cats naturally infected with feline immunodeficiency virus. Vet Immunol Immunopathol 57:153, 1997.
26. Pedersen NC, et al: Feline leukemia virus infection as a potentiating cofactor for the primary and secondary stages of experimentally induced feline immunodeficiency virus infection. J Virol 64(2):598, 1990.
27. Courchamp F, et al: Dynamics of two feline retroviruses (FIV and FeLV) within one population of cats. Proc R Soc Lond B Biol Sci 264:785, 1997.
28. Hosie MJ and Flynn JN: Feline immunodeficiency virus vaccination: Characterization of the immune correlates of protection. J Virol 70:7561, 1996.
29. Pu R, et al: Mechanism(s) of FIV vaccine protection. Leukemia 11(Suppl 3):98, 1997.
30. Flynn JN, et al: Vaccination with a feline immunodeficiency virus multiepitopic peptide induces cell-mediated and humoral immunity, but does not confer protection. J Virol 71:7586, 1997.
31. Barr MC: FIV, FeLV, and FIPV: Interpretation and misinterpretation of serological test results. Semin Vet Med Surg (Small Anim) 11:144, 1996.

CHAPTER 91

FIP-RELATED DISEASE

Rosalind Gaskell and Susan Dawson

Feline infectious peritonitis (FIP) is a slowly progressive, fatal disease of cats that occurs in two forms. The first is the classic effusive or "wet" form, characterized by the accumulation of fluid in one or both body cavities, particularly the abdomen. The second is the noneffusive or "dry" form, in which there are granulomatous lesions present in a variety of body organs and clinical signs are related to the organ most affected. Although FIP was first described as a clinical entity in the 1960s, many aspects of the disease are still an enigma, and despite some advances, treatment, prevention, and control remain problematic.

ETIOLOGY

The disease is caused by feline coronavirus (FCoV). FCoV is closely related antigenically and in genome organization to some coronaviruses of other species, including transmissible gastroenteritis virus (TGEV) of pigs, the recently emerged porcine respiratory coronavirus, and canine coronavirus (CCV), which causes enteritis in dogs. Cross-species transmission of these viruses has been shown to occur, and they are considered host range mutants of the same virus.[1, 2] Cats may be infected experimentally with CCV,[3] and CCV has induced lesions in cats typical of effusive FIP.[4] There is also evidence that FIP-like lesions were induced in dogs by a modified live CCV vaccine.[5, 6]

There are two recognized biotypes of FCoV: feline infectious peritonitis virus (FIPV) and feline enteric coronavirus (FECV). They are morphologically and antigenically indistinguishable, although their biologic behavior is different. Experimentally, FIPV generally induces FIP, whereas FECV generally induces only a mild enteritis from which cats recover. However, there is overlap between the two, and evidence is accumulating that FIPV is a mutation of FECV. Thus FIPVs and FECVs isolated from the same group of cats are much more closely related genetically than are FIPVs and FECVs obtained from geographically separate areas.[7, 8] Cats from households seropositive for FCoV are just as likely to develop FIP whether or not there is a history of the disease in the colony.[9]

Precisely where in the genome relevant mutations occur to account for these virulence variants has not yet been elucidated. Like other RNA viruses, coronaviruses have various mechanisms that may enhance adaptation to differing biologic selection pressures. A number of differences have been found among strains of FCoVs, including deletions in certain genes, some of which may relate to cell culture adaptation.[7, 10] However, conclusive evidence for the underlying genetic basis of differences in pathogenicity among FCoVs awaits the development of infectious clones.

The origin of the more virulent, FIP-inducing mutant virus in an individual cat is not clear. It appears that mutants may arise within an FCoV-infected cat at a low level.[8, 11] However, it is likely that FIP-inducing viruses can also spread from cat to cat. In experimental transmission studies, such mutants appear to retain their capacity to induce FIP, at least in the short term.[8] Additionally, in the field, clusters of cases may sometimes occur, suggesting horizontal spread.[12, 13] Whatever the precise origin of the FIP virus, it has been suggested that it is the ability of the mutant virus to replicate in macrophages and thus escape the gut that leads to the development of FIP.[12, 14]

Feline coronaviruses have also been classified on the basis of their serotype. All FCoVs, regardless of their biotype, are considered to belong to serotype I or II.[12] In contrast to serotype II viruses, type I isolates appear to predominate in the field, are not neutralized by antisera to CCV, and do not grow well in cell culture. It has been suggested that type II FCoVs may have arisen as recombinants between type I viruses and CCV.[7]

PATHOGENESIS

The main route of infection with FCoV is oronasal from contact with infected feces. Following infection, virus replicates initially in oropharyngeal tissues and in the enterocytes at the tips of the intestinal villi.[15, 16] In most cases, infection is inapparent, but mild enteritis and diarrhea may occur. Subsequently, the outcome of infection depends on the result of complex interactions among the strain and dose of virus; the route of infection; and the age, genotype, immune competence, and immune status of the cat.

In an individual cat in which both FIPV-like strains and the correct predisposing factors are present, dissemination of the virus in macrophages will occur, and the classic pyogranulomatous lesions of FIP may develop. Lesions can occur in a variety of tissues. In wet FIP they typically consist of fibrinous deposits and small pyogranulomas on the omentum and serosal surfaces of most abdominal organs; lesions also tend to occur in mesenteric lymph nodes, liver, and spleen. In dry FIP the granulomatous lesions are usually much larger and surrounded by more fibrosis; they are often found outside the abdomen and thorax, particularly in the central nervous system (CNS) and eye. A characteristic feature of FIP is perivascular cuffing, where infected macrophages and other cells tend to congregate around small venules.[17]

Although cats generally mount a high-level humoral antibody response to FCoV infection, this does not appear to be protective, because virus present within macrophages is inaccessible. Therefore, it is the cat's ability to mount a strong cell-mediated immune response that is thought to influence the clinical consequences of infection.[12] A strong cell-mediated and local immune response help restrict virus largely to the intestinal mucosa and mesenteric lymph nodes, leading to eventual recovery and virus elimination. Noneffusive or granulomatous FIP is thought to develop when there is a moderate cell-mediated immune response and the virus is partially contained; effusive FIP develops when the cell-mediated response is minimal. In some cats the response may be sufficient to effect clinical recovery, but they may retain small foci of infection, leading to the development of an asymptomatic carrier state. In the longer term, some of these animals may develop recrudescent disease.

The pathogenesis of FIP is further complicated by the phenomenon of antibody-dependent enhancement (ADE). It has been shown in experimental studies that cats with preexisting antibody to FCoV, either actively or passively acquired, develop enhanced, accelerated disease after challenge, compared with coronavirus-naive cats.[18, 19] However, there is little evidence to suggest that ADE occurs in the field.[20–22] This may be because naturally infected cats are exposed to lower doses, possibly by "trickle exposure" to low-level infection; alternatively, there may be differences between naturally passaged virus and virus grown in cell culture.[23]

The mechanisms behind ADE are complex. Although infected cats produce large amounts of antibody that can neutralize virus in cell culture, in cats with FIP, antibody actually increases the uptake of virus into macrophages through binding of the antibody-virus complex to the Fc receptor; it is possible that complement-binding receptors may be involved as well.[2, 14, 24] The second component to ADE is that immune complexes are deposited in the walls of small blood vessels in the target tissues. The complement cascade is activated, blood coagulation occurs, and various cytokines are released, all of which contribute to the perivasculitis and leakage of fluid that are so characteristic of FIP.[25, 26]

CLINICAL SIGNS

FECV Infection. Feline coronavirus–induced enteritis is usually mild or subclinical and is most common in kittens just after weaning.[27] However, transient vomiting and mild to occasionally more severe diarrhea may occur for up to several days in some animals.

FIP. The initial signs of wet and dry FIP are similar but nonspecific.[17] They include pyrexia, depression, inappetence, lethargy, and sometimes diarrhea. The more characteristic signs of FIP then develop over a period of days to months. Wet FIP, in general, is more rapidly progressive than is dry FIP. In both forms of the disease there is a chronic, fluctuating, unresponsive fever; anorexia; and weight loss. In dry FIP the fever may be more persistent. Kittens with FIP may show stunted growth.[12]

As the disease progresses, at least 75 per cent of cats with wet FIP have ascites.[12] Pleural and sometimes pericardial effusion occurs in about 25 per cent of affected cats, and these cats may be dyspneic and have muffled heart sounds.[26] In intact males, the scrotum may be enlarged. Hepatic involvement leading to jaundice may also occur, especially in the later stages of the disease.

In dry FIP, granulomatous lesions develop in a variety of organs. Clinical signs reflect the organs involved. The abdomen is most frequently affected, with lesions in the liver, the mesenteric lymph nodes, and, less commonly, the kidneys. Other common sites include the CNS and eyes. A variety of neurologic signs may be seen, including ataxia, paresis, behavioral changes, disorientation, nystagmus, seizures, hyperesthesia, and peripheral neuropathies. Ocular lesions typically involve inflammation of the uveal tract, with iritis, anterior uveitis, and chorioretinitis sometimes being the only clinical manifestation of the disease.

Although wet and dry FIP are usually described as two discrete syndromes, some cats have an overlap of the two conditions. Thus a small proportion (about 10 per cent) of cats with wet FIP have CNS or eye lesions, and some cats with dry FIP have a small amount of fluid in the abdomen. In addition, some cats with dry FIP progress to the wet form of the disease.

DIAGNOSIS

FECV Infection. It is difficult to confirm a diagnosis of mild transient enteritis in kittens due to FECV infection, because the clinical signs may be related to a number of other causes. Electron microscopy of feces, though not routinely available, may be used to detect the presence of FCoV or other possible viral causes of enteritis. Virus isolation is difficult and therefore is not a practicable means of diagnosis. Although rising antibody titers to FCoV may indicate recent infection, interpretation of FCoV serology is problematic. Polymerase chain reaction (PCR) is available in some laboratories and may be used to detect FCoV in feces.[28, 29] However, viral RNA may also be detected in the feces of asymptomatic cats, making positive results difficult to interpret.

FIP. The only definitive method for diagnosing FIP is by histopathologic examination of diseased tissues taken either at biopsy or at necropsy. However, a diagnosis of FIP can often be achieved through a combination of clinical and laboratory findings. A weighted scoring system has been described that can be used as an aid to clinical diagnosis (Table 91–1).[12] Nevertheless, a number of other conditions may present with clinical signs similar to those seen in FIP (Table 91–2).

Wet FIP is easier to diagnose than dry FIP because of the presence of fairly characteristic abdominal or pleural fluid.

TABLE 91–1. A WEIGHTED SCORING SYSTEM FOR FIP DIAGNOSIS

A score is given for each of the following factors, and the total score is used to assess the likelihood that the cat has FIP. Cats scoring less than 75 are unlikely to have FIP; 75 to 200, FIP should be considered as a differential diagnosis; greater than 200, FIP should be at the top of the diagnostic list.

1. Antibiotic-resistant, persistent, spiking fever	10
2. Abdominal effusion	10
3. Pleural effusion	5
4. Above effusions yellowish, mucinous, high protein, fibrin tags; moderate numbers macrophages and polymorphonuclear neutrophil leukocytes	15 × sign 2 or 3
5. Icteric serum	5
6. Palpable or visual masses in mesenteric lymph nodes, kidneys, ileocecocolic area	5
7. Aspirates or biopsy of above masses shows granulomatous inflammation	15 × sign 6
8. Neurologic abnormalities	15
9. Anterior uveitis/retinitis	10
10. Anterior uveitis with keratitic precipitates	25
11. Characteristic complete blood count	10
12. Elevated serum globulin	10
13. Characteristic serum electrophoresis	15
14. FCoV antibody titer negative to 1:25	0
15. FCoV antibody titer 1:100–1:400	5
16. FCoV antibody titer 1:1600	10
17. FCoV antibody titer 1:3200 or greater	20

Total the above points and multiply by the following:

a. The cat comes from a pure breed cattery or from a large multiple-cat environment (pound, shelter, pet store, multipet household)	3 × total points
b. The cat is from 3 months to 3 years of age	2 × total points

Adapted from Pedersen NC: An overview of feline enteric coronavirus and infectious peritonitis virus infections. Feline Pract 23:14, 1995.

The fluid is typically straw-colored and viscous; it has a high protein content, froths easily on shaking, and may clot if left standing. It contains moderate numbers of inflammatory cells, including macrophages and neutrophils. In cats

TABLE 91–2. FELINE INFECTIOUS PERITONITIS: SOME DIFFERENTIAL DIAGNOSES

Abdominal Fluid

Lymphocytic/plasmacytic cholangiohepatitis
Bacterial peritonitis
Neoplasia
Heart failure
Pancreatitis
Hypoproteinemia

Pleural Fluid

Exudative pleurisy (pyothorax)
Neoplasia
Chylous effusions/chylothorax
Heart failure
Diaphragmatic rupture

Neurologic/Ocular Signs

Feline leukemia virus
Feline immunodeficiency virus
Neoplasia
Toxoplasma gondii
Feline spongiform encephalopathy
Idiopathic encephalomyelitis/meningitis
Feline "staggering disease"

with CNS or ocular disease, increased amounts of protein and cells are sometimes found in cerebrospinal fluid and aqueous humor.

No single clinicopathologic test is diagnostic for FIP, although certain changes may support a diagnosis.[12, 30–32] Serum protein concentrations are typically increased owing to a polyclonal gammopathy. Other biochemical parameters such as bilirubin, blood urea nitrogen, or liver enzymes may be increased. Hematologic changes are fairly nonspecific but are similar in both forms of the disease. In general, cats have a leukocytosis with neutrophilia but a lymphopenia and a mild nonregenerative anemia.

Because virus isolation is difficult in FIP, serology has been used to aid diagnosis. However, serologic tests cannot differentiate between infection with a more virulent FIP-inducing strain and infection with a less virulent enteric strain of FCoV. Serology also cannot distinguish between past and present infection.[17, 33] A large proportion of clinically healthy cats, particularly in multicat households, are seropositive for FCoV but never develop FIP-related disease. Therefore, cats should not be euthanized because of a positive antibody titer to FCoV. Vaccinated cats may also have a low titer to FCoV.

Serologic tests used for FIP are generally based on immunofluorescent antibody or ELISA-based techniques. However, antibody titers may vary among laboratories. In some studies, high antibody titers were shown to be a risk factor for FIP, but there is considerable overlap in titers in cats with and without FIP.[13] Many cats with high titers never develop FIP, and some cats with FIP have only low or even undetectable levels of FCoV antibody.[28, 34] Therefore, although a high titer to FCoV may be compatible with a diagnosis of FIP (see Table 91–1), definitive diagnosis should always be based on other criteria.

Nucleic acid probes[35] and PCR[28, 29] have now been applied to FIP diagnosis. Viral RNA was detected by PCR in the tissues, body fluids, and feces of cats with FIP, but plasma and feces from asymptomatic cats and cats with non-FIP-related disease have also been found to be positive.[28, 29] This technique is useful for studying the epidemiology of FCoV infection, but for diagnosis it has the same limitations as serology. Eventually, when the precise mutation or mutations associated with FIPV are known, it may be possible to develop probes or PCR techniques specific for FIP. Some laboratories are currently offering PCR-based tests for FIP that are said to be associated with a genomic sequence invariably associated with the disease, although to date there are no published data to support this.[36]

TREATMENT

There is no effective treatment at present for FIP, and most therapy is based on supportive care. As the disease has an immunologic basis, drugs such as corticosteroids and cyclophosphamide have been used for their immune-suppressive and anti-inflammatory properties.[37] Although not curative, in a few cats they may have prolonged life.[38] A number of immunomodulating drugs have been tested in vitro,[39] and of these, interferon, *Propionibacterium acnes*, and thioproline (Promodulin) have been tested in cats.[37, 40] There is limited evidence that some of these treatments delay the onset of clinical signs or prolong life.[37, 38] However, most clinical cases are seen too late in the course of infection for these drugs to have full effect.

The antiviral agents ribavirin and adenine arabinoside have been shown to be effective against FIPV in vitro.[41] In addition, ribavirin has been tested in vivo, but its usefulness is limited owing to toxicity at therapeutic doses.[42] Combination therapies of both immunomodulating and antiviral drugs appear promising in vitro but have not shown good results in cats.[38]

EPIDEMIOLOGY

Serologic surveys show that infection with FCoV is widespread: approximately 75 to 100 per cent of cats from breeding catteries and 25 per cent of household pets have FCoV antibody.[12, 43] Kittens usually lose their maternally derived antibodies by 8 weeks of age, and most kittens have become infected and seroconvert by 10 weeks of age.[9, 44, 45] The majority of infections are asymptomatic, although diarrhea and stunted growth may occur.

FIP usually occurs in younger cats, peaking between 6 months and 2 years of age; there may be a slight increase again in animals older than 13 years of age.[13, 32, 46] The overall mortality to FIP in household pets is approximately 1:5000, although in some countries it may be higher; in colony cats it is generally about 5 per cent.[12, 21, 22, 47–49] Mortality rates in catteries are often higher the first few months after infection, occasionally reaching 40 per cent. Thereafter, epidemics (>10 per cent mortality/year) may periodically occur.[13]

Several factors may influence development of FIP. Larger catteries appear to have increased risk compared with smaller households,[46] and there may also be a seasonal effect.[13] Breed and other genetic influences, such as specific bloodlines and matings, have been implicated as risk factors.[46, 49] In a recent study of purebred cats that took account of environmental factors, FIP susceptibility appeared to be a partially heritable trait.[49] Similarly a genetic predisposition has been suggested although this hypothesis for cheetahs has recently been questioned.[50, 51]

Stresses such as pregnancy in younger queens, surgery, or intercurrent infections may play a role in precipitating FIP. Kittens often develop the disease after weaning and moving to a new home. Infection with feline leukemia virus (FeLV) or feline immunodeficiency viruses may also precipitate the disease in cats infected with FCoV.[8, 52] However, FeLV has largely been eradicated from many cat populations and no longer plays a significant role.

Cats may be infected with FCoV from a variety of sources (Fig. 91–1). They may be infected by kittens undergoing a primary infection. These cats are probably most infectious in the first few weeks after infection and before clinical signs develop.[8, 15, 53] It was always thought that FCoVs are relatively fragile in the external environment, but there is now evidence that the infectious virus may persist dried on a surface for as long as seven weeks.[54]

Clinically healthy carrier cats are an important source of virus, particularly in endemically infected colonies. The proportion of infected cats that become carriers, the amounts of virus shed, and the duration of the carrier state in an individual animal are not entirely clear. Epidemiologic studies on seropositive queens isolated with their kittens suggested that approximately one in three queens is a carrier that transmits virus to her kittens.[44] In more recent studies, fecal shedding patterns have been monitored by PCR. Thirty-five to 70 per cent of cats in private multicat households were found to be shedding virus at any one time over a one-year period, although it is likely that some, particularly the

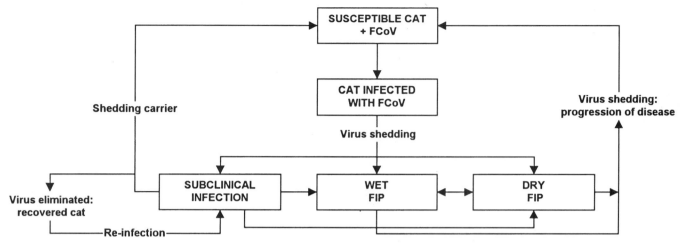

Figure 91–1. Algorithm demonstrating spread of FIP between cats.

intermittent shedders, were undergoing reinfection.[13, 45] In studies with a closed breeding colony, individual cats appeared to resist superinfection by closely related FCoVs.[55] This latter study also formally confirmed the existence of a carrier state, in that virus shedding in an isolated cat continued for up to seven months.[55] From epidemiologic studies it appears that most cats stop shedding FCoV within a year.[9] Studies using PCR show that the major site of virus persistence and replication in FCoV carrier cats appears to be the intestinal tract, although the virus may also be detected at a low level in other tissues.[55]

PREVENTION AND CONTROL

It is difficult to be categoric in terms of advice on prevention and control of FIP-related disease, because so many factors may influence the outcome of infection. Essentially, both management and, where available, vaccination can play a role.

VACCINATION

Vaccination against FIP has been attempted by various methods, including both conventional and recombinant vaccines.[2, 56–58] The results of these experiments were diverse; protection was often unpredictable, and in some studies ADE was seen after challenge. An intranasal, temperature-sensitive mutant FIPV vaccine, derived from strain DF2 (serotype II), has been developed and is now widely marketed in many parts of the world.[59, 60] The vaccine virus replicates only in the tissues of the upper respiratory tract and is thought to work by inducing both strong local mucosal IgA and cell-mediated immune responses. Laboratory-based safety studies, together with extensive field use, suggest that the vaccine is safe and does not seem to induce ADE.[48, 60, 61] The vaccine appeared to be reasonably efficacious in a number of experimental challenge studies using seronegative animals, including challenge with a heterologous serotype I FCoV.[59–61] Field studies also demonstrated some evidence of efficacy in seronegative cats entering a cat shelter and in a household pet population, but not in catteries with endemic disease.[21, 22, 48] In the household pet study, efficacy was demonstrable only in the longer term, possibly because in the early stages some cats were already incubating the disease.

In contrast, some experimental challenge studies have shown a lack of efficacy, and also evidence of ADE.[23, 62, 63] It is not clear why this phenomenon may occur under laboratory conditions but does not appear to occur in the field. However, overall, the vaccine appears to be safe under natural conditions and is probably most useful for seronegative animals going into a high-risk situation.

The vaccine is recommended for use only in kittens 16 weeks or older. Although its use has been reported in 6-week-old kittens during an outbreak of FIP, under experimental conditions it does not appear to be efficacious in such young animals.[12] Clearly this age restriction limits the vaccine's usefulness. On the more positive side, the vaccine appears to reduce fecal shedding after challenge with FECV, and this may reduce the chances of it mutating to the more virulent FIPV.[64]

MANAGEMENT

Household Pets. FIP is uncommon in household pets. Exceptions are new kittens obtained from colonies infected with FCoV. Sometimes the stress of weaning and entering a new home precipitates development of FIP. Ideally, household pets should be obtained from a source where there are few cats and no history of disease. In some circumstances, it may be appropriate to obtain kittens known to be seronegative for FCoV.

Generally, if household pets are kept singly or in small stable groups and have no contact, direct or indirect, with catteries, they are unlikely to become infected with FCoV. It is probably unnecessary to vaccinate household pets kept at home. Exposure to FCoV may occur if the cat enters a boarding cattery or perhaps a veterinary hospital. Most cats in a boarding cattery, however, will be household pets and therefore unlikely to be shedding FCoV. If hygiene is good, exposure is likely to be minimal. However, depending on the circumstances, vaccination may be advisable.

Cattery With Endemic FIP. In catteries with a history of FIP, two management approaches have been advocated: eradicating infection, or taking measures to try to reduce the incidence of disease. Eradication of infection has been achieved by isolating queens one to two weeks prepartum and then early weaning of their kittens into isolation.[9, 44, 65] Strict quarantine measures are required, and kittens should be tested to ensure freedom from infection at 12 to 16 weeks of age. Infection may be eradicated from adult cats by keeping them isolated in small groups (three to four cats) and monitoring their antibody titers over time; decreasing titers indicate freedom from infection. High-titered animals are more likely to shed virus than are low-titered animals.[66]

Although it is possible to eradicate infection, it requires good facilities and substantial effort, and it is easier to achieve in small catteries. However, probably because most breeders have some contact with other groups of cats that may be infected, reinfection is common. The virus is readily transmissible via contaminated litterboxes, bedding, feeding and cleaning utensils, and personnel. Extensive precautions are required in terms of protective clothing and hygiene and disinfection procedures. Hot water and soap or detergent solution can be used, followed by disinfection with a 1:32 dilution of sodium hypochlorite.

Eradication is often difficult. In some situations it may be preferable to accept infection but to try and reduce the incidence of FIP by minimizing exposure to the virus and to those factors known to predispose to the disease.[65] Cats should be kept in stable households with adequate facilities for housing, good hygiene (especially for litterboxes), and separation during parturition and lactation. Overcrowding should be avoided: 8 to 10 cats is the maximum number for a simple breeding program in one home. Greater numbers require additional facilities and commitment.[65]

New entrants to such a colony pose a risk because they may be FCoV carriers and may reinfect other cats, possibly with a new virus strain. Because FCoV carriers tend to shed virus for some months, short-term quarantine is probably not indicated. Serologic or PCR testing can be carried out, but there are limitations, as previously discussed. An individual cat entering a high-risk household should probably be vaccinated. Cat shows and stud cats are also possible sources of infection, although hygiene at cat shows is probably sufficient to minimize this.

Cattery With No History of FIP. In most cases, the FCoV status of cats is unknown. It is questionable whether, in the absence of disease, owners should be encouraged to test their cats. Nevertheless, some catteries may contain either cats known to be seronegative for FCoV or cats with serologic evidence of previous exposure but with low titers, suggesting that they are no longer shedding virus. In these cases, reasonable hygiene precautions and barrier measures should be taken to minimize the risk of infection being introduced. If a new cat enters the colony, it should be tested for antibody to FCoV.

Alternatively, a cattery with no history of FIP may contain cats that are infected with FCoV, but factors involved in precipitating the disease may be reduced or absent. Clearly in such cases it is important to try to retain the status quo in terms of number of cats and management procedures, and new entrants should probably be vaccinated.

Rescue Catteries. Similar measures apply with respect to minimizing exposure to virus through good hygiene and other management practices and reducing stress factors such as overcrowding that are known to precipitate disease. Cats should be housed individually or, if this is not possible, batched on arrival and kept in stable groups. Vaccination is indicated.

REFERENCES

1. Horzinek MC, et al: Antigenic relationships among homologous structural polypeptides of porcine, feline, and canine coronaviruses. Infect Immun 37:1148, 1982.
2. Olsen CW: A review of feline infectious peritonitis virus: Molecular biology, immunopathogenesis, clinical aspects, and vaccination. Vet Microbiol 36:1, 1993.
3. Stoddart CA, et al: Attempted immunisation of cats against feline infectious peritonitis using canine coronavirus. Res Vet Sci 45:383, 1988.
4. McArdle F, et al: Induction and enhancement of feline infectious peritonitis by canine coronavirus. Am J Vet Res 53:1500, 1992.
5. Martin ML: Canine coronavirus enteritis and a recent outbreak following modified live vaccination. Comp Contin Ed 7:1012, 1985.
6. Wilson RB, et al: A neurologic syndrome associated with use of a canine coronavirus-parvovirus vaccine in dogs. Comp Contin Ed 8:117, 1986.
7. Vennema H, et al: A comparison of the genomes of FECVs and FIPVs and what they tell us about the relationships between feline coronaviruses and their evolution. Feline Pract 23:40, 1995.
8. Poland AM, et al: Two related strains of feline infectious peritonitis virus isolated from immunocompromised cats infected with a feline enteric coronavirus. J Clin Microbiol 34:3180, 1996.
9. Addie DD, Jarrett O: Control of feline coronavirus infections in breeding catteries by serotesting, isolation, and early weaning. Feline Pract 23:92, 1995.
10. Horzinek MC, et al: Perspectives on feline coronavirus evolution. Feline Pract 23:34, 1995.
11. Pedersen NC: Virologic and immunologic aspects of feline infectious peritonitis virus infection. Adv Exp Med Biol 218:529, 1987.
12. Pedersen NC: An overview of feline enteric coronavirus and infectious peritonitis virus infections. Feline Pract 23:7, 1995.
13. Foley JE, et al: Risk factors for feline infectious peritonitis among cats in multiple-cat environments with endemic feline enteric coronavirus. JAVMA 210:1313, 1997.
14. Stoddart CA, Scott FW: Intrinsic resistance of feline peritoneal macrophages to coronavirus infection correlates with in vivo virulence. J Virol 63:436, 1989.
15. Pedersen NC, et al: Pathogenicity studies of feline coronavirus isolates 79-1146 and 79-1683. Am J Vet Res 45:2580, 1984.
16. Stoddart ME, et al: The sites of early viral replication in feline infectious peritonitis. Vet Microbiol 18:259, 1988.
17. Stoddart ME, Bennett M: Feline coronavirus infections. In Chandler EA, Gaskell CJ, Gaskell RM (eds): Feline Medicine and Therapeutics. Oxford, Blackwell Scientific Publications, 1994, pp 506–514.
18. Pedersen NC, Boyle JF: Immunologic phenomena in the effusive form of feline infectious peritonitis. Am J Vet Res 41:868, 1980.
19. Weiss R, Scott F: Antibody-mediated enhancement of disease in feline infectious peritonitis: Comparisons with dengue haemorrhagic fever. Comp Immunol Microbiol Infect Dis 4:175, 1981.
20. Addie DD, et al: Risk of feline infectious peritonitis in cats naturally infected with feline coronavirus. Am J Vet Res 56:429, 1995.
21. Fehr D, et al: Evaluation of the safety and efficacy of a modified live FIPV vaccine under field conditions. Feline Pract 23:83, 1995.
22. Fehr D, et al: Placebo-controlled evaluation of a modified live virus vaccine against feline infectious peritonitis: Safety and efficacy under field conditions. Vaccine 15:1101, 1997.
23. McArdle F, et al: Independent evaluation of a modified live FIPV vaccine under experimental conditions (University of Liverpool experience). Feline Pract 23:67, 1995.
24. Hohdatsu T, et al: A study on the mechanism of antibody-dependent enhancement of feline infectious peritonitis virus infection in feline macrophages by monoclonal antibodies. Arch Virol 120:207, 1991.
25. Jacobse-Geels HE, et al: Antibody immune complexes and complement activity fluctuations in kittens with experimentally induced feline infectious peritonitis. Am J Vet Res 43:666, 1982.
26. Olsen CW: Feline viral diseases; feline coronavirus infections. In Ettinger SJ, Feldman EC (eds): Textbook of Veterinary Internal Medicine, 4th ed. Philadelphia, WB Saunders, 1995, pp 421–425.
27. Pedersen NC, et al: An enteric coronavirus infection of cats and its relationship to feline infectious peritonitis. Am J Vet Res 42:368, 1981.
28. Herrewegh AAPM, et al: Detection of feline coronavirus RNA in feces, tissues, and body fluids of naturally infected cats by reverse transcriptase PCR. J Clin Microbiol 33:684, 1995.
29. Addie DD, et al: Feline coronavirus in the intestinal contents of cats with feline infectious peritonitis. Vet Rec 139:522, 1996.
30. Sparkes AH, et al: Feline infectious peritonitis: A review of clinicopathological changes in 65 cases, and a critical assessment of their diagnostic value. Vet Rec 129:209, 1991.
31. Sparkes AH, et al: An appraisal of the value of laboratory tests in the diagnosis of feline infectious peritonitis. J Am Anim Hosp Assoc 30:345, 1994.
32. Wolf AM: Feline infectious peritonitis, part 1. Feline Pract 25:26, 1997.
33. Pedersen NC: The history and interpretation of feline coronavirus serology. Feline Pract 23:46, 1995.
34. Sparkes AH, et al: Coronavirus serology in healthy pedigree cats. Vet Rec 131:35, 1992.
35. Martinez ML, Weiss RC: Detection of feline infectious peritonitis virus infection in cell cultures and peripheral blood mononuclear leukocytes of experimentally infected cats using a biotinylated cDNA probe. Vet Microbiol 34:259, 1993.
36. Telford D, et al: PCR-based diagnosis of feline infectious peritonitis. Vet Rec 140:379, 1997.
37. Weiss RC: Treatment of feline infectious peritonitis with immunomodulating agents and antiviral drugs: A review. Feline Pract 23:103, 1995.
38. Wolf AM: Feline infectious peritonitis, part 2. Feline Pract 25:24, 1997.

INF

39. Weiss RC, et al: Inhibition of feline infectious peritonitis virus replication by recombinant human leukocyte α interferon and feline fibroblastic (β) interferon. Am J Vet Res 49:1329, 1988.
40. Weiss RC, et al: Effect of interferon or *Propionibacterium acnes* on the course of experimentally induced feline infectious peritonitis in specific pathogen-free and random-source cats. Am J Vet Res 51:726, 1990.
41. Barlough JE, Scott FW: Effectiveness of three antiviral agents against FIP virus in vitro. Vet Rec 126:556, 1990.
42. Weiss RC, et al: Evaluation of free or liposome-encapsulated ribavirin for antiviral therapy of experimentally induced feline infectious peritonitis. Res Vet Sci 55:162, 1993.
43. Pedersen NC: Serologic studies of naturally occurring feline infectious peritonitis. Am J Vet Res 37:1449, 1976.
44. Addie DD, Jarrett O: A study of naturally occurring feline coronavirus infections in kittens. Vet Rec 130:133, 1992.
45. Foley JE, et al: Patterns of feline coronavirus infection and fecal shedding from cats in multiple-cat environments. JAVMA 210:1307, 1997.
46. Kass PH, Dent TH: The epidemiology of feline infectious peritonitis in catteries. Feline Pract 23:27, 1995.
47. Addie DD, et al: The risk of typical and antibody enhanced feline infectious peritonitis among cats from feline coronavirus endemic households. Feline Pract 23:24, 1995.
48. Postorino Reeves N: Vaccination against naturally occurring FIP in a single large cat shelter. Feline Pract 23:81, 1995.
49. Foley JE, Pedersen NC: The inheritance of susceptibility to feline infectious peritonitis in purebred catteries. Feline Pract 24:14, 1996.
50. O'Brien SJ, et al: Genetic basis for the species vulnerability in the cheetah. Science 227:1428, 1985.
51. Spencer JA: Lymphocyte blast transformation responses and restriction fragment length analysis in the cheetah. Onderstepoort J Vet Res 60:211, 1993.
52. Pedersen NC, Floyd K: Experimental studies with three new strains of feline infectious peritonitis virus FIPV-UCD2, FIPV-UCD3, and FIPV-UCD4. Comp Contin Educ Pract Vet 7:1001, 1985.
53. Stoddart ME, et al: Virus shedding and immune response in cats inoculated with cell culture-adapted feline infectious peritonitis virus. Vet Microbiol 16:145, 1988.
54. Scott FW: The immune responses to FIP in cats. Feline Health Topics 3:1, 1989.
55. Herrewegh AAPM, et al: Persistence and evolution of feline coronavirus in a closed cat-breeding colony. Virology 234:349, 1997.
56. Pedersen NC, Black JW: Attempted immunization of cats against feline infectious peritonitis using either avirulent live virus or sublethal amounts of virulent virus. Am J Vet Res 44:229, 1983.
57. Vennema H, et al: Early death after feline infectious peritonitis challenge due to recombinant vaccinia virus immunization. J Virol 64:1407, 1990.
58. Vennema H, et al: Primary structure of the membrane and nucleocapsid protein genes of feline infectious peritonitis virus and imunogenicity of recombinant vaccinia viruses in kittens. Virology 181:327, 1991.
59. Gerber JD, et al: Protection against feline infectious peritonitis by intranasal inoculation of a temperature-sensitive FIPV vaccine. Vaccine 8:536, 1990.
60. Gerber JD: Overview of the development of a modified live temperature-sensitive FIP virus vaccine. Feline Pract 23:62, 1995.
61. Hoskins JD, et al: Independent evaluation of a modified live FIPV vaccine under experimental conditions (Louisiana experience). Feline Pract 23:72, 1995.
62. Scott FW, et al: Evaluation of the safety and efficacy of Primucell-FIP vaccine. Feline Health Topics 7:6, 1992.
63. Scott FW, et al: Independent evaluation of a modified live FIPV vaccine under experimental conditions (Cornell experience). Feline Pract 23:74, 1995.
64. Hoskins JD, et al: The potential use of a modified live FIPV vaccine to prevent experimental FECV infection. Feline Pract 23:89, 1995.
65. Pedersen NC, et al: Recommendations from working groups of the international feline enteric coronavirus and feline infectious peritonitis workshop. Feline Pract 23:108, 1995.
66. Hickman A, et al: Elimination of feline coronavirus infection from a large experimental specific pathogen-free cat breeding colony by serologic testing and isolation. Feline Pract 23:96, 1995.

CHAPTER 92

OTHER FELINE VIRAL DISEASES

Alice M. Wolf

FELINE PARVOVIRUS (PANLEUKOPENIA)

Feline parvovirus (FPV) infection most commonly affects young, unvaccinated cats and results in an acute or peracute systemic and enteric infection characterized by fever, vomiting, diarrhea, anorexia, and malaise. The viral effects on bone marrow cause severe panleukopenia that has given this infection its common name. FPV infection is frequently fatal in young kittens, but adults are likely to recover.

FPV is a small, single-stranded DNA virus that is very similar morphologically and antigenically to canine parvovirus (CPV) type 2, mink enteritis virus, and raccoon parvovirus.[1] Most people believe that FPV is the ancestor virus for CPV and current strains of CPV can infect cats as well as dogs.[2]

EPIZOOTIOLOGY

The host range for FPV includes wild and domestic felids and some of the Procyonidae, Mustelidae, and Viverridae.[3]

FPV is shed in secretions and excretions from infected animals for weeks to months following infection. It is very stable in organic debris in the environment and may remain viable at room temperature for over one year. FPV is resistant to most common quaternary ammonium, iodine, and phenolic disinfectants but is inactivated by 4 per cent formalin solutions, 1 per cent glutaraldehyde, or a 1:32 dilution of bleach (sodium hypochlorite).[4]

Vaccines currently available against FPV are very effective, and clinical disease is almost nonexistent in appropriately vaccinated pet cats. Feral cats, unvaccinated cats in multiple-cat environments, and wild felids are at high risk for infection.[3]

PATHOGENESIS

Infection with FPV is usually acquired through the oronasal route from direct contact with an infected cat or contact with infectious materials from the environment. The virus initially replicates in oropharyngeal lymphoid tissue. The viral replication cycle is aborted at this point in immune hosts. In susceptible individuals, the virus escapes and spreads systemically. FPV can replicate in most body tissues, but rapidly dividing cells in the intestinal crypts, bone marrow, and lymphoid organs are most severely affected. In fetal and neonatal kittens, cells of the cerebellum and retina also have a high mitotic rate and are affected by FPV.

CLINICAL DISEASE

The clinical manifestations of FPV infection are dependent on the immunologic status and age of the cat at the time of infection. FPV infection in pregnant queens may cause abortion, fetal resorption, fetal mummification, and other reproductive problems. If fetuses are born alive, they usually have cerebellar hypoplasia and/or retinal dysplasia, as do kittens infected after birth but before 3 to 4 weeks of age. Older kittens generally show classic gastrointestinal and systemic signs of infection. Peracute FPV is rapidly progressive and often fatal within 24 hours owing to secondary bacteremia and endotoxemia associated with severe intestinal damage and panleukopenia. Signs include abdominal pain, severe depression, and subnormal body temperature. Because of the rapid progression to death in peracute disease, more typical gastrointestinal signs may not be observed, and the diagnosis is often made retrospectively in these animals during histopathologic examination. Classic signs of acute FPV infection include dehydration, vomiting, abdominal pain, hemorrhagic diarrhea, and fever. Owners may describe the cat as "hanging over the water bowl," which is probably reflective of thirst associated with dehydration counteracted by abdominal pain discouraging the desire to drink. Adult cats are usually less severely affected and have either mild gastroenteric symptoms and fever that are self-limited and resolve within a few days or inapparent illness. Recovered cats probably develop solid, lifelong immunity against reinfection with FPV.

DIAGNOSIS

Clinical Diagnosis

FPV infection should be suspected in kittens or cats with a questionable vaccination history, potential for exposure to this agent, typical clinical signs, and physical findings. Kittens with cerebellar hypoplasia usually have no other evidence of disease at the time of examination. Physical findings in cats with acute disease include fever or subnormal rectal temperature, dehydration, and abdominal pain. Affected cats often vomit or retch when abdominal palpation is performed.

Laboratory Diagnosis

Laboratory findings include evidence of dehydration and variable degrees of leukopenia, primarily neutropenia with or without lymphopenia. Electrolyte abnormalities may be present secondary to persistent vomiting and diarrhea. Infection can be confirmed by electron microscopic examination for FPV in feces. Although not approved for this use, fecal enzyme-linked immunosorbent assay (ELISA) tests for CPV antigen appear to detect FPV and can be used as a more rapid method for detecting FPV in feces. Because FPV and CPV are shed by healthy cats, identification of fecal parvovirus may not confirm the illness.

Gross pathologic findings in cats dying from acute or peracute disease occur primarily in the intestine and bone marrow. The intestinal mucosa is edematous and inflamed, and the bowel lumen is often filled with hemorrhagic fluid. The serosal surface may be covered with fibrinous exudate in severe cases. Mesenteric lymph nodes are enlarged, edematous, and occasionally hemorrhagic. The bone marrow may grossly appear liquid or gelatinous. Histopathologic examination reveals intestinal crypt necrosis with blunting, fusing, or sloughing of the intestinal villi. There is lymphoid depletion in mesenteric lymph nodes. Eosinophilic intranuclear inclusion bodies produced by FPV can be seen in some infected cells.

TREATMENT

Affected cats should be given no oral food or water to avoid exacerbating vomiting, decrease intestinal cell replication, and decrease the bacterial content of the intestine. Supportive care should be provided with vigorous intravenous fluid therapy to restore deficits, provide maintenance, and replace additional fluids lost in vomitus or diarrhea. Electrolyte levels should be monitored and additives used to maintain appropriate balance. Broad-spectrum antibiotics should be administered parenterally to help prevent and combat bacterial invasion from the compromised intestine. Plasma or other colloid replacement may be beneficial in selected animals. Antiemetic drugs can be used in cats with frequent or severe vomiting. Intestinal protectants (e.g., kaolin, bismuth) are probably of little value but are not likely to be harmful.

PROGNOSIS

Kittens with cerebellar hypoplasia have stable disease and may be suitable pets if kept in a protected environment. Cats with acute FPV tend to either die or recover more quickly than dogs with CPV infection. The prognosis is guarded, but with proper, aggressive supportive care, the majority of these cats will recover.

PREVENTION

Currently, both killed and modified live virus (MLV) parenteral FPV vaccines are available. Newer FPV vaccine types are under development, including subunit and poxvirus vectored recombinant vaccines. Among the products currently available, MLV vaccines are generally preferred but should not be given to kittens younger than 4 weeks of age because of the risk of vaccine-associated cerebellar hypoplasia. Signs of panleukopenia occurred in cats infected with feline immunodeficiency virus (FIV) that were vaccinated with an MLV FPV vaccine.[5] The need for booster immunizations following appropriate kittenhood vaccination against FPV is a subject of much debate in the veterinary community. The immunity stimulated by appropriate parenteral vaccination is quite solid and may be lifelong. Cats with access to the outdoors will encounter wild-type virus in the environment, and their immune status may also be kept active by natural exposure. If revaccination is performed, cats should require parenteral revaccination against panleukopenia no more frequently than every three years.[6] FPV antigen is usually contained in a combination product with feline herpesvirus (FHV-1), feline calicivirus (FCV), and occasionally other antigens.

MLV FPV antigen is also combined with FHV-1 and FCV in an intranasal vaccine. Intranasal administration of FPV antigen has no immunologic advantage over parenteral administration, and the duration of immunity when it is given by this route is unknown (see later).

FELINE HERPESVIRUS TYPE 1

Feline herpesvirus type 1 (FHV-1) is most commonly a clinical problem in catteries, multiple-cat households, and shelter or animal rescue environments.[7] Typical signs of FHV-1 infection include keratoconjunctivitis, upper respiratory disease, and abortion.[8] FHV-1 is one of the viruses associated with the feline upper respiratory disease complex and is commonly referred to as rhinopneumonitis. Clinical disease in young kittens is more severe than in older animals.

FHV-1 is a double-stranded DNA virus with a worldwide distribution. It can affect both wild and domestic felids.[3]

Unlike human respiratory illness and contrary to popular beliefs, FHV-1 is rarely acquired by aerosol exposure. Transmission usually requires direct contact between affected and unaffected cats or contact with infectious secretions or excretions. Therefore, appropriate husbandry, disinfection, and animal handling techniques can markedly limit the impact of FHV-1 in multicat environments. FHV-1 can remain infectious at room temperature for more than 30 days but is readily inactivated by most common detergents and disinfectants.[4]

Currently available vaccines against FHV-1 do not prevent infection with the virus but are generally effective in limiting the clinical signs of illness. Overt clinical disease is most common and severe in group-housed cats regardless of their vaccination status. Crowding, poor husbandry, and the presence of chronic FHV-1 carriers in these environments contribute to the high incidence.

PATHOGENESIS

Infection with FHV-1 is acquired by oronasal exposure to infectious secretions and excretions from acutely or chronically infected cats. Acutely infected cats can shed large amounts of virus in their nasal and ocular discharges and saliva for several weeks. Chronic carrier cats may be completely asymptomatic and shed smaller amounts of virus intermittently, often when stressed. Infected queens may transmit FHV-1 to kittens in utero. More often, kittens become infected at 4 to 6 weeks of age, when their maternal antibody wanes, during grooming by or contact with the shedding queen. Acutely infected kittens then spread the virus horizontally to littermates or other in-contact cats.

FHV-1 replicates best at slightly below normal core body temperature. For this reason, infection is usually limited to the more superficial epithelial tissues of the eyes, mouth, and upper respiratory system. Severe infection of the nasal tissues may result in necrosis and distortion of the turbinates, predisposing these cats to chronic secondary bacterial infections. Infection of the tracheal mucosa occurs occasionally, but involvement of the lower respiratory tree and pulmonary tissue is uncommon. Viremia can occur in some individuals, resulting in generalized systemic infection. Genital infection may cause vaginitis or cervicitis and result in temporary reproductive failure.

CLINICAL DISEASE

Acute primary infection or recrudescent infection in pregnant queens may or may not produce typical clinical signs of upper respiratory disease in the queen. Affected fetuses may die in utero and be aborted. If delivered normally, they may develop respiratory symptoms or a wasting illness ("fading kittens") and usually die in the early perinatal period. Postmortem examination of these kittens reveals upper respiratory infection, pneumonia, and occasionally liver necrosis.

Kittens infected at or after weaning and susceptible adult cats usually develop more typical signs of FHV-1, including sneezing, oculonasal discharge, rhinitis, conjunctivitis, fever, and anorexia. The discharges are initially serous but become mucopurulent owing to secondary bacterial invasion of ulcerated epithelial surfaces. Hair loss may occur on skin around the eyes and nose as a result of the irritative effects of the exudates. Ulcerations of the dorsal surface of the tongue and hard palate cause oral pain and hypersalivation in a few individuals. Infection may be relatively mild and self-limited and resolve within a few days, or signs may persist for several weeks, depending on the general health and immunocompetence of the affected cat.

Herpetic keratitis is a unique problem associated with FHV-1. The classic lesion is a linear dendritic type ulcer, but by the time most animals are seen clinically, corneal ulceration is often more generalized and severe.[9] Secondary bacterial infection of the corneal epithelium may cause deeper ulceration and possible desmetocele formation or corneal perforation. Epithelial proliferation and fibrous tissue formation associated with healing corneal and conjunctival ulcers can produce adhesions between the conjunctival and corneal epithelium (symblepharon). Infection may spread to the deeper tissues of the eye, resulting in panophthalmitis and a phthisical, nonfunctional globe. Corneal sequestration may occur in some affected cats, particularly if topical corticosteroids are applied to the eye.[9]

Following recovery from acute infection, many cats become chronic carriers of FHV-1. Virus is shed periodically from these individuals. Episodes of viral shedding are often associated with stress or corticosteroid administration. Clinical signs of illness are often absent in chronic FHV-1 carriers, so they are difficult to identify but may be a source of infectious virus for in-contact cats. Some chronic carriers intermittently have signs of keratitis/conjunctivitis or mild rhinitis during a recrudescence of viral activity.

An additional problem associated with FHV-1 is chronic bacterial rhinosinusitis secondary to viral damage to the nasal turbinates in cats affected early in life. These "chronic snufflers" have a history of an early episode of upper respiratory illness. They continue to have sinus and nasal cavity congestion and discharge following recovery from the viral component of the illness. The turbinates and nasal epithelium in these cats are damaged and distorted. Because of the abnormal nasal cavity anatomy and disruption of the normal mucosal defense mechanisms, this area is susceptible to bacterial overgrowth and chronic infection. Most bacteria isolated from animals with chronic rhinosinusitis are part of the normal nasal flora rather than invasive pathogens.

DIAGNOSIS

Specific clinical diagnosis of FHV-1 infection may be difficult, because several different pathogens in the feline upper respiratory disease complex (herpesvirus, calicivirus, *Chlamydia, Mycoplasma, Bordetella*) may be present in the same environment. Clinical signs associated with several of these agents may be similar, and often more than one agent is involved in producing the cat's signs of respiratory disease. The presence of keratitis and corneal ulceration is a specific diagnostic clue that strongly implicates the involvement of FHV-1.

Routine hematology and biochemical profiles are not helpful in the diagnosis of FHV-1 infections and usually reflect the general debilitating effects of the viral illness. Leukocytosis with neutrophilia may occur during the first week of infection; lymphocytosis may be found during the recovery phase. Virus isolation is best performed on conjunctival or pharyngeal swabs from acutely affected cats. Attempts to isolate virus from chronic carrier cats may be disappointing, because FHV-1 is shed only intermittently.[7] Conjunctival and nasal scrapings or biopsies can be evaluated for typical intranuclear herpesvirus inclusions by cytologic or histologic examination or by immunofluorescent antibody testing. The polymerase chain reaction (PCR) test is a more specific and sensitive method for detecting FHV-1 infection in both acutely infected and chronic carrier cats.[9, 10]

TREATMENT

Because FHV-1 is highly contagious, affected cats should be strictly isolated. Treatment of acutely affected cats with upper respiratory disease is symptomatic. The cat's eyes and nose should be gently cleaned frequently to remove irritating discharges and improve breathing. Systemic broad-spectrum antibiotics should be administered. Doxycycline may be effective against the secondary upper respiratory disease agents *Chlamydia, Mycoplasma,* and *Bordetella*. Doxycycline causes less gastroenteric distress and dental enamel staining in young animals than does tetracycline. Parenteral fluid therapy should be given to cats that are not eating and/or drinking in order to maintain hydration and to help keep oculonasal secretions from becoming inspissated. Highly palatable, soft textured foods should be offered frequently. Cats that remain anorectic for more than three to four days should receive nutritional support by force feeding or by nasopharyngeal, esophagostomy, or pharyngostomy tube feeding. Environmental humidification with a vaporizer or nebulizer may assist in reducing the tenacity of secretions and aid in their expulsion. Pediatric-strength nasal decongestants may be used on a short-term basis (three to four days) to help reduce nasal congestion and improve breathing. Maintaining a higher than normal environmental temperature may also reduce the replication rate of FHV-1.

In addition to cleaning discharge from the eyes, ophthalmic ointment containing chloramphenicol, oxytetracycline, or chlortetracycline is recommended, because these antibiotics are effective against *Chlamydia, Mycoplasma,* and *Bordetella*. These organisms may be secondarily involved in the upper respiratory disease process. Ophthalmic products containing corticosteroids must be avoided. If herpetic keratitis is present, specific antiherpetic ophthalmic treatment is recommended. Ophthalmic preparations containing idoxuridine, trifluridine, or vidarabine should be used topically at least four to six times daily.[9] These agents are irritating, and cats frequently resist repeated treatments. Oral administration of recombinant human interferon alfa is sometimes used as an adjunct to specific antiviral therapy[8, 11] Some ophthalmologists also recommend giving oral lysine to aid in healing herpetic corneal ulcers.[12]

The use of systemic antiviral therapy to treat FHV-1 infections is controversial. Acyclovir is very efficacious in the treatment of human herpes simplex, however, in vitro studies demonstrate that FHV-1 is relatively resistant to its effects. The doses of acyclovir required to suppress FHV-1 may be nephrotoxic.[13] Acyclovir in combination with low doses of recombinant human interferon alfa may improve clinical efficacy and reduce the risk of toxicity, but clinical studies have not yet been reported. Another antiherpetic drug, valacyclovir, does not have good efficacy against FHV-1 and causes renal, hepatic, and bone marrow toxicosis in cats.[14]

The treatment of chronic bacterial rhinosinusitis secondary to pediatric FHV-1 infection is particularly frustrating for the animal, the owner, and the clinician. These cats usually have a history of acute upper respiratory infection at an early age, or if the early history is unknown, the cat usually has had nasal discharge since being acquired by the owner. Clinical signs typically resolve during a course of antibiotic therapy but recur after treatment is discontinued. Humidification and short-term decongestant therapy may be used in combination with antibiotics if signs are severe. Surgical approaches have not been successful. Clinical signs of chronic rhinosinusitis persist for life in most cats, and complete resolution is unlikely.

PREVENTION

FHV-1 vaccines do not completely prevent viral infection but are effective in reducing clinical signs of illness.[15] Parenteral vaccines are available as either MLV or killed virus preparations. MLV vaccines have the advantage of having a reduced antigen mass and may not require an adjuvant. Side effects from parenteral MLV FHV-1 vaccines are uncommon, but they may cause clinical signs of FHV-1 infection if aerosolized or accidentally sprayed on the skin and ingested orally by the cat. MLV upper respiratory vaccines have also been implicated in outbreaks of clinical signs of upper respiratory infection in catteries.[16] Killed vaccines must contain high levels of antigen and an adjuvant in order to have efficacy similar to that of MLV products. At least two doses of parenteral FHV-1 vaccine are given to kittens at a three- to four-week interval. Current laboratory evidence suggests that the duration of immunity provided to cats by modern parenteral FHV-1 vaccines may be as long as four to five years.[6] Cats under high levels of stress and exposure to FHV-1 in crowded environments may need revaccination more frequently than household pets.

Intranasal MLV FHV-1 vaccine can be used to provide more rapid onset of good local mucosal immunity. The FHV-1 intranasal vaccine strain is temperature-sensitive so that it replicates only at the cooler temperatures of the upper respiratory mucosa. Intranasal vaccines are particularly suited for use in catteries, animal shelters, and humane organizations where cats of differing ages and disease and immunologic status are kept in close contact and often under less than ideal conditions of husbandry. Local immunity stimulated by intranasal vaccines is developed within 48 to 96 hours of administration but is of relatively short duration. Systemic immunity following intranasal vaccination develops within 7 to 10 days and, if vaccination is repeated within three to four weeks, provides good systemic protection against disease symptoms. Mild upper respiratory signs (sneezing, serous ocular and nasal discharge) occur within three to four days in a small proportion of cats vaccinated and owners should be warned about the occurrence of these symptoms. Physical resistance to intranasal instillation of the product also occurs in some individuals.

Intranasal FHV-1 and calicivirus vaccine can be used in early vaccination and weaning programs to help reduce the incidence of chronic rhinosinusitis in catteries with endemic upper respiratory infectious disease. Kittens should be vaccinated with several drops of intranasal vaccine instilled in the conjunctival sac and nasal cavity at 10 to 14 days of age when their eyes open. MLV panleukopenia antigen should not be included in vaccines given to kittens younger than 3 weeks of age. The kittens are weaned from the queen at 4 to 6 weeks of age and raised in isolation from other cats until their vaccination series is complete. Because the local immune response to intranasal vaccines is not blocked by maternal antibody, this regimen may stimulate early local immunity that will prevent the kitten from becoming infected with virulent virus shed from the queen during these early weeks of life. Isolation prevents further viral exposure until the kittens have developed solid, active systemic immunity. This same early weaning and isolation program is also helpful for reducing coronavirus exposure and infection in cattery-raised kittens.

FELINE CALICIVIRUS

Feline calicivirus (FCV), like FHV-1, is primarily a problem in multiple-cat environments. FCV infection most commonly affects the upper respiratory tract (pneumotropic form) and occasionally causes joint pain and lameness (rheumatic form).[17] Recent studies suggest that the difference in clinical disease manifestations is not related to any identifiable feature of the virus subtypes.[17, 18] It may be due to the unique response of a specific cat to the virus.

ETIOLOGY

FCV is a single-stranded RNA virus with a worldwide distribution. There is one serotype with multiple subtypes of varying degrees of antigenic cross-reactivity. FCV affects domestic felids and a few wild felid species.[3, 19]

Infection is acquired by ingestion or inhalation of infectious virus present in saliva and excretions or secretions from affected cats. Like FHV-1, the oral route of infection is most important, and direct contact with infected cats or virus-contaminated fomites is the primary method of transmission rather than aerosolized particulates. Husbandry methods to prevent cat-to-cat contact and cross-contamination during cleaning and feeding procedures are very important to prevent the spread of FCV in a population of cats. FCV is relatively stable in the environment and is not susceptible to inactivation by lipid solvents or disinfectants or quaternary ammonium compounds. Inactivation of FCV can be achieved with 1:32 sodium hypochlorite solution.[4]

Like FHV-1, vaccines currently available to protect against FCV usually prevent severe signs of disease but do not provide complete protection against viral infection.[20] FCV is most likely to occur in young cats in multiple-cat environments. Coinfection with FHV-1 and other feline upper respiratory disease agents increases the severity of clinical signs. Crowding, stress, and poor husbandry also contribute to the incidence of disease and the severity of signs.

PATHOGENESIS

FCV infection is acquired predominantly via ingestion, and initial viral replication occurs in the oropharyngeal tissues. Subsequent viremia spreads the virus primarily to the epithelial tissues of the nasal cavity, oral cavity, tongue, conjunctiva, and palate.

CLINICAL DISEASE

Kittens are more likely to be affected than adult cats. Experimentally, clinical disease caused by FCV alone is typically mild. Aerosol exposure with the pneumotropic subtypes causes fever and low-grade conjunctivitis and rhinitis within three days of infection.[21, 22] Keratitis is not a feature of FCV disease. Vesicles and erosions of the tongue, hard palate, and nasal planum occur in many affected cats, but these are superficial and heal rapidly.[18, 19, 22] Coughing is not a prominent clinical sign, but histologic examination of the lung from acutely affected cats demonstrates areas of patchy viral pneumonitis. Illness is self-limited and resolves within 10 to 14 days. In reports of naturally occurring FCV infection in catteries and multiple-cat households, clinical signs are typically described as much more severe. This is most likely because FCV is not acting alone but in combination with other upper respiratory disease agents and secondary bacterial invaders in these environments.

The rheumatic form of illness is often referred to as "limping kitten syndrome."[17, 22] Affected kittens exhibit fever greater than 104°F, joint swelling and pain, and muscle soreness. Oral ulcers may appear at the same time as signs of lameness.[22] Kittens may maintain a good appetite in spite of fever but are reluctant to walk and exhibit pain on palpation of bones and joints.[22] These signs resolve spontaneously after two to four days without specific treatment. Similar rheumatic signs have also been described subsequent to MLV calicivirus vaccination in a few cats.[22]

Recovered cats often remain lifelong carriers of FCV and are a continuing source of infectious virus for susceptible individuals in multiple-cat environments. FCV is shed continuously from the oral cavity irrespective of health status or stress.[23] Recrudescence of clinical signs of upper respiratory disease usually does not occur in these chronic carriers. New antigenic variants may provide a wider spectrum of subtypes available for dissemination to susceptible cats in the environment.

Lymphoplasmacytic stomatitis and gingivitis have been linked to chronic carriage of calicivirus in some cats.[23, 24] It is postulated that the presence of FCV causes chronic immune stimulation in the oropharyngeal tissues that leads to abnormal accumulation and proliferation of lymphocytes and plasma cells in these locations.

TREATMENT

Like FHV-1, FCV is highly contagious by contact among affected cats, and acutely infected individuals should be isolated. Symptomatic treatment for FCV upper respiratory disease should generally follow the guidelines described in the previous section for FHV-1. Viral keratitis is not a feature of FCV, but symptomatic treatment of conjunctivitis with tetracycline-type ointments is recommended to combat potential secondary *Chlamydia* or *Mycoplasma* infections. Oral antiviral agents are not recommended. Interferon inhibits the replication of FCV in vitro.

The rheumatic form of FCV infection is self-limited and resolves within two to three days. Treatment is directed at maintaining hydration and nutritional status during this time. A low dose of aspirin may be beneficial to help decrease fever and reduce joint pain.

Treatment of lymphoplasmacytic stomatitis is very difficult and often unrewarding. If persistent FCV is the underlying cause of lymphoid proliferation, it will remain a problem for the life of the cat. Treatment usually involves immune-suppressive doses of corticosteroids and/or other immune-suppressive drugs. Antibiotics are often included in the protocol and seem to help some animals by decreasing secondary bacterial involvement in the inflammatory process.

PREVENTION

Both killed parenteral and MLV parenteral or intranasal vaccines are available to prevent FCV infection. Recently, genetic analysis of viral subtypes isolated from FCV outbreaks in multiple-cat environments suggested that clinical disease resulted from the use of MLV FCV vaccine.[20] Some clinicians recommend using only killed FCV products.

Because of the large number of viral subtypes, the viral strains used in FCV vaccine production provide cross-protection against most, but not all, subtypes of FCV.[20] Therefore, significant morbidity due to FCV may occur in an apparently well-vaccinated cat because of exposure to a strain against which the vaccine provides no protection.

In addition, a recent study demonstrates that there has been an antigenic shift in clinically relevant subtypes of FCV isolated from naturally infected cats.[25] This study suggests that some FCV subtypes used in vaccine production may now be less protective because of these antigenic changes over time.

RABIES

Feline rabies is an important public health concern because cats continue to have the highest rabies incidence of any domesticated animal.[26, 27] This may be because cats are more likely than other species to have nonfatal interactions with important wildlife reservoirs of rabies virus such as raccoons, skunks, and bats.[26, 28] Because of the variability of the clinical manifestations of rabies in the cat and the intimate interactions between cats and human beings, the impact of feline rabies on human health care is considerable.[29] In one single incident, a rabid pet-store kitten exposed at least 665 people who subsequently received antirabies prophylaxis at an estimated health care cost of more than $1.1 million.[29] In endemic areas, rabies should be considered as a differential diagnosis for any cat with unexplained changes in behavior and/or signs of central or peripheral nervous system disease.

ETIOLOGY

Rabies is caused by an enveloped RNA virus of the family Rhabdoviridae. This virus is endemic in most parts of the world. Wildlife tends to be the major reservoir and vector of disease in industrialized countries with good pet vaccination programs.[26, 28] Domesticated animals, particularly dogs and cats, are a significant reservoir and vector of disease to human beings in less developed areas that lack rabies vaccination programs.

EPIZOOTIOLOGY

All warm-blooded animals can be infected with rabies virus, but susceptibility to disease is highly variable. The course of illness following infection of wildlife reservoirs is generally unknown. The subclinical carrier period can apparently be quite long in some species, such as the striped skunk, but it is believed that most affected animals will eventually die from their disease. The major reservoirs of sylvatic rabies in the United States are the striped skunk; red, grey, and arctic fox; raccoon; and bat. Coyote rabies introduced from Mexico has recently become a major concern in Texas and the Southwest. Although rodents are highly susceptible to rabies virus, they are unlikely to be significant reservoirs or vectors because their encounters with larger mammalian carriers are usually fatal.

Cats are naturally highly resistant to rabies virus infection. Feline rabies is acquired through contact with infected wildlife reservoirs, usually due to a bite wound. Raccoons and skunks have also been observed eating from food bowls left outdoors for cats and/or feeding alongside them. If there is an open wound in the oral cavity, rabies virus could be introduced during contact with infected saliva during communal feeding. Rarely, ingestion of rabies-infected tissue has been suspected as the source of exposure. Killed rabies virus vaccines have replaced MLV products, thereby eliminating postvaccinal rabies.

Rabies virus is sensitive to sunlight and heat, and infectious saliva is unlikely to survive long outside the host. Virus may remain viable in the tissues of dead animals for several days. Phenols, chlorine, formalin, and quaternary ammonium compounds are effective disinfectants.

The incidence of feline rabies in the United States continues to slowly increase, whereas the incidence of dog rabies continues to decline. These trends are likely due to feline interactions with wildlife reservoirs and more aggressive vaccination programs for dogs. Most affected cats are younger than 3 years of age, and males predominate.

PATHOGENESIS

Introduction of rabies virus occurs through a bite wound or contamination of an existing wound with infectious virus. Rabies virus initially replicates in local myocytes, then travels retrograde via the neuromuscular junction and peripheral nerves to the dorsal root ganglia and spinal root ganglia of the central nervous system (CNS). This phase of rabies virus migration generally takes at least 21 days but may be shorter or longer, depending on the amount and strain of rabies virus inoculated, the amount of innervation at the inoculation site, the distance from the inoculation site to the CNS, the immunologic status of the host, and other factors.

Following replication in the spinal ganglia, rabies virus undergoes general dissemination to and replication in the CNS. Clinical signs usually begin to appear at about this time. Virus then travels back out from the CNS to other body tissues via peripheral, motor, and sensory nerves. When the salivary glands are involved, the affected animal is infectious to others.

The incubation period before CNS signs appear following naturally occurring rabies infection is highly variable. The usual range for cats is one and a half to eight weeks, but incubation up to one year has been reported.

Infectious virus may be shed in saliva for several days before the appearance of clinical signs of illness, and shedding continues until the animal dies. Rabies virus remains viable for several days in a carcass at room temperature and for long periods in infected tissues kept under refrigeration or frozen.

CLINICAL DISEASE

The development of clinical rabies has been divided into three stages: prodromal, excitatory or furious, and paralytic or dumb. These divisions are somewhat arbitrary, and not every cat exhibits these distinctive signs at each stage of the illness.

Prodromal signs of rabies in cats usually manifest as changes in behavior. Some cats may become shy, withdrawn, irritable, and resistant to restraint or handling. Others may become outgoing, attentive, and affectionate. Physical examination during this time may demonstrate a low-grade fever, pupillary dilatation, or impaired corneal reflexes. The prodromal period in cats is typically very short, lasting only a day or two.

The furious phase of rabies in cats lasts two to four days, and clinical signs are most dramatic during this time. Physical signs include muscle twitching or tremors and muscle weakness with ascending hind limb incoordination. Extreme, unpredictable, vicious behavior and aggression directed against both animate and inanimate objects characterize this phase. Pharyngeal muscle dysfunction causes dysphagia and extreme ptyalism. Generalized major motor seizures may also occur during the furious phase.

The final paralytic or dumb phase of rabies lasts one to four days. Cats may occasionally progress to this phase without exhibiting obvious "furious" signs. In this phase, neurologic dysfunction progresses from paresis to generalized paralysis, coma, respiratory arrest, and death. Signs of mandibular and laryngeal paralysis resulting in jaw drop are less common in cats than in dogs.

DIAGNOSIS

Clinicians residing in endemic areas should keep a high index of suspicion for rabies in any cat with unexplained behavioral or neurologic signs. Routine laboratory diagnostic studies are not helpful in making the diagnosis, and there are no specific in-clinic tests to detect rabies virus. The diagnosis of rabies is made postmortem by examination or evaluation of CNS tissues. It is very important to handle potentially rabies-infected tissues with caution. Specimens should be refrigerated, not frozen, and sent to the testing laboratory promptly to preserve tissue architecture and enhance diagnostic accuracy. Histologic examination for Negri bodies (viral inclusion bodies) and mouse inoculation tests are still used occasionally. More recently, immunofluorescent antibody (IFA), ELISA, electron microscopic examination, and PCR tests have replaced these techniques.[30, 31] Monoclonal antibody testing can also be performed to determine which wildlife strain of rabies was the infecting agent.[27] It is important to remember that none of these tests has a reliability of 100 per cent. Regardless of a negative test result, if there is a history of potential rabies exposure and clinical signs are characteristic, appropriate physician-directed rabies prophylactic measures should be recommended for any human beings that may have been exposed to this animal.[32]

TREATMENT

Rabies is a fatal disease, and because of the human health risk involved in handling a clinically affected cat, treatment cannot be recommended. Potential rabies-exposed animals and rabies suspects should be handled in accordance with local and state health department regulations.

PREVENTION

Vaccination with killed rabies virus products is highly effective in preventing clinical rabies in cats and is safe for retrovirus-infected cats.[33] Newer subunit and recombinant rabies vaccine products have recently been introduced. The initial vaccination is given at 12 weeks of age and then repeated in one year. The appropriate revaccination interval after that is determined by the vaccine's duration of immunity and the local and state regulations governing rabies control measures. Although some communities do not require rabies vaccination of cats, it should be strongly recommended to clients. Keeping cats confined indoors where they will not contact wildlife reservoirs and not leaving food accessible to wildlife will also help prevent potential exposure to this serious feline and human health hazard.

POXVIRUS (CATPOX, COWPOX)

Poxvirus (cowpox and cowpox-like virus) infections in domestic and exotic cats are relatively infrequent and occur primarily in Western Europe.[34] Cats are accidental hosts and are infected from contact with reservoir hosts such as wild rodents and small mammals.[34, 35] There appears to be a seasonal incidence of the disease, with most cases occurring between June and November. The virus typically produces skin papules or nodules that progress to vesicles that rupture, leaving an ulcerated or scabbed surface.[34] The head, neck, and limbs are most frequently affected, but lesions may appear anywhere on the body. Clinical signs of malaise, fever, and anorexia or a more severe form of fatal systemic infection with bronchoalveolar pneumonia and exudative pleuritis can result. The diagnosis is confirmed by IFA or electron microscopic identification of poxvirus within affected tissues.[34] Treatment is nonspecific and supportive and consists of maintaining hydration and nutritional intake. Broad-spectrum antibiotics should be administered. Corticosteroids worsen the disease. Most cats with mild cutaneous pox lesions recover within four to six weeks; those with extensive dermal lesions and immunocompromised cats frequently succumb. No preventive measures exist for this disease other than avoiding contact between cats and affected wildlife reservoirs. Cowpox infection has been transmitted from infected cats to human beings, causing life-threatening systemic illness.[36]

BORNA DISEASE VIRUS

Borna disease virus (BDV) is an enveloped RNA virus in the family Bornaviridae with a worldwide distribution.[37] Natural infection with BDV in cats causes a widespread nonsuppurative meningoencephalomyelitis. Clinical signs of acute disease include a staggering gait, hind limb ataxia, and paresis, giving the infection its common name of "staggering disease."[38] Subclinical infection with BDV is probably common in cats, because serologic surveys reveal large numbers of clinically normal, seropositive cats in Borna disease–endemic areas. Diagnosis is presumptive, based on signs and physical findings. Cerebrospinal fluid analysis should reveal nonsuppurative inflammation. No specific treatment for BDV is available, and acutely affected cats may recover.[38] Confirmation of the diagnosis is made on postmortem examination through immunodiagnostic or PCR identification of BDV in brain tissues.[38] There does not appear to be any risk of direct transmission of this agent from cats to people.

FELINE SPONGIFORM ENCEPHALOPATHY

Although not classically caused by a virus, transmissible spongiform encephalopathies, or prion diseases, are of considerable concern in many parts of the world.[39] Feline spongiform encephalopathy (FSE) caused by the bovine spongiform encephalopathy (BSE) agent has been reported in wild and domestic cats.[40] It is suspected that the infection was introduced into these animals through inadequately processed BSE-infected meat and bone meal used in animal feeds. Affected cats have progressive neurologic symptoms affecting locomotor and sensory responses, and many have abnormal behavior patterns. The diagnosis of FSE is confirmed by histopathologic examination that reveals typical spongiform encephalopathy and the presence of fibrils and modified PrP protein in the brain. There is no effective treatment for FSE, and affected cats usually die or are euthanized. The BSE agent is restricted to the brain, spinal cord, and intestine of infected cattle, and prevention consists of avoiding ingestion of BSE-infected tissues.[39] BSE eradication programs and changes in processing procedures for animal feeds should eliminate this disease in domestic companion animals, although wildlife reservoirs may persist for a while in some areas. There is no direct transmission of the agent between cats and human beings.[39]

ASTROVIRUS

Astroviruses are small, single-stranded RNA viruses that can cause diarrhea in cats.[41] Several naturally infected cats had a protracted course of watery diarrhea associated with weight loss, anorexia, and poor condition.[41, 42] Most astrovirus infections in cats are either inapparent or are mild and self-limited. Treatment is symptomatic. There are currently no vaccines. Affected cats are not considered a hazard to human health.

ROTAVIRUS

The rotaviruses are a group of highly interrelated, enveloped RNA viruses that can cause diarrhea in many species.[43] Rotavirus infection is widespread in cats, and virus has been isolated from the feces of both normal and diarrheic animals.[43] Clinical descriptions of disease caused by rotavirus in companion animals are lacking. Experimental rotavirus infection of cats causes inapparent disease or only mild, self-limited diarrhea.[44] Treatment for cats with rotavirus diarrhea is symptomatic and supportive. Recent studies demonstrated significant homology among some feline, canine, and human rotavirus genogroups.[45] Although zoonotic transmission of rotavirus has not been confirmed, there is concern because humans and animals apparently share closely related viral strains.[45]

REOVIRUS

Reoviruses are double-stranded DNA viruses that inhabit the upper respiratory and gastrointestinal tracts of many species. Three reovirus isotypes have been isolated from healthy and diseased cats and in general do not appear to be significantly pathogenic. Experimental infection of kittens with two strains of feline reovirus type 2 caused either inapparent infection with seroconversion or mild, self-limited diarrhea without signs of systemic illness.[46] Natural infections are reported to cause diarrhea and protrusion of the nictitating membranes.[46] In experimental studies, reovirus type 3 caused serous or mucopurulent conjunctivitis in some infected kittens, but its role in naturally occurring upper respiratory disease in cats is unclear. Reovirus infection is apparently widespread in the cat population.[46] One seroepidemiologic survey revealed that antibodies against serotype 3 were most prevalent; antibodies against serotype 2 were the least prevalent.[46] Diagnosis of reovirus infection is made through virus isolation from conjunctival swabs or feces. There is no specific treatment, and affected cats recover spontaneously with minimal supportive care. There are currently no measures available to prevent feline reovirus infections.

PSEUDORABIES

Pseudorabies virus is a member of the herpes family of DNA viruses and affects many domestic species, including cattle, sheep, swine, dogs, and cats.[47] Cats may become infected through contact with infected swine or by eating infected pork products. Rats may be temporary hosts for pseudorabies virus, and feline infection may also occur from eating carrier rodents.[47]

The incubation period for pseudorabies in cats ranges from one to nine days. The characteristic form of infection causes peracute illness and death within 36 hours. Initial clinical signs include malaise, lethargy, depression, agitation, aggression, and resistance to handling. Subsequent signs develop rapidly and include hypersalivation, exaggerated swallowing efforts, retching, vomiting, and aimless vocalization.[47] More severe neurologic manifestations appear during the terminal stages of illness and include hyperesthesia, face rubbing, and severe pruritus resulting in self-mutilation.[47, 48] Atypical pseudorabies occurs in 40 per cent of affected cats. In these animals, the illness is of longer duration and lacks the more classic pruritic signs of "mad itch."[47] Depression, weakness, gulping, and swallowing are the most prominent signs. Rhythmic tail movements, facial muscle twitching, and anisocoria occur with both forms of the disease.

Pseudorabies is invariably fatal in infected cats. Because of the rapid progression of the disease, clinical pathologic examination is unlikely to be useful. Antemortem diagnosis is usually based on exposure history and clinical signs. Because prominent clinical signs include hypersalivation and aggression, the major differential diagnosis for feline pseudorabies is rabies virus infection. Postmortem diagnosis of pseudorabies is confirmed by identification of intranuclear inclusion bodies in or isolation of pseudorabies virus from CNS tissues.[48]

Prevention of pseudorabies in cats is based on eradicating the disease in swine and not feeding uncooked or inadequately cooked infected pork products to cats. Because of the peracute and fatal nature of feline infection and restriction of pseudorabies virus to feline nervous tissue, there is no risk of cat-to-cat transmission.[48] Human beings are resistant to pseudorabies virus, and infected cats do not pose a risk to public health.

FELINE SYNCYTIUM-FORMING VIRUS (FOAMY VIRUS)

Syncytium-forming viruses are enveloped RNA viruses in the retrovirus family that cause persistent and apparently benign infections in primates, cats, and cattle.[49] Feline syncytium-forming virus (FeSFV) infection is widespread in the feline population.[49]

Although some earlier reports attempted to link FeSFV infection with various neoplastic and other disease conditions in cats, this work was done before the discovery of FIV. Seroepidemiologic surveys have demonstrated that FIV-infected cats are commonly co-infected with FeSFV.[50] Transmission of both of these viral infections is believed to occur primarily via bite wounds. Experimental studies have demonstrated that FeSFV does not enhance FIV susceptibility, progression, or severity.[50] It is therefore most likely that the association between FIV and FeSFV is coincidental and due to a similar mode of transmission in an at-risk population of cats. The only significant disease condition still ascribed to FeSFV is feline chronic progressive polyarthritis. Most cats with this severe, deforming joint disorder are co-infected with FeLV, so the true pathogenic role, if any, of FeSFV in these animals is unclear.

FeSFV causes a persistent but benign infection of no clinical consequence. Treatment is not available, and preventive measures are not necessary. Detection of serum virus-neutralizing antibody against FeSFV is diagnostic for infection.[49] Although humans have their own foamy virus infection, FeSFV is not transmissible to human beings or other mammals.[51]

MORBILLIVIRUS

Canine distemper virus (CDV) is a negative-stranded RNA virus of the genus *Morbillivirus,* family Paramyxoviridae. Recent attention has been focused on this virus as a pathogen of large cats because of lion mortality attributed to CDV in the Serengeti.[52–54] Retrospective studies have confirmed CDV-associated deaths in captive large cats from North America and Europe as early as 1972.[54, 55] These findings suggest that CDV infection of large cats is older and more widespread than previously thought. Studies were conducted using a CDV isolate from a fatal natural infection in a Chinese leopard from a North American zoo.[53] Specific pathogen-free cats inoculated with this leopard isolate developed transient CDV viremia and pronounced lymphopenia but did not show any clinical symptoms of illness. Another study attempting to isolate viruses from the CNS of cats demonstrated eosinophilic intranuclear and intracytoplasmic inclusions in co-cultured cells from the CNS of three cats.[56] Although no virus was isolated, on electron microscopic examination, these structures were similar in morphology to paramyxovirus nucleocapsids.[56]

CDV can cause fatal pneumonia and CNS disease in large, nondomestic felids. Domestic cats may acquire CDV infection but are apparently more resistant to clinical signs of illness. However, as we have seen with FPV, it may require only a small genetic change to alter the host spectrum of this agent. Presently, there are no approved vaccines available to protect cats from this viral infection. Should a CDV mutant become more pathogenic for the domestic cat population, a serious epidemic of disease might result. Therefore, veterinarians should be alert for signs of CDV-like illness in domestic cats.

Equine morbillivirus (EMV) is a newly recognized respiratory pathogen that affects primarily horses and human beings.[57] At present, the virus has been identified only in Australia. In experiments evaluating the infectivity of EMV for other species, domestic cats were found to be highly susceptible to this virus.[57] Cats could be infected with EMV by subcutaneous inoculation, intranasal exposure, oral ingestion, and direct contact with affected cats.[57] The incubation period for all routes of infection ranges from four to eight days. Clinical signs of illness include dyspnea, tachypnea, fever, malaise, anorexia, and lethargy.

Affected cats develop respiratory system lesions, including hydrothorax, severe pulmonary edema and congestion, and enlarged, edematous pulmonary lymph nodes.[57] Histologic changes include severe interstitial pneumonia, serofibrinous alveolar edema, intra-alveolar hemorrhage, thrombosis of small veins, alveolar wall necrosis, and syncytial cell formation in pulmonary tissue and the endothelium of pulmonary vessels. Some cats also have gastroenteric lesions consisting of congested ceca and edematous mesenteric lymph nodes. Syncytial cells are seen in the intestinal lymph nodes, spleen, and Peyer's patches.[57]

Clinical diagnosis of EMV infection is usually presumptive and based on a history of exposure and appropriate clinical signs. There is no specific therapy; treatment is symptomatic and supportive, but mortality is high. Confirmation of EMV infection is made by finding characteristic syncytia in small pulmonary blood vessels and other organs on histopathologic examination.[57]

Because the geographic distribution of this virus is limited and disease outbreaks are quite small and sporadic, it is unlikely that a vaccine will be developed against this agent.

REFERENCES

1. Truyen U, et al: Evolution of the feline-subgroup of parvoviruses and control of canine host range in vivo. J Virol 69:4702, 1995.
2. Spitzer AL, et al: Tropic determination for canine and feline panleukopenia virus functions through the capsid protein VP2. J Gen Virol 78:925, 1997.
3. Hofmann-Lehmann R, et al: Prevalence of antibodies to feline parvovirus, calicivirus, herpesvirus, coronavirus, and immunodeficiency virus and of feline leukemia virus and the interrelationship of these viral infections in free-ranging lions in east Africa. Clin Diagn Lab Immunol 3:554, 1996.
4. Kennedy MA, et al: Virucidal efficacy of the newer quaternary ammonium compounds. J Am Anim Hosp Assoc 31:254, 1995.
5. Buonavoglia C, et al: Use of a feline panleukopenia modified live virus vaccine in cats in the primary-stage of feline immunodeficiency virus infection. Zentralbl Veterinarmed 40:343, 1993.
6. Scott FW, et al: Duration of immunity in cats vaccinated with an inactivated feline panleukopenia, herpesvirus, and calicivirus vaccine. Feline Pract 25:12, 1997.
7. Hickman MA, et al: An epizootic of feline herpesvirus, type 1 in a large specific pathogen-free colony and attempts to eradicate the infection by identification and culling of carriers. Lab Anim 28:320, 1994.
8. Stiles J: Treatment of cats with ocular disease attributable to herpesvirus infection: 17 cases (1983–1993). JAVMA 207:599, 1995.
9. Stiles J, et al: Comparison of nested polymerase chain reaction, virus isolation, and fluorescent antibody testing for identifying feline herpesvirus in cats with conjunctivitis. Am J Vet Res 58:804, 1997.
10. Stiles J, et al: Use of nested polymerase chain reaction to identify feline herpesvirus in ocular tissue from clinically normal cats and corneal sequestra or conjunctivitis. Am J Vet Res 58:338, 1997.

11. Weiss RC: Synergistic antiviral activities of acyclovir and recombinant human leukocyte (alpha) interferon on feline herpesvirus replication. Am J Vet Res 50:1672, 1989.

12. Flodin NW: The metabolic roles, pharmacology, and toxicology of lysine. J Am Coll Nutr 16:7, 1997.

13. Owens JG: Pharmacokinetics of acyclovir in the cat. J Vet Pharmacol Ther 19:488, 1996.

14. Nasisse MP, et al: Effects of valacyclovir in cats infected with feline herpesvirus-1. Am J Vet Res 58:1141, 1997.

15. Sussman MD, et al: Vaccination of cats for feline rhinotracheitis results in a quantitative reduction of virulent feline herpesvirus-1 latency load after challenge. Virology 228:379, 1997.

16. Pedersen NC: Feline herpesvirus. In Pedersen NC (ed): Feline Infectious Diseases. Goleta, CA, American Veterinary Publications, 1988, p 26.

17. TerWee J, et al: Comparison of the primary signs induced by experimental exposure to either a pneumotropic or "limping" strain of feline calicivirus. Vet Microbiol 56:33, 1997.

18. Geissler K, et al: Genetic and antigenic heterogeneity among feline calicivirus isolates from distinct disease manifestations. Virus Res 48:193, 1997.

19. Kadoi K, et al: A strain of calicivirus isolated from lions with vesicular lesions on the tongue and snout. New Microbiol 20:141, 1997.

20. Radford AD, et al: The use of sequence analysis of a feline calicivirus (FCV) hypervariable region in the epidemiological investigation of FCV related disease and vaccine failures. Vaccine 15:1451, 1997.

21. Reubel GH, et al: Effect of chronic feline immunodeficiency virus infection on experimental feline calicivirus-induced disease. Vet Microbiol 39:335, 1994.

22. Dawson S, et al: Acute arthritis of cats associated with feline calicivirus infection. Res Vet Sci 56:133, 1994.

23. Dick CP, et al: Sites of persistence of feline calicivirus. Res Vet Sci 47:367, 1989.

24. Waters L, et al: Chronic gingivitis in a colony of cats infected with feline immunodeficiency virus and feline calicivirus. Vet Rec 132:340, 1993.

25. Lauritzen A, et al: Serological analysis of feline calicivirus isolates from the United States and United Kingdom. Vet Microbiol 56:55, 1997.

26. Patronek GJ: Free-roaming feral cats—their impact on wildlife and human beings. JAVMA 212:218, 1998.

27. Krebs JW, et al: Rabies surveillance in the United States during 1996. JAVMA 211:1525, 1997.

28. Rupprecht CE: The ascension of wildlife rabies: A cause for public health concern or intervention? Emerg Infect Dis 1:107, 1995.

29. Noah DL, et al: Mass human exposure to rabies in New Hampshire: Exposures, treatment, and cost. Am J Public Health 86:1149, 1996.

30. Tepsumethanon V, et al: Fluorescent antibody test for rabies: Prospective study of 8,987 brains. Clin Infect Dis 25:1459, 1997.

31. Jayakumar R, et al: Detection of rabies virus antigen in animals by avidin-biotin dot ELISA. Zentralbl Bakteriol 285:82, 1996.

32. Presutti RJ, et al: Bite wounds: Early treatment and prophylaxis against infectious complications. Postgrad Med 101:243, 1997.

33. Reubel GH, et al: Effects of incidental infections and immune activation on disease progression in experimentally feline immunodeficiency virus–infected cats. J Acquir Immune Defic Syndr 7:1003, 1994.

34. Canese MG, et al: Feline poxvirus infection: A case report. Schweiz Arch Tierheilkd 139:454, 1997.

35. Naidoo J, et al: Characterization of orthopox viruses isolated from feline infections in Britain. Arch Virol 125:261, 1992.

36. Stolz W, et al: Characteristic but unfamiliar—the catpox infection, transmitted by a domestic cat. Dermatology 193:140, 1996.

37. Durrwald R, et al: Borna disease virus (BDV) a (zoonotic) worldwide pathogen: A review of the history of the disease and the virus infection with a comprehensive bibliography. Zentralbl Veterinarmed 44:147, 1997.

38. Lundgren AL, et al: Neurological disease and encephalitis in cats experimentally infected with Borna disease virus. Acta Neuropathol 93:391, 1997.

39. Narang H: Origin and implications of bovine spongiform encephalopathy. Proc Soc Exp Biol Med 211:306, 1996.

40. Fraser H, et al: Transmission of feline spongiform encephalopathy to mice. Vet Rec 134:449, 1994.

41. Kurtz JB, et al: Astroviruses: Human and animal. Ciba Found Symp 128:92, 1987.

42. Harbour DA, et al: Natural and experimental astrovirus infection of cats. Vet Rec 120:555, 1987.

43. Mochizuki M, et al: Isolation from diarrheal and asymptomatic kittens of three rotavirus strains that belong to the AU-1 genogroup of human rotaviruses. J Clin Microbiol 35:1272, 1997.

44. Snodgrass DR, et al: A rotavirus from kittens. Vet Rec 104:222, 1979.

45. Vonsover A, et al: Identification of feline- and canine-like rotaviruses isolated from humans by restriction fragment length polymorphism assay. J Clin Microbiol 31:1783, 1993.

46. Muir P, et al: Reovirus type 2 in domestic cats: Isolation and experimental transmission. Vet Microbiol 30:309, 1992.

47. Pedersen NC: Pseudorabies. In Pedersen NC (ed): Feline Infectious Diseases. Goleta, CA, American Veterinary Publications, 1988, p 29.

48. Card JP, et al: Differential tropism of pseudorabies virus for sensory neurons in the cat. J Neurovirol 3:49, 1997.

49. Winkler IG, et al: A rapid streptavidin-capture ELISA specific for the detection of antibodies to feline foamy virus. J Immunol Methods 207:69, 1997.

50. Zenger E, et al: Evaluation of cofactor effect of feline syncytium-forming virus on feline immunodeficiency virus infection. Am J Vet Res 54:713, 1993.

51. Winkler I, et al: Characterization of the genome of feline foamy virus and its proteins shows distinct features different from those of primate spumaviruses. J Virol 71:6727, 1997.

52. Harder TC, et al: Phylogenetic evidence of canine distemper in Serengeti's lions. Vaccine 13:521, 1995.

53. Harder TC, et al: Canine distemper virus from diseased large felids: Biological properties and phylogenetic relationships. J Gen Virol 77:397, 1996.

54. Myers DL, et al: Distemper: Not a new disease in lions and tigers. Clin Diagn Lab Immunol 4:180, 1997.

55. Appel MJ, et al: Canine distemper epizootic in lions, tigers, and leopards in North America. J Vet Diagn Invest 6:277, 1994.

56. Wilcox GE, et al: Recovery of viral agents from the central nervous system of cats. Vet Microbiol 9:355, 1984.

57. Hooper PT, et al: The lesions of experimental equine morbillivirus disease in cats and guinea pigs. Vet Pathol 34:323, 1997.

CHAPTER 93

SYSTEMIC MYCOSES

Joseph Taboada

Systemic mycoses are fungal infections that disseminate from a single portal of entry. The respiratory system serves as the portal of entry for most systemic fungi that affect the dog and cat, but the gastrointestinal system is occasionally implicated. Whereas opportunistic fungi can cause a number of systemic fungal infections (sporotrichosis, aspergillosis, candidiasis, zygomycosis, hyalohyphomycosis, and phaeohyphomycosis), blastomycosis, cryptococcosis, histoplasmosis, and coccidioidomycosis are the most common systemic my-coses seen in small animal practice in North America (Fig. 93–1). Aspergillosis and candidiasis, two common systemic mycotic infections in people, are relatively rare in dogs and cats. Aspergillus most often causes infiltrative nasal and frontal sinus disease rather than systemic infection in dogs and cats. Pythiosis, a gastrointestinal infection caused by Pythium insidiosum, and prototothecosis, a systemic infection caused by Prototheca spp., are protistan-caused infections that mimic the systemic mycoses (see Chapter 87). Because

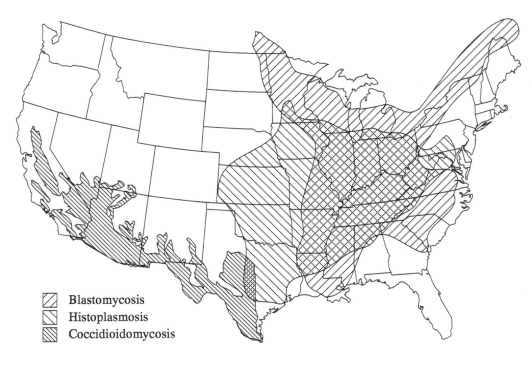

Figure 93–1. Areas in the United States endemic for blastomycosis, coccidioidomycosis, and histoplasmosis.

Blastomycosis
Histoplasmosis
Coccidioidomycosis

Pythium insidiosum is a hyphal organism in infected tissue, it is often confused with other opportunistic invaders (such as the Zygomycetes), even after histologic evidence of infectious disease has been noted.

Systemic mycoses have become a problem of growing importance in human medicine because of immune-suppressive diseases such as AIDS and the expanded use of immune-suppressive therapy for cancer and immune-mediated diseases. Immune suppression does not play as important a role in veterinary patients, but the growing importance of such diseases in humans has led to tremendous pharmacologic advances in the treatment of fungal infections over the past decade. These advances have changed the way we treat systemic mycoses in dogs and cats.[1, 2]

Systemic fungal infections cause disease, the clinical signs of which are dependent on which systems are involved (Table 93–1). Weight loss, lymphadenopathy, and fever are typical of most systemic mycoses. Because the respiratory system is the typical portal of entry, clinical signs such as cough, dyspnea, and exercise intolerance are common. If the gastrointestinal system is the portal of entry, as may occur with histoplasmosis, malabsorption often leads to severe diarrhea and weight loss.

In most cases, diagnosis of a systemic mycosis is dependent on demonstrating the presence of the organism in tissue. For yeasts such as *Cryptococcus* or *Candida* or for dimorphic fungi that have a yeast phase in tissue such as *Blastomyces dermatitidis* or *Histoplasma capsulatum*, the diagnosis can usually be made cytologically. For other fungi that grow as hyphal organisms in infected tissue, the diagnosis is usually dependent on histopathology or culture. Serology is used extensively in practice for the diagnosis of fungal infections, but with the exception of tests for cryptococcal antigen, most commercially available assays determine the presence of antibody and may indicate only previous exposure. As polymerase chain reaction (PCR) techniques become more readily available and undergo rigorous evaluation to determine specificity and sensitivity, the diagnostic evaluation of animals suspected of having fungal disease will likely change dramatically.

Many treatment regimens have been reported for the management of various systemic mycoses, but few veterinary studies have been performed that have critically evaluated these agents in a prospective manner, and studies comparing treatment regimens are practically nonexistent. A lack of controlled observations has led to recommendations that are based primarily on anecdotal information, extrapolation from what is done in people, and small retrospective studies. The "best" treatment regimen for any given systemic fungal infection is therefore largely a matter of opinion.

The principal antifungal agents are antibiotics produced by microorganisms (e.g., amphotericin B and griseofulvin) and synthetic agents (e.g., potassium iodide, flucytosine, azole derivatives, allylamine derivatives, and chitin synthesis inhibitors). The options for treatment of fungal infections increased substantially during the 1990s with the Food and Drug Administration's approval of the azole derivatives fluconazole and itraconazole. Clinical trials have been performed using itraconazole,[3–6] and case reports and retrospective reviews documenting the use of both drugs have started to appear in the veterinary literature. The high cost of most antifungal agents and the long treatment protocols required affect the number of cases that are treated, both limiting and probably epidemiologically biasing the data that have been generated to date. Adding to the difficulty of assessing the efficacy of antifungal agents are that the pharmacologic principles of antifungal therapy are only partially understood, in vitro testing of fungi for resistance to antifungal agents provides little clinically useful information, susceptibility testing yields variable results, and tissue distribution of antifungal agents correlates variably with the clinical outcome.

ANTIFUNGAL AGENTS

AMPHOTERICIN B

Amphotericin B is a polyene macrolide antibiotic produced by the aerobic actinomycete *Streptomyces nodosus*. It

TABLE 93–1. DIFFERENTIAL DIAGNOSES FOR SYSTEMIC MANIFESTATIONS OF SYSTEMIC MYCOSES

Multisystemic granulomatous, neoplastic, and immune-mediated diseases must be differentiated from disseminated systemic mycoses

Differential Diagnosis for Nodular Skin Disease

BACTERIAL SKIN DISEASE

Actinomycosis
Mycobacteriosis
Botryomycosis
Brucellosis
Rhodococcus equi infection

MYCOTIC AND MISCELLANEOUS INFECTIOUS SKIN DISEASE

Cryptococcosis
Coccidioidomycosis
Sporotrichosis
Basidiobolomycosis
Conidiobolomycosis
Phaeohyphomycosis
Hyalohyphomycosis
Eumycotic mycetoma
Dermatophytic mycetoma
Protothecosis
Pythiosis
Nodular leishmaniasis

NONINFECTIOUS PYOGRANULOMATOUS SKIN DISEASE

Foreign body reaction
Idiopathic nodular panniculitis
Sebaceous adenitis (nodular form)
Canine cutaneous sterile pyogranuloma/granuloma syndrome

NEOPLASIA

Squamous cell carcinoma
Cutaneous lymphoma
Mycosis fungoides (cutaneous T-cell lymphoma)
Cutaneous histiocytosis

MISCELLANEOUS DISEASES

Systemic lupus erythematosus
Systemic vasculitis
Cutaneous embolic disease

Differential Diagnosis for Chorioretinitis, Exudative Retinal Detachment, and Panophthalmitis

FUNGAL

Cryptococcosis
Coccidioidomycosis
Geotrichosis
Histoplasmosis
Aspergillosis

NEOPLASIA

Lymphosarcoma
Metastatic neoplasia

MISCELLANEOUS INFECTIOUS CAUSES

Protothecosis
Brucellosis
Toxoplasmosis
Neosporum caninum infection
Leishmaniasis

Lymphadenopathy must be differentiated from numerous causes, including lymphosarcoma, other fungal infections, rickettsial diseases, brucellosis, mycobacteriosis, protothecosis, and leishmaniasis

Solitary bone lesions must be differentiated from primary or metastatic bony neoplasia and other fungal or bacterial osteomyelitis

---

was discovered in the 1950s and was one of the first antifungal agents found to be widely useful in treating systemic fungal infections. It has become the gold standard against which the efficacy of new antifungal agents is compared, and despite significant toxicity and poor oral bioavailability, it remains the drug of choice for the treatment of many invasive mycoses. The traditional formulation of amphotericin B is a desoxycholate preparation (Fungizone) that, after intravenous administration, is highly protein bound (91 to 95 per cent), primarily to lipoproteins, erythrocytes, and cholesterol in the plasma, and then is redistributed from the blood to the tissues. Penetration into the cerebrospinal fluid (CSF) is poor. Tissue accumulation accounts for the majority of drug disposition. Only 5 to 10 per cent of amphotericin B is excreted in the urine and bile. Although great care should be used when treating animals in renal or hepatic failure, no modification of the dosage is necessary unless the renal or hepatic damage is attributable to the drug. Amphotericin B acts by binding to sterols in cell membranes, especially ergosterol in fungal cell membranes. Binding alters membrane permeability, causing leakage of sodium, potassium, and hydrogen ions and eventually leading to cell death. Amphotericin B also probably has important immunostimulatory effects by oxidation-dependent stimulation of host macrophages.[7] Stimulation of macrophages may play an important role in the treatment of some systemic fungal infections with amphotericin B. Toxic effects are attributable to affinity for sterols such as cholesterol in mammalian cell membranes.

Amphotericin B has been effective in the treatment of blastomycosis, histoplasmosis, coccidioidomycosis, crypto-coccosis, systemic candidiasis, zygomycosis, and pythiosis (in horses). It is administered as a series of intravenous infusions (0.22 to 0.5 mg/lb [0.5 to 1 mg/kg] every 48 hours to a cumulative dose of 2 to 4 mg/lb [4 to 8 mg/kg] or until azotemia occurs). Bolus dosing over 5 to 10 minutes is common, but renal toxicity can be reduced by infusing the drug in 5 per cent dextrose over 1 to 5 hours. Nephrotoxicity is the most significant adverse effect and is dose-dependent.[8] Generally, renal azotemia is reversible, and renal function returns to normal following cessation of therapy. However, return to pretreatment values may take several months. Irreversible renal dysfunction is more likely in animals with preexisting azotemia or in those receiving other nephrotoxic agents such as aminoglycosides. Blood urea nitrogen (BUN) should be monitored before each administration of amphotericin B. If the BUN is greater than 50 mg/dL, the drug should be discontinued until the azotemia has resolved. Nephrotoxicity is thought to be caused by disruption of renal tubular epithelial cell permeability resulting in increased delivery of chloride ions to the distal tubule, with subsequent decreased glomerular filtration rate (GFR) being the result of tubuloglomerular feedback. This feedback is amplified by sodium depletion and suppressed by sodium loading. Administration of 0.9 per cent sodium chloride (5 to 10 mL/lb) before amphotericin B administration decreases the incidence of nephrotoxicity in people. Other possible mechanisms of nephrotoxicity include decreased renal blood flow and direct renal cellular toxicity. Tumor necrosis factor may also play a role in mediating amphotericin B–induced azotemia. Pentoxifylline, a hemorrheologic drug, seems to exert protective effects in people and rats. Mannitol and dopamine have also been shown to decrease nephrotoxicity in experimental situations. Other possible toxic effects include thrombophlebitis, pyrexia (usually ameliorated by pretreatment with nonsteroidal anti-inflammatory drugs or a low dose of prednisone), hypokalemia, distal renal tubular acidosis, hypomagnesemia, cardiac arrhythmias, and nonregenerative anemia.

In dog studies, lipid-complexed amphotericin B was determined to be 8 to 10 times less nephrotoxic than conventional amphotericin B.[9] The decreased toxicity is due to decreased renal cell uptake, reduced tubular toxicity, reduced free amphotericin in solution in plasma, and a selective transfer of amphotericin directly to fungal cell membranes. The reduced toxicity allows higher cumulative doses to be used, which increases drug efficacy. This increase in efficacy is also thought to be related to rapid uptake of lipid complexes by phagocytic cells of the reticuloendothelial (RE) system, which allows sites of inflammation and organs with high RE system activity such as liver, spleen, and lung to receive higher doses of amphotericin B despite minimal renal uptake.[10]

There are currently three lipid formulations of amphotericin B that are marketed for clinical use in human patients: amphotericin B lipid complex (ABLC; Abelcet), a mixture of two phospholipids and amphotericin B; amphotericin B colloidal dispersion (Amphotec), a cholesterol sulfate complexed to amphotericin B; and liposome-encapsulated amphotericin B (AmBisome).[11] Clinical trials in people have documented improvement in treatment outcomes for *Candida, Aspergillus, Cryptococcus, Mucor, Histoplasma, Blastomyces*, and *Coccidioides* infections. ABLC has been used successfully to treat blastomycosis in dogs without significant nephrotoxicity being noted.[12] ABLC can be used in dogs at a dose of 0.5 to 1 mg/lb (1 to 2 mg/kg) intravenously three times a week to a cumulative dose of 11 mg/lb. Azotemia is rare.

ORAL AZOLE ANTIFUNGAL DRUGS

The azoles are classified as imidazoles (ketoconazole [Nizoral]) or triazoles (fluconazole [Diflucan] and itraconazole [Sporanox]), according to whether they contain two or three nitrogen atoms, respectively, in the five-member azole ring. Ketoconazole and itraconazole have similar pharmacologic profiles, but fluconazole is unique because of its comparatively small molecular size and low lipophilicity. The azole antifungal agents act by inhibiting ergosterol synthesis through interaction with 14-α-demethylase, a cytochrome P-450 enzyme that is necessary for the conversion of lanosterol to ergosterol. Similar interaction in mammalian cells with enzymes dependent on cytochrome P-450 also mediates some of the major toxic effects. The imidazoles are much more potent inhibitors of mammalian cell cytochrome P-450 than are the triazoles. Other antifungal effects include inhibition of endogenous respiration, toxic interaction with membrane phospholipids, and inhibition of morphogenetic transformation of yeasts to the mycelial forms. Some of the azole antifungal drugs, especially itraconazole and ketoconazole, are potent immune-suppressive agents, suppressing T-lymphocyte proliferation in vitro. Ketoconazole has anti-inflammatory properties that are probably mediated through inhibition of 5-lipoxygenase activity.

Ketoconazole and itraconazole are weak bases that require an acid environment for maximal oral absorption. Antacid administration inhibits oral bioavailability, and the bioavailability of itraconazole is two to three times higher when taken with food. Fluconazole is not affected by gastric pH, and food does not affect its oral bioavailability. Peak plasma concentrations of itraconazole and fluconazole do not occur until 6 to 14 days after treatment is begun. This may account for the clinical lag time. A loading dose can be given for the first three days of treatment to reduce the time until steady-state concentrations are attained. Ketoconazole and itraconazole are extensively bound to plasma proteins (>99 per cent), but because of their lipophilicity, both drugs distribute well throughout most tissues, but concentrations in urine and CSF are typically very low. Neither drug crosses the blood-brain, blood-prostate, or blood-ocular barrier well. Despite this, central nervous system (CNS), prostatic, and ocular fungal infections respond well to treatment with itraconazole. Itraconazole is concentrated in the skin, with delivery being via sebum. Sebum concentrations are 5 to 10 times higher than plasma concentrations, and detectable amounts persist for up to 14 days after the drug is discontinued. Detectable concentrations can be found in the hair and stratum corneum for up to four weeks. This property makes itraconazole ideal for treating dermatophyte infections and other fungal infections with cutaneous manifestations. Fluconazole is minimally protein-bound and highly water-soluble and distributes similarly to free water. High concentrations can be found in urine, CSF, and ocular fluids, and the drug crosses the blood-brain, blood-prostate, and blood-ocular barriers well. Ketoconazole and itraconazole are extensively metabolized in the liver and excreted in the bile and, to a lesser extent, in the urine. In contrast, fluconazole is minimally metabolized, and approximately 80 per cent is excreted unchanged in the urine; consequently, the dose of fluconazole should be reduced in animals with decreased GFR.

The azole antifungal agents are widely used in veterinary medicine for treating systemic fungal infections.[3, 5, 6, 13] Ketoconazole has been effective as a sole therapeutic agent in the management of blastomycosis, histoplasmosis, cryptococcosis, and coccidioidomycosis. However, with the possible exception of coccidioidomycosis, ketoconazole is probably not as effective as amphotericin B. Ketoconazole is primarily used in conjunction with amphotericin B when managing systemic infections, allowing lower doses of amphotericin B to be used and thus limiting nephrotoxicity. Itraconazole and fluconazole are more effective than ketoconazole and can be used as sole agents in the management of most systemic mycoses. Itraconazole appears to be more effective than fluconazole in most situations, but fluconazole may be superior in the management of cryptococcosis and CNS, prostatic, and urinary tract infections. Itraconazole is the treatment of choice for blastomycosis in dogs and probably cats and is the primary treatment for systemic aspergillosis in people. Itraconazole has recently proved very effective as a sole treatment agent for histoplasmosis in cats.[5] The author has found itraconazole to be effective in treating about 20 per cent of dogs with gastrointestinal pythiosis, despite the fact that *Pythium insidiosum* does not contain significant concentrations of membrane ergosterol. In treating most systemic fungal infections, there is a lag between the initiation of treatment and clinical improvement. In severely affected animals, amphotericin B should probably be used initially or in conjunction with the triazole during this lag period.

The dose of ketoconazole is 4.5 to 13.6 mg/lb (10 to 30 mg/kg) divided twice a day. Side effects are often limiting, especially at higher doses. Fluconazole (1 to 4.5 mg/lb; 2.5

to 10 mg/kg) and itraconazole (2.2 to 4.5 mg/lb; 5 to 10 mg/kg) are usually better tolerated. Pharmacokinetic studies of itraconazole have been performed in cats.[14] Based on these studies, the oral itraconazole solution is preferred to the capsules, with a 24-hour dosing interval being sufficient at 4.5 mg/lb (10 mg/kg). Steady-state concentrations take up to three weeks to achieve. Most adverse effects of itraconazole are related to high serum concentrations, and animals that exhibit adverse effects usually do well on half the original dose. Adverse effects of the azole antifungal agents are similar across the class. Ketoconazole is the least tolerated, and itraconazole appears to be the best. Dose-related gastrointestinal side effects (anorexia and vomiting) are most common, especially in cats. When these occur, dividing the dose into two treatments or reducing the dose may be of benefit. Azole-induced anorexia in cats is often ameliorated by the use of appetite stimulants such as oxazepam or cyproheptadine. Liver enzymes should be periodically monitored in animals being treated with azole antifungals. Asymptomatic increases in transaminase concentrations are seen in about half of animals treated with itraconazole, but this does not necessitate a change in therapy unless the animal also has anorexia, vomiting, depression, or abdominal pain. Enzyme concentrations often return to normal over time without intervention. Symptomatic hepatotoxicity is occasionally seen with ketoconazole use but is unusual following fluconazole or itraconazole administration. Cutaneous reactions are seen in approximately 7 per cent of dogs receiving itraconazole at a dose of 4.5 mg/lb (10 mg/kg).[3] A local ulcerative dermatitis due to a cutaneous vasculitis (Fig. 93–2) usually resolves shortly after the drug is discontinued. More severe reactions such as erythema multiforme or toxic epidermal necrolysis are rare. Thrombocytopenia has been associated with fluconazole use in people but has not been documented in animals. Adrenal insufficiency is possible with ketoconazole use. Azole interference with the activity of hepatic microsomal enzymes can lead to increased concentrations of coadministered drugs such as cyclosporine, digoxin, phenytoin, sulfonylureas, and warfarin.

FLUCYTOSINE

Flucytosine is a synthetic antifungal drug with activity attributed to disruption of protein synthesis by inhibition of DNA and RNA synthesis. The drug is synergistic with amphotericin B and is used almost exclusively as an adjunct to amphotericin B in the treatment of cryptococcosis. Flucytosine has good oral bioavailability. It is widely distributed and crosses the blood-brain barrier. The most common side effects are diarrhea, anorexia, and vomiting. Dose-dependent bone marrow suppression manifesting as neutropenia, thrombocytopenia, or pancytopenia is a less common but more significant toxicity. Cutaneous or mucocutaneous drug eruptions consisting of depigmentation followed by ulceration, exudation, and crust formation, occurring most frequently on the scrotum and nasal planum, have been described in a series of dogs.[15] Flucytosine is used in cats primarily as adjunctive therapy in the treatment of cryptococcosis. The dose of flucytosine used in cats is 125 to 250 mg orally divided two to four times a day.

ALLYLAMINES

Terbinafine is a synthetic allylamine antifungal drug that interferes with squalene epoxidase and is a potent inhibitor of ergosterol biosynthesis.[16] Squalene accumulation in the fungal cell may account for the drug's fungicidal activity. Most of the side effects in people are gastrointestinal, hepatobiliary dysfunction, and cutaneous reactions. Terbinafine is primarily used to treat dermatophytosis, sporotrichosis, dimorphic fungal infection, and aspergillosis. The drug dose ranges from 4.5 to 9 mg/lb (10 to 20 mg/kg) once a day.

CHITIN AND GLUCAN SYNTHESIS INHIBITORS

Drugs that inhibit the synthesis of chitin or glucan, two substances important to the structural and functional integrity of the fungal cell wall, hold promise as antifungal therapeutic agents. Chitin synthetase inhibitors, such as drugs in the nikkomycin class, and the lipopeptide inhibitors of fungal glucan synthase, such as the echinocandin and pneumocandin classes, are important investigational areas in antifungal research.[17] The only drug with a similar mechanism that has been evaluated in veterinary patients is lufenuron, a nonspecific inhibitor of chitin synthesis. In a pilot study, 17 dogs with coccidioidomycosis were treated with lufenuron at either 4.5 mg/lb (10 mg/kg) or 2.2 mg/lb (5 mg/kg) for 16 weeks. Response to therapy was generally slow, but dogs treated for 16 weeks remained free of symptoms for the one-year follow-up period.[1]

Figure 93–2. *A*, Lesion on the prepuce of a dachshund being treated for blastomycosis with itraconazole. The lesion is caused by an itraconazole-induced cutaneous vasculitis. *B*, Paronychial lesion caused by an itraconazole-induced cutaneous vasculitis in a Doberman pinscher.

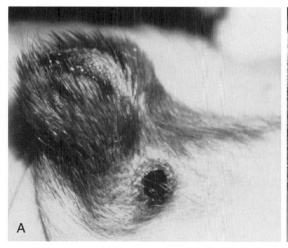
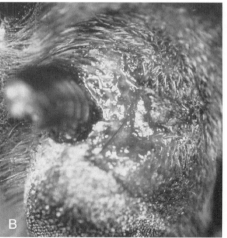

SPECIFIC SYSTEMIC MYCOSES

BLASTOMYCOSIS

Blastomycosis is a systemic fungal infection that usually originates in the lungs and then disseminates to the lymphatics, skin, eyes, bones, and other organs. The infection is seen in a wide variety of mammalian species, but the dog is most commonly affected. Young, male, large breed dogs (especially sporting breeds and hounds) living near water are at an increased risk.[18] The dog has been used as a sentinel animal for disease in humans, as the incidence in dogs is about 10 times higher than that in people. In endemic areas, blastomycosis usually occurs as a sporadic event, but outbreaks are occasionally observed in both dogs and people.[19–21] Epidemiologically, outbreaks can often be traced back to a common point source of exposure to a focal area in the environment from which infective spores had been aerosolized for a short time. Confirmation of the source is rarely achieved by organism isolation because of the transient nature of the environmental contamination and the difficulties inherent in laboratory isolation.

The dimorphic fungus *Blastomyces dermatitidis* is the causative agent of blastomycosis. In infected tissue or when cultured at 37°C, the organism is a thick-walled yeast that reproduces by budding. Most often, organisms in tissue have a single bud, attached to the mother cell by a broad base. When cultured at 25°C, mold colonies are characterized by a white cottony growth that may become tan as the colony ages. The colonies grow slowly and contain branching, septate 1- to 2-μm mycelia that form round to piriform 2- to 10-μm conidia resembling the microconidia of *Histoplasma capsulatum*. In nature, *Blastomyces dermatitidis* is probably a soil saprophyte, but the reservoir remains unresolved because the organism can rarely be cultured from the environment. In those unusual situations in which the organism is found, it is usually cultured from wet, acidic or sandy soil containing decaying wood, animal feces, or other organic enrichment.[22] Moisture appears to be important to growth and transmission.

Disease occurrence is reported primarily in a geographically restricted distribution that follows the Mississippi, Ohio, Missouri, Tennessee, and St. Lawrence Rivers, the southern Great Lakes, and the southern mid-Atlantic states. Within these geographic regions, infections are generally limited to smaller geographic pockets, with most affected animals living within a quarter of a mile of water.[21, 23] It is not unusual for one veterinary practice within an endemic area to diagnose blastomycosis commonly while another practice located within the same county rarely encounters the infection.

Pathophysiology

Blastomycosis is not a contagious disease. It follows contact with the organism in the environment. Infection usually occurs via a respiratory route after the host inhales infective conidiophores. Rarely, disease may be seen following direct inoculation.[24] The incubation period varies from 5 to 12 weeks. Rain, dew, fog, or mist may play a critical role in liberating conidiophores from the environment. In addition, activities that disrupt the soil such as digging or construction may play a role in the aerosolization of spores. After inhalation, conidia are phagocytized by alveolar macrophages and transform from the mycelial phase to the yeast phase. The yeasts stimulate local cell-mediated immunity, which results in a marked suppurative to pyogranulomatous inflammatory response. In some cases, the cell-mediated immune response controls the infection locally; in others, phagocytized yeasts are transported into the pulmonary interstitium, where they gain access to both the lymphatics and the vascular system. Hematogenous and lymphatic dissemination then results in multisystemic pyogranulomatous disease. Although dissemination can be to any organ system, the lymph nodes, eyes, skin, bones, subcutaneous tissues, and prostate are common organs affected in dogs; skin, subcutaneous tissues, eyes, CNS, and lymph nodes are most commonly affected in cats.[3, 23, 25, 26] It is unknown whether subclinical infection occurs in dogs and cats.

The immune response determines the severity of clinical disease, but blastomycosis is not considered an opportunistic infection. Antibody production occurs in most but not all cases, with the highest titers usually found in dogs with severe disseminated disease. Antibodies are not considered protective but can be used as a clinical marker of recent exposure or current disease. Recovery from infection is dependent on cell-mediated immunity. An adequate immune response may result in mild respiratory disease that resolves spontaneously. If dissemination has occurred, disease may be obvious in other organ systems, even without apparent pulmonary involvement. A poor immune response may result in severe pulmonary and disseminated disease.

Clinical Signs

Bluetick coonhounds, treeing-walker coonhounds, Pointers, and Weimaraners have the highest risk of infection.[18] Males are affected more commonly than females, and although any age dog can be affected, those in the 2- to 4-year age group have the highest incidence of disease. Exposure to possible environmental sources of infection, close proximity to water, and the likelihood of being housed in outdoor kennels probably explains the breed association. Clinical findings in animals with blastomycosis vary greatly because of the multisystemic nature of the disease. One or more organ systems may be involved.

Nonspecific signs such as anorexia, depression, weight loss, cachexia, and fever are common. Approximately 40 per cent of dogs are febrile, and dogs with chronic pulmonary disease are most likely to be cachectic. Because the lungs serve as the portal of entry for the *Blastomyces* organism, it is not surprising that pulmonary signs are seen in 65 to 85 per cent of affected dogs. Signs of pulmonary involvement range from mild respiratory distress when exercised to severe dyspnea at rest. Hypoxemia resulting in cyanosis is seen in the most severely affected cases and has a negative prognostic significance.[3] A dry, hacking cough is common. Mildly affected dogs may initially be diagnosed as having kennel cough. Enlarged perihilar lymph nodes compressing primary bronchi, as well as infiltrative bronchointerstitial and alveolar disease, contribute to the cough. Rapid, shallow respiratory efforts may be noted and can be caused by pleural effusion or pleuritic pain. Chylothorax and solid granulomatous masses are uncommonly reported complications of blastomycosis.

Diffuse lymphadenopathy is seen in about 40 to 60 per cent of dogs with blastomycosis. The lymph node enlargement can be marked and may be mistaken for lymphosarcoma if cytology or histopathology is not performed.

Cutaneous signs are reported in about 30 to 50 per cent of affected dogs and are also commonly noted in affected cats. Reported prevalences of skin disease in cases of blasto-

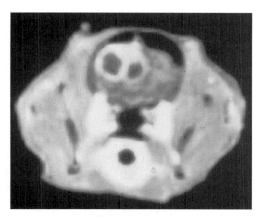

Figure 93–3. Cross-sectional magnetic resonance image revealing a contrast-enhancing mixed-intensity lesion in the rostral portion of the right cerebral cortex in a cat with blastomycosis.

mycosis may underestimate the actual prevalence, because lesions are sometimes small and easily overlooked unless a thorough dermatologic examination is performed. In experimental studies, over 70 per cent of dogs had cutaneous involvement. Typical skin lesions are characterized by single or multiple papules, nodules, or plaques that can ulcerate and drain a serosanguineous to purulent exudate. The nodular lesions are often quite small in dogs, but large abscesses occasionally occur, especially in cats. Paronychia is common in dogs, so the feet and nail beds should be closely examined.

Ocular involvement is noted in 20 to 50 per cent of cases. Posterior segment disease, characterized by chorioretinitis, retinal separation, subretinal granulomas, and vitreitis, usually occurs initially. Approximately 50 per cent of affected dogs have bilateral ocular involvement. Optic neuritis is occasionally noted and may signify more diffuse CNS involvement and a poorer prognosis. Anterior segment disease is usually, but not always, secondary to the posterior segment involvement. It may be characterized by conjunctivitis, keratitis, iridocyclitis, and eventually anterior uveitis and endophthalmitis. Secondary glaucoma is common in dogs with anterior segment disease. Long-term effects on vision are common, even in dogs that are aggressively treated. Dogs that have vision and only posterior segment disease at the time of diagnosis have a better prognosis for vision than dogs with anterior segment disease or endophthalmitis. It is unlikely that dogs with severe visual impairment at the time of diagnosis will regain vision, even with complete response to therapy.

Lameness caused by fungal osteomyelitis or painful paronychia is noted in about 25 per cent of dogs with blastomycosis. Fungal osteomyelitis is noted in about 10 to 15 per cent of dogs with blastomycosis. The pain and swelling are usually noted over epiphyseal regions below the elbow or stifle. Single lesions are more common than multiple lesions. Fungal mono- or polyarthritis is a rare cause of lameness.

The reproductive system is affected in approximately 5 to 10 per cent of affected dogs. Orchitis was noted in 16 per cent of 61 intact male dogs with blastomycosis seen at Louisiana State University. Fungal prostatitis or mastitis is reported in less than 5 per cent of affected dogs.

The nervous system is affected in less than 5 per cent of canine cases but is commonly affected in feline cases (Fig. 93–3). Advanced CNS imaging such as computed tomography (CT) or magnetic resonance imaging (MRI) should be considered in any cat diagnosed with blastomycosis, even if obvious neurologic signs are not apparent. The clinical signs associated with nervous system involvement are dependent on which parts of the CNS are involved, but often neurologic localization indicates diffuse or multifocal disease. Other potential sites of infection include liver, spleen, kidney, and nasal cavity.

Feline blastomycosis is less common than canine blastomycosis. The veterinary literature contains only scattered case reports and small case series.[26] Most of the clinical signs observed in dogs are also noted in cats. The main differences are that large abscesses are more common in cats than in dogs, and neurologic involvement is often noted.

Diagnosis

Blastomycosis is usually fairly easy to diagnose because of the large numbers of characteristic yeasts found within lesions, especially within infected skin, eyes, and lymph nodes.[23, 27]

Hematology is generally not helpful in the diagnosis. Complete blood count (CBC) results are often normal. When abnormal, a mild nonregenerative anemia and mature neutrophilia or neutrophilia with mild left shift may be seen. Clinical chemistry results are also often unremarkable. Hypoalbuminemia is the most consistent abnormality on serum chemistries. Hypercalcemia is noted in up to 10 per cent of cases.[23] The hypercalcemia is most often mild, but severe hypercalcemia requiring treatment is occasionally seen.

Radiographic assessment can be very helpful in the diagnostic evaluation of a dog or cat suspected of having blastomycosis (Figs. 93–4 to 93–6). Thoracic radiographs may reveal an interstitial pattern in about 70 per cent of canine cases. Although a nodular interstitial pattern is classically observed (41 per cent of cases), diffuse interstitial (24 per cent) and bronchointerstitial (5 per cent) patterns may also be prominent findings. An alveolar or mixed interstitial-alveolar pattern is observed in about 20 per cent of canine cases, and tracheobronchial lymphadenopathy is noted in about 30 per cent. Radiographic patterns mimicking other diseases such as mediastinal mass (8 per cent) or solitary pulmonary mass (8 per cent) are not as common. Pleural effusion (7 per cent) is rarely observed and when present may obscure pulmonary parenchymal changes. Pneumothorax induced by pulmonary blastomycosis is rare. Bone lesions may be noted on radiographs of long bones, especially those in the distal limbs. Most lesions occur on the extremi-

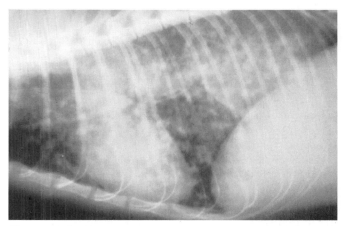

Figure 93–4. Lateral thoracic radiograph revealing a diffuse nodular interstitial pattern in a cat with blastomycosis.

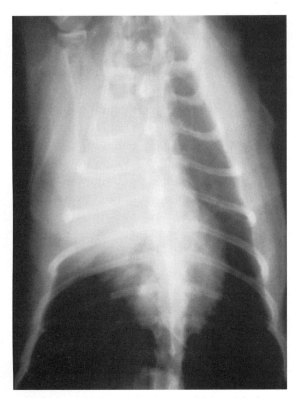

Figure 93–5. Consolidation of the right cranial lung lobe in a cat with blastomycosis. Consolidating and abscessing lesions are often seen in cats with systemic fungal infections.

ties, with most of the observed lesions being solitary foci of osteomyelitis. Lesions are osteolytic and typically occur at the ends of the long bones (Fig. 93–7). The forelimbs are affected more commonly than the rear limbs, with most extremity lesions being below the elbow or the stifle. Periosteal proliferation and soft tissue swelling are noted in about 50 per cent of lesions.

Definitive diagnosis is made by organism identification. This can be done by cytology, histopathology, or fungal culture. Cytology from affected tissue typically reveals pyogranulomatous or suppurative inflammation, often with thick-walled yeasts (8 to 12 μm in diameter, with 0.5- to 0.75-μm-thick walls) that bud to form daughter cells from a broad base (Fig. 93–8).[27] The yeast cells lack a capsule, helping to differentiate them from *Cryptococcus*. If the skin is affected, it yields organisms about 80 per cent of the time. This is the easiest and most useful source organism. Impression smears, skin scrapings, and fine-needle aspirate of nodular lesions can be used. Vitreal aspirates yield organisms from almost all affected eyes, and lymph node aspirates yield organisms approximately 60 per cent of the time. Bone and lung aspirates, transtracheal wash cytology, and bronchoalveolar lavage each yield organisms less than 50 per cent of the time.[23, 28] Urinalysis or prostatic wash cytology rarely reveals organisms. Rarely, organisms may be coughed up and swallowed and appear in the stool on fecal examination.[29] Care must be taken when handling samples that may contain yeast cells. Direct inoculation of organisms from needle-stick injury may result in localized cutaneous disease.[30] This is seen as an occupational hazard in laboratory workers who handle infective material and cultures and in veterinary personnel who sample infected tissue via fine-needle aspirate or biopsy. Local inoculation is probably rare as a cause of subcutaneous disease in dogs and cats.

Histopathology is generally characterized by purulent to pyogranulomatous lesions in infected tissue, with broad-based organisms usually being apparent. Special stains such as periodic acid–Schiff (PAS), Gridley's fungal, and Gomori's methenamine silver stain are best for demonstrating organisms.

Culture is not needed for definitive identification in clinical cases. If tissue is cultured, mycelial growth on Sabouraud's dextrose agar may take one to four weeks at 37°C, whereas yeast will grow on blood or brain-heart infusion agar in one to two weeks at 25°C. Culturing the organism from the environment is rarely achieved. The microbiology lab should be alerted if blastomycosis is suspected, as viable cultures of *Blastomyces dermatitidis* present a potential danger of infection for laboratory personnel if the plates are handled inappropriately.[31]

Serology should be used diagnostically only when a high degree of suspicion for blastomycosis exists and repeated attempts have failed to demonstrate the organisms. Several different types of serologic tests have been evaluated, including agar-gel immunodiffusion (AGID), complement fixation, enzyme-linked immunosorbent assay (ELISA), counterimmunoelectrophoresis, and agar-gel precipitin tests. An AGID test is most commonly used. This test detects antibodies directed against the fungal organism and has a sensitivity and specificity of approximately 90 per cent. Serology may be negative early in the disease course, and in some cases it may revert back to negative as the disease progresses. Antibody titers have not proved useful as an assessment tool in following response to therapy.

Treatment

Spontaneous recovery from symptomatic blastomycosis has been reported in people but rarely occurs in dogs and has not been reported in cats. Therefore, all cases of symptomatic blastomycosis in dogs and cats should be treated. Itraconazole is presently considered the treatment of choice, except in cases of moderate to severe hypoxemia, when amphotericin B should still be considered the drug of first choice.[3] Clinical cures can be expected in 70 to 75 per cent of treated cases. Treatment failure is most likely in dogs that are hypoxemic or have three or more systems affected. The dose of itraconazole that has proved effective is 2.2 mg/lb (5 mg/kg) orally once a day or divided twice a day. The drug should be continued for two to three months or until active disease is not apparent. Response to itraconazole treatment is minimal during the initial one to two weeks. A loading dose of 4.5 mg/lb (10 mg/kg) daily for the first three days of treatment may minimize this lag time. Treatment for an extra month after signs have resolved does not appear to reduce the likelihood of recurrence. Recurrence occurs in approximately 20 per cent of treated dogs from months to years after treatment has been discontinued.[3, 23] Thoracic radiographs are an insensitive tool in monitoring recovery, as significant radiographic abnormalities continue to improve for months after itraconazole treatment has been discontinued. Cats require 4.5 mg/lb (10 mg/kg) once a day or divided twice a day, and longer courses of treatment are usually required.

Ketoconazole is effective in less than 50 per cent of cases at an oral dose of 4.5 to 13.6 mg/lb (10 to 30 mg/kg) divided twice daily for a minimum of three months. The response rate is much lower, and the relapse rate is higher when compared with treatment with itraconazole; in addition, dogs generally have to be treated longer. Toxicity is more likely

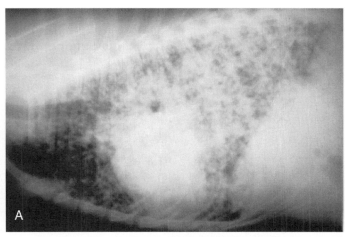

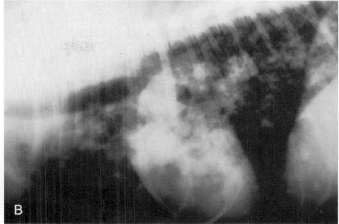

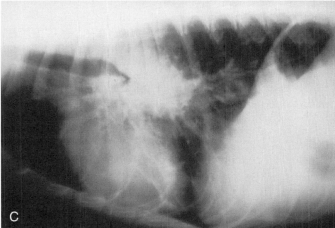

Figure 93–6. *A*, Lateral thoracic radiograph from a dog with blastomycosis revealing the classic "snowstorm" appearance of the nodular interstitial pattern commonly seen in systemic mycotic infections. *B*, Lateral thoracic radiograph from a dog with blastomycosis showing multiple large, ill-defined nodules and a bronchointerstitial pattern. *C*, Lateral thoracic radiograph from a dog with blastomycosis showing perihilar lymphadenopathy and a patchy interstitial pattern. Perihilar lymphadenopathy is common in systemic fungal infections, especially histoplasmosis and coccidioidomycosis.

with ketoconazole. Fluconazole has not been investigated for the treatment of blastomycosis in dogs and cats. The author's clinical impression is that it is not as effective as itraconazole, and fluconazole is more expensive. Fluconazole has been used successfully at high doses to treat blastomycosis in people.[32] Because fluconazole does not require a low gastric pH for maximal bioavailability and is not affected by the presence or lack of food, it may be a better initial choice in animals that will not eat. Because it is excreted in the urine and crosses the blood-brain, blood-ocular, and blood-prostatic barriers well, it may be a more appropriate treatment choice for urinary tract, prostatic, and CNS infections. Studies evaluating efficacy in these situations in dogs and cats have not been performed, however. The availability of a parenteral form of fluconazole makes it useful for treating severely affected or hypoxemic animals in which amphotericin B is not an appropriate option.

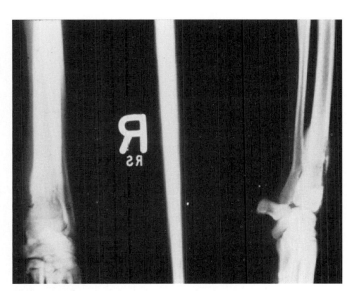

Figure 93–7. Lateral and anteroposterior view of the distal radius, ulna, and carpus from a Brittany spaniel with *Blastomyces* osteomyelitis. Note the bony lysis and periosteal proliferation involving the distal aspect of the proximal radius.

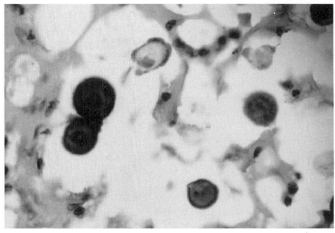

Figure 93–8. Impression smear from a dog with cutaneous lesions revealing thick-walled, budding yeast typical of *Blastomyces dermatitidis*.

Amphotericin B has very good efficacy against *Blastomyces* organisms. It is recommended that amphotericin B be used in combination with itraconazole or ketoconazole for severely affected or hypoxemic animals. Reconstituted, amphotericin B is mixed with 5 per cent dextrose in water (D5W) and administered as a rapid infusion over 10 minutes or as a longer infusion over one to six hours. The longer infusion is less likely to cause toxicity. The dose used is 0.22 mg/lb (0.5 mg/kg) for dogs, 0.1 mg/lb (0.25 mg/kg) for cats, intravenously every other day to a total dose of 1.8 mg/lb (4 mg/kg) when used in combination with azole antifungal drugs. A higher dose of 0.22 to 0.45 mg/lb (0.5 to 1 mg/kg) to a total dose of 3.6 mg/lb (8 mg/kg) is recommended if amphotericin B is the sole treatment agent. The BUN or creatinine should be monitored before each treatment, and amphotericin B should be discontinued if the dog or cat becomes azotemic (BUN >50 mg/dL, creatinine >3 mg/dL). The efficacy of amphotericin B when combined with ketoconazole or itraconazole is equal to that seen with itraconazole alone, but side effects are much more likely.

ABLC (Abelcet) allows higher total doses to be used, with decreased toxicity.[12] A dose of 0.45 to 0.9 mg/lb (1 to 2 mg/kg) intravenously every other day to a total dose of 5.4 to 10.9 mg/lb (12 to 24 mg/kg) has been recommended for dogs with blastomycosis. ABLC is expensive when compared with the deoxycholate form, but the author considers it the treatment of choice for severely affected dogs.

Ancillary therapy in hypoxemic animals should include oxygen, bronchodilators, and possibly antibiotics. Anterior uveitis should be treated with topical steroids and atropine; secondary glaucoma with dichlorphenamide (0.9 to 1.8 mg/lb [2 to 4 mg/kg] orally two to three times a day). Atropine should not be used in animals with glaucoma.

Approximately 70 to 75 per cent of dogs treated with either itraconazole or ketoconazole–amphotericin B combination respond completely to therapy. Dogs that die are usually those with severe respiratory disease and hypoxemia. Dogs that live through the first 10 days of therapy generally do well. Hypoxemia and the involvement of three or more systems are poor prognostic factors.[3] Relapse occurs in 15 to 20 per cent of treated dogs. It usually occurs in the first six months after treatment but can occur after a year or more. Relapses should be treated as new infections and are no less likely to respond.

Public Health Significance

Blastomycosis is not likely to be transmitted from animal to animal or from animal to person. Localized *Blastomyces* infections have occurred following needle-stick injuries when obtaining fine-needle aspirate from infected lesions, and laboratory workers can potentially be infected from fungal cultures.[30, 31] Outbreaks in which both people and dogs are affected are due to exposure to a common environmental source rather than to zoonosis.

HISTOPLASMOSIS

Histoplasmosis is a systemic fungal infection that usually originates in the lungs and potentially the gastrointestinal tract and then disseminates to the lymphatics, liver, spleen, bone marrow, eyes, and other organs. A wide variety of mammalian species can be affected, and cats may be more susceptible to infection than dogs. As with most systemic fungal diseases, animals younger than 4 years old are at an increased risk, but any age can be affected.

Histoplasmosis is caused by the dimorphic fungus *Histoplasma capsulatum*. In infected tissue or when cultured at 30 to 37°C, the organism is a yeast. The organism is found primarily intracellularly in infected tissue. When cultured at 25°C, the organism grows as a white cottony or buff-brown mold. The colonies take 7 to 10 days to grow. In the environment, *H. capsulatum* is a soil saprophyte that survives a wide range of moistures and temperatures. Nitrogen-rich soils, especially those containing bird or bat guano, appear ideal for supporting growth. The fungus is endemic throughout most of the temperate and subtropical regions of the world. Most cases of histoplasmosis in the United States occur in the central states, with the geographic distribution following the Mississippi, Ohio, and Missouri Rivers. The geographic distribution is wider than that of blastomycosis.

Pathophysiology

Histoplasmosis is not a contagious disease. Infection is probably via inhalation or ingestion of infective conidia from the environment. The respiratory system is likely the primary route of infection in cats, humans, and dogs, but the gastrointestinal system (following ingestion of conidia) may also be an important route in the dog.

After inhalation or ingestion, conidia transform from the mycelial phase to the yeast phase and are phagocytized by cells of the macrophage monocyte system, where they grow as facultative intracellular organisms. Hematogenous and lymphatic dissemination results in multisystemic disease. Although dissemination can be to any organ system, resulting in a granulomatous inflammatory response, the lungs, gastrointestinal system, lymph nodes, liver, spleen, bone marrow, eyes, and adrenal glands are common organs affected in dogs; lungs, liver, lymph nodes, eyes, and bone marrow are most commonly affected in cats. The incubation period is 12 to 16 days in dogs and humans.

The cell-mediated immune response determines the severity of clinical disease, with subclinical infection probably being common. Most cases of infection are sporadic events, but point-source outbreaks of disease are occasionally reported in both dogs and humans. Epidemiologically, these outbreaks are usually associated with exposure to areas heavily contaminated with *Histoplasma* organisms such as chicken coops, bat habitats, or starling roosts.

Clinical Signs

Feline histoplasmosis occurs most commonly in cats younger than 4 years of age. There is no breed or sex predilection. Disease in cats is usually insidious in onset and nonspecific, with clinical findings varying greatly because of the multisystemic nature of the infection. Depression, anorexia, fever, pale mucous membranes, and weight loss are common. Pulmonary involvement, as evidenced by dyspnea, tachypnea, or abnormal lung sounds, is seen in about 50 per cent of affected cats. Cough is uncommon. Hepatomegaly, splenomegaly, or lymphadenopathy is noted in about a third of affected cats. Ocular involvement may result in abnormal retinal pigment proliferation, retinal edema, granulomatous chorioretinitis, anterior uveitis, panophthalmitis, or optic neuritis. Retinal detachment and secondary glaucoma are less common than in animals affected with blastomycosis. Fungal osteomyelitis may cause lameness in one or more limbs. Cutaneous lesions consisting of multiple small nodules that may ulcerate and drain or crust over are noted less commonly than in animals affected with blastomycosis.

Gastrointestinal signs other than anorexia are uncommon in cats with histoplasmosis. Oral and lingual ulceration has been reported as an unusual manifestation. Icterus is occasionally seen in cats with hepatic involvement.

Canine histoplasmosis is also most commonly seen in dogs younger than 4 years of age. Male dogs are affected 1.2 times as frequently as female dogs, and Pointers, Weimaraners, and Brittany spaniels may be overrepresented. The clinical findings are related to the route of infection and the extent of systemic dissemination. Clinically inapparent infection is probably common following inhalation of organisms. In those dogs showing clinical signs, findings vary greatly, but gastrointestinal signs are most common (Table 93–2). Large-intestinal diarrhea with tenesmus, mucus, and fresh blood is most common early in the disease course. Small-intestinal diarrhea that may be voluminous and associated with malabsorption and/or protein-losing enteropathy may become apparent as the disease progresses. Nonspecific clinical signs such as fever, anorexia, depression, and severe weight loss are common and may be caused by elaboration of inflammatory mediators such as tumor necrosis factor and interleukin-1. Abnormal lung sounds with or without coughing, tachypnea, or dyspnea are seen in less than 50 per cent of affected dogs. Pleural effusion is seen in rare cases and may contribute to respiratory signs.[33] Splenomegaly, hepatomegaly, and lymphadenopathy are occasionally seen.

Diagnosis

A normocytic-normochromic nonregenerative anemia is the most common CBC abnormality. It is caused by chronic inflammation, gastrointestinal blood loss, and bone marrow infection. Neutrophilia and monocytosis are often seen, but leukocyte counts are variable. Neutropenia and/or pancytopenia is noted in a minority of affected animals, especially in cats. The CBC rarely results in a definitive diagnosis, as Histoplasma organisms are only occasionally seen in monocytes or neutrophils and rarely in eosinophils. Thrombocytopenia due to increased utilization or platelet destruction is seen in as many as half of affected dogs and a third of affected cats. Serum chemistry abnormalities are nonspecific. Hypoalbuminemia is the most consistent abnormality. Increases in serum alanine aminotransferase (SALT), serum aspartate aminotransferase (SAST), alkaline phosphatase, and total bilirubin may indicate hepatic involvement. Hypercalcemia, although not as common as in dogs with blastomycosis, has been reported. Hypercalcemia is more common in cats than in dogs.[5] It should be noted that hypoalbuminemia lowers total serum calcium and may mask subtle hypercalcemia. Feline leukemia virus (FeLV) and feline immunodeficiency virus (FIV) tests are usually negative in cats.

Thoracic radiographs often reveal a diffuse interstitial or linear interstitial pattern that tends to coalesce to a nodular interstitial pattern (Fig. 93–9). Alveolar infiltrates are rarely reported. Hilar lymphadenopathy is common in dogs but unusual in cats. Calcified pulmonary infiltrates or hilar lymph nodes may indicate inactive disease in dogs. Osseous lesions consisting of osteolysis, periosteal new bone formation, and subperiosteal bone proliferation are rarely noted. Bones of the distal appendicular skeleton, especially carpal and tarsal bones, are affected most commonly.

Organism identification is required for definitive diagnosis. The most common means of organism identification is cytology. Cytology from affected tissue reveals pyogranulomatous inflammation, often with numerous small, round to oval intracellular yeast cells (2 to 4 μm in diameter) characterized by a basophilic center and a light halo caused by shrinkage of the cell from the cell wall during fixation (Fig. 93–10). Whereas multiple Histoplasma organisms are usually found within phagocytic cells of the mononuclear phagocyte system, a small number of the organisms are released from cells during slide preparation and may be seen free on the slides stained with a Wright-Giemsa–type stain. Samples for cytology should be collected from tissue with apparent abnormalities. In the cat, aspiration cytology from bone marrow or lymph nodes or cytology from tracheal wash or bronchoalveolar lavage is most likely to yield organisms. In the dog, cytology from rectal scrapings or biopsies and aspiration cytology from bone marrow, liver, lymph nodes, spleen, or tracheal wash or bronchoalveolar lavage are most likely to yield organisms. Buffy coat smears, cytology of pleural or peritoneal effusions, aspirates of lytic bone lesions, and aspirates or impression smears of nodular skin lesions may also yield organisms.

If organisms are not cytologically apparent, histopathology may be diagnostic. Pyogranulomatous lesions with multiple intracellular organisms are usually apparent. Histoplasmosis should be ruled out when granulomatous hepatitis or

TABLE 93–2. DIFFERENTIAL DIAGNOSIS FOR GASTROINTESTINAL SIGNS SEEN IN DOGS AND OCCASIONALLY CATS WITH HISTOPLASMOSIS

Large-Intestinal Disease

Diet-associated colitis
  Dietary hypersensitivity
  Foreign material–induced colitis
Idiopathic colitis
  Lymphocytic-plasmacytic colitis
  Eosinophilic colitis
  Granulomatous colitis
  Histiocytic ulcerative colitis of Boxer dogs
  Suppurative colitis
Parasitic and protozoal colitis
  Trichuriasis (whipworms)
  Ancylostomiasis (hookworms)
  Strongyloidiasis
  Entamebiasis
  Balantidiasis
  Giardiasis
Bacterial colitis
  Salmonella sp.
  Campylobacter jejuni
  Yersinia enterocolitica, Y. pseudotuberculosis
  Mycobacteria
  Clostridium perfringens, C. difficile
Candidiasis
Gastrointestinal pythiosis
Protothecosis
Cecocolic or ileocolic intussusception
Pancreatitis-associated colitis

Chronic Small-Intestinal Disease

Idiopathic inflammatory bowel disease
  Lymphocytic-plasmacytic enteritis
  Eosinophilic enteritis
  Granulomatous enteritis
Intestinal lymphosarcoma
Parasitic enteritis (ancylostomiasis, toxocariasis)
Chronic giardiasis
Small-intestinal bacterial overgrowth
Gastrointestinal pythiosis
Lymphangiectasia
Exocrine pancreatic insufficiency
Partial intestinal obstruction
Chronic enteropathy of Shar Peis
Immunoproliferative enteritis of basenjis

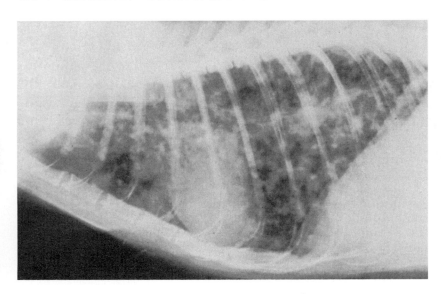

Figure 93–9. Lateral thoracic radiograph of an 8-year-old Siamese cat with a two-week history of dyspnea caused by *Histoplasma capsulatum* infection. This coalescing pattern of interstitial infiltrates is commonly seen in cats with pulmonary histoplasmosis.

other granulomatous or pyogranulomatous disease is seen on biopsy.[34] The yeast does not stain well with routine hematoxylin-eosin (H&E) stains, so special stains such as PAS, Gridley's fungal, and Gomori's methenamine silver stain are often used to demonstrate organisms.

Fungal culture from affected tissue can be used for diagnosis but is rarely needed in clinical cases. The organism grows as buff-brown mycelial growth on Sabouraud's dextrose agar. It usually takes 7 to 10 days to grow at room temperature. The yeast produces white, moist colonies on blood agar when grown at 30 to 37°C. The cultured organism is of pathogenic potential, which precludes culture attempts in a practice setting.

Serology is presently an ineffective method of diagnosis. Both false-positive and false-negative results are common. Poor correlation between necropsy findings and complement-fixation tests has been seen in multiple studies.

Treatment

Pulmonary histoplasmosis may be self-limited, but antifungal treatment is still recommended because of the potential for chronic dissemination. Dogs or cats with other systemic findings indicative of disseminated histoplasmosis usually die without treatment. Treatment protocols are similar to those described for blastomycosis, although they have not been as well studied. Longer treatment times are probably needed in most cases, but this is highly variable, depending on the severity of the infection and the response of the animal.

Itraconazole (4.5 mg/lb [10 mg/kg] orally once a day or divided twice a day) is considered the treatment of choice for feline histoplasmosis. At least two to four months of therapy is required. There are few studies that have evaluated the efficacy of itraconazole treatment, but in one study, all eight of eight cats treated were cured.[5] Ketoconazole is effective in about one third of affected cats. The addition of amphotericin B to ketoconazole treatment regimens may improve the efficacy, especially in severely affected cats. Fluconazole is likely effective but has not been well studied.

In dogs with histoplasmosis, ketoconazole has been described as the treatment of choice. Amphotericin B should be added to the protocol in fulminant cases. Itraconazole or fluconazole is safer and may result in better efficacy than ketoconazole, but evaluation has been minimal. For dogs with gastrointestinal disease, ancillary therapy should be considered along with antifungal therapy. A highly digestible diet should be fed to dogs with small-intestinal involvement, and fiber may be useful in dogs with signs of colitis. Small-intestinal bacterial overgrowth is probably common in dogs with histoplasmosis and should be treated with tylosin (4.5 to 9 mg/lb [10 to 20 mg/kg] orally twice a day), metronidazole (3.4 to 4.5 mg/lb [7.5 to 10 mg/kg] orally two to three times a day), tetracycline (6.8 to 9 mg/lb [15 to 20 mg/kg] orally three times a day), or amoxicillin (4.5 to 9 mg/lb [10 to 20 mg/kg] orally twice a day). Nonspecific therapy for diarrhea can include loperamide (0.045 to 0.09 mg/lb [0.1 to 0.2 mg/kg] orally twice a day) for small-intestinal diarrhea and sulfasalazine (4.5 to 13.6 mg/lb [10 to 30 mg/kg] orally two to three times a day) for large-intestinal diarrhea. Ancillary respiratory therapy may include oxygen and bronchodilators in hypoxemic animals and antibiotics in dogs with secondary bacterial pneumonia.

Resolution of clinical signs is the best means of patient monitoring. Rechecks should be performed monthly while dogs or cats are being treated and should include physical and ocular examinations as well as a chemistry panel to evaluate liver enzymes in animals receiving azole antifungals. Treatment should be continued for one month beyond resolution of clinical signs, and animals should be reevalu-

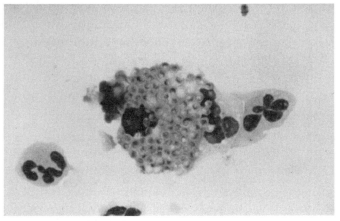

Figure 93–10. Cytology from a bronchoalveolar lavage sample revealing a macrophage containing many round to oval-shaped *Histoplasma* organisms in a cat with histoplasmosis. (Courtesy of Dr. Jan VanSteenhouse.)

ated three and six months after discontinuing therapy to assess for relapse. Serology is not useful in monitoring response to therapy or evaluating for relapse.

The prognosis is good for dogs with only pulmonary signs, but dogs with gastrointestinal or severe dissemination have a guarded prognosis. The prognosis is fair to good for cats treated with itraconazole, although long-term therapy may be required. Severely debilitated cats have a guarded prognosis.

COCCIDIOIDOMYCOSIS

Coccidioidomycosis is a systemic fungal infection that, like blastomycosis and histoplasmosis, typically originates in the lungs and may disseminate.[35] Other terms that have been used to describe coccidioidomycosis include valley fever and San Joaquin Valley fever. The disease can occur in most mammals and has been reported in cold-blooded vertebrates. Dogs appear to be affected more commonly than cats. Young (<4 years old) large and medium-size male dogs housed outside are most commonly affected, with the likelihood of infection decreasing with increasing age. The Boxer, Pointer, Australian shepherd, beagle, Scottish terrier, Doberman pinscher, and cocker spaniel may be at increased risk. There does not appear to be an age, breed, or sex predilection in cats.

Epidemics may occur in endemic areas when rainy periods are followed by drought conditions resulting in dust storms. Dust storms, earthquakes, or other conditions that spread arthrospores from the soil into the air contribute to outbreak conditions. A 10-fold increase in cases in California in 1992 and 1993 is best explained by this pattern of rain and drought, and increased numbers of cases in Los Angeles in 1993 may be attributable to soil disturbances associated with the 1993 earthquake and cleanup activities.[36]

Coccidioidomycosis is caused by the geophilic dimorphic fungus *Coccidioides immitis*. In infected tissue or when cultured at 37°C, the organism grows as a large spherule that gradually enlarges to 20 to 200 μm and is pathognomonic for coccidioidomycosis. Endospores are produced by cleavage from the wall of the spherule. In the environment or when cultured at 25°C, the organism grows as a mycelium that forms square to rectangular (2 to 4 μm by 3 to 10 μm) multinucleate arthrospores. The organism is easily cultured, but the mycelial form cannot be easily identified as *C. immitis*.

Coccidioides immitis is a soil saprophyte that grows only in areas with sandy alkaline soils, semiarid conditions, high summer and moderate winter temperatures, and low geographic elevations (sea level to a few hundred feet). In the United States the organism is endemic to the desert Southwest, including parts of California, Arizona, Texas, New Mexico, Nevada, and Utah. It is also prevalent in Mexico and Central America and parts of South America.

Pathophysiology

Coccidioidomycosis is not a contagious disease. Infection is usually via inhalation of infective arthrospores from the environment. Direct inoculation of arthrospores can cause localized cutaneous infection. During periods of high temperature and low rainfall, the mycelia lie dormant below the soil surface. Following a period of rain, the organism returns to the surface, sporulates, and releases large numbers of arthrospores that can be disseminated by the wind. After periods of drought, large numbers of arthrospores may be released, which may result in disease epidemics.

It takes very few arthrospores to cause infection; inhalation of less than 10 arthrospores will produce disease. Following inhalation, arthrospores move from the peribronchial tissue to the subpleural area. Spherules form and produce endospores, which in turn produce more spherules. Following endospore formation, an intense inflammatory response may ensue that results in respiratory signs. The incubation period varies from one to three weeks in dogs. Hematogenous and lymphatic dissemination occurs uncommonly compared with other systemic mycoses, but when it occurs, multisystemic disease may be the result. Although dissemination can be to any organ system, bones and joints, spleen, liver, kidneys, heart, reproductive organs, eyes, brain, and spinal cord are affected most commonly.[35] The skin is commonly affected in cats.[37]

The immune response determines the severity of clinical disease. Whereas recovery is dependent on cell-mediated immunity, humeral response is common and serves as a marker of exposure or previous infection. Antibodies can be found in most dogs living in endemic areas. An adequate immune response may result in subclinical or mild respiratory disease that resolves spontaneously. Most cases in dogs and cats are probably subclinical. A poor immune response may result in severe pulmonary and/or disseminated disease. Recovered humans are considered immune. It is unknown whether the same immunity occurs in dogs and cats.

Clinical Signs

Most affected dogs and cats probably show no or only mild respiratory signs before mounting an effective immune response that results in spontaneous recovery. A small subset of animals does not develop an effective immune response, which can lead to more obvious respiratory signs or disseminated multisystemic disease.

Cats are resistant to infection in comparison to dogs and people. Nonspecific clinical signs such as depression, anorexia, fever, and weight loss typify feline coccidioidomycosis, but findings vary greatly because of the multisystemic nature of the disease.[37] Typically, signs are present for less than a month before diagnosis. The skin is the most common organ system affected in cats. Cutaneous lesions are seen in more than 50 per cent of affected cats and may include draining skin lesions, subcutaneous masses, and abscesses. Localized lymphadenopathy is noted in about a third of cats with skin lesions. Pulmonary involvement, as evidenced by dyspnea, tachypnea, or abnormal lung sounds, is seen in about 25 per cent of affected cats, and lameness in one or more limbs caused by osseous involvement is noted in approximately 20 per cent. Proliferative and lytic long bone lesions and soft tissue swelling are commonly found in cats that present for lameness. Ocular involvement is noted in approximately 10 per cent of affected cats. Ocular infection may be characterized as granulomatous chorioretinitis with retinal detachment, uveitis, and panophthalmitis. CNS involvement is uncommon and may result in signs referable to the localization of the fungal granulomas within the nervous system.

In dogs, the clinical findings are related to the severity of pulmonary involvement and the extent of systemic dissemination. Clinically inapparent infection is common following inhalation of organisms. When clinical signs develop, they are often present for one to six months before a diagnosis is made. The most common presenting complaint is chronic cough. Nonspecific clinical signs such as chronic waxing and waning fever, anorexia, depression, and weight loss are also typical. Lameness caused by osteomyelitis and painful periarticular swelling is a common presenting complaint. Multiple osseous lesions may be seen in as many as 65 per cent of dogs with coccidioidomycosis. As in other systemic mycoses, the distal portions of long bones are affected most commonly. Approximately 20 per cent of dogs have cutaneous signs characterized by nodules, abscesses, ulcers, and draining tracts. Skin lesions in dogs usually occur as an extension from an infected bony lesion. Primary skin and subcutaneous infections following direct cutaneous inoculation can occur but are considered rare. Regional lymphadenopathy associated with cutaneous or osseous lesions is common, but generalized peripheral lymphadenopathy is unusual. Visceral organ involvement may result in icterus, signs of renal failure with renomegaly, or gastrointestinal signs. Cardiac involvement may result in right- or left-sided congestive heart failure or pericardial effusion. Myocardial infection can result in arrhythmias, which may cause syncope or contribute to cardiac failure.

Seizures, ataxia, behavior changes, and coma have been associated with CNS involvement, with the clinical signs being related to the part of the CNS affected. Ocular lesions often involve both the posterior and the anterior segments but are not as common as with other systemic fungal infections. Anterior segment disease, characterized by iritis and granulomatous uveitis, usually as an extension of posterior segment disease, is most common. Lesions are usually unilateral, but bilateral disease may be seen. Glaucoma has been reported in almost half of affected eyes. Granulomatous chorioretinitis with or without bullous retinal detachment is common but may not be apparent because of the severity of the anterior segment disease.

Diagnosis

Hematology commonly reveals a mild normocytic-normochromic nonregenerative anemia; moderate neutrophilia, often with a left shift; and monocytosis. Serum chemistry findings are variable, depending on the organ systems affected. Hypoalbuminemia and hyperglobulinemia are consistent abnormalities. Increases in SALT, SAST, alkaline phosphatase, and total bilirubin may indicate hepatic involvement, and azotemia and hyperphosphatemia may indicate renal involvement. Hypercalcemia has been reported but is not as common as in dogs with blastomycosis or cats with histoplasmosis.

Thoracic radiographs often reveal an ill-defined, diffuse interstitial or peribronchiolar pattern. Alveolar infiltrates are uncommon. The hilar and central lung regions are usually affected, and the peripheral lung regions are affected less commonly. Hilar lymphadenopathy is seen in approximately 80 per cent of affected dogs (Fig. 93–11). Mediastinal widening due to mediastinal lymph node enlargement is less common. Because of the subpleural site of spherule formation, pleural involvement, as evidenced by pleural thickening or effusion, is seen in almost 65 per cent of dogs. Osseous lesions consisting of periosteal and endosteal new bone formation and osteolysis are noted in approximately 20 per cent of dogs with coccidioidomycosis (Fig. 93–12). Affected animals usually have multiple osseous lesions, with bones of the distal appendicular skeleton being affected about three times more frequently than bones of the axial skeleton. The distal diaphysis, metaphysis, and epiphysis are affected most often. Hypertrophic osteopathy may occur secondary to the pulmonary or hilar lymph node involvement.

Organism identification is required to definitively diagnose coccidioidomycosis. Cytology can be useful, but low numbers of spherules make cytologic demonstration more difficult than demonstration of yeast forms in other systemic fungal infections. Exudate from draining skin lesions and pleural fluid are most likely to yield organisms. Tracheal wash or bronchoalveolar lavage samples, lymph node aspirates, or aspirates from other affected tissues yield organisms less commonly, and bone aspirates do not yield organisms often. When seen, spherules appear as large (20 to 200 µm), round, double-walled structures containing many endospores (Fig. 93–13). The walls appear refractile on wet preps or KOH preps and stain blue when H&E-type stains are used. They stain deep red to purple with PAS, and the endospores stain bright red. With Papanicolaou's stain, the walls stain purple-black, the cytoplasm stains yellow, and the endospores stain red-brown. Histopathology is more likely to demonstrate organisms than cytology (Fig. 93–14). Multiple biopsy samples should be taken when coccidioidomycosis is suspected to increase the likelihood of finding organisms.

Coccidioides immitis grows readily on a wide variety of

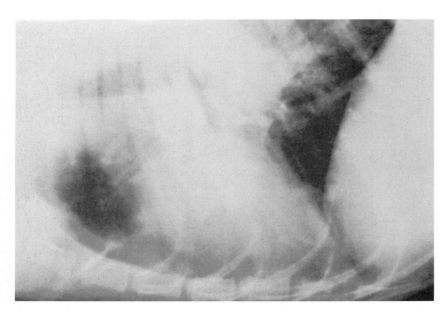

Figure 93–11. Lateral thoracic radiograph of a 2-year-old English Pointer with severe hilar lymphadenopathy associated with pulmonary coccidioidomycosis.

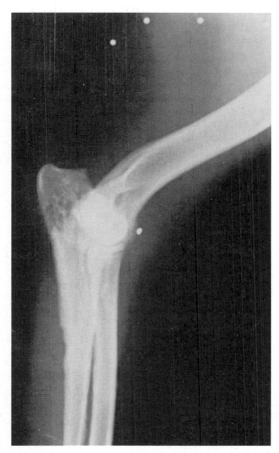

Figure 93-12. Lateral radiograph of the elbow of an 8-year-old English Pointer with osseous coccidioidomycosis. Lytic areas are present in the proximal ulna; productive periosteal and endosteal change is seen in the ulnar metaphysis. Metallic densities present in the soft tissue are lead shot that was acquired while hunting.

agars at room temperature as a white cotton-like mold that changes to tan or brown with age. Definitive identification requires inoculation into animals to induce spherule formation, special culture conditions, or detection of extracellular coccidioidal antigens produced by the growing culture. Lab-

oratory personnel must handle cultures with caution, as arthrospores from cultures are highly infectious.

Serology is used in dogs and cats from endemic areas to make a presumptive diagnosis of coccidioidomycosis when clinical signs are suggestive but organisms cannot be demonstrated. Precipitin antibodies are thought to represent IgM and are detectable two to four weeks after infection. An AGID test allows detection of precipitin antibodies. This test may become negative after four to five weeks and then positive again in those animals in which dissemination has occurred. False-negative results may be seen in animals with early infections, fulminant disease, or chronic infections and in those that are significantly immune suppressed. Complement-fixing (CF) antibodies are thought to represent IgG and are detectable shortly after precipitin antibodies. The AGID test can be used to estimate CF antibodies. A CF test can also be used to detect CF antibodies. The CF titer generally increases with the severity of disease. Low titers (<1:16) may indicate early, chronic, localized, or past infection; titers greater than 1:32 are suggestive of active, disseminated disease; higher titers are generally seen in more severe disease.

Treatment

Although many cases are subclinical or resolve spontaneously, treatment should be initiated in all cases severe enough to be recognized. Ketoconazole (4.5 to 13.6 mg/lb [10 to 30 mg/kg] orally divided twice a day) or itraconazole (2.2 to 4.5 mg/lb [5 to 10 mg/kg] orally once a day) is considered the treatment of choice, but studies rigorously evaluating different treatment protocols in dogs and cats are lacking. Ketoconazole is generally preferred because it is less expensive, but side effects are more likely. Ketoconazole treatment should be continued for at least two months beyond clinical remission. Most animals need to be treated for at least 6 to 12 months. Itraconazole treatment may allow shorter treatment courses, but there has been limited study in dogs to date. Chronic low-dose therapy beyond the initial treatment course may be necessary to keep some animals in remission. Coccidioidomycosis is less responsive to amphotericin B than are other systemic fungal infections, but am-

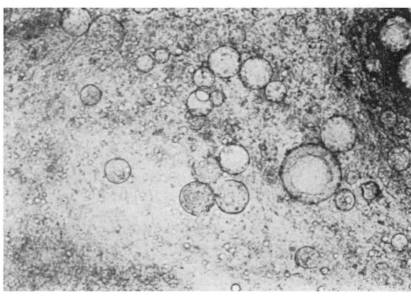

Figure 93-13. Potassium hydroxide wet mount of *Coccidioides immitis* spherules present in exudate from a draining cutaneous lesion, demonstrating the distinctive double-walled appearance of the large, variably sized spherules. (Magnification: 40×.)

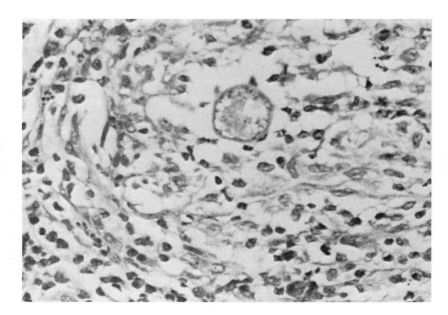

Figure 93–14. Coccidioidal granuloma within a prostatic biopsy from a 7-year-old cocker spaniel. (H&E; magnification: 40×.)

photericin B therapy is still considered the gold standard of therapy in people.

Resolution of clinical signs is the best means of patient monitoring. Rechecks should be performed monthly while dogs or cats are being treated and should include a chemistry panel to evaluate liver enzymes in dogs receiving azole antifungals. Treatment should be continued for two months beyond resolution of clinical signs, and animals should be reevaluated three and six months after discontinuing therapy to assess for relapse. Serology has been used to monitor response to therapy or evaluate for relapse, but CF titers may stay elevated for a year or more following therapy. CF titers should be less than 1:16 when therapy is discontinued and will often increase with relapse of clinical disease.

The prognosis is considered good when only pulmonary signs are apparent but is guarded for dogs and cats with disseminated disease. Most disseminated cases respond well initially but relapse when treatment is discontinued. If left untreated, disseminated disease is usually fatal.

Public Health Significance

Direct transmission of *Coccidioides immitis* from animal to animal or animal to person is not likely. However, caution should be used when handling animals with draining cutaneous wounds and when changing bandages, as fungal spherules present in exudate may revert to the mycelial phase and produce infectious arthroconidia at the lower temperatures on the surface of the bandage. Laboratory workers can potentially be infected from fungal cultures.

CRYPTOCOCCOSIS

Cryptococcosis is an opportunistic systemic fungal infection of worldwide significance that usually originates in the nasal cavity, paranasal tissues, or lungs. It can then disseminate, most commonly to the skin, eyes, or CNS. Disease occurs in a wide variety of mammalian species. Among domestic animals, it occurs most commonly in the cat, in which it is the most common of the systemic mycoses. Unlike the other systemic mycoses, cryptococcosis does not follow strict geographic boundaries but is most common in the southeastern and southwestern United States, southern California, and the east coast of Australia.[13, 38]

Cryptococcosis is caused by *Cryptococcus neoformans*, a saprophytic, round, yeastlike organism with a restricted ecologic niche. *Cryptococcus neoformans* var. *neoformans* is the subspecies that most commonly causes disease and is environmentally associated with pigeon droppings or other avian habitats. *Cryptococcus neoformans* var. *gattii* is a second subspecies that is capable of causing disease and is associated with bark and leaf litter of certain eucalyptus trees. In infected tissue, and often when cultured, the organism is a variable-sized yeast (3.5 to 7 µm) with a large heteropolysaccharide capsule (1 to 30 µm). Both subspecies have been shown to cause disease in cats and humans. *Cryptococcus neoformans* reproduces primarily by budding from a narrow base. Under controlled laboratory conditions, the organism undergoes sexual reproduction, but most infections are thought to be caused by environmental exposure to the yeastlike phase.

The pigeon is thought to be the most important vector of *Cryptococcus neoformans*. The *Cryptococcus* organism can be found in high numbers in pigeon roosts, barn lofts, and hay mows and along cupolas and cornices where pigeons often sit. In the desiccated state, the *Cryptococcus* organism may be no larger than 1 µm and may survive up to two years.

Pathophysiology

Cryptococcosis is not a contagious disease. Infection occurs most commonly via inhalation of yeast from the environment. Debris and droppings in and around avian habitats, especially pigeon habitats, contain the largest numbers of *Cryptococcus* organisms. Most yeasts are probably too large to be inhaled into the lungs and settle out in the nasal cavity or nasopharynx, where they can produce disease or result in animals becoming asymptomatic carriers of the organism. In one study, cryptococcal organisms could be cultured from nasal washings in 14 per cent of asymptomatic dogs and 7 per cent of asymptomatic cats.[39] The small, desiccated forms of the yeast are also infective and can be inhaled into the small airways and alveoli, leading to pulmonary disease. After inhalation into the nasal cavity, paranasal sinuses, or lungs, cell-mediated immune response results in granuloma formation. Dissemination can occur by either direct extension or hematogenous spread. Direct extension from the nasal cavity through the cribriform plate to the CNS or to the paranasal soft tissues and skin is common. Although dissemination can be to any organ system, the skin, eyes, and CNS are affected most commonly.

Lesions consist of either granulomatous inflammation with few organisms or gelatinous masses of organisms with little inflammation. The large capsule surrounding the cryptococcal organism contributes to pathogenicity by inhibiting phagocytosis, plasma cell function, and leukocyte migration. As with the other systemic mycoses, the immune response determines the severity of clinical disease. Antibodies are readily produced by the humoral immune system but are not considered protective. Recovery, therefore, is dependent on cell-mediated immunity. Most human cases of cryptococcosis are associated with immune suppression, especially lymphoreticular neoplasia and AIDS. However, immune suppression has not been as apparent in most affected cats and dogs. An association with FeLV and FIV infections in cats has been reported, and chronic glucocorticoid use has been implicated as a predisposing factor in both cats and dogs.[6, 40–42]

Clinical Signs

Cats are more commonly affected by cryptococcosis than dogs. There is no apparent breed, sex, or age predilection in cats. Clinical findings are usually related to upper respiratory, nasopharyngeal, cutaneous, ocular, or CNS involvement.[5, 6, 13, 40, 43] Nonspecific signs such as depression and anorexia are common in chronic cases, but fever is uncommon. Upper respiratory signs related to nasal cavity involvement are seen in 50 to 80 per cent of affected cats. In these cats, sneezing and snuffling are common, and unilateral or bilateral mucopurulent nasal discharge with or without blood is typically seen. Proliferative soft tissue masses or ulcerative lesions within the nasal cavity or over the bridge of the nose are seen in approximately 70 per cent of cases with upper respiratory involvement (Fig. 93–15). Oral ulcerations are occasionally noted but are not common. Nasopharyngeal mass lesions causing snoring, stertor, and inspiratory dyspnea are occasionally noted.[43] These cats usually have caudal nasal cavity disease as well. Unlike in other systemic mycoses, the lungs are not commonly affected. The skin or subcutaneous tissues are affected in approximately 40 to 50 per cent of infected cats. Primary lesions include papules or

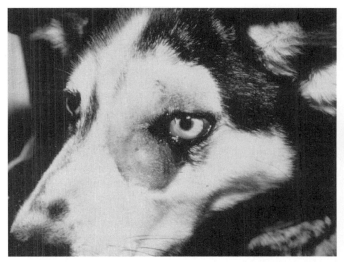

Figure 93–16. Periocular swelling in a female Siberian husky caused by cryptococcal infection.

nodules that may ulcerate and drain. Multiple lesions are typical, and regional lymphadenopathy is common. Hematogenous spread from the respiratory system may result in lameness secondary to osteomyelitis, renal failure secondary to renal disease, and generalized lymphadenopathy.

The eyes are affected in 20 to 25 per cent of infected cats, especially those with CNS involvement. Granulomatous chorioretinitis with or without exudative retinal detachment is the most common ocular manifestation and can lead to panophthalmitis. Less often, optic neuritis can be seen, resulting in blindness. Anterior uveitis is not as common as posterior segment disease. CNS involvement is reported in approximately 20 per cent of affected cats. This may be an underrepresentation of the actual number of cases with nervous system involvement.[42] The forebrain is most commonly affected, as invasion through the cribriform plate is thought to be common. Signs may include depression, behavior changes, seizures, circling, ataxia, blindness, head pressing, cranial nerve deficits and paresis. Cats with concurrent FeLV or FIV infection tend to be more severely affected and may be more likely to develop neurologic or ophthalmic signs.

Canine cryptococcosis is typically seen in dogs younger than 4 years of age. There is no apparent sex predilection, and American cocker spaniels, Labrador retrievers, Great Danes, and Doberman pinschers appear to be overrepresented. In dogs, clinical findings are most often related to CNS, upper respiratory, ocular, or cutaneous involvement.[44] As in cats, depression and anorexia are common, but fever is not. CNS involvement is reported in approximately 50 to 80 per cent of affected dogs. The brain is affected in most dogs.[45, 46] The spinal cord may be affected along with the brain, and rarely the spinal cord alone is affected, causing signs consistent with either meningitis or an extradural compressive lesion.[47] Signs of nervous system involvement may include mental depression, vestibular syndrome, ataxia, cranial nerve deficits (especially cranial nerves V, VII, and VIII), seizures, paresis, blindness, hypermetria, and cervical pain. In dogs with CNS signs, other systems are usually affected as well, reflecting multisystemic dissemination.

The upper respiratory system or perinasal tissues are affected in approximately 50 per cent of dogs with cryptococcosis (Fig. 93–16).[44] The caudal nasal cavity and frontal sinuses are affected more commonly than the rostral nasal

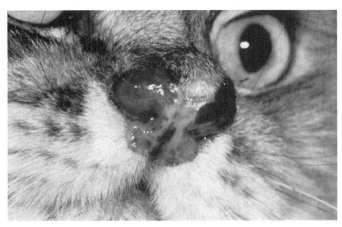

Figure 93–15. Nasal cryptococcosis in a cat. (Courtesy of Dr. Carol Foil.)

cavity. Signs may include upper airway stridor, nasal discharge and sneezing, epistaxis, or firm swellings over the bridge of the nose or affecting the periorbital tissues. The eyes or periorbital tissues are affected in approximately 20 to 40 per cent of dogs with cryptococcosis. Granulomatous chorioretinitis with or without exudative retinal detachment is the most common ocular manifestation and can lead to panophthalmitis. In addition to chorioretinitis, fundic examination may reveal retinal hemorrhage or retinal scarring. Optic neuritis may be noted as a cause of blindness. As with the other systemic mycoses, anterior uveitis is less common than posterior segment disease. The skin is affected in approximately 10 to 20 per cent of dogs with cryptococcosis. Subcutaneous nodules with ulcerative draining lesions, often on the head, footpads, nail beds, and mucous membranes of the mouth, occur most commonly. Proliferative lesions in the ear canals may result from cryptococcal otitis externa. Direct extension from the ears to the CNS may result. Multiorgan dissemination is more common in dogs than in cats. Disease may be subclinical or may result in clinical signs referable to the organ systems affected.

Diagnosis

Hematology and clinical chemistries are often normal in animals with cryptococcosis. Mild nonregenerative anemia and mature neutrophilia or neutrophilia with a mild left shift may be seen. Because the nervous system is so commonly affected, CSF tap for culture and cytology should be considered. CSF commonly yields increased opening pressure, increased protein, and mixed mononuclear and neutrophilic pleocytosis. Organisms are visualized in approximately 90 per cent of dogs with CNS cryptococcosis.[48]

Nodular infiltrates, an interstitial pattern, pleural effusion, and tracheobronchial lymphadenopathy have occasionally been reported. Nasal radiographs may demonstrate increased soft tissue density and bone destruction in the nasal passages and frontal sinuses.

Organism identification allows for definitive diagnosis and can usually be made cytologically or histologically. Cytology from affected tissue is the quickest and easiest means of identifying cryptococcal organisms. Nasal swabs, exudate from cutaneous lesions, aspirates of masses, subretinal or vitreal aspirates, and CSF often reveal organisms. Organisms are apparent in approximately 75 per cent of cases. The large capsule makes identification easy (Fig. 93–17). Gram's

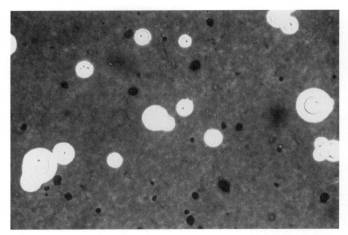

Figure 93–18. India ink preparation revealing cryptococcal organisms. (Courtesy of Dr. Carol Foil.)

stain is useful in looking for cryptococcal organisms, as the cells retain the crystal violet and the capsule stains lightly red with the safranin. If India ink is used, the organism and capsule appear unstained and silhouetted against the black background (Fig. 93–18). Care must taken in interpreting India ink preparations, as lymphocytes, fat droplets, and aggregated ink particles may be confused with the organism. Budding is occasionally noted. The thin wall and the large capsule differentiate *Cryptococcus* from *Blastomyces*.

Histopathology should be used if cytology fails to identify organisms. Nodular to diffuse granulomatous lesions or areas of degeneration with little inflammation are seen in infected tissue. Yeastlike organisms are usually numerous. Special stains such as PAS, Gridley's fungal, and Gomori's methenamine silver stain are best at demonstrating organisms. Mucicarmine stains best demonstrate the capsule.

Cryptococcal organisms grow readily when cultured. The organism can be cultured from infected tissue, exudate, CSF, urine, joint fluid, and blood if large enough samples are submitted. Yeastlike growth occurs in two days to six weeks on Sabouraud's dextrose agar. Hyphae rarely grow, even at 37°C. Care must be taken in interpreting positive cultures from the nasal cavity, as 14 per cent of asymptomatic random-source dogs and 7 per cent of asymptomatic random-source cats were culture-positive in one study.[39] Cultures from nasal swabs need to be interpreted together with other supportive clinical data. Animals in the above-mentioned study were all negative on serum latex agglutination tests and did not have macroscopic or microscopic findings supportive of cryptococcal infection.

Serology is useful as an inexpensive and noninvasive diagnostic test when cytology has failed to demonstrate organisms. Latex agglutination procedures are used to detect cryptococcal capsular antigen. Antibody titers are not useful diagnostically, because most infected animals do not mount a humeral immune response.[49] The commercially available latex cryptococcal antigen agglutination tests can be used on serum, urine, or CSF. CSF is the best sample to use in animals with neurologic signs, and serum is the best sample to use in animals with upper respiratory or cutaneous signs but without neurologic signs. Most cases are positive with titers between 1:10 and 1:100,000. The median titer in infected cats in one study was 1:1000.[49] False-negative antigen titers are rare but may occasionally be seen in localized disease. False-positive antigen titers are uncommon and are usually related to technique or interfering substances such

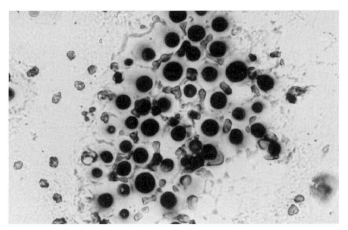

Figure 93–17. Cryptococcal organisms noted on fine-needle aspirate cytology from the dog in Figure 93–16. Note the large capsules surrounding the organisms and the minimal inflammatory response.

as rheumatoid factor. The laboratory can treat samples with pronase to eliminate interference factors and improve the sensitivity of the test. The latex agglutination antigen titer tends to correlate well with the extent of disease but does not correlate well with prognosis.[50] It may be used to evaluate the treatment progress.

Treatment

Amphotericin B is the most effective drug in vitro against cryptococcal isolates, but both itraconazole and fluconazole have proved to be equally efficacious in treating CNS cryptococcosis in people. There is little information evaluating amphotericin B in the treatment of cryptococcal infections in dogs and cats. Amphotericin B is synergistic with flucytosine. Flucytosine can be used at a dosage of 11.4 to 22.7 mg/lb (25 to 50 mg/kg) orally four times a day and has been used in dogs and cats. The combination of amphotericin B and flucytosine may be especially useful for treating CNS infections. Cryptococcal organisms may rapidly develop resistance to flucytosine, so it has limited efficacy as a sole treatment agent. The dose of flucytosine should be adjusted downward in animals with concurrent renal failure. Toxicity to flucytosine includes ulcerative drug eruptions on the skin (especially on the face) and mucocutaneous junctions, enterocolitis, leukopenia, and thrombocytopenia. Amphotericin B has also been effective when combined with azole antifungal agents.

Subcutaneously administered amphotericin B in combination with azole antifungals or flucytosine has been used to successfully treat both feline and canine cryptococcosis.[51] Amphotericin B (0.22 to 0.36 mg/lb; 0.5 to 0.8 mg/kg) is diluted in 0.45 per cent saline containing 2.5 per cent dextrose (400 mL for cats, 500 mL for dogs less than 20 kg, 1000 mL for dogs greater than 20 kg) and administered subcutaneously two to three times per week. This protocol may allow larger cumulative doses of amphotericin B to be given with reduced toxicity. Concentrations greater than 20 mg/L of amphotericin B resulted in local irritation and sterile abscess formation, so more concentrated formulations of amphotericin B should not be used subcutaneously.

Ketoconazole is variably effective as a sole treatment agent but is ineffective in cases with CNS involvement. There were only scattered reports of successful treatment of cryptococcal infections in dogs and cats before the availability of the triazole antifungals, but since they became available, successful treatment has been reported more commonly. Fluconazole (50 mg/cat orally twice a day; 2.2 mg/lb [5 mg/kg] orally once to twice a day for dogs) is very effective and is the treatment of choice for cryptococcosis in cats and probably dogs.[13, 44] Itraconazole (4.5 mg/lb [10 mg/kg] orally daily) is effective in cats and dogs but appears to be less effective than fluconazole.[6, 48] Controlled trials in people have revealed the two drugs to be equally efficacious. Ketoconazole (4.5 to 13.6 mg/lb [10 to 30 mg/kg] orally twice a day) is even less effective but can be used if other drugs are unavailable.

Resolution of clinical signs is the best means of patient monitoring, but serially monitoring latex agglutination antigen titers can significantly augment the clinician's clinical observations.[40, 50] Rechecks should be performed monthly while dogs or cats are being treated and should include a chemistry panel to evaluate liver enzymes in animals receiving azole antifungals and a latex agglutination antigen titer. Sequential titers should differ by two or more dilutions before they are considered significantly different. A decline

of two- to fourfold per month during the initial few months of antifungal therapy generally corresponds to an adequate clinical response. Ideally, treatment should be continued until the titer is negative or for at least two months beyond resolution of clinical signs. In some animals, detectable cryptococcal polysaccharide antigen persists in the circulation long after the infection has been successfully treated. This is thought to be caused by continued elimination of unviable organisms and capsular material from infected tissues and macrophages. Most of these animals have low titers, and high residual titers may indicate insufficient therapy and thus persistence of viable organisms.[40] One author's recommendation is to continue antifungal drug treatment to a titer of less than 1.[50] In cases in which there has been a 32-fold decrease and resolution of clinical signs, treatment may be discontinued, but titers should be reevaluated periodically to ensure that the titer continues to decline or at least remains stable. Animals should be reevaluated at least three and six months after discontinuing treatment to assess for relapse. Negative antigen titers are occasionally seen in animals with localized disease, so they do not always indicate clinical cure.

The prognosis is good for cats with extraneural disease. The prognosis is guarded for dogs with any form of the disease and for cats with CNS involvement.

SPOROTRICHOSIS

Sporotrichosis is a chronic granulomatous disease of worldwide significance caused by the dimorphic saprophytic fungus *Sporothrix schenckii*. The organism lives as a mycelium in the soil and when cultured at room temperature, and as a yeast at body temperature. The mycelia are thin, finely branched, and septate. They produce clusters of conidiophores, which are the infective stage. The yeast form exists in infected tissue and is characterized as pleomorphic round, oval, or cigar-shaped cells that measure 2 by 3 μm to 3 by 10 μm (Fig. 93–19). The yeast is fairly characteristic, and a diagnosis can usually be made from a cytologic preparation. Both dogs and cats can be infected. Dogs are infected less commonly and usually have only cutaneous or subcutaneous disease. Cats are infected more frequently and commonly have systemic dissemination.

Pathophysiology

Infection with *Sporothrix schenckii* in dogs and cats usually follows trauma that results in inoculation of infective

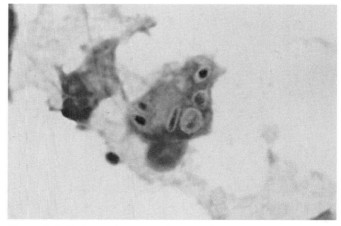

Figure 93–19. Impression smear from a skin lesion on a cat revealing pleomorphic organisms characteristic of sporotrichosis.

conidiophores. Yeast from cutaneous lesions can be infective and is a potential zoonotic source of infection via contamination of wounds or via scratches or bites. The skin is the primary organ system affected, but dissemination via lymphatics is common in cats and less common in dogs. Immune suppression predisposes to infection and increases the likelihood of dissemination.

Sporotrichosis occurs in three primary forms: cutaneous, cutaneolymphatic, and disseminated disease. In the dog, the infection is usually cutaneous or cutaneolymphatic. Disseminated disease is rare and usually follows immune suppression with corticosteroids when the disease is misdiagnosed. The cutaneolymphatic form is common in the cat, and dissemination is seen in greater than 50 per cent of feline cases. The lesions in cats are characterized by large numbers of yeasts, making zoonotic transmission more likely from cats than from dogs.

Clinical Signs

Most affected cats are younger than 4 years of age, and males are affected approximately twice as commonly as females.[52] Young hunting dogs may be predisposed. The cutaneous form of the disease is characterized by multiple subcutaneous or dermal nodular lesions that occur most commonly on the head, neck, trunk, and distal limbs. The tail base may also be involved in cats. The nodules typically ulcerate, drain a purulent exudate, and crust over (Fig. 93–20). They are often confused with bite wound abscesses or cellulitis. Lesions on the distal limbs commonly result in regional lymphadenitis, which is manifested as linear ulcerating lesions and regional lymphadenopathy. Lesions in cats may be associated with extensive areas of necrosis. Otitis externa has been reported.

Dissemination may occur and be subclinical or may result in serious systemic disease. Too few cases have been reported to develop a clear picture of a dissemination pattern, but internal lymph nodes, spleen, liver, lungs, eyes, bones, muscles, and CNS have all been affected. Signs may be nonspecific or may correspond to a specifically affected site, such as lameness in a dog with dissemination causing osteomyelitis.

Diagnosis

Cytology from skin lesions is the most common means of diagnosis. Lesions from cats contain large numbers of organisms, making diagnosis fairly easy; lesions from dogs usually contain very few organisms. The organisms may be seen intracellularly within macrophages or neutrophils or may be present extracellularly. Culture can be used to make a definitive diagnosis. Material for culture should include exudate from deep within a draining tract and tissue samples from biopsy specimens. Cultured organisms pose a serious threat to persons working in the laboratory, so the laboratory should be notified whenever a sample is submitted from a dog or cat with suspected sporotrichosis. Histopathology reveals pyogranulomatous inflammation. Numerous organisms are commonly seen in lesions from cats even when stained with H&E. Fungal stains such as PAS or immunofluorescent techniques may aid in finding organisms in dogs. Immunofluorescent testing can be performed by the Centers for Disease Control and Prevention in Atlanta, Georgia.

Therapy

Traditionally, sporotrichosis has been treated with potassium iodide, ketoconazole, or combinations of the two. Approximately 55 per cent of treated cats in the literature responded to one or both of these drugs.[52] Recently, itraconazole has become the treatment of choice in people and is effective in dogs and cats. It is especially valuable in cats because of the species' tendency to develop iodism on potassium iodide.

The response to itraconazole treatment in cutaneous and cutaneolymphatic cases is generally good. The prognosis must be guarded for disseminated disease, but too few cases have been reported to give a well-informed likelihood of response.

Public Health Significance

Canine sporotrichosis is of minimal zoonotic potential, but feline sporotrichosis is a significant zoonotic disease. Veterinarians and veterinary assistants are at the highest risk of infection.[53] Care should be taken to limit contact with exudate and lesions from infected cats. Gloves should always be worn when handling cats suspected of having sporotrichosis, and owners should be advised of the possibility of infection and the need for strict hygiene. Following any contact, gloves should be removed carefully and disposed of, and hands, wrists, and arms should be washed thoroughly with either chlorhexidine or povidone-iodine scrub.

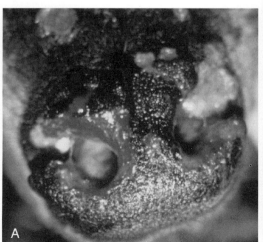
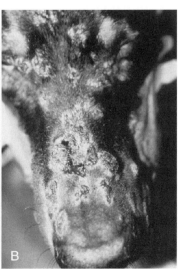

Figure 93–20. *A* and *B,* Sporotrichosis affecting the skin and nasal mucosa of a Doberman pinscher.

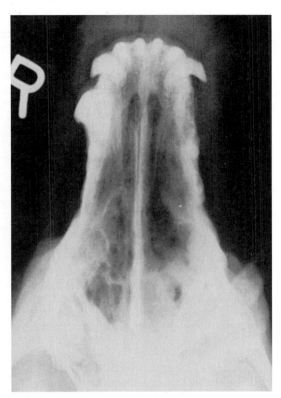

Figure 93–21. Ventrodorsal, open-mouth radiograph of an 11-year-old mixed breed dog with unilateral nasal aspergillosis. The left side of the nasal cavity demonstrates loss of the normal turbinate pattern and punctate bone lysis anteriorly; increased soft tissue density is seen in the posterior part of the nasal cavity.

ASPERGILLOSIS

Aspergillosis is a disease of dogs and occasionally cats caused by several species of *Aspergillus*. *Aspergillus fumigatus* is the most commonly implicated species. It is a ubiquitous saprophyte with worldwide distribution that typically causes disease localized to the nasal cavity and paranasal sinuses of immunocompetent dogs. Only occasionally does the species cause disease elsewhere in the animal, usually in the lower respiratory tract. Other species of *Aspergillus*, including *A. terreus, A. deflectus*, and *A. flavipes*, tend to cause disseminated disease in immunocompromised dogs. Disseminated disease is much less common than nasal disease in dogs. Both forms of the disease are rare in cats.

In the environment, *Aspergillus fumigatus* grows most abundantly in decaying vegetation, sewage, compost, decomposing wood chips, and moldy hay. It can be cultured from the normal nasal cavity of dogs. *Aspergillus terreus* and *A. deflectus* are primarily soil inhabitants. The fungus grows as a mycelium both in the environment and in infected tissue. In the environment, it produces large numbers of small spores that can become airborne and inhaled into the nasal cavity and occasionally the lower parts of the respiratory tract. After spores are inhaled, local immune responses involving IgA and macrophages usually prevent fungal colonization.

Nasal Aspergillosis

Nasal aspergillosis is a common cause of nasal disease in dogs, accounting for 12 to 34 per cent of chronic nasal disease diagnoses. It typically occurs in healthy, apparently immunocompetent dogs (although lymphocyte blastogenesis studies have been suppressed in some dogs). Most cases occur in young to middle-age male dogs, but any age and both sexes can be affected. Brachycephalic breeds are underrepresented, and dolichocephalic breeds may be overrepresented. Golden retrievers were predisposed in one study when compared with the hospital control population. The clinical signs are those found with any chronic nasal disease, but epistaxis and nasal pain are often prominent findings. Nasal discharge is usually chronic (median 3.5 months) and may be bilateral or start unilaterally and become bilateral. Local disease can be very destructive, resulting in turbinate destruction and frontal sinus osteomyelitis. Occasionally, invasion through the cribriform plate is seen.

Diagnosis is based on demonstration of the organism in diseased tissue. Radiology is usually performed as part of the evaluation of an animal with chronic nasal disease. Open-mouth ventrodorsal views generally reveal significant turbinate lysis and increased radiolucency, usually as a mixed pattern, but rarely increased radiopacity (Fig. 93–21). CT is ideal for showing the turbinate destruction and has become the imaging technique of choice for the evaluation of animals with suspected nasal aspergillosis.[54, 55]

Cytology can be used to confirm suspected aspergillosis. Cytology from nasal discharge, swabs, or nasal flush material does not usually reveal the fungal hyphae but is accurate when it does (Fig. 93–22). Biopsies are a more reliable source of cytologic material than nasal discharge. Histopathology usually reveals pyogranulomatous inflammation and necrosis with numerous fungal hyphae. The inflammation can be more widespread than the fungal colony formation, and a diagnosis of nonspecific rhinitis may be read off of biopsy material if no fungal organisms are seen. Fungal culture can be used to demonstrate the organism, but unfortunately it can be misleading, because 30 to 40 per cent of normal dogs and dogs with nasal neoplasia yield growth of *Aspergillus* or *Penicillium* spp. on culture.

Rhinoscopy is a valuable diagnostic technique in the evaluation of animals with suspected nasal aspergillosis. Rhinoscopic visualization usually reveals white to greenish-grey fungal colonies, which are very characteristic. Visualization improves the likelihood of histologic diagnosis through selection of a more representative biopsy site. Indeed, a diagnosis of nasal aspergillosis is often made from the rhinoscopic appearance of the lesions, allowing treatment to be initiated under the same anesthesia.

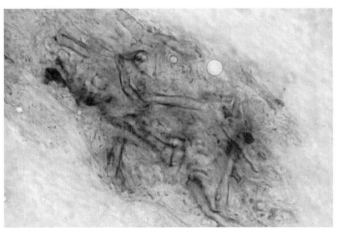

Figure 93–22. Nasal discharge cytology from a dog with nasal aspergillosis revealing *Aspergillus* organisms.

Serology can be used as a diagnostic aid in the evaluation of animals with nasal aspergillosis. AGID and ELISA tests are commercially available. Both false-positives (5 to 15 per cent) and false-negatives are reported.

Topical therapy is presently the preferred method of treatment.[55–59] Systemic therapy has been used in the past to manage dogs with nasal aspergillosis, but it is expensive and is generally less efficacious than topical therapy. Fluconazole and itraconazole can be used but must be given for months and are probably effective in only slightly more than 50 per cent of cases. Initial studies reported success using surgically placed indwelling frontal sinus catheters and repeated infusions of povidone-iodine or enilconazole. More recently, single infusions of clotrimazole or enilconazole have been described.

Clotrimazole is presently considered the treatment of choice. It is a synthetic imidazole with high efficacy against *Aspergillus* infections when used topically. Fungicidal concentrations of clotrimazole seem to remain at topical sites for a number of days after application. The cure rate after first-time administration is approximately 80 per cent. Few side effects were observed in over 70 dogs treated from one institution.[59] The most common side effects are sneezing and bloody nasal discharge that may worsen for a few days following treatment. If trephination is used to place administration tubes, subcutaneous emphysema occurs in about 25 per cent of cases. An occasional dog shows acute onset of neurologic signs following clotrimazole administration. This may be caused by CNS exposure to the drug in animals with invasion through the cribriform plate, resulting in a drug-induced meningoencephalitis. One dog was reported that developed severe pharyngeal swelling and upper airway obstruction following clotrimazole administration.[60] The vehicle used in the solution was polyethylene glycol and ethanol rather than polypropylene glycol, which may have contributed to the irritation. The dog also was very slow to recover from anesthesia. The authors speculated that this may have been caused by clotrimazole-induced delay in hepatic metabolism of barbiturate anesthesia.

Clotrimazole can be administered through indwelling tubes introduced into the frontal sinuses via trephination, but administration via the nares has recently been advocated and results in fewer complications.[57] For nares administration, 1 g (100 mL) of clotrimazole is given. Half is placed in the left naris, and half is placed in the right. The dog is placed in dorsal recumbency, and a large (20 French or larger) Foley catheter is placed behind the soft palate. The balloon is inflated, and gauze sponges are packed around the balloon to prevent nasopharyngeal loss of the solution. Two red rubber catheters (10 French) are inserted through the nares into the medial meatus to the level of the medial canthus of the eye, and a smaller Foley is inserted in each nostril behind each red rubber tube. The 3-cc balloon is partially inflated and pulled back to give a snug fit in each naris. The clotrimazole solution is infused through the red rubber tubes into each side until it starts to drip out through the Foley catheters. Each Foley is then clamped, and the remainder of the clotrimazole is slowly infused over an hour. The dog is placed in dorsal recumbency with the nose parallel to the table for 15 minutes, then in left lateral recumbency for 15 minutes, then in right lateral recumbency for 15 minutes, and then in ventral recumbency for the final 15 minutes. Any leaks can be occluded with cotton swabs. There is only an approximately 20 per cent recurrence after the single infusion, with no difference between dogs with indwelling tubes and those with nares administration. There is a marked

increase in morbidity associated with indwelling tubes as compared with nares treatment. Follow-up single treatments may be curative in many but not all dogs with recurrence. Approximately 85 per cent of dogs will be cured by this technique. If perinasal soft tissue, such as periorbital tissue, is affected, the topical treatment alone will not be effective, and systemic therapy with itraconazole or terbinafine should also be used.

Enilconazole is an imidazole with very poor oral bioavailability. It has been used most extensively as a topical agent in other countries and is not approved for use in the United States as a topical agent. It is available as a poultry product, but the vehicle is different from that used in medical-grade enilconazole in Europe. Results of reported studies are based on the nonapproved medical-grade product available in Europe.[58] Enilconazole is administered as a 100 mg/mL solution in a propylene glycol vehicle. An emulsion is made by mixing this solution 1:1 with water or saline. The emulsion must be used within five minutes, or it hardens. In most studies, the emulsion has been instilled into the nasal cavity through two indwelling tubes, implanted bilaterally through trephine holes in each frontal sinus, to lie in the midnasal chambers. An additional tube is implanted in the frontal sinus of dogs with fungal sinusitis. The diseased tissue is not removed via rhinotomy before treatment. The dose is 4.5 mg/lb (10 mg/kg) instilled twice a day for 7 to 14 days. Complications include premature removal of the tubes (20 per cent), subcutaneous emphysema, and anorexia. In a recent case report, enilconazole was administered as a one-hour infusion through tubes endoscopically placed through the internal nares.[56] In another study, 24 dogs were treated with enilconazole alone; 20 of 24 were clinically free of disease 6 to 39 months after treatment, but the follow-up was not extensive in 8 of the dogs.[58] Four dogs did not respond to treatment; two of these four had extensive periorbital soft tissue invasion. The author has noted anaphylactic-like reactions (possibly associated with aspiration) in two dogs treated with enilconazole.

Disseminated Aspergillosis

Disseminated aspergillosis is most often caused by *A. terreus*; *A. deflectus*, *A. flavipes*, and *A. fumigatus* have also been reported, in decreasing order of frequency. The portal of entry is thought to be the respiratory tract, with subsequent hematogenous spread. Immune suppression or immunodeficiency may predispose to dissemination. The German shepherd is predisposed, possibly owing to defects in mucosal immunity such as IgA deficiency.[61, 62] Cats are often co-infected with FeLV or feline infectious peritonitis (FIP) or feline panleukopenia virus.

The disease typically involves multiple organ systems and develops over several months. In dogs, the most consistent clinical feature is vertebral pain and progressive paraparesis or lameness. Swelling and draining tracts may develop over areas of osteomyelitis.[63] While discospondylitis may be seen without other system involvement, the infection often causes multiple small granulomas and fungal thrombi in multiple organs. The kidneys and spleen are commonly affected, but any site may be involved. In animals without intervertebral or bone involvement causing pain, clinical signs are usually nonspecific. The gastrointestinal system is rarely involved in dogs but is occasionally affected in cats.

Blood work is generally nonspecific. A CBC may reveal a neutrophilic leukocytosis and a nonregenerative anemia. A chemistry panel may reveal azotemia and increased liver enzymes. It is important to perform a urinalysis, including sediment examination, in animals suspected of having disseminated aspergillosis, because fungal hyphae are often present in the urine secondary to renal involvement.[64]

Few reports of treatment are available. The prognosis is generally very poor, but long-term survival was reported in four dogs treated with long-term itraconazole. The infection was eliminated in only one of the four dogs, however.

CANDIDIASIS

Candida spp. are normal inhabitants of the gastrointestinal, genitourinary, and upper respiratory systems. *Candida* may overgrow in cases of immune suppression or prolonged broad-spectrum antibiotic use, especially in wounds, the oropharynx, or the gastrointestinal tract. Animals with neutropenia are especially predisposed to infection. Infections may be localized, or dissemination may occur via a hematogenous route, resulting in microabscesses at multiple sites.

Localized candidiasis is usually characterized as a nonhealing ulcer covered by a whitish-grey plaque in the oral cavity, in the gastrointestinal tract, or on the genitourinary mucosa. Chronic moist, exudative lesions may occur on the skin or at the nail beds.

Disseminated disease is typified by fever and the acute appearance of multiple raised erythematous skin lesions in dogs. In dogs, pain is often caused by myositis and osteomyelitis, and other signs are referable to the systems affected. Cats are less likely to have multiple skin lesions. The CBC in systemically affected animals is often characterized by leukopenia and thrombocytopenia. Renal involvement is common, and yeast may be found in the urine, especially in cats.

Itraconazole and ABLC are considered the treatments of choice, but few reports of successful treatment are available.

ZYGOMYCOSIS

Zygomycetes rarely cause disease in dogs and cats. Organisms in the order Mucorales, including *Rhizopus*, *Mucor*, *Mortierella*, and *Absidia*, are ubiquitous fungi that are common contaminants of cultures. These fungi may be opportunistic invaders, causing disseminated disease in immunocompromised animals. Clinical signs are nonspecific, and many reported cases were diagnosed at necropsy. The gastrointestinal tract may be involved, mimicking gastrointestinal pythiosis. *Conidiobolus* and *Basidiobolus* are two genera in the order Entomophthorales that may also cause disease that mimics pythiosis. Gastrointestinal and pharyngeal infection is probably most common. Large subcutaneous lesions may also be seen. Successful treatment has not been reported.

HYALOHYPHOMYCOSIS AND PHAEOHYPHOMYCOSIS

The term hyalohyphomycosis is used to encompass all opportunistic infections caused by nondematiaceous (nonpigment-forming) fungi whose basic tissue form is hyaline hyphal elements. Aspergillosis and penicilliosis are included in this group. Disease is rare and is generally seen in immunocompromised hosts.[65] Other organisms in this group include *Paecilomyces*, *Chrysosporium*, *Pseudallescheria*, *Geotrichum*, *Acremonium*, and *Pseudallescheria*.

Phaeohyphomycosis is the term used to describe infections caused by saprophytic opportunistic dematiaceous (pigment-forming) fungi. Organisms in this group include *Cladosporium*, *Drechslera*, *Exophiala*, *Moniliella*, *Phialemonium*, *Phialophora*, *Pseudomicrodochium*, *Stemphylium*, *Alternaria*, and *Scolecobasisium*. Most of these organisms cause subcutaneous disease, but CNS or disseminated disease is rarely seen.

TABLE 93–3. DRUG APPENDIX

GENERIC	TRADE	DOSE	ROUTE	FREQUENCY
Amphotericin B	Fungizone	Dog: 0.22–0.5 mg/lb/day (0.5–1 mg/kg/day) Cat: 0.11–0.25 mg/lb/day (0.25–0.5 mg/kg/day)	IV	q48 h
		Dog/cat: 0.22–0.36 mg/lb/day (0.5–0.8 mg/kg/day) diluted in 0.45% NaCl and 2.5% dextrose	SQ	q48 h
Lipid formulations of amphotericin B	Abelcet	Dog: 0.5–1 mg/lb/day (1–2 mg/kg/day)	IV	q48 h
Flucytosine	Ancobon	Dog: 11.4–22.7 mg/lb/day (25–50 mg/kg/day)	PO	q6 h
Ketoconazole	Nizoral	Dog: 4.5–13.6 mg/lb/day (10–30 mg/kg/day)	PO	q12 h
Itraconazole	Sporanox	Dog: 2.2–4.5 mg/lb (5–10 mg/kg) Cat: 4.5 mg/lb (10 mg/kg)	PO	q24 h
Fluconazole	Diflucan	Dog/cat: 1–4.5 mg/lb (2.5–10 mg/kg)	PO	q12 h
Enilconazole		Dog: 4.5 mg/lb (10 mg/kg)	Intranasal	q12 h
Clotrimazole	Lotrimin	Dog: 1 g	Intranasal	Once
Sodium iodide		Dog: 20 mg/lb/day (44 mg/kg/day) Cat: 10 mg/lb/day (22 mg/kg/day)	PO	q8 h
Terbinafine		Dog/cat: 4.5–9 mg/lb (10–20 mg/kg)	PO	q24 h
Lufenuron	Program	Dog: 2.2–4.5 mg/lb (5–10 mg/kg)	PO	q24 h

REFERENCES

1. Greene RT, Burtsch RC: New antifungal therapies: Chitin synthesis inhibitors. 15th Annual Veterinary Medical Forum of the American College of Veterinary Internal Medicine, 1997, p 520.
2. Taboada J, Merchant SR: Treatment of fungal diseases: Antifungal agents used in the treatment of systemic disease. 13th Annual Veterinary Medical Forum of the American College of Veterinary Internal Medicine, 1995, p 800.
3. Legendre AM, et al: Treatment of blastomycosis with itraconazole in 112 dogs. J Vet Intern Med 10:365, 1996.
4. Brooks DE, et al: The treatment of canine ocular blastomycosis with systemically administered itraconazole. Prog Vet Comp Ophthalmol 1:263, 1991.
5. Hodges RD, et al: Itraconazole for the treatment of histoplasmosis in cats. J Vet Intern Med 8:409, 1994.
6. Medleau L, et al: Itraconazole for the treatment of cryptococcosis in cats. J Vet Intern Med 9:39, 1995.
7. Mozaffarian N, et al: Enhancement of nitric oxide synthesis by macrophages represents an additional mechanism of action for amphotericin B. Antimicrob Agents Chemother 41:1825, 1997.
8. Sawaya BP, et al: Amphotericin B nephrotoxicity: The adverse consequences of altered membrane properties. J Am Soc Nephrol 6:154, 1995.
9. Janoff AS, et al: Amphotericin B lipid complex (ABLC): A molecular rationale for the attenuation of amphotericin B related toxicities. J Liposome Res 3:451, 1993.
10. Szoka FCJ, Tang T: Amphotericin B formulated in liposomes and lipid based systems: A review. J Liposome Res 3:363, 1993.
11. Hiemenz JW: Lipid formulations of amphotericin B: Recent progress and future directions. Clin Infect Dis 22:S133, 1996.
12. Krawiec DR, et al: Use of amphotericin B lipid complex for treatment of blastomycosis in dogs. JAVMA 209:2073, 1996.
13. Malik R, et al: Cryptococcosis in cats: Clinical and mycological assessment of 29 cases and evaluation of treatment using orally administered fluconazole. J Med Vet Mycol 30:133, 1992.
14. Boothe DM, et al: Itraconazole disposition after single oral and intravenous and multiple oral dosing in healthy cats. Am J Vet Res 58:872, 1997.
15. Malik R, et al: Suspected drug eruption in seven dogs during administration of flucytosine. Aust Vet J 74:285, 1996.
16. Gupta AK, et al: Antifungal agents: An overview. Part II. J Am Acad Dermatol 30:911, 1994.
17. Kurtz MB, Douglas CM: Lipopeptide inhibitors of fungal glucan synthase. J Med Vet Mycol 35:79, 1997.
18. Rudmann DG, et al: Evaluation of risk factors for blastomycosis in dogs; 857 cases (1980–1990). JAVMA 201:1754, 1992.
19. Morgan MW, Salit IE: Human and canine blastomycosis: A common source infection. Can J Infect Dis 7:147, 1996.
20. Baumgardner DJ, et al: Blastomycosis in dogs: A fifteen year survey in a very highly endemic area near Eagle River, Wisconsisn. Wilderness Environ Med 7:1, 1996.
21. Baumgardner DJ, et al: The epidemiology of blastomycosis in dogs: North central Wisconsin, USA. J Med Vet Mycol 33:171, 1995.
22. Cote E, et al: Blastomycosis in six dogs in New York state. JAVMA 210:502, 1997.
23. Arceneaux KA, Taboada J: Blastomycosis in dogs: 115 cases (1980–1995). JAVMA 213:658, 1998.
24. Marcellin-Little DJ, et al: Chronic localized osteomyelitis caused by atypical infection with *Blastomyces dermatitidis* in a dog. JAVMA 209:1877, 1996.
25. Bloom JD, et al: Ocular blastomycosis in dogs: 73 cases, 108 eyes (1985–1993). JAVMA 209:1271, 1996.
26. Miller PE, et al: Feline blastomycosis: A report of three cases and a literature review (1961–1988). J Am Anim Hosp Assoc 26:417, 1990.
27. Garma-Avina A: Cytologic findings in 43 cases of blastomycosis diagnosed antemortem in naturally-infected dogs. Mycopathologia 131:87, 1995.
28. Hawkins EC, DeNicola DB: Cytologic analysis of tracheal wash specimens and bronchoalveolar lavage fluid in the diagnosis of mycotic infection in dogs. JAVMA 197:79, 1990.
29. Baumgardner DJ, Paretsky DP: Identification of *Blastomyces dermatitidis* in the stool of a dog with acute pulmonary blastomycosis. J Med Vet Mycol 35:419, 1997.
30. Ramsey DT: Blastomycosis in a veterinarian. JAVMA 205:968, 1994.
31. Cote E, et al: Possible transmission of *Blastomycosis dermatitidis* via culture specimen. JAVMA 210:479, 1997.
32. Pappas PG, et al: Treatment of blastomycosis with higher doses of fluconazole. Clin Infect Dis 25:200, 1997.
33. Kowalewich N, et al: Identification of *Histoplasma capsulatum* organisms in the pleural and peritoneal effusions of a dog. JAVMA 202:423, 1993.
34. Chapman BL, et al: Granulomatous hepatitis in dogs: Nine cases (1987–1990). JAVMA 203:680, 1993.
35. Davidson AP: Canine coccidioidomycosis update. 13th Annual Veterinary Medical Forum of the American College of Veterinary Internal Medicine, 1995, p 808.
36. Stevens DA: Coccidioidomycosis. N Engl J Med 332:1077, 1995.
37. Greene RT, Troy GC: Coccidioidomycosis in 48 cats: A retrospective study (1984–1993). J Vet Intern Med 9:86, 1995.
38. Richter KP: Feline cryptococcosis. 13th Annual Veterinary Medical Forum of the American College of Veterinary Internal Medicine, 1995, p 804.
39. Malik R, et al: Asymptomatic carriage of *Cryptococcus neoformans* in the nasal cavity of dogs and cats. J Med Vet Mycol 35:27, 1997.
40. Jacobs GJ, et al: Crytococcal infection in cats: Factors influencing treatment outcome, and results of sequential serum antigen titers in 35 cats. J Vet Intern Med 11:1, 1997.
41. Walker C, et al: Analysis of leucocytes and lymphocyte subsets in cats with naturally-occuring cryptococcosis but differing feline immunodeficiency virus status. Aust Vet J 72:93, 1995.
42. Gerds-Grogan S, Dayrell-Hart B: Feline cryptococcosis: A retrospective evaluation. J Am Anim Hosp Assoc 33:118, 1997.
43. Malik R, et al: Nasopharyngeal cryptococcosis. Aust Vet J 75:483, 1997.
44. Malik R, et al: Cryptococcosis in dogs: A retrospective study of 20 consecutive cases. J Med Vet Mycol 33:291, 1995.
45. Berthelin CF, et al: Cryptococcosis of the nervous system in dogs. Part 1: Epidemiologic, clinical, and neuropathologic features. Prog Vet Neurol 5:88, 1994.
46. Tiches D, et al: A case of canine central nervous system cryptococcosis: Management with fluconazole. J Am Anim Hosp Assoc 34:145, 1998.
47. Kerwin SC, et al: Cervical spinal cord compression caused by cryptococcosis in a dog and successful treatment with surgery and fluconazole. J Am Anim Hosp Assoc 34:523, 1998.
48. Berthelin CF, et al: Cryptococcosis of the nervous system in dogs. Part 2: Diagnosis, treatment, monitoring, and prognosis. Prog Vet Neurol 5:136, 1994.
49. Flatland B, et al: Clinical and serologic evaluation of cats with cryptococcosis. JAVMA 209:1110, 1996.
50. Malik R, et al: A latex cryptococcal antigen agglutination test for diagnosis and monitoring of therapy for cryptococcosis. Aust Vet J 74:358, 1996.
51. Malik R, et al: Combination chemotherapy of canine and feline cryptococcosis using subcutaneously administered amphotericin B. Aust Vet J 73:124, 1996.
52. Davies C, Troy GC: Deep mycotic infections in cats. J Am Anim Hosp Assoc 32:380, 1996.
53. Reed KD, et al: Zoonotic transmission of sporotrichosis: Case report and review. Clin Infect Dis 16:384, 1993.
54. Codner EC, et al: Comparison of computed tomography with radiography as a noninvasive diagnostic technique for chronic nasal disease in dogs. JAVMA 202:1106, 1993.
55. Mathews KG, et al: Computed tomographic assessment of noninvasive intranasal infusions in dogs with fungal rhinitis. Vet Surg 25:309, 1996.
56. McCullough SM, et al: Endoscopically placed tubes for administration of enilconazole for treatment of nasal aspergillosis. JAVMA 212:67, 1998.
57. Richardson EF, et al: Distribution of topical agents in the frontal sinuses and nasal cavity of dogs: Comparison between current protocols for treatment of nasal aspergillosis and a new noninvasive technique. Vet Surg 24:476, 1995.
58. Sharp NJ, et al: Treatment of canine nasal aspergillosis with enilconazole. J Vet Intern Med 7:40, 1993.
59. Davidson A, Mathews KG: Nasal aspergillosis: Treatment with clotrimazole. J Am Anim Hosp Assoc 33:475, 1997.
60. Caulkett N, et al: Upper-airway obstuction and prolonged recovery from anesthesia following intranasal clotrimazole administration. J Am Anim Hosp Assoc 33:264, 1997.
61. Berry WL, Leisewitz AL: Multifocal *Aspergillus terreus* discospondylitis in two German shepherd dogs. J S Afr Vet Assoc 67:222, 1996.
62. Butterworth SJ, et al: Multiple discospondylitis associated with *Aspergillus* species infection in a dog. Vet Rec 136:38, 1995.
63. Moore AH, Hanna FY: Mycotic osteomyelitis in a dog following nasal aspergillosis. Vet Rec 137:349, 1995.
64. Starkey RJ, McLoughlin MA: Treatment of renal aspergillosis in a dog using nephrostomy tubes. J Vet Intern Med 10:336, 1996.
65. Matsumoto T, et al: Developments in hyalohyphomycosis and phaeohyphomycosis. J Med Vet Mycol 32:S329, 1994.

SECTION V

CANCER

CHAPTER 94

TUMOR BIOLOGY

Cheryl London

Over the past several years, tremendous advances have been made in our understanding of tumor biology. This has, in large part, been because of rapid advances in molecular techniques that have permitted the identification of genes involved in the processes of carcinogenesis and metastasis. With this knowledge has come greater opportunity for the development of novel therapeutics, such as antiangiogenic agents. This chapter focuses on the events that transform a normal cell into a malignant cell capable of replicating in an uncontrolled manner, invading local tissues, and spreading to distant sites in the body. By definition, benign tumors consist of abnormal cells that remain clustered together in a single mass often compressing, but never invading, the surrounding tissues. Benign tumors are often curable by simple surgical excision. By comparison, malignant tumors are made up of cells that possess the ability not only to invade adjacent tissues but also to break loose, enter the bloodstream or lymphatic vessels, and form secondary tumors (metastases) at distant locations. The term *cancer* refers to a malignant tumor.

THE BIOLOGY OF CARCINOGENESIS

It is now known that in most instances, a tumor arises from a single cell that has undergone a series of genetic mutations affecting the mechanisms that regulate growth and differentiation. Although two genetic alterations may be sufficient, as many as five may be necessary for malignant transformation. In most instances, the genes affected by such mutations are either proto-oncogenes or tumor suppressor genes.

PROTO-ONCOGENES AND TUMOR SUPPRESSOR GENES

Oncogenes were initially identified as components of acutely transforming retroviruses (discussed later). Further work determined that they were actually altered genes derived from eukaryotic chromosomes, and their normal counterparts were thus termed proto-oncogenes. Proto-oncogenes regulate cellular responses to external signals that stimulate growth and differentiation.[1, 2] The gene products of proto-oncogenes include growth factors, growth factor receptors, cytoplasmic tyrosine and serine-threonine kinases, guanine nucleotide binding proteins, and nuclear transcription factors (Table 94–1). In normal cells, the expression of proto-oncogenes is extremely well regulated, leading to coordinated control of cell functions, including gene expression, DNA synthesis, and cellular metabolism.

Several different kinds of mutations can affect the function of a proto-oncogene, such as point mutation, deletion, translocation, or amplification, all of which may result in constitutive expression or activation of the resultant protein.

For example, a mutation in the proto-oncogene c-*kit*, a tyrosine kinase growth factor receptor, may lead to constitutive phosphorylation (and activation) of the receptor in the absence of growth factor binding. This, in turn, leads to the affected cell or cells receiving an inappropriate signal, which may result in uncontrolled growth. Such activating mutations have been demonstrated in canine mast cell tumors, although their role in development of these tumors remains to be defined.[3] Therefore, oncogenes are positive effectors of malignant transformation, and mutations affecting them lead to a gain of function.

In contrast, tumor suppressor genes encode proteins that restrict or inhibit cell proliferation. Thus, tumor suppressor genes are negative regulators of transformation, and loss of function may lead to uncontrolled growth and the development of a tumor. The classic example of a tumor suppressor gene is p53, which has been found to be mutated in as many as 60 per cent of human tumors (as well as some spontaneous animal tumors).[4–6] p53 is expressed after cells experience some form of DNA damage, leading to an arrest in the cell cycle. If the DNA damage is severe, p53 will act to promote death of the cell, thereby eliminating potentially harmful mutations. In the absence of p53, such mutations will be allowed to persist in the cell, as well as its progeny, potentially leading to the development of a malignancy. Recently, another p53 family member, p73, has been identified and appears to possess functions like that of p53.[7, 8] Its role in spontaneous tumor development remains to be seen. Unlike oncogenes, tumor suppressor gene mutations may be carried in the germ line, leading to a predisposition for the development of tumors in affected offspring. Such is the case for the retinoblastoma gene (RB1, a regulator of cell cycle progression). Offspring carrying a mutation in RB1 have a 95 per cent chance of developing retinoblastoma, compared with the relatively rare incidence in the population not inheriting the mutated gene.[9]

Other nonclassic tumor suppressor genes include those that regulate cell-cell contact. In nonhematopoietic tissues, cell survival is often dependent on cell contact with either the basement membrane or adjacent cells. Loss of this contact often leads to cell death, thus ensuring the organized structure and function of tissues. It has become increasingly evident that cells often lose this contact-dependent growth inhibition via mutations in genes that mediate such adhesions. One such group of proteins are the cadherins, transmembrane glycoproteins that mediate calcium-dependent cellular interactions. Loss of cadherin-mediated cell adhesion (particularly E-cadherin) has been demonstrated to be an important step in malignant transformation and the development of invasive potential for several epithelial malignancies.[10, 11] Another example is the adenomatous polyposis coli (APC) gene, mutations in which lead to the development of familial colon cancer and are associated with the majority of cases of sporadic colorectal cancer, as well as gastric cancer and malignant melanoma. The APC protein regulates

TABLE 94–1. CATEGORIES OF PROTO-ONCOGENE PRODUCTS

CATEGORY	FUNCTION	EFFECT OF ABERRANT PRODUCT	EXAMPLES
Growth factors	Proteins/peptides that bind to receptors on the cell surface; binding initiates cell signals that maintain cell viability or stimulate proliferation/ differentiation	Excessive production may give cells a growth advantage, predisposing them to further genetic alteration	*INT-2, SIS, HST/KS*
Growth factor receptors	When stimulated, they generate intracellular signals that may alter cell viability and/or cell cycling	Either an absence of appropriate signaling or excessive signaling can result in loss of normal growth control	*FMS, KIT, ERBB-2, PDGFR, TRK, RET*
Cytoplasmic tyrosine kinases	Function in signal transduction within the cell; after activation by growth factor receptors, they phosphorylate the amino acid tyrosine in target proteins within the cytoplasm, allowing propagation of the intracellular signal	Disruption of normal intracellular signaling, leading to alterations in cell growth and survival	*ABL, LCK, SRC, YES*
Serine-threonine kinases	Function in signal transduction within the cell; after activation, they phosphorylate the amino acids serine and threonine in target proteins within the cytoplasm	Disruption of normal intracellular signaling, leading to alterations in cell growth and survival	*AKT, RAF, MOS*
Guanine nucleotide binding proteins	Function in signal transduction within the cell, often activating cytoplasmic kinases in response to signals generated by growth factor receptors or cytoskeletal elements	Disruption of normal intracellular signaling, leading to alterations in cell growth and survival	*RAS, BC, NF-1,*
Nuclear proteins	Directly control the transcription of genes	Mutations can lead to aberrant expression of genes responsible for the control of growth and differentiation	*JUN, FOS, MYC, BRCA, REL*

the activity of a molecule called β-catenin, which in turn is regulated by cadherins.[12] Inactivation of APC results in the accumulation of β-catenin, its association with nuclear transcription factors, and the promotion of tumor growth.

MECHANISMS OF DNA REPAIR

Other proteins known to play a role in malignant transformation include enzymes responsible for the repair of DNA.[2, 13] When DNA is damaged by such things as ultraviolet radiation or chemicals, or double strand breaks occur during the normal process of immunoglobulin or T-cell receptor gene rearrangement, DNA repair enzymes are used to correct mutations and/or re-anneal the strand breaks. Two such genes have been identified as key players in hereditary human tumor syndromes. Xeroderma pigmentosa (XP) is a disease in which individuals are extraordinarily sensitive to ultraviolet light, developing severe blistering and eventually skin cancers.[2] It is now clear that mutations in the XP gene family are responsible for this disorder. The XP genes encode enzymes responsible for the excision repair of pyrimidine dimers known to be induced by exposure to ultraviolet irradiation. Another example is the Mut gene family (MutS and L), which encodes enzymes responsible for DNA mismatch repair.[13] Mutations in these genes are responsible for a major hereditary form of colon cancer, hereditary nonpolyposis colorectal cancer. Therefore, mutations that impair the ability of cells to recover from DNA damage can

enhance the spontaneous mutation rate and lead to malignant transformation.

Another potential connection between genomic instability and the development of tumors is the telomere. As cells undergo repeated cell division, the ends of the chromosomes (telomeres) become increasingly shorter. This has led to the belief that telomere length may act as an internal cellular clock that limits the life span of a dividing cell; once the telomeres become sufficiently shortened, the cell dies. Such a role for telomeres is supported by the finding that immortalization of cell lines in tissue culture is accompanied by the activation of the enzyme telomerase, the function of which is to actively maintain telomere length during periods of cell division.[14, 15] It has also been reported that many spontaneous tumors express telomerase, whereas the normal tissues from which the tumor is derived do not. Presumably, telomerase would promote the stability of telomere length in malignant cells, thereby preventing cell death. However, more careful examination has revealed that many normal tissues may express telomerase at low levels. Furthermore, tumor formation is completely unaffected in mice genetically deficient in telomerase.[15] Therefore, the exact role that telomerase plays in malignant transformation is still unclear.

APOPTOSIS AND CARCINOGENESIS

Mutations in genes that contribute to the process of malignant transformation are often critical in regulating cell death. Apoptosis is a process of cell death that is programmed into the cell machinery and is often triggered during normal tissue homeostasis.[17, 18] For example, in the intestinal epithelium, which is renewed every five to seven days, the outer layer of epithelium must die to be replaced by a new set of cells. Another example is that of the hematopoietic system, in which neutrophils and lymphocytes undergo apoptosis regularly. Unlike necrosis, in which cells die owing to some extreme injury (such as ischemia), apoptosis is not associated with inflammation or leakage of cell contents. Rather, after apoptosis has been triggered, cell condensation occurs, and DNA is cleaved into fragments that are then enclosed in membrane-bound vesicles to form apoptotic bodies. Apoptotic bodies are often phagocytosed by monocytes and macrophages, or sometimes by neighboring cells.

Although apoptosis occurs during normal tissue homeostasis, it is equally important in the elimination of damaged cells, especially in the case of gene mutations. When DNA damage takes place owing to exposure to radiation or chemicals or as a natural "mistake" during mitosis, the cell is arrested at the G1/S interface of the cell cycle. The process of cell cycle arrest is caused by the rapid expression of p53 in response to the DNA injury. p53 is a transcription factor that induces the expression of other molecules that function to block cyclin-dependent kinases critical for cell division.[19, 20] It is also a transcriptional repressor of the proto-oncogene bcl-2, the gene product of which acts to promote cell survival and directly inhibit apoptosis.[21, 22] If possible, the DNA damage will be repaired, and the cell will then resume cycling. However, when significant DNA disruption occurs, the cell undergoes apoptosis. Therefore, apoptosis is a critical regulator of the survival of cells containing mutated DNA. When apoptosis is disrupted, through either aberrant expression of proteins that inhibit cell death or dysfunction of proteins that promote cell death, potentially dangerous genetic mutations may be allowed to persist. This is supported by the extremely high frequency of p53 mutations found in human tumors. Furthermore, many therapeutic modalities kill neoplastic cells by inducing DNA damage (chemotherapy, radiation therapy). Cells defective in apoptotic mechanisms would likely be resistant to such therapies.

MULTI-STEP CARCINOGENESIS

With the exception of acutely transforming retroviruses, most cancers are believed to arise through the process of multi-step carcinogenesis, in which mutations accumulate over time, eventually allowing the outgrowth of neoplastic cells.[23–26] The first step, termed *initiation*, induces a permanent and irreversible mutation in the affected cell. This mutation alone is usually not sufficient to result in malignant transformation. Moreover, initiated cells cannot be distinguished from the surrounding normal cells, as no obvious phenotypic abnormality is exhibited. Such initiated cells may then be affected by *promoting agents* that induce reversible tissue and cellular changes. Promoting agents are not capable of generating neoplastic transformation unless they act on previously initiated cells. They can enhance the outgrowth of initiated cells, causing changes in cellular morphology, mitotic rate, and degree of terminal differentiation, but they do not alter the genome itself. Rather, they expand the population of initiated cells and alter its phenotype, increasing the probability of further genetic damage taking place. Hormones may act as promoting agents, expanding the population of initiated cells during a normal physiologic process, such as lactation. Either initiated cells or cells affected by promoting agents may be acted on by a *progressing agent*. These agents induce significant alterations in the genome that may affect cell growth rate and invasiveness, thereby leading to the development of cells exhibiting a malignant phenotype and metastatic potential. The process of progression is irreversible, usually occurring in a stepwise fashion, gradually increasing the malignant potential of the cell until a mature neoplasm is formed. In summary, malignant transformation requires more than one genetic alteration (initiation). Promotion increases the likelihood that initiated cells will undergo further genetic alteration (progression).

MECHANISMS OF DNA DAMAGE

Multi-step carcinogenesis may take place in several different ways, and more than one mechanism may contribute to the generation of a particular tumor. Point mutation, chromosomal translocation, or gene amplification may occur as a spontaneous event in any cell population, especially those that are actively dividing. Inadequate or inefficient DNA repair mechanisms may result in permanent changes, and in a cycling cell population, the number of affected cells may expand greatly. This spontaneous process of gene mutation is referred to as *passive carcinogenesis*. In such cases, it is probable that mutations accumulate over a lifetime, providing some explanation as to why many cancers develop in older individuals.[27]

There are several neoplastic diseases in humans that have been demonstrated to be the result of an inherited genetic defect *(heritable carcinogenesis)*. Moreover, many new genes have recently been identified that predispose individuals to certain types of cancers, such as BRCA mutations and the development of breast cancer.[28, 29] Most of these involve tumor suppressor genes and exhibit recessive inheritance patterns. The classic example is that of the previously discussed mutation in RB1, in which approximately 95 per cent of individuals receiving the mutated gene develop retinoblastoma. The high incidence of tumors in individuals with inherited mutations occurs because the initial mutation is present in the germ line, and every cell in that line is essentially in an initiated state from birth. Therefore, there is a large number of potential target cells, making it highly probable that one or more cells will experience at least one additional mutation, eventually leading to malignant transformation. Although no breed-specific genetic alterations predisposing to the development of tumors have been identified in domestic animals, Boxers, German shepherds, Scottish terriers, and golden retrievers (and possibly rottweilers) do have a higher incidence of cancer than other breeds. Intensive breeding practices may have inadvertently selected for populations of purebred dogs with defects in tumor suppressor genes, DNA repair mechanisms, or deficient immunosurveillance.

There are several biologic agents capable of contributing to the development of or directly causing cancer *(biologic carcinogenesis)*. These include viruses, certain hormones (estrogen and mammary tumors in dogs and cats), and some parasites (*Spirocerca lupi* and esophageal fibrosarcoma and osteosarcoma in dogs). Perhaps best studied are the RNA retroviruses, as research on these led to the initial discovery of oncogenes.[30, 31] Upon entering the cell, retroviruses convert their RNA to DNA and integrate into the host chromosome as a provirus. New virus is generated by transcription of the provirus and budding of virus particles from the cell membrane. Acutely transforming retroviruses contain an oncogene derived from a eukaryotic chromosome. At some point during evolution of the virus, integration occurred close to or at the location of a proto-oncogene. Subsequently, the gene was incorporated into the new virus particles as a consequence of new virus production. However, the virus has almost always lost a portion of its own vital genes in the process, making it replication-deficient (with the exception of the Rous sarcoma virus) and necessitating the presence of a replication-competent helper virus for the production of complete virus particles. The portion of eukaryotic DNA obtained by the virus is either expressed at an inappropriate level, having lost all control mechanisms normally present in the chromosome, or mutated, leading to aberrant function of the resultant protein. Acutely transforming viruses tend to transform cells rapidly, as every infected cell expresses the oncogene. Some examples include the simian sarcoma virus, the Abelson murine leukemia virus, and the feline sarcoma virus, which requires help from the feline leukemia virus to complete replication. In comparison to acutely transforming retroviruses, slow-acting retroviruses do not contain an oncogene and remain replication-competent. They induce malignant transformation by insertion of provirus into the chromosome adjacent to a proto-oncogene, or within the gene itself. This may disrupt normal gene regulation or generate a truncated protein that exhibits constitutive activation. As this is a random process, such viruses tend to induce tumors after a long latency period. Examples include the feline leukemia virus, mouse mammary tumor virus, and avian leukosis virus.

DNA tumor viruses are much more complicated than their retroviral counterparts.[30, 32] They often contain many more genes and exhibit intricate regulation of viral production. Specific DNA viruses have been identified as the causative agents of several human cancers. These include Epstein-Barr virus and Burkitt's lymphoma, herpesvirus 8 and Kaposi's sarcoma, human papillomavirus and cervical cancer, and hepatitis B and C viruses and hepatocellular carcinoma. In veterinary medicine, both bovine and canine papillomaviruses have been linked to the development of squamous cell carcinoma.[32, 33] Several genes have been identified within DNA tumor viruses that are capable of disrupting normal growth regulatory proteins. These viral gene products may bind to and inhibit endogenous RB1 and p53, with the same consequence as inactivating mutations that affect these genes, or they may mimic the function of bcl-2, thereby promoting cell survival. In either case, these viral proteins interfere with the regulation of apoptosis, contributing to malignant transformation.

A large number of chemical compounds have been identified, both naturally occurring and synthetic, that are capable of inducing malignant neoplasia (chemical carcinogenesis). In most cases, chemical carcinogens require repeated exposure to cause DNA damage, the effects being additive over a lifetime.[25, 34] As some of these chemicals accumulate in body fat, they may be slowly released over many years. Therefore, there is often a long latency between exposure and tumor development. Furthermore, the carcinogenic potential of various chemicals may be influenced by several factors, including species, age, and sex. Some examples include pyrrolizidine alkaloids (plant derived), which induce liver cancer, nitrates and nitrites used as preservatives in foods, pesticides, and polychlorobiphenyls (PCBs). Chemotherapy agents are often mutagens, inducing DNA damage that can lead to the development of secondary neoplasms after treatment.

Physical carcinogens capable of inducing malignancy include ultraviolet and ionizing radiation, as well as foreign bodies and fibers, such as asbestos.[35, 36] Ultraviolet radiation induces pyrimidine dimers and point mutations in DNA. It is known to be a cause of several different cancers in animals and humans, including squamous cell carcinoma (cats, dogs, cows, humans), melanoma (humans), and cutaneous hemangiosarcoma (dogs).[37–39] Physical carcinogens include electromagnetic radiation (X-rays, gamma rays), particulate radiation (electrons, protons, neutrons, alpha particles), and heavy ions. These agents induce strand breaks, point mutations, deletions, and chromosomal fragmentation. In human medicine, chronic leukemias, thyroid tumors, and breast cancer, as well as others, have been linked to radiation exposure. Radiation-induced tumors have also been recognized in dogs after treatment of primary tumors with radiation therapy.[40, 41]

THE BIOLOGY OF METASTASIS

Whereas most primary tumors can be eliminated by surgical excision, metastatic disease remains the most formidable obstacle to a cure. Much cancer research has focused on elucidating the mechanisms of metastasis in an effort to provide opportunities for the development of new therapeutic strategies. Perhaps one of the most important discoveries has been that metastasis is an active process, not necessarily the result of random events. In fact, fewer than 0.01 to 0.1 per cent of cells that leave the primary tumor actually survive.[42, 43]

Most tumor cells metastasize via the lymphatic or vascular system, although some cancers can also spread along or through tissue planes. Although not absolute, different tumor types tend to exhibit preferential routes of metastasis, with sarcomas more likely to spread via blood vessels, and carcinomas more likely to travel through the lymphatics. In 1889, Paget formulated the seed and soil hypothesis, proposing that specific interactions occur between metastatic cells and the target organ, and that tumor cells (seed) will not survive unless the necessary environmental conditions (soil) are present in the organ.[44] Alternatively, it was hypothesized that tumor cells metastasize randomly, becoming trapped in the first capillary bed encountered, thereby facilitating spread to the target organ. It now appears as if both these mechanisms are correct; although circulatory anatomy relative to the primary tumor plays an important role in the distribution of metastases, it cannot fully explain the metastatic patterns of some tumors.

For tumor cells to metastasize, they must induce the growth of new blood vessels, invade the surrounding extracellular matrix (ECM) and enter the circulation or lymphatics, survive in the circulation long enough to adhere to endothelial basement membrane, invade the surrounding tissue, proliferate, and then induce neovascularization again (Fig. 94–1). These steps are interdependent, and failure to complete any one of them will impair the metastatic process. Furthermore, all these steps constitute normal physiologic events, such as those that occur during migration of leukocytes in and out of the vasculature and lymphatics, during wound healing, and as part of the embryonic development itself; malignant cells simply use the properties of normal cells to promote pathologic events.

ANGIOGENESIS

Before a primary or metastatic tumor can grow beyond 1 to 2 mm in diameter, it must develop a blood supply to bring

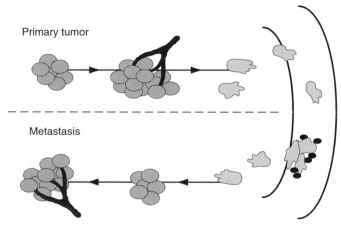

Primary tumor

Metastasis

Figure 94–1. For a primary tumor to generate metastatic disease, several steps must be successfully completed. For a primary tumor to grow beyond a few millimeters in size, it must first induce the ingrowth of new blood vessels (angiogenesis). Tumor cells must then migrate through the extracellular matrix and basement membrane into the vasculature. If they survive potential mechanical and immune-mediated destruction, they can attach to the endothelium and begin to leave the vasculature. The formation of tumor emboli and the binding of platelets to neoplastic cells facilitate both survival and attachment. Next, tumor cells must migrate into the surrounding parenchyma. If the cells are unable to induce angiogenesis or the surrounding microenvironment does not possess the necessary growth factors, secondary tumors (metastatic disease) will not form.

oxygen and nutrients to the tumor cells.[43, 45] The induction of angiogenesis requires proliferation of endothelial cells, breakdown of the ECM, migration of endothelial cells into the tumor, and formation of capillaries. This process is facilitated by multiple growth factors produced by both tumor cells and host cells, including endothelial cells, epithelial cells, mesothelial cells, and leukocytes. Unlike vascular networks in normal tissue, newly formed blood vessels in tumors are often disorganized and exhibit differences in cellular composition, including decreased endothelial cell contact, large fenestrations, and poorly formed basement membranes, thereby facilitating the process of metastasis.[43, 45] Moreover, several recent studies have demonstrated that the angiogenesis index (extent of tumor neovascularization) is a useful prognostic factor for many different tumors such as breast, prostate, ovarian, and gastric carcinomas in humans, and mammary tumors in dogs; the greater the extent of angiogenesis, the greater the likelihood that metastatic disease has occurred.[43, 46]

The process of angiogenesis has received much attention, as it represents a common therapeutic target for almost all tumors. Moreover, as the newly formed vessels are derived from noncancerous tissue (normal endothelial cells), resistance to therapeutics is much less likely to develop, as the endothelial cells are not subject to the genomic instability found in malignant cells. It was recently demonstrated that administration of the antiangiogenic agent endostatin was capable of inducing the regression of several different types of tumors in mice.[47, 48] Perhaps most startling was the finding that although the tumors grew back after discontinuation of therapy, they always remained responsive to the effects of endostatin, even after multiple cycles of tumor growth and regression. Moreover, after multiple cycles, the tumors appeared to regress and enter a state of dormancy even after the therapy was discontinued. Therefore, as predicted, drug resistance did not develop. The ability of such inhibitors to act on spontaneous tumors and established metastatic disease

remains to be seen, but the prospects for effective therapy are exciting.

INVASION

In order for tumor cells to effectively enter blood vessels or lymphatics, they must first migrate through the surrounding ECM and basement membrane. This is accomplished through a combination of a decrease in cell-to-cell contact between tumor cells, the destruction of matrix proteins by tumor-derived enzymes, and an increase in tumor cell motility.[10, 49, 50] The attachment of tumor cells to each other and to ECM molecules regulates the ability of cells to leave a tumor mass and migrate into vessels. Loss or mutation of specific cellular adhesion molecules such as E-cadherin and integrins (cell surface receptors that bind matrix molecules) can facilitate local invasion by promoting detachment. Alternatively, the expression of certain types of integrins may allow tumor cells to more effectively migrate by binding vitronectin, fibronectin, laminin, and other matrix proteins that can induce motility.[10]

Basement membranes and ECM are composed of collagens, elastin, glycoproteins, and proteoglycans. Degradation of these substances is necessary for tumor cells to reach lymphatic and blood vessels. To facilitate this process, tumor cells can produce any number of different enzymes capable of digesting matrix components. Matrix metalloproteinases (MMPs) constitute a family of at least 16 zinc-binding enzymes that digest basement membrane and matrix molecules.[49, 51] They are secreted as proenzymes, requiring extracellular activation. It is now clear that production of MMPs, either by tumor cells or by host cells in response to the tumor, correlates with the ability of tumor cells to invade and metastasize. Moreover, both the number of different MMP family members that can be detected and the relative level of any individual MMP tend to increase with progression of the tumor.[49, 51] While MMP activity was initially believed to be critical for tumor cell invasion, the production of MMPs may be equally important in promoting angiogenesis at sites of metastasis by facilitating endothelial cell migration, as well as regulating tumor growth, perhaps by altering the local composition of the ECM.[51]

The MMPs are susceptible to inhibition by a family of proteins termed the tissue inhibitors of metalloproteinases (TIMPs).[49, 51] There are currently four members of the TIMP family, all of which inhibit MMP activity by forming a complex with the active enzyme; however, they differ in their pattern of tissue expression. Experimental models have demonstrated that TIMPs can modulate MMP activity, altering the ability of malignant cells to invade tissue and reducing or preventing the metastasis of tumor cells. However, inhibition of MMP activity may not be the only biologic function of the TIMPs, as they have also been shown to stimulate the proliferation of certain tumor cell lines both in vitro and in vivo.[51] It is therefore possible that factors such as the relative concentrations of specific MMPs and/or TIMPs, as well as the local composition of the ECM, may all influence the manner in which a tumor cell responds to alterations in TIMP expression.

Tumor cells often exhibit altered cytoskeletal elements and responses to motility factors (tumor and host cell derived), all of which contribute to an increased capacity to move through tissue. At least 11 autocrine motility factors have been identified, including autotaxin, hepatocyte growth factor, and insulin-like growth factor.[49] During the process of migration, cells extend pseudopodia into the surrounding matrix, releasing proteases at the leading edge while simultaneously detaching from the trailing edge. As the cell moves into the zone of lysis, it must stop active proteolysis, attach to the ECM, and pull itself forward.

LYMPHATIC VERSUS HEMATOGENOUS METASTASIS

Migration of cells into the lymphatics may occur through direct entry of lymphatic channels or through passage from blood back into the lymphatic system. Tumor emboli may become trapped in the first draining lymph node encountered, or they may skip local lymph nodes to form distant nodal metastases. It is clear that the presence of lymph node metastasis is a negative prognostic factor for survival, and in some instances (melanoma, colorectal cancer), elective removal of draining lymph nodes is associated with an increase in the cure rate.[43]

Typically, tumor cells invade into capillaries or thin-walled venules that offer little resistance to penetration. The vast majority of tumor cells that enter the circulation are rapidly eliminated, either through mechanical trauma or destruction by immunologic mechanisms. The survival of cells in the vasculature is promoted by the formation of tumor emboli, around which fibrin and platelets aggregate.[42, 52, 53] Indeed, some tumors produce factors (such as thromboplastin) that may directly induce platelet aggregation and coagulation.[43] Experimentally, metastatic disease can be reduced by the administration of anticoagulants, although such agents have not been as successful in the treatment of spontaneous malignancies.[42]

ARREST, EXTRAVASATION, AND GROWTH

Once in the circulation, mechanical trapping of tumor emboli in the microvasculature may occur, leading to local hypoxia and tissue damage, thereby facilitating movement of cells out of the vasculature. Alternatively, tumor cells may first attach to the internal surface of capillaries or postcapillary venules, then migrate through the vessel walls into the surrounding tissue. This initial adherence may be facilitated by the presence of platelets and fibrin, both of which normally stick to the endothelial surface, especially if it has been damaged.[52, 53] Firm adhesion of tumor cells is also mediated by a number of molecules normally used by leukocytes during migration to sites of inflammation, including selectins and their ligands, integrins, and the receptor for hyaluronic acid, CD44.[10] After arrest and attachment, tumor cells extravasate into the surrounding tissue using the same mechanisms as those employed during the initial invasion into vessels.

After migration into sites of metastasis, tumor cells must now begin the process of establishing new growth. Recent evidence suggests that this step is the most important determinant of whether metastasis will occur, as it has been demonstrated that tumor cells can reach the microvasculature of many organs, but growth occurs in only a select few. Proliferation of metastatic cells is regulated by both the local microenvironment and factors produced by the tumor cells (seed and soil hypothesis). Organ-derived factors such as transforming growth factor–alpha (TGF-α) and hepatocyte growth factor are known to promote the growth of certain malignancies.[43] Additionally, tumor cells must induce angiogenesis to successfully grow beyond a few millimeters in size. Production of both basic fibroblast growth factor and interleukin-8 (IL-8) promotes angiogenesis, while interferon-alpha (IFN-α) and perhaps IL-1 and TGF-β act to inhibit neovascularization.[49] As discussed earlier, it is likely that the level and diversity of expression of MMPs by tumor cells also influence the establishment of metastatic disease. Moreover, there is experimental evidence that certain tissue-derived factors can affect the production of these MMPs, thereby altering the ability of cells to invade.[51] Lastly, recent evidence suggests that the local tumor microenvironment may regulate the response of metastatic cells to certain chemotherapeutic agents by inducing multidrug resistance in the tumor cells.[43]

TUMOR HETEROGENEITY

As malignant tumors consist of a population of rapidly dividing cells that are often subject to errors in DNA repair, it is not surprising that gene mutation occurs frequently in neoplastic cells. Consequently, cells within a given tumor often differ widely in their growth rate, morphology, karyotype, cell surface receptors, sensitivity to radiation or chemotherapy, and ability to metastasize. Evidence suggests that the heterogeneity of tumors is an acquired trait. Initially, malignant cells in a given tumor exhibit similar characteristics. However, by the time most tumors become clinically evident, the malignant cells are already endowed with diverse biologic characteristics. Moreover, the heterogeneity within tumors often increases as a malignancy progresses, leading to an increased propensity for metastasis. It is exactly this heterogeneity that frustrates clinicians, as it is extremely difficult to standardize treatment protocols when malignant cells are constantly altering their characteristics. Furthermore, the response of a primary tumor to a certain therapeutic modality may not predict the response of metastatic disease to the same treatment.

CONCLUSIONS

Clearly, our understanding of the mechanisms responsible for carcinogenesis and metastasis has improved dramatically over the past several years. As a result, new therapeutic strategies are emerging, some of which hold great promise for markedly advancing our ability to detect cancers at very early stages and to effectively treat established metastatic disease.

REFERENCES

1. Minden MD, Pawson AJ: Oncogenes. In Tannock IF, Hill RP (eds): The Basic Science of Oncology, 2nd ed. New York, McGraw-Hill, 1992, p 61.
2. Perkins AS, Stern DF: Molecular biology of cancer: Oncogenes. In DeVita VT, Hellman S, Rosenberg SA (eds): Cancer: Principles and Practice, 5th ed., vol 1. Philadelphia, Lippincott-Raven Press, 1997, p 79.
3. London CA, Helfand SC, Galli SJ, Geissler EN: Spontaneous canine mast cell tumors express tandem duplications in the proto-oncogene c-kit. Submitted for publication.
4. Van Leeuwen IS, Hellmen E, Cornelisse CJ, et al: p53 mutations in mammary tumor cell lines and corresponding tumor tissues in the dog. Anticancer Res 16:3737, 1996.
5. Teifke JP, Lohr CV: Immunohistochemical detection of p53 overexpression in paraffin wax-embedded squamous cell carciomas of cattle, horses, cats, and dogs. J Comp Pathol 114:205, 1996.
6. Gamblin RM, Sagartz JE, Couto CG: Overexpression of p53 tumor suppressor protein in spontaneously arising neoplasms of dogs. Am J Vet Res 58:857, 1997.
7. Jost CA, Marin MC, Kaelin WG: p73 is a human p-53-related protein that can induce apoptosis. Nature 389:191, 1997.

ONC

8. Oren M: Lonely no more: p53 finds its kin in a tumor suppressor haven. Cell 90:829, 1997.
9. Squire J, Phillips RA: Genetic basis of cancer. *In* Tannock IF, Hill RP (eds): The Basic Science of Oncology, 2nd ed. New York, McGraw-Hill, 1992, p 41.
10. Price JT, Bonovich MT, Kohn EC: The biochemistry of cancer dissemination. Crit Rev Biochem Mol Biol 32:175, 1997.
11. St. Croix B, Kerbel RS: Cell adhesion and drug resistance in cancer. Curr Opin Oncol 9:549, 1997.
12. Gumbiner BM: A balance between β-catenin and APC. Curr Biol 7:R443, 1997.
13. Eshleman JR, Markowitz SD: Mismatch repair defects in human carcinogenesis. Hum Mol Genet 5:1489, 1996.
14. Shay JW: Telomerase in human development and cancer. J Cell Physiol 173:266, 1997.
15. Kipling D: Mammalian telomerase: Catalytic subunit and knockout mice. Hum Mol Genet 6:1999, 1997.
16. Blasco MA, Lee HW, Hande MP, et al: Telomere shortening and tumor formation by mouse cells lacking telomerase RNA. Cell 91:25, 1991.
17. Wyllie AH: Apoptosis and carcinogenesis. Eur J Cell Biol 73:189, 1997.
18. Green DR, Bissonette RP, Cotter TG: Apoptosis and cancer. *In* DeVita VT, Hellman S, Rosenberg SA (eds): Important Advances in Oncology 1994. Philadelphia, JB Lippincott, 1994, p 37.
19. Symonds H, Krall L, Remington L, et al: p53-dependent apoptosis suppresses tumor growth and progression in vivo. Cell 78:703, 1994.
20. Prokocimer M, Rotter V: Structure and function of p53 in normal cells and their aberrations in cancer cells: Projections on the hematologic cell lineages. Blood 84:2391, 1994.
21. Korsmeyer SJ: Programmed cell death: Bcl-2. *In* DeVita VT, Hellman S, Rosenberg SA (eds): Important Advances in Oncology 1993. Philadelphia, JB Lippincott, 1993, p 19.
22. Cory S: Regulation of lymphocyte survival by the Bcl-2 gene. Ann Rev Immunol 13:513, 1995.
23. Barrett JC: Mechanisms of multistep carcinogenesis and carcinogen risk assessment. Environ Health Perspect 100:9, 1993.
24. Farber E: The multistep nature of cancer development. Cancer Res 44:4217, 1984.
25. Archer MC: Chemical carcinogenesis. *In* Tannock IF, Hill RP (eds): The Basic Science of Oncology, 2nd ed. New York, McGraw-Hill, 1992, p 102.
26. Beckmann MW, Niederacher D, Schnurch HG, et al: Multistep carcinogenesis of breast cancer and tumor heterogeneity. J Mol Med 75:429, 1997.
27. Ershler WB, Longo DL: Aging and cancer: Issues of basic and clinical science. J Natl Cancer Inst 89:1489, 1997.
28. Kent P, O'Donoghue JM, O'Hanlon DM, et al: Linkage analysis and the susceptibility gene (BRCA-1) in familial breast cancer. Eur J Surg Oncol 21:240, 1995.
29. Brugarolas J, Jacks T: Double indemnity: p53, BRCA and cancer. p53 mutation partially rescues developmental arrest in Brca1 and Brca 2 null mice, suggesting a role for familial breast cancer genes in DNA damage repair. Nat Med 3:721, 1997.
30. Benchimol S: Viruses and cancer. *In* Tannock IF, Hill RP (eds): The Basic Science of Oncology, 2nd ed. New York, McGraw-Hill, 1992, p 88.
31. Poeschla EM, Wong-Staal F: Etiology of cancer: RNA viruses. *In* DeVita VT, Hellman S, Rosenberg SA (eds): Cancer: Principles and Practice, 5th ed., vol 1. Philadelphia, Lippincott-Raven Press, 1997, p 153.
32. Howley PM, Ganem D, Kieff E: Etiology of cancer: DNA viruses. *In* DeVita VT, Hellman S, Rosenberg SA (eds): Cancer: Principles and Practice, 5th ed., vol 1. Philadelphia, Lippincott-Raven Press, 1997, p 168.
33. Shimada A, Shinya K, Awakura T, et al: Cutaneous papillomatosis associated with papillomavirus infection in a dog. J Comp Pathol 108:103, 1993.
34. Yuspa SH, Shields PG: Etiology of cancer: Chemical factors. *In* DeVita VT, Hellman S, Rosenberg SA (eds): Cancer: Principles and Practice, 5th ed., vol 1. Philadelphia, Lippincott-Raven Press, 1997, p 185.
35. Rauth AM: Radiation carcinogenesis. *In* Tannock IF, Hill RP (eds): The Basic Science of Oncology, 2nd ed. New York, McGraw-Hill, 1992, p 119.
36. Hall EJ: Etiology of cancer: Physical factors. *In* DeVita VT, Hellman S, Rosenberg SA (eds): Cancer: Principles and Practice, 5th ed., vol 1. Philadelphia, Lippincott-Raven Press, 1997, p 203.
37. Nikula KJ, Benjamin SA, Angleton GM, et al: Ultraviolet radiation, solar dermatosis, and cutaneous neoplasia in beagle dogs. Radiat Res 129:11, 1992.
38. Dorn CR, Taylor D, Schneider R: Sunlight exposure and the risk of developing cutaneous and oral squamous cell carcinoma in white cats. J Natl Cancer Inst 46:1973, 1971.
39. Madewell BR, Conroy JD, Hodgkins EM: Sunlight–skin cancer association in the dog: A report of 3 cases. J Cutan Pathol 8:434, 1981.
40. Thrall DE, Goldschmidt MH, Biery DN: Malignant tumor formation at the site of previously irradiated acanthomatous epulides in four dogs. JAVMA 178:127, 1981.
41. Thrall DE, Goldschmidt MH, Evans SM, et al: Bone sarcoma following orthovoltage radiotherapy in two dogs. Vet Rad 24:169, 1983.
42. Hill RP: Metastasis. *In* Tannock IF, Hill RP (eds): The Basic Science of Oncology, 2nd ed. New York, McGraw-Hill, 1992, p 178.
43. Fidler IJ: Molecular biology of cancer: Invasion and metastasis. *In* DeVita VT, Hellman S, Rosenberg SA (eds): Cancer: Principles and Practice, 5th ed., vol 1. Philadelphia, Lippincott-Raven Press, 1997, p 135.
44. Paget S: The distribution of secondary growths in cancer of the breast. Lancet 1:571, 1889.
45. Hanahan D, Folkman J: Patterns and emerging mechanisms of the angiogenic switch during tumorigenesis. Cell 86:353, 1996.
46. Weidner N: Intratumor microvessel density as a prognostic factor in cancer. Am J Pathol 147:9, 1995.
47. Boehm T, Folkman J, Browder T, et al: Antiangiogenic therapy of experimental cancer does not induce acquired drug resistance. Nature 390:404, 1997.
48. Kerbel RS: A cancer therapy resistant to resistance. Nature 390: 335, 1997.
49. Woodhouse EC, Chuaqui RF, Liotta LA: General mechanisms of metastasis. Cancer 80: 1529, 1997.
50. Mundy GR: Mechanisms of bone metastasis. Cancer 80:1546, 1997.
51. Chambers AF, Matrisian LM: Changing views of the role of matrix metalloproteinases in metastasis. J Natl Cancer Inst 89:1260, 1997.
52. Gasic GJ: Role of plasma, platelets, and endothelial cells in tumor metastasis. Cancer Metastasis Rev 3:99, 1984.
53. Zacharski LR, Rickles RF, Henderson WG, et al: Platelets and malignancy. Am J Clin Oncol 5:593, 1982.

CHAPTER 95

PRINCIPLES OF CHEMOTHERAPY

Antony S. Moore and Angela E. Frimberger

Chemotherapy is the principal modality used to treat systemic cancers such as hematologic malignancies and metastatic carcinomas or sarcomas. The main obstacles to the use of chemotherapy in veterinary medicine are the preconceptions and misconceptions of owners and veterinarians regarding the toxicity of chemotherapeutic drugs. The goal of chemotherapy in human oncology is to cure the patient, whereas in veterinary medicine, palliation is a more appropriate goal. Thus, the drug dosages and schedules used are less likely to result in side effects. In palliative treatment the primary goal is to improve quality of life, which in veterinary medicine may result in an owner delaying euthanasia. Just as quality of life for humans depends largely on preservation of body image as well as essential organ function, owners interpret their pets' well-being in terms of their own expectations and beliefs. Communication between the veterinarian and the owner is therefore essential. Options for treatment should never be limited by the veterinarian's interpretation of the owner's finances or preferences; rather, open and honest dialogue allows an owner to make an informed decision and ultimately creates a team approach to chemotherapeutic treatment of the pet's cancer.

In general, chemotherapy drugs are most active against cells that are actively dividing and in a particular phase of the cell cycle. In brief, cells may be in mitosis or undergoing RNA and protein synthesis (G1 and G2 phase) or DNA synthesis (S phase, which occurs between G1 and G2). Cells may also enter G0, during which time they are dormant and may not be affected by chemotherapy. While most tumor cells are in active cell cycle phases, only a small percentage of normal cells are actively dividing. Normal tissues can be classified as static (nerve, striated muscle), in which the capacity for mitosis is limited; expanding (organs, glands), in which mitosis can be induced; and renewing (hematopoietic cells, mucosa, epidermis, gametes, fetal tissues), in which the proliferating proportion approaches that of tumor tissue. Toxicity from chemotherapy is most common in tissues that are renewing. Toxicity is usually related to drug dosage. This has implications for both the animal (toxicity and efficacy) and the owner and veterinary staff (safety in handling drugs during administration and follow-up care).

Most chemotherapeutic agents are both toxic and mutagenic. Organ damage and increased risk of fetal loss have been reported in persons handling and administering chemotherapy with inadequate attention to personal safety. Precautions should be taken when handling chemotherapy drugs during any phase of preparation, administration, and disposal of drugs or waste. Ideally, a vertical laminar flow biologic safety cabinet should be used to prepare all chemotherapy drugs. If this is not available, protective eyewear, a respirator mask, a disposable gown with closed-cuff sleeves, and latex (not vinyl) gloves should be worn. All these items can be purchased specifically for chemotherapy administration. Hydrophobic filters that insert into chemotherapy drug vials prevent aerosolization of drugs during preparation for dosing. If a filter is not used, alcohol-moistened gauze should be wrapped around the vial top and the needle to protect from aerosolized drug. When administering drugs either parenterally or orally, latex gloves should be worn. During parenteral administration, Luer-lok syringes should be used to decrease the risk of drug leakage or spills. Breaking of pills should be avoided. If owners are administering drugs orally, gloves and a waste bag should be provided. The gloves and drug vial can be returned in the waste bag for appropriate disposal. For drugs that are excreted in the urine (particularly cisplatin), the pet should be encouraged to urinate on soil where urine will drain quickly, and any urine in other areas should be handled and disposed of as chemotherapy for approximately 48 hours following administration.

By dosing chemotherapy on a metabolic basis, the risk of toxicity to a pet is decreased. Although imperfect, current dosage recommendations are based on body surface area (BSA), measured in square meters (m²). This scheme implies that smaller animals have a higher metabolic rate and therefore should receive a higher dosage on a body weight basis. For some drugs (e.g., doxorubicin), dosage based on BSA is imperfect, and small dogs and cats should be dosed at a lower rate than larger dogs (Table 95–1). Until further guidelines are available, the veterinarian should use a BSA conversion table and become familiar with the individual drugs that require lower dosages for small pets.

The concept of dose intensity is important. It is defined as milligrams per square meter of drug per week of therapy and should be the highest dose tolerated by the animal with minimal toxicity. For example, in the dosing of myelosuppressive drugs, because there is individual variation in the metabolism of drugs and in the sensitivity of normal tissues, the aim should be to deliver doses that produce a neutrophil nadir of between 1500 and 1000 cells per microliter. There is ample evidence in both human and veterinary oncology that optimal dose intensity improves the outcome for chemotherapy.

TOXICITY FOLLOWING CHEMOTHERAPY

Myelosuppression is a general term applied to the toxic effects of chemotherapy on bone marrow (Table 95–2). The most chemosensitive cells in the bone marrow are the proliferating hematopoietic progenitors and precursors, which are starting to commit to a particular lineage but are still immature. The more differentiated cells form a nonproliferating pool of maturing hematopoietic cells that will be unaffected by chemotherapy and will provide mature cells for 5 to 10 days. This means that the nadir (or low point) of peripheral cell counts occurs at this time. The time at which the nadir occurs also depends on the life span of the hematopoietic cell. Neutrophils live only hours in both dogs and cats, and their nadir occurs at 5 to 10 days after chemotherapy; platelets live for approximately 10 days, and their nadir occurs 1 to 2 weeks after chemotherapy; erythrocytes live for 120 days in the dog and 70 days in the cat, and although anemia may occur over a prolonged course of chemotherapy, it is rarely clinically significant. Like the maturing cells, hematopoietic stem cells are largely nonproliferating and so are relatively resistant to chemotherapy toxicity. However, they are stimulated to divide by the loss of proliferating precursor cells and rapidly replace the lost cells, so that nadirs following chemotherapy rarely last more than several days. This

TABLE 95–1. DOSAGES OF DRUGS THAT ARE NOT ACCURATELY DETERMINED BY BODY SURFACE AREA

DRUG	LARGE DOGS	SMALL DOGS (< 10 kg)	CATS
Doxorubicin	30 mg/m²	1 mg/kg	1 mg/kg **or** 25 mg/m²
Cisplatin	70 mg/m²	50 mg/m²	**Do not use**
Carboplatin	350 mg/m²	300 mg/m²	210 mg/m²

All dosages are given every three weeks.

TABLE 95–2. MYELOSUPPRESSIVE POTENTIAL OF SOME COMMONLY USED CHEMOTHERAPEUTIC AGENTS

HIGHLY MYELO-SUPPRESSIVE	MODERATELY MYELO-SUPPRESSIVE	MILDLY MYELO-SUPPRESSIVE
Doxorubicin	Melphalan	L-asparaginase*
Vinblastine	Vincristine (0.75 mg/m²)*	Vincristine (0.5 mg/m²)*
Cyclophosphamide	Methotrexate	Corticosteroids

*L-asparaginase slows the hepatic metabolism of vincristine, leading to a prolonged half-life; hence the combination is highly myelosuppressive.

also has implications for the interval between administrations of myelosuppressive drugs. If these drugs are given when the stem cell pool is dividing (i.e., soon after the previous administration), severe prolonged myelosuppression owing to stem cell destruction may occur. The usual timing for myelosuppressive drug administrations is every two to three weeks. Some drugs (such as lomustine and carboplatin) may have delayed or prolonged nadirs, and dosing intervals are longer for these drugs.

When administering chemotherapy, a complete blood count (CBC), including a platelet count, should be collected at the expected neutrophil nadir, usually one week after administration (Fig. 95–1). The absolute neutrophil count (not the total leukocyte count) should be evaluated. Although many animals have low neutrophil counts without clinical signs, a count of less than 1000 cells per microliter is sufficient reason to reduce all subsequent dosages of that myelosuppressive drug. A dosage reduction of 25 per cent is a good rule of thumb. In addition, a CBC should be evaluated immediately before each chemotherapy treatment. If the neutrophil count is less than 3000 cells per microliter at the time myelosuppressive chemotherapy is due, it is best to delay administration by one week or until the count is greater than 3000 cells.

Owners should be instructed in the use of a rectal thermometer and take the pet's temperature twice a day during the period around the neutrophil nadir. A fever or any other sign of sepsis should be treated as an emergency, and the veterinarian should provide systemic support consisting of intravenous fluids and broad-spectrum antibiotics (cephalosporin and gentamicin are good choices, but fluid support must be provided before gentamicin is administered).

Thrombocytopenia rarely causes clinical signs; however, at counts less than 50,000, the risk of bleeding increases, and the veterinarian should be alert to petechiation, ecchymoses, or mucosal bleeding. Myelosuppressive chemotherapy should not be administered if the platelet count is less than 100,000 cells per microliter.

The gastrointestinal mucosa is another site of renewing tissue, and toxicoses may occur anywhere in the gastrointestinal system. Clinical signs include nausea, vomiting, inappetence, anorexia, or diarrhea. The management of these toxicoses depends on the severity of signs. For inappetence, tempting with palatable foods or appetite stimulants such as cyproheptadine may be used. For occasional or mild vomiting, withholding food for 24 hours and then introducing multiple small feedings of a bland diet is usually sufficient. Metoclopramide may reduce the severity of vomiting; for diarrhea, subsalicylate may be therapeutic. For severe gastrointestinal signs, intravenous fluid support and parenteral antiemetic treatment should be considered. Antiemetics include metoclopramide infused at a constant rate; chlorpromazine; or ondansetron, a serotonin antagonist that has shown promise in veterinary patients and is an excellent antiemetic in people. Cisplatin is a powerful emetic, and the prophylactic administration of butorphanol immediately following cisplatin administration reduces both the incidence and the severity of vomiting. Ondansetron may also be used in the same setting. If vomiting occurs following cisplatin treatment, and particularly if it is prolonged or associated with anorexia, intravenous fluids should be administered, as dehydration exacerbates the nephrotoxic effects of cisplatin. Severe hemorrhagic colitis following doxorubicin administration increases the risk of subsequent sepsis, owing to breakdown of the protective mucosal barrier to gram-negative intestinal bacteria at a time when the animal is myelosuppressed. Antibiotics should be administered to these animals, in addition to supportive and symptomatic care.

In veterinary oncology, cardiotoxicity is clinically a problem only with doxorubicin chemotherapy. Although both cats and dogs show histologic cardiac changes, dogs appear to be more sensitive to clinical cardiac damage than are cats. Cardiotoxicity is a chronic toxicity related to the total cumulative dose of doxorubicin rather than the amount of each individual dose. The end result resembles dilated cardiomyopathy and may progress to congestive heart failure. Although cardiotoxicity in dogs can occur at any cumulative dosage, it is most frequent at dosages above 180 mg/m^2, and doxorubicin should not be given above this level without echocardiographic monitoring. Electrocardiograph changes are inconsistent and a poor indicator of early cardiac damage. Echocardiographic changes usually precede clinical signs, but the damage progresses even after doxorubicin has been discontinued. Breeds susceptible to dilated cardiomyopathy, particularly Doberman pinschers, appear to be more sensitive to this toxicity, and pretreatment cardiac evaluation, as well as close monitoring, is strongly recommended in these dogs. The risk of cardiotoxicity is reduced by delivering the drug as a continuous infusion over several hours, by using liposome-encapsulated doxorubicin, or by pretreatment with the

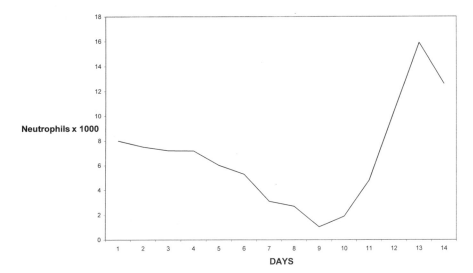

Figure 95–1. The neutrophil nadir for doxorubicin occurs between 7 and 10 days following administration. Notice that the neutrophil and white blood cell (WBC) counts "rebound" within a few days of the nadir. This is due to release of cells from the marrow owing to cytokine stimulation, but it could be misinterpreted as a sign of infection.

cardioprotectant drug dexrazoxane. These options are yet to be fully evaluated in clinical veterinary practice.

Nephrotoxicity is the primary dose-limiting toxicity of cisplatin and depends on both the individual and the cumulative dosage. Cisplatin should not be administered to dogs with preexisting renal disease and should be used with caution in dogs with urinary tract tumors. It is important to monitor the serum creatinine concentration before each cisplatin treatment. Cisplatin should not be administered if the serum creatinine is above the normal range. In addition, cisplatin should always be delivered with appropriate saline diuresis (Table 95–3). Doxorubicin has been anecdotally associated with nephrotoxicity in cats.

Urothelial toxicity (sterile hemorrhagic cystitis) is associated with cyclophosphamide and ifosfamide administration. This toxicity is uncommon following cyclophosphamide administration, but it will occur after ifosfamide treatment unless the urothelial protectant mesna is given concurrently. Clinical signs of stranguria, dysuria, and hematuria can be severe and prolonged over many weeks. This toxicosis should be distinguished from infectious cystitis by bacterial culture; however, even if bacteria are isolated and signs resolve with antibiotic administration, the drug should not be administered again, as infectious cystitis may have been secondary to the toxicity. Chlorambucil is usually substituted for cyclophosphamide if urothelial toxicity occurs in lymphoma patients. If urothelial toxicity occurs, steroidal or nonsteroidal anti-inflammatory drugs may reduce the severity of signs. In persistent cases, intravesicular instillation of 20 mL of 25 per cent DMSO for 20 minutes may help reduce signs, and may be repeated weekly.

Extravasation is rarely a problem if chemotherapy is administered carefully through a "first-stick" intravenous catheter. The catheter should be tested with a saline flush both before the drug is administered and after infusion is complete. Although a butterfly catheter is acceptable for volumes less than 1 mL, larger volumes should be administered through a secure over-the-needle catheter. If any drug is extravasated, aspirate as much drug as possible before removing the catheter. If vincristine is extravasated, the area should be infused with 10 mL of 0.9 per cent sodium chloride and warm compresses applied. The resulting reaction is rarely severe and can be reduced further by preventing self-trauma. If doxorubicin is extravasated, ice compresses should be applied for 6 to 12 hours. Dilution of the drug will only increase the area affected. Doxorubicin slough can be severe, and surgical resection or debridement may be necessary. The full extent of the reaction may not be apparent for three to four weeks.

Hypersensitivity reactions may occur during doxorubicin administration owing to histamine release from mast cells. This effect occurs only with rapid administration and is not a problem if the drug is given as a slow infusion or an intravenous injection at a rate of 1 mL per minute. A similar but more severe reaction occurs following administration of etoposide and paclitaxel owing to "carrier" solutions in these formulations. Both carriers cause massive histamine release, the effects of which are only partly prevented by pretreatment with antihistamines and corticosteroids. True anaphylaxis may occur following L-asparaginase administration, particularly by the intravenous or the intraperitoneal route. This toxicity occurs rarely if L-asparaginase is administered intramuscularly or subcutaneously. If anaphylaxis occurs, treatment with corticosteroids and antihistamines plus any necessary supportive measures should be instituted. The pet should not receive any further L-asparaginase. Attachment of polyethylene glycol (PEG) conjugates to the L-asparaginase abrogates the immune response and extends its half-life while preserving efficacy.

Hair loss is rarely a problem in pets that have fur. However, in dog breeds with hair (e.g., poodles, terriers, Old English sheepdogs), alopecia can be significant, although regrowth usually occurs in four to eight weeks. In addition, dog breeds with "feathers" will lose these (e.g., golden retrievers). Cats will lose whiskers and sometimes body fur and may experience haircoat color changes. These problems are cosmetic and rarely of consequence to an adequately prepared owner.

Specific cat toxicities may occur with chemotherapy. Cisplatin causes a fatal acute pulmonary edema in cats and should not be administered systemically. Intralesional administration of a colloidal suspension of cisplatin may be safe in cats, but care should be taken if this route is used. Topical and systemic administration of 5-fluorouracil causes acute fatal neurotoxicity in cats, and products containing this drug should not be used.

The major dose-limiting toxicity in veterinary cancer chemotherapy is myelosuppression. Recombinant hematopoietic growth factors and autologous bone marrow transplantation are widely available in human oncology practice and are in the initial stages of evaluation in veterinary oncology. Such techniques may allow the use of higher dose intensity without increasing the risk of myelosuppression; however, species specificity may limit the utility of growth factors. Similarly, advances that are being made in the treatment of pain and nausea, and in the prevention of toxicities such as cystitis (mesna with ifosfamide or cyclophosphamide), will reduce the incidence of other toxicities. These advances will improve the ability of veterinary oncologists to deliver adequate chemotherapy doses and will result in better quality of life for pets with cancer.

CHEMOTHERAPEUTIC STRATEGIES IN VETERINARY PRACTICE

Tumors grow most rapidly when they are small. As they grow larger, the growth rate decreases owing to a decrease in the proportion of cells in active phases of the cell cycle, increased loss of cells, and cell death due to poor circulation, lack of nutrition, and hypoxia. Larger tumors may also have a poor blood supply; thus chemotherapy drugs may not be delivered to cancer cells at cytotoxic levels. In addition, resistance to chemotherapy can occur through spontaneous mutations in the tumor cells. The likelihood that mutation has occurred is related to the number of cell divisions that have occurred; therefore, resistance to chemotherapy is more likely in large tumors. In general, chemotherapy will be most

TABLE 95–3. CISPLATIN DIURESIS PROTOCOLS

PROTOCOL	DRUG	RATE (mL/kg/h)	DURATION
Six-Hour Protocol			
Prediuresis	0.9% sodium chloride	18.3	4 hours
Chemotherapy	Cisplatin 50–70 mg/m^2		20 minutes
Postdiuresis	0.9% sodium chloride	18.3	2 hours
Four-Hour Protocol			
Prediuresis	0.9% sodium chloride	25	3 hours
Chemotherapy	Cisplatin 50–70 mg/m^2		20 minutes
Postdiuresis	0.9% sodium chloride	25	1 hour

active against small tumors, either following early detection or following a cytoreductive (debulking) procedure such as surgery or radiation therapy. Chemotherapy is rarely effective or curative for large, bulky tumors. The exceptions to this rule would be vincristine treatment for canine transmissible venereal tumor and combination chemotherapy for lymphoma. Early therapeutic trials for the treatment of lymphoma using single-agent chemotherapy drugs such as vincristine or cyclophosphamide produced dramatic clinical responses in both dogs and cats. However, these responses were often of short duration, and further treatment using the same drug did not provide further response. In other words, these animals had resistant tumors. Tumor resistance to chemotherapy is common even before treatment is started, and tumor cells acquire resistance rapidly after drug exposure owing to their high mutation rates.

Combination chemotherapy may overcome some of these problems by affecting different metabolic pathways in cells that are resistant to other drugs in the combination. Although combination chemotherapy could potentially be more toxic to normal cells, patterns of toxicity vary among drugs, and judicious scheduling of chemotherapeutic agents so that their toxicities do not overlap appears to improve tumor kill without compounding toxicity. For example, drugs that do not produce significant bone marrow suppression (such as vincristine or L-asparaginase) may be scheduled to be given one week after a myelosuppressive agent (doxorubicin, cyclophosphamide) or even on the same day in combination. Although combination chemotherapy may circumvent individual drug resistance, it does not avoid the problem of cross-resistance to multiple unrelated chemotherapy drugs. The transmembrane pump protein (P-glycoprotein) is present at increased levels in some tumor cells, and both the level and the prevalence increase with exposure to chemotherapy. This phenomenon of multiple-drug resistance occurs between anthracyclines (such as doxorubicin), vinca alkaloids (vincristine), and other drugs such as actinomycin D, paclitaxel, and etoposide. In practical terms, this means that a dog with lymphoma that is resistant to the combination of vincristine, cyclophosphamide, and prednisone may not respond to doxorubicin treatment. To reduce the risk of drug resistance occurring, it is important not to administer drugs at subtherapeutic dosages; the highest dose intensity possible should be delivered. It is also important not to modify the planned dosages or schedule in anticipation of a toxicity that has not occurred. For example, a dog that became neutropenic after receiving doxorubicin is not at increased risk for myelosuppression from other chemotherapeutics such as cyclophosphamide, so the dosages should not be reduced. It is also important not to change the protocol for short-term or non-life-threatening toxicities such as emesis or diarrhea. If there is tumor growth, however, it is not good practice to continue the same treatment protocol at the same dosages; rather, an alternative, non-cross-resistant regimen should be used.

Whereas bacterial culture and sensitivity testing appears to be reliable, similar tests for chemotherapeutic sensitivity using tumor cells do not appear to have the same power of prediction. Such tests can predict drug resistance and may have a role in identifying agents that could cause side effects without palliation of the tumor. However, because the ability of such tests to predict tumor sensitivity is low, combination chemotherapy is recommended over single agents suggested by assays.

Adjuvant chemotherapy is used following resection of a primary tumor when the animal is at significant risk for recurrence or metastasis. The most obvious veterinary example is the effectiveness of adjuvant cisplatin, doxorubicin, or carboplatin in the treatment of canine osteosarcoma. The effectiveness of adjuvant chemotherapy is based on experimental evidence that tumors are most sensitive to chemotherapy at the earliest stages of growth. When a primary tumor is resected, micrometastatic foci of tumor cells have a high growth fraction and a low number of resistant cells. As the tumor grows, the growth fraction decreases; the cell cycle time increases; cellular heterogeneity increases, leading to a higher level of spontaneous resistance; and areas of poor vascular perfusion increase. Therefore, adjuvant chemotherapy is best administered soon after surgery. The disadvantage of adjuvant chemotherapy is that some animals may be cured with surgery, and they will be exposed to needless risks of toxicity. For tumors such as osteosarcoma and hemangiosarcoma in dogs, and mammary tumors in cats, this percentage is small, but for animals with other tumors, the decision may be more difficult. Neoadjuvant chemotherapy is used before localized treatment modalities such as surgery or radiation therapy, with the objectives of reducing the size of the primary tumor and reducing the scope and side effects of other definitive treatment.

Although the majority of chemotherapy is delivered either intravenously or orally, drugs such as cisplatin have been delivered to veterinary patients as an intracavitary infusion into the pleural or peritoneal cavities to successfully control malignant effusions; intralesionally, in a collagen or oil-based vehicle, to control localized tumors; and intra-arterially and intrathecally for specific treatment protocols.

COMMONLY USED CHEMOTHERAPY DRUGS

Alkylating Agents. Alkylating agents create cross-links in DNA, causing strand breaks. An interesting feature of this class of drugs is the apparent lack of cross-resistance between different alkylating agents. Cyclophosphamide is used primarily in combination chemotherapy for lymphoma in dogs and cats and also has efficacy against some carcinomas and sarcomas, usually in combination with doxorubicin. The splitting of Cytoxan tablets is discouraged, because the non-scored tablet consists of active ingredient sealed within a compression coating. Splitting of tablets is therefore inherently inaccurate and exposes the handler to increased risk. An oral suspension may be made by dissolving the injectable form of cyclophosphamide in aromatic elixir, which can be stored in a glass container, refrigerated, for up to 14 days. Other alkylating agents used include chlorambucil, melphalan, nitrogen mustard, procarbazine, lomustine, carmustine, and ifosfamide.

Antitumor Antibiotics. Antitumor antibiotics act by interfering with topoisomerases, DNA intercalation, and other mechanisms. These drugs usually exhibit cross-resistance with others in their class and with drugs in other classes such as vincristine, paclitaxel, and etoposide. Doxorubicin is the most active single agent in the treatment of lymphoma in dogs. It also has broad-spectrum efficacy in the treatment of solid tumors, particularly osteosarcoma. It is also used at a low dose for "sensitization" of tumor cells to radiation therapy. Other antitumor antibiotics used in veterinary medicine include mitoxantrone, actinomycin D, bleomycin, epirubicin, methoxymorpholino-doxorubicin, daunorubicin, idarubicin, and 9-aminocamptothecin.

Mitotic Inhibitors. Mitotic inhibitors act to inhibit assembly (vinca alkaloids) or disassembly (paclitaxel) of the mitotic spindle. Vincristine is a highly efficacious drug for the treatment of lymphoma in dogs and cats and can be considered curative for transmissible venereal tumor in dogs. Another mitotic inhibitor is vinblastine. Paclitaxel and etoposide are rarely used in veterinary medicine owing to the severe hypersensitivity reactions to the delivery vehicles used for these drugs.

Platinum Compounds. Platinum compounds create cross-links in DNA. These drugs are similar to alkylating agents, and there is no cross-resistance with other classes of chemotherapeutic drugs. Cisplatin is the drug of choice for osteosarcoma and many carcinomas. It has intracavitary use for palliation of mesothelioma and carcinomatosis, and intralesional use for local control for some carcinomas and sarcomas. *Do not* use cisplatin in cats. For intralesional use, the lyophilized form is dissolved in sterile water to a dilution of 10 mg/mL. Each milliliter of this solution is added to 2 mL of sterile sesame oil and injected into the tumor at a dose of 1 mL/cm^3 of tissue. Carboplatin has similar efficacy to cisplatin without renal toxicity or vomiting but is more myelosuppressive. It is more expensive than cisplatin; how-

ever, this may be offset by the lower cost of administration, as no hospitalization is required. Carboplatin is safe for cats.

Antimetabolites. Antimetabolites are analogs of normal metabolites and are incorporated into DNA, where they interfere with enzyme activity or transcription or translation. These drugs often have significant toxicity with low efficacy at veterinary dosages. Methotrexate and cytosine arabinoside are examples used in veterinary medicine. The drug 5-fluorouracil can be neurotoxic in dogs and *should not* be used in cats.

Other Chemotherapy Agents. L-asparaginase is a useful drug for the treatment of lymphoma and lymphoblastic leukemia. Hydroxyurea is a drug used for the treatment of primary erythrocytosis and chronic granulocytic leukemia.

FURTHER READING

1. Ogilvie GK, Moore AS: Managing the Veterinary Cancer Patient: A Practice Manual. Trenton, NJ, Veterinary Learning Systems, 1995.
2. London CA, Frimberger AE: Principles of oncology. *In* Morgan RV (ed): Handbook of Small Animal Practice. Philadelphia, WB Saunders, 1997, pp 745–760.
3. Frimberger AE: Anticancer drugs—new drugs or applications for veterinary medicine. *In* Bonagura JD, Kirk RW (eds): Current Veterinary Therapy XIII. Philadelphia, WB Saunders, in press.

ONC

CHAPTER 96

PRACTICAL RADIATION THERAPY

Alain Théon

Radiation therapy refers to the use of ionizing radiation for local and regional treatment of patients with malignant tumors and, occasionally, selected benign diseases. It is a consultative discipline in which veterinary radiation oncologists evaluate animals referred by other veterinarians. The objective of radiation therapy is tumor eradication with preservation of normal tissue structure and function. Access to modern equipment and the evolution of veterinary oncology into a multidisciplinary specialty have led to an increasing role for radiation therapy in the management of cancer in small animals. It can be used alone or in combination with surgery or chemotherapy. The increased application of radiation therapy has led to a progressive decrease in the need for radical surgery in many common cancers.

BIOLOGIC PRINCIPLES OF RADIATION THERAPY

BIOLOGIC EFFECT OF RADIATION

The main requirement of the type of radiation used in radiation therapy is that it be sufficiently energetic to cause

ionization and excitation of atoms and molecules in cells, resulting in a variety of short-lived ions and chemically unstable free radicals. With therapeutic radiation doses, the molecular damage most detrimental to cell survival is that involving the structure and function of genomic DNA.[1] Most of the damage to DNA results indirectly from interaction of DNA with free radicals derived from the ionization of cellular water, which is the most common molecule in cells. Although the vast majority of DNA damage can be repaired, heterologous DNA double-strand breaks are most often irreparable and represent lethal damage. Radiation repair is usually more efficient in normal cells than in tumor cells.

The mechanisms of radiation-induced cell death vary among cell types. The injury may be lethal through interruption of the cell's capacity to reproduce indefinitely (reproductive death) or, less commonly, through structural degeneration independent of the reproductive cycle (interphasic death) by apoptosis in response to unrepaired DNA damage. Because less genetic injury is required for loss of reproductive integrity than for loss of most other cellular functions, cells usually die a reproductive death while attempting to divide. Cell death—in terms of loss of reproductive integrity—is particularly relevant to radiotherapy of tumors, because one of the most important characteristics of a tumor cell is its ability to divide indefinitely. Radiation damage prevents DNA from replicating normally but does not result in immediate cell death. After radiation exposure, reproductively dead cells may appear physically intact and progress through a few cycles of DNA replication and mitosis, during which the number of chromosomal aberrations and genomic dysfunctions increase, leading to metabolic failure and cell lysis.[1]

TISSUE RESPONSE

The degree and speed of tumor regression, called radiosensitivity, are determined by many factors. These factors include susceptibility to ionizing radiation related to tumor type; tumor cell kinetics, namely, the rate of cellular proliferation, cell death, and cell loss, and the proportion of clonogenic cells; and the amount of vasculoconnective tissues in or about the tumor.[2] Radiosensitivity is not a reliable index of tumor curability, but slow regression of a tumor type that usually regresses quickly is often associated with an unfavorable prognosis. Tumors such as mast cell tumors in dogs and oral squamous cell carcinomas in cats that regress quickly and completely may also recur quickly. Incomplete tumor regression at the completion of treatment does not necessarily indicate treatment failure. Some soft tissue sarcomas, meningiomas, and pituitary adenomas may remain detectable for weeks or even months after the course of radiotherapy is finished yet ultimately disappear and never recur. Tumor disappearance may also be delayed when bony changes associated with bone invasion are present. Anatomic deformity caused by tumors with an abundant intercellular stroma may be slow to resolve and may be interpreted as a treatment failure. Slowly regressing oral epulides in dogs are in fact one of the few highly curable tumors with radiation therapy. A practical implication of the complex reasons for different rates of tumor response is that only persistent or continual growth is a reliable sign of treatment failure. Therefore, as long as a tumor is regressing after radiotherapy, biopsy is contraindicated. A prematurely positive result from a biopsy specimen may lead to unnecessary salvage surgery, and repeated biopsies interfere with the healing of normal tissues.

The effects of radiation on normal tissues are restricted to the treatment site. Chronologically, the clinical effects of irradiation are subdivided into acute effects occurring during or immediately after (first three months) treatment and late effects occurring months to years after treatment completion. The rate of appearance of injury depends not only on the proliferative activity of the stem cells but also on the lifetime of the differentiating progeny of these cells.

Acute effects result primarily from radiation-induced stem cell depletion that exceeds cell production in actively proliferating parenchymal tissues. The most common acute radiation reactions involve the skin and mucous membranes and result from inadequate stem cell proliferation required to maintain the epithelial surface. The acute effects of radiation therapy always accompany curative radiotherapy, because to some extent they mirror the damage done to tumor tissue. Although acute effects may be temporarily painful and require supportive therapy, they are not complications but normal tissue reactions that are usually self-limited and resolve naturally after treatment. Acute reactions of the skin (skin desquamation and epilation) and oral mucosa (mucositis) may be lessened by cleansing the tissue with a 1:1 solution of hydrogen peroxide and normal saline and using antibiotics and systemic corticosteroids to minimize infection and inflammation.

Late effects are considered complications of radiation therapy. They are caused primarily by damage to the vasculoconnective stroma and slowly proliferating parenchymal tissues such as the kidneys, cartilage, bone, or lungs. Clinically, radiation complications appear to be less severe in cats than in dogs. In cats, feline immunodeficiency virus (FIV) infection may be associated with a higher risk for radiation complications. Unlike acute effects, radiation complications are not self-limited, tend to be progressive, and are usually irreversible. In practice, with appropriate treatment techniques, the risk of severe complications is low and should be weighed against the probability of tumor control. Radiation complications are usually managed conservatively. Occasionally, severe complications, including chronic ulcers, radionecrosis of soft tissues or bone, intestinal or rectal stenosis, or cystitis, may require surgical resection of the involved tissue or organ.

RADIOCURABILITY

Technically, any cancer can be locally destroyed by radiation if the dose is sufficient. In clinical practice, the dose of radiation that can be delivered to a tumor is limited by the response of normal tissue adjacent to the tumor that is included in the irradiated volume. Normal tissue in the radiation field is said to be dose-limiting with respect to the maximal dose that can be safely administered. Thus, a radiocurable tumor is one that can be eradicated by a dose of radiation well tolerated by surrounding normal tissues. A practical implication is that a tumor that is curable in one anatomic site may be incurable in another if normal tissue surrounding the tumor cannot tolerate a curative radiation dose. The art of clinical radiotherapy is to determine a radiation dose that will potentially cure or control the disease and result in a probability of serious complications of less than 5 per cent for bone or soft tissue necrosis and less than 1 per cent for spinal cord injury.

Because curative radiation doses are often close to the maximal dose tolerated by normal tissues, the radiation dose must be planned and delivered accurately to the tumor with little radiation dose to uninvolved normal structures. Accurate tumor localization with modern imaging technology (computed tomography and magnetic resonance imaging) and optimal use of radiation therapy techniques allow delivery of a high radiation dose to tumors relative to surrounding normal tissue. The choice of a treatment technique depends on the location, size, and extension of the tumor and adjacent normal structures. Each technique exploits specific differences in patterns of dose distribution in tissues according to the type (photon vs. electron) and energy of radiation and the distance from the source of radiation to the lesion to be treated. In teletherapy (external beam therapy), the distance (50 to 100 cm) between the source of radiation and the patient allows delivery of a relatively uniform dose of radiation to a large volume of tissue. The higher the energy of the radiation, the more significant is the sparing of superficial structures (skin and subcutaneous tissues) and the greater is the penetration of the beam. Medium-energy (200 to 300 kV) X-rays produced by orthovoltage units are useful for the treatment of superficial tumors because their limited penetration in tissue minimizes radiation dose to deeper uninvolved tissues. High-energy radiation (>1 MV $= 1$ million electron-volt), including X-rays produced by linear accelerators and gamma rays produced by telecobalt units, are used in the treatment of large and deep-seated tumors. The availability of high-energy radiation therapy units in veterinary medicine has expanded the number and type of cancers that can be cured with irradiation. High-energy electrons produced by a linear accelerator have a tissue penetration range of a few centimeters, which allows complete sparing of the underlying tissues. Electron beams are useful for the treatment of superficially located tumors or tumors overlying radiosensitive normal tissue (spinal cord, brain, lung, gastrointestinal tract).

Brachytherapy is a technique in which sealed radioactive sources are applied directly to the area to be treated. The short distance between the source of irradiation and the tumor provides a rapid decrease in dose as distance from the radiation source increases. This allows delivery of a high radiation dose to the tumor-bearing structures while sparing uninvolved adjacent normal tissues. When radioactive sources (usually iridium-192) are implanted directly into the tissues (Fig. 96–1), the technique is called interstitial brachytherapy or curietherapy. It is used for small lesions that cannot be completely excised and for operable cutaneous tumors with indistinct margins that have a high probability of recurrence. It may also be used in combination with teletherapy to boost the radiation dose to a specific area. When radioactive sources (usually strontium-90) are applied to the tumor surface (Fig. 96–2), the technique is called surface brachytherapy or plesiotherapy. Treatment is curative for superficial lesions of the skin, including carcinoma in situ and squamous cell carcinomas less than 2 mm thick. It may also be used as a primary or ancillary treatment for superficial fibrovascular infiltrates of the cornea that are not responsive to medical treatment. The shortest distance between the radiation source and tumor cells is achieved by use of organ-seeking radiopharmaceuticals that are administered systemically. Irradiation is then selective to the tissue that concentrates the radioisotope. Clinical applications of systemic radiotherapy include radioactive iodine-131 for the treatment of feline hyperthyroidism and functional thyroid cancer in dogs and cats; phosphorus-32 for myelo- and lymphoproliferative diseases, such as polycythemia vera and essential thrombocythemia[3]; and samarium-153 or strontium-89 for metastatic bone tumors.[4]

Another way to achieve uncomplicated cure with radiation therapy is to divide a dose into a series of equal-size doses given over several weeks, a process called fractionation. Fractionated irradiation allows selective regeneration of normal tissues, owing to their greater ability to repair radiation injury between treatments and repopulate during the course of radiotherapy relative to the majority of tumors. As a result, curative treatment may be given while not exceeding the tolerance of the surrounding normal tissues. Clinical data, essentially in people, indicate that large doses per fraction are preferentially damaging to slowly proliferating tissues responsible for radiation complications. As a rule, when the dose of radiation per fraction decreases, the risk of radiation complications decreases, which allows the use of higher total doses and inclusion of a larger volume of normal tissue. In people, standard fractionation for external beam therapy includes daily (five days a week) dose fractions of 1.8 to 2.0 Gy (1 Gy $=$ 100 rad). In teletherapy, various treatment schedules have evolved over the years,

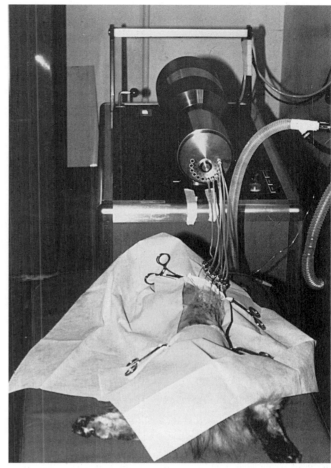

Figure 96–1. Setup for interstitial brachytherapy using a remote afterloader for postoperative irradiation of an interscapular fibrosarcoma in a cat. The technique is ideal for this location, because a high radiation dose can be delivered while sparing normal tissue, including the spinal cord and lungs. The treatment is done on an outpatient basis with no radiation hazard to personnel. The head of the remote afterloader (Gammamed IIi, RTS Technology, Inc., North Andover, MA), containing a radioactive source (10 Ci iridium-192) in a shielded container, is connected by source guide tubes to plastic needles implanted in the tumor bed below the skin. When all personnel have left the treatment room, the afterloader is activated from a shielded control room and drives the radioactive source throughout the array of applicators to deliver the planned dose. When treatment is completed, the radioactive source returns to the shielded container, and personnel can safely enter the treatment room.

with dose fractions decreasing from 4 Gy given on an alternate-day (Monday, Wednesday, Friday) schedule to 3 Gy given on a daily (five days a week) schedule, and total radiation doses have increased from 40 to 60 Gy. Current recommendations for curative treatment are delivery of daily (5 days a week) radiation doses of 3 Gy or less in an overall treatment time that is as short as is consistent with acute reactions (over three to four weeks). Longer overall treatment times or intertreatment times (three fractions/week) increase the risk of "tumor escape" through accelerated repopulation. The benefit of daily treatments compared with alternate-day treatments has been shown in cats with oral carcinomas[5] and in dogs with mast cell tumors.[6] Fractionation with larger doses per fraction may be used for interstitial brachytherapy (five doses of 5 to 7.5 Gy given once a week) or plesiotherapy (one or two doses of 150 to 200 Gy) without serious complications, because the treatment volumes include small amounts of normal tissue.

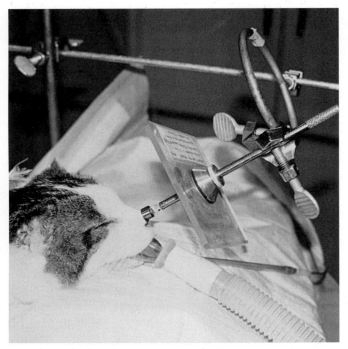

Figure 96–2. Cat undergoing surface brachytherapy for early-stage squamous cell carcinoma of the nasal plane. The strontium-90 radioactive source at the tip of the applicator is a fission by-product with a half-life of 30 years, which produces an electron beam (2.3 MeV maximum energy). Electrons have a shallow penetration in tissues, which allows delivery of high radiation doses to the tumor without exposure to the underlying normal tissues. The dose is 100 per cent at the surface and decreases rapidly with depth: 40 per cent at 1 mm, 20 per cent at 2 mm, and less than 1 per cent at the surface of the nasal cartilage. The applicator is carefully placed directly on the surface of the lesion. The Lucite shielding protects the operator's hands from scattered electrons. Because each application takes three to four minutes, the applicator is held with a stand during treatment to minimize radiation exposure to personnel. The surface dose ranges from 200 to 250 Gy. Usually one treatment is sufficient.

CLINICAL RADIATION THERAPY

The basic principle of clinical radiation therapy is that treatment should always have potential benefit for the patient, even though the treatment outcome may not be entirely predictable. The selection of patients for radiation therapy should involve consultation with a radiation oncologist, preferably in a multidisciplinary clinic setting. The only contraindication for radiation therapy in dogs and cats is the inability to tolerate the multiple anesthesias necessary for positioning and immobilization during treatment. Concurrent diseases, particularly those of heart and liver, may be more limiting to survival than cancer.

TREATMENT GOALS

After evaluation of the extent (staging) and pathologic characteristics of the tumor, the objective of radiation therapy must be defined based on the likelihood of tumor spread, expected cure rate, and treatment morbidity. The treatment goal should be defined at the onset of formulating the therapeutic strategy, because it affects the selection of appropriate treatment modalities (irradiation alone or in combination with other modalities) and the radiation treatment plan (technique and target volume). A correct assessment of the treatment goal is one of the most important decisions in radiation therapy. Overly aggressive treatment plans can expose animals that are not curable to needless morbidity, prolonged and expensive treatment, and unnecessary radiation effects. Therapeutic decisions that are too pessimistic deprive the animal of a small but real chance for cure.

Curative Radiotherapy. Radiation therapy is most commonly used with curative intent when there is no evidence of widespread dissemination of metastases. Animals are treated with curative intent when it is expected that there is a finite probability of destroying the tumor after adequate therapy, even if that chance is low. Radiation therapy given with curative intent is called definitive therapy if it is used for a localized, primary tumor that has been biopsied or incompletely resected. Radiation therapy is called adjuvant therapy if it is applied to primary tumor or sites of potential spread when the malignant cell burden is microscopic or below the level detectable by current imaging methods.

Local and regional tumor control is an absolute necessity for cure of an animal with a solid tumor. Tumor control refers to the complete eradication of the tumor at the primary site and in adjacent involved tissues and lymphatics. Failure to achieve control results in an increased likelihood of metastases and death. Tumors that are diagnosed and treated at an early stage before distant metastases have occurred are often curable by radiation therapy. Tumors arising from or involving organs highly vulnerable to radiation injury, and tumors with a high propensity to develop distant metastases, are rarely cured with radiation therapy alone.

The probability of tumor control depends on several clinical factors, including tumor size and extent, histologic grade, proliferative activity, location, and history of previous treatment. Other factors such as species, gender, age, and performance status may also affect tumor control. One of the most important factors affecting the probability of local control is tumor size and extension. An inverse relationship between the probability of local control and the tumor volume has been shown for mast cell tumors,[7] oral tumors (squamous cell carcinomas, fibrosarcomas, melanomas, and epulides),[8, 9] and soft tissue sarcomas[10] in dogs; squamous cell carcinomas of the nasal plane in cats[11]; and intranasal tumors (carcinomas, chondrosarcomas) in dogs.[12] Although invasion of bone or cartilage is not a contraindication to irradiation, local control rates are higher when the tumor is confined to the site of origin.

Histologic identification and grading of tumors are useful pretreatment predictors of biologic behavior. In practice, some tumors are easily controlled with low radiation doses (e.g., round cell tumors), but most of the common tumors (carcinomas and soft tissue sarcomas) that can be cured with radiation require high doses. A few tumor types (e.g., glial tumors) are rarely cured, even with high doses. Usually, microscopic tumor deposits of any histologic type can be cured with moderate doses of radiation.[13] Histologic grading and tumor cell kinetics have been shown to be prognostic factors. High histologic grades are associated with a poorer prognosis after irradiation for mast cell tumors[7] and soft tissue sarcomas.[14] A high tumor growth fraction is associated with a poorer prognosis for squamous cell carcinomas of the nasal plane, meningiomas in dogs, and oral squamous cell carcinomas in cats.[5, 11, 15]

Tumors of similar histologic types arising from different anatomic sites possess different biologic characteristics. In some instances, cancers arising from sites only 1 or 2 cm distant from one another show markedly different responses that are not explainable by current knowledge. For example, in cats, squamous cell carcinoma of the facial skin is curable with radiation therapy alone, but squamous cell carcinoma of the oral cavity is rarely controlled. Paradoxically, in dogs, squamous cell carcinoma of the oral cavity is radiocurable, but squamous cell carcinoma of the nasal plane cannot be controlled with irradiation.

Palliative Radiotherapy. When cure is not possible owing to extensive disease or distant metastases, treatment is aimed at palliation. Palliation, defined as noncurative treatment, can be subdivided into growth restraint and local control and symptom control. Palliation should not be viewed as an unworthy goal, as many animals may live for long periods in comfort with residual tumor or metastasis.

For animals that have good prospects of prolonged survival and limited lesions with metastases (or a high probability of metastases) or in animals with extensive locoregional disease without demonstrable metastases, the goal of palliative radiation therapy is to achieve lasting local control and improve duration and quality of survival. In this setting, control indicates that the local disease can be kept within bounds for extended periods. In dogs with large intracranial tumors (gliomas, pituitary adenomas, meningiomas) or inoperable soft tissue sarcomas, the treatment goal is to control the growth of the tumor and extend the dog's survival. In this setting, the radiation therapy technique and dose are similar to those in curative radiation therapy.

For animals with extensive and rapidly progressive tumors and anticipated short survival, radiation therapy may be used to slow the local progression of the disease or to relieve distressing symptoms. In this setting, the treatment course is as short as possible, using larger dose fractions and lower total doses.[16] Pain, compression of vital structures such as the brain, ulcerating skin lesions, and bone tumors or bone metastases in weight-bearing bones susceptible to fracture can be managed effectively with palliative radiation. Dogs with appendicular osteosarcoma that are not candidates for amputation may benefit from palliative radiation therapy.[17]

CLINICAL ROLE OF RADIATION THERAPY

Ideally, the radiation oncologist should be involved at the time of diagnosis and initial decision making so that if and when radiation therapy is used, he or she will have knowledge of all the factors necessary for treatment planning. Seeing the intact, untouched lesion before surgery can be of immense help in planning definitive treatment. The best results are achieved by an initial multidisciplinary plan tailored to the particular animal's circumstances rather than by ad hoc attempts to rescue the failures of one modality by the other. Treatment of localized tumors involves the use of surgery, radiation therapy, or a combination of the two (Fig. 96–3). Treatment of tumors with high probability or evidence of metastasis at the time of diagnosis involves a combination of local treatment and systemic chemotherapy.

Primary Radiation Therapy. Radiation therapy plays an important role in the curative treatment of small malignant solid tumors. It is also used in the management of benign tumors, including adenomas of the pituitary and perianal glands and oral epulides in dogs and thyroid adenomas in cats. Whereas surgery is essentially a local treatment, radiotherapy offers locoregional treatment covering a wider area, which is less constrained by anatomic boundaries and surgical techniques. Local control rates of radiation therapy are equivalent to those of surgery for small localized tumors (2 to 4 cm) in many sites, and radiation therapy has the advantage of controlling the disease in situ, thus avoiding disruption of anatomic structure and preserving function. In

practice, radiation therapy is used for lesions that are technically difficult to completely resect without excessive functional and cosmetic mutilation. Radiation therapy is particularly well suited for lesions of the facial skin, including carcinomas of the nose, eyelids, ear canals, or pinnae, and certain more extensive lesions of the forehead and cheeks. Radiation therapy may be preferred at specific sites on the trunk or extremities for tumors that have extended near or around critical structures such as the spinal cord, nerves, large vessels, or tendons. For certain early-stage lesions situated in less strategic locations, surgery can be carried out expediently and effectively and is therefore preferred. For example, surgery is preferred for oral tumors that are rostrally located, where a wide excision is possible. Radiation therapy is preferred for caudally located tumors when a high risk of oral incompetence is anticipated following radical excision or when regional lymph node involvement is observed or anticipated.

Less frequently, primary radiotherapy is employed for tumors that are highly radiocurable or technically unresectable. Tumors of any size, including transmissible venereal tumors at all sites, localized mycosis fungoides of the oral mucosa in dogs, and extranodal solitary lymphomas (stage I), can be cured with radiation therapy alone. Radiation therapy is the mainstay of treatment for central nervous system tumors and intranasal tumors, because most such lesions are inoperable. Radiation therapy is also used as primary treatment for palliation of advanced, invasive, inoperable cancers of the head and extremities. Re-irradiation of recurrent tumors that are unresectable owing to their strategic locations may be used in selected cases to prolong survival.[18] Because of the poor radiation tolerance of previously irradiated adjacent normal tissues, recurrences are best managed by resection when feasible.

Combination Surgery and Radiation Therapy for Advanced Locoregional Disease. Radiation therapy and surgery may be equally beneficial for the treatment of small lesions, but they are mutually beneficial for the treatment of advanced tumors. The goals of a combined approach are to preserve function and cosmetic appearance and to reduce the chance of local failure when probability of cure by either modality alone is low. The timing and dose of radiotherapy and its sequencing with surgery relate to (1) resectability—preoperative irradiation may be used if complete resection is not feasible, (2) the dose desired—high doses must follow surgery, and (3) the extent of planned surgery—extensive procedures must precede radiotherapy. The interval between the application of each treatment method should be planned to minimize additive complications without losing any advantage in tumor control. When radiation therapy is given preoperatively, the optimal time interval between irradiation and surgery is usually three weeks. This allows resolution of acute radiation reactions and is not long enough for fibrosis to develop. When radiation therapy is given postoperatively, an interval of two to three weeks after surgery allows satisfactory wound healing in most cases. Depending on the operability of the tumor, two settings for combining these modalities can be identified: (1) planned irradiation used as adjuvant therapy to wide surgical resection, and (2) a sequential combined modality treatment in which one technique is used as a "rescue" when the other has proved incomplete or inadequate.

Adjuvant Radiation Therapy. Adjuvant radiation therapy is used to improve local control and functional results for operable tumors. A tumor is considered operable if it is highly likely that all gross disease can be resected, leaving

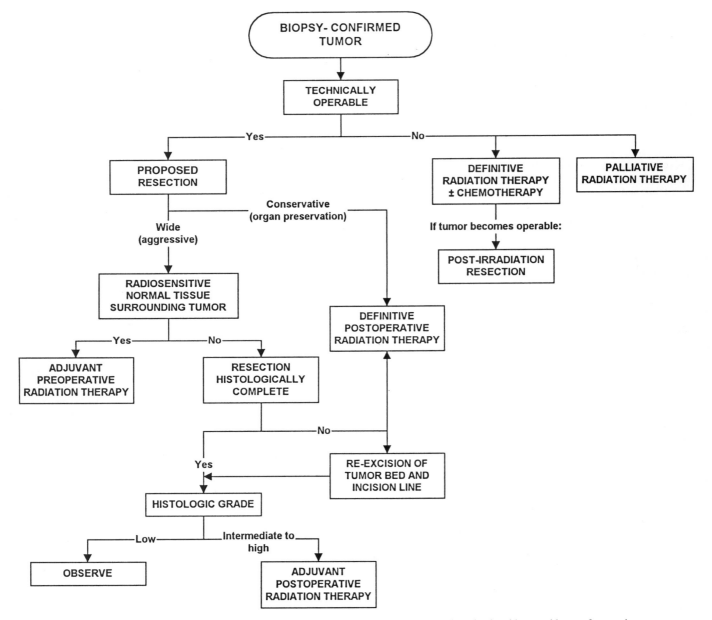

Figure 96–3. Integration of radiation therapy in the management of solid tumors in animals with no evidence of systemic disease. Definitive RT refers to radiation therapy given at full dose when gross disease is present, and adjuvant RT refers to radiation therapy given at moderate dose for treatment of microscopic or subclinical disease.

at most microscopic disease. Operable tumors include accessible medium-size or advanced tumors in locations where a wide resection is possible. Adjuvant radiation therapy is used in such cases to improve local control and functional results. In this setting, clinically apparent disease is surgically resected, and irradiation is given to eliminate tumor microextension at the periphery of the gross tumor and in regional lymph nodes. In clinical practice, animals with resectable tumors are treated with postoperative irradiation when histopathologic evidence of microscopic residual disease (close or positive surgical margins) is present, or when the risk of local recurrence is high after surgery because of extensive tumor invasion and high histologic grade. Clean surgical margins are not a guarantee that all tumor cells have been removed, as cell aggregates greater than $10^6/cm^3$ or higher are required for histopathologic detection. Aggressive intermediate or high-grade fibrosarcomas, hemangiopericyto-

mas, cutaneous hemangiosarcomas, infiltrative lipomas and liposarcomas, myxosarcomas, synovial cell sarcomas, and mast cell tumors resected with clean surgical margins benefit from adjuvant postoperative irradiation.

For large operable tumors with anticipated extensive regional microextensions, or those that arise from or are located close to radiosensitive normal tissue (brain, spinal cord, lung, abdominal cavity), there is an advantage in using adjuvant preoperative irradiation. In contrast to postoperative irradiation, preoperative treatment can be given to a smaller treatment volume with lower radiation doses, resulting in comparable tumor control with a lower risk of radiation complications. In this setting, irradiation is followed by wide-margin surgical resection according to the original extent of the disease. This treatment combination is effective for most operable cutaneous soft tissue sarcomas in dogs and cats. The benefits of this approach have been demonstrated for the treatment of feline fibrosarcomas at vaccination sites overlying the spinal cord and lungs.[19]

Sequential Combination of Surgery and Radiation Therapy. In clinical practice, the sequential combination of irradiation followed by surgery is reserved for situations in which either the tumor is initially thought to be unresectable or the original boundaries are obscured. It is used for technically inoperable advanced tumors, because irradiation may result in partial tumor regression, improving its resectability. In this setting, a definitive dose of radiation is used, followed by limited surgical resection to eliminate the residual gross disease that has not been sterilized by irradiation. This approach has been found effective, with minimal surgical morbidity in expert hands, for advanced lesions arising from the head (carcinomas and soft tissue sarcomas of the face and oral cavity) and neck region (thyroid carcinomas) and the extremities (fibrosarcomas, hemangiopericytomas, and mast cell tumors).

Unfortunately, radiation therapy is too frequently used after a partial resection with gross residual disease present. This is when the treatment combination is the least effective. Irradiation is most effective for the treatment of microscopic or subclinical residual disease.[13] Partial removal of gross disease (surgical debulking) gives very little therapeutic advantage. For example, a surgical excision that removes 99 per cent of a tumor containing 10^{10} cells (approximately 10 g of tissue) leaves 10^8 tumors cells. In fact, subtotal resection may lessen the chance of cure by irradiation in some situations, because tumor cells may be disseminated throughout the surgical bed and may be implanted in relatively hypoxic scar tissue, where they are less sensitive to irradiation. In addition, reduction of tumor volume may result in a compensatory burst of accelerated tumor repopulation, which can decrease the efficacy of radiation therapy.

Surgical Procedures Helpful for Radiation Therapy. Because the most common treatment combination is irradiation given after surgery, the surgeon has a critical role in treatment. Unless the primary tumor can be removed in toto, it is usually preferable to perform a biopsy of the site, visualize the extent of the tumor, and then end the procedure and reconsider the treatment options rather than doing heroic surgical procedures that will compromise the efficacy of radiation therapy. Because the radiation treatment field must incorporate all areas that have potentially been contaminated by surgical dissection, single incisions, as opposed to multi-branched ones, should be performed. Drain sites should be positioned close to the wound to be included in the treatment field. Good communication between the radiation oncologist and the surgeon is imperative. Information regarding the total extent of tissue involvement, the estimated volume of residual tumor, and the quality of the surgical margins is required for radiation treatment planning. To excise the tumor evidence and refer the animal for radiation therapy imposes a severe handicap on the therapist. The location of the cutaneous surgical scar, palpable postoperative induration, owner recollection, and surgical notes are usually inadequate to determine the location of the tumor bed. Radiation treatment fields based primarily on the location of the skin incision are associated with a risk of geographic treatment miss. In order to deliver the radiation dose precisely to the tumor confines as identified at the surgical procedure, the surgeon should place radiopaque markers (surgical hemostatic clips or wire) during the surgical procedure to document the boundaries of the tumor bed and residual disease. Radiographic documentation of the clips is used to localize the entire tumor volume for treatment planning and to verify

that the treatment setup provides adequate coverage of the entire tumor volume (Fig. 96–4). If clips are not present for guidance, the radiation oncologist must use larger than usual fields to decrease the likelihood of inadequate coverage, with subsequent increased risk of complications.

Integration of Radiation Therapy, Surgery, and Chemotherapy for Inoperable or Metastatic Disease. The use of combinations of radiation therapy and chemotherapy has increased over the past few years. Radiation therapy alone or in combination with surgery is usually directed at primary tumor masses and involved regional nodes, whereas systemic treatment is aimed at distant metastases.

Radiation therapy and chemotherapy play an important role in the management of metastases that are either documented (radiographically, histopathologically, or cytologically) or suspected (subclinical disease). Radiation therapy is effective for the treatment of subclinical disease in the regional lymphatics and in the treatment of clinically positive lymph nodes. For tumors with a high potential for regional spread (invasive tumors with intermediate or high histologic grades), a large treatment field is used to include the first-echelon lymph nodes along with the primary lesion. The benefit of large-field irradiation can be demonstrated by the lower rate of metastasis observed in dogs with malignant oral tumors treated with irradiation when compared with dogs treated with surgery.[8] When clinically positive nodes are present, the radiation field includes the gross disease (primary and positive nodes) and contiguous nodes that are at risk. In this setting, radiation therapy is often used with palliative intent.

Adjuvant chemotherapy is used for the treatment of subclinical disease after effective local treatment (surgery and/or irradiation) has been done. The initial decision whether to use local treatment alone or to use both a local and a systemic approach depends on the risk of occult distant disease and the availability of effective chemotherapy. As local treatment becomes more effective, animals live longer, and a higher number of them develop metastasis. This pattern of failure is seen with some tumors that previously had the reputation of low metastatic rates, including squamous cell carcinomas of the oral cavity, fibrosarcomas in any location, and hemangiopericytomas. As a result, chemotherapy may have a bigger part to play as an adjuvant to local treatment. Adjuvant chemotherapy with cisplatin, carboplatin, or doxorubicin is indicated for control of subclinical disease in tumors with a high risk of distant failure, including osteogenic sarcomas and high-grade soft tissue sarcomas.

For the treatment of locally advanced unresectable disease, concomitant chemoradiotherapy is the most promising approach. Schedules of concomitant chemoradiotherapy can be synchronous, with both modalities administered close together, or alternating, with the treatments administered in a nonoverlapping fashion. Giving radiotherapy and chemotherapy concomitantly is a dose-intensive approach that exploits the independent complementary activity of radiotherapy locally and chemotherapy distantly (spatial cooperation) and the potentially enhanced local activity (within the radiotherapy field). In cats with mediastinal lymphoma and severe respiratory compromise secondary to pleural effusion, radiation therapy may be used along with induction chemotherapy to improve the likelihood of rapid and complete remission. The beneficial effects of concurrent chemotherapy and radiation therapy result from the added toxic effects of the two modalities in the treatment field, with less than additive

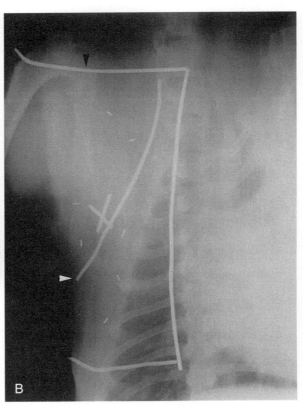

Figure 96–4. Dog with a mast cell tumor in the axillary region treated postoperatively with two orthogonal radiation fields. *A,* Lateral view. *B,* Dorsoventral view. The tumor bed is defined by radiopaque surgical hemostatic clips. The clinical setup was based on the location of the scar and surgical induration, the surgeon's recollection of the tumor location, and the surgical report, which provided anatomic landmarks (rib number) and measurements of tumor extension. Postoperative radiographic films were taken to verify treatment setup. The radiation fields marked with solder wire *(black arrowhead)* were determined clinically *(X* at the center of the treatment field). Although the skin incision was done almost directly over the tumor, the location of the skin incision marked with solder wire *(white arrowhead)* was not immediately above the tumor, because the position of the underlying tissues was different on the treatment table than it was on the operating table. The ventrodorsal radiation field *(B)* was barely adequate. The lateral field *(A)* was clearly inadequate, because surgical clips *(black arrows)* extended outside the dorsal border of the radiation field. Correction of the treatment setup would not have been possible without demarcation of the tumor volume with surgical clips. The geographic treatment miss would have resulted in tumor recurrence.

effects against dose-limiting normal tissues. Cisplatin and carboplatin are ideal agents for concomitant chemoradiotherapy. They have established single-agent activity, as well as synergistic interaction but nonoverlapping toxicities with radiotherapy. The drugs may be used predominantly as a systemic cytotoxic agent in addition to irradiation or predominantly as a radiosensitizer administered as small, frequent doses systemically[20] or intratumorally.[21] The benefit of adding chemotherapy with cisplatin to irradiation has been shown in dogs with appendicular osteosarcomas, whether they are resectable[22] or not,[23] and in a variety of other carcinomas and soft tissue sarcomas.[21] Several clinical trials are under way to test the efficacy of irradiation combined with carboplatin and mitoxantrone for the treatment of advanced tumors in dogs and cats.

ROLE OF RADIATION THERAPY IN MANAGEMENT OF CANCER PATIENTS

Radiation therapy can be used in the clinical management of virtually every type of solid tumor in dogs and cats. Table 96–1 outlines the role of radiotherapy for specific tumors, results obtained, and possible treatment complications that should be discussed with owners before treatment. It is not intended for use as a manual of radiation therapy. Most of

the results are given as local control rates at two years, because in general, the risk of local failure two years after irradiation is very low in animals that have survived disease-free. As a result, the two-year local control rate represents a reliable estimate of the cure rate in dogs and cats that have no evidence of metastasis before treatment. The local control rates given here represent a lower limit, because they were obtained with treatment protocols that may not have been optimal. It is anticipated that the current use of higher radiation doses given with effective fractionation schemes and optimal irradiation techniques will result in higher local control rates. Specific results according to tumor size, location, and other prognostic factors are given in the other chapters of this section.

A great improvement in the treatment of cancer could be achieved immediately if all animals received what is currently acknowledged as the best available treatment. This requires that individual veterinarians appreciate the potential of available treatment modalities, and especially the advantage of multidisciplinary consultation at the time of initial diagnosis and treatment.

The role of radiation therapy for the treatment of brain tumors, and in combination with surgery for mammary and salivary gland adenocarcinomas, thymomas, and intra-abdominal carcinomas (prostate, bladder, and rectum), needs to be established in animals because of its important role in people.

TABLE 96–1. ROLE OF RADIATION THERAPY IN THE TREATMENT OF SPECIFIC NEOPLASTIC DISEASES

ANATOMIC SITE	ROLE OF RADIOTHERAPY	RESULTS	ACUTE REACTIONS	COMPLICATIONS
Skin/Subcutaneous Tissue				
Squamous cell carcinoma	Curative treatment alternative to surgery for carcinomas not invading bone; treatment of choice for lesions of the eyelids, of the nasal plane in cats, and over cartilage; performed preoperatively for advanced tumors; palliative treatment with modest increase in survival for carcinoma of nasal plane in dogs	Nasal plane in cats: 2-year LCR: 77% for lesions <2 cm, 37% for advanced lesions[11]; comparable results for tumors of pinnae and forehead	Erythema, moist desquamation, epilation; rarely ulceration	Permanent epilation, skin atrophy, subcutaneous fibrosis; rarely soft tissue necrosis
Mast cell tumor (dogs)	Primary treatment for small lesions, postoperatively for microscopic or gross residual disease; adjuvant postoperative treatment for completely resected grade II or III lesions; preoperative treatment for unresectable tumors	2-year LCR: 70–92% for microscopic disease, 50–85% for lesions <2 cm, 20–58% for large tumor and gross residual tumor[6, 7, 24]; low histologic grade and location on an extremity are favorable prognostic factors	Same as above	
Soft tissue sarcomas	For operable tumors: postoperative treatment when there is a risk of surgical complication owing to tumor size or location; preoperative treatment when there is an increased risk of radiation complications owing to radiosensitive normal tissue (brain, spinal cord, lung, guts) in the treatment field. For advanced inoperable lesions: primary treatment followed by limited resection if rendered operable	In dogs, 2-year LCR: 33%[16] for primary radiotherapy for all histologic types and sizes; 41–51% for hemangiopericytoma (HPA)[11, 25] and 30% for fibrosarcoma (FSA)[11] after subtotal resection; 76% for FSA and 100% for HPA after microscopically incomplete resection.[11] In cats with cutaneous FSA at vaccination sites, 2-year LCR: 55%[19] with preoperative treatment.		
Perianal gland	Postoperative treatment for adenocarcinomas; primary treatment for large adenomas	1-year LCR: 47% of perianal adenomas/carcinomas[26]	Same as above	
Head and Neck				
Oral cavity	In dogs: Curative radiotherapy for small caudally located squamous cell carcinoma (SCC), mycosis fungoides (MF), fibrosarcoma (FSA) of the gingiva/palate or buccal mucosa; alternative to surgery for small rostrally located SCC, plasmacytoma of the gingiva/palate and floor of the mouth, and epulides; postoperatively for advanced resectable SCC and FSA; used alone or combined with chemotherapy to improve survival for advanced unresectable lesions; palliation for advanced melanomas (MMA) and tumors of the base of the tongue and tonsils. In cats: Palliation of symptoms for SCC, with modest increase in survival.	In dogs: 2-year LCR for small lesions (<2 cm): 100% for epulides, 74% for SCC, 67% for FSA, and 54% for MMA[8, 9, 10]; comparable results for postoperative treatment of advanced resectable (2–4 cm) epulides, SCC, and FSA; prolongation of survival for advanced SCC (median survival, 7.5 months) and FSA (median survival, 7.1 months), palliation of symptoms for advanced MMA (median survival, 7–8 months)[8, 16]	Painful mucositis resulting in dysphagia, xerostomia, weight loss	Persistent xerostomia, dental decay; rarely fistula, bone exposure and osteoradionecrosis of mandible and maxilla
Nasal cavity/ paranasal sinuses	Primary treatment to improve survival for carcinomas and sarcomas; combination with surgery may not increase survival; curative for localized lymphoma	Median survival for nonlymphoproliferative tumors: 13 months in dogs[12] and 12 months in cats[27]	Nasal and oral mucositis, conjunctivitis ± keratitis for eye in radiation field, skin epilation	Loss of smell, chronic keratitis, cataract, keratoconjunctivitis; rarely bone necrosis
Ear canal	Primary treatment alternative to surgery for small ceruminous adenocarcinoma or squamous cell carcinomas; postoperatively for advanced lesions	In dogs and cats, 2-year LCR: 56%[28]	Otitis, dysphagia	Damage to middle and inner ear and cranial nerves (Horner's syndrome)
Thyroid	In dogs: Postoperative treatment after subtotal resection for adenocarcinomas; preoperatively for inoperable lesions followed by limited resection if rendered operable. In cats: Primary treatment with radioiodine for functional adenomas and adenocarcinomas; postoperative treatment after subtotal resection of nonfunctional tumors.	In dogs treated with teletherapy: 2-year survival rate: 66% after subtotal resection in dogs with no evidence of metastasis.[29] In cats treated with radioiodine, 2-year-cure rate for adenomas: 92%[30]; median survival for postoperative treatment of adenocarcinomas: 20.5 months[31]	Teletherapy: skin epilation, dysphagia (esophagitis), hoarseness, and cough (tracheitis)	Teletherapy: subcutaneous fibrosis; rarely spinal cord damage
Central Nervous System				
Pituitary gland	Effective in controlling signs of mass effects in dogs with macroadenoma/carcinomas and no or mild neurologic signs; used in combination with medical treatment for pituitary-dependent hyperadrenocorticism (PDH); ineffective for dogs with severe neurologic signs	1-year survival in dogs with pituitary Cushing's disease and no neurologic signs: 100%[32]; with mild neurologic signs: 73%[13]	Hair loss, skin erythema, otitis, dullness (brain edema)	Hearing loss, cataract formation if eye in field; rarely brain necrosis
Intracranial meningioma	Postoperative irradiation after incomplete resection for cure and primary treatment for inoperable lesions	Postoperative irradiation 2-year LCR: 73%[15]	Same as above	
Spinal cord	Postoperative treatment to improve neurologic signs and survival	Median survival for postoperative irradiation of meningiomas: 17 months[34]		Rarely irreversible spinal cord myelopathy
Bone				
Primary bone tumors	For appendicular osteosarcomas (OSA): preoperative treatment combined with chemotherapy (cisplatin/carboplatin) for limb-sparing procedure; palliative treatment as alternative to amputation or for pain relief in advanced disease. For axial and skull tumors: postoperative treatment ± chemotherapy.	Median survival of dogs with OSA treated with limb-sparing surgery, irradiation, and cisplatin: 9 months[22]; irradiation and cisplatin: 5 months[23]; palliative irradiation alone: 4 months[17]	Skin erythema, dry/moist desquamation	Subcutaneous fibrosis, ankylosis, distal edema; rarely bone/soft tissue necrosis
Metastatic bone tumors	Palliative local treatment or systemic administration of bone-seeking radioisotopes (Sm-153) for pain relief	Overall 1-year survival rate in dogs: 17%[4]	Depression of platelet and white blood cell count	

LCR = local control rate.

ONC

REFERENCES

1. Fuks Z, Weichselbaum RR: Radiation therapy. *In* Mendelsohn J, Howley PM, Israel MA (eds): The Molecular Basis of Cancer. Philadelphia, WB Saunders, 1995, p 401.
2. Withers HR, McBride WH: Biologic basis of radiation therapy. *In* Perez CA, Brady LW (eds): Principles and Practice of Radiation Oncology, 3rd ed. Philadelphia, Lippincott-Raven, 1998, p 79.
3. Smith M, Turrel J: Radiophosphorus (³²P) treatment of bone marrow disorders in dogs: 11 cases. JAVMA 194:98, 1989.
4. Lattimer JC, Corwin LA, Stapelton J, et al: Clinical and clinicopathological response of canine bone tumor patients to treatment with samarium-153-EDTMP. J Nucl Med 31:1316, 1990.
5. Théon AP, Griffey S, Metzger L: Radiation therapy of carcinomas of the oral cavity in cats: Influence of tumor proliferation. Vet Radiol Ultrasound 37:469, 1996.
6. LaDue T, Price GS, Dodge R, et al: Radiation therapy for incompletely resected canine mast cell tumors. Vet Radiol Ultrasound 39:57, 1998.
7. Turrel JM, Kitchell BE, Miller LM, Théon AP: Prognostic factors for radiation treatment of mast cell tumors in 85 dogs. JAVMA 193:936, 1988.
8. Théon AP, Rodriguez JC, Madewell BR: Analysis of prognostic factors and patterns of failure in dogs with malignant oral tumors treated with megavoltage irradiation. JAVMA 210:778, 1997.
9. Théon AP, Rodriguez JC, Griffey SM, Madewell BR: Analysis of prognostic factors and patterns of failure in dogs with periodontal tumors treated with megavoltage irradiation. JAVMA 210:785, 1997.
10. McChesney SL, Withrow SJ, Gillette EL, et al: Radiotherapy of soft tissue sarcomas in dogs. JAVMA 194:60, 1989.
11. Théon AP, Madewell BR, Shearn V, Moulton B: Prognostic factors associated with radiotherapy of squamous cell carcinoma of the nasal plane in cats. JAVMA 206:991, 1995.
12. Théon AP, Madewell BR, Harb MF, Dungworth DL: Megavoltage irradiation of neoplasms of the nasal and paranasal cavities in 77 dogs. JAVMA 202:1469, 1993.
13. Théon AP: Indications and applications of radiation therapy. *In* Bonagura JD (ed): Kirk's Current Veterinary Therapy XII, Small Animal Practice. Philadelphia, WB Saunders, 1995, p 467.
14. Gillette SM, Dewhirst MW, Gillette EL, et al: Response of canine soft tissue sarcomas to radiation or radiation plus hyperthermia: A randomized phase II study. Int J Hyperthermia 8:309, 1992.
15. Théon AP, Griffey S, Lecouteur RA, Carr E: Radiation therapy of incompletely resected meningiomas: Influence of tumor cell proliferation and sex hormone receptors. JAVMA (submitted).
16. Bateman KE, Catton PA, Pennock PW, et al: 0-7-21 Radiation therapy for the palliation of advanced cancer in dogs. J Vet Intern Med 8:267, 1994.
17. McEntee MC, Page RL, Novotney CA, et al: Palliative radiotherapy for canine appendicular osteosarcoma. Vet Radiol Ultrasound 34:367, 1993.
18. Turrel JM, Théon AP: Reirradiation of tumors in cats and dogs. JAVMA 193:936, 1988.
19. Cronin K, Page RL, Spodnick G, et al: Radiation therapy and surgery for fibrosarcoma in 33 cats. Vet Radiol Ultrasound 39:51, 1998.
20. Larue SM, Withrow SJ, Powers BE, et al: Limb-sparing treatment of osteosarcoma in dogs. JAVMA 195:1734, 1989.
21. Théon AP, Madewell BR, Ryu J, Castro J: Concurrent irradiation and intratumoral chemotherapy with cisplatin: A pilot study in dogs with spontaneous tumors. Int J Radiat Oncol Biol Phys 29:1027, 1994.
22. Withrow SJ, Thrall DE, Straw RC, et al: Intra-arterial cisplatin with or without radiation in limb-sparing for canine osteosarcoma. Cancer 71:2484, 1993.
23. Heidner GL, Page RL, McEntee MC, et al: Treatment of canine appendicular osteosarcoma using cobalt 60 radiation and intraarterial cisplatin. J Vet Intern Med 5:313, 1991.
24. Frimberger AE, Moore AS, LaRue SM, et al: Radiotherapy of incompletely resected, moderately differentiated mast cell tumors in the dog: 37 cases. J Am Anim Hosp Assoc 33:320, 1997.
25. Evans SM: Canine hemangiopericytomas. A retrospective analysis of response to surgery and orthovoltage radiation. Vet Rad 28:13, 1987.
26. Gillette EL: Radiation therapy of canine and feline tumors. J Am Anim Hosp Assoc 12:359, 1976.
27. Théon AP, Peaston AE, Madewell BR, Dungworth DL: Irradiation of non-lymphoproliferative neoplasms of the nasal cavity and paranasal sinuses in 16 cats. JAVMA 204:78, 1994.
28. Théon AP, Barthez PE, Madewell BR, Griffey S: Radiation therapy of ceruminous gland carcinomas in dogs and cats. JAVMA 205:566, 1994.
29. Théon AP, Marks SL, Feldman ES: Analysis of prognostic factors and patterns of failure in dogs with thyroid carcinomas treated with megavoltage irradiation. JAVMA (submitted).
30. Théon AP, Van Vechten MK, Feldman E: Prospective randomized comparison of intravenous versus subcutaneous administration of radioiodine for treatment of hyperthyroidism in cats. Am J Vet Res 55:1734, 1994.
31. Guptill L, Scott-Moncrieff CR, Janovitz EB, et al: Response to high-dose radioactive iodine administration in cats with thyroid carcinoma that had previously undergone surgery. JAVMA 207:1055, 1995.
32. Goossens MM, Feldman E, Théon AP, Koblik P: Effectiveness of cobalt-60 radiation therapy in canine pituitary dependent hyperadrenocorticism. JAVMA 212:374, 1998.
33. Théon AP, Feldman E: Megavoltage irradiation of pituitary macrotumors in dogs with neurologic signs. JAVMA 213:225, 1998.
34. Siegel S, Kornegay JN, Thrall DE: Postoperative irradiation of spinal cord tumors in 9 dogs. Vet Radiol Ultrasound 37:150, 1996.

CHAPTER 97

PARANEOPLASTIC SYNDROMES

Gregory K. Ogilvie

Tumors commonly induce clinical signs directly by invading, destroying, or obstructing structures or interfering with function in that part of the body, or indirectly by producing changes at a site distant from the tumor or its metastases. These distant effects of malignancy are known as paraneoplastic syndromes. In many cases, the clinical signs of the paraneoplastic syndrome are more devastating than the effect of the underlying malignancy. Paraneoplastic syndromes may be the first sign of a malignancy, and the syndrome may be so severe that appropriate therapy for the underlying cancer is not initiated. The best-known and best-characterized paraneoplastic syndromes are those produced by tumors that secrete hormone-like substances such as parathormone or insulin. These tumor-produced hormones or hormone-like substances are distributed by the circulation and act on target organs at sites distant from the tumor or its metastases. Generally, removal or destruction of the tumor eliminates the production of the hormone or other substance

Supported in part by grants from the National Cancer Institute (#2 CA 29582). The contents are solely the responsibility of the author and do not necessarily represent the official views of the National Cancer Institute.

that induces the paraneoplastic syndrome. In veterinary medicine, the etiology of many paraneoplastic syndromes remains elusive.

The purpose of this chapter is to briefly review what is known about the most common and clinically important paraneoplastic syndromes in veterinary medicine. These include cancer cachexia, hypercalcemia, hypocalcemia, hypoglycemia, erythrocytosis, hypertrophic osteopathy, anemia, leukocytosis, thrombocytopenia, hypergammaglobulinemia, fever, and neurologic abnormalities. Other paraneoplastic conditions such as mucocutaneous, rheumatic and connective tissue, and renal syndromes are covered elsewhere.

CANCER CACHEXIA

CLINICAL IMPORTANCE

Cancer cachexia is arguably the most common paraneoplastic syndrome in veterinary medicine.[1-4] This syndrome is characterized clinically by anorexia, wasting, weight loss, weakness, fatigue, poor performance status, and impaired immune function, which are not resolved by adequate nutritional intake. This paraneoplastic syndrome occurs with a variety of malignancies in dogs and cats. Cancer cachexia is the result of profound alterations in carbohydrate, protein, and lipid metabolism.[1-11] These metabolic alterations are possibly secondary to a hormone (e.g., toxohormone) or a cytokine (e.g., tumor necrosis factor, interleukin-1, interleukin-6, interferons alfa and gamma). This clinically important syndrome occurs in up to 87 per cent of hospitalized human cancer patients and is suspected to affect a similar percentage of veterinary patients.[1-4] These profound alterations in carbohydrate, protein, and lipid metabolism have been documented in dogs with cancer, even before evidence of cancer cachexia was clinically apparent.[1-11]

PATHOPHYSIOLOGY

Cancer and Carbohydrate Metabolism. Significant alterations in carbohydrate metabolism result in a net energy gain by the tumor and a net energy loss by the host.[1-5] Essentially, the tumor grows at the expense of the host. In tumor cells, glucose is the preferred substrate for energy production. Relative insulin resistance has been reported in both human and canine cancer patients.[1] Data suggest that in dogs with lymphoma, this insulin resistance may be the result of a postreceptor defect. Therefore, dietary therapy may be effective in abating this problem.[1]

When dogs with untreated lymphoma without clinical evidence of cancer cachexia were compared with controls using an intravenous glucose tolerance test, lactate and insulin concentrations were significantly higher in the former. However, the increased lactate levels did not normalize after a complete remission was obtained with doxorubicin chemotherapy.[5] After dogs came out of remission and began to show evidence of cachexia, they had even higher lactate levels. In addition, the hyperinsulinemia did not abate after remission induction with doxorubicin chemotherapy. The same findings in lactate and insulin metabolism were observed in 90 dogs with a wide variety of nonhematopoietic malignancies before and after these solid tumors were surgically excised.[12] These alterations in carbohydrate metabolism result partially because tumors preferentially metabolize glucose, use anaerobic glycolysis for energy, and form lactate as an end product of metabolism. These results parallel those observed in similar human patients.[3, 12, 13]

The impact of hyperlactatemia and hyperinsulinemia in dogs with lymphoma is far reaching. Research is under way to determine whether these findings should alter the choice of fluids as well as enteral and parenteral feeding products. In one study, the hyperlactatemia that was observed in dogs with lymphoma became more pronounced when lactated Ringer's solution was administered.[6] Because hyperlactatemia was present after a simple intravenous glucose tolerance test,[7] fluids that contain dextrose may further increase lactate levels. It can be hypothesized that when parenteral and enteral nutrients that are high in simple carbohydrates are given as the primary source of calories, clinically significant hyperlactatemia and hyperinsulinemia may result in dogs with cancer. Because the host must convert the majority of the lactate back to glucose, this results in a net energy gain by the tumor and an energy loss by the host. Thus, if the increase in already elevated lactate concentrations lasts for several hours, this may worsen the animal's cachectic state. A group of 22 dogs with lymphoma was studied to determine whether a diet high in simple carbohydrates was detrimental. These dogs were randomized and fed isocaloric amounts of a high-fat diet or a high-carbohydrate diet before and after remission was attained with up to five dosages of doxorubicin chemotherapy. Mean insulin and lactate levels from the dogs fed the high-carbohydrate diet were significantly higher than the levels from the dogs fed the high-fat diet, both at the time the dogs were started on the diets and at the time they went into remission with chemotherapy. Dogs fed the high-fat diet were more likely to go into remission. This study showed that diet was effective in influencing response to therapy and select aspects of carbohydrate metabolism in dogs with lymphoma.[14]

Cancer and Protein Metabolism. In cancer cachexia, protein degradation often exceeds protein synthesis, resulting in a negative nitrogen balance.[1-8] Net protein loss in cancer cachexia results in decreased cell-mediated and humoral immunity, gastrointestinal function, and wound healing. Loss of body protein is manifested clinically as atrophy of skeletal muscle, hypoalbuminemia, decreased rate of healing, and frequent infections. Because fatty acids cannot serve as gluconeogenic precursors for the cancer, amino acids are the primary substrate for gluconeogenesis in cancer cachexia. Plasma amino acid profiles in both human cancer patients and tumor-bearing laboratory animals reveal a pronounced decrease in amino acids that are used as gluconeogenic substrates, but no decrease in leucine, the only amino acid that cannot serve as a gluconeogenic precursor. Many of the same alterations in amino acid profiles have been identified in dogs with lymphoma that were identified previously in people and laboratory animals with cancer.[1, 2] Dogs with lymphoma have significant decreases in threonine, glutamine, glycine, valine, cystine, and arginine[4] but significantly increased isoleucine and phenylalanine levels. These alterations do not improve with remission. Therefore, animals with cancer have alterations in protein metabolism that may result in serious health risks. Correcting some of the abnormalities in amino acid levels may have a profound clinical impact. For example, supplementation with arginine has been shown to improve the immune function of arginine-deficient animals. Glutamine supplementation decreases the severity of chemotherapy-induced damage to the gastrointestinal tract of cats.[4]

Cancer and Fat Metabolism. Most weight loss in dogs

and people with cancer cachexia is due to depletion of body fat.[1-4] Patients with cancer cachexia have increased fat breakdown, which correlates with increased levels of free fatty acids and certain plasma lipoproteins. Knowledge that tumor cells have difficulty using lipids as a fuel may be of value clinically, especially because host tissues can continue to oxidize lipids for energy. Because insulin normally increases triglyceride synthesis in adipose tissue and decreases lipolysis, the insulin resistance identified in people and dogs with cancer favors the decreased lipid synthesis and increased lipolysis that occur in cancer cachexia. Insulin supplementation in tumor-bearing laboratory animals results in decreased fat loss. Dogs with lymphoma have significantly higher free fatty acid, total triglyceride, and very-low-density lipoprotein concentrations in their serum when compared with controls.[8] Their high-density lipoprotein cholesterol levels were significantly lower than those of controls. After treatment with doxorubicin, the dogs with lymphoma developed significantly elevated total cholesterol levels, as is also noted in people with cancer.

Experimentally, specific types of triglycerides and fatty acids have minimized cancer cachexia and, in some circumstances, have had anticancer effects. Medium chain triglycerides and 3-hydroxybutyrate reduce weight loss and tumor size in rodents.[1-4] Diets that are high in fish oils and rich in the omega-3-type polyunsaturated fatty acids eicosapentaenoic acid (EPA, 20:5, omega-3) and docosahexaenoic acid (DHA, C22:6, omega-3) are also effective for promoting weight gain and have an anticancer effect.[12]

CLINICAL CONSEQUENCES

The metabolic manifestations of cancer occur before clinical evidence of cancer cachexia is ever noted. These metabolic changes appear to continue even after clinical remission is achieved or the cancer has been surgically removed. The consequences of cancer cachexia are obvious: decreased quality of life and decreased therapeutic response and enhanced toxicity to radiation, surgery, chemotherapy, and supportive drugs or procedures.[12, 13] Cachexia and hypoalbuminemia are poor prognostic indicators.

TREATMENT

Enteral and Parenteral Therapy. Nutritional manipulation in human cancer patients shows promise for minimizing clinically apparent cancer cachexia and abating some metabolic alterations. Detrimental effects, such as increased rate of tumor growth or rate of metastasis, have not been demonstrated after nutritional support of people with cancer cachexia. Nutrient profiles that contain 30 to 50 per cent of nonprotein calories as fat instead of carbohydrate decrease glucose intolerance, fat loss, and tumor growth while host weight, nitrogen, and energy balance increase. Simply changing the fat content may decrease the degree of cancer cachexia in dogs with cancer. Dogs with lymphoma that were fed high-fat diets were much more likely to go into remission, whereas dogs fed a high-carbohydrate diet had a shorter disease-free interval.[9, 13]

The addition of medium chain fatty acids and omega-3 fatty acids may be beneficial in treating dogs with cancer.[15] Polyunsaturated n-3 fatty acids and arginine have been shown in vitro and in rodent models to inhibit the growth and metastasis of tumors. These observations had never been documented in an outbred species with spontaneously occurring cancer. A recent study evaluated the hypothesis that polyunsaturated n-3 fatty acids and arginine can improve metabolic parameters, decrease chemical indices of inflammation, enhance quality of life, and extend disease-free interval and survival time in dogs treated for lymphoblastic lymphoma. In that study, dogs fed the experimental diet had higher serum levels of the n-3 fatty acids docosahexaenoic acid (C22:6) and eicosapentaenoic acid (C20:5), as well as arginine, when compared with controls. Higher serum levels of C22:6 and C20:5 were associated with lower (P<0.05) plasma lactic acid responses to intravenous glucose and diet tolerance testing. Increasing C22:6 levels were associated with longer disease-free interval and survival time for dogs with stage III lymphoma. It is reasonable to suggest that n-3 fatty acids may be of value when treating dogs with lymphoma with chemotherapy.

Another study was designed to determine the effect of a diet supplemented with n-3 fatty acids and arginine on irradiated skin and oral mucosa, carbohydrate metabolism, and quality of life in a group of dogs with nasal tumors.[16] Dogs fed the experimental diet supplemented with n-3 fatty acids and arginine had significantly higher serum levels of the n-3 fatty acids C22:6 and C20:5, as well as arginine, when compared with controls. These dogs had lower plasma lactic acid responses to intravenous glucose and diet tolerance testing. Increasing C22:6 and C20:5 levels were associated with lower concentrations of inflammatory mediators, decreased resting energy expenditure, improved performance scores, less histologic damage to irradiated skin and oral mucosa, and normalization of blood lactic acid. In a dose-dependent manner, n-3 fatty acids resulted in decreased histologic evidence of radiation damage to skin and mucosa and improved performance scores in dogs with malignant nasal tumors. These results may be a basis for dietary intervention with long chain n-3 fatty acids for pets with cancer.

Until more information is available, the following guidelines are suggested.[1-4, 11]

- Treat the associated symptoms such as nausea, vomiting, and diarrhea.
- Consider pharmacologic support to enhance appetite early before weight loss is recorded. Fresh aromatic foods that are warmed to body temperature, diazepam derivatives, cyproheptadine for cats, and megestrol acetate may effectively enhance an animal's appetite. Metoclopramide can be invaluable in animals that are nauseated. Dronabinol may be of value in some cases.
- Provide increased nutritional support. Consider diets that have moderate amounts of highly bioavailable protein, modest amounts of simple carbohydrates, arginine, and increased levels of n-3 fatty acids. Hills Patented Prescription Diet Canine N/D is one such food.
- Increase the fiber content in those diets with restricted fiber content.
- Whenever possible, provide nourishment by regular feeding practices.[1-4, 11] When that is not possible, tube feeding is valuable. Enteral products that are fed to animals through nasogastric, esophagostomy, gastrostomy, or jejunostomy tubes should contain high-quality protein, and carbohydrate caloric sources should be minimized until more information is available. Parenteral feeding techniques should be employed when the gastrointestinal tract cannot be

used. Most cancer patients are thought to be hypermetabolic, but recent research may suggest otherwise. Each animal should be assessed and fed as an individual. Some animals with cancer may need considerably more nutrients than normal animals. As an example, to calculate the number of calories needed for a dog with cancer, the basal energy requirement (kcal/day) is determined by multiplying 70 by the animal's weight in $kg^{0.75}$ and then multiplying by 1.2 to 2. A simpler formula is multiplying 30 by the animal's weight in kg and then adding 70. The protein requirement for dogs without renal disease is approximately 4 to 6 g/kg/day.

- Lactate- and glucose-containing parenteral fluids should be avoided in critically ill animals with cancer that require acute, intensive fluid therapy.

ENDOCRINE SYNDROMES OF CANCER

Cancer may manifest itself by the production of cytokines, protein hormones, or hormone precursors that may result in dramatic and dominant clinical syndromes. These endocrine syndromes of cancer are caused by one of three mechanisms:[17] cancer production of cytokines, cancer metabolism of cytokines, or cancer metabolism of precursor steroids to bioactive steroids.

Cancers do not produce an ectopic syndrome by synthesizing and secreting steroids, catecholamines, or thyronines unless the tumor is directly derived from a gland that normally produces these hormones. It has been hypothesized that peptide hormones are produced in small quantities by most or all normal tissues and act in a paracrine fashion. Neoplasms derived from these tissues produce the same hormones but in much larger quantities and result in significant systemic effects. Hormone precursors produced by neoplasms in pets are limited, but in people the list is extensive, including proopiomelanocortin, corticotropin-releasing hormone, chorionic gonadotropin, vasopressin, cytokine growth factors, parathyroid hormone–related protein, parathormone, erythropoietin, eosinophilopoietin, growth hormone, prolactin, gastrin, gastrin-releasing peptide, secretin, glucagon, calcitonin, renin, prorenin, vasoactive intestinal peptide, somatostatin, hypophosphatemia-producing factor, and endothelin-1.[17]

HYPERCALCEMIA

Clinical Importance. Cancer is the most common cause of hypercalcemia in the dog and cat (Fig. 97–1).[18–21] This electrolyte abnormality can result in polyuria, polydipsia, depression, weakness, renal failure, encephalopathy, coma, and death. Any neoplastic process has the potential to cause an elevated calcium level. As many as 30 per cent of human cancer patients develop this paraneoplastic syndrome sometime during the course of their disease.[17] Whereas lymphoma is the most common cause of hypercalcemia in dogs and cats, carcinomas of the lung, thymus, pancreas, and thyroid are the most common causes in people.[17] Fifty per cent of women with breast cancer have hypercalcemia.[17]

Pathophysiology. Two mechanisms have been described to explain malignancy-associated hypercalcemia. The first, local osteolytic hypercalcemia, results from invasion of bone or bone marrow by malignant cells.[17, 21] The hypercalcemia results from locally acting bone-resorbing factors such as ectopic tumor-produced parathormone (PTH) or parathormone-related protein (PTH-rP), prostaglandins (PGE_1, PGE_2), 1,25-dihydroxycholecalciferol vitamin D, osteoclast-activating factor, lymphotoxin, and interleukin-1.[17, 19] The tumors associated with local osteolytic hypercalcemia in veterinary medicine include multiple myeloma, lymphoma, and mammary neoplasia.[17] The most common mechanism of malignancy-associated hypercalcemia is humoral hypercalcemia.[18] In this form of the paraneoplastic syndrome, the tumor induces circulating factors that stimulate osteoclastic bone resorption and possibly increase renal calcium reabsorption. Several studies indicate that the factor responsible for humoral hypercalcemia is PTH-rP.[18–20] PTH-rP has been purified from lymphomas and apocrine cell adenocarcinomas of the anal sac.[20] The cDNA of PTH-rP was cloned and found to encode a 16,000-dalton protein that has 8 of 13 N-terminal amino acids identical to PTH. Ectopic secretion of 1,25-dihydroxycholecalciferol vitamin D from malignant lymphocytes[17, 21] is another potential mechanism of malignancy-associated hypercalcemia. Hypercalcemia is reviewed in Chapter 149.

Clinical Aspects. In the veterinary patient, alterations in renal function are the most common clinical manifestations of hypercalcemia caused by malignant disease.[2, 19] The first sign is an inability to concentrate urine owing to decreased

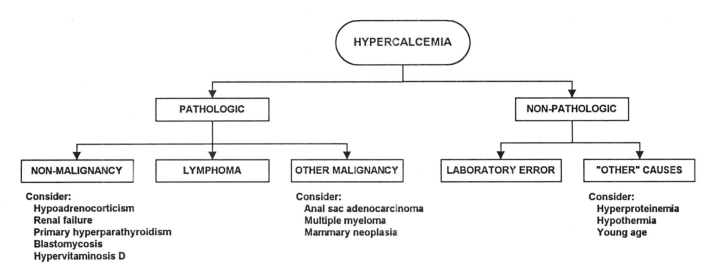

Figure 97–1. Hypercalcemia is commonly seen in dogs and cats with cancer. This illustrates the most common differential diagnoses of this electrolyte disorder in the veterinary patient.

sensitivity of the distal convoluted tubules and collecting ducts to antidiuretic hormone (ADH). The progressive renal disease manifests clinically as polyuria, polydipsia, vomiting, hyposthenuria, and dehydration. Calcium can also directly affect the gastrointestinal, cardiovascular, and neurologic systems, causing anorexia, vomiting, constipation, bradycardia, hypertension, skeletal muscle weakness, depression, stupor, coma, and seizures. Therefore, hypercalcemic animals can have few signs or can constitute a metabolic emergency. Differential diagnosis, diagnosis, and treatment of hypercalcemia are reviewed in Chapter 149.

HYPOCALCEMIA

Clinical Importance. Hypocalcemia is a rare complication in veterinary and human cancer patients. In veterinary medicine, only a few possible etiologies have been mentioned.

Pathophysiology. Hypocalcemia of magnesium deficiency can occur from prolonged intestinal drainage procedures, parenteral hyperalimentation without magnesium supplementation, cisplatin therapy, and severe liver disease. Hypomagnesemia impairs the effect of PTH on its target organs, resulting in hypocalcemia. The tumor lysis syndrome[22] also may be associated with hypocalcemia secondary to increases in serum phosphate concentrations that cause tissue calcium precipitation.

Clinical Aspects. The clinical signs associated with hypocalcemia can be divided into acute and chronic syndromes. Acute decreases in calcium can result in depression, weakness, twitching, and seizures that can be terminal. Chronic hypocalcemia can be associated with weakness, depression, behavioral changes such as irritability and confusion, gastrointestinal disturbances, and muscular weakness.

Treatment. The underlying cause should be identified and treated as soon as possible. Although rare, when hypocalcemia is associated with clinical signs, intravenous administration of calcium should be initiated, followed by oral calcium supplements and vitamin D if needed (see Chapter 149).

HYPOGLYCEMIA

Clinical Importance. Insulinoma is the most common malignancy associated with hypoglycemia (blood glucose < 70 mg/dL) in the dog and cat.[2, 22, 24] Many other non–islet cell tumors can cause hypoglycemia, including hepatocellular carcinoma, hepatoma, plasmacytoid tumor, lymphoma, leiomyosarcoma, oral melanoma, hemangiosarcoma, and salivary gland adenocarcinoma.[23, 24]

Pathophysiology. In contrast to insulinomas that produce excessive quantities of insulin, hypoglycemia of extrapancreatic tumors in the dog has been associated with low to low-normal insulin levels.[23] Possible mechanisms of hypoglycemia secondary to extrapancreatic tumors include secretion of an insulin-like substance, accelerated utilization of glucose by the tumor, and failure of gluconeogenesis and/or glycogenolysis by the liver.[23, 24] The most common differential diagnoses of nonmalignant causes of hypoglycemia include hyperinsulinism, hepatic dysfunction, adrenocortical insufficiency, hypopituitarism, extrapancreatic tumor, starvation, sepsis, and laboratory error.

Clinical Aspects. Animals with hypoglycemia secondary to malignancy usually have neurologic signs.[2, 23, 24] Clini-

cal signs associated with hypoglycemia that occur in companion animals are generally seen when the blood glucose is less than 45 mg/dL. Neurologic signs predominate, because carbohydrate reserve is limited in neural tissue and brain function depends on an adequate quantity of glucose. The neurologic signs include weakness, disorientation, and seizures that may progress to convulsions, coma, and death. Hypoglycemia is a potent stimulus for the release of catecholamines, growth hormone, glucocorticoids, and glucagon. These substances compensate for hypoglycemia by promoting glycogenolysis. It may be difficult to identify the cause of hypoglycemia in dogs or cats with extrapancreatic tumors. Insulin-producing tumors are diagnosed by identifying inappropriate (normal or elevated) insulin concentrations at the time of low blood glucose concentrations. The identification of malignancy-associated hypoglycemia in some cases may require periodic sampling during a 72-hour fast. The diagnosis is made when the blood glucose is dramatically reduced but insulin levels are elevated.

Polyneuropathies and polymyopathies have been documented in dogs with insulin- secreting pancreatic beta-cell neoplasia. Some of these dogs have profound muscle weakness resulting in an inability to walk or, in some, to stand. Surgical removal of the pancreatic tumor and resolution of the hypoglcemia often allow transient resolution of the weakness. The cause of this paraneoplastic syndrome is not known.

Treatment. Surgery may be the treatment of choice for tumors that cause hypoglycemia. Because many of these tumors are malignant, surgery may not be curative. Insulinoma is reviewed in Chapter 152.

ERYTHROCYTOSIS

Clinical Importance. Erythrocytosis is an uncommon condition that can result in vague, often confusing clinical signs. Often, increased red blood cell numbers are a clue to an underlying malignancy.

Pathophysiology. Erythrocytosis can be caused by increased production of erythropoietin or by tumor-induced hypoxia, which triggers production of erythropoietin. Erythropoietin is normally produced by the kidney in dogs and cats and from the carotid bodies in cats. Thus it is not surprising that some renal and other tumors produce erythropoietin. These uncommon tumors include renal cell tumors, lymphoma, and hepatic tumors.[2, 25] When erythrocytosis is secondary to elevated erythropoietin concentrations, four possible mechanisms may be responsible[2, 25]: (1) tumor production of erythropoietin; (2) induction of hypoxia by tumor mass effect, where vascular obstruction or hypoxia subsequently induces increased erythropoietin; (3) elaboration of a tumor-induced factor that stimulates the release of erythropoietin; or (4) tumor-induced change in metabolism of erythropoietin. Other causes of erythrocytosis include dehydration, pulmonary and cardiac disorders, venoarterial shunts, Cushing's disease, the chronic administration of adrenocortical steroids, and polycythemia vera.[2, 25] Polycythemia vera is a myeloproliferative disorder that results from clonal proliferation of red blood cell precursors. Erythrocytosis of paraneoplastic origin can be distinguished from polycythemia vera by the absence of pancytosis or splenomegaly, and from secondary polycythemia by the absence of decreased arterial oxygen saturation.[2, 25]

Clinical Aspects. Dogs and cats with erythrocytosis have vague clinical signs that include lethargy, depression, anorexia, polyuria, and polydipsia.

Treatment. Surgical removal of the erythropoietin-producing tumor or the tumor that induces regional or systemic hypoxia is the treatment of choice. Phlebotomies may temporarily reduce the red blood cell load. The chemotherapeutic agent hydroxyurea (18 to 23 mg/lb, or 40 to 50 mg/kg, orally, divided, twice a day), can be used to induce reversible bone marrow suppression by inhibiting DNA synthesis without inhibiting RNA or protein synthesis.[2, 25]

OTHER SYNDROMES OF ECTOPIC HORMONE PRODUCTION

SYNDROME OF INAPPROPRIATE SECRETION OF ANTIDIURETIC HORMONE

Clinical Importance. Inappropriate secretion of ADH is one of the best-characterized and most frequently encountered ectopic hormone syndromes in human medicine.[2, 22] Although recognized in a variety of cancers in humans, it occurs infrequently in veterinary oncology.[2] Diagnostic criteria for the syndrome of inappropriate secretion of ADH include hypo-osmolality and hyponatremia of extracellular fluids, urine that is less than maximally dilute, absence of volume depletion, sustained renal excretion of sodium, and normal renal and adrenal function.

Pathophysiology. The cause of inappropriate secretion of ADH is the production of an ADH-like molecule from a tumor. In addition, many drugs (including barbiturates, chlorpromazine, thiazides, and vincristine) can induce biochemical and physiologic changes identical to this syndrome.

Clinical Aspects. The clinical signs result from excess retention of water, with clinical manifestations of weakness and lethargy that may progress to seizures, coma, and death.

Treatment. Treatment is directed at elimination of the underlying malignancy or drug. In addition, water restriction to normalize the serum osmolality may be helpful in mild to moderate cases. Severe cases can be treated with domeclazine therapy and the intravenous administration of hypertonic saline.

ECTOPIC PRODUCTION OF ADRENOCORTICOTROPIC HORMONE

Clinical Importance. The ectopic production of adrenocorticotropic hormone (ACTH) or related polypeptides has been described for a variety of cancers in humans, including small cell lung cancer, bronchial carcinoid, islet cell tumor of the pancreas, thyroid medullary carcinoma, and pheochromocytoma.[2, 25] This condition was reported in one dog with a primary lung tumor.[26]

Pathophysiology. The syndrome results from excessive production of steroids from normal adrenal glands that are under the influence of the ectopic production of ACTH or ACTH-like substances.

Clinical Aspects. Clinical signs are the same as those of Cushing's disease (see Chapter 154). The tumors are rarely suppressible with dexamethasone.[17]

Treatment. Eliminate the underlying cause.

HYPERTROPHIC OSTEOPATHY

Clinical Importance. Hypertrophic osteopathy is a disorder that occurs primarily in bones of the extremities in dogs and, rarely, in cats. This paraneoplastic syndrome is often associated with primary and metastatic lung tumors and may cause lameness or painful swellings of affected bones.[2] Other neoplastic and non-neoplastic conditions associated with hypertrophic osteopathy include esophageal sarcoma, rhabdomyosarcoma of the urinary bladder, pneumonia, heartworm disease, congenital and acquired heart disease, and focal lung atelectasis.[2] The disease results in increased peripheral blood flow and periosteal proliferation of new bone along the shafts of long bones, often beginning with the digits and extending as far proximally as the femur and humerus. Initially there is soft tissue proliferation, followed by production of osteophytes that tends to radiate from the cortices at 90 degrees (Fig. 97–2).

Pathophysiology. The cause of this unique syndrome is unknown, but successful treatment by vagotomy suggests a neurovascular mechanism that may involve a reflex emanating from the tumor or nearby pleura carried through afferent vagal fibers.[2]

Clinical Aspects. Dogs and cats with hypertropic osteopathy have painful, swollen extremities that are warm to the touch. Long-standing cases may have deformed, thickened extremities that can alter function after the underlying etiology is eliminated.

Treatment. Glucocorticoid therapy offers temporary improvement in clinical signs and may reduce the extent of swelling. Removal of the tumor can result in resolution of clinical signs and regression of the bony changes. Other treatments such as unilateral vagotomy on the side of the lung lesion, incision through the parietal pleura, subperiosteal rib resection, bilateral cervical vagotomy, and the use of analgesics have been suggested.

ANEMIA

Clinical Importance. Anemia occurs frequently in veterinary cancer patients.[2] This paraneoplastic syndrome may impact quality of life, response to therapy, and overall survival time.

Pathophysiology. Causes include anemia of chronic disease, bone marrow invasion by tumor cells, blood loss, marrow suppression by chemotherapy, hypersplenism, immune-mediated disease, megaloblastic anemia, vitamin and iron deficiency, microangiopathic hemolytic anemia, and pure red cell aplasia (Fig. 97–3).[2, 22, 27] In most animals, a clear cause of anemia is not found, and the diagnosis of anemia of chronic disease is made. Anemia of chronic disease is commonly seen in animals with metastatic or disseminated tumors and is caused by or associated with a shortened erythrocyte life span, disordered iron metabolism, depressed bone marrow response, and disordered iron storage.[2, 22, 27]

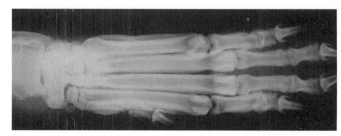

Figure 97–2. Hypertrophic osteopathy frequently causes lameness, as well as hot and painful extremities. Although any bones can be involved, those of the distal extremities are most commonly affected. Radiographically, there is subtle periosteal new bone formation in the involved bones.

ONC

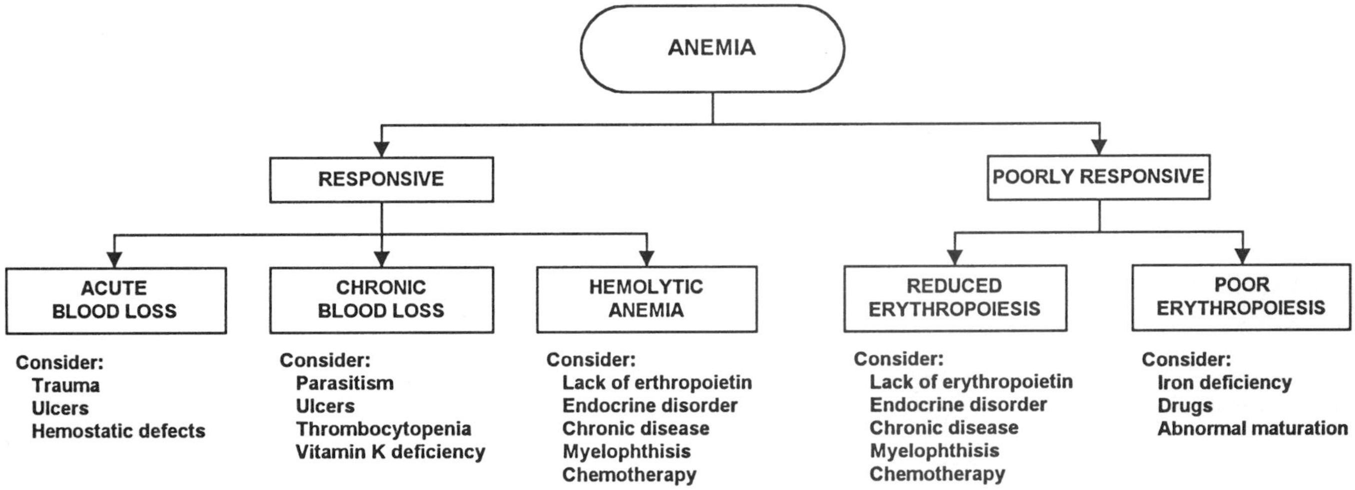

Figure 97–3. Anemia can be due to a number of different etiologies in the veterinary cancer patient. The most common differential diagnoses are identified in this algorithm.

The cause of blood-loss anemia as a paraneoplastic syndrome is not clearly understood. The blood loss may be obvious (bleeding superficial tumors) or inapparent (bladder or gastrointestinal tumors). Microangiopathic hemolytic anemia, commonly seen in dogs with splenic hemangiosarcoma, occurs secondary to hemolysis in the arteriolar circulation, which may result from damage to arteriolar endothelium or from fibrin deposition within the artery.[27] Disseminated intravascular coagulation (DIC) is an important cause of this type of anemia and is commonly seen in cases of hemangiosarcoma. Immune-mediated hemolytic anemia, which results in premature destruction of red blood cells by immune mechanisms,[2, 27] is sometimes triggered by tumors of animals.

Chemotherapy-induced nonregenerative anemia is seen commonly in animals. The condition is frequently associated with chronic drug therapy. Histologically, chemotherapy-induced changes are noted as bone marrow hypoplasia of erythroid or other cell lines, which subsequently results in decreased red cell mass, normal erythrocytic indices, and inadequate reticulocytosis.[2, 27] Chemotherapeutic agents frequently cause a reduction of white blood cells and platelets. The degree of anemia associated with the administration of chemotherapeutic agents is generally mild and without clinical signs.

Other less likely causes of cancer-induced anemia include leukoerythroblastic anemia, hematopoietic dysplasia, hypersplenism, erythrophagocytosis, megaloblastic anemia, and red cell aplasia.[2, 27] Many of the mechanisms work alone or in concert to induce a decrease in red blood cell numbers. Clinical signs that relate to anemia may be overshadowed by manifestations of the underlying neoplastic condition, but the clinical signs can limit the quality of life of the animal.

Clinical Aspects. Clinically, anemia of chronic disease is recognized by normocytic, normochromic red blood cells; normal bone marrow cellularity; depressed iron metabolism; and reticuloendothelial iron sequestration. Blood-loss anemia is recognized clinically when the red blood cells are microcytic and hypochromic owing to decreased hemoglobin synthesis.[2, 22, 27] Poikilocytosis, microleptocytosis, inadequate reticulocytosis, increased total iron binding capacity, decreased serum iron concentrations, and elevated platelet counts may also be seen in this condition. Hemolysis and schistocytosis are the hallmarks of microangiopathic hemolytic anemia.

Although hemangiosarcoma is the most common cause of this type of anemia, it can be seen with a variety of neoplastic diseases. Removal of the tumor and appropriate supportive care (e.g., intravenous fluids) may be beneficial in this type of anemia. The diagnosis of immune-mediated disease–induced anemia is based on finding antibody or complement on the surface of the animal's red blood cells through a Coombs' test or slide agglutination test, as well as the presence of spherocytosis and regenerative anemia.

Treatment. Treatment of all causes of anemia is directed at elimination of the neoplastic condition. Transfusions of compatible blood are rarely needed in most types of paraneoplastic disease–induced anemia. Neither is therapy with recombinant erythropoietin. The marked decrease in serum iron concentration seen in blood-loss anemia may be treated with ferrous sulfate (10 to 20 mg daily, orally), along with appropriate steps to eliminate the tumor.[2] Medical management of immune-mediated hemolytic anemia with prednisone ≤ 0.9 mg/lb, or 2 mg/kg, daily, orally) and azathioprine (0.9 mg/lb, or 2 mg/kg, daily for four days, then 0.23 to 0.45 mg/lb, or 0.5 to 1 mg/kg, every other day, orally) may be indicated if rapid resolution of the underlying neoplastic condition is not possible.[2, 27, 28] Cyclophosphamide may have limited value in treating immune-mediated hemolytic anemia and associated conditions in the dog.[2]

LEUKOCYTOSIS

Clinical Importance. Increases in white blood cell count have been seen in a variety of canine tumors, including lymphoma and hemangiosarcoma.[2, 24, 27]

Pathophysiology. The mechanism of the elevated white blood cell count is obscure but may involve elaboration of hematopoietic growth factors (e.g., granulocyte colony stimulating factor, granulocyte-macrophage colony stimulating factor, or interleukin-3) or be a result of tissue necrosis and granulocyte breakdown, with a positive feedback that initiates increased production of neutrophils.[2, 27]

Clinical Aspects. There are no clinical signs clearly attributed to this condition. Generally, the condition is not clinically significant, but it can be incorrectly attributed to sepsis. If the leukocytosis is caused by malignancy-induced production of hematopoietic growth factors, bone pain may be noted owing to bone marrow "packing" of hematopoietic precursors that are actively dividing.

Treatment. Eliminate the underlying neoplastic condition.

THROMBOCYTOPENIA

Clinical Importance. Thrombocytopenia is a serious condition regardless of its etiology. Thrombocytopenia has been commonly recognized as a direct effect or as a paraneoplastic syndrome associated with malignant disease.

Pathophysiology. Mechanisms associated with decreased platelet numbers in dogs with cancer include decreased platelet production from the bone marrow; sequestration of platelets in capillaries; increased platelet consumption, such as in DIC; increased platelet destruction; and reduction in the presence of hematopoietic growth factors.

Clinical Aspects. Platelet consumption is the most significant hemostatic abnormality in tumor-bearing dogs.[2, 28] Decreased platelet numbers and elevated plasma fibrinogen concentrations are often seen in animals with extensive tumors that involve spleen or marrow.[2, 27] DIC, a common cause of platelet consumption, is seen in 39 per cent of all dogs with the condition.[27] If DIC is suspected, prolongation of clotting times (ACT, OSPT, APTT) and elevated fibrinogen may be identified along with the thrombocytopenia. The acute and chronic forms of DIC have slightly different clinical and laboratory presentations (Table 97–1). Immune-mediated thrombocytopenia is also a significant cause of decreased platelet numbers in dogs with cancer.[2, 27] This condition is diagnosed by demonstration of antibodies against bone marrow megakaryocytes.

Treatment. In all cases of malignancy-induced thrombocytopenia, elimination of the underlying neoplastic condition is the treatment of choice. DIC can be treated with intravenous fluids, whole blood or platelet-rich plasma transfusions, and heparin. Immune-mediated thrombocytopenia has been successfully resolved in dogs by elimination of the tumor and treatment with immune-suppressive drugs such as prednisone ≤ 0.9 mg/lb, or 2 mg/kg, daily) and azathioprine (0.9 mg/lb, or 2 mg/kg, daily for four days, then 0.23 to 0.46 mg/lb, or 0.5 to 1 mg/kg, every other day).[2, 27–29] Vincristine (0.5 to 0.75 mg/m²) can be used to temporarily increase platelet numbers.

TABLE 97–1. CLINICAL AND LABORATORY PARAMETERS USED TO DIAGNOSE DISSEMINATED INTRAVASCULAR COAGULOPATHY (DIC)

TESTS/ OBSERVATIONS	ACUTE DIC	CHRONIC DIC
Clinical signs	Clinically evident coagulopathies	Few clinical signs evident
Onset and duration	Rapid onset, quick progression	Insidious, prolonged
PT, APTT, ACT	Prolonged	Normal to slightly decreased
Platelets	Decreased	Often normal
FDP	Very high	High
Fibrinogen	Decreased to normal	Normal
Antithrombin III	Reduced	Normal
Prognosis	Grave	Good

PT = prothrombin time; APPT = activated partial prothrombin time; ACT = activated clotting time; FDP = fibrin degradation products.

HYPERGAMMAGLOBULINEMIA

Clinical Importance. M-component disorders or hyperviscosity syndromes have been diagnosed in animals with a variety of malignancies, especially multiple myeloma.[2, 27, 30]

Pathophysiology. These diseases are the result of excessive secretion of a monoclonal line of immunoglobulin-producing cells. IgG, IgA, IgM, and light chain protein classes are produced in large quantities and may be identified by performing protein immunoelectrophoresis on serum. In addition, Bence Jones proteins (light chains) are rarely identified in the urine. Approximately 75 per cent of dogs with plasma cell tumors have M-component disorders. The prevalence of this condition in cats with myeloma is unknown but is probably approximately the same. Other tumors associated with this syndrome include lymphoma, lymphocytic leukemia, and primary macroglobulinemia.[2, 30]

Clinical Aspects. Clinical signs associated with M-component disorders result from elevated globulins and from direct effect of the tumor. Bleeding disorders, commonly noted clinically as epistaxis, are the result of elevated proteins interfering with normal platelet function.[28] A hyperviscosity syndrome becomes clinically apparent as elevated protein decreases fluidity of the blood, which results in central nervous system signs, retinopathies, visual disturbances, and congestive heart failure. Renal decompensation also may occur from development of renal amyloidosis or Bence Jones proteinuria, and because increased serum viscosity causes a decrease in renal perfusion and impaired concentrating ability. Neurologic signs (e.g., seizures, ataxia, nystagmus) occur secondary to central nervous system tissue hypoxia caused by altered blood flow and diminished delivery of oxygen to neural tissue. A hypertrophic cardiomyopathy-like state may occur, followed by generalized cardiac failure caused by excessive cardiac workload secondary to the high volume of hyperviscous blood. Myocardial hypoxia may also occur.

Treatment. The treatment of M-component disorders revolves around appropriate antitumor and supportive therapy. Multiple myeloma has responded to melphalan (0.045 mg/lb, or 0.1 mg/kg, daily for 10 days, then 0.23 mg/lb, or 0.5 mg/kg, daily, orally) and prednisone (0.46 mg/lb, or 0.5 mg/kg, daily, orally) therapy with a median survival time of 18 months.[2, 24] Radiation therapy and surgery may also be of value in select cases. Lymphoma is best treated with a variety of protocols such as doxorubicin as a single agent or with combination chemotherapy using cyclophosphamide, vincristine, prednisone, and doxorubicin. The hyperviscosity syndrome may require immediate therapy directed toward reduction of protein levels in the blood. Plasmapheresis rapidly reduces protein levels in cases that exhibit signs associated with the hyperviscosity syndrome.[24] Supportive care involves fluid therapy to treat dehydration. Antibiotics are often indicated because myeloma cells secrete an immune-suppressive substance that suppresses macrophage and lymphocyte function.

FEVER

Clinical Importance. Fever is a common complication of cancer and infections. Although other noninfectious causes (e.g., drug toxicity) have been associated with fever, some neoplastic diseases cause an elevated body temperature as a paraneoplastic syndrome.[2] Tumor-associated fever usually is defined as unexplained fever that coincides with the growth or elimination of a tumor.

TABLE 97–2. PARANEOPLASTIC SYNDROMES OF THE NERVOUS SYSTEM

SITE INVOLVED	SYNDROME
Brain	Cerebellar degeneration
	Optic neuritis
	Progressive multifocal leukoencephalopathy
Spinal cord	Subacute necrotic myelopathy
	Subacute motor neuropathy
Peripheral nerve	Sensory neuropathy
	Peripheral neuropathy
	Autonomic gastrointestinal neuropathy
Muscle and neuromuscular junction	Dermatomyositis and polymyositis
	Myasthenic syndrome (Eaton-Lambert syndrome)
	Myasthenia gravis

Pathophysiology. Tumor-induced fevers may result from the release of pyrogens from tumor cells, normal leukocytes, or other normal cells. These tumor-elaborated pyrogens may act on the hypothalamus to reset the body's temperature regulation. Although the incidence of cancer-associated fever is unknown in animals, fever of unknown origin is found to be caused by cancer in up to 40 per cent of people.[2, 22]

Clinical Aspects. Tumor-induced fever can be quite debilitating and impacts quality of life, response to therapy, and survival time. Anorexia, depression, malaise, and other ill-defined clinical signs are often seen in these animals. Occasionally, the animal acts normally despite high body temperature.

Treatment. Fever that is directly related to malignant disease can be treated symptomatically with antipyretics or nonsteroidal anti-inflammatory agents. Resolution of the underlying malignant condition usually results in disappearance of the fever.

NEUROLOGIC ABNORMALITIES

Clinical Importance. The remote effect of cancer on the nervous system is an unrecognized condition in veterinary medicine.

Pathophysiology. The cause of these neurologic syndromes in veterinary and human medicine is not well understood. They involve a number of different anatomic sites and induce a wide variety of syndromes (Table 97–2).[33]

Clinical Aspects. There are several reports in the veterinary literature of cancer-induced peripheral neuropathies, including a case of trigeminal nerve paralysis and Horner's syndrome in the dog.[2, 31, 32] Animals also exhibit neurologic signs secondary to endocrine, fluid, and electrolyte disturbances caused by neoplasia. Hypercalcemia, hyperviscosity syndrome, and hepatoencephalopathy are common examples. The neurologic syndromes of myasthenia gravis (e.g., megaesophagus, acetylcholinesterase-responsive neuropathy) secondary to thymoma are well described in the literature.

Treatment. Elimination of the neoplastic condition may result in resolution of these neurologic syndromes.

REFERENCES

1. Ogilvie GK, Vail DM: Nutrition and cancer: Recent developments. *In* Couto GM (ed): Clinical Management of the Cancer Patient. Vet Clin North Am 20:1, 1990.
2. Ogilvie GK, Moore AS: Paraneoplastic syndromes. *In* Managing the Veterinary Cancer Patient: A Practice Manual. Trenton, NJ, Veterinary Learning Systems, 1995, pp 197–222.
3. Puccio M, Nathanson L: The cancer cachexia syndrome. Semin Oncol 24:277, 1997.
4. Ogilvie GK: Metabolic alterations and nutritional therapy for the veterinary cancer patient. Compend Contin Educ Pract Vet 15:925, 1993.
5. Ogilvie GK, Vail DM, Wheeler SJ, et al: Effect of chemotherapy and remission on carbohydrate metabolism in dogs with lymphoma. Cancer 69:233, 1992.
6. Vail DM, Ogilvie GK, Fettman MJ, et al: Exacerbation of hyperlactatemia by infusion of LRS in dogs with lymphoma. J Vet Intern Med 4:228, 1990.
7. Vail DM, Ogilvie GK, Wheeler SL, et al: Alterations in carbohydrate metabolism in canine lymphoma. J Vet Intern Med 4:8, 1990.
8. Ogilvie GK, Ford RD, Vail DM: Alterations in lipoprotein profiles in dogs with lymphoma. J Vet Intern Med 8:62, 1994.
9. Ogilvie GK, Walters LM, Fettman MJ, et al: Energy expenditure in dogs with lymphoma fed two specialized diets. Cancer 71:3146, 1993.
10. Ogilvie GK, Walters L, Salman MD, et al: Alterations in carbohydrate metabolism in dogs with nonhematopoietic malignancies. Am J Vet Res 58:277, 1997.
11. Ogilvie GK, Vail DM: Unique metabolic alterations associated with cancer cachexia in the dog. *In* Kirk RW (ed): Current Veterinary Therapy XI. Philadelphia, WB Saunders, 1992, pp 433–438.
12. Proceedings, adjuvant nutrition in cancer treatment symposium, Tulsa, OK, November 6–7, 1992, pp 9–103.
13. Krishnaswamy K: Effects of malnutrition on drug metabolism and toxicity in humans. Nutritional Toxicol 2:105, 1987.
14. Anderson KE: Influences of diet and nutrition on clinical pharmacokinetics. Clin Pharmacokinet 14:325, 1988.
15. Ogilvie GK, Fettman MJ, Mallinckrodt CH, et al: Effect of fish oil and arginine on remission and survival time in dogs with lymphoma. Cancer (submitted 1998).
16. Anderson CR, Ogilvie GK, LaRue SM, et al: Effect of fish oil and arginine on acute effects of radiation injury in dogs with neoplasia: A double blind study. Proceedings, Veterinary Cancer Society, 1997, pp 33–34.
17. Odell WD: Endocrine/metabolic syndromes of cancer. Semin Oncol 24:299, 1997.
18. Meuten DJ: Hypercalcemia. Vet Clin North Am 14:891, 1984.
19. Weir EC, Burtis WJ, Morris CA, et al: Isolation of a 16,000-dalton parathyroid hormone–like protein from two animal tumors causing humoral hypercalcemia of malignancy. Endocrinology 123:2744, 1988.
20. Weir EC, Nordin RW, Matus RE, et al: Humoral hypercalcemia of malignancy in canine lymphosarcoma. Endocrinology 122:602, 1988.
21. Kruger JM, Osborne CA, Polzin DJ: Treatment of hypercalcemia. *In* Kirk RW (ed): Current Veterinary Therapy IX. Philadelphia, WB Saunders, 1986, pp 75–90.
22. Bienzle D, Jacobs RM, Lumsden JH: Relationship of serum total calcium to serum albumin in dogs, cats, horses and cattle. Can Vet J 34:360, 1993.
23. Leifer CE, Peterson ME, Matus RE, Patnaik AK: Hypoglycemia associated with nonislet cell tumors in 13 dogs. JAVMA 186:53, 1985.
24. Leifer CE, Peterson ME: Hypoglycemia. Vet Clin North Am 14:873, 1984.
25. Staszaski H: Hematological paraneoplastic syndromes. Semin Oncol 24:329, 1997.
26. Ogilvie GK, Haschek WA, McKiernan B, et al: Classification of primary lung tumors in dogs: 210 cases (1975–1985). JAVMA 195:106, 1989.
27. Meyer DJ, Coles EH, Rich LJ: Veterinary Laboratory Medicine. Interpretation and Diagnosis. Philadelphia, WB Saunders, 1992, pp 12–26.
28. Helfand SC, Couto CG, Madewell BR: Immune-mediated thrombocytopenia associated with solid tumors in dogs. J Am Anim Hosp Assoc 21:787, 1985.
29. Ogilvie GK, Felsberg PJ, Harris SW: Short term effect of cyclophosphamide and azathioprine on the selected aspects of the canine immune system. J Vet Immunol Immunopathol 18:119, 1988.
30. Matus RE, Leifer CE: Immunoglobulin-producing tumors. Vet Clin North Am 15:741, 1985.
31. Carpenter JL, King NW, Abrams KL: Pheochromocytoma in dogs: 13 cases. JAVMA 191:1594, 1987.
32. Shahar R, Rosseau C, Steiss J: Peripheral polyneuropathy in a dog with functional islet B-cell tumor and widespread metastases. JAVMA 187:175, 1985.
33. Dalmau JO, Posner JB: Paraneoplastic syndromes affecting the nervous system. Semin Oncol 24:318, 1997.

CHAPTER 98

HEMATOPOIETIC TUMORS

David M. Vail

LYMPHOMA

Lymphoma (lymphosarcoma) is the most common hematopoietic tumor affecting dogs and cats and is defined as a proliferation of malignant lymphoid cells that primarily affects lymph nodes or solid visceral organs such as the liver or spleen. The management of lymphoma is initially quite gratifying in both species, as response rates approach 90 per cent in dogs and 70 per cent in cats treated with a variety of chemotherapeutic approaches. However, most animals eventually succumb to relapse of chemotherapy-resistant disseminated tumors.

ETIOLOGY

The etiology of lymphoma in companion animals is, for the most part, unknown. Whereas certain varieties of lymphoma in cats have been directly and indirectly associated with feline leukemia virus (FeLV) and feline immunodeficiency virus (FIV), respectively, no strong evidence exists for a retroviral origin of lymphoma in dogs. A weak to moderate association between lymphoma in dogs and the use of pesticides or exposure to strong magnetic fields has been observed in preliminary epidemiologic studies.[1-3] More thorough studies are necessary to evaluate these associations further. Occasional clustering of lymphoma in related dogs has suggested a familial component in limited instances.[4]

CLASSIFICATION

Classification schemes for lymphoma have been evaluated and include those based on anatomic site, World Health Organization (WHO) clinical stage (Table 98–1), histologic/cytologic phenotype, and immunophenotype.

Canine Classification. In the dog, 80 to 85 per cent of cases are of the multicentric anatomic type and present as WHO stage III or IV.[5-7] Alimentary (about 7 per cent),

TABLE 98–1. WORLD HEALTH ORGANIZATION CLINICAL STAGING FOR DOMESTIC ANIMALS WITH LYMPHOMA

STAGE	CRITERIA
I	Single lymph node
II	Multiple lymph nodes in a regional area
III	Generalized lymphadenopathy
IV	Liver and/or spleen (with or without stage III)
V	Bone marrow or blood involvement and/or any nonlymphoid organ (with or without stage I to IV)
Substage	
a	Without clinical signs of disease
b	With clinical signs of disease

From World Health Organization: TNM Classification of Tumors in Domestic Animals. Geneva, World Health Organization, 1980.

cutaneous (about 6 per cent), mediastinal (about 3 per cent), and miscellaneous extranodal sites (central nervous system, bone, heart, nasal cavity, primary ocular) are less frequently encountered. Regardless of the histologic classification scheme used (e.g., Kiel, NCI Working Formulation), the majority (80 per cent) correspond to medium- and high-grade non-Hodgkin's lymphoma in people.[8-10] The majority of canine lymphoma is of the B-cell immunophenotype, with approximately 20 to 30 per cent being of T-cell derivation.[5, 8-10]

Feline Classification. In the cat, a definite and repeatable shift in anatomic type, immunophenotypic derivation, and retroviral association has occurred concomitant with the initiation of widespread FeLV testing and vaccination programs over the last 10 to 15 years.[11, 12] Studies before this era reported that the mediastinal and multicentric forms of lymphoma predominated and that these represented younger, FeLV-positive cats. Newer reports document that at the present time, lymphoma affects primarily older, FeLV-negative cats and that the alimentary form predominates (Table 98–2). Only 10 to 20 per cent of cases are now associated with FeLV antigenemia, compared with 60 to 70 per cent of cases published before FeLV test and vaccine availability. As one would predict, along with a shift away from FeLV antigen–associated tumors has come a shift away from traditional signalment and relative frequency of anatomic sites. The median age of 9 to 10 years reported now is considerably older than the 4- to 6-year medians reported prior to this era. The median age of cats within various anatomic tumor groupings has not changed, however, and sites traditionally associated with FeLV (i.e., mediastinal and multicentric) are still affected in younger, FeLV-antigenemic cats. Similarly, the alimentary form occurs most often in older, FeLV-negative cats. Whether this change in the epidemiology of lymphoma in cats is owing to FeLV vaccination itself, or whether the procedure of FeLV antigen testing before vaccination has allowed separation of potentially infective cats from the susceptible population, is unclear. Either situation would result in a reduction in the number of FeLV-positive lymphomas.

A distinct class of lymphoma in cats has been reported.[13-15] This represents a granulated round cell tumor that has been termed either globule leukocyte tumor or large granular lymphocyte lymphoma, although they are likely variations of the same disease. This tumor usually involves the intestinal tract and abdominal viscera, with widespread metastasis being the norm. Affected cats are generally FeLV-negative.

CLINICAL PRESENTATION AND SIGNS

Canine Multicentric Lymphoma. Lymphoma affects primarily middle-aged to older dogs. No sex predilection is observed, and many different breeds are represented. Only

TABLE 98–2. CHARACTERISTICS OF FELINE LYMPHOMA BY ANATOMIC SITE

ANATOMIC SITE	RELATIVE FREQUENCY (%)	AGE	T-CELL ASSOCIATION	FeLV-POSITIVE
Alimentary	50–70	Aged (10–14 years)	Low	Low (≤5%)
Multicentric	10–25	Depends on FeLV status*	Depends on FeLV status*	Approximately one third
Mediastinal/thymic	10–20	Young	High	High (>80%)
Nasal	About 10	Aged	Low	Low
Renal	5–10	Middle-aged	Low to moderate	Low to moderate
Other	5–25	Mixed	Mixed	Mixed

*FeLV-positive cats tend to be younger and more commonly have lymphoma of T-cell derivation.

10 to 20 per cent of dogs are clinically ill at presentation (WHO substage b),[5–7] therefore, the majority of cases present as healthy dogs with incidental generalized lymphadenopathy. In substage b dogs, the clinical signs are nonspecific and can include inappetence, anorexia, weight loss, and lethargy. Paraneoplastic hypercalcemia may result in a presentation of polyuria and polydipsia. In stage V disease, if bone marrow involvement is marked, peripheral cytopenias may result in presentations reflecting neutropenic sepsis, thrombocytopenic hemorrhage, or anemia.

Canine Lymphoma of Other Sites. The presentation and associated clinical signs reflect the anatomic form present in each individual case. Alimentary forms present with signs specific to the gastrointestinal tract, including vomiting, diarrhea (with or without blood), weight loss, and inappetence. Mediastinal forms may present with respiratory signs, including dyspnea, and muffled heart sounds. Mediastinal lymphoma may also present with precaval syndrome, characterized by pitting edema of the head, neck, and forelimbs secondary to tumor compression or invasion of the vena cava (Fig. 98–1). Because nearly half of mediastinal lymphomas are associated with paraneoplastic hypercalcemia,[16] polydipsia and polyuria are common presenting complaints for this anatomic form.

Cutaneous lymphoma has been termed the great imitator, owing to its ability to present in many varying forms. Single or multiple cutaneous lesions can occur, which may appear as mild eczematous plaques or more impressive nodular tumors (Fig. 98–2). Lesions may or may not be pruritic and can occur anywhere on the skin and in the oral cavity.

Miscellaneous sites result in signs attributable to the location (e.g., lameness for bone lesions, neurologic compromise for central nervous system lymphoma).

Feline Lymphoma. No breed or sex predilections have been identified. Age and its association with FeLV status have been discussed previously. In general, cats are more likely than dogs to present with clinical illness; 75 per cent or more present with substage b signs.[11, 12] The clinical presentation of lymphoma in cats is dependent on the anatomic sites involved. Cats with alimentary lymphoma or large granular lymphocyte lymphoma present with varying degrees of weight loss, unkempt haircoat, inappetence, chronic diarrhea, and vomiting. Cats with mediastinal disease are often in severe respiratory distress owing to the effects of an intrathoracic mass or the presence of significant pleural effusion. Cats with renal lymphoma may present with polyuria and polydipsia owing to secondary renal failure. In the case of nasal lymphoma, chronic serosanguineous nasal discharge, exophthalmos, and facial deformity are common presentations. Cats with FeLV-associated lymphoma are more likely to present with pale mucous membranes due to anemia.

DIAGNOSIS

Physical Examination. A thorough physical examination should include palpation of all assessable lymph nodes, including a rectal examination in the dog. Inspection of mucous membranes for pallor or petechia indicative of anemia or thrombocytopenia secondary to myelophthisis, and evidence of major organ failure, including the appearance of icterus or uremic ulcers, should be undertaken. Abdominal palpation may reveal organomegaly, intestinal wall thickening, or mesenteric lymphadenopathy. The presence of a mediastinal mass and/or pleural effusion can be suspected following thoracic compression in cats and auscultation in both dogs and cats. An ocular examination, including fun-

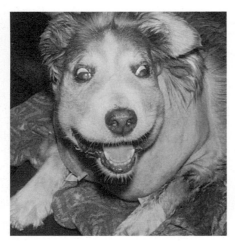

Figure 98–1. Precaval syndrome in a dog with mediastinal lymphoma. Pitting edema of the head and neck is noted.

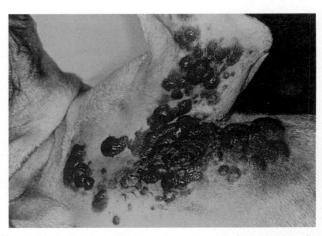

Figure 98–2. Cutaneous T-cell lymphoma (mycosis fungoides) in a dog.

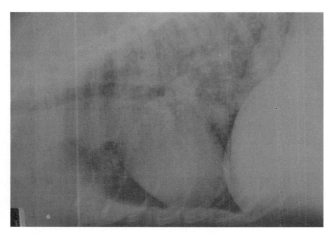

Figure 98–3. A lateral thoracic radiographic projection of a dog illustrating interstitial pulmonary infiltration with tumor typical of lymphoma at this site.

duscopic assessment, reveals abnormalities (e.g., uveitis, hemorrhage, ocular infiltration) in approximately one third to one half of dogs with lymphoma.[17]

Hematologic Abnormalities. A complete blood count (CBC), including a platelet count, is a necessary part of any evaluation of dogs or cats suspected of having lymphoma. Hematologic abnormalities occur in the majority of cases with multicentric lymphoma.[18] Anemia, when present, is usually normocytic, normochromic, and nonregenerative, reflecting anemia of chronic disease. Regenerative anemias may reflect concomitant blood loss or hemolysis. Cats with FeLV-associated disease may have a macrocytic anemia. If significant myelophthisis is present, the anemia may be accompanied by thrombocytopenia and leukopenia. Circulating atypical lymphocytes may be indicative of bone marrow involvement and leukemia. It is important to differentiate multicentric lymphoma with bone marrow involvement (i.e., stage V disease) from primary lymphoblastic leukemia (discussed later in this chapter), as the prognosis for each is entirely different. Hypoproteinemia is more commonly observed in animals with alimentary lymphoma.

Bone marrow aspiration is recommended for staging, because of the prognostic significance of marked marrow involvement, and in those cases in which lymphoma is suspected but not yet documented. In addition to neoplastic infiltration, increased myeloid-erythroid ratios may be observed.

Serum Biochemical Abnormalities. These often reflect the anatomic site involved. In addition, approximately 15 per cent of dogs with lymphoma (40 per cent of those with mediastinal involvement) have hypercalcemia secondary to a paraneoplastic syndrome.[16, 18] In cases of hypercalcemia of unknown origin, lymphoma should always be high on the differential disease list, and thorough diagnostics directed at this possibility should be undertaken. In addition, the presence of hypercalcemia can serve as a marker for response to therapy. Elevations in blood urea nitrogen and serum creatinine can occur secondary to renal infiltration with tumor, hypercalcemic nephrosis, or prerenal dehydration. Liver-specific enzyme or bilirubin elevations may result from hepatic parenchymal infiltration. Serum globulin elevations, usually monoclonal in nature, occur infrequently with B-cell-derived lymphoma.

Retroviral Status. In the cat, retroviral screening (for FeLV and FIV) is important from a diagnostic and prognostic

standpoint. The relative frequency of FeLV associations is presented in Table 98–2.

Imaging. Imaging (radiography, ultrasonography, or computed tomography) may be important for diagnosis, especially in those cases lacking peripheral lymphadenopathy or limited to intracavitary or extranodal sites. Imaging is equally important for clinical staging (i.e., determining extent of disease), as results may significantly impact the overall prognosis and alter the caregiver's willingness to pursue therapy.

Abnormalities on thoracic radiographs are noted in approximately two thirds to three quarters of dogs with lymphoma[19, 20]; this includes one third with evidence of pulmonary infiltrates (Fig. 98–3) and two thirds with thoracic lymphadenomegaly. Importantly, 20 per cent of dogs present with cranial mediastinal lymphadenopathy, which correlates negatively with both remission and survival duration.[19] Abdominal radiographs or ultrasound investigation may reveal evidence of sublumbar lymph node, spleen, or liver involvement in approximately 50 per cent of cases in dogs. Abdominal ultrasonography is most important in cats when intestinal lymphoma is suspected. Special studies, including contrast studies of the gastrointestinal tract, computed tomography (CT) or myelographic studies of the central nervous system (CNS), and skeletal surveys, are reserved for those cases in which the appropriate anatomic site is suspected.

In the author's practice, for typical cases of multicentric lymphoma in dogs, imaging is limited to thoracic radiographs, as there is no prognostic difference between dogs with stage III and those with stage IV disease (i.e., liver and spleen involvement). However, cranial mediastinal lymphadenopathy is of prognostic significance.[19]

Cytologic and Histopathologic Diagnosis. Microscopic confirmation of lymphoma is the cornerstone of diagnosis in both cats and dogs. Fine-needle aspirate (FNA) cytologic assessment by a skilled clinical pathologist may be adequate to make a diagnosis of lymphoma in dogs, but conclusive histologic confirmation is recommended. Predominance of a homogenous population of immature lymphoid cells is suggestive of lymphoma (Fig. 98–4). Avoidance of nodes draining reactive areas (e.g., submandibular nodes in the presence of periodontal disease) is recommended, as reactive hyperplasia may mask (or mimic) the true neoplastic condition.

In the cat, FNA assessment alone is not sufficient in most

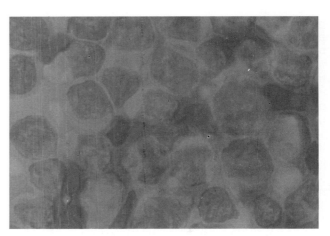

Figure 98–4. Fine-needle aspirate cytology (Wright's-Giemsa stain, 1000×) of a peripheral lymph node in a dog with high-grade lymphoma. The node is effaced with a homogenous population of immature lymphoid cells.

cases, owing to difficulties encountered in distinguishing lymphoma from benign hyperplastic lymph node syndromes unique to the species, including idiopathic peripheral lymphadenopathy, plexiform vascularization of lymph nodes, and peripheral lymph node hyperplasia of young cats.[21-24] In these cases, whole lymph node excision is preferred, as the orientation, invasiveness, and architectural abnormalities may be necessary for diagnosis.

In addition to confirming a diagnosis of lymphoma, histologic and cytologic samples can be analyzed by various histochemical and immunohistochemical techniques to determine immunophenotype (B versus T cell), tumor proliferation rates (e.g., Ki-67, proliferating cell nuclear antigen [PCNA], argyrophilic nucleolar organizer regions [AgNOR]), and histologic subtype (high-, intermediate-, or low-grade tumors).[5, 8, 10, 25-27] The availability of such analysis is increasing, but at present, only immunophenotype in dogs is consistently predictive of prognosis. Histologic assessments of markers of multidrug resistance and apoptotic pathways (e.g., P-glycoprotein, p53) are currently being evaluated in dogs with lymphoma, but their significance requires further evaluation.[28-31]

Additional site-specific cytologic or histologic assessments may be warranted when extranodal sites are suspected. Thoracocentesis and cytologic evaluation of pleural fluid are often diagnostic in cats with mediastinal lymphoma but are less likely to be of value in dogs with effusions secondary to mediastinal involvement. Conversely, cerebrospinal fluid (CSF) analysis is more commonly helpful in dogs than in cats with CNS lymphoma, as the more common spinal form of lymphoma in cats is generally extradural.[32, 33] In cats suspected of having CNS lymphoma, bone marrow and renal involvement is often present, and cytologic assessment of these organs is generally more easily attainable than is assessment of spinal sites.

DIFFERENTIAL DIAGNOSIS

The differential diagnosis for lymphoma varies with the anatomic form of the disease and is presented in Table 98–3.

THERAPY

Untreated dogs and cats generally live an average of 4 to 6 weeks once a diagnosis is established. In general, lymphoma is a systemic disease and requires a systemic approach to therapy (i.e., chemotherapy). Exceptions to this occur in cases of solitary site or extranodal lymphoma, where local therapy involving either surgery or radiotherapy may be indicated.

Systemic Chemotherapy in Dogs With Lymphoma. There are almost as many chemotherapy protocols for dogs with lymphoma as there are veterinary oncologists. This likely reflects our inability to achieve cure in the majority of cases. Lymphoma in the dog can be an initially gratifying disease to treat, as remission rates approach 80 to 90 per cent with available combination chemotherapy protocols, and quality of life is generally excellent during the period of remission.[34] However, the majority of dogs eventually succumb to multidrug-resistant recurrence of their disease, on average, one year after diagnosis.

Owing to the large and ever-increasing number of available chemotherapeutic protocols, several factors should be considered and discussed with caregivers when choosing the

TABLE 98–3. COMMON DIFFERENTIAL DIAGNOSIS FOR LYMPHOMA

ANATOMIC FORM	DIFFERENTIAL LIST
Generalized lymphadenopathy	Disseminated infections (e.g., bacterial, viral, rickettsial, parasitic, fungal) Immune-mediated disorders (e.g., lupus, polyarthritis, vasculitis, dermatopathy) Other hematopoietic tumors (e.g., leukemia, multiple myeloma, malignant or systemic histiocytosis) Tumors metastatic to nodes In cats, many benign reactive hyperplastic syndromes (see text)
Alimentary	Infiltrative enteritis (e.g., lymphocytic, plasmacytic enteritis) Nonlymphoid intestinal neoplasms Granulomatous enteritis Granulated round cell tumors in cats Gastrointestinal mast cell tumor in cats
Cutaneous	Infectious dermatitis (e.g., advanced pyoderma) Immune-mediated dermatitis (e.g., pemphigus) Other cutaneous neoplasms
Mediastinal	Thymoma Heart base tumor (chemodectoma) Ectopic thyroid tumor Pulmonary lymphomatoid granulomatosis Granulomatous disease (e.g., hilar lymphadenopathy with blastomycosis)

protocol to be used. These factors include the cost, time commitment, efficacy, and toxicity of the protocols in question, as well as the clinician's experience with them. With the availability of generic drugs, protocols are becoming affordable to a larger segment of veterinary clientele. In general, more complex combination chemotherapy protocols are more expensive, more time consuming (e.g., repeated office visits, closer monitoring), and more likely to result in toxicity than are simpler, single-agent protocols. However, as a general rule, more complex combination protocols result in longer remission and survival durations than do single-agent protocols. A complete listing of all available protocols for dogs with lymphoma is beyond the scope of this chapter, and the reader is referred to a recent review and reports.[7, 8, 34] The combination protocol used by the author and the most widely used single-agent protocol are presented here.

Most complex combination protocols are modifications of CHOP protocols initially designed for human use. CHOP represents combinations of cyclophosphamide (C), doxorubicin (H, hydroxydaunorubicin), vincristine (O, Oncovin), and prednisone (P). Regardless of which CHOP-based protocol is used, overall median remission and survival times are approximately 8 and 12 months, respectively.[34] Approximately 20 to 25 per cent of treated dogs will be alive two years or longer after initiation of these protocols. Response rates and length of response vary according to the presence or absence of prognostic factors discussed later in this chapter. Historically, following an intensive induction portion of the protocol, when drugs are given weekly, treatment intervals are slowly spread out and drugs are given less frequently in what is termed the maintenance phase of the protocol. One important question that is yet to be answered in veterinary medicine is how long chemotherapy should be continued after complete remission is achieved; that is, how long the maintenance phase should last or, for that matter, whether maintenance therapy should be used at all. In most human

TABLE 98–4. COMBINATION CHEMOTHERAPY PROTOCOL FOR DOGS WITH LYMPHOMA

TREATMENT WEEK	DRUG, DOSAGE, AND ROUTE
1	Vincristine 0.5–0.7 mg/m², IV
	L-Asparaginase 400 U/kg, SC
	Prednisone 2 mg/kg, PO
2	Cyclophosphamide 200 mg/m², IV
	Prednisone 1.5 mg/kg, PO
3	Vincristine 0.5–0.7 mg/m², IV
	Prednisone 1 mg/kg, PO
4	Doxorubicin 30 mg/m², IV
	Prednisone 0.5 mg/kg, PO
6	Vincristine 0.5–0.7 mg/m², IV
7	Cyclophosphamide 200 mg/m², IV
8	Vincristine 0.5–0.7 mg/m², IV
9*	Doxorubicin 30 mg/m², IV
11	Vincristine 0.5–0.7 mg/m², IV
13	Cyclophosphamide 200 mg/m², IV
15	Vincristine 0.5–0.7 mg/m², IV
17	Doxorubicin 30 mg/m², IV
19	Vincristine 0.5–0.7 mg/m², IV
21	Cyclophosphamide 200 mg/m², IV
23	Vincristine 0.5–0.7 mg/m², IV
25†	Doxorubicin 30 mg/m², IV

*If in complete remission at week 9, continue to week 11.
†If in complete remission at week 25, therapy is discontinued and monthly reevaluations are instituted.
IV = intravenously; SC = subcutaneously; PO = orally.

protocols, following a six-month induction phase, no benefit to continued maintenance therapy has been shown, and no further therapy is given until such time as recurrence is observed. In veterinary medicine, no definitive studies exist as to the benefit of maintenance therapy. Presently, the author prefers a modified version of the University of Wisconsin–Madison (UW-M) lymphoma protocol[6] outlined in Table 98–4. In this protocol, chemotherapy is discontinued at six months if the dog is in complete remission at that time. This protocol achieves remission in approximately 90 per cent of dogs treated, and remission and survival lengths are similar to those historically observed when long-term maintenance is used. Dogs are reevaluated by physical examination monthly after therapy is discontinued, with special attention to lymph node size. If recurrence is suspected, the diagnostic steps outlined earlier are revisited.

The most effective and commonly used single-agent chemotherapy protocol for dogs with lymphoma is doxorubicin,[7, 35, 36] given at a dose of 30 mg/m² intravenously every three weeks for five treatments. Response is observed in 75 to 80 per cent of cases, and median remission and survival durations of approximately five and seven months, respectively, are reported. This single-agent protocol has the advantages of being less time consuming and requiring fewer hospital visits. Because only one drug is used, any side effects encountered are attributable to that drug.

If financial or other client concerns preclude the use of more aggressive systemic chemotherapy, prednisone therapy (2 mg/kg a day, orally) alone often results in short-lived remissions of approximately one to two months. In these cases, it is advisable to educate clients that if they decide to pursue more aggressive therapy at a later date, dogs with prior prednisone therapy may be more likely to develop multiple drug resistance and experience shorter remission and survival durations with subsequent combination protocols. This is especially true following long-term prednisone use or in dogs that have experienced a recurrence while on prednisone.[37] Therefore, the earlier clients opt for aggressive

therapy, the more likely it is that a durable response will result.

Modifications in chemotherapy dose and/or frequency may be necessary under conditions of excess toxicity, as discussed in Chapter 95. When hypercalcemia is present, if the dog is substage a and continues to eat and drink, ancillary therapy for hypercalcemia is usually unnecessary, as initiation of chemotherapy will result in eucalcemia within a few days. If, however, the animal is ill, azotemic, or showing signs attributable to hypercalcemia, therapy directed specifically at hypercalcemia (see Chapter 97) concurrent with the initiation of systemic chemotherapy is warranted.

Systemic Chemotherapy in Cats With Lymphoma. Several combination chemotherapy protocols for cats have been reported and reviewed previously.[11, 12, 34, 38] It has become clear that the addition of doxorubicin to COP-based protocols (C, cyclophosphamide; O, vincristine [Oncovin]. P, prednisone) has shown superior results to COP alone in the cat.[11, 38] In general, cats do not enjoy as high a response rate or remission and survival duration as dogs with lymphoma. Complete response rates vary between 50 and 70 per cent, and overall median remission and survival durations are approximately four and six months, respectively. However, a larger proportion of cats (30 to 40 per cent) that achieve a complete response with combination chemotherapy enjoy more durable (i.e., ≥ 2 years) overall remission and survival times than do dogs. Response rates and length of response vary according to the presence or absence of prognostic factors discussed later in this chapter. The modified CHOP-based protocol preferred by the author for cats is represented in Table 98–5. Cats with granular cell lymphoma or globule leukocyte tumors tend to respond poorly to chemotherapy, but durable responses have been reported.[15]

Reinduction or Rescue Therapy. Ultimately, most

TABLE 98–5. COMBINATION CHEMOTHERAPY PROTOCOL FOR CATS WITH LYMPHOMA

TREATMENT WEEK	DRUG, DOSAGE, AND ROUTE
1	Vincristine 0.5–0.7 mg/m², IV
	L-Asparaginase 400 U/kg, SC
	Prednisone 2 mg/kg, PO
2	Cyclophosphamide 200 mg/m², IV
	Prednisone 2 mg/kg, PO
3	Vincristine 0.5–0.7 mg/m², IV
	Prednisone 1 mg/kg, PO
4	Doxorubicin 25 mg/m², IV
	Prednisone 1 mg/kg, PO*
6	Vincristine 0.5–0.7 mg/m², IV
7	Cyclophosphamide 200 mg/m², IV
8	Vincristine 0.5–0.7 mg/m², IV
9†	Doxorubicin 25 mg/m², IV
11	Vincristine 0.5–0.7 mg/m², IV
13	Chlorambucil 1.4 mg/kg, PO
15	Vincristine 0.5–0.7 mg/m², IV
17	Methotrexate 0.5–0.8 mg/kg IV
19	Vincristine 0.5–0.7 mg/m², IV
21	Chlorambucil 1.4 mg/kg, PO
23	Vincristine 0.5–0.7 mg/m², IV
25‡	Doxorubicin 25 mg/m², IV

*Prednisone is continued (1 mg/kg PO) every other day from this point on.
†If in complete remission at week 9, continue to week 11.
‡If in complete remission at week 25, therapy is continued at 3-week intervals following the same sequence of drugs used in week 11 through 25 until week 51. If in complete remission at week 51, continue treatments at 4-week intervals using the same sequence of drugs, with the exception that methotrexate substitutes for doxorubicin from this point forward.
IV = intravenously; SC = subcutaneously; PO = orally.

dogs and cats that have been successfully treated with chemotherapy have a relapse of their lymphoma. Often this represents a recrudescence of the tumor in a more drug-resistant form. Evidence suggests that recurrent lymphoma in dogs is more likely to express the gene encoding the P-glycoprotein transmembrane drug pump that is often associated with multiple drug resistance.[28–30] At the first recurrence of lymphoma, it is recommended that reinduction be attempted by reintroducing the induction protocol that was initially successful. In general, the likelihood of a response and the length of the response are half that encountered in the initial therapy; however, a subset of animals will enjoy long-term reinductions.

If reinduction fails or the dog or cat did not respond to the initial induction, the use of so-called rescue agents or rescue protocols can be attempted. These are drug or drug combinations that are typically not found in the standard CHOP protocol and are withheld for use in the drug-resistant setting. A number of rescue protocols have been reported in the veterinary literature and have previously been reviewed.[34, 39] The most common protocols used in dogs include single-agent or combination use of actinomycin D, mitoxantrone, doxorubicin (if doxorubicin was not part of the original induction protocol), a doxorubicin-dacarbazine combination, and MOPP (M, mechlorethamine; O, Oncovin; P, procarbazine; P, prednisone). Mitoxantrone, doxorubicin, and MOPP have also been advocated in cats with resistant relapse. In general, overall rescue response rates of 40 to 50 per cent are reported, but these responses are usually not durable, with median responses of one and a half to two months being the norm. A small subset of animals will enjoy longer rescue durations.

Therapy for Extranodal Lymphoma. If extranodal involvement is part of a more generalized or multicentric disease process, systemic therapies previously discussed should be instituted. Conversely, if the extranodal site is solitary and not part of a multicentric presentation, local therapy may be performed without institution of systemic chemotherapy. In these latter cases, strict adherence to staging diagnostics, including bone marrow evaluation and radiographic and ultrasonographic imaging of the thorax and abdomen, is warranted to ensure that the process is localized. If the disease is confined, local surgery and/or radiotherapy is often effective (Fig. 98–5). Clients should be informed that in these cases, systemic lymphoma is likely to occur months to years later, and a regular recheck schedule should be instituted. It is the author's opinion that systemic therapy should be withheld until systemic disease is documented.

In cases in which CNS involvement is part of a more generalized process, the penetration of chemotherapy through the blood-brain barrier may be of concern, and additional therapies are recommended. In standard CHOP protocols, only prednisone consistently penetrates the blood-brain barrier. The addition of cytosine arabinoside, which does achieve therapeutic CSF levels, to a CHOP-based protocol is recommended in such cases. Radiotherapy directed either to the entire neural axis in the case of multifocal CNS lymphoma or to specific CNS locations in the case of solitary central or spinal lymphoma can also be effective. Cytoreductive surgery has been attempted in a small number of cases of extradural lymphoma in both cats and dogs with mixed results.[32, 33, 40]

Cutaneous lymphoma in solitary sites has been effectively treated with local surgery or radiotherapy; however, the likelihood of ultimate systemic spread is high. Multiple cutaneous lesions are more commonly encountered (see Fig.

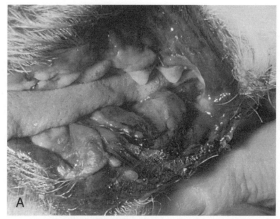
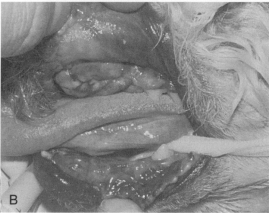

Figure 98–5. *A,* Solitary gingival lymphoma in a dog staged negative for systemic involvement. *B,* The same dog six months following external beam radiation therapy (48 Gy total dose). A complete response and long-term survival were achieved.

98–2), and systemic therapy is necessary. In general, cutaneous lymphoma tends to be less responsive to chemotherapy than multicentric lymphoma, and clinical signs can wax and wane considerably over time. Responses have been reported with oral *cis*-retinoic acid therapy (Accutane 1 to 3 mg/kg divided, twice a day, orally), Doxil (a liposome-encapsulated form of doxorubicin), L-asparaginase, dacarbazine, topical nitrogen mustard, and standard CHOP-based protocols.[41–43] Response rates, however, are approximately 40 to 50 per cent, and long-term survival is uncommon.

PROGNOSIS

Prognostic Factors in Dogs. A listing of factors known or suspected to affect remission rates and/or remission and survival durations in dogs with lymphoma is presented in Table 98–6. Age, body weight, and breed do not affect duration of remission or survival, and most studies fail to correlate clinical stage to prognosis, except for dogs with marked stage V disease—that is, if bone marrow is heavily infiltrated, if gross leukemia is present, or if peripheral cytopenias exist secondary to myelophthisis. The two factors that most consistently correlate with prognosis in dogs with lymphoma are immunophenotype and WHO substage status.[5–9, 19] Many reports have confirmed that dogs with CD3 immunoreactive tumors (i.e., T-cell derivation) are associated with significantly shorter remission and survival durations (Fig. 98–6). Similarly, dogs presenting with sub-

TABLE 98–6. FACTORS KNOWN OR SUSPECTED TO AFFECT PROGNOSIS IN DOGS WITH LYMPHOMA

FACTOR	STRENGTH OF ASSOCIATION	COMMENTS	REFERENCE
WHO clinical stage	Weak	Likely to be predictive of outcome only in stage V disease with marked marrow involvement	8
WHO substage	Strong	Dogs with substage b experience shorter remission and survival durations	5–7, 9
Immunophenotype	Strong	Dogs with T-cell lymphoma experience shorter remission and survival durations than dogs with B-cell tumors	5, 8, 9, 19
Hypercalcemia	Moderate	Poorer prognosis is not independent; more likely due to T-cell association	6, 7
Prolonged steroid pretreatment	Moderate	Most studies show previous steroid use shortens response durations	37
Sex	Moderate	Several large studies report that males experience shorter remission and survival durations; other reports are contradictory	5, 6, 19, 44
Proliferation rate	Moderate	High proliferation may confer better response; other reports are contradictory	5, 25
Cranial mediastinal lymphadenomegaly	Moderate to strong	Large compilation of cases reports association with shorter remission and survival durations; other reports are contradictory	16, 19
Histologic grade	Weak	Low-grade tumors less likely to respond	8
P-glycoprotein expression	Moderate	Associated with poor response rates and shorter remission and survival durations	29, 30

WHO = World Health Organization.

stage b disease (i.e., clinically ill) also do poorly when compared with dogs with substage a disease (Fig. 98–7).

Other factors reported to correlate with prognosis are less consistent; that is, they are not found to correlate in all studies, they are based on preliminary reports, or there are contradictory reports in the literature. Some correlate following univariate analysis but are no longer significant when they are scrutinized by multivariate analysis (in which all factors are considered together). An example is the presence of hypercalcemia. In several reports, the presence of hypercalcemia is associated with a poor prognosis; however, if multivariate analysis is performed, it is no longer predictive, primarily because dogs with hypercalcemia are more likely to have T-cell-derived lymphoma, which is a much stronger correlate.

Prognostic Factors in Cats. Unlike in the dog, CD3 immunoreactivity has not been established as a negative prognostic indicator in the cat.[11] This may reflect the wider variations in frequency of the different anatomic forms of lymphoma encountered in cats and the difficulty in separating out differences. It appears that the factors most strongly associated with a more positive prognosis in cats are com-

plete response to therapy (which, unfortunately, cannot be determined before therapy), negative FeLV status, early clinical stage, substage a, and the addition of doxorubicin to the treatment protocol.[11, 38, 45] Early reports may contradict more recent studies, partly because FeLV-associated lymphoma is declining, and populations in the early literature may not equate to more recent populations studied. In general, FeLV-negative cats that achieve a complete response on CHOP-based protocols have a high likelihood of long-term survival, with approximately 35 per cent alive one and a half years after diagnosis. Cats with nasal lymphoma, overall, have the best prognosis, as local radiotherapy (or chemotherapy, if radiotherapy is not available) results in excellent control, with median survivals approaching one and a half years.

The Future of Lymphoma Therapy. Based on the similarity of results reported in the various combination chemotherapy protocols, it appears that we have gone about as far as we can using available chemotherapeutics. All combination protocols reported to date stop short of the same 10- to 12-month median survival "brick wall." Advances in remission and survival durations await the development of new chemotherapeutics or novel treatment modalities. Mech-

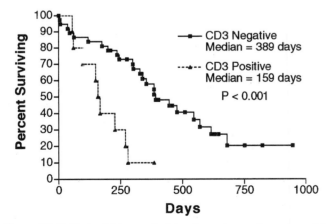

Figure 98–6. Kaplan-Meier survival duration estimates for a group of 55 dogs with lymphoma treated with an identical CHOP-based combination chemotherapy protocol at the University of Wisconsin. Dogs with CD3 immunoreactive (T-cell) lymphoma had significantly shorter survival durations.

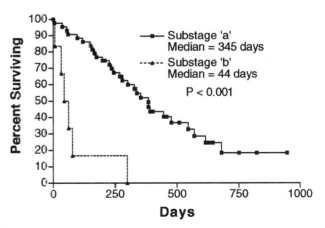

Figure 98–7. Kaplan-Meier survival duration estimates for a group of 55 dogs with lymphoma treated with an identical CHOP-based combination chemotherapy protocol at the University of Wisconsin. Dogs with substage b disease (i.e., clinically ill) had significantly shorter survival durations.

anisms of avoiding or abrogating multidrug resistance, enhancing tumor apoptosis (programmed cell death), targeting treatments with immunoconjugates (i.e., antibody-directed therapies), and novel immunomodulatory therapies are all active areas of investigation in both human and veterinary medicine.

LYMPHOID LEUKEMIA

Leukemia is defined as a proliferation of neoplastic cells in the bone marrow. An important distinction is that, by definition, the malignant cells may or may not be present in the peripheral blood circulation. A categorization of lymphoid leukemia into acute lymphoblastic leukemia (ALL) and chronic lymphocytic leukemia (CLL) is important from a diagnostic, prognostic, and therapeutic standpoint (Fig. 98–8). Both forms are relatively rare in companion animals.[46–50]

ACUTE LYMPHOBLASTIC LEUKEMIA

ALL is characterized by proliferations of morphologically immature lymphoblasts in the bone marrow or peripheral blood. It may be confused with multicentric lymphoma in dogs that have advanced stage V disease (i.e., secondary bone marrow infiltration). The primary component of ALL is leukemia, and the clinical course is rapid, progressive, and poorly responsive to therapy.[46, 48, 50]

No breed or sex predilection exists for dogs with ALL. Middle-aged to older dogs are typically affected. Cats with ALL are usually younger and FeLV antigenemic.[49] Presentations are nonspecific and commonly include lethargy, weight loss, intermittent pyrexia, hepatosplenomegaly, and nonspecific abdominal pain. Neurologic signs, both central and peripheral, have been reported. The majority of affected animals are anemic, and varying degrees of thrombocytopenia and leukocytopenia are commonly present.

Diagnosis is confirmed following documentation of marked lymphoblast proliferation within the bone marrow or peripheral blood. Bone marrow aspirate or core biopsy and CBC are usually all that is required for diagnosis. Aspiration cytology of lymph nodes and involved organs and confirmation of retroviral status in cats may be contributory. The presence of 30 per cent or more lymphoblasts within the bone marrow is considered diagnostic. Approximately 10 per cent of cases are classified as aleukemic leukemia, owing to the presence of bone marrow infiltration and the absence of peripherally circulating lymphoblasts. ALL may be further differentiated clinically from stage V multicentric lymphoma by its more rapid progression, lack of significant lymphadenopathy in approximately 50 per cent of cases, poor chemoresponsiveness, and short survival time.

Prognosis is generally poor for dogs and cats with ALL.[46, 48–50] Combination chemotherapy protocols designed to treat lymphoma result in remission in approximately 25 per cent of cases, but the length of remission is usually very short, and survival times of more than a few months are rare. A short-term response to low-dose cytosine arabinoside (10 mg/m^2 subcutaneously, twice a day) has been reported in a cat.[51]

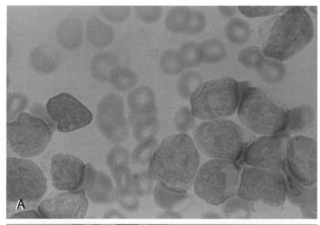

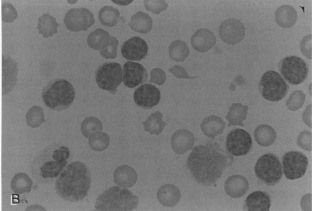

Figure 98–8. *A,* Peripheral blood smear (Wright's-Giemsa stain, 1000×) of a dog with acute lymphoblastic leukemia (ALL). Note morphologically immature lymphoblasts characteristic of ALL. *B,* Peripheral blood smear (Wright's-Giemsa stain, 1000×) of a dog with chronic lymphocytic leukemia (CLL). Note morphologically mature lymphocytes characteristic of CLL. (Photomicrograph courtesy of Dr. Karen Young, University of Wisconsin.)

CHRONIC LYMPHOCYTIC LEUKEMIA

CLL is characterized by the proliferation of phenotypically mature lymphocytes rather than lymphoblasts. It is reported primarily in older dogs and cats. Clinical presentations are nonspecific and can include lethargy, organomegaly, pyrexia, polyuria and polydipsia, hemorrhage (from thrombocytopenia), intermittent lameness, and collapse.[47] The majority of dogs present with mild to moderate lymphadenopathy, splenomegaly, and pale mucous membranes. Some dogs and cats are asymptomatic and a diagnosis is found incidentally following routine blood work.

Hematologically, a normocytic, normochromic, nonregenerative anemia usually accompanies a marked mature peripheral lymphocytosis, which may range from 10,000 to 300,000/μL or more. Thrombocytopenia and neutropenia may be present, owing to myelophthisis. Although a minority of cases present with hyperglobulinemia, following immunoelectrophoresis, approximately half have evidence of a monoclonal gammopathy, often with Bence Jones proteinuria, indicative of a B-cell derivation. No association with FeLV infection has been documented in the cat.

Unlike ALL, CLL can have a protracted clinical course and is usually initially responsive to chemotherapy.[47] Treatment is not instituted unless significant clinical signs, organomegaly, or peripheral cytopenias (anemia, neutropenia, thrombocytopenia) are present that impact or threaten the animal's quality of life. Animals with CLL have been followed without treatment for many months. If therapy is indicated, chlorambucil (0.2 mg/kg/day, orally, in the dog; 2 mg/cat, every other day, orally) is combined with prednisone (2 mg/kg/day, orally). Dosage is adjusted based on response. Approximately 75 per cent of animals will respond and enjoy a normal quality of life, with a median survival of approximately one year. Although the prognosis is good in the short term, eventually CLL becomes resistant to therapy or progresses to ALL. When this happens, lymphoblasts replace mature lymphocytes as the abnormally proliferating population, and survival is short.

NONLYMPHOID LEUKEMIAS AND MYELOPROLIFERATIVE DISORDERS

Myeloproliferative disorders (MPDs) are defined as a group of nonlymphoid bone marrow cell disorders in which proliferation of one, several, or all of the marrow cell lines is present. They can represent preneoplastic or neoplastic conditions that may have a benign or malignant course. These are rare conditions in companion animals. With few exceptions (see Polycythemia Vera later), the veterinary literature regarding MPDs is sparse and composed almost entirely of single case reports. Our experience with MPDs is, therefore, almost exclusively anecdotal, and specific characterizations and recommendations are lacking.

CLASSIFICATION

In general, MPDs are classified first on the derivation of the cell in question and second on the degree of cellular differentiation. If the proliferating cell population is mature or microscopically typical of a well-differentiated bone marrow cell line, the MPD is termed chronic. If the proliferating population represents an immature or poorly differentiated cell line, the MPD is classified as acute. Table 98–7 lists the MPDs reported in the veterinary literature. Because pluripotent bone marrow stem cells are involved, one MPD may evolve into another, and more often than not, more than one cell line is involved in the same disorder.

CLINICAL PRESENTATION

Animals with chronic MPDs may be without clinical signs until organ proliferation or bone marrow myelophthisis results in systemic disease. Clinical signs in dogs with late-stage chronic MPDs or acute MPDs are generally nonspe-

cific. These can include organomegaly, pallor, sepsis, and hemorrhage from thrombocytopenia. Most MPDs have been associated with FeLV infection in cats.

DIAGNOSIS

Diagnosis of MPDs is based on documentation of the proliferating cell line in the absence of non-neoplastic diseases associated with bone marrow hyperplasia or hypoplasia. The differential diagnosis, therefore, includes chronic inflammatory diseases (e.g., ehrlichiosis), multicentric lymphoma, estrogen toxicity, lead poisoning, and, in the case of essential or primary thrombocytosis, iron deficiency. Because many of the acute MPDs represent poorly differentiated cell lineage and/or combinations of cell lineage, light microscopic morphology is often not sufficient to determine the specific cellular derivation. Histochemical and immunohistochemical stains are necessary in many instances for precise classification. Several private and academic laboratories perform these analyses; a complete listing of available tests is beyond the scope of this chapter and can be found elsewhere.[78]

THERAPY

The acute MPDs are generally poorly responsive to single-agent or combination chemotherapy protocols, and the prognosis is therefore grave. Several agents and combinations have been tried, including doxorubicin, cytosine arabinoside, 6-thioguanine, and CHOP-based protocols.[48, 50, 59] Response rates are low, and overall survival is generally short. If chemotherapy is pursued, aggressive supportive therapy is necessary and may include whole blood or blood-component therapy to address cytopenias secondary to myelophthisis, antibiotic support, and aggressive fluid therapy.

Chronic MPDs carry a guarded prognosis; however, initial durable responses to therapy are more likely than with acute MPDs. Therapy is not required until clinical signs or significant peripheral cytopenia develops. Hydroxyurea has been used successfully for treating several types of chronic MPD, in particular polycythemia vera (see later), essential thrombocythemia, basophilic leukemia, and chronic myelogenous leukemia (CML).[65, 67, 69, 70, 78] In dogs with CML, hydroxyurea is used at an initial dose of 20 to 25 mg/kg orally, twice daily. This dosage is continued until the leukocyte count drops to less than 20,000 cells/μL, at which time the dose is reduced to 10 to 15 mg/kg daily or switched to

TABLE 98–7. MYELOPROLIFERATIVE DISORDERS (MPDS) REPORTED IN DOGS AND CATS

CLASSIFICATION	CELL LINEAGE	REFERENCE
Acute MPD		
Acute myelogenous leukemia	Myeloblasts	48–50
Acute myelomonocytic leukemia	Myeloblasts/monoblasts	48–50, 52–54
Acute monocytic leukemia	Monoblasts	48–50, 55
Acute megakaryoblastic leukemia	Megakaryoblasts	56–62
Erythroleukemia	Erythroblasts	49, 63
Chronic MPD		
Chronic myelogenous leukemia	Neutrophils, late precursors	64–66
Primary thrombocythemia	Platelets	67, 68
Basophilic leukemia	Basophils and precursors	69, 70
Eosinophilic leukemia	Eosinophils and precursors	71, 72
Polycythemia vera	Erythrocytes	68, 73–77

50 mg/kg orally given once every two to three weeks. A common side effect of hydroxyurea therapy in dogs is onychomadesis (sloughing of the claw or toe nail). In dogs responding to hydroxyurea therapy, survival of many months has been reported. Ultimately, many of the chronic MPDs shift into a terminal phase or "blast crisis," in which a fatal acute leukemic crisis is observed.

POLYCYTHEMIA VERA (PRIMARY ERYTHROCYTOSIS)

Polycythemia vera (PV) is defined as an abnormal proliferation of erythroid precursors in the bone marrow that occurs independent of erythropoietin (EP) and follows a normal, orderly pattern of maturation. The result is abnormally elevated packed cell volume, erythroid count, and blood hemoglobin levels. It must be differentiated from so-called relative polycythemia or secondary polycythemia. Relative polycythemia is a result of hemoconcentration secondary to severe dehydration, body fluid shifts, or acute splenic contraction in dogs. It is readily corrected with fluid-based therapies. Secondary polycythemia is defined as EP-mediated erythrocytosis. Conditions associated with secondary polycythemia include right-to-left cardiac shunts, congestive heart failure, severe chronic pulmonary disease, some forms of renal disease, and neoplasms that secrete EP or EP-like substances.

Middle-aged dogs and cats are typically affected.[68, 73–77] Clinical signs and physical examination findings associated with PV include hyperemic mucous membranes, injected scleral and retinal vessels, weakness, exercise intolerance, frank hemorrhage (epistaxis, hematuria, melena), neurologic signs (dementia, seizures, paralysis, ataxia), and occasional splenomegaly. Cardiac and renal compromise may also be present. The majority of signs reported are secondary to hyperviscosity syndrome, discussed at length in the plasma cell tumor section of this chapter.

Diagnosis follows the documentation of significant erythrocytosis (60 to 75 per cent hematocrit) with normal to decreased serum EP levels and the absence of conditions associated with relative or secondary polycythemia. Thoracic and abdominal radiography, abdominal ultrasonography, arterial blood gas, bone marrow aspirate, and serum EP levels should be procured to rule out differentials. Erythroid hyperplasia with relatively normal patterns of maturation are found on bone marrow cytology. Radioactive chromium determinations of red blood cell mass may contribute to the diagnosis.

Therapy for PV involves reduction in the red blood cell mass and suppression of erythroid production in the bone marrow. Reduction of red blood cell mass can easily be achieved by phlebotomy (15 to 20 cc/kg body weight) and reinfusion of the animal's own plasma once the red blood cells have been removed.[74–76] Several techniques can be used to suppress erythroid production, including the use of radioactive phosphorus (^{32}P) or more commonly available chemotherapy.[68, 78] The chemotherapy of choice is hydroxyurea, although alkylating agents such as melphalan, cyclophosphamide, and busulfan have also been used with mixed results. Hydroxyurea is instituted at 20 to 25 mg/kg orally twice a day in dogs (10 to 15 mg/kg in cats). Once the hematocrit is below 60 per cent, hydroxyurea is reduced to every-other-day therapy. Careful observation of CBCs should be undertaken to monitor potential myelosuppression of other cell lineages. The majority of cases respond to therapy, and survival for a year or longer is the norm. Progression to leukemia is reported in some people with PV.

PLASMA CELL NEOPLASMS

Plasma cell neoplasms are defined as neoplastic proliferations of cells of the B-lymphocyte plasma cell lineage. This population is believed in most instances to be monoclonal (i.e., derived from a single cell), as they typically produce homogenous immunoglobulin. Plasma cell neoplasms include multiple myeloma, IgM (Waldenström's) macroglobulinemia, and solitary plasmacytoma (including solitary osseous plasmacytoma and extramedullary plasmacytoma). Multiple myeloma is the most important plasma cell neoplasm based on incidence and severity.

MULTIPLE MYELOMA

Multiple myeloma (MM) is responsible for approximately 8 per cent of all hematopoietic tumors.[79, 80] The true incidence of MM in the cat is unknown, but it is a much rarer diagnosis than in the dog.[81, 82]

In MM, malignant plasma cells produce an overabundance of a single type or component of immunoglobulin, referred to as the M component. Rarely, biclonal immunoglobulin production has been reported.[83] The M component can represent any class of immunoglobulin or only a portion of the molecule such as the light chain (Bence Jones protein) or heavy chain (heavy chain disease) of the molecule.

Etiology

The etiology of MM is, for the most part, unknown. Genetic predispositions, viral infections, chronic immune stimulation, and exposure to carcinogens have all been suggested as contributing factors.[84–86] MM has not been associated with either FeLV or FIV infection.

Pathophysiology

A wide array of pathologic abnormalities and related clinical syndromes can occur owing to tumor infiltration of various organs systems, presence of high levels of circulating M component, or a combination thereof.

Hyperviscosity syndrome (HVS) represents one of a constellation of clinicopathologic abnormalities resulting from greatly increased serum viscosity. The magnitude of HVS is related to the type, size, shape, and concentration of the M component in the blood. It is more common with IgM macroglobulinemias because of their high molecular weight, however, IgA- and IgG-associated HVS can occur, albeit less frequently.[79, 87, 88] High serum viscosity occurs in approximately 20 per cent of dogs with MM and can result in bleeding diathesis, neurologic signs (e.g., dementia, depression, seizure activity, coma), ophthalmic abnormalities (e.g., dilated and tortuous retinal vessels, retinal hemorrhage, retinal detachment), and increased cardiac workload with the potential for subsequent development of cardiomyopathy.[79, 87–91] These consequences are thought to be a result of sludging of blood in small vessels, ineffective delivery of oxygen and nutrients, and coagulation abnormalities. HVS is less common in cats but has been reported in association with IgG-, IgA-, and IgM-secreting tumors.[82, 87, 92–95]

Renal disease is present in 30 to 50 per cent of dogs with MM.[79] This can ensue as a result of Bence Jones (light chain) proteinuria, tumor infiltration into renal tissue, hypercalcemia, amyloidosis, diminished perfusion secondary to HVS, dehydration, or ascending urinary tract infection.

Bence Jones proteinuria occurs in approximately 25 to 40 per cent of dogs with MM, but its true incidence in cats is not well established.

Hypercalcemia occurs in 15 to 20 per cent of dogs with MM and is thought to result primarily from the production of osteoclast activating factor or other cytokines by neoplastic cells.[79, 87] In two dogs with MM and hypercalcemia, serum elevations in circulating N-terminal parathyroid hormone–related protein were noted, although the relative contribution to hypercalcemia is unknown.[96] Hypercalcemia may also be exacerbated by associated renal disease. Hypercalcemia is rare in cats with MM.[97]

Susceptibility to infection and immunodeficiency are often the ultimate cause of death in animals with MM. Normal immunoglobulin levels are usually severely depressed, and leukopenias may be present secondary to marrow infiltration (myelophthisis).

Variable cytopenias may be observed in association with MM. A normocytic, normochromic, nonregenerative anemia is encountered in approximately two thirds of dogs.[79, 87] This can result from myelophthisis, blood loss from coagulation disorders, anemia of chronic disease, or increased erythrocyte destruction secondary to high serum viscosity. Similar factors lead to thrombocytopenia and leukopenia in 25 to 30 per cent of affected dogs.

Bleeding diathesis can result from one or a combination of events. M components may interfere with coagulation by inhibition of platelet aggregation and the release of platelet factor 3, adsorption of minor clotting proteins, generation of abnormal fibrin polymerization, and a functional decrease in calcium.

Cardiac disease, if present, is usually the result of excessive cardiac workload and myocardial hypoxia secondary to hyperviscosity. Myocardial infiltration with amyloid and anemia may be complicating factors.

Clinical Presentation and Signs

MM occurs in aged dogs and cats, and no breed or sex predilection has been consistently reported. Clinical signs are variable owing to the wide range of possible pathologic effects and may be present up to one year before diagnosis.[79] The most common clinical signs in decreasing order of frequency are lethargy and weakness, lameness, hemorrhage, polyuria and polydipsia, and neurologic deficits. Bleeding diathesis is usually represented by epistaxis and gingival bleeding. CNS signs may include dementia, seizure activity, and deficiencies in midbrain or brain stem localizing reflexes secondary to HVS or extreme hypercalcemia. Signs reflective of transverse myelopathies secondary to vertebral column infiltration, pathologic fracture, or extradural mass compression can also occur.

In the cat, anorexia and weight loss are the most common clinical signs.[82, 98] A history of chronic respiratory infections may be present. Skeletal lesions are uncommon in cats; however, organomegaly is more commonly seen owing to organ infiltration. Epistaxis, pleural and peritoneal hemorrhagic effusions, retinal hemorrhage, and central neurologic signs have been reported.[82, 87, 92–95] Polydipsia and polyuria can occur secondary to renal disease, and dehydration may develop. Hind limb paresis secondary to osteolysis of lumbar vertebral bodies has been reported in a cat.[99]

Diagnosis

The diagnosis of MM usually follows the demonstration of bone marrow plasmacytosis, osteolytic bone lesions (primarily in the dog), and serum or urine myeloma proteins (M component). In the absence of osteolytic bone lesions, a diagnosis can also be made if marrow plasmacytosis is associated with a progressive increase in the M component.

All animals suspected of plasma cell tumors should receive a CBC, platelet count, serum biochemistry profile, and urinalysis. Particular attention is paid to renal function and serum calcium levels. Serum electrophoresis and immunoelectrophoresis are performed to determine the presence of a monoclonal spike (Fig. 98–9) and to categorize the class of immunoglobulin involved. In the dog, the M component is usually that of IgG or IgA in nearly equal incidence.[79, 87] If IgM constitutes the M component, the term macroglobulinemia (Waldenström's) is applied. Biclonal gammopathy has also been reported.[83, 100] In the cat, MM is usually associated with IgG elevations, with only a few reports of IgA or IgM gammopathies.[82, 87, 92–95] Occasionally, cryoglobulinemia has been reported in dogs with MM.[87, 101, 102] Cryoglobulins are paraproteins that are insoluble at temperatures below 37°C; thus blood collection and clotting must be performed at 37°C prior to serum separation. If Bence Jones proteinuria is suspected, heat precipitation and electrophoresis of urine are necessary, as commercial urine dipstick methods are not capable of this determination.

Definitive diagnosis usually requires a bone marrow aspirate or core biopsy. Normal marrow contains less than 5 per cent plasma cells, whereas myelomatous marrow often greatly exceeds this level. Malignant plasma cells can have a varied microscopic appearance, and the degree of differentiation can range from that of normal plasma cells to those in early stages of differentiation.

Skeletal survey radiographs are recommended to determine the presence and extent of osteolytic lesions, which may have diagnostic, prognostic, and therapeutic implications. Rarely, biopsy of osteolytic lesions (i.e., Jamshidi core biopsy) is necessary for diagnosis. Bone lesions can be isolated, discrete lesions (including pathologic fractures) or

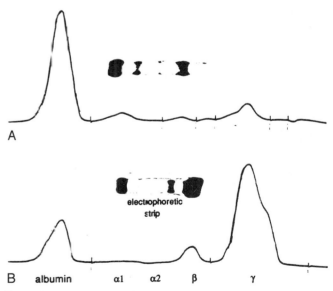

Figure 98–9. *A,* Serum protein electrophoresis from a normal dog. Stained cellulose acetate electrophoretic strip with accompanying densitogram. *B,* Serum protein electrophoresis from a dog with multiple myeloma. Note large M component spike (representing an IgA monoclonal gammopathy) present in the γ region. (From Vail DM: Plasma cell neoplasms. *In* Withrow SJ, MacEwen EG [eds]: Small Animal Clinical Oncology, 2nd ed. Philadelphia, WB Saunders, 1996, p 512.)

diffuse osteopenias (Fig. 98–10). Approximately 25 to 30 per cent of dogs with MM have evidence of bony lysis or diffuse osteoporosis.[79, 87] Bones engaged in active hematopoiesis are more commonly affected (e.g., vertebrae, ribs, pelvis, skull, and proximal long bones). Skeletal lesions are rare in cats with MM and dogs with IgM (Waldenström's) macroglobulinemia.[82, 87, 98] In macroglobulinemia, malignant cells often infiltrate the spleen, liver, and lymph tissue rather than bone.[87, 102]

If clinical hemorrhage is present, a coagulation assessment (e.g., platelet count, prothrombin time, partial thromboplastin time) and serum viscosity measurements should be undertaken. Nearly half of such cases will have abnormal prothrombin and partial thromboplastin times.

All animals should undergo a careful funduscopic examination; abnormalities may include retinal hemorrhage, venous dilatation with sacculation and tortuosity, retinal detachment, and blindness.

Differential Diagnosis

Disease syndromes other than MM can be associated with monoclonal gammopathies and should be considered in any list of differentials. These include other lymphoreticular tumors (lymphoma, chronic and acute lymphocytic leukemia), chronic infections (e.g., ehrlichiosis, leishmaniasis, feline infectious peritonitis), and monoclonal gammopathy of un-

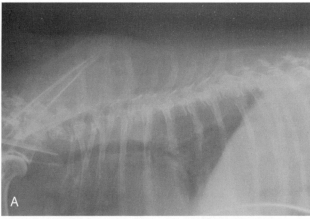

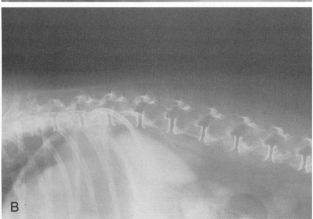

Figure 98–10. Lateral thoracic (*A*) and lumbar (*B*) vertebral radiographs of a dog with multiple myeloma. There are multiple expansile, lytic lesions in the axial skeleton, most apparent in the spinous processes of the vertebrae, but also in the ribs. Note the overall decreased opacity of the lumbar vertebrae, which is secondary to diffuse marrow involvement with tumor, causing a loss of bone trabeculae and thinning of cortices. (Photograph courtesy of Dr. Lisa Forrest, University of Wisconsin.)

known significance (MGUS). MGUS (i.e., benign, essential, or idiopathic monoclonal gammopathy) is a benign monoclonal gammopathy that is not associated with osteolysis, bone marrow infiltration, or Bence Jones proteinuria.[103, 104]

Therapy

Initial Therapy. Therapy should be directed at both the tumor cell mass and the secondary systemic effects. Chemotherapy is highly effective at reducing myeloma cell burden, relieving bone pain, initiating skeletal healing, and reducing levels of serum immunoglobulins.[79, 87] Its use significantly extends and improves the quality of most animals' lives. Complete elimination of neoplastic myeloma cells is rarely achieved, however, and although MM remains a gratifying disease to treat, eventual relapse is to be expected.

Melphalan, an alkylating agent, in combination with prednisone, is the treatment of choice. In the dog, the initial starting dose is 0.1 mg/kg orally once a day for 10 days; then it is reduced to 0.05 mg/kg once a day continuously. Prednisone is initiated at a dosage of 0.5 mg/kg orally once a day for 10 days, then reduced to 0.5 mg/kg every other day. Therapy is continued until clinical relapse occurs or myelosuppression necessitates a dose reduction. The most clinically significant toxicity of melphalan is myelosuppression, particularly thrombocytopenia. CBCs, including platelet counts, should be performed biweekly for two months following initiation of therapy and monthly thereafter. If significant myelosuppression occurs, reduction of the dose or treatment frequency may be necessary. An alternative pulse dosing regimen for melphalan (7 mg/m² orally once a day for five consecutive days every three weeks) has been used successfully at the University of Wisconsin in a small number of cases in which myelosuppression was limiting more conventional continuous low-dose therapy. Melphalan and prednisone therapy can also be used in cats with MM, although the results are less rewarding.

Cyclophosphamide can be used as an alternative alkylating agent, or sometimes in combination with melphalan, but there is no evidence that it is superior. In the author's practice, cyclophosphamide is used only in those cases presenting with severe hypercalcemia or with widespread systemic involvement, when a faster-acting alkylating agent may more quickly alleviate systemic effects of the disease. Cyclophosphamide is initiated at a single dosage of 200 mg/m² intravenously at the same time oral melphalan therapy is started. Chlorambucil, another alkylating agent, has been used successfully for the treatment of IgM macroglobulinemia in dogs at a dosage of 0.2 mg/kg orally once a day.[87] In nine dogs with IgM macroglobulinemia, response to chlorambucil occurred in the majority, and a median survival of 11 months was reported.[87]

Evaluation of Response to Therapy. Response is based on improvement in clinical signs and clinicopathologic parameters and radiographic improvement of skeletal lesions. Subjective improvement in bone pain, lameness, lethargy, and anorexia should be evident within three to four weeks. Objective laboratory improvement, including reduction in serum immunoglobulin or Bence Jones proteinuria, is usually noted within three to six weeks. Radiographic improvement in osteolytic bone lesions may take months, and resolution may be only partial.

As previously discussed, complete resolution of MM rarely occurs, and a good response is defined as a reduction in measured M component (i.e., immunoglobulin or Bence Jones proteins) to at least 50 per cent of pretreatment values.[87] For routine follow-up, quantification of serum immunoglobulin or urine Bence Jones protein is performed monthly until a good response is noted and then every two to three months thereafter. Repeat bone marrow aspiration is performed if warranted.

Therapy Directed at Complications. The long-term control of complications of MM, including hypercalcemia, HVS, bleeding diathesis, renal disease, immune suppression, and pathologic skeletal fractures, depends on controlling the tumor mass. Therapy directed more specifically at these complications may, however, be indicated in the short term.

If hypercalcemia is marked and significant clinical signs exist, standard therapies are indicated (see Chapter 97). Moderate hypercalcemia typically resolves within two to three days following initiation of melphalan and prednisone chemotherapy.

HVS is best treated in the short term by plasmapheresis. Whole blood is collected from the animal and centrifuged to separate plasma from packed cells. Packed red cells are resuspended in normal saline and reinfused into the animal. Bleeding diathesis usually resolves along with HVS; however, platelet-rich plasma transfusions may be necessary in the face of thrombocytopenia.

Renal impairment may necessitate aggressive fluid therapy. Careful attention to secondary urinary tract infections and appropriate antimicrobial therapy are indicated. Animals with MM can be thought of as immunologic cripples, and prophylactic antibiotic therapy in dogs with MM has been recommended[87]; in people, however, this approach has shown no benefit over diligent monitoring and aggressive antimicrobial management when indicated.[105] Antimicrobials with low nephrotoxic potential are preferred.

Pathologic fractures of weight-bearing long bones and vertebrae resulting in spinal cord compression may require immediate intervention in conjunction with systemic chemotherapy. Orthopedic stabilization of fractures should be undertaken and may be followed by external beam radiotherapy.

Rescue Therapy. At the time of relapse, or in cases initially resistant to melphalan, rescue therapy may be attempted. The author has had success with a combination of doxorubicin (30 mg/m^2 intravenously every 21 days), vincristine (0.7 mg/m^2 intravenously on days 8 and 15), and prednisone (1 mg/kg orally daily), given in 21-day cycles. Although most dogs initially respond to the rescue protocol, the duration of response tends to be short, lasting only a few months. High-dose cyclophosphamide (300 mg/m^2 intravenously every seven days) has also been used with limited success as a rescue agent. A durable rescue with liposome-encapsulated doxorubicin has been reported in a dog with MM.[106]

Prognosis

The prognosis for dogs with MM is good for initial control of tumor and return to a good quality of life. In a group of 60 dogs with MM, 43 per cent achieved a complete remission (i.e., serum immunoglobulins normalized), 49 per cent achieved a partial remission (i.e., immunoglobulins < 50 per cent of pretreatment values), and only 8 per cent did not respond to melphalan and prednisone chemotherapy.[79] Long-term survival is the norm, with a median of 540 days reported. Hypercalcemia, Bence Jones proteinuria, and extensive bony lysis are known negative prognostic indices in the dog. The long-term prognosis for dogs is poor, as recurrence is expected. Eventually, the tumor is no longer respon-

sive to available chemotherapeutics, and death follows from renal failure, sepsis, or euthanasia for intractable bone or spinal pain.

The prognosis for MM in the cat is not as favorable as in the dog.[82, 94, 98] Although most cats transiently respond to melphalan and prednisone or cyclophosphamide protocols, responses are not durable, and most cats succumb within two to three months. One long-term survivor has been reported in the cat.[97]

SOLITARY PLASMACYTOMA

Solitary collections of monoclonal plasmacytic tumors can originate in bone or soft tissues and are referred to as solitary osseous plasmacytoma (SOP) and extramedullary plasmacytoma (EMP), respectively. In the majority of cases, SOP eventually progresses to systemic MM.[107, 108] Cutaneous EMP, including oral cavity EMP, is typically a benign disorder in dogs. Conversely, the natural behavior of noncutaneous EMP appears to be much more aggressive. Gastrointestinal EMP has been reported to involve the esophagus, stomach, and small and large intestines.[109-114] Metastasis to associated lymph nodes is common in these cases, but bone marrow involvement and monoclonal gammopathies are less commonly encountered. One report exists of subcutaneous EMP in a cat with IgG gammopathy that progressed to lymph node disease and distant metastasis.[115]

Clinical Signs

Clinical signs associated with solitary plasmacytomas relate to the location of involvement; in those rare cases with high levels of M component, HVS may occur. SOP is usually associated with pain and lameness if the appendicular skeleton is affected or with neurologic signs if vertebral bodies are involved. Cutaneous EMP usually has a benign course with no related clinical signs. Gastrointestinal EMP, however, typically presents with relatively nonspecific signs that may suggest alimentary involvement. One case of ataxia and seizure activity in a dog with EMP secondary to tumor-associated hypoglycemia has been reported.[116]

Diagnosis

The diagnosis of SOP and EMP requires tissue biopsy. It is important to thoroughly stage such cases using bone marrow aspirate, serum electrophoresis, and skeletal survey radiographs to ensure that disease is confined to a local site before initiation of therapy. In the case of poorly differentiated solitary plasmacytic tumors, immunohistochemical studies directed at detecting immunoglobulin, light and heavy chains, and thioflavin T may be helpful in confirming a diagnosis.

Therapy

Animals with solitary forms of plasma cell tumors may be treated with local therapy in the absence of systemic chemotherapy, provided thorough clinical staging does not reveal systemic involvement. Effective local control has been achieved with surgical excision or external beam radiotherapy alone or in combination. Most dogs with SOP and EMP eventually develop systemic MM, and there is controversy among veterinary oncologists whether systemic chemotherapy should be initiated at the time of local therapy. Systemic

ONC

spread may not occur for many months to years after diagnosis in people, and studies in humans reveal no benefit from the initiation of systemic chemotherapy before documentation of systemic spread.[105] Long-term follow-up of animals with solitary plasmacytoma is indicated in order to recognize both recurrence of disease and systemic spread.

Prognosis

Dogs with cutaneous plasmacytomas are usually cured following surgical excision. Dogs with SOP or EMP of the alimentary tract treated by surgical excision in combination with systemic chemotherapy (once systemic disease is documented) enjoy long-term survival in the majority of cases.

HISTIOCYTIC DISORDERS

A number of histiocytic disorders have been reported in dogs and, more rarely, in cats.[117–130] These disease entities remain a fairly confusing area of veterinary medicine, as several different syndromes have been documented that may or may not be variations of the same disease or related to a similar cell of origin. Indeed, literally dozens of histiocytic syndromes have been described in people and continue to be a topic of debate among oncologists. Continued development and application of reliable histochemical and immunohistochemical markers are necessary to unravel the relationships among the various syndromes described. Cutaneous histiocytoma, a benign entity affecting primarily young dogs, is not discussed in this chapter (see Chapter 99).

The histiocytic diseases of dogs can generally be separated into four syndromes. In order of apparent clinical aggressiveness, they are periadnexal multinodular granulomatous dermatitis (PMNGD), cutaneous histiocytosis (CH), systemic histiocytosis (SH), and malignant histiocytosis (MH). All involve a predominance of proliferations of cells representing the histiocyte or monocyte-macrophage lineage. Microscopic criteria of malignancy are generally demonstrated only in MH, where atypical, pleomorphic mononuclear cells make up the tumor mass. Confirmation of a histiocytic origin can be attempted histochemically and immunohistochemically. Cells of the histiocyte or monocyte-macrophage lineage are generally positive for lysozyme, human alpha-1 antitrypsin, alpha-1 antichymotrypsin, mac387, cathepsin B, and CD18.[117, 118, 122, 124, 125, 129, 130] They should be negative for both T- and B-lymphocyte markers.

Periadnexal Multinodular Granulomatous Dermatitis. In PMNGD, multiple benign lesions are confined exclusively to cutaneous tissues.[117] They arise most commonly on the head and microscopically have a periadnexal pattern. There is no strong sex or breed predilection. PMNGD occurs at a median age of 6 years, but animals as young as 8 months have been reported. This is a benign entity and may be an autoimmune proliferation of cells. Attempts at finding an infectious etiology have been negative. Lesions have been reported to regress spontaneously in some cases; however, most are readily responsive to corticosteroid therapy. In some reports, continuous, intermittent low-dose corticosteroid therapy was required to prevent recrudescence of disease.

Cutaneous Histiocytosis. CH represents a benign, diffuse infiltration of histiocytes that grow rapidly into infiltrating nodules and plaques that occur in multiple locations on the skin. Microscopically, the histiocytes form sheetlike aggregations that, unlike PMNGD, do not have a periadnexal

association. They often occur in younger dogs. In the author's experience, golden retrievers and German shepherds are overrepresented. The clinical behavior is similar to that of PMNGD, in that CH is highly responsive to corticosteroid therapy. Long-term maintenance therapy may be required to prevent recurrence.

Systemic Histiocytosis. SH is a distinct proliferative disorder of histiocytes occurring predominantly in middle-aged Bernese Mountain Dogs but is not exclusive to that breed.[119, 121, 125] SH may represent a variant manifestation of MH. Like MH, there is strong evidence of a familial association for SH in Bernese Mountain Dogs, and inheritance is reportedly of a polygenic mode.[119] In Bernese Mountain Dogs, SH and MH together constitute approximately one quarter of all tumors reported in that breed. SH has also been observed in golden retrievers, rottweilers, and Doberman pinschers.

SH is classically described as a nodular disease confined to the cutaneous tissues, peripheral lymph nodes, and, to a lesser extent, ocular sites (e.g., conjunctiva and episcleral tissues). Cutaneous lesions more frequently involve the flank, muzzle, nasal planum, eyelid, and scrotum. Although most gross disease is confined to skin and lymph nodes, widespread microscopic infiltration of many organ systems has been discovered at necropsy. The histiocytes constituting SH do not exhibit the degree of malignant atypia found in MH. Although initial reports stated a significant male predilection (thereby suggesting sex-linked inheritance), larger, more recent studies have observed equal male-female representation or only a slight male overrepresentation.

The clinical course of SH is that of a waxing and waning chronic syndrome that is characterized by periods of relative lesion-free remission followed by recrudescence of lesions and symptoms. In addition to cutaneous lesions, clinical signs are typically nonspecific and include lethargy, inappetence, and weight loss. Cutaneous manifestations may include conjunctivitis with marked chemosis, uveitis, and occasionally glaucoma. Any Bernese Mountain Dog with ocular lesions should be considered a candidate for SH. The disease is rarely fatal in and of itself, but euthanasia is ultimately performed in the majority of cases owing to the chronic debilitating nature of the disease. SH is poorly responsive to therapy, including corticosteroid and/or cytotoxic chemotherapy. Survival durations have been reported from 2 to 48 months, with medians of approximately 9 to 10 months.[119, 121, 125]

Malignant Histiocytosis. MH is a rapidly progressive, widely metastatic proliferation of atypical malignant histiocytes.[118, 122, 124, 126] Classically, histiocytes present in MH have a high degree of microscopic atypia and appear as large, round, individualized cells with abundant cytoplasm. Multinucleated cells, erythrophagia, and, to a lesser extent, leukophagia are commonly observed. Once again, the Bernese Mountain Dog is overrepresented, and a polygenic mode of inheritance has been established, with autosomal and sex-linked inheritance all but ruled out.[119] Most larger studies do not corroborate the male overrepresentation reported in earlier studies. In addition to Bernese Mountain Dogs, golden retrievers, rottweilers, and Doberman pinschers have been reported to be at increased risk. The median age of affected dogs is 6 years.

Presenting signs are nonspecific and include lethargy, inappetence, weight loss, dyspnea, and neurologic signs. Anemia is often present and may be due to erythrophagia. Widespread dissemination of disease is revealed following radiographic and ultrasonographic evaluation.[120, 123] Lung parenchyma, mediastinal lymphadenopathy, and hepatosplenomegaly are common findings. Pulmonary changes can include complete consolidation, nodular opacities, or diffuse interstitial infiltrations (Fig. 98–11). Pleural effusion and osteolytic bone lesions less commonly accompany the disease. Diagnosis is confirmed by cytologic and histologic assessment of lesions. Bone marrow and CSF involvement is often confirmatory. Hyperferritinemia has been reported and may be associated with the erythrophagocytic nature of the tumor.

The clinical course of MH is rapid and uniformly fatal. At necropsy, lung, lymph node, liver, and spleen are most commonly affected; however, bone, CNS, heart, skin, and adrenal gland involvement is not unusual. Prognosis is grave, and response to combination chemotherapy (usually doxorubicin based) has been generally unrewarding, at best resulting in short-term palliation. The author has observed several responses, including a reported complete response, using single-agent Doxil (liposomal doxorubicin); however, most have been short-lived. Recently, a small group of dogs with MH responded to novel immunotherapy involving treatment with a human cytotoxic T-cell line, TALL-104. These results, though promising, are preliminary.[127]

To further complicate the classification of histiocytic disease in dogs, a recently reported, large compilation of cases describes a possible association between MH and malignant fibrous histiocytosis (MFH).[118] MFH has generally been described as a soft tissue sarcoma. However, in 263 dogs, three categories of histologic classification were described: MH (29 per cent), MFH (42 per cent), and tumors with microscopic characteristics of both (28 per cent). A comparison of breed and organ involvement in all cases was remarkably similar, suggesting either a similar undifferentiated precursor or the possibility that one or both of these diseases can differentiate toward the phenotype of the other. At the University of Wisconsin, we have observed a similar phenomenon involving primarily retriever breeds (e.g., golden, Labrador, and flat-coated). In these cases, wide dissemination of disease typical of MH is observed, with a uniformly fatal conclusion. Immunohistochemical analysis of some samples was consistent with MH criteria.

At least two cases of MH-like disease have been reported in cats.[128, 129] Both were aged cats (13 years) who presented with nonspecific signs typical of MH in the dog. Anemia was present in both cats. Pulmonary and splenic involvement was present in one, and splenic, hepatic, and bone marrow involvement in the other. In both cases, erythrophagocytosis by the neoplastic infiltration was observed. In one, immunohistochemical markers were consistent with a diagnosis of MH.

REFERENCES

1. Hayes HM, et al: Case-control study of canine malignant lymphoma: Positive association with dog owner's use of 2,4-dichlorophenoxyacetic acid herbicides. J Natl Cancer Inst 83:1226, 1991.
2. Zahm SH, Blair A: Pesticides and non-Hodgkin's lymphoma. Cancer Res (Suppl) 52:5485s, 1992.
3. Reif JS, et al: Residential exposure to magnetic fields and risk of canine lymphoma. Am J Epidemiol 141:352, 1995.
4. Teske E, et al: Clustering in canine malignant lymphoma. Vet Q 16:134, 1994.
5. Vail DM, et al: Assessment of potential doubling time (Tpot), argyrophilic nucleolar organizer regions (AgNOR), and proliferating cell nuclear antigen (PCNA) as predictors of therapy response in canine non-Hodgkin's lymphoma. Exp Hematol 24:807, 1996.
6. Keller ET, et al: Evaluation of prognostic factors and sequential combination chemotherapy for canine lymphoma. J Vet Intern Med 7:289, 1993.
7. Valerius KD, et al: Doxorubicin alone or in combination with asparaginase, followed by cyclophosphamide, vincristine, and prednisone for treatment of multicentric lymphoma in dogs: 121 cases (1987–1995). JAVMA 210:512, 1997.
8. Teske E, et al: Prognostic factors for treatment of malignant lymphoma in dogs. JAVMA 205:1722, 1994.
9. Greenlee PG, et al: Lymphomas in dogs. Cancer 66:480, 1990.
10. Fournel-Fleury C, et al: Cytohistological and immunological classification of canine malignant lymphomas: Comparison with human non-Hodgkin's lymphomas. J Comp Path 117:35, 1997.
11. Vail DM, et al: Feline lymphoma (145 cases): Proliferation indices, CD3 immunoreactivity and their association with prognosis in 90 cats receiving therapy. J Vet Intern Med 12:349, 1998.
12. Mauldin GE, et al: Chemotherapy in 132 cats with lymphoma: 1988–1994 (abstract). Proceedings of the 15th annual conference of the Veterinary Cancer Society. Tucson, AZ, 1995.
13. McEntee MF, et al: Granulated round cell tumor of cats. Vet Pathol 30:195, 1993.
14. Wellman ML, et al: Lymphoma involving large granular lymphocytes in cats: 11 cases (1982–1991). JAVMA 201:1265, 1992.
15. Drobatz KJ, et al: Globule leukocyte tumor in six cats. J Am Anim Hosp Assoc 29:391, 1993.
16. Rosenberg MP, et al: Prognostic factors in dogs with lymphoma and associated hypercalcemia. J Vet Intern Med 5:268, 1991.
17. Krohne SDG, et al: Ocular involvement in canine lymphoma, a retrospective study (abstract). Proceedings of the 7th annual conference of the Veterinary Cancer Society, Madison, WI, 1987.
18. Madewell BR: Hematological and bone marrow cytological abnormalities in 75 dogs with malignant lymphoma. J Am Anim Hosp Assoc 22:235, 1986.
19. Starrak GS, et al: Correlation between thoracic radiographic changes and remission/survival duration in 270 dogs with lymphosarcoma. Vet Radiol Ultrasound 38:411, 1997.
20. Blackwood L, et al: Radiographic abnormalities in canine multicentric lymphoma: A review of 84 cases. J Small Anim Pract 38:62, 1997.
21. Moore FM, et al: Distinctive peripheral lymph node hyperplasia of young cats. Vet Pathol 23:386, 1986.
22. Mooney SC, et al: Generalized lymphadenopathy resembling lymphoma in cats: Six cases (1972–1976) JAVMA 190:897, 1987.
23. Lucke VM, et al: Plexiform vascularization of lymph nodes: An unusual but distinctive lymphadenopathy in cats. J Comp Pathol 97:113, 1987.
24. Kirkpatrick CE, et al: Argyrophilic, intracellular bacteria in some cats with idiopathic peripheral lymphadenopathy. J Comp Pathol 101:345, 1989.
25. Fournel-Fleury C, et al: Growth fractions in canine non-Hodgkin's lymphoma as determined in situ by the expression of the Ki-67 antigen. J Comp Pathol 117:61, 1997.
26. Vail DM, et al: Application of rapid CD3 immunophenotype analysis and argyrophilic nucleolar organizer region (AgNOR) frequency to fine needle aspirate specimens from dogs with lymphoma. Vet Clin Pathol 26:66, 1997.
27. Teske E, et al: DNA ploidy and cell kinetic characteristics in canine non-Hodgkin's lymphoma. Exp Hematol 21:579, 1993.
28. Moore AS, et al: The expression of P-glycoprotein in canine lymphoma and its association with multidrug resistance. Cancer Invest 13:475, 1995.
29. Bergman PJ, et al: Monoclonal antibody C219 immunohistochemistry against P-glycoprotein: Sequential analysis and predictive ability in dogs with lymphoma. J Vet Intern Med 10:354, 1996.
30. Lee JJ, et al: P-glycoprotein expression in canine lymphoma. Cancer 77:1892, 1996.
31. Gamblin RM, et al: Overexpression of p53 tumor suppressor protein in spontaneously arising neoplasms of dogs. Am J Vet Res 58:857, 1997.
32. Lane SB, et al: Feline spinal lymphosarcoma: A retrospective evaluation of 23 cats. J Vet Intern Med 8:99, 1994.
33. Spodnick GJ, et al: Spinal lymphoma in cats: 21 cases (1976–1989). JAVMA 200:373, 1992.

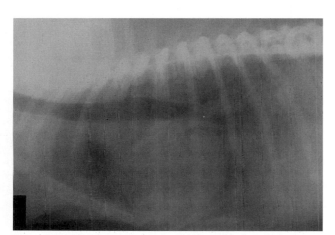

Figure 98–11. A lateral thoracic radiographic projection of a Bernese Mountain Dog with malignant histiocytosis. Multiple poorly defined soft tissue opacity nodules are seen scattered throughout the pulmonary fields. A small amount of free pleural effusion is also noted.

34. Vail DM: Recent advances in chemotherapy for lymphoma of dogs and cats. Comp Contin Educ Pract Vet 15:1031, 1993.
35. Carter RF, et al: Chemotherapy of canine lymphoma with histopathological correlation: Doxorubicin alone compared to COP as first treatment regimen. J Am Anim Hosp Assoc 23:587, 1987.
36. Postorino NC, et al: Single agent therapy with adriamycin for canine lymphosarcoma. J Am Anim Hosp Assoc 25:221, 1989.
37. Price GS, et al: Efficacy and toxicity of doxorubicin/cyclophosphamide maintenance therapy in dogs with multicentric lymphosarcoma. J Vet Intern Med 5:259, 1991.
38. Moore AS, et al: A comparison of doxorubicin and COP maintenance of remission in cats with lymphoma. J Vet Intern Med 10:372, 1996.
39. Mauldin GE, et al: MOPP chemotherapy as rescue for cats with refractory lymphoma (abstract). Proceedings of the annual conference of the American College of Veterinary Radiology and Veterinary Cancer Society, Chicago, IL, 1997.
40. Couto CG, et al: Central nervous system lymphosarcoma in the dog. JAVMA 184:809, 1984.
41. Beale K, Bolon B: Canine cutaneous lymphosarcoma: Epitheliotropic and non-epitheliotropic, a retrospective study. In Ihrke PJ, Mason IS, White SD (eds): Advances in Veterinary Dermatology, Vol 2. Oxford, Pergamon Press, 1993, p 273.
42. White SD, et al: Use of isotretinoin and etretinate for the treatment of benign cutaneous neoplasia and cutaneous lymphoma in dogs. JAVMA 202:387, 1993.
43. Vail DM, et al: Preclinical trial of doxorubicin entrapped in sterically stabilized liposomes in dogs with spontaneously arising malignant tumors. Cancer Chemother Pharmacol 39:410, 1997.
44. MacEwen EG, et al: Evaluation of some prognostic factors for advanced multicentric lymphosarcoma in the dog: 147 cases (1978–1981). JAVMA 190:564, 1987.
45. Mooney SC, et al: Treatment and prognostic factors in lymphoma in cats: 103 cases (1977–1981). JAVMA 194:696, 1989.
46. Matus RE, et al: Acute lymphoblastic leukemia in the dog: A review of 30 cases. JAVMA 183:859, 1983.
47. Leifer CE, Matus RE: Chronic lymphocytic leukemia in the dog: 22 cases (1974–1984). JAVMA 189:214, 1986.
48. Couto CG: Clinicopathologic aspects of acute leukemias in the dog. JAVMA 186:681, 1985.
49. Grindem CB, et al: Morphological classification and clinical and pathological characteristics of spontaneous leukemia in 10 cats. J Am Anim Hosp Assoc 21:227, 1985.
50. Grindem CB, et al: Morphological classification and clinical and pathological characteristics of spontaneous leukemia in 17 dogs. J Am Anim Hosp Assoc 21:219, 1985.
51. Helfand SC: Low-dose cytosine arabinoside–induced remission of lymphoblastic leukemia in a cat. JAVMA 191:707, 1987.
52. Jain NC, et al: Clinical-pathological findings and cytochemical characterization of myelomonocytic leukemia in 5 dogs. J Comp Pathol 91:17, 1981.
53. Raskin RE, Krehbiel JF: Myelodysplastic changes in a cat with myelomonocytic leukemia. JAVMA 187:171, 1985.
54. Graves TK, et al: A potentially misleading presentation and course of acute myelomonocytic leukemia in a dog. J Am Anim Hosp Assoc 33:37, 1997.
55. Latimer KS, Dykstra MJ: Acute monocytic leukemia in a dog. JAVMA 184:852, 1984.
56. Cain R, et al: Platelet dysplasia associated with megakaryoblastic leukemia in a dog. JAVMA 188:529, 1986.
57. Harvey JW, et al: Myeloproliferative disease with megakaryocytic predominance in a dog with occult dirofilariasis. Vet Clin Pathol 11:5, 1982.
58. Messick J, et al: Identification and characterization of megakaryoblasts in acute megakaryoblastic leukemia in a dog. Vet Pathol 27:212, 1990.
59. Hamilton TA: Cytosine arabinoside chemotherapy for acute megakaryocytic leukemia in a cat. JAVMA 199:359, 1991.
60. Colbatzky F, Hermanns W: Acute megakaryoblastic leukemia in one cat and two dogs. Vet Pathol 30:186, 1993.
61. Pucheu-Haston CM, et al: Megakaryoblastic leukemia in a dog. JAVMA 207:194, 1995.
62. Miyamoto T, et al: A case of megakaryoblastic leukemia in a dog. J Vet Med Sci 58:177, 1996.
63. Liu S, Carb AV: Erythroblastic leukemia in a dog. JAVMA 152:1511, 1968.
64. Thomsen MK, et al: Enhanced granulocyte function in a case of chronic granulocytic leukemia in a dog. Vet Immunol Immunopathol 28:143, 1991.
65. Leifer CE, et al: Chronic myelogenous leukemia in the dog. JAVMA 183:686, 1983.
66. Pollet L, et al: Blastic crisis in chronic myelogenous leukemia in a dog. J Small Anim Pract 19:469, 1978.
67. Hammer AS, et al: Essential thrombocythemia in a cat. J Vet Intern Med 4:87, 1990.
68. Smith M, Turrel JM: Radiophosphorus (^{32}P) treatment of bone marrow disorders in dogs: 11 cases (1970–1987). JAVMA 194:98, 1989.
69. Mears EA, et al: Basophilic leukemia in a dog. J Vet Intern Med 11:92, 1997.
70. MacEwen EG, et al: Treatment of basophilic leukemia in a dog. JAVMA 166:376, 1975.
71. Swenson CL, et al: Eosinophilic leukemia in a cat with naturally acquired feline leukemia virus infection. J Am Anim Hosp Assoc 29:497, 1993.
72. Lewis MG, et al: Retroviral-associated eosinophilic leukemia in the cat. Am J Vet Res 46:1066, 1985.
73. Peterson ME, Randolph JF: Diagnosis of canine primary polycythemia and management with hydroxyurea. JAVMA 180:415, 1982.
74. Evans LM, Caylor KB: Polycythemia vera in a cat and management with hydroxyurea. J Am Anim Hosp Assoc 31:434, 1995.
75. Meyer HP, et al: Polycythaemia vera in a dog treated by repeated phlebotomies. Vet Q 14:108, 1993.
76. Holden AR: Polycythemia vera in a dog. Vet Rec 120:473, 1987.
77. Watson ADJ, Yeats JA: Primary polycythaemia in a dog. Aust Vet J 61:61, 1984.
78. Jain NC: Cytochemistry of normal and leukemic leukocytes. In Schalm's Veterinary Hematology, 4th ed. Philadelphia, Lea & Febiger, 1986, p 909.
79. Matus RE: Prognostic factors for multiple myeloma in the dog. JAVMA 188:1288, 1986.
80. Liu S-K, et al: Primary and secondary bone tumors in the dog. J Small Anim Pract 18:313, 1977.
81. Engle GC, Brodey RS: A retrospective study of 395 feline neoplasms. J Am Anim Hosp Assoc 5:21, 1969.
82. Carpenter JL, et al: Tumors and tumor like lesions. In Holzworth J (ed): Diseases of the Cat. Medicine and Surgery, Philadelphia, WB Saunders, 1987, p 406.
83. Larsen AE, Carpenter JL: Hepatic plasmacytoma and biclonal gammopathy in a cat. JAVMA 205:708, 1994.
84. Potter M, et al: Induction of plasmacytomas with silicone gel in genetically susceptible strains of mice. J Natl Cancer Inst 86:1058, 1994.
85. Imahori S, Moore GE: Multiple myeloma and prolonged stimulation of RES. N Y State J Med 72:1625, 1972.
86. Porter DD: The development of myeloma-like condition in mink with Aleutian disease. Blood 25:736, 1967.
87. MacEwen EG, Hurvitz AI: Diagnosis and management of monoclonal gammopathies. Vet Clin North Am Small Anim Pract 7:119, 1977.
88. Shull RM, et al: Serum hyperviscosity syndrome associated with IgA multiple myeloma in two dogs. J Am Anim Hosp Assoc 14:58, 1978.
89. Hurvitz AI, et al: Macroglobulinemia with hyperviscosity syndrome in a dog. JAVMA 157:455, 1970.
90. Center SA, Smith JF: Ocular lesions in a dog with hyperviscosity secondary to an IgA myeloma. JAVMA 181:811, 1982.
91. Kirschner SE, et al: Blindness in a dog with IgA-forming myeloma. JAVMA 193:349, 1988.
92. Hawkins EC, et al: Immunoglobulin A myeloma in a cat with pleural effusion and serum hyperviscosity. JAVMA 188:876, 1986.
93. Williams DA, Goldschmidt MH: Hyperviscosity syndrome with IgM monoclonal gammopathy and hepatic plasmacytoid lymphosarcoma in a cat. J Small Anim Pract 23:311, 1982.
94. Forrester SD, et al: Serum hyperviscosity syndrome associated with multiple myeloma in two cats. JAVMA 200:79, 1992.
95. Hribernik TN, et al: Serum hyperviscosity syndrome associated with IgG myeloma in a cat. JAVMA 181:169, 1982.
96. Rosol TJ, et al: Parathyroid hormone (PTH)–related protein, PTH, and 1,25-dihydroxyvitamin D in dogs with cancer associated hypercalcemia. Endocrinology 131:1157, 1992.
97. Sheafor SE, et al: Hypercalcemia in two cats with multiple myeloma. J Am Anim Hosp Assoc 32:503, 1996.
98. Drazner FH: Multiple myeloma in the cat. Comp Contin Educ Pract Vet 4:206, 1982.
99. Mitcham SA, et al: Plasma cell sarcoma in a cat. Can Vet J 26:98, 1985.
100. Jacobs RM, Couto CG, Wellman ML: Biclonal gammopathy in a dog with myeloma and cutaneous lymphoma. Vet Pathol 23:211, 1986.
101. Braund KG, et al: Neurologic complications of IgA multiple myeloma associated with cryoglobulinemia in a dog. JAVMA 174:1321, 1979.
102. Hurvitz AI, et al: Monoclonal cryoglobulinemia with macroglobulinemia in a dog. JAVMA 170:511, 1977.
103. Hoenig M, O'Brien JA: A benign hypergammaglobulinemia mimicking plasma cell myeloma. J Am Anim Hosp Assoc 24:688, 1988.
104. Dewhirst MW, et al: Idiopathic monoclonal (IgA) gammopathy in a dog. JAVMA 170:1313, 1977.
105. Anderson K: Plasma cell tumors. In Holland JF, Frei E, Bast RC, et al (eds): Cancer Medicine, 3rd ed. Philadelphia, Lea & Febiger, 1993, p 2075.
106. Kisseberth WC, et al: Response to liposome-encapsulated doxorubicin (TLC D-99) in a dog with myeloma. J Vet Intern Med 9:425, 1995.
107. MacEwen EG, et al: Nonsecretory multiple myeloma in two dogs. JAVMA 184:1283, 1984.
108. Meis JM, et al: Solitary plasmacytomas of bone and extramedullary plasmacytomas. Cancer 59:1475, 1987.
109. Hamilton TA, Carpenter JL: Esophageal plasmacytoma in a dog. JAVMA 204:1210, 1994.
110. MacEwen EG, et al: Extramedullary plasmacytoma of the gastrointestinal tract in two dogs. JAVMA 184:1396, 1984.
111. Brunnert SR, et al: Gastric extramedullary plasmacytoma in a dog. JAVMA 200:1501 1992.
112. Jackson MW, et al: Primary IgG secreting plasma cell tumor in the gastrointestinal tract of a dog. JAVMA 204:404, 1994.
113. Lester SJ, Mesfin GM: A solitary plasmacytoma in a dog with progression to a disseminated myeloma. Can Vet J 21:284, 1980.
114. Trevor PB, et al: Metastatic extramedullary plasmacytoma of the colon and rectum in a dog. JAVMA 203:406, 1993.
115. Carothers MA, et al: Extramedullary plasmacytoma and immunoglobulin-associated amyloidosis in a cat. JAVMA 195:1593, 1989.
116. DiBartola SP: Hypoglycemia and polyclonal gammopathy in a dog with plasma cell dyscrasia. JAVMA 180:1345, 1982.

117. Carpenter JL, et al: Idiopathic periadnexal multinodular granulomatous dermatitis in twenty-two dogs. Vet Pathol 24:5, 1987.
118. Kerlin RL, Hendrick MJ: Malignant fibrous histiocytoma and malignant histiocytosis in the dog—convergent or divergent phenotypic differentiation? Vet Pathol 33:713, 1996.
119. Padgett GA, et al: Inheritance of histiocytosis in Bernese Mountain Dogs. J Small Anim Pract 36:93, 1995.
120. Schmidt ML et al: Clinical and radiographic manifestations of canine malignant histiocytosis. Vet Q 14:117, 1993.
121. Paterson S, et al: Systemic histiocytosis in the Bernese Mountain Dog. J Small Anim Pract 36:233, 1995.
122. Hayden DW, et al: Disseminated malignant histiocytosis in a golden retriever: Clinicopathologic, ultrastructural, and immunohistochemical findings. Vet Pathol 30:256, 1993.
123. Shaiker LC, et al: Radiographic findings in canine malignant histiocytosis. Vet Radiol 32:237, 1991.
124. Rosin A, et al: Malignant histiocytosis in Bernese Mountain Dogs. JAVMA 188:1041, 1986.
125. Moore PF: Systemic histiocytosis of Bernese Mountain Dogs. Vet Pathol 21:554, 1984.
126. Wellman ML, et al: Malignant histiocytosis in four dogs. JAVMA 187:919, 1985.
127. Visonneau S, et al: Successful treatment of canine malignant histiocytosis with the human major histocompatibility complex nonrestricted cytotoxic T-cell line TALL-104. Clin Cancer Res 3:1789, 1997.
128. Court EA, et al: Malignant histiocytosis in a cat. JAVMA 203:1300, 1993.
129. Walton RM, et al: Malignant histiocytosis in a domestic cat: Cytomorphologic and immunohistochemical features. Vet Clin Pathol 26:56, 1997.
130. Moore PF: Utilization of cytoplasmic lysozyme immunoreactivity as a histiocytic marker in canine histiocytic disorders. Vet Pathol 23:757, 1986.

ONC

CHAPTER 99

TUMORS OF THE SKIN

Susan A. Kraegel and Bruce R. Madewell

ANATOMY

Skin is composed of two layers. The outer layer or epidermis contains layers of keratinocytes with melanocytes, Langerhans cells, and Merkel cells. The inner layer or dermis contains connective tissue cells (fibroblasts), tissue hematopoietic cells (mast cells, histiocytes), epidermal appendages (hair follicles, sweat glands, sebaceous glands), nerves, blood vessels, and lymph vessels. Other cells found in the skin include granulocytes, lymphocytes, monocytes, and plasma cells. Primary tumors can arise from any cell normally found in the skin (Table 99–1).

GENERAL APPROACH TO SKIN TUMORS

HISTORY AND PHYSICAL EXAMINATION

Papules, nodules, or masses in the skin are common reasons for owners to seek veterinary care. Masses may be epidermal, dermal, or hypodermal in origin or span more than one layer. All masses should be carefully palpated, measured, and recorded. The record should include the location, size, appearance (alopecia, color, ulceration), borders (circumscribed, infiltrative), consistency (firm, soft, mixed), and attachments (movable, fixed). Lymph nodes draining the lesion should be assessed for changes in texture, size, and mobility.

BIOPSY

Skin masses should be biopsied prior to therapy to allow the clinician to select a rational and definitive treatment. For many skin masses, fine-needle aspiration provides a diagnosis. When cytology is nondiagnostic, formal biopsy is performed for all but the smallest of masses. Suboptimal surgery for a mass that is malignant and that is not diagnosed preoperatively may subject an animal to needless surgery or preclude the chance of later surgical cure. Abnormal lymph nodes should also be aspirated for cytologic interpretation.

Fine-Needle Aspiration (FNA). FNA for cytology requires only a 27- to 22-gauge needle, a syringe, and glass slides. Smaller needles (27 or 25 gauge) are less painful and decrease blood contamination of specimens while still providing a diagnostic sample. The procedure is as follows: immobilize the lesion with one hand, advance the needle

TABLE 99–1. COMMON SKIN TUMORS

Epithelial Tumors

Epidermal tumors
  Papilloma
  Squamous cell carcinoma
  Basal cell tumors
  Intracutaneous cornifying epithelioma
Follicular tumors
  Trichoepithelioma
  Pilomatricoma
Sebaceous gland tumors
Sweat gland tumors
Perianal gland tumors (see Chapter 139)
Anal sac apocrine gland tumors (Chapters 97, 149)
Ceruminous gland tumors

Spindle Cell Tumors

Soft tissue sarcoma (Chapter 100)

Round Cell Tumors

Canine cutaneous histiocytoma
Mast cell tumor
Plasmacytoma
Lymphoma
Transmissible venereal tumor (see Chapter 163)

Neuroendocrine Tumors

Melanocytic tumors

into the mass, apply suction with the syringe, move the needle back and forth through the mass in several directions while maintaining constant suction, release the suction, withdraw the needle, detach the needle from the syringe, fill the syringe with air, and reattach the syringe to the needle to expel the contents of the needle onto the slide.

Needle Biopsy. A variety of manual and automated biopsy needles yielding 12- to 20-gauge, 1- to 2-cm specimens can be used to biopsy the center of any mass that can be visualized, palpated, or imaged. These instruments require only a local anesthetic and a 2-mm stab incision to pass the needle through the skin.

Shave Biopsy. For superficial, exophytic lesions, a shave biopsy may be adequate. The blade is held parallel to the surface of the mass, and a small piece of tissue is removed by slicing horizontally.

Punch Biopsy. For diffuse, superficial lesions, 2- to 8-mm punch biopsy specimens are taken at several sites.

Incisional Biopsy. Incisional biopsy is useful when neither cytology nor needle biopsy yields diagnostic information. The incision should be carefully positioned so that uninvolved tissue planes are not entered and contaminated with tumor cells. The incision should be logically oriented so that the entire biopsy tract will be easily included in any subsequent excision. Using sterile technique, a wedge of tissue is taken.

Excisional Biopsy. For small, freely movable dermal masses that are not diagnosed cytologically, excisional biopsy provides both a diagnostic and therapeutic procedure. An elliptical incision, parallel to the stress lines of the body, should be made around the entire mass.

HISTOPATHOLOGY

Entire surgical specimens should be submitted for histopathologic evaluation. Even when the diagnosis is known prior to surgery, histopathology of the final specimen may provide additional information useful for treatment planning. Besides providing a histologic diagnosis, the pathologist can report the degree of differentiation or tumor grade. For undifferentiated tumors, immunohistochemistry or special stains assist in determining histogenesis. Pathologists should also report the nearest approach of the tumor to the surgical margin and the completeness of excision. Applying India ink to the cut surfaces of a tumor prior to fixation in formalin is a simple way to ensure that the pathologist can distinguish surgical margins from preparation artifacts. There are possibilities for error at all levels of the biopsy process; each report must be evaluated in light of all clinical information.

SQUAMOUS CELL CARCINOMA (SCC)

EPIDEMIOLOGY AND PATHOGENESIS

SCC can affect any cutaneous site in the dog or cat. The risk for cutaneous SCC increases with age and peaks at about 10 to 11 years of age. A syndrome of multifocal SCC in situ has been reported for cats and in one dog and is often referred to by the human eponym Bowen's disease.

Sunlight. SCC that occurs in sparsely haired, unpigmented, or lightly pigmented sites is believed to be induced by sunlight. In white-faced cats, the most common locations are unpigmented portions of the pinnae, nasal plane, and eyelids. In lightly pigmented or white dogs, sites exposed by sunbathing in dorsal recumbency are the most common—abdominal and inguinal skin.

Ultraviolet irradiation (UVR) in sunlight acts as a carcinogen in the formation of skin cancer. UVR induces photochemical reactions that activate inflammatory pathways, alter the immune system, and directly damage DNA. This combination of events results in improper repair of DNA photoproducts, permanent mutations in regulatory genes, and clonal expansion of premalignant cells. Histologically, lesions progress from preneoplastic epidermal hyperplasia with dysplasia to actinic keratosis (carcinoma in situ) to neoplastic SCC.

UVR damage is cumulative and dose-dependent. It is determined by hair thickness, skin color, length of sunlight exposure, geographic location, and environment. Higher cumulative lifetime doses can be expected in animals that are older, sparsely haired or white, and kept outdoors in sunny, high-altitude, or Southern locations.

Papillomavirus. The cause of SCC in non–sun-exposed sites is undetermined, but papillomavirus may be one initiating factor. SCC has developed at canine oral papillomavirus vaccination sites, and positive immunohistochemical staining for papillomavirus occurs in or near some canine SCC and feline Bowen's lesions.[1, 2]

BIOLOGIC BEHAVIOR

SCCs infiltrate locally. The metastatic route is first to regional lymph nodes and later to lungs. The biologic behavior of sunlight-associated carcinoma is usually less aggressive than non–sunlight-associated carcinoma. In one study of 61 cats with SCC of the face, only one cat developed regional lymph node involvement.[3] In the dog, squamous cell carcinoma of the nasal plane should not be considered a solar-induced tumor. It is locally aggressive and occurs in both pigmented and unpigmented dogs. Because Bowen's disease is confined to the epithelium, it is considered a premalignant dermatosis. Invasion of some lesions, however, is reported.

HISTORY AND PHYSICAL EXAMINATION

General. A mass, thickening, or ulcer of the skin is the most frequent presenting complaint. Enlarged lymph nodes may be secondary to inflammation or metastasis.

Sunlight-Associated. For sunlight-associated carcinomas, signs may progress slowly or wax and wane over months. Small lesions are frequently mistaken by owners for nonhealing wounds. Preneoplastic lesions appear as thickened, erythematous regions of surface scaling with small crusts and scabs. SCC may be proliferative or ulcerative; ulcerative lesions often have a rim of erythematous, thickened skin surrounding the erosion or ulcer.

Nasal Plane of the Dog. Clinical signs include epistaxis or sneezing, and ulceration or swelling of the nasal plane.

Bowen's Disease. In cats, lesions are found in haired, pigmented skin as multifocal or solitary, nodular plaques.

DIAGNOSIS AND STAGING

Biopsy is the diagnostic procedure. Enlarged lymph nodes should be aspirated to distinguish reactive from metastatic lesions. Thoracic radiography to search for metastases is recommended for animals with non–sunlight-associated SCC. In animals with sunlight-induced SCC and normal lymph nodes, thoracic radiographs are not required. CT or MRI scan results are used to delineate margins of large infiltrative lesions to assist in treatment planning.

THERAPY

Overview. Preneoplastic and small superficial lesions can be effectively treated with surgery, radiotherapy, hyperthermia, cryosurgery, photodynamic therapy, or topical chemotherapy. For larger lesions, surgery is most effective. For deep, invasive lesions that are not surgically accessible, radiation teletherapy or intralesional chemotherapy may provide local tumor control. An important adjunct for sunlight-associated tumors is the elimination of further UVR exposure by keeping the animal out of direct sunlight.

Surgery. Surgical excision is a rapid and effective therapy for accessible SCC. One advantage of surgery is that the surgical margins can be examined microscopically to ensure complete excision. For SCC of the pinna, eyelid, and small nasal plane lesions, total pinnectomy, eyelid resection, or nasal plane amputation may provide the longest survival times with the least morbidity. In cats with nasal plane resection and/or pinnectomy, the median survival in one study was 673 days.[3] For dogs with nasal plane SCC, nasal plane resection or combined nasal plane and premaxilla resection is the only therapy documented to result in survival times greater than 6 months.[4, 5]

Chemotherapy. Chemotherapy for SCC may be administered topically, intralesionally, or systemically. Topical 5-fluorouracil (5 per cent) may control preneoplastic lesions in some dogs. 5-Fluorouracil is contraindicated in cats, owing to neurotoxicity. For control of nonresectable SCC, intratumoral injection of an antineoplastic drug in a slow-release formulation gives high sustained local drug levels. Injection of collagen gel with cisplatin or 5-fluorouracil induced complete remissions in 50 per cent of dogs with SCC.[6] In cats with SCC of the nasal plane, carboplatin in sterile sesame oil yielded a 73 per cent complete response rate.[7] Systemic chemotherapy is used to provide palliation for dogs and cats with widespread or metastatic lesions. The synthetic retinoid etretinate at 1 mg/kg twice a day in dogs or 10 mg/cat/day causes regression of some preneoplastic lesions.[8] Piroxicam, cisplatin, mitoxantrone, and bleomycin may have activity in SCC.

Radiotherapy. Radiotherapy is effective for solar-induced SCC and may also have activity in non–solar-associated SCC. Dogs with SCC of the nasal plane, however, show little, if any, response to radiation therapy. For shallow lesions, strontium-90 plesiotherapy gives a high dose of radiation in one treatment. For 25 cats with superficial nasal plane tumors treated with strontium, the median disease-free interval was 34 months.[9] For larger lesions, teletherapy with either orthovoltage or megavoltage is given over 3 to 4 weeks. In one study of 90 cats irradiated for SCC of the nasal plane, tumor control was 60 per cent at 1 year and 10 per cent at 5 years; the cure rate for cats with noninvasive tumors less than 2 cm in diameter was estimated to be 56 per cent.[10] In another study, the median survival for 11 cats treated with radiotherapy was 361 days.[3]

Photodynamic Therapy (PDT). With PDT, a photosensitizing drug that preferentially localizes in tumor cells is given either systemically or locally and activated with laser light. Although PDT is effective for cats with small, mini-

mally invasive carcinomas of the face, only a few facilities have lasers available for clinical veterinary use.

CANINE DIGITAL TUMORS

Epidemiology and Pathogenesis. SCC and malignant melanoma are the first and second most common digital tumors in the dog, respectively. There appears to be an increased risk for digital SCC in large-breed dogs with black coats.

Biologic Behavior. Subungual carcinomas are locally invasive, with radiographic evidence of bone lysis and/or periosteal new bone in 80 per cent of affected dogs.[11,12] Radiographic changes can also accompany non-neoplastic, inflammatory lesions but are rarely observed with digital melanoma. The metastatic rate for subungual SCC is low.[11] For digital melanomas, over one half of dogs ultimately develop pulmonary metastasis.[12]

History and Physical Examination. Dogs with digital tumors frequently have a swollen, painful digit, resembling an infection. A mass may not be evident. Nail deformity or loss and signs of chronic inflammation are common.

Treatment and Prognosis. Wide amputation of the digit is recommended for all dogs with digital tumors and no evidence of metastasis. Complete excision may require disarticulation at the metacarpophalangeal or metatarsophalangeal level or higher. Following excision, the median survival for dogs with subungual SCC is greater than 2 years versus only 1 year for melanoma.[12]

OTHER EPITHELIAL SKIN NEOPLASMS

Papilloma. Papillomas are benign tumors sometimes associated with canine papillomavirus infection.[1] They are solitary or multicentric papules usually with a verrucous appearance. Many will spontaneously regress.[13] Surgical excision is curative.

Intracutaneous Cornifying Epithelioma (Keratoacanthoma). This canine tumor appears as a dermal or subcutaneous mass with a dilated pore, often containing keratin, opening to the skin surface. Solitary masses are cured with excision. Certain breeds, particularly the Norwegian elkhound, are predisposed to the development of multiple tumors. The retinoid etretinate (1 mg/kg twice a day) may prevent the development of new tumors.[8]

Basal Cell Tumor. Basal cell tumors arise from uncommitted basal reserve cells of the epidermis and/or adnexa. In the dog the majority occur on the head and neck, whereas in the cat there is no site predilection. Hyperpigmentation can cause these tumors to resemble melanomas. Surgical excision is curative.

Follicular Tumors. The common hair follicular tumors, pilomatrixoma (or pilomatricoma) and trichoepithelioma, are benign; surgical excision is curative.

Sebaceous Tumors. Tumors of the sebaceous glands occur commonly in dogs, most often on the head, and rarely in cats. Most tumors are benign, and the therapy for both adenomas and adenocarcinomas is surgical excision.

Sweat Gland Tumors. Apocrine adenomas and adenocarcinomas are uncommon tumors in the dog and cat; they appear as solid, circumscribed, raised masses. Some carcinomas resemble an ulcerative, inflammatory dermatitis rather than a tumor. For adenomas and nodular adenocarcinomas, the prognosis is good to excellent with complete surgical excision.[14] Local recurrence or regional and distant metastases may complicate management of high-grade or inflammatory adenocarcinomas.

MELANOMAS

Dermal melanomas are usually solitary, pigmented tumors. The head is the most common location, the ear predominating in the cat and the eyelid in the dog. In the cat, ear tumors are benign whereas eyelid tumors are malignant.[15] In the dog, most tumors, including those of the eyelid, are benign. In both species, melanomas of the lip are often malignant. Although histology aids in differentiating benign from malignant melanoma, criteria are not absolute. In one study of cats, 9 per cent of the original diagnoses did not correlate with the clinical behavior of the tumor.[15] For benign tumors, surgical excision is curative. Malignant tumors may be locally invasive and have the potential to metastasize to lymph nodes, lungs, and distant sites. Wide surgical excision of the primary tumor may improve quality of life or survival time, but the prognosis is guarded. Effective chemotherapy for metastases has not been described.

MAST CELL TUMORS

CANINE MAST CELL TUMOR

Epidemiology and Pathogenesis

Dogs have a uniquely high risk for cutaneous mast cell tumors. The median age is 8 to 10 years, but tumors have been reported in dogs 0.3 to 16 years of age.[16] Breeds at high risk have historically included dogs of bulldog ancestry, but others, including Labrador retrievers, Chinese Shar Peis, and Bernese Mountain Dogs, may also have an increased risk.

The propensity for dogs to develop mast cell tumors is unexplained and is most likely multifactorial. Breed predilections imply underlying genetic determinants. Antigenic stimulation of mast cell proliferation leading to neoplasia has also been hypothesized as a contributing factor. Alteration of the c-*kit* receptor, a modulator of mast cell development and function, in about one half of canine mast cell tumors suggests that derangement of normal regulation may be one step in carcinogenesis.[17]

Biologic Behavior

Mast cells are connective tissue hematopoietic cells derived from bone marrow progenitor cells. Their major role is to mediate the inflammatory response to foreign antigens. When activated, mast cells release histamine, heparin, proteases, and other mediators from preformed cytoplasmic granules. Mast cells also synthesize and release lipid mediators and cytokines.

Because they can release biologically active mediators, mast cell tumors produce a wide range of local and systemic effects. Local release of proteases, histamine, and heparin along with cytokine recruitment of other inflammatory cells manifests clinically as erythema, pruritus, swelling, ulceration, delayed healing, and hemorrhage. Increased plasma histamine concentrations occur in dogs with mast cell tumors regardless of tumor stage, grade, or size.[18] Hyperacidity secondary to parietal cell H_2 receptor stimulation is indicated by decreased gastrin levels and may cause occult or overt gastrointestinal ulceration. Clinically significant H_1 stimulation resulting in hypotension and shock may occur following manipulation or treatment of large tumors.

The clinical behavior of canine mast cell tumors is variable and unpredictable, but all are potentially malignant. Tumors can arise in the dermis and/or subcutis. They may be solitary or multiple; multiple tumors may arise de novo or represent metastatic spread. Tumors often have a prolonged, indolent course but can also grow rapidly with tissue invasion from the onset. The potential for regional and widespread systemic metastasis always exists. It is rare, however, to have clinically detectable systemic mast cell tumor without local lymph node involvement. Besides regional lymph nodes, other sites of metastasis include the spleen, liver, and bone marrow.

History and Physical Examination

Dogs with mast cell tumors usually have a skin mass, present from weeks to years. Owners may describe the mass as pruritic or as waxing and waning in size. The clinical appearance is variable. Cutaneous mast cell tumors are typically firm, circumscribed, raised, erythematous, dermal masses with alopecia or ulceration. Other clinical features, however, are relatively common; the tumor may be poorly demarcated, infiltrative, subcutaneous, soft to gelatinous in consistency, attached to the dermis by a stalk, or have a dimpled appearance. Mast cell tumors may swell with manipulation. Soft, subcutaneous tumors may be impossible to differentiate from hemangiopericytomas or lipomas on physical palpation. Involved regional lymph nodes may feel normal, firm, or enlarged.

Diagnosis and Staging

Aspiration of all dermal and subcutaneous masses prior to surgery is the best method of ensuring preoperative diagnosis; mast cell tumors usually exfoliate readily and have a distinctive cytologic appearance. They are recognized by a predominance of round cells with blue to purple cytoplasmic granules using most cytologic stains. The cells may be homogeneous or pleomorphic and contain variable numbers and sizes of granules. Aspiration of regional lymph nodes should always be attempted, even if the node palpates normally. Small numbers of well-differentiated mast cells can be found in normal canine lymph nodes, but high numbers of mast cells or poorly differentiated mast cells likely indicate regional metastasis.[19]

Therapeutic decisions for mast cell tumors depend on accurately distinguishing locally confined tumors from metastatic tumors. For dogs with small, well-differentiated dermal mast cell tumors and negative lymph node aspirates, an extensive work-up is unlikely to detect systemic spread. Complete staging evaluation includes lymph node cytology; buffy coat smear; abdominal ultrasonography to evaluate the liver, spleen, and internal lymph nodes; and bone marrow cytology. As splenic metastasis is more common than bone marrow metastasis, splenic aspiration and cytology may be an appropriate staging procedure. Occasional, normal-appearing mast cells in splenic aspirates, buffy coat smears, and bone marrow aspirates must be interpreted with caution. They may be a normal finding in some dogs, particularly those with inflammatory diseases.

Grading of mast cell tumors in the dog is confounded by the existence of two opposite grading systems. That of Bostock labels Grade 1 tumors poorly, Grade 2 tumors intermediately, and Grade 3 tumors well differentiated.[20] That of Patnaik labels well-differentiated tumors confined to the dermis Grade 1, moderately pleomorphic tumors infiltrating lower dermal and subcutaneous tissues Grade 2, and pleomorphic tumors that replace the subcutaneous and deep tissues Grade 3.[21] Because the system of Patnaik conforms to the accepted nomenclature of assigning the most well-differentiated tumor the lowest grade, it is more often used.

Therapy and Prognosis

Overview. For solitary mast cell tumors with no evidence of metastasis, treatment is surgical excision. Incompletely excised tumors should be either immediately reexcised or irradiated. Treatment of multicentric or metastatic mast cell tumors is less straightforward; the morbidity of locoregional therapy must be weighed against the likelihood of deterioration secondary to systemic disease. Multiple slowly growing tumors may be multifocal rather than metastatic and respond to excision. Some dogs with early lymph node involvement may respond to surgery and postoperative radiotherapy to the regional lymph nodes. For dogs with nonresectable tumor, complete lymph node effacement, or metastases to skin or internal organs, palliative therapy with H_2 blockers and corticosteroids is recommended.

Surgery. Mast cell tumors require wide surgical margins. The current recommendation is en bloc excision with at least 3-cm margins in all directions, including deep to the tumor. Close approach or actual extension of malignant mast cells to the surgical borders on histopathology is an indication that a tumor is likely to recur. If feasible, an immediate, second excision to include the previous surgical site along with additional margins in all directions is the simplest option.

Radiotherapy. For incompletely excised tumors that are not amenable to additional surgery, radiation therapy to the tumor bed is also effective. The prognosis for dogs receiving adjuvant radiotherapy for postsurgical microscopic disease of Grade 2 tumors is very good with survival rates of over 90 per cent at 3 to 5 years.[22, 23] Radiation therapy as the sole modality for mast cell tumors is less effective.[24]

Chemotherapy. Optimum chemotherapy for dogs with non-resectable or metastatic mast cell tumors is undetermined. Glucocorticoids may have both anti-inflammatory and antineoplastic effects in mast cell tumors and are widely used. Clinical trials of single-agent prednisone at 1 mg/kg/day or vincristine at 0.75 mg/M^2 weekly for 4 weeks in dogs with advanced mast cell tumors showed response rates of 20 per cent and 7 per cent, respectively.[25, 26] Most responses were partial and transient. The toxicity with vincristine (32 per cent) was considered unacceptable. A variety of other agents, including chlorambucil, L-asparaginase, cyclophosphamide, and vinblastine, have been reported anecdotally to have anticancer activity against mast cell tumors. Responses are uncommon and of short duration. Drug combinations containing prednisone are advocated but have not been compared with prednisone alone in controlled trials.

Prognosis. No single prognostic factor can reliably predict recurrence or metastasis; dogs with apparently identical tumors may have very different clinical outcomes. Prognosis following therapy is statistically linked, however, to a variety of factors including tumor grade, stage, proliferation markers, duration, and location. Survival times decrease with increasing Patnaik Grade with 4-year survival rates following surgery of 93 per cent, 50 per cent, and 6 per cent for dogs with Grade 1, 2, and 3 tumors, respectively.[21] Early-stage tumors, those confined to a solitary cutaneous site, have a good prognosis. A high number of agrophilic nucleolar organizer regions (AgNORs) or a high cellular proliferation index (based on proliferating cell nuclear antigen [PCNA] immunohistochemistry) in the biopsy specimen indicates a high growth rate and is associated with short survival time.[27] Tumors present for over 7 months before surgery are associated with a good prognosis, probably reflecting a slow growth rate.[20] Tumors on the extremities are associated with longer survival times than those on the trunk.[24]

FELINE MAST CELL TUMOR

Mast cell tumors affect cats less frequently than dogs. Affected cats range from less than 1 year to over 19 years of age, and Siamese cats are overrepresented.[13] Tumor location can be anywhere, although the head is the most frequent site.

Cutaneous mast cell tumor in the cat generally appears as an intracutaneous nodule. Occasional tumors appear as diffuse swellings. The most common location for metastasis is to regional lymph nodes. Progression of cutaneous tumors to viscera as is seen in dogs is uncommon.[28]

Diagnosis is by cytology or histopathology. The regional lymph node should be palpated carefully and aspirated for cytologic examination if enlarged. Further staging is recommended only for cats with positive lymph nodes, signs of systemic illness, or palpable intra-abdominal abnormalities.

Treatment is surgical excision. Local recurrence is rare, but one third of cats develop new tumors at other sites.[28] Although radiation and chemotherapy are occasionally used in cats with nonresectable mast cell tumors, published data are absent. Overall, the mortality rate for cats with cutaneous mast cell tumors is low. The canine mast cell grading systems do not provide prognostic information for the cat.[28]

OTHER ROUND CELL TUMORS

CANINE CUTANEOUS HISTIOCYTOMA

Histiocytoma is a common canine tumor. The majority of affected dogs are under 3 years of age, and the head is the most common site. Histiocytomas, however, can occur at any age and at any site. Tumors arise rapidly and appear as solitary, raised, alopecic, dome-shaped nodules that subsequently ulcerate and regress. Multicentric tumors are occasionally described. Immunohistochemistry has demonstrated that this tumor is an epidermotropic Langerhans cell histiocytosis and that regression is mediated by CD8+ T cells.[29] Treatment is rarely needed, but surgical excision is advised for lesions that do not regress or when the diagnosis is in doubt.

CUTANEOUS PLASMACYTOMA

Cutaneous plasmacytomas appear as alopecic, hyperemic, raised masses in middle-aged to old dogs. Common cutaneous locations are the skin of the digits, lips, and ears. Dogs that have systemic signs of illness should be evaluated for multiple myeloma, but in almost all dogs the tumor is limited to the skin. Simple excision is curative for these benign neoplasms.[30, 31]

CUTANEOUS LYMPHOMA

Epitheliotropic Cutaneous Lymphoma. Epitheliotropic lymphoma is a specific histologic subtype of lymphoma characterized by distinctive infiltration of the epidermis and adnexal structures by malignant lymphocytes, either diffusely or in pathognomonic aggregates termed Pautier's microabcesses. It is the most common form of cutaneous lymphoma in dogs but is rare in cats. It is also known as mycosis fungoides, owing to similarities to the disease in humans. These tumors arise from T lymphocytes.[32] Affected animals may have erythema, depigmentation, exfoliative dermatitis, alopecia, ulceration, pruritus, plaques, or nodules. Erythema, ulcers, or plaques also occur in the oral cavity. Lesions are often slowly progressive and present for months before diagnosis. Metastases to lymph nodes and internal organs occur in advanced stages. Surgery or radiation therapy may control solitary or regionally confined tumors. For diffuse or multifocal skin involvement, corticosteroids, retinoids (isotretinoin or etretinate at 1 mg/kg twice a day), antiseborrheic and antibacterial shampoos, and antibiotics may provide symptomatic palliation.[8] Although clinical responses to combination chemotherapy have been reported, it is unclear whether treatment prolongs survival.

Non-epitheliotropic Cutaneous Lymphoma. Non-epitheliotropic cutaneous lymphoma may be either a primary or metastatic tumor. Immunophenotyping suggests that the majority of these tumors are of T-cell origin in both dogs and cats.[32] Animals usually have solitary to multiple, erythematous, frequently ulcerated, dermal nodules. Progression is rapid. Complete clinical staging, including aspiration of lymph nodes, thoracic radiography, abdominal ultrasonography, and bone marrow cytology, is performed prior to making treatment decisions. Localized tumors may be treated with surgical excision or irradiation. For widespread tumor, combination chemotherapy, as used for the treatment of multicentric lymphoma, induces remissions in some cases, but overall response rates and survival times are poor.

REFERENCES

1. Schwegler K, Walter JH, Rudolph R: Epithelial neoplasms of the skin, the cutaneous mucosa and the transitional epithelium in dogs: An immunolocalization study for papillomavirus antigen. Zentralbl Veterinarmed A 44(2):115, 1997.
2. LeClerc SM, Clark EG, Haines DM: Papillomavirus infection in association with feline cutaneous squamous cell carcinoma in situ. 13th Proceedings of AAVD/ACVD Meeting, 1997, p 125.
3. Lana SE, Ogilvie GK, Withrow SJ, et al: Feline cutaneous squamous cell carcinoma of the nasal planum and the pinnae: 61 cases. J Am Anim Assoc 33:329, 1997.
4. Rogers KS, Helman RG, Walker MA: Squamous cell carcinoma of the canine nasal planum: Eight cases (1988–1994). J Am Anim Hosp Assoc 31:373, 1995.
5. Kirpensteijn J, Withrow SJ, Straw RC: Combined resection of the nasal planum and premaxilla in three dogs. Vet Surg 23:341, 1994.
6. Kitchell BK, Orenberg EK, Brown DM et al: Intralesional sustained-release chemotherapy with therapeutic implants for treatment of canine sun-induced squamous cell carcinoma. Eur J Cancer 31A(12):2093, 1995.
7. Théon AP, VanVechten MK, Madewell BR: Intratumoral administration of carboplatin for treatment of squamous cell carcinomas of the nasal plane in cats. Am J Vet Res 57:205, 1996.
8. Power HT, Ihrke PJ: The use of synthetic retinoids in veterinary medicine. In Bonagura JD, Kirk RW (eds): Current Veterinary Therapy XII, Small Animal Practice. Philadelphia, WB Saunders, 1995, p 585.
9. VanVechten MK, Théon AP: Strontium-90 plesiotherapy for treatment of early squamous cell carcinomas of the nasal planum in 25 cats. Veterinary Cancer Society Proceedings, 1993, p 107.
10. Théon AP, Madewell BR, Shearn VI, Moulton JE: Prognostic factors associated with radiotherapy of squamous cell carcinoma of the nasal plane in cats. JAVMA 206(7):991, 1995.
11. O'Brien MG, Berg J, Engler SJ: Treatment by digital amputation of subungual squamous cell carcinoma in dogs: 21 cases (1987–1988). JAVMA 201(5):759, 1992.
12. Marino DJ, Matthiesen DT, Stefanacci JD, et al: Evaluation of dogs with digit masses: 117 cases (1981–1991). JAVMA 207(6):726, 1995.
13. Goldschmidt MH, Shofer FS: Skin Tumors of the Dog and Cat. Oxford, Pergamon Press, 1992.
14. Kalaher KM, Anderson WI, Scott DW: Neoplasms of the apocrine sweat glands in 44 dogs and 10 cats. Vet Record 127:400, 1990.
15. Goldschmidt MH, Liu SM, Shofer FS: Feline dermal melanoma: A retrospective study. In Ihrke PJ, Mason IS, White SD (eds): Advances in Veterinary Dermatology, Vol. 2. Oxford, Pergamon Press, 1993, p 285.
16. Miller D: The occurrence of mast cell tumors in young Shar-Peis. J Vet Diagn Invest 7:360, 1995.
17. London CA, Helfand SC, Galli SJ, et al: Spontaneous canine mast cell tumors express mutations in c-kit. Veterinary Cancer Society Meeting Proceedings, Pacific Grove, CA, 1996, p 91.
18. Fox LE, Rosenthal RC, Twedt DC, et al: Plasma histamine and gastrin concentrations in 17 dogs with mast cell tumors. J Vet Intern Med 4:242, 1990.
19. Bookbinder PF, Butt MT, Harvey HJ: Determination of the number of mast cells in lymph node, bone marrow, and buffy coat cytologic specimens from dogs. JAVMA 200(11):1648, 1992.
20. Bostock DE: The prognosis following surgical removal of mastocytomas in dogs. J Small Anim Pract 14:27, 1973.
21. Patnaik AK, Ehler WJ, MacEwen EG: Canine cutaneous mast cell tumor: Morphologic grading and survival time in 83 dogs. Vet Pathol 21:469, 1984.
22. Frimberger AE, Moore AS, LaRue SM, et al: Radiotherapy of incompletely resected moderately differentiated mast cell tumors in the dog: 37 cases (1989–1993). J Am Anim Hosp Assoc 33:320, 1997.
23. Al-Sarraf R, Mauldin GN, Patnaik A, et al: A prospective study of radiation therapy for the treatment of grade 2 mast cell tumors in 32 dogs. J Vet Intern Med 10:376, 1996.
24. Turrel JM, Kitchell BE, Miller LM, et al: Prognostic factors for radiation treatment of mast cell tumor in 85 dogs. JAVMA 193:936, 1988.
25. McCaw DL, Miller MA, Ogilvie GK, et al: Response of canine mast cell tumors to treatment with oral prednisone. J Vet Intern Med 8:406, 1994.
26. McCaw DL, Miller MA, Bergman PJ, et al: Vincristine therapy for mast cell tumors in dogs. J Vet Intern Med 11:375, 1997.
27. Simoes JP, Schoning P, Butine M: Prognosis of canine mast cell tumors: A comparison of three methods. Vet Pathol 31:637, 1994.
28. Buerger RG, Scott DW: Cutaneous mast cell neoplasia in cats: 14 cases (1975–1985). JAVMA 11:1440, 1987.
29. Moore PF, Schrenzel MD, Affolter VK, et al: Canine cutaneous histiocytoma is an epidermotropic Langerhans cell histiocytosis that expresses CD1 and specific β_2-integrin molecules. Am J Pathol 148(5):1699, 1996.
30. Rakich PM, Latimer KS, Weiss R, et al: Mucocutaneous plasmacytomas in dogs: 75 cases (1980–1987). JAVMA 194(6):803, 1989.
31. Baer KE, Patnaik AK, Gilbertson SR, et al: Cutaneous plasmacytomas in dogs: A morphologic and immunohistochemical study. Vet Pathol 26:216, 1989.
32. Day M: Immunophenotypic characterization of cutaneous lymphoid neoplasia in the dog and the cat. J Comp Pathol 112(1):79, 1995.

CHAPTER 100

SOFT TISSUE SARCOMAS AND HEMANGIOSARCOMAS

Rodney L. Page and Donald E. Thrall

The term soft tissue sarcoma refers to a group of tumors of mesenchymal origin that includes numerous histologic types (Table 100–1). It is more clinically relevant, however, to subcategorize soft tissue sarcomas by histologic grade (degree of malignancy).[1] The grade designation of soft tissue sarcomas is based on morphologic criteria that include assessment of mitotic index (number of mitotic figures per 10 40× fields), degree of necrosis, and extent of differentiation.[2,3] Some mesenchymal neoplasms are not included within the soft tissue sarcoma designation owing to unique clinical behavior (hemangiosarcoma, mast cell tumors) or insufficient information to document the clinical relevance of the histologic grading schemes (leiomyosarcoma, rhabdomyosarcoma). Although grading schemes have been proposed that seemingly correlate with clinical behavior in dogs, similar schemes have not yet been evaluated for feline sarcomas. Recommendations for feline sarcoma management are based on limited data; therefore, such recommendations may change as additional data are acquired. Management of canine hemangiosarcoma is discussed here, whereas mast cell tumors are reviewed elsewhere (see Chapter 98).

Canine sarcomas are common (15/100,000 dogs at risk). The incidence of injection-site sarcomas in cats is not accurately known, although an estimate of 1 to 3 per 10,000 vaccinated cats has been made.[4] In addition, simple resection of sarcomas in both dogs and cats is associated with a high local recurrence rate and substantial morbidity and mortality.

This chapter addresses initial diagnostic considerations, biopsy recommendations, staging, and treatment options. The goal is to provide a comprehensive, algorithm-based method for management of soft tissue sarcomas and hemangiosarcomas in dogs. Distinctions in management decisions for feline sarcomas are made to clarify the unique biology of injection-site tumors.

BIOLOGIC BASIS OF ONCOGENESIS

Evidence exists that genetic alterations, viral transformation, transformation following injection, and radiation exposure may result in sarcomas in either dogs or cats. In addition, there are anecdotal reports in which it is suggested that sarcomas may arise at sites of prior necrosis or inflammation.

TABLE 100–1. HISTOLOGIC CLASSIFICATION OF SOFT TISSUE SARCOMAS

Hemangiopericytoma	Fibrosarcoma
Neurofibrosarcoma	Malignant fibrous histiocytoma
Myxosarcoma	Synovial cell sarcoma
Liposarcoma	Undifferentiated sarcoma

Mutated p53 has been identified in approximately 40 per cent of soft tissue sarcomas. Mutation of this tumor suppressor gene makes it possible for such cells to escape cellular senescence pathways and become immortalized. Mutation of the p53 gene results in apparent overexpression of the associated protein in approximately 35 to 50 per cent of soft tissue sarcomas in dogs.[5] A second genetic aberration in human sarcomas is overexpression of the MDM2 protein.[6] This is a p53 nuclear binding protein that is thought to inactivate normal p53. No reports of this phenomenon exist in dogs or cats.

The feline sarcoma virus (FeSV) is an acutely transforming retrovirus that requires concurrent feline leukemia virus (FeLV) infection for tumorigenesis. Sarcomas in FeSV-positive cats, although rare, are particularly significant, because FeSV can cause transformation of human cells. Young, FeLV-positive cats in which a sarcoma arises should be tested for FeSV and isolated.

High-dose radiation exposure can induce sarcoma formation, such as following irradiation of a tumor. However, the incidence of radiation-induced tumors is low (<5 per cent) in animals receiving contemporary irradiation schedules, and tumors do not develop until years after irradiation. The benefits of tumor control are greater than the risk of a radiation-induced sarcoma.

Causes for the development of postinjection sarcomas in cats are not well understood. Original associations between aluminum adjuvant particles and cancer have not been confirmed. A role of the immune system in transformation of fibroblasts around the injection site has been proposed. Many cats develop injection-site reactions following vaccination, and when they are removed, those reaction sites appear to be granulomatous in nature. No correlation between postvaccination granulomatous reaction and tumor development has been established. Much remains to be learned about the development of tumors following vaccination in cats. It is likely that host as well as vaccine factors will be found to play a role.

From a comparative perspective, it is interesting that the incidence of soft tissue sarcomas and hemangiosarcomas in companion animals is much greater than that in humans. Even before the increase in the incidence of tumors following vaccine injection, sarcomas in cats occurred at a higher incidence than in humans. The reasons underlying these observations are unknown. Certain breeds of dogs are known to be predisposed to the development of sarcomas. German shepherd dogs and golden retrievers are at higher risk for development of hemangiosarcoma than are other breeds. Retrievers are also frequently diagnosed with soft tissue sarcomas. The question of whether the higher relative incidence of tumors in retrievers is due to a breed-specific problem or their popularity has not been resolved.

PRESENTATION, DIAGNOSIS, AND STAGING

Soft tissue sarcomas are palpable, semifirm to firm lumps found in the dermis, subcutaneous tissue, or deeper muscular and musculofascial compartments. The most common owner observation is that of a progressively enlarging mass. The size at presentation is determined by whether the mass is superficial or deep, location, type of hair-coat, and owner awareness and concern. Superficial and peripherally located sarcomas are often detected at smaller sizes than are those in less accessible locations, and this may be correlated with a favorable response. Oral sarcomas have a better prognosis if they are located rostrally rather than caudally in the oral cavity, because the tumor is often detected at a smaller size. Feline sarcomas that arise at injection sites may be difficult to detect at an early stage if they develop intramuscularly in the thigh or deep within the interscapular space.

Numerous differential diagnoses exist for such masses, including non-neoplastic conditions (abscess, granuloma) and other tumors (benign and malignant). Figure 100–1 illustrates an approach to diagnosis of superficial masses based on initial fine-needle aspiration and tissue biopsy. Fine-needle aspiration is most useful for diagnosis of round

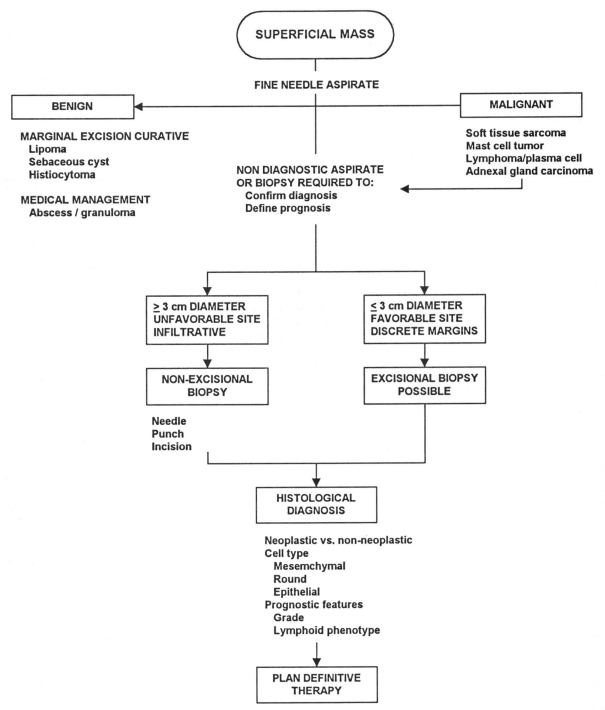

Figure 100–1. Initial diagnostic algorithm for any superficial or palpable mass, including soft tissue carcinoma.

cell tumors (mast cell tumors, lymphoma) and to identify benign skin tumors or non-neoplastic diseases. Fine-needle aspiration biopsy is not usually recommended for mammary neoplasia owing to low diagnostic sensitivity or for oronasal neoplasia owing to difficult tumor access. Cytologic diagnosis of neoplasia should be followed by biopsy to provide confirmation of diagnosis and to identify any prognostic variables, such as grade, before treatment planning. Sequential measuring, mapping, and biopsy of palpable masses is the best way to determine whether significant changes are occurring. A topographic map should be a part of every pet's medical record.

Hemangiosarcomas develop most often within the spleen or liver. Clinical signs relate to hemorrhage, either episodic or acute in nature. Superficial hemangiosarcomas are single or multiple erythematous masses in the epidermis or subcutis, with an apparent predilection for the ventral abdominal skin. Hemangiosarcomas may be either cystic or solid, and obtaining a definitive diagnosis from fine-needle or tissue-cutting needle biopsy may be difficult. Incisional biopsy or dermal punch at the normal tissue–mass interface is often necessary, with confirmation by special staining techniques (Factor VIII–related antigen). Hemangiosarcomas can also arise in other sites such as heart, bone, and central nervous system.

The biopsy procedure is critical to the successful management of animals with soft tissue sarcoma. The type and placement of a biopsy should be considered carefully. In Figure 100–1, guidelines are given for the use of excisional versus nonexcisional biopsies of superficial tumors. Excisional biopsy should be conducted only when the mass is small, epidermal or dermal, and located in a region where reasonable margins (2 to 3 cm) can be obtained in all directions. Too often an excisional biopsy is considered to be a definitive therapeutic procedure. Nonexcisional biopsies, when adequately performed, provide the same information as excisional biopsies but do not disrupt the normal tissue bed or risk contamination of adjacent musculofascial compartments with tumor cells. This is of particular importance for feline soft tissue sarcomas in the interscapular space. A successful biopsy should provide knowledge of (1) whether the mass is neoplastic, (2) the type of neoplasm (at least round cell, epithelial, or mesenchymal designation), and (3) prognostic factors (grade, phenotype).

Imaging of the primary tumor and potential regional or distant metastatic sites must precede treatment planning. Survey radiographs of the thorax and primary tumor should be included in the minimal database. Survey radiographs may not define the tumor boundaries accurately. Computed tomography (CT) or magnetic resonance imaging (MRI) better establish normal tissue margins for complete resection. This is particularly helpful when the tumor is clinically invasive and potentially difficult to resect without normal tissue damage. The use of CT or MRI is also important for radiation treatment planning. More complete tumor damage is expected if accurate radiation dose to the tumor can be accomplished with minimal normal tissue exposure. Ultrasonographic evaluation of a primary tumor can be helpful in determining proximity of the tumor to large vessels or cavitation. Abdominal ultrasonography is generally recommended on any intermediate- or high-grade sarcoma occurring in the lumbar epaxial region, pelvic region, or pelvic limbs to evaluate the medial iliac lymph node size and other potential sites of metastasis within the abdomen.

Abdominal ultrasound examination has become a routine procedure for many clinical problems, and as a result, small splenic nodules that would not be detectable by physical examination or survey radiographs are more commonly identified. Definitive diagnosis of such incidental nodules is often not possible with ultrasound-guided biopsy techniques, and the clinical signs may not warrant exploratory laparotomy. Reevaluation of the nodule four to eight weeks later for evidence of progression may lead to a stronger rationale for a definitive diagnostic procedure. Breeds at high risk (German shepherd dog, golden retriever) require closer monitoring or attention. Careful measurement of the nodule is essential, because a 1-cm^3 mass must increase only to 1.2 cm in diameter to double in volume, and rapid increases in nodule size should be pursued with a biopsy.

Gallium[67] is a radioisotope that has been reported to help differentiate sarcoma from surrounding normal fibrous tissue in humans. A recent study in dogs with sarcomas reported localization of the radionuclide within tumor tissue.[7] Initial staging and evaluation for evidence of recurrence may be more accurately detected with such selective strategies than with conventional imaging and physical examination.

TREATMENT OF SOFT TISSUE SARCOMAS

The importance of an accurate histologic diagnosis, staging, and determination of the extent of invasion and spread is emphasized for soft tissue sarcomas. Initial attempts at tumor management represent the best chance for successful control. Failure of surgery to control many sarcomas is usually related to incomplete excision or a high-grade malignancy that may have occult extension or metastasis at the time of surgery. Therefore, knowing the extent of surgery required for long-term control and any requirements for adjuvant therapy before the initial resection is essential (Fig. 100–2). Decisions about therapeutic options are made after considering three critical issues: (1) Can the animal tolerate treatment? (2) Is the tumor resectable with or without multimodality therapy? (3) Is therapy planned to be curative or palliative?

SURGICAL CONSIDERATIONS

Sarcomas are usually located in subcutaneous tissues or in musculoaponeurotic structures and are therefore difficult to remove without substantial soft tissue disruption. Local extension of sarcomas is usually by longitudinal growth along intermuscular fascial planes. However, sarcomas rarely cross major muscular septa (compartments) early in their development. Iatrogenic compartmental disruption has been associated with increased recurrence in humans following incomplete resection due to contamination or extension of tumor beyond the gross tumor boundary.

Sarcomas often appear to be encapsulated and thus easy to resect. In fact, this pseudocapsule is a mixture of compressed tumor and normal tissue that affords no barrier to tumor extension. Careful histologic evaluation typically reveals microscopic extension beyond the pseudocapsule.

Complete surgical resection depends on the site of the tumor, the size and nature of its margins (infiltrative vs. discrete), and the skill of the surgeon. In addition, the histologic grade of the sarcoma should be considered in surgical treatment planning. High-grade sarcomas have greater risk of recurrence following marginal resection.[2] The effect of grade on recurrence was not observed when more substantial

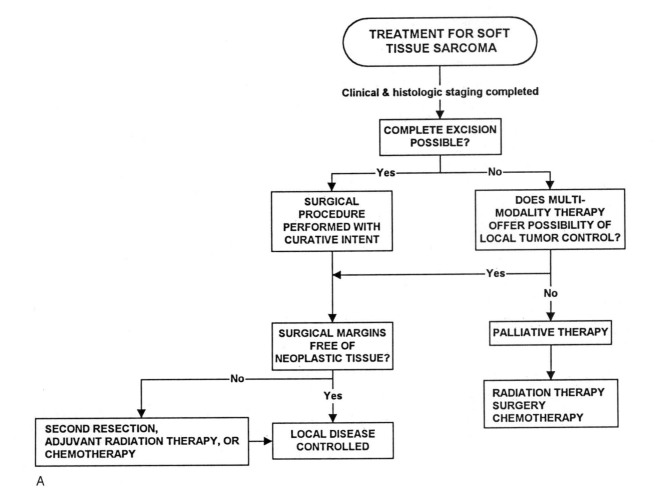

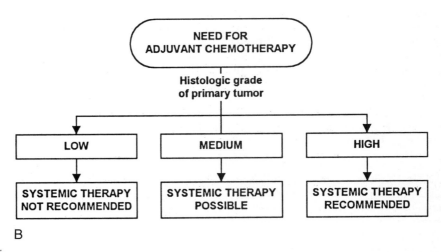

Figure 100–2. *A,* Algorithm for treatment of soft tissue sarcoma. *B,* Algorithm to determine need for adjuvant chemotherapy.

surgical removal of normal tissue around the sarcoma was performed.[3] Therefore, aggressive normal tissue resection is indicated and may obviate the effect of grade on local recurrence. However, high-grade sarcomas are more likely to metastasize than low- or intermediate-grade sarcomas. (Table 100–2).

Several techniques for normal tissue preservation are available that make it possible to consider more aggressive local tumor resection. These include tissue expanders, which permit closure of extensive defects, and new grafting techniques that speed healing following reconstruction. Such techniques and expertise likely require referral of the animal to a specialist. Referral is encouraged when it is clear that adequate surgical resection is not possible without special skills and equipment.

Aggressive or radical surgical management of feline injection-site sarcomas must be considered. Current recommendations include removal of wide normal tissue margins and routine removal of adjacent osseous structures that limit obtaining tumor-free margins, such as vertebral spinous processes and sections of scapula or pelvis. Without such an aggressive approach, recurrence is likely (>50 to 75 per cent). In several recent reports it was suggested that radical surgical resection may decrease the incidence of recurrence, particularly if performed when the mass is first recognized.[8] Long-term control, however, may require adjuvant treatment in addition to surgery.[9]

Following tumor removal, tissue margins should be evaluated for completeness of excision. The excised tissue should be marked on the cut surface with India ink or tagged so that the cut surface can be identified more easily for evaluation after fixation. Areas that are of particular concern, such as the deep margin, may be carefully noted with additional tagging or marking. All sites requiring careful evaluation by the pathologist should be clearly communicated. It has recently been confirmed that normal tissue margins that are contaminated with neoplastic cells predispose to recurrence in both dogs and cats.[3, 10]

In general, drains should be avoided in tumor sites. Drainage tracts have been a source of tumor contamination and regrowth. If radiation is to be used postoperatively, the entire path of the drain and the entire incision must be included in the radiation field. This necessitates use of larger radiation fields, resulting in increased risk of complications. Careful consideration of incision directions, complete subcutaneous closure, and the prudent placement of drains should be part of the presurgical planning process.

A tumor may be beyond surgical removal if the tumor volume is too large or if it is invasive into critical organs, nerves, or vessels as determined by physical examination or CT or MRI. In many instances the use of planned multimodality therapy may offer the possibility of local tumor control

when surgery alone is not likely to be successful. Numerous strategies exist for the use of combined modality therapy. The most common includes radiation combined with surgery.

RADIATION THERAPY

Contemporary radiation treatment schedules involve the use of CT-based treatment plans and higher total radiation doses delivered in a more biologically relevant schedule than used previously. Although improved responses may result from such changes, it is unlikely that all sarcomas in dogs and cats will be controlled with radiation therapy alone, owing to the advanced size of the tumors at diagnosis or presentation to the radiation oncologist.

Several strategies have been evaluated to enhance the response of sarcomas to radiation therapy. Hyperthermia combined with radiation therapy is based on the concept that heat cytotoxicity is related to factors independent of those conferring radiation resistance (energy status, cell cycle) and the ability of hyperthermia to increase radiation sensitivity. Hyperthermia combined with radiation has been evaluated in several prospective clinical studies, and it has resulted in improved tumor control relative to radiation alone.[11] Currently, the use of hyperthermia is limited by access to the technology and nonuniform thermal dose delivery to biologically heterogeneous tissues.

Radiation combined with surgery may be a logical strategy for improved long-term control of sarcomas that are not amenable to single-modality therapy. Radiation may be combined with surgery in several ways. Adjuvant radiation therapy is often recommended after histopathologic examination confirms the presence of tumor cells at the margin of the resected tumor. In this situation, the entire surgical field and incision must be irradiated. Adjuvant radiation therapy has been reported to extend disease-free intervals in dogs with incompletely resected sarcomas (>80 per cent of dogs free of disease 3 to 5 years after treatment).[12, 13] Although these results are good, definitive multimodality preplanning would result in better surgical incision planning, marking of the predicted radiation field with steel clips, and more substantial subcutaneous closure so that less normal tissue is irradiated and fewer complications develop.

Preoperative radiation can be used in an attempt to sterilize the margins of the mass and "downstage" the tumor to make surgery easier and more cosmetic. A group of cats treated with preoperative radiation therapy was recently reported. Most cats treated in this manner have undergone multiple resections of the primary tumor.[10] Radiation therapy consisted of 16 daily fractions of 3 Gy for a total dose of 48 Gy. Aggressive surgical removal of the tumor and adjacent tissue was accomplished two to four weeks later. Bone resection adjacent to the site was conducted as needed. Eight of the 33 cats (26 per cent) developed metastasis with or without local regrowth. Eleven cats developed local regrowth only. If no tumor cells were detected at the margin of the resected tissue, median tumor-free survival was 23 months, and 35 to 40 per cent of cats were tumor-free at three, four, and five years. We have modified our treatment protocol based on these initial data and currently recommend chemotherapy and increased radiation field sizes where possible, based on critical surrounding normal tissue. It is hoped that such changes will reduce the possibility that clonogenic tumor cells exist at the edge of the radiation field. In situations in which the radiation field size is limited by normal tissue, more complex radiation plans such as shrinking fields may be necessary.

TABLE 100–2. MEDIAN SURVIVAL OF DOGS WITH SOFT TISSUE SARCOMAS FOLLOWING WIDE SURGICAL RESECTION AS A FUNCTION OF MITOTIC INDEX

MITOTIC INDEX*	SURVIVAL (DAYS)	% METASTASES
<10	1444	13
10–19	532	7
>19	236	41

*Mitotic figures per 10 40× fields.

Data abstracted from Kuntz CA, Dernell WS, Powers BE, et al: Prognostic factors for surgical treatment of soft-tissue sarcomas in dogs: 75 cases (1986–1996). JAVMA 211:1147, 1997.

FELINE SARCOMAS

Our current recommendations for owners of cats that have injection-site sarcomas include (1) removal of persistent (>2 months) vaccine reactions; (2) use of a nonexcisional biopsy to diagnose subcutaneous masses greater than 1 cm in diameter to avoid accidental contamination of adjacent normal tissue; and (3) early, aggressive treatment. Aggressive treatment recommendations include wide surgical resection of small (<2 cm diameter) tumors, including any closely associated bone. Multimodality therapy should be considered for tumors larger than this or for tumors that have recurred. The surgical removal of the mass should be conducted by someone familiar with the aggressive techniques required in these cats. The margins of the normal tissue should be carefully checked for tumor contamination. Carboplatin or doxorubicin chemotherapy should be considered in large tumors (>2 cm diameter) or tumors that have recurred to potentially delay the onset of metastasis.

CHEMOTHERAPY

The protocol most commonly used in dogs with sarcomas includes doxorubicin. A partial or complete response is achieved in approximately 30 to 40 percent of these dogs.[14] The duration of response is not known, and it is not certain whether survival is prolonged. Doxorubicin-based protocols may also be used as an adjuvant or as a neoadjuvant prior to surgery in a planned multimodality strategy. There are no data on the results of such treatment in dogs with sarcomas, but the strategy can be initiated without substantial initial risk and evaluated for success at frequent intervals to determine whether treatment should be continued. Chemotherapy has the added potential advantage of addressing metastases that may occur in dogs with high-grade sarcomas.[3] Other compounds such as the platinum agents have begun to be evaluated, and other techniques such as intralesional chemotherapy may be useful for individual situations.

CURATIVE VERSUS PALLIATIVE TREATMENT

Curative therapy is used when the likelihood of long-term tumor control is sufficiently high to warrant the associated expense and risk. If, because of size, location, impairment of critical functions, or metastasis, a tumor is clearly beyond the stage at which long-term local control is likely, palliative therapy should be considered. Palliative therapy is designed to alleviate clinical signs without regard for prolongation of life. Palliative management consists of using appropriate oral or parenteral (e.g., dermal patch) pain medication, surgery, chemotherapy, and radiation.[15] Palliative use of radiation therapy has become popular in the last three to five years owing to the rapid relief of pain and the low likelihood of acute radiation effects. Several treatment schedules exist, but all involve the use of three to six relatively large fractions (e.g., 6 to 10 Gy). This approach typically results in few acute normal tissue reactions, but late effects may be accentuated.[16]

Palliative radiation therapy has been successfully employed for sarcomas in both dogs and cats. Improved function and/or pain reduction occurs in about 50 per cent of sarcoma patients following palliative therapy. This treatment, combined with newer parenteral pain medications, has had a significant positive impact on the quality of life for pets with cancer.

TREATMENT OF HEMANGIOSARCOMAS

Cutaneous hemangiosarcomas may be staged according to the depth of invasion into the cutaneous structures. Stage I includes tumors limited to the epidermis, stage II tumors are located in the hypodermis with or without involvement of the epidermis, and stage III tumors have invaded underlying muscle. Treatment of stage I tumors with complete excision is considered curative, whereas adjuvant therapy with doxorubicin-based protocols following surgery is recommended for stage II and III tumors. Outcomes are not known for cutaneous hemangiosarcomas treated with chemotherapy, but median survival of dogs with stage II and III tumors is 225 to 275 days following surgery alone, and most dogs died of recurrence or metastases.[17] Radiation therapy to localized stage II and III cutaneous tumors may also be considered.

Splenic hemangiosarcoma can also be staged according to extent of invasion. Stage I hemangiosarcoma is confined to the spleen, stage II is the presence of a ruptured spleen with or without lymph node invasion, and stage III is distant lymph node or other metastases (e.g., liver, bowel). Splenectomy has value as a palliative procedure. Hemoperitoneum or splenic rupture is associated with a negative outcome compared with dogs without rupture. Supportive therapy for dogs undergoing splenectomy for hemangiosarcoma can be significant (e.g., blood products for control of hemostatic abnormalities), and intensive postoperative monitoring should continue for at least 3 to 5 days to control potential hemorrhage or cardiac arrhythmias. Median survival time for all dogs with splenic hemangiosarcomas following surgery is approximately three months. The use of adjuvant doxorubicin-based protocols may extend the median survival time to five to six months.[18] Dogs with stage I and II tumors are routinely treated with chemotherapy at our hospital, and dogs with stage III are treated with two complete courses of therapy and reevaluated. If significant response has occurred, treatment is continued. Treatment is stopped or another agent is used if tumor progression occurs. Dogs with stable disease are treated with an additional two courses of therapy and reevaluated for response. Treatment with an immunostimulant, liposomally encapsulated muramyl tripeptide, was recently reported to prolong survival of dogs with stage I and II hemangiosarcoma following surgery and chemotherapy.[19] However, this compound is not available commercially.

POST-TREATMENT EVALUATION

Treatment results must be evaluated as critically as are staging, planning, and therapeutic procedures. We routinely evaluate each animal at monthly intervals for three months, followed by bimonthly evaluations for another six months, and then evaluations every three months thereafter. At each evaluation, tumor measurements, abdominal ultrasonograms, and survey radiographs are obtained. Relapse is characterized by progressive enlargement (generally over a two- to four-week period) of a mass in the primary site or regional lymph node. Suspicious masses should be biopsied to confirm recurrence. However, biopsy of residual tissue after irradiation is often misleading histologically, because cells sterilized by treatment may appear clonogenic. Appropriate treatment decisions can be made after recurrence is documented based on the health of the pet. Equally important is the accurate assessment of the previous treatment so that future adjustments can be made if needed.

SUMMARY

Soft tissue sarcomas and hemangiosarcomas are responsible for a significant proportion of the morbidity and mortality associated with neoplasia in companion animals. Prevention, early diagnosis, and aggressive intervention (curative or palliative) are necessary to improve the management of these tumors. The feline sarcoma task force has made recommendations for the judicious use of feline rabies and FeLV vaccines, which may reduce the future impact of postinjection sarcomas.[20] The routine examination of geriatric pets (>7 years old) with the intent of better screening for cancer is required for early diagnosis. Thoracic radiographs and abdominal ultrasound evaluations should become part of the annual (or even semiannual) screening of elderly pets. Diagnosis of small or incidental splenic lesions would increase treatment options and likely prolong survival of dogs with hemangiosarcoma. Thorough evaluation and staging of the animal with a soft tissue sarcoma are mandated by the frequent failure of simple surgical resection and the need to offer more sophisticated alternatives. Aggressive intervention that offers a higher chance for permanent control is clearly more cost-effective than multiple insufficient procedures. The use of palliative radiation offers the possibility of pain relief and symptom management for pets with non-curable tumors. This treatment should be used more extensively, along with appropriate oral and parenteral pain medication to reduce the discomfort and pain associated with cancer in companion animals.

REFERENCES

1. Coindre J, Trogani M, Contesso G, et al: Reproducibility of a histopathologic grading system for adult soft tissue sarcoma. Cancer 58:306, 1986.
2. Bostock DE, Dye MT: Prognosis after surgical excision of canine fibrous connective tissue sarcomas. Vet Pathol 17:581, 1980.
3. Kuntz CA, Dernell WS, Powers BE, et al: Prognostic factors for surgical treatment of soft-tissue sarcomas in dogs: 75 cases (1986–1996). JAVMA 211:1147, 1997.
4. Kass P, Spangler W, Chomel B, et al: Epidemiologic evidence for a causal relation between vaccination and fibrosarcoma tumorigenesis in cats. JAVMA 205:396, 1994.
5. Gamblin RM, Sagartz JE, Couto CG: Overexpression of p53 tumor suppressor protein in spontaneously arising neoplasms of dogs. Am J Vet Res 58:857, 1997.
6. Oliner JD, Kinzler KW, Meltzer PS, et al: Amplification of a gene encoding a p53-associated protein in human sarcomas. Nature 358:80, 1992.
7. Poteet BA, King GK, Bergman PB, et al: Clinical evaluation of 67-gallium scintigraphy in small animal soft tissue sarcomas. Personal communication, 1997.
8. Davidson EB, Gregory CR, Kass PH: Surgical excision of soft tissue fibrosarcomas in cats. Vet Surg 26:265, 1997.
9. Hershey AE, Sorenmo K, Hendrick M, et al: Feline fibrosarcoma: Prognosis following surgical treatment: A preliminary report. Personal communication, 1997.
10. Cronin KL, Page RL, Spodnick G, et al: Radiation therapy and surgery for fibrosarcoma in 33 cats. Vet Radiol Ultrasound 39:51, 1988.
11. Page RL, Thrall DE: Contributions from spontaneously arising neoplasms in animals to the understanding of hyperthermic biology and medicine. In Vivo 8:851, 1994.
12. Mauldin GN, Maleo KA, Burk RL, et al: Radiation for the treatment of incompletely resected soft tissue sarcomas in dogs: 21 cases. Proceedings, Vet Cancer Society, Columbus, OH, 1993.
13. Forrest LJ, Vail DM, Chun R, et al: Postoperative radiotherapy in dogs with soft tissue sarcomas. Personal communication, 1997.
14. Hammer AS, Couto CG: Adjuvant chemotherapy for sarcomas and carcinomas. Vet Clin North Am Small Anim Pract 20:1015, 1990.
15. Hardie EM, Kyles AE: Pharmacologic management of pain and infection in the surgical oncology patient. Vet Clin North Am Small Anim Pract 25:77, 1995.
16. Thrall DE: Biologic basis of radiation therapy. Vet Clin North Am Small Anim Pract 27:21, 1997.
17. Ward H, Fox LE, Calderwood-Mays MB, et al: Cutaneous hemangiosarcoma in 25 dogs: A retrospective study. J Vet Intern Med 8:345, 1994.
18. Hammer AS, Couto CG, Filippi J, et al: Efficacy and toxicity of VAC chemotherapy (vincristine, doxorubicin and cyclophosphamide) in dogs with hemangiosarcoma. J Vet Intern Med 5:160, 1991.
19. Vail DM, MacEwen EG, Kurzman ID, et al: Liposome-encapsulated muramyl tripeptide phosphatidylethanolamine adjuvant immunotherapy for splenic hemangiosarcoma in the dog: A randomized multi-institutional clinical trial. Clin Cancer Res 1:1165, 1995.
20. 1998 Report of the American Association of Feline Practitioners and Academy of Feline Medicine Advisory Panel on Feline Vaccines. JAVMA 212:227, 1998.

ONC

CHAPTER 101

BONE AND JOINT TUMORS

Rodney C. Straw

Dogs and cats with tumors involving bones and joints usually present with lameness and a regional mass. Initial evaluation involves interpretation of good-quality radiographs of the local site taken in lateral and craniocaudal projections. Special views may be necessary. The overall radiographic abnormality of bone affected by cancer varies from osteolysis to osteogenic changes. An entire spectrum of changes between these two extremes can be seen. There are some features that are commonly seen with bone and joint cancer. Cortical lysis is common and may be severe enough to leave obvious areas of discontinuity of the cortex leading to pathologic fracture. There is often soft tissue extension with an obvious soft tissue swelling, and a palisading pattern of new bone radiating from the axis of the cortex may be seen. A triangular-appearing deposition of dense new bone on the cortex at the periphery of the lesion called Codman's triangle is often noted, but this is not pathognomonic for cancer. Bone tumors do not directly cross articular cartilage, and primary lesions usually remain monostotic. A notable exception is synovial sarcoma. Tumors may extend into periarticular soft tissues, however, and adjacent bones are at risk because of extension through adjacent soft tissue structures. Other radiographic changes seen with bone tumors include loss of the fine trabecular pattern in the metaphysis, a vague transition zone at the periphery of the medullary extent of the lesion (rather than a sharp sclerotic margin), and areas of fine punctate lysis. Any one or combinations of these changes may be seen depending on the size, histology, location, and duration of the lesion.

Differential diagnoses of lytic, proliferative, or mixed pattern aggressive bone lesions include primary bone tumor (osteosarcoma, chondrosarcoma, fibrosarcoma, hemangiosarcoma); joint tumor (synovial sarcoma and other soft tissue sarcomas); bone cyst; osteochondroma; multinodular osteochondrosarcoma; multiple cartilaginous exostoses; metastatic bone cancer; multiple myeloma or lymphoma of bone; systemic mycosis with bony localization; and bacterial osteomyelitis. Signalment and history can help narrow the diagnostic possibilities; however, a definitive diagnosis must be based on histopathology.

Bone biopsy may be performed as open incisional, or a closed needle or trephine biopsy. The advantage of the open techniques is that a large sample of tissue is procured. Disadvantages include an involved operative procedure with risk of postsurgical complications such as hematoma formation, wound breakdown, infection, local seeding of tumor, and pathologic fracture. Although closed biopsy with a Michelle trephine yields a diagnostic accuracy rate of 93.8 percent, there is increased risk of creating pathologic fracture than with a smaller gauge needle.[1] Jamshidi needle biopsy has an accuracy rate of 91.9 percent for detecting tumor versus other disorders and an 82.3 percent accuracy rate for diagnosis of specific tumor subtype.[2] The risk of problems seen with other techniques of biopsy are minimized by using a Jamshidi needle. The radiographic center of the lesion is chosen, and two to three samples are taken via the same small skin incision. Always perform biopsies in such a way that the entire biopsy tract can be removed by the definitive surgical procedure. Diagnostic accuracy is clearly improved when a pathologist thoroughly familiar with bone cancer evaluates samples. After tumor removal, histology should be performed on a larger specimen to confirm the preoperative diagnosis, establish histologic grade where this is applicable, and evaluate completeness of resection.

Examination for evidence of spread of the disease is important. Regional lymph nodes should be palpated and fine-needle cytology performed on any enlarged node. Sites of bone metastasis may be detected by a careful orthopedic examination. Organomegaly may be detected by abdominal palpation. Usually pulmonary metastases are undetectable by clinical examination, but careful thoracic auscultation is important to detect intercurrent cardiopulmonary disorders. High-detail thoracic radiographs should be taken during inspiration with the patient awake and should include three views: a ventrodorsal view or a dorsoventral view and both right and left lateral views. Pulmonary computed tomography (CT) is more sensitive than plain radiography but is rarely performed in veterinary medicine. Bone survey radiography can be used to detect occult skeletal lesions.[3] Nuclear scintigraphy (bone scan) can also be used for clinical staging. Nuclear bone scan can be a useful tool for the detection and localization of bone metastasis. Nuclear bone scans are very sensitive but not specific for identifying sites of skeletal tumor. Computed tomography may be useful to plan primary tumor resection, especially for tumors located in the axial skeleton. Magnetic resonance imaging can also be used to stage local disease.

CANINE OSTEOSARCOMA

Osteosarcoma (OS) accounts for approximately 85 percent of malignancies originating in the canine skeleton.[4] This tumor usually affects middle-aged to older dogs, with a median age of 7 years. Young dogs may be affected, especially with rib primaries. There is a predilection for large and giant breeds. Males are reported to be slightly more frequently affected than females. Approximately 75 percent of OS occur in the appendicular skeleton. The metaphyseal region of long bones is the most common primary site. Front limbs are affected twice as often as rear limbs, and the distal radius and proximal humerus are the two most common locations. OS may arise in any bone, although it is rare for OS to be primarily located in bones adjacent to the elbow. Usually only one bone is affected, and multicentric OS at the time of initial diagnosis occurs in less than 10 percent of all cases.[3] OS of extraskeletal sites is rare, but primary OS has been reported in many and varied soft tissue sites.[5]

OS is a malignant mesenchymal tumor of primitive bone cells that produce an extracellular matrix of osteoid. There are subclasses of OS based on the type and amount of matrix and characteristics of the cells: osteoblastic, chondroblastic, fibroblastic, poorly differentiated, and telangiectatic OS. It has not been demonstrated that there is a difference in the biologic behavior of the different subclasses in dogs.

OS is very aggressive, causing severe disruption of the affected bone. Metastasis is very common and arises early in the course of the disease. Although less than 5 percent of dogs have radiographically detectable pulmonary metastasis at presentation, approximately 90 percent will die of metastatic disease, usually to the lungs, within 1 year when amputation is the only treatment.[6] Metastasis via the hematogenous route is most common; however, on rare occasions, extension to regional lymph nodes may occur. Although the lung is the most commonly reported site for metastasis, tumor spread to bones or other soft tissue sites occurs. The biologic behavior of OS of the mandible is an exception. Dogs with OS of the mandible treated with mandibulectomy alone have approximately a 70 percent 1-year survival rate.[7]

Excluding dogs with mandibular primaries, occult metastatic disease is present 90 percent of the time at presentation and the median survival is only 3 to 4 months if surgery is the only treatment; therefore, some form of systemic therapy is necessary if survival is to be improved. With no treatment at all, dogs experience great pain because of extensive destruction of bone and surrounding tissue, and most owners elect euthanasia for their pets soon after diagnosis. Dogs presenting with stage III disease (measurable metastases) have a very poor prognosis, and all attempts so far have failed to control extensive disease. However, carefully selected dogs that develop pulmonary metastases sometime after treatment may be helped with surgery.[8]

Cisplatin (Platinol), used either alone or in combination with doxorubicin (Adriamycin), or liposome-encapsulated muramyl tripeptide-phosphatidylethanolamine, has improved survival of dogs with osteosarcoma.[9–12] It is recommended that adjuvant chemotherapy be administered as close to the time of surgery as possible. Between three and six doses of cisplatin at 70 mg/M^2 body surface area has been safely administered to dogs with OS after amputation or limb sparing on a 21-day schedule. The median survival was 392 days, with a 1-year survival rate of 52 percent and a 2-year survival of 31 percent.[4] Saline diuresis helps prevent nephrotoxicity, which is the dose-limiting toxicity in dogs.[13]

Carboplatin (Paroplatin) is less nephrotoxic than cisplatin. In a study of dogs with appendicular OS treated with amputation and up to four doses of carboplatin, the median survival was 321 days, and 35.4 percent of dogs were alive at 1 year.[14] One of the advantages with carboplatin is that it can be given intravenously without the saline diuresis necessary for cisplatin administration. The drug can be given at amputation and every 21 days, provided there are no signs of severe bone marrow suppression. The dose for use in dogs is 300 mg/M[2] administered every 3 weeks for four treatments; however, the maximum tolerated cumulative dose has not been described.

Doxorubicin has been shown to be a useful drug when given intravenously at a dosage of 30 mg/M[2] every 2 weeks for five treatments. This was performed perioperatively to amputation and resulted in 1- and 2-year survival rates of 50.5 and 9.7 percent, respectively.[15]

A drug delivery system that has undergone extensive evaluation but remains investigational is a biodegradable polymer called open cell polylactic acid containing cisplatin (OPLA-Pt).[16] This form of chemotherapy shows promise as an adjuvant and as an intraoperative form of drug delivery.

Work continues to find better protocols using various drugs, delivery systems, biologic response modifiers, radiation therapy, gene therapy, and other methods to improve these results.

Although it is clear that surgery alone rarely cures canine OS, surgery still remains important in managing this disease. Amputation of the affected limb is the standard surgical treatment for canine appendicular OS. Even large and giant breed dogs can function well after limb amputation, and most owners are pleased with their pets' mobility and quality of life after surgery. Severe preexisting orthopedic or neurologic conditions may cause poor results in some cases, and careful preoperative examination is important.

Although most dogs function well with amputation, there are some situations where limb sparing would be preferred over amputation, such as dogs with severe preexisting orthopedic or neurologic disease, or dogs with owners who absolutely will not permit amputation. Limb sparing usually involves marginal (or rarely wide) tumor removal including a large section of the affected bone. Reconstruction usually involves cortical allografts and bone plates. Limb-sparing procedures can result in excellent outcomes in selected cases. There is no significant difference in survival rates for dogs treated with amputation and cisplatin compared with dogs treated with limb sparing and cisplatin.[17] For properly selected dogs, approximately 90 percent will attain good to excellent function after limb sparing.[17]

Dogs suitable for limb sparing have relatively small tumors with minimal soft tissue extension and less than 50 percent of the bone affected. It is recommended that dogs treated with limb sparing receive either some form of preoperative treatment, (IA cisplatin, IV cisplatin, radiotherapy to the tumor bone, or a combination of radiotherapy with IV or IA cisplatin) or OPLA-Pt implantation at surgery. Adjuvant chemotherapy is also recommended after surgery.[18] The most suitable cases for limb sparing are dogs with tumors in the distal radius or ulna. Work with limb-sparing surgery in dogs demonstrated a 1-year local recurrence–free rate around 75 per cent.[17] Local disease control was improved with pretreatment with moderate doses of radiation, intra-arterial cisplatin, or both or when OPLA-Pt was implanted at the time of tumor removal. Limb sparing is a complicated process and requires a supply of allografts (bone bank) and, more importantly, a coordinated team effort among surgical and medical oncologists, radiologists, pathologists, and technical staff. Limb sparing requires a dedicated owner and clinical team. Complications can arise in any or all phases of treatment. The major complications related mainly to surgery are recurrent local disease and allograft infection. Infection rates

can be as high as 40 per cent. The majority of dogs with infected allografts may be adequately managed with antibiotics. Many dogs, however, continue to have evidence of infection, but their function is usually not severely affected. In severe and uncontrolled infections, allografts may have to be removed and, as a last resort, amputation may be necessary. As an unexpected finding, dogs with allograft infections appear to be twice as likely to survive compared with dogs with limb sparings without infected allografts. The reason for this remains unclear but is the subject of continued work.

Bone tumors originating in proximal sites of the scapula can be successfully removed by partial scapulectomy.[19] Dogs function well with partial scapulectomy; however, gait abnormalities may occur after scapulectomy by disarticulation at the scapulohumeral joint. Mandibulectomy and maxillectomy are appropriate surgeries for bone tumor primaries of oral sites.[20, 21] Tumors of periorbital sites can be removed by orbitectomy.[22] Rib tumors can be removed by thoracic wall resection and the defect reconstructed with polypropylene mesh* with plastic plates† for large defects, or by diaphragmatic advancement for caudally located defects.[23] Small primary tumors of the ulna can be removed by partial ulnectomy. Certain primary bone tumors of the pelvis can be removed by techniques of hemipelvectomy.[24]

It appears that radiation therapy can cause considerable necrosis of primary OS in dogs.[18, 25] Palliative radiation for primary OS has been described.[4] This may be a treatment option for dogs presented with stage III disease or where the owner does not want to pursue any attempts at permanent local control.

BONE SURFACE OSTEOSARCOMA

OS usually originates from elements within the medullary canal of bones (classic, intraosseous OS); however, there are forms of this cancer that originate from the outside surface of bones. Periosteal OS is a high-grade form of surface OS and seems to arise from the periosteal surface but has invasive characteristics. There is cortical lysis with extension of the tumor into the bone and surrounding soft tissues. These tumors are histologically similar to intraosseous OS and have similar aggressive biologic behavior. Parosteal OS, or juxtacortical OS, arises from the periosteal surface of bones but appears less aggressive than periosteal OS both radiographically and in terms of biologic behavior. Parosteal osteosarcomas are relatively uncommon and are moderately well circumscribed. The tumors grow out from the periosteal side of a cortex, and cortical lysis is usually very mild. Histologically, these tumors look more benign compared with intraosseous or periosteal osteosarcoma. Histologic specimens must be evaluated carefully because it is often easy to miss the areas of tumor cells and misdiagnose the lesion as osteoma, chondroma, or reactive bone.

Parosteal OS is usually slow growing but can induce pain at the local site. Metastases can occur, but the prognosis for survival is much better than for intraosseous OS.[26, 27] Control of parosteal OS can be achieved by en bloc resection of the tumor with the adjacent cortical bone.[26] The margins of resection must be carefully evaluated for signs of tumor infiltration. Extension of malignant cells up to the cut edge signifies the need for either further surgery (removal of more cortical bone with the entire previous surgical field or limb amputation) or perhaps adjuvant radiation or chemotherapy.

*Marlex mesh, CR Bard Inc., Billerica, MA.
†Lubra plates, Fort Collins, CO.

MULTILOBULAR OSTEOCHONDROSARCOMA

Multilobular osteochondrosarcoma (MLO) is an uncommon tumor that generally arises from the skull of dogs. Characteristically, the borders of the tumor are sharply demarcated with limited lysis of adjacent bone and there is a coarse granular mineral density throughout seen on radiographs. Histologically, these tumors are composed of multiple lobules each centered on a core of cartilaginous or bony matrix that is surrounded by a thin layer of spindle cells: A histologic grading system has been described.[28] These tumors have the potential to recur locally following incomplete resection, and metastasis can occur. The average age of affected dogs is 7.5 years, and there is no breed or sex predilection. A little over half the dogs may develop metastases after treatment, with a median time to metastasis of 14 months. The median survival time is 21 months. Local tumor recurrence and metastasis after treatment appears to be partially predicted by histologic grade. When metastatic lesions are identified by thoracic radiography, dogs may remain asymptomatic for their lung disease for a year or more. Local tumor excision with histologically complete surgical margins appears to offer good opportunity for long-term tumor control.

CHONDROSARCOMA

Chondrosarcoma (CS) is the second most common primary tumor of bone in dogs and accounts for approximately 5 to 10 percent of all canine primary bone tumors.[29] CS is characterized histologically by anaplastic cartilage cells that elaborate a cartilaginous matrix. There is a spectrum of differentiation and maturation of the cells within and between each tumor. Histologic grading systems have been devised.[30] The etiology is generally unknown, although CS can arise in dogs with multiple cartilaginous exostosis. In a clinicopathologic study of 97 dogs with CS, the mean age was 8.7 years (range, 1 to 15 years) and golden retrievers were at a higher risk of developing CS than any other breed.[31] There was no sex predilection, and 61 percent of the tumors occurred on flat bones. CS can originate in the nasal cavity, ribs, long bones, pelvis, extraskeletal sites (such as the mammary gland, heart valves, aorta, larynx, trachea, lung, and omentum), vertebrae, facial bones, digits, and os penis. The nasal cavity is the most common site for canine chondrosarcoma.[30, 31]

CS is generally considered to be slow to metastasize. Tumor location rather than histologic grade was prognostic in one study.[30] The median survival of dogs with nasal CS ranges from 210 days to 510 days with various treatments including radiation therapy. Metastatic disease is not a feature of nasal CS in dogs. The reported median survival for dogs with CS of ribs treated with en bloc resection is 1080 days.[23] The reported median survival for dogs with CS of long bones treated by amputation alone is up to 540 days.[31] Death is usually associated with metastatic disease. A reliable adjuvant chemotherapeutic agent is not known for canine CS.

HEMANGIOSARCOMA

Primary hemangiosarcoma (HS) of bone is rare and probably accounts for less than 5 percent of all bone tumors. This disease generally affects middle-aged to older dogs and can occur in dogs of any size. This is a highly metastatic tumor, and virtually all dogs affected will develop measurable metastatic disease within 6 months of diagnosis. Metastases can be widely spread throughout various organs such as lungs, liver, spleen, heart, skeletal muscles, kidney, brain, and other bones. Dogs can present with multiple lesions, making it difficult to determine the site of primary disease. There is profound bone lysis, and the malignant cells aggressively invade adjacent normal structures. The lesion, however, may be confused with telangiectatic OS, especially if the diagnosis is based on small tissue samples. Often the dominant radiographic feature is lysis; however, HS does not have a unique radiographic appearance, and diagnosis is based on histopathology.

If HS is diagnosed, the dog must be thoroughly staged with thoracic and abdominal films, bone survey radiography or bone scintigraphy, and ultrasonographic evaluation particularly of the heart and abdominal organs. Right atrial HS may be present without clinical or radiographic signs of pericardial effusion. The prognosis is very poor, and even dogs with HS clinically confined to one bony site have less than a 10 percent probability of surviving 1 year if the tumor can be completely excised. Cyclophosphamide, vincristine, and doxorubicin have been used in combination as an adjuvant protocol, and the reported median survival for dogs with nonskeletal HS is 172 days.[32] Doxorubicin as a single-agent adjuvant seems to be as effective as the combination of drugs with some long-term survivors, although the overall survival prognosis is still poor.[33]

FIBROSARCOMA

Primary fibrosarcoma (FS) is also a rare tumor of dogs and probably accounts for less than 5 percent of all primary bone tumors. It is difficult to distinguish FS from fibroblastic OS histologically, especially from small tissue samples. Complete surgical resection of the primary lesion is recommended for dogs with FS clinically confined to the primary site. This treatment may be curative, although metastatic potential may be considerable. There is no good evidence that adjuvant chemotherapy is of any benefit in preventing metastatic disease. It has been postulated that primary FS of bone has a propensity to metastasize to such sites as heart, pericardium, skin, and other bones rather than to the lung.[34]

METASTATIC TUMORS OF BONE

Almost any malignant tumor with the capacity to metastasize can spread to bone via the hematogenous route. The lumbar vertebrae and the pelvis are common sites for cancer spread, especially for urogenital malignancies such as prostate, bladder, urethral, and mammary cancer. Metastatic lesions in long bones frequently affect the diaphysis probably because of the proximity to the nutrient foramen. Nuclear scintigraphy is a very sensitive technique to detect bone metastasis. A whole skeleton bone scan is recommended when metastatic bone cancer is suspected because multiple sites of bone metastasis may exist even if the patient is symptomatic for tumor in only one bone.

JOINT TUMORS OF DOGS

The most common tumor affecting canine joints is the synovial cell sarcoma. The tumor is thought to arise from precursor mesenchymal cells outside the synovial membrane of articular structures. However, because joint spaces all had evidence of bone lysis in one study, the tumor was thought to perhaps arise from within the joint, although this has not been proven.[35] Metastases to the regional lymph nodes and lungs can occur. With amputation, the median survival is longer than 3 years. Limb-sparing techniques have not been useful, and attempts at local excision have not been successful. A histologic grading system has been described.[36] High-grade (grade III) tumors carried a poor prognosis. Other prognostic indicators that negatively impacted survival are advanced clinical stage and positive cytokeratin staining of the tumor cells.[36]

Other tumors reported to affect joints include fibrosarcoma, rhabdomyosarcoma, malignant fibrous histiocytoma, hemangiosarcoma, liposarcoma, melanoma, mast cell tumor, squamous cell carcinoma, undifferentiated sarcoma, and osteosarcoma.[35] Many of these tumors appear radiographically similar to synovial cell sarcoma. Histologic diagnosis is essential to differentiate joint tumors.

OSTEOMA

Osteomas are benign tumors of bone. Radiographically, these are well-circumscribed dense bony projections that are usually not painful to palpation. Histologically, they are composed of tissue almost indistinguishable from bone. The diagnosis is made after considering physical examination, radiographic, and histologic findings. The most important differential diagnosis is MLO when the lesion occurs on the skull. Treatment for osteoma is simple surgical excision, which is usually curative.

MULTIPLE CARTILAGINOUS EXOSTOSES

Multiple cartilaginous exostoses (MCE) is considered a developmental condition of growing dogs. The condition may be heritable. Lesions occur by the process of endochondral ossification when new bone is formed from a cartilage cap analogous to a physis. Lesions are located on bones that form from endochondral ossification, and lesions stop growing at skeletal maturity. Malignant transformation can occur, but generally lesions remain as unchanged, mature, bony projections from the surface of the bone from which they arose.

Radiographically, there is a bony mass on the surface of the affected bone, which has quite a benign appearance with fine trabecular pattern in the body of the mass. To obtain a histologic diagnosis, biopsy material must be collected so that sections can include the cartilaginous cap and the underlying stalk of bone. Histologically, this cartilaginous cap gives rise to an orderly array of maturing bone according to the sequence of endochondral ossification. The cortical bone surfaces of the mass and the adjacent bone are confluent. A strong presumptive diagnosis is made by evaluation of the physical findings, history, and radiographic findings.

Treatment involves conservative surgical excision, but this is necessary only if lameness does not resolve after the dog is skeletally mature. Because of the likelihood of a heritable etiology, affected dogs should not be bred. Owners should also be advised of the possibility of late malignant transformation. Dogs with a previous history of MCE should be carefully evaluated for bone malignancy if signs return later in life.

BONE CYSTS

Cysts are rare, benign lesions of bone. Affected animals are often young and present because of mild or moderate lameness; however, pathologic fracture can occur through cystic areas of long bones leading to severe lameness. There appears to be a familial tendency in Doberman pinschers and Old English sheepdogs. The only true cyst of primary intraosseous origin is a simple bone cyst (SBC, or unicameral bone cyst). These lesions are usually in metaphyseal regions of long bones, and they can adjoin an open growth plate. Sometimes, however, unicameral bone cysts can be diaphyseal or epiphyseal. Neither the etiology nor the pathogenesis is known, but it is speculated that during fetal development a rest of synovial or presynovial tissue becomes misplaced or incorporated into the adjacent osseous tissue. Cysts have been described to occur in bone just below articular cartilage (subchondral bone cysts or juxtacortical bone cysts). In these, it has often been possible to demonstrate direct communication with the articular synovial membrane. Malignant transformation of SBC is not known to occur in small animals. Radiographically, SBCs are single or, more commonly, multilocular, sharply defined, centrally located, radiolucent defects in the medullary canal of long bones. Variable degrees of thinning of the cortices with symmetric bone expansion are often radiographic features. The diagnosis cannot, however, be reliably made from interpretation of radiographs. Lytic OS can be misdiagnosed as a cyst. Diagnosis of a SBC relies on the histologic finding of a thin fibrous wall lined by flat to slightly plump layers of mesothelial or endothelial cells. Treatment consists of meticulous curettage and autogenous bone grafting.

Aneurysmal bone cysts (ABC) are spongy, multiloculated masses filled with free-flowing blood. The walls of an ABC are rarely lined by epithelium, and the lesion is probably an arteriovenous malformation. A proposed pathogenesis of ABC is that a primary event such as trauma or a benign bone tumor occurs within the bone or periosteum. This event disrupts the vasculature, resulting in a rapidly enlarging lesion with anomalous blood flow, which damages the bone mesenchyme. The bone reacts by proliferating. As the vascular anomaly becomes stabilized, the reactive bone becomes more consolidated and matures. It is important to differentiate these lesions from OS or other malignant lesions of bone. The age of affected dogs ranges from 2 to 14 years. Treatment can be achieved by en bloc resection and reconstruction, but extensive curettage with packing of the defect with autogenous bone graft can be effective.

FELINE OSTEOSARCOMA

Cancer involving bones of cats is rare. Tumors occur in long bones approximately twice as often as in axial skeleton sites, and the hind limbs are affected nearly twice as often as the front limbs. OS generally affects older cats (mean 10.2 years with a range of 1 to 20 years). OS of cats is composed of mesenchymal cells embedded in malignant osteoid, but there may be a considerable amount of cartilage matrix with numerous multinucleate giant cells. Tumors are invasive; however, some surrounding soft tissue may be compressed rather than infiltrated. Osteosarcomata in cats can be of the juxtacortical type. The disease is far less metastatic than in dogs. In cats with OS of a limb where there are no clinically detectable metastatic lesions, amputation alone may be curative. In one study of 15 cats, the median survival after amputation alone was 24 months.[37]

MULTIPLE CARTILAGINOUS EXOSTOSES IN CATS

MCE is a disease that occurs after skeletal maturity in cats. This is in contrast to dogs, where exostoses develop before closure of growth plates. Also, in contrast to dogs, the lesions seldom affect long bones, are rarely symmetric, and are probably of viral rather than familial origin. Cats with MCE have rather rapidly progressing, conspicuous, hard swellings over affected sites causing pain and loss of function. Common sites for lesion development are the scapula, vertebrae, and mandible; however, any bone can become affected. Radiographically, the lesions are either sessile or pedunculated protuberances from bone surfaces with indistinct borders with the normal bone. There may be a loss of smooth contour with evidence of lysis, particularly if there is malignant transformation. Affected cats range in age from 1.3 to 8 years (mean 3.2 years). Virtually all cats with MCE will test positive for the FeLV. The lesions are composed of hard, irregular exostoses with fibrous and cartilaginous caps. Endochondral ossification occurs from the cartilage caps and extends to a variable thickness. The caps tend to blend with adjacent tissue, making surgical removal difficult. Cats usually develop multiple sites of disease, and there is a potential for malignant transformation and metastasis.

Cats with MCE have a guarded prognosis. Lesions may be removed surgically for palliation; however, local recurrences are common or new, painful, debilitating lesions may occur. No reliably effective treatment is known for this condition in cats.

REFERENCES

1. Wykes PM, Withrow SJ, Powers BE: Closed biopsy for diagnosis of long bone tumors: Accuracy and results. J Am Anim Hosp Assoc 21:489, 1985.
2. Powers BE, LaRue SM, Withrow SJ, et al: Jamshidi needle biopsy for diagnosis of bone lesions in small animals. JAVMA 193:205, 1988.
3. LaRue SM, Withrow SJ, Wrigley RH: Radiographic bone surveys in the evaluation of primary bone tumors in dogs. JAVMA 188:514, 1986.
4. Straw RC. Tumors of the skeletal system. *In* Withrow SJ, MacEwen EG (eds): Small Animal Clinical Oncology, 2nd ed. Philadelphia, WB Saunders, 1996, pp 287–315.
5. Patnaik AK: Canine extraskeletal osteosarcoma and chondrosarcoma: A clinico-pathological study of 14 cases. Vet Pathol 27:46, 1990.
6. Spodnick GJ, Berg RJ, Rand WM, et al: Prognosis for dogs with appendicular osteosarcoma treated by amputation alone: 162 cases (1978–1988). JAVMA 200:995, 1992.
7. Straw RC, Powers BE, Klausner J, et al: Canine mandibular osteosarcoma: 51 cases (1980–1992). J Am Anim Hosp Assoc 32:257, 1996.
8. O'Brien MG, Straw RC, Withrow SJ, et al: Resection of pulmonary metastases in canine osteosarcoma: 36 cases (1983–1992). Vet Surg 22:105, 1993.
9. Straw RC, Withrow SJ, Richter SL, et al: Amputation and cisplatin for treatment of canine osteosarcoma.. J Vet Intern Med 5:205, 1991.
10. MacEwen EG, Kurzmann ID, Rosenthal RC: Therapy for osteosarcoma in dogs with intravenous injection of liposome-encapsulated muramyl tripeptide. J Natl Cancer Inst 81:935, 1989.
11. Mauldin GN, Matus RE, Withrow SJ: Canine osteosarcoma treatment by amputation versus amputation and adjuvant chemotherapy using doxorubicin and cisplatin. J Vet Intern Med 2:177, 1988.
12. Shapiro W, Fossum TW, Kitchell BE: Use of cisplatin for the treatment of appendicular osteosarcoma in dogs. JAVMA 4:507, 1988.
13. Ogilvie GK, Krawiec DR, Gelberg HB: Evaluation of a short-term saline diuresis protocol for the administration of cisplatin. Am J Vet Res 49:1076, 1988.
14. Bergman PJ, MacEwen EG, Kurzman ID, et al: Amputation and carboplatin for treatment of dogs with osteosarcoma: 48 cases (1991–1993). J Vet Intern Med 10(2):76, 1996.
15. Berg J, Weinstein MJ, Springfield DS, et al: Response of osteosarcoma in the dog to surgery and chemotherapy with doxorubicin. JAVMA 206(10):1555, 1995.
16. Straw RC, Withrow SJ, Douple EB, et al: The effects of *cis*-diaminedichloroplatinum II released from d,l,-polylactic acid implanted adjacent to cortical allografts in dogs. J Orthop Res 12:871, 1994.
17. Straw RC, Withrow SJ: Limb-sparing surgery versus amputation for dogs with bone tumors. Vet Clin North Am 26(1):135, 1996.
18. Withrow SJ, Thrall DE, Straw RC, et al: Intra-arterial cisplatin with or without radiation in limbsparing for canine osteosarcoma. Cancer 71:2484, 1993.
19. Kirpensteijn J, Straw RC, Pardo AD, et al: Partial and total scapulectomy in the dog. J Am Anim Hosp Assoc 30:313, 1994.
20. Schwarz PD, Withrow SJ: Mandibulectomy. *In* Bojrab MJ (ed): Current Techniques in Small Animal Surgery. Philadelphia, Lea & Febiger, 1994, pp 850–861.
21. Schwarz PD, Withrow SJ: Maxillectomy and premaxillectomy. *In* Bojrab MJ (ed): Current Techniques in Small Animal Surgery. Philadelphia, Lea & Febiger, 1990, pp 861–870.
22. O'Brien MG, Withrow SJ, Straw RC, et al: Total and partial orbitectomy for the treatment of periorbital tumors in 24 dogs and 6 cats: A retrospective study. Vet Surg 25:471, 1996.
23. Pirkey-Ehrhart N, Withrow SJ, Straw RC, et al: Primary rib tumors in 54 dogs. J Am Anim Hosp Assoc 31:65, 1995.
24. Straw RC, Withrow SJ, Powers BE: Partial or total hemipelvectomy in the management of sarcomas in seven dogs and two cats. Vet Surg 21:183, 1992.
25. Thrall DE, Withrow SJ, Powers BE, et al: Radiotherapy prior to cortical allograft limb sparing in dogs with osteosarcoma: A dose response assay. Int J Rad Onc Biol Phys 18:1354, 1990.
26. Banks WC: Parosteal osteosarcoma in a dog and a cat. JAVMA 158:1412, 1971.
27. Withrow SJ, Doige CE: En bloc resection of a juxtacortical and three intra-osseous osteosarcomas of the zygomatic arch in dogs. J Am Anim Hosp Assoc 867:872, 1980.
28. Straw RC, LeCouteur RA, Powers BE, et al: Multilobular osteochondrosarcoma of the canine skull: Sixteen cases. JAVMA 195:1764, 1989.
29. Brodey RS, Riser WH, van der Heul RO: Canine skeletal chondrosarcoma: A clinicopathological study of 35 cases. JAVMA 165:68, 1974.
30. Sylvestre AM, Brash ML, Atilola MAO, et al: A case series of 25 dogs with chondrosarcoma. Vet Comp Orthop Traumatol 5:13, 1992.
31. Popovitch CA, Weinstein MJ, Goldschmidt MH, Shofer FS: Chondrosarcoma: A retrospective study of 97 dogs (1987–1990). J Am Anim Hosp Assoc 30:81, 1994.
32. Hammer AS, Couto CG, Filippi J, et al: Efficacy and toxicity of VAC chemotherapy (vincristine, doxorubicin, and cyclophosphamide) in dogs with hemangiosarcoma. J Vet Intern Med 5:160, 1991.
33. Ogilvie GK, Powers BE, Mallinckrodt CH, et al: Doxorubicin chemotherapy and surgery for hemangiosarcoma in the dog. Proc 14th Ann Vet Cancer Soc, 39–40, 1994.
34. Wesselhoeft Ablin L, Berg J, Schelling SH. Fibrosarcoma in the canine appendicular skeleton. J Am Anim Hosp Assoc 27:303, 1991.
35. Whitelock RG, Dyce J, Houlton JEF, et al: A review of 30 tumours affecting joints. Vet Comp Orthop Traumatol 10:146, 1997.
36. Vail DM, Powers BE, Getzy DM, et al: Evaluation of prognostic factors for dogs with synovial sarcoma: 36 cases (1986–1991). JAVMA 205:1300, 1994.
37. Turrel JM, Pool RR: Primary bone tumors in the cat: A retrospective study of 15 cats and a literature review. Vet Radiol 23:152, 1982.

CHAPTER 102

TUMORS OF UROGENITAL SYSTEM AND MAMMARY GLANDS

Deborah W. Knapp, David J. Waters, and Bradley R. Schmidt

BLADDER CANCER

Bladder cancer is uncommon in the dog, comprising less than 1 per cent of all reported canine malignancies.[1] Transitional cell carcinoma (TCC) is the most common neoplasm of the canine urinary bladder, with squamous cell carcinoma, adenocarcinoma, undifferentiatied carcinoma, rhabdomyosarcoma, and other mesenchymal tumors being reported less frequently.[1, 2] In a report of 115 dogs with bladder or urethral tumors, median age was 10 years, and the female:male ratio was 1.95:1.[1] Scottish terriers, Shetland sheepdogs, and West Highland white terriers are at increased risk.[1, 3–5] Although the cause of TCC is not known, it has been associated with the use of flea control products and with cyclophosphamide therapy.[6]

TCC can be papillary or nonpapillary and is typically infiltrative.[2] The majority of canine TCCs are aneuploid, and approximately 50 per cent have immunoreactivity for tumor-associated glycoproteins.[7] Dogs with TCC of the bladder have elevated concentrations of basic fibroblast growth factor (bFGF) in the urine compared with normal dogs and dogs with urinary tract infection.[8] TCC is often trigonal in location and can result in partial or complete urinary tract obstruction. In recent studies, more than 50 per cent of TCC involved the urethra. Thirty-seven per cent of dogs with TCC had metastasis at the time of diagnosis.[1]

DIAGNOSIS AND CLINICAL STAGING

Clinical signs in dogs with TCC of the urinary bladder include hematuria, dysuria, pollakiuria, and less commonly lameness due to bone metastasis or hypertrophic osteopathy.[1] Signs may have been present for weeks to months and may have partially responded to antibiotic therapy. Physical examination, including a rectal examination, may reveal thickening of the urethra and trigone region of the bladder, enlargement of iliac lymph nodes, and in some cases, a mass in the bladder or a distended bladder. Physical examination was normal in 30 per cent of dogs with urethral and bladder tumors.[1]

Evaluation of dogs suspected of having TCC should include a complete blood count, serum biochemistry profile, urinalysis, urine culture, contrast cystography, urethrography, and ultrasonography. Caution must be taken when passing a urinary catheter during diagnostic procedures to avoid penetration of the diseased urethra or bladder wall. Diagnosis of TCC requires histologic confirmation. Although neoplastic cells may be present in the urine of 30 per cent of dogs with TCC,[1] neoplastic cells are often indistinguishable from reactive epithelial cells associated with inflammation. Methods of obtaining tissue for histopathologic diagnosis include cystotomy, cystoscopy, and traumatic catheterization. The measurement of specific tumor markers shed in urine has been reported to improve early disease detection in people with TCC using a qualitative, rapid, latex agglutination, dipstick test (Bard) on voided urine. This test has also been used in canine urine samples.[8a] Routine evaluation of geriatric dogs or those with clinical signs related to the lower urinary tract may help in early detection of TCC, especially as newer generation tumor marker analyses are developed.

Once a diagnosis of TCC has been confirmed, abdominal and thoracic radiography should be performed to complete clinical staging. Abdominal ultrasonography is useful to assess the extent of metastasis, and cystosonography[3] along with contrast cystography has been useful in quantifying the extent of bladder lesions.

TREATMENT

Because trigonal location or urethral involvement occurs frequently, complete surgical excision of TCC is usually not possible. Additionally, many dogs appear to develop multifocal tumors of the urinary bladder. In humans with bladder cancer, the concept of the entire bladder lining undergoing malignant change has been considered,[9] although this has not been investigated in the dog. Surgery has been used as an emergency, palliative procedure to debulk nonresectable tumors in dogs with urinary tract obstruction. Whole bladder intraoperative radiation therapy has been evaluated in 11 dogs with TCC and 2 dogs with other bladder tumors.[10] Although 1-year and 2-year survival rates were 69 per cent and 23 per cent, respectively, complications included pollakiuria, urinary incontinence, cystitis, and stranguria.[10] Medical management of TCC is indicated in dogs with nonresectable or metastatic tumors.

Chemotherapy

In a retrospective study of 18 dogs with measurable, histologically confirmed TCC of the bladder treated with cisplatin at a dosage of 60 mg/M^2 IV, tumor responses were as follows: 0 complete remissions (CR), 3 partial remissions (PR, greater than or equal to 50 per cent decrease in tumor volume), and 4 stable disease (SD, less than 50 per cent change in tumor volume) at 42 days on therapy.[4] Cisplatin toxicity included seizures and death in one dog and progressive azotemia in two dogs. Median survival was 130 days.[4] Similar results were reported by Moore et al. in a retrospective study of 15 dogs using a lower cisplatin dose.[11]

Carboplatin, a cisplatin analogue with less renal toxicity, has been investigated in canine TCC.[3] Although there have been anecdotal reports of carboplatin activity against TCC, results of a phase II trial were disappointing.[3] In this trial, 14 dogs with TCC were treated with 300 mg/M[2] carboplatin IV at 3-week intervals. Remission did not occur in any of 12 dogs with evaluable tumor follow-up.

Regarding other forms of chemotherapy, partial remission occurred in one of six dogs treated with mitoxantrone,[12] and in one of three dogs treated with actinomycin D.[13] Combined cyclophosphamide and doxorubicin has also been reported.[14]

Piroxicam Therapy

Piroxicam, a nonsteroidal anti-inflammatory drug, had antitumor activity in dogs with TCC of the urinary bladder in phase I and II clinical trials.[5, 15] In 34 dogs treated with piroxicam (0.3 mg/kg PO every 24 hours), tumor responses were 2 CR, 4 PR, 18 SD, and 10 progressive disease (PD). Two dogs with CR died of nontumor-related causes more than 2 years after onset of piroxicam therapy and were free of tumor on postmortem examination. Median survival of all dogs was 181 days.[5] Piroxicam therapy was generally well tolerated. Gastrointestinal toxicity (anorexia, melena, vomiting) occurred in 6 of 34 dogs; these signs resolved with discontinuation of piroxicam.[5] In 2 of the 6 dogs, piroxicam was reinstituted and was well tolerated when given with misoprostol.

In an attempt to improve response to therapy, a phase III, randomized clinical trial comparing cisplatin alone to cisplatin combined with piroxicam was performed in dogs with TCC.[16] Cisplatin combined with piroxicam induced remission more frequently than cisplatin alone, but renal toxicity in dogs treated with combined therapy was more severe and was dose limiting. Until strategies are developed to decrease or prevent the renal toxicity, we do not recommend cisplatin combined with piroxicam.

Supportive Care

Urinalysis and urine culture should be performed regularly to detect secondary bacterial infection, and antibiotics should be given as needed. Urination should be monitored closely. If urinary tract obstruction occurs, temporary catheterization, definitive anticancer therapy, antibiotics to reduce inflammation associated with secondary bacterial infection, or surgical debulking could be considered. As a palliative procedure, prepubic catheters have been maintained for several months in dogs with bladder or urethral TCC.[17]

FELINE BLADDER TUMORS

Bladder cancer is rare in cats. A series of 27 feline bladder tumors included 15 carcinomas, 5 benign mesenchymal tumors, 5 malignant mesenchymal tumors, and 2 lymphosarcomas.[18] Most cats were elderly (20 males and 7 females).[18] Partial cystectomy was performed in 9 cats, and 4 cats (2 with leiomyoma, 1 with hemangiosarcoma, and 1 with leiomyosarcoma) survived greater than 6 months.[18]

URETHRAL TUMORS

Most urethral tumors are malignant epithelial tumors (TCC or squamous cell carcinoma), while smooth muscle tumors are reported less frequently.[19] It is important to distinguish urethral tumors from granulomatous urethritis.[20] Urethral tumors are often inoperable, although urinary diversion techniques, such as vaginourethroplasty, have been described.[20, 21] The response of urethral TCC to chemotherapy and piroxicam appears similar to that of bladder TCC.[4, 5, 16]

RENAL TUMORS

Primary renal tumors are uncommon in dogs, accounting for less than 2 per cent of all tumors, whereas tumors that have metastasized to the kidneys are more common.[22] A series of 54 primary renal tumors in dogs included 35 renal tubular cell carcinoma (RCC), 5 TCC, 3 renal transitional cell papilloma, and smaller numbers of anaplastic carcinoma, anaplastic sarcoma, fibroma, hemangiosarcoma, lymphoma, and nephroblastoma.[22] Approximately half of RCC are bilateral.

Clinical signs in dogs with renal tumors include anorexia, depression, and weight loss. Fibrous cutaneous masses occur in German shepherds affected with hereditary multifocal renal cystadenocarcinoma.[23] Laboratory findings with renal tumors include azotemia and, rarely, polycythemia.[24] Clinical staging should include radiography of the thorax and abdomen, and abdominal ultrasonography. Excretory urography and CT may facilitate surgical planning. Nephrectomy is considered appropriate for unilateral tumors that have not metastasized. In a series of 9 dogs with RCC that survived at least 22 days after nephrectomy, median survival was 8 months.[22] Survival times of 3 dogs with TCC of the kidney undergoing nephrectomy were 3, 5, and 25+ months.[22]

Lymphoma is the most common renal neoplasm of cats.[25] Renal lymphoma typically involves both kidneys and other organs. Renal lymphoma may respond to chemotherapy[25] but is usually not curable.

CANINE PROSTATE CANCER

Dogs and humans are the only two species in which prostate cancer occurs with any appreciable frequency. The true incidence of prostate cancer in dogs is unknown, although the prevalence of clinically latent carcinoma and premalignant lesions in elderly male dogs may be relatively high.[26] Benign prostatic hyperplasia is not considered to be a precursor of prostate cancer in dogs or humans.

The close association between high-grade prostatic intraepithelial neoplasia (HGPIN) and invasive carcinoma in dogs and men supports the concept that prostatic carcinogenesis is a multistep process.[27, 28] Basal cell layer disruption, microvessel density, and proliferative index of canine HGPIN are intermediate between benign epithelium and invasive carcinoma.[27] This suggests that HGPIN is evolutionarily conserved as an intermediate in the apparent progression from benign to invasive carcinoma.

The vast majority of prostatic neoplasms are carcinomas, with adenocarcinoma, transitional cell (urothelial) carcinoma, and undifferentiated carcinoma being most common. Mesenchymal neoplasms (osteosarcoma, hemangiosarcoma, fibrosarcoma, leiomyosarcoma) account for less than 2 per cent of canine prostatic neoplasms.[29] Analysis of a large case series indicates that many primary tumors concurrently display features of glandular, urothelial, and squamoid differentiation.[30]

Prostate carcinoma is most frequently diagnosed in elderly

dogs; median age at diagnosis is 10 years.[30–32] When the chronologic age of dogs is converted to physiologic age in human year equivalents, the mean age at prostate cancer diagnosis in dogs and humans is strikingly similar (67 and 70 years, respectively).[33] No breed predisposition for prostate cancer has been identified. Prostate carcinoma occurs in sexually intact and castrated dogs.[32, 34] In a large retrospective study, approximately half of dogs with prostate carcinoma were surgically castrated prior to prostate cancer diagnosis.[30] Median age at castration was 5 years, and only 6 per cent of dogs were castrated prior to 6 months of age. It is not known whether the metastatic capacity is different between the prostate carcinomas of castrated dogs and tumors that arise in sexually intact dogs.[32] In one study, castrated dogs were more likely to have lung metastases than sexually intact dogs.[32] In a larger series, however, no difference in biologic behavior was detected between the prostate carcinomas of sexually intact dogs compared with those castrated before 12 months of age.[30]

Canine prostate carcinoma exhibits aggressive biologic behavior; advanced disease is often present at the time of diagnosis. In one study, 80 per cent of dogs had metastases at necropsy and mean time from diagnosis to necropsy was 2 to 3 weeks.[30] Regional lymph node and lung are the most frequent metastatic sites. As is the case in humans with prostate cancer, canine prostate carcinoma has a high propensity for skeletal metastasis (DJ Waters, unpublished data; see also references 31, 35). Of 129 dogs with prostate carcinoma that underwent necropsy, 24 per cent had skeletal metastases (DJ Waters, unpublished data). Skeletal metastasis was the initial clinical manifestation of malignancy in 16 of 29 dogs (55 per cent). Lumbar vertebrae and pelvis are the most frequently affected skeletal sites. Metastases seldom arise in skeletal sites distal to the elbow or stifle. Osteoproductive and mixed (osteolytic and osteoproductive) lesions are common, in contrast to the high percentage of lytic skeletal metastases associated with other canine malignancies.

DIAGNOSIS AND CLINICAL STAGING

Clinical signs of prostatic neoplasia are usually referable to the urinary tract (dysuria, urethral obstruction), gastrointestinal tract (tenesmus), or musculoskeletal system (abnormal gait, myelopathic signs). Systemic signs of anorexia, weight loss, and depression are present in approximately one third of dogs.

Evaluation of dogs suspected to have prostate cancer should include thoracic and abdominal radiography, ultrasonography, prostate cytology, and prostate biopsy. Prostate carcinoma must be distinguished from other non-neoplastic prostatic diseases including abscess, paraprostatic cyst, acute or chronic prostatitis, and benign hyperplasia.[36] In some dogs, carcinoma and non-neoplastic disease coexist within the prostate. Thus, diagnosis of paraprostatic cyst does not exclude the possibility of concurrent prostate carcinoma. Rectal palpation usually reveals a firm or hard asymmetric prostate. Mineralization within the prostatic parenchyma seen on radiographs is suggestive of prostate carcinoma. Ultrasound usually shows hyperechoic foci.[37] Retrograde distention urethrography may demonstrate irregularity of the prostatic urethra.[38]

Cytologic evaluation of a prostatic aspirate or fluid collected before and after prostatic massage may reveal cancer cells. Aspirates may be obtained transabdominally (with or without ultrasound guidance) or perirectally.[39] Abscessation

and acute prostatitis have been considered probable contraindications for prostatic aspirate. However, at some institutions, ultrasound-guided aspiration of cysts or abscesses has been used for cytology and culture.

Results of physical examination, imaging, and clinical pathology may strongly support a diagnosis of prostate carcinoma. However, definitive diagnosis requires histopathologic confirmation. Prostatic tissue can be obtained using closed (perirectal or transabdominal approach) or open (surgical biopsy at laparotomy) techniques.

TREATMENT

Prognosis for dogs with prostate carcinoma is guarded. Early cancers are difficult to detect, owing in part to the lack of a serum biochemical marker. Local tumor control has been reported following prostatectomy[40, 41] or radiotherapy.[42] These therapeutic approaches, however, are associated with complications including urinary incontinence as a sequela to surgical trauma or radiation-induced bladder fibrosis. In most dogs, metastases are present at the time of diagnosis. Currently, no therapeutic agent has documented effectiveness against extraprostatic metastases. It is not known whether antiandrogens, such as ketoconazole, flutamide, and finasteride, or surgical castration can downstage local disease (making radical prostatectomy more likely to be curative) or suppress distant metastases.

TESTICULAR TUMORS

Collectively, canine testicular tumors are the second most common tumor of male dogs. Sertoli cell tumor, seminoma, and interstitial cell tumor are the most common histopathologic types.[43] Mixed germ cell–stromal cell tumors and other tumors have also been reported.[44] Multiple tumors may be present within the testis. Cryptorchid dogs have a 13.6 times increased risk for developing seminoma or Sertoli cell tumor compared with dogs with scrotal testes.[43]

Most dogs with testicular tumors are elderly dogs, although a bimodal peak in the age distribution at diagnosis has been described.[45] Clinical signs in dogs with Sertoli cell tumor or seminoma may include scrotal or inguinal enlargement, abdominal mass, or signs of hyperestrogenism.[46] Up to 50 per cent of Sertoli cell tumors and rarely seminoma produce estrogen.[47] Interstitial cell tumors are usually small, do not produce hormones, and are often an incidental finding.

Evaluation of dogs with suspected testicular tumors should include a complete blood count, platelet count, thoracic and abdominal radiography, and abdominal ultrasound. Histopathologic confirmation is required for diagnosis of testicular tumors. The metastatic frequency is less than 15 per cent for Sertoli cell tumors and less than 5 per cent for seminoma.[48] Metastasis to abdominal viscera, lung, mediastinum, brain, and other sites may occur. Metastasis of interstitial cell tumor has not been reported.

Castration with or without scrotal ablation is usually curative if metastasis has not occurred. Limited information exists on the medical treatment of testicular tumors. One dog with a metastatic Sertoli cell tumor was reported to respond to methotrexate, vinblastine, and cyclophosphamide.[49] Recently, one with metastatic seminoma that we treated had partial remission with carboplatin followed by tumor progression, and then partial remission with doxorubicin.

Dogs with estrogen-induced myelosuppression may need fresh whole blood or platelet-rich plasma, especially if surgery is planned. Blood counts may improve 2 to 3 weeks after tumor removal, but normalization may take up to 5 months.[49] Prognosis is guarded to poor for dogs with significant myelosuppression.

Testicular tumors are rare in cats. Carcinoma, interstitial cell tumor, malignant seminoma, and malignant Sertoli cell tumors have been reported.[49, 50] The biologic behavior and treatment of feline testicular tumors remain to be defined.

MAMMARY GLAND TUMORS

CANINE MAMMARY NEOPLASMS

Epidemiology and Biologic Behavior

Neoplasms of the mammary gland account for approximately 50 per cent of tumors of female dogs, and breed-related susceptibility has been reported.[51] Early ovariohysterectomy has a protective effect on mammary tumor development.[52] Compared with sexually intact female dogs, the risk of mammary cancer development is 0.05 per cent for dogs undergoing ovariectomy prior to the first estrus and 8 per cent for dogs undergoing ovariectomy prior to the second estrus.[52] These data suggest the importance of steroid hormones in the early events of canine mammary carcinogenesis. Obesity may also influence risk for mammary cancer. A decreased risk for mammary carcinoma was reported in spayed female dogs that had thin body condition at 9 to 12 months of age.[53]

Collectively, canine mammary tumors represent a histologically diverse and biologically heterogeneous group of neoplasms. Adenomas and benign mixed tumors account for nearly one half of all canine mammary tumors, with the remaining tumors being usually classified as carcinomas and adenocarcinomas.[54] Sarcomas (fibrosarcoma, osteosarcoma, chondrosarcoma) account for less than 5 per cent of canine mammary tumors. Metastases most frequently involve regional lymph nodes and lung, and less commonly involve kidney, heart, liver, adrenal gland, bone, and brain.[55, 56]

Because benign tumors lack metastatic capacity, local tumor control with surgery is curative. The prognosis for malignant canine mammary neoplasms is variable, with disease-related mortality ranging from 18 to 63 per cent.[57, 58] Median survival after surgical excision of mammary carcinoma ranges from 7 to 16 months.[59, 60] A particularly poor prognosis has been reported for two subsets of malignant mammary tumors: sarcoma and inflammatory carcinoma. Median survival for dogs with sarcoma of the mammary gland was 3 months in one study.[60] In dogs with inflammatory carcinoma, local tumor control is often difficult, and metastases are frequently present at the time of diagnosis.[61]

Potentially important prognostic factors in dogs with mammary carcinoma include tumor size,[62, 63] invasiveness,[57] regional lymph node status,[63] nuclear differentiation,[66] lymphoid infiltration,[66] S phase rate and DNA ploidy,[64] tumor microvessel density,[65] and steroid hormone receptor status.[67, 68] In many instances, however, the prognostic utility of these factors remains controversial owing to (1) the multifocality of canine mammary tumors resulting in multiple tumors in the same dog that exhibit different biologic behavior; (2) lack of consensus in histopathologic classification owing to intratumoral and intertumoral heterogeneity, and as a result, no single classification scheme has been universally accepted; (3) lack of uniform criteria used in clinical staging; and (4) lack of uniformity in surgery used to achieve local tumor control.

Diagnosis and Treatment

Thorough palpation of the entire mammary chain is indicated to determine if the index tumor is accompanied by other mammary nodules. Inflammatory carcinomas are typically diffuse, rather than discrete, and are often associated with painful swelling. Thoracic radiographs should be obtained to evaluate for evidence of pulmonary metastases. With the exception of dogs with suspected inflammatory carcinoma, fine-needle aspiration is seldom indicated because of the poor predictive value of this technique to distinguish between benign and malignant disease.[69] Instead, definitive diagnosis is usually achieved through excisional biopsy.

Surgery is the mainstay in the treatment of canine mammary neoplasms. Currently, there are no data that suggest that a survival advantage is conferred by increased "surgical dose" (i.e., unilateral or bilateral mastectomy) compared with more conservative surgery (i.e., lumpectomy, partial mastectomy).[57, 58, 70–72] Decisions regarding surgical dose should take the following into consideration: (1) overall health status, (2) location of the tumor, and (3) multifocality. A clear beneficial effect of concurrent ovariohysterectomy has not been demonstrated.[73] However, ovariohysterectomy is indicated in reproductively inactive, sexually intact female dogs to prevent pyometra.

There are no data to suggest whether adjuvant cytotoxic chemotherapy enhances the likelihood of local tumor control or improves overall survival. Activity of doxorubicin against canine mammary carcinoma has been reported.[74] Failure of adjuvant therapy with tamoxifen[75] may reflect this compound's species-specific and target tissue–specific antiestrogen/estrogen agonist activity.

FELINE MAMMARY NEOPLASMS

Mammary tumors represent 15 to 20 per cent of the neoplasms of female cats. The vast majority (>80 per cent) of feline mammary tumors are malignant, and most are adenocarcinomas. The majority of affected cats are sexually intact females, and the protective effect of ovariohysterectomy on the development of mammary cancer is apparently less dramatic in cats than in dogs.[76] Regional lymph node and lung are the most frequent sites of metastasis. Unlike its human and canine counterparts, feline mammary carcinoma infrequently metastasizes to the skeleton.[77] Tumor size is an important prognostic factor in feline mammary carcinoma.[77, 79]

Treatment of feline mammary tumors is initially directed at local tumor control. The invasive nature of these tumors may necessitate aggressive surgery (e.g., en bloc excision of mammary tissue and body wall) in order to attain tumor-free margins. Increased surgical dose has not been shown to offer a survival advantage.[79] Median survival after surgical treatment was 13 months in one study.[78] Cytotoxic chemotherapy (doxorubicin, cyclophosphamide) induced partial or complete response in some cases.[80, 81]

OVARIAN TUMORS

Ovarian tumors are uncommon in dogs and cats. Ovarian tumors have been categorized as epithelial (adenoma, adenocarcinoma), germ cell (dysgerminoma, teratoma, teratocarcinoma), and sex cord (granulosa cell tumor, interstitial cell tumor, luteoma, thecoma) tumors.[82, 83] Epithelial tumors comprise 40 to 50 per cent of canine ovarian tumors and may be bilateral. Approximately half of epithelial tumors are malignant, and half of malignant tumors have already metastasized at the time of diagnosis.[83, 84] Germ cell tumors account for approximately 10 per cent of canine ovarian tumors, and sex cord stromal tumors comprise most of the remaining ovarian tumors.[83] Up to 30 per cent of germ cell and sex cord tumors have already metastasized at the time of diagnosis.[33, 84] Sites of metastasis include abdominal viscera, lung, lymph nodes, and bone. Epithelial and granulosa cell tumors may be associated with widespread peritoneal implantation and malignant effusion.

Epithelial and granulosa cell tumors are most common in middle-aged and older dogs. Teratomas may occur in young dogs.[83] Signs of ovarian tumors are usually not present until large tumors have developed. Dogs with epithelial tumors often have a space-occupying mass or malignant effusion in the abdomen or thorax at presentation. Dogs with germ cell tumors may have signs of an abdominal mass or hormonal dysfunction (persistent proestrus/estrus). Sex cord stromal tumors also produce estrogen, progesterone, and, less commonly, androgens.

Evaluation of dogs suspected to have ovarian tumors should include a complete blood count, platelet count, thoracic and abdominal radiography, and abdominal ultrasound. Diagnosis requires histopathology. Transabdominal needle biopsy is not recommended because of possible tumor cell seeding of the needle tract.

Surgical resection is the treatment of choice for localized ovarian tumors, and ovariohysterectomy is recommended. Care must be taken during surgery to prevent seeding of the peritoneal cavity with tumor cells. Limited survival data are available, but survival times up to 6 years have been reported.[83] Myelosuppresion may resolve with removal of the tumor, but prolonged supportive care may be required. Reports of intraperitoneal cisplatin or bleomycin with or without systemic chemotherapy have been published with survival times of 10 months to 5 years.[85–87]

Granulosa cell tumors are the most common ovarian neoplasm of cats.[84] These tumors are usually unilateral, and hyperestrogenism is commonly reported.

UTERINE, VAGINAL, AND VULVAR TUMORS

Uterine tumors are rare in dogs and cats. Affected animals are usually middle-aged or elderly.[88] The majority of canine uterine tumors are benign mesenchymal tumors; 85 to 90 per cent of tumors are leiomyomas.[88] Uterine leiomyomas are generally noninvasive and slow growing. The majority of feline uterine tumors are adenocarcinomas that arise from the endometrium. Clinical signs may be absent, or may include vaginal discharge or signs related to compression of adjacent viscera by the tumor. While ovariohysterectomy has been recommended for dogs and cats with uterine tumors,[83] the efficacy of other therapies remains undefined.

Vulvar and vaginal tumors comprise approximately 2 to 3 per cent of canine neoplasms.[88] Most are leiomyomas that develop in elderly, sexually intact dogs. Fibromas and fibroleiomyomas have also been described.[88] These tumors may be hormone-dependent.[88] Clinical signs usually include a slow-growing perineal mass, a mass that protrudes out of the vulva, or, less frequently, vulvar bleeding or discharge. Conservative surgical excision with ovariohysterectomy is often curative for benign tumors.

TRANSMISSIBLE VENEREAL TUMORS

Transmissible venereal tumor (TVT) is a naturally occurring, contagious (via a cellular mode of transmission) tumor of dogs that is usually transmitted at coitus.[89] TVT occurs most frequently in sexually intact stray dogs in wet temperate climates.[90] TVT is a discrete, undifferentiated round cell tumor of suspected reticuloendothelial origin with a standard karyotype of 59 chromosomes. TVT is antigenic, and immune response is thought to play a crucial role in "spontaneous regression" of some TVT. Metastasis is uncommon but has been reported in lymph nodes, skin, eye, liver, and brain.[89]

Clinical signs of TVT include a large friable mass affecting the vagina, penis, or, less commonly, the oral cavity, eye, or nose. These tumors are sensitive to radiation therapy and to chemotherapy.[91] Vincristine results in cure in 90 per cent of dogs; doxorubicin should be considered in resistant tumors.[91]

REFERENCES

1. Norris AM, et al: Canine bladder and urethral tumors: A retrospective study of 115 cases (1980–1985). J Vet Intern Med 6:145, 1992.
2. Valli VE, et al: Pathology of canine bladder and urethral cancer and correlation with tumour progression and survival. J Comp Pathol 113:113, 1995.
3. Chun R, et al: Phase II clinical trial of carboplatin in canine transitional cell carcinoma of the urinary bladder. J Vet Intern Med 11:279, 1997.
4. Chun R, et al: Cisplatin treatment of transitional cell carcinoma of the urinary bladder in dogs: 18 cases (1983–1993). JAVMA 209:1588, 1996.
5. Knapp DW, et al: Piroxicam therapy in 34 dogs with transitional cell carcinoma of the urinary bladder. J Vet Intern Med 8:273, 1994.
6. Glickman LT, et al: Epidemiologic study of insecticide exposures, obesity, and risk of bladder cancer in household dogs. J Toxicol Environ Health 28:407, 1989.
7. Clemo FAS, et al: Immunoreactivity of canine transitional cell carcinoma of the urinary bladder with monoclonal antibodies to tumor-associated glycoprotein 72. Vet Pathol 32:155, 1995.
8. Allen DK, et al: Elevated levels of basic fibroblast growth factor in urine of dogs with bladder cancer. J Vet Intern Med 10:231, 1996.
8a. Borjesson D, et al: Detection of canine transitional cell carcinoma using a bladder tumor antigen urine dipstick test. JAVMA, in press.
9. Fair WR, et al: Cancer of the bladder. In DeVita VT, Hellman S, Rosenberg SA (eds): Principles and Practice of Oncology, 4th ed. Philadelphia, JB Lippincott, 1993, p 1052.
10. Walker M, Breider M: Intraoperative radiotherapy of canine bladder cancer. Vet Radiol 23:200, 1987.
11. Moore AS, et al: Cisplatin (cisciamminedichloroplatinum) for treatment of transitional cell carcinoma of the urinary bladder or urethra. A retrospective study of 15 dogs. J Vet Intern Med 4:148, 1990.
12. Ogilvie GK, et al: Efficacy of mitoxantrone against various neoplasms in dogs. JAVMA 198:1618, 1991.
13. Hammer AS, et al: Treatment of tumor-bearing dogs with actinomycin D. J Vet Intern Med 8:236, 1994.
14. Helfand SC, et al: Comparison of three treatments for transitional cell carcinoma of the bladder in the dog. J Am Anim Hosp Assoc 30:270, 1994.
15. Knapp DW, et al: Phase I trial of piroxicam in 62 dogs bearing naturally occurring tumors. Cancer Chemother Pharmacol 29:214, 1992.
16. Knapp DW, et al: In vivo synergistic activity between cisplatin and piroxicam in canine transitional cell carcinoma of the urinary bladder, a model of human invasive bladder cancer. Proc Am Assoc Cancer Res 38:430, Abst 2880, 1997.
17. Smith JD, et al: Placement of a permanent cystostomy catheter to relieve urine outflow obstruction in dogs with transitional cell carcinoma. JAVMA 206:496, 1995.
18. Schwarz PD, et al: Urinary bladder tumors in the cat: A review of 27 cases. J Am Anim Hosp Assoc 21:237, 1985.
19. Davies JV, Read HM: Urethral tumours in dogs. J Small Anim Pract 31:131, 1990.
20. Moroff SD, et al: Infiltrative urethral disease in female dogs: 41 cases (1980–1987). JAVMA 199:247, 1991.
21. White RN, et al: Vaginourethroplasty for treatment of urethral obstruction in the bitch. Vet Surg 25:503, 1996.
22. Klein MK, et al: Canine primary renal neoplasms: A retrospective review of 54 cases. J Am Anim Hosp Assoc 24:443, 1988.

ONC

23. Lium B, Moe L: Hereditary multifocal renal cystadenocarcinomas and nodular dermatofibrosis in the German shepherd dog: Macroscopic and histopathologic findings. Vet Pathol 22:447, 1985.

24. Waters DJ, Prueter JC: Secondary polycythemia associated with renal disease in the dog: Two case reports and review of literature. J Am Anim Hosp Assoc 24:109, 1988.

25. Mooney SC, et al: Renal lymphoma in cats: 28 cases (1977–1984). JAVMA 191:1473, 1987.

26. Waters DJ, Bostwick DG: Prostatic intraepithelial neoplasia occurs spontaneously in the canine prostate. J Urol 157:713, 1997.

27. Waters DJ, et al: Prostatic intraepithelial neoplasia in dogs with spontaneous prostate cancer. Prostate 30:92, 1997.

28. Bostwick DG: High grade prostatic intraepithelial neoplasia: The most likely precursor of prostate cancer. Cancer (Suppl) 75:1823, 1995.

29. Hayden DW, et al: Prostatic leiomyosarcoma in a dog: Clinicopathologic and immunohistochemical findings. J Vet Diag Invest, in press, 1998.

30. Cornell KK, et al: Canine prostate carcinoma: Clinicopathologic findings in 168 cases. Proc Vet Cancer Soc, p 86, 1997.

31. Leav I, Ling GV: Adenocarcinoma of the canine prostate. Cancer 22:1329, 1968.

32. Bell FW, et al: Clinical and pathologic features of prostatic adenocarcinomas in sexually intact and castrated dogs: 31 cases (1970–1987). JAVMA 199:1623, 1991.

33. Waters DJ, et al: Comparing the age at prostate cancer diagnosis in humans and dogs. J Natl Cancer Inst 88:1686, 1996.

34. Obradovich J, et al: The influence of castration on the development of prostatic carcinoma in the dog. J Vet Intern Med 1:183, 1987.

35. Durham SK, Dietze AE: Prostatic adenocarcinoma with and without metastasis to bone in dogs. JAVMA 188:1432, 1986.

36. Stone EA, Barsanti JA: Urologic Surgery of the Dog and Cat. Philadelphia, Lea & Febiger, 1992.

37. Feeney DA, et al: Canine prostatic disease—comparison of ultrasonographic appearance with morphologic and microbiologic findings: 30 cases (1981–1985). JAVMA 190:1027, 1987.

38. Feeney DA, et al: Canine prostatic disease—comparison of radiographic appearance with morphologic and microbiologic findings: 30 cases (1981–1985). JAVMA 190:1019, 1987.

39. Barsanti JA, Finco DR: Prostatic diseases. In Ettinger SJ, Feldman EC (eds): Textbook of Veterinary Internal Medicine, 4th ed. Philadelphia, WB Saunders, 1995, p 1662.

40. Basinger RR, et al: Urodynamic alterations associated with clinical prostatic diseases and prostatic surgery. J Am Anim Hosp Assoc 25:385, 1989.

41. Hardie EM, et al: Complications of prostatic surgery. J Am Anim Hosp Assoc 20:50, 1984.

42. Turrel JM: Intraoperative radiotherapy of carcinoma of the prostate gland in 10 dogs. JAVMA 190:48, 1987.

43. Hayes HM, Pendergrass TW: Canine testicular tumors: Epidemiologic features of 410 dogs. Int J Cancer 18:482, 1976.

44. Patnaik AK, Mostofi FK: A clinicopathologic, histologic, and immunohistochemical study of mixed germ cell–stromal tumors of the testis in 16 dogs. Vet Pathol 30:287, 1993.

45. Looijenga LHJ, et al: Seminomas of the canine testis, counterpart of spermatocytic seminoma of men? Lab Invest 74:490, 1994.

46. Lipowitz AJ, et al: Testicular neoplasms and concomitant clinical changes in the dog. JAVMA 163:1364, 1973.

47. Grootenhuis AJ, et al: Inhibin, gonadotrophins and sex steroids in dogs with Sertoli cell tumours. J Endocrinol 127:235, 1990.

48. Withrow SJ and Reeves NP: Tumors of the male reproductive tract. In Withrow SJ, MacEwen EG (eds): Small Animal Clinical Oncology, 2nd ed. Philadelphia, WB Saunders, 1996, p 373.

49. Theilen GH, Madewell BR: Tumors of the urogenital tract. In Theilen GH, Madewell BR (eds): Veterinary Cancer Medicine. Philadelphia, Lea & Febiger, 1979, p 357.

50. Carpenter JL, et al: Tumors and tumor-like lesions. In Holzworth J (ed): Diseases of the Cat. Philadelphia, WB Saunders, 1987, p 406.

51. Cohen D, et al: Epidemiological analysis of the most prevalent sites and types of canine neoplasia observed in a veterinary hospital. Cancer Res 34:2859, 1974.

52. Schneider R, et al: Factors influencing canine mammary cancer development and postsurgical survival. J Natl Cancer Inst 43:1249, 1969.

53. Sonnenschein EG, et al: Body conformation, diet and risk of breast cancer in pet dogs: A case-control study. Am J Epidemiol 133:694, 1991.

54. Brodey RS, et al: Canine mammary gland neoplasms. J Am Anim Hosp Assoc 19:61, 1983.

55. Fidler IJ, Brodey RS: A necropsy study of canine malignant mammary neoplasms. JAVMA 151:710, 1967.

56. Krook L: A statistical investigation of carcinoma in the dog. Acta Pathol Microbiol Scand 35:407, 1954.

57. Allen SW, Mahaffey EA: Canine mammary neoplasia: Prognostic indicators and response to surgery. J Am Anim Hosp Assoc 25:540, 1989.

58. Misdorp W, Hart AAM: Prognostic factors in canine mammary cancer. J Natl Cancer Inst 56:779, 1976.

59. Bostock DE: The prognosis following the surgical excision of canine mammary neoplasms. Eur J Cancer 11:389, 1975.

60. Else RW, Hannant D: Some epidemiologic aspects of mammary neoplasia in the bitch. Vet Rec 104:296, 1979.

61. Susaneck SJ, et al: Inflammatory mammary carcinoma in the dog. J Am Anim Hosp Assoc 19:971, 1983.

62. Bostock DE: Canine and feline mammary neoplasms. Br Vet J 142:506, 1986.

63. Kurzman ID, Gilbertson SR: Prognostic factors in canine mammary tumors. Semin Vet Med Surg 1:25, 1986.

64. Hellmen E, et al: Prognostic factors in canine mammary tumors: A multivariate study of 202 consecutive cases. Vet Pathol 30:20, 1993.

65. Allen K, et al: Tumor microvessel density as a prognostic factor in dogs with mammary carcinoma. Proc Vet Cancer Soc, p 75, 1997.

66. Gilbertson SR, et al: Canine mammary epithelial neoplasms: Biological implications of morphologic characteristics assessed in 232 dogs. Vet Pathol 20:127, 1983.

67. Sartin EA, et al: Estrogen and progesterone receptor status of mammary carcinomas and correlation with clinical outcome. Am J Vet Res 53:2196, 1992.

68. Rutteman GR, et al: Oestrogen (ER) and progestin receptors (PR) in mammary tissue of the female dog: Different receptor profile in nonmalignant and malignant states. Br J Cancer 58:594, 1988.

69. Allen SW, et al: Cytologic differentiation of benign from malignant canine mammary tumors. Vet Pathol 23:649, 1986.

70. MacEwen EG, et al: Evaluation of effects of levamisole and surgery on canine mammary cancer. J Biol Resp Mod 4:418, 1985.

71. Misdorp W, Hart AAM: Canine mammary cancer. I. Prognosis. J Small Anim Pract 20:385, 1979.

72. Misdorp W, Hart AAM: Canine mammary cancer. II. Therapy and causes of death. J Small Anim Pract 20:395, 1979.

73. Yamagami T, et al: Influence of ovariectomy at the time of mastectomy on the prognosis for canine malignant mammary tumours. J Small Anim Pract 37:462, 1996.

74. Hahn KA, et al: Canine malignant mammary neoplasia: Biologic behavior, diagnosis, and treatment alternatives. J Am Anim Hosp Assoc 28:251, 1992.

75. Morris JS, et al: Use of tamoxifen in the control of mammary neoplasia. Vet Rec 133:539, 1993.

76. Hayes HM, et al: Epidemiological features of feline mammary carcinomas. Vet Rec 108:476, 1981.

77. Waters DJ, et al: Skeletal metastasis in feline mammary carcinoma: Case report and literature review. J Am Anim Hosp Assoc 34:103, 1998.

78. Weijer K, et al: Feline malignant mammary tumors I. Morphology and biology: Some comparisons with human and canine mammary carcinomas. J Natl Cancer Inst 49:1697, 1972.

79. MacEwen EG, et al: Prognostic factors for feline mammary tumors. JAVMA 185:201, 1984.

80. Jeglum KA, et al: Chemotherapy of advanced mammary adenocarcinoma in 14 cats. JAVMA 187:157, 1985.

81. Ogilvie GK, et al: Phase II evaluation of doxorubicin for treatment of various canine neoplasms. JAVMA 195:1580, 1989.

82. Nielsen SW, et al: Tumours of the ovary. Bull WHO 53:203, 1976.

83. Klein MK: Tumors of the female reproductive system. In Withrow SJ, MacEwen EG (eds): Small Animal Clinical Oncology, 2nd ed. Philadelphia, WB Saunders, 1996, p 347.

84. Patnaik AK, Greenlee PG: Canine ovarian neoplasms: A clinicopathologic study of 71 cases including histology of 12 granulosa cell tumors. Vet Pathol 24:509, 1987.

85. Moore AS, et al: Intracavitary cisplatin chemotherapy experience with six dogs. J Vet Intern Med 5:227, 1991.

86. Olsen J, et al: Cytoreductive treatment of ovarian carcinoma. J Vet Intern Med 8:133, 1994.

87. Greene JA, et al: Ovarian papillary cystadenocarcinoma in a bitch: Case report and literature review. J Am Anim Hosp Assoc 15:351, 1979.

88. Brodey RS, Roszel JF: Neoplasms of the canine uterus, vagina, vulva: A clinicopathologic survey of 90 cases. JAVMA 151:1294, 1967.

89. Richardson RC: Canine transmissible venereal tumors. Compend Contin Educ Pract Vet 31:951, 1981.

90. Higgins DA: Observations on the canine transmissible venereal tumor as seen in the Bahamas. Vet Rec 79:67, 1966.

91. MacEwen EG: Transmissible venereal tumor. In Withrow SJ, MacEwen EG (eds): Small Animal Clinical Oncology, 2nd ed. Philadelphia, WB Saunders, 1996, p 533.

SECTION VI

THE NERVOUS SYSTEM

CHAPTER 103

NEUROLOGIC MANIFESTATIONS OF SYSTEMIC DISEASE

Michael Podell

GENERAL PRINCIPLES

Systemic diseases can induce a variety of neurologic manifestations affecting the central nervous system (CNS) and peripheral nervous system (PNS) in small animals. Typically, identification of a systemic illness as the underlying cause of neurologic signs is diagnostically simple, with historical signs suggesting a multiorgan problem that can be quickly identified with appropriate laboratory tests. However, when the neurologic signs are the sole manifestation of the illness, or when an unrelated, coincidental metabolic disease is present, the diagnosis of a systemic disease as the underlying cause can be more challenging. The purpose of this chapter is to help clinicians identify the presence of a systemic disease associated with preceding neurologic signs and to realize the potential neurologic complications associated with systemic illnesses. The goal is to develop more efficient diagnostic plans to provide rapid reversal of many of the neurologic signs resulting from metabolic derangement before permanent deficits occur.

Metabolic-induced neurologic disorders (MINDs) of the CNS (metabolic encephalopathies [MEs]) or PNS (myopathies and/or neuropathies) are syndromes that are not caused by primary structural problems in that part of the nervous system. Overall, the underlying mechanisms are the inability to generate energy, the inability to use energy in a normal fashion, changes in baseline excitability of the membrane potential, or direct toxic effects. Differential sensitivity exists, however, among animals and within the nervous system of each animal. This selective vulnerability is most apparent in the brain. Here, the more metabolically active regions are most susceptible to injury, so that grey matter is more vulnerable than white matter, and within the grey matter, layers 3, 5, and 6 of the neocortex and portions of the hippocampus, amygdala, thalamus, and basal ganglia are highly sensitive to the effects of metabolic derangement. Although the brain constitutes only 2 per cent of body mass, it receives 20 per cent of the cardiac output and oxygen supply. Seventy-five per cent of this oxygen is consumed by the grey matter for aerobic glycolysis.[1] Over 60 per cent of the body's glucose is used in the brain, with the majority of this energy going to preserve normal ionic gradients responsible for maintaining the delicate balance between excitation and inhibition of the nervous system.

In general, early clinical signs of MINDs are diffuse, not fixed in time, and reversible. The onset of clinical signs of MEs ranges from peracute (hypoxia) to chronic (hepatic encephalopathy). Waxing-waning behavior changes are the predominant early clinical signs in the majority of small animal MEs. Aimless wandering, nondirectional circling, and disorientation are common early changes.[2] As the disease continues, clinical signs progress in a rostral (cerebro-cortical) to caudal (brain stem) fashion. Over time, animals can develop stupor or coma with untreated MEs. Oculomotor abnormalities are common, ranging from symmetric, reactive miosis in early MEs to symmetric, fixed mydriasis with prolonged hypoxia. Marked motor abnormalities are unusual early in the course of MEs, with the exception of epileptic seizure activity. As more brain stem involvement occurs, ataxia and paresis can be seen. Respiratory pattern irregularities are common with MEs. Diffuse cortical disease can result in an irregular cycle of hyperventilation followed by apnea (Cheyne-Stokes respiration). The presence of ataxic breathing (irregular inspiratory and expiratory patterns) indicates caudal brain stem involvement, a poor prognostic sign.

In the PNS, similar abnormalities are responsible for loss of function. Long and large-diameter nerve fibers are affected first via disruption in axonal transport of integral substances necessary for nerve viability. Nerves then undergo a dying back process, with degeneration of the axons in a distal to proximal fashion.[3] The clinical signs include a chronic systemic disease, preferential lower and pelvic limb involvement, sensory loss prior to motor loss, muscle wasting, and slow return to normal with treatment. In contrast, the proximal muscles are typically affected, muscle mass is preserved, and muscles may be painful with myopathies. Because muscle contraction and relaxation are both energy-dependent activities, failure to maintain normal ionic gradients is a common mechanism for myopathies associated with systemic illness.

Five major classifications of systemic diseases are listed in Table 103–1. Examples of the more common systemic diseases associated with neurologic manifestations in the cat and dog are presented, with emphasis placed on pathophysiology and identification of the disease process.

FUEL DEPRIVATION

Oxygen Deprivation. Hypoxic-ischemic encephalopathy is the result of decreased cerebral oxygen supply through either decreased arterial oxygen tension (Pao_2 <50 mmHg) or reduced or absent cerebral blood flow. Irreversible brain injury occurs within 20 seconds after anoxia and two to four minutes after hypoxia-ischemia. A common cause of hypoxia-ischemia in small animals is an anesthetic complication. Surviving animals may initially be comatose with fixed and dilated pupils, followed by dementia, cortical blindness,

TABLE 103–1. CLASSIFICATION OF SYSTEMIC DISEASES WITH NEUROLOGIC MANIFESTATIONS

I. Fuel deprivation
  A. Oxygen
    1. Hypoxia
      a. Primary pulmonary disease
      b. Decreased O_2 transport
    2. Vascular disease
      a. Ischemia
        i. Decreased peripheral vasomotor tone (shock)
        ii. Decreased cardiac output
        iii. Thromboembolic disease
      b. Hemorrhage
        i. Hypertension
        ii. Coagulopathies
        iii. Vasculitis
  B. Glucose utilization (hypoglycemia)
    1. Increased uptake
      a. Hyperinsulinemia
        i. Islet cell tumors
        ii. Insulin overdose
      b. Non–islet cell neoplasia (hepatoma, leiomyoma)
      c. Excessive metabolism (breed-, activity-related)
    2. Decreased output
      a. Primary liver disease
      b. Malnutrition
      c. Thiamine deficiency
    3. Increased uptake of amino acids by extrahepatic tissues

II. Water and ionic imbalances
  A. Water
    1. Hypoosmolar states (retention of free water)
      a. Hyponatremia
    2. Hyperosmolar states (loss of free water)
      a. Hypernatremia (diabetes insipidus)
      b. Hyperglycemia (diabetes mellitus)
  B. Ions (excess or deficiency)
    1. Potassium
    2. Calcium

III. Endogenous neurotoxins
  A. Renal failure
  B. Hepatic disease
  C. Endocrine dysfunction
    1. Adrenal
      a. Cushing's disease
      b. Addison's disease
    2. Thyroid
      a. Hypothyroidism (myxedema)
      b. Thyrotoxicosis

IV. Exogenous neurotoxins and injury
  A. Sedative-depressant drugs (e.g., antiepileptic drugs)
  B. Plant toxicity and poisons
  C. Heat stroke

V. Neurologic complications of cancer
  A. Metastases to the nervous system
  B. Vascular accidents and infections
  C. Adverse effects from therapy
  D. Paraneoplastic syndromes

and motor abnormalities. Because the degree of necrotic neuronal death is proportional to the lack of oxygen, the prognosis is greatly dependent on the total duration of the hypoxic injury. Therapy consists of reversing the underlying event and providing supportive care to reintroduce energy to the brain by instituting proper ventilation and oxygenation, maintenance of normal hydration, and early enteral nutritional support. Steroid therapy does not improve neurologic recovery in people[4] and increases metabolic demand on the body. Steroids produce adverse effects and have minimal benefit to the brain. Many animals may become functional pets over time, taking several weeks to recover.

Cerebrovascular disease resulting in focal lesions is often related to underlying systemic illness in the cat and dog.[5]

Historical signs may be vague initially (e.g., lethargy, inappetence), progressing to acute, focal cerebrocortical signs. Thromboembolic disease from sepsis, tumor metastasis, atherosclerotic disease, and hemorrhage from systemic causes of hypertension have been documented.

Glucose Deficiency. Hypoglycemia is a common cause of neurologic signs associated with systemic diseases. The brain requires an average of 100 g of glucose per day to function. A blood glucose below 40 mg/dL induces a stress response to release counterregulatory hormones and induce gluconeogenesis. Progressive and/or persistent hypoglycemia results in cerebrovascular constriction, thus reducing oxygen delivery. Eventually, neuronal cell death occurs. Neuroglycopenic effects range from behavior changes (withdrawn) and weakness early, progressing to tremors, partial and generalized seizures, blindness, and unresponsiveness.

The most common cause of hypoglycemia in small animals is increased uptake or decreased output. Increased uptake is seen with insulinoma, non–islet cell tumors, excessive exogenous insulin, and excess metabolism in certain toy and sporting breed dogs. Most dogs with pancreatic islet cell tumors have clinical signs for several months consisting of episodic weakness or seizures interspersed with periods of being normal. No correlation exists between severity or frequency of clinical signs, degree of hypoglycemia, and survival time after treatment.[6] Non–islet cell tumors arising from the liver, smooth muscle, and other areas can produce insulin-like growth factor or other counterregulatory hormones, resulting in reversible hypoglycemia once the tumor is removed.[7] Insulin overdose is a common complication of diabetes mellitus management. This problem appears to be more common in heavier cats receiving more than 6 U/injection of insulin, regardless of type.[8] Persistent cortical blindness and epileptic seizures after restoration of euglycemia may occur.

Thiamine Deficiency. Thiamine (vitamin B_1) is essential for the oxidative decarboxylation of pyruvic acid in the Krebs cycle. Failure to complete this cycle results in decreased gluconeogenesis. Thiamine deficiency occurs in cats and dogs fed primarily diets of overcooked meats or fish containing thiaminase, or in those with prolonged anorexia. Clinical signs are related to a progressive, bilateral, symmetric polioencephalomalacia involving predominantly the subcortical grey matter. Cats can initially develop central vestibular disease, head tremor, mydriasis, and cervical ventroflexion, which may progress to opisthotonos, coma, and death. In dogs, ataxia, paresis, vestibular signs, and seizures have been observed. Parenteral administration of thiamine (10 to 20 mg intramuscularly for cats; 25 to 50 mg intramuscularly for dogs) resolves clinical signs early in the course of the disease.

WATER AND IONIC IMBALANCES

Hypoosmolality With Hyponatremia. Hyponatremic encephalopathy is the result of an osmotic shift between extracellular fluid and brain cells, resulting in a net movement of water into the brain and associated cerebral edema. Whereas the cause of hyponatremia may differ depending on the animal's volume status, the clinical signs are more dependent on the onset of the osmolar shift. Acute hyponatremia (hours) can lead to pressure necrosis of the cerebral hemispheres after an expansion 5 per cent or greater, followed by brain herniation.[9] Little intracranial compensation can occur during the acute stage. With chronic (days) hyponatremia, the brain compensates with a loss of cation to lower intracellular osmolality with minimum water gain and few to no clinical signs. A rapid correction in serum sodium of 20 mEq/L or greater of hyponatremia (< 130 mEq/L) over 24 to 48 hours can lead to a potentially fatal demyelination of the brain stem, known as central pontine myelinolysis.[10] Sodium replacement with 0.9 per cent sodium chloride (NaCl) in volume-depleted animals is calculated by the equation: Na deficit (mEq) = 0.3 × body weight in kg × (normal Na − animal's Na).[11] Appropriate volume correction is simultaneously administered.

Hyperosmolality. Acute plasma hyperosmolality leads to shifting of intracellular water into the extracellular space, resulting in disruption of the neuronal ionic gradients, cell shrinkage, brain shrinkage, and tearing of arachnoid blood vessels, with intracranial bleeding. With chronic hyperosmolar shifts, the brain adapts by de novo synthesis of idiogenic osmoles to increase intracellular osmolarity. Rapid correction of the resultant hypernatremia can lead to cerebral edema, as the brain becomes hyperosmolar to the plasma. Common causes of plasma hyperosmolality with neurologic signs include central or nephrogenic diabetes insipidus (free water loss) and diabetes mellitus (hypotonic fluid loss). Antecedent clinical signs include intense polydipsia and polyuria. Because central diabetes insipidus may cause similar neurologic signs indirectly through fluids shifts or directly from a pituitary mass, brain imaging is recommended after diagnosis of this disease in middle-age to old dogs.[12]

Neurologic complications associated with diabetes mellitus can be caused by hyperosmolality, electrolyte imbalances, or metabolic acidosis and by PNS changes with chronic inability to maintain Na-K ATPase activity in the nerve membranes. Diabetic neuropathy is typically a subclinical, electrophysiologic phenomenon in the dog[13] but results in a pronounced tibial neuropathy in the cat. These cats have a marked, symmetric plantigrade stance with pelvic limb weakness. Many cats improve after sustained euglycemia.

Initial correction of hypernatremia to replace total body water can be calculated with the formula: water deficit = body weight in kg × [animal's Na/normal Na) − 1].[11] The deficit should be corrected over a 48-hour period to prevent cerebral edema. The initial fluid should be 0.45 per cent NaCl/2.5 per cent dextrose solution. A 5 per cent dextrose in water solution can be used if serum sodium is not declining adequately.

Ionic Imbalances. Potassium and calcium imbalances have a direct effect on muscle membrane stability. Hypokalemia (≤ 3 mEq/L) from excessive urine loss or dietary depletion decreases membrane excitability, leading to episodic weakness, cervical ventroflexion, and bizarre postures in the cat (Fig. 103–1)[14]; this can also be seen in the dog. Clinical signs resolve with appropriate potassium supplementation. Oral potassium gluconate supplement at an initial dose of 5 to 10 mEq/day is preferable, as parenteral supplementation may exacerbate the hypokalemia through volume expansion and enhanced potassium diuresis.

Generalized weakness with or without tetanic muscle contractions is commonly seen with hypocalcemia (ionized calcium < 5 mg/dL in dogs and < 4.5 mg/dL in cats), owing to increased membrane excitability. The more acute the onset, the more severe the clinical signs; progression to status epilepticus is possible. Initial treatment consists of 10 per cent calcium gluconate intravenously at a dosage of 0.5 to 1.5 mL/kg over 10 to 20 minutes while monitoring heart rate.[15] Identification and treatment of the underlying cause are essential to prevent recurrence.

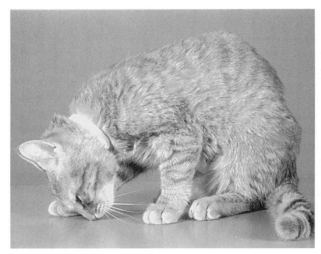

Figure 103–1. Cervical ventroflexion in a 2-year-old female spayed domestic shorthair cat with hypokalemic polymyopathy secondary to potassium-losing nephropathy.

ENDOGENOUS NEUROTOXINS

The blood-brain barrier is a highly specialized, integrated network of capillaries and glial cells that maintains the internal environment of the brain and cerebrospinal fluid. Certain endogenous neurotoxins and/or consequences of systemic diseases have been identified that alter the brain's neurochemical balance by either bypassing the blood-brain barrier or causing direct changes in neurotransmitter activity.

Uremic Encephalopathy. Neurologic clinical signs associated with acute or chronic renal failure can be seen when the glomerular filtration rate decreases below 10 to 20 per cent of normal. Some data suggest that parathyroid hormone is the putative neurotoxin, although this is controversial.[16] Clinical signs in cats and dogs include depression, stupor, myoclonic movements, generalized weakness, and partial and generalized seizures. Animals may not have prolonged antecedent mental depression before more pronounced neurologic signs, as occurs in people.[17] Calcitriol (1,25-dihydroxyvitamin D 1.5 to 3.5 mg/kg/day) reverses the neurologic depression in the majority of chronically treated uremic small animals by lowering parathyroid hormone serum concentration.[16]

Hepatic Encephalopathy. Advanced congenital or acquired liver disease can produce a complex of neurologic signs known as hepatic encephalopathy (HE). Waxing-waning bizarre, unpredictable behavior; dementia; progressive loss of arousability; myoclonus; and seizures can all occur. Clinical signs can worsen after protein digestion. There are several possible mechanisms for the pathogenesis of the neurologic syndrome of HE, including hyperammonemia, synergistic neurotoxins, altered monoamine (tryptophan) and "false" neurotransmitter synthesis, alterations in amino acid neurotransmitters, and increased cerebral concentrations of an endogenous benzodiazepine.[18] Medical therapy should reduce the by-products of protein metabolism and subsequent neurotoxins. Surgical correction of congenital portocaval shunts is most successful in dogs younger than 2 years of age for reduced mortality[19] and neurologic morbidity. Generalized seizures may persist after ligation, despite lack of other evidence of HE.[20] The recommended antiepileptic drug therapy for these dogs is potassium bromide at an initial oral loading dose of 100 mg/kg orally four times a day for 24 hours, followed by maintenance therapy at 30 mg/kg a day. Bromide is a renal-excreted, non-protein-bound drug with good antiepileptic properties in the cat and dog. Benzodiazepine therapy should be avoided to prevent potentiation of inhibitory neurotransmission in the brain.

Thyroid Diseases. Primary hypothyroidism is a common endocrinopathy of the older dog with multiple neurologic manifestations. The most severe form is the extremely rare condition called myxedema, associated with bradycardia, hypothermia, dementia, stupor or coma, generalized lower motor neuron weakness, and possible seizures. Concurrent complications of hyponatremia, hypoventilatory hypoxia, and cerebral ischemia make this a life-threatening condition. Treatment consists of gradual rewarming, correction of serum sodium and osmolarity, steroid therapy (sodium prednisolone succinate 10 mg/kg intravenously three times a day for 24 hours), and levothyroxine replacement (100 to 200 μg intravenously once), followed by maintenance thyroid supplementation. Marked improvement is usually seen within 24 hours.

Chronic, progressive peripheral or central vestibular disease can also occur in hypothyroid dogs.[21] These dogs are typically older (>7 years), with progressive ataxia and head tilting as primary signs. Other clinical syndromes are related to motor unit dysfunction. Generalized lower motor neuron weakness with exercise intolerance can be the result of hypothyroid neuromyopathy. Concurrent or separate signs of megaesophagus and facial and/or laryngeal paralysis may be present. Many, but not all, dogs will improve with appropriate thyroid supplementation.[22]

Thyrotoxicosis (hyperthyroidism) in cats can produce multiple neurologic abnormalities. Predominant behavior changes include irritability, hyperactivity, aggression, and reduced sleep cycles. Some cats may exhibit a paradoxic "apathy," characterized by excessive dullness. Progressive neuromuscular weakness with cervical ventroflexion, exercise intolerance, and loss of jumping ability can be seen with more advanced disease and associated muscle wasting. Signs are reversible with appropriate treatment of the underlying hyperthyroid condition.

Adrenal Diseases. Adrenal hormonal excess or deficiency has been associated with a variety of neurologic disturbances. Signs attributed to hypoadrenocorticism (Addison's disease) include episodic, progressive lethargy, dullness, tremors, vomiting, and possible acute collapse.[23] Glucocorticoid-deficient hypoglycemia may exacerbate these signs. Rapid reversal of neurologic signs is seen with mineral and/or glucocorticoid replacement and restoration of metabolic homeostasis.

Cushing's disease (hyperadrenocorticism) can produce CNS and PNS abnormalities through direct or indirect mechanisms. Direct compression of a pituitary macroadenoma onto the brain results in early signs of dullness and dementia, with progression to obtundation, tetraparesis and ataxia, visual impairment, and seizures. Up to 35 per cent of dogs with pituitary-dependent Cushing's with a visualized (computed tomography or magnetic resonance imaging scan) tumor of greater than 4 mm may develop neurologic signs.[24] Cerebrovascular accidents may also occur secondary to systemic arterial hypertension or thromboembolic disease. In the PNS, an irreversible, progressive fibrosing myopathy can occur, regardless of duration, severity, or onset of treatment, with canine Cushing's disease. A progressive stiff gait leading to inability to flex the limbs is characteristic of this condition. This is an extremely rare condition.

Pheochromocytoma can induce neurologic signs in approximately 10 per cent of clinically symptomatic dogs.[25] Generalized weakness, pelvic limb weakness, focal forebrain signs, and seizures may develop. Signs can be the result of direct intracranial metastasis or secondary intracranial hemorrhage due to hypertension.

EXOGENOUS NEUROTOXINS AND INJURY

A variety of environmental or iatrogenic substances can produce diffuse forebrain disturbances. More common conditions are toxic reactions to antiepileptic drugs, rodenticides, and heat stroke. Removal of the inciting cause and appropriate supportive care are often corrective.

NEUROLOGIC COMPLICATIONS OF CANCER

More neurologic complications secondary to systemic cancer are being observed with the advancement of diagnostic and treatment capabilities in veterinary oncology. These complications can be serious to life-threatening and may be diagnostically challenging, yet early treatment can be quite beneficial. Moreover, the nervous system problems are unique, in that small lesions can create major clinical signs (as compared with the liver), heterogeneous function is present, barriers must be kept intact for proper function, and damage to CNS tissue has limited capacity to repair itself, so that clinical signs may be irreversible.[26]

Direct and extensional metastases to the nervous system are the most common neuro-oncologic complications in the cat and dog. Hemangiosarcoma, mammary and thyroid carcinoma, and melanoma spread preferentially to the end-arterial vasculature of the grey-white matter regions of the cerebrum.[27] Clinical signs are related to tumor location and the secondary effects. Dogs with intracranial extension of nasal carcinoma may present only with CNS signs. Chemotherapy and radiation therapy can indirectly or directly affect the nervous system. Paraneoplastic effects cause mainly PNS changes, including neuropathy (e.g., secondary to insulinoma, carcinoma, sarcoma) and myasthenia gravis (e.g., secondary to thymoma, osteogenic sarcoma).

REFERENCES

1. Arieff AI, Griggs RC: General considerations in metabolic encephalopathies and systemic disorders of the nervous system. In Arieff AI, Griggs RC (eds): Metabolic Brain Dysfunction in Systemic Disease. Boston, Little, Brown, 1992, p 1.
2. O'Brien DP, Kroll RA: Metabolic encephalopathies. In Kirk RW, Bonagura JD (eds): Current Veterinary Therapy XI. Philadelphia, WB Saunders, 1992, p 998.
3. Schaumberg HH, et al: Disorders of peripheral nerve. In Plum F (ed): Contemporary Neurology Series, 2nd ed, vol 36. Philadelphia, FA Davis, 1992, p 348.
4. Norris JW, Pappiu HM: Cerebral water and electrolytes: Effect of asphyxia, hypoxia, and hypercapnia. Arch Neurol 23:248, 1970.
5. Joseph RJ, et al: Canine cerebrovascular disease: Clinical and pathological findings in 17 cases. J Am Anim Hosp Assoc 24:569, 1988.
6. Melhaff CJ, et al: Insulin-producing islet cell neoplasms: Surgical considerations and general management in 35 dogs. J Am Anim Hosp Assoc 21:607, 1985.
7. Leifer CE, et al: Hypoglycemia associated with nonislet cell tumor in 13 dogs. JAVMA 186:53, 1985.
8. Whitley NT, et al: Insulin overdose in dogs and cats: 28 cases (1986–1993). JAVMA 211:326, 1997.
9. Garcia JH, et al: Post-ischemic brain edema: Quantitation and evolution. In Cervos-Navarro J, Ferszt R (eds): Brain Edema: Pathology, Diagnosis, and Therapy. New York, Raven, 1980, p 147.
10. Laureno R: Central pontine myelinolysis following rapid correction of hyponatremia. Ann Neurol 13:232, 1983.
11. DiBartola SP: Disorders of sodium and water: Hypernatremia and hyponatremia.

CNS

In DiBartola SP (ed): Fluid Therapy in Small Animal Practice. Philadelphia, WB Saunders, 1992, p 57.

12. Harb MF, et al: Central diabetes insipidus in dogs: 20 cases (1986–1995). JAVMA 209:1884, 1996.

13. Steiss JE, et al: Electrodiagnostic analysis of peripheral neuropathy in dogs with diabetes mellitus. Am J Vet Res 42:2061, 1981.

14. Dow SW, et al: Potassium depletion in cats: Hypokalemic polymyopathy. JAVMA 191:1563, 1987.

15. Chew DJ, Meuten DJ: Disorders of calcium and phosphorus metabolism. Vet Clin North Am 12:411, 1983.

16. Nagode LA, et al: Benefits of calcitriol therapy and serum phosphorus control in dogs and cats with chronic renal failure. Vet Clin North Am 26:1293, 1996.

17. Wolf A: Canine uremic encephalopathy. J Am Anim Hosp Assoc 16:735, 1980.

18. Maddison JE: Hepatic encephalopathy: Current concepts and pathogenesis. J Vet Intern Med 6:341, 1992.

19. Lawrence D, et al: Results of surgical management of portosystemic shunts in dogs: 20 cases (1985–1990). JAVMA 201:1750, 1992.

20. Matushek KJ, et al: Generalized motor seizures after portosystemic shunt ligation in dogs: Five cases (1981–1988). JAVMA 196:2014, 1990.

21. Bichsel P, et al: Neurologic manifestations associated with hypothyroidism in four dogs. JAVMA 192:1745, 1988.

22. Jaggy A, et al: Neurological manifestations of hypothyroidism: A retrospective study of 29 dogs. J Vet Intern Med 8:328, 1994.

23. Peterson ME, et al: Pretreatment clinical and laboratory findings in dogs with hypoadrenocorticism: 225 cases (1979–1993). JAVMA 208:85, 1996.

24. Betroy EH, et al: One-year follow-up evaluation of magnetic resonance imaging of the brain in dogs with pituitary-dependent hyperadrenocorticism. JAVMA 208:1268, 1996.

25. Gilson SD, et al: Pheochromoctyoma in 50 dogs. J Vet Intern Med 8:228, 1994.

26. Posner JB: Neurologic Complications of Cancer. Philadelphia, FA Davis, 1995, p 1.

27. Fenner WR: Metastatic neoplasms of the central nervous system. *In* Murtaugh RJ (ed): Seminars in Veterinary Medicine and Surgery (Small Animal). Philadelphia, WB Saunders, 1990, p 253.

CHAPTER 104

DISEASES OF THE BRAIN

William R. Fenner

In most patients, only one brain area will be affected by a disease (focal disorders); however, with certain disorders, such as encephalitis, multiple brain areas will be involved simultaneously (diffuse disorders). The cerebrum is also highly susceptible to metabolic changes, so many systemic disorders, e.g., hypoglycemia or hyperviscosity syndromes, may present with predominantly neurologic manifestations.

First ask, "where is the problem," then "what is causing the problem," and finally "what can be done to resolve the problem." The neurologic examination generally answers the first question. The second is answered by integrating the lesion's location, the patient's history, and diagnostic test results. The third answer is derived by past experience, consulting reference texts, and consulting colleagues.

Identifying the disease process causing a patient's clinical signs requires that you first obtain a complete history of the patient's illness. The clinical signs' speed of onset, when considered with their rate and order of progression, will generally allow you to establish a differential diagnosis. This differential diagnosis is further defined by the lesion's location and the patient species. Diagnostic tests are chosen to distinguish between the rank-ordered differential diagnoses; thus establishing a diagnosis becomes possible (Fig. 104–1).

DIAGNOSTIC APPROACH TO PATIENTS

Historical Review and Client Complaints. Although the neurologic examination localizes a patient's problem within the nervous system, the primary complaint and the natural history of an illness provide the most information about the cause. A history has two components; a general history of the patient's previous care and a specific history that expands on the primary complaint to fully investigate the present illness. The information obtained from a history can be subdivided into three broad categories: anatomic, etiologic, and prognostic.

Anatomically, a history provides two types of information. The history may determine if a patient actually has a dysfunction of the nervous system. Epilepsy, narcolepsy, and myasthenia gravis are examples of nervous system diseases in which the neurologic examination may be normal. In those disorders, the history is crucial to establishing the presence of a nervous system disorder. Historical information may aid in localizing a problem within the nervous system. Back pain, for example, both localizes a lesion to the spinal column and tells a clinician that the problem is extramedullary. With epilepsy, the history confirms the presence of CNS dysfunction and localizes it to the cerebrum.

The most valuable historical information is a more complete etiologic understanding of a patient's problem. If diseases are classified according to the DAMNIT system, conditions in each major disease category tend to follow a historical pattern common to all diseases in that category (Table 104–1). Degenerations are slow in onset but relent-

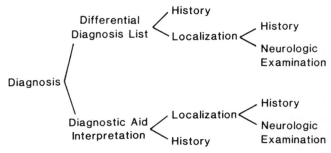

Figure 104–1. Diagnostic approach to patients with neurologic disease.

TABLE 104–1. THE DAMNIT SYSTEM

D egenerative
A nomalous
M etabolic, Malformations
N utritional, Neoplastic
I nflammatory, Immune, Ischemic (Vascular)
T oxic, Traumatic

lessly progressive. Isolated trauma, on the other hand, is acute in onset, but then has a static or improving course. The history allows ranking diseases most resembling the patient's historical course high on the diagnostic list, while eliminating other disorders from consideration. The etiologic information also helps choose and interpret diagnostic aids. Trauma, neoplasia, and vascular injuries to the CNS may produce an elevation of cerebrospinal fluid (CSF) albumin without elevating the white blood cell (WBC) count. When the CSF results are considered in light of the patient's history, the results are easier to interpret, as these conditions have different natural histories.

Obtaining the History. A thorough review includes current health: past illnesses, vaccination status, and body systems. With long-standing patients, this information will already be part of your medical records. With new patients, this general information may be critical to a successful diagnosis. Prior illness, injury, or medical or surgical problems may have resulted in permanent neurologic damage that would confuse the current neurologic examination. Prior knowledge prevents your chasing an unlikely diagnosis.

Certain diseases, such as globoid cell leukodystrophy in Cairn terriers and spinal muscular atrophy of Brittany spaniels, are known to have both age and breed predilections. The animal's use may determine the extent of diagnosis and therapy acceptable to a client (e.g., epilepsy may be acceptable in a companion animal, but not in a guide dog). Inquire about the environment, diet, exposure to toxins, or nutritional deficiencies.

Ask clients to describe what they actually notice, not what they think is causing the problem. For example, a client might say, "My dog is blind." If you let it go at that, the conclusion becomes, "There is a visual deficit." However, if you ask, "Why do you think the dog is blind? What do you see happening?" you may find the owner suspects blindness because the pet loses its balance and bumps into objects while falling. The patient has a vestibular, not a visual problem. Your job is to separate clinical fact from clinical fiction.

Ask how, when, and where the problem started; then what happened next. Most disorders fall into one of three patterns: acute, subacute, or chronic (Fig. 104–2). With acute disorders, the signs develop rapidly, often reaching their maximal intensity within 24 hours. Peracute disorders may reach maximal intensity within minutes of onset. Examples of acute or peracute disorders include trauma, some toxic or metabolic injuries, and vascular disorders. Acute exacerbations may develop in the course of a more chronic disorder, such as brain herniation during the course of a brain tumor.

Signs in subacute disorders usually develop progressively over days to weeks. Examples of subacute disorders include most inflammatory, many metabolic, and some neoplastic processes. In chronic disorders, signs continue to develop over months to years. Examples of chronic disorders include degenerations, nutritional disorders, some metabolic disorders (especially intrinsic ones, e.g., lysosomal storage disorders), and tumors.

Clinical progression is related to onset. Have the signs changed and, if so, how? Static signs do not change since initial onset, implying an anomaly, or possibly nervous system trauma or infarct. Progressive signs increase in severity of the disorder over time. Progression may reflect increasing severity of the initial signs and/or addition of new signs.

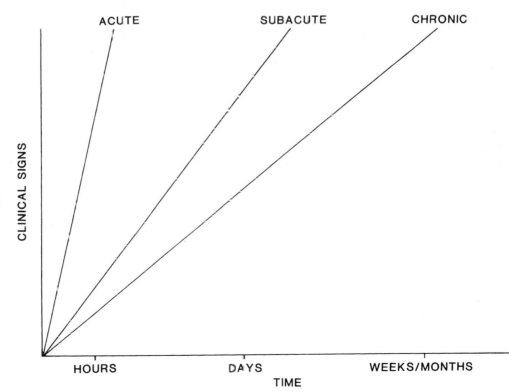

Figure 104–2. Time/sign graph demonstrating onset of neurologic signs.

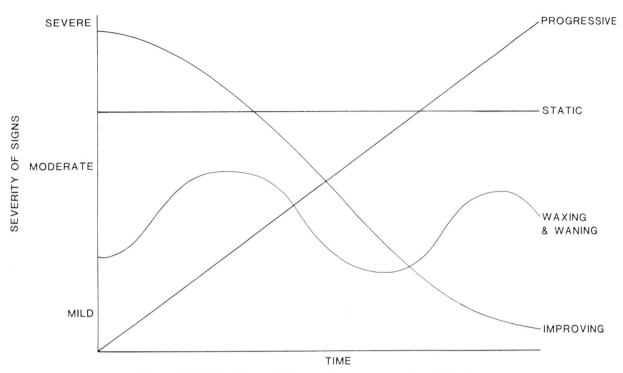

Figure 104–3. Time/sign graph demonstrating progression of neurologic signs.

Clinical worsening is characteristic of inflammations, degenerations, and neoplasms. If the disease process continues to damage the initially affected tissues but also begins to compress adjacent tissues, e.g., tumors, additional signs develop. In many degenerations, where the pathology is confined to a functional group of cells within the nervous system, e.g., cerebellar abiotrophies, the worsening is largely confined to increasing severity of the initial signs.

The clinical course may also improve and signs present at the onset of illness may lessen in severity or resolve. An improving course is most typical of vascular and traumatic injuries to the nervous system. Finally, the signs may vary in intensity over time—i.e., they wax and wane. Waxing and waning patterns are especially characteristic of metabolic disorders, e.g., hepatoencephalopathy, spinal instabilities, immune disorders, or incompletely treated CNS inflammatory diseases. Combining information about the onset and progression of a patient's signs is often sufficient to determine a probable disease category in a patient (Fig. 104–3).

A disorder's anatomic course reflects how it spreads to involve other portions of the nervous system. Do the signs represent a logical progression or a random change? A logical progression is seen in disorders in which the signs change because of progressive involvement of anatomic areas adjacent to the initial site. With an improving disorder, the first area to improve should be the most peripheral area of the injury. Logically progressive disorders are usually expanding mass lesions, which include neoplasms, abscesses, granulomas, and edema fluid around trauma. Logical improvement usually results when masses decrease in size, e.g., resolving hematomas, infarcts, and edema fluid around trauma (Fig. 104–4). A special variant of logical progression is seen with systems degenerations, e.g., spinal muscular atrophy of Brittany spaniels or cerebellar abiotrophies. In these conditions, the problem affects groups of functionally related cells, e.g., lower motor neurons or Purkinje cells,

which may be widely scattered throughout the nervous system. Most of these conditions are chronic, and the clinical picture is steady worsening of a single complex of signs—e.g., in spinal muscular atrophy, the patients have progressive weakness and atrophy of muscles.

With random progression, signs do not appear in a logical order; rather, they appear in unrelated portions of the nervous system, without rhyme or reason to the sequence in which they appear. This is most typical in inflammatory diseases, especially those caused by infectious agents. This pattern may also be seen with some toxic, nutritional, and metabolic disorders, as well as with metastatic neoplasms (Fig. 104–5).

In some disorders, there is widespread, symmetric involvement of the nervous system from the earliest stage of the illness. This diffuse pattern is similar to that seen with systems disturbances. Diffuse clinical signs are characteristic of metabolic, toxic, nutrition, and degenerative disorders (Fig. 104–6).

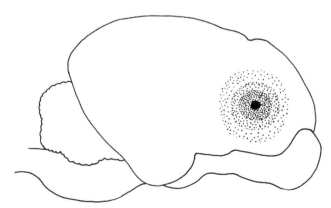

Figure 104–4. Anatomic representation of a logical progression/regression of neurologic disease.

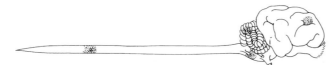

Figure 104–5. Anatomic representation of a random progression of a neurologic disorder.

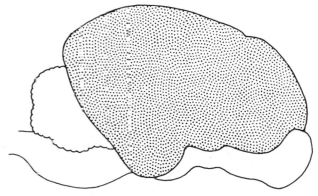

Figure 104–6. Anatomic representation of a diffuse neurologic disorder.

Inquire about aggravating factors. Do signs worsen with exercise, excitement, or stress, as they would in a patient with narcolepsy, myasthenia gravis, and/or cardiac syncope? Are the signs worsened by a meal (metabolic disorders)? Is there any history that shows the signs dependent on a specific event? Consider what type of disorder would do this.

Investigate the effects of previous therapy. Have any therapies been tried already? What duration, dosage, and route of administration, and what clinical effect? If possible, have the client keep a record of the times that drugs are given and their effect on the patient's illness.

Organizing the Information. The history allows you to make a time/sign graph that can be used to determine the major disorders that may be generating the patient's signs. Each major disease category tends to have a historical pattern that runs true for that pathologic process, across species and specific etiologic lines (Fig. 104–7). The following is a brief summary of those patterns.

DISEASE CATEGORIES

Toxic Injuries. Exposure to an injurious chemical may result in clinical nervous system disorders. Environmental exposure (e.g., lead, mercury, organophosphate) is most common, but microorganisms may also generate toxins (e.g., tetanus or botulism). Toxins may affect the nervous system by impairing neuronal respiration or axon transport, by impairing release of neurotransmitter, by enhancing the action of neurotransmitter, or by mimicking the action of neurotransmitter. Toxic effects that affect neurotransmitters are frequently reversible if exposure to the toxin is ended. Toxic

effects that impair neuronal respiration or axon transport may be irreversible, as they may result in either the neuron's or axon's death. Clinical signs of toxic injuries are generally acute in onset, with the signs diffuse from the onset. Anatomic involvement may be restricted to a functional system (tetanus = inhibitory interneurons) or to a morphologic region (lead poisoning = cerebrum). Patients with toxic injuries usually begin improving shortly after exposure to the toxin is ended or the toxin is successfully removed from the body, e.g., with chelation in lead poisoning. Most toxic illnesses are monophasic if correctly diagnosed and treated (acute onset, rapid stabilization, then improvement and recovery).

Metabolic and Nutritional Injuries. Metabolic and nutritional injuries occur when the nervous system either is deprived of a factor essential for survival or is exposed to toxic metabolic by-products that persist in the body as a result of failure of another organ system. A deficiency state may be due to the lack of a nutrient in the diet (e.g., thiamine deficiency); an inherited enzyme deficiency (e.g., lysosomal storage disorders); or a patient's inability to maintain an adequate nutrient supply (e.g., hypoglycemia owing to insulin excess). Toxic metabolic states usually reflect damage to one of the organ systems responsible for removing toxic by-

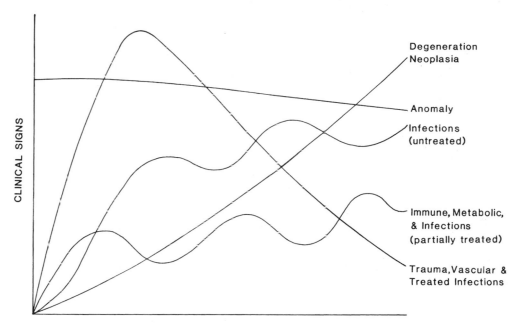

Figure 104–7. Time/sign graph demonstrating the onset and progression of common pathogenetic mechanisms of neurologic disease.

CLINICAL SIGNS

Degeneration
Neoplasia

Anomaly

Infections
(untreated)

Immune, Metabolic,
& Infections
(partially treated)

Trauma, Vascular &
Treated Infections

TIME

products of metabolism from the systemic circulation, e.g., the kidneys or liver. The clinical onset of metabolic encephalopathies is quite variable. Acute onset of signs is rare and usually seen with substrate deficiencies, e.g., hypoglycemia. Subacute clinical onset appears most common in patients with metabolic and nutritional disorders, and chronic onset is relatively uncommon. All metabolic and nutritional diseases tend to be diffuse at onset, with a widespread, symmetric involvement of the nervous system from the earliest state of the illness. Most of these conditions wax and wane, although some patients with enzyme deficiencies have chronically progressive signs.

Trauma. Traumatic nervous system injuries generally have an acute clinical onset. The trauma produces local swelling, loss of blood supply, nervous system hypoxia, and necrosis. When these secondary processes stabilize, the nervous system begins to repair itself. The severity of the initial injury and whether or not there is residual compression from the initiating process (e.g., a herniated intervertebral disk) determine the success of the repairs. If repair occurs, the signs of traumatic nervous system injury are generally focal and improve in a logical pattern. If there is instability associated with the injury (e.g., with spinal fractures or vertebral instabilities), the clinical signs might wax and wane. If repairs are unsuccessful, the patient will have an acute onset, but then a static clinical course.

Vascular. Vascular injury to the nervous system may result from loss of blood supply (ischemia/infarct) or from hemorrhage into the nervous system. In most cases, the initial process is focal, regardless of type. It is possible with systemic bleeding disorders to have multifocal or diffuse hemorrhage, with subsequent multifocal onset. The onset is almost always acute, with a logical progression, then logical improvement of focal signs. Vascular patients usually improve, resulting in a monophasic illness. Rarely (e.g., in the case of bleeding disorders), the signs may be progressive.

Malformations and Anomalies. Malformations and anomalies may cause nervous system dysfunction in one of two ways, each having a different clinical course. If the anomaly or malformation is in the substance of the nervous tissue itself (e.g., congenital syringomyelia or spinal dysraphism), the clinical signs are usually apparent at birth and there is little progression of the disease. A notable exception is hydrocephalus, which is often progressive. If the malformation is in the tissues that support the nervous system—for example, the skull or spine—the abnormality may not cause signs until late in the course of the animal's life if at all (e.g., hemivertebrae, occipital dysplasia). This late onset occurs because, in most cases, the signs result from nervous tissue compression. The compression may take months or years to develop, often resulting from joint instability. Regardless of the onset with malformations and anomalies, the signs are usually logical in their progression and represent a local injury.

Tumors. Tumors generally produce signs as a result of compression and replacement of nervous tissue parenchyma by proliferating neoplastic tissue. The nervous system may also suffer vascular compromise (ischemia), bleeding, edema, and inflammation around the tumor site. These secondary changes often produce as many clinical signs as the primary tumor itself. Normally in CNS tumors, the signs are subacute or chronic in onset, with a logical progression of local signs. Metastatic tumors may have a random progression and be more rapid in their onset. Patients with secondary events (e.g., ischemia) may also have acute exacerbations of their more chronic condition.

Inflammations. Inflammations may be either focal or disseminated. Focal inflammations are the least common in the nervous system and may reflect a focal abscess or solitary granuloma. A brain abscess, which is a local region of necrosis and suppuration that usually occur in response to bacterial infection, is relatively uncommon in dogs and cats. The clinical signs reflect a rapidly expanding mass lesion produced by the inflammatory process and its associated tissue edema. The signs are typically acute to subacute in onset, with a logical progression of local signs. If the patient has received inadequate therapy, the signs may wax and wane rather than progress. Solitary granulomas, which represent an accumulation of inflammatory cells, intermingled with a fibrotic reaction, are also seen rarely in the nervous system. They are usually the result of the body's attempts to remove or neutralize some chronic irritant, e.g., a fungal organism, a protozoal organism, a foreign body, or a parasite. The predominant cell type seen in the granuloma is a reflection of the chronicity of the process as well as the initiating agent. Depending on the etiology, granulomas may be focal (foreign body) or multifocal (disseminated), such as occurs with an infection. Granulomas tend to be slower in onset and progression than abscesses; they are usually subacute to chronic. Focal granulomas are logically progressive in most cases, representing expansion of a local mass.

Disseminated inflammations may result from infectious causes or immune disorders, or the cause may be unknown. In all cases, there is a widespread nervous system infiltration with inflammatory cells whose type is determined by the specific etiology. Frequently there is edema of adjacent tissue, secondary reaction to inflammatory by-products, and vascular compromise in addition to the primary inflammation. Disseminated inflammations cause widespread nervous system failure. Inflammations are generally subacute but may occur acutely or chronically, depending on the specific cause. Random progression is likely, although in some cases the signs may wax and wane. In some patients (e.g., dogs with granulomatous meningoencephalitis), the initial signs may appear focal, then as additional granulomas manifest themselves, the true disseminated nature of the illness becomes apparent.

THE NEUROLOGIC EXAMINATION

A careful neurologic examination is the basis for localizing a lesion in the CNS.[1-3] Localizing a lesion is somewhat like working a jigsaw puzzle; neuroanatomy is the illustration on the box cover that allows you to place the examination pieces together.

The examination includes observation, watching the gait, carefully palpating for abnormal muscle tone and mass, performing tests of reflexes and reactions in that patient, and finally interpreting the information in order to answer a series of questions about that patient.

The neurologic examination cannot be understood without at least some knowledge of neuroanatomy. Morphologically, the nervous system may be subdivided two ways: into functional systems and into anatomic regions. The functional systems are composed of those cells and their processes concerned with a specific function: examples are the motor system, the pain perception (nociceptive) system, the system of consciousness (reticular activating system), and the balance (special proprioceptive) system. These functional systems extend through many different focal anatomic regions, but not all anatomic regions contain cells for every functional system. An example would be the cerebrum, which does not contain cells from the unconscious proprioceptive system; therefore, cerebral disorders rarely cause ataxia. The cerebellum does not contain fibers from the motor system; therefore, cerebellar disorders do not cause weakness. Focal anatomic regions are discrete sections of the nervous system (such as the brain stem, cerebrum, and cerebellum in the brain) organized around certain functions or reflexes unique to that specific area. As an example, the cerebrum is concerned with memory, higher order function, and vision. The brain stem is concerned with vegetative functions of the body, e.g., heart rate and respiration. Each focal anatomic region contains fibers or cells from one or more functional systems.

The major functional systems are consciousness, motor, nociception, proprioception (unconscious = muscle stretch, conscious = joint perception and position, special = balance and orientation to gravity), and the autonomic system. The major anatomic regions are cerebrum (including diencephalon), cerebellum, brain stem (including midbrain, pons, and medulla), spinal cord, and peripheral nervous system. When the anatomic regions with their unique feature and their functional systems are combined, they are distinguished as follows: *cerebrum* = consciousness, voluntary motor regulation, pain localization, joint perception, vision, learning, behavior, and some cranial nerve response; *cerebellum* = muscle stretch perception, balance, and fine motor coordination; *brain stem* = consciousness, postural motor regulation, pain recognition, joint perception, muscle stretch perception, balance, the autonomic systems, cranial nerve reflexes, and vegetative functions; *spinal cord* = motor regulation, pain perception, joint perception, muscle stretch perception, balance (cranial cervical cord), the autonomic system, and spinal reflexes; the *peripheral nervous system (PNS)* is concerned with motor regulation, pain recognition, joint perception, muscle stretch perception, the autonomic systems, and reflexes. These combinations yield a brief summary of the clinical signs expected with lesions in each local anatomic region (Table 104–2). The neurologic examination allows the clinician to test the various functional systems and local reflexes to pinpoint the disease process.

Conduct the examination in a logical, methodical, and consistent manner. Develop a specific sequence and follow it on all patients. Start with the general and advance to the specific, leaving painful portions of the examination until the end. Remember that all reactions and responses require both sensory input and motor output. Clinicians often assume an abnormality reflects a lesion on the motor side of the reflex arc, when the converse is true. A classic example is the depressed patellar reflexes seen in about 50 per cent of dogs with old dog degenerative myelopathy. These dogs generally also manifest the presence of crossed extensors on examination. The crossed extensors confirm that the motor pathways of the reflex arc are intact. The depressed tendon reflexes in these patients are the result of injury to the dorsal nerve roots.

Make a list of all abnormal findings in the patient as the examination is conducted. The best way to do this is to use a standard neurologic examination form, either copied from a text or created on your own (Fig. 104–8). When the examination is completed, try to explain all of the findings with a lesion confined to a single focus within the nervous system. If all the signs can be explained with such a single lesion, the cause is probably a focal disease such as an infarct or a neoplasm. If you cannot explain all the signs with a single lesion, the patient probably has a disseminated

TABLE 104–2. SUMMARY OF CLINICAL SIGNS WITH LESIONS IN ANATOMIC REGIONS

ANATOMIC REGION	CLINICAL SIGNS
Cerebrum	Mentational changes Visual deficits (normal pupils) Circling Weakness (hemi- or tetraparesis) Seizures Abnormal (delayed) postural reactions
Cerebellum	Ataxia Intentional tremors Normal strength Abnormal (ataxic) postural reactions Head tilt (variable) Menace deficit (rare) Torticollis (rare) Pathologic nystagmus
Brain stem	Cranial nerve deficits Pathologic nystagmus Weakness Abnormal (delayed) postural reactions Ataxia Head tilts Circling Depressed mental state Respiratory depression Cardiac arrhythmias
Vestibular injury	Pathologic nystagmus Abnormal (ataxic) postural reactions Ataxia Head tilts Circling Falling or rolling Positional strabismus Abnormal muscle tone
Spinal cord injury	Weakness Abnormal (delayed) postural reactions Ataxia Abnormal spinal reflexes Pain Bladder and bowel paralysis Horner's syndrome (rarely) Respiratory distress (rarely)
Peripheral spinal nerve injury	Weakness Depressed (absent) spinal reflexes Abnormal (delayed) postural reactions Hypotonia Atrophy Analgesia Pain
Peripheral cranial nerve injury	Loss of affected cranial nerve function

disorder, such as an inflammation or degeneration. In this sense, the neurologic examination also helps to determine the etiology of a problem.

Normal findings are as important as the abnormal in arriving at a localization. Take, for example, a tetraparetic dog whose sole findings on neurologic examination are weakness and exaggerated limb reflexes in all four limbs. A lesion involving both cerebral hemispheres, the brain stem, or the cranial cervical spinal cord could result in such a weakness. However, the cerebral and brain stem injury would each cause additional signs, such as changes in mental status or cranial nerve function. It is the absence of such deficits that allows you to localize this patient's injury to the cervical spinal cord. Secondary objectives achieved by performing the neurologic examination include determining the extent of nervous system involvement, guidance when choosing diagnostic aids, and assistance in arriving at a prognosis.

NEUROLOGY CONSULTATION FORM

The Ohio State University Veterinary Teaching Hospital

OSU case: CLIENT NAME DATE

CLINICIAN BREED DOB SEX

STUDENT CAGE/STALL

Clinical questions:

Patient history:

Current therapy:

NEUROLOGIC EXAMINATION

General observations

Mental status:

Gait/Stance:

Level of ataxia/wkns

Cranial Nerve Exam:

	LEFT	RIGHT
Menace reaction		
PLR (OS stimulated)		
PLR (OD stimulated)		
Pupil size		
Pupil symmetry		
Strabismus		
Pathologic nystagmus		
Nystagmus description		

	LEFT	RIGHT
Oculovestibular reflex		
Facial reflex		
Palpebral reflex		
Retractor Oculi		
Facial Sensation		
Facial symmetry		
Gag reflex		
Tongue function		

Limb Exam:

	Thoracic limbs LEFT	Thoracic limbs RIGHT	Pelvic Limbs LEFT	Pelvic Limbs RIGHT
Postural reaction				
Hopping				
Hemistanding				
Flexor reflex				
Triceps reflex				
Biceps reflex				
Patellar reflex				
Cranial tibial reflex				
Crossed extensor reflex				
Babinski reflex				

Anal reflex:

Bladder size/tone:

Nociceptive exam:

NEUROLOCALIZATION:

ASSESSMENT AND RECOMMENDATIONS:

EXAMINER

Figure 104–8.

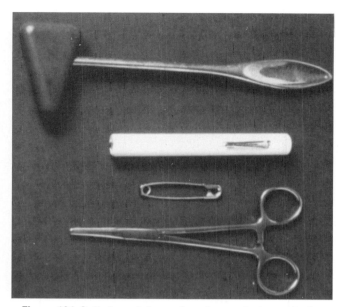

Figure 104–9. Tools needed to perform the neurologic examination.

The tools required to perform the neurologic examination on a patient are simple and inexpensive. The include an instrument for striking tendons, such as a reflex hammer or bandage scissors; a strong light source; a pair of hemostats; and a safety pin. With these tools, a clinician should be able to perform a complete neurologic examination (Fig. 104–9).

TECHNIQUE OF THE EXAMINATION

The author divides the neurologic examination into six parts: general observations, gait and stance, postural reaction testing, cranial nerve examination, spinal reflex examination, and pain perception evaluation. The general observations, gait and stance, and postural reactions all evaluate general functional systems. The cranial nerve examination primarily tests local anatomic regions, while the spinal reflex examination and evaluation of pain perception test both functional systems and local anatomic regions.

GENERAL OBSERVATIONS

The general observations include mental status, head posture, head coordination, and the tendency to circle. Observe the patient from a distance before putting the animal on the examination table or handling the animal (Table 104–3).

Mental Status. Is the patient alert, aware of its surroundings, and oriented to gravity (mental status examination)? The mental status examination evaluates primarily the cerebrum and brain stem, although the vestibulo-cerebellar system is also partially evaluated. Normal animals are alert and aware of their surroundings. Patients with disorders that affect either brain stem or cerebrum may have disorders of consciousness. Injury to the rostral brain stem may damage the reticular activating system (RAS), the portion of the brain that controls level of consciousness and regulates sleep-wake cycles. RAS injury depresses the level of consciousness, which, depending on the severity of the change in consciousness, may be classified as depression, stupor, or coma. The RAS regulates consciousness by modulating cerebral activity. Thus cerebral disorders may also depress the level of consciousness. Generally, to decrease the level of consciousness, a cerebral injury must involve both cerebral hemispheres and be rapid in onset. Examples of conditions which can affect the cerebrum in such a manner include metabolic disorders (e.g., hepatoencephalopathy, hypoglycemia) plus inflammatory disorders (e.g., encephalitis). Some patients with cerebral disorders have a hyperalert state (delirium) or sleep-wake cycle reversal rather than a depressed level of consciousness.

Injuries to the cerebrum may change the content of consciousness as well. Such a change is referred to as dementia. Affected animals have loss of self-awareness; they may wander aimlessly, head-press, or display other inappropriate behaviors. Any cerebral injury is capable of causing dementia, with or without associated stupor.

Since loss of balance will create a profound disorientation, patients with vestibulo-cerebellar disorders may appear to have an abnormal mental state. This is not a true mental status abnormality, but can appear so to the client. True consciousness disorders are always a sign of brain dysfunction.

Head Posture. Does the patient have normal head and neck posture, or does it have a head tilt or other abnormality (vestibulo-cerebellar examination)? In a normal patient, the head is parallel to the ground and the neck is straight. In patients with vestibular disorders, the head is often tilted (usually toward the side of the lesion) (Fig. 104–10). These patients may also have torticollis (a twisted neck). Patients with cervical spinal injuries may also have torticollis, but without the associated head tilt of vestibular injury. Is the patient able to elevate the head? If the animal is unable to raise its head, the examiner should be suspicious of neck

TABLE 104–3. GENERAL OBSERVATIONS

OBSERVATION	SYSTEM EVALUATED	NORMAL FINDING	ABNORMAL FINDING
Mental status	Reticular activating system (rostral brain stem)	Alert	Depression, stupor, or coma
	Cerebrum	Alert and appropriate	Dementia, delirium, depression, stupor, or coma
	Vestibulo-cerebellar	Oriented	Loss of balance
Head posture	Vestibulo-cerebellar	Head parallel to ground	Head tilt
	Motor system to neck	Neck aligned with body	Torticollis
		Normal elevation of head	Unable to raise neck
Gait and stance	Proprioceptive system		
	Conscious	Limbs normal position	Limbs knuckle under
	Unconscious	Smooth gait	Ataxia, hypermetria
	Special	Limbs normal position	Broad-based stance, ataxia
	Motor system	Normal strength	Weakness

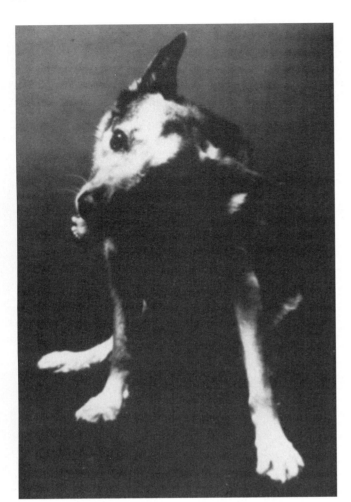

Figure 104–10. A patient demonstrating a head tilt.

weakness. Inability to raise the head has been seen with feline hypokalemic polymyopathy, occipital dysplasia in the dog, botulism, cervical vertebral malformations, and feline thiamine deficiency. The key to evaluating disorders of head posture is to look for limb changes or cranial nerve deficits that will indicate a central localization of the injury.

Head Coordination. The head is coordinated primarily by the cerebellum, with some input from the vestibular system. Disturbances of head coordination typically appear as head tremor, which implies a cerebellar (or a cerebellar peduncular) lesion. Such tremor is often exaggerated when the animal attempts purposeful movement, such as eating or drinking (intention tremor).

Circling. Does the patient walk in a straight line, or tend to circle? If the patient circles, is it always in the same direction? Many patients with injuries to the brain will tend to circle. The mere presence of circling does not localize the injury to a specific brain region, but generally the patient does circle toward the side of the injury. Patients with vestibular system injuries usually have concomitant head tilts and also are more likely to circle in only one direction. Patients with cerebral injuries rarely have head tilts and may circle in both directions (wander aimlessly) (Fig. 104–11).

STANCE AND GAIT

Does the patient have normal limb position at rest and a normal gait (proprioceptive and motor system examination)?

A normal animal stands with its thoracic limbs at approximately shoulder width and its pelvic limbs at about hip width, with the palmar aspect of the thoracic limbs and the plantar aspect of the pelvic limbs in contact with the ground. Patients may assume an abnormal stance as a result of weakness, loss of position sense, or pain. Animals with lesions of the conscious proprioceptive system will often stand "knuckled over," with the dorsal aspect of their paws in contact with the ground. Knuckling may be seen with injuries to the PNS, spinal cord, brain stem, or cerebrum. In a patient with cranial nerve deficits, knuckling is strong evidence of a brain disorder. Animals with special proprioceptive (vestibulo-cerebellar) dysfunction tend to have a broad-based stance. Without other abnormalities on the neurologic examination, a broad-based stance is not sufficient to make a central localization for a patient's problem. Holding up a limb or carrying a limb is generally a sign of pain. If the pain is neural in origin, it usually implies an injury to peripheral nerve, nerve root, or meninges.

A normal animal's gait should be smooth and well coordinated. Gaiting requires normal function of almost all parts of the nervous system. Loss of coordination (gait ataxia) tends to be manifested as irregular length of stride or an irregular rhythm of limb movement. Look carefully at an animal's nails for abnormal wear, which may suggest a gait disturbance not observed during the examination. Observe the gait in an area with good footing, such as on short-clipped grass or on carpeting. If there are steps or curbs available, make the patient go up and down them; this increases the demands on the nervous system, allowing subtle abnormalities to be detected.

Characterize the abnormalities present in the gait and which limbs are affected. While observing the gait, try to grade the severity of dysfunction in each limb so that improvement or worsening of the condition can be quantitated on follow-up examinations. Ataxia (an unconscious proprioceptive sign) may appear as swaying, veering, crossing over of the limbs, scuffing of the toes, etc. Ataxia may be seen with cerebellar, brain stem, spinal cord, or PNS injuries (of spinal nerves or cranial nerve VIII). Cerebral lesions rarely cause ataxia. Weakness is characterized by stumbling, falling, tripping, or inability to initiate or sustain an activity. Weakness may be caused by injury to the cere-

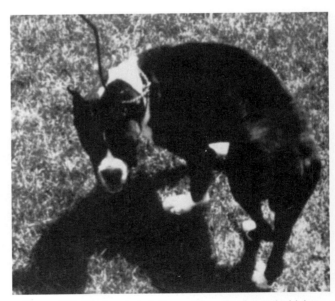

Figure 104–11. A patient circling as the result of a cerebral injury.

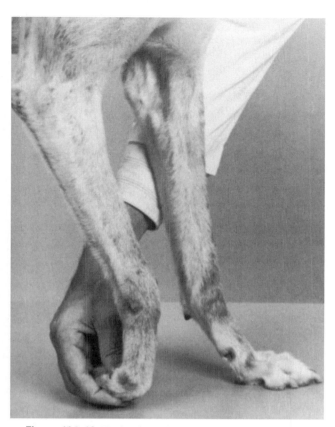

Figure 104–12. Testing for deficits in conscious proprioception.

brum, brain stem, spinal cord, or peripheral spinal nerve. Cranial nerve injuries and cerebellar injuries will not result in limb weakness.

In addition to the gait, observe muscle tone. Spasticity (an increase in muscle tone) may affect the gait, making it rigid and choppy. Spasticity may be seen with injuries to the cerebrum, brain stem, or spinal cord. Since spasticity indicates a lesion of an upper motor neuron (UMN), it confirms a central (CNS) lesion. Dysmetria is an abnormal length of stride, with the limb movements either exaggerated in length (hypermetria) or foreshortened (hypometria). Dysmetria may be seen with injury to the cerebellum, spinal cord, brain stem, peripheral spinal nerves, and cranial nerve VIII.

ATTITUDINAL AND POSTURAL REACTIONS

After evaluating the gait, test the attitudinal and postural reactions (A&P reactions). These reactions examine the proprioceptive fibers of peripheral nerves, spinal cord, brain stem, cerebrum, and cerebellum. Some test special proprioception as well, thus also testing the inner ear. These reactions also test the long motor pathways of the UMNs and their connections to the lower motor neurons (LMNs).

One technique is to place a patient's limb in an abnormal position to see if the patient returns the limb to a normal position. You may also make the patient carry more weight on a limb than normal and see if the limb can still be used normally.

These reactions are good screening tools for the detection of nervous system injury, but not particularly valuable in precise lesion localization. However, knowing which limbs are abnormal along with the type of abnormality seen may give a clue to the location of the lesion. Cerebral injuries

depress the A&P reactions. The clinical deficit is normally seen in both thoracic and pelvic limbs on the opposite side of the body from the damaged hemisphere (contralateral). With brain stem injuries, the reactions are depressed or absent. With brain stem injuries, the clinical signs are usually bilateral, but more severe on the same side of the body as the side of the brain stem injury (ipsilateral). With cerebellar injuries, the A&P reactions are usually still present, but ataxic. With peripheral vestibular injuries, the A&P reactions are preserved, but the patient tends to lean, fall, and roll to the affected side when the maneuvers are performed. With lesions in the spinal cord and peripheral spinal nerves, the A&P reactions tend to be depressed or absent on the side of the nervous system injury.

Proprioceptive Positioning. In this test, a limb is abnormally abducted or adducted, or the paw is knuckled under (Fig. 104–12). If the A&P reactions are intact, the patient briskly and smoothly brings the limb back to a normal resting position.

Hemihopping/Hemistanding/Hemiwalking. In this test, the patient's limbs on one side are held off the ground, while the patient is forced to walk sideways on its two remaining limbs (Fig. 104–13). This is an excellent test of strength. A normal animal has no trouble maintaining itself during this test. Weak animals sag and/or collapse on the abnormal side. This test is also excellent at detecting subtle asymmetries not detected on observation of gait.

Wheelbarrowing. In this test, first the patient's thoracic and then its pelvic limbs are held off the ground, while the patient is walked forwards and backwards on its two weight bearing limbs (Fig. 104–14). A normal animal has no trouble supporting itself during this test. Generally, the limbs move

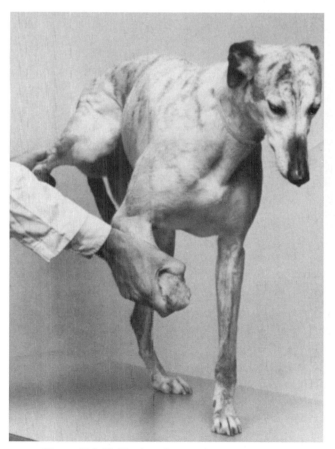

Figure 104–13. Hemistanding a patient to test strength.

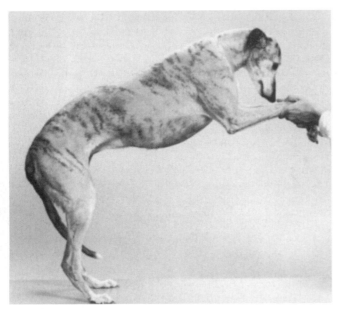

Figure 104–14. Wheelbarrowing an animal.

symmetrically. Animals tend to wheelbarrow forward better on the thoracic limbs, so differences between abilities going forward and abilities going backwards are less significant than differences between left and right limbs. This test is also good for detecting subtle limb deficits not seen during evaluation of the gait.

Hopping. In this test, the clinician supports all limbs except one, making the patient hop on the one weight-bearing limb (Fig. 104–15). The patient should be made to bear as much of its weight as possible on the limb being tested. This test is excellent for detecting subtle loss of strength, as well as for detecting left-to-right asymmetry between paired limbs.

Additional A&P Reactions. These include the extensor postural thrust reaction, righting reaction (which tests special proprioception), visual placing reactions, tactile placing reactions, and tonic neck reaction. Each test evaluates similar pathways, although each individual test may evaluate one portion of the nervous system more completely than another. These tests are all well described in standard neurology texts.[1, 2] In most patients, performing two or three of these tests is sufficient. Be certain to record which tests are performed and the abnormalities found so that on future examination, the same tests can be repeated for comparison.

CRANIAL NERVE EXAMINATION

During the routine cranial nerve examination, you will evaluate the function of cranial nerves II–X and cranial nerve XII. Cranial nerves I and XI are difficult to test as part of a routine examination. Normally, except for Horner's syndrome, a cranial nerve deficit indicates a lesion above the foramen magnum. A cranial nerve deficit, in combination with limb signs, is generally sufficient to confirm a brain injury. In most cases, the cranial nerve abnormalities will provide fairly precise localization of a lesion.

Anatomic Review

Animals have 12 pairs of cranial nerves, two of which originate in the cerebrum (including diencephalon). Nine

pairs originate in the brain stem, and one pair originates in both spinal cord and brain stem. All cranial nerves exit through foramina in the skull, thus the classification as cranial nerves.

The olfactory nerve (cranial nerve I) originates in the cerebrum, is sensory, and provides the sense of smell. This nerve is difficult to test, and clinical disorders of smell are rarely recognized in veterinary practice.

The optic nerve (cranial nerve II) also originates in the cerebrum (diencephalon), is sensory, and is concerned with vision and light perception. This nerve is tested using the menace response, which tests vision; by observation of pupil size; and via the pupillary light reflex, which tests pupillary accommodation to light.

Cranial nerve III (oculomotor nerve) originates in the brain stem (mesencephalon) and provides motor innervation to the eyeball. It has a parasympathetic division, which constricts the pupil in response to light (pupillary accommodation); and a somatic division, which moves the eyeball via the extraocular muscles. There is also some innervation of periorbital muscles, so damage to cranial nerve III may produce ptosis (a drooping of the upper eyelid). Cranial nerve III is tested with the pupillary light reflex, by observing pupil size and symmetry, by observing ocular position, and by observing ocular motility (the vestibulo-ocular reflexes).

Cranial nerve IV (trochlear) originates in the brain stem (mesencephalon) and provides motor innervation to the eyeball. It moves the eyeball via the extraocular muscles. Test this nerve by observing ocular position and ocular motility (the vestibulo-ocular reflexes).

Cranial nerve V (trigeminal) is both motor and sensory. It originates in the brain stem (metencephalon) and provides pain and proprioceptive information from the head, as well as motor innervation to the muscles of mastication. The sensory (nociceptive) information is carried to the contralateral cerebral hemisphere via the thalamus and generates avoidance responses to pain. This nerve is tested by corneal reflex, palpebral reflex, retractor oculi reflex, evaluation of jaw tone, and noxious stimulation of the face.

Cranial nerve VI (abducens) originates in the brain stem (myelencephalon) and provides motor innervation to the

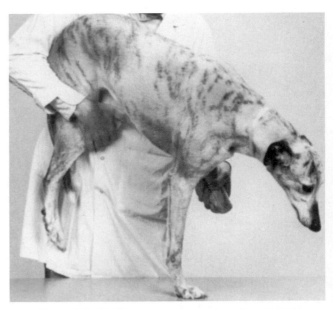

Figure 104–15. Hopping an animal, using a thoracic limb.

eyeball. It moves the eyeball via the extraocular and retractor oculi muscles. This nerve is tested by observing ocular position, by the retractor oculi reflex, and by observing ocular motility (the vestibulo-ocular reflexes).

Cranial nerve VII (facial) originates in the brain stem (myelencephalon) and provides both motor and sensory functions. It is motor to the muscles of facial expression, lacrimal glands, and salivary glands. It is sensory (taste) to the rostral third of the tongue. This nerve is tested by observing facial symmetry, the palpebral and corneal reflexes, and monitoring tear production. Testing of taste is crude and probably stimulates nociceptors of the tongue (cranial nerve V) in addition to cranial nerve VII.

Cranial nerve VIII (vestibulocochlear) originates in the brain stem (myelencephalon) and is sensory. This nerve is responsible for hearing, changes in posture relative to gravity, detection of angular (rotational) movement, and regulation of extraocular muscle tone. It is tested by observing extraocular motility, head posture, gait, balance, and vestibulo-ocular reflexes, and by electrical testing of hearing.

Cranial nerve IX (glossopharyngeal) originates in the caudal brain stem (myelencephalon). It provides sensory innervation (taste) to the caudal two thirds of the tongue, sensation to the pharynx, and motor innervation to the pharynx, palate, larynx, and some salivary glands. This nerve is tested by observing the gag reflex and swallowing motions. Under light sedation, the movement of the palate and arytenoids with respiration can be detected.

Cranial nerve X (vagus) originates in the brain stem (myelencephalon) and has predominately autonomic and some somatic motor functions. It regulates gastrointestinal motility, has regulatory functions over the heart, provides motor function for swallowing (along with cranial nerve IX), and regulates esophageal motility. It is tested by observing the gag reflex and swallowing behavior.

Cranial nerve XI (spinal accessory) originates in caudal brain stem (myelencephalon) and cranial cervical spinal cord. It is concerned with motor innervation to the elevators of the shoulder and to a lesser extent the head. It is a difficult nerve to test without electromyography.

Cranial nerve XII (hypoglossal) originates in the brain stem (myelencephalon) and is responsible for motor innervation of the tongue. This nerve can be tested indirectly by observing the tongue for voluntary movement and atrophy. Direct testing requires electromyography.

Unlike spinal nerves, some cranial nerves are purely sensory and others purely motor; thus testing a cranial nerve reflex usually tests more than one cranial nerve, e.g., the palpebral reflex tests both cranial nerves V (sensory) and VII (motor). This is unlike most spinal reflexes where a single spinal reflex tests a single peripheral nerve, e.g., patellar reflex tests femoral nerve (both motor and sensory). Additionally, many brain stem cranial nerve reflexes are modulated by the cerebrum. As such, testing a cranial nerve reflex usually tests two peripheral cranial nerves, one motor and one sensory; a central connection (usually in the brain stem); and a higher regulatory center (usually in the cerebrum).[4]

Tests of Cranial Nerve Function

The Menace Response. The menace response tests cranial nerves II (sensory), VII (motor), and their central connections in the brain stem and cerebrum (Fig. 104–16). Perform the test by making a menacing gesture toward an animal. The normal response is an avoidance behavior—for

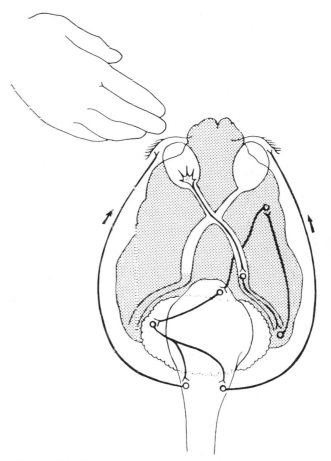

Figure 104–16. Anatomic representation of the menace pathways.

example, an eye blink on the side being menaced or turning the head away from the menacing gesture. Diminution or loss of the menace reaction normally indicates a lesion in one of the following sites: retina (ipsilateral), optic nerve (ipsilateral), optic tract (contralateral), cerebrum (contralateral), brain stem (ipsilateral), or facial nerve (ipsilateral). Some animals with cerebellar pathology may have an ipsilateral absence of the menace response as well.[5]

False-positive menace responses may also occur. The most common cause of a false-positive response is air currents produced by the hand that generates a corneal reflex. Vision requires normal consciousness, so the menace response is often absent or diminished in animals with a depressed level of consciousness, even when the visual pathways are anatomically intact.

The Pupillary Light Reflex (PLR). This reflex tests the reflex portion of cranial nerve II and the visceral (parasympathetic) function of cranial nerve III (Fig. 104–17). Perform the test by illuminating one eye with a bright light source. Normally both pupils constrict equally and rapidly. The pupillary constriction in the eye being illuminated is called the direct pupillary response, while the constriction in the opposite pupil (the one being illuminated indirectly) is called the consensual response. The PLR is abnormal when one or both pupils fail to constrict. An optic nerve (cranial nerve II) lesion will interfere with the light reflex. With such a lesion, neither pupil will constrict when the abnormal eye (cranial nerve II) is illuminated, i.e., there will be loss of both the direct pupillary light reflex in the affected eye and the consensual light reflex in the opposite eye. When the

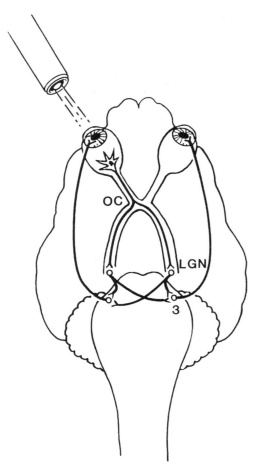

Figure 104–17. Anatomic representation of the pathways of the pupillary light reflex. OC = optic chiasm; LGN = lateral geniculate nucleus; and 3 = cranial nerve III.

will dilate more slowly than the normal eye in a dark room (poor dark adaptation). A number of ophthalmic disorders, including glaucoma, iritis, uveitis, and synechia, may produce anisocoria. Because of this, all patients with anisocoria should have a complete ophthalmic examination.

Pupil Size. The size of the pupil is determined by the amount of ambient light (cranial nerve II) and the integrity of the pupillary muscles (cranial nerve III and sympathetic nerve). Abnormally large pupils may be seen with excitement (sympathetic stimulation), bilateral cranial nerve II injury, cranial nerve III injury, and/or ophthalmic disease. Abnormally small pupils may be seen with loss of sympathetic tone (Horner's syndrome), excess parasympathetic tone, and ophthalmic disease.

Ocular Position. In normal dogs and cats, both eyes should appear to be looking ahead and in the same direction. Normal resting ocular position is determined by the influence of the cerebrum and cranial nerve VIII on the extraocular muscles, via cranial nerves III, IV, and VI (Fig. 104–18).[6] If one or more of these cranial nerves are not functioning, deviations from this parallel position (strabismus) may be seen. A lesion of cranial nerve III or cranial nerve VIII may result in a ventrolateral strabismus. A lesion to cranial nerve IV will produce intorsion (rotation) of the eye, which can only be detected on retinal examination in the dog. A lesion of cranial nerve VI will produce a medial strabismus. If the cerebrum is injured, there may be a gaze deviation rather than a strabismus. In this case, both eyes are looking in the same direction, but looking off to one side. Gaze deviations are uncommon in veterinary patients, generally reflecting an acute and severe cerebral injury. Animals with retrobulbar

eye with the normal cranial nerve II is illuminated, both pupils constrict as motor function is spared.

With an efferent lesion (a lesion of cranial nerve III or its nucleus in the brain stem), the affected (denervated) pupil will not constrict regardless of which eye is illuminated. In this case, the unaffected (normal) pupil will constrict normally as each eye is illuminated. Thus, with an efferent lesion, when the affected side is illuminated, there is an absent direct pupillary response, but a normal consensual in the opposite eye. When the normal eye is illuminated, it has a normal direct PLR, but there is now an absent consensual PLR in the opposite (diseased) eye.

Because non-neurologic disorders (e.g., posterior synechia, iris atrophy, glaucoma, and other ophthalmic diseases) may cause an abnormal PLR, a thorough ocular examination is essential in patients with abnormal pupils. Other causes of a sluggish PLR include excessive sympathetic tone (excitement), a weak light source, and prior administration of cycloplegic drugs.

Pupillary Symmetry. If the oculomotor nerve (parasympathetic) and sympathetic nerve to the eye are each normal, the two pupils will be equal in size. Unequal pupils (anisocoria) indicate possible damage to one of those two nerves. If the oculomotor nerve is abnormal, the denervated pupil will be larger than normal and the PLR will be absent or depressed in the affected eye. If the sympathetic nerve is abnormal, the affected pupil will be smaller than normal, the PLR will be preserved in both eyes, but the affected eye

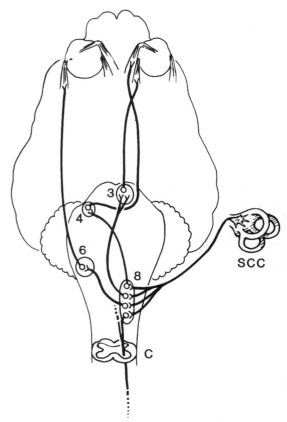

Figure 104–18. Anatomic representation of the pathways for ocular position. SCC = semicircular canal; C = cervical spinal cord; 3 = cranial nerve III; 4 = cranial nerve IV; 6 = cranial nerve VI; and 8 = cranial nerve VIII.

masses may show a strabismus if the mass physically displaces the eyeball.

Ocular Motility (Voluntary and Involuntary). *Voluntary* eye movement is initiated by cerebral stimulation of the pontine gaze centers, which in turn stimulate cranial nerves III, IV, and VI. As the patient looks around the examination room, see if it is able to move its eyes in all directions. With cerebral lesions, both eyes are involved and there is a tendency for the eyes to look toward the side of the diseased cerebral hemisphere (conjugate gaze deviation). With a cranial nerve lesion, only one eye is involved. That eye tends to have a strabismus at rest and lack the ability to move.

Clinicians can initiate *involuntary,* rhythmic oscillations of the eye, known as nystagmus, by turning the head. This maneuver stimulates cranial nerve VIII, which in turn stimulates cranial nerves III, IV, and VI, which innervate the extraocular muscles. This involuntary, reflex eye movement is known as "physiologic nystagmus" and the test is the vestibulo-ocular reflex (also sometimes referred to as the "doll's eye"). The normal patient will manifest a rhythmic oscillation of both eyes; first the eyes will tonically (slowly) deviate from the direction of head movement, followed by a rapid (saccadic) eye movement in the direction of head movement. Nystagmus is named for the direction of the fast (saccadic) component; thus in the vestibulo-ocular reflex, the nystagmus is in the direction of head movement. This slow-rapid, slow-rapid oscillation continues as long as the head is being turned. A lesion of cranial nerve VIII or its central connections can result in loss of the ability to initiate this physiologic nystagmus. With such a vestibular injury, physiologic nystagmus will not be seen in either eye when the head is turned toward the abnormal cranial nerve VIII. A lesion of cranial nerve III or VI will paralyze the eyeball on the side of the lesion. In that patient, there will be loss of physiologic nystagmus in the affected eye, regardless of direction of head movement, but the other (normal) eye will be normal.

Pathologic Nystagmus. A normal animal, whose head is stationary, will not have spontaneous nystagmus. If nystagmus is present in such an animal, it is considered abnormal and is referred to as pathologic nystagmus. Pathologic nystagmus usually results from an imbalance in the special proprioceptive system, which includes the inner ear, cranial nerve VIII, the brain stem, and the cerebellum. A lesion of any of those four structures can cause pathologic nystagmus. By noting the direction(s) of the nystagmus, whether or not the direction changes, and in what head positions the nystagmus is elicited, some conclusions may be drawn about the patient's lesion.

In horizontal nystagmus, the eyes move in a plane parallel to the animal's head (the eyes move from side to side). Horizontal nystagmus is most commonly seen in patients with peripheral vestibular injuries. The fast component (direction) of the nystagmus is typically away from the diseased side. In vertical nystagmus, the eyes move in a plane perpendicular to the animal's head (the eyes move up and down). This type of nystagmus is most commonly seen in patients with central vestibular disease. With rotatory nystagmus, the eyes rotate in a clockwise or counterclockwise manner in the orbit. Rotatory nystagmus has components of both horizontal and vertical movement and is not localizing; it may be seen with a lesion anywhere in the special proprioceptive system.

Pathologic nystagmus is also classified by whether it is present at all times (resting) or must be elicited by placing the head in an abnormal position (positional). Resting nystagmus is seen when the patient's head is at rest (not moving) and in a normal position. This type of nystagmus is most characteristic of peripheral vestibular disease. Nystagmus found only when the patient's head is at rest but in an abnormal position, such as turned on its side or upside down, is positional. Positional nystagmus is most characteristic of central vestibular dysfunction (e.g., brain stem and cerebellar lesions) but is also seen during the compensation phase of peripheral vestibular diseases.

Finally, pathologic nystagmus is classified by whether or not it persists or can be reproduced for more than 2 weeks after its onset. Most pathologic nystagmus resulting from an injury to the peripheral vestibular system spontaneously resolves during the 10 to 14 days following the initial injury. After the nystagmus has resolved, it can only be reinitiated by new damage to the vestibular system. The nystagmus appears to resolve from CNS compensation for the original injury. Few patients can compensate for brain stem or progressive cerebellar injuries; as a result, the pathologic nystagmus persists over time.

Cranial Muscle Symmetry. The superficial muscle of the head can be divided into two major groups. The first are the muscles of facial expression. These muscles are innervated by cranial nerve VII and include the muscles of the eyelid and lip. The second group contains the muscles of mastication, which are innervated by cranial nerve V and includes the temporal and masseter muscles. Facial muscle paralysis may result from injury to the contralateral cerebrum, ipsilateral brain stem, or ipsilateral cranial nerve VII. Clinically, drooping of the lip, deviation of the nasal philtrum, an increase in palpebral fissure width (pseudoptosis), and, in some, true ptosis (drooping of the eyelid) are seen. The diminished muscle function can be confirmed by testing the facial (palpebral and/or corneal) reflexes. Masticatory muscle paralysis may result from ipsilateral injury to the brain stem or peripheral cranial nerve V. The clinical appearance is loss of muscle mass and weakness of the jaw, often manifested as a dropped jaw and inability to close the mouth.

Facial Reflexes

Palpebral Reflex. This reflex tests the maxillary division of cranial nerve V and its brain stem connection to cranial nerve VII. The reflex is initiated by touching the palpebral margins, which produces an eye blink (Fig. 104–19). Reflex injury is generally manifested as loss of the eye blink. In

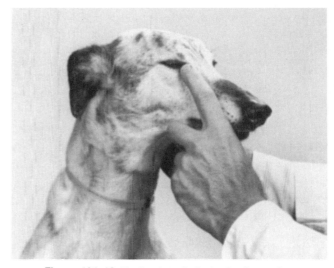

Figure 104–19. Testing the palpebral reflex in a patient.

some animals with incomplete paresis of cranial nerve V or VII, lagophthalmos, which is incomplete closure of the palpebral margins, may be seen.

Corneal Reflex. This reflex tests the ophthalmic division of cranial nerve V and its brain stem connection to cranial nerve VII. The reflex is initiated by lightly touching the cornea, which produces an eye blink. Reflex injury is generally manifested as loss of the eye blink. In some animals with incomplete paresis of cranial nerve V or VII, lagophthalmos may be seen.

Retractor Oculi Reflex. This reflex tests the ophthalmic division of cranial nerve V and its brain stem connection to cranial nerve VI. The reflex is initiated by lightly touching the cornea, which produces retraction of the globe in the orbit. Lack of the reflex is generally the result of neurologic dysfunction. In some animals with loss of the retrobulbar fat pad, the eye may be enophthalmic and incapable of retraction; in others, a retrobulbar mass may prevent retraction.

Facial Sensory Examination. This test examines cranial nerve V and its cerebral connections. It is performed by lightly stimulating the nasal mucosa, which should produce an avoidance response such as head turning. The nasal mucosa is a more reliable site for stimulation than the lips. Injury to the pathways is manifested as absence of the avoidance response.

The Oral Cavity

Gag Reflex. This reflex tests cranial nerves IX and X and their brain stem connections. To initiate the reflex, lightly stimulate the oropharynx, which should produce a swallowing reflex. Loss of the reflex usually implies brain stem or peripheral nerve dysfunction.

Oral Examination. The oral examination evaluates the tongue (cranial nerve XII) and completes the evaluation of cranial nerves IX and X. Look for atrophy of the tongue, which can be produced by brain stem or PNS injury to cranial nerve XII. Also look for deviation of the tongue, which can be caused by cerebral injuries as well as brain stem and PNS injuries. Examine the pharynx for evidence of paralysis of the soft palate, and look at the larynx for evidence of laryngeal paralysis. Either of these conditions may result from brain stem or PNS injuries.

Summary

Most cranial nerve reflexes and responses evaluate more than one cranial nerve, as well as evaluate the CNS connections between the two nerves. Abnormalities of each test may reflect an injury to the PNS or CNS. In many cases, CNS injuries to either brain stem or cerebrum may decrease the responsiveness of a cranial nerve reflex. Only a few cranial nerve reflexes are affected by injuries to the cerebellum. Table 104–4 lists the cranial nerve reflexes discussed, their sensory and motor nerves, normal responses, and which portions of the CNS are tested by each.

When evaluating the examination completed to this point, it may help to divide the brain into its local subdivisions and consider each one's major functional categories. The cerebrum is concerned with "brain" functions, so if it is damaged, abnormalities of learning, behavior, and vision are seen in addition to cranial nerve deficits. These patients will also have limb signs, which will be discussed next. The brain stem is concerned with "head" function and is further subdivided into the midbrain, pons, and medulla. If the midbrain is abnormal, there is abnormal eyeball function. If the pons is abnormal, the face does not function properly. If the medulla is abnormal, the mouth, tongue, and throat do not function normally. With brain stem diseases, there may also be disturbances of vegetative functions (e.g., consciousness, heart rate, and respiration), as well as limb signs. Finally, there is the cerebellum, which is concerned with coordinating movement of the whole body. If it is diseased, dysregulation of voluntary motor coordination, with associated tremors of head and body, will occur, along with limb ataxia. Refer back to Table 104–2 for specific signs.

SPINAL SEGMENTAL REFLEXES

After completing the cranial nerve examination, proceed to the spinal reflex examination. The spinal segmental reflexes directly test reflex arcs of the spinal cord. They also indirectly test brain centers that regulate spinal reflexes. Injuries within a reflex arc can cause reflex dampening or total reflex loss. Discovering a diminished reflex precisely localizes a lesion to the reflex arc tested. Since the efferent portion of the reflex arc is a lower motor neuron (LMN), such a change in reflex activity is called an LMN sign or an LMN reflex change. If a lesion occurs cranial to a reflex arc, it disconnects the tested reflex from its brain or upper motor neuron (UMN) regulation. This regulation tends to be inhibitory, so loss of UMN regulation results in disinhibition with reflex exaggeration. Reflex exaggeration is referred to as a UMN sign or UMN reflex change. UMN changes confirm the presence of a CNS lesion but are not as precisely localizing as LMN reflexes. Spinal reflexes may be divided into types based on the type of stimulation required to elicit them or the special circumstances needed for them to be present. There are proprioceptive reflexes, nociceptive reflexes, and special (released) reflexes.

Proprioceptive Reflexes

These are reflexes initiated by the stretching tendons or muscle spindles. They are strongly influenced by the UMN, so are likely to be exaggerated by CNS lesions cranial to the reflex arc. Thus, brain diseases, especially cerebrum and brain stem, are commonly associated with UMN changes of proprioceptive reflexes in limbs. Grading the strength of these reflexes allows for follow-up of a patient's condition. A standard grading scale is as follows: 0 = absent reflex, 1 = diminished reflex, 2 = normal reflex, 3 = increased reflex, 4 = increased reflexes with clonus. Reflex attenuation is the most important change to recognize, as that change both indicates the presence of nervous system dysfunction and precisely localizes the injury. Exaggerated proprioceptive reflexes are the next most important change, since it confirms the presence of central nervous system dysfunction, but only localizes the injury to a region cranial to the reflex being tested. Normal proprioceptive reflexes are the least helpful finding, as mild injuries to either LMN or UMN may fail to change the reflexes. Of course, normal reflexes are also seen in patients with a normal nervous system. As part of the evaluation of proprioceptive reflexes, evaluate the muscle tone of each limb. Injuries in the reflex arc (LMN injuries) produce hypotonia of the limb, while injuries of the UMN pathways produce a hypertonia or spasticity of the affected limbs. Proprioceptive reflexes and muscle tone are best evaluated in a relaxed animal in lateral recumbency.

Thoracic Limb Reflexes. Thoracic limb reflexes are summarized in Figure 104–20.

Triceps Reflex. This reflex tests the radial nerve, which

TABLE 104–4. CRANIAL NERVE REFLEX EVALUATION

MANUEVER	SENSORY NERVE	MOTOR NERVE	NORMAL RESPONSE	CNS PORTION TESTED
Menace	II	VII	Eye blink, head turn	Cerebrum
Pupillary light reflex (FLR)	II	III	Pupil constriction	Midbrain
Pupillary symmetry	—	III	Pupils equal in size	Midbrain
		Sympathetic		Cervical spinal cord
Pupillary size	II	III	Pupils midrange	Midbrain
		Sympathetic		Cervical spinal cord
Ocular position	VIII	III/IV/VI	Normal conjugate position	Brain stem
Oculo-vestibular reflex	VIII	III/IV/VI	Physiologic nystagmus	Brain stem
Pathologic nystagmus	VIII	III/IV/VI	Eyes remain at rest	Brain stem, cerebellum
Palpebral reflex	V	VII	Eye blink	Brain stem, cerebrum
Corneal reflex	V	VII	Eye blink	Brain stem, cerebrum
Retractor oculi reflex	V	VI	Eyeball retraction	Brain stem
Temporal muscle tone and size		V	Full, symmetric muscles Good jaw tone	Brain stem
Nasal sensory examination	V	VII and muscles of neck	Lip retracts, head pulls away	Brain stem, cerebrum
Gag reflex	IX/X	IX/X	Normal swallowing	Brain stem
Tongue examination	V	XII	Normal movement, position, no atrophy	Brain stem

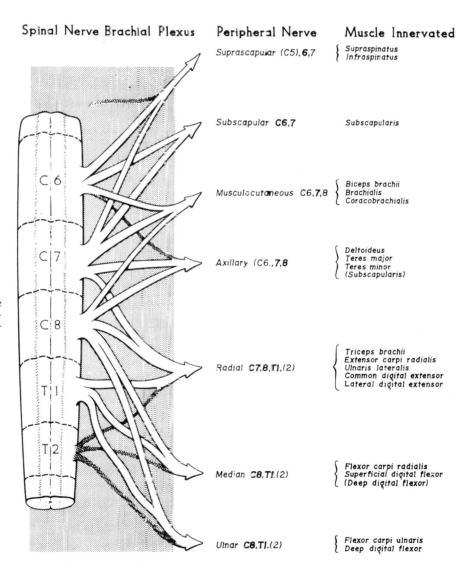

Figure 104–20. An anatomic representation of the thoracic limb reflexes. (From DeLahunta A: Veterinary Neuroanatomy and Clinical Neurology. Philadelphia, WB Saunders, 1983, p 63.)

Spinal Nerve Brachial Plexus   Peripheral Nerve   Muscle Innervated

Suprascapular (C5),6,7 — { Supraspinatus / Infraspinatus

Subscapular C6,7 — Subscapularis

Musculocutaneous C6,7,8 — { Biceps brachii / Brachialis / Coracobrachialis

Axillary (C6.,7,8 — { Deltoideus / Teres major / Teres minor / (Subscapularis)

Radial C7,8,T1,(2) — { Triceps brachii / Extensor carpi radialis / Ulnaris lateralis / Common digital extensor / Lateral digital extensor

Median C8,T1,(2) — { Flexor carpi radialis / Superficial digital flexor / (Deep digital flexor)

Ulnar C8,T1,(2) — { Flexor carpi ulnaris / Deep digital flexor

Flexor reflex: Sensory: varies with area stimulated
Motor: musculocutaneous, axillary, median, ulnar, radial
Biceps reflex: Sensory and Motor: musculocutaneous
Triceps reflex: Sensory and Motor: radial

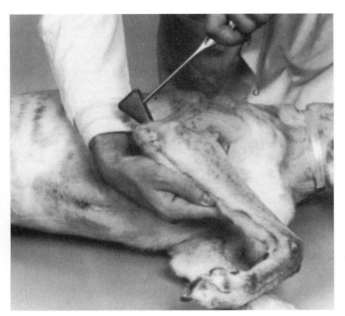

Figure 104–21. Testing the triceps reflex in a patient.

arises from spinal cord segments C7–T1(T2). The reflex is elicited by striking the tendon of insertion of the triceps muscle (Fig. 104–21). A normal response is a slight extension of the limb at the elbow. The reflex is often difficult to obtain in normal animals and, when present, is hard to interpret.

Extensor Carpi Radialis Reflex. This reflex tests the radial nerve, and thus also tests spinal cord segments C7–T1(T2). The reflex is elicited by striking the muscle belly of the extensor carpi radialis muscle, which results in extension of the carpus. This reflex is easier to elicit in many animals than the triceps reflex tests but is also difficult to interpret.

Biceps Reflex. This reflex evaluates the musculocutaneous nerve, which arises from spinal cord segments C6–C8. The reflex is initiated by striking a finger, which is placed on the tendon of insertion of the biceps muscle (Fig. 104–22). A normal response is a slight flexion of the elbow. This reflex is more difficult to obtain that the triceps reflex and is also difficult to interpret.

Pelvic Limb Reflexes. Pelvic limb reflexes are summarized in Figure 104–23.

Patellar Reflex. This reflex tests the femoral nerve, which arises from spinal cord segments L4–L6. The reflex is elicited by striking the patellar tendon, which produces extension of the stifle (Fig. 104–24). This reflex is probably the most reliable tendon reflex in veterinary medicine. With this reflex, a phenomenon known as a *false localizing sign* arises in patients with sciatic nerve paralysis. The functional loss of the antagonist muscles of the quadriceps may result in an excessively brisk patellar reflex, which falsely resembles a UMN reflex change.

Anterior Tibialis Reflex. This reflex tests the peroneal branch of the sciatic nerve, which originates from spinal cord segment L6–S1(S2). The reflex is initiated by striking the belly of the cranial tibial muscle (Fig. 104–25). The normal response is flexion of the tarsus. The author does not consider this reflex to be very reliable, but it can usually be elicited in a patient.

Gastrocnemius Reflex. This reflex tests the tibial branch of the sciatic nerve, which originates form spinal cord segment L6–S1(S2). The reflex is initiated by striking either the belly of the gastrocnemius muscle or its tendon of insertion just proximal to the tuber calcaneus. The expected normal response is extension of the tarsus; however, in the author's experience, many patients will have tarsal flexion instead. The author does not believe this reflex is reliable.

Nociceptive Reflexes

These reflexes are initiated by nociceptive (painful) stimuli, such as pinching, compression of digits, or pinpricks. Regardless of the stimulus used, it is important to realize that these reflexes test only the spinal reflex arc integrity. A preserved reflex tells nothing about the health of the nociceptive pathways traveling cranially to the brain. These reflexes do not have a large UMN influence; therefore, they are not normally exaggerated in patients with UMN lesions. The most significant change seen is loss of a nociceptive reflex, which indicates an LMN lesion.

Flexor Reflexes. These reflexes are initiated by compressing a digit. The normal response is limb withdrawal from the stimulus source (Fig. 104–26). The thoracic limb flexor response uses all peripheral nerves of the thoracic limb and tests spinal cord segments C6–T2. The pelvic limb flexor reflex tests primarily the sciatic nerve and its branches. It tests L6–S2 nerve roots, as their fibers compose the sciatic nerve. Reflex loss indicates a lesion in the reflex arc.

Perineal Reflexes. These reflexes are normally initiated by lightly pricking the perianal region; they test the perineal and pudendal nerves, spinal cord segments S1–S3, and the cauda equina (Fig. 104–27). The expected response is anal sphincter constriction and tail flexion. If a mild weakness is suspected, the best way to test the reflex is during a digital rectal examination so that the examiner can feel the sphincter's contracture strength.

Panniculus Reflex (Cutaneous Trunci Reflex). This reflex is initiated by stimulating truncal skin with a pin or hemostat. The clinician should be able to obtain the reflex over the entire thoracic trunk and the cranial lumbar trunk. The stimulus is carried to the CNS by the dorsal root that supplies the dermatome being stimulated and travels cranially in the CNS to synapse on the lateral thoracic nerve's

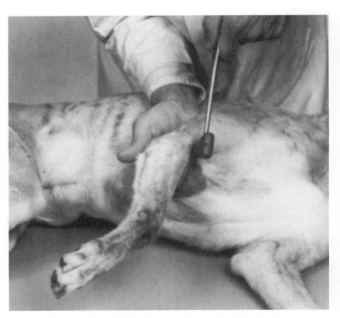

Figure 104–22. Testing the biceps reflex in a patient.

CNS

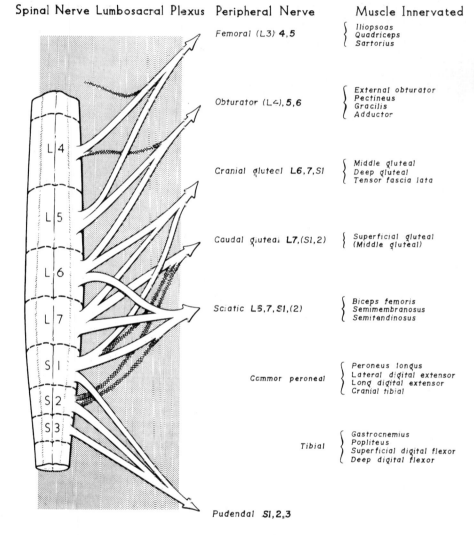

Figure 104–23. An anatomic representation of the pelvic limb reflexes. (From DeLahunta A: Veterinary Neuroanatomy and Clinical Neurology. Philadelphia, WB Saunders, 1983, p 64.)

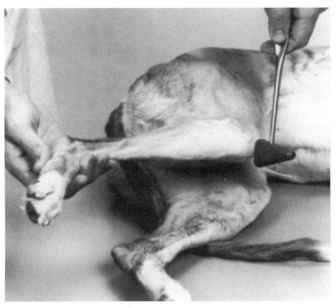

Figure 104–24. Testing the patellar reflexes in a patient.

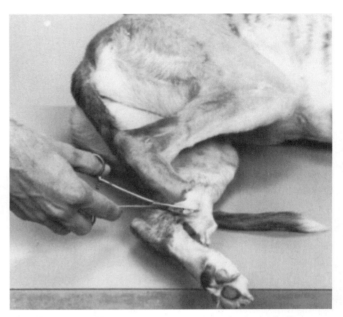

Figure 104–26. Testing the flexor reflexes in the pelvic limb.

LMNs (C8–T1 spinal cord segments). This reflex helps localize transverse spinal cord lesions when there is a clear demarcation between an area of absent reflex and a zone of normal reflex activity. The reflex also helps distinguish between injuries to the brachial plexus (reflex should be present) and injuries to the thoracic limb nerve roots (reflex often absent). In some normal animals, this reflex may not be present, so it must be interpreted cautiously.

Special (Released) Reflexes

These are reflexes that are suppressed by the UMNs of normal, adult animals. If there is a disconnection between the reflex arc and the UMN, these reflexes become released or disinhibited. The ability to elicit these reflexes in an adult animal indicates loss of UMN inhibition to a reflex arc and the presence of a CNS lesion.

Babinski Reflex. This reflex is elicited only in the pelvic limbs. It is elicited by lightly stroking the plantar aspect of the metatarsus. In normal animals, the toes either do nothing or flex slightly. In the presence of UMN disease, the toes spread apart and elevate (dorsiflex), which is known as a positive Babinski. The presence of a positive Babinski reflex is considered an indication of damage to the UMN pathways to the pelvic limb.

Crossed Extensor Reflex. This reflex may be seen in any limb. It is elicited by performing a flexor reflex. In a normal, recumbent animal, the limb being stimulated flexes (a normal flexor reflex) and the contralateral, paired limb does nothing. In the face of a UMN injury, when the stimulated limb flexes, the contralateral paired limb involuntarily extends (Fig. 104–28). This "crossed extension" is a consistent and reliable sign that the limb that extends has lost some or all of its UMN regulation. This reflex change then,

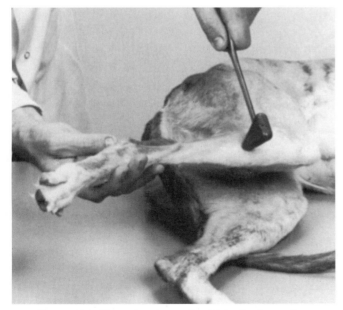

Figure 104–25. Testing the anterior tibial reflex in a patient.

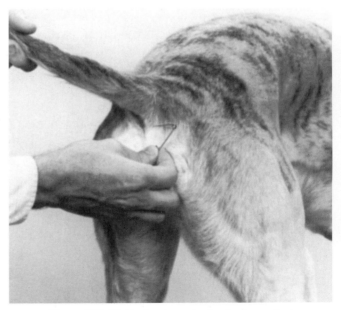

Figure 104–27. Testing the perineal reflex in a patient.

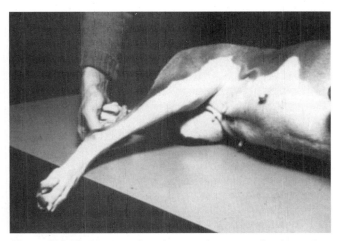

Figure 104–28. Demonstration of a crossed extensor reflex in a patient.

CNS

is one method of differentiating the patient with stupor from the patient in coma. This nociceptive evaluation tests peripheral nerve, spinal cord, brain stem, and cerebrum. The cerebellum is not involved in the nociceptive pathways. Peripheral nerve lesions usually cause focal sensory loss, confined to the distribution of the involved nerve(s). Spinal cord lesions cause a bilateral, symmetric sensory loss that is apparent caudal to the injury level. Brain stem lesions rarely produce detectable analgesia, since a brain stem lesion severe enough to affect nociception would result in the patient's death. Cerebral lesions produce only hypalgesia. Detectable sensory deficits with most cerebral injuries are unilateral and contralateral to the diseased hemisphere. This is because bilateral cerebral injuries depressing nociception depress consciousness as well.

Exaggerated Responsiveness to Pain. This is tested by digital manipulation of the paraspinal region with a hemostat, safety pin, or similar device. The objective is to produce a recognizable stimulus that does not bother a normal patient. Repeat the stimulus up and down the spine, searching for an area where the patient shows an unusually acute response to the stimulus (Fig. 104–29). An exaggerated response normally indicates a nerve root or meningeal lesion, e.g., a herniated disk or meningitis. This test is most valuable in localizing spinal cord lesions.

confirms the presence of CNS injury. It is important that the patient be carefully observed during flexor reflex testing, so that voluntary extension of the contralateral limb and/or struggling by the patient is not confused with a true crossed extension reflex. Table 104–5 reviews the spinal reflexes.

Nociceptive Evaluation

Animals may have two types of sensory disturbance. First is a decreased ability to perceive pain. A mild decrease is called hypalgesia or hypesthesia; total loss is referred to as analgesia or anesthesia. The second type of sensory disturbance is an increased sensitivity or exaggerated responsiveness to pain. Hyperesthesia refers to increased sensitivity; hyperpathia is an exaggerated response to pain. In veterinary patients, it is impossible to distinguish between the two.

Diminished Pain Perception. Test for this by producing enough pain to initiate cerebral recognition and response. This is normally done by compressing the digits vigorously; the expected response is turning of the head and/or vocalization. Pain perception evaluation is most successful in patients with a normal level of consciousness, although creating pain

INTERPRETATION OF FINDINGS

Begin by making a list of the abnormal findings, along with a list of the anatomic regions of the nervous system. Mark each anatomic region where a lesion could produce the listed signs (Fig. 104–30). Then ask several questions. Does the patient have a neurologic disease? If there are pluses after any listed sign, this question is answered in the affirmative. Is the disease in the CNS or PNS? If the animal has cranial nerve deficits, the evaluation of the limbs and mental status can be used to answer this question. If there are cranial nerve deficits with no other signs, the lesion is probably in the PNS. If there are both cranial nerve deficits and limb signs present, the lesion is probably in the CNS (with the exception of peripheral vestibular injuries, which

TABLE 104–5. SPINAL REFLEX TESTING

REFLEX TESTED	PNS TESTED	CNS SEGMENTS TESTED	RESPONSE	INTERPRETATION
Triceps	Radial nerve	**C7, C8, T1,** (T2)	Exaggerated	UMN lesion
			Normal	± No lesion
			Diminished	LMN lesion
Biceps	Musculocutaneous nerve	C6, **C7, C8**	Exaggerated	UMN lesion
			Normal	± No lesion
			Diminished	LMN lesion
Thoracic flexor	Musculocutaneous, axillary, median, ulnar, and radial nerves	C6, **C7, C8** T1, (T2)	Normal	± No lesion
			Diminished	LMN lesion
Patellar	Femoral nerve	L4, **L5,** L6	Exaggerated	UMN lesion
			Normal	± No lesion
			Diminished	LMN lesion
Cranial tibial	Sciatic nerve	**L6, L7, S1,** (S2)	Exaggerated	UMN lesion
			Normal	± No lesion
			Diminished	LMN lesion
Pelvic flexor	Primarily sciatic nerve	**L6, L7, S1,** (S2)	Normal	± No lesion
			Diminished	LMN lesion
Perineal	Pudendal nerve	**S1, S2, S3**	Normal	Normal
			Diminished	LMN lesion
Crossed extensor		**UMN** to limb	Absent	Normal
			Present	UMN lesion

Bold = essential to reflex; plain text = always supplies axons to nerve, not essential to reflex; ( ) = supplies axons to reflex in some animals, not essential to reflex.

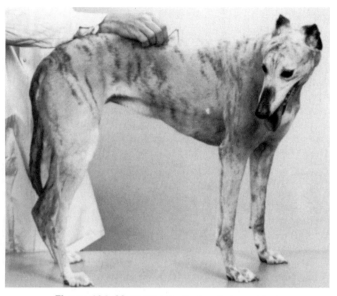

Figure 104–29. Testing for back pain in a patient.

may cause limb ataxia). If the disease is below the foramen magnum and there are UMN reflex changes present, the lesion is in the CNS. If all spinal reflexes are LMN, the lesion is probably in the PNS.

Is the disease above or below the foramen magnum? If the patient has abnormal cranial nerve reflexes, historical seizures, abnormal head posture, abnormal head coordination, or an abnormal level of consciousness, the lesion is above the foramen magnum. If the lesion involves the limbs alone, the lesion is likely below the foramen. After you have localized the pathologic process to above or below the foramen and to CNS or PNS, you can try to localize the lesion more precisely to a specific anatomic area of brain, e.g., brain stem.

There are several benefits to be gained by localizing the patient's lesion. You as a clinician now know whether the problem is focal or disseminated. The localization may automatically eliminate some differentials from your diagnosis. As an example, you would not list an intervertebral disk extrusion among the differentials for a dog with signs consistent with a focal cerebral mass. Finally, localization helps a clinician choose diagnostic aids. Certain diagnostic tools are of value only with lesions in certain anatomic regions. An example is the electroencephalogram, which is primarily helpful in patients with cerebral injuries. By having a rank-ordered differential diagnosis, you can choose your diagnostic tests in the order of greatest potential yield for your patient.

DIAGNOSTIC TESTING

The ability to diagnose disorders of the brain has increased dramatically in the last several years. Not only are standard diagnostic tests, such as cerebrospinal fluid (CSF) evaluation and electroencephalography (EEG), yielding more information, but also enhanced imaging techniques, such as magnetic resonance imaging (MRI), is becoming available to veterinarians, both in referral institutions and in general practice.[7–16] Ultrasound of the cranial vault is being investigated, and brain biopsy is now an accepted procedure.[17–21] All of these advances have allowed clinicians to diagnose diseases of the brain with much greater accuracy.

CEREBROSPINAL FLUID EVALUATION

CSF bathes the entire CNS, both internally (the ventricles and central canal) and externally (the subarachnoid space). Many nervous system diseases, especially inflammations and neoplasms, will affect CSF composition. The ease of sample collection and the value of the information gained have made CSF evaluation a mainstay in the diagnosis of CNS disease. The CSF changes frequently confirm that structural pathology is present, determine the pathology's general nature, and occasionally determine a specific etiology.[7, 12] Routine CSF analysis also allows a clinician to monitor the effectiveness of therapy.[10]

Some patients will have false-negative or false-positive CSF results. A disease must involve either the ventricular system or the subarachnoid space for cells to be shed into the CSF. Many CNS disorders, especially neoplasms, only involve deeper parenchyma. Those deeply seated processes may disrupt the blood-brain barrier (BBB), allowing protein leakage, without shedding cells into CSF. Some noninflammatory diseases, including neoplasms, may produce inflammatory changes in the CSF.[22, 12] With inflammations, there is also a possibility for error if CSF is not collected in the acute stages of the disease. As inflammations become more chronic, both the number and nature of cells shed into the CSF change. In some patients, the BBB may open transiently during an epileptic seizure, leading to artifactual changes in CSF.

Spinal Fluid Collection

CSF for analysis may be collected either at the cerebellomedullary cistern or by lumbar puncture. The lumbar space is more difficult to enter, yields smaller fluid volumes, and has a higher sample blood contamination rate. The cerebellomedullary cistern is easier to enter and yields larger fluid volumes, generally with less blood contamination.

To collect CSF, you need a small-gauge (20- or 22-gauge) spinal needle, a fluid container, and a three-way stopcock and manometer if you are going to measure pressure. All patients should be under general anesthesia during CSF collection to minimize the potential for injury from a patient moving during collection. Complications of CSF collection include anesthetic misadventures, CNS damage from the spinal needle, and/or brain herniation. Although clinical brain herniation is uncommon, it is generally fatal. If during the CSF collection, the pressure appears to be elevated, stop the collection and wake the patient. If a patient appears to

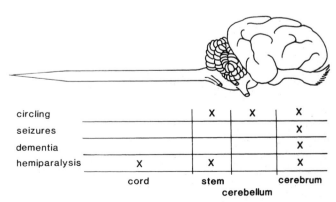

	cord	stem	cerebellum	cerebrum
circling			X	X	X
seizures					X
dementia					X
hemiparalysis		X	X		X

Figure 104–30. Demonstration of using signs to localize a lesion.

be in danger of herniation, hyperventilation with O_2 may decrease the intracranial pressure (ICP) sufficiently to avoid problems.

Cerebellomedullary Collection. Prior to anesthesia, clip the cranial portion of the patient's dorsal neck and back of the skull from between the pinnae caudally to the second or third cervical vertebra. Anesthetize and intubate the patient. If concerned about elevated intracranial pressures, hyperventilate the patient. Under anesthesia, place the patient in lateral recumbency and scrub the clipped area for a sterile procedure. Place the patient's spine parallel to the table, with the head at 90 degrees to the long axis of the body. Do not overflex the neck, as occluding the jugular veins will artifactually elevate the ICP and increase the potential for brain herniation.

The landmarks used for cerebellomedullary CSF collection are the wings of the atlas (C1) and the occipital protuberance. Use the occipital protuberance to find the midline. Make a "T," with the line between the two wings of the atlas forming one bar and the midline of the neck forming the other. Insert the needle at the intersection of the two lines. A 1.5-inch needle is sufficient for cerebellomedullary collections in both dogs and cats. Face the needle bevel craniad. Advance the needle slowly on a line approximately perpendicular to the long axis of the spine. A sudden loss of resistance occurs when the needle advances into the subarachnoid space. When the change in resistance is felt, remove the stylet and look for CSF. To prevent accidental needle movement, continue holding the needle with thumb and forefinger each time the stylet is removed. If no fluid appears after a few seconds, replace the stylet and advance the needle further. If you are certain you are in the subarachnoid space and there is still no flow of fluid, try occluding the jugular veins. After that, if there is still no flow, there is a strong possibility the animal has suffered a brain herniation that is blocking the flow of CSF. Hyperventilate the patient and discontinue the procedure.

If the needle hits bone, move the needle tip a few millimeters cranial, then caudal. If you still cannot find the interspace between occiput and C1, remove the needle and start the entire process over. After fluid begins to flow, allow it to drip into a container. If the fluid is going to be stored for any length of time, collect it in a plastic container, since WBCs adhere to glass. Adherence affects cytology results. Immediately refrigerate CSF to be stored in order to slow cellular degradation.

Complications of CSF Collection

Blood contamination is the most common CSF collection complication. This generally results from meningeal vessel penetration. If the fluid appears bloody at the onset of collection, replace the stylet and leave the needle in place for 30 to 60 seconds. Often the blood will clear. If blood is still present, collect the first and second portions of the sample in separate containers. Often the contamination will diminish during the collection, leaving a second sample that is adequate for interpretation. If the CSF flow is insufficient for spontaneous collection, you may need to aspirate the fluid carefully with a syringe. This increases the potential for blood contamination.

The most serious complication of CSF collection is brain herniation. In the face of elevated intracranial pressure, the pressure shift created by the CSF removal may precipitate a shift in intracranial contents. This sudden movement of intracranial contents (brain herniation) may result in the

patient's death, although it may also be asymptomatic.[23] Brain herniation in dogs and cats has occurred in association with CSF collection and anesthesia.[24] In reports of anaerobic bacterial infections, three of four patients had CNS herniation, although it appears that the herniation occurred prior to CSF collection rather than as a result of collection.[25] Progressive sensory and motor paralysis, pupillary size changes, sudden onset of pathologic nystagmus, and reflex abnormalities signal brain herniation is occurring. The actual relationship between herniation and CSF collection is not as conclusive as once believed, so fear of herniation should not prevent collecting CSF in a patient unless that patient's clinical condition is deteriorating rapidly.[23]

CSF Analysis

Spinal fluid analysis should include pressure measurement, gross visual examination, cytologic analysis, biochemical analysis, and fluid culture. You may also want to perform serology on the CSF if an infectious cause is suspected. As normal values for fluid collected from cerebellomedullary and lumbar spaces differ slightly, it is important to note where the fluid was collected. CSF from the cerebellomedullary cistern tends to have slightly more cells and lower protein than the fluid from the lumbar space.[26]

Pressure. Opening pressure (OP) is measured at the beginning of CSF collection, using a manometer. Only pressure elevations are considered significant. Simpson showed that normal values for the dog are dependent on body weight (BW) in kilograms.[27] His published formula for calculating normals based on body size is: $OP = 46.5 + 3.83 \, (BW) \times 0.048 \, (BW)^2$. Normal pressures in dogs ranged from 50 to 140 mm H_2O, depending on body size. Typically CSF pressures elevate when either CSF flow or resorption is impaired. Obstructed flow is typical with mass lesions, such as neoplasms, hematomas, and granulomas. Impaired CSF resorption is more common with inflammatory processes, especially meningitis. Patients with meningitis will have moderate to severe elevations of CSF pressure above the normal. Patients with tumors are more likely to have massive elevations of CSF pressure.

Gross Evaluation. Normal CSF should be clear and colorless on gross visual examination. Increased white cell numbers and/or protein elevation generally causes CSF to become turbid and assume an off-white to grayish color. Turbid CSF indicates a cell count elevation above 500/dL. Spinal fluid may assume a pink coloration from blood contamination. Spin down a small sample of the CSF and examine the supernatant. If the pink color persists, it indicates free hemoglobin. Free hemoglobin suggests previous subarachnoid hemorrhage rather than contamination during fluid collection. Yellow-orange (xanthochromic) CSF generally indicates breakdown of hemoglobin from previous hemorrhage or severe elevations of CSF protein (>100 mg/dL). Xanthochromia may also be seen in some cases of protracted icterus.

Cytologic Evaluation. The cytologic evaluation should begin with a total cell count on unconcentrated fluid. A slide should then be prepared using a cell concentration technique for evaluation of cell morphology and differential cell counts. The two most common slide preparation techniques are cytocentrifugation and sedimentation. In cytocentrifugation, the CSF is centrifuged at 1500 × g for 10 minutes. The supernatant is pipetted off and the cells resuspended by adding a drop of normal serum or 20 per cent albumin to the sediment. The protein is added to provide better cell adherence to the slide and prevent drying artifact. Dry and stain the slide, generally with a Wright-Giemsa stain. In sedimentation, you mix CSF and normal serum in a 50:50 ratio. Place the mixture in a cylinder attached to a slide and allow time for the cells to sediment onto the slide. Pipette off the liquid, then dry and stain the slide. Some CSF volume is lost to further evaluation because you add the extra protein. The sedimentation technique may preserve cell architecture better than centrifugation methods. For the general practitioner, the sedimentation technique is easiest and reliable. Membrane filtration is a third, less commonly used cell-concentrating technique. Cytologists need to be experienced in reading membrane filtration cytology for reliable results.

The total cell count and slide preparation should be completed as soon as possible, since CSF cells undergo degeneration rapidly. WBCs degrade more rapidly than RBCs in CSF.[28] Such a differential degradation would greatly alter your interpretation of the CSF if the slides were not prepared in a timely manner. Refrigeration slows WBC lysis, so when slides cannot be prepared immediately, refrigerate the sample.

There should be less than 5 WBC/dL in normal CSF, regardless of collection site. Cell numbers may increase with inflammations, tumors, necrosis, trauma, and vascular injuries to the CNS. Cytology is most changed with inflammations. Typically with CNS inflammations, WBC numbers increase in CSF. The type and number of cells reflect the cause of the inflammation, providing further etiologic information. Deeply seated inflammations may disrupt the BBB, allowing protein leakage without cell migration into the CSF. In such patients, even though cell numbers may be normal, cytologic examination may reveal abnormal cell distribution.[8] In patients with noninflammatory diseases, proportions of cells in CSF may change, even though total cell numbers remain within normal limits.[29] CSF cytology is most reliable in acute, untreated CNS infections. As diseases become more chronic and various therapies are tried, CSF no longer accurately reflects the etiology.

Some inflammatory diseases and many neoplasms are associated with normal CSF cytology; therefore, normal cell counts and distributions do not exclude the possibility of an infectious or neoplastic process. With blood contamination, there may be WBC in the CSF from the blood. Elevations of WBC are probably significant even in the face of mild blood contamination.[30] It is my experience that severe contamination makes most CSF uninterpretable.

Suppurative meningitis is diagnosed if there are predominately polymorphonuclear leukocytes (PMNs) in CSF. Suppurative meningitis is a pathologic response to bacterial infection; acute, severe viral encephalitis; and presumed immune vasculitis/meningitis of young dogs. Suppurative meningitis may also be seen following myelography, and with some tumors, especially meningiomas.[22, 31–33]

When the CSF cells are composed of multiple cell types, including macrophages, lymphocytes, neutrophils, and sometimes plasma cells, a mixed inflammation is diagnosed. Mixed cytology is generally the result of a granulomatous inflammation, such as occurs with fungal, protozoal, and some idiopathic diseases. Mixed cytology may also be seen in inadequately treated chronic bacterial infections and in response to foreign bodies. Nonsuppurative inflammation is diagnosed if the cell numbers are increased and primarily mononuclear cells, especially lymphocytes. Nonsuppurative inflammation is most characteristic of viral and rickettsial infections but is also seen with neoplasms. Although nonsuppurative CSF is unlikely to result from an acute bacterial infection of the nervous system, it may be seen.[34] Table 104–6 provides an overview of CSF cytologic changes in various inflammatory diseases.

Because CSF cytology normally changes during the progression of any illness, the most reliable diagnostic evaluation would consist of serial CSF collections. Serial CSF will also evaluate the patient's response to therapy.[10] The need for anesthesia makes serial CSF collection uncommon in managing canine and feline CNS diseases.

In any inflammatory process, but especially one with visible organisms, CSF should be cultured. Negative cultures, even when organisms are seen, may result from small

TABLE 104–6. COMPARATIVE CSF RESULTS IN INFLAMMATORY DISEASES

DISEASE	NUMBER OF WBCs	WBC TYPE	TOTAL PROTEIN LEVEL	ALBUMIN LEVELS	GLOBULIN LEVELS	CSF ANTIBODIES DETECTED	ORGANISMS SEEN
Bacterial meningitis	+ + +	PMN (mixed)	+ + (+)	+ +	+ +	Varies	Yes (Varies)
Steroid-responsive meningitis/arteritis	+ + +	PMN (mixed)	+ +	+ +	+ (+)	No (IgA)	No
Tumor (meningioma)–associated pleocytosis	+ (+)	PMNs (mixed)	+ (+)	+ (+)	WNL	No	No
Granulomatous meningoencephalitis	+ + (+)	Mixed (PMN or mono)	+ + (+)	+ +	+ +	No	No
Feline infectious peritonitis	+ + +	Mixed (PMNs or mono)	+ + +	+ +	+ +	Yes (?)	No
Fungal meningoencephalitis	+ +	Mixed (PMN + eos)	+ +	+ +	+ (+)	Varies	Varies
Protozoal meningoencephalitis	+ (+)	Mixed (PMN + eos)	+ (+)	+	+ (+)	Variable	Rarely
Rocky Mountain spotted fever	+	Mixed	+	+	+	?	No
Eosinophilic meningitis	+ (+)	Eosinophils	+	+	+	No	No
Other viral encephalitis	+	Mononuclear	+ (+)	WNL	+	?	No
Canine distemper	+	Monocellular (lymphocytes)	+	WNL	+	Yes	No

WNL = within normal limits; + = mild elevation; + + = moderate elevation; + + + = marked elevation; symbols in parentheses indicate variations, for example, + (+) indicates that typically the test results are mildly elevated but in some patients are moderately elevated.
From Fenner WR: Bacterial infections of the CNS. *In* Green C (ed): Infectious Diseases of the Dog and Cat, 2nd ed. Philadelphia, WB Saunders Co, 1998, p 652.

numbers of organisms in the CSF, improper sample storage or transport, improper choice of culture technique, or inadequate nutrients in normal CSF to support growth.

Biochemical Evaluation. Although CSF contains essentially the same constituents as plasma, they are present in different concentrations than in plasma. Generally those levels are lower than the plasma levels. The two biochemical constituents most commonly measured are protein and glucose. The CSF protein concentration is generally quite low compared with plasma proteins. In dogs and cats, protein from a cerebellomedullary cisternal tap is generally less than 25 mg/dL, whereas that from a lumbar puncture may be as high as 45 mg/dL. This is in contrast to the 5 to 8 g/dL of protein seen in plasma. Storage of CSF does not significantly affect protein content, so CSF may be sent to an outside laboratory for protein evaluation.

CSF protein is elevated in many diseases of the nervous system, including encephalitis, meningitis, neoplasms, trauma, and infarcts.[29] About 75 per cent or greater of CSF protein should be albumin. Protein elevation may result from increased BBB permeability, local immunoglobulin production, or a combination of both. Total protein quantitation and protein electrophoresis should be performed on all CSF samples. Electrophoresis allows a clinician to discern the protein source.[35, 36] In noninflammatory BBB disruptions, e.g., neoplasms and infarcts, most CSF protein will still be albumin. If the elevated protein is predominantly globulin, the source is likely to be local (intrathecal) immunoglobulin production. This is most consistent with an inflammatory process of the CNS (encephalitis).[37, 38] In patients with a combination of elevated albumin and globulin in CSF, an inflammatory process that affects both CNS and meninges, e.g., feline infectious peritonitis (FIP), should be suspected.[37, 39] The ability to quantitate proteins is essential in attempting to distinguish the meningioma with an inflammatory CSF cytology from other causes of inflammatory CSF cytologic changes.

The second chemical measurement performed on CSF is glucose concentration. Normal CSF glucose is about 60 to 80 per cent of blood levels. In humans, the ratio between blood glucose and CSF glucose is routinely lowered in bacterial infections. A similar relationship between bacterial encephalitis and decreased CSF glucose does not appear in the dog. The plasma glucose can drop dramatically in the presence of septicemia and bacteremia. A meningitic patient that was also bacteremic would be expected to have a concomitant drop in CSF glucose.

Other Tests on CSF. Spinal fluid may be examined serologically for antibodies against infectious agents, as well as for bacterial antigens. In normal animals, there should be little or no antibody present. Intrathecal antibodies indicate local immunoglobulin production. This serves as evidence that the organism against which the antibodies are found is the cause of the encephalitis. False-positive antibody levels may result from plasma protein leakage into CSF. Fever may transiently open the BBB, so many systemically ill patients will have some antibodies in CSF. Those antibodies present may be the result of previous infections, not the current illness. Increased albumin on your CSF electrophoresis would support a false-positive diagnosis, as it indicates an increased BBB permeability. Measuring simultaneous serum antibody titers is also helpful. If both serum and CSF titers are elevated, there is a greater possibility of the CSF titer being the result of leakage. If only CSF titers are elevated, it is most likely intrathecal production. A second limitation

of CSF serology is that you must wait for paired titers for greatest accuracy.

ELECTRODIAGNOSTIC EVALUATIONS

Electroencephalography (EEG). Electroencephalography is the graphic recording of shifts in resting membrane potential of the dendritic network of the superficial cerebral cortical layers. This network is influenced and modulated by subcortical nuclear activity, such as the reticular formation. EEG is a noninvasive, relatively inexpensive diagnostic tool. Frequently EEGs can be recorded without chemical restraint. In spite of this, EEG tracings are often difficult to interpret, limiting this technique's use to referral institutions. The EEG is often helpful in localizing mass effects in the CNS.[13] The EEG is helpful in confirming the presence of cerebral diseases, and sometimes in establishing a differential category. EEG does not allow a clinician to establish a precise etiologic diagnosis. When evaluating the EEG, a clinician looks for changes in frequency, amplitude, shape, and distribution of potentials. Abnormal potentials that persist are more significant than those that are transient. There are three basic changes seen on EEG: slowing, paroxysms, and depression of normal rhythms. EEG changes are most likely to be seen with metabolic diseases, inflammatory diseases, and mass lesions. EEG does not replace other diagnostic tests.

Brain Stem Auditory Evoked Response (BAER, BER). The BAER is a signal-averaged technique designed to test the auditory pathways. Subcutaneous recording electrodes are placed on the patient at the vertex of the skull and near the ear at the petrous bone. An earphone is used to deliver a series of clicks to the ear of the patient. A signal averager is triggered by the clicks and records all brain activity that occurs during a set time (generally 100 msec) following the sound. About 1000 recordings are stored, then the patterns compared mathematically by a signal averager. Random waveforms are removed by this averaging process, leaving the "common" waveforms. This averaged response is assumed to have been generated by the sound and is the BAER.[40] The BAER has proved to be highly useful in the evaluation of deafness.[41–43] The BAER will also be altered by brain stem and some cerebral lesions, so it is a useful tool in confirming the presence of a central lesion in patients with vestibular dysfunction.[44]

Visual Evoked Potentials (VEP). This procedure also generates a signal-averaged response; however, the visual system is being tested rather than the auditory. The stimulus is light, and recording electrodes are over occipital cortex and skull vertex.[45, 45] As the VEP is testing visual pathways, it evaluates cerebral pathways rather than brain stem pathways. Data on this technique's use remain spotty in veterinary medicine.

RADIOGRAPHIC AND ALTERNATE IMAGING EVALUATION

Positioning is critical when attempting to use any imaging technique of the brain or skull; therefore, general anesthesia is required. In most patients, the imaging technique is performed during the same anesthetic procedure used to collect CSF.

Routine Radiographic Procedures

Survey skull radiographs are primarily useful in patients with suspected bony or cartilaginous changes. Examples would be patients with head trauma, suspected deformations of the calvarium, suspected hydrocephalus, and slowly growing brain tumors. Plain skull radiographs are also of value in suspected disorders of the middle and inner ear. Normally, a patient should have a ventrodorsal (VD) or dorsoventral (DV) radiograph taken, along with a lateral radiograph. In patients with suspected foramen magnum deformities, an open mouth, frontal view is indicated. In patients with vestibular disorders, oblique views should be taken to visualize the osseous bulla. The clinician reviews the films for evidence of changes in density of the bony skull. Thinning of the skull may be produced by chronic pressure, e.g., hydrocephalus or meningiomas. Some brain tumors may calcify, as will some arteriovenous malformations. In patients with head trauma, the films are reviewed for fractures. In general, plain skull films are of limited value in patients with brain disease.

Contrast Radiography

Arteriography and Angiography. A positive contrast study of the brain's arterial circulation can be made by injecting an iodinated contrast agent into either the internal carotid or vertebral arteries. Internal carotid procedures evaluate the arterial circle, rostral cerebral arterial circulation, and middle cerebral arterial circulation. Vertebral arterial studies evaluate the basilar arterial, caudal cerebral arterial, and cerebellar arterial circulation. These procedures require a rapid cassette changer for complete studies. Although valuable in identifying vascular lesions or highly vascular mass lesions, these procedures' cost and difficulty have limited their use in veterinary medicine.

Venography. The cavernous sinus provides venous drainage for the cranial vault floor. The cavernous sinus passes on each side of the pituitary. Fibers of cranial nerves II, III, IV, V, and VI all pass through the cavernous sinus. Mass lesions may compress these nerves, distort the cavernous sinus, and be detected by *cavernous sinus venography.* The angularis oculi vein is catheterized and an iodinated contrast agent injected. This procedure does not require film changers, so it can be performed in many practices, but interpretation is difficult.[47]

Ultrasonography. In most patients, ultrasound has little value in brain imaging, since bone reflects sound. The skull normally prevents a sound beam from reaching the brain. In patients with an open fontanelle, however, the ultrasound beam has a port for entry to brain. In these patients, ultrasound has been of great value in the diagnosis of hydrocephalus.[17–19, 47] If a patient is having a brain biopsy or a craniotomy performed, ultrasonography can be used intraoperatively to assist in directing the biopsy needle or localizing a mass for surgical removal.[48, 49] The ultrasonographic procedure will not only help with the biopsy, but will also further clarify the extent of a mass lesion.

Computed Tomography (CT Scans). In computed tomography, multiple radiographic projections of an object are subjected to digital analysis, which allows reconstruction of the object's internal composition. CT's great advantage is that it allows a clinician to image brain tissue, rather than simply the supporting, e.g., bony skull, structures. By scanning a patient at multiple, sequential levels, a clinician is able to create a three-dimensional image of the object being analyzed. Although CT has slightly lower spatial resolution than conventional radiography, it does provide better contrast resolution. This means that CT can display images that have only a slightly different density than the surrounding objects.

When iodinated contrast agents are used to enhance subject contrast, the differences between normal and abnormal tissue are accentuated. Intravenous contrast agents allow a clinician to detect damage to the BBB, such as occurs with many neoplasms.[47, 50] As CT filters out scatter radiation to a greater extent than conventional radiography, it also provides a cleaner image.[51, 52] CT scanning has become routine in veterinary neurology, allowing for antemortem localization of mass lesions, granulomas, and inflammatory disorders.[15, 21] Owing to secondary changes (e.g., ventricular shifts, edema), CT may not distinguish between neoplasms and focal inflammation. CT is very effective at localizing lesions and providing guidance for biopsies.[53]

Magnetic Resonance Imaging (MRI). A magnetic resonance image is derived from radio wave signals produced by body tissue protons. The radio signal is detected by a radiofrequency receiver; the signal is analyzed by a computer and an image produced. The most common proton used for MRI imaging is the hydrogen nucleus, since it is the most abundant proton in the body. The patient is exposed to a short pulse of radiofrequency electromagnetic energy. Energy from this pulse will be absorbed by protons, changing their magnetic axes. When the pulse is terminated, the protons will revert to their original axes, releasing their energy. This released energy is the radio wave detected by the receiver and analyzed to produce the image. The chemical composition of a tissue will determine the rate at which a tissue both absorbs and releases the radiofrequency energy. By using different pulse sequences, magnetic resonance techniques can detect subtle differences between tissues and produce images that reflect these differences. MRI is especially efficient at detecting differences in water content between tissues. Many pathologic processes affect the BBB. The abnormal tissue will have different water content than adjacent normal tissue. These differences are detected by MRI and reproduced as tissue differences on the images.[47, 51] MRI is also able to visualize brain tissue, so it can produce a three-dimensional image of the brain. MRI's ability to detect subtle differences in tissues make it ideal for early neoplasm detection. MRI also recognizes inflammatory diseases with greater reliability than CT scans, potentially including early meningitis.[54] In addition, use of certain ions, e.g., gadolinium, may alter the rate at which protons release energy. Administering one of these ions intravenously allows it to act as a contrast agent to detect alterations in the BBB. In focal granulomatous meningoencephalitis (GME), the MRI changes may closely resemble those of a neoplasm, accentuating the importance of a complete battery of diagnostic aids.[55] In general, except for cranial disorders secondarily affecting the brain, MRI offers many advantages over CT for brain imaging.[53] These advantages include superior tissue contrast, ability to view several planes, the absence of ionizing radiation, absence of bone artifact, and vascular imaging capability.[53]

BRAIN BIOPSY

As localizing techniques have become more effective, the use of brain biopsy has become more widespread at referral institutions. Brain biopsy may be performed as part of a surgical exploratory, may be ultrasound guided through a small burr hole, or may be guided by landmarks of CT scans or MRI images.[20, 21, 56] Brain biopsies have been beneficial in the antemortem diagnosis of brain tumors and when choosing therapy. Perhaps the greatest benefit of biopsy has been in inflammatory diseases which may mimic neoplasms, especially GME.[15] In GME, early diagnosis and treatment allow for a greatly improved quality and length of life.

PRINCIPLES OF THERAPY

Treatment of brain diseases has two components: first is to treat the specific disease, if it is amenable to therapy; the second is to provide supportive care and prevent life-taking complications such as brain edema. Thus successful therapy of CNS disorders requires accurate diagnosis. After you know the disease, you can choose the therapeutic agent that will provide the most effective therapy. There will be some cases where presumptive therapy is instituted prior to a final diagnosis, e.g., treating brain edema in a patient with suspected brain tumors. When this is done, remember the treatment may alter the results of your diagnostic tests. Use of glucocorticosteroids, for example, may normalize CSF cytology and stabilize the BBB, affecting MRI and CT scan results.

The BBB affects the ability to obtain and maintain therapeutic blood levels of your drug when treating CNS diseases. The BBB provides both an anatomic and physiologic barrier to the movement of materials into the CNS. This barrier limits the entry of therapeutic agents into the CNS. This limited entry may cause significant discrepancies between serum and CSF drug concentrations, with subsequent decreased drug effectiveness. Macromolecules are prevented from crossing this barrier, which means you want a drug with low albumin binding (a high free fraction). Drugs such as the penicillins have a high level of albumin binding, limiting their ability to enter the CNS. Find a drug with a low ionization at physiologic pH and high lipid solubility, since these factors will allow the drug to more readily cross the BBB. Within drug families, there are some agents that will cross the BBB and some that will not. For example, esterified ampicillins are more lipophilic than are nonesterified ampicillins, so they penetrate the BBB with greater ease. Both chloramphenicol and trimethoprim are relatively lipophilic, so they penetrate even a normal BBB readily. Inflamed meninges are more permeable than normal meninges, increasing all drugs' ability to cross the BBB. This may lead to a 5- to 10-fold increase in the CSF concentrations of a drug. If the BBB stabilizes, CSF drug concentrations drop.

Choose a drug that will achieve sufficient concentrations in the CNS to produce a clinical response throughout the period of therapy. Some drugs are actively removed from the CNS by a facilitated transport system. In meningitis, this transport system is disrupted, artificially elevating CSF drug concentration. If steroids stabilize the BBB or the meningitis is treated, the drug concentrations may drop. When choosing a specific agent to use for a given patient, attempt to use the single, least toxic, most effective drug.

Treatment of Edema/Elevated Intracranial Pressure. Untreated brain edema harms the brain by compressing axons and elevating ICP. The ICP elevations compress cerebral venous sinuses, impairing CSF resorption, further increasing ICP. A vicious cycle can develop, ultimately leading to brain herniation and the patient's death. Several methods are used to alleviate brain edema and/or lower ICP. There is a direct relationship between CO_2 levels and intracranial blood volume. As CO_2 levels lower, intracranial volume decreases, lowering ICP. *Hyperventilation* is a simple and effective means of lowering a patient's CO_2 level.

Diuretics lower ICP, by both removing edema and de-

creasing intracranial volume. *Mannitol* is an osmotic diuretic commonly used to lower elevated ICP. Administer the mannitol as a 20 per cent solution, at a rate of 1 mL/lb/minute. You want to raise the patient's serum osmolality slowly, till clinical signs alleviate. *Furosemide* may also be used. Furosemide appears to decrease CSF production, decreasing intracranial contents. Furosemide is given at 0.3 mg/lb as an intravenous bolus, which should be repeated in 4 hours. If furosemide is administered in conjunction with mannitol, both drugs' effects are enhanced.[57]

Corticosteroids have been successfully used to treat the edema associated with brain tumors. More recently, there is evidence that corticosteroids may also alleviate edema following CNS injury, provided they are administered in high doses and within 8 hours of trauma. Experimentally, patients receiving a bolus of prednisolone sodium succinate at 13.6 mg/lb, then given 0.045 mg/lb of dexamethasone twice daily for the next 3 days, had significantly better outcomes than patients with other treatments. Although there may be a high incidence of complications (e.g., diarrhea, melena, vomiting) with this drug protocol, the complications do not appear to be serious.[58]

Anti-inflammatory Therapy. CNS inflammations are characterized by increased blood flow, exudation of fluids, and leukocyte migration into the affected area, with altered function of the involved portions of the nervous system. Inflammatory cells may damage the nervous system, stripping axons of myelin and phagocytizing neurons. The nervous system effects of inflammation include edema, necrosis, mass effects, vasculitis, hypoxia, and direct toxic effects of neutrophils on the CNS. CNS inflammations are intensely destructive phenomena, even when the nervous system is not the primary target organ. The most effective therapy for inflammations is the judicious use of corticosteroids. Since many clinical signs in encephalitis are inflammation more than organism related, even patients with infections may be treated initially with steroids.[31, 39, 59, 60] Further discussion appears in the section on infections of the CNS later in this chapter.

Anticonvulsant Therapy. This topic is discussed in detail in Chapters 43 and 103. The basic principle of anticonvulsant therapy is to initiate long-term, oral drug therapy with an agent known to be effective against seizures. Drugs currently available for treatment of epilepsy in the dog and cat include phenobarbital, bromide, clonazepam, clorazepate, and, in the cat, primidone. Choice of a drug should be based on the ability to achieve and maintain therapeutic levels, with minimal side effects. None of the drugs currently in use are ideal; each has the potential for causing toxicity. In general, if the epilepsy is idiopathic, about 80 per cent of patients may be treated effectively. In patients with symptomatic epilepsy, the ability to effectively treat the seizures will depend on the ability to treat the underlying etiology.[61-64]

Antineoplastic Therapy. Brain tumor therapy may consist of surgical removal, chemotherapy, radiation therapy, or a combination of two or more methods. Concomitant with the tumor treatment is treatment of secondary effects, such as edema. Both radiation therapy and surgery have shown promise in veterinary medicine. In general, they increase the length of a patient's life and preserve or improve the quality of life.[65] Although there are selected cases in which chemotherapy has benefitted a patient, it has not shown the promise of radiation or surgery.[10, 60, 66-73] There may be evidence that some forms of chemotherapy will enhance the effects of radiation therapy, creating an adjunct role for them in brain tumor treatment.[74]

DISEASES OF THE BRAIN

CLINICAL PRESENTATION

Patients with brain diseases generally present with both head and limb abnormalities, regardless of which portion of the brain is involved. This combination of head and limb signs may also occur in other clinical settings, most commonly in the patient with peripheral vestibular injury, e.g., otitis interna/media, in which affected patients have head signs (head tilts, pathologic nystagmus, facial weakness, and/or Horner's syndrome) in combination with limb signs (ataxia, abnormal muscle tone). Another setting is patients with diffuse neuromuscular disorders, e.g., myasthenia gravis or acute idiopathic polyradiculoneuritis, where affected patients will have head signs (weakness of facial muscles) in combination with limb signs (weakness of limbs, abnormal muscle tone, and/or abnormal spinal reflexes). A third setting is the patient with a cervical cord injury causing head signs (Horner's syndrome) and limb signs (weakness, ataxia).

Brain injuries may be focal or disseminated. Focal diseases are limited to one brain region, e.g., cerebrum, cerebellum, or brain stem. Disseminated diseases involve more than one brain region, and in many cases will also involve spinal cord and/or PNS.

FOCAL DISEASES

These conditions are confined to one brain region. The neurologic examination allows you to localize the injury precisely. Knowing the brain region involved is more important for establishing a prognosis and predicting complications than for arriving at a diagnosis. This is because every brain region tends to be subject to similar pathologic processes, e.g., a neoplasm may occur in any brain region. Prognosis varies significantly with brain region. The brain stem is crucial to life, i.e., it controls the vegetative centers of the body, and difficult to approach surgically. Thus, regardless of cause, brain stem diseases tend to carry poor prognoses. On the other hand, many cerebellar masses are amenable to surgical therapy, cause less devastating signs, and are associated with a high quality of life. Cerebral diseases are intermediate in gravity between brain stem and cerebellar injuries. The seizures and mental status changes seen with many cerebral diseases discourage many clients and may result in a client's unwillingness to continue therapy.

Cerebral disorders tend to cause changes in mental status and vision, and cause seizures. Many patients with cerebral diseases will circle. Most patients with cerebral diseases have weakness of limbs, with increased spinal reflexes and decreased postural reactions.

Cerebellar disorders tend to cause ataxia of head and limbs. These patients may have tremor of the head, as well as postural tremor of the trunk when the patient is standing. Many patients with cerebellar diseases will have head tilts and pathologic nystagmus. If the lesion involves the cerebellar peduncles, the patient may also have torticollis, usually to the side of the lesion. Patients with diffuse disorders of myelin (e.g., dysmyelinogenesis) will have similar signs.[75]

Brain stem disorders tend to cause cranial nerve deficits and weakness of limbs. Most brain stem disorders cause vestibular signs. Rostral brain stem lesions often depress consciousness. Caudal brain stem lesions often result in an abnormal heart rate and rhythm or respiratory distress.

FOCAL BRAIN DISEASES OF RAPID ONSET

These diseases tend to be caused by one of four major disease categories: head trauma, vascular injuries, idiopathic disorders, or neoplasms. Of these, neoplasms tend to be rapid in onset as a result of secondary changes, such as obstruction of CSF flow, leading to secondary hydrocephalus. In those cases, the rapid onset of signs is often a terminal event. Head trauma, vascular injuries, and idiopathic disorders are discussed in this section. Neoplasms are discussed under focal diseases of chronic onset.

Head Trauma

Traumatic injuries to the CNS are by definition rapid in onset. Many traumatized patients have head injuries, but not all of them suffer CNS damage. Those patients that do sustain damage to the CNS are defined as having craniocerebral trauma (CCT), regardless of the injury's precise location within the brain. Patients with CCT frequently die or suffer severe disability. The clinician's goal is to reverse any reversible injuries, while preventing further injuries from occurring. The most common cause of CCT is a motor vehicle accident. Other causes include blunt trauma, falls, animal fights, and gunshot wounds.

Traumatic nervous system injuries not only produce immediate and direct injury to nervous tissues (primary events); they also initiate a secondary, metabolic cascade of events that worsen the neurologic disease as well as produce systemic and metabolic derangements.[76] These secondary events may be related to sympathetic nervous system activation.[77] Increased ICP, systemic hypertension, myocardial necrosis, cardiac arrhythmias, pulmonary edema, and increased nutritional requirements all occur after CCT.[76] Other secondary events result from endogenous opiate release, excitatory neurotoxin release, free radical production, free fatty acid release, loss of high-energy phosphates, CNS acidosis, and CNS ion imbalance. Each of these factors' relative importance remains unknown, as does knowledge of how long it takes these secondary events to produce irreversible CNS injury.

Primary Events. The primary events occur at the time of injury and are predominantly mechanical in nature. Fiber tracts are mechanically disrupted and cell membranes injured. These mechanical disruptions may not be reparable. This immediate physical injury is a contusion. There may also be a reversible physiologic disruption of some cells, a concussion. Concussions are completely reversible.

Secondary Events

Pressure Changes. ICP rises in most patients with CNS trauma, usually as a result of brain edema and intracranial hemorrhage. The elevated ICP decreases cerebral blood flow by compressing dural veins, further elevating ICP. If untreated, the elevated ICP may result in brain herniation. Treat elevated ICP with diuretics, osmotic agents, and steroids. CSF production may also be decreased with diuretics and osmotics. Intracranial blood volume is decreased by hyperventilation and elevating the head. You may attempt to decrease cerebral metabolic rate by cooling the head or, in some cases, by anesthetizing the patient.

Edema. Brain edema may be either cytotoxic or vasogenic. Cytotoxic edema accumulates in cells, particularly neurons and astrocytes, and usually arises from cellular hypoxia. Vasogenic edema is extracellular and arises from leakage across a damaged BBB. Vasogenic edema primarily affects white matter and is more amenable to therapy than the cytotoxic variety.

Hypoxia. Significant CNS hypoxia occurs in most CCT patients, usually as a consequence of elevated ICP. The hypoxic patients may also be hypercapnic, further elevating ICP.

Seizures. Many patients with CCT will have seizures, either immediately or as a delayed sequela to the trauma.

Diagnostic Approach. Step one in treating CCT patients is to stabilize life-threatening, non-neural injuries. Treat shock and evaluate for evidence of pneumothorax and cardiac arrhythmias. If the abdomen is tense or painful, radiograph and ultrasound the patient, searching for a ruptured viscus or lacerated abdominal organ. When the patient's general medical condition is stable, evaluate the intracranial injury.

First, localize the lesion (Fig. 104–31). This establishes a database that allows you to determine the initial therapeutic course, monitor therapy, and establish a prognosis. Determine whether the patient has CNS injury or PNS injury, as there are differences in therapy and prognosis. Few patients with PNS injury require therapy (e.g., patients with peripheral vestibular injuries may appear profoundly disoriented, but have an injury requiring little therapy and carrying a good prognosis). In contrast, patients who have CNS injury frequently require vigorous therapy and have poor outcomes (e.g., patients with brain stem injury have a poor prognosis even with therapy).

Patients with PNS injury usually survive without serious sequela. In contrast, patients with CNS injury may not survive and those that do survive may have serious sequela including epilepsy, personality changes, and severe paralysis of limbs. The distinction between PNS and CNS injury is based on the neurologic examination of the patient.

Therapeutic Approach

Medical Therapy. Once the initial evaluation is complete, initiate medical therapy (Fig. 104–32). Elevate the head, facilitating passive venous sinus emptying decreasing ICP, enhancing CSF resorption, and helping to maintain cerebral blood flow.

As CO_2 increases, so does vasodilatation, which increases intracranial volume, directly elevating ICP. *Oxygen* lowers CO_2, lowering ICP. Oxygen can be delivered via a nasal oxygen line, via an oxygen chamber, or, if the patient is comatose, intubating the patient. Intubation and *hyperventilation* is the quickest way to reverse both hypercapnia and hypoxia in a stuporous or comatose patient. Oxygen also acts to prevent or reverse cerebral edema.

Steroids reduce edema and stabilize cell membranes.[59, 78, 79] Steroids also stabilize the BBB, preventing further edema from developing. Steroids lessen the inflammatory response that results from tissue necrosis, decreasing the secondary demyelination that occurs 1 to 5 days following CCT. Steroid use should be of short duration, because they may inhibit remyelination. Steroids should be started intravenously. Treatment regimens differ, based on when the patient presents relative to the time of trauma.

If the patient is presented within 1 hour of trauma and has a depressed level of consciousness, there are two possible protocols:

1. Administer methylprednisolone 14 mg/lb as an intravenous bolus, then give repeat boluses at 2 and 6 hours. These are followed by continuous infusion of methylprednisone at a rate of 1.2 mg/lb/hour for 48 hours. After this, discontinue the steroids.

2. Administer prednisone sodium succinate 14 mg/lb intravenously; repeat the dose at 2 and 6 hours. Then administer prednisolone sodium succinate as a continuous IV infusion at a rate of 2.2 mg/lb/hour for the next 48 hours.

If the patient is presented more than 1 hour, but less than 8 hours, post injury, or is not in coma: administer a bolus of prednisolone sodium succinate at 14 mg/lb, then give dexamethasone at a dose of 0.045 mg/lb twice daily for 3 days.

Several *diuretics*[57, 80] reverse brain edema, including os-

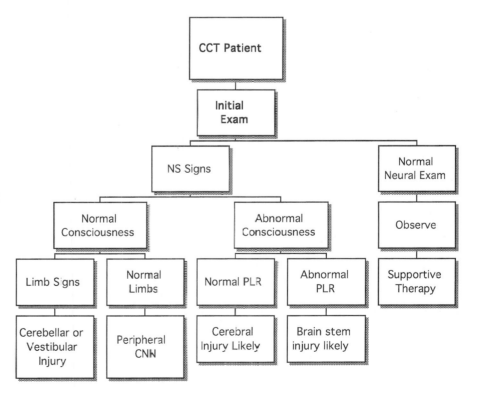

Figure 104–31. Algorithm for evaluation of craniocerebral trauma patient.

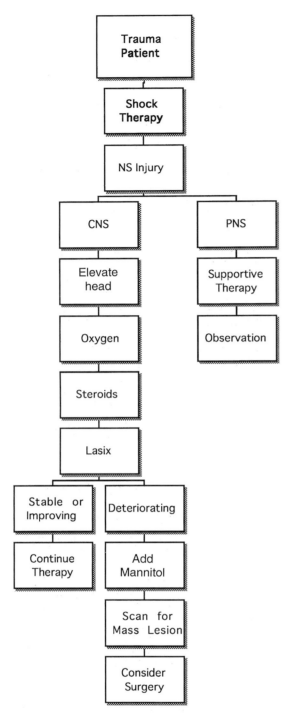

Figure 104–32. Medical therapy algorithm for the patient with craniocerebral trauma.

motic diuretics (e.g., mannitol), carbonic anhydrase inhibitors, and furosemide. Administer furosemide at 0.3 mg/lb, as an IV bolus. Repeat the dose every 4 hours. Furosemide appears to decrease the production of CSF and facilitate resorption of brain edema.

If the patient has decreased consciousness, administer a single (0.5 gm/lb) bolus of mannitol intravenously or over a period of time as a 20 per cent solution at a rate of 1 mL/lb/minute. Administer the mannitol in conjunction with the furosemide, as the clinical effects of each are lengthened and the potential for rebound edema is lessened when given together.[57]

Calcium blockers, vasodilators, narcotic antagonists, prostacyclin, and antiprostaglandins such as aspirin have all been advocated to prevent posttraumatic vascular impairment by preventing vasospasm or preventing development of arteriolar microthrombi.[81, 82] I do not routinely use these drugs in CCT patients.

In patients that experience *seizures,* administer intravenous benzodiazepines such as diazepam or lorazepam to control active seizures. Place these patients on oral anticonvulsants. Anticonvulsant therapy may be tapered off and discontinued if the patient remains seizure-free for 6 months.

Surgical Therapy. Surgery is rarely needed following CCT unless the patient has depressed skull fractures compressing neural tissue or an open wound that may introduce an infection. Surgical exploration for hematomas is advocated by some authors in deteriorating patients. I have not seen any beneficial outcomes in patients with blind explorations. With MRI and CAT scans available, surgery should be reserved for patients with documented mass lesions.

Supportive Therapy. Proper supportive therapy is essential. This includes fluids, frequent turning to prevent bed sores, and careful electrolyte monitoring. Institute hyperalimentation if the patient is unable to eat as soon as feasible.

Prognosis. Prognosis in CCT depends on injury severity and location. With injuries confined to the PNS, the prognosis is usually good. Generally patients in coma greater than 48 hours will not recover. After those two generalizations, the prognosis is best determined by whether the signs are stable or deteriorating and where the injury is in the CNS. Patients with deteriorating injuries do poorly. Clinical features of deterioration in CCT include rapidly declining mentation, dilating pupils, progressive paresis, bradycardia, and/or loss of vestibulo-ocular nystagmus. Such signs usually indicate brain herniation. Patients with *cerebral* injuries often have a fair prognosis. Although many patients with cerebral injury will improve, they may have persistent behavioral deficits.[83] *Brain stem* injuries usually carry a poor prognosis. *Cerebellar* injuries generally carry a fair to good prognosis.

The degree of sympathetic nervous system activation is a major prognostic determinant in patients with CCT.[77] Measuring circulating catecholamines has increased prognostic accuracy in humans with CCT. Patients with markedly elevated levels of norepinephrine (NE) had a much poorer prognosis that those with normal NE levels.[77]

A prognostic scale for use in veterinary medicine has been proposed (Table 104–7).[76, 84, 85]

Vascular Disorders

Nervous system vascular injury may result from loss of blood supply (ischemia) or from bleeding into the nervous tissue (hemorrhage).[86, 87] In most cases, the initial CNS injury is focal, regardless of cause; although multifocal or diffuse CNS hemorrhage does occur with systemic bleeding disorders. In those latter patients, the clinical signs will be multifocal at the onset. Nervous system vascular injury may result from a variety of causes, including neoplasms, CNS infection, aneurysms, atherosclerosis, arteriovenous malformations, cardiogenic emboli, vasospasm, atrial fibrillation, mitral stenosis, hematologic disorder, and vasculitis (secondary to parvoviral infection, Rocky Mountain spotted fever, dirofilariasis, or other infections).[88–90] Other causes of neurovascular disease include polycythemia, hyperviscosity syndromes (plasma cell myeloma, macroglobulinemia), bleeding disorders, immune disease, uremia, sepsis, disseminated in-

TABLE 104–7. CLINICAL RATING SCALE FOR EVALUATION OF CRANIOCEREBRAL TRAUMA (CCT)

CRITERIA	SCORE
Motor Activity	
Normal gait, normal reflexes	6
Hemiparesis, tetraparesis, or decorticate activity	5
Recumbent with intermittent extensor rigidity	4
Recumbent with constant extensor rigidity	3
Recumbent with intermittent extensor rigidity/ opisthotonos	2
Recumbent, hypotonic with depressed-absent spinal reflexes	1
Brain Stem Reflexes	
Normal pupillary light reflex and oculovestibular reflexes (OVRs)	6
Slow PLR and normal to reduced oculovestibular reflexes	5
Bilateral/unresponsive miosis and normal to reduced OVRs	4
Pinpoint pupils and reduced to absent OVRs	3
Unilateral/unresponsive mydriasis and reduced to absent OVRs	2
Bilateral/unresponsive mydriasis and reduced to absent OVRs	1
Level of Consciousness	
Occasionally alert and responsive	6
Depressed/delirious, but capable of response to stimulus	5
Obtunded/stupor, but responds to visual stimuli	4
Obtunded/stupor, but responds to auditory stimuli	3
Obtunded/stupor, but responds to noxious stimuli	2
Comatose and unresponsive to noxious stimuli	1

Total Score	Prognosis
3–8	Grave
9–14	Poor to guarded
15–18	Good

travascular coagulation (DIC), vascular tumors, and cardiomyopathy.[91] Most reported intracranial vascular injuries are associated with a systemic illness such as sepsis, hypothyroidism, bleeding disorders, or septicemia.[89] In humans, there is an increased incidence of cardiovascular anomalies, such as patent foramen ovale, in patients with ischemic strokes.[92] Ischemic and hemorrhagic events appear to occur with about equal frequency. Ischemia secondary to atherosclerotic disease (the classic human "stroke") is rare in small animals, which has led to the misperception that veterinary patients do not have vascular accidents. Vascular accidents occur regularly, but not from atherosclerosis. Additionally, secondary ischemic events occur in patients with CCT as discussed in the preceding section.

Clinical Presentation. In most patients, clinical signs of vascular system injury are *acute* in onset. Generally, the pathology and signs remain confined to one anatomic region of the nervous system *(focal)*. In ischemic injuries, the signs develop over a fixed period (usually less than a day), then stabilize and begin to improve within several days. In patients with hemorrhage into the nervous system, the course is less predictable. If the underlying cause for the bleeding cannot be identified and corrected, the patient may continue to bleed and the clinical signs will be progressive. When bleeding results from systemic illness, the bleeding may be multifocal within the CNS and the signs mimic inflammation. Subarachnoid hemorrhage produces a sterile meningitis and fever. Feline ischemic encephalopathy occurs more frequently in late summer, but may be seen at any time of year.[87, 93] None of the other vascular disorders appear to be seasonal.

Clinical signs reflect the brain portion damaged. Brain stem or cerebellar peduncular injuries develop torticollis. Some patients with vascular injuries, especially if to the brain stem, will have brain-heart syndrome and cardiac arrhythmias. It is not clear if the cardiac arrhythmias are the cause or the result of the CNS insult.

In patients with vascular disease, most neurologic signs are asymmetric. Idiopathic ischemia tends to be a disease of middle to old age. Other causes do not have age predilections. There is no breed or sex predilection in patients with CNS vascular accidents. Based on location and history, the differential diagnoses for these patients include abscesses, neoplasms, aberrant parasite migration, granulomatous diseases, and CCT.

Diagnostic Approach. Did the vascular accident result from a primary intracranial or extracranial disorder? Evaluate extracranial disorders. Hypothyroidism may predispose to atherosclerosis and infarction in dogs.[87] Screen for leukemia virus–related disease in cats. Evaluate all patients for bleeding disorders with a bleeding panel. Serum protein electrophoresis will rule out hyperviscosity syndrome. An electrocardiogram and echocardiogram should be performed to evaluate for myocardial disease, especially if there are auscultable arrhythmias. An ophthalmic examination, looking for chorioretinitis, hemorrhages, or vascular changes, may provide clues to an underlying etiology.

CSF evaluation is indicated. With a mass effect, expect increased CSF pressure. Many patients will have increased CSF protein, primarily albumin. With subarachnoid or intraventricular hemorrhage, there will also be free blood in the early stages following the bleed. Shortly you will find evidence of *erythrophagocytosis* by neutrophils and macrophages and, several days later, xanthochromia. In patients with severe necrosis and malacia, there may be an increase in the number of WBCs in the CSF. The primary cell types are mononuclear lymphocytes and macrophages, resulting in a diagnosis of nonsuppurative inflammation. The lack of organisms and the presence of predominantly albumin on CSF electrophoresis will distinguish this inflammatory response from that seen in patients with CNS infections.

Enhanced Imaging. CT scan, MRI, and/or scintigraphy may demonstrate the vascular lesion. In infarctions, there will often be massive disruption of the BBB, with edema but no blood in the neurophil. With hemorrhage, the BBB will be disrupted and free blood will be present in CNS. In either case, imaging will confirm a mass effect.

Therapy. The key elements needed to treat strokes were elegantly summarized by Caplan in 1997. A clinician needs to know the following: the nature and location of the lesion; the mechanism of the injury (e.g., hypoperfusion, embolism, vasoconstriction); the status of blood components that relate to coagulability, viscosity, and blood flow; and finally the state of the brain—is it normal, reversibly ischemic, or infarcted?[94]

Develop a therapeutic plan aimed at essential disorders, while also supporting the patient. Unless the patient is in shock, moderate fluid restriction is indicated to prevent worsening of the brain edema. Monitor and treat cardiac arrhythmias. Nutritional support is often needed in the early stages following acute vascular injuries. There may be a marked decline in systemic albumin levels as the patient enters a catabolic state. Systemic electrolyte disturbances may develop that warrant therapy especially sodium imbalances.

If an underlying disease is detected, treat that disease.

CNS

Give corticosteroids to decrease CNS inflammation and edema, using the same protocols for treating head injury. If the MRI or CT scan identifies both extracellular and intracellular edema, add furosemide to the therapy. If the patient is actively experiencing seizures, administer anticonvulsants, preferably diazepam because it is less sedative. Thrombolysis for stroke has not been explored in veterinary medicine, partially owing to limited initial diagnostics. It is not generally known within the first 8 hours whether a patient has an occlusive disease. The use of neuroprotective drugs is under active investigation experimentally and may improve treatment of both stroke and trauma patients in the future.[94]

A postischemic but prenecrotic period of several hours to days exists in patients with transient cerebral ischemia.[95] In that postischemic cerebral tissue, there is a persistent relative hypermetabolism using glycolysis rather than oxidative metabolism that is especially prominent during the reperfusion period. This glycolysis is believed to be detrimental because it increases brain lactic acid levels. Since brain glucose levels reflect the plasma levels, systemic hyperglycemia will produce moderate brain glucose elevations, facilitating glycolysis. Based on those findings, mild hypoglycemia during the postischemic interval might reduce the degree of necrosis in the brain. Clinical experience shows that postischemic hyperglycemia increases the morbidity and mortality of stroke patients.[96, 97] Another study did not find the same clinical effects.[98] It appears that hypoxia-ischemia in conjunction with hyperglycemia can result in infarction, whereas hypoxia-ischemia alone may only injure neurons in selectively vulnerable areas of the brain.[99]

Prognosis. The prognosis depends both on which brain portion is involved and the etiology. Brain stem injuries carry a poor prognosis, regardless of cause. However, patients with cerebral and cerebellar vascular injuries often recover. Patients with "idiopathic" cerebral and cerebellar vascular injuries usually have a fair to good prognosis for functional recovery. Some patients with cerebral injuries have permanent behavioral changes, especially patients with feline ischemic encephalopathy. If a cause is found, the prognosis depends on the ability to correct the underlying etiology. If cardiovascular emboli are suspected, drugs that affect platelet adhesion granulomatous meningoencephalitis may prevent future strokes. In the rare patient with bacterial emboli, antibiotics are the best prevention. Many patients with cerebrovascular disease ultimately have a poor prognosis, because their underlying disorder is untreatable.

Aberrant Parasite Migration

A number of metazoal parasites may localize in the CNS as part of aberrant migration or if the dog or cat serves as an aberrant host. Most commonly found are *Dirofilaria immitis* and Cuterebridae. Other parasites include *Toxocara, Ancylostoma, Taenia, Baylisascaris,* and *Angiostrongylus.*[87] In each of these cases, the signs are referable to the portion of the CNS involved. The signs are focal and progressive, resulting from necrosis and malacia along the migratory tract of the parasite. On CSF evaluation, esosinophils are seen. A definitive diagnosis rests on necropsy. There is no effective therapy.[100]

Idiopathic Disorders

Idiopathic Epilepsy. This subject is covered in Chapters 43 and 103.

Idiopathic Vestibular Disease. Seen in both cats and dogs, the signs are usually acute to peracute in onset, often peaking in less than 24 hours. In cats, the disease occurs most frequently in late spring, summer, and early fall, but may occur any time of year.[101, 102] There is no age predilection in cats, but in dogs it is usually a problem of middle or older age.[103] For this reason, it is also called geriatric or senile vestibular syndrome in the dog. There is no sex predilection in either species. This is a common cause of peripheral vestibular disease, accounting for 39 per cent of all canine cases.[103] The clinical signs include loss of balance, severe (often incapacitating) disorientation, ataxia, nystagmus, and head tilt.[101–103] Nausea may be seen initially, and many patients (about 25 per cent in my experience) vomit during the first 24 hours. The nausea may persist, making patients anorectic for several days. Clinical signs stabilize rapidly, and the nystagmus disappears over several days. The ataxia gradually resolves over 3 to 6 weeks. No other signs should be seen on physical examination, but, rarely, affected animals will have other cranial nerve signs. The pathologic nystagmus is constant and rotary or horizontal. Diagnostic testing is generally normal, with the possible exception of the brain stem evoked response. The diagnosis is one of exclusion.

Treatment does not alter the disease course, but supportive therapy to prevent self-injury and maintain good nutrition is important.

The prognosis is generally excellent in these patients. There is rarely any sequela (occasionally a mild head tilt), and recovery occurs in all patients. If the patient does not recover, you should reexamine your initial diagnosis.[102]

Idiopathic Trigeminal Neuropathy (Canine Dropped Jaw Syndrome). This is a condition of unknown pathogenesis that produces a motor dysfunction of cranial nerve V in dogs. The patient appears unable to close its mouth, and the owner may complain the patient appears dysphagic. Other motor cranial nerves, especially the sympathetic innervation to the eye, are affected on rare occasions. Clinical signs are acute to peracute in onset. Sensory abnormalities are rare in affected patients. No age, breed, or sex predilection has been described. Atrophy of the masticatory muscles is uncommon. Most patients recover rapidly and completely. The lack of atrophy and rapid recovery suggest the problem is more a disorder of myelin than axons. Since the disease is confined to the PNS, limb strength and spinal reflexes appear normal. The disease occurs more frequently in the autumn. Motor nerve conduction velocities are slowed in these patients. If there is axonal involvement, the EMG may be abnormal. All other diagnostic tests are generally normal in this condition. The primary therapy is supportive care. Teach the owner to feed the dog with the head elevated. Steroids do not alter the course of the disease and tend to increase the appetite, making the patient appear worse. The prognosis is generally excellent, as all reported cases recovered. The normal duration of signs is 4 to 6 weeks, with extremes of 8 weeks.

Idiopathic Facial Paralysis. This is a disorder of unknown cause associated with either unilateral or bilateral paralysis of cranial nerve VII. Although the signs are primarily referable to cranial nerve VII, with careful testing other (often subclinical) cranial nerve involvement may also be found. Some degree of cranial nerves V, IX, and X involvement is seen in humans. An association with recent viral illness, especially influenza, is also common in humans.

Affected animals have an acute onset of facial paralysis (unilateral or bilateral), including loss of eye blink, drooping of lip, and sagging of the ear. Owners often complain of excessive salivation, because of the diminished lip tone. If the lacrimal gland is denervated, the eye on the affected side will be dry, as will the nostril on the same side.

Clinically this condition has been associated with endocrine dysfunction (hypothyroidism and Cushing's disease primarily) and toxins such as lead poisoning. A causal relationship between these conditions has not been clarified. At present, pure isolated facial paralysis appears idiopathic.

An evaluation for endocrine disease should be performed, especially thyroid function. Thyroid-stimulating hormone stimulation rather than measuring resting hormone levels is preferred. An EMG will confirm localization and rule out involvement of other nerves. If neoplasia or middle ear infection is a serious differential diagnosis, skull films should be obtained. Otherwise, skull radiographs are rarely beneficial in this condition.

If an associated disorder is found, treat it specifically. Otherwise, treat only secondary symptoms such as dry eye (keratoconjunctivitis sicca). In humans, steroid treatment is routinely used for the idiopathic form of facial paralysis. There is no agreement in the veterinary literature on the benefits of steroids.

With idiopathic facial paralysis, expect functional recovery over 1 to 2 months.

FOCAL DISEASES OF INTERMEDIATE ONSET

Inflammatory disorders are the most common cause of subacute focal brain injury. Examples of focal inflammations include focal empyema (brain abscess) and focal granulomas. Brain abscesses are most likely to occur at the cerebellopontine angle from otitis media/interna progression into the cranial vault. Granulomas may be seen with GME, fungal infections (e.g., cryptococcosis), protozoal infections (e.g., neosporosis), foreign bodies (e.g., grass awns), and aberrant parasite migrations. Most inflammatory disorders are multifocal, even when the initial localization suggests a focal process. All inflammations other than brain abscesses and otitis interna are discussed as a group later in this chapter in the section on disseminated disorders. The other common focal disease of intermediate progression is neoplasia, covered in the next section.

Focal Inflammations

Brain Abscesses. Brain abscesses are uncommon focal accumulations of pus in the CNS with clinical signs of a steadily progressive mass lesion.

Signs in patients with brain abscesses generally begin subacutely. The signs are usually focal in nature and referable to the part(s) of the nervous system involved. There is often a history of inner ear, respiratory, or oral infection. Brain abscesses usually progress steadily unless they are being treated.[25]

CSF analysis and enhanced imaging are the tests of choice for the diagnosis of brain abscesses. The most common CSF finding is an increased number of WBCs, usually PMNs. You may see phagocytized organisms in the WBC. CSF cultures may be positive, and Gram stains may reveal the organism in the CSF. CSF protein is usually elevated, with local globulin production. If the abscess is extradural, CSF may be normal. Image-enhancing techniques (CT/MRI) accurately localize an abscess. The abscess may resemble hemorrhage or neoplasia, so CSF combined with enhanced imaging is needed to definitively establish the diagnosis.

Abscesses localized to the brain stem nearly always arise by direct extension, in contrast to those of hematogenous origin, which are frequently multiple and occur in any part of the brain. Most brain stem abscesses are cerebellopontine in location and arise from otogenic infections. They are usually unilateral, but if the ear infection is bilateral, the abscess may be as well. Brain abscesses are actually large suppurative foci, with necrosis and edema of the adjacent nervous tissue contributing to the size of the lesion. Owing to a lack of CNS fibrous tissue, there is little walling off or true abscess formation. Necrosis of tissue adjacent to an abscess is common. Cerebellar herniation is often seen as a terminal event in patients with unsuccessfully treated brain abscesses.

Therapy. Antimicrobials are the basis of therapy.[25] The drug should be chosen based on its ability to penetrate the BBB and its availability in both parenteral and oral forms. Use your Gram stain to choose the most appropriate drug. If no organism is seen, use a broad-spectrum antimicrobial. It is preferable to choose a bactericidal drug over a bacteriostatic drug. In CNS infections, the levels of antibiotics used are often higher than for other infections. In small animals, surgical drainage may become feasible as localization techniques improve, but the hallmark of therapy remains antimicrobials. Some references suggest that a single bolus of steroids should be given prior to antimicrobial therapy.[33, 104-108] Although there is much inflammation associated with brain abscesses, long-term steroid use appears contraindicated. Not only do steroids impair the patient's immune system, they also normalize the BBB, thus diminishing the ability of antimicrobial drugs to penetrate the CNS. Nonsteroidal anti-inflammatory drugs—i.e., aspirin—may be beneficial in these cases. In addition, proper fluid therapy and nutritional support are essential.[109]

In most cases of brain abscess, the prognosis appears to be very grave. This may be because of slow diagnosis, inability to surgically drain the abscess, or some other, undetermined factor(s).

FOCAL DISEASES OF SLOW ONSET

The major examples of chronically progressive, focal brain disorders are brain tumors. Some granulomas may be quite slow in their progression, but most inflammations have clearly become multifocal by the time they can accurately be classified as chronic.

Neoplastic Disorders

Brain tumors produce clinical signs when proliferating neoplastic tissues compress and/or replace normal neural parenchyma. This results in a gradual progression of focal neurologic impairment. Tumor expansion may secondarily damage the vascular supply to adjacent nervous tissue, leading to vascular compromise (ischemia) or bleeding. This secondary vascular injury may present acutely. Other common secondary changes include edema and inflammation around the tumor site and ventricular obstruction with secondary hydrocephalus. Such secondary changes often produce as many clinical signs as the primary tumor itself. In patients with (metastatic) neoplasms, the signs may be multifocal, since tumors may arise in multiple, separate locations either simultaneously or over time. Metastatic sites are generally at the periphery of a brain region's arterial supply, often referred to as a watershed zone. Primary CNS tumors may spread distally in the nervous system via the CSF pathways, e.g., choroid plexus tumors and ependymomas. As most tumors grow slowly, signs normally progress gradually. With metastatic tumors, the clinical signs are less predictable. Primary brain tumors are typically solitary. The major exceptions to this rule are meningiomas in cats, where there will be more than one tumor present in over one third of cases. Secondary tumors may be solitary or multiple.

Clinical Presentation. Although seen in very young animals, tumors are most commonly seen in middle-aged and older animals.[110–112] The clinical signs typically reflect the location of the tumor. Signs in patients with brain tumors are often transiently steroid-responsive but otherwise constantly progressive without appropriate therapy. In some patients, the first clinical sign is loss of vision.[113]

Seizures are among the most commonly reported first sign in patients with cerebral neoplasms. At Ohio State University (OSU), over 50 per cent of our patients with cerebral neoplasms have seizures as their first clinical sign.[111] Animals with brain tumors may have endocrine signs, e.g., polydipsia or polyuria; gonadal atrophy; unexplained obesity; or an abnormal hair coat, especially with pituitary neoplasms.[114] Contralateral attention deficits may be seen in hemispheric mass lesions.[115]

The most common early sign in patients with brain stem neoplasms are vestibular signs, which are usually acute in onset. Generally patients with extramedullary tumors (e.g., meningiomas) survive longer than patients with intramedullary (e.g., astrocytomas) or metastatic tumors (e.g., hemangiosarcomas). With extramedullary neoplasms, cranial nerve deficits are often the principal early clinical sign.[116, 117] With mass lesions at the cerebellopontine angle, you may see *paradoxic vestibular syndrome*. With paradoxic vestibular syndrome, the patient's head tilt and/or circling will be away from the side of the injury.[118]

Sudden death from respiratory paralysis may occur in patients with brain stem neoplasms, usually as a result of brain herniation. Tremor, ataxia, and vestibular signs are the hallmark of cerebellar neoplasms. Table 104–8 provides an overview of tumor incidence in dogs and cats.

Diagnostic Approach. The history of CNS signs in middle-aged or older dogs or cats should raise the possibility of neoplasm. Seizures with no other signs in any animal over the age of 7 should place neoplasm first on the list of differentials. A progressive, focal CNS disease is the initial clue to the presence of a brain tumor in many other patients. Confirmation of the diagnosis rests on laboratory testing.

All patients suspected of having a brain tumor should be thoroughly screened for primary tumors in other organs. The incidence of metastatic neoplasms is rising in veterinary medicine, especially as patients with systemic neoplasms are being treated. Historically, the incidence of CNS metastasis

has been considered to be lower than that of primary neoplasia in the CNS. However, reports in human patients suggest that the incidence of metastasis now exceeds that of primary neoplasia.[119] Pathology records at OSU College of Veterinary Medicine support this increased incidence of metastases. In the 35-year period ending in 1986, 71 per cent of all pathologically confirmed intracranial neoplasms diagnosed at OSU were primary CNS tumors. Since 1986, those figures have almost reversed, with 55 per cent of pathologically confirmed intracranial tumors being metastatic in origin.[120] It now appears that CNS metastasis occurs in about 20 to 30 per cent of human patients with systemic neoplasms. The most common site for such metastasis is the brain in both veterinary patients and humans. Reasons for this changed incidence of primary and metastatic intracranial tumors can be attributed to several factors. First, improved chemotherapy results in longer patient survival. The longer a patient survives, the greater the possibility of tumor entry into the CNS. The BBB, which limits tumor entry into the CNS, also limits the entry of antineoplastic agents. The CNS becomes a "safe harbor" for metastases. Thus paradoxically, the barrier that once was responsible for the low incidence of CNS metastases may now account for the increased incidence. This factor may be especially important with lymphoreticular neoplasms, as lymphocytes can cross the BBB. A second reason for increased recognition of CNS metastasis is improved diagnostic capabilities. With the advent of improved imaging techniques and routine screening of the CNS in patients with systemic neoplasia, CNS metastases are now being found prior to the onset of clinical signs of CNS disturbance. A third reason for the increased recognition of CNS metastases may be increased awareness on a clinician's part that a CNS metastasis may be the initial source of clinical signs in patients with systemic neoplasia. Previously, many animals with CNS mass lesions were never examined for non-neural primary tumors. Those cases may have been misdiagnosed as primary nervous system tumors, when in fact the CNS mass was a metastatic neoplasm. Careful antemortem or post-mortem screening of patients with CNS mass lesions may uncover a primary tumor in another organ. This same screening may reveal evidence of metastasis from a primary CNS neoplasm.[121] Table 104–9 shows routes of metastasis to CNS.

CSF Tap. Most patients with brain tumors have abnormal CSF (Table 104–10). The classically described CSF changes in patients with brain tumors are elevated pressure and albumin, with a normal WBC count. This combination actually occurs in less than 50 per cent of patients with intracranial neoplasms.[122] A significant number of tumor patients will have some form of inflammatory CSF response, charac-

TABLE 104–8. CNS NEOPLASMS OF DOGS AND CATS

TUMOR TYPE	INCIDENCE	BREED PREDILECTION	AGE AT ONSET
Astrocytoma	Common	Brachycephalic	Old
Oligodendroglioma	Common	Brachycephalic	Old
Choroid plexus	Common	None	Middle–old
Meningioma	Common	Dolichocephalic	Old
Primary lymphoma	Common	None	Middle–old
Pituitary adenoma	Common	Brachycephalic	Old
Glioblastoma	Rare	Brachycephalic	Old
Ependymoma	Rare	None	Middle–old
Medulloblastoma	Rare	None	Young–middle
Epidermoid	Rare	None	Young (dermoids)
Metastatic tumors	Common	None	Middle–old

TABLE 104–9. ROUTES OF SECONDARY CNS NEOPLASIA

MODE	EXAMPLE
Metastasis	
Hematogenous	Brain metastasis
Lymphatics	Perineural lymphatics to leptomeninges
Body fluids	CSF spread from CNS neoplasms
Direct Extension	
From tumor itself	Nasal carcinoma invades through cribriform plate into cranial vault
From lymph node	Spinal lymphoma in cats or metastasis to an epidural lymph node
From a metastasis	Skeletal metastasis of a neoplasm, e.g. osteosarcoma
Perineural growth	Tumor in an organ invades nerve sheath and grows along sheath into CNS

Adapted from Posner JB: Neurologic Complications of Cancer. Contemporary Neurology Series, Vol 45. Philadelphia, FA Davis 1995, p 16.

terized by mild to severe elevations of WBCs.[29, 117, 123] Meningiomas and choroid plexus tumors were the most likely to have changes in CSF WBC, including neutrophilia.[22, 122] You may also see an elevated WBC in lymphoma (lymphocytes and macrophages).

Elevated CSF pressure is seen in most patients with intramedullary tumors. Extramedullary tumors may produce little change in CSF pressure until the late stages of the disease. In general, posterior fossa tumors affect intracranial pressure less than tumors of the middle and cranial fossa. Elevated CSF protein is generally seen with intramedullary tumors, especially in choroid plexus tumors and CNS lymphoma. With extramedullary neoplasms, there may be little or no protein elevation. On electrophoresis, the protein elevations should be primarily albumin. Table 104–10 reviews the expected CSF changes in patients with brain tumors.

Electroencephalography (EEG). The EEG is helpful in confirming the presence of a localized process in about two thirds of patients with brain tumors.[15, 124] In cerebral neoplasms, it may provide evidence that the patient is developing a seizure disorder and provide evidence of anticonvulsant therapies' effects. No pathognomonic EEG pattern has been found for any tumor type or location. Most animals with brain tumors have slow-wave activity observed in the EEG. Asymmetric amplitudes or frequencies are observed, but these changes do not identify tumor type or precise location.[13] EEG is less helpful than diagnostic imaging procedures, which allow therapeutic decisions to be made based on test results.

Ophthalmic Examination. Some patients with elevated intracranial pressure will have optic nerve edema visualized on ocular fundus examination. Optic nerve edema does not confirm a diagnosis of neoplasia, as inflammatory disease such as granulomatous meningoencephalitis may produce similar changes. Optic nerve edema does warn a clinician that CSF collection poses an increased risk of brain herniation. Rarely, tumor infiltration of the optic nerve can be visualized on the ophthalmic examination.

Imaging Techniques. Plain skull films are usually normal except for patients with bony tumors or meningiomas. Angiography is not routinely performed in veterinary patients, but might be helpful.

CT and MRI, especially when combined with contrast enhancement, have proved to be the diagnostic tools of choice in CNS mass lesions.[13, 14, 21, 50, 51, 67] These tests identify the mass location, clarify the BBB involvement, identify the feasibility of biopsy, and allow you to choose the best surgical approaches.[21] Sequential imaging identifies the rate of tumor growth and determines the effects of therapy. Steroid use prior to imaging may increase the chance of a false-negative result, as it stabilizes the BBB. Low-grade gliomas often fail to enhance. Ultrasonography has been used to help localize tumors during biopsy procedures.[48]

Therapeutic Approach. There are two components to successfully treating patients with brain tumors. First, clinical signs are alleviated with palliative therapy. Unless the clients' initial complaints are addressed, it is unlikely that they will be willing to tolerate the time or expense required for definitive therapy. Second, definitive therapy is directed at removal or destruction of the neoplasm itself.

Palliative therapy usually consists of administering glucocorticosteroids and anticonvulsants if needed. Corticosteroids' clinical effect appears to be directed at tumor capillaries, decreasing their permeability. Steroids decrease blood to tumor transport by 29 per cent within 6 hours of administration. They further decrease tumor blood volume by 21 per cent within 24 hours.[125] These changes will result in a reduced intracranial pressure, decreased brain edema, and a reduction in clinical signs. The second form of palliative therapy is anticonvulsant therapy in patients with secondary epilepsy. These patients are treated as all other epileptics, but tend to be less responsive to anticonvulsant therapy.

Primary therapy of the neoplasm itself may consist of surgical removal, radiation therapy, chemotherapy, or a combination of one or more of those modes of therapy.[10, 60, 65, 67–71, 73, 74, 126] Surgical removal of superficial mass lesions (e.g., meningiomas) has been remarkably successful. Symptom-free survivals of 13 months to 2 years without additional therapy may be seen in many patients. Patients with bony tumors may respond favorably to decompression followed by radiation therapy of the tumor site. If the mass is benign, surgical excision alone can be curative. With improved techniques, surgical excision of deeper extramedullary tumors (e.g., meningiomas around the brain stem) may become practical. Currently, surgical decompression is performed in

TABLE 104–10. CSF CHANGES IN BRAIN TUMORS OF DOGS

TUMOR TYPE	WBC ELEVATION ($\geq$5/μL)	PROTEIN ($\geq$25 mg/dL)	PRESSURE ELEVATION ($\geq$170 mm H$_2$O)
Astrocytoma	5/26 (19.2%)	13/25 (52%)	12/21 (57.1%)
Choroid plexus tumors	10/16 (62.5%)	15/15 (100%)	7/10 (70%)
Ependymoma	3/6 (50%)	5/6 (83.3%)	6/6 (100%)
Meningioma	12/20 (60%)	13/20 (65%)	13/18 (72.2%)
Oligodendroglioma	1/7 (14.3%)	4/6 (66.7%)	1/4 (25%)
All tumor types	31/75 (41.3%)	50/72 (69.4%)	39/59 (66.1%)

Data from Bailey CS, Higgins RS: Characteristics of cisternal cerebrospinal fluid associated with primary brain tumors in the dog: A retrospective study. JAVMA 188:414, 1986.

these patients, but cures are uncommon. Patients with surgically removed tumors may also have either chemotherapy or radiation therapy following surgery to delay the return of the tumor. Similarly, debulking of intramedullary tumors has benefitted some patients.

If the tumor is superficial, biopsy it, even if it does not appear to be amenable to surgical removal. Megavoltage or orthovoltage radiation without surgery has increased both survival and quality of life in several reports. Many patients receiving radiation therapy will remain both steroid- and anticonvulsant-dependent, but their mean survival is dramatically increased over those patients not being irradiated.[65, 70]

Despite these reports, it is difficult to provide the client with accurate information regarding probable response to therapy without a biopsy. The probable increase in the patient's lifespan warrants initiating the therapy, even if the client does not allow biopsy but does elect radiation therapy.

Brain tumor chemotherapy should not be performed without a tissue diagnosis. If the patient appears to have metastatic disease or a primary CNS lymphoma, chemotherapy may be rewarding. If the tumor is glial or meningeal in origin, the results of therapy are less rewarding. Cytosine arabinoside or BCNU/CCNU are the most widely used drugs for chemotherapy of brain tumors. They are chosen because of their ability to cross the BBB, as well as their cytopathic effects.

DISSEMINATED DISEASES

Disseminated diseases are those conditions that affect multiple parts of the CNS at the same time. Diffuse disorders are a subgroup that tend to be widespread and symmetric in their effects. Frequently these conditions are limited to one major anatomic region (e.g., the brain), or to a functional system (e.g., the cerebellar abiotrophies). In contrast to the diffuse disorders are the multifocal diseases, in which there are many discrete lesions within the nervous system. The prototype multifocal disorder is encephalitis.

DISSEMINATED DISEASES OF RAPID ONSET

These conditions tend to be toxic, metabolic, and nutritional in etiology. Most congenital anomalies are detected shortly after birth with no antecedent period of normalcy for comparison. Inflammatory disorders may be rapid in onset, so are included in the differential diagnosis of this group; however, they are more likely to have a subacute clinical onset.

Thiamine Deficiency (Feline and Canine). Thiamine is an essential, water-soluble B vitamin (B_1) that is a cofactor in the decarboxylation of pyruvate and alpha-ketoglutarate. Both these reactions are essential for aerobic metabolism. Deficiency of this nutrient blocks CNS aerobic metabolic pathways. Thiamine cannot be manufactured by mammals; therefore, it must be provided in the diet. Some fish (tuna and salmon) contain the enzyme thiaminase; if raw fish is prepared at home, cats may develop thiamine deficiency.

Hypoglycemia. The CNS relies on a large and sustained supply of glucose for its metabolism.[127] The CNS is also effectively isolated behind the BBB, which limits (prevents) entry of water-soluble substances such as glucose into the CNS. To meet the nutrient requirements of the CNS, there is a glucose transport system. This system, located in the endothelial cells of the brain capillary system, is saturable, stereospecific, nonconcentrative, not energy-dependent, and not influenced by insulin[128]; glucose under 50 mg/dL is abnormal.[129]

Hepatoencephalopathy. Hepatoencephalopathy (HE), owing to portosystemic encephalopathy (PSE), is a neurologic condition associated with the liver's failure to remove toxins and digestive by-products from the systemic circulation. HE may result from shunting of portal blood directly into the systemic circulation, from structural liver disease, or from a deficiency of urea cycle enzymes.[130]

Hypocalcemia. Calcium is essential for normal cell membrane and neuromuscular function. Decreased calcium is capable of causing profound neurologic symptoms. As with hypoglycemia, the clinical syndrome's severity depends on the rate, degree, and duration of calcium decline. Causes of calcium abnormalities are reviewed in Chapter 63.

Hypoxia and Anoxia. Oxygen deprivation of the CNS produces a series of changes in function that, if allowed to persist, result in clouding of consciousness, confusion, and varying degrees of ataxia. Signs are acute and, except with cerebrovascular accidents, occur in a known clinical setting.

Renal Failure. There is no correlation between the severity of CNS signs and the degree of uremia.

Hyperthyroidism. The hallmarks of hyperthyroidism are systemic signs, but there are described CNS manifestations in cats[131] that display both CNS and neuromuscular signs.

Metronidazole Intoxication. Metronidazole, a nitronidazole antibiotic used to treat anaerobic bacterial and certain protozoal infections, may also produce CNS intoxication as a result of overdosage.[132, 133] The drug crosses the BBB readily, accumulating in CNS. The mechanism of CNS intoxication is not understood but appears to be dose related.[132, 133]

Both cats and dogs are reported to develop CNS signs as a result of metronidazole intoxication.[132, 133] The clinical signs included ataxia, weakness, disorientation, diminished postural reactions, seizures, and apparent blindness. Metronidazole had been administered for periods ranging from 5 days to 10 months prior to the onset of signs. In all cases, the signs were acute in onset. Laboratory testing will probably be normal. The diagnosis is based on the history of metronidazole being administered in excessive doses and clinical response to cessation of therapy.

The treatment of metronidazole intoxication consists of stopping the metronidazole and providing supportive therapy. The patient improves within 48 hours, and a complete recovery should be expected.

Lead Poisoning. Intoxication with lead impairs neuronal respiration. Intoxication causes primarily a cerebral disturbance with seizures and behavioral changes, although megaesophagus has been seen. Diarrhea is common.[134-136]

Lead poisoning, seen at any age, is more common in younger animals and intact males.[134]

Approximately half of affected patients will have nucleated RBCs on the complete blood count, and 25 per cent will have basophilic stippling. Blood lead levels above 40 μg/mL are abnormal (see Chapter 80).

DEVELOPMENTAL DEFECTS

Anomalies and Malformations. Malformations and anomalies result from pathologic nervous system development. Defects may be acquired (e.g., the result of an in utero viral exposure) or genetic.[87] The clinical course will partly be determined by whether the defect causes all its damage during gestation or whether the change results in continued nervous system deterioration post partum. In cases where all damage to the neuropil occurs in utero, the signs are usually static, i.e., they do not worsen over time. In cases where continued tissue deterioration occurs, the clinical signs will worsen as well.

Clinical progression is also affected by which tissue is abnormal. If the nervous tissue is anomalous or malformed (e.g., syringomyelia), the clinical signs are apparent at birth or shortly after and worsen slightly. If the malformation is to the nervous system's supporting tissues (e.g., the skull and spine), signs may not become apparent until later in the animal's life. These conditions are late in onset and progressive.

In most patients with CNS malformations, the signs are present at birth or immediately after. In those with delayed onset of signs, clinical abnormalities generally develop in young animals. The signs are usually symmetric, i.e., the left and right side of the patient are equally involved. In those patients in which clinical worsening takes place, the progression is generally a logical progression based on involvement of contiguous structures.

Hydrocephalus. Hydrocephalus is a pathologic accumulation of fluid within the ventricular system of the brain. It may be congenital or acquired postnatally. It may be a passive condition in which the extra CSF is filling voids in CNS tissue, referred to as compensatory hydrocephalus or hydrocephalus ex vacuo. It may also be due to obstruction of CSF flow, either in the ventricular system or at the point of resorption, e.g., arachnoid granulations. Hydrocephalus, especially compensatory hydrocephalus, does not always result in clinical signs. It may be seen in both dogs and cats.[2, 87, 137]

Congenital hydrocephalus is most frequently obstructive. When compensatory, it is due to other congenital defects, e.g., cerebellar hypoplasia. Some congenital cases of hydrocephalus are apparently due to failure of the arachnoid villi to resorb CSF at an adequate rate. Other cases of congenital hydrocephalus involve a narrowed mesencephalic aqueduct with obstruction to CSF flow. This may be due to inherited defects or to inflammatory occlusion of the mesencephalic aqueduct. Unilateral cases may involve obstruction of the foramen of Monro. Although congenital hydrocephalus appears hereditary in some breeds (e.g., Yorkshire terriers), it is a spontaneous malformation in others. The highest incidence is in toy breeds (Chihuahua, Yorkshire terrier, Manchester terrier, Pomeranian, toy poodle) and in brachycephalic breeds (e.g., English bulldog, Boston terrier, Pekingese, Lhasa apso). The most common clinical findings in patients with hydrocephalus include seizures, visual deficits, slowed learning, and dementia. Some, but not all, congenital hydrocephalics have an open fontanelle. The presence of an open fontanelle should never be considered as diagnostic of hydrocephalus because it may occur as a normal variant in otherwise healthy dogs. Many congenital hydrocephalics have a dome-shaped, prominent calvarium. Some affected patients have a bilateral divergent strabismus, referred to as a "setting sun sign." Although the clinical course in congenital hydrocephalus is usually slowly progressive, some patients appear to stabilize. A small number of patients with hydrocephalus will have a sudden, catastrophic worsening of their condition. When these patients are necropsied, intraventricular hemorrhage and internal capsular tears are commonly found. The pathogenesis of these secondary changes remains unknown.

Secondary obstructive (adult onset) hydrocephalus results from postnatally acquired impairments in CSF movement. This may be from ventricular obstruction, e.g., secondary to neoplasms or due to impaired CSF resorption at the arachnoid villi, usually as a consequence of inflammation. Infectious causes of hydrocephalus may also result in narrowing of the mesencephalic aqueduct; inflammatory changes may no longer be present at the time of post-mortem examination. Affected animals often have a history of recent inflammatory CNS disease or traumatic head injury. Hypovitaminosis A causes hydrocephalus by altering CSF resorption at the arachnoid granulations. Secondary hydrocephalus is often rapidly progressive and is associated with massive elevations of ICP. It is difficult in these patients to distinguish between the signs resulting from the primary pathologic process and those from the hydrocephalus.

In congenital hydrocephalus, skull radiographs may demonstrate a thin calvarium. These same patients will lose the radiographic, bony gyral pattern. Contrast ventriculography will definitively diagnose this condition but is rarely performed, owing to improved diagnostic imaging techniques. If an affected patient has an open fontanelle, ultrasound of the ventricles may be used to demonstrate the ventricular enlargement.[17, 19] This is most useful in congenital hydrocephalus. Enhanced imaging techniques, such as MRI or CT scanning, confirm the presence of hydrocephalus (whether congenital or adult onset) and may reveal the underlying cause in secondary obstructive hydrocephalus. CSF collection has been used to measure pressure increases. Increased pressure is an inconsistent finding in congenital hydrocephalus, and collecting CSF in patients with secondary obstructive hydrocephalus may be dangerous because the elevations in pressure may result in brain herniation.

Therapy of hydrocephalus depends on whether the patient has congenital or adult onset hydrocephalus. If adult onset, decrease ICP, then treat the underlying etiology. In both cases, decrease CSF production or increase CSF resorption. Medical treatment with steroids is known to increase CSF resorption, and there are some data noting that steroids also diminish the rate of production of CSF. Steroids may be used in either congenital or secondary obstructive hydrocephalus. There has been limited success in the long-term therapy of congenital hydrocephalus with maintenance prednisone. If a mass lesion is causing the obstructive hydrocephalus, the steroids may restore CSF flow. Diuretics, such as furosemide, diminish CSF production. Short term, they decrease ICP, but their long-term use may be associated with systemic electrolyte disturbances.

Surgical drainage has been of benefit in some cases. This requires permanent placement of a ventriculovenous (or ventriculoperitoneal) shunt.[2] In very young patients, the complications of surgery can be quite high.

The prognosis in hydrocephalus depends on whether it is congenital or secondary obstructive. In congenital hydrocephalus, the prognosis appears to be fair if the condition is diagnosed early and treated appropriately. Affected animals may always be dull and have limited ability to learn, but may make acceptable pets. The prognosis is generally worse in patients with secondary hydrocephalus and is generally determined by the underlying cause of the hydrocephalus.

Cerebellar Hypoplasia. Cerebellar hypoplasia results from a failure of cerebellar development in utero. The condition may be seen in dogs but is more common in cats. The condition may be heritable, result from in utero viral or toxic injury, or may not have a known cause. Inherited cerebellar hypoplasia has been reported in the Airedale, Irish setter, and chow chow. Bull terriers, Weimaraners, dachshunds, and Labradors have also been reported to have cerebellar hypoplasia, although the inheritance in those breeds has not been shown.[13, 81, 39]

In cerebellar hypoplasia, clinical signs are present at birth. In the cat and dog, where continued cerebellar development occurs after parturition, the degree of disability may not be apparent until cerebellar maturation has occurred. At that point, affected animals can be compared with their littermates that have developed normally, and the clinical impairment becomes obvious. In most patients, the signs are static, as this is not a progressive condition. Not all animals in a litter will be affected.

The principal clinical sign seen in this condition is cerebellar tremor. This tremor affects both head and limbs. The tremors worsen with excitement or stress and abate during rest. Some patients with cerebellar hypoplasia lose their menace reaction, but this is an inconsistent finding. In some animals, other CNS malformations occur from the same in utero infection, which result in additional signs.

Cerebellar hypoplasia is a diagnosis of exclusion.[13, 39, 81, 138, 139] Enhanced imaging techniques will demonstrate a small cerebellum in many affected patients, but not all. Some canine patients with cerebellar hypoplasia may also have *occipital dysplasia,* an anomalous development of the foramen magnum. In those cases, plain skull radiographs will demonstrate the associated bony malformation. All other diagnostic aids will be normal in cerebellar hypoplasia patients. The lack of clinical progression of a pure cerebellar disorder is often the basis for diagnosis.

Currently no therapy is available, either to promote normal cerebellar maturation or to alleviate the clinical signs. The prognosis is often determined by the animal's expected use and degree of disability. If the animal is an indoor pet, it may function quite nicely even though it does not generally show any clinical improvement. Affected animals should not be bred, owing to the condition's possible heritable nature.

Lissencephaly. This is a condition in which there is retention of the early fetal pattern of the telencephalon as a result of restricted growth of the primordial cells.[2, 100] The gyri and sulci fail to form, and the brain surface is nearly smooth. Paradoxically, the grey matter of the cortex is thicker than normal, but the periventricular grey matter may appear attenuated as a result of the much smaller total number of axons. This rare condition is most widely reported in the dog, especially Lhasa apsos, wire-haired fox terriers, and Irish setters.[87] The disease is characterized by dementia, seizures, and blindness. Affected animals have severe behavior changes. Most affected animals are symptomatic at birth or shortly after. The diagnosis is established at necropsy, and there is no effective therapy.

Hypomyelinogenesis-Dysmyelinogenesis. This is a group of diffuse disorders that preferentially affect the fiber tracts of the general proprioceptive system. The condition is most commonly seen in dogs. Myelination begins about the middle of gestation in most domestic species and extends into postnatal life. Myelination proceeds in an orderly fashion in the brain and spinal cord, and its completion confers functional maturation on the tissue. Because of the prolonged periods involved, disorders of myelination (genetic and otherwise) may affect the mitosis of oligodendroglia or inhibit the production of myelin. Surviving neonates may be able to compensate for the damage by continued slow myelination, becoming more normal with time. Oligodendroglial cells may be present in reduced numbers, or normal-appearing cells may fail to produce myelin. Since myelin in the peripheral nerves is under separate genetic control, it will be unaffected. Hypomyelination may result from prenatal viral infection following infection of oligodendroglial cells. Myelin reduction is often most extensive in the spinal cord but also occurs in the cerebellum and brain stem.[75] Inherited hypomyelination is seen in chow chows. Other affected breeds include Samoyeds, lurchers, Weimaraners, Dalmatians, Australian silkie terriers, springer spaniels, and schnauzers.[87]

Since the pathology affects primarily proprioceptive fibers, affected patients' clinical signs closely resemble those of patients with cerebellar disease. Since hypomyelinogenesis usually occurs in neonates, it is easily confused with cerebellar hypoplasia. At birth or when the animals first experience tremors (myoclonus) of the limbs and head, a base wide stance and rocking horse gait are present. Ataxia is pronounced, but there is no weakness. The tremors are enhanced with excitement and movement but usually abate with rest and sleep. Some animals in affected litters appear more ataxic than others. This disease usually affects multiple animals in a given litter. The signs are not usually progressive. Rather, many patients improve over several weeks to months, even becoming normal in some cases. Unless the neonate cannot nurse, the physical examination is usually normal. If it cannot nurse, you will see cachexia.

Known causes of hypomyelinogenesis/dysmyelinogenesis include inheritance and in utero infections.

Clinically, the diagnosis rests on the history with confirmation depending on histology and histochemistry. No therapy is currently available, but many patients will improve. Since many animals will recover with time, the prognosis is generally quite good.

Scotty Cramp. This is a hyperkinetic syndrome associated with episodes of spasticity and alternating hyperflexion/hyperextension of the limbs. Evidence suggests that there is a deficiency of serotonin available in these patients. Although resting levels are normal, there is not adequate serotonin for utilization during stress.[2]

The disease appears limited to the Scottish terrier breed. Clinical signs first appear at 6 weeks to 18 months of age. Typically the signs are induced by exercise or excitement and will disappear with rest. The signs last 1 to 30 minutes and are primarily characterized by a goose-stepping gait. An affected animal's mental status is normal during these events.

The history and signs are often enough to establish a diagnosis. The methysergide challenge, a provocative test, blocks the effects of serotonin. Administer 0.14 to 0.28 mg/lb of methysergide. Within 2 hours, there should be an increase in the frequency and severity of the clinical events. The drug's effects last about 8 hours. Side effects of the drug include nausea, vomiting, and diarrhea.

Diazepam, a centrally acting muscle relaxant, may reduce the severity of the signs. The drug should be given at a dose of 0.2 to 1 mg/lb intravenously for emergency situations. Vitamin E has been shown to decrease the frequency of the events. Try to avoid stress, and use behavior modification to reduce anxiety. Avoid antiprostaglandins—e.g., aspirin, indomethacin, phenylbutazone, banamine, and penicillin—which will all exacerbate the disease.

IDIOPATHIC DISORDERS

Seizure Disorders. These are covered in Chapter 33.

Diffuse Diseases of Slow Onset. Diffuse diseases of slow onset include both degenerations and most inflammations. These processes affect multiple CNS areas at the same time and are almost always progressive. Degenerations tend to be more symmetric than inflammations and are less likely to be associated with a febrile response.

DEGENERATIVE DISORDERS

Lysosomal Storage Diseases. Lysosomes are single, membrane-bound, cytoplasmic particles containing hydrolytic enzymes that are present in all cells. They are responsible for degradation of protein, polysaccharides, and nucleic acids. They require an acid pH environment for proper functioning. They function in two ways. Intracellularly, they function by fusing with vacuoles containing cellular material to be degraded or engulfed foreign material. These vacuoles are referred to as *secondary lysosomes,* and it is here that enzymatic digestion occurs. The second method of function is to fuse with the cell membrane to release enzymes extracellularly. The lysosomal storage disorders represent a group of inherited defects that result in abnormal lysosomal function.[2] In most of these conditions, there is secondary lysosomal engorgement with undegraded material. The cell's metabolic function is compromised because of lysosomal hypertrophy that crowds out normal organelles and impairs cellular respiration. The waste product build-up injures the cell. Sphingolipids, mucopolysaccharides, and glycoproteins comprise the bulk of the substrates that accumulate. Distended cells represent the basic cellular pathology. Intracellular storage material may or may not be demonstrable histopathologically, depending upon its solubility in solutions used during histopathologic preparation. Ultrastructurally the material is contained within membrane-bound structures. Pathologically, the gangliosidoses and ceroid-lipofuscinoses are characterized by swollen, vacuolated neurons, while the leukodystrophies are characterized by dysmyelination and degeneration of the white matter.

Clinically, there are certain similarities to the entire group. All these disorders are rare. All known disorders are inherited by an autosomal recessive pattern, so they are most likely to be seen in pure breed animals, especially from highly inbred lines. Generally, affected patients are normal at birth. Most of them fail to thrive and do not develop concomitantly with the rest of the litter. As with most recessive disorders, usually only one or at most a couple of members from a litter will be affected (Table 104–11). These are progressive disorders, which usually result in death of affected animals within 4 to 6 months after the onset of clinical signs. The age of onset and speed of progression vary but are often related. Typically the younger an animal is affected, the more rapidly the signs will progress. Tibetan mastiffs are an example of a breed with adult onset of signs. More than one body system may be affected in these conditions, which may allow diagnosis by biopsy of tissues other than the nervous system. There is no therapy for these conditions. The definitive diagnosis requires necropsy confirmation of the disease. Population control and genetic counseling are important.[16, 140–145]

Cerebellar Abiotrophy. These are a group of generally inherited, slowly progressive, degenerative diseases of the cerebellum reported in many species and breeds, including dogs (Kerry blue terriers, Gordon setters, rough-coated collies, Australian kelpies, Airedales, Bernese Running Dogs, Bernese Mountain Dogs, Finnish harriers, Brittany spaniels, Border collies, beagles, Samoyeds, wire-haired fox terriers, Labrador retrievers, golden retrievers, Great Danes, chow chows, Rhodesian ridgebacks, as well as mixed breeds) and cats.[87]

In most animals, signs begin at 2 months of age or older. Normally the disease is confined to the cerebellum, so affected animals show only cerebellar signs. Clinical signs are normally slowly progressive, eventually incapacitating the animal.

This condition is also a diagnosis of exclusion. All diagnostic aids are normal, including alternate imaging techniques. Brain biopsy may be attempted to confirm the diagnosis if antemortem diagnosis is essential. The history is the tool used to establish this diagnosis. This condition is generally easy to separate from hypoplasia at necropsy, since cerebellar abiotrophies reflect cell dysfunction and death in a previously normal tissue. In instances where the lesions are present at birth, neuronal attrition has begun in utero. It is believed that there is some metabolic defect in the cerebellar neurons that results in their premature degeneration and death. Cerebellar abiotrophies are fairly homogeneous within a given kindred or breed, but between breeds or species, there may be overlaps and inconsistencies. Macroscopic lesions are variable, but there is usually minimal reduction in cerebellar size. Microscopically, there is degeneration/loss of the Purkinje cells. Symmetric degeneration of extrapyramidal neurons is also present in some types and follows a pattern characteristic for each condition. The olivary and pontine nuclei are most commonly involved, but the caudate, putamen, and substantia nigra can also be affected in some types.

Neuroaxonal Dystrophies (NADs). These are inherited CNS degenerations of both dogs and cats. Known breeds affected with NADs include rottweilers, collies, Jack Russell terriers, Chihuahuas, and tricolor cats.[100, 146] NADs may reflect disturbances in axon transport. They are characterized by membrane-filled swellings of axons, both distally and near the neuron cell body.

In most patients, clinical signs begin at an early age and progress steadily. The predominant signs are cerebellar, including tremor and ataxia. Progression in rottweilers is slow (taking up to 6 years); in all other breeds, it is more rapid.

All ancillary diagnostic tests are normal. Confirming this diagnosis requires histopathology, leaving this an antemortem diagnosis of exclusion.

Bull Mastiff Cerebellar Degeneration and Hydrocephalus. Bull mastiff puppies in Great Britain and the United States have been seen with an inherited cerebellar degeneration and hydrocephalus.[100] The clinical signs include ataxia, tremor, visual deficits, behavior changes, and depression seen as the disease progresses. The signs begin at 1 to 2 months of age.

Diagnostic tests are normal; enhanced imaging confirms the hydrocephalus. No treatment is successful, and the prognosis is poor.

Rottweiler Leukoencephalomyelopathy. This is a progressive, heritable, white matter degeneration of rottweilers.[100] Affected patients have symmetric limb ataxia and weakness without cranial nerve deficits. Signs typically begin between 1.5 and 3.5 years of age, then slowly progress. All diagnostic tests are normal, and no therapy has been reported effective.

Pathologically, there is widespread symmetric demyelination of the spinal cord, brain stem, and cerebellum.

Other Degenerations. Various degenerations have been reported in Dalmatians (Dalmatian leukodystrophy), Labrador retrievers (fibrinoid leukodystrophy and leukoencephalomalacia), miniature poodles (demyelinating myelopathy), Egyptian mau cats (spongioform degeneration), Australian

TABLE 104–11. LYSOSOMAL STORAGE DISORDERS

SPECIES/BREED	AGE ONSET	DURATION	SIGNS/PATHOLOGY
Neuronal Disorders			
GM₁ GANGLIOSIDOSIS (BETAGALACTOSIDASE DEFICIENCY)			
Feline Siamese, Korat, mixed breeds	4–6 months	6–10 months	Ataxia, tremors, paresis, visual loss, seizures, behavior changes. Corneal and retinal lesions. CNS, liver, pancreatic acinar cells involved
Canine Beagle/mixed	2–4 months	4–6 months	Visual signs, tremors, dysmetria, paresis, behavior changes. CNS, liver, kidney, spleen, lymph nodes
Canine German short-haired pointers	6 months	18 months	Behavior changes, seizures, ataxia, weakness, visual signs, coma. CNS
Feline DSH	4–10 weeks		Tremors, dysmetria, ataxia, paresis. Dwarfism, corneal opacity. CNS, liver, endothelium, bone marrow, spleen, kidney
SPHINGOMYELIN LIPIDOSIS (SPHINGOMYELINASE DEFICIENCY)			
Cats Siamese, DSH	3–6 months	3–6 months	Stunted growth, ataxia, dysmetria, tremors. CNS, liver, lung, spleen, lymph nodes, kidney, bone marrow, adrenal gland
GLUCOCEREBROSIDOSIS (GLUCOCEREBROSIDASE DEFICIENCY)			
Dogs Sidney silkie	7 months	1 month	CNS, liver
MANNOSIDOSIS (ALPHA-MANNOSIDASE DEFICIENCY)			
NEURONAL CEROID LIPOFUSCINOSIS			
Dogs English Setters	14–18 months	8–12 months	Visual, mental, behavioral changes, cerebellar signs, seizures. CNS, lymph nodes, salivary gland, prostate, kidney
Cats			
Leukodystrophies			
GLOBOID CELL			
Canine Cairns and West Highland whites, beagles, blue tick hound, poodle	11–30 weeks	2–3 months	Tremor, dysmetria, paresis, muscle atrophy, visual changes, mental changes.
Feline			CNS, PNS
METACHROMATIC LEUKODYSTROPHY			
Cavitating leukodystrophy Canine			
Dalmatians	3–6 months		Decreased vision, ataxia, paresis

cattle dogs (polioencephalomyelopathy), domestic short-haired cats (encephalomyelopathy,) and Irish setters (hereditary quadriplegia and amblyopia).[87, 147–149] These conditions are all rare and with limited data. They are degenerative and diffusely progressive, and the diagnosis requires histopathologic confirmation.

INFLAMMATORY DISORDERS

CNS inflammations may be caused by infections, parasitic infestations, immune disorders, or idiopathic mechanisms. Such inflammation is described as encephalitis, myelitis, or meningitis based on whether the inflammatory process affects brain, spinal cord, or meninges, respectively. Nervous system inflammations usually produce subacute, multifocal lesions. Although they may occur in animals of any age, they are most common in the young. Some causes of CNS inflammation may be seasonal.

Some CNS inflammations may be controlled or cured with appropriate therapy.

Untreated, progression is random, often a clue to an inflammatory process.

Inflammations may be infectious or noninfectious.[31] In comparison with the frequency of infections involving other organ systems, CNS infections are uncommon in animals. One report ranked the frequency for the various causes of meningoencephalitis in dogs as, in decreasing order of frequency: viral (e.g., canine distemper, parainfluenza encephalitis, etc.); presumed immune meningitis (steroid-responsive meningitis-arteritis, juvenile polyarteritis/meningitis); protozoal (neosporosis, toxoplasmosis); idiopathic (granulomatous meningoencephalitis, pug encephalitis); bacterial; and rickettsial.[150] In that paper, two of the six leading causes of meningoencephalitis (granulomatous meningoencephalitis and steroid-responsive meningitis) were noninfectious. Many causes of encephalitis, such as rickettsial, are seasonal. Most infections are more likely to be sporadic than epidemic in a population, especially bacterial infections.

The low prevalence of CNS infections results from the CNS being afforded better protection by its barriers rather than a scarcity of infectious agents capable of attacking the CNS. Supporting evidence is provided by the awareness that either an organism must find a way to elude the host's barrier system (e.g., canine distemper via lymphocytes) or the host's barrier system must be disrupted (e.g., CNS ischemia with vasculitis) for CNS infections to occur.[33, 151, 152] More infections result from an organism's ability to bypass the CNS' defense mechanisms than occur as a result of an organism's unique neurotropism.

CNS inflammations are characterized by increased blood flow, exudation of fluids, leukocyte migration into the affected area, and altered CNS function. In addition to infections and idiopathic and immune disorders, CNS inflammation may result from trauma and some neoplasms.[31, 33, 153, 154]

Inflammations may be localized or disseminated. The most common focal inflammation is an abscess. An abscess is a local region of necrosis and suppuration, usually in response to bacterial infection. The clinical signs reflect a rapidly expanding mass lesion produced by the inflammatory process and its associated tissue edema. Abscesses are usually rapid in onset, have local progression, and mimic the behavior of rapidly progressive neoplasms. Granulomas are accumulations of inflammatory cells intermingled with a fibrotic reaction. Granulomas result from the body's attempt to remove or make harmless some chronic irritant, e.g., fungi, protozoa, foreign bodies, or parasites. A granuloma's predominant cell type will reflect the process's chronicity as well as the initiating agent. Depending on the etiology, granulomas may be focal (solitary), e.g., foreign body; or multifocal (disseminated) e.g., fungal infection. Granulomas tend to develop more slowly than abscesses and are generally progressive. Disseminated inflammations may result from infectious causes, which are frequently hematogenous in origin; immune disorders; or may be of unknown cause. There is widespread CNS infiltration with inflammatory cells, whose type is determined by the etiology. Adjacent tissue becomes edematous, secondary reactions to inflammatory by-products occur, and vascular supply to adjacent tissue becomes compromised as a result of inflammation. Disseminated inflammations are usually subacute in onset, although some viral infections may be acute in onset.

Meningitis is a meningeal inflammation, whereas *meningism* is the clinical manifestation of pain in the meningocortical region of the brain, marked by excitation followed by depression, generally associated with fever. Meningism is generally the result of meningitis, but not always. *Myelitis* is a spinal cord inflammation, while *encephalitis* refers to brain inflammation. If more than one CNS portion is inflamed, the root words are combined, e.g., an inflammation of both brain and spinal cord would be an *encephalomyelitis*. A brain abscess is the focal accumulation of pus in the parenchyma of the brain. Most brain abscesses appear to be associated with contiguous infections, such as progression of otitis interna, but may arise from hematogenous spread of organisms as well. There appears to be an association with septic embolization and brain abscessation in humans, suggesting a need for an ischemic injury to allow the infection to become established. Brain abscesses appear uncommon in the dog and cat. Epidural abscesses develop outside the parenchyma of the nervous system, adjacent to the dura mater. Spinal epidural abscesses are more common than are cranial epidural abscesses because of the greater available space in the spinal canal.

An infection's location in the nervous system will be determined by interplay of factors including etiologic agent, its entry route into CNS, and the character of the immune response to the infection. To gain entry to the CNS, an organism must first colonize the host, cross the mucous membrane barrier, and escape the host defenses. The patient's age and organism magnitude and virulence all play

a role here. The most common infection routes include hematogenous, via the systemic circulation; direct invasion; contiguous or parameningeal spread; and entry along a nerve root.

In most cases, if an infection is able to seat itself in the CNS, one of the CNS's protective barriers has been disrupted. The principal barrier to hematogenous entry is the BBB, which provides both an anatomic and physiologic barrier between the systemic circulation and the parenchyma of the CNS. For a hematogenous infection to occur, the organism must get past this barrier. In viral infections, this occurs when infected lymphocytes are transported across the BBB. In bacterial infections, successful infection generally requires that the BBB be disrupted.

Barriers to direct, contiguous, and parameningeal infections include the meninges, spinal column, and skull. Direct invasion by microorganisms requires prior trauma, which provides access across these protective membranes. In the dog and cat, transneuronal spread of organisms appears relatively rarely. Organisms that may use this route are rabies, herpes suis, and *Listeria monocytogenes*.

In review, successful CNS pathogens must pass a host's mucosal epithelium; invade, then survive in the intravascular space; cross the BBB; and, ultimately, survive and reproduce in the CNS or CSF.[33] Systemic infections, including splenic abscesses, pleuritis, lung abscesses, vegetative endocarditis, bite wounds, urinary tract infections, pneumonia, infected cranial sinuses, and middle ear infections, may predispose a patient to CNS bacterial infections.[150, 151, 155–158] The circumstances that facilitate establishing a CNS infection include a sustained bacteremia, bacterial adhesion to BBB components and/or transport within phagocytes that have the capacity to cross the BBB, injury to the BBB or meningeal barrier system (e.g., head trauma), immune deficiency states, vasculitis, parameningeal localization of infections, and the virtual absence of host humoral defense mechanisms inside the CNS.[150, 151]

The anatomy that protects the CNS from infection may increase the damage once infection is present. The meninges and bony indentations of the skull and spine may trap inflammatory products, promoting local abscess formation. The BBB may limit the ingress of phagocytes, antibodies, and antibiotics, thus delaying attempts to control the infection.[151, 159]

The organism itself may play a role in the production of clinical signs. Organism factors include whether or not the organism produces toxins (e.g., *Clostridium botulinum*), vasculitis (e.g., *Rickettsia rickettsii*), or is neurotrophic (e.g., rabies). Many bacteria are toxin producers. These toxins may produce more CNS injury than the infecting organism, resulting in severe injury even in the presence of low-grade infections. *Rickettsia* and other inflammations produce vasculitis within the CNS. Vasculitis may lead to local tissue infarction, a phenomenon seen in the steroid-responsive meningitis/arteritis syndrome of young dogs.[160–162] If the organism is cytopathic, there will be actual destruction of neural elements caused by the organism itself, e.g., rabies encephalitis.

The local accumulations of WBCs may produce significant pathology. This includes fibrin deposition, thrombosis of veins, and arteritis, all of which increase the sequelae of encephalitis. Vasculitis can also result from degeneration of leukocytes. These degenerating leukocytes release toxins that produce vasospasm, local ischemia, and tissue edema. CSF pleocytosis may on its own lead to further chemotactic attraction for additional leukocytes, creating a positive feedback cycle with worsening disease. The brain edema appears to be induced by the free unsaturated fatty acids found in membranes of neutrophils (PMNs). During meningitis, there is marked resistance to the outflow of CSF through the arachnoid granulations. The resistance may be due to granulocytes occluding the outflow pathways for CSF. This resistance is associated with elevations of CSF pressure and can be decreased with the use of corticosteroids. The resistance to outflow persists for up to 2 weeks after the CSF becomes sterile.[31, 33] Ventricular inflammation may also lead to obstructed CSF flow with secondary hydrocephalus, a phenomenon well demonstrated in FIP meningoencephalitis of cats and parainfluenza meningoencephalitis in dogs.

The CNS defenses against infections include an intact anatomic barrier between the CNS and the rest of the body, adequate blood flow, a healthy immune system, and finally overall good health. The local host defenses in the nervous system itself are generally inadequate to reverse most infections unassisted. Even in the CSF of patients with meningitis, the concentrations of immunoglobulins and complement are relatively low. This lack of host defenses in the CNS is largely responsible for the ineffectiveness of the CNS defenses against encapsulated organisms.[33, 154]

The majority of phagocytic cells present in CNS inflammations are of plasma origin. The WBCs appear as a result of the presence of the chemotactic component of complement (C5a). The peak inflammatory response occurs about 72 hours after infection begins. Although local production of antibody in the CSF appears to take place, it is produced by blood-derived plasma cells that migrate into the CNS. There is also increased passive movement of antibodies into the CSF from blood, which occurs in low to nonexistent levels in the face of a normal BBB.

Clinical Features of CNS Inflammation. Many patients with CNS infections will also be systemically ill. Fever is common, generally the result of exogenous and endogenous pyrogens. Patients with tremors or seizures may be hyperthermic from exertion. Many patients will have ophthalmic signs, including retinitis, choroiditis, uveitis, and vasculitis of retinal vessels. There may be abnormalities of heart rate and rhythm, either as a result of elevated intracranial pressures or from direct involvement of the brain stem. There may also be direct injury to the myocardium as a result of acute CNS injuries, with myocardial necrosis and death. In advanced disease, with severe brain edema or mass effect, brain herniation with acute respiratory insufficiency may be seen.[31, 104, 105, 153, 154]

The specific signs seen in a given patient with a CNS infection first depend on the location of infection. Classic meningitis causes paraspinal discomfort, paraspinal muscle rigidity, and decreased vertebral mobility, combined with a stiff, short-strided gait.[155] Frequently, hyperesthesia on muscle palpation or traction on limbs is found. Vomiting, photophobia, nuchal rigidity, and depressed mental status may be seen. Additional signs of neurologic dysfunction vary according to the CNS area(s) involved. Forebrain diseases are principally characterized by behavioral or personality changes and seizures. Other findings with cerebral diseases include circling, menace deficits, partial facial muscle weakness, reduced facial pain sensation, and abnormal postural reactions. Brain stem involvement is manifested by depressed consciousness, head tilt, loss of balance, ataxia, limb weakness, and multiple cranial nerve deficits, especially pathologic nystagmus. Cerebellar disorders are usually characterized by ataxia, tremor, and pathologic nystagmus. Spinal cord involvement results in limb ataxia and weakness.

There are large differences in clinical appearance between the patient with meningitis (pain and fever), meningoencephalitis (pain, fever, and CNS dysfunction), and encephalitis or myelitis alone (CNS dysfunction).

Inflammations tend to involve multiple portions of the CNS at one time. On neurologic examination, it may appear the patient has a focal disease.[150] Even when the history or initial examination suggest primarily a focal CNS disease, a careful neurologic examination will reveal involvement of additional portions of the nervous system in most patients.

In summary, encephalitis and/or meningitis should be suspected in any patient who presents with progressive CNS dysfunction without localizing signs. The presence of fever, emesis, photophobia, nuchal rigidity, and altered mental state lend support to such a diagnosis.

Treatment of CNS infections has two components: first is to treat the specific causative agent; the second is to provide supportive care and prevent life-taking complications such as brain edema.

Antimicrobial Therapy. When choosing a specific antimicrobial agent to use for a given patient, attempt to use the single, least toxic, most effective, bactericidal drug. The properties that you are seeking in your drug include ability to reverse the disease process without injury to the patient, capacity to achieve therapeutic levels in the CNS, and persistence of therapeutic levels until the disease is cured. Table 104–12 presents the properties of specific antimicrobial drugs.

Drug Administration. (Table 104–13) The major variable determining efficacy of an appropriate antimicrobial drug is peak CSF concentration. If the peak concentration is grater than 10 times the minimum bactericidal concentration, a cure will be seen in greater than 90 per cent of bacterial meningitis patients.[163] There is no agreement on how long to treat a meningitic patient. Ten to 14 days of therapy following resolution of the signs is recommended.

Supportive Therapy. First, direct supportive therapy at treating or preventing brain edema. Many complications of meningitis arise from the inflammatory process, not the infection itself or the organism's direct effects. Adjunct corticosteroid therapy has become increasingly advocated. Administering a dose of dexamethasone at 0.07 mg/lb at 15 to 20 minutes prior to initiating antimicrobial therapy, then continuing the dexamethasone at the same dosage four times daily for up to 4 days, has been associated with lower intracranial pressures, lower CSF cytokine concentrations, less CNS inflammation (as measured by normalization of CSF glucose levels), and fewer neurologic sequelae when dexamethasone-treated patients are compared with patients not receiving dexamethasone.[107, 108, 151, 164, 165] These studies looked primarily at patients with *Haemophilus* infections, but preliminary reports in other bacterial infections suggest similar benefits.

Dexamethasone use raises the question whether such steroid use will affect CSF antimicrobial concentrations or the speed with which CSF becomes sterile.[166] Steroid use does not appear to affect CSF antibiotic concentrations during the first 24 hours of therapy.[106] More importantly, steroid use did not affect the rate at which CSF became sterile.

Steroid's beneficial effects were not seen if steroid use was delayed for 12 or more hours after the first antimicrobial dose.[107] Empiric steroid treatment prior to diagnostics remains contraindicated. The steroids may affect CSF values, obscuring your diagnosis. More importantly, although many patients may benefit from steroid use, patients with viral, fungal, protozoal, and rickettsial meningoencephalitis may

TABLE 104–12. TABLE OF ANTIMICROBIAL DRUGS

DRUG	PROPERTY	CNS PENETRATION	ORGANISMS
Penicillin	Microbicidal	Intermediate (except in meningitis)	Gram-positives, *Bacteroides*, anaerobes
Ampicillin	Microbicidal	Intermediate	Gram-positive, *Enterococcus*, *Pasteurella*
Carboxypenicillins (ticarcillin)	Microbicidal	Intermediate	*Proteus, Pseudomonas*
Ureido penicillins (mezlocillin)	Microbicidal	Intermediate	*Proteus, Pseudomonas*
Isoxazolyl penicillins (cloxacillin, flucloxacillin, oxacillin)	Microbicidal	Intermediate to poor	Gram-positives
Vancomycin	Microbicidal	Intermediate to poor	Gram-positives
Chloramphenicol	Microbistatic	Good	Gram-negatives (*Pseudomonas, Salmonella, Staphylococcus*
Cephalosporins—new generation (moxalactam, cefotaxime, ceftizoxime, ceftazidime, ceftriaxone)	Microbicidal	Intermediate-good	Gram-negatives
Sulfonamide-trimethoprim in combination	Microbicidal-microbistatic	Good	Pneumococci, meningococci, *Listeria, Haemophilus, Staphylococcus*, gram-negatives
Metronidazole	Microbicidal	Good	Anaerobes
Aminoglycosides	Microbicidal	Poor	Gram-negatives
Amphotericin-B	Microbicidal	Poor	Systemic fungi
Ketoconazole	Microbistatic	Intermediate	Systemic fungi
Flucytosine	Microbicidal	Intermediate	Systemic fungi

be worsened by their use. As such, steroids should only be used in patients where you are confident the benefits outweigh the risks. If you are still suspicious of brain edema, diuretics may be indicated if the patient deteriorates. Fluid restriction does not appear to be helpful in preventing brain edema and may be contraindicated for systemic illness.[109] The risk of brain edema appears lower than the sequela of fluid restriction, and so if appropriate, maintenance fluid therapy should be used.[167]

If the patient is febrile, antipyrogen use is recommended. If the patient is hyperthermic from tremors or seizures, cold water, ice packs, or alcohol baths should be sufficient. If the patient develops seizures, they should be treated with anticonvulsants. If a waterbed is available, recumbent ani-

TABLE 104–13. DRUG DOSAGES FOR USE IN NERVOUS SYSTEM DISEASES

DRUG	DOSE	ROUTE	FREQUENCY (HR)	INDICATION
Antimicrobial Drug Dosages for CNS Infections				
Penicillin (aqueous)	$10–22 \times 10^3$ U/kg	Intravenous	4–6	
Ampicillin	5–22 mg/kg	Intravenous	6	
Carbenicillin	10–30 mg/kg	IV/IM	4–6	
Oxacillin	8.8–20 mg/kg	Intravenous or per os	4–8	
Cloxacillin				
Gentamicin	2 mg/kg	Intravenous or intramuscular	8	
Chloramphenicol	10–15 mg/kg	Per os	4–6	
Cefalexin	20 mg/kg (10–30)	Per os	8	
Cephapirin	20–30 mg/kg	Intravenous/IM	8	
Amphotericin B	0.15–0.50 mg/kg	Intravenous	48	
Flucytosine	50 mg/kg	Per os	8	
Rifampin	10–20 mg/kg	Per os	8–12	
Metronidazole	10–15 mg/kg	Per os	8	
Cefotaxime	6–40 mg/kg	IM/IV	4–6	
Anti-inflammatory Drugs				
Dexamethasone	1 mg/kg	IV or per os	q12–24h	Steroid-responsive meningitis, antiedema CNS dose
Prednisone	1–2 mg/kg	Per os	q24h	GME, steroid-responsive meningitis, antiedema CNS dose
Methylprednisone	30 mg/kg	IV	Bolus, repeat at 2 and 6 hours	Brain trauma
	2.5 mg/kg	IV	Infusion for 48 hours	Brain trauma
Prednisone sodium succinate	30 mg/kg	IV	Bolus, repeat at 2 and 6 hours	Brain trauma
	5 mg/kg/hr	IV	Infusion for 48 hours	Brain trauma
Diuretics				
Mannitol	1 g/kg	IV	Once	Brain edema
Furosemide	0.7–1 mg/kg	IV	q4h	Brain edema
Miscellaneous				
Thiamine	1–25 mg	IM	q24h	Deficiency states

mals should be kept on it. Frequent turning to prevent decubital ulcers and passive pulmonary congestion is essential. If the patient has an altered mental status, the bladder may need to be expressed and suppositories used to prevent constipation.

Meningitic patients frequently develop systemic sequelae including shock and disseminated intravascular coagulation (DIC).

The most common (or significant) causes of encephalitis in cats include rabies, FIP, toxoplasmosis, neosporosis, feline immunodeficiency virus (FIV), and the systemic fungal diseases.[2, 31, 100]

The most common (or significant) causes of encephalitis in dogs include rabies, GME, canine distemper, toxoplasmosis, neosporosis, and systemic fungal diseases.[2, 31, 100, 150]

Diagnostic Tests. CSF analysis remains the diagnostic test of choice in CNS inflammations. Normally, CSF WBC numbers will be elevated. The highest WBC counts are seen with granulomatous diseases (e.g., FIP and GME) and bacterial meningitis. With systemic fungal, protozoal, and parasitic infections, eosinophils may also be present in the CSF. You may see bacteria and fungi on CSF cytologic examination. CSF protein levels should be increased with globulin elevations. In some viral diseases, the protein elevation may be minimal, for example, in canine distemper and rabies. CSF analysis is discussed in greater detail at the beginning of the chapter.

Serologic testing of blood and CSF may identify the specific causative agent of the CNS inflammation. Serology's principal limitation is the delay for the test results to become available. CSF serologic results are a more reliable indicator of CNS involvement than serum results.

Computed Tomography/MRI. These image enhancing techniques are better at identifying mass lesions than disseminated inflammations; however, with GME or other focal inflammations, they are beneficial in establishing a definitive diagnosis.[15, 168–170] Imaging may also be helpful if there is abscess formation or edema production.

Treatment. Therapy should be directed primarily at the causative agent if one can be identified. This therapy should be longer than for a similar non-CNS infection. When choosing drugs, be certain to consider the ability of the drug to cross the BBB. General supportive therapy should accompany the etiology-specific therapy.

Listeriosis (Circling Disease). This is a bacterial meningoencephalitis normally seen in adult animals, caused by *Listeria monocytogenes. Listeria* is a gram-positive organism, which normally resides in soil and silage. The disease is usually seen in ruminants but may occur in cats and dogs. The route of entry appears to be the oral cavity. Abrasions of the mucous membranes allow penetration by the organism. The bacteria then travels via a cranial nerve to the brain stem. The clinical signs will center around the nerve traveled; usually cranial nerves V, VII, IX, and X are involved. The disease is infectious but not contagious.

Clinical Picture. Young adults are the most likely to be affected. Generally the signs start acutely, then slowly progress. The neurologic signs are generally confined to the brain stem and include asymmetric cranial nerve deficits, limb weakness, depression, and vestibular dysfunction. Torticollis, circling, head tilts, ataxia, and weakness are other common signs. As the disease progresses, brain herniation may result.

Diagnosis. CSF analysis remains the diagnostic test of choice. The pressure should be normal to increased. The WBC count should be increased, with a predominately monocellular pleocytosis. A few neutrophils are generally

seen, but they comprise a small percentage of the cell population. Usually there will be an elevated protein as well. Cultures of the CSF are generally unrewarding, and the organism is rarely seen on Gram stain.

Therapy. Vigorous therapy with chlortetracycline or high doses of penicillin is indicated. Fluid therapy should be administered if the animals are having trouble eating or drinking.

Prognosis. If treated early and vigorously, the prognosis is good. Residual signs, including head tilts, may be seen for several weeks following treatment but usually resolve.

Rabies Encephalitis. Rabies is a viral CNS infection caused by one of several related Lyssaviruses in the rhabdovirus family, which can affect any warm-blooded animal, including humans. Once the CNS is infected, the disease appears to be invariably fatal. Transmission is normally through bite wounds; however, aerosol transmission and absorption through mucous membranes are reported. Virus may be shed a few days before the onset of clinical signs, which is the basis for the 10-day to 2-week observation period enforced following animal bites. The virus is destroyed by lipid solvents and low pH. There appear to be antigenic differences between the rabies viruses found in dogs, bats, foxes, and some other reservoirs. It is also now known that there are several rabies-related but antigenically distinct members of the Lyssavirus family that cause rabies-like diseases in humans and animals. Since 1983, there has been more cat rabies in the United States than dog rabies, making the importance of vaccinating cats more apparent. There are also now two confirmed cases of cats acquiring rabies from hunting bats.[171–173]

Clinical Presentation. Rabies is clinically unpredictable.[173–175] The incubation following either aerosol exposure or inoculation from the bite of a rabid animal varies tremendously. Although incubations longer than 12 months have been documented, in most cases signs develop within 25 days of exposure. Since the virus travels via peripheral nerves, the bite location plays a role in the incubation period. It is presumed that bites about the face will have shorter incubations than bites on the limbs, as the virus has a shorter distance to migrate to CNS. The clinical disease has classically been divided into three syndromes. Affected animals may display all three syndromes or have combinations of signs from all three syndromes simultaneously.

The prodromal stage is usually seen in all patients. These animals may be febrile. Affected patients display vague, nonspecific signs including apprehension, restlessness, anorexia, vomiting, and excess salivation. These signs may last up to 5 days before the animal develops new signs or dies.

The acute neurologic or furious stage follows the prodromal stage. Wandering, viciousness, dementia, and seizures are seen in the furious stage. This is the most common form in cats.[175] Death typically follows in less than 8 days after the onset of furious rabies.

The third stage is the terminal or dumb form of rabies. Progression of spinal paralysis to brain stem signs characterizes this form of rabies. This is an ascending disease. Death usually occurs in less than 5 days after the onset of dumb rabies. Dumb rabies may occur immediately after the prodromal stage or after the furious stage. Dumb rabies may be associated with anal paralysis and urinary incontinence.

Rabies does not respond to any therapy, and death occurs within 2 weeks of clinical onset. Although the signs of rabies are variable, the virus has a predilection for the brain stem. As a result, the terminal events usually center around the brain stem with death occurring from respiratory paralysis.

Diagnostic Considerations. Rabies should be a differential diagnosis in all cases of progressive brain disease. Consider the animal's vaccination history, the incidence of rabies in your community, and the potential for exposure of the patient to rabies as you rank your differentials.

CSF Analysis. Spinal fluid is usually normal or, at best, there might be a mild, nonsuppurative inflammation in rabid patients.

Post-mortem Diagnosis. The definitive diagnosis of rabies still rests on post-mortem tissue examination and virologic studies. Fluorescent antibody test on the brain is the most rapid and reliable test.

Animal Restraint. Any animal that bites a human must be observed for 10 days for signs of rabies. If the animal dies, the head should be shipped to the State Health Department for rabies testing.

Therapy. No treatment has been reported effective in veterinary patients with rabies. There are reports of human recoveries, after extensive supportive care. Serologic evidence suggests that spontaneous recoveries might occur in some species of animals, including dogs, cats, and skunks.

Prognosis. The prognosis is grave; consider this an invariably fatal disease.

Prevention. Current evidence suggests that current vaccines, when properly administered, are safe and effective.[173] An oral vaccine is now being used successfully in Europe to control rabies in feral foxes, and one is under consideration for use in raccoons.[176]

Postvaccinal Rabies. This is a progressive CNS and PNS disease that follows vaccination of dogs or cats for rabies with attenuated vaccines. There are no reports of this condition occurring following vaccination with killed virus vaccines. Serologic testing confirmed that affected animals had vaccine-induced rabies. At present, none have been reported to shed virus.

Clinical Picture. All affected animals developed a progressive caudal paresis beginning 12 to 17 days after vaccination with a modified live virus (MLV) rabies vaccine. The signs usually start unilaterally in the vaccinated limb. Over time, the signs will progress to involve the brain stem. The affected animals almost never have a furious phase. The signs in affected limbs may be either UMN or LMN, since the disease starts in the LMN then progresses up to the UMN. The signs are rapidly progressive, and death is inevitable. These animals should be handled exactly as one would handle animals with naturally occurring rabies.

Diagnostic Tests

CSF ANALYSIS. Affected animals had a nonsuppurative encephalitis, characterized by increased numbers of mononuclear cells with an increased CSF protein.

OTHER TESTS. Sixty per cent of the cats with vaccine-induced rabies are feline leukemia virus (FeLv)–positive. The significance of that finding is unknown.

Aujeszky's Disease (Pseudorabies). This is a herpesvirus disease, whose reservoir is pigs but which may occur in dogs and cats.[177] Outbreaks are usually sporadic in nature. The etiology is unusual for a herpesvirus because of its lack of host specificity. Dogs and cats usually acquire the infection by ingesting infected tissue. Following exposure, the virus spreads centripetally along nerves until it reaches a ganglion; it then enters the spinal cord or brain and spreads throughout the CNS. The viral infection of the ganglion and spinal cord segment initiates the localized or generalized pruritus so characteristic of this disease. There is no macroscopic pathology associated with pseudorabies, excepting

that of automutilation, which may be quite severe and localized to the site of infection.

Clinical Picture. The disease is rapidly lethal in carnivores. It is usually seen in pet animals from farms. Most dogs and cats are found dead by their owners, often with the owner believing the patient was poisoned. If found alive, the affected patients show a profound dementia, pain, seizures, and self-mutilation that progresses quickly to death.

Diagnostic Approach and Therapy. Normally there will be increased numbers of mononuclear cells in the CSF. Post mortem, the disease is diagnosed by serology, mouse inoculation, and histopathology. There is no effective therapy, and the prognosis is quite poor.

Infectious Canine Distemper Virus Encephalitis (CDVE). Infectious canine distemper is caused by a morbillivirus of the paramyxovirus family. This virus is antigenically similar to human measles and bovine rinderpest viruses. Canine distemper virus has the capacity for infecting many tissues, including the CNS. In CNS, the virus invades glia to produce destruction of white matter. CDVE is the most common cause of encephalitis in the dog.[178–180] Although CDVE may occur in any age dog, it is most common in dogs less than 1 year of age. In puppies, systemic illness is frequent, in addition to encephalitis. CDVE involves meninges as well as neuraxis with lesions involving both grey and white matter. The clinical disease differs based on the patient's age and immunocompetence, as well as virus biotype, and other unknown host factors.[181–183] CDV may also cause encephalitis in sea lions, tigers, and lions. The neurologic form of CDV may occur in well-vaccinated animals, without systemic signs.[184, 178–180]

Infection is principally through aerosol inoculation. The virus replicates in tonsils and bronchial lymph nodes, then infects lymphocytes, which are responsible for spreading the virus. If antibodies fail to develop, clinical disease will occur. Normally, antibodies develop about 9 days following infection. CNS infection appears to occur 14 to 18 days post infection. If there is an appropriate immune response, the CNS may be spared. Without an immune response, infected lymphocytes enter the CNS either by crossing the BBB or by entering CSF and then crossing the CSF-brain barrier. Once in the CNS, virus exits lymphocytes and enters CNS neurons and glia. In the glia, the virus replicates and by some unknown mechanism produces demyelination. Some dogs survive the initial infection and then develop partial immunity. These dogs are at risk for later CNS injury from immunopathologic damage to white matter and secondary inflammation.[181–183, 185] Thus, it is apparent that dogs with CDV infection may have direct, virus-induced damage to the CNS as well as later indirect damage as a result of developing immunity. Several factors will affect the development of CDVE and its sequelae. Most important is age at the time of infection. Very young puppies are more likely to have grey matter infection, severe neuronal necrosis, minimal inflammation, and a high mortality. This is probably related to the development of immunocompetence. Older animals are more likely to develop an inflammatory white matter disease. Different strains of the distemper virus will produce different clinical syndromes. There now appear to be strains that are tropic for neurons that produce polioencephalitis; strains with tropism for astrocytes that produce demyelination; and strains that produce chronic (persistent) CNS infections.[181]

Young dogs (6 to 12 weeks of age) typically have a neuronal disease. This is also the form usually seen in postvaccinal distemper. Clinical signs include seizures, dementia, severe personality changes, weakness, and ataxia. The postvaccinal disease occurs 7 to 10 days after vaccination and is only seen in immature dogs. Pathologic changes in the neuronal disease primarily affect the cerebrum and brain stem. In the postvaccinal form, they are especially seen in the pons. This is the form of the disease most likely to produce distemper myoclonus.[186, 178]

A chronic progressive multifocal CNS disease may occur in adult animals, regardless of age. This is primarily a white matter disease, which often has predominantly cerebellar vestibular signs with spinal cord and brain involvement. These patients undergo a chronic, inflammatory demyelination as a result of viral persistence.[182, 183] This condition and GME have many clinical similarities, based on location and progression of clinical signs.[186, 178]

Old dog encephalitis (ODE) appears to be a variant of chronic CDV infection. In spite of the name, this disease may occur at any age. The most prominent clinical sign is dementia, with ataxia and central blindness. Patients with ODE rarely experience seizures. This disease is most characterized by how severely abnormal the animals behave and walk, yet how unremarkable their neurologic examination remains.[178]

In multisystemic distemper, there are generally no diagnostic challenges. Affected patients will have respiratory signs, chorioretinitis, and CNS disease. In mature patients, the diagnosis is often less certain. Many affected patients will be lymphopenic during the acute phase of illness. CSF is often normal in affected patients. There may be a mild increase in the number of WBCs, primarily mononuclear cells. There may also be a mild increase in protein, which is usually either IgG or IgM.[38, 37, 187] CSF serology may be helpful but not conclusive in vaccinated patients. Antibodies against CDV should not be present in CSF even in vaccinated dogs unless there is local infection. Severe injury to the BBB could allow serum antibodies to leak into the CSF. Testing the cells in CSF for CDV antigen will allow for a specific diagnosis if the results are positive.

If present, myoclonus is suggestive of CDVE, but myoclonus is not always present. In addition, other conditions (e.g., hypocalcemia) may produce movement disorders that mimic myoclonus. Epithelial inclusions from the vagina, prepuce, and conjunctiva are rarely present in the CNS form of CDV.

At present, no therapy, including steroids, is known to be effective in the treatment of CDVE. The prognosis for the CNS form of CDV is guarded, and a small percentage of patients recover but are left with sequelae. Myoclonus is usually permanent. If the patient is left with seizures, they may be controlled in some instances. The other neural deficits may improve as the inflammation resolves. However, some animals progress regardless of therapy.

***Herpes canis* Encephalitis.** This is a virus encephalitis that is occasionally seen in nursing puppies and is often fatal. It also has been incriminated as producing a nonsuppurative meningoencephalitis and cerebral signs in immunosuppressed adult dogs. Clinically, the patients have predominantly brain stem and cerebellar signs. Although the route of entry is hematogenous, some patients have a trigeminal ganglioneuritis. If the virus has an axonal route of entry to the CNS, as do other herpesviruses, it would explain the brain stem localization. If patients survive the initial systemic illness, the neurologic disease appears to be self-limiting.[2, 100]

Parvovirus Encephalitis. This is an encephalitis consisting of vasculitis and leukomalacia of the CNS in the dog. Unlike in the cat, the pathology and clinical signs are not confined to the cerebellum. In many patients, the disease is rapidly progressive and fatal.[2, 100]

Feline Infectious Peritonitis (FIP). In addition to peritoneal and pleural effusions, the virus also produces a nonsuppurative meningoencephalitis in about 63 per cent of cases, with resultant clinical signs in about 29 per cent of cases. This is the most common cause of encephalitis in cats.[2, 100, 188, 189]

This condition may occur in cats of any breed, age, or sex, mostly in cats less than 3 years of age. Signs begin acutely to subacutely and are multifocal and slowly progressive.

In the neurologic form of FIP, the general physical examination is often abnormal. Patients display fever, chorioretinitis, keratic precipitates, and/or anterior uveitis. Cats with FIP encephalitis rarely have pleural or peritoneal effusions; however, many have renal involvement with irregular kidney size. Affected patients are often anemic and hyperglobulinemic.

The neurologic examination in these patients typically displays clear, multicentric CNS dysfunction. The predominant signs are referable to the posterior fossa (brain stem and cerebellum), with lesser signs referable to other CNS regions.[188]

The CSF is consistent with a granulomatous inflammation—increased lymphocytes or neutrophils and a markedly increased protein. The CSF protein levels may be so high that CSF is too viscous to flow through a spinal needle. In those patients, CSF will not be collected. Serology is less helpful. It is probable that FIP infects most cats early in life and remains latent, escaping the host's ability to check its replication at some later time. Rising antibody titers merely reflect this event. The role of antiviral antibody in initiating the lesions of FIP is at present unknown, except that attempts at vaccination may result in severe lesions, suggesting an immune-mediated basis of the disease. There is no effective therapy for FIP encephalitis, and the prognosis is poor.

Protozoal Encephalitis. Several coccidian protozoa are now known to have the capacity to invade and colonize the CNS. The most widely reported are *Toxoplasma gondii* and *Neosporum caninum,* which both infect cats and dogs.[87, 190–203]

Infection with these coccidian protozoa may occasionally produce neurologic signs, but most cases are subclinical or have systemic illness. At necropsy, most patients with systemic protozoal infection will have evidence of CNS involvement, without clinical evidence of that involvement. In patients with neurologic signs, there are two different illnesses based on age. Adults show a multifocal histiocytic inflammation and CNS malacia. Clinical infections in adults are uncommon.[87, 200–203] In animals under 6 months of age, a generalized inflammatory muscle disease (polymyositis) and widespread nerve root inflammation (polyradiculoneuritis) are more likely to result. The juvenile form of the clinical neurologic disease is most common. Protozoal illness is often seen in conjunction with concurrent immunosuppressive illness, e.g., cancer or immunosuppressive therapy.[196, 204] FIV is not thought to predispose a cat to activation of latent CNS protozoal infections.[193]

Any age, breed, or sex may be involved. Toxoplasmosis is acquired via carnivorous behavior, fecal contamination, or congenitally in dogs.

Respiratory illness, icterus, and pneumonia may be seen with toxoplasmosis. Muscle pain, uveitis, and chorioretinitis are also common in protozoal infections. Neurologic examination reveals multifocal disease.[193]

The diagnosis is based on evidence of a multifocal disease, especially if there is concomitant evidence of systemic illness. Serologic confirmation for the appropriate parasite is the definitive antemortem diagnostic tool. In cases of suspected feline toxoplasmosis, a fecal examination should be performed. This test is reliable only in cats, as they are the only species known to shed *T. gondii* oocysts in the feces. Accurate identification requires a parasitologist. CSF may demonstrate an increased number of cells and increased protein if active inflammation is present.

Mycotic Encephalitis. Fungal encephalomyelitis (*Cryptococcus neoformans* [the most frequent]; *Coccidioidomyces immitis; Histoplasma capsulatum; Blastomyces dermatitidis; Aspergillus* spp.; *Mucor* spp.; *Prototheca,* an achlorophyllous alga; and phaeohyphomycosis) may occur in any animal. Fungal organisms can cause encephalitis and chorioretinitis.[205] Cryptococcosis is the most frequent mycotic encephalitis, and most patients with cryptococcosis will have neurologic signs.[206–209]

Fungal encephalitis may be seen at any age, most commonly in adults. There is a slowly progressive illness, often with sytemic signs.[210] With CNS histoplasmosis, there may be an antecedent history of colitis or vague weight loss. With cryptococcal infection, chronic rhinitis is common. With blastomycosis, a draining wound or tract may be seen. If there is a draining wound or rhinitis, the organism may be seen on cytology of exudates. In many patients, it is cytology of the extraneural site that establishes a diagnosis.[210] Neurologic signs include depression, dementia, ataxia, weakness, cranial nerve deficits, and LMN paralysis.[211] In most patients, multifocal signs will be seen; however, focal encephalitis may occur in some patients.[212]

When CSF is examined, the organism may be seen on cytologic examination, especially with cryptococcal infections. There will be increased numbers of WBCs and increased CSF protein, including elevated globulins. With cryptococcal infections, eosinophils will be seen on CSF analysis and help to distinguish fungal infections from other granulomatous meningitis and encephalitis, especially the specific condition referred to as GME. The protein elevations may be so great as to cause the CSF to become gelatinous. Serologic assays are available to test both for antigen of the organism and patient antibody against the organism.

There are few reports of successful treatment of fungal encephalitis.[206] Currently available drugs include amphotericin B, flucytosine, ketoconazole, itraconazole, and fluconazole.[206, 210, 213–215] Ketoconazole, itraconazole, and fluconazole are more expensive, but safer for the patient.[207] Of these drugs, fluconazole has the best ability to cross the BBB.[210] Therapy should continue at least 6 weeks longer than remission of clinical signs. Even in cases that initially have a positive outcome, you may be unable to clear the organism from the CNS. In such cases, late relapses are common.[216] Immunosuppresive conditions, such as FIV- or FeLV-positive cats, are associated with a worse outcome.[217]

Meningitis. This represents bacterial infection of the meninges as a result of septicemia and bite wounds. Viral and miscellaneous protozoal infections are also seen, but these are rare. Immune-mediated meningitis is suspected but not proven. A sterile suppurative vasculitis/meningitis has been reported in young dogs, along with a sterile eosinophilic meningitis.[31, 218]

Dogs and cats of any age, breed, or sex may develop meningitis. The primary complaint is hyperesthesia, neck pain, depression, and fever. A history of systemic illness,

bite wounds near the spine, infections of sinuses and inner ears, or other contiguous infections may be uncovered.

Physical examination reveals nonspecific illness including fever (103 to 106°F), depression, anorexia, and hyperesthesia to touch over the entire body. The neurologic examination is usually not very abnormal, with mild ataxia in all four limbs to mild paresis in all limbs; the spinal reflexes are normal, but hyperesthesia and neck pain are severe.

Clinical laboratory testing may show leukopenia in viral infections. Radiographs will be normal (unless the meningitis is secondary to bony infection of spine). CSF should show normal to increased pressure, normal to increased cell number (the cell type will reflect the cause of meningitis), and increased protein. Organisms may be found. In the sterile suppurative meningitis of young dogs, the predominant cell type will be mature, healthy-appearing neutrophils without organisms. In bacterial meningitis, the neutrophils are often toxic and organisms will be seen.[31, 33, 154, 218]

If bacterial meningitis is confirmed, 4 to 6 weeks of appropriate antibiotic therapy as determined by CSF culture and sensitivity is essential.[163] Therapy should be continued even after resolution of signs. There is some evidence that treatment with steroids for the first 24 hours of treatment with antibiotics will both hasten and improve the degree of recovery.[104] If the meningitis is immune or sterile, use of immunosuppressive doses of corticosteroids is indicated.

The prognosis is generally guarded for patients with bacterial infections and potentially good for immune vasculitis.[150]

Granulomatous Meningoencephalitis (GME, Inflammatory Reticulosis). GME is an inflammatory disease of the CNS with a diffuse, white matter, perivascular orientation. This may actually be a fairly homogeneous group of diseases, rather than a single disease. Some patients have apparent neoplastic transformation of cells in the inflammatory lesion, while others do not. Neoplastic reticulosis, which is a form of primary CNS lymphoma, was at one time considered a variant of this disease. Antibodies against different IgG classes, against alpha$_1$-trypsin, and against lysozyme were used to further classify this condition and confirm its difference from GME. Those results suggest that many cases previously diagnosed as neoplastic reticulosis were in fact B-cell lymphomas. Those cases of inflammatory reticulosis with disseminated pathology were shown to be true inflammatory lesions with a polyclonal immunoglobulin-producing cell population.[219–221] A few cases of focal reticuloses were also found to be inflammatory. Based on this evidence, it now appears that what were once considered to be the reticuloses are in fact at least two separate diseases: one, an inflammatory condition now called granulomatous meningoencephalitis (GME); and the other, a primary CNS lymphoma. There are cases that cannot be classified in either group, so it is possible that a distinct third group of conditions will be named in the future.

GME is a nonsuppurative inflammatory disease of the CNS of dogs and less commonly cats associated with a marked perivascular proliferation of reticuloendothelial (RE) cells. Although lesions may occur in any portion of the CNS, there appears to be a predilection for the cerebrum and the cerebellopontine angle. The lesions tend to coalesce, so appear as focal or multifocal masses.

GME is probably the second most common inflammatory disease of the canine nervous system after CDVE.[87, 150] The disease tends to occur more in female, toy breed dogs. It is mostly a disease of young to middle-aged dogs (1 to 8 years), but may occur at any age. The onset is usually rapid, although indolent cases have been reported. Without treatment, the disease progresses to death within several months, although long-term survivals are documented. The clinical signs vary, but can be grouped into three categories.[37, 221–223]

Ocular Form. The ocular form is relatively uncommon. It is characterized by acute visual loss in the affected eye(s) with loss of the pupillary light reflex if the affected eye is illuminated (optic neuritis). This disease is the slowest to progress, often remaining static for months. The principal differential for this condition is the syndrome of acute retinal degeneration (SARD), which is also seen in toy breeds of dogs. With the passage of time, lesions of GME become more disseminated in the CNS, and at necropsy multiple lesions are found.

Focal Form. The focal form mimics an expanding mass, with the signs reflecting the site of the granuloma.[15, 224, 225] The most common sites of localization are the forebrain (cerebrum) and cerebellopontine angle.[226] This form is intermediate in progression, with signs partially responsive to therapy. The duration of the illness may be up to 6 months but is usually shorter. Although the signs are referable to the largest mass, at necropsy the disease is usually more widespread.

Disseminated Form. The final form is the disseminated form. Here the patient obviously has diffuse disease from the beginning. These patients have meningitis, with neck pain and fever. This is the most rapidly progressive form of the disease. Because this is a multifocal disease, any neurologic sign can be seen.

Diagnosis. The diagnosis can only be confirmed at necropsy or by brain biopsy; however, with improved diagnostic techniques, a reliable tentative diagnosis can be made without histopathology. The principal diagnostic aid is CSF analysis. There should be an elevated WBC consisting of a mixture of cell types, but predominantly mononuclear cells. The range of cell numbers is great, but high cell numbers are common. There should be about 10 to 20 per cent PMNs in the CSF, 10 to 20 per cent monocytes and macrophages, and 60 to 80 per cent lymphocytes and plasma cells.[37, 219] Eosinophils are rarely seen in CSF of patients with GME; if present, consider alternative diagnoses. In some cases, large anaplastic-looking mononuclear cells may be seen. These cells are considered diagnostic of this condition. The protein will generally be elevated (40 to 1000 mg/dL), with significant elevation of IgG on electrophoresis.[11, 36] CSF pressure is usually normal. CSF normalizes rapidly with steroid therapy, so avoid treating with steroids before collecting CSF. Because other inflammatory diseases may cause similar CSF changes, cultures, fungal titers, and toxoplasmosis titers should also be performed on CSF.

Treatment. Standard treatment consists of administering immunosuppressive drugs, administering radiation therapy, or a combination. The factors most associated with increased survival time in published studies are a focal localization and treatment with radiation therapy.[226] The immunosuppressive drug most often used is prednisolone (0.5 to 1 mg/lb/day); however, other drugs such as cytoxan and azathioprine are used. We treat GME patients with combination immunosuppressive therapy with successful survivals of over 3 years. In spite of current advances, therapy is limited to remission rather than cure.

All confirmed cases of GME have tissue diagnoses. That highlights one of the frustrations when trying to accurately evaluate therapy. Any case that is cured by therapy, but not biopsied, automatically has GME eliminated from the differential list and becomes classified as an idiopathic inflammatory disease. Until more cases are biopsied, accurate therapeutic trials cannot be performed.

Pug/Maltese/Yorkshire Terrier Encephalitis. Pug encephalitis is a chronic granulomatous meningoencephalitis in adult pugs. This bears many similarities to GME histologically, except that there is more malacia and eosinophils may be found in the lesions. The disease affects all brain regions. A familial tendency for this condition is suggested. Possible immunosuppression, with secondary CNS infection, is suspected in most cases. The onset of CNS signs is 9 months to 4 years. The disease is multifocal; however, cerebral signs, including seizures and dementia, are often the earliest complaint. Circling, head tilts, nystagmus, and other brain stem signs are common in the later stages of the disease. Cerebellar signs may be seen in some patients.[227] Similar clinical and pathologic conditions have now been reported in Maltese dogs and Yorkshire terriers.[228, 229] In each case, the clinical picture was of a relentlessly progressive encephalitis. The pathology is subtly different enough in each species to investigate them as separate disorders.

The diagnosis is based on abnormal CSF, with a mixed inflammatory picture. We have seen eosinophils in the CSF of some affected patients at OSU.

Corticosteroids may alleviate the clinical signs for short periods, and antimicrobials have no effect. This appears to be an invariably fatal disease. At least one patient developed brain-heart syndrome.[230]

Feline Polioencephalomyelitis. This is a slowly progressive chronic disease of cats without an age predilection. The signs involve the spinal cord or cerebellum; rarely the brain stem or cerebrum is affected. Many of these animals have nonregenerative anemias.

Rickettsial Diseases. Several rickettsial diseases, including Rocky Mountain spotted fever and ehrlichiosis, can produce meningoencephalitis in dogs.[31, 100, 231, 232] The neurologic signs are the result of vasculitis-induced meningoencephalitis. The most common neurologic signs are vestibular signs and/or neck pain, but any portion of the neuraxis may be affected clinically or pathologically. Affected patients are generally systemically ill. Many patients will have thrombocytopenia, leukocytosis, and other hematologic evidence of vasculitis. CSF may reveal a mild, nonsuppurative response. The definitive test is serologic evaluation.

Treatment with tetracycline appears effective at resolving both systemic and neurologic signs of rickettsial infection.

OTHER DIFFUSE DISORDERS

Tremor Syndromes (Idiopathic Tremor/White Dog Shaker Syndrome/Steroid-Responsive Tremor Syndrome; Mycotoxin Ingestion; and Inflammatory Tremor Syndrome). These three conditions all present with dogs being brought to the hospital for acute, severe, generalized tremor. Although tremor is normally a cerebellar sign, based on the nature and severity of signs, these patients probably have a more diffuse CNS disorder.[233, 234] It may be a diffuse demyelinating disorder or possibly a generalized neurotransmitter deficiency, on the order of Parkinson's disease or Huntington's chorea in humans.

The signs are usually acute in onset in all three conditions. For unknown reasons, idiopathic tremor is frequently seen in (but not limited to) young to middle-aged small dogs with white hair coats; especially the Maltese, West Highland white terrier, bichon frisé, and poodle.[234–236] Mycotoxin ingestion and inflammatory tremor are seen in any breed. The principal clinical sign is diffuse tremor of the entire body. There is usually no other history of note. On general physical examination, the patients may be hyperthermic from the tremors. Chaotic, random eye movements (opsoclonus) are a characteristic feature of this condition on neurologic examination. Opsoclonus resembles a severe but uncoordinated pathologic nystagmus. The body tremors are often so severe that the animal is disabled.

The principal differentials for diffuse tremors are mycotoxin ingestion, inflammatory tremors, and idiopathic tremors; ask about access to moldy foods. CSF evaluation in all cases without documented mold ingestion is essential. CSF in idiopathic patients will be normal, while with inflammatory tremor there will frequently be a mild mixed or mononuclear inflammatory response.[234] In most patients, CSF proteins are normal, but there may be mild elevations.

For mycotoxin ingestion, the only therapy is supportive therapy and time. This is a self-limiting condition. Steroids are generally effective in reversing the clinical disease in both inflammatory and idiopathic tremor. The patients generally require treatment for several weeks, with slowly tapering doses of prednisone. If the drug is discontinued too early, the signs may recur. Response to therapy is slower in inflammatory disorders than with idiopathic tremor, but ultimately both groups respond well.[234] Diazepam, a centrally acting skeletal muscle relaxant, may be needed in some patients. Diazepam appears to abort the tremors, allowing the nervous system to recover.

Feline Spongioform Encephalopathy. A progressive neurologic disease was identified in five cats in Great Britain, which has characteristics similar to scrapie. Affected cats had ataxia of limbs, especially the pelvic limbs, behavior changes, hyperesthesia, head tremor, muscle fasciculations, and hypersalivation. Histopathologically, the cats' nervous systems consisted of discrete vacuoles in grey matter, scattered throughout the CNS. The lesions appeared identical to those of scrapie and bovine spongioform encephalopathy (BSE). The geographic pattern in the affected cats is similar to that of BSE, but a connection between the two conditions has not been established.[237]

Feline Immunodeficiency Virus (FIV). It appears that up to 30 per cent of cats infected with FIV may develop neurologic signs, not related to secondary infections.[238] The principal changes reflect cerebral injury and include depression, behavior changes, dementia, loss of toilet training, and aggression. Focal signs are not seen in affected cats. The clinical signs are similar to those of a metabolic encephalopathy.[239]

Diagnostic testing should include serologic testing for the FIV virus, CSF evaluation, and a complete metabolic screen. At present, diagnosing CNS signs from FIV infection requires that you prove both that FIV is present in the affected patient and that there are no other well-established causes of neurologic disease present in the patient concurrently. CSF of affected cats may show mild elevations in leukocytes. The presence of FIV antibodies is considered diagnostic of CNS infection, providing there was no blood contamination of the CSF.[238]

Several drugs are being investigated in the treatment of FIV encephalopathy: azidothymidine (AZT), human recombinant alpha-interferon, and phosphonomethoxyethyl adenine (PMEA). The prognosis for FIV encephalopathy is poor.[238]

REFERENCES

1. DeLahunta A: Veterinary Neuroanatomy and Clinical Neurology, 2nd ed. Philadelphia, WB Saunders, 1983, p 471.
2. Oliver JE, Hoerlein BF, Mayhew IG (eds): Veterinary Neurology. Philadelphia, WB Saunders, 1987.
3. Braund KG: Symposium on diagnosing neurologic disease. Vet Med 90:139–179, 1995.
4. Brodal A: Neurological Anatomy: In Relation to Clinical Medicine, 3rd ed. New York, Oxford University Press, 1981, p 1053.
5. Holliday TA: Clinical signs of acute and chronic experimental lesions of the cerebellum. Vet Sci Commun 3:259–278, 1980.
6. Baloh RW, Honrubia V: Clinical Neurophysiology of the Vestibular System, 2nd ed. Philadelphia, FA Davis, 1990, p 301. (Plum F, Baringer JR, Gilman S, [eds]: Contemporary Neurology Series, Vol 32.)
7. Chrisman CL: Cerebrospinal fluid analysis. Vet Clin North Am Small Anim Pract 22:781–810, 1992.
8. Christopher MM, Perman V, Hardy RM: Reassessment of cytologic values in canine cerebrospinal fluid by use of cytocentrifugation. JAVMA 192:1726–1729, 1988.
9. Latimer KS: Cytologic Examination of Cerebrospinal Fluid. Veterinary Medical Forum. Washington, DC, American College of Veterinary Internal Medicine, 1993, pp 36–38.
10. Russack V, Kim S, Chamberlain MC: Quantitative cerebrospinal fluid cytology in patients receiving intracavity chemotherapy. Ann Neurol 34:108–112, 1993.
11. Sorjonen DC, Golden DL, Levesque DC, et al: Cerebrospinal fluid protein electrophoresis: A clinical evaluation of a previously reported diagnostic technique. ProgVet Neurol 2:261–268, 1991.
12. Thomson CE, Kornegay JN, Stevens JB: Analysis of cerebrospinal fluid from the cerebellomedullary and lumbar cisterns of dogs with focal neurologic disease: 145 cases (1985–1987). JAVMA 196:1841–1844, 1990.
13. Steiss JE, Cox NR, Knecht CD: Electroencephalographic and histopathologic correlations in eight dogs with intracranial mass lesions. Am J Vet Res 51:1286–1291, 1990.
14. Shores A: Magnetic resonance imaging. Vet Clin North Am Small Anim Pract 23:437–459, 1993.
15. Speciale J, Van Winkle TJ, Steinberg SA, Wortman JA: Computed tomography in the diagnosis of focal granulomatous meningoencephalitis: Retrospective evaluation of three cases. J Am Anim Hosp Assoc 28:327–332, 1992.
16. Schunk KL: Disorders of the vestibular system. Vet Clin North Am Small Anim Pract 18:641–665, 1988.
17. Hudson JA, Simpson ST, Buxton DF, et al: Ultrasonographic diagnosis of canine hydrocephalus. Vet Radiol 31:50–58, 1990.
18. Cartee RE, Hudson JA, Finn BS: Ultrasonography. Vet Clin North Am Small Anim Pract 23:345–377, 1993.
19. Rivers WJ, Walter PA: Hydrocephalus in the dog: Utility of ultrasonography as an alternate diagnostic imaging technique. J Am Anim Hosp Assoc 28:333–343, 1992.
20. Niebauer GW, Dayrell-Hart BL, Speciale J: Evaluation of craniotomy in dogs and cats. JAVMA 198:89–95, 1991.
21. Harari J, Moore MM, Leathers CW, et al: Computed tomographic–guided, free-hand needle biopsy of brain tumors in dogs. ProgVet Neurol 4:54–59, 1993.
22. Carillo JM, Sarfaty D, Greenlee P: Intracranial neoplasm and associated inflammatory response from the central nervous system. J Am Anim Hosp Assoc 22:367–373, 1986.
23. Speciale J: Brain Herniation. 14th ACVIM Forum. San Antonio, American College of Veterinary Internal Medicine, 1996, pp 673–675.
24. Kornegay J, Oliver J, Gorgacz E: Clinicopathologic feature of brain herniation in animals. JAVMA 182:1111–1116, 1983.
25. Dow SW, LeCouteur RA, Henik RA: Central nervous system infection associated with anaerobic bacteria in two dogs and two cats. J Vet Intern Med 2:171–176, 1988.
26. Bailey CS, Higgins RJ: Comparison of total white blood cell count and total protein content of lumbar and cisternal cerebrospinal fluid of healthy dogs. Am J Vet Res 46:1162–1165, 1985.
27. Simpson ST, Reed RB: Manometric values for normal cerebrospinal fluid in dogs. J Am Anim Hosp Assoc 23:629–632, 1987.
28. Chow G, Schmidley JW: Lysis of erythrocytes and leukocytes in traumatic lumbar punctures. Arch Neurol 41:1084–1085, 1984.
29. Rand J, Parent J, Percy D, Jacobs R: Clinical, cerebrospinal fluid, and histological data from thirty-four cats with primary noninflammatory disease of the central nervous system. Can Vet J 35:174–181, 1994.
30. Hurtt A, Smith M: Effects of iatrogenic blood contamination on results of cerebrospinal fluid analysis in clinically normal dogs and dogs with neurologic disease. JAVMA 211:866–867, 1997.
31. Meric JM: Canine meningitis: A changing emphasis. J Vet Intern Med 2:26–35, 1988.
32. Widmer WR, DeNicola DB, Blevins WE, et al: Cerebrospinal fluid changes after iopamidol and metrizamide myelography in clinically normal dogs. Am J Vet Res 53:396–401, 1992.
33. Quagliarello V, Scheld WM: Bacterial meningitis: Pathogenesis, pathophysiology, and progress. N Engl J Med 327:864–872, 1992.
34. Powers WJ: Cerebrospinal lymphocytosis in acute bacterial meningitis. Am J Med 79:216–220, 1985.
35. Bichsel P, Vandevelde M, Vandevelde E, et al: Immunoelectrophoretic determination of albumin and IgG in serum and cerebrospinal fluid in dogs with neurologic disease. Res Vet Sci 1:101–107, 1984.
36. Sorjonen DC: Total protein, albumin quota, and electrophoretic patterns in cerebrospinal fluid of dogs with central nervous system disorders. Am J Vet Res 48:310–315, 1987.

37. Sarfaty D, Carillo JM, Greenlee PG: Differential diagnosis of granulomatous meningoencephalomyelitis, distemper, and suppurative meningoencephalitis in the dog. JAVMA 188:387–392, 1986.

38. Johnson GC, Fenner WR, Krakowka S: Production of immunoglobulin G and increased antiviral antibody in cerebrospinal fluid of dogs with delayed-onset canine distemper encephalitis. J Neuroimmunol 17:237–251, 1988.

39. Pumarola M: Canine granulomatous meningoencephalitis (CGME). Vet Int 4:25–31, 1992.

40. Holliday TA, TeSelle ME: Brain stem auditory-evoked potentials of dog: Wave forms and effects of recording electrode positions. Am J Vet Res 46:845–849, 1985.

41. Holliday TA, Nelson HJ, Williams DC, Willits N: Unilateral and bilateral brain stem auditory-evoked response abnormalities in 900 Dalmatian dogs. J Vet Intern Med 6:166–174, 1992.

42. Strain GM, Kearney MT, Gignac IJ, et al: Brain stem auditory-evoked potential assessment of congenital deafness in Dalmatians: Associations with phenotypic markers. J Vet Intern Med 6:175–182, 1992.

43. Marshall AE: Use of brain stem auditory-evoked response to evaluate deafness in a group of Dalmatian dogs. JAVMA 188:718–721, 1986.

44. Kawasaki Y: Extra- and intracranial components contributing to brain stem auditory evoked potentials in dogs and the binaural interaction. Prog Vet Neurol 7:153–158, 1996.

45. Strain GM, Jackson RM, Tedford BL: Visual evoked potentials in the clinically normal dog. J Vet Intern Med 4:222–225, 1990.

46. Bichsel P, Oliver JJ, Coulter DB, Brown J: Recording of visual-evoked potentials in dogs with scalp electrodes. J Vet Intern Med 2:145–149, 1988.

47. Bailey MQ: Diagnostic imaging of intracranial lesions. Semin Vet Med Surg Small Anim 5:232–236, 1990.

48. Knake JE, Chandler WF, McGillicuddy JE, et al: Intraoperative sonography for brain tumor localization and ventricular shunt placement. Am J Neuroradiol 3:425–430, 1982.

49. Gallagher J, Penninck D, Boudrieau R, et al: Ultrasonography of the brain and vertebral canal in dogs and cats: 15 cases (1988–1993). JAVMA 207:1320–1324, 1995.

50. Turrell JM, Fike JR, LeCouteur RA, et al: Computed tomographic characteristics of primary brain tumors in 50 dogs. JAVMA 188:851–856, 1986.

51. Wortman JA: Principles of X-ray computed tomography and magnetic resonance imaging. Semin Vet Med Surg Small Anim 1:176–184, 1986.

52. Berland LL: Practical CT. Technology and Techniques. New York, Raven Press, 1987.

53. Kortz G: Brain Imaging—CT or MR—Which One and Why. ACVIM Forum. San Diego, American College of Veterinary Internal Medicine, 1998, pp 290–291.

54. Runge V, Wells J, Williams N, et al: Detectability of early brain meningitis with magnetic resonance imaging. Invest Radiol 30:484–495, 1995.

55. Lobetti R, Pearson J: Magnetic resonance imaging in the diagnosis of focal granulomatous meningoencephalitis in two dogs. Vet Radiol Ultrasound 37:424–427, 1996.

56. LeCouteur R, Koblik P, Higgins R, et al: Computed Tomography–Guided Stereotactic Brain Biopsy in 25 Dogs and 10 Cats Using the Pelorus Mark III Biopsy System. 16th ACVIM Forum. San Diego, American College of Veterinary Internal Medicine, 1998, p 697.

57. Pollay M, Fullenwider C, Roberts PA, Stevens FA: Effect of mannitol and furosemide on blood-brain osmotic gradient and intracranial pressure. J Neurosurg 59:945–950, 1983.

58. Culbert L, Marino D, Baule R, Knox V: Complications associated with high-dose prednisolone sodium succinate therapy in dogs with neurologic injury. J Am Anim Hosp Assoc 34:129–34, 1998.

59. Bracken MB, Shepard MJ, Collins WF, et al: A randomized controlled trial of methylprednisolone or naloxone in the treatment of acute spinal-cord injury. N Engl J Med 322:1405–1411, 1990.

60. Parker AJ: Treatment of brain tumors and encephalitis in the dog and cat. Prog Vet Neurol 1:133–136, 1990.

61. Engel J: Seizures and Epilepsy. Philadelphia, FA Davis, 1989, p 536. (Plum F, Gilman S, Martin JB [eds]: Contemporary Neurology Series, Vol 31.)

62. Lane SB, Bunch SE: Medical management of recurrent seizures in dogs and cats. J Vet Intern Med 4:26–39, 1990.

63. Pearce LK: Potassium bromide as an adjunct to phenobarbital for the management of uncontrolled seizures in dogs. ProgVet Neurol 1:95–101, 1990.

64. Shell LG: Introduction: Seizures in dogs and cats: Taking a logical approach to an age-old problem. Vet Med 88:620–621, 1993.

65. Gallagher J, Berg J, Knowles K, et al: Prognosis after surgical excision of cerebral meningiomas in cats: 17 cases (1986–1992). JAVMA 203:1437–1440, 1993.

66. Black PM: Brain tumors (Part One). N Engl J Med 324:1471–1476, 1991.

67. Iwamoto KS, Norman A, Freshwater DB, et al: Diagnosis and treatment of spontaneous canine brain tumors with a CT scanner. Radiother Oncol 26:76–78, 1993.

68. Moore MP, Gavin PR, Weidner JP, Bagley RS: Boron Neutron Capture Therapy for Brain Tumors. Veterinary Medical Forum. Washington, DC: American College of Veterinary Internal Medicine, 1993, pp 725–727.

69. Packer RJ: Chemotherapy for medulloblastoma/primitive neuroectodermal tumors of the posterior fossa. Ann Neurol 28:823–828, 1990.

70. Thrall DE, Heidner GL, Kornegay JN, Page RL: Analysis of survival in a retrospective study of 86 dogs with brain tumors. J Vet Intern Med 5:219–226, 1991.

71. Vecht CJ, Haaxma-Reiche H, Noordijk EM, et al: Treatment of single brain metastasis: Radiotherapy alone or combined with neurosurgery? Ann Neurol 33:583–590, 1993.

72. Evans SM, Dayrell-Hart B, Powlis W, et al: Radiation therapy of canine brain masses. J Vet Intern Med 7:216–219, 1993.

73. Theon A, Feldman E: Megavoltage irradiation of pituitary macrotumors in dogs with neurologic signs. JAVMA 213:225–231, 1998.

74. Chamberlain M, Barba D, Kormanik P, et al: Concurrent cisplatin therapy and iodine 125 brachytherapy for recurrent malignant brain tumors. Arch Neurol 52:162–167, 1995.

75. Duncan ID: Abnormalities of myelination of the central nervous system associated with congenital tremor. J Vet Intern Med 1:10–23, 1987.

76. Shores A: Cranio-Cerebral Trauma: Emergency Management and Prognosis. ACVIM Forum. San Diego, American College of Veterinary Internal Medicine, 1988, pp 3–5.

77. Hamill RW, Woolf PD, McDonald MD, et al: Catecholamines predict outcome in traumatic brain injury. Ann Neurol 21:438–443, 1987.

78. Dewey CW, Budsberg SC, Oliver JE Jr: Principles of head trauma management in dogs and cats: Part 1. Comp Continuing Ed 14:199–207, 1992.

79. Colter S, Rucker NC: Acute injury to the central nervous system. Vet Clin North Am Small Anim Pract 18:545–563, 1988.

80. Cottrell JE, Marlin AE: Furosemide and human head injury. J Trauma 21:805–806, 1981.

81. Lindsberg PJ, Hallenbeck JM, Feuerstein G: Platelet-activating factor in stroke and brain injury. Ann Neurol 30:117–129, 1991.

82. Hallenbeck JM, Jacobs TP, Faden AI: Combined PGI$_2$, indomethacin, and heparin improves neurological recovery after spinal trauma in cats. J Neurosurg 58:749–754, 1983.

83. O'Brien D: Brain Damage and Behavior. Veterinary Medical Forum. Washington, DC, American College of Veterinary Internal Medicine, 1993, pp 542–545.

84. Shores A: Small Animal Coma Scale Revisited. Tenth ACVIM Forum. San Diego, American College of Veterinary Internal Medicine, 1992, pp 748–749.

85. Diringer M, Edwards D: Does modification of the Innsruck and the Glasgow Coma Scales improve their ability to predict functional outcome? Arch Neurol 54:606–611, 1997.

86. Raichle ME: The pathophysiology of brain ischemia. Ann Neurol 13:2–10, 1983.

87. Summers B, Cummings J, DeLahunta A: Veterinary Neuropathology. St. Louis, CV Mosby, 1995, p 527.

88. Norton F: Cerebral infarction in a dog. ProgVet Neurol 3:120–125, 1992.

89. Joseph RJ, Greenlee PG, Carillo JM, Kay WJ: Canine cerebrovascular disease: Clinical and pathologic findings in 17 cases. J Am Anim Hosp Assoc 24:569, 1988.

90. Frank JR, Nutter FB, Kyles AE, et al: Systemic arterial dirofilariasis in five dogs. J Vet Intern Med 11:189–194, 1997.

91. Forrester SD, Greco DS, Relford RL: Serum hyperviscosity syndrome associated with multiple myeloma in two cats. JAVMA 200:79–82, 1992.

92. Petty GW, Khandheria BK, Chu C-P, et al: Patent foramen ovale in patients with cerebral infarction. Arch Neurol 54:819–822, 1997.

93. Shell L: Feline ischemic encephalopathy (cerebral infarct). Feline Pract 24:32–33, 1996.

94. Caplan L: New therapies for stroke. Arch Neurol 54:1222–1224, 1997.

95. Voll CL, Auer RN: The effect of postischemic blood glucose levels on ischemic brain damage in the rat. Ann Neurol 638–646, 1988.

96. Pulsinelli WA, Levy DE, Sigsbee B, et al: Increased damage after ischemic stroke in patients with hyperglycemia with or without diabetes mellitus. Am J Med 74:540–544, 1983.

97. Kushner M, Nencini P, Reivich M, et al: Relation of hyperglycemia early in ischemic brain infarction to cerebral anatomy, metabolism, and clinical outcome. Ann Neurol 28:129–135, 1990.

98. Hattori H, Wasterlain CG: Posthypoxic glucose supplement reduces hypoxic-ischemic brain damage in the neonatal rat. Ann Neurol 28:122–128, 1990.

99. Montgomery DL: Astrocytes: Form, functions, and roles in disease. Vet Pathol 31:145–167, 1994.

100. Greene CE, Braund KG: Diseases of the brain. In Ettinger SJ (ed): Textbook of Veterinary Internal Medicine, 3rd ed, Vol 1. Philadelphia, WB Saunders, 1989, pp 578–623.

101. Burke EE, Moise NS, DeLahunta A, Erb HN: Review of idiopathic feline vestibular syndrome in 75 cats. JAVMA 187:941–943, 1985.

102. Shell LG: Idiopathic vestibular disease. Feline Pract 23:27, 1995.

103. Schunk KL: Diseases of the vestibular system. ProgVet Neurol 1:247–254, 1990.

104. Pfister H-W, Feiden W, Einhaupl K-M: Spectrum of complications during bacterial meningitis in adults: Results of a prospective clinical study. Arch Neurol 50:575–581, 1993.

105. Pomeroy SL, Holmes SJ, Dodge PR, Feigin RD: Seizures and other neurologic sequelae of bacterial meningitis in children. N Engl J Med 323:1651–1657, 1990.

106. Gaillard J, Abadie V, Cheron G, et al: Concentrations of ceftriaxone in cerebrospinal fluid of children with meningitis receiving dexamethasone therapy. Antimicrob Agents Chemother 38:1209–1210, 1994.

107. Jafari H, McCracken GJ: Dexamethasone therapy in bacterial meningitis. Pediatr Ann 23:82–88, 1994.

108. Schaad U, Kaplan S, McCracken GJ: Steroid therapy for bacterial meningitis. Clin Infect Dis 20:685–690, 1995.

109. Singhi S, Singhi P, Srinivas B, et al: Fluid restriction does not improve the outcome of acute meningitis. Pediatr Infect Dis J 14:495–503, 1995.

110. Palmer AC: Clinical signs associated with intracranial tumours in dogs. Res Vet Sci 2:326–339, 1961.

111. Foster ES, Carillo JM, Patnaik AK: Clinical signs of tumors affecting the rostral cerebrum in 43 dogs. J Vet Intern Med 2:71, 1988.

112. Triolo A, Howard M, Miles K: Oligodendroglioma in a 15-month-old dog. JAVMA 205:986–988, 1994.

113. Davidson MG, Nasisse MP, Breitschwerdt EB, et al: Acute blindness associated with intracranial tumors in dogs and cats: Eight cases (1984–1989). JAVMA 199:755–758, 1991.

114. Miller WH Jr: Parapituitary meningioma in a dog with pituitary-dependent hyperadrenocorticism. JAVMA 198:444–446, 1991.

115. Ohler C, Mughannam A, Reinke J, et al: Transient hemi-inattention in a dog with metastatic renal hemangiosarcoma. J Am Anim Hosp Assoc 30:207–212, 1994.

116. Hobbs SL, Cobb MA, Langley-Hobbs S: A cranial neuropathy associated with multicentric lymphosarcoma in a dog. Vet Rec 127:525–526, 1990.

117. Bagley R, Wheeler S. Klopp L, et al: Clinical features of trigeminal nerve-sheath tumor in 10 dogs. J Am Anim Hosp Assoc 34:19–25, 1998.

118. Adamo PF, Clinkscales JA: Cerebellar meningioma with paradoxical vestibular signs. ProgVet Neurol 2:137–142, 1991.

119. Posner JB: Neurologic Complications of Cancer. Philadelphia, FA Davis, 1995, p 482. (Contemporary Neurology Series, Vol 45.)

120. Fenner WR: Metastatic neoplasms of the central nervous system. Semin Vet Med Surg Small Anim 5:253–261, 1990.

121. Schulman FY, Ribas JL, Carpenter JL, et al: Intracranial meningioma with pulmonary metastasis in three dogs. Vet Pathol 29:196–202, 1992.

122. Bailey CS, Higgins RS: Characteristics of cisternal cerebrospinal fluid associated with primary brain tumors in the dog: A retrospective study. JAVMA 188:414–417, 1986.

123. Brehm DM, Vite CH, Steinberg HS, et al: A retrospective evaluation of 51 cases of peripheral nerve sheath tumors in the dog. J Am Anim Hosp Assoc 31:349–359, 1995.

124. Steiss JE: EEG findings in dogs with confirmed neurologic disease. Veterinary Medical Forum. Washington, DC: American College of Veterinary Internal Medicine, 1993, pp 739–741.

125. Jarden JO, Dhawan V. Moeller JR, et al: The time course of steroid action on blood-to-brain and blood-to-tumor transport of 82Rb: A positron emission study. Ann Neurol 25:239–245, 1989.

126. Chamberlain MC, Levin VA: Adjuvant chemotherapy for primary lymphoma of the central nervous system. Arch Neurol 47:1113–1116, 1990.

127. Seiber FE, Traystman RJ: Special issues: Glucose and the brain. Crit Care Med 20:104–114, 1992.

128. Kalaria RN, Gravina SA, Schmidley JW, et al: The glucose transporter of the human brain and the blood-brain barrier. Ann Neurol 24:747, 1988.

129. Howerton TL, Shell LG: Neurologic manifestations of altered serum glucose. ProgVet Neurol 3:57–64, 1992.

130. Bunch SE: Hepatic encephalopathy. ProgVet Neurol 2:287–296, 1991.

131. Joseph RJ, Peterson ME: Review and comparison of neuromuscular and central nervous system manifestations of hyperthyroidism in cats and humans. ProgVet Neurol 3:114–119, 1992.

132. Dow SW, LeCouteur RA, Poss ML, Beadleston D: Central nervous system toxicosis associated with metronidazole treatment of dogs: Five cases (1984–1987). JAVMA 195:365–368, 1989.

133. Saxon B, Magne ML: Reversible central nervous system toxicosis associated with metronidazole therapy in three cats. ProgVet Neurol 4:25–27, 1993.

134. Morgan RV, Moore FM, Pearce LK, Rossi T: Clinical and laboratory findings in small companion animals with lead poisoning: 347 cases (1977–1986). JAVMA 199:93–97, 1991.

135. Morgan RV, Pearce LK, Moore FM. Rossi T: Demographic data and treatment of small companion animals with lead poisoning: 347 cases (1977–1986). JAVMA 199:98–102, 1991.

136. Maddison JE, Allan GS: Megaesophagus attributable to lead toxicosis in a cat. JAVMA 197:1357, 1990.

137. Shell LG: Congenital hydrocephalus. Feline Pract 24:10–11, 1996.

138. Kornegay JN: Ataxia, dysmetria, tremor. Cerebellar diseases. Probl Vet Med 3:409–416, 1991.

139. O'Brien D: Hereditary Cerebellar Ataxia. Veterinary Medical Forum. Washington, DC, American College of Veterinary Internal Medicine, 1993, pp 546–549.

140. Alroy J, Schelling SH, Thalhammer JG, et al: Adult onset lysosomal storage disease in a Tibetan terrier: Clinical, morphological and biochemical studies. Acta Neuropathol Berl 84:658–663, 1992.

141. Braund KG, Amling KA: Muscle biopsy samples for histochemical processing: Alterations induced by storage. Vet Pathol 25:77–82, 1988.

142. Cuddon PA, Higgins RJ, Duncan ID, et al: Polyneuropathy in feline Niemann-Pick disease. Brain 112:1429–1443, 1989.

143. Kuwamura M, Awakura T, Shimada A, et al: Type C Niemann-Pick disease in a boxer dog. Acta Neuropathol Berl 85:345–348, 1993.

144. Shell LG, Potthoff AI, Carithers R, et al: Neuronal-visceral GM₁ gangliosidosis in Portuguese water dogs. J Vet Intern Med 3:1–7, 1989.

145. Sisk DB, Levesque DC, Wood PA, Styer EL: Clinical and pathologic features of ceroid lipofuscinosis in two Australian cattle dogs. JAVMA 197:361–364, 1990.

146. Sacre BJ, Cummings JF, DeLahunta A: Neuroaxonal dystrophy in a Jack Russell terrier pup resembling human infantile neuroaxonal dystrophy. Cornell Vet 83:133–142, 1993.

147. Brenner O, DeLahunta A, Summers B, et al: Hereditary polioencephalomyelopathy of the Australian cattle dog. Acta Neuropathol 94:54–66, 1997.

148. Neer T, Kornegay J: Leucoencephalomalacia and cerebral white matter vacuolar degeneration in two related Labrador Retriever puppies. J Vet Intern Med 9:100–104, 1995.

149. Palmer A, Cavanagh J: Encephalomyelopathy in young cats. J Small Anim Pract 36:57–64, 1995.

150. Tipold A: Diagnosis of inflammatory and infectious diseases of the central nervous system in dogs: A retrospective study. J Vet Intern Med 9:304–314, 1995.

151. Martin JB, Tyler KL, Schelc WM: Bacterial meningitis. In Tyler KL, Martin JB (eds): Infections of the CNS. Philadelphia, FA Davis, 1993, pp 176–187. (Contemporary Neurology Series, Vol 41.)

152. Johnson R: Viral Infections of the Nervous System. New York, Raven Press, 1982.

153. Whitley RJ: Viral encephalitis. N Engl J Med 323:242–250, 1990.

154. Greenlee JE: Bacterial meringitis. In Johnson RT (ed): Current Therapy in Neurologic Disease. Philadelphia, BC Decker, 1985, pp 123–128.

155. Sorjonen D: Myelitis and meningitis. Vet Clin North Am Small Anim Pract 22:951–964, 1992.

156. Elwood C, Cobb M, Stepier R: Clinical and echocardiographic findings in 10 dogs with vegetative bacterial endocarditis. J Small Anim Pract 34:420–427, 1993.

157. Bachur R, Caputo G: Bacteremia and meningitis among infants with urinary tract infections. Pediatr Emerg Care 11:280–284, 1995.

158. Kornegay JN: Multiple neurologic deficits. Inflammatory diseases. Probl Vet Med 3:426–439, 1991.

159. Seebach J, Bartholdi D, Frei K, et al: Experimental Listeria meningoencephalitis, macrophage inflammatory protein–1 alpha and –2 are produced intrathecally and mediate chemotactic activity in cerebrospinal fluid of infected mice. J Immunol 155:4367–4375, 1995.

160. Snyder P, Kazcos E, Scott-Moncrieff J, et al: Pathologic features of naturally occurring juvenile polyarteritis in Beagle dogs. Vet Pathol 32:337–345, 1995.

161. Tipold A, Jaffy A: Steroid responsive meningitis-arteritis in dogs: Long-term study of 32 cases. J Small Animal Pract 35:311–316, 1994.

162. Irving G, Chrisman CL: Long-term outcome of five cases of corticosteroid-responsive meningomyelitis. J Am Anim Hosp Assoc 26:324–328, 1990.

163. Whitby M, Finch R: Bacterial meningitis. Rational selection and use of antibacterial drugs. Drugs 31:266–278, 1986.

164. Bell W, McGuinness G: Antibacterial and antifungal therapy for CNS infections. In Tyler KL, Martin JB (eds): Infections of the CNS. Philadelphia, FA Davis, 1993. pp 305–353. (Contemporary Neurology Series, Vol 41.)

165. Schaad U, Lips U, Gnehm H, et al: Dexamethasone therapy for bacterial meningitis in children. Swiss Meningitis Study Group. Lancet 342:457–461, 1993.

166. Rockowitz J, Tunkel A: Bacterial meningitis. Practical guidelines for management. Drugs 50:838–853, 1995.

167. Brown L, Feigin R: Bacterial meningitis: Fluid balance and therapy. Pediatr Ann 23:93–98, 1995.

168. Dzyban LA, Tidwell AS: Imaging diagnosis: Granulomatous meningoencephalitis. Vet Radiol 37:428–430, 1996.

169. Lobetti RG, Pearson J: Magnetic resonance imaging in the diagnosis of focal granulomatous meningoencephalitis in two dogs. Vet Radiol Ultrasound 37:424–427, 1996.

170. Buback J, Schultz K, Walker M, Snowden K: Magnetic resonance imaging of the brain for diagnosis of neurocysticercosis in a dog. JAVMA 208:1846–1848, 1996.

171. Uhaa IJ, Mandel EJ, Whiteway R, Fishbein DB: Rabies surveillance in the United States during 1990. JAVMA 200:920–929, 1992.

172. Brass DA: Insectivorous bats as reservoirs of rabies. Compend Contin Ed 15:33–40, 1993.

173. Rupprecht C, Childs J: Feline rabies. Feline Pract 24:15–19, 1996.

174. Eng TR, Fishbein DB, the National Study Group on Rabies: Epidemiologic factors, clinical findings, and vaccination status of rabies in cats and dogs in the United States in 1988. JAVMA 197:201–209, 1990.

175. Fogelman V, Fischman HR, Horman JT, Grigor JK: Epidemiologic and clinical characteristics of rabies in cats. JAVMA 202:1829–1833, 1993.

176. Uhaa IJ, Dato VM, Sorhage FE, et al: Benefits and costs of using an orally absorbed vaccine to control rabies in raccoons. JAVMA 201:1873–1882, 1992.

177. Fagan JG: Aujeszky's disease in a pack of foxhounds. Irish Vet J 43:126. 1990.

178. Thomas WB, Sorjonen DC, Steiss JE: A retrospective evaluation of 38 cases of canine distemper encephalomyelitis. J Am Anim Hosp Assoc 29:129–133, 1993.

179. Shell LG: Canine distemper. Comp Contin Ed 12:173–179, 1990.

180. Raw ME, Pearson GR, Brown PJ, Baumgartner W: Canine distemper infection associated with acute nervous signs in dogs. Vet Rec 130:291–293, 1992.

181. Higgins RJ, Child G, Vandevelde M: Chronic relapsing demyelinating encephalomyelitis associated with persistent spontaneous canine distemper virus infection. Acta Neuropathol Berl 77:441–444, 1989.

182. Zurbriggen A, Vandevelde M: The pathogenesis of nervous distemper. ProgVet Neurol 5:109–115, 1995.

183. Muller C, Fatzer R, Beck K, et al: Studies on canine distemper virus persistence in the central nervous system. Acta Neuropathol 89:438–445, 1995.

184. McCandlish IA, Cornwell HJ, Thompson H, et al: Distemper encephalitis in pups after vaccination of the dam. Vet Rec 130:27–30, 1992.

185. Botteron C, Zurbriggen A, Griot C, Vandevelde M: Canine distemper virus–immune complexes induce bystander degeneration of oligodendrocytes. Acta Neuropathol Berl 83:402–407, 1992.

186. Tipold A, Vandevelde M, Jaggy A: Neurological manifestations of canine distemper virus infection. J Small Animal Pract 33:466–470, 1992.

CNS

187. Sorjonen DC, Cox NR, Swango LJ: Electrophoretic determination of albumin and gamma globulin concentrations in the cerebrospinal fluid of dogs with encephalomyelitis attributable to canine distemper virus infection: 13 cases (1980–1987). JAVMA 195:977–980, 1989.

188. Baroni M, Heinold Y: A review of the clinical diagnosis of feline infectious peritonitis viral meningoencephalomyelitis. ProgVet Neurol 6:88–94, 1995.

189. Wolf A: Feline infectious peritonitis, Part 1. Feline Pract 25:26–29, 1997.

190. Dubey JP, Lindsay DS, Lipscomb TP: Neosporosis in cats. Vet Pathol 27:335–339, 1990.

191. Dubey JP: Neosporosis. Veterinary Medical Forum. Washington, DC, American College of Veterinary Internal Medicine, 1993, pp 710–712.

192. Hay WH, Shell LG, Lindsay DS, Dubey JP: Diagnosis and treatment of *Neospora caninum* infection in a dog. JAVMA 197:87–89, 1990.

193. Lappin MR, Greene CE, Winston S, et al: Clinical feline toxoplasmosis. Serologic diagnosis and therapeutic management of 15 cases. J Vet Intern Med 3:139–143, 1989.

194. Lappin MR, Greene CE, Prestwood AK, et al: Prevalence of *Toxoplasma gondii* infection in cats in Georgia using enzyme-linked immunosorbent assays for IgM, IgG, and antigens. Vet Parasitol 33:225–230, 1989.

195. Jacobson LS, Jardine JE: *Neospora caninum* infection in three Labrador littermates. J S Afr Vet Assoc 64:47–51, 1993.

196. Thulin JD, Granstrom DE, Gelberg HB, et al: Concurrent protozoal encephalitis and canine distemper virus infection in a raccoon *(Procyon lotor)*. Vet Rec 130:162–164, 1992.

197. Dubey JP, Higgins RT, Smith JH, O'Toole TD: *Neospora caninum* encephalomyelitis in a British dog. Vet Rec 126:193–194, 1990.

198. Dubey JP, Fenner WR: Clinical segmental myelitis associated with an unidentified *Toxoplasma*-like parasite in a cat. J Vet Diagn Invest 5:472–480, 1993.

199. Cuddon P, Lin D-S, Bowman D, et al: *Neosporum caninum* infection in English Springer Spaniel littermates: Diagnostic evaluation and organism isolation. J Vet Intern Med 6:325–332, 1992.

200. Jackson W, DeLahunta A, Adaska J, et al: *Neospora caninum* in an adult dog with progressive cerebellar signs. ProgVet Neurol 4:124–127, 1995.

201. Dubey J: Toxoplasmosis. JAVMA 205:1593–1598, 1994.

202. Barber J, Payne-Johnson C, Trees A: Distribution of *Neospora caninum* within the central nervous system and other tissues of six dogs with clinical neosporosis. J Small Animal Pract 37:568–574, 1996.

203. Ruehlmann D, Podell M, Oglesbee M, Dubey J: Canine neosporosis: A case report and literature review. J Am Animal Hosp Assoc 31:174–182, 1995.

204. O'Neil SA, Lappin MR, Reif JS, et al: Clinical and epidemiological aspects of feline immunodeficiency virus and *Toxoplasma gondii* coinfections in cats. J Am Animal Hosp Assoc 27:211–220, 1991.

205. Davies C, Troy G: Deep mycotic infections in cats. J Am Anim Hosp Assoc 32:380–391, 1996.

206. Gelb LD: Infections: Bacteria, fungi and parasites. *In* Pearlman A, Collins RC (eds): Neurobiology of Disease. New York, Oxford University Press, 1990, pp 417–434.

207. Medleau L, Greene CE, Rakich PM: Evaluation of ketoconazole and itraconazole for treatment of disseminated cryptococcosis in cats. Am J Vet Res 51:1454–1458, 1990.

208. Rudmann DG, Coolman BR, Perez CM, Glickman LT: Evaluation of risk factors for blastomycosis in dogs: 857 cases (1980–1990). JAVMA 201:1754–1759, 1992.

209. Burtch M: Granulomatous meningitis caused by *Coccidioides immitis* in a dog. JAVMA 212:827–829, 1998.

210. Berthelin C, Bailey C, Kass P, et al: Cryptococcosis of the nervous system in dogs. Part 1: Epidemiologic, clinical, and neuropathologic features. ProgVet Neurol 5:88–97, 1995.

211. Gerds-Grogan S, Dayrell-Hart B: Feline cryptococcosis: A retrospective evaluation. J Am Anim Hosp Assoc 33:118–122, 1997.

212. Glass E, DeLahunta A, Kent M, et al: A cryptococcal granuloma in the brain of a cat causing focal signs. J Vet Intern Med 7:137–140, 1996.

213. Greene R, Troy G: Coccidioidomycosis in 48 cats: A retrospective study (1984–1993). J Vet Intern Med 9:86–91, 1995.

214. Medleau L, Jacobs G, Marks M: Itraconazole for the treatment of cryptococcosis in cats. J Vet Intern Med 9:39–42, 1995.

215. Legendre AM, Rohrbach BW, Toal RL, et al: Treatment of blastomycosis with itraconazole in 112 dogs. J Vet Intern Med 10:365–371, 1996.

216. Tiches D, Vite CH, Dayrell-Hart B, et al: A case of canine central nervous system cryptococcosis: Management with fluconazole. J Am Anim Hosp Assoc 34:145–151, 1997.

217. Jacobs G, Medleau L, Calvert C, Brown J: Cryptococcal infection in cats: Factors influencing treatment outcome, and results of sequential antigen titers in 35 cats. J Vet Intern Med 11:1–4, 1997.

218. Smith-Maxie LL, Parent JP, Rand J, et al: Cerebrospinal fluid analysis and clinical outcome of eight dogs with eosinophilic meningoencephalomyelitis. J Vet Intern Med 3:167–174, 1989.

219. Bailey CS, Higgins RJ: Characteristics of cerebrospinal fluid associated with canine granulomatous meningoencephalitis. JAVMA 188:418–421, 1986.

220. Sorjonen DC: Clinical and histopathological features of granulomatous meningoencephalomyelitis in dogs. J Am Anim Hosp Assoc 26:141–147, 1990.

221. Thomas JB, Eger C: Granulomatous meningoencephalomyelitis in 21 dogs. J Small Anim Pract 30:287–293, 1989.

222. Braund KG: Granulomatous meningoencephalitis. JAVMA 186:138–141, 1985.

223. Sorjonen DC: Granulomatous Meningoencephalomyelitis: Clinical and Histopathologic Correlations. ACVIM Forum. San Diego, American College of Veterinary Internal Medicine, 1987, pp 848–850.

224. Murtaugh RJ, Fenner WR, Johnson GC: Focal granulomatous meningoencephalomyelitis in a pup. JAVMA 187:835–836, 1985.

225. Gearhart MA, DeLahunta A, Summers BA: Cerebellar mass in a dog due to granulomatous meningoencephalitis. J Am Anim Hosp Assoc 22:683–686, 1985.

226. Munana K, Luttgen P: Prognostic factors for dogs with granulomatous meningoencephalomyelitis: 42 cases (1982–1996). JAVMA 212:1902–1906, 1998.

227. Cordy DR, Holliday TA: A necrotizing meningoencephalitis of pug dogs. Vet Pathol 26:191–194, 1989.

228. Jull B, Merryman J, Thomas W, McArthur A: Necrotizing encephalitis in a Yorkshire Terrier. JAVMA 211:1005–1007, 1997.

229. Stalis I, Chadwick B, Dayrell-Hart B, et al: Necrotizing meningoencephalitis of Maltese dogs. Vet Pathol 32:230–235, 1995.

230. Bradley GA: Myocardial necrosis in a Pug dog with necrotizing meningoencephalitis. Vet Pathol 28:91–93, 1991.

231. Firneisz GD, Cochrane SM, Parent J, Houston DM: Canine ehrlichiosis in Ontario. Can Vet J 31:652–653, 1990.

232. Maretzki C, Fisher D, Greene C: Granulocytic ehrlichiosis and meningitis in a dog. JAVMA 205:1554–1556, 1994.

233. Cuddon PA: Tremor syndromes. ProgVet Neurol 1:285–299 1990.

234. Wagner S, Podell M, Fenner W: Generalized tremors in dogs: 24 cases (1984–1995). JAVMA 211:731–735, 1997.

235. Bagley RS: Clinical Evaluation of Dogs with Tremors. Veterinary Medical Forum. Washington, DC, American College of Veterinary Internal Medicine, 1993, pp 870–872.

236. Bagley RS, Kornegay JN, Wheeler SJ, et al: Generalized tremors in Maltese: Clinical findings in seven cases. J Am Anim Hosp Assoc 29:141–145, 1993.

237. Wyatt JM, Pearson GR, Smerdon TN, et al: Naturally occurring scrapie-like spongiform encephalopathy in five domestic cats. Vet Rec 128:233–236, 1991.

238. Dow SW, Dreitz MJ, Hoover EA: Exploring the link between feline immunodeficiency virus infection and neurologic disease in cats. Vet Med 87:1181–1184, 1992.

239. Hurtrel M, Ganiere JP, Guelfi JF, et al: Comparison of early and late feline immunodeficiency virus encephalopathies. AIDS 6:399–406, 1992.

CHAPTER 105

MULTIFOCAL NEUROLOGIC DISEASE

Rodney S. Bagley

Many diseases occur primarily or exclusively in specific areas within the nervous system, allowing the clinician to localize the lesion to discrete areas based on clinical signs. Some disease processes, however, concurrently affect the nervous system in a number of anatomically and functionally distinct areas (Table 105–1). In this instance, the clinical signs are more diffuse in nature. The more clinically important diseases that result in multifocal or diffuse clinical signs are reviewed herein. It is taken for granted that more than one disease can be present within the nervous system at one time (e.g., a brain tumor and a cervical disk extrusion).

INFLAMMATORY DISEASES

Encephalitis and meningitis often exist concurrently in dogs and cats and are the most common diseases that result in multifocal nervous system signs.[1-3] Etiologies include both infectious and noninfectious causes. Infectious agents associated with encephalitis and meningitis include viral (distemper, parvovirus, parainfluenza, herpes, feline infectious peritonitis, pseudorabies, rabies), bacterial, rickettsial (Rocky Mountain spotted fever, ehrlichiosis), spirochetal (Lyme disease, leptospirosis), fungal (blastomycosis, histoplasmosis, cryptococcosis, coccidioidomycosis, aspergillosis), protozoal (toxoplasmosis, neosporosis), parasitic, and unclassified organisms (prototheocosis). The incidence of infectious agents causing meningitis varies with geographic location.

As these diseases often affect the nervous system at multiple levels, a focal neuroanatomic localization may not be possible. Intracranial signs (behavior changes, mental status abnormalities, visual deficits), including cranial nerve dysfunction and spinal cord signs (paresis, ataxia), are common. Neck pain is a prominent clinical feature of meningitis but may be less obvious with pure parenchymal involvement (e.g., myelitis). Pain may be assessed by vocalization during direct palpation or by reluctance to move the head and neck. Diffuse spinal pain is also common, lending information about the diffuse nature of these diseases. Some animals react as if pain is caused by minimal touching throughout the body, especially on the limbs and face. Other animals become irritable and uncharacteristically aggressive. Because chorioretinitis is often present concurrently, fundic examination may yield important clues to the polysystemic nature of the problem.

For diagnosis, imaging studies such as magnetic resonance (MR) imaging and computed tomography (CT) scans are helpful for defining structural lesions (Fig. 105–1).[4] Multifocal lesions are visible, especially after intravenous contrast medium administration. Cerebrospinal fluid (CSF) analysis is extremely valuable for diagnosis. Increased numbers of nucleated cells and increased protein concentrations are common (Fig. 105–2). Nucleated cell types can vary, depending on the etiology; mononuclear cells and neutrophils are most typical. If concurrent hemorrhage has occurred, erythrophagocytosis may be noted. Evidence of inflammation on CSF evaluation alone, however, is not specific for primary encephalitis, because other central nervous system (CNS) diseases (e.g., neoplasia) may result in CSF pleocytosis and increased protein concentrations. Evaluation of serum or CSF titers for the aforementioned infectious diseases is often necessary to establish associated infectious diseases.

Treatment of meningitis is ideally directed at a specific causative organism. Without a definable specific cause, the best treatment success is achieved with multiple-drug therapies rather than single-agent protocols and by treating earlier rather than later in the disease course. Trimethoprim-sulfadiazine (30 mg/kg every 12 hours), clindamycin (20 to 25 mg/kg every 12 hours), and corticosteroids (prednisone 1 to 4 mg/kg every 12 hours) are used in combination. Although corticosteroids may seem contraindicated with infectious diseases, they are often beneficial in the acute treatment of brain inflammation and edema. These associated pathophysiologic events are more often the cause of the neurologic deterioration than is primary cell death from the organism itself. If rickettsial diseases are suspected, doxycycline (5 to 20 mg/kg orally every 12 hours) or, less ideally, chloramphenicol (15 to 25 mg/kg orally every 8 hours) can be substituted or added to the regimen. If the animal is receiving phenobarbital, *do not* use chloramphenicol, as this drug decreases the metabolism of the barbiturate, and the dog or cat could become comatose and possibly die.

INFECTIOUS DISEASES

Bacterial Meningitis. Bacterial meningitis is rare in dogs and cats.[1] Often, a concurrent disease that results in persistent bacteremia is present. Notable examples in dogs are endocarditis and pyometra. Extension of a local bacterial disease process, most commonly from the nasal passages or middle ear, is also possible (Fig. 105–3). Dogs and cats with bacterial meningitis usually have rapidly progressing clinical signs, and the disease is often fatal. Abscesses may form, resulting in focal clinical signs.[5] A variety of causative organisms is possible.

Diagnosis is aided primarily by CSF analysis. Although attempts have been made to classify CSF changes commonly associated with septic inflammatory CNS diseases, the degree of crossover in CSF nucleated cell counts and types makes it difficult to presumptively diagnose a specific inflammatory disease solely from CSF results. One clue to the presence of a bacterial component is decreased CSF glucose

TABLE 105–1. DISEASES THAT COMMONLY RESULT IN MULTIFOCAL NERVOUS SYSTEM SIGNS

Degenerative
  Storage disease
  Multineuronal degeneration
Anomalous
  Hydrocephalus, syringomyelia/hydromyelia complex
Metabolic
  Hepatic
  Renal
  Hypoglycemia
  Thyroid (hypo and hyper)
  Hyperadrenocorticism
  Hyperosmolar syndromes
    Adipsia
Neoplastic
  Lymphoma
  Leukemias
  Metastatic tumors
Nutritional
  Thiamine
Inflammatory
  Infectious
    Viral
      Distemper
      Herpes
      Parvo
      Parainfluenza
      Feline infectious peritonitis
      Feline immunodeficiency virus
    Bacterial
      Tetanus
    Fungal
      Cryptococcosis
      Blastomycosis
      Coccidioidomycosis
      Candidiasis
      Aspergillosis
    Protozoal
      Toxoplasmosis
      Neosporosis
    Parasitic
      Toxocariasis
    Rickettsial
      Rocky Mountain spotted fever
      Ehrlichiosis
    Unclassified
      Prototheocosis
  Noninfectious
    Granulomatous meningoencephalitis
    Pug encephalitis
    Maltese encephalitis
    Spinal cord vasculitis
    Nonclassified
      Steroid-responsive meningitis
Idiopathic
  Dysautonomia
Toxins
Vascular disease
  Thromboembolism
  Hypertension
  Cerebral hemorrhage

concentration as compared with plasma, presumably due to consumption of glucose by the organism. If bacterial encephalitis is suspected, additional CSF should be collected in a sterile container without fixative or other chemicals for culture and sensitivity testing. Glass tubes containing EDTA, commonly used for submission of CSF for cytologic analysis, are not appropriate for culture, as EDTA is bacteriostatic and may hinder organism growth. The number of organisms in CSF can be small, so the greater the amount of CSF cultured, the more likely it is that an organism will be isolated.

Because identification of the organism may take a few days and the clinical signs can be rapidly progressive, treatment is often initiated before culture analysis. Before a specific cause is identified, the author uses trimethoprim-sulfadiazine, clindamycin, and corticosteroids in combination to treat CNS inflammation or infection. If the animal is unable to swallow, methylprednisolone sodium succinate (30 mg/kg) can be administered intravenously. If it can swallow effectively, prednisone/prednisolone can then be initiated at anti-inflammatory dosages. Surgical decompression of a focal abscess should occur as soon as possible after detection.

Tetanus. Another bacterial disease with initially confusing clinical signs is tetanus. Tetanus is caused by a neurotoxin secreted by the organism *Clostridium tetani*. This toxin binds to interneurons and inhibits the release of inhibitory neurotransmitter (glycine) in inhibitory interneurons (Renshaw cells). The organism gains access to the body through a wound. Cats are more resistant to the disease than dogs. Wounds on a dog may be undetectable but on cats are usually obvious. Clinical signs include extensor rigidity, inability to open the mouth, salivation, prolapsed nictitating membrane, inability to urinate, and seizures. Bradycardia,[6] megaesophagus, and hiatal hernia[7] may be seen. Tetanus localized to one part of the body is occasionally found. Diagnosis is based on clinical signs. Anaerobic culturing of a wound may reveal the organism. A serum test for antibodies has occasionally been useful but is not readily available. Treatment includes wound debridement, antitoxin (administered once intravenously), penicillin, muscle relaxants, enteral or parenteral nutrition support, a quiet environment, and good supportive care. Anticonvulsants are given if seizures occur.

Canine Distemper. Canine distemper is caused by a paramyxovirus. Clinical signs can occur in dogs of any age, regardless of vaccination status. Most commonly, however, young dogs with inadequate vaccinations are affected. The disease is characterized pathologically by two main forms: neuronal and glial cell death (polioencephalomyelopathy) and demyelination (leukoencephalomyelopathy).[3, 8–10] It has been suggested that those animals with a poorer antibody response to the virus tend to have the former form, and those with an adequate immune response to the virus tend to have the latter, immune-mediated demyelination. Any region of the nervous system can be involved. Myoclonus, a rhythmic, shocklike contraction of one muscle or a group of muscles, is usually the result of previous or concurrent distemper infection and lends a clue to the virus's presence. Muscles of the limbs are commonly involved, but other muscles, including the tongue, may be affected.[11] Clinical signs of a prior or concurrent systemic illness (respiratory, gastrointestinal) are not always found in dogs with distemper-caused neurologic signs. Diagnosis is suggested by finding inclusion bodies in pathologic specimens. Increased CSF antibody titer (IgG and IgM) against distemper virus is supportive of a diagnosis, especially if concurrent serum distemper titers are not elevated or if a CSF electrophoresis suggests intrathecal antibody production. Occasionally, dogs with CNS distemper do not have positive CSF distemper titers.[12] No specific treatment is effective against the distemper virus. Corticosteroids, although seemingly contraindicated, may decrease inflammation and improve clinical signs in some dogs.

Other viruses of dogs that result in encephalitis or meningitis do so primarily in young animals. Examples include herpesvirus, parvovirus, and parainfluenza virus. Occasionally, these viruses cause encephalitis or meningitis in adult

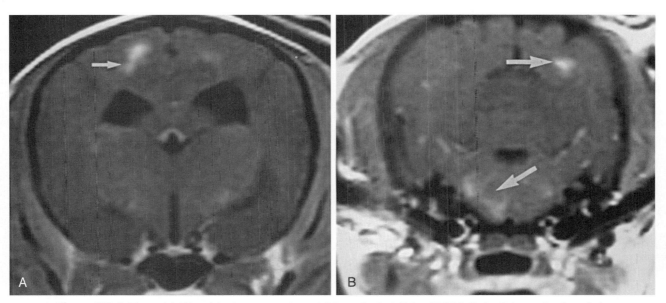

Figure 105–1. Transaxial, T1-weighted, contrast-enhanced (Magnevist [gadolinium DTPA], Berlex Laboratories, Inc., Cedar Knolls, NJ) MR at the level of the thalamus *(A)* and brain stem *(B)* from a dog with multifocal clinical signs. Multifocal lesions are present in the cortex and brain stem *(arrows)*. Diagnosis was granulomatous meningoencephalitis.

dogs. Parainfluenza virus has a propensity for causing hydrocephalus.

Feline Infectious Peritonitis (FIP). FIP results from a coronavirus-induced vasculitis in cats. This disease can involve various areas of the nervous system, primarily the intracranial structures and spinal cord. Young and, conversely, geriatric cats seem predisposed.[13] Of the two FIP forms, the "dry" form most commonly affects the nervous system. This viral infection results in an immune complex vasculitis that is responsible for most of the pathologic effects. CSF analysis may show pleocytosis, with either mononuclear cells or neutrophils as the predominant cell type. No specific treatment is effective. Immune-suppressive therapy may result in short-term improvement of clinical signs.

Feline Immunodeficiency Virus (FIV). FIV has re-

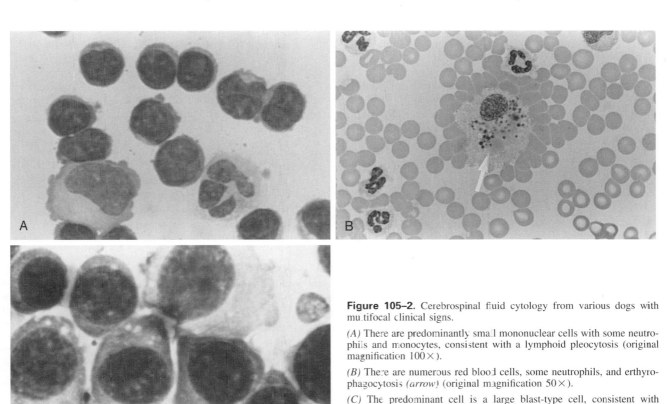

Figure 105–2. Cerebrospinal fluid cytology from various dogs with multifocal clinical signs.

(A) There are predominantly small mononuclear cells with some neutrophils and monocytes, consistent with a lymphoid pleocytosis (original magnification 100×).

(B) There are numerous red blood cells, some neutrophils, and erythrophagocytosis *(arrow)* (original magnification 50×).

(C) The predominant cell is a large blast-type cell, consistent with lymphosarcoma (original magnification 100×).

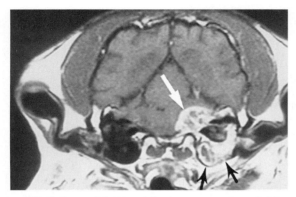

Figure 105–3. Transaxial, T1-weighted, contrast-enhanced (Magnevist [gadolinium DTPA], Berlex Laboratories, Inc., Cedar Knolls, NJ) MR at the level of the vestibular area from a snow leopard with seizures and a head tilt. A brain abscess is present extending from the middle/inner ear to the brain stem *(arrows)*. A surgical biopsy and culture found that both fungal and bacterial organisms were present.

cently been associated with nervous system signs, including behavior changes, seizures, anisocoria, and muscle twitching.[3] As the clinical spectrum of this disease evolves, it may represent an important CNS pathogen of cats.

Protozoal Infections. *Toxoplasma gondii* and *Neospora caninum* are protozoal organisms that can affect any area of the nervous system and cause encephalitis, myelitis, peripheral neuropathy, or myositis.[14] A classic sign of infection in young animals is hyperextended pelvic limbs. CSF analysis often reveals pleocytosis and increased protein concentration. Diagnosis is based on the presence of IgM or rising IgG titers to the organism (toxoplasmosis) or visualization of the protozoan in biopsy specimens (both toxoplasmosis and neosporosis).[15] Clinical distinction between the two organisms is not always possible but is increased by awareness of *Neospora,* special staining, and electron microscopic characteristics. Treatment for toxoplasmosis currently is clindamycin[16]; however, this drug is often used in combination with a potentiated sulfa drug in immune-suppressed humans with toxoplasmosis.[17] A similar treatment is used for neosporosis, but few cases with definitive treatment success have been reported.[18]

Rickettsial Infections. Infection with the rickettsial organisms associated with Rocky Mountain spotted fever (RMSF) and ehrlichiosis commonly involve the brain stem, particularly the vestibular system.[19] With RMSF there is often a history of systemic illness (usually with a thrombocytopenia) 5 to 10 days before the development of neurologic signs. As the animal's fever is decreasing, neurologic signs appear. Diagnosis is based on lack of mass lesion on intracranial imaging studies and pleocytosis on CSF evaluation. Occasionally, increased contrast enhancement is noted in the choroid plexus area in affected dogs. This must be differentiated from the degree of contrast enhancement normally seen in these structures. CSF usually contains milder increases in nucleated cells (<50 nucleated cells/μL; normal, <5 nucleated cells/μL) and milder increases in protein concentration (<50 mg/dL; normal, <25 mg/dL). Diagnosis is supported by increasing serum titers to the organism, but results often are available after the disease has progressed. Prognosis is dependent primarily on the severity of clinical signs before treatment. Dogs that are severely obtunded before treatment are less likely to recover. Dogs with clinical features of vestibular disease after a systemic febrile illness associated with thrombocytopenia should be treated with

tetracycline or doxycycline before establishing a definitive diagnosis with titers.

Fungal Infections. Of the fungal diseases that can affect the nervous system, cryptococcosis, blastomycosis, coccidioidomycosis, candidiasis, and aspergillosis are most common. [2, 3] Immunodeficiency may play a role in these uncommon nervous system infections. Definitive diagnosis is made through viewing the organism in CSF or biopsy samples and fungal culture of infected nervous tissues. Treatment can be attempted with antifungal agents; however, the presence of an intact blood-brain barrier may hinder the drug's ability to reach therapeutic concentrations in CNS tissue. Fluconazole and itraconazole hold the most promise for treating fungal encephalitis or meningitis. These drugs are rather expensive, and owner financial constrains often limit their use in long-term therapy.

NONINFECTIOUS DISEASES

Most meningitis syndromes (about 60 per cent) in dogs do not have a definable infectious cause. Noninfectious disease of the supratentorial structures include some specific diseases such as granulomatous meningoencephalitis (GME) and pug encephalitis. There are also many nonspecific entities. GME, an idiopathic condition, can occur as a disseminated disease, a focal mass lesion, or a primary ocular disease.[1] Some dogs that were thought to have this disease were later shown to have had lymphoma. CSF usually shows a mononuclear pleocytosis. Occasionally, the CSF is normal or contains increased protein concentrations. CT or MRI scans may show diffuse inflammatory changes or a mass lesion.[4] Biopsy is needed for definitive diagnosis. Treatment options include immune suppression (corticosteroids, azathioprine), surgery (for a focal mass), or radiation therapy. The latter has shown the most promise for definitive treatment of this disease.[20] Most dogs with GME die within six months to one year after diagnosis unless radiation therapy is used.

Pug encephalitis usually occurs in young pugs but has been reported in dogs as old as 7 years of age. The disease is characterized histologically by forebrain inflammation and necrosis, primarily of the cerebral hemispheres.[21] Initial clinical signs may be neck pain, mimicking primary spinal cord disease. This disease has been uniformly fatal, and therapy (corticosteroids) has not altered its course. A similar disease has been described in Maltese terriers.[22]

Other inflammatory diseases that do not have a definitive cause are often grouped together under the term "steroid-responsive meningitis." [2, 3] Almost assuredly, multiple diseases exist within this group. Younger, large breed dogs are more often affected. Clinical signs usually include cervical pain. Additionally, there is a syndrome of spinal cord vasculitis that occurs in beagles and Bernese Mountain Dogs. Other dogs such as German shorthaired pointers have an apparent breed-associated meningitis syndrome.[2, 3] Clinical signs are similar to those mentioned for other meningitis syndromes. Corticosteroid therapy may also benefit these dogs.

GENERALIZED TREMORS

Generalized tremor syndrome occurs in numerous breeds of dogs.[23, 24] Diffuse, low-amplitude tremors are the norm. Many dogs are initially thought to be hypothermic or apprehensive. Historically, dogs with white haircoats have been affected ("white shakers"). Dogs with a variety of haircoat colors, however, can be affected. Clinical signs usually occur in dogs that are 1 to 4 years old and include generalized tremor, ocular muscle tremor, vestibular signs (head tilt, ataxia), cerebellar signs, and seizures. The disease is often associated with a mild encephalitis. CSF from affected animals usually contains mild increases in nucleated cell counts and normal to slightly increased protein content. No obvious cause of the encephalitis has been found. Clinical signs usually respond to immune-suppressive dosages of corticosteroids. After the clinical signs have initially resolved, the corticosteroid dosage can be slowly decreased (over weeks to months) to prevent recurrence. The disease in some dogs remains in remission only with continual corticosteroid administration, similar to other autoimmune diseases.

METABOLIC DISEASES

Many metabolic diseases may affect the nervous system at multiple areas and result in diffuse or multifocal clinical signs.[25] Hypoglycemia secondary to insulinoma can result in CNS signs (depression, seizures, tremors) as well as peripheral dysfunction (weakness, decreased spinal reflexes, muscle atrophy).[26–31] The dichotomy of seizures (a supratentorial sign) and decreased to absent reflexes (a lower motor neuron sign) may initially result in confusion during neuroanatomic localization. Clinical signs of weakness with insulinomas are often attributed to hypoglycemia, and the concurrent neuropathy is often overlooked.

Hyperthyroidism of cats has been associated with both central and peripheral nervous system abnormalities.[32] CNS signs include restlessness, hyperexcitability, irritability, aggression, wandering, pacing, circling, insomnia, and seizures. Apathy, lethargy, and depression occur infrequently. Focal neurologic deficits may result from associated cerebrovascular accidents, most likely secondary to hypertension. Clinical signs of peripheral nervous system involvement include generalized weakness, neck ventroflexion, muscle tremors, gait abnormalities, and muscle atrophy. Muscle weakness often manifests as a decreased ability to jump. Neck ventroflexion may occur with other diseases, including myasthenia gravis, polymyopathy (including hyperkalemic polymyopathy), and organophosphate toxicity.

Hypothyroidism has also been associated with various nervous system abnormalities in dogs.[33] Whether these signs reflect a primary metabolic disturbance or secondary structural abnormalities associated with underlying vascular disease cannot always be determined. Cranial (vestibular, facial, trigeminal) and appendicular peripheral nerves may be abnormal. Morphologic changes in nerves include demyelination, remyelination, and axonal necrosis. These changes, however, are not specific for hypothyroid neuropathy.

Hyperadrenocorticism may result in abnormalities of the muscle and peripheral nervous system.[34] Affected dogs have stiff gait, most obvious in the pelvic limbs. An associated pseudomyotonic state has been described. Whether this is primarily a myopathy or a neuropathy has not been determined. Extremely rarely, dogs with hyperadrenocorticism have acute pelvic limb dysfunction resulting from aortic thromboembolism. The hypercoagulability associated with hyperadrenocorticism is suspected to be the cause of the thrombosis. If the disease is the result of a pituitary tumor, clinical signs of intracranial disease are also possible. Macroadenomas may enlarge dorsally from the sella and compress the diencephalon (see Chapter 154).

NEOPLASIA

Tumors of the nervous system include primary and secondary (metastasis) neoplasms.[35] Often tumors of the nervous system result in focal clinical signs. Some tumors, however, are diffuse and therefore result in diffuse clinical signs. Prominent examples include lymphosarcoma and carcinomatosis. Multiple cranial nerves (III, IV, V, VI, VII) may be involved with hematogenous neoplasia (leukemias) owing to direct involvement with the tumor cells.[36] Choroid plexus tumors, which often arise within the ventricles of the brain, may metastasize within the neural axis through the CSF.[37] If the spinal cord is affected, clinical signs of spinal dysfunction may occur concurrent with intracranial signs from the primary tumor. Diagnosis is aided by advanced imaging and CSF analysis.

Neoplasia secondarily can involve the brain via metastasis or via direct extension from extraneural sites.[38, 39] Clinical signs may be localized or multifocal, depending on the number and location of metastases and associated pathophysiologic sequelae such as hemorrhage and edema.[38]

OTHER DISEASES

Many degenerative neurologic diseases of dogs and cats are inherited or congenital and therefore are seen primarily in young animals.[1] Storage diseases are prominent examples. Diseases that involve the neuronal cell body are more likely to have cerebral, cranial nerve, or peripheral nerve signs, whereas diseases that primarily involve myelin are more likely to result in ataxia and paresis of the limbs.[1] The storage diseases and other degenerative diseases of dogs and cats have been reviewed previously.[1]

Numerous toxins can affect the nervous system, often at multiple sites.[40, 41] Examples of primary toxins include organophosphates, metaldehyde, lead, and bromethalin. Diagnosis can be difficult if exposure has not been documented historically. Treatment is directed toward the specific toxin.

Vascular disease involving the supratentorial structures is uncommon in animals as compared with human beings.[42] Thrombosis, infarction, and hemorrhage can occur secondary to drug therapy (L-asparaginase, anticoagulants), thrombocytopenia and other bleeding disorders, trauma, hypertension (hyperthyroidism, hyperadrenocorticism), atherosclerosis from hypothyroidism, and infection (septic emboli). Clinical signs are usually acute in onset and may be initially progressive as the vascular event results in secondary brain disease and edema. Hemorrhage and infarction may be seen with CT and MRI scans. Acutely, the associated mass effect and edema can mimic other intracranial structural diseases such as tumor. Diagnosis is supported by cerebral angiography; however, this is uncommonly performed in dogs and cats. The application of newer, noninvasive technologies such as MRI angiography and transcranial Doppler ultrasonography may aid in the diagnosis of these diseases in animals in the future.

REFERENCES

1. Oliver JE Jr, Lorenz MD, Kornegay JN: Systemic or multifocal signs. In Handbook of Veterinary Neurology, 3rd ed. Philadelphia, WB Saunders, 1997, pp 341–402.
2. Meric SM: Canine meningitis: A changing emphasis. J Vet Intern Med 2:26, 1986.
3. Muñana KR: Encephalitis and meningitis. Vet Clin North Am 26:857, 1996.
4. Plummer SB, Wheeler SJ, Thrall D E, et al: Computed tomography of primary

inflammatory brain disorders in dogs and cats. Vet Rad Ultrasound 33:307, 1992.

5. Dow SW, LeCouteur RA, Henik RA, et al: Central nervous system infection associated with anaerobic bacteria in two dogs and two cats. J Vet Intern Med 2:171, 1988.

6. Panciera D, Baldwin CJ, Keene BW: Electrocardiographic abnormalities associated with tetanus in two dogs. JAVMA 192:225, 1988.

7. Dieringer TM, Wolf AM: Esophageal hiatal hernia and megaesophagus complicating tetanus in two dogs. JAVMA 199:87, 1991.

8. Zurbriggen A, Vandevelde M: The pathogenesis of nervous distemper. Prog Vet Neurol 5:109, 1994.

9. Thomas WB, Sorjonen DC, Steiss JE: A retrospective evaluation of 38 cases of canine distemper encephalomyelitis. J Am Anim Hosp Assoc 29:129, 1993.

10. Guilford WG, Shaw DP, O'Brien DP, et al: Fecal incontinence, urinary incontinence, and priapism associated with multifocal distemper encephalomyelitis in a dog. JAVMA 197:90, 1990.

11. Silver GM, Bagley RS, Moore MP: Myoclonus of the tongue muscles in a dog. Prog Vet Neurol 7:137, 1996.

12. Sorjonen DC, Cox NR, Swango LJ: Electrophoretic determination of albumin and gamma globulin concentrations in cerebrospinal fluid of dogs with encephalomyelitis attributable to canine distemper virus infection: 13 cases (1980–1987). JAVMA 195:977, 1989.

13. Kornegay JN: Feline infectious peritonitis: The central nervous system form. J Am Anim Hosp Assoc 14:580, 1978.

14. Hass JA, Shell L, Saunders G: Neurological manifestations of toxoplasmosis: A literature review and case summary. J Am Anim Hosp Assoc 5:253, 1989.

15. Lappin MR, Greene CE, Prestwood AK, et al: Diagnosis of recent *Toxoplasma gondii* infection in cats by use of an enzyme-linked immunosobent assay for immunoglobulin M. Am J Vet Res 50:1580, 1989.

16. Greene CE, Cook JR Jr, Mahaffey EA: Clindamycin for treatment of toxoplasma polymyositis in a dog. JAVMA 187:631, 1985.

17. Rolston KVI, Hoy J: Role of clindamycin in the treatment of central nervous system toxoplasmosis. Am J Med 83:551, 1987.

18. Hoskins JD, Bunge MM, Dubey JP, et al: Disseminated infection with *Neospora caninum* in a ten-year-old dog. Cornell Vet 81:329, 1991.

19. Greene CE, Burgdorfer W, Cavagnolo R, et al: Rocky Mountain spotted fever in dogs and its differentiation from canine ehrlichiosis. JAVMA 186:465, 1985.

20. Sisson AF, LeCouteur RA, Dow SW, et al: Radiation therapy of granulomatous meningoencephalomyelitis of dogs (abstract 26). Proceedings of the Seventh Annual ACVIM Forum, San Diego, 1989, p 1031.

21. Cordy DR, Holliday TA: A necrotizing meningoencephalitis of pug dogs. Vet Pathol 26:191, 1989.

22. Van Winkle T, Stalis I, Summers B: Necrotizing meningoencephalitis in Maltese dogs: A comparison with pug encephalitis. Vet Pathol 29:446, 1992.

23. Bagley RS: Tremor syndromes in dogs: Diagnosis and treatment. J Small Anim Pract 33:485, 1992.

24. Bagley RS, Kornegay JN, Wheeler SJ, et al: Generalized tremors in Maltese terriers: Clinical finding in 7 cases (1984–1990). J Am Anim Hosp Assoc 29:141, 1993.

25. Cuddon PA: Metabolic encephalopathies. Vet Clin North Am 26:893, 1996.

26. Howerton TL, Shell LG: Neurologic manifestations of altered serum glucose. Prog Vet Neurol 3:57, 1992.

27. Shahar R, Rousseaux C, Steiss J: Peripheral polyneuropathy in a dog with functional islet B-cell tumor and widespread metastasis. JAVMA 187:175, 1985.

28. Bergman PJ, Bruyett DS, Coyne BE, et al: Canine clinical peripheral neuropathy associated with pancreatic islet cell carcinoma Prog Vet Neurol 5:57, 1994.

29. Braund KG, Steiss JE, Amling KA, et al: Insulinoma and subclinical peripheral neuropathy in two dogs. J Vet Intern Med 1:86, 1987.

30. Dyer KR, Messing A: Peripheral neuropathy associated with functional islet cell adenomas in SV40 transgenic mice. J Neuropathol Exp Neurol 48:399, 1989.

31. Schrauwen E, Van Ham L, Hoorens J: Peripheral polyneuropathy associated with insulinoma in the dog: Clinical, pathological, and electrodiagnostic features. Prog Vet Neurol 7:16, 1996.

32. Joseph RJ, Peterson ME: Review and comparison of neuromuscular and central nervous system manifestations of hyperthyroidism in cats and humans. Prog Vet Neurol 3:114, 1992.

33. Jaggy A, Oliver JE, Ferguson DC, et al: Neurological manifestations of hypothyroidism: A retrospective study of 29 dogs. J Vet Intern Med 8:328, 1994.

34. Feldman EC, Nelson RW: Canine hyperadrenocorticism. *In* Feldman EC, Nelson RW (eds): Canine and Feline Endocrinology and Reproduction, 2nd ed. Philadelphia, WB Saunders, 1996, pp 187–265.

35. Bagley RS, Kornegay JN, Page RL, et al: Central nervous system neoplasia. *In* Slatter DH (ed): Textbook of Small Animal Surgery, 3rd ed. Philadelphia, WB Saunders, 1992, pp 2137–2166.

36. Carpenter JL, King NW Jr, Abrams KL: Bilateral trigeminal nerve paralysis and Horner's syndrome associated with myelomonocytic neoplasia in a dog. JAVMA 191:1594, 1987.

37. McGrath JT: Neurologic Examination of the Dog, 2nd ed. Philadelphia, Lea & Febiger, 1960, pp 164–165.

38. Fenner WR: Metastatic neoplasms of the central nervous system. Semin Vet Med Surg 5:253, 1990.

39. Waters DJ, Hayden DW, Walter PA: Intracranial lesions in dogs with hemangiosarcoma. J Vet Intern Med 3:222, 1989.

40. Dorman DC, Fikes JD: Diagnosis and therapy of neurotoxicological syndromes in dogs and cats: General concepts, part 1. Prog Vet Neurol 4:95, 1993.

41. Dorman DC: Diagnosis and therapy of neurotoxicological syndromes in dogs and cats: Selected syndromes induced by pesticides, part 2. Prog Vet Neurol 4:111, 1993.

42. Thomas WB: Cerebrovascular disease. Vet Clin North Am 26:925, 1996.

CHAPTER 106

DISEASES OF THE SPINAL CORD

Richard A. LeCouteur and Jacqueline L. Grandy

MECHANISMS OF DISEASE

Spinal cord diseases may be divided into two groups.[1] The first group comprises diseases that affect both the nervous system and other organ systems. The second group includes diseases that are unique to the nervous system, such as disorders of myelin, neurons, or supporting cells (glial cells and the like). Categories of disease that may be included in either of these two groups include congenital and familial disorders, toxicities, nutritional disorders, degenerations, neoplasia, and idiopathic disorders.

The localization of specific functions in the nervous system has important effects on the clinical presentation and progression of spinal cord diseases. Localization of function in the spinal cord causes a similar pathologic process to result in many different clinical presentations, depending on the part(s) of the spinal cord it affects. For example, a spinal cord neoplasm located at the level of the C3 vertebra may result in tetraparesis, whereas the identical neoplasm located at the level of the T13 vertebra may result in paraparesis with the thoracic limbs unaffected. Furthermore, localization of function in the spinal cord renders it inherently vulnerable to focal lesions that, in other organs (where function is more uniformly distributed), might not result in detectable clinical signs. For example, a small infarction of the cervical spinal cord may result in tetraplegia, whereas a similar lesion occurring in hepatic parenchyma probably would not compromise liver function.[1]

The unique susceptibility of the nervous system to a localized lesion is compounded by its strictly limited capacity to restore function in damaged tissue. The pathologic reactions of the spinal cord to disease are to a degree nonspecific, so that various disorders may induce a somewhat similar histologic appearance.[2, 3]

Clinical syndromes affecting the spinal cord may be characterized by a single focal lesion (transverse myelopathy) or by several focal lesions (multifocal disorders). Myelopathies may be extrinsic, in which spinal cord dysfunction is secondary to diseases of the vertebrae, meninges, or epidural space; or may be intrinsic, in which the disease begins as an intramedullary lesion. Extrinsic myelopathies are almost always transverse myelopathies.

Because the nervous system can respond in only a limited number of ways to the numerous causes of myelopathies, it is necessary to follow a systematic diagnostic approach in an animal with a spinal cord disorder.

APPROACH TO A SPINAL CORD PROBLEM

DIAGNOSIS

Signalment

Accurate diagnosis of a spinal cord disorder must include consideration of an animal's age, breed, and sex. Diseases may be specific to certain species and breeds.[4-8]

History

An accurate and complete history constitutes the initial step in the diagnosis of all neurologic problems. Important aspects of history include rapidity of onset of the problem and the nature of its progression. This information may be helpful in determining the cause of a problem. For example, neoplastic diseases affecting the spinal cord often result in focal signs that have an insidious onset and a gradual progression. In contrast, vascular disorders such as infarction or hemorrhage may produce an acute onset of focal signs without evidence of progression. Inflammatory, degenerative, or metabolic disorders generally cause a diffuse distribution of signs that have an insidious onset and gradual progression. Traumatic and congenital diseases may result in either a focal or multifocal distribution of signs, most often with an acute onset and without progression, although such diseases may have a progressive course.

While careful consideration of these factors is helpful in determining the cause of a spinal cord problem, there are so many exceptions to general statements that such information must be used with caution. For example, an acute onset of signs does not rule out neoplasia as a potential cause of myelopathy, as a neoplasm may be associated with rapid decompensation of neural tissue, particularly if vascular factors such as infarction or hemorrhage are involved.

Physical Examination

A physical examination consists of a series of observations that provides information regarding the general health of all body systems. Results of this examination are used to supplement information collected in the history and may implicate involvement of body systems other than the nervous system. For example, an animal suspected as having spinal pain may in fact have abdominal pain. A thorough orthopedic examination should be completed in any dog or cat suspected of having a spinal cord disorder. Particular attention should be paid to the examination of joints. Rupture of anterior cruciate ligaments bilaterally or bilateral patellar luxations may mimic paraparesis as a result of a neural disorder.

Neurologic Examination

A neurologic examination is an extension of a physical examination. When spinal cord disease is suspected, it is essential to complete a thorough, comprehensive, and unbiased examination of the nervous system. Errors in diagnosis commonly occur when only the region of an obvious neurologic deficit is examined and more subtle alterations in other parts of the nervous system are overlooked. The objectives of the neurologic examination are to detect the presence of and to determine the location and extent of a disorder of the nervous system.[4-8]

Problem List and Differential Diagnosis

A complete list of problems should be compiled following completion of physical and neurologic examinations. All identified problems should be included, despite the fact that some may not appear to be directly related to the presenting complaint. A list should be compiled of possible causes for each problem included on the problem list. The most probable causes should be listed first. Ranking of differential diagnoses is based on information collected in the history regarding signalment, nature of onset and progression of signs, and on results of the physical and neurologic examinations.

Minimum Database

Initial clinicopathologic tests include a complete blood count, blood chemistry profile, and urinalysis. Results of initial blood and urine tests may support a diagnosis of a metabolic, toxic, or infectious disorder that is either producing or complicating signs of spinal cord dysfunction. Additional diagnostic tests may be required to investigate disorders suspected on the basis of results of initial screening tests. For example, hyperglobulinemia detected in a cat with signs of myelopathy may support completion of a serum feline infectious peritonitis (FIP) virus titer.

Thoracic radiographs should be obtained as part of the minimum database in dogs or cats with a spinal cord disorder. This is especially necessary in older animals, in animals in which abnormalities of cardiovascular or respiratory function are suspected, or in animals in which neoplasia is included on a list of differential diagnoses. Abdominal radiography or abdominal ultrasound should also be obtained.

Ancillary Diagnostic Investigations

The recommended essential procedures for diagnosis of a myelopathy in advised order of completion are noncontrast vertebral radiography, cerebrospinal fluid (CSF) analysis, and myelography. Additional procedures such as electrophysiologic testing or advanced imaging (computed tomography [CT] or magnetic resonance imaging [MRI]) may be added to this list, depending on the nature of the problem being investigated.

Noncontrast Vertebral Radiography. Noncontrast vertebral radiography is essential in the accurate diagnosis of a disorder affecting the spinal cord.[4-8] Owing to the limitations of a neurologic examination in outlining multiple lesions of the spinal cord, and for the purpose of comparison if problems related to other regions of the vertebral column occur in the future, the entire vertebral column must be radiographed. Correct technique, exact positioning, and use of appropriate projections are essential.[9-12] Further diagnostic investigations may be indicated on the basis of results of initial interpretation of noncontrast vertebral radiographs. For example, a finding of discospondylitis may be followed by culture and sensitivity testing of blood, urine, or an aspirate from an infected disk, or by serologic testing for *Brucella canis.* Differentiation of an infectious lesion from a vertebral neoplasm may be difficult on the basis of results of noncontrast vertebral radiography. In such cases, a biopsy by means of needle aspiration or surgical excision may be indicated.

Cerebrospinal Fluid Analysis. CSF collection and analysis are essential when noncontrast vertebral radiographs do not completely define location, nature, and extent of a spinal cord disorder.[13] Collection of CSF may be accomplished by means of a cisternal or a lumbar subarachnoid puncture. It has been recommended that CSF be collected from a cisternal site if cervical spinal cord disease is suspected and from a lumbar location if a thoracolumbar disorder is involved. However, a lumbar collection site (most often between L4 and L5 or L5 and L6 vertebrae) may be used for most dogs or cats with a spinal cord disorder regardless of the suspected location of the problem. Precautions must be used in the collection of CSF from animals in which an increased intracranial pressure is suspected.

Analysis of CSF collected from a dog or cat with a spinal cord disorder should always include a total red blood cell count, total and differential white blood cell count, and a quantitative estimation of protein content. Results for CSF from normal dogs and cats have been published.[14-17] It should be noted that normal values differ in CSF collected from lumbar and cisternal collection sites.[17, 18]

Results of CSF analysis may support further examination of CSF such as bacterial or fungal culture and sensitivity testing, completion of titers, or CSF protein electrophoresis and determination of the IgG index.[19-21]

Myelography. Myelography is the radiographic examination of the spinal cord and emerging nerve roots following injection of contrast material into the subarachnoid space. It should be done when results of noncontrast vertebral radiography and CSF analysis do not fully define a disorder affecting the spinal cord, or when spinal surgery is contemplated.[11, 12] Patterns of myelographic alteration may be used to differentiate intramedullary, intradural-extramedullary, and extradural space-occupying lesions.[11, 12]

Myelography should only be considered if positive findings are essential for diagnosis and prognosis, or to determine a precise site for surgery, as it is a difficult procedure to complete and may result in undesirable consequences.[22-24] A lumbar injection site is preferred for dogs or cats with spinal cord disease at any level of the vertebral column. Use of dynamic radiographic techniques and completion of oblique projections may augment diagnostic information gained from a myelographic study.

Electrophysiology. The role of electrophysiologic testing in the diagnosis of spinal cord disease is limited. Abnormal findings on electromyographic (EMG) examination are seen only when the lower motor neurons in the ventral horn of the spinal cord, or their axons in the ventral root, are affected by a pathologic process. EMG examination may be used to define the extent of a lesion affecting the brachial or lumbar enlargement of the spinal cord by mapping the distribution of EMG abnormalities caused by denervation and correlating this information with the spinal nerve root origins of the nerves supplying the affected muscles.[1] Electrophysiologic findings may be valuable in precisely defining location and extent of a spinal cord lesion, as EMG may help to distinguish between disuse atrophy and atrophy secondary to denervation.[25, 26]

Determination of sensory or motor nerve conduction velocities of the thoracic or pelvic limbs may aid in the identification of the nerve roots affected by a spinal cord disorder. Spinal cord potentials (cord dorsum potentials) evoked by stimulation of a peripheral sensory nerve may be used in combination with sensory nerve conduction velocities to determine involvement of sensory nerve roots proximal to the dorsal root ganglia. Evoked spinal cord potentials are of limited usefulness for localization, determination of the severity and prognosis, and evaluation of the response to therapy by animals with spinal cord disorders.[25, 26]

A variety of pressure, flow, and electrophysiologic techniques have been developed to assess the function of the lower urinary tract.[5] Cystometry, profile recording of urethral closure pressure, electromyography of urethral sphincter, uroflowmetry, and evoked spinal cord potential measurements following pudendal nerve stimulation have all been investigated in dogs or cats.[5] Combinations of these electrophysiologic tests may provide the information needed regarding the functional status of spinal cord segments involved in micturition.

CLINICAL SIGNS OF SPINAL CORD DISEASES

Assessment of an animal's gait and posture, postural reactions, spinal reflexes, cranial nerve function, and state of consciousness is essential in determining the presence or absence of spinal cord disease, the most likely location(s) of a spinal cord lesion, and whether a focal, multifocal, or disseminated disease process is present involving the spinal cord and/or other parts of the nervous system.[1]

Five groups of clinical signs are seen to a varying degree in all animals that have a disease affecting the spinal cord. These clinical signs are depression or loss of voluntary movement, alteration of spinal reflexes, changes of muscle tone, muscle atrophy, and sensory dysfunction. Careful assessment of these groups of clinical signs in an animal suspected of having a disease affecting the spinal cord facilitates lesion localization and diagnosis. Neurologic disorders that result in loss of either voluntary movement alone or sensory dysfunction alone are unlikely to be spinal cord disorders, as the majority of spinal cord diseases do not affect selected tracts while sparing anatomically adjacent pathways.

Diseases of the spinal cord may also result in dysfunction of bladder, urethral sphincter, and anal sphincter, and in loss of voluntary control of urination and defecation. This may be due to interruption of spinal cord pathways connecting brain stem and cerebrum to bladder and rectum that are important in normal detrusor reflex function and voluntary control of micturition and defecation, or may be due to interruption of the parasympathetic nerve supply to the bladder and urinary and anal sphincters (L7–S3 spinal cord segments and spinal nerves). Spinal cord diseases also indirectly interfere with excretory functions by impairing the ability of an animal to assume the posture necessary for normal defecation or urination.

Voluntary Movement. Loss of voluntary movements due to interruption of motor pathways at any point from cerebrum to muscle fibers is referred to as paralysis (plegia). Lesser degrees of motor loss are referred to as paresis. The terms tetraplegia (or quadriplegia) and tetraparesis (or quadriparesis) refer to absence of voluntary movements in thoracic and pelvic limbs and depression of movements in thoracic and pelvic limbs, respectively. The terms paraplegia and paraparesis describe absence of voluntary movements and depression of voluntary movements in only the pelvic limbs. Hemiplegia and hemiparesis refer to paralysis or motor dysfunction, respectively, of a pelvic limb and a thoracic limb on the same side.

Voluntary movements must be differentiated from reflex movements on the basis of neurologic examination findings and general observations.

Ataxia (incoordination) is seen in association with paresis and probably occurs as a result of interference with both ascending and descending spinal cord pathways. Many ascending spinal cord tracts contribute to the transmission of sensory information to the cerebrum for coordination of voluntary movements; however, interference with the spinocerebellar tracts probably causes a large part of the ataxia seen in association with spinal cord disease in animals. Observation of gait is the only means available for clinical testing of these pathways.

Spinal Reflexes. Spinal reflexes are stereotyped involuntary actions that are independent of brain input, and may be elicited consistently by specific stimuli. The central nervous system (CNS) components of spinal reflex arcs are located entirely within the spinal cord. Disturbance of spinal reflexes occurs in almost all animals with spinal cord disease. A spinal reflex may be normal, depressed (hyporeflexia), absent (areflexia), or exaggerated (hyperreflexia). Classification of spinal reflexes into one of these categories is helpful for localization of a spinal cord lesion.

Depression of a spinal reflex in association with spinal cord disease most frequently occurs as a result of involvement by a pathologic process of spinal cord segments mediating the reflex. It must be remembered that involvement of motor nerves arising from, or sensory nerves traveling to, such spinal cord segments, or abnormalities of the effector organ (muscle), may also result in depression of spinal reflexes.

Exaggeration of a spinal reflex in association with spinal cord disease occurs when a lesion affects the spinal cord cranial to segments that mediate a reflex. Neural mechanisms that result in spinal reflex exaggeration are not completely understood. The concept that reflex exaggeration simply results from interruption of descending inhibitory pathways is useful in the exercise of lesion localization; however, other factors are likely to be involved, such as collateral axonal sprouting or the development of denervation supersensitivity. Exaggeration of a reflex may result from a brain lesion as well as from a spinal cord lesion.

Spinal cord lesions that affect both grey and white matter may result in depression of spinal reflexes mediated by spinal cord segments involved in a pathologic process, and in exaggeration of spinal cord reflexes mediated by spinal

cord segments caudal to a lesion. This is useful in lesion localization, particularly for a lesion that affects the cervical enlargement (C6–T2 spinal cord segments), where thoracic limb hyporeflexia and pelvic limb hyperreflexia may be present.

Interpretation of reflex abnormalities must be approached with the knowledge that two (or more) lesions located within the same anatomic division of the spinal cord may result in reflex changes identical to those produced by a single lesion. For example, two lesions between T3 and L3 spinal cord segments cause hyperreflexia in the pelvic limbs that is indistinguishable from that resulting from a solitary lesion in this location. Further, hyporeflexia produced by one spinal cord lesion may mask hyperreflexia that would otherwise result from a second lesion in a more cranial location. For example, a lesion in the lumbar enlargement (L4–S3 spinal cord segments) causes hyporeflexia in the pelvic limbs that masks the hyperreflexia that otherwise results from a second lesion cranial to the L4 spinal cord segment.

Depression of spinal reflexes caudal to a lesion may be seen for several days following spinal cord injury in humans or primates and is called spinal shock. Spinal shock may occur in quadrupeds; however, it is too brief in duration to be of clinical significance. Hyporeflexia observed immediately following spinal cord injury should be attributed to damage to spinal cord segments mediating the reflexes, or to other systemic complications, such as hypovolemic shock, that frequently accompany spinal cord trauma.

Muscle Tone. Maintenance of normal muscle tone is a function of spinal reflexes (tonic muscle stretch reflexes). Alterations of muscle tone are therefore interpreted in a similar fashion to that for alterations in spinal reflexes described above. Abnormal muscle tone may be depressed (hypotonia), absent (atonia), or exaggerated (hypertonia), depending on the location of a spinal cord lesion.

Muscle Atrophy. Two types of muscle atrophy may occur in association with a spinal cord disease. Denervation atrophy is seen when lower motor neurons (LMNs) that innervate a muscle are damaged by a lesion affecting their spinal cord segment(s) of origin. Denervation atrophy is evident within a week of injury, usually is severe, and is associated with EMG abnormalities. Disuse atrophy may be seen in muscles innervated by LMNs caudal to a spinal cord lesion. Disuse atrophy usually is slower in onset and progression than denervation atrophy, most often is less severe in character, and most often is not associated with EMG alterations.

Sensory Dysfunction. Abnormalities of sensory (ascending) pathways of the spinal cord contribute to the ataxia of spinal cord disease; however, specific clinical tests of their function do not exist. Perception in animals must be inferred from certain behavioral responses that indicate ascending sensory signals have reached the cerebral cortex (e.g., aversive response to a noxious stimulus). Interruption of sensory signals at any point between (and including) sensory receptors in the periphery and cerebral cortex may depress or obliterate normal sensory function. Therefore, results of clinical examination for signs of sensory dysfunction alone may not be of value in localizing a lesion to the spinal cord. However, when combined with results of other parts of a neurologic examination, signs of sensory dysfunction may provide important diagnostic and prognostic information.

Proprioceptive positioning (perception of body position or movement) and pain perception are tested during a neurologic examination. Proprioceptive positioning is a sensitive indicator of spinal cord function, and depression or loss of proprioceptive positioning frequently is the sign first produced by a myelopathy.

Pain perception may be normal, depressed (hypesthesia), absent (anesthesia), or exaggerated (hyperesthesia). Two types of pain perception may be distinguished in animals. Cutaneous ("superficial") pain perception is manifested by a response to pricking or pinching of the skin, and deep pain perception is manifested by reaction to pinching the toes or tail across bone with hemostatic forceps. Areas of decreased or absent cutaneous pain perception may aid in identification of specific nerves, nerve roots, and spinal cord segments involved in a pathologic process. This technique of cutaneous mapping is especially useful in lesions that affect the cervical or lumbar enlargements.

Deep pain perception appears to be the sensory function that is most resistant to a spinal cord disease and is the last spinal cord function to disappear in myelopathies of any type. An animal with a complete bilateral loss of deep pain perception due to a transverse myelopathy is necessarily paralyzed caudal to the lesion. Therefore, loss of deep pain perception is a grave prognostic sign.

Hyperesthesia in association with a spinal cord disease may indicate nerve root or spinal nerve involvement, or may be consistent with meningeal irritation. A focal area of hyperesthesia over the vertebral column may indicate the location of a spinal cord lesion.

LOCALIZATION OF SPINAL CORD DISEASES

Motor, sensory, reflex, and sphincter abnormalities may be used to determine the location of a lesion within one of four major longitudinal divisions of the spinal cord. The divisions are cervical (C1 to C5 spinal cord segments), cervical enlargement (C6 to T2), thoracolumbar (T3 to L3), and lumbar enlargement (L4 to Cd5). It is essential to remember that these divisions refer to spinal cord segments, not vertebrae, and that spinal cord segments do not correspond exactly with vertebrae of the same number. Some variations may be encountered as a result of slight differences between animals in segments that form cervical and lumbar enlargements. The diseases most commonly associated with neurologic signs referable to each of these four regions are listed in Tables 106–1 through 106–4.

A disorder of each of the four regions of the spinal cord results in a combination of neurologic signs that is specific for the region involved.[6] Recognition of these clinical signs allows accurate localization of a spinal cord lesion. The presence of neurologic deficits indicative of involvement of more than one region of the spinal cord is highly suggestive of multifocal or disseminated spinal cord disease.

The functional differences between upper motor neurons (UMNs) and LMNs may be used to localize lesions to one of the longitudinal regions of the spinal cord. Cell bodies of spinal cord LMNs are located in the spinal cord grey matter. Their axons leave the spinal cord via the ventral nerve roots to become part of a peripheral nerve, and to terminate in a muscle. The LMNs of the thoracic limb have their cell bodies in C6 to T2 spinal cord segments that form the cervical enlargement, whereas LMNs of the pelvic limb arise from the L4 through S1 spinal cord segments of the lumbar enlargement. Anal and urethral sphincter LMNs originate from S1 through S3 spinal cord segments. Signs of LMN dysfunction, which in diseases affecting the spinal cord

TABLE 106–1. DISEASES AFFECTING THE CERVICAL REGION (SPINAL CORD SEGMENTS C1–C5)*

Hereditary/congenital	*Atlantoaxial subluxation*
	Congenital vertebral anomalies
	Spina bifida
	Myelodysplasia
	Syringomyelia/hydromyelia
	Globoid cell leukodystrophy
	Hereditary ataxia
	Pilonidal sinus/epidermoid cyst/ dermoid cyst
	Spinal stenosis
Degenerative	*Intervertebral disk disease*
	Cervical spondylomyelopathy
	Leukoencephalomyelopathy of rottweilers
	Neuroaxonal dystrophy of rottweilers
	Spondylosis deformans
	Dural ossification
	Synovial cyst
Inflammatory/infectious	*Discospondylitis*
	Corticosteroid responsive meningitis- arteritis
	Granulomatous meningoencephalomyelitis
	Distemper myelitis
	Feline infectious peritonitis meningitis/ myelitis
	Bacterial/fungal/rickettsial/protothecal meningitis/myelitis
	Protozoal myelitis
	Feline polioencephalomyelitis
	Spinal nematodiasis
Neoplastic	*Neoplasia*
Traumatic	*Spinal cord trauma*
Vascular	*Ischemic myelopathy*
	Progressive hemorrhagic myelomalacia
	Hemorrhage
	Vascular malformations and benign vascular tumors
Nutritional	Hypervitaminosis A in cats
Idiopathic	Spinal intra-arachnoid cysts
	Osteochondromatosis
	Calcinosis circumscripta

*Common causes are listed in italics.

reflect damage to the spinal cord segment(s) from which LMNs originate, are decreased or absent voluntary motor activity; decreased or absent muscle tone; normal, decreased, or absent segmental spinal reflexes; and rapid, severe atrophy of an affected muscle due to denervation.

UMNs arise from cell bodies located in the brain. Their axons form descending pathways of the spinal cord and terminate on interneurons that in turn synapse with LMNs. Lesions affecting UMNs result in UMN signs. These UMN signs result from an increase in the excitatory state of LMNs. UMN signs include depression or loss of voluntary motor activity, normal or exaggerated segmental spinal reflexes, appearance of abnormal spinal reflexes (e.g., crossed extensor reflex), increased muscle tone, and muscle atrophy due to disuse.

Unilateral signs resulting from spinal cord disease are unusual; however, signs frequently are asymmetric. In the majority of cases, a lesion resulting in asymmetric signs is located on the side of greater motor and sensory deficit.

Cervical (C1 to C5). Fatal respiratory paralysis resulting from interruption of descending respiratory motor pathways or damage to motor neurons of the phrenic nerve (C5 to C7 spinal cord segments) occurs in a complete transverse

TABLE 106–2. DISEASES AFFECTING THE CERVICAL ENLARGEMENT (SPINAL CORD SEGMENTS C6–T2)*

Hereditary/congenital	*Congenital vertebral anomalies* Spina bifida Myelodysplasia Syringomyelia/hydromyelia Globoid cell leukodystrophy Hereditary ataxia Pilonidal sinus/epidermoid cyst/ dermoid cyst Spinal stenosis
Degenerative	*Intervertebral disk disease* *Cervical spondylomyelopathy* Spondylosis deformans Dural ossification Synovial cyst
Inflammatory/infectious	*Discospondylitis* Distemper myelitis FIP meningitis/myelitis Bacterial/fungal/rickettsial/protothecal meningitis/myelitis Protozoal myelitis Feline polioencephalomyelitis Granulomatous meningoencephalomyelitis Spinal nematodiasis
Neoplastic	*Neoplasia*
Traumatic	*Spinal cord trauma*
Vascular	*Ischemic myelopathy* Progressive hemorrhagic myelomalacia Hemorrhage Vascular malformations and benign vascular tumors
Nutritional	Hypervitaminosis A in cats
Idiopathic	Spinal intra-arachnoid cysts Osteochondromatosis

*Common causes are listed in italics.

myelopathy. Lesions that are less than complete may not affect respiration, but other signs may be detectable.

Ataxia and paresis of all four limbs usually are seen. Tetraplegia rarely is seen, as lesions of sufficient severity to cause tetraplegia also produce respiratory paralysis. Hemiparesis occasionally may be present in association with a cervical lesion. Lesions of the cervical spinal cord may result in paraparesis with minimal neurologic deficits in thoracic limbs. The reasons for this are poorly understood.

Spinal reflexes and muscle tone are intact in all limbs and may be normal or exaggerated. Muscle atrophy generally is not present; however, disuse atrophy may develop in cases that have a chronic course. Anal reflexes are intact, and anal tone usually is normal. Bladder dysfunction may occur as a result of detrusor muscle areflexia, with normal or increased urinary sphincter tone and loss of voluntary control of micturition. Reflex dyssynergia may also be seen. Although voluntary control of defecation may be lost, reflex defecation occurs when feces are present in the rectum. Horner's syndrome (ptosis, miosis, and enophthalmos) rarely may be present in an animal with a severe destructive cervical lesion. Proprioceptive positioning and other postural reactions usually are depressed or absent in all limbs. Complete loss of proprioceptive positioning may occur without detectable loss of pain perception.

Cervical hyperesthesia ("spasms," apparent pain on palpation, cervical rigidity, and abnormal neck posture) may be seen in some animals with cervical myelopathy. It should be noted that apparent cervical pain may also be seen in association with lesions affecting the brain stem and cerebrum.

Occasionally an animal may hold a thoracic limb in a partially flexed position, a posture that may be consistent with C1 to C5 nerve root or spinal nerve entrapment ("root signature"), although this posture is seen more commonly with a disorder affecting the cervical enlargement.

Disorders that affect the cervical region of the spinal cord must be differentiated from brain lesions that result in tetraparesis. This may be accomplished by performing a complete neurologic examination; however, occasionally this distinction may be difficult. In most circumstances, a cervical lesion does not result in neurologic deficits attributable to involvement of the medulla oblongata; however, there are several notable exceptions to this rule. Positional strabismus, resulting from loss of the vertebral joint proprioceptive input to the attitudinal reflexes, may be seen in association with a cranial cervical lesion (C1 to C3 spinal cord segments). A cranial cervical lesion may also cause facial hypesthesia as a result of involvement of the spinal nucleus and tract of the trigeminal nerve. Cranial cervical trauma often results in clinical signs referable to injury of the caudal brain stem (head tilt, pharyngeal paresis, facial paresis) or cerebellum.

The Schiff-Sherrington sign (syndrome or phenomenon) consists of hypertonicity of thoracic limb muscles and hyperextension of the neck, and is seen in association with spinal cord lesions caudal to the cervical enlargement. It is essential to differentiate this sign from thoracic limb hypertonicity resulting from a cervical lesion.

Cervical Enlargement (C6 to T2). Ataxia and paresis

TABLE 106–3. DISEASES AFFECTING THE THORACOLUMBAR REGION (SPINAL CORD SEGMENTS T3–L3)*

Hereditary/congenital	*Congenital vertebral anomalies* Spina bifida Myelodysplasia Syringomyelia/hydromyelia Mucopolysaccharidosis Globoid cell leukodystrophy Pilonidal sinus/epidermoid cyst/ dermoid cyst Spinal stenosis
Degenerative	*Intervertebral disk disease* *Degenerative myelopathy* Spondylosis deformans Dural ossification Synovial cyst Diffuse idiopathic skeletal hyperostosis
Inflammatory/infectious	*Discospondylitis* Distemper myelitis FIP meningitis/myelitis Bacterial/fungal/rickettsial/protothecal meningitis/myelitis Protozoal myelitis Feline polioencephalomyelitis Spinal nematodiasis Granulomatous meningoencephalomyelitis
Neoplastic	*Neoplasia*
Traumatic	*Spinal cord trauma*
Vascular	*Ischemic myelopathy* Progressive hemorrhagic myelomalacia Hemorrhage Vascular malformations and benign vascular tumors
Idiopathic	Osteochondromatosis Spinal intra-arachnoid cyst Calcinosis circumscripta

*Common causes are listed in italics.

TABLE 106–4. DISEASES AFFECTING THE LUMBAR ENLARGEMENT (SPINAL CORD SEGMENTS L4–Cd5) AND CAUDA EQUINA*

Hereditary/congenital	Spina bifida
	Sacrocaudal dysgenesis
	Congenital vertebral anomalies
	Myelodysplasia
	Syringomyelia/hydromyelia
	Globoid cell leukodystrophy
	Pilonidal sinus/epidermoid cyst/ dermoid cyst
	Spinal stenosis
Degenerative	*Intervertebral disk disease*
	Lumbosacral vertebral canal stenosis
	Spondylosis deformans
	Dural ossification
	Diffuse idiopathic skeletal hyperostosis
	Synovial cyst
Inflammatory/infectious	*Discospondylitis*
	Protozoal myelitis
	Distemper myelitis
	FIP meningitis/myelitis
	Bacterial/fungal/rickettsial/protothecal meningitis/myelitis
	Feline polioencephalomyelitis
	Spinal nematodiasis
	Granulomatous meningoencephalomyelitis
Neoplastic	*Neoplasia*
Traumatic	*Spinal cord trauma*
Vascular	*Ischemic myelopathy*
	Progressive hemorrhagic myelomalacia
	Hemorrhage
	Vascular malformations and benign vascular tumors
Idiopathic	Osteochondromatosis
	Spinal intra-arachnoid cyst

*Common causes are listed in italics.

of all four limbs usually are present. Occasionally paresis of thoracic limbs and paralysis of pelvic limbs may be seen.

Spinal reflexes and muscle tone may be normal or decreased in thoracic limbs, and normal or exaggerated in pelvic limbs. The nature of thoracic limb reflex alterations depends on the exact craniocaudal location of a lesion within this region. Muscle atrophy often is severe in thoracic limbs. Panniculus reflex may be depressed or absent unilaterally or bilaterally as a result of interruption of the LMNs involved in this reflex (C8 and T1 spinal cord segments). If bladder dysfunction occurs, it is similar to that observed with a lesion in the cervical region, with loss of voluntary control of urination. Anal reflexes and anal tone most often are normal, although voluntary control of defecation may be absent. Unilateral Horner's syndrome is commonly observed with a spinal cord lesion of the cervical enlargement, particularly a lesion involving T1 to T3 spinal cord segments or nerve roots.

Proprioceptive positioning and other postural reactions usually are depressed in all four limbs. Alterations in these functions may be more pronounced in the pelvic limbs than in thoracic limbs. Occasionally, proprioceptive positioning is absent only in a thoracic and pelvic limb on the same side. Severe depression or loss of pain perception rarely is seen in association with a lesion of the cervical enlargement, except in intrinsic myelopathies (e.g., ischemic myelopathy). There may be hyperesthesia at the level of a lesion of the cervical enlargement, thoracic limb lameness, or apparent neck pain.

Thoracolumbar (T3 to L3). The majority of spinal cord lesions of dogs or cats occur in this region. Typically thoracic limb gait is normal, and paresis and ataxia, or paralysis, are seen in pelvic limbs. Thoracic limb spinal reflexes are normal. Pelvic limb spinal reflexes and muscle tone are normal to exaggerated, depending on the severity of the lesion. Muscle atrophy is not seen in thoracic limbs. Pelvic limb muscle atrophy, if present, is the result of disuse and is seen in animals with a severe, chronic lesion.

Anal reflexes and anal tone usually are normal or exaggerated. Voluntary control of defecation may be lost. Reflex defecation occurs when the rectum is filled with feces; however, it may not be at an appropriate time or place. Degree of bladder dysfunction varies, depending on the severity of a spinal cord lesion. There may be loss of voluntary control of urination, detrusor muscle areflexia with normal or increased urinary sphincter tone, or reflex dyssynergia in which initiation of voiding occurs and is stopped by involuntary contraction of the urethral sphincter. The bladder can be manually expressed in some animals, but not in others as a result of increased tone of the urinary bladder sphincter. This is often referred to as a "UMN bladder." Although "overflow" incontinence may occur with lesions of the spinal cord in this region secondary to overfilling of the bladder, detrusor muscle tone and urinary sphincter tone are present, distinguishing this type of incontinence from that due to lesions of the lumbar enlargement and cauda equina ("LMN bladder").

Proprioceptive positioning and other postural reactions are normal in the thoracic limbs, and depressed or absent in the pelvic limbs. Pain perception is normal in the thoracic limbs and may be normal, depressed, or absent in the pelvic limbs. Panniculus reflex may be reduced or absent caudal to a lesion. In the lumbar region, the panniculus reflex may be present in lesions caudal to L3 as a result of the pattern of cutaneous innervation of lumbar spinal nerves.[1] There may be an area of hyperesthesia at the level of a lesion. The Schiff-Sherrington sign may be seen with a lesion in this region. Usually it is an indication of an acute and severe spinal cord lesion, although such a lesion may be reversible.

Lumbar Enlargement (L4 to Cd5) and Cauda Equina. Involvement of this region by a pathologic process results in varying degrees of pelvic limb paresis and ataxia, or paralysis, and is often accompanied by dysfunction of bladder and by paresis or paralysis of anal sphincter and tail. Thoracic limb function is normal. Pelvic limb reflexes and muscle tone are reduced or absent. Muscle atrophy often is present in pelvic limbs. Conscious proprioception and other postural reactions may be reduced or absent in pelvic limbs.

Anal tone and anal reflexes are reduced or absent. The rectum and colon may become distended with feces, and fecal incontinence, with continual leakage of feces, is often seen. Constipation may result from the inability to void feces. Paresis or paralysis of the urethral sphincters and detrusor muscle result in overfilling of the bladder and "overflow" incontinence. Affected animals have a large residual volume of urine in the bladder, and the bladder is easily expressed manually ("LMN bladder"). The Schiff-Sherrington sign occasionally may be seen with an acute lesion affecting this region of the spinal cord.

The term cauda equina is used to describe the lumbar, sacral, and caudal nerve roots and spinal nerves as they extend caudally from the caudal tip (conus medullaris) of the spinal cord within the vertebral canal. Lesions that affect the cauda equina result in clinical signs that are indistinguishable from lesions that affect the spinal cord segments from which the nerves of the cauda equina arise (L6 to Cd5).

ALPHABETICAL LISTING OF DISEASES

ATLANTOAXIAL SUBLUXATION (ATLANTOAXIAL INSTABILITY) AND MALFORMATIONS OF THE ODONTOID PROCESS

Etiology and Pathogenesis. Subluxation, instability, or malformation of the atlantoaxial joint that permits excessive flexion of the joint may result in compression of the spinal cord as a result of dorsal displacement of the cranial portion of the body of the axis into the vertebral canal. These conditions may result from congenital or developmental abnormalities, trauma, or a combination.[9, 10, 27, 28]

Agenesis or hypoplasia of the dens, non-union of the dens with the axis, absence of the transverse ligament of the atlas, and dorsal angulation of the odontoid process with compression of the spinal cord have been associated with atlantoaxial instability in dogs.[29, 30] Traumatic atlantoaxial luxation may occur in any breed of dog or cat and usually results from rupture of the atlantoaxial ligaments or fracture of the dens at its junction with the axis. Onset of signs is usually acute and coincides with the trauma; however, occasionally the onset of signs is delayed.

Clinical Findings. Congenital or developmental malformations occur most frequently in small dog breeds.[31] Animals with congenital atlantoaxial joint abnormalities usually develop clinical signs during the first year of life. Occasionally a dog with a congenital atlantoaxial abnormality may be normal until trauma occurs at an older age, at which time clinical signs may occur.

Clinical signs associated with congenital atlantoaxial instability may have an acute onset, may be slowly progressive, or may be intermittent. Signs are indicative of a transverse myelopathy between C1 and C5, and vary from mild cervical pain to tetraparesis or tetraplegia and possibly death as a result of respiratory paralysis. Occasionally, signs of brain stem dysfunction may follow an atlantoaxial luxation (e.g., dysphagia, facial paralysis, or vestibular deficits).

Atlanto-occipital luxation results in trauma to the medulla oblongata and clinical signs indicative of a caudal brain stem or cranial cervical spinal cord injury. Severe injuries may result in respiratory paralysis and death.

Diagnosis. Atlantoaxial instability is best demonstrated by means of radiography. Radiographically, the body of the axis is displaced dorsally and cranially into the vertebral canal and the distance between the dorsal arch of the atlas and spinous process of the axis is increased. If lateral views are not diagnostic, slight flexion of the head may be necessary. Extreme care must be taken when manipulating an animal suspected of having atlantoaxial instability under anesthesia or during radiography, as flexion of the animal's neck may result in further spinal cord compression. Splinting the animal's neck and head in extension prior to anesthesia may help in preventing excessive flexion of the head during induction of anesthesia, intubation, and positioning for radiography. Abnormalities of the dens may be seen on ventrodorsal views or slightly oblique lateral views such that the wings of the atlas are not superimposed on the dens (Fig. 106–1). An open mouth view may show agenesis, non-union, or fracture of the dens; however, the degree of cervical flexion required for completion of this view may result

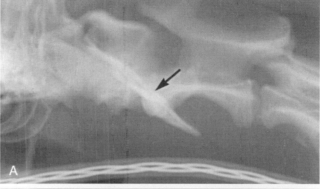
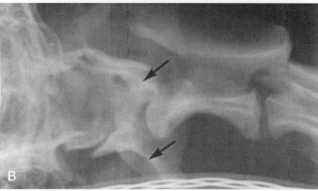

Figure 106–1. Atlantoaxial subluxation and agenesis of the dens. Lateral (A) and oblique (B) radiographs of the cranial cervical vertebrae of a 10-month-old female miniature dachshund that was tetraparetic after a minor trauma. In the lateral projection (A), the wings of the atlas are superimposed (arrow), obscuring the cranial aspect of the axis. In the oblique projection (B), the cranial aspect of the axis is visible as the wings of the atlas (arrows) are rotated out of the primary area of interest, and absence of the dens is confirmed.

in further spinal cord compression. Therefore, obtaining an open mouth view usually is not recommended.

Animals with congenital or developmental abnormalities of C2 may have additional vertebral abnormalities such as shortening of C1 or abnormal atlanto-occipital articulation. Agenesis or malformation of the dens may be an incidental finding and is probably not of clinical significance unless associated with radiographic findings of atlantoaxial instability. However, spinal cord compression associated with hypoplasia of the dens without radiographic evidence of atlantoaxial instability has been reported in a dog. Similarly, abnormal angulation of the dens may cause spinal cord compression. In these cases, myelography or advanced imaging (especially CT) may be necessary to demonstrate spinal cord compression (Fig. 106–2).

Treatment. Animals with an acute onset of neurologic deficits resulting from atlantoaxial instability or traumatic atlanto-occipital luxation should be treated medically, as described for other forms of spinal cord trauma. In addition, the head and neck should be splinted in extension. Animals with mild luxations and cervical pain only or with minimal neurologic deficits, or animals with multiple vertebral abnormalities such as atlantoaxial instability and shortening of the body of C1, may respond to splinting of the head and neck in extension and strict cage rest for at least 6 weeks. Casting material or a metal metacarpal splint may be used for this purpose. Care must be taken to ensure that respiration is not compromised. Splinting the head and neck may permit formation of fibrous tissue to stabilize the atlantoaxial joint,

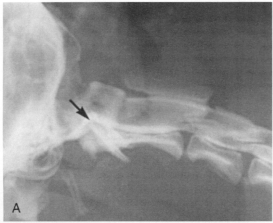

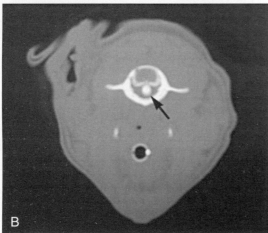

Figure 106–2. Dorsal angulation of the dens. Lateral myelogram *(A)* and transverse computed tomography (CT) image *(B)* taken after myelography of the cranial cervical vertebrae of a 3-year-old male Chihuahua that had an acute onset of tetraparesis and generalized ataxia. The myelogram *(A)* confirms ventral compression of the spinal cord (arrow) in the region of the dens. The CT image *(B)* confirms that the dens (arrow) is causing compression of the overlying spinal cord.

and is most successful in small dogs. However, clinical signs may recur.

Surgical stabilization and/or decompression is indicated in animals with moderate to severe neurologic deficits, or recurrent episodes of neck pain unresponsive to medical therapy or splinting, and in animals in which angulation of the dens results in spinal cord compression. Various surgical techniques have been described, utilizing either a dorsal or a ventral approach.[32–34]

The prognosis for animals with atlantoaxial instability varies depending on the severity of spinal cord injury that occurs. Prognosis is fair to good for those with mild to moderate neurologic deficits, and guarded for those with an acute onset of tetraplegia.

BACTERIAL, FUNGAL, RICKETTSIAL, OR PROTOTHECAL MENINGOMYELITIS

Etiology and Pathogenesis. Dogs and cats are affected infrequently by bacterial or fungal meningitis and/or myelitis.[3–6, 35, 36] Several routes of infection exist. Direct implantation of organisms may occur following a bite wound, spinal puncture, or surgery, or may accompany migration of a foreign body such as a grass awn. Extension

may occur from a focus of infection such as a paravertebral infection, discospondylitis, or dermoid sinus, or from infection following tail docking. Infection may also result from hematogenous spread of systemic infection such as endocarditis. Because clinical signs produced by bacterial or fungal agents depend more on the neural structures affected than on the agent responsible, these agents are discussed together.

Meningitis may be accompanied by infection of the underlying parenchyma of the spinal cord (myelitis). Meningitis and/or myelitis may be focal, multifocal, or disseminated in distribution and is frequently accompanied by meningoencephalitis. Pathologically, meningitis is characterized by infiltration of inflammatory cells into the leptomeninges. Inflammation may occur throughout the entire subarachnoid space of the brain and spinal cord. Myelitis is characterized by necrosis and infiltration of inflammatory cells within spinal cord parenchyma.

Bacteria that have been isolated from cats or dogs with meningitis and myelitis include *Staphylococcus aureus, S. epidermidis, S. albus, Pasteurella* spp., *Actinomyces,* and *Nocardia.* Fungal infections have been caused by *Cryptococcus neoformans, Blastomyces dermatitidis, Histoplasma capsulatum,* and *Coccidioides immitis. Cryptococcus neoformans* is found ubiquitously and frequently causes infection in immunosuppressed animals. Cryptococcosis is more common in cats than in dogs, and infection may result from extension of nasal infection through the cribriform plate. *Blastomyces, Histoplasma,* and *Coccidioides* infections are found in certain geographic areas in the United States, and in such cases the CNS is infected by hematogenous spread.[1]

Focal epidural infections have been reported to occur, generally as a result of migrating grass awns or penetrating wounds.[37] Proliferation of inflammatory tissue may result in an extradural space-occupying lesion causing spinal cord compression and clinical signs of a transverse myelopathy.[38] Abscessation may occur within the spinal cord and may have the radiographic appearance of an intramedullary mass.[39]

Rickettsial or protothecal infections may cause meningomyelitis similar in clinical presentation to that resulting from bacterial or fungal infection of the CNS. Ehrlichiosis *(Ehrlichia canis* infection) and Rocky Mountain spotted fever (RMSF, caused by *Rickettsia rickettsii)* may cause meningoencephalitis or meningomyelitis in dogs. Rocky Mountain spotted fever is transmitted primarily by two outdoor ticks *(Dermacentor variabilis* and *D. andersoni),* while ehrlichiosis is transmitted by a tick that is frequently found inside houses *(Rhipicephalus sanguineus).* Acutely, both diseases may induce immune-mediated vasculitis in a variety of tissues including the CNS. Borreliosis caused by *Borrelia burgdorferi* has been reported to occur in dogs and may be expected to cause meningomyelitis as it does in humans.[40] *Prototheca wickerhamii* and *Prototheca zopfii,* species of ubiquitous, colorless unicellular algae, have been isolated from pyogranulomatous lesions of the spinal cord and other organs. Protothecosis rarely occurs, and infection may depend on inadequate host immune response.[40]

Clinical Findings

Bacterial or Fungal Infections. Clinical signs of meningitis include apparent spinal pain, hyperesthesia, and cervical or thoracolumbar rigidity, occasionally manifested as a "sawhorse" posture.[40] Irritation of the numerous nerve endings in the meninges results in reflex muscle spasms when affected animals are stimulated. Fever is intermittent and is more likely to occur in association with concurrent bacteremia or disseminated fungal infection. Fever may occur in association with primary CNS infections as a result of the presence of leukocytic pyrogens in the CSF or in the hypothalamic circulation.

Neurologic deficits are indicative of associated myelitis or radiculitis, and abnormalities depend on the location and extent of infection. Focal myelitis may result in signs of transverse myelopathy. Disseminated bacterial meningomyelitis often is associated with meningoencephalitis, and clinical signs usually are acute and rapidly progressive. Focal bacterial meningitis and/or myelitis and fungal meningomyelitis may be associated with development of more slowly progressive clinical signs.

Paraparesis and pelvic limb ataxia are common in animals with cryptococcal meningitis and/or myelitis. Progressive paralysis of a single pelvic limb has been reported in two cats with cryptococcal infection of the lumbar spinal cord. Cats with CNS cryptococcal infections may show an acute onset of clinical signs despite chronic destruction of nervous tissue.

Clinical signs of bacterial or fungal meningitis and myelitis are indistinguishable from other causes of meningitis and myelitis in animals. Other causes include granulomatous meningoencephalitis (GME), corticosteroid-responsive meningitis and necrotizing vasculitis of the meningeal arteries, distemper virus myelitis of dogs, and CNS toxoplasmosis and FIP meningomyelitis in cats. The differential diagnosis of meningitis also includes intervertebral disk protrusion (especially in the cervical spine), spinal fracture, discospondylitis, polymyositis, and polyarthritis.

Rickettsial Infections. Central depression is the most consistent clinical finding in dogs with rickettsial infection. Other abnormalities indicative of spinal cord and/or meningeal involvement include paraparesis, tetraparesis, ataxia, and generalized or localized hyperesthesia.[41, 42] Cervical rigidity and apparent pain may occur in animals with RMSF.[1] Neurologic abnormalities indicative of cerebral involvement include vestibular disturbances, seizures, cerebellar abnormalities, and coma. Other clinical signs that occur in dogs with rickettsial infections include listlessness, depression, fever, anorexia, lymphadenopathy, dyspnea, diarrhea, vomiting, hemorrhagic diathesis, and joint pain. Dogs of all ages may be infected, and clinical signs are often indistinguishable from those of systemic viral infections (especially canine distemper), septicemia, and immune-mediated disorders.

Prototothecal Infections. Clinical signs reported in dogs with CNS prototothecosis have included ataxia, circling, and paresis or paralysis. Only the cutaneous form of this disease has been reported in cats.[40]

Diagnosis

Bacterial or Fungal Infections. A diagnosis of bacterial or fungal meningitis and/or myelitis is made on the basis of results of CSF analysis and isolation of a causative organism by culture of CSF. Clinical signs may reflect meningeal irritation or myelopathy that may be indistinguishable from signs caused by other noninfectious myelopathies, such as intervertebral disk disease. Presence of fever or abnormal hemogram cannot be relied upon for diagnosis of meningitis/myelitis, as neither may be present in affected animals.

Bacterial or fungal meningitis has been reported to result in moderate to severe CSF pleocytosis, reflecting the degree of leptomeningeal or ependymal involvement.[13] More than 5000 white blood cells/μL may be present in some cases. Polymorphonuclear (PMN) cells predominate. Mixed mono-

nuclear and PMN pleocytosis occurs with fungal meningitis, and eosinophils may be present, especially in cases of cryptococcal meningitis. The CSF appears turbid if the cell count is greater than 500 white blood cells/μL. Disseminated bacterial meningomyelitis is rarely recognized antemortem in dogs or cats. Focal bacterial epidural, meningeal, or parenchymal infections more commonly occur.

CSF protein may be moderately to markedly increased as a result of increased capillary permeability and leakage of serum proteins into the CSF, and probably also owing to local production of immunoglobulins.[13, 43] If CSF protein content is high, fibrin clots may develop. CSF pressure is usually normal but occasionally increased, especially in animals with cryptococcal meningitis. Hemorrhage into the CSF may occur; a red or pink supernatant is indicative of recent hemorrhage. Xanthochromia develops if more than 48 hours have elapsed following hemorrhage. CSF glucose content may be decreased (CSF glucose is normally 60 to 80 per cent of a simultaneously determined plasma glucose concentration) as a result of glucose utilization by microorganisms and possibly by PMN leukocytes. However, low CSF glucose concentration is not a consistent finding in animals with bacterial meningitis.

Bacteria or fungal organisms may be identified by Gram stain or acridine orange stain of sedimented or centrifuged CSF. Cryptococcal organisms often are observed in cell preparations of CSF and can be identified by staining with Wright's stain or Gram stain, or using a wet mount preparation with India ink.

CSF from all animals with CSF abnormalities consistent with meningitis should be submitted for both aerobic and anaerobic bacterial culture, and antibiotic sensitivity testing of any cultured bacterial isolates. CSF fungal culture may also be performed. Negative CSF culture results are common, even in those animals in which bacteria or fungal organisms have been identified in CSF. Culturing the sediment of centrifuged CSF, or filtering CSF and culturing the filter, may increase the likelihood of obtaining a positive CSF culture. Causative organisms may be isolated from blood cultures of animals that are bacteremic or have systemic fungal infection. *Histoplasma* organisms may be found in buffy coat or bone marrow neutrophils or monocytes. It is recommended that a large volume of CSF, preferably 2 or 3 mL, be collected for bacterial and/or fungal culture. If a delay in processing of a CSF sample is anticipated, CSF may be aseptically inoculated into a blood culture bottle for submission to a diagnostic laboratory.

Serology may also be useful in diagnosis of CNS fungal infections. The titer of antibody-coated latex agglutination to cryptococcal (capsular) antigen may be useful in supporting a diagnosis of cryptococcal meningitis and in assessing the response to therapy. The latex cryptococcal agglutination titer (LCAT) is more sensitive than the indirect fluorescent antibody test and may be used on CSF. However, animals with localized CNS infection may have a negative titer.[44]

Focal epidural inflammatory lesions may appear as an extradural mass on myelography. Chronic focal meningitis may result in obstruction of CSF flow and blockage of contrast material on myelography owing to arachnoid adhesions.

Rickettsial Infections. The characteristic histopathologic lesions of RMSF are necrotizing vasculitis, perivascular accumulation of PMN cells, and lymphoreticular cell infiltration in most tissues of the body including the meninges and CNS. The histopathologic lesion occurring in canine ehrlichiosis is generalized lymphoid and plasma cell accumulation in bone marrow, meninges, kidney, and other organs. Results of CSF analysis of dogs with RMSF may be normal or may show a mild increase in protein (<60 mg/dL) and nucleated cells (<80 cells/μL) with lymphocytes being the predominant cell type. Currently, there is little information on the expected CSF findings in animals with ehrlichiosis. In one reported case, CSF protein and nucleated cells were increased, with lymphocytes being the predominant cell type. Diagnosis of both diseases is based on serology[45] (see Chapter 86).

Prototothecal Infections. Neutrophilic or eosinophilic leukocytes often are increased in CSF of animals with protothecosis. Culture of CSF on fungal media may result in isolation of the organism. Rectal scrapings should also be performed. Fluorescent antibody examination may demonstrate the organism in tissue sections.[40]

Treatment

Bacterial Infections. In treating bacterial meningitis and/or myelitis, it is desirable to use an antimicrobial that is specific for the causative organism and that crosses the blood-brain barrier (or blood–spinal cord barrier) in therapeutic concentrations, in order that drug concentrations may be maintained after the acute phase of inflammation has subsided[46] (Table 106–5). The blood–brain, blood–spinal cord, and blood–CSF barriers are most permeable to antimicrobials with high lipid solubility, low ionization potential, and low protein-binding affinity.[41, 46, 47] Antibiotics may be administered to animals with suspected bacterial meningitis prior to obtaining results of culture and sensitivity testing. Selection should be based on tentative organism identification (by Gram stain or acridine orange stain) from CSF, the suspected source of infection, and the ability of an antibiotic to reach effective tissue concentrations in CNS. High-dose intravenous therapy with a bactericidal drug should be used when possible, although many bactericidal drugs penetrate poorly into the CSF. Penicillin and penicillin derivatives in high doses have been recommended for the treatment of

TABLE 106–5. PENETRATION OF ANTIBIOTICS INTO THE CEREBROSPINAL FLUID[46]

Good Levels Without Meningeal Inflammation

Chloramphenicol
Sulfonamides
Metronidazole
Trimethoprim-sulfamethoxazole
Isoniazid
Rifampin
Pyrazinamide

Therapeutic Levels With Meningeal Inflammation

Penicillin
Ampicillin
Nafcillin
Oxacillin
Cefotaxime
Ceftriaxone
Ceftizoxime
Vancomycin

Poor or No Penetration Even With Meningeal Inflammation

Aminoglycosides
Erythromycin
Tetracycline
Clindamycin
First-generation cephalosporins

From Gormley WB, et al: Cranial and intracranial bacterial infections. *In* Youmans JR (ed): Neurological Surgery, 4th ed. Philadelphia, WB Saunders, 1996, p 3191.

CNS infections caused by gram-positive cocci (e.g., penicillin G 10,000 to 20,000 U/lb IV every 6 hours for at least 7 days). Oxacillin may be used for the treatment of meningitis caused by penicillin-resistant strains of *Staphylococcus.*

Most cephalosporins penetrate poorly into the CNS.[48] Several third-generation cephalosporins (e.g., cefotaxime) reach effective CNS concentrations and are considered the drugs best suited for treatment of gram-negative meningitis. First- and second-generation[48, 49] cephalosporins do not reach effective CSF concentrations and should not be used in treatment of CNS infections.

Metronidazole is useful for treatment of most anaerobic infections, is bactericidal, and diffuses well into all tissues including the CNS.[50] Metronidazole has had an increasing role in the therapy of brain abscesses of humans and is used in combination with high doses of penicillin when aerobes are present. Toxicity (central vestibular signs and cerebellar dysfunction) has been reported in dogs treated with metronidazole.[51] Chloramphenicol reaches higher CSF concentrations than most other antibiotics; however, it is bacteriostatic, and many strains of *Staphylococcus* have been shown to be resistant to this drug.[52] Most sulfonamides penetrate effectively into the CSF. Sulfadiazine (which is less protein-bound than other sulfonamides) penetrates into the CSF and nervous tissue better than sulfamethoxazole and is effective if given orally. Data are not available regarding the concentration of trimethoprim in CSF of dogs. Intrathecal administration of antibiotics has been used in humans. Although possible for use in dogs or cats, multiple CSF punctures, each requiring anesthesia, are needed. Some drugs are toxic when directly introduced into the CNS (e.g., penicillin may cause seizures), and drugs may not diffuse freely through CSF, especially if there is a blockage of CSF flow.

Treatment with antibiotics should be started as soon as possible after submission of CSF for culture. After results of culture and sensitivity are known, therapy may be altered. Treatment is continued for 4 to 6 weeks; however, treatment for longer periods is often necessary and relapses are possible. It is also important to identify possible sources of infection outside the CNS (endocarditis, discospondylitis, paravertebral abscess). Localized spinal cord or meningeal infections that are well encapsulated may be resistant to antibiotic therapy. Surgical exploration is indicated if focal meningeal or epidural infection refractory to medical therapy is suspected.

Use of corticosteroids in cases of bacterial meningitis and myelitis is controversial. Corticosteroids may decrease inflammation and thereby decrease the resulting spinal cord and nerve root damage; however, such treatment may also decrease host defense mechanisms, and in turn may result in worsening of clinical signs and in a higher incidence of relapse.

Prognosis in cases of bacterial meningitis and myelitis depends both on the ability to eliminate the causative organism, and on the extent of neurologic deficits. Neurologic deficits occurring as a result of spinal cord or nerve root inflammation may be permanent.

Fungal Infections. Fungal infection of the CNS of dogs or cats is extremely difficult to eliminate.[40, 41] The disease is often multisystemic and is seldom recognized in the early stages of CNS involvement. Amphotericin B is frequently used to treat systemic fungal infections, although it is poorly absorbed into the CSF and nervous tissue. Intrathecal administration of amphotericin B has been recommended, especially in animals with *Coccidioides immitis* meningitis, but may result in arachnoiditis and cranial nerve toxicity.

Combinations of drugs have been recommended. Amphotericin B, ketoconazole (poor CNS penetration), and flucytosine (good CNS penetration) are the main agents used. Rifampin has been used to enhance amphotericin B activity. Combined treatment with amphotericin B and 5-fluorocytosine (5-FU) has been recommended for use in cases of cryptococcosis. Long-term, high-dose ketoconazole therapy is reported to be effective for treatment of cryptococcosis in cats.[53] Sequential LCAT determinations may provide a quantitative indication of clinical response to treatment of cryptococcosis.[44, 54]

Because of the difficulty in obtaining therapeutic concentrations of antifungal agents within nervous tissue, the prognosis for CNS mycotic infections is poor.[55] Newer generation azole antifungal agents (e.g., fluconazole, itraconazole) are currently under investigation for treatment of fungal infections of the CNS.[56–60]

Rickettsial Infections. Rickettsial organisms appear to be extremely sensitive to tetracyclines (10 mg/lb orally three times a day for 14 days).[40] Tetracyclines are bacteriostatic, and elimination of the organisms from the body depends on the immunocompetence of an affected animal. Doxycycline has better CNS penetration than that seen with oxytetracycline or tetracycline and is used in animals with meningitis or myelitis resulting from RMSF or ehrlichiosis. Chloramphenicol is used in place of tetracycline to treat young dogs prior to the eruption of permanent teeth. Severely affected dogs, especially those with neurologic involvement, may die despite therapy. Neurologic deficits may be permanent in affected dogs. Recovery may be prolonged, and pancytopenia persistent, in dogs with chronic ehrlichiosis.

Protothecal Infections. Treatment of cutaneous protothecosis in a dog using a 6-month course of oral ketoconazole has been reported.[61] Effective therapy for disseminated protothecosis has not been described.

CALCINOSIS CIRCUMSCRIPTA

Calcinosis circumscripta is usually an idiopathic condition that results in circumscribed single or multiple calcium deposits, often in periarticular connective tissue.[62] It occurs mainly in young dogs of large breeds, with an apparently high incidence in German shepherd dogs.[53–65] Clinical signs of spinal cord compression caused by these slow-growing deposits will vary depending on the location of the mass. Diagnosis is made on the basis of radiography. Myelography usually reveals a solitary, rounded, mineralized mass dorsal to the spinal cord, resulting in extradural spinal cord compression (Fig. 106–3). Advanced imaging (CT or MRI) may further delineate the extent of mass lesions. Complete surgical removal of the mass provides long-term resolution of clinical signs in affected dogs.[62–64]

CERVICAL SPONDYLOMYELOPATHY

Etiology and Pathogenesis. Several terms have been used to describe this disease of the cervical vertebral column of Great Danes, Doberman pinschers, and other large breeds of dog.[66–71] These terms include "wobbler" syndrome, caudal cervical malformation-malarticulation, cervical spondylopathy, cervical vertebral instability, and cervical vertebral stenosis. The term "wobbler" is nonspecific, describing a dog with generalized ataxia and tetraparesis that may be seen with a variety of cervical myelopathies. The number

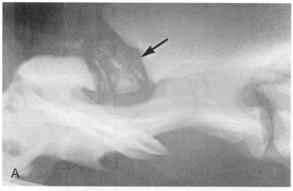
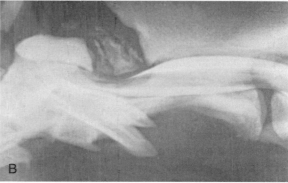

Figure 106–3. Calcinosis circumscripta. Lateral radiograph *(A)* and myelogram *(B)* of the cranial cervical vertebrae of a 10-month-old neutered male German shepherd dog with signs of worsening tetraparesis and generalized ataxia. The radiograph *(A)* confirms a focal area of soft tissue mineralization between the dorsal arch of C1 and the spinous process of C2 (arrow). The myelogram *(B)* shows dorsal spinal cord compression caused by this mass.

of different terms that have been used reflects the many unanswered questions that remain regarding etiology and pathogenesis of this condition. The term cervical spondylomyelopathy accurately reflects the complexity of the syndrome, and has therefore become widely accepted. Although the etiology remains undetermined, the high incidence of this syndrome in certain breeds of dog suggests that heredity is a contributing factor. Osteochondrosis resulting from overnutrition and rapid growth may also be a factor.[66–71] In humans, stenosis of the vertebral canal may be clinically "silent" as long as it is not complicated by other factors such as vertebral instability or intervertebral disk protrusion.

Vertebral instability, either alone or in combination with vertebral malformation and/or soft tissue stenosis, has been suggested as an initiating cause of spinal cord compression and associated neurologic abnormalities.[68] Histopathologic alterations seen in the spinal cord are characteristic of chronic compression and usually involve both white and grey matter. White matter degeneration is noted in tracts cranial and caudal to the level of focal compression. Myelin degeneration appears to predominate over axonal degeneration.

Cervical spondylomyelopathy occurs most frequently in young (<2 years of age) Great Danes, and middle-aged or older (3 to 9 years of age) Doberman pinschers.[66–71] Other breeds of dog that have been reported to be affected include the Saint Bernard, Weimaraner, Labrador retriever, German shepherd, Boxer, basset hound, Rhodesian ridgeback, Dalmatian, Samoyed, Old English sheepdog, and bull mastiff. Males appear to be affected more frequently than females. The C5–C6 and C6–C7 vertebrae and disks appear to be affected most commonly, although alterations consistent with a diagnosis of cervical spondylomyelopathy may be seen at the level of C4–C5, and less frequently at C3–C4. Spinal cord compression may be present at more than one site in the cervical spine. Stenosis of the vertebral canal of basset hounds has been reported to occur at C2–C3. Although the lesions seen in all breeds of dog of all age groups are similar, certain pathologic changes are more characteristic of each particular group. Younger Great Danes frequently have dorsal spinal cord compression as a result of elongation of the cranial aspect of the dorsal arch of affected vertebrae. Older Doberman pinscher dogs frequently have severe ventral spinal cord compression centered over the anulus fibrosus of the affected intervertebral disk.

Clinical Findings. The clinical signs reflect chronic compression of the cervical spinal cord. Clinical signs are most often gradually progressive over several months or years; however, less frequently clinical signs may develop acutely, perhaps following an apparently insignificant traumatic episode. Gait deficits are frequently noted initially in the pelvic limbs. A mild pelvic limb ataxia progresses in severity until a wide-based, crouching stance and dragging or knuckling of the toes of the pelvic limbs may be seen. Abnormalities may be more easily observed when an affected dog rises from a lying position, turns, or negotiates stairs or a curb.

Neurologic abnormalities that may be noted in the pelvic limbs include depression or loss of proprioceptive positioning reactions and exaggerated spinal reflexes. Thoracic limb abnormalities most often occur after the development of neurologic deficits in pelvic limbs, and thoracic limb deficits seldom progress to the level of severity of pelvic limb abnormalities. Thoracic limb deficits usually are of mild severity and may be evident only during intensive evaluation of postural reactions, particularly thoracic limb hopping reactions. Neurogenic atrophy of supraspinatus or infraspinatus muscles may be detected; however, widespread lower motor neuron involvement in thoracic limbs rarely is seen. In dogs with a chronic course, a stiff, "choppy" thoracic limb gait may be seen, often in combination with a rigid flexion of the neck. Although affected dogs may resist extension of the neck, apparent neck pain, as seen frequently with an acute cervical disk protrusion, seldom is elicitable.

Diagnosis. Radiography is the most accurate method for delineating the pathologic alterations of cervical spondylomyelopathy.[72, 73] Diagnosis of cervical vertebral canal stenosis has been made on the basis of noncontrast lateral radiographs of the cervical spine; however, numerous studies have emphasized that noncontrast radiographs of the cervical spine may be normal in affected dogs. Abnormalities that may be present on noncontrast radiographs include malalignment of vertebrae, remodeling of vertebrae with cranial stenosis of the vertebral canal, new bone formation (spondylosis deformans), narrowing or collapse of one or more intervertebral disk spaces, calcification of the nucleus pulposus of one or more intervertebral disks, sclerosis of vertebral endplates, and degenerative changes of vertebral articular facets. It is important to note that features such as vertebral remodeling with spondylosis deformans, narrowing of intervertebral disk spaces, and asymmetry of articular facets may not be associated with clinically significant vertebral canal stenosis. "Tilting" between adjacent vertebrae that may be apparent on plain spinal radiographs may be within normal limits.

Myelography is essential to determine the location(s), nature, and extent of spinal cord compression. Myelography findings are essential in considering treatment options and

any surgical repair that is to be attempted. The importance of ventrodorsal projections in defining lateral spinal cord compression, and dynamic or "stressed" radiographs in outlining dorsal spinal cord compression, in combination with myelography, has been emphasized by several authors. Lateral and ventrodorsal "traction" radiographs are recommended as a method of showing the dynamic nature of a lesion.[68–71]

The myelographic abnormality most frequently recognized in Doberman pinschers is ventral spinal cord compression resulting from a hypertrophied, hyperplastic, or "redundant" dorsal anulus fibrosus. Other findings include dorsal spinal cord compression resulting from hypertrophied or hyperplastic ligamentum flavum, dorsolateral spinal cord compression resulting from malformed articular processes, and spinal cord compression resulting from malformed or malaligned vertebrae.

Dynamic or "stress" radiography, following myelography, may be of value in demonstrating instability, ventral spinal cord compression as a result of dorsally protruding intervertebral disks, or dorsal spinal cord compression as a result of ventrally protruding interarcuate ligament or joint capsule. A dorsal extended view is appropriate for demonstration of dorsal spinal cord compression due to interarcuate ligament hypertrophy/hyperplasia. It has been reported, however, that routine use of "stressed" views is not warranted because of the possibility of misinterpretation of alterations, and the risk of further injury to a spinal cord that may already be severely compromised.

"Traction" radiography, whereby firm traction is placed on the cervical spine during exposure of a lateral or ventrodorsal radiograph, may further delineate the dynamic nature of a lesion. By means of this technique, spinal cord compression resulting from "redundant" or protruding anulus fibrosus may be relieved by the procedure. Failure to relieve the compression by means of "traction" may indicate a static lesion such as a disk protrusion. It should be noted that "traction" may relieve the compression evident on lateral radiographs, while the lateral compression seen on ventrodorsal radiographs may remain. "Traction" views in both the lateral and ventrodorsal projections are recommended following myelography, as they do not appear to increase spinal cord compression and provide information that is useful in the selection of an appropriate surgical technique.

Advanced imaging modalities such as CT or MRI may be useful in further defining the nature and extent of spinal cord and nerve root involvement in caudal cervical spondylomyelopathy, and in differentiating this condition from other causes of caudal cervical spinal cord compression.[74]

Treatment. Numerous treatment regimens have been recommended for the management of dogs with cervical spondylomyelopathy.[66–78] Treatment is directed either toward the relief of clinical signs by means of medical treatment and management practices or toward surgical relief of spinal cord compression. The large number of recommended treatments reflects the variety of lesions demonstrated by various diagnostic techniques, the variable results achieved by investigators, and the personal bias of individual surgeons. In most dogs the disease course is chronic and progressive, and prognosis in the absence of treatment is considered guarded to poor.

Medical therapy consists of use of anti-inflammatory medications and management procedures that reduce neck movement, such as close confinement or use of a neck brace.[68–71] Some affected dogs may be maintained at an acceptable level of neurologic function for months to years by means of corticosteroid administration. In some dogs, corticosteroid therapy may be discontinued during periods of improved neurologic function and reestablished during periods of relapse of neurologic abnormalities. Adverse effects of long-term corticosteroid therapy must be considered, and it must be remembered that this approach does not address the underlying sustained spinal cord compression in most cases.

Techniques for surgical management attempt to correct the underlying spinal cord compression.[66–82] The high potential for morbidity and postoperative complications associated with surgical management of cervical spondylomyelopathy must be considered prior to recommending surgery. These considerations must be balanced with the present knowledge of the natural progression of the disease. Surgical procedures may use either a dorsal or ventral approach to the vertebral column. The primary objectives of all surgical procedures is decompression of the spinal cord, stabilization of affected vertebrae, or both.

Prognosis for dogs with cervical spondylomyelopathy is difficult to determine. In general, medical therapy may be expected to provide clinical improvement for a variable period of time (weeks to years). Medical therapy does not alter sustained and often progressive spinal cord compression. Surgical therapy that relieves spinal cord compression may be associated with postoperative complications; however, the following statements may be made. The prognosis for dogs with a chronic history of worsening signs is not as favorable as for dogs with acute onset of signs. Mildly affected dogs have a fair prognosis for recovery. Dogs with a single level of compression appear to have a better prognosis after surgery than those with multiple-level compressions. Long-term follow-up of dogs treated by fusion reveals that up to 19 per cent of dogs develop spinal cord compression at an adjacent interspace an average of 20 months after surgery.[83] Overall, prognosis for long-term resolution of clinical signs must be considered guarded, regardless of the type of therapy.

CONGENITAL VERTEBRAL ANOMALIES

Etiology and Pathogenesis. Vertebral anomalies frequently occur in cats or dogs as a result of disturbances in embryonic development.[31, 84, 85] The majority of such anomalies are not clinically significant. If a vertebral anomaly causes instability or deformity of the vertebral canal, or spinal cord or nerve root compression, clinical signs may result. Multiple spinal anomalies may occur in a single dog or cat.

The most frequently recognized vertebral anomalies are alteration in location of the anticlinal vertebrae, anomalies of articular processes, variations in numbers of vertebrae, transitional vertebrae, butterfly vertebrae, block vertebrae, nonfusion of sacral vertebrae, or hemivertebrae. Of these anomalies, hemivertebrae are the most significant as a cause of neurologic abnormalities.[31]

Hemivertebrae. Hemivertebrae are wedge shaped, and the apex may be directed dorsally, ventrally, or medially across the midline.[31] Hemivertebrae may be associated with moderate to severe angulation of the spine and may be displaced dorsally during growth by pressure from adjacent vertebrae. Hemivertebrae occur most commonly in the thoracic spine of "screw-tailed" brachycephalic breeds (French and English bulldogs, pugs, and Boston terriers) but may occur at any location in any breed of dog. Thoracic hemivertebrae are inherited (autosomal recessive) in German shorthaired pointers. Kinked tails result from development of caudal

hemivertebrae. Kyphosis, scoliosis, and lordosis are commonly associated with hemivertebrae.

Block Vertebrae. Block vertebrae may involve the vertebral bodies, vertebral arches, dorsal spinous processes, or entire vertebrae, at any level of the vertebral column. The sacrum is considered a "normal" block vertebra. Block vertebrae may be the same length as the number of involved vertebrae, or may be shorter, and can result in abnormal angulation of the spine. Partial "blockage" of vertebral bodies may occur, allowing partial development of an intervertebral disk.

Butterfly Vertebrae. Butterfly vertebrae result from persistence of the notochord. In some instances, sagittal cleavage of the notochord may result in a sagittal cleft dorsoventrally through the vertebral body. On a dorsoventral radiograph, such vertebrae resemble a butterfly with wings spread. Compensatory growth of the adjacent normal vertebrae often fills in the funnel-shaped depression of the vertebral endplates. Butterfly vertebrae are most commonly seen in brachycephalic "screw-tailed" breeds.

Transitional Vertebrae. Dogs may have variations in the number of cervical, thoracic, lumbar, or sacral vertebrae. Furthermore, congenital absence or alteration in the shape of vertebral articular processes and variation in the location of the anticlinal (usually T11) and diaphragmatic (usually T10) vertebrae may occur. Vertebrae that have the characteristics of two major divisions of the vertebral column are referred to as transitional vertebrae. Observed alterations include transverse processes of C7 resembling a rib, a transverse process on the most caudal thoracic vertebra in place of a rib, the first sacral vertebra having a transverse process, and the last lumbar vertebra having a transverse process that has fused with the ilium. These alterations may be accompanied by alteration in size and shape of the vertebral body, or the plane of the vertebral body or intervertebral disk.

Clinical Findings, Diagnosis, and Treatment. Congenital vertebral anomalies frequently occur; however, clinical signs related to anomalous vertebrae are not present in the majority of affected animals. In most animals in which clinical signs develop, trauma to the spinal cord has occurred secondary to vertebral instability or progressive deformity with growth. Diagnosis of a vertebral anomaly is made by means of radiographs of the vertebral column (Fig. 106–4). Radiographically, hemivertebrae and adjacent vertebrae appear to be formed of normal bone, and disk spaces are usually normal or widened. Vertebral bodies appear to have a portion absent and do not appear to be compressed. Adjacent vertebrae frequently have an altered shape that conforms to the defect found in the congenitally affected segment. Vertebral endplates are smooth and of normal thickness. Hemivertebrae should be differentiated from vertebral compression due to a traumatic fracture, pathologic fracture as a result of vertebral neoplasia, or osteomyelitis. In most cases, myelography is necessary to determine the presence of spinal cord compression resulting from a congenital anomaly. Advanced imaging (CT or MRI) may be useful in further defining extent of vertebral and spinal cord involvement. Vertebral anomalies resulting in spinal cord compression and instability of the vertebral column may be treated by means of surgical decompression, vertebral realignment, and stabilization.[86]

CORTICOSTEROID-RESPONSIVE MENINGITIS-ARTERITIS

Etiology and Pathogenesis. Corticosteroid-responsive meningitis-arteritis occurs in young, medium- to large-breed

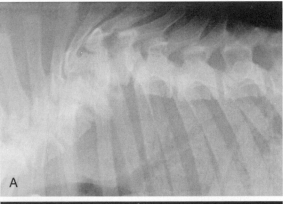

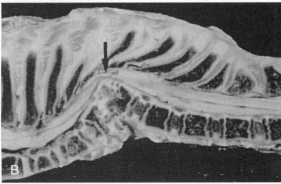

Figure 106–4. Hemivertebrae. Lateral radiograph (*A*) of the midthoracic region of the vertebral column of a 3-month-old male Malamute that had a history of inability to use the pelvic limbs since birth. Pain perception was absent in the pelvic limbs. Note the kyphosis associated with hemivertebrae affecting three midthoracic vertebrae. Severe spinal cord compression (arrow) is seen in a gross necropsy specimen (*B*) of the vertebral column sectioned in the midsagittal plane.

dogs, and may be the most frequently occurring form of meningitis.[87–89] The etiology is unknown; however, immunopathologic mechanisms are suspected, as IgA seems to play a central role in the pathogenesis.[21, 90–92] It has been suggested that repeated vaccinations with multivalent modified live vaccines may be a cause. The clinical and clinical pathologic findings associated with this disease are similar to those seen in dogs with necrotizing vasculitis of the spinal meningeal arteries.[49, 93–98]

Clinical Findings. Affected dogs are usually 7 to 16 months of age. Clinical signs include reluctance to move, arched back, stiff gait, apparent cervical and/or thoracolumbar pain, fever, muscle rigidity or spasms, apparent pain on opening the mouth, and, less commonly, neurologic deficits such as decreased proprioceptive positioning, paraparesis, or tetraparesis. Optic neuritis has been reported in an affected animal.[87] Clinical signs are indistinguishable from those of meningitis and myelitis due to other causes (bacterial, fungal, viral) and necrotizing vasculitis of spinal meningeal arteries. Clinical signs may be acute in onset and progressive, or may have a waxing and waning course over a period of weeks or months.

Diagnosis. Diagnosis is made on the basis of increased white blood cells in the CSF, failure to isolate an infectious agent from the CSF, and response to therapy with corticosteroids. The majority of affected dogs may have a mature neutrophilia in peripheral blood. The CSF white blood cell count may be normal, or may range from 50 to more than 3000 cells/μL, with predominantly mature neutrophils. Bacteria or fungi are not seen within white blood cells. Protein

concentration in the CSF most often is increased (40 to 350 mg/dL). Bacterial (aerobic and anaerobic) and fungal cultures of the CSF, urine, and blood are negative. It may be difficult to distinguish this disease from granulomatous meningoencephalomyelitis (GME) on the basis of CSF analysis. Examination of the IgG index and IgM and IgA contents of CSF may be useful in distinguishing corticosteroid-responsive meningitis from other causes of meningitis such as chronic distemper encephalitis or GME of dogs.[21]

Treatment. Early diagnosis is essential for successful treatment.[92] Initially, a corticosteroid is given at a dose sufficient to produce a remission of clinical signs (prednisone 1 to 2 mg/lb per day). Corticosteroids are reduced slowly over several months to the lowest dose necessary to maintain remission of clinical signs. Maintenance treatment using every other day dosage is preferred. Approximately 50 per cent of affected animals have recurrence of clinical signs following discontinuation of corticosteroid therapy. Increasing the corticosteroid dose may be necessary if clinical signs recur. Therapy for up to 6 months may be necessary to prevent recurrence of clinical signs. Ideally, CSF analysis results should be within normal limits prior to cessation of therapy.[92] Prognosis for eventual resolution of clinical signs is good. Treatment with antibiotics may be indicated initially if the diagnosis is uncertain and bacterial meningitis is suspected.

DEGENERATIVE MYELOPATHY

Etiology and Pathogenesis. Degenerative myelopathy is characterized by slowly progressive ataxia and paresis of the pelvic limbs. Histologically, there is demyelination, axonal degeneration, and astrocytosis in the white matter of the spinal cord. These changes are found throughout the spinal cord and are most severe in thoracic spinal cord segments, especially in dorsolateral and ventromedial funiculi.[99–101] Etiology of degenerative myelopathy is unknown in dogs.[102, 103] Dural ossification, spondylosis deformans, chronic intervertebral disk protrusion, or infectious or vascular disorders may occur concurrently with degenerative myelopathy. The occurrence of degenerative myelopathy predominantly in German shepherd dogs suggests a genetic basis for the disease, although direct evidence to support this does not exist.

Clinical Findings. Degenerative myelopathy generally occurs in dogs 6 years of age or older, although a similar condition has been reported in German shepherd dogs 6 and 7 months of age.[104] Males are affected more often than females. It has been reported most commonly in German shepherd dogs and German shepherd mixed breed dogs, although it does occur in other large and medium breeds.[99–101]

Affected dogs usually have a slowly progressive paraparesis and pelvic limb ataxia. Onset of clinical signs is gradual. Neurologic deficits often are more noticeable when the dog walks on smooth surfaces. Affected dogs may have worn pelvic limb toenails. Although neurologic deficits are most often present bilaterally, they may be asymmetric. Paraparesis and ataxia progressively worsen, so that most affected dogs become nonambulatory within several months to 1 year after neurologic deficits are first detected. Paralysis of the pelvic limbs rarely occurs, probably because most large dogs undergo euthanasia if they become nonambulatory.

Apparent pain or discomfort is not evident in affected dogs. Voluntary control of urination and defecation is retained, although affected dogs may not be able to urinate or defecate in an appropriate place owing to severe paraparesis or inability to assume a voiding posture. This is important, as some dogs have apparent incontinence in the house, which may suggest a lesion of the cauda equina or sacral spinal cord segments. Muscle atrophy is not severe in the initial stages of the disease but may become noticeable in later stages; it is due to disuse rather than denervation. Cutaneous and deep pain perception remain intact throughout the course of the disease.

Neurologic examination findings usually are indicative of a transverse myelopathy between T3 and L3. Abnormalities include decreased or absent conscious proprioception and placing reactions in the pelvic limbs, normal to exaggerated patellar reflexes, normal to exaggerated withdrawal reflexes in the pelvic limbs, normal anal sphincter tone and anal reflex, normal muscle tone in the tail, and in some cases crossed extensor reflexes in the pelvic limbs. The panniculus reflex usually is normal bilaterally. It is important to note that patellar reflexes may be decreased or absent unilaterally or bilaterally in some cases, possibly as a result of degeneration of the dorsal root ganglia or dorsal grey matter of the lumbar spinal cord (i.e., an afferent rather than a LMN lesion).

Diagnosis. Diagnosis of degenerative myelopathy is based on clinical findings, age and breed of the dog, and the ruling out of all other causes of a transverse myelopathy in the T3 to L3 region of the spinal cord. Diseases to be considered in the differential diagnosis include discospondylitis, myelitis, spinal cord compression due to type II intervertebral disk protrusion, and spinal neoplasia. Radiographs of the vertebral column may be normal, or may demonstrate degenerative changes such as dural ossification, spondylosis deformans, or narrowed intervertebral disk spaces. An increased protein content (40 to 100 mg/dL) is often found in CSF collected from the lumbar subarachnoid space. The CSF protein level is usually normal in samples collected from the cisternal subarachnoid space. The white blood cell count is normal in both lumbar and cisternal CSF. Significant myelographic abnormalities are not found.

Treatment. Effective treatment has not been reported, and affected dogs usually progress to severe nonambulatory paraparesis within a year of initial diagnosis. Therapy with vitamin supplementation, ϵ-aminocaproic acid (EACA), N-acetylcysteine, and exercise has been recommended by one author.[99–101] However, to date there are no controlled studies to show that this therapeutic regimen is of any benefit.

DIFFUSE IDIOPATHIC SKELETAL HYPEROSTOSIS (DISH)

Etiology and Pathogenesis. DISH is a diffuse ossifying condition of young dogs (predominantly large and giant breeds) or cats.[105, 106] It has been suggested that four of the following five criteria be present for confirmation of DISH in dogs: (1) flowing calcification and ossification along ventral and lateral aspects of three contiguous vertebral bodies leading to segmental bony ankylosis; (2) relative preservation of disk width within involved areas, and absence of extensive radiographic changes of degenerative disk disease, such as endplate sclerosis, nuclear calcification, or localized spondylosis deformans; (3) periarticular osteophytes surrounding true vertebral joints; (4) formation of pseudoarthrosis between the bases of spinous processes; and (5) periarticular osteophytes and calcification and ossification of soft tissue attachments (enthesiophytes) in both axial

and peripheral skeleton.[105] Other associated findings may include periarticular osteophytes, sclerosis and ankylosis of sacroiliac joints, and bony ankylosis of the symphysis pubis.

The etiology of this condition is obscure. DISH is a disease entity that most likely represents a "vulnerable state" in which extensive vertebral ossification results from some stimulus that causes only modest new bone formation in most animals. These "bone formers" have a high incidence of associated extraspinal hyperostosis at the sites of ligament or tendon attachment. The pathologic alterations in DISH include findings consistent with spondylosis deformans; however, DISH differs quantitatively and qualitatively from spondylosis deformans and represents a regional ossification encompassing ligaments, paraspinal connective tissue and anulus fibrosus, and periosteal new bone formation on the ventral surface of the vertebrae.[107–109] Spinal rigidity of several vertebrae resulting from DISH may result in syndromes caused by "dynamic overload" of an adjacent "mobile segment" of the vertebral column. Typically, a rigid fusion of several lumbar vertebrae may result in degenerative changes (sclerosis, spondylosis deformans, disk protrusion) affecting the "overloaded" disk immediately cranial to the fused segments. The degenerative changes in the adjacent disk may result in clinical signs associated with spinal cord compression or nerve root entrapment.

Clinical Findings. Clinical signs may be minimal compared with the dramatic radiographic changes and include mild apparent spinal pain, stiff or stilted gait, and difficulty in jumping. Rarely clinical signs of spinal cord compression resulting from extreme bony proliferation and spinal canal stenosis may result in a transverse myelopathy between T3 and S3. Nerve entrapment may result from bony proliferation at the level of the intervertebral foramen.

Diagnosis and Treatment. Diagnosis is based on radiographic confirmation of the diagnostic criteria listed above (Fig. 106–5).[105] Analysis of CSF and myelography are necessary to rule out other disorders that may result in similar clinical signs. Advanced imaging (CT or MRI) may be of use in accurately investigating the possibility of spinal cord compression or nerve root entrapment resulting from bony proliferation.

Treatment for DISH has not been described. Conservative

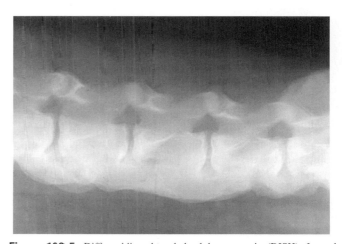

Figure 106–5. Diffuse idiopathic skeletal hyperostosis (DISH). Lateral radiograph of the lumbar region of a 4-year-old neutered male Akita. Note the smooth proliferative laminar bridging of the ventral aspects of L4 through L7, consistent with a diagnosis of DISH. The intervertebral disks in this region do not appear to be narrowed. Spondylosis deformans is present at L7–S1. Proliferative remodeling changes are observed at multiple articular facets along the lumbar spine.

(medical) management is recommended, unless clinical signs of spinal cord compression or nerve root entrapment are present, in which case surgical decompression may be considered.

DISCOSPONDYLITIS (SPONDYLITIS, VERTEBRAL OSTEOMYELITIS)

Etiology and Pathogenesis. Bacterial or fungal infection of the intervertebral disks and adjacent vertebral bodies (discospondylitis), or of only the vertebral bodies (spondylitis), may result in extradural spinal cord or cauda equina compression as a result of granulation tissue, bony proliferation, or pathologic fracture or luxation. Less commonly, discospondylitis may lead to diffuse or focal meningitis and myelitis.[110–113] These conditions result from implantation of bacteria or fungi introduced by migrating plant awns (grass seeds, foxtails), hematogenous spread, extension of a paravertebral infection, a penetrating wound, or previous disk or vertebral surgery.

Discospondylitis and spondylitis occur more commonly in dogs in areas where grass awn infections are a problem. Several theories exist to explain migration of grass awns to the vertebral column. Awns may be swallowed and migrate through the bowel wall (possibly at the caudal duodenal flexure), through the mesentery to the attachment to ventral epaxial muscles, and to the vertebral column. Evidence of scarring, however, has not been found in the gut or abdomen of dogs with discospondylitis. Because dogs with discospondylitis thought to be due to plant awn migration have lesions most commonly in the cranial lumbar spine (L2–L4), it has been suggested that awns may be inhaled and migrate through the lungs to the diaphragm and lodge at the crural insertion on the lumbar vertebrae. Plant awns may also migrate through skin and paravertebral or abdominal muscles to the vertebral column. Grass seeds are able to travel long distances owing to the direction of the barbs. Forward progress may be aided by muscle movements.

Hematogenous spread of bacteria or fungi is probably the most common cause of discospondylitis. Sources of infection include bacterial endocarditis, dental disease, and urinary tract infections. Retrograde flow in the vertebral veins has been suggested as a possible route of infection to the vertebral column. Whether discospondylitis associated with urinary tract infection is due to venous or arterial dissemination of bacteria, or whether there is a direct causal relationship between urinary tract infection and discospondylitis, has not been established. Many dogs with discospondylitis have concurrent urinary tract infection. Discospondylitis due to *Brucella canis* infection most likely results from bacteremic spread from a genital infection.

Affected intervertebral disks may have evidence of degeneration (collapsed disk space, spondylosis deformans) or trauma (traumatic disk protrusion, vertebral luxation). Discospondylitis may occur with increased frequency in immunocompromised animals.[114–116] The organisms most commonly isolated from blood, affected vertebrae, and urine of dogs with discospondylitis are coagulase-positive *Staphylococcus* spp. *(aureus, intermedius),* although a number of other organisms have been identified.[110–112, 116–120]

Discospondylitis has been reported to occur in cats.[121]

Clinical Findings. Discospondylitis may occur in dogs or cats of any age; however, it is most commonly seen in giant and large breeds of dog. Any level of the vertebral column may be affected by discospondylitis, and multiple lesions may be seen, in either adjacent vertebrae or nonadjacent vertebrae. Discospondylitis occurs more commonly in the thoracic and lumbar spine than in the cervical spine. The lumbosacral disk space frequently is involved.

Clinical findings depend on the location of the affected vertebra or vertebrae. The most common clinical signs are weight loss, anorexia, depression, fever, reluctance to run or jump, and apparent spinal pain (which may be severe). Hyperesthesia may be present only over the site of the lesion or may be poorly localized, especially with involvement of multiple sites.[110]

Diagnosis. Diagnosis may be difficult, as clinical signs often are nonspecific. Discospondylitis should always be considered in an animal with fever of unknown origin. If the lumbosacral intervertebral disk is involved, dogs often show a stilted, short-strided pelvic limb gait and shifting pelvic limb lameness. Clinical signs may be present for several weeks or months before diagnosis.

Neurologic deficits associated with spinal cord or cauda equina compression may be present and may reflect either a transverse or a multifocal myelopathy. Neurologic deficits associated with a transverse myelopathy (T3–L3) occur most commonly and include paraparesis, decreased conscious proprioception, exaggerated spinal reflexes, and, much less commonly, paraplegia. Cervical lesions most commonly cause only apparent cervical pain, and lumbosacral lesions may cause neurologic deficits due to compression of nerves of the cauda equina. Rarely, animals may demonstrate clinical signs of diffuse suppurative meningitis associated with extension of infection to involve the spinal meninges. Dogs may have a history of draining tracts in the paravertebral area associated with grass seed migration. Discospondylitis has been described in dogs with osteomyelitis in other sites (femur and sternum).

Affected animals may have a normal or elevated peripheral WBC count. Typical radiographic findings are destruction of the bony endplates adjacent to an infected disk, collapse of the intervertebral disk, and varying degrees of new bone production. Early lesions may consist only of lytic areas in affected vertebral endplates. More advanced lesions show a mixture of bone lysis and extensive new bone production, with osteophytes bridging adjacent vertebrae containing a central destructive focus (Fig. 106–6). Affected vertebral bodies may be shortened, and bony proliferation may result in fusion of one or more vertebrae. Discospondylitis may be superimposed on other vertebral abnormalities including fracture and associated callus formation, spondylosis deformans, or a surgical site.

Discospondylitis may be present in more than one site in the vertebral column; therefore, it is important to radiograph the entire spine in animals suspected of having discospondylitis. Occasionally, clinical signs may occur before characteristic radiographic changes are evident. Tomography may also be a useful method for radiographic diagnosis of discospondylitis, particularly at the lumbosacral junction (Fig. 106–7). Bone scintigraphy may be useful either for detection of early lesions prior to development of radiographically evident lesions, or in animals in which it is uncertain whether lesions are due to infection or to other causes (e.g., severe spondylosis deformans). Advanced imaging (CT or MRI) may be useful in identification of subtle vertebral lesions.[110, 122]

Collection of CSF is indicated in animals with neurologic deficits. CSF may be normal or may have an increased white cell count and/or protein content when discospondylitis lesions cause extradural compression of the spinal cord or result in meningitis and/or myelitis. Myelographic findings

CNS

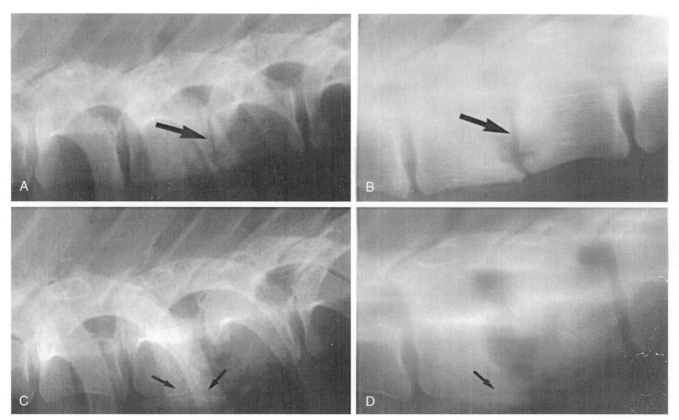

Figure 106–6. Discospondylitis. Lateral radiograph *(A)* and linear tomogram *(B)* of the midthoracic vertebral column of a 1-year-old female Doberman pinscher 8 weeks following the onset of apparent back pain. Note the collapse of the T6–T7 disk (large arrow), destruction of the vertebral endplates, and well-delineated lysis of the T6 and T7 vertebral bodies. These changes are easily observed on the tomogram, where superimposed ribs are not a factor. Lateral radiograph *(C)* and linear tomogram *(D)* of the midthoracic vertebrae completed 3 months following *(A)* and *(B)*. The dog had received a 4-week course of a broad-spectrum antibiotic that resulted in clinical improvement following the initial radiographic examination; however, signs of spinal pain had returned. Note progression of the radiographic changes seen 3 months earlier, and the presence of bony proliferation (small arrows) at T6–T7. Following surgical biopsy and culture of the T6–T7 disk, therapy with an appropriate antibiotic drug was commenced. Complete radiographic resolution of the discospondylitis and fusion of the T6–T7 vertebrae were apparent after 6 months of continued antibiotic therapy.

usually indicate extradural compression that results from extension of granulation tissue and bony proliferation within the spinal canal. Clinical signs do not always correlate well with the degree of compression seen on myelography and depend on factors such as rate and duration of compression as well as degree of compression. Aerobic, anaerobic, and fungal cultures of blood and urine should be done prior to treatment in an attempt to isolate causative organisms. Some authors consider any organism other than S. *intermedius* cultured from the urine unlikely to be the causative organism unless it is also cultured from blood or a vertebral lesion. Cultures of CSF are indicated if the WBC count is elevated. Cultures of fluid from draining sinuses may also be performed. Efforts should be made to diagnose *B. canis* infection in all dogs with discospondylitis.[117]

Surgical biopsy may be indicated in affected dogs in which a causative organism is not isolated from blood or urine, and/or animals that are unresponsive to treatment with broad-spectrum antibiotics. Fluoroscopy-guided needle aspiration of lesions is possible in some animals.[123] However, cultures of samples collected in this way are often negative, especially if animals have been treated with antibiotics prior to completion of a biopsy.

Treatment. Treatment consists of long-term use of an antimicrobial that is effective against the causative organism(s) determined by results of blood and/or urine cultures. If an organism is not cultured, dogs without severe neuro-logic deficits may be treated empirically, assuming infection with the most common organism isolated from animals with discospondylitis (coagulase-positive *Staphylococcus* spp.). Antibiotics that are most effective for this purpose are cepha-losporins, or beta-lactamase–resistant penicillins such as ox-acillin and cloxacillin. A trimethoprim/sulfonamide combination or chloramphenicol is less effective but is less expensive and may be effective in some cases.

Clinical signs may recur if the infection is not completely eliminated prior to cessation of antibiotic therapy, and repeated cultures of blood and urine and ongoing treatment with an appropriate antibiotic may be necessary. Treatment is continued for at least 6 weeks, and vertebral radiographs are taken every 2 to 3 weeks to monitor progression/regression of a lesion, and to monitor for development of new lesions. Antibiotic administration may be necessary for up to 6 months before radiographic evidence of resolution of lesions is seen. Clinical improvement in animals with disco-spondylitis (resolution of fever, improved appetite, reduction of apparent spinal pain) should be seen within 2 weeks of starting antibiotic therapy. Surgical exploration of a lesion should be considered in animals that are unresponsive to treatment or have persistent draining tracts suggestive of grass seed migration. Objectives of surgery are curettage of lesions and harvesting of material for bacterial and fungal culture. A cancellous bone graft has been recommended following curettage of a disk space. Decompressive surgery

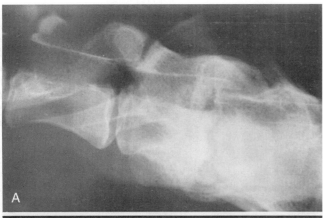

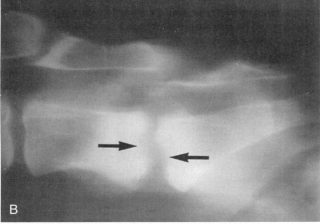

Figure 106–7. Discospondylitis. Lateral radiograph *(A)* and linear tomogram *(B)* of the lumbosacral region of the vertebral column of a 4-year-old German shepherd dog that had a 1-month history of apparent pain and pelvic limb weakness. Note sclerosis of the vertebral endplates, spondylosis deformans, new bone formation, and collapsed disk seen on the radiograph of L7–S1. A tomogram of this region confirms the presence of bone lysis (arrows) consistent with a diagnosis of discospondylitis. *Staphylococcus aureus* was cultured from urine, blood, and material obtained from the L7–S1 disk by means of needle aspiration.

is indicated if evidence of spinal cord compression is found on myelography and if animals show severe or progressive neurologic deficits. Surgical stabilization of the vertebrae may be necessary following decompression.[124]

DISTEMPER MYELITIS

Etiology and Pathogenesis. Canine distemper (CD) virus is a neurotropic virus that may cause focal or diffuse demyelination in both grey and white matter of the CNS.[125] The mechanism by which demyelination occurs is not known, but it may be due to a primary effect of the virus on glial cells, or may occur secondary to immunologic mechanisms. The white matter of the cerebellum, cerebellar peduncles, optic nerves, optic tracts, and spinal cord are most severely affected. Focal or diffuse demyelination may occur in the white matter of the spinal cord.[126, 127] Further histopathologic changes seen in the spinal cord and throughout the CNS include perivascular cuffing by mononuclear cells, gliosis, microglial proliferation, inflammatory cell infiltration of the pia-arachnoid, and neuronal changes (nuclear pyknosis, chromatolysis, shrunken cells, and neuronophagia). Intranuclear and intracyloplasmic inclusions may or may not be present.

Clinical Findings. Affected animals may or may not have a history of systemic illness. Dogs of any age may be affected, but those with myelitis due to CD infection are usually less than 3 years of age. Dogs that have been vaccinated according to recommended schedules may be affected. Clinical signs of CD myelitis reflect the location of the lesion(s), which may be focal or diffuse, at any location in the spinal cord. The T3–L3 spinal cord segments are affected most often, and clinical signs indicative of a transverse myelopathy in this region are seen. Neurologic abnormalities include paraparesis or paraplegia and normal to exaggerated reflexes in the pelvic limbs. Neurologic deficits are progressive and are bilateral; however, they may be asymmetric. Affected dogs may have clinical signs indicative of current or previous systemic CD infection. Neurologic deficits commonly seen in dogs with CD infection are vestibular and/or cerebellar abnormalities and visual deficits.[128] Self-mutilation occasionally is seen in dogs with CD infection. The limbs and tail are the common sites of mutilation. Paresis or paralysis of the limbs may also be present.

Distemper Myoclonus. Myoclonus is the rhythmic twitching of a muscle or muscle group and is most often associated with CD infection.[129] Any muscles may be involved, including the facial and masticatory muscles or limb muscles. The pathogenesis of myoclonus is unknown. It is thought to result from an abnormality in the motor neuron and interneuron pools of the medulla and spinal cord. Animals may recover from systemic CD infection, and occasionally from CNS infection; however, myoclonus may persist. Myoclonus is generally permanent and may persist during sleep. Myoclonus may be alleviated by oral therapy with procainamide.

Diagnosis. Antemortem diagnosis often is difficult.[130] Clinical signs of multifocal CNS disease, particularly neurologic deficits indicative of spinal cord and cerebellovestibular disease, are highly suggestive of CD infection (see Chapter 88). Hematologic findings in dogs with CD infection are nonspecific. Abnormalities of CSF may be useful in diagnosis of CD infection; however, CSF may be normal. The CSF white blood cell count and protein content are usually mildly to moderately increased. Cells seen in CSF are predominantly lymphocytes (10 to 60 cells/μL). The presence of interferon in CSF appears to be a reliable indicator of virus persistence.[129] CSF electrophoresis may also be performed and is useful in predicting the histopathologic changes in dogs with CD encephalomyelitis.[131] Determination of the IgG index may also aid in diagnosis of CD encephalomyelitis.[126]

Increased CD virus–specific antibody titers in CSF may be useful in the diagnosis of CD infection. Increased anti–CD virus antibody in CSF may offer evidence for chronic CD infection, because antibody is produced locally in the CNS and significant levels of increased titers have rarely been present in vaccinated dogs or in dogs with systemic CD infection without CNS involvement. Cerebrospinal CD antibody may be artifactually increased if whole blood contamination of CSF occurs during collection. Negative CD antibody results do not rule out a diagnosis of CD.[40, 129]

Treatment. Clinical signs of CD myelitis may be either rapidly or more slowly progressive. Periods of apparent improvement may be seen followed by progression of clinical signs. A specific antiviral drug having an effect on CD in dogs is not currently available. Favorable results have been reported by some investigators with short-duration (1 to 3 days) corticosteroid therapy.[40] Intravenous administration of modified live vaccine in dogs with CD is effective only if given before clinical signs appear. Treatment of CD myelitis is almost always unrewarding. The prognosis is poor for recovery. In dogs that recover from CD infection, residual signs such as myoclonus or optic neuritis may improve with time. Immunization by vaccination is the only effective approach to CD prevention.[126]

DURAL OSSIFICATION

Etiology and Pathogenesis. Dural ossification is the formation of bony plaques on the inner surface of the dura mater.[6] Bony plaques are found most commonly in the cervical and lumbar spine and may occur laterally, ventrally, or dorsally. Dural ossification is found in over 40 per cent of large and small breeds of dog over 2 years of age, and in over 60 per cent of dogs 5 years of age or older. Although many dogs with dural ossification also have spondylosis deformans, a direct correlation between the two conditions does not exist. The etiology of dural ossification is unknown.
Clinical Findings. Dural ossification rarely results in neurologic deficits or apparent spinal pain in dogs. Other causes of spinal cord disease should be ruled out before attributing clinical significance to dural ossification.
Diagnosis and Treatment. Radiographically, bony plaques appear as thin radiopaque lines (linear shadows), which are most easily viewed at the site of intervertebral foramina. These linear shadows need to be distinguished from calcified herniated disk material within the spinal canal, vertebral osteophytes, and the accessory processes of the lumbar vertebrae. There is not a specific treatment for dural ossification; however, surgical removal of a bony plaque from the vicinity of a nerve root rarely may be necessary to alleviate apparent pain due to nerve root compression.

FELINE INFECTIOUS PERITONITIS, MENINGITIS, AND MYELITIS

Etiology and Pathogenesis. Feline infectious peritonitis (FIP) is a serious, almost always fatal disease caused by a coronavirus (see Chapter 91).[132-137] Pyogranulomatous meningitis and myelitis may occur in cats with FIP. FIP is most commonly seen in younger cats between 6 months and 5 years of age. Meningeal and spinal cord lesions are probably the result of immune complex–mediated vasculitis. Involvement of the CNS is more frequently observed in the noneffusive (dry) form than in the effusive (wet) form of FIP.
Clinical Findings. Focal, multifocal, or diffuse involvement of the spinal cord, brain, and meninges may occur with FIP, and clinical signs reflect the location of these lesions. The most commonly recognized neurologic signs are pelvic limb ataxia, hyperesthesia (especially over the back), and generalized ataxia.[137] Affected animals usually manifest other clinical signs indicative of disseminated disease such as persistent fever (frequently >105°F), weight loss, enlarged kidneys, chorioretinitis, panophthalmitis, or anterior uveitis.[137]
Diagnosis. Histopathologic examination of biopsy specimens is the only conclusive method for the diagnosis of FIP. Short of this, a variety of factors may be considered to support a diagnosis of FIP (see Chapter 91).[138-140] CSF usually is abnormal with an elevated white blood cell count and protein level. The differential CSF white blood cell count is variable, but PMN cells, lymphocytes, and monocytes usu-

ally are present. Polymorphonuclear cells may be the predominant cell type in CSF. Protein concentration may be high (>2000 mg/dL), and CSF may be viscous and may clot. This should be taken into consideration when a CSF puncture is performed, as fluid may flow into the needle slowly. Results of cytologic examination of CSF depend on the degree of meningeal involvement. Meningeal inflammation may be extensive, and CSF in these cases is generally highly abnormal. In the presence of focal or parenchymal inflammation, CSF may be normal.
Treatment. Prognosis for cats with FIP of the CNS is poor. The feline leukemia virus (FeLV) status of cats suspected of having FIP should be determined prior to commencing treatment because the prognosis for cats with both viruses is hopeless.[141] The most effective treatment protocols combine high levels of corticosteroids (prednisolone 1 to 2 mg/lb orally once daily in the evening), cytotoxic drugs (either cyclophosphamide 1 mg/lb orally once daily for 4 consecutive days of each week, or melphalan 1 mg orally every third day), and broad-spectrum antibiotics (ampicillin 10 mg/lb orally every 8 hours), together with maintenance of nutrient intake and electrolyte balance. Cats receiving cytotoxic drugs should be routinely monitored for evidence of kidney dysfunction or bone marrow suppression. If a positive response to therapy is seen, treatment should be continued for at least 3 months.[141]

FELINE POLIOENCEPHALOMYELITIS (FELINE NONSUPPURATIVE MENINGOENCEPHALOMYELITIS)

Feline polioencephalomyelitis is a chronic, slowly progressive encephalomyelitis of unknown etiology described in immature and mature cats.[40, 142] A viral etiology is suspected on the basis of the histopathologic changes, although a specific viral agent has not been isolated. The chronic clinical course, distribution of lesions, and lack of inclusions distinguish this disease from rabies, pseudorabies, and FIP. It has been proposed that a tick-borne virus may be the causative agent in Sweden.[143-146]
Clinical signs include ataxia, paraparesis, tetraparesis, hypermetria, head tremors, and localized hyperesthesia. Spinal reflexes, pupillary light reflexes, and postural reactions may be normal or depressed. Clinical signs usually are indicative of multifocal CNS disease but may be suggestive of focal transverse myelopathy in the thoracolumbar region or lumbar enlargement. Clinical signs are slowly progressive over several months. Antemortem diagnosis is difficult, and is made by ruling out other multifocal CNS diseases. Treatment of affected cats has not been reported.

GLOBOID CELL LEUKODYSTROPHY (KRABBE-TYPE LEUKODYSTROPHY)

Etiology and Pathogenesis. Globoid cell leukodystrophy is an inherited lysosomal storage disease that results from a deficiency of galactocerebrosidase (GALC) activity.[6, 147] Globoid cell leukodystrophy is characterized by bilaterally symmetric demyelination of the white matter of the brain, spinal cord, spinal nerve roots, and peripheral nerves, and by accumulation, especially perivascularly, of large phagocytic cells with foamy-appearing cytoplasm (globoid cells). Globoid cell leukodystrophy is inherited as an autosomal recessive trait in Cairn terriers and West Highland white terriers, and findings in other breeds of dog suggest a recessive factor. The condition may not be inherited as a simple autosomal recessive trait in cats. Cloning of the GALC cDNA has been completed, and the disease-causing mutation identified, in both West Highland white terriers and Cairn terriers.[147]

Clinical Findings. Clinical signs generally are first seen between 2 and 6 months of age and are progressive. However, neurologic abnormalities were not evident in an affected basset hound until 4 years of age. Affected cats usually show abnormalities by 6 weeks of age. Progressive paraparesis and paraplegia predominate in some affected animals, while in others cerebellar signs predominate. Spinal reflexes in the pelvic limbs may be normal or exaggerated, indicative of T3–L3 transverse myelopathy. Neurologic signs in affected animals usually progress to quadriparesis, dysmetria, head tremor, behavioral changes, and/or blindness. Spinal reflexes may be decreased or absent and muscle atrophy may be evident in some animals, indicative of LMN disease. Clinical signs usually progress over a period of 2 to 6 months, although clinical signs were observed to progress for 2 years in one dog. Clinical signs in cats with globoid cell leukodystrophy are generally more indicative of cerebellar disease and are more rapidly progressive than in dogs.

Diagnosis. Diagnosis is made on the basis of age, breed, and presence of progressive neurologic deficits and by ruling out other causes of progressive myelopathy such as canine distemper myelitis. CSF may contain phagocytic cells containing PAS-positive material (globoid cells), and CSF protein content may be increased. In some animals, CSF may be normal. Brain and/or peripheral nerve biopsy may show characteristic demyelination and globoid cell accumulation and may be done to confirm a diagnosis of globoid cell leukodystrophy. A rapid test for the identification of the genotype at the cDNA position 473 has been developed.[147] Results of this test may permit breeders to screen their dogs for this problem and may result in elimination of this disease in the future.

Treatment. Treatment for globoid cell leukodystrophy has not been described.[6] Selective breeding based on genetic testing may eliminate this disease in the future.[147]

GRANULOMATOUS MENINGOENCEPHALOMYELITIS (GME)

Etiology and Pathogenesis. GME is a nonsuppurative meningoencephalomyelitis of undetermined etiology in dogs.[6, 148–150] It is characterized histopathologically by large perivascular accumulations of mononuclear cells throughout the brain, spinal cord, and meninges. A recent immunomorphologic study suggested that inflammatory lesions in canine GME consist of a heterogeneous population of major histocompatibility complex (MHC) class II antigen–positive macrophages and predominantly CD3 antigen–positive lymphocytes.[151] These data suggest a T-cell–mediated delayed-type hypersensitivity of an organ-specific autoimmune disease.[151]

Clinical Findings. A higher incidence of GME has been found in female dogs, small breed dogs, poodles, poodle mixed breed dogs, and Airedale terriers. Affected dogs usually are between 1 and 9 years of age, although dogs may be affected at any age. Clinical signs may indicate focal or multifocal cerebral, brain stem, cerebellar, and/or spinal cord involvement. GME may involve the spinal cord at any level; however, lesions appear to be most severe in the cervical spinal cord, and clinical findings are often indicative of cervical spinal cord disease. Findings include apparent cervi-cal pain, rigidity, reluctance to move, hyperesthesia, cervical paraspinal muscle spasms, exaggerated spinal reflexes, decreased conscious proprioception, paraparesis, tetraparesis, and paraplegia. Affected animals usually have an acute onset of clinical signs that are progressive over several days to months.[148, 149]

Diagnosis. Antemortem diagnosis is difficult and usually is made on the basis of clinical findings and results of CSF analysis. Dogs with GME may have intermittent fever. Complete blood count and spinal and skull radiographs frequently are within normal limits. The CSF is abnormal in most affected dogs. The CSF white blood cell count is usually increased (may be greater than 1000 WBC/μL). Mononuclear cells predominate. The percentage of lymphocytes and monocytes varies considerably. Polymorphonuclear cells may also be present and constituted 0 to 62 per cent of the differential white blood cell count in one study.[152] In the same study, less than 1 per cent of the differential white blood cell count consisted of macrophages with ingested debris, plasma cells, and cells undergoing mitosis. The total and differential CSF white blood cell counts do not reflect the severity of meningeal involvement or the degree of necrosis. Protein concentration in CSF is usually elevated, while CSF pressure may be normal or increased. Alterations in CSF were similar in untreated and corticosteroid-treated dogs in one study.[152] Meningeal lesions may render CSF collection from cisternal puncture difficult. Although CSF collected from the lumbar subarachnoid space of affected dogs may have fewer white blood cells than cisternal CSF, it is of use in diagnosis. The difference in white blood cell counts probably reflects a greater distance of the lumbar subarachnoid space from the site of the majority of lesions. Bacterial and fungal cultures are negative, and organisms are not identified in CSF cell preparations. Noncontrast radiography, myelography, and advanced imaging (CT or MRI) may confirm an intramedullary space-occupying lesion of the spinal cord.

Treatment. GME is either continuously or episodically progressive, and the prognosis is poor for recovery of affected animals. Treatment with corticosteroids may result in improvement of clinical signs for several days to several months or years. Immunosuppressive doses of corticosteroids should be given, and therapy must be sustained indefinitely. The corticosteroid regimen used for treatment of corticosteroid-responsive meningitis should be used for therapy of dogs with GME. Clinical remissions of greater than 1 year occur in some cases; however, clinical signs usually recur with discontinuation of treatment with corticosteroids. Radiation therapy may be an effective treatment for dogs with focal GME.[150] Alternative immunomodulatory drugs may also have a role in the treatment of GME in the future.[153]

HEMORRHAGE

Etiology and Pathogenesis. Intramedullary, intrameningeal, or epidural hemorrhage may be due to coagulopathies including thrombocytopenia, clotting factor deficiencies, disseminated intravascular coagulation, and anticoagulant poisonings (warfarin and the like).[154] Acute hemorrhage may also occur in association with tumors, vascular malformations, acute intervertebral disk protrusion, trauma, parasitic migration, or meningitis (Fig. 106–8). Spontaneous intramedullary hemorrhage with hematoma formation has been reported in the cervical spinal cord of a dog.[155] Spontaneous subperiosteal vertebral hemorrhage and hematoma formation

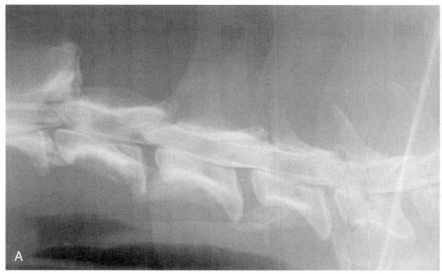

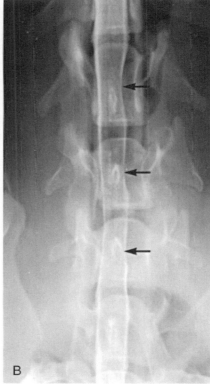

CNS

Figure 106–8. Hemorrhage. Lateral *(A)* and ventrodorsal *(B)* myelogram of the cervical vertebrae of a 10-year-old neutered male mixed breed dog with an acute onset of tetraparesis. There is narrowing of the C5–C6 intervertebral disk. The lateral myelogram *(A)* demonstrates inconsistent filling of the subarachnoid space. The ventrodorsal projection confirms lateral deviation of the right contrast column and attenuation of the left contrast column (arrows), owing to an extradural space-occupying mass. Exploratory surgery demonstrated that the extradural compression was caused by hemorrhage that had occurred secondary to the acute C5–C6 disk extrusion.

associated with spinal cord compression and transverse myelopathy have been reported in dogs.

Clinical Findings. Neurologic deficits depend on the location of the hemorrhage and usually indicate a focal or multifocal myelopathy. Clinical signs most often are acute in onset, and neurologic deficits may be severe. Extensive grey matter necrosis may occur with intramedullary hemorrhage, resulting in LMN signs over a relatively large area of the spinal cord, especially if the cervical or lumbosacral spinal cord is involved. Subarachnoid hemorrhage may result in clinical signs suggestive of meningitis, including cervical rigidity, hyperesthesia, and increased body temperature.

Diagnosis. Animals with coagulopathies may have evidence of hemorrhage elsewhere in the body. Diagnostic tests for coagulopathies should be undertaken. Subarachnoid CSF puncture may be contraindicated in animals with a coagulopathy because of the high probability of inducing further hemorrhage. Red blood cells may be present in CSF for a short time following subarachnoid hemorrhage, and CSF supernatant may be red or pink in color. Xanthochromia may be present in CSF 48 hours or more after the hemorrhage has occurred. CSF white blood cell count and protein may also be elevated.

Myelography is indicated in cases in which epidural hemorrhage is suspected to be the cause of spinal cord compression and in which noncontrast radiographs and results of CSF analysis are normal and evidence of coagulopathy is not found. Epidural hemorrhage is not distinguishable from other extradural space-occupying lesions on myelography. Hemorrhage may be secondary to other abnormalities such as intervertebral disk extrusion, as a result of laceration of a vertebral venous sinus.

Treatment. Treatment is directed at the underlying cause in animals with coagulopathies. Epidural and intramedullary hematomas not associated with coagulopathy may be removed surgically. Prognosis depends on the severity of neurologic deficits present at the time of diagnosis.

HEREDITARY ATAXIA (ATAXIA IN SMOOTH-HAIRED FOX TERRIERS AND JACK RUSSELL TERRIERS)

Etiology and Pathogenesis. An inherited, progressive, generalized ataxia has been reported to occur in young smooth-haired fox terriers and Jack Russell terriers. This disease is characterized pathologically by demyelination bilaterally throughout the dorsolateral and ventromedial white matter of the spinal cord. In Jack Russell terriers, widespread wallerian-type degeneration in the white matter of the brain and degenerative changes in the central auditory pathways and peripheral nerves may be seen. Hereditary ataxia is inherited as an autosomal recessive trait in smooth-haired fox terriers. Etiology of ataxia in Jack Russell terriers is not known; however, clinical and pathologic findings suggest it may be congenital. Degenerative myelopathies have been described in several breeds of dogs other than fox terriers and Jack Russell terriers, including English foxhounds, harriers, beagles,[156-158] Boxer dogs,[1] German shepherd dogs,[99-104] poodles,[1] Afghan hounds,[1] a Pyrenean mountain dog,[159] a Cairn terrier,[160] Dutch Kooiker dogs,[161] and Australian cattle dogs.[152] The pathogenesis of these conditions is unclear.

Clinical Findings, Diagnosis, and Treatment. Both males and females are affected. Neurologic abnormalities are first seen between 2 and 6 months of age and include pelvic limb ataxia and swinging of the hindquarters. Ataxia becomes progressively worse over 6 months to 2 years and involves all four limbs. Affected animals often have a prancing pelvic limb gait. Dysmetria may be severe, and affected dogs fall to the ground with slight change in position. Diagnosis is made on the basis of age, breed, and clinical findings. Treatment is not effective. Affected animals are eventually unable to walk.

HYPERVITAMINOSIS A OF CATS

Etiology and Pathogenesis. Hypervitaminosis A in cats is characterized by extensive confluent exostosis that is most prominent in the cervical and thoracic spine.[6, 7, 163] It is caused by a chronic excess of dietary vitamin A and is usually a result of feeding a diet consisting largely of liver. Exostosis may extend to involve the entire spine, ribs, and pelvic and thoracic limbs with complete fusion of the spine and joints. Compression of spinal nerve roots or nerves may occur if new bone formation extends into intervertebral foramina.

Clinical Findings, Diagnosis, and Treatment. Clinical signs in affected cats include apparent cervical pain and rigidity, thoracic limb lameness, ataxia, reluctance to move, paralysis, and hyperesthesia or anesthesia of the skin of the neck and forelimbs. The three most proximal diarthrodial joints of the cervical spine are almost always first affected. Osseous lesions develop insidiously, and clinical disease usually is advanced in cats older than 2 years of age before significant clinical features are recognized. Radiographic evidence of extensive exostosis of the cervical vertebral column and a history of excessive dietary intake of vitamin A or liver are necessary for diagnosis. Reduction of dietary intake of vitamin A prevents the development of further exostosis; however, it may be difficult to persuade affected cats to eat anything other than liver.

INTERVERTEBRAL DISK DISEASE

Etiology and Pathogenesis. Degeneration of intervertebral disks may result in protrusion or extrusion of disk material into the spinal canal, causing spinal cord compression and clinical signs ranging from apparent pain to complete transverse myelopathy. Degenerative changes may occur in any of the intervertebral disks; however, they occur most commonly in the cervical, caudal thoracic, and lumbar spine. The intervertebral disks between T1 and T11 are stabilized dorsally by the intercapital ligaments, and as a result disk protrusion or extrusion is less likely in this region.[164–166]

Two types of disk herniation (type I and type II) have been reported to occur in dogs.[167] Type I disk herniation occurs with degeneration and rupture of the dorsal anulus fibrosus and extrusion of nucleus pulposus into the spinal canal. Type I disk extrusion is most commonly associated with chondroid disk degeneration (Fig. 106–9). Although they occur most commonly in chondrodystrophoid breeds (dachshund, beagle, Pekingese, Lhasa apso, Shih Tzu) and breeds with chondrodystrophoid tendencies (miniature poodle and cocker spaniel), chondroid disk degeneration and type I disk extrusion may occur in any breed, including large breeds of dog. Type II disk protrusion is characterized by bulging of the intervertebral disk without complete rupture of the anulus fibrosus. Type II disk protrusion is most commonly associated with fibroid disk degeneration (Fig. 106–10). Chondroid metaplasia of the nucleus pulposus, chondroid disk degeneration, and type I disk extrusion may occur in any breed, including large breeds of dog. This author (RAL) has noted an unusually high incidence of type I disk extrusion in Doberman pinschers. The smaller lumbar epidural space in dachshunds may explain the occurrence of severe clinical signs seen in this breed in association with apparently small amounts of extruded disk material. It is also possible that the larger epidural space present in large breeds of dog may account for the fact that small amounts of extruded disk material within the spinal canal in these breeds may not cause spinal cord compression and associated clinical signs.[168]

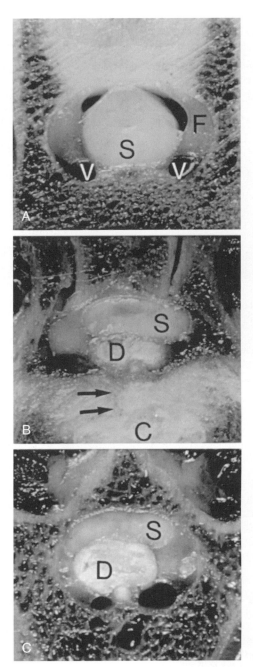

Figure 106–9. Type I disk extrusion. Gross necropsy specimens from a 4-year-old male dachshund that had an acute onset of pelvic limb paralysis. Pain perception was absent in the pelvic limbs. Myelography confirmed acute disk extrusion at T11–T12 that had caused severe spinal cord compression. *A,* Transverse section of the T12 vertebral canal 1 cm caudal to the extruded T11–T12 disk. Note the normal appearance of the spinal cord (S) within the spinal canal. Epidural fat (F) and internal vertebral venous plexus or vertebral sinuses (V) are also present within the spinal canal. *B,* Transverse section of the vertebral canal at the level of the T11–T12 disk. Calcified material (C) is present within the nucleus pulposus. A fissure (arrows) is present within the dorsal anulus fibrosus, and calcified material from the nucleus pulposus (D) has extruded through the fissure into the spinal canal. Dorsal displacement and compression of the spinal cord (S) have occurred. *C,* Transverse section of the vertebral canal 5 mm cranial to *B.* Extruded calcified material (D) from the nucleus pulposus is compressing the spinal cord (S) at this level.

Chondroid degeneration of disks is characterized by an increase in collagen content of the disk, alteration of specific glycosaminoglycan concentration of the nucleus pulposus, and a decrease in water content of the disk. The normally

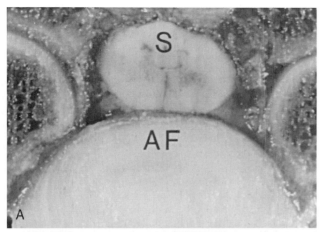

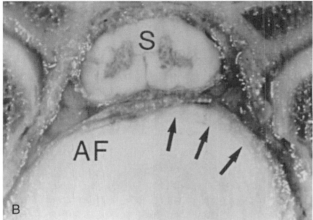

Figure 106–10. Type II disk protrusion. Gross necropsy specimens from a 7-year-old female Doberman pinscher that had a history of progressively worsening tetraparesis and generalized ataxia. Myelography confirmed type II disk protrusion at C6–C7. The disk protrusion appeared to be predominantly on the left. *A,* Transverse section of the vertebral canal at the level of the C5–C6 disk. Note the normal appearance of the spinal cord (S) within the spinal canal, and the close anatomic relationship of the dorsal anulus fibrosus (AF) to the spinal cord. *B,* Transverse section of the vertebral canal at the level of the C6–C7 disk. Note the compression of the left spinal cord (S) that is resulting from dorsal bulging *(arrows)* of the anulus fibrosus (AF) at this level.

gelatinous nucleus pulposus becomes progressively more cartilaginous and granular and eventually may mineralize (calcify). Extrusion of degenerative nucleus pulposus occurs through fissures in, or rupture of, the anulus fibrosus. In chondrodystrophoid breeds of dog, 75 to 100 per cent of all disks undergo chondroid metaplasia by 1 year of age.[169]

Fibroid disk degeneration occurs in older dogs of all breeds but is most often recognized as a clinical problem in older, large breed, nonchondrodystrophoid dogs and is characterized by fibrous metaplasia of the nucleus pulposus. An increase in the noncollagenous glycoprotein content of intervertebral disks occurs in nonchondrodystrophoid breeds of dog with aging. Calcification of the disk may occur but is rare. Protrusion of the disk occurs with a bulging of the anulus fibrosus as a result of partial rupture of the anular bands. Rupture of the anulus fibrosus and extrusion of nucleus pulposus (characteristic of type I disk extrusion) uncommonly is seen in association with type II disk protrusion.

Intervertebral disk protrusion or extrusion may occur in a ventral, dorsal, or lateral direction. In most instances, only dorsal protrusions or extrusions are of clinical significance as meningeal irritation and nerve root and/or spinal cord

compression may occur. Occasionally a lateral disk protrusion or extrusion may result in nerve root or spinal nerve compression with associated clinical signs. The cause of intervertebral disk degeneration is unknown. Trauma does not appear to play a major role, and mechanical and anatomic factors are probably important. Disk extrusions are most common in the cervical and T11 to L3 regions of the vertebral column. Genetic factors probably have a role.

Type I disk extrusion often results in more severe clinical signs than type II protrusion, although the mechanical distortion and compression of the spinal cord caused by type II protrusion may be greater. Nucleus pulposus is most often extruded into the spinal canal acutely (minutes to hours) or subacutely (days) from disks undergoing chondroid degeneration, whereas slowly progressive spinal cord compression most often accompanies protrusion of disks undergoing fibroid degeneration as the bulging fibrous mass increasingly enlarges within the spinal canal. The spinal cord changes seen in acute versus chronic spinal cord compression differ, and are reflected in the difference in clinical signs and response to treatment seen in these different types of intervertebral disk disease. The severity of spinal cord injury depends on the velocity at which the compressive force is applied, the degree of compression, and the duration of the compression. Vascular factors, as well as mechanical distortion of the spinal cord as a result of herniated disk material, are important in the pathogenesis of resulting spinal cord lesions. Severe spinal cord lesions may be found without evidence of compression, presumably as a result of vascular changes.

Hemorrhage, edema, and necrosis of spinal cord grey and white matter are characteristic of acute spinal cord injury associated with acute type I disk extrusion. Hemorrhage and edema are not a major feature of chronic spinal cord compression in which white matter changes such as demyelination, focal malacia, vacuolization, and loss of axons are seen. Type I disk extrusions often are associated with rupture of vertebral venous sinuses, and hemorrhage into the epidural space may increase the degree of spinal cord compression. Pulmonary emboli arising from the nucleus pulposus have been described in three chondrodystrophoid dogs with acute thoracolumbar transverse myelopathies as a result of type I disk extrusions, presumably as a result of disk material entering the vertebral venous sinuses. Nucleus pulposus may also penetrate the dura mater. Traumatic rupture of the anulus fibrosus and extrusion of normal nucleus pulposus may occur, resulting in spinal cord compression and an acute onset of clinical signs indicative of a transverse myelopathy.[170, 171]

Degenerative disk disease also occurs in cats,[7, 170, 171] although the incidence of clinical signs associated with disk protrusion is low. Degenerative changes, distribution of disk protrusions, and clinical signs are similar to type II disk protrusions in nonchondrodystrophoid dogs. Type I disk extrusion associated with a calcification of intervertebral disks and an acute onset of neurologic deficits may occur in cats.

Clinical Findings. Chondroid degeneration and type I disk extrusion most commonly occur in dogs 3 years of age and older. Fibroid degeneration and type II disk protrusion most commonly occur in dogs older than 5 years of age. Clinical signs seen in association with type I disk extrusion include apparent pain and/or motor and/or sensory deficits. These clinical signs usually develop rapidly, within minutes or hours of disk extrusion. However, clinical signs may progress slowly over several days or manifest periods of improvement and subsequent worsening over weeks or months. These findings are probably associated with extrusion of small amounts of disk material into the spinal canal over a period of time.

Clinical signs associated with type I disk extrusion in the cervical spine usually are less severe than those associated with extrusions in the thoracolumbar region because the vertebral canal in this region is larger in diameter in relation to the spinal cord than is the case in the thoracolumbar region. Apparent neck pain is the most common clinical finding in dogs with cervical disk extrusion. Affected dogs often hold the head and neck rigidly and cry out when moved, and may show spasms of cervical musculature. Neurologic deficits indicative of a cervical myelopathy such as proprioceptive deficits, tetraparesis, or tetraplegia are seen less commonly.

Ipsilateral Horner's syndrome and hyperthermia have been described in cases of acute, severe, dorsolateral cervical disk extrusions. Lower motor neuron deficits in the thoracic limbs may be seen in caudal cervical disk extrusions. Thoracic limb lameness may also be seen in caudal cervical disk extrusions as a result of nerve root compression, particularly from lateral disk extrusions where disk material enters an intervertebral foramen.

Clinical findings in animals with thoracolumbar type I disk extrusion depend on the severity of spinal cord injury and range from apparent back or abdominal pain to complete paraplegia and loss of deep pain perception. Neurologic deficits usually are indicative of a transverse myelopathy between T3 and L3, as most disk extrusions in this region occur between T11 and L3. Lower motor neuron signs may be seen in the pelvic limbs if disk extrusion occurs caudal to L3 as a result of compression of the lumbosacral spinal cord or nerves of the cauda equina. Lower motor neuron signs also may be seen in paraplegic animals with progressive hemorrhagic myelomalacia (PHM).

The panniculus reflex may be depressed or absent caudal to the site of disk extrusion. The site of a lesion is usually one or two vertebral spaces cranial to the loss or depression of panniculus reflex. The Schiff-Sherrington sign may be seen in animals with acute type I disk extrusion caudal to T2.

Clinical signs seen in both cervical and thoracolumbar type I disk extrusion may be asymmetric, especially if extrusion occurs dorsolaterally within the spinal canal.[172, 173] Apparent pain associated with disk extrusions results from inflammation and/or ischemia caused by compression of meninges and/or spinal nerve roots. Extruded disk material initiates an extradural inflammatory reaction that results in fibrous adhesions between the dura mater and extruded disk material. Pain may also arise from stimulation of sensory nerve endings in the anulus fibrosus and dorsal longitudinal ligament. The nucleus pulposus of each disk does not contain nerve fiber endings.

Clinical signs associated with type II disk protrusion generally are slowly progressive over a period of months. Clinical signs, however, may develop acutely over days in some animals. Neurologic deficits usually are indicative of a cervical or thoracolumbar myelopathy. Paraparesis or tetraparesis, depending on the site of the lesion, is the most common clinical finding, and deficits may be asymmetric. In the cervical spine, type II protrusions most commonly occur in caudal cervical disks. In some cases, caudal cervical type II disk protrusion may be part of the spectrum of abnormalities associated with cervical spondylomyelopathy. Apparent neck or back pain may or may not be a feature of type II disk protrusion.

Diagnosis. A tentative diagnosis of type I disk protrusion or extrusion may be made on the basis of age, breed, history, and clinical signs; however, other causes of transverse myelopathy or apparent pain should be considered in the differential diagnosis. It must be remembered that apparent spinal pain is seen in animals with meningitis. Dogs with thoracolumbar disk extrusions may appear to have abdominal pain. The differential diagnosis in animals with type II disk protrusion includes other causes of progressive transverse myelopathy, the most likely being neoplasia or degenerative myelopathy.

Spinal radiographs and, in almost all cases, CSF analysis and myelography are necessary to confirm a diagnosis of disk extrusion or protrusion. General anesthesia is required to achieve the precise positioning needed to obtain radiographs of diagnostic value. Foam wedges or sandbags are usually needed to align the vertebral column parallel to the table top for lateral projections. Care must be taken, however, in anesthetizing and positioning animals that have acute type I disk extrusions, as further extrusion of disk material and further spinal cord compression may occur with manipulation and movement of the spine.

Calcification of the nucleus pulposus is best seen on lateral radiographic views and usually is seen in one or more disks of most chondrodystrophoid dogs more than 1 year of age. Calcified disks also may be seen in older nonchondrodystrophoid breeds of dog. Calcified material within the nucleus pulposus is indicative of disk degeneration, but alone is not of clinical significance.

The disk space of an extruded disk may be narrower than adjacent disk spaces and may be wedge shaped with a decrease in the width of the disk space dorsally. However, positioning is important because some disk spaces (C7–T1, T9–T10 or T10–T11, and L7–S1) are normally narrower than adjacent spaces, and cervical and lumbosacral disks are normally wedge shaped on hyperextension and flexion of the spine. "Spikes" of calcified material suggestive of disk extrusion may extend dorsally from a disk. Calcified material may be present within the vertebral canal but often is difficult to visualize as a result of overlying vertebral articular processes or ribs. Intervertebral foramina are larger in the lumbar spine, and calcified material often is easily visualized in the spinal canal in this region. Disk material within the spinal canal may appear as a hazy, indistinct shadow or as a dense mass with distinct margins. In many cases of disk extrusion, calcified material is not visualized within the spinal canal, as disk material is probably not sufficiently mineralized to be visible on radiographs. Ventrodorsal views, and in some cases oblique views, are important in determining laterality of any visible mineralized material within the spinal canal. Vertebral osteophytes and vertebral endplate sclerosis may be seen associated with chronic disk degeneration and extrusion or, in cases of chronic disk degeneration, without disk extrusion or protrusion.

Type II disk protrusion may be associated with narrowing of the disk space, osteophyte production, and endplate sclerosis. Calcification of disk material rarely is seen in association with type II disk protrusion. In some animals with type I or type II disk herniation, obvious abnormalities are not seen on noncontrast vertebral radiographs (Fig. 106–11).

Myelography is almost always necessary to confirm that disk material has herniated into the spinal canal resulting in spinal cord compression.[173–175] Myelography is most important in determining the site (or sites) of disk herniation and in lateralization of disk material within the spinal canal prior to surgical decompression.[176] Myelography is necessary as a means of distinguishing disk protrusion from other

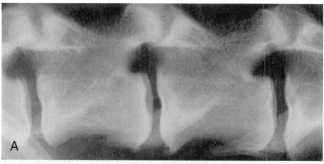

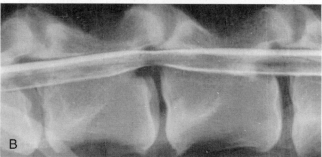

Figure 106–11. Type II disk protrusion. Lateral radiograph *(A)* and myelogram *(B)* of the midlumbar vertebral column of a 7-year-old castrated male Great Dane with a 3-month history of corticosteroid-responsive back pain. The dog was neurologically normal at the time of this study. Slight narrowing of the L2–L3 disk and mild ventral spondylosis deformans are seen on the lateral radiograph. The myelogram confirms severe ventral spinal cord compression at the level of L2–L3 associated with a type II disk protrusion.

causes of slowly progressive transverse myelopathy such as spinal neoplasia and degenerative myelopathy.

CSF should be collected and analyzed prior to myelography to rule out inflammatory or infectious disease of the spinal cord and/or meninges.[177] Clinical signs in animals with GME, distemper myelitis, FIP, spinal lymphoma, and other disorders may mimic those of cervical or thoracolumbar disk disease.

The characteristic myelographic findings in both type I and type II disk herniation into the spinal canal are extradural compression of the spinal cord with displacement of the spinal cord and narrowing of the subarachnoid space on lateral and/or ventrodorsal views, depending on the location of the compressive mass. Type II, and most type I, disk herniations result in a ventral or ventrolateral epidural mass that causes dorsal displacement of the spinal cord. Disk material may extend over more than one vertebral segment in type I extrusions and may result in deviation or narrowing of contrast columns over more than one vertebral length. Disk material may completely encircle the spinal cord. Acute type I disk extrusions often are accompanied by spinal cord edema and swelling, and occasionally dural laceration.[178] The spinal cord may be widened over several spinal cord segments, and the myelographic appearance is similar to that of an intramedullary mass, making precise determination of the site of disk extrusion difficult. In some animals, disk material is scattered along the spinal canal without obvious mechanical distortion of the spinal cord.

Rarely, in the cervical region, type I disk extrusion may occur laterally or intraforaminally, resulting in neck pain or thoracic limb pain due to nerve root compression. In such cases, myelograms may be normal; however, increased density associated with calcified disk material may be visualized intraforaminally on ventral oblique radiographs of the cervical spine. Traumatic disk protrusion is usually associated with narrowing of the intervertebral disk space on radiographs. Other abnormalities such as vertebral fracture, luxation, or instability also may be seen. Myelography is useful in determining the presence or absence of spinal cord compression in such cases, and therefore whether surgical decompression is indicated.

The use of advanced imaging techniques, such as CT or MRI, may aid in the exact localization of intervertebral disc extrusions, particularly in cases of intraforaminal disk extrusion.[179–181]

Treatment

Type I Disk Extrusion. The appropriate treatment for animals with type I disk extrusion depends on an individual animal's neurologic status. Medical treatment directed at decreasing spinal cord edema by means of corticosteroids is indicated only in those animals with an acute onset of neurologic deficits that are examined within 8 hours of the injury. The recommended agents and dosages are as desribed for spinal cord trauma. The use of corticosteroids in dogs with type I disk extrusion has been associated with pancreatitis, gastrointestinal bleeding, and colonic perforations.

Nonsurgical (medical or conservative) treatment is recommended for animals with apparent pain only or animals that have mild neurologic deficits but are ambulatory and have not had previous clinical signs associated with disk disease. These animals should be strictly confined to a small area such as a hospital cage or a quiet place away from other pets for at least 2 weeks, and walked (on a leash or harness) only to urinate and defecate. The objective of confinement is to allow fissures in the anulus fibrosus to heal, thus preventing further extrusion of disk material and allowing resolution of the inflammatory reaction caused by small amounts of extruded disk material.

Use of analgesics, muscle relaxants, or nonsteroidal anti-inflammatory agents is not recommended in most cases because it is believed that their use encourages animals to exercise and risk further disk extrusion. Cautious use of analgesics or nonsteroidal anti-inflammatory agents occasionally may be indicated; however, strict confinement followed by a period of restricted exercise is imperative. Owners should also be warned that an animal's neurologic status may deteriorate owing to extrusion of further disk material despite this treatment. If the neurologic status worsens, an animal's treatment should be reevaluated immediately. Owners should also be warned that a recurrence of clinical signs is common as a result of further disk extrusion at the same or a different site, and subsequent episodes may be more severe, especially in the thoracolumbar spine.

Animals with severe cervical pain frequently do not respond to cage rest. These dogs often have large amounts of disk material within the spinal canal, and dogs that do not show improvement after 7 to 10 days of confinement should be evaluated further by means of radiographs and myelography, and ventral cervical decompression should be considered.

Surgical disk fenestration has been recommended as a prophylactic measure to prevent further extrusion of disk material into the spinal canal.[182, 183] Fenestration of the disks most likely to herniate (C2–C3 through C6–C7 in the cervical spine and T11–T12 through L3–L4 in the thoracolumbar spine) is recommended in animals that have had one or more episodes of apparent neck or back pain and have evidence of intervertebral disk disease on radiographs. Various surgical techniques have been described.[164–166] Fenestration of disks does not remove disk material from the spinal canal and therefore is not recommended as the sole surgical procedure in dogs that have evidence of disk material within the spinal canal and spinal cord compression on radiographs and myelography.

The role of disk fenestration in the management of intervertebral disk disease is controversial.[182-185] Disk fenestration in the thoracolumbar region is not easily accomplished, and complications such as scoliosis, pneumothorax, and hemorrhage may occur. Disk fenestration in the cervical region is achieved more easily and rarely is associated with such complications. Fenestration does not prevent recurrence of disk extrusion in all animals. The effectiveness of fenestration depends largely on the amount of nucleus pulposus removed. Completion of disk fenestration is recommended at the time of spinal cord decompression.

Animals with neurologic deficits such as paresis or paralysis with deep pain perception intact, animals with recurrent bouts of apparent back or neck pain, or animals with apparent back or neck pain (or mild neurologic deficits) that is unresponsive to strict confinement should be evaluated by means of spinal radiographs, CSF analysis, and myelography. Surgical decompression of the spinal cord and removal of disk material from the spinal canal should be considered. Although many dogs with moderate or severe paresis improve neurologically if treated with cage rest, neurologic recovery is often more rapid and more complete in animals following surgical decompression of the spinal cord. In addition, the neurologic status of some dogs with type I disk extrusion, especially in the thoracolumbar spine, suddenly worsens over a period of hours or days despite medical treatment. Such deterioration usually results from further disk extrusion that may result in irreversible spinal cord damage and permanent paralysis. This progression of signs always is a risk with medical treatment of animals with thoracolumbar disk disease. Progression is impossible to predict on the basis of history, clinical signs, or radiography. Owners should be made aware of treatment options and offered the opportunity of referral to an appropriate surgical facility when animals are initially presented. Surgical decompression should be performed as soon as possible to prevent further spinal cord damage incurred as a result of sustained compression or further extrusion of disk material. In addition, if surgery is delayed 2 to 3 weeks, disk material hardens and becomes adherent to dura mater, and becomes difficult or impossible to remove from the spinal canal.

Prognosis for neurologic recovery in animals that retain deep pain perception postsurgically is fair to very good. The major factors that correlate with the degree of neurologic improvement seen postsurgically are the animal's neurologic status prior to surgery, the rapidity of onset of clinical signs, and the time interval between onset of clinical signs and surgical decompression. Animals that have severe neurologic signs, a rapid onset of clinical signs (hours), and a long period of time before surgery generally have a prolonged recovery period and may have varying degrees of permanent neurologic deficit.

The incidence of recurrence of clinical signs due to disk extrusion is greater in nonsurgically than surgically treated dogs. One author found that one third of dogs with type I disk herniation that were treated nonsurgically had a recurrence of clinical signs, and generally showed greater severity of neurologic deficits at the time of recurrence.[1] Another author reported a recurrence rate of 40 per cent in nonsurgically treated dogs.[1]

The advantages and disadvantages of various techniques for spinal cord decompression have been discussed.[125-127] Surgical treatment is not without risks. Anesthesia is necessary, and surgery occasionally results in further spinal cord damage as a result of surgical manipulation. Nonsurgical treatment should be attempted in animals that are poor anesthesia or surgical candidates or if surgical treatment is not possible financially.

In animals with clinical signs of a complete transverse myelopathy, without deep pain perception for a period of more than 24 hours, the prognosis for return of spinal cord function is poor despite medical or surgical treatment. Some of these animals may improve neurologically if given sufficient time; however, it is a matter of controversy whether surgical treatment increases the probability of improvement. In cases in which deep pain perception has been absent for less than 24 hours, the prognosis for return of spinal cord function is poor; however, surgical treatment may increase the likelihood of neurologic improvement.

Regardless of whether medical or surgical treatment is instituted, animals that are paretic or paralyzed require intensive nursing care.[186] Neurologic improvement may take weeks or months, and this requires owner cooperation and enthusiasm regarding care and physical therapy. Manual expression, intermittent catheterization, and/or indwelling catheterization of the bladder is often required to ensure emptying of the bladder. Weekly urinalysis, especially in animals that do not have voluntary control of micturition, is important in monitoring for urinary tract infection. It is also important to keep animals well padded, clean, and dry to prevent formation of pressure sores, and to ensure that caloric and water intake is adequate. Physical therapy does not result in neurologic improvement but helps to prevent disuse muscle atrophy associated with paraplegia or tetraplegia. Physical therapy should not be attempted in animals treated medically for at least the first 2 weeks following onset of signs, as further extrusion of disk material may occur.[140]

Type II Disk Protrusion. Treatment with corticosteroids may result in neurologic improvement for variable periods of time in animals with type II disk protrusion. However, corticosteroid therapy is not curative. The reason for this improvement is not clear, as intramedullary hemorrhage and edema seen in cases of acute spinal cord injury are not a feature of chronic spinal cord compression. In the thoracolumbar spine, surgical removal of protruded disk material may result in clinical improvement; however, the neurologic status of some dogs is worsened permanently despite careful surgical technique. The reasons for this are not known, but increased vascular permeability has been described in the spinal cord associated with release of chronic spinal cord compression and this probably plays a role in this phenomenon. Ventral decompression in the cervical spine allows removal of protruded type II disk material, and neurologic improvement may occur over several months; however, some dogs, especially those with moderate to severe neurologic deficits prior to surgery, may manifest temporary or permanent worsening of clinical signs postoperatively.

Acupuncture. The use of acupuncture for the treatment of intervertebral disk extrusion in dogs is controversial. Acupuncture may be an excellent adjunctive therapy in nonsurgical management of affected dogs.[187] However, the use of acupuncture as an alternative to surgery for dogs that have severe spinal cord compression resulting from disk extrusion is not recommended.

Chemonucleolysis. Injection of the proteolytic enzyme chymopapain into the nucleus pulposus of intervertebral disks to cause discolysis has been used infrequently in veterinary medicine.[81, 188-191] The precise mechanism by which chymopapain causes dissolution of the nucleus pulposus is unknown. In one study in dogs, dissolution of the nucleus pulposus was demonstrated histologically in all cervical intervertebral disks injected with chymopapain via a ventral surgical approach. Similar pathologic findings were found in lumbar disks of dogs injected with chymopapain transcutaneously under fluoroscopic guidance via a lateral approach. Significant postoperative clinical complications were not seen. Radiographic narrowing of the intervertebral disk spaces was found in both the cervical and lumbar chymopapain-injected spaces. Cervical injection resulted in a more noticeable narrowing than lumbar injection. However, successful injection as determined histologically was not always detected radiographically. These studies have described only the acute response to chymopapain. However, another study has shown chymopapain injection results in progressive dissolution of nucleus pulposus and eventual regeneration of nuclear ground material.

Chemonucleolysis may be of benefit in animals with intervertebral disk disease when the nucleus pulposus is still contained within an intact or partially ruptured anulus fibrosus. Dissolution of the nucleus pulposus in these cases may relieve pressure of the protruding disk on the spinal cord and nerve roots. Chemonucleolysis may also be useful as a prophylactic measure in animals with evidence of intervertebral disk degeneration to prevent acute type I disk extrusion.

Chemonucleolysis is not indicated in cases of type I disk extrusion, as the enzyme is unable to reach sequestered nucleus pulposus within the spinal canal. Chemonucleolysis has been used in the treatment of type II disk protrusion in the cervical spine of large breeds of dog. The majority of dogs in one study improved clinically despite persistence, or only slight decrease, in the degree of spinal cord compression on myelography. Injection of chymopapain via a surgical approach to the intervertebral disks is recommended to prevent inadvertent intrathecal injection or accidental penetration of the vertebral arteries, spinal arteries, or spinal nerve roots. Further evaluation of the effect of chemonucleolysis in dogs with intervertebral disk disease is needed; however, it seems likely that this technique may have advantages over the methods used at present for surgical disk fenestration.

ISCHEMIC MYELOPATHY DUE TO FIBROCARTILAGINOUS EMBOLISM

Etiology and Pathogenesis. Ischemic myelopathy results from ischemic necrosis of spinal cord grey and white matter associated with fibrocartilaginous emboli that occlude arteries and/or veins of the leptomeninges and spinal cord parenchyma of dogs[192-194] or cats.[195, 196] This disease is characterized by an acute onset of neurologic deficits and is generally nonprogressive after several hours. In most cases, the substance occluding spinal cord arteries and veins has histologic and histochemical properties similar to fibrocartilage of intervertebral disks and is presumed to originate from the nucleus pulposus of an intervertebral disk. Pathogenesis of this fibrocartilaginous embolism is not known. Acute spinal cord infarction has been reported secondary to neoplastic emboli and intravascular coagulation.[197] The majority of affected animals do not have evidence of degenerative intervertebral disk disease and are breeds of dog that have a low incidence of degenerative disk disease and type I disk extrusion.

Clinical Findings. Ischemic myelopathy most commonly occurs in large and giant breeds of dog, generally between 1 and 9 years of age, of either sex, but has also been described in many breeds including smaller dogs such as miniature schnauzers and Shetland sheepdogs.[192-194] It has also been described in cats.[195-196]

Ischemic myelopathy is characterized by an acute onset of neurologic deficits that may be severe. Clinical signs may progress over several hours but are generally not progressive after 12 hours. Affected animals usually do not have a history or evidence of trauma but may have a history of exercise prior to the onset of clinical signs. Apparent pain usually is not present at the time of examination or during the course of the disease, although dogs are often reported to "cry out" at the onset of clinical signs.

Neurologic deficits usually are bilateral and are often (but not always) asymmetric. Clinical signs seen to depend on the location and extent of the spinal cord lesion. Many spinal cord segments may be involved, and the neurologic deficits present may indicate extensive grey and white matter necrosis. If fibrocartilaginous embolism occurs in the cervical enlargement, unilateral or bilateral LMN signs in the thoracic limbs and UMN signs in the pelvic limbs are seen. The absence of a panniculus reflex unilaterally or bilaterally often is noted in lesions involving the T1 spinal cord segment. An ipsilateral Horner's syndrome commonly is seen in dogs with fibrocartilaginous embolism of the cervical enlargement as a result of damage to preganglionic sympathetic cell bodies in the spinal cord segments T1 and T2. A Horner's syndrome may also be seen in severe lesions in the cervical spinal cord, owing to interruption of the tecto-tegmental spinal tract.

Fibrocartilaginous embolism in the lumbosacral spinal cord causes unilateral or bilateral LMN signs in the pelvic limbs, anal and urinary sphincters, and tail. Lesions may also occur in the C1 to C5 and T3 to L3 spinal cord segments and result in symmetric or asymmetric UMN signs to all four limbs or pelvic limbs, respectively. Neurologic deficits may range from decreased conscious proprioception and mild paresis to complete paralysis and analgesia in affected limbs.

Diagnosis. Ischemic myelopathy should be suspected in any dog (especially large and giant breeds of dog) with an acute onset of nonprogressive neurologic deficits that are not associated with apparent spinal pain, especially if deficits are asymmetric or indicate that at least several spinal cord segments are involved. A diagnosis is made by ruling out other causes of myelopathy. Spinal radiographs are normal. CSF may be normal or may have an elevated protein concentration as a result of leakage of protein through damaged vascular endothelium. Xanthochromia may be present 48 hours or more after a subarachnoid hemorrhage. Appearance on a myelogram usually is normal, although mild intramedullary swelling as a result of spinal cord edema may be seen for as long as 24 hours after the onset of clinical signs.

Treatment. Corticosteroids (as recommended for spinal trauma) may be given initially to reduce any secondary spinal cord edema; however, after several days, edema usually is resolved. Good nursing care is essential in recumbent animals to prevent pressure sores, urinary tract infections, and contracture of denervated muscles. Prognosis depends on the severity of an animal's neurologic deficits. Animals that retain pain perception in affected limbs and tail usually regain neurologic function, although recovery may take several weeks to months and LMN signs may persist (muscle atrophy and/or paresis). Animals with absent pain perception

CNS

for 24 hours are likely to have irreversible spinal cord damage and have a poor prognosis for return of function in affected limb or limbs. Many animals show improvement within 2 weeks of onset of signs, unless extensive grey matter destruction has occurred.

LEUKOENCEPHALOMYELOPATHY OF ROTTWEILER DOGS

Etiology and Pathogenesis. Leukoencephalomyelopathy is a demyelinating disorder of the brain and spinal cord that has been reported to occur in rottweilers. It is characterized by progressive tetraparesis and hypermetria, especially of the thoracic limbs. Leukoencephalomyelopathy has been reported in 2 dogs in the United States.[198] A similar disorder has been reported in 16 rottweilers in the Netherlands.[199]

Histopathologic examination demonstrated demyelination in white matter of the spinal cord, brain stem, and cerebellum, with intact naked axons and thinly myelinated axons accompanied by reactive astrogliosis. The spinal cord lesions were found in the lateral funiculi and occasionally the dorsal funiculi, predominantly in the cervical and thoracic spinal cord, and tended to be bilaterally symmetric. The lack of neuronal fiber degeneration makes primary demyelination more likely than secondary demyelination.

Etiology of this disease is unknown. It may be the result of an acquired primary demyelinating disease, but whether the lesions seen are due to a single demyelinating event or the result of repeated demyelination and remyelination is not known. Because the lesions are bilaterally symmetric, toxic, metabolic, and nutritional mechanisms may be involved. Infectious causes, such as CD virus, may also result in demyelination. Vascular mechanisms may also be involved, as lesions have a segmental distribution; however, axon degeneration would be expected. An inherited condition in which myelin formation is defective and cannot be maintained (leukodystrophy) is also possible. The two dogs in the United States report were related, as were the 16 dogs reported in the Netherlands.

Other leukodystrophies have been reported in young animals, although an adult-onset leukodystrophy has not been described in dogs. The relationship of this disease to neuroaxonal dystrophy of rottweilers is not known.[200] Histopathologic lesions and clinical findings differ from those described in dogs with neuroaxonal dystrophy; however, a dog related to a dog with leukoencephalomyelopathy was diagnosed as having neuroaxonal dystrophy.

Clinical Findings. Both males and females have been reported to be affected. Clinical findings reported were tetraparesis, hypermetria (especially of the forelimbs), decreased conscious proprioception (especially of the pelvic limbs), and exaggerated spinal reflexes. Clinical signs became apparent between 18 months and 42 months of age, and abnormalities were slowly progressive over several months to 1 year. Neurologic abnormalities were consistent with a transverse myelopathy of the cervical spinal cord. Neurologic deficits referable to structures rostral to the foramen magnum were not detected.

Diagnosis and Treatment. Diagnosis may be made on the basis of age and breed of an affected dog, and by ruling out other causes of cervical myelopathy such as CD myelitis, granulomatous meningoencephalomyelitis, cervical spondylomyelopathy, or spinal neoplasia. Results of radiography, CSF analysis, and myelography were normal in dogs reported. Treatment of leukoencephalomyelopathy of rottweilers has not been effective.

LUMBOSACRAL VERTEBRAL CANAL STENOSIS

Etiology and Pathogenesis. Lumbosacral vertebral canal stenosis (also called lumbosacral instability, lumbosacral malformation/malarticulation, lumbar spinal stenosis, lumbosacral spondylolisthesis, and cauda equina syndrome) is a term that encompasses a spectrum of disorders that result in narrowing of the lumbosacral vertebral canal with resulting compression of the cauda equina. The term *cauda equina syndrome* describes a group of neurologic signs that result from compression, destruction, or displacement of those nerve roots and spinal nerves that form the cauda equina by a variety of causes, including lumbosacral vertebral canal stenosis (Table 106–6).[201]

The term lumbosacral vertebral canal stenosis is defined as an acquired disorder of large-breed dogs that results from several or all of the following: type II disk protrusion (dorsal bulging of the anulus fibrosus), hypertrophy and/or hyperplasia of the interarcuate ligament, thickening of vertebral arches or articular facets, and (infrequently) subluxation/instability of the lumbosacral junction. It is likely that several separate disorders currently are included within this definition. Other terms have been used to describe this syndrome, including lumbosacral spondylolisthesis, lumbar spinal stenosis, and lumbosacral instability. In humans, the term spondylolisthesis refers specifically to a forward (anterior) movement of a lower lumbar vertebra relative to a lumbar vertebra or sacrum directly below it. This problem rarely occurs in dogs, in which the most frequently encountered problem is a ventral "slippage" of the sacrum relative to the body of the L7 vertebra. The term retrolisthesis has been proposed to describe this "reverse spondylolisthesis" of dogs. Lumbar spinal stenosis is a term that perhaps is best used to describe a congenital ("idiopathic") syndrome reported to occur in young dogs. Lumbosacral instability is a misleading term, as instability is not demonstrated consistently in association with lumbosacral vertebral canal stenosis.

Certain similarities between vertebral and soft tissue alterations seen in dogs with lumbosacral vertebral canal stenosis and in Doberman pinscher dogs with caudal cervical spondylomyelopathy have been noted. As the etiology and pathogenesis for both conditions are incompletely understood, such comparisons are of little significance at the present time. An association has been reported between lumbosacral

---

TABLE 106–6. DISORDERS THAT RESULT IN SIGNS OF CAUDA EQUINA DYSFUNCTION IN DOGS

Congenital Disorders

Vertebral and/or nerve root anomalies (e.g., spina bifida)
Idiopathic lumbar stenosis

Acquired Disorders

Infections (e.g., discospondylitis)
Neoplasia (e.g., malignant nerve sheath neoplasia)
Intervertebral disk disease
Iatrogenic stenosis (e.g., postsurgical scarring)
Lumbosacral vertebral canal stenosis (with/without "retrolisthesis")

Combined Disorders

Combination of congenital and acquired disorders (e.g., disk degeneration and lumbosacral vertebral canal stenosis)

stenosis and transitional vertebrae in German shepherd dogs.[204] In another report, more than 30 per cent of German shepherd dogs with clinical signs of cauda equina compression had radiographic and pathologic abnormalities consistent with osteochondrosis of the sacral endplate.[205]

Clinical Findings. Acquired degenerative lumbosacral vertebral canal stenosis occurs most commonly in large-breed dogs, especially German shepherd dogs.[206] Males appear to be affected more frequently than females. Dogs with the congenital ("idiopathic") form appear to be of the smaller breeds. Affected dogs in both categories are between 3 and 7 years of age, although the problem may occur at any age. Degenerative lumbosacral vertebral canal stenosis rarely is recognized in cats.[7, 106, 171]

Signs of cauda equina compression seen frequently in affected dogs include the following: apparent pain on palpation of the lumbosacral region, on caudal extension of the pelvic limbs, or on elevation of the tail; difficulty in rising; pelvic limb lameness (often unilateral); pelvic limb muscle atrophy; paresis of the tail; scuffing of the toes; urinary and/or fecal incontinence, or "inappropriate" voiding as a result of an inability to assume a voiding posture; self-mutilation of the perineum, tail, or pelvic limbs; and rarely, paraphimosis. These signs most often are insidious in onset and progress gradually over months, and they are easily confused with those of hip dysplasia or degenerative myelopathy.[202, 203, 206]

Abnormalities detected on neurologic examination include gait deficits related to sciatic nerve paresis (e.g., dragging of toes). Depression or loss of conscious proprioception, normal or slightly exaggerated patellar reflexes ("pseudoexaggeration" related to loss of antagonism to femoral nerve–innervated muscles by sciatic nerve–innervated muscles), depressed or absent flexion reflexes in pelvic limbs, decreased anal tone and anal sphincter reflexes, atonic bladder, hypesthesia of the perineum and tail, and muscle atrophy may be seen. These abnormalities relate to deficits of the sciatic, pudendal, caudal, and pelvic nerves, whose nerve roots comprise the cauda equina.[202, 203, 206]

Diagnosis. Characteristic clinical findings may be consistent with a diagnosis of degenerative lumbosacral vertebral canal stenosis. Careful mapping of areas of loss of cutaneous sensation may assist in determining involved nerve roots. However, presence of this syndrome must be confirmed by means of plain radiographs and special radiographic procedures.[207] Rarely can this condition be diagnosed on the basis of plain radiographic findings alone. Plain radiographic findings include spondylosis deformans ventral and lateral to the lumbosacral articulation, sclerosis of vertebral endplates, "wedging" or narrowing of the L7–S1 disk space, and secondary degenerative joint disease in the region of L7–S1 articular facets (Fig. 106–12). Ventral displacement of the sacrum with respect to L7 ("retrolisthesis") and diminished dorsoventral dimensions of the lumbosacral spinal canal may be seen; however, such findings must be interpreted with caution, as they may be seen in normal dogs in association with slight rotation of the vertebral column on lateral radiographs. General anesthesia is mandatory for obtaining radiographs of the lumbosacral vertebral column. A ventrodorsal projection also is recommended.

"Stressed" plain radiographic projections (flexed and extended views), completed with careful attention to avoid rotation, often assist in determining the presence of instability or "retrolisthesis." Several attempts to separate normal dogs from dogs with lumbosacral vertebral canal stenosis by means of objective measurements made from radiographs

have not been successful.[208] Appearance on plain radiographs helps to eliminate other causes of cauda equina syndrome (e.g., discospondylitis or vertebral neoplasia). Linear tomography, when available, may provide specific information regarding the diameter of the lumbosacral vertebral canal that cannot be obtained from plain radiographs.

Electromyography may complement information available from a neurologic examination and from plain spinal radiographs by confirming denervation in muscles innervated by the nerves of the cauda equina. Motor nerve conduction velocity determinations in sciatic and tibial nerves and measurement of evoked spinal cord potentials may also provide indirect evidence of cauda equina dysfunction.[209, 210] Several contrast radiographic techniques exist for examination of the lumbosacral vertebral canal. Use of such techniques is necessary for demonstration of soft tissue vertebral canal stenosis.[209, 211] Myelography most often is useful in the diagnosis of lumbosacral problems, as the terminal portion of the subarachnoid space of dogs may fill with contrast material at this level. Transosseous vertebral sinus venography (filling of vertebral sinuses with contrast material) and epidurography (filling of the lumbosacral epidural space with contrast material) have been used by many investigators in an attempt to outline soft tissue stenosis of the lumbosacral vertebral canal. Results obtained with either of these techniques must be interpreted cautiously, as falsely positive studies occur with both.

A technique that is useful for confirmation of lumbosacral soft tissue stenosis is discography.[209, 212] Discography consists of radiography completed following the injection of contrast material into the nucleus pulposus of an intervertebral disk (Fig. 106–13). This technique has special application to the lumbosacral disk space.

CT, either alone or combined with the contrast techniques listed above, and MRI may provide further information regarding soft tissue stenosis of the lumbosacral vertebral canal, particularly with regard to the L7–S1 intervertebral foramen.[213–217]

Surgical exploration may be indicated in dogs (with appropriate history and clinical signs) in which results of ancillary diagnostic tests do not provide a definite diagnosis of soft tissue stenosis.

Treatment. Some affected dogs in which clinical signs are mild or in which apparent lumbosacral pain is the sole problem improve temporarily after strict confinement and restricted leash exercise for a period of 4 to 6 weeks. Use of analgesic drugs or corticosteroids has been recommended; however, their use must be accompanied by strict confinement.

Clinical signs commonly recur in affected dogs treated only by means of medical therapy. Dogs with recurrence of signs, or dogs that are moderately to severely affected at the time of initial presentation (especially those with urinary/fecal incontinence), should be considered candidates for surgery. Dorsal decompressive laminectomy of L7 and S1 vertebrae is recommended. This procedure may be combined with foraminotomy or facetectomy in dogs in which compression of spinal nerves at the level of the intervertebral foramina is suspected. In animals with radiographically confirmed instability or significant retrolisthesis, fusion of the lumbosacral articulation may be necessary. A dorsal approach for fusion has been recommended.[218]

Dogs should be confined for 2 to 4 weeks postoperatively. Postoperative complications include seroma formation at the surgical site and formation of a laminectomy scar at the site of the laminectomy. Both may be avoided by use of appro-

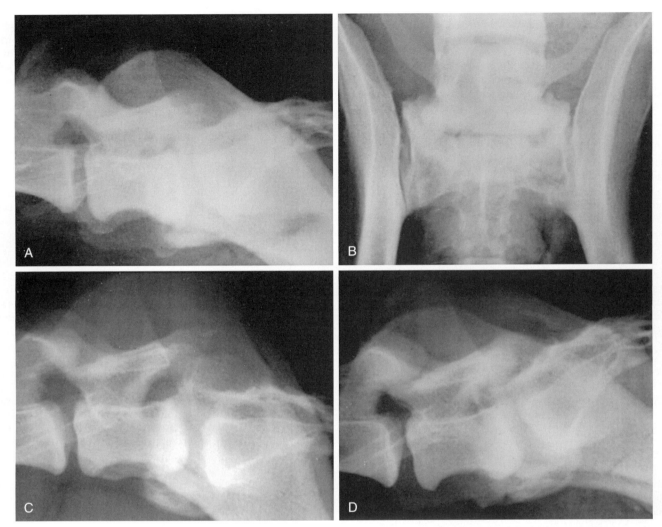

Figure 106–12. Lumbosacral vertebral canal stenosis. Lateral *(A)* and ventrodorsal *(B)* radiographs of the lumbosacral region of the vertebral column of a 7-year-old female Vizsla. The dog had a history of apparent spinal pain, hypotonic tail, urinary incontinence, and pelvic limb paresis. Sclerosis of vertebral endplates of L7 and S1, L7–S1 spondylosis deformans, "wedging" of the L7–S1 disk, and malalignment of L7–S1 are evident on the neutrally positioned lateral projection. Spondylosis deformans is seen lateral to the L7–S1 vertebral articulation on the ventrodorsal projection. A flexed lateral projection *(C)* confirms the presence of "retrolisthesis" with excessive ventral movement of the sacrum with respect to the body of L7. Instability of the lumbosacral articulation is further suggested by the extended projection *(D)*, where "wedging" of the L7–S1 disk is seen. Use of these stressed projections is essential for confirmation of instability in association with lumbosacral vertebral canal stenosis.

priate surgical technique and postoperative patient management.

Attention to bladder emptying may be necessary in dogs with bladder atony prior to surgery. The bladder should be manually expressed three times daily in such dogs. Urine should be submitted for culture and sensitivity testing prior to and 2 weeks after completion of surgery, and appropriate antibiotic therapy instituted as indicated by results.

Prognosis for affected dogs is dependent on the severity of signs prior to surgery. Return to normal function may be expected in dogs that are mildly affected prior to surgery. Dogs with bladder atony or a flaccid anal sphincter prior to surgery have the poorest prognosis.

MUCOPOLYSACCHARIDOSIS

Etiology and Pathogenesis. The mucopolysaccharidoses are a group of genetic diseases that result from defects in the metabolism of glycosaminoglycans. Two subclasses have been recognized in cats, and paraparesis associated

with spinal cord compression has been reported in Siamese cats with mucopolysaccharidosis VI (MPS VI).[6, 7] Mucopolysaccharidosis VI is the result of a deficiency of the lysosomal enzyme arylsulfatase B and, in addition to causing characteristic physical deformities, can result in skeletal changes, including fusion of the cervical vertebrae, variable fusion of thoracic and lumbar vertebrae, bony proliferation and bony protrusion into the vertebral canal in the thoracic and lumbar spine causing compression of the spinal cord, and bony proliferation in the intervertebral foramina causing nerve root compression.[219] Bony proliferative changes and associated spinal cord compression occur prior to, or at the time of, epiphyseal closure (about 9 months of age) and are probably nonprogressive after this time. Mucopolysaccharidosis VI is an inherited abnormality and has an autosomal recessive mode of inheritance.

Mucopolysaccharidosis I due to a deficiency in alpha-L-iduronidase has been reported in a domestic shorthaired cat. The clinical features were similar to those of MPS VI, but bony proliferative changes and associated spinal cord compression were not found. Although vacuolar changes

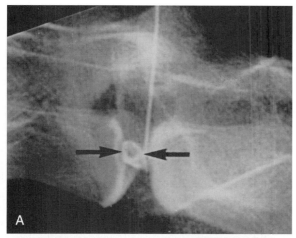

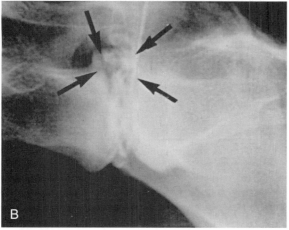

Figure 106–13. Lumbosacral vertebral canal stenosis. *A,* Discogram at L7–S1 in a normal 5-year-old male Saint Bernard. Note the placement of a spinal needle in the nucleus pulposus of the L7–S1 disk. Contrast material (0.2 mL) is confined to the region of the nucleus pulposus (arrows). *B,* Discogram at L7–S1 in a 6-year-old male Great Dane with a history of apparent spinal pain and self-mutilation of the right side of the tail. Note the irregular pattern of contrast filling of the disk and the "dome-shaped" region of contrast material that has accumulated within the vertebral canal (arrows). This abnormal discogram is consistent with a diagnosis of L7–S1 disk degeneration with bulging of the dorsal anulus fibrosus into the vertebral canal. This diagnosis was confirmed following a dorsal laminectomy completed over this site.

were observed in neurons of brain and cervical spinal cord, presumably as a result of storage of glycosaminoglycans, neurologic deficits were not found clinically. Mucopolysaccharidosis I probably has an autosomal recessive mode of inheritance.

Clinical Findings. The characteristic physical findings in cases of MPS VI are small head, flat broad face, widely spaced eyes, corneal clouding, small ears, depressed bridge of the nose, large forepaws, and concave deformity of the sternum. Affected kittens are smaller than normal littermates, and physical deformities are noticeable by 8 weeks of age. Neurologic deficits due to skeletal changes and spinal cord compression are seen between 4 and 7 months of age and progress over 2 to 4 weeks. Neurologic findings are indicative of a transverse myelopathy between T3 and L3 and include absent conscious proprioception, normal to exaggerated pelvic limb reflexes, and decreased pain perception in the pelvic limbs. The thoracic limb gait may be normal, or affected cats may have a crouching posture. Spinal reflexes in the thoracic limbs are normal.

Diagnosis. Radiographs of the spine show vertebral fusion and bony protrusions into the spinal canal and intervertebral foramina of the thoracolumbar spine.[219] However, bony proliferation is not an indication of neurologic dysfunction. Myelography is necessary to demonstrate spinal cord compression. Subarachnoid CSF puncture may be difficult, owing to proliferative changes around the vertebrae. MPS VI can be confirmed by measurement of arylsulfatase B activity in leukocytes.

Treatment. As skeletal changes are nonprogressive after about 9 months of age, decompressive surgery may result in improvement in neurologic signs. However, spinal cord compression may be present at more than one site. The underlying lysosomal enzyme deficit is not amenable to treatment at present. Bone marrow transplantation is being investigated as a possible therapy for MPS VI.[220]

MYELODYSPLASIA

Etiology and Pathogenesis. The term myelodysplasia describes a number of malformations of the spinal cord believed to result from incomplete closure or development of the neural tube.[6, 7, 221] Malformations identified histopathologically include anomalies of the central canal (hydromyelia, duplication of the central canal, or absence of the central canal); anomalies of the central grey matter, ventral median fissure, and dorsal median septum; grey matter ectopias, chromatolysis, and loss of nerve cell bodies; and syringomyelia, usually in the dorsal columns. Lesions are found throughout the spinal cord but are more severe in the lumbar region.

Myelodysplasia is considered to be an inherited condition in the Weimaraner, transmitted by a mutant gene.[222] Both males and females are affected. Myelodysplasia has been described in other breeds of dogs and cats, including a Dalmatian, a rottweiler, a West Highland white terrier, an English bulldog, mixed breed dogs, and Manx cats.[7, 221, 223] Etiology and pathogenesis of the condition in these animals are unknown.

Clinical Findings. Clinical signs vary in severity and usually are referable to a transverse myelopathy between T3 and L3. Clinical abnormalities usually are evident at 4 to 6 weeks of age, when puppies become ambulatory, although abnormal reflexes have been reported in affected newborn puppies. The major clinical finding in affected dogs is a symmetric "bunny-hopping" pelvic limb gait. Other clinical findings are crouching stance, abduction or overextension of one or both pelvic limbs, decreased conscious proprioception in the pelvic limbs, scoliosis, and in one case, torticollis. Spinal reflexes and pain perception usually are normal. In Weimaraner dogs, other findings include abnormal hair "streams" in the dorsal neck region, koilosternia (gutter-like depression in the chest), and occasionally, a head tilt.

Diagnosis. Diagnosis is made on the basis of history, signalment, clinical signs, plain radiography, CSF analysis, and myelography. Advanced imaging techniques such as CT and MRI have also been used.[223]

Treatment. There is not an effective treatment. In Weimaraner dogs and probably in other dogs or cats, clinical signs are not progressive and affected animals may be acceptable pets.

NEOPLASIA

Etiology and Pathogenesis. The spinal cord may be a site of primary or metastatic neoplasia, or may be compressed or invaded by primary or metastatic tumors arising from the vertebrae and surrounding tissues.[224–227] Primary neural tumors include astrocytoma, glioma, ependymoma, neuroepithelioma, malignant nerve sheath neoplasm (schwannoma, neurofibroma, neurofibrosarcoma), meningioma, meningeal sarcoma, and reticulum cell sarcoma. Primary lymphosarcoma of the spinal cord also has been reported in a dog.

Tumors of spinal nerves that extend into the spinal canal or spinal nerve roots may cause extradural or intradural compression of the spinal cord.[228] These tumors may also invade the spinal cord parenchyma. The distinction between schwannoma, Schwann cell sarcoma, neurofibroma, and neurofibrosarcoma is difficult to make histologically, but all have similar features clinically and on gross pathology.[224] The term malignant nerve sheath neoplasm has been proposed for this tumor.[224] These tumors may involve any cranial or spinal nerve or dorsal or ventral nerve root and commonly spread to involve adjacent nerves and nerve roots. Malignant nerve sheath tumors commonly arise from nerve roots or spinal nerves contributing to the brachial plexus. These tumors may arise from more than one site. Lymphosarcoma may also involve peripheral nerves and extend along spinal nerves and nerve roots into the spinal canal, resulting in clinical signs of spinal cord disease.[229] Meningeal sarcomatosis is a rare condition characterized by diffuse infiltration of the leptomeninges by neoplastic mesenchymal cells.

The spinal cord may also be compressed by tumors originating from surrounding structures. Most commonly these tumors arise from bone, cartilage, fibrous tissue, and blood vessels of vertebrae, and less commonly from the hemopoietic elements of bone and tissue outside the vertebral column including muscle, fat, and paraganglia.[224] Primary vertebral tumors, which may cause compression of the spinal cord as a result of either extension of tumor mass into the spinal canal or pathologic fracture of the vertebra, include osteosarcoma, chondrosarcoma, fibrosarcoma, hemangioma, hemangiosarcoma, plasma cell myeloma, giant cell sarcoma (arising from primitive stromal elements of bone marrow), and undifferentiated sarcomas.[224] Tumor metastases from sites elsewhere in the body may also be found in vertebrae, epidural space, meninges, and rarely the parenchyma of the spinal cord. Secondary tumors result from hematogenous or lymphatic spread of tumor emboli and include hemangiosarcoma, lymphosarcoma, mammary adenocarcinoma, pulmonary carcinoma, prostatic carcinoma, and malignant melanoma. Clinical signs associated with secondary spinal tumors may occur early or late in the course of the disease. With the prolonged survival times that accompany recent therapeutic regimens for osteosarcoma of long bones, an increased frequency of vertebral metastases can be expected, particularly in cranial thoracic vertebrae. Embolic tumor cells may pass directly to the lumbar vertebrae from tumors in the pelvic area by reversal of blood flow in the vertebral veins with increases in central venous pressure.

Retrospective studies have shown the most commonly occurring spinal tumors in dogs to be primary and secondary bone tumors, and tumors of spinal nerves and nerve roots. Primary intramedullary tumors occur less commonly than extradural or intradural-extramedullary tumors. Spinal tumors of all types occur more frequently in large breeds of dog. Epidural lymphosarcoma is the most commonly occurring spinal tumor in cats.[229–233] Primary intramedullary tumors rarely occur in cats. Etiology of vertebral and spinal cord tumors is unknown. Lymphosarcoma in cats may be associated with FeLV or feline immunodeficiency virus (FIV) infection; however, not all cats with spinal lymphosarcoma test positive for FeLV or FIV.[230]

Spinal tumors may occur in animals of any age. Although tumors more commonly occur in animals more than 5 years of age, spinal cord blastoma (nephroblastoma) in dogs[234] and lymphosarcoma in cats are found most commonly in young animals. Spinal cord blastoma has been reported in large breeds of dog aged 6 months to 3 years. German shepherd dogs have a higher incidence of this tumor than other breeds. These tumors are generally located in an intradural and extramedullary location, closely associated with the pia mater of the spinal cord and separated from the spinal cord by a thin band of connective tissue. The tumor may replace most of the spinal cord and may also have an intramedullary component. These tumors occur in T10–L2 spinal cord segments and may be the result of neoplastic transformation of remnants of embryonic medullary (neuro)epithelium in this region of the spinal cord. However, immunocytochemical studies do not support a neuroectodermal origin for these tumors. The mixed epithelial and mesenchymal patterns seen in these tumors are similar to nephroblastomas.[234]

Metastatic spinal tumors have also been reported to occur in dogs.[226] Primary spinal cord, meningeal, and nerve root tumors rarely metastasize outside the spinal canal; however, tumors may arise from multiple sites or may metastasize along CSF pathways (meningioma, ependymoma). Primary vertebral tumors commonly metastasize to other organ systems.

Clinical Findings. Clinical signs depend on the location of the tumor. Tumors may involve more than one spinal cord segment and more than one spinal tumor may be present, resulting in multifocal signs. However, most animals have clinical signs referable to a transverse myelopathy. Tumors may occur anywhere within the spinal cord or spinal canal and usually result in progressive neurologic deficits. The duration of clinical signs may vary considerably (from 1 week to 1 year in one study). Animals may have the following signs: acute onset of severe neurologic deficits associated with pathologic fracture of a vertebra, resulting in spinal cord compression; epidural, subarachnoid, or intramedullary hemorrhage; or spinal cord ischemia associated with tumor expansion. Neurologic deficits are usually bilateral but may be asymmetric.

Tumors of nerves of the brachial plexus initially cause progressive LMN signs in the ipsilateral thoracic limb, including muscle atrophy and paresis. The affected limb is often painful on palpation or movement; cutaneous sensation generally remains intact.[224] If the tumor extends into the spinal canal, UMN signs to the pelvic limbs may become apparent. Tumors of nerves of the cauda equina or lumbosacral plexus, with extension into the spinal canal, may cause unilateral or bilateral LMN signs in the pelvic limbs, tail, perineum, urinary bladder, and anal sphincter.

Apparent pain is a common finding associated with extradural and intradural tumors[227] and was the predominant clinical sign in a study of dogs with vertebral tumors. Apparent pain may be intractable, especially in animals with a tumor affecting spinal nerve roots. This may be due to stretching or inflammation of the meninges surrounding the expanding tumor. Intramedullary tumors are reported to cause a more rapid progression of clinical signs and are much less likely to be painful than extradural or intradural-extramedullary tumors. In general, however, extradural, intradural-extramedullary, and intramedullary tumors cannot be distinguished on the basis of clinical findings.

Diagnosis. A tentative diagnosis of spinal tumor can be made on the basis of radiographic, CSF, and myelographic findings. Definitive diagnosis can only be made after biopsy of a suspected lesion.

Radiography. Bone lysis with a cortical break is the most common radiographic finding in animals with vertebral tumors. Other radiographic findings include destruction of vertebral endplates, collapse of an adjacent disk space, collapse and shortening of a vertebral body, pathologic fracture, bone sclerosis and bony production, cystlike expansile lesions, and adjacent soft tissue masses. Bone tumors most commonly occur in the vertebral body but may also be found in the dorsal spinous processes, transverse processes, and articular facets. Primary and secondary bone tumors or specific tumor types cannot be distinguished radiographically. Primary bone tumors usually (but not always) involve one vertebra. More than half of the secondary bone tumors in one study involved more than one vertebra. Rarely, metastatic tumors (e.g., carcinoma) may arise within a disk space. Such tumors may have a radiographic appearance that resembles that of discospondylitis. Metastases from intrapelvic soft tissue tumors often produce periosteal new bone on the ventral aspect of multiple lumbar vertebral bodies in association with paravertebral soft tissue mass formation. Vertebral lesions of multiple myeloma are characterized by "punched out" lytic lesions.

Vertebral lesions may also occur with spread of tumors from surrounding soft tissues into the vertebrae. Bone tumors are not always easily detected by means of radiography, owing to inconsistent vertebral shape, overlying rib and soft tissue shadows, and improper positioning. Other diseases, such as bacterial or fungal discospondylitis, spondylitis, or vertebral osteomyelitis, must be considered in the differential diagnosis of vertebral tumors.

Expanding tumors within the spinal canal may result in widening of the vertebral canal and loss of bone density as a result of ischemia and necrosis of overlying bone. Similarly, tumors of spinal nerves extending into the spinal canal may cause widening of intervertebral foramina.

CSF Analysis. CSF may be normal or may have an increased protein concentration and/or white blood cell count.[13] A mild to moderate increase in CSF white blood cell count may occur in animals with tumors arising from or invading the leptomeninges. Polymorphonuclear cells may predominate, probably as a result of meningeal inflammation and necrosis. Tumor cells rarely are found in CSF, except in CSF from animals with lymphosarcoma, in which abnormal lymphocytes are often present in association with meningeal infiltration. Collection of CSF from the lumbar subarachnoid space may yield more cells than cisternal collection, owing to probable caudal flow of CSF in animals. Inability to demonstrate tumor cells in CSF may be the result of the methods used to analyze CSF. The use of cell-concentrating techniques that yield a greater percentage of cells present in CSF may result in the preservation of more neoplastic cells. Xanthochromia, suggesting previous subarachnoid hemorrhage, occasionally is present. CSF protein concentration may be increased owing to abnormal permeability of blood–spinal cord or blood-meningeal barrier, as a result of extradural compression or meningeal or parenchymal tumor infiltration.

Myelography. Myelography may be helpful in differentiating intramedullary, intradural-extramedullary, and extradural tumors. Cisternal and lumbar injection of contrast material may be necessary to outline both the cranial and caudal extent of a tumor. It is important to obtain survey radiographs of the entire vertebral column prior to and after injection of contrast, as more than one tumor may be present and the neurologic deficits of one tumor may "mask" those produced by another. Several radiographic views (at least lateral and ventrodorsal) are necessary to determine whether a tumor is intramedullary, intradural-extramedullary, or extradural. Tumors may have a mixed myelographic appearance, with extradural, intradural, and/or intramedullary components (e.g., nerve root tumors, meningioma, and spinal cord blastoma). Myelographic findings may also be misleading, as extradural tumors may appear intramedullary on some views, or spinal cord edema associated with acute extradural compression may appear the same as an intramedullary mass. Other mass lesions resulting in spinal cord compression, intramedullary swelling, and intradural lesions must be considered in the differential diagnosis of spinal tumors.

Both CT (Fig. 106–14) and MRI aid in exact determination of location and extent of spinal tumors.[235, 236] Use of these advanced imaging modalities aids in precise surgical planning and radiation therapy planning.

Biopsy. Biopsy of suspected lesions is necessary to differentiate neoplasms from other vertebral and spinal cord abnormalities and to determine histologic type.[237]

Treatment. The majority of vertebral tumors are not surgically resectable, owing to their malignant characteristics and the decreased stability of the vertebral column that may result from extensive surgery. Surgical decompression of the spinal cord and debulking of tumor mass may be palliative in some cases. Some tumors within the spinal canal are surgically resectable, including some tumors that appear intramedullary on myelography, such as spinal cord blastoma.[238] Surgical exploration of solitary tumors within the spinal canal is recommended for animals with clinical signs that are indicative of an incomplete transverse myelopathy, even those in which myelographic findings are consistent with an intramedullary mass.[231] Intradural nerve root tumors are rarely completely surgically resectable, and recurrence rate is high. Resection of ventral nerve roots contributing to the brachial or lumbosacral plexus may necessitate amputation of the affected limb.[224]

There is not a direct relationship between tumor size and rate of progression or severity of clinical signs. The spinal cord is able to compensate for pressure applied gradually,

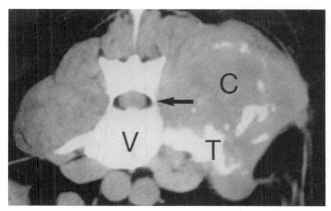

Figure 106–14. Vertebral neoplasia. Transverse CT image of the vertebral column of a 13-year-old spayed female Old English sheepdog at the level of the L4 vertebral body (V). Note the chondrosarcoma (C) arising from the transverse process (T) of L4. There are areas of calcification within the neoplasm. The tumor involves the lateral lamina (arrow) of L4. Exact determination of location and extent of a neoplasm is possible by means of CT.

and animals with spinal tumors may remain ambulatory despite having little normal spinal cord tissue remaining. Compression applied to the spinal cord rapidly, such as may occur with a pathologic fracture, may cause severe and irreversible spinal cord damage.

Corticosteroids may decrease spinal cord edema associated with spinal cord tumors and result in clinical improvement for a variable period of time. Radiation therapy and chemotherapy may be helpful in animals with spinal lymphosarcoma. Most chemotherapeutic agents do not cross the blood–spinal cord or blood-CSF barrier in concentrations sufficient to eliminate tumor cells in the meninges or spinal cord. Several chemotherapeutic agents, including methotrexate and cytosine arabinoside, may be given intrathecally and have been used in the treatment of meningeal lymphosarcoma and leukemic meningitis. Complications of intrathecal use of chemotherapeutic agents include arachnoiditis and seizures. Chemotherapy may be helpful in the treatment of plasma cell myeloma.

Chemotherapy and radiation therapy have not been used in the treatment of a sufficient number of primary spinal cord, nerve root, or meningeal tumors to assess results; however, initial experience suggests that further use of radiation therapy is warranted.[239] Various chemotherapeutic regimens have been used in the treatment of bone tumors and tumors that metastasize to bone, generally with poor results. Chemotherapy regimens in the future may offer more hope in the treatment of vertebral tumors. In general, the prognosis for animals with nonresectable spinal tumors is poor.

NEUROAXONAL DYSTROPHY OF ROTTWEILER DOGS

Etiology and Pathogenesis. Neuroaxonal dystrophy is a disease of rottweilers characterized by the accumulation of axonal spheroids throughout the neuraxis.[200, 240, 241] Clinically, affected animals have progressive ataxia in all limbs and severe hypermetria, especially of the thoracic limbs. Histologically, axonal spheroids are found in massive numbers throughout the brain and spinal cord, especially in the dorsal horns of the spinal cord and nucleus gracilis and nucleus cuneatus. The cerebellum is mildly atrophic in some dogs. Afferent fibers entering the sensory nuclei in the spinal cord, brain stem, and diencephalon are primarily affected. Electron microscopy has shown axonal spheroids to be enlarged distal portions of axons and synaptic terminals, containing accumulations of smooth membrane-bound vesicles, membranous lamellae, dense bodies, and other organelles. Histologic lesions may be mild in young dogs.

A recessive mode of inheritance with variable penetrance in rottweilers is suspected from preliminary breeding studies. Etiology and pathogenesis of distal membranous axonopathies are not understood, but location of lesions suggests a derangement in the presynaptic portion of neurons or abnormalities in axonal transport. Axonal dystrophies have been associated with toxins, nutritional deficiency, aging, and genetic disorders in other species and humans. A progressive neuroaxonal dystrophy has been reported to occur in a Jack Russell terrier pup, with pathologic alterations similar to those reported in rottweilers.[242]

Clinical Findings. Affected dogs may be clumsy as puppies, or clinical signs may not be seen until dogs are more than 12 months of age. Both male and female dogs are affected. Clinical signs may progress slowly over several years. The initial clinical finding is progressive ataxia of all limbs. Paresis or abnormalities in conscious proprioception

have not been found in affected dogs. Patellar reflexes may be exaggerated; however, other reflexes are normal. These findings are consistent with a transverse myelopathy of the cervical spinal cord or multifocal spinal cord disease. As the disease progresses, other signs become apparent, including hypermetria (especially of the thoracic limbs), incoordination, tremors of the head, positional nystagmus, decreased menace response, and crossed extensor reflexes. Thoracic limb hypermetria may be severe in older dogs, especially when climbing stairs. The neurologic deficits seen in older dogs are predominantly referable to abnormalities in the cerebellum or input to the cerebellum.

Diagnosis. Diagnosis is made on the basis of age, breed, and neurologic findings and by ruling out other causes of cervical spinal cord and cerebellar disease. This disease is unusual in that it is slowly progressive over several years, but in the initial stages may appear clinically similar to other causes of a cervical myelopathy, including CD myelitis and cervical spondylomyelopathy. Cerebrospinal fluid may have an elevated protein concentration (40 mg/dL was reported in one dog[240]). Spinal radiographs and myelograms are normal.

Treatment. Currently, treatment is not effective. Clinical improvement has not been detected during treatment with corticosteroids. Owing to the slow progression of the disease, affected dogs may be acceptable pets for several years. Affected dogs should not be used for breeding, although a diagnosis of neuroaxonal dystrophy may not be made until after these dogs have produced litters.

OSTEOCHONDROMATOSIS (MULTIPLE CARTILAGINOUS EXOSTOSES)

Etiology and Pathogenesis. A skeletal osteochondroma is a cartilage-capped exostosis arising from the surface of a bone formed by endochondral ossification. An animal with a monostotic lesion has a solitary osteochondroma. Polyostotic skeletal involvement is called osteochondromatosis (synonyms: multiple cartilaginous exostoses, hereditary multiple exostoses, multiple osteochondromatosis, diaphyseal aclasis, dyschondroplasia, and hereditary deforming chondrodysplasia). There are consistent differences between cats and dogs regarding age of onset of lesions, patterns of skeletal involvement, and pathogenesis.[243, 244]

The incidence of feline osteochondromatosis is unknown.[7] Feline osteochondromatosis is characterized by an initial appearance of lesions in the skeleton of mature cats (2 to 4 years of age). Growth of the lesions is progressive. The disease has no apparent sex or breed predilection in cats, and a hereditary pattern has not been demonstrated in cats. Malignant transformation to osteosarcoma has been reported to occur in an osteochondroma of a cervical vertebra in a cat.

The incidence of osteochondromatosis in dogs remains undetermined. The disease is frequently demonstrated in the skeleton of dogs radiographed for unrelated reasons. Onset of clinical disease is usually in dogs less than 18 months of age.[245] Onset in mature dogs is infrequently recognized.[246] A hereditary basis has been indicated in dogs, although a sex or breed predilection is not apparent. Continued growth or reactivation of growth of exostoses in dogs is suggestive of neoplastic transformation.

The etiology of canine osteochondromatosis is unknown. The current view regarding pathogenesis of feline osteochondromatosis is that the disease is virus related and probably virus induced. The random distribution of lesions is compatible with a hematogenous distribution of a virus. The virus may be FeLV, feline fibrosarcoma virus acting in an atypical manner, or another member of the feline retrovirus family.

Clinical Findings. Osteochondromatosis may occur anywhere in the vertebral column but most commonly is found in the thoracic and lumbar spine. The disease may result in spinal cord compression and clinical signs indicative of a progressive transverse myelopathy between T3 and L3. Neurologic deficits are often asymmetric.

Diagnosis. Radiographically, vertebral lesions tend to be circular and smooth, with sclerotic borders. Lesions are usually multiple and may be cystic or proliferative, with an increased radiodensity. Myelography is necessary to demonstrate associated spinal cord compression. Extension of exostoses into the spinal canal results in extradural compression of the spinal cord. Surgical biopsy is necessary to differentiate osteochondromatosis from benign bone tumors (osteomas), neoplastic lesions, or infectious processes.

Treatment. Treatment of canine osteochondromatosis affecting the vertebral column is unnecessary unless a lesion results in clinical sequelae. An osteochondroma should be removed if it impinges on the spinal cord, or if malignant transformation is suspected. Surgical excision of cartilaginous exostoses and spinal cord decompression are the recommended treatments for lesions causing spinal cord compression and neurologic deficits. Intraoperative spinal stabilization may be indicated following lesion removal.[247] The prognosis for dogs that have stopped growing is good; however, the prognosis for animals that are still growing is guarded, as lesions may continue to expand and subsequently result in spinal cord compression.

Treatment of feline osteochondromatosis is complicated by the association with FeLV and the progressive nature of lesions in cats. It seems that at best the surgical removal of a lesion may provide only temporary relief to a cat, because of the tendency for excised lesions to recur and for new lesions to develop.

PILONIDAL SINUS, EPIDERMOID CYST, AND DERMOID CYST (DERMOID SINUS, PILONIDAL CYST)

Etiology and Pathogenesis. A pilonidal sinus is an invagination of the skin dorsal to the spine, extending below the skin to variable depths and in some cases as far as the dura mater, where it may communicate with the subarachnoid space. The formation of pilonidal sinuses is related to failure of complete separation of the neural groove from the epidermis during embryonic development. Pilonidal sinuses may occur anywhere along the dorsal midline from cervical to sacrocaudal regions and may be single or multiple. Purebred and crossbred Rhodesian ridgeback dogs are most commonly affected, although other breeds of dogs may be affected.[248] There have not been reports of sinuses occurring along the ridge of hair of Rhodesian ridgebacks. The sinuses contain inspissated sebum, hair, and exfoliated cells and commonly become inflamed or infected. If sinuses communicate with the subarachnoid space, extension of infection results in meningitis or myelitis. Pilonidal sinuses are likely to occur as a hereditary defect in Rhodesian ridgebacks, but the mode of inheritance is not definitely known.[6]

Dermoid cysts have been reported to occur in the brain and spinal cord of dogs and cats.[249] In one report, a dermoid cyst in the spinal cord of a cat at the level of T3 was considered a congenital anomaly.[1]

Epidermoid cysts have been reported to occur in the brain and spinal cord of dogs.[191] Such cysts are thought to arise from entrapment and subsequent growth of primordial epithelial cells during closure of the neural tube. Morphologically similar cysts have developed in humans following injury or after repeated lumbar subarachnoid punctures for CSF collection, presumably from mechanical implantation of epidermal cells. An intramedullary spinal epidermoid cyst reported in a dog was thought to have a congenital cause. Apparently, spinal epidermoid cysts rarely occur in dogs.[250]

Clinical Findings. Clinical signs of meningitis and myelitis may be seen in animals as a result of extension of infection from a pilonical sinus to the subarachnoid space. Localized or generalized spinal pain and rigidity may be seen associated with meningitis. Neurologic deficits indicative of a transverse or diffuse myelopathy may be seen as a result of myelitis. Signs resulting from a spinal dermoid or epidermoid cyst depend on its location.

Diagnosis. A pilonidal sinus may be palpable as a cord of fibrous tissue under the skin of the dorsal midline. Palpation may be painful if the sinus is infected. An opening in the skin on the dorsal midline is usually found, and hair may or may not be seen protruding from this opening. CSF in animals with meningitis or myelitis is generally abnormal and indicative of bacterial infection. Fistulography performed by injecting a radiographic contrast material such as metrizamide, which is not an irritant to nervous tissue, into the sinus demonstrates whether pilonidal sinuses are continuous with the subarachnoid space. Myelography may also demonstrate communication.

Diagnosis of a spinal dermoid or epidermoid cyst is based on clinical signs and results of plain spinal radiography, CSF analysis, and myelography. Typically an epidermoid cyst should be suspected in the presence of an intramedullary, expansile lesion on myelography in a young dog with progressive neurologic deficits. Diagnosis is confirmed by means of an open surgical biopsy, which may provide the only means to rule out spinal neoplasia (e.g., spinal cord blastoma). Advanced imaging (CT or MRI) may be useful in fully delineating the extent and location of these cystic structures.

Treatment. Animals with meningitis and/or myelitis associated with a pilonidal sinus should be treated as an animal with meningitis and myelitis due to another cause. Antibiotic therapy should be selected on the basis of CSF culture, culture of the contents of the pilonidal sinus, and sensitivity testing. Complete surgical excision of the pilonidal sinus is essential.[251] Laminectomy may be necessary to remove portions of a pilonidal sinus from within the spinal canal. Recurrence of infection is likely in dogs in which a pilonidal sinus is incompletely removed. Prognosis depends on the severity of neurologic deficits prior to surgery, the response to antibiotic therapy, and whether or not the pilonidal sinus is removed completely. Complications of surgical removal include wound dehiscence and seroma formation. Affected animals should not be used for breeding.

Treatment of spinal dermoid or epidermoid cysts of dogs has not been reported. Surgical excision may be possible in some animals.

PROGRESSIVE HEMORRHAGIC MYELOMALACIA

Etiology and Pathogenesis. Acute, severe spinal cord injury may result in progressive ascending and descending infarction and hemorrhagic necrosis of the spinal cord parenchyma. Progressive hemorrhagic myelomalacia (PHM) occurs infrequently and usually follows peracute explosive extrusion of a thoracolumbar disk, but may also be seen in animals after other types of spinal cord trauma.[6] This condition previously has been termed "hematomyelia." The majority of dogs with thoracolumbar disk extrusions have evidence of a localized myelopathy affecting up to four spinal cord segments. In animals with PHM, hemorrhagic necrosis of a large number of spinal cord segments may occur over a period of hours to days. Etiology of this syndrome is not known; however, spinal cord pathology indicates severe ischemia.

Clinical Findings. Clinical signs depend on the location of the lesion; however, most affected animals initially have clinical signs indicative of a transverse myelopathy between T3 and L3. Neurologic deficits usually are severe (paraplegia and absent deep pain perception in pelvic limbs) and peracute in onset (over several hours). Clinical signs indicating a diffuse myelopathy progress over a period of hours to 1 to 2 days. As infarction and hemorrhagic necrosis of the spinal cord progress caudally, LMN signs may be seen in the pelvic limbs and anus. As PHM progresses cranially, the level of cutaneous anesthesia and LMN signs in intercostal muscles extend cranially until thoracic limbs exhibit LMN signs. The Schiff-Sherrington sign may be present prior to involvement of the spinal cord cranial to T3. Diaphragmatic paralysis and bilateral Horner's syndrome may be seen with involvement of the cervical spinal cord. Affected animals often are in extreme pain, are anxious, and have an increased body temperature.

Diagnosis. A diagnosis is made on the basis of progressive clinical signs indicative of a diffuse myelopathy. Any animal with an acute onset of paraplegia due to a lesion between T3 and L3 that shows LMN signs in the pelvic or thoracic limbs should be suspected of having more than one lesion, or PHM.

Treatment. In most cases, PHM is fatal within 24 to 48 hours as a result of respiratory paralysis. Effective medical or surgical treatments do not exist, and euthanasia is recommended. Difficulty often arises when treating animals that have an acute onset of paraplegia, with or without deep pain perception, within hours after the onset of clinical signs. Ideally, if decompressive surgery is indicated, it should be performed as soon as possible; however, a small percentage of these cases may show clinical signs of PHM after surgery. Hemorrhagic myelomalacia in some cases may not progress to involve the cervical cord, and affected animals may survive; however, the spinal cord damage incurred and associated severe neurologic deficits are permanent.

PROTOZOAL MYELITIS

Etiology and Pathogenesis. *Toxoplasma gondii* is an obligate intracellular coccidian parasite. Cats are the only known definitive host of the organism and, as such, pass environmentally resistant oocysts in feces. The seroprevalence of infection varies by region but is approximately 30 per cent in cats in the United States. Despite this high seroprevalence, clinical disease caused by *T. gondii* is rare.[252, 253]

T. gondii infection may cause a focal or disseminated myelopathy in dogs or cats.[6] Animals are infected after ingesting meat containing toxoplasma bradyzoites and/or tachyzoites, after ingesting cat feces containing sporulated oocysts, or by transplacental or congenital infection. The infective organism is spread hematogenously to most organs of the body, including the CNS. Although the incidence of disease associated with *T. gondii* is low, opportunistic infection in immunosuppressed animals may be more widespread than previously reported. Immaturity and concurrent CD virus infection may result in an increased susceptibility of dogs to toxoplasmosis. In dogs with systemic toxoplasmosis, the incidence of CNS involvement is high. In cats, concurrent infection with FeLV or FIV or administration of corticosteroids may predispose to the development of clinical signs of toxoplasmosis through immunosuppression and reactivation of latent infection.[254–256]

Neospora caninum is a recently discovered, cyst-forming coccidium in the phylum Apicomplexa that is structurally similar to, but distinct from, *T. gondii*.[257–264] This protozoal parasite is associated most commonly with natural infection in dogs and cattle. The organism forms meronts in many tissues of dogs, especially brain and spinal cord, resulting in meningoencephalomyelitis. Clinical signs result from host cell death following rapid intracellular multiplication of the parasite and ensuing inflammatory response of the host. Cats have been infected experimentally and have been shown to develop clinical disease. *N. caninum* organisms do not react to *Toxoplasma* immunoperoxidase staining techniques, and the life cycle is unknown. Clinically, this protozoal disease appears similar to toxoplasmosis; however, CNS signs (progressive ascending paralysis) and myositis are seen more commonly than in toxoplasmosis, and *T. gondii* almost always has been associated with concurrent disease in dogs (e.g., canine distemper infection), whereas *N. caninum* appears to be a primary pathogen.

Clinical Findings. Animals with CNS involvement by *T. gondii* usually have clinical signs of progressive multifocal or disseminated disease. Clinical signs indicating a focal transverse or diffuse myelopathy may be seen initially. Neurologic deficits depend on site of involvement and may be UMN or LMN. If lower motor neurons are involved, denervation may result in severe muscle atrophy.

In dogs less than 1 year of age, a syndrome of progressive paralysis and rigid extension of one or both pelvic limbs may be seen in association with *T. gondii* infection. Muscle atrophy and contracture of affected limbs are seen, and limbs cannot be flexed. Muscle changes may be the result of myositis and myonecrosis and/or denervation as a result of myelitis or radiculitis in the caudal lumbar and sacral spinal cord segments. Animals with CNS toxoplasmosis may or may not have other clinical signs indicative of systemic infection (fever, lymphadenopathy, pneumonia, apparent muscle pain, gastrointestinal tract disease, iritis, or chorioretinitis).

Overall, neosporosis is an increasingly prevalent infectious disease that merits consideration in juvenile and adult dogs with progressive paraparesis. Neosporosis may cause fatal disease in dogs of all ages (several weeks to 15 years). Puppies are affected more severely than older dogs. Young dogs develop an ascending paralysis, with pelvic limbs affected more severely than thoracic limbs. Other signs of dysfunction include difficulty in swallowing, paralysis of the jaw, muscle flaccidity, and muscle atrophy.

Diagnosis. Antemortem confirmation of CNS toxoplasmosis or neosporosis in dogs or cats is extremely difficult and may be tentatively based on all of the following: (1) demonstration of serologic evidence of infection, (2) clinical signs of disease referable to toxoplasmosis or neosporosis, (3) exclusion of other common causes of these clinical signs, and (4) positive response to appropriate treatment (see Chapters 84 and 87).

Treatment. Several antibacterial agents have been recommended for treatment of toxoplasmosis and neosporosis in dogs and cats (see Chapter 87).

SACROCAUDAL DYSGENESIS IN MANX CATS

Etiology and Pathogenesis. Manx cats have varying degrees of taillessness associated with sacral and/or caudal vertebral deformities.[6, 7, 267] Some tailless cats have a normal sacrum, spinal cord, and cauda equina. Others show varying dysgenesis or agenesis of the sacral and/or caudal vertebrae that may be associated with spina bifida and/or malformations of the terminal spinal cord and/or cauda equina. Spinal cord malformations include absence or partial development of sacral and caudal spinal cord segments or cauda equina, myelodysplasia, meningocele, meningomyelocele, diastematomyelia of sacral segments (duplication), myeloschisis (cleft within the spinal cord), syringomyelia in the lumbar and sacral spinal cord segments, shortening of the spinal cord, and subcutaneous cyst formation. These spinal cord and cauda equina malformations are associated with a variety of neurologic deficits.

Sacrocaudal dysgenesis is inherited as an autosomal dominant trait and may be lethal in some homozygote cats. Sacrocaudal dysgenesis and associated malformations have been recognized in most breeds of cats, many not of true Manx breeding.

Clinical Findings. Clinical signs are variable depending on the degree of spinal cord and cauda equina malformation and include paraparesis, paraplegia, megacolon, atonic bladder, absent anal and urinary bladder sphincter tone, absent anal reflex, urinary and fecal incontinence, and perineal analgesia. Affected cats often walk plantigrade in the pelvic limbs with a "bunny-hopping" gait. Vertebral abnormalities may be palpable in the lumbosacral region, and in some cats a meningocele, congenital or the result of necrosis of the overlying skin, may exit through the skin and drain CSF.

Clinical signs usually are evident soon after birth and may remain static or may be progressive. Worsening of neurologic deficits may be due to progressive syringomyelia in the lumbar and sacral spinal cord.

Diagnosis. Diagnosis is made on the basis of clinical findings and radiographic findings indicative of dysgenesis or agenesis of the sacral and caudal vertebrae. Myelography may demonstrate meningocele or attachment of spinal cord to subcutaneous tissues in the lumbosacral region. The degree of spinal deformity does not always correspond with the degree of neurologic impairment. Clinical findings are the most important factors to consider in determining prognosis.

Treatment. Prognosis for severely affected cats is hopeless, and treatment is not available. Cats with urinary and fecal incontinence may be managed with manual bladder expression and fecal softening agents; however, recurrent urinary tract infection, megacolon, and chronic constipation are common problems. Meningocele in cats with minimal neurologic deficits may be surgically correctable. Many tailless cats do not have neurologic deficits, and sacral and caudal deformities often are an incidental radiographic finding.

SPINA BIFIDA

Etiology and Pathogenesis. Spina bifida occurs in both dogs and cats and describes a group of developmental defects characterized by failure of fusion of the vertebral arches with or without protrusion or dysplasia of the spinal cord and meninges.[6, 7] This defect is part of the complex of spinal dysraphism and is the most commonly occurring dysraphic defect. Dysraphism (*raphe* [Greek], seam) means defective fusion of parts that normally unite. Spina bifida is the absence of a portion of the dorsal elements of the vertebrae. The spinal cord and meninges may be normal (spina bifida occulta), or may be abnormal and there may be protrusion of the meninges and/or spinal cord through the vertebral defect.

Myelodysplasia consisting of hydromyelia, syringomyelia, anomalies of the dorsal septum, anomalies of the central grey matter, abnormal position of the central grey matter, anomalies of the dorsal and ventral horns, and myeloschisis (cleft in the dorsal part of the spinal cord) may occur in association with spina bifida. The most severe defects involve myelorachischisis, with superficial location of the neuroectoderm that is continuous with the skin. Spina bifida with myelorachischisis has been reported to occur in dogs and cats.

Etiology of spina bifida is unknown and probably multifactorial with genetic and environmental components. The relatively high incidence of spina bifida in some breeds of animals (e.g., bulldogs and Manx cats) suggests a heritable basis to the disorder. Teratogenic compounds, nutritional deficiencies, and environmental changes during pregnancy are also known to induce this defect.

Clinical Findings. Spina bifida is usually an incidental radiographic finding; however, if associated with spinal cord malformations, it may result in clinical signs of spinal cord or cauda equina dysfunction. There is a high incidence of spine bifida in English bulldogs. Spina bifida may occur anywhere in the spinal column but occurs most commonly in the caudal lumbar spine where clinical signs are indicative of a transverse myelopathy from L4 to S3 spinal cord segments. Clinical signs usually become evident when affected animals start to walk.

Spina bifida also has been reported in the thoracic spine of a dog and may be associated with other spinal deformities such as scoliosis. Other associated anomalies include dimpling of the skin or "streaming" (abnormal direction) of the haircoat over the affected region or a palpable abnormality in the spinal column. Meningoceles may cause necrosis of the overlying skin and drainage of CSF. Meningoceles may be present in the absence of clinical signs associated with spinal cord malformation.

Diagnosis. Radiographically, absence of the vertebral arch or failure of fusion of the spinous processes in one or more vertebrae may be seen (Fig. 106–15). Myelography may demonstrate meningocele. Advanced imaging (CT or MRI) may be used to accurately define location and extent of bony and soft tissue abnormalities in animals with spina bifida.

Treatment. Treatment of spina bifida rarely is attempted. Treatment is not effective for affected animals with clinical signs of spinal cord malformation. Meningocele may be amenable to surgery if neurologic abnormalities are not evident. Treatment is not necessary for animals with vertebral defects in the absence of spinal cord dysfunction. In planning therapy, the potential for additional spinal cord malformations (e.g., hydromyelia) seen in association with spina bifida must be considered.

SPINAL INTRA-ARACHNOID CYSTS

Etiology and Pathogenesis. Intra-arachnoid cysts are intra-arachnoid membrane accumulations of CSF that may

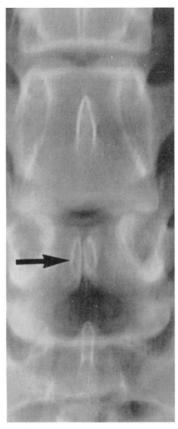

Figure 106–15. Spina bifida. Ventrodorsal radiograph of the caudal lumbar vertebral column of an 8-year-old spayed female chow. A deficit in fusion of the embryologic neural tube has resulted in nonfusion of the spinous process of L7 (arrow). This congenital defect was an incidental finding in this dog.

occur in any location along the cerebrospinal axis of cats or dogs.[268–273] The intra-arachnoid accumulation of CSF within the cyst results in expansion of the cyst between the overlying dura mater and underlying pia mater, causing compression of the spinal cord. Intra-arachnoid cysts may be congenital in origin or may occur secondary to trauma, infection, inflammation, or subarachnoid hemorrhage.

Clinical Findings. A single intra-arachnoid cyst has been described in either the cranial cervical or caudal thoracic spinal canal. This author (RAL) has diagnosed multiple intra-arachnoid cysts in the caudal cervical region of three rottweiler dogs. Neurologic deficits were indicative of a progressive transverse myelopathy in either the C1–C5 or T3–L3 spinal cord region. Apparent cervical pain and spasms of the cervical muscles were a feature of cervical lesions; however, apparent pain was not evident in dogs with thoracic lesions. Neurologic deficits may be asymmetric.

Diagnosis. Diagnosis is made on the basis of results of myelography or advanced imaging (CT or MRI). Surgical findings and histopathologic examination of excised tissues are used for confirmation of the diagnosis.

Plain radiographs of the spine may be normal or may show enlargement of the vertebral canal with smooth cortical margins presumably as a result of pressure atrophy of bone overlying the cyst. Abnormalities in CSF analysis have not been reported. Care should be taken in attempting a cisternal subarachnoid puncture in an animal suspected of having a cervical arachnoid cyst, as lesions may be located on the dorsal midline. One reported dog was injured inadvertently during attempted cisternal puncture.

On myelography, pooling of contrast material within the subarachnoid space, resulting in a characteristic widening of the subarachnoid space and spinal cord compression, may be seen (Fig. 106–16). In all reported cases, lesions have been intradural-extramedullary and located on the dorsal midline. This author (RAL) has seen intra-arachnoid cysts in dorsolateral and ventral locations in the cervical region of dogs. Lesions may extend over more than one spinal cord segment.

Advanced imaging (CT or MRI) may be used to fully delineate intra-arachnoid cysts. Although intra-arachnoid cysts have a characteristic appearance on advanced imaging, they must be differentiated from other cystic lesions (e.g., cystic neoplasms or cysts associated with infections).

Treatment. Surgical exploration is necessary to confirm a diagnosis of intra-arachnoid cyst and to decompress the spinal cord. Complete surgical excision of an intra-arachnoid cyst usually is not possible. Partial excision of an intra-arachnoid cyst (also called surgical fenestration) may result

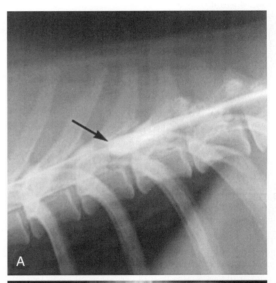

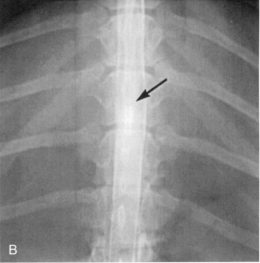

Figure 106–16. Spinal intra-arachnoid cyst. Lateral *(A)* and ventrodorsal *(B)* projections of a myelogram of the mid-thoracic region of a 2-year-old toy poodle that had a 1-year history of progressive pelvic limb paresis and ataxia. Note widening of the dorsal subarachnoid contrast column present at T9–T10 on the lateral projection (arrow). There is apparent intramedullary expansion of this area on the ventrodorsal projection (arrow). An intra-arachnoid cyst was removed by means of a dorsal laminectomy.

in decompression of the spinal cord and permanent clinical improvement.

SPINAL NEMATODIASIS

Etiology and Pathogenesis. Aberrant migration and growth of parasites within the spinal canal rarely occur in dogs or cats. The route of migration of most parasites that enter the CNS is unknown, with the exception of hematogenous-borne *Dirofilaria immitis*. Parasites may cause extensive damage to neural parenchyma as a result of infarction, spinal cord compression, or granuloma formation. Parasites reported to occur in CNS of dogs include *D. immitis, Toxocara canis* larvae, *Angiostrongylus cantonensis* (rat lungworm of Australia), *Ancylostoma caninum* (Australia),[274-276] *Baylisascaris* sp.,[277] and *Spirocerca lupi*.[278]

Clinical Findings. Clinical signs depend on location of the migrating parasite. Lesions may be focal or multifocal. Spinal nematodiasis usually is seen in immature animals, with the exception of *D. immitis*. Clinical signs often have an acute onset and usually are progressive. Clinical signs rarely occur with aberrant *Toxocara* migration in dogs; however, a single *Toxocara* larva has been found in the cauda equina of a dog. Clinical signs reported associated with *Angiostrongylus cantonensis* in the dog include paraparesis, paraplegia, urinary and fecal incontinence, paralysis of the tail, and apparent pain. *Ancylostoma caninum* migration in the spinal cord has been reported to result in paraparesis, apparent neck pain, and tetraplegia.

Diagnosis. Definite diagnosis is difficult antemortem because it requires isolation or demonstration of the parasite within the CNS.

An increase in white blood cell count, especially eosinophils, and/or protein may be present in the CSF.[275] Affected animals usually have a large parasite burden, and nematode eggs or larvae may be found in the feces. Dogs with *D. immitis* infestation may have circulating microfilaria. Lesions may be located by means of myelography or advanced imaging (CT or MRI).

Treatment. Prognosis for animals with spinal nematodiasis depends on the severity of resulting neurologic deficits, and usually is poor. Medical therapy often is ineffective in eliminating parasites in the CNS. Surgical removal of *Dirofilaria immitis* adults from the spinal epidural space has been reported.

SPINAL CORD TRAUMA

Etiology and Pathogenesis. Acute spinal cord injuries of dogs or cats result most commonly from direct physical trauma such as missile injury or vertebral fracture or luxation. Also, spinal cord trauma is the underlying cause of neurologic signs in numerous myelopathies (e.g., intervertebral disk disease). Chronic spinal cord compression usually is seen in association with chronic progressive diseases such as neoplasia or type II disk protrusion.[279] Following injury, the spinal cord may undergo sustained compression, distraction, or both. The severity of a spinal cord injury, as determined by the eventual degree and quality of recovery, is related to three factors: the *velocity* with which the compressive force is applied, the *degree* of compression (transverse deformation), and the *duration* of the compression. An understanding of differences between acute and chronic spinal cord injury is essential for effective management and determination of prognosis in cats or dogs with spinal trauma.[280]

Acute Spinal Cord Injury. Blunt traumatic injury to the spinal cord causes neurologic deficits through both *direct* and *indirect* mechanisms. The direct effects are due to immediate mechanical disruption of neural pathways and have been considered by most investigators not to be amenable to therapy. Indirect effects develop during the first few hours following injury and result in delayed secondary injury to the spinal cord. It is likely that they result in part from release of endogenous pathophysiologic factors in response to the initial trauma and that such factors produce injury by reducing spinal cord blood flow or by altering the local metabolic environment within injured spinal cord tissue. The spinal cord remains physically intact but is functionally deranged. A common feature of acute spinal cord injury is early, often progressive hemorrhage in the central region of the injured spinal cord, especially in the grey matter. Direct mechanical disruption of vessels at the site of injury is expected; however, the loss of circulation spreads for a considerable distance cranial and caudal to the site of injury. Angiographic studies have consistently shown that the large arteries remain patent and the major loss of microcirculation involves capillaries and venules. The secondary damage has been considered potentially reversible through the use of either physical (e.g., hypothermia) or pharmacologic interventions.

Trauma to the spinal cord triggers a series of progressive, autodestructive events that lead to varying degrees of tissue necrosis, depending on the severity of the injury.[280] In spite of extensive investigation, the mechanisms responsible for the initiation and propagation of these pathophysiologic and biochemical events remain undetected. Recent evidence suggests, however, that the overall initiator of this autodestructive cascade of events is mechanical deformation of any type (i.e., impact or compression injury), and that the primary sites of injury are the cellular and subcellular membranes of glia, neurons, and vascular endothelial cells. Lipid peroxidation and activation of membrane lipases, with release of fatty acids leading to production of eicosanoids, are the earliest mechanically stimulated biochemical events described.

Within 5 minutes of spinal cord injury, postcapillary venules become congested. This is followed by opening of endothelial gap junctions here and at the capillary level, resulting in diapedesis of red blood cells and extravasation of fluid proteins and electrolytes through the "leaky" vasculature. Within 30 minutes of injury, microscopic hemorrhages appear in the central grey matter and coalesce over the following several hours (central hemorrhagic necrosis). Vacuolization develops within endothelial cells, indicating a profound ischemic or hypoxic insult, that subsequently leads to coagulative necrosis of the neuronal population. Adjacent white matter is relatively less severely affected; however, periaxonal swelling and retraction balls may be observed. These events may lead to autodissolution of the spinal cord within 24 hours, even in the absence of ongoing mechanical compression.

These phenomena would appear to have an ischemic basis, and considerable effort has been expended in characterizing the associated microcirculatory alterations. Causes of the ischemia include direct mechanical irritation causing vasospasm and biochemical damage due to release of glutamate, intracellular calcium, catecholamines, and prostaglandins. Other studies point to intravascular thrombosis, possibly owing to release of thromboxane, as an additional cause of posttraumatic ischemia. One of the most damaging biochemical alterations to the injured spinal cord is the accumulation of the excitatory amino acid neurotransmitter glutamate. Glutamate also causes an elevation of intracellular calcium that may in turn cause activation of calcium-dependent proteases or lipases, leading to further breakdown of cytoskeletal components.

A special feature of acute spinal cord injury is progressive hemorrhagic myelomalacia. This condition may occur following spinal cord injury, and appears to be a progression of central hemorrhagic necrosis and edema to areas of the spinal cord not directly involved in the initiating injury.

Chronic Spinal Cord Compression. It has been shown experimentally that when slow compression of the spinal cord is compared with rapid compression of an equal amount, the extent of spinal cord dysfunction is determined by the contact velocity of compression. The major pathologic substrate for neural dysfunction after slow balloon compression is thought to be physical injury to the neural membranes, irrespective of blood flow changes, and the ability of that membrane to recover appears to be related to rapidity and duration of compression. Clinical observations support the conclusion that spinal cord conduction is resistant to slow compression. Further, it has been demonstrated that levels of compression that do not have an effect when applied slowly cause an immediate loss of conduction through the injured site when applied rapidly.[281]

Chronic spinal cord compression results either from a slowly developing lesion (e.g., neoplasia), or from an acute compression that is sustained. In contrast to acute spinal cord injury, chronic compression injury affects white matter more severely than it affects grey matter. Hemorrhage and edema, the major findings of acute trauma, are not significant in chronic compression. Characteristic lesions are degeneration of myelin, focal areas of malacia, vacuolization, and loss of white matter axons. Mechanical deformation is likely to be the major factor in pathogenesis of these lesions; however, ischemia and venous obstruction also may be important considerations.

Clinical Findings

Acute Spinal Cord Injury. Dogs or cats with a spinal injury frequently have serious injuries to other organ systems. A primary concern is to balance the relative urgency of non-neurologic injuries (hemorrhage, shock, airway obstruction, or limb fractures) and the need for early treatment of spinal cord injury.[279]

A complete neurologic examination is performed to localize the site(s) of injury and to determine severity. Careful palpation of the vertebral column may aid in identification of a vertebral fracture or luxation. Administration of tranquilizers or analgesic drugs should be delayed until completion of the neurologic examination, as such medications may alter an animal's responses. A neurologic examination should be performed with care to prevent further injury resulting from excessive movement of a vertebral instability.

Several aspects of the neurologic examination are of special importance in assessment of a dog or cat with a spinal cord injury. Recognition of the Schiff-Sherrington sign is important. Following trauma, this sign must be differentiated from other postures associated with cranial injury (e.g. decerebrate rigidity or decerebellate posture). Both deep and cutaneous pain perception should be assessed, as results of these tests are important in determining prognosis. It should be remembered that vertebral column injuries may be multiple, and that a neurologic examination may not indicate presence of a second lesion.

Chronic Spinal Cord Compression. Clinical signs of chronic spinal cord compression may progress over weeks or months, or may be seen to occur acutely. Acute onset of neurologic signs with chronic spinal cord compression frequently is seen in association with such disorders as spinal neoplasia or type II disk protrusion. Sudden onset of signs may accompany pathologic fracture of a vertebra, and spinal cord hemorrhage or infarction. In some cases, sudden decompensation of a chronically compressed spinal cord may occur in the absence of pathologic changes. In these cases, it is assumed that compensatory mechanisms within the spinal cord are exhausted, and that sudden decompensation has occurred.

Diagnosis

Acute Spinal Cord Injury. Results of a neurologic examination are used to determine the site and severity of a spinal injury. Radiographs of the entire spinal column should be taken. Two radiographic views are essential only when ventrodorsal views may be accomplished by means of a horizontal beam. The objectives of radiographic examination of an animal following acute spinal trauma are the following: precise determination of location and extent of a lesion, demonstration of multiple lesions that may not be apparent on the basis of a neurologic examination, and assessment of the need for surgical therapy and determination of the most appropriate surgical procedure to be used. Accurate interpretation of radiographs depends on a knowledge of results of a neurologic examination.

Completion of a myelogram is recommended in animals that have sustained spinal trauma. Results of a myelogram may determine the extent of spinal cord swelling resulting from concussion in animals without evidence of a spinal fracture or luxation, and may confirm that surgical decompression by means of laminectomy is not necessary in animals with a fracture that is evident on plain radiographs. In the diagnosis of intervertebral disk disease, a myelogram is essential prior to surgery.

The use of advanced imaging (CT or MRI) in acute spinal cord injury patients may be reserved for those patients in which results of the above diagnostic techniques do not fully explain results of a neurologic examination.

Chronic Spinal Cord Compression. Methods for diagnosis of chronic spinal cord compression are the same as for acute spinal cord injury. A myelogram is considered essential in all such cases.

Treatment. Management of an animal with spinal trauma follows a list of priorities, with the focus of treatment being prevention of secondary spinal cord damage that occurs after the initial injury. Immediate treatment of non-neural injuries is limited to those problems that are life-threatening, such as shock or hemorrhage.

Acute Spinal Cord Injury. Treatment of acute spinal cord trauma should always be instituted as soon as possible following injury. The specific objectives of therapy are relief of edema, control of intra- or extramedullary hemorrhage, relief of spinal cord compression, and, in cases of vertebral fracture/luxation, removal of bone fragments from the spinal canal and realignment and stabilization of the vertebral column. Treatment of acute spinal cord trauma may be medical, surgical, or a combination of both. The goal of medical therapy is to control the chemical and vascular changes that result in secondary spinal cord injury. Numerous drugs have been described for the treatment of spinal cord injury; however, the efficacy of many of these drugs in the treatment of spinal cord injury remains undetermined.

Corticosteroids are routinely and widely used in the treatment of acute spinal cord injury. Despite a positive clinical impression that corticosteroids have beneficial effects, their use is controversial. Some studies have failed to demonstrate significant improvement of neurologic recovery in association with corticosteroid administration. The use of low versus high doses of corticosteroids in the treatment of spinal trauma also has yielded conflicting results. The use of corticosteroids may result in complications leading to increased morbidity and mortality (e.g., gastrointestinal bleeding, pancreatitis, colonic perforation).

The only corticosteroid with proven efficacy in the management of spinal cord injury is methylprednisolone sodium succinate (MPSS). MPSS has been studied intensely in both the research and clinical setting for the past 10 years.[282-289] The drug must be administered as soon as possible after injury, and the effective dose range and time after injury when the drug may be given are narrow. Spinal cord uptake of MPSS rapidly decreases with time after injury, probably owing to secondary post-traumatic tissue loss and progressive blood flow decrease to the injury site. The molecular mechanism of action of MPSS may involve intercalation into the cell membrane and suppression of lipid peroxidation and hydrolysis. The inhibition of injury-induced lipid peroxidation results in attenuation of progressive post-traumatic ischemia and hypoxia, together with reversal of intracellular calcium accumulation. MPSS also directly retards secondary neuronal degeneration. The beneficial effects of antioxidant doses of MPSS support the contention that post-traumatic lipid peroxidation is a critical degenerative mechanism that may be interrupted with an antioxidant agent.

Current recommendations in people are that patients with acute spinal cord injury that receive MPSS (30 mg/kg administered over 15 minutes) within 3 hours of injury be maintained on an infusion of 5.4 mg/kg per hour for 24 hours, and those that receive the initial bolus 3 to 8 hours post injury receive the infusion for 48 hours. Higher doses, and initiation of treatment more than 8 hours after injury, may exacerbate spinal cord damage. Complications include an increase in the incidence of pneumonia (2.6-fold in people) and gastrointestinal hemorrhage and perforation. While some experimental and clinical studies have found an improved recovery in research animals and people treated with MPSS following spinal cord injury, a number of other studies have not found a significant improvement. One of the conclusions of the Third National Acute Spinal Cord Injury Randomized Controlled Trial[284] was that although the improvements in spinal cord injury patients following MPSS treatment were statistically significant, the actual functional differences were relatively small and benefited upper body function as opposed to actual locomotion.

The 21-aminosteroid tirilazad mesylate is a potent inhibitor of lipid peroxidation. In the Third National Acute Spinal Cord Injury Randomized Controlled Trial,[284] tirilazad (2.5 mg/kg every 6 hours for 48 hours) administration (following an initial 30 mg/kg bolus of MPSS) to spinal cord injury patients resulted in motor recovery rates equivalent to those of patients who received MPSS for 24 hours. Reasons cited for the failure of the 48-hour tirilazad regimen to improve neurologic recovery as much as 48-hour MPSS included the possibility that there are important mechanisms other than lipid peroxidation in spinal cord injury and that a less than optimal dose was used. Another randomized controlled trial of the drug in spinal cord injured people is currently underway.

One of the most damaging effects of spinal cord injury is the accumulation of intracellular calcium in injured neurons,

and neuronal death is closely related to the rise in intracellular calcium. The administration of the calcium channel antagonists nimodipine or flunarizine following spinal cord injury has provided mixed results.

A decision regarding surgical therapy must be made as soon as non-neural injuries have been treated and medical management has been instituted. Ideally, this is within 2 hours of injury. Indications for surgery following spinal cord injury are moderate to severe paresis, or paralysis, associated with myelographic evidence of spinal cord compression; progressive worsening of neurologic signs despite adequate medical therapy; and luxation or fracture of the vertebral column in association with distraction, malalignment, instability, or myelographic evidence of spinal cord compression. Any animal with sustained compression of the spinal cord following injury, regardless of the cause, must be considered a candidate for surgical decompression of the spinal cord. In general, it is best to initiate surgical therapy in any animal in which there is uncertainty regarding the indications for surgical versus medical therapy. Neurosurgical procedures require specialized knowledge and equipment, and prompt referral to a qualified surgeon may be indicated.

The major objectives of surgical management of spinal trauma are decompression of sustained spinal cord compression and realignment and stabilization of vertebrae if necessary. Laminectomy alone is not sufficient for decompression in most cases, and the compressing mass (e.g., disk material, hematoma, bone fragments) should be removed when possible. In cases in which spinal cord swelling is the major source of compression, or in which there is discoloration of the spinal cord, durotomy or myelotomy may be combined with laminectomy.

Satisfactory methods of external fixation of spinal fractures in cats and dogs do not exist.[290] Use of polymethyl methacrylate and Steinmann pin fixation for the majority of spinal fractures or luxations is favored by this author (RAL).[291, 292] Surgical management of spinal cord injury of animals provides the best opportunity for rapid and complete recovery in animals with sustained compression or instability and facilitates postinjury care, as the risk of further injury resulting from movement of an unstable vertebral column is minimized. However, conservative management, including strict confinement for 4 to 6 weeks, may be efficacious in animals with minimal neurologic deficits and without myelographic evidence of sustained spinal cord compression or vertebral displacement or instability.

Regardless of the type of stabilization used, strict confinement is recommended for 6 weeks after surgery. Potential complications encountered in dogs or cats with a spinal injury include development of a urinary tract infection and pressure sores. Careful attention to nursing care is essential regardless of the type of therapy.[293]

Prognosis for an animal with an acute spinal cord injury depends on numerous factors; however, results of a neurologic examination should be the main determinant. Assessment of pain perception is essential for accurate prognosis. Perception of a painful stimulus must be differentiated from reflex activity that is mediated at the level of the spinal cord. Owners of affected animals should be made aware at the outset of therapy of factors such as prognosis, expense involved, expected time from treatment to recovery, and the need for prolonged physical therapy in most cases. Following a severe spinal injury, an animal may require many months to recover, and residual neurologic deficits may persist.

Chronic Spinal Cord Compression. The approach to treatment of chronic spinal cord compression is different from that for acute spinal cord injury. As previously stated, hemorrhage and edema usually are not prominent factors in chronic compression. Therefore, medical management by means of corticosteroids would not be expected to be efficacious; however, many animals with chronic spinal cord compression improve clinically following corticosteroid administration. The reason for such a response is undetermined; however, it may be due to effects of corticosteroids at the membrane level resulting in improved conduction in remaining axons. Occasionally, animals may be maintained for months or years by means of corticosteroid therapy alone.

Surgical decompression and stabilization should be considered in dogs or cats that have neurologic deficits associated with chronic spinal cord compression. Surgical decompression in such animals should be approached cautiously, as pathologic alterations within the spinal cord may be irreversible, and the most that may be achieved is to arrest progression of neurologic deficits. In some cases, compensation for the irreplaceable loss of neural tissue may occur. Neurologic status may be worsened by surgical decompression, even with meticulous surgical technique. Such deterioration may be the result of reactive hyperemia that follows decompression, which in turn results in vascular protein leakage in the affected spinal cord segments.

SPINAL STENOSIS

Etiology and Pathogenesis. Spinal stenosis is a term indicating a narrowed vertebral canal, which may produce a variety of neurologic syndromes.[31] Stenosis may be *focal*, *segmental* (affecting several adjacent vertebrae), or *generalized* (throughout the vertebral column). Spinal stenosis may result either from bony impingement on neural elements (congenital stenosis, developmental stenosis resulting from inborn errors in skeletal growth, idiopathic developmental stenosis, or acquired stenosis), or from compression of neural tissue by nonosseous components of the walls of the vertebral canal (hypertrophy of the dorsal longitudinal ligament or ligamentum flavum, or disk extrusion/protrusion).

Congenital Spinal Stenosis. Congenital stenosis may occur as a primary lesion, or may be seen in association with other congenital anomalies of the spinal cord or vertebral column.[294, 295] In dogs, congenital stenosis may occur in association with block vertebrae or hemivertebrae.[31] Congenital spinal stenosis has been reported in association with transitional vertebrae, especially at the lumbosacral junction of dogs.[31, 204] Despite the congenital origin of this stenosis, initial manifestation of clinical signs may not be seen until after an animal has reached skeletal maturity.

Thoracic Vertebral Canal Stenosis. Segmental vertebral stenosis frequently occurs in the cranial thoracic spine of several breeds of dog (e.g., Doberman pinscher).[31] Vertebrae T7 through T7 are affected most frequently. A decrease in the dorsoventral diameter of the vertebral canal (as compared with adjacent vertebrae) is seen, and spinal cord compression may be seen. Mild lordosis, kyphosis, or scoliosis may be seen in association with the stenosis.

Developmental Stenosis Resulting from Inborn Errors in Skeletal Growth. This condition has been reported to occur in dogs.[168] The term "inborn errors" indicates incoordination of ossification and bone growth as a result of hereditary transmission or fresh mutation of a normal gene.[31] The errors are based on metabolic or other disturbances of cells involved in skeletal development. The disproportionate

bone growth is already present at birth; however, the causative agents remain active during maturation. Therefore, the term "developmental" is used to distinguish this group from the congenital stenoses. These conditions result in generalized spinal stenosis, which is more pronounced in the lumbar vertebral column. The vertebrae have a narrowed vertebral canal; however, the spinal cord and cauda equina are of normal size. This results in a disproportion between the dimensions of the vertebral canal and the volume of its contents. The relative spinal stenosis of chondrodystrophic breeds of dog may contribute to the increased incidence of disk extrusions in these breeds. As with congenital stenosis, clinical signs may not develop until later in life and may be related to only a single level of the stenotic vertebral canal.

Idiopathic Developmental Stenosis. A genetic disturbance in which pathologic effects are apparent in their entirety only when growth is complete, and the vertebrae have attained full size, is termed "developmental."[31] Clinical signs of spinal stenosis may result should some additional factor (e.g., disk protrusion) compromise the available diameter of the spinal canal in adult life. Hypertrophy of bone of the vertebral arch or ligamenta flava may be present in this condition. This condition had been reported to occur in dogs.

Hypertrophy of the Nonosseous Components of the Vertebral Canal. Spinal stenosis resulting from ligamentous proliferation at C2–C3 has been reported in young rottweilers.[31, 296]

Clinical Findings. Clinical signs of spinal stenosis reflect the location of the lesion, regardless of the precise cause.

Diagnosis. The diagnosis of spinal stenosis is made primarily by radiography. Myelography is essential for the precise localization of spinal stenosis. Other contrast-enhanced radiographic techniques may be used to define stenosis affecting the lumbosacral junction. Advanced imaging (CT or MRI) may aid in the determination of location and extent of lesions associated with spinal stenosis.

Treatment. Treatment of spinal stenosis may be either medical or surgical. Relief of apparent pain by means of analgesic or anti-inflammatory drugs, combined with exercise restriction, may be adequate in dogs with mild clinical signs. In animals in which apparent pain persists or the stenotic condition worsens, decompressive surgery is indicated. Surgery is best performed early in the course of the disease. Internal spinal stabilization or fusion may be necessary in animals with instability evident on stress radiography, or in animals after extensive decompressive procedures.

SPONDYLOSIS DEFORMANS

Etiology and Pathogenesis. Spondylosis deformans is characterized by the formation of osteophytes (bony spurs) around the margins of vertebral endplates.[297] Osteophytes may form at one or multiple intervertebral disk spaces and may appear to bridge or almost bridge intervertebral disk spaces. The radiographic appearance of solid bony bridges may represent only an interdigitation of the adjacent osteophytes. Osteophyte production in spondylosis deformans is the noninflammatory bony response to degenerative changes in the intervertebral disks. These degenerative changes involve the anulus fibrosus and lead to the formation of intradiskal fissures.

The incidence and size of vertebral osteophytes increase with age. All breeds of dog are affected, although large canine breeds may have a higher incidence of spondylosis deformans.[298] The caudal thoracic, lumbar, and lumbosacral spinal segments are affected most frequently. Because these segments are areas of greatest spinal mobility, dynamic and mechanical factors may play a role in osteophyte formation. Spondylosis deformans is uncommon in the cervical and cranial thoracic segments in dogs. In cats, the incidence of spondylosis deformans forms a bell-shaped curve with the highest incidence at the level of T7–T8.

The terms ankylosing spondylosis or ankylosing spondylitis have been used by some authors to describe spondylosis deformans, despite the fact that it is not an inflammatory condition and ankylosis is uncommon.

Clinical Findings. In most affected animals, spondylosis deformans is not of clinical significance. Rarely, bony spurs may project into the spinal canal or intervertebral foramina, resulting in compression of spinal cord or spinal nerves. In such affected animals, clinical signs depend on the location of the lesion and include apparent spinal pain, lameness, and signs of transverse myelopathy or peripheral neuropathy. Other causes of spinal cord disease, peripheral nerve disease, and apparent spinal pain should be investigated and ruled out before attributing an animal's clinical signs to spondylosis deformans. Localized pain or lameness is reported to occur in animals with fracture of vertebral osteophytes.

Diagnosis. A diagnosis of spondylosis deformans is based on results of radiographs of the spine (Fig. 106–17). Bony osteophytes associated with spondylosis deformans may be seen at one or multiple intervertebral disk spaces ventral to the vertebral bodies on lateral projections and lateral to the vertebral bodies on ventrodorsal views. These osteophytes have a curved, "beak-like" appearance with smooth ventral and lateral borders. Osteophytes range in size from small bony spurs to those that equal the dorsoventral dimensions of the vertebral body. Spurs from adjacent vertebrae may interdigitate. Osteophytes form predominantly around the ventral and lateral margins of the vertebral endplates, and those apparent on lateral radiographs appear to be projecting dorsally into the spinal canal. Such osteophytes generally are located lateral to the spinal canal. Extensive osteophyte production dorsolateral to the vertebral body may compress spinal nerves at the level of the intervertebral foramina.

Bone may form in the mass of connective tissue formed between developing osteophytes and remain unattached to the vertebral bodies. These apparently free bone fragments are usually seen ventral to the intervertebral disk and may eventually become incorporated into developing osteophytes. These bone fragments may appear radiographically to be fractured osteophytes, but in fact they are not formed as a result of trauma.

Vertebral osteophytes may occur at either normal or nar-

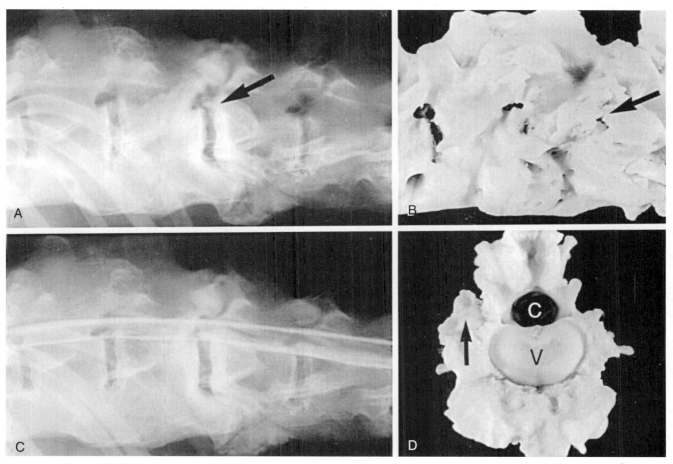

Figure 106–17. Spondylosis deformans. Lateral radiograph (A), gross pathologic specimen (B), and lateral myelogram (C) of the cranial lumbar vertebral column of a 12-year-old male golden retriever. Note the extensive spondylosis deformans that is present in the absence of myelographic abnormalities. Osteophytes (arrow) may appear to project into the vertebral canal on the lateral projection; however, these are actually dorsolateral and do not result in spinal cord compression. The typical location of osteophytes is seen in (D), where the spinal canal (C) of the L2 vertebra (V) is not encroached upon by the ventrally and laterally located osteophytes. The arrow in (D) indicates osteophytes located in close proximity to the intervertebral foramen. This dog was neurologically normal.

rowed disk spaces. Dorsally or dorsolaterally projecting osteophytes need to be distinguished from calcified disk material on lateral radiographs. Vertebral osteophytes may also form as a result of instability between adjacent vertebrae as a result of vertebral fracture or luxation, discospondylitis, congenital vertebral malformations, and surgery such as disk fenestration. However, the term spondylosis deformans is used specifically to define the formation of vertebral osteophytes secondary to disk degeneration. Disk protrusion may occur at the same site as spondylosis deformans, resulting in spinal cord compression. Myelography or advanced imaging (CT or MRI) is necessary to determine whether disk protrusion or dorsal vertebral osteophyte formation is causing spinal cord compression.

Treatment. Spondylosis deformans rarely results in spinal cord compression. However, should spinal cord compression or nerve root entrapment be demonstrated in an animal with neurologic deficits, surgical decompression may result in clinical improvement. Analgesics may be of benefit in animals with evidence of pain suspected to be the result of spinal nerve compression by vertebral osteophyte production. In most animals, spondylosis deformans is not of clinical significance and treatment is not necessary.

SYNOVIAL CYSTS

Spinal synovial cysts may arise from the articular facets and surrounding connective tissues of cervical and thoracolumbar vertebrae of dogs. These cysts may result in progressive extradural compression of the spinal cord. The etiology of synovial cysts is unknown; however, both degenerative changes and trauma have been suggested as likely causes.[299, 300] Clinical signs resulting from compression of the spinal cord by a synovial cyst reflect the location of the cyst (or cysts) and are usually slowly progressive. The diagnosis of synovial cyst is made primarily by means of radiography. Myelography is essential for precise localization. Advanced imaging techniques, particularly CT, may further delineate location and extent of a synovial cyst. Surgical decompression of the spinal cord and excision of the cyst appear to provide long-term resolution of clinical signs in affected dogs.

SYRINGOMYELIA AND HYDROMYELIA

Etiology and Pathogenesis. Syringomyelia (cavitation of the spinal cord) and hydromyelia (dilatation of the central canal) result in similar signs of spinal cord dysfunction. Syringomyelia may occur secondary to hydromyelia (communicating syringomyelia) or may not communicate with the central canal (noncommunicating syringomyelia). Syringomyelia may be associated with spinal cord tumors, myelitis, meningitis, and spinal cord trauma. The cause of syringomyelia is not known, but the condition may result from venous obstruction or distention, or may be due to mechanical disruption or shearing of spinal cord tissue planes.

Hydromyelia with or without syringomyelia may be associated with congenital malformations such as myelodysplasia; meningomyelocele or hydrocephalus; or lesions resulting in obstruction of CSF flow into the spinal subarachnoid space at the foramen magnum such as chronic arachnoiditis, trauma, congenital malformations, and vascular malformations; or it may be idiopathic.[301–304] Hydromyelia and syringomyelia in these animals probably results from

intracranial and spinal cord venous or arterial pressure changes and associated CSF pressure changes.

Syringomyelia in Weimaraners with myelodysplasia may be the result of progressive hydromyelia, abnormalities in the central canal, or abnormal vascular patterns in local areas of the spinal cord leading to low-grade ischemia, degeneration, rarefaction, and cavitation in the spinal cord.

Regardless of the cause, cavitation may be progressive, probably along planes of structural weakness such as the grey matter of the dorsal horns, and subsequent necrosis and edema of spinal cord parenchyma around such a cavitation (or dilated central canal) can result in the onset and progression of clinical signs.

Clinical Findings. Clinical signs depend on the location of the lesion and whether or not other spinal cord lesions are present. Clinical findings include progressive spinal deformity (scoliosis, torticollis); LMN or UMN signs, depending on location; and apparent spinal pain (Fig. 106–18). Clinical signs may be acute or may be progressive over weeks to several years. In Weimaraners with myelodysplasia, clinical signs do not appear to be progressive.

Diagnosis. Myelography may show obstruction of the flow of CSF at the foramen magnum if hydromyelia or syringomyelia is due to chronic arachnoiditis or arachnoid adhesions. Cisternal puncture for the collection of CSF is contraindicated in these animals, owing to likely inadvertent puncture of the spinal cord. Lumbar CSF may show evidence of chronic inflammation. Myelography in other cases may be normal or may show intramedullary swelling of the spinal cord. Advanced imaging (CT or MRI) is extremely useful in identifying the location and extent of cavitary lesions of the spinal cord.[305]

Treatment. Treatment of scoliosis in a dog has been reported, following drainage of an intraspinal cystic lesion.[306] Surgical drainage of cavitary lesions in humans has resulted in improvement in some cases.

VASCULAR MALFORMATIONS AND BENIGN VASCULAR TUMORS

Etiology and Pathogenesis. Spinal arteriovenous malformations and benign vascular tumors (hemangioma, cavernous angioma) have been reported to occur in dogs. Arteriovenous malformations consist of one or more anomalous arteries arising from radicular arteries that drain without a capillary bed into one or more veins communicating with veins on the surface of the spinal cord, resulting in the formation of tangles of tortuous distended vessels on or within the spinal cord. These malformations may be extramedullary, intramedullary, or both. Hemangioma is regarded as a benign neoplasm of endothelium that consists of discrete masses of tangled capillaries with or without cavernous or solid areas. Multiple hemangiomas may occur and are predominantly extramedullary, but may be intramedullary. These tumors may arise from the meninges.

Clinical Findings. Arteriovenous malformations and vascular tumors may occur anywhere in the spinal canal, and clinical signs usually reflect a progressive transverse myelopathy. An acute onset or sudden worsening of clinical signs may occur as a result of hemorrhage or thrombosis associated with abnormal vasculature of the malformation or tumor. Clinical signs may be the result of spinal cord compression or ischemia.

Diagnosis. CSF may be normal or may have an elevated protein concentration. CSF may be xanthochromic, and the

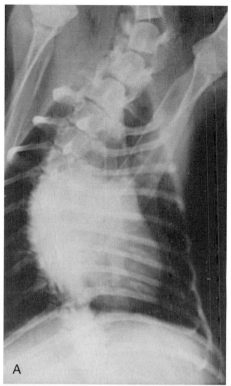

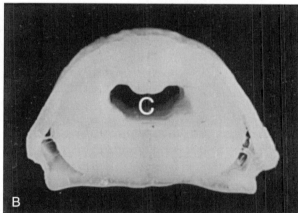

Figure 106–18. Hydromyelia and scoliosis. Ventrodorsal radiograph *(A)* of the caudal cervical and thoracic vertebral column of a 1-year-old female beagle. Note the scoliosis of the vertebral column. The spinal cord throughout the region of scoliosis *(B)* had an enlarged central canal (C) consistent with a diagnosis of hydromyelia.

white blood cell count may be mildly elevated if subarachnoid hemorrhage has occurred or a meningeal inflammatory response is associated with tumor growth.

Myelography may show evidence of an intradural or intramedullary mass. Advanced imaging (CT or MRI) may be used to further define these lesions. Surgical biopsy is necessary to distinguish these lesions from other neoplasms, subarachnoid cysts, and other intradural and intramedullary lesions.

Treatment. Surgical removal of a vascular malformation or vascular tumor may be possible.

REFERENCES

1. LeCouteur RA, Child G: Diseases of the spinal cord. *In* Ettinger SJ, Feldman EC (eds): Textbook of Veterinary Internal Medicine, 4th ed. Philadelphia, WB Saunders, 1995, p 629.
2. Kornegay JN: Pathogenesis of diseases of the central nervous system. *In* Slatter DH (ed): Textbook of Small Animal Surgery, 2nd ed. Philadelphia, WB Saunders, 1993, p 1022.
3. Summers BA, et al: Veterinary Neuropathology. Philadelphia, Mosby–Year Book, 1995.
4. Wheeler SJ: Manual of Small Animal Neurology, 2nd ed. Gloucestershire, BSAVA, 1995.
5. Oliver JE Jr, et al: Handbook of Veterinary Neurology, 3rd ed. Philadelphia, WB Saunders, 1997.
6. Braund KG: Clinical Syndromes in Veterinary Neurology, 2nd ed. Baltimore, Williams & Wilkins, 1994.
7. Kornegay JN: Feline neurology. *In* Kay WJ, Brown NO (eds): Problems in Veterinary Medicine, Vol 3. Philadelphia, JB Lippincott, pp 309–451.
8. Moore MP: Approach to the patient with spinal cord disease. Vet Clin North Am 22:751, 1992.
9. Wheeler SJ, Sharp NJH: Small Animal Spinal Disorders. Philadelphia, Mosby-Wolfe, 1994.
10. Jeffery ND: Handbook of Small Animal Spinal Surgery. Philadelphia, WB Saunders, 1995.
11. Sande RD: Radiology, myelography, computed tomography, and magnetic resonance imaging of the spine. Vet Clin North Am 22:811, 1992.
12. Brawner WR: Neuroradiology. *In* Slatter DH (ed): Textbook of Small Animal Surgery, 2nd ed. Philadelphia, WB Saunders, 1993, p 1008.
13. Bailey CS, Vernau W: Cerebrospinal fluid. *In* Kaneko JJ, Harvey JW, Bruss ML (eds): Clinical Biochemistry of Domestic Animals. San Diego, Academic Press, 1997.
14. Chrisman CL: Cerebrospinal fluid analysis. Vet Clin North Am 22:781, 1992.
15. Rand JS, et al: Reference intervals for feline cerebrospinal fluid: Cell counts and cytologic features. Am J Vet Res 51:1044, 1990.
16. Rand JS, et al: Reference intervals for feline cerebrospinal fluid: Biochemical and serologic variables, concentration electrophoretic fractionation. Am J Vet Res 51: 1049, 1990.
17. Bailey CS, Higgins RJ: Comparison of total white blood cell count and total protein content of lumbar and cisternal cerebrospinal fluid of healthy dogs. Am J Vet Res 46:1162, 1985.
18. Thomson CE, et al: Analysis of cerebrospinal fluid from the cerebellomedullary and lumbar cisterns of dogs with focal neurologic disease: 145 cases (1985–1987). JAVMA 196:1841, 1990.
19. Sorjonen DC, et al: Cerebrospinal fluid protein electrophoresis: A clinical evaluation of a previously reported diagnostic technique. Prog Vet Neurol 2:261, 1991.
20. Tipold A, et al: Determination of the IgG index for the detection of intrathecal immunoglobulin synthesis in dogs using an ELISA. Res Vet Sci 54:40, 1993.
21. Tipold A, et al: Intrathecal synthesis of major immunoglobulin classes in inflammatory diseases of the canine CNS. Vet Immunol Immunopathol 42:149, 1994.
22. Lewis DG, Hosgood G: Complications associated with the use of iohexol for myelography of the cervical vertebral column in dogs: 66 cases (1988–1990). JAVMA 200:1381, 1992.
23. Widmer WR, Blevins WE: Veterinary myelography: A review of contrast media, adverse effects, and technique. J Am Anim Hosp Assoc 27:163, 1991.
24. Carroll GL, et al: Asystole associated with iohexol myelography in a dog. Vet Radiol Ultrasound 38:284, 1997.
25. Holliday TA: Electrodiagnostic examination: Somatosensory evoked potentials and electromyography. Vet Clin North Am 22:833, 1992.
26. Poncelet L, et al: Study of spinal cord evoked injury potential by use of computer modeling and in dogs with naturally acquired thoracolumbar spinal cord compression. Am J Vet Res 59:300, 1998.
27. Jaggy A, et al: Occipitoatlantoaxial malformation with atlantoaxial subluxation in a cat. J Small Anim Pract 32:366, 1991.
28. McCarthy RJ, et al: Atlantoaxial subluxation in dogs. Compend Contin Educ 17:215, 1995.
29. Wheeler SJ: Atlantoaxial subluxation and absence of the dens in a rottweiller. J Small Anim Pract 33:90, 1992.
30. DeCamp CE, et al: Traumatic atlantooccipital subluxation in a dog. J Am Anim Hosp Assoc 27:415, 1991.
31. Bailey CS, Morgan JP: Congenital spinal malformations. Vet Clin North Am 22:985, 1992.
32. Thomas WB, et al: Surgical management of atlantoaxial subluxation in 23 dogs. Vet Surg 20:409, 1991.
33. Schulz KS, et al: Application of ventral pins and polymethylmethacrylate for the management of atlantoaxial instability: Results in nine dogs. Vet Surg 26:317, 1997.
34. Thomson MJ, Read RA: Surgical stabilisation of the atlantoaxial joint in a cat. VCOT 9:36, 1996.
35. Foil CS: Fungal diseases. Clin Dermatol 12:529, 1994.
36. Munana KR: Encephalitis and meningitis. Vet Clin North Am Small Anim Pract 26:857, 1996.
37. Dewey CW, et al: Spinal epidural empyema in two dogs. J Am Anim Hosp Assoc 34:305, 1998.
38. Kraus KH, et al: Paraparesis caused by epidural granuloma in a cat. JAVMA 194:789, 1989.
39. Lobetti RG: Subarachnoid abscess as a complication of discospondylitis in a dog. J Small Anim Pract 35:480, 1994.
40. Greene CE: Infectious Diseases of the Dog and Cat. Philadelphia, WB Saunders, 1990.

CNS

41. Sorjonen DC: Myelitis and meningitis. Vet Clin North Am 22:951, 1992.
42. Maretzki CH, et al: Granulocytic ehrlichiosis and meningitis in a dog. JAVMA 205:1554, 1994.
43. Tipold A: Diagnosis of inflammatory and infectious diseases of the central nervous system in dogs: A retrospective study. J Vet Intern Med 9:304, 1995.
44. Malik R, et al: A latex cryptococcal antigen agglutination test for diagnosis and monitoring of therapy for cryptococcosis. Aust Vet J 74:358, 1996.
45. Egenvall AE, et al: Clinical features and serology of 14 dogs affected by granulocytic ehrlichiosis in Sweden. Vet Rec 140:222, 1997
46. Gormley WB, et al: Cranial and intracranial bacterial infections. In Youmans JR (ed): Neurological Surgery, 4th ed. Philadelphia, WB Saunders, 1996, p 3191.
47. Fenner WR: Bacterial infections of the central nervous system. In Greene CE (ed): Infectious Diseases of the Dog and Cat. Philadelphia, WB Saunders, 1990, p 184.
48. The choice of antimicrobial drugs. Med Lett Drug Ther 30:33, 1988.
49. Meric SM: Canine meningitis—a changing emphasis. J Vet Intern Med 2:26, 1988.
50. Scully BE: Metronidazole. Med Clin North Am 72:613, 1988.
51. Dow SW, et al: Central nervous system toxicosis associated with metronidazole treatment for dogs: Five cases (1984–1987). JAVMA 195:365, 1989.
52. Franke EL, Neu HC: Chloramphenicol and tetracyclines. Med Clin North Am 71:1155, 1987.
53. Hansen BL: Successful treatment of severe feline cryptococcosis with long-term high doses of ketoconazole. J Am Anim Hosp Assoc 23:193, 1987.
54. Flatland B, et al: Clinical and serologic evaluation of cats with cryptococcosis. JAVMA 209:1110, 1996.
55. Gerds-Grogan S, Dayrell-Hart B: Feline cryptococcosis: A retrospective evaluation. J Am Anim Hosp Assoc 33:118, 1997.
56. Medleau L, et al: Evaluation of ketoconazole and itraconazole for treatment of disseminated cryptococcosis in cats. Am J Vet Res 51:1454, 1990.
57. Tiches D, et al: A case of canine central nervous system cryptococcosis: Management with fluconazole. J Am Anim Hosp Assoc 34:145, 1998.
58. Berthelin CF, et al: Cryptococcosis of the nervous system of dogs. Part II. Diagnosis, treatment, monitoring and prognosis. Progr Vet Neurol 5:136, 1994.
59. Legendre A, Berthelin C: How do I treat? Central nervous system cryptococcosis in dogs and cats. Progr Vet Neurol 6:32, 1995.
60. Medleau L: Itraconazole for the treatment of cryptococcosis in cats. J Vet Intern Med 9:39, 1995.
61. Ginel PJ, et al: Cutaneous protothecosis in a dog. Vet Rec 140:651, 1997.
62. Lewis DG, Kelly DF: Calcinosis circumscripta in dogs as a cause of spinal ataxia. J Small Anim Pract 31:36, 1990.
63. McEwan JD, et al: Thoracic spinal calcinosis circumscripta causing cord compression in two German shepherd dog littermates. Vet Rec 130:575, 1992.
64. Marks S, et al: Resolution of quadriparesis caused by cervical tumoral calcinosis in a dog. J Am Anim Hosp Assoc 27:72, 1991.
65. Bichsel P, et al: Solitary cartilaginous exostoses associated with spinal cord compression in three large-breed dogs. J Am Anim Hosp Assoc 21:619, 1985.
66. Burbidge HM: A review of wobbler syndrome in the Doberman pinscher. Aust Vet Practit 25:147, 1995.
67. Bruecker KA: Caudal cervical spondylomyelopathy in large breed dogs. In Bojrab MJ (ed): Current Techniques in Small Animal Surgery, 4th ed. Philadelphia, Williams & Wilkins, 1998, p 828.
68. VanGundy TE: Disc-associated wobbler syndrome in a Doberman pinscher. Vet Clin North Am 18:667, 1988.
69. Bruecker KA, Seim HB III: Caudal cervical spondylomyelopathy. In Slatter DH (ed): Textbook of Small Animal Surgery, 2nd ed. Philadelphia, WB Saunders, 1993, p 1056.
70. Lincoln JD: Cervical vertebral malformation/malarticulation syndrome in large dogs. Vet Clin North Am 22:923, 1992.
71. Seim HB III, Bruecker KA: Caudal cervical spondylomyelopathy: Wobbler syndrome. In Bojrab MJ (ed): Disease Mechanisms in Small Animal Surgery. Philadelphia, Lea & Febiger, 1993, p 899.
72. Lewis DG: Cervical spondylomyelopathy ("wobbler" syndrome) in the dog: A study based on 224 cases. J Small Anim Pract 30:657, 1989.
73. Lewis DG: Radiological assessment of the cervical spine of the doberman with reference to cervical spondylomyelopathy. J Small Anim Pract 32:75, 1991.
74. Sharp NJH, et al: Radiological evaluation of "wobbler" syndrome–caudal cervical spondylomyelopathy. J Small Anim Pract 33:491, 1992.
75. Seim HB III: Wobbler syndrome in the doberman pinscher. In Kirk RW (ed): Current Veterinary Therapy X: Small Animal Practice. Philadelphia, WB Saunders, 1989, p 858.
76. Bruecker KA, et al: Caudal cervical spondylomyelopathy: Decompression by linear traction and stabilization with Steinmann pins and polymethyl methacrylate. J Am Anim Hosp Assoc 25:677, 1989.
77. McKee WM: Vertebral distraction-fusion for cervical spondylopathy using a screw and double washer technique. J Small Anim Pract 31:22, 1990.
78. Goring RL, et al: The inverted cone decompression technique: A surgical treatment for cervical vertebral instability "wobbler syndrome" in doberman pinschers. Part I. J Am Anim Hosp Assoc 27:403, 1991.
79. Lyman R: Continuous dorsal laminectomy is the procedure of choice. Progr Vet Neurol 2:143, 1991.
80. Chambers JN, et al: Update on ventral decompression for caudal cervical disk herniation in Doberman pinschers. J Am Anim Hosp Assoc 22:775, 1986.
81. Bailey CS: Chymopapain chemonucleolysis. In Kirk RW, Bonagura JD (eds): Current Veterinary Therapy XI: Small Animal Practice. Philadelphia, WB Saunders, 1992, p 1018.
82. Dixon BC, et al: Modified distraction-stabilization technique using an interbody polymethyl methacrylate plug in dogs with caudal cervical spondylomyelopathy. JAVMA 208:61, 1996.
83. Wilson ER, et al: Observation of a secondary compressive lesion after treatment of caudal cervical spondylomyelopathy in a dog. JAVMA 205:1297, 1994.
84. Colter SB: Congenital anomalies of the spine. In Bojrab MJ (ed): Disease Mechanisms in Small Animal Surgery. Philadelphia, Lea & Febiger, 1993, p 950.
85. Coates JR, Kline KL: Congenital and inherited neurologic disorders in dogs and cats. In Bonagura JD, Kirk RW (eds): Kirk's Current Veterinary Therapy XII: Small Animal Practice. Philadelphia, WB Saunders, 1995, p 1111.
86. Shell LG, et al: Spinal dysraphism, hemivertebra, and stenosis of the spinal canal in a rottweiler puppy. J Am Anim Hosp Assoc 24:341, 1988.
87. Meric SM, et al: Corticosteroid-responsive meningitis in ten dogs. J Am Anim Hosp Assoc 21:677, 1985.
88. Irving G, Chrisman C: Long-term outcome of five cases of corticosteroid-responsive meningomyelitis, J Am Anim Hosp Assoc 26:324, 1990.
89. Meric SM: Two recently described canine meningitis syndromes. Aust Vet Practit 20:106, 1990.
90. Tipold A, et al: Neuroimmunological studies in steroid-responsive meningitis-arteritis in dogs. Res Vet Sci 58:103, 1995.
91. Tipold A, et al: Is there a superantigen effect on steroid-responsive meningitis-arteritis in dogs? Tierarztl Prax 24:514, 1996.
92. Tipold A, Jaggy A: Steroid responsive meningitis-arteritis in dogs: Long-term study of 32 cases. J Small Anim Pract 35:311, 1994.
93. Meric SM, et al: Necrotizing vasculitis of the spinal pachyleptomeningeal arteries in three Bernese mountain dog littermates. J Am Anim Hosp Assoc 22:459, 1986.
94. Presthus J: Aseptic suppurative meningitis in Bernese mountain dogs. Norsk Veterinaertidsskrift 101:169, 1989.
95. Scott-Moncrieff JCR, et al: Systemic necrotizing vasculitis in nine young beagles JAVMA 201:1553, 1992.
96. Kemi M, et al: Histopathology of spontaneous panarteritis in beagle dogs. Nipon-Juigaku-Zasshii 52:55, 1990.
97. Gerhardt A, et al: Necrotizing vasculitis of the cerebral and spinal leptomeninges in a Bernese mountain dog. DTW Dtsch Tierarzl Wochenschr 105:139, 1998.
98. Snyder PW, et al: Pathologic features of naturally occurring juvenile polyarteritis in Beagle dogs. Vet Pathol 32:337, 1995.
99. Clemmons RM: Degenerative myelopathy. In Kirk RW (ed): Current Veterinary Therapy X: Small Animal Practice. Philadelphia, WB Saunders, 1989, p 830.
100. Clemmons RM: Degenerative myelopathy. Vet Clin North Am 22:965, 1992.
101. Clemmons RM: Degenerative myelopathy. In Bojrab MJ (ed): Disease Mechanisms in Small Animal Surgery. Philadelphia, Lea & Febiger, 1993, p 984.
102. Toenniessen JG, Morin DE: Degenerative myelopathy: A comparative review. Compend Contin Educ 17:271, 1995.
103. Barclay KB, Haines DM: Immunohistochemical evidence for immunoglobulin and complement deposition in spinal cord lesions in degenerative myelopathy in German shepherd dogs. Can J Vet Res 58:20, 1994.
104. Longhofer SL, et al: A degenerative myelopathy in young German shepherd dogs. J Small Anim Pract 31:199, 1990.
105. Morgan JP, Stavenborn M: Disseminated idiopathic skeletal hyperostosis (DISH) in a dog. Vet Radiol 32:65, 1991.
106. Morgan JP: Radiographic and myelographic diagnosis of spinal disease. In JR August (ed): Consultations in Feline Medicine, 3rd ed. Philadelphia, WB Saunders, 1997, p 425.
107. Resnick D, Niwayama G: Radiographic and pathologic features of spinal involvement in diffuse idiopathic skeletal hyperostosis (DISH). Radiology 119:559, 1976.
108. Hoffman LE, et al: Diffuse idiopathic skeletal hyperostosis (DISH): A review of radiographic features and report of four cases. J Manipulative Physiol Ther 18:547, 1995.
109. Rotes-Querol J: Clinical manifestations of diffuse idiopathic skeletal hyperostosis (DISH). Br J Rheumatol 35:1193, 1996.
110. Kornegay JN: Discospondylitis. In Slatter DH (ed): Textbook of Small Animal Surgery, 2nd ed. Philadelphia, WB Saunders, 1993, p 1087.
111. Moore MP: Discospondylitis. Vet Clin North Am 22:1027, 1992.
112. Walker TL: Vertebral osteomyelitis and discospondylitis. In Bojrab MJ (ed): Disease Mechanisms in Small Animal Surgery. Philadelphia, Lea & Febiger, 1993, p 971.
113. Jaffe MH, et al: Canine discospondylitis. Compend Contin Educ 19:551, 1997.
114. Turnwald GH, et al: Diskospondylitis in a kennel of dogs: Clinicopathologic findings. JAVMA 188:178, 1986.
115. Carpenter JL, et al: Tuberculosis in five basset hounds. JAVMA 192:1563, 1988.
116. Watt PR, et al: Disseminated opportunistic fungal disease in dogs: 10 cases (1982–1990). JAVMA 207:67, 1995.
117. Kerwin SC, et al: Discospondylitis associated with Brucella canis infection in dogs: 14 cases (1980–1991). JAVMA 201:1253, 1992.
118. Butterworth SJ, et al: Multiple discospondylitis associated with Aspergillus species infection in a dog. Vet Rec 136:38, 1995.
119. Dallman MJ, et al: Disseminated aspergillosis in a dog with discospondylitis and neurologic deficits. JAVMA 200:511, 1992.
120. Berry WL, Leisewitz AL: Multifocal Aspergillus terreus discospondylitis in two German shepherd dogs. J S Afr Vet Assoc 67:222, 1996.
121. Malik R, et al: Bacterial discospondylitis in a cat. J Small Anim Pract 31:404, 1990.
122. Kraft SL, et al: Magnetic resonance imaging of presumptive lumbosacral discospondylitis in a dog. Vet Radiol Ultrasound 39:9, 1998.

CNS

123. Fischer A, et al: Fluoroscopically guided percutaneous disc aspiration in 10 dogs with discospondylitis. J Vet Intern Med 11:284, 1997.

124. McKee WM, et al: Surgical treatment of lumbosacral discospondylitis by a distraction-fusion technique. J Small Anim Pract 31:15, 1990.

125. Muller CF, et al: Studies on canine distemper virus persistence in the central nervous system. Acta Neuropathol 89:438, 1995.

126. Tipold A, et al: Neurological manifestations of canine distemper virus infection. J Small Anim Pract 33:466, 1992.

127. Shell LG: Canine distemper. Compend Contin Educ 12:173, 1990.

128. Raw ME, et al: Canine distemper infection associated with acute nervous signs in dogs. Vet Rec 130:291, 1992.

129. Appel MJG: Canine Distemper. In Barlough JE (ed): Manual of Small Animal Infectious Diseases. New York, Churchill Livingstone, 1988, p 49.

130. Thomas WB, et al: A retrospective evaluation of 38 cases of canine distemper encephalomyelitis. J Am Anim Hosp Assoc 29:129, 1993.

131. Sorjonen DC, et al: Electrophoretic determination of albumin and gamma globulin concentrations in the cerebrospinal fluid of dogs with encephalomyelitis attributable to canine distemper virus infection: 13 cases (1980–1987). JAVMA 195:977, 1989.

132. McReynolds C, Macy D: Feline infectious peritonitis. Part I. Etiology and diagnosis. Compend Contin Educ 19:1007, 1997.

133. McReynolds C, Macy D: Feline infectious peritonitis. Part II. Treatment and prevention. Compend Contin Educ 19:1111, 1997.

134. Zenger E: FIP, FeLV, FIV: Making a diagnosis. Proc. 16th ACVIM Forum, San Diego, 1998, p 407.

135. Vennema H, et al: Feline infectious peritonitis viruses arise by mutation from endemic feline enteric coronaviruses. Virology 243:150, 1998.

136. Foley JE, et al: Risk factors for feline infectious peritonitis among cats in multiple-cat environments with endemic feline enteric coronaviruses. JAVMA 210:1313, 1997.

137. Kline KL, et al: Feline infectious peritonitis with neurologic involvement: Clinical and pathological findings in 24 cats. J Am Anim Hosp Assoc 30:111, 1994.

138. Sparkes AH, et al: An appraisal of the value of laboratory tests in the diagnosis of feline infectious peritonitis. J Am Anim Hosp Assoc 30:345, 1994.

139. Barr MC: FIV, FeLV, and FIPV: Interpretation and misinterpretation of serological test results. Semin Vet Med Surg 11:144, 1996.

140. Zenger E: Newer diagnostic testing methodology for infectious agents. In August JR (ed): Consultations in Feline Internal Medicine, 3rd ed. Philadelphia, WB Saunders, 1997, p 37.

141. Evermann JF, et al: Feline infectious peritonitis. JAVMA 206:1130, 1995.

142. Lundgren AL: Feline non-suppurative meningoencephalomyelitis. A clinical and pathological study. J Comp Pathol 107:411, 1992.

143. Lundgren AL: Feline meningoencephalomyelitis (Vingelsjuka) in Sweden. Suomen-Elainlaakarilehti 97:321, 1991.

144. Lundgren AL, et al: Immunoreactivity of the central nervous system in cats with a Borna disease–like meningoencephalomyelitis (staggering disease). Acta Neuropathol 90:184, 1995.

145. Lundgren AL, et al: Staggering disease in cats: Isolation and characterization of the feline Borna disease virus. J Gen Virol 76(Pt 9):2215, 1995.

146. Lundgren AL, et al: Neurological disease and encephalitis in cats experimentally infected with Borna disease virus. Acta Neuropathol 93:391, 1997.

147. Victoria T, et al: Cloning of the canine GALC cDNA and identification of the mutation causing globoid cell leukodystrophy in West Highland White and Cairn terriers. Genomics 33:457, 1996.

148. Sorjonen DC: Clinical and histopathological features of granulomatous meningoencephalomyelitis in dogs. J Am Anim Hosp Assoc 26:141, 1990.

149. Thomas JB, Eger C: Granulomatous meningoencephalomyelitis in 21 dogs. J Small Anim Pract 30:287, 1989.

150. Munana KR, Luttgen PJ: Prognostic factors for dogs with granulomatous meningoencephalomyelitis: 42 cases (1982–1996). JAVMA 212:1902, 1998.

151. Kipar A, et al: Immunohistochemical characterization of inflammatory cells in brains of dogs with granulomatous meningoencephalitis. Vet Pathol 35:43, 1998.

152. Bailey CS, Higgins RJ: Characteristics of cerebrospinal fluid associated with canine granulomatous meningoencephalomyelitis: A retrospective study. JAVMA 188:418, 1986.

153. Sturges BK, et al: Leflunomide for the treatment of inflammatory or malacic lesions in three dogs. J Vet Intern Med 12:207, 1998.

154. Stokol T, et al: Hematorrhachis associated with hemophilia A in three German shepherd dogs. J Am Anim Hosp Assoc 30:239, 1994.

155. Martin RA, et al: Focal intramedullary spinal cord hematoma in a dog. J Am Anim Hosp Assoc 22:545, 1986.

156. Sheahan BJ, et al: Structural and biochemical changes in a spinal myelinopathy in twelve English foxhounds and two Harriers. Vet Pathol 28:117, 1991.

157. Palmer AC, et al: Spinal cord degeneration in hound ataxia. J Small Anim Pract 25:139, 1984.

158. Palmer AC, Medd RK: Hound ataxia. Vet Rec 122:263, 1988.

159. Wright JA, Brownlie S: Progressive ataxia in a Pyrenean mountain dog. Vet Rec 116:410, 1985.

160. Cummings JF, et al: Multisystemic chromatolytic neuronal degeneration in Cairn terriers. J Vet Intern Med 5:91, 1991.

161. Mandigers PJJ, et al: Hereditary necrotizing myelopathy in Kooiker dog. Res Vet Sci 54:118, 1993.

162. Brenner O, et al: Hereditary polioencephalomyelopathy of the Australian cattle dog. Acta Neuropathol 94:54, 1997.

163. Goldman AL: Hypervitaminosis A in a cat. JAVMA 200:1970, 1992.

164. Braund KV: Intervertebral disk disease. In Bojrab HJ (ed): Disease Mechanisms in Small Animal Surgery. Philadelphia, Lea & Febiger, 1993, p 960.

165. Toombs JP: Cervical intervertebral disk disease in dogs. Comp Contin Educ 14:1477, 1992.

166. Toombs JP, Bauer MS: Intervertebral disc disease. In Slatter DH (ed): Textbook of Small Animal Surgery, 2nd ed. Philadelphia, WB Saunders, 1993, p 1070.

167. Burbidge HM, Bray JP: The canine intervertebral disc: Part two. Degenerative changes—nonchondrodystrophoid versus chondrodystrophoid disks. J Am Anim Hosp Assoc 34:135, 1998.

168. Morgan JP, et al: Vertebral canal and spinal cord mensuration: A comparative study of its effect on lumbosacral myelography in the Dachshund and German shepherd dog. JAVMA 191:951, 1987.

169. Morgan JP, Miyabayashi T: Degenerative changes in the vertebral column of the dog: A review of radiographic findings. Vet Radiol 29:72, 1988.

170. Kornegay JN: Paraparesis, tetraparesis, urinary/fecal incontinence. Probl Vet Med 3:363, 1991.

171. Grevel V: Lähmungen der Hintergliedmaßen bei der Katze. Berl Munch Tierarztl Wochenschr 102:253, 1989.

172. Morgan PW, et al: Cervical pain secondary to intervertebral disc disease in dogs: Radiographic findings and surgical implications. Progr Vet Neurol 4:76, 1993.

173. Dallman MJ, et al: Characteristics of dogs admitted for treatment of cervical intervertebral disk disease: 105 cases (1972–1982). JAVMA 200:2009, 1992.

174. Kirberger RM, et al: The radiological diagnosis of thoracolumbar disc disease in the Dachshund. Vet Radiol Ultrasound 33:255, 1992.

175. Slocum B, et al: Myelography of disc disease. In Bojrab MJ (ed): Current Techniques in Small Animal Surgery, 4th ed. Philadelphia, Williams & Wilkins, 1998, p 803.

176. Smith JD, et al: Incidence of contralateral versus ipsilateral neurological signs associated with lateralized Hansen type II disc extrusion. J Small Anim Pract 38:495, 1997.

177. Thomson CE, et al: Canine intervertebral disc disease: Changes in the cerebrospinal fluid. J Small Anim Pract 30:685, 1989.

178. Roush JK, et al: Traumatic dural laceration in a racing greyhound. Vet Radiol Ultrasound 33:22, 1992.

179. Burk RL: Problems in the radiographic interpretation of intervertebral disc disease in the dog. Probl Vet Med 1:381, 1989.

180. Hara Y, et al: Usefulness of computed tomography after myelography for surgery on dogs with cervical intervertebral disc protrusion. J Vet Med Sci 56:791, 1994.

181. Schulz KS, et al: Correlation of clinical, radiographic, and surgical localization of intervertebral disc extrusion in small-breed dogs: A prospective study of 50 cases. Vet Surg 27:105, 1998.

182. Creed JE, Yturraspe DJ: Intervertebral disc fenestration. In Bojrab MJ (ed): Current Techniques in Small Animal Surgery, 4th ed. Philadelphia, Williams & Wilkins, 1998, p 835.

183. Bojrab MJ, Constantinescu GM: Prophylactic thoracolumbar disc fenestration. In Bojrab MJ (ed): Current Techniques in Small Animal Surgery, 4th ed. Philadelphia, Williams & Wilkins, 1998, p 839.

184. McKee WM: A comparison of hemilaminectomy (with concomitant disc fenestration) and dorsal laminectomy for the treatment of thoracolumbar disc protrusion in dogs. Vet Rec 130:296, 1992.

185. Fingeroth JM: Fenestration: Pros and cons. Probl Vet Med 1:445, 1989.

186. Sikes R: Postoperative management of the neurosurgical patient. Probl Vet Med 1:467, 1989.

187. Janssens LA: Acupuncture for the treatment of thoracolumbar and cervical disc disease in the dog. Probl Vet Med 4:107, 1992.

188. Atilola MAO, et al: Cervical chemonucleolysis in the dog: A surgical technique. Vet Surg 17:135, 1988.

189. Atilola MAO, et al: Canine chemonucleolysis: An experimental radiographic study. Vet Radiol 29:168, 1988.

190. Fry TR, Johnson AL: Chemonucleolysis for treatment of intervertebral disk disease. JAVMA 199:622, 1991.

191. Biggart JF: Discolysis. In Bojrab MJ (ed): Current Techniques in Small Animal Surgery, 4th ed. Philadelphia, Williams & Wilkins, 1998, p 855.

192. Neer TM: Fibrocartilaginous emboli. Vet Clin North Am 22:1017, 1992.

193. Dyce J, Houlton JEF: Fibrocartilaginous embolism in the dog. J Small Anim Pract 34:332, 1993.

194. Cauzinille L, Kornegay JN: Fibrocartilaginous embolism of the spinal cord in dogs: Review of 36 histologically confirmed cases and retrospective study of 26 suspected cases. J Vet Intern Med 10:241, 1996.

195. Turner PV, et al: Fibrocartilaginous embolic myelopathy in a cat. Can Vet J 36:712, 1995.

196. Scott HW, O'Leary MT: Fibrocartilaginous embolism in a cat. J Small Anim Pract 37:228, 1996.

197. Little PB: Central nervous system rendezvous—canine acute posterior paresis. Can Vet J 35:517, 1994.

198. Gamble DA, Chrisman CL: A leukoencephalomyelopathy of rottweiler dogs. Vet Pathol 21:274, 1984.

199. Wouda W, van Nes JJ: Progressive ataxia due to central demyelination in rottweiler dogs. Vet Q 8:89, 1986.

200. Chrisman CL: Neurological diseases of rottweilers: Neuroaxonal dystrophy and leukoencephalomalacia. J Small Anim Pract 33:500, 1992.

201. Palmer RH, Chambers JN: Canine lumbosacral diseases. Part I. Anatomy, pathophysiology, and clinical presentation. Comp Contin Educ 13:61, 1991.

202. Palmer RH, Chambers JN: Canine lumbosacral diseases. Part II. Definitive diagnosis, treatment, and prognosis. Comp Contin Educ 13:213, 1991.

203. Watt PR: Degenerative lumbosacral stenosis in 18 dogs. J Small Anim Pract 32:125, 1991.
204. Morgan JP, et al: Lumbosacral transitional vertebrae as a predisposing cause of cauda equina syndrome in German shepherd dogs: 161 cases (1987–1990) JAVMA 202:1877, 1993.
205. Lang J, et al: A sacral lesion resembling osteochondrosis in the German shepherd dog. Vet Radiol Ultrasound 33:69, 1992.
206. Ferguson HR: Conditions of the lumbosacral spinal cord and cauda equina. Semin Vet Med Surg 11:254, 1996.
207. Ness MG: Degenerative lumbosacral stenosis in the dog: A review of 30 cases. J Small Anim Pract 35:185, 1994.
208. Schmid V, Lang J: Measurements on the lumbosacral junction in normal dogs and those with cauda equina compression. J Small Anim Pract 34:437, 1993.
209. Sisson AF, et al: Diagnosis of cauda equina abnormalities by using electromyography, discography, and epidurography in dogs. J Vet Intern Med 6:253, 1992.
210. Fischer A, et al: Electromyographic findings in dogs with lumbosacral disease. Proceedings WSAVA World Congress, Berlin, 1993, p 382.
211. Morgan JP, Bailey CS: Cauda equina syndrome in the dog: Radiographic evaluation. J Small Anim Pract 31:69, 1990.
212. Biggart JF: Discography for diagnosis of neurologic disease. In Bojrab MJ (ed): Current Techniques in Small Animal Surgery, 4th ed. Philadelphia, Williams & Wilkins, 1998, p 809.
213. Wheeler SJ: Lumbosacral disease. Vet Clin North Am 22:937, 1992.
214. De Haan JJ, et al: Magnetic resonance imaging in the diagnosis of degenerative lumbosacral stenosis in four dogs. Vet Surg 22:1, 1993.
215. Jones JC, et al: Computed tomographic morphometry of the lumbosacral spine of dogs. Am J Vet Res 56:1125, 1995.
216. Chambers JN, et al: Diagnosis of lateralized lumbosacral disc herniation with magnetic resonance imaging. J Am Anim Hosp Assoc 33:296, 1997.
217. Adams WH, et al: Magnetic resonance imaging of the caudal lumbar and lumbosacral spine in 13 dogs (1990–1993). Vet Radiol Ultrasound 36:3, 1995.
218. Slocum B, Slocum TD: L7–S1 fixation-fusion technique for cauda equina syndrome. In Bojrab MJ (ed): Current Techniques in Small Animal Surgery, 4th ed. Philadelphia, Williams & Wilkins, 1998, p 861.
219. Konde LJ, et al: Radiographically visualized skeletal changes associated with mucopolysaccharidosis VI in cats. Vet Radiol 28:223, 1987.
220. Wenger DA, et al: Bone marrow transplantation in the feline model of arylsulfatase B deficiency. In Krivit W, Paul NW (eds): Bone Marrow Transplantation for Treatment of Lysosomal Storage Diseases. March of Dimes Birth Defects Foundation, Birth Defects Original Article Series. New York, AR Liss, Vol 2, p 177, 1986.
221. Malik R, et al: Abnormal control of urination and defaecation in a dog with myelodysplasia. Aust Vet Practit 21:178, 1991.
222. Broek AHM van den, et al: Spinal dysraphism in the Weimaraner. J Small Anim Pract 32:258, 1991.
223. Brunetti A, et al: Meningomyelocele and hydrocephalus in a bulldog. Prog Vet Neurol 4:54, 1993.
224. LeCouteur RA: Nervous system neoplasia. In Withrow SJ, MacEwen EG (eds): Clinical Veterinary Oncology, 2nd ed. Philadelphia, WB Saunders, 1996, p 393.
225. Bagley RS, et al: Central nervous system. In Slatter DH (ed): Textbook of Small Animal Surgery, 2nd ed. Philadelphia, WB Saunders, 1993, p 2137.
226. Waters DJ, Hayden DW: Intramedullary spinal cord metastasis in the dog. J Vet Intern Med 4:207, 1990.
227. Fenner WR: Metastatic neoplasms of the central nervous system. Semin Vet Med Surg 5:253, 1990.
228. Brehm DM, et al: A retrospective evaluation of 51 cases of peripheral nerve sheath tumors in the dog. J Am Anim Hosp Assoc 31:349, 1995.
229. Sponick GJ, et al: Spinal lymphoma in cats: 21 cases (1976–1989). JAVMA 200:373, 1992.
230. Barr MC, et al: Spinal lymphosarcoma and disseminated mastocytoma associated with feline immunodeficiency virus infection in a cat. JAVMA 202:1978, 1993.
231. Levy MS, et al: Spinal tumors in 37 dogs: Clinical outcome and long-term survival (1987–1994). J Am Anim Hosp Assoc 33:307, 1997.
232. Noonan M, et al: Lymphoma of the central nervous system: A retrospective study of 18 cats. Compend Contin Educ 19:497, 1997.
233. Lane SB, et al: Feline spinal lymphosarcoma: A retrospective evaluation of 23 cats. J Vet Intern Med 8:99, 1994.
234. Ribas JL: Thoracolumbar spinal cord blastoma: A unique tumor of young dogs. J Vet Intern Med 4:127, 1990.
235. Drost WT, et al: Comparison of radiography, myelography and computed tomography for the evaluation of canine vertebral and spinal cord tumors in sixteen dogs. Vet Radiol Ultrasound 376:28, 1996.
236. Hopkins AL, et al: Spinal meningeal sarcoma in a rottweiler puppy. J Small Anim Pract 36:183, 1995.
237. Irving G, McMillan MC: Fluoroscopically guided percutaneous fine-needle aspiration biopsy of thoracolumbar spinal lesions in cats. Prog Vet Neurol 1:473, 1990.
238. Ferretti A: Surgical treatment of a spinal cord tumor resembling nephroblastoma in a young dog. Prog Vet Neurol 4:84, 1993.
239. Bell FW, et al: External beam radiation therapy for recurrent intraspinal meningioma in a dog. J Am Anim Hosp Assoc 28:319, 1992.
240. Chrisman CL, et al: Neuroaxonal dystrophy of rottweiler dogs. JAVMA 184:464, 1984.
241. Evans MG, et al: Neuroaxonal dystrophy in a rottweiler pup. JAVMA 192:1560, 1988.
242. Sacre BJ, et al: Neuroaxonal dystrophy in a Jack Russell terrier pup resembling human infantile neuroaxonal dystrophy. Cornell Vet 83:133, 1993.
243. Pool RR: Osteochondromatosis. In Bojrab MJ (ed): Disease Mechanisms in Small Animal Surgery. Philadelphia, Lea & Febiger, 1993, p 821.
244. Pool RR: Tumors of bone and cartilage. In Moulton JE (ed): Tumors in Domestic Animals, 3rd ed. Berkeley, University of California Press, 1990.
245. Ness MG: Osteochondroma causing progressive posterior paresis in a Lakeland terrier puppy. Vet Rec 132:608, 1993.
246. Jacobson LS, Kirberger RM: Canine multiple cartilaginous exostoses: Unusual manifestations and review of the literature. J Am Anim Hosp Assoc 32:45, 1996.
247. Santen DR, et al: Thoracolumbar vertebral osteochondroma in a young dog. JAVMA 199:1054, 1991.
248. Selcer EA, et al: Dermoid cyst in a Shih Tzu and a boxer. J Am Anim Hosp Assoc 20:634, 1984.
249. Henderson JP, et al: Dermoid cyst of the spinal cord associated with ataxia in a cat. J Small Anim Pract 34:402, 1993.
250. Tomlinson J, et al: Intraspinal epidermoid cyst in a dog. JAVMA 193:1435, 1988.
251. Marks SL, et al: Dermoid sinus in a Rhodesian ridgeback. J Small Anim Pract 34:356, 1993
252. Dubey JP: Toxoplasmosis. JAVMA 205:1593, 1994.
253. Lappin MR: Feline toxoplasmosis. Waltham Focus 4:2, 1994.
254. Heidel JR, et al: Myelitis in a cat infected with Toxoplasma gondii and feline immunodeficiency virus. JAVMA 196:316, 1990.
255. Patton S, et al: Concurrent infection with Toxoplasma gondii and feline leukemia virus. J Vet Intern Med 5:199, 1991.
256. Lappin MR, et al: Effect of feline immunodeficiency virus infection on Toxoplasma gondii–specific humoral and cell-mediated immune responses of cats with serologic evidence of toxoplasmosis. J Vet Intern Med 7:95, 1993.
257. Dubey JP, et al: Neosporosis in cats. Vet Pathol 27:335, 1990.
258. Dubey JP: Neospora caninum: A look at a new Toxoplasma-like parasite of dogs and other animals. Comp Contin Educ 12:653, 1990.
259. Hoskins JD, et al: Disseminated infection with Neospora caninum in a ten-year-old dog. Cornell Vet 81:329, 1991.
260. Cuddon P, et al: Neospora caninum infection in English springer spaniel littermates. J Vet Intern Med 6:325, 1992.
261. Ruehlmann D, et al: Canine neosporosis: A case report and literature review. J Am Anim Hosp Assoc 31:174, 1995.
262. Barber JS, Trees AJ: Clinical aspects of 27 cases of neosporosis in dogs. Vet Rec 139:439, 1996.
263. Barber JS, et al: Distribution of Neospora caninum within the central nervous system and other tissues of six dogs with clinical neosporosis. J Small Anim Pract 37:568, 1996.
264. Dubey JP, Lindsay DS: A review of Neospora caninum and neosporosis. Vet Parasitol 67:1, 1996.
265. Lappin MR, et al: Serologic evidence of selected infectious diseases in cats with uveitis. JAVMA 201: 1005, 1992.
266. Lappin MR, et al: Detection of Toxoplasma gondii antigen-containing immune complexes in the serum of cats. Am J Vet Res 54:415, 1993.
267. Kroll RA, Constantinescu GM: Congenital abnormalities of the spinal cord and vertebrae. In August JR (ed): Consultations in Feline Internal Medicine, 2nd ed. Philadelphia, WB Saunders, 1994, p 413.
268. Grevel V, et al: Eine Arachnoidzyste bei der Katze. Kleintierpraxis 34:55, 1989.
269. Dyce J, et al: Canine "arachnoid cysts." J Small Anim Pract 32:433, 1991.
270. Bentley JF, et al: Spinal arachnoid cyst in a dog. J Am Anim Hosp Assoc 27:549, 1991.
271. Vernau KM, et al: Magnetic resonance imaging and computed tomography characteristics of intracranial intra-arachnoid cysts in 6 dogs. Vet Radiol Ultrasound 38:171, 1997.
272. Shamir MH, et al: Subarachnoid cyst in a cat. J Am Anim Hosp Assoc 33:123, 1997.
273. Cambridge AJ, et al: Radiographic diagnosis: Arachnoid cyst in a dog. Vet Radiol Ultrasound 38:434, 1997.
274. Mason KV: Canine neural angiostrongylosis: The clinical and therapeutic features of 35 natural cases. Aust Vet J 64:201, 1987.
275. Mason KV: Haematological and cerebrospinal fluid findings in canine neural angiostrongylosis. Aust Vet J 66:152, 1989.
276. Collins GH, et al: Angiostrongylosis in dogs in Sydney. Aust Vet J 69:170, 1992.
277. Thomas JS: Encephalomyelitis in a dog caused by Baylisascaris infection. Vet Pathol 25:94, 1988.
278. Smith DA, Knottenbelt DC: Spirocerca lupi localization in the spinal cord of a dog. Zimbabwe Vet J 18:19, 1989.
279. LeCouteur RA: Central nervous system trauma. In Kornegay JN (ed): Neurologic Disorders. Contemporaray Issues in Small Animal Practice, Vol 5. New York, Churchill Livingstone, 1986, p 147.
280. Kraus KH: The pathophysiology of spinal cord injury and its clinical implications. Semin Vet Med Surg 11:201, 1996.
281. Vandevelde M, Wolf M: Spinal cord compression. In Bojrab MJ (ed): Disease Mechanisms in Small Animal Surgery. Philadelphia, Lea & Febiger, 1993, p 1140.
282. Young W. Methylprednisolone treatment for acute spinal cord injury study. J Neurotrauma 8(Suppl 1):S43, 1991.
283. Tator CH: Update on the pathophysiology and pathology of acute spinal cord injury. Brain Pathol 5:407, 1995.
284. Bracken MB, et al: Results of the Third National Acute Spinal Cord Injury Randomized Controlled Trial. JAMA 277:1597, 1997.

285. Heary RF, et al: Steroids and gunshot wounds to the spine. Neurosurgery 41:576, 1997.
286. Ross IB, et al: Effect of nimodipine or methylprednisolone on recovery from acute experimental spinal cord injury in rats. Surg Neurol 40:461, 1993.
287. Ross IB, Tator CH: Spinal cord blood flow and evoked potential responses after treatment with nimodipine or methylprednisolone in spinal cord-injured rats. Neurosurgery 33:470,1993.
288. DeLey G, Leybaert L: Effect of flunarizine and methylprednisolone on functional recovery after experimental spinal injury. J Neurotrauma 10:25, 1993.
289. Young W, Bracken MB: The second national acute spinal cord injury study. J Neurotrauma 9(Suppl 1):S397, 1992.
290. Patterson RH, Smith GK: Backsplinting for treatment of thoracic and lumbar fracture/luxation in the dog: Principles of application and case series. VCOT 5:179, 1992.
291. Bruecker KA, Seim HB III: Spinal fracture and luxations. In Slatter DH (ed): Textbook of Small Animal Surgery, 2nd ed. Philadelphia, WB Saunders, 1993, p 1110.
292. Brueker KA: Principles of vertebral fracture management. Semin Vet Med Surg 11:259, 1996.
293. Longshore RC, O'Brien DP: Medical care of the neurosurgical patient. Semin Vet Med Surg 11:208, 1996.
294. Stigen O, et al: Stenosis of the thoracolumbar vertebral canal in a Basset hound. J Small Anim Pract 31:621, 1990.
295. Wheeler SJ: Vertebral abnormalities in dogs. J Small Anim Pract 32:149, 1991.
296. Baum F III, et al: Cervical fibrotic stenosis in a young rottweiler. JAVMA 201:1222, 1992.
297. Morgan JP, Biery DN: Spondylosis deformans. In Newton CD, Nunamaker DH (eds): Textbook of Small Animal Orthopedics. Philadelphia, JB Lippincott, 1985, p 733.
298. Langeland M, Lingaas F: Spondylosis deformans in the boxer: Estimates of heritability. J Small Anim Pract 36:166, 1995.
299. Bougie JD, et al: An unusual cause for lumbar radiculopathy: A synovial facet joint cyst of the right L5 joint. J Manipulative Physiol Ther 19:48, 1996.
300. Kotilainen E, Marttila RJ: Paraparesis caused by a bilateral cervical synovial cyst. Acta Neurol Scand 96:59, 1997.
301. Schmahl W, Kaiser E: Hydrocephalus, syringomyelia, and spinal cord angiodysgenesis in a Lhasa-apso dog. Vet Pathol 21:252, 1984.
302. Child G, et al: Acquired scoliosis associated with hydromyelia and syringomyelia in two dogs. JAVMA 189:909, 1986.
303. Tamke PG, et al: Acquired hydrocephalus and hydromyelia in a cat with feline infectious peritonitis: A case report and brief review. Can Vet J 29:997, 1988.
304. Johnson L, et al: Syringomyelia and hydrocephalus in two dogs. Prog Vet Neurol 3:82, 1992.
305. Kirberger RM, et al: Hydromyelia in the dog. Vet Radiol Ultrasound 38:30, 1997.
306. Bagley RS, et al: Scoliosis and associated cystic spinal cord lesion in a dog. JAVMA 211:573, 1997.

CNS

CHAPTER 107

NEURO-OPHTHALMOLOGY— PUPILS THAT TEACH

B. Keith Collins

Pupil abnormalities are common and can be the most prominent manifestation of ocular disease. Changes in pupil size, shape, and response to light stimulation may all indicate pupillary dysfunction.

The pupil is the central aperture of the iris. Changes in pupil size regulate the amount of light entering the eye and also affect depth perception, which is greatest when the pupil is small. In this manner, the pupil (and iris) is somewhat analogous to the iris diaphragm of a camera. Pupil movement is mediated by two smooth muscles with antagonistic functions, the iris sphincter (or constrictor) and the iris dilator muscles.

Contraction of the iris sphincter muscle causes a decrease in pupil size, or miosis. Contraction of the iris dilator muscle causes an increase in pupil size, or mydriasis. The normal pupil is round in the dog. In domestic cats, the pupil is slitlike when constricted, vertically oval when semidilated, and circular when widely dilated. It has been suggested that the eyes of animals with slitlike pupils are more sensitive to light stimulation than are the eyes of animals with round pupils.[1]

The iris musculature, and therefore pupil mobility, is controlled primarily by the autonomic nervous system. The iris sphincter muscle is considered the stronger of the two muscles and is under parasympathetic innervation. Light stimulation of the eye acts via the pupillary light reflex pathways to cause an endogenous release of acetylcholine and subsequent pupillary constriction. Exogenously applied cholinergic drugs, such as pilocarpine, likewise stimulate pupillary constriction.

The iris dilator muscle is under sympathetic innervation. Endogenous norepinephrine is released in response to psychosensory stimuli including pain, fear, or excitement, and the result is pupillary dilatation. The transient mydriasis that may occur in excited animals is mediated by adrenaline and is part of the so-called fight or flight response.

Pupil motion is not entirely dependent on autonomic innervation and can be affected by inflammatory ocular conditions such as uveitis. Prostaglandins and, to a lesser extent, histamines are important chemical mediators of ocular inflammation and stimulate the iris constrictor muscle directly, resulting in miosis.[2, 3]

NEUROANATOMY

PUPILLARY LIGHT REFLEX

Afferent Pathway

The afferent arc of the pupillary light reflex (PLR) is a three-neuron pathway.[4] It begins when light stimulates photoreceptor cells of the outer retina. This reaction is converted to a neurologic impulse and relayed to the first-order bipolar cells of the retina. The photoreceptor cells and bipolar cells together constitute the retinal chain neuron. The signal continues in the second-order ganglion cells of the inner retina. The long axons of the ganglion cells converge centripetally and then turn posteriorly at the optic disk to form the optic nerve (Fig. 107–1).

The optic nerve passes through the orbit and enters the cranium via the optic foramen. A percentage of fibers within the optic nerve crosses over (or decussates) at the optic chiasm to enter the optic tract of the opposite side. The percentage of decussation is approximately 65 per cent for the cat and 75 per cent for the dog.[5] Decussating nerve fibers arise in the nasal (or medial) retina, whereas those arising from the far temporal (or lateral) retina remain ipsilateral. The net effect is to have sensory input from the right or left half of a visual field of each eyeball conveyed to the opposite visual cortex.

The nerve fibers responsible for vision, and the pupillomotor fibers that mediate the PLR, have a common pathway to the level of the optic tract. Pupillomotor fibers exit the optic tract via the superior brachium of the rostral (superior) colliculus to enter the midbrain, where they synapse on third-order neurons in the pretectal nuclei. Most of the third-order axons that arise from each pretectal nucleus decussate again via the caudal commissure and synapse in the parasympathetic component of the oculomotor nucleus of the opposite side. This completes the afferent arc of the PLR.

Second-order nerve fibers that remain in the optic tract are responsible for vision. They are projected to the lateral geniculate body (LGB) of the thalamus, the optic radiations, and finally the occipital (or visual) cortex, where the initial light stimulus is ultimately perceived as vision.

It is important to note that fibers that mediate the PLR and those that are projected for vision are separate after the level of the optic tract. Therefore, lesions confined to the LGB, the optic radiations, or the visual cortex will cause

blindness but will not affect the PLR. Blindness with a normal PLR is characteristic of a central (cortical) lesion.

Efferent Pathway

The efferent arc of the PLR is a two-neuron pathway mediated by the parasympathetic component of the oculomotor nerve (cranial nerve III).[4] In contrast to the afferent pathway, the efferent nerve fibers are uncrossed and project to the ipsilateral iris.

The parasympathetic nucleus is located in the rostral portion of the oculomotor nucleus of the midbrain (see Fig. 107–1). Preganglionic axons, which arise from cell bodies in the nucleus, enter the orbit through the orbital fissure and synapse on the ciliary ganglion lateral to the optic nerve. Postganglionic cell bodies in the ciliary ganglion send their axons via the short ciliary nerves to innervate the iris and ciliary body musculature. In the dog, there are five to eight short ciliary nerves. Cats have only two short ciliary nerves, referred to as the medial (nasal) and lateral (malar) nerves.[4]

SYMPATHETIC SYSTEM

The ocular sympathetic tract is a three-neuron pathway.[4] The central, or upper motor neuron (UMN), pathway begins in the hypothalamus. Psychosensory information is relayed from the hypothalamus and higher cortical centers to the midbrain, where it descends in the spinal cord through the lateral tectotegmentospinal tract to synapse on the lower motor neuron (LMN). Preganglionic LMN cell bodies are located in the intermediate grey matter of spinal cord segments T1–T3. Their axons exit the spinal cord and join the thoracic sympathetic trunk ventrolateral to the vertebral column. From this point, sympathetic fibers course craniad through the cervicothoracic and middle cervical ganglions without synapse and join the vagosympathetic trunk. Next, sympathetic fibers diverge from the vagus and synapse on postganglionic cell bodies located in the cranial cervical ganglion caudomedial to the tympanic bullae.

Postganglionic axons continue rostrad to enter the cranium, pass through the middle ear and the cavernous sinus, and finally enter the orbit through the orbital fissure with the ophthalmic branch of the trigeminal nerve (cranial nerve V). Sympathetic fibers are distributed to the dilator muscle of the iris and also to smooth muscle of the periorbita, eyelids, and third eyelid.

OCULAR EXAMINATION

Primary ocular disease is a common cause of pupillary dysfunction, and a complete ocular examination is a prerequisite to consideration of neurologic deficits. Diseases that cause mechanical or structural abnormalities of the iris and that might cause pupillary dysfunction must be identified (Table 107–1). Some pupillary abnormalities are more evident in ambient light and should be noted at this time. Recognition of concurrent visual deficits is important in the diagnosis of afferent neurologic lesions. Testing of menace reflexes, observation of the animal's ability to follow cotton balls thrown in the air, and possibly observation of the animal's ability to negotiate an obstacle course may all be useful in evaluating vision.

The remainder of the examination is performed in dark or dim light conditions using, preferably, the Finnoff transillu-

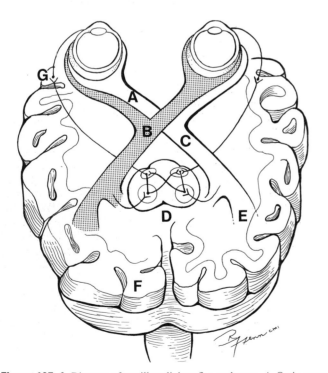

Figure 107–1. Diagram of pupillary light reflex pathways. *A*, Optic nerve; *B*, optic chiasm; *C*, optic tract; *D*, midbrain with pretectal nuclei *(large circles)* and parasympathetic oculomotor nuclei *(small ovals)*; *E*, lateral geniculate body of the thalamus; *F*, visual cortex; *G*, efferent parasympathetic pathway.

TABLE 107–1. NON-NEUROLOGIC CAUSES OF ANISOCORIA

CONDITION	PUPIL	ASSOCIATED SIGNS
Anterior uveitis	Usually miotic, sluggish PLR	Conjunctival hyperemia, aqueous flare, corneal edema, decreased intraocular pressure
Glaucoma	Mydriatic, sluggish to unresponsive PLR	Episcleral vascular injection, corneal edema, elevated intraocular pressure
Posterior synechiae	Variable shape, slow to unresponsive	Pigment clumps on anterior lens surface, with or without anterior uveitis
Iris atrophy	Variable shape, slow to unresponsive	Pupil margin often irregular, tapetal reflection may be seen through iris stroma or around pupillary margin, usually occurs in older animals
Iris hypoplasia	Variable shape, slow to unresponsive	Large areas of iris stroma may be absent, tapetal reflection may be seen through iris stroma, usually recognized in young animals as a congenital defect, may be associated with coat color dilution
Pharmacologic blockade	Mydriatic, absent direct and indirect PLR	History of prior atropine use or exposure to toxic plants
Pharmacologic stimulation	Miotic or mydriatic, variable PLR	History of parasympathomimetic drugs (e.g., pilocarpine) or sympathomimetic drugs (e.g., phenylephrine)

PLR = pupillary light reflex.

minator as a light source. The examiner stands approximately an arm's length from the animal but level with the animal's head. The pupils are then retroilluminated by directing light toward the bridge of the animal's nose in such a manner as to illuminate both eyes simultaneously. The observed fundic reflection provides a ready assessment of disparities in pupil size (i.e., anisocoria). Care is taken not to stimulate one pupil more than the other with the light source. After the pupils are assessed for symmetry, the light source is moved to within a few centimeters of the eye for assessment of the PLR.

EVALUATION OF THE PUPILLARY LIGHT REFLEX

A strong focal light source such as the Finnoff transilluminator should be used to evaluate the PLR. The animal should be calm but alert when assessing PLR. A brief period may be required for the animal to acclimate to the examination room. Excited or anxious animals with excessive sympathetic stimulus often have bilaterally dilated pupils that are relatively unresponsive to light.

Pupillary light reflexes are assessed using the "swinging flashlight" test. This is a simple procedure whereby a given eye is illuminated for two to four seconds before redirecting the light source toward the opposite eye for an equal period of time.[2, 4] The examiner notes during this time whether the pupil constricts, dilates, or fails to respond. The test can be performed in light or dark conditions but is more sensitive when performed in the dark, because pupillary excursions are greater.[2]

In the eye into which light is directed, constriction of the pupil is called the direct or ipsilateral response. Simultaneous constriction of the opposite pupil is called the indirect or consensual response. Each pupil should be freely mobile and constrict in both a direct and an indirect manner.

Upon moving the light source from one eye to the next during the swinging flashlight test, the newly illuminated pupil should already be in a semiconstricted position. If this pupil suddenly dilates while receiving direct illumination, the eye is abnormal and is said to have a positive swinging flashlight test or Marcus Gunn's sign.[2, 4] This finding is considered pathognomonic of a prechiasmal (i.e., retinal or optic nerve) lesion. Following evaluation of the PLR, the

examination is completed by ophthalmoscopic assessment of the retina and optic nerve.

PHARMACOLOGIC TESTING

Pharmacologic testing facilitates the differentiation of central, preganglionic, and postganglionic efferent autonomic lesions. The conditions in which testing may be beneficial include disorders of the sympathetic system (e.g., Horner's syndrome) and disorders of the parasympathetic system (e.g., oculomotor nerve paralysis).[6]

Pharmacologic localization of a lesion is possible because of denervation supersensitivity. This is a phenomenon whereby the denervated muscle cells become supersensitive to the neurotransmitter, and it occurs to a much greater extent with lesions of the postganglionic neuron. The net effect is an exaggerated response to what, in a normal eye, would be an ineffective concentration of an exogenously applied neurotransmitter. Following application of the drug, the pupillary response of the denervated eye occurs sooner and to a greater extent and persists for a longer time when compared with the normal eye.

With unilateral lesions, both eyes are tested in an identical manner. With bilateral lesions, only one eye is tested. In each instance, the opposite eye allows for comparison of response. Both direct- and indirect-acting drugs can be used to differentiate a pre- from a postganglionic lesion. Clinical response to the indirect-acting drugs is less predictable; therefore, only the direct-acting drugs are presented here.

Testing for Sympathetic Lesions. Miosis is the abnormal finding, and mydriasis is the anticipated response to the drugs. A dilute solution of a direct-acting drug, 1 per cent phenylephrine (stock 10 per cent solution diluted 1:10 with saline), is applied to the eye or eyes. This drug stimulates the denervated and supersensitive muscle cells directly. If the lesion is postganglionic, the affected eye will dilate quickly (usually within 20 minutes). In the case of a preganglionic lesion, the eye may also dilate but should take longer (30 to 40 minutes). The normal eye does not respond to these weak concentrations.

Testing for Parasympathetic Lesions. Mydriasis is the abnormal finding, and miosis is the anticipated response to the drugs. A dilute solution of a direct-acting drug, 0.1 per cent pilocarpine (stock 1 per cent solution diluted 1:10

TABLE 107–2. NEUROLOGIC CAUSES OF ANISOCORIA

CONDITION	PUPIL	ASSOCIATED SIGNS
Unilateral retinal disease	Mydriatic, sluggish to absent direct PLR, normal indirect PLR	Pupils dilate symmetrically in darkness, abnormal funduscopic exam and/or ERG, positive swinging flashlight test, visual deficits
Unilateral optic neuritis	Mydriatic, sluggish to absent direct PLR, normal indirect PLR	Pupils dilate symmetrically in darkness, funduscopic evidence of optic neuritis unless retrobulbar lesion, normal ERG, positive swinging flashlight test, visual deficits, with or without other neurologic disease
Optic chiasmal lesions*	Mydriatic, absent PLR	Pupils dilate symmetrically in darkness, normal funduscopic exam, visual deficits, with or without other neurologic disease
Unilateral optic tract lesion	Slightly mydriatic contralateral pupil, intact PLR	Pupils dilate symmetrically in darkness, normal funduscopic exam, normal ERG, negative swinging flashlight test, visual deficits, with or without other neurologic disease
Horner's syndrome	Miotic, PLR intact	Anisocoria increases in darkness, with or without ptosis, enophthalmos, and third eyelid prolapse; vision normal
Oculomotor nerve palsy	Mydriatic, absent direct and indirect PLR	Anisocoria increases in light, ptosis, reduced ocular mobility, strabismus if external ophthalmoplegia also present, vision normal
Midbrain lesion	Variable	Miosis often occurs with acute trauma and may progress to mydriasis
Cerebellar syndrome	Ipsilateral miosis	Menace deficit with normal vision, intention tremors, hypermetric gait, other neurologic signs
Feline spastic pupil syndrome[4, 14]	Static anisocoria	Eyes are visual and are not inflamed, cat is usually seropositive for feline leukemia virus
Dysautonomia[15]	Static mydriasis	Occurs in dogs and cats, additional ocular signs may include third eyelid prolapse, dry eye

*Anisocoria present only if lesion is asymmetric.
PLR = pupillary light reflex; ERG = electroretinogram.

with saline), is applied to the eye or eyes. Pilocarpine is a structural analogue of acetylcholine and stimulates the denervated muscle cells directly. If the lesion is postganglionic, the affected eye will constrict quickly (usually within 20 minutes), whereas the normal eye, or an eye with a central or preganglionic lesion, will generally not respond at all to this weak concentration. A negative response may also indicate pharmacologic blockade with a drug such as atropine, assuming the mechanical and structural integrity of the iris was determined to be normal during the initial ophthalmic examination. An iris of normal integrity will constrict following a single application of 1 or 2 per cent pilocarpine, irrespective of neurologic status. A continued negative response confirms pharmacologic blockade. Repeated applications of these higher concentrations will eventually cause the pupil to constrict, because pilocarpine is an atropine antagonist.

DIFFERENTIAL CONSIDERATIONS OF PUPILLARY DYSFUNCTION

Pupillary dysfunction may present as unilateral or bilateral persistent (or static) miosis or mydriasis, inequality of pupil size (anisocoria), abnormal pupil shape (dyscoria), abnormal placement (corectopia), or simply a decreased responsiveness to light. Lesions of the sympathetic or PLR pathways cause abnormal pupillary responses and/or anisocoria.

Anisocoria[7] is probably the most common finding with pupillary disease, although bilateral and symmetric lesions do not manifest as anisocoria. Recognition of anisocoria is usually simple, but it can be challenging to determine which is the abnormal pupil. When evaluating the PLR, if only one pupil is slow to respond, it is abnormal.[8] Both pupils may be slow to respond if the lesion is bilateral. Pupillary responses may remain intact with some causes of anisocoria, including optic tract lesions and Horner's syndrome. Anisocoria may be more pronounced in light conditions (e.g., with oculomotor paralysis) or dark conditions (e.g., with Horner's syndrome), and this should be noted. Concurrent visual deficits usually implicate an afferent lesion.

Although this chapter is concerned primarily with neurologic dysfunction of the pupil, primary or secondary ocular disease is important in the differential diagnosis (see Table 107–1). A complete ophthalmic examination is necessary to determine whether the pupillary dysfunction is neurologic or the result of non-neurologic ocular disease.

AFFERENT LESIONS

The hallmark signs of an afferent lesion are blindness in one or both eyes and maximal and symmetric mydriasis during dark room examination (Table 107–2). Pupils that do not dilate in this manner suggest a lesion elsewhere. Afferent lesions include those affecting the retina, optic nerve, optic chiasm, or optic tract. Unilateral afferent lesions may result in subtle anisocoria noticeable in ambient light because of differential light stimulation of the contralateral eye.

EFFERENT LESIONS

Horner's Syndrome

Ocular sympathetic denervation causes the clinical condition known as Horner's syndrome. Clinical signs include miosis, drooping of the upper eyelid (ptosis), narrowing of the palpebral fissure, enophthalmos, and protrusion of the third eyelid (Fig. 107–2).[9–12] Miosis and, less consistently, third eyelid prolapse are suggested as the most common signs.[9, 10] Anisocoria is more pronounced on dark examination, as the affected pupil has an inability to dilate more than a few millimeters. The affected eye retains an intact PLR, and vision is normal. In bright light, the normal pupil is also constricted; thus the pupils may appear nearly equal in size.

Damage anywhere along the sympathetic pathway may cause Horner's syndrome, but LMN lesions are most common in animals.[11] The two most common causes of postganglionic Horner's syndrome are otitis media and orbital disease.[9–11] Concurrent clinical signs are important to note and often help to localize the site of the lesion. In two reviews,

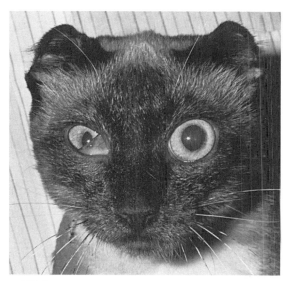

Figure 107–2. Horner's syndrome in a cat. Note miosis, third eyelid prolapse, and ptosis in the right eye. (The editors thank Drs. Richard and Jacqueline LeCouteur for this photo.)

the cause for Horner's syndrome was undetermined in approximately 50 per cent of the cases.[10, 11]

Internal Ophthalmoplegia

Internal ophthalmoplegia refers to paralysis of the intraocular muscles (i.e., iris sphincter and ciliary body muscles).[4, 13] Such an eye has a persistently dilated pupil that is unresponsive to direct or indirect light, whereas the fellow eye has normal direct and indirect reflexes. The afferent pathways are normal, and the eye is visual. Anisocoria is more pronounced in lighted conditions when the normal pupil is constricted.

Pharmacologic blockade with atropine or similar compounds is a common cause of internal ophthalmoplegia. It is important to elucidate in the history whether atropine or a similar parasympatholytic agent has been applied to the eye. The pupil may remain dilated for several weeks after discontinuation of the drug. Additional causes of internal

ophthalmoplegia include orbital disease, cavernous sinus syndrome, midbrain lesions, and idiopathic causes.

Because the cat has only two short ciliary nerves, each of which innervates half of the iris, aberrant pupil shapes may occur. If only the medial (nasal) short ciliary nerve is damaged, the clinician will observe a "D" pupil if the right eye is affected and a "reverse D" if the left eye is affected. Conversely, if only the lateral (malar) nerve is damaged, a "D" pupil occurs if the left eye is affected and a "reverse D" if the right eye is affected.[4]

Miscellaneous Considerations

Additional causes of anisocoria include feline spastic pupil syndrome; dysautonomia, which occurs in both dogs and cats; effects of various drugs; brain trauma; and cerebellar syndrome. The reader is referred to Table 107–2 for salient features of these disorders.

CNS

REFERENCES

1. Prince JH: Comparative Anatomy of the Eye. Springfield, IL, Charles C Thomas, 1956.
2. Thompson HS: The pupil. *In* Moses RA, Hart WM (eds): Adler's Physiology of the Eye, 8th ed. St. Louis, CV Mosby, 1987, pp 311–338.
3. Yoshitomi T, Ito Y: Effects of indomethacin and prostaglandins on the dog iris sphincter and dilator muscles. Invest Ophthalmol 29:127, 1988.
4. Scagliotti R: Current concepts in veterinary neuro-ophthalmology. Vet Clin North Am 10:417, 1980.
5. Slatter DH, De Lahunta A: Neuro-ophthalmology. *In* Slatter DH (ed): Fundamentals of Veterinary Ophthalmology, 1st ed. Philadelphia, WB Saunders, 1981, pp 587–661.
6. Collins BK, O'Brien D: Autonomic dysfunction of the eye. Semin Vet Med Surg (Small Anim) 5:24, 1990.
7. Neer TM, Carter JD: Anisocoria in dogs and cats: Ocular and neurologic causes. Comp Contin Educ 9:817, 1987.
8. Thompson HS, Pilley SFJ: Unequal pupils. A flow chart for sorting out the anisocorias. Surv Ophthalmol 21:45, 1976.
9. Neer TM: Horner's syndrome: Anatomy, diagnosis, and causes. Comp Contin Educ 6:740, 1984.
10. Kern TJ, Aromando MC, Erb HN: Horner's syndrome in dogs and cats: 100 cases (1975–1985). JAVMA 195:369, 1989.
11. Morgan RV, Zanotti SW: Horner's syndrome in dogs and cats: 49 cases (1980–1986). JAVMA 194:1096, 1989.
12. van den Broek AHM: Horner's syndrome in cats and dogs: A review. J Small Anim Pract 28:929, 1987.
13. Gerding PA, Brightman AH, Brogdon JD: Pupillotonia in a dog. JAVMA 11:1477, 1986.
14. Brightman AH, Macy DW, Gosselin Y: Pupillary abnormalities associated with the feline leukemia complex. Fel Pract 11:24, 1977.
15. Canton DD, Sharp NJH, Aguirre GD: Dysautonomia in a cat. JAVMA 192:1293, 1988.

CHAPTER 108

PERIPHERAL NERVE DISORDERS

Karen Dyer Inzana

The peripheral nervous system can be defined as those portions of the nervous system that reside partially or entirely outside the central nervous system (CNS) and are invested by a unique set of glial elements, Schwann cells, fibroblasts, and satellite cells. Using this definition, the peripheral nervous system includes cranial nerves III through XII, all the spinal nerves with their roots, peripheral nerves, and the peripheral components of the autonomic nervous system.[1] Collectively, they function to relay information about the environment to the CNS and in turn provide motor control of peripheral structures. Because peripheral nerves are the sole neural structure that controls skeletal muscle, they provide the most elemental level of motor control by the nervous system. It is impossible to clinically evaluate the CNS if the peripheral nervous system is nonfunctional.

Structurally, peripheral nerves are collections of neuronal cell processes enveloped in fibrous connective tissue (Fig. 108–1).[2] There are three distinct supportive tissue sheaths—the endoneurium, perineurium, and epineurium—that surround individual axons, fascicles of axons, or the entire peripheral nerve, respectively. Neurons are the principal cells that make up the peripheral nerves.[2, 3] Cell bodies are located in the brain stem and spinal cord (motor neurons) or in clusters of cells (ganglia—sensory and autonomic) located in the periphery. Cell bodies extend processes (axons) outside the nervous system that either receive information from sensory receptors (sensory or afferent neurons) or transmit information regarding movement to peripheral muscles (motor or efferent neurons). All axons are invested with a Schwann cell covering. In most axons 1μm or more in diameter, the Schwann cell also generates a myelin sheath that facilitates propagation of action potentials along the axon. Motor axons terminate on multiple skeletal muscle end plates, whereas sensory axons either terminate in secondary neurons, many of which form connections with the motor axons of the same or nearby peripheral nerves, or continue uninterrupted to the brain stem as sensory spinal tracts.

Functionally, information is transmitted along axons electrically in the form of an action potential.[4, 5] The action potential is created by ion influxes, primarily sodium, that change the electrical gradient across the axonal cell membrane. In myelinated axons, sodium ion channels are concentrated at nodes of Ranvier, and action potentials are propagated along the axon from node to node (saltatory conduction). Ion channels are uniformly located along the entire length of nonmyelinated axons, and conduction is continuous along the cellular membrane. Information is transmitted to muscles or other neurons most commonly chemically, by the physical release of a neurotransmitter at the axon terminal that interacts with receptors linked to additional ion channels on the receptor surface.

METHODS OF EVALUATION

There are three main methods of evaluating the peripheral nervous system: clinically, electrophysiologically, and histologically. Clinically, the hallmarks of peripheral nerve dis-

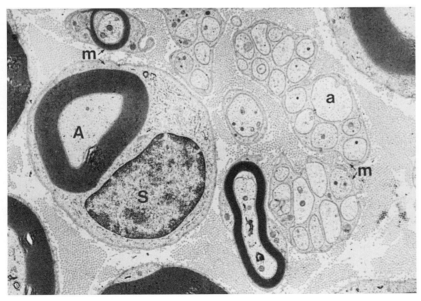

Figure 108–1. Electron micrograph of a peripheral nerve magnified 12000×. Cross-sections of both myelinated (A) and unmyelinated (a) axons are present surrounded by Schwann cell membranes (m). The section of the medium-sized myelinated axon in the center was taken through the Schwann cell nucleus (S).

ease are motor deficits ranging from weakness to paralysis, hypotonic muscles with rapid muscle atrophy, and diminished or absent spinal reflexes. Sensation may be altered if sensory nerves are affected by the disease process. These clinical signs may be diffuse, or they may be confined to one or more peripheral nerves or cranial nerves. The clinical signs attributed to individual peripheral nerve or cranial nerve injury are outlined in Tables 108–1 and 108–2. Most peripheral neuropathies are diffuse in clinical presentation. Weakness is often more pronounced in the pelvic limbs, and with the exception of the recurrent laryngeal, hypoglossal, and vagus nerves, the cranial nerves are usually affected only in more severe cases. Clinical signs of laryngeal paralysis including stridor, inspiratory dyspnea, voice change, and exercise intolerance may be an early sign of a more diffuse peripheral neuropathy.[6, 7] Similarly, dysphagia and megaesophagus have been associated with generalized peripheral nerve disease.[8] In rare cases in which the sensory nerves are affected alone, weakness is less apparent than poor coordination. Muscle atrophy is less marked, but spinal reflexes are uniformly depressed.

Measuring the electrical activity of skeletal muscle via needle electromyography (EMG) is useful to confirm suspicions of peripheral nerve or muscle disease, as well as to map the distribution of injury.[9] A variety of spontaneous electrical potentials may be recorded from denervated or otherwise injured skeletal muscle. These spontaneous potentials have been broken down into several characteristic potentials, including fibrillation potentials, positive sharp waves, and high-frequency discharges.[10, 11] The distinction between denervation and primary muscle diseases is not easily established by the type of abnormal electrical activity. There is a tendency for denervation to produce more fibrillations, whereas high-frequency discharges are seen more often in primary muscle disease. Because we are not able to attribute clinical significance to the different types of abnormal electrical potentials, they are referred to simply as spontaneous activity.

CNS

TABLE 108–1. CLINICAL SIGNS OF PERIPHERAL NERVE OR CRANIAL NERVE INJURIES

NERVE	SPINAL CORD SEGMENTS	MUSCLES INNERVATED	SPINAL REFLEX ALTERATIONS WITH INJURY	MOTOR FUNCTION	CUTANEOUS DISTRIBUTION	CLINICAL SIGNS OF DYSFUNCTION
Brachial Plexus						
Suprascapular	C6–C7	Supraspinatus, infraspinatus	None	Extension and lateral support of the shoulder	None	Little gait abnormality
Axillary	C6–C8	Deltoid	No deficits or incomplete withdrawal reflex	Flexion of shoulder	Dorsolateral brachium—behind scapular spine	Little gait abnormality
Musculo-cutaneous	C6–C8	Biceps brachii	Decreased or absent biceps tendon reflex, no elbow flexion with withdrawal reflex	Flexion of elbow	Medial forelimb—medial humeral condyle	Little gait abnormality, unable to raise paw to table top (flex elbow)
Radial	C6–T2	Triceps brachii, extensor carpi radialis, ulnaris lateralis, common and lateral digital extensors	Decreased or absent triceps tendon reflex and extensor carpi radialis response	Extension of elbow, carpus, and digits	Dorsolateral forelimb—dorsal surface of paw	Loss of weight bearing, unable to fix limb in extension
Median and ulnar	C8–T2	Flexor carpi radialis, superficial digital and deep digital flexors, flexor carpi ulnaris	Decreased or absent flexion of carpus and digits during withdrawal reflex	Flexion of carpus and digits	Palmar surface of paw, caudal forelimb	Little gait abnormality
Pelvic Plexus						
Obturator	L4–L6	Pectineus, gracilis	None	Adduction of pelvic limb	None	Little gait abnormality, limb may slide laterally on slick floor
Femoral	L3–L6	Quadriceps femoris	Decreased or absent patellar reflex	Extension of stifle	Saphenous branch supplies medial thigh and digit	Inability to extend stifle
Sciatic	L6–S3	Gluteus, semimembranosus, semitendinosus, all muscles innervated by peroneal and tibial nerves	Decreased or absent withdrawal reflex	Flexion and extension of hip	Caudal and lateral surfaces of limb	Cannot flex or extend digits and hock or flex stifle
Peroneal	L6–S3	Peroneus longus, cranial tibial, lateral and long digital extensor	Decreased or absent cranial tibial response	Flexion of hock, extension of digits	Dorsal aspect of paw, hock, and distal limb	Cannot extend paw, therefore knuckles on dorsum, poor hock flexion
Tibial	L6–S3	Gastrocnemius, superficial and deep digital flexors	Decreased or absent gastrocnemius tendon reflex	Extension of hock, flexion of paw	Plantar surface of paw	Unable to fix hock in extension

TABLE 108–2. CRANIAL NERVES

CRANIAL NERVE	ANATOMIC COURSE	FUNCTION	EVALUATION
I: olfactory	Sensory ending in nasal mucosa, enter cribiform plate to olfactory bulb of pyriform cortex	Smell	Not routinely evaluated
II: optic	Retinal ganglion cells form optic nerve, which traverses optic foramen to optic chiasm and optic tracts in diencephalon	Vision and pupillary light reflexes	Menace reaction, pupillary light reflexes, avoids objects
III: oculomotor	Cell bodies in mesencephalon send processes through the orbital fissure to extraocular eye muscles and iris	Motor to extraocular eye muscles, parasympathetic to eye	Eye movement, pupillary light reflexes; damage causes ventrolateral strabismus and mydriasis
IV: trochlear	Cell bodies in mesencephalon, processes cross in rostral medullary velum, pass through orbital fissure to extraocular eye muscles	Motor to dorsal oblique muscle, which rotates globe	Not routinely tested in dogs; damage causes rotational deviation of globe
V: trigeminal	Motor bodies in metencephalon; sensory cell bodies in trigeminal ganglion terminate on metencephalic neurons; axons divide into mandibular, maxillary, and ophthalmic branches, which pass through oval foramen, round foramen, and orbital fissure, respectively	Motor to muscles of mastication including masseter, temporal, pterygoids, rostral digastricus, and myohyoid; sensory to the face	Jaw tone masticatory muscle mass, sensation to face
VI: abducent	Cell bodies in metencephalon, taking a long intracranial course to exit the orbital fissure to the eye	Motor to extraocular eye muscles, including lateral rectus and retractor bulbi	Eye movement; damage causes ventromedial strabismus
VII: facial	Cell bodies in myelencephalon, pass through internal acoustic meatus, petrous temporal bone to stylomastoid foramen	Motor to muscles of facial expression; sensory to small area of pinna; parasympathetic innervation to lacrimal glands, mandibular and sublingual salivary glands	Ability to blink, retract lip, move ear, produce tears
VIII: vestibulocochlear	Sensory neurons arise from receptors in inner ear, traverse internal acoustic meatus to myelencephalon	Balance, linear acceleration, hearing	Body posture, eye movement, hearing; damage causes positional strabismus and nystagmus
IX: glossopharyngeal	Cell bodies in myelencephalon exit external jugular foramen	Sensory and motor to the pharynx; parasympathetic innervation to zygomatic and parotid salivary glands	Gag reflex, swallowing
X: vagus	Cell bodies in myelencephalon exit external jugular foramen	Sensory and motor to pharynx; parasympathetic to cardiac, pulmonary, and gastrointestinal systems	Gag reflex, swallowing, oculocardiac reflex
XI: accessory	Cell bodies in myelencephalon and rostral spinal cord, exit external jugular foramen	Motor to larynx, trapezius, and sternobrachiocephalicus	Vocalization, muscle tone
XII: hypoglossal	Cell bodies in myelencephalon exit hypoglossal canal	Motor to tongue muscles	Tongue movement

Because nervous tissue is electrically excitable, the functional integrity of specific regions can be evaluated by measuring their ability to conduct an action potential evoked by electrical stimulus or stimulation of specific receptors. Using a combination of neuroanatomic and physiologic principles, any region of the central and peripheral nervous systems can be electrophysiologically evaluated. The techniques most useful for peripheral nerve disease include motor and sensory nerve conduction, brain stem auditory evoked potentials, and occasionally spinal cord evoked potentials. These have been described in detail elsewhere.[9–11] Briefly, in demyelinating neuropathies, motor and sensory nerve conduction is slowed, but the evoked action potential remains near normal in amplitude and duration. With axonal loss, significant reduction in nerve conduction velocity is not seen, but the evoked action potential is often reduced in amplitude and prolonged. The distinction between axon loss and myelin loss is not as readily apparent in central conduction studies. Instead, either conduction block or changes in the evoked potentials are simply an indication of disease.

The peripheral nervous system can be evaluated histologically without creating marked functional impairment. Muscle biopsies described in Chapter 86 are extremely useful at distinguishing denervation from primary muscle disease. Denervated skeletal muscles develop characteristic changes of angular atrophy. By evaluating histologic types of muscle fibers in unfixed, frozen samples, both type grouping and large grouped atrophy can be useful indicators of chronicity of disease and regenerative attempts.[12] Fascicular biopsies of peripheral nerves can be obtained from both motor and sensory nerves.[12, 13] The peripheral nerve to be sampled is surgically isolated, and a thin strip, less than one third the nerve diameter and extending 2 to 3 cm, is excised. Nerve samples should then be secured in a stretched position before fixation in 2.5 per cent glutaraldehyde. Samples may then be sent to a laboratory that specializes in neuromuscular evaluation, where they will usually be osmicated and embedded in plastic for both light and electron microscopy. Post-osmicated peripheral nerve biopsies can also be suspended in resin and individual fibers teased apart so that the pathology of successive internodes can be appreciated.[12]

MECHANISMS OF DISEASE

Because at least a portion of most peripheral nerves reside in the CNS, they can be affected by CNS diseases. However, this chapter concentrates on diseases unique to the peripheral nervous system and neuromuscular junction. Before considering individual diseases, it is useful to understand some of the complex interrelationships between neurons, axons, and Schwann cells that might contribute to disease processes.

The neuron is a specialized cell whose cell body possesses an unusually large surface area that aids in recognition of synaptic inputs from adjacent cells. The neuron contains many of the typical cellular organelles, including a single nucleus, one or more nucleoli, Golgi apparatus, and mitochondria. Under most conditions, the cytoplasm of neuronal cell bodies contains abundant rough endoplasmic reticulum or Nissl substance.[2, 3] Unlike most cells, neurons must support cellular processes that often extend great distances from the cell body. Damage to a neuron results in degeneration of all its cellular processes and dissolution of the myelin sheath produced by Schwann cells. Unlike damage to other peripheral nerve structures, regeneration is extremely limited in neuronopathies. Histologically, in earlier stages of acute neuronal death, neurons may be initially vacuolated, followed by cell shrinkage, pyknosis, and phagocytosis by macrophages. In sublethal injury, neurons may undergo a number of metabolic alterations, usually characterized by dissolution of Nissl substance or chromotolysis. Central chromotolysis is a classic feature of the "axon reaction," changes in the neuronal cell body as a consequence of damage to axonal processes of the cell body, but it can be a feature of inherited and toxic neuronopathies as well.[14, 15] Cytoplasmic inclusions may occur in neurons as a consequence of aging, or they may be a feature of metabolic storage disease or viral infections. Neurofilament accumulations may be seen in several inherited neuronopathies. The consequences of these changes on the remainder of the peripheral nervous system vary with their severity and with the neuron's ability to provide support for its processes despite these accumulations.

The axon is the most prominent cellular process of the neuron. Within the axon cylinder are cytoskeletal elements, microfilaments, neurotubules, and a microtrabecular matrix, which provide the structural framework for the neuron. Within this filamentous matrix, the axon also contains many organelles, including mitochondria, smooth endoplasmic reticulum, lysosomes, and a variety of tubovesicular structures, some of which contain newly synthesized proteins and lipids. Notably, the axon lacks any structures associated with protein synthesis or assembly such as ribosomes, rough endoplasmic reticulum, or Golgi bodies. Therefore, axons are dependent on protein synthesis in the cell body for maintenance of its structural and functional needs. Specialized processes have been developed to transport materials from the cell body to the nerve terminal (anterograde transport). Transported material travels at rates that vary from 0.25 mm/day for cytoskeletal elements to 400 mm/day for membranous structures. Once substances reach the nerve terminal,

there is a brief turnaround time, and then material is transported back to the cell body (retrograde transport) at approximately 200 mm/day for recycling. Nerve growth factor, tetanus toxoid, and several infectious agents probably use retrograde axonal transport to reach the CNS.

Damage to the axon results in wallerian degeneration of all distal sections no longer in contact with the cell body. Histologically, this appears initially as dissolution of the myelin sheath, with some clumping of the cytoskeletal elements and degenerating organelles within the axon. This is followed by progressive loss of axonal contents. Schwann cells survive, but peripheral nerve myelin degenerates with the axon. Complete severance of the axon and attendant wallerian degeneration are not difficult to identify histologically. More subtle lesions that result from metabolic alterations of the neuron or its ability to supply constitutive elements to the distal axon are more problematic. Much work has involved identifying disease processes that affect axonal transport. The clearest example of a disease caused by injury to axonal transport stems from the fact that agents that depolymerize tubulin, such as the vinca alkaloids, disrupt the neurotubulin cytoskeleton that provides the framework for fast axonal transport. Other associations have been less clear. Focal accumulations of microfilaments or other cytosolic organelles are characteristic features of several inherited and toxic neuropathies and may be the result of failure in the transport of these materials.[15, 16] Many believe that distal neuropathies may arise from a metabolic derangement within the axon or neural cell body, perhaps affecting the transport of necessary materials. The observation in many neuropathies that larger and longer axons are preferentially affected in distal segments, and that degeneration gradually extends to proximal axons over time (the "dying back" neuropathies), supports an inability to supply trophic substances to distal areas.[16]

Schwann cells are the primary supportive cells of the peripheral nervous system. They form an intimate relationship with all peripheral axons, both myelinated and unmyelinated. Through a series of cellular adhesion molecules located in their plasma membrane and growth factors secreted into the extracellular matrix, Schwann cells and neurons maintain extensive intracellular communication.[17] Schwann cells receive the signal to begin myelination from axons and require axonal contact to produce the extracellular matrix that constitutes the endoneurium. In turn, they not only produce peripheral nerve myelin, which is important in facilitating impulse propagation along the axon, but also direct the localization of voltage-dependent sodium channels to the nodal gap between Schwann cells. Schwann cells produce trophic factors that support the survival of axons, and they express surface ligands that direct growth and regeneration of axon sprouts. Schwann cells even regulate the diameter of axons, probably through regulation of the degree of phosphorylation of neurofilaments.[18] As previously mentioned, axonal integrity is a requirement for the maintenance of the myelin sheath. Any disease process that injures the axon will cause secondary demyelination. However, there are examples of neuropathies that target primarily Schwann cells. In cross section, myelin degeneration appears first as vacuolation, followed by separation of lamellae and finally removal of myelin debris by macrophages. This is usually associated with attempts at remyelination by surviving Schwann cells. Inappropriately thin myelin sheaths surrounding large axons or numerous "onion bulbs"— concentric layers of Schwann cell membranes surrounding demyelinated or remyelinated axons—are indications of remyelination.[15, 16] Often primary demyelination is best identified in teased fiber specimens, where individual denuded internodes or multiple short "intercalated" internodes over single internodal areas are considered characteristic. We have not advanced to the stage of understanding demyelinating neuropathies on the molecular basis, although rapid advancement is occurring in this and other areas of basic neurobiology. Some of the primary demyelinating neuropathies in veterinary patients include acute polyradiculoneuritis, which is an example of an immune-mediated attack on peripheral nerve myelin, and Schwann cells are the targets of several hereditary disorders of lipid metabolism.

The pathophysiologic mechanisms of most peripheral neuropathies in veterinary patients are not well understood. A discussion of what is known about individual diseases follows. They are grouped first by the proposed mechanism, and then by the predominant pathology. It should be noted that any grouping of diseases is somewhat arbitrary. As we learn more about the molecular basis for these diseases, more similarities or differences might be found.

DEVELOPMENTAL AND CONGENITAL DISORDERS

Developmental or congenital disorders are peripheral neuropathies that occur in specific breeds with a predictable clinical course and characteristic pathology. A genetic basis is likely. The age of onset, specific clinical signs, and rate of progression vary from disease to disease. Developmental disorders should be suspected in any young, purebred dog that develops lower motor neuron signs.

DEVELOPMENTAL DISORDERS CHARACTERIZED BY LOSS OF MOTOR NEURON (NEURONAL ABIOTROPHY)

Progressive Neuronopathy in Cairn Terriers

Also known as multisystemic chromatolytic neuronal degeneration, progressive neuronopathy has been reported in both male and female young Cairn terriers in the United Kingdom, Australia, and North America.[19–21] Clinical signs of rear limb weakness usually begin around 4 months of age. The disease is progressive, with tetraparesis, patellar hyporeflexia, generalized hypermetria, and head tremors developing within one to two months. One dog also developed cataplectic attacks responsive to imipramine.[21] Histologically, central and peripheral chromatolysis was present in dorsal and ventral horns of the spinal cord and brain stem, especially within the cuneate, glossopharyngeal, vagal, and trigeminal mesencephalic nuclei. Chromatolytic changes were also observed in the cerebrum, autonomic, and myenteric ganglia. Myelomalacia was present symmetrically in the funicular white matter segment of the thoracolumbar spinal cord, in proximity of the dorsal horns in one case.[21] Other cases showed only mild wallerian degeneration in peripheral nerves and white matter tracts in the spinal cord. The pathogenesis is unknown. Both genetic and toxic causes have been suggested.

Focal Spinal Muscular Atrophy in German Shepherd Dogs

Asymmetric loss of ventral horn cells in the cervical spinal intumescence has been reported in two German shepherds.[22] Forelimb weakness was first noted between 12 and 14 days of age and was followed by brachial and antebrachial muscle loss, resulting in valgus deformity and flexion of the carpal joints. The paresis progressed to inability to rise in one dog. The other dog was successfully treated with surgical tenotomy and carpal splinting. Histologically, asymmetric degeneration of the somatic motor neurons with peripheral chromatolysis was reported. These changes were confined to the cervical intumescence, with wallerian degeneration of peripheral nerves in the forelimbs and secondary muscle atrophy. The etiology is unknown. A genetic basis was speculated, based on similarities to focal spinal muscular atrophies in humans.

Hereditary Progressive Spinal Muscle Atrophy in English Pointers

A progressive neuropathy has been reported in English pointer dogs in Japan.[23–25] Clinical signs of generalized weakness began between 4 and 5 months of age and progressed to tetraplegia and areflexia over the following 3 to 4 months. Dysphonia and muscle fasciculations were common clinical features of the disease. Electrophysiologically, spontaneous activity developed in epaxial, proximal, and distal limb muscles. Motor nerve conduction was reduced, but sensory nerve conduction remained relatively normal.[25] Histologically, skeletal muscle changes were compatible with chronic denervation, and peripheral nerves showed only wallerian degeneration. Ventral horn cells were normal in number but contained lipidlike granular accumulations that ultrastructurally consisted of multilamellar structures arranged concentrically or in parallel. These membranous bodies were confined to cells within the ventral horn of the spinal cord and in the hypoglossal and spinal accessory nuclei of the brain stem. Breeding studies indicated that the disease can be reproduced in successive generations. An autosomal recessive mode of inheritance is theorized.

Spinal Muscular Atrophy in Rottweilers

This is a lower motor neuron disorder reported in both male and female rottweilers.[26, 27] Clinical signs began between 4 and 8 weeks of age with regurgitation and generalized weakness. Clinical signs rapidly progressed to tetraplegia within weeks. Spinal reflexes were diminished, and there was generalized muscle atrophy and pelvic limb rigidity. Megaesophagus was usually present radiographically. Histologically, changes consisted of central chromatolysis and marked swelling of the cell body in predominantly large motor neurons throughout the spinal cord. Chromatolytic neurons were are also present in cranial nerve nuclei, including oculomotor, trigeminal motor, and ambiguous nuclei, and in the red nucleus. Ultrastructurally, swollen cell bodies exhibited increased concentrations of neurofilaments and prominent Golgi complexes. Peripheral axons were undergoing various stages of wallerian degeneration. A genetic cause was speculated.

Neuronal Abiotrophy in Swedish Lapland dogs

Neuronal abiotrophy is an autosomal recessive trait reported in Swedish Lapland dogs.[28, 29] Clinical signs began abruptly between 5 and 7 weeks of age. Weakness initially began in either the thoracic or the pelvic limbs but rapidly progressed to tetraplegia with diminished to absent spinal reflexes 7 to 14 days after the onset of clinical signs. Rapid muscle atrophy that was more prominent in distal muscles ensued. Electrophysiologically, spontaneous activity was noted in limb muscles. Motor nerve conduction was slowed, and the evoked muscle response was markedly reduced. Histologically, the disease was characterized by neuronal degeneration and both central and peripheral chromatolysis of ventral horn cells throughout the spinal cord and dorsal root ganglion. Purkinje's neurons in the cerebellum were also markedly affected. Whereas degenerating axons were found throughout the brain stem, degenerating neurons were present only in the nucleus of the mesencephalic tract of the trigeminal nerve.

Spinal Muscle Atrophy in Brittany Spaniels

This is an autosomal dominant condition with variable penetrance. Three forms of the disease have been recognized: accelerated, intermediate, and chronic.[30–33] The accelerated form appears in dogs homozygous for the trait; heterozygotes develop the intermediate or chronic form of the disease.[30] With the accelerated form, clinical signs of weakness develop between 4 and 6 weeks of age and progress to severe tetraparesis within 2 to 3 months. Later features include respiratory muscle paresis, causing dyspnea and ineffective thermoregulation, and cranial nerve involvement, causing difficulty prehending and swallowing food. The intermediate form is the most common, with clinical signs developing between 4 and 12 months of age. The condition progresses from weakness to severe tetraparesis by 2 to 3 years of age. Progressive muscle atrophy is observed in proximal pelvic limbs, paraspinal muscles, and intercostal muscles. The chronic form is relatively rare, with mild weakness that begins during adulthood and is gradually progressive.

Histologically, the three syndromes are characterized by varying degrees of neuronal chromatolysis and proximal axonal swellings containing maloriented neurofilaments. Neurofilaments are also present in the cell body and proximal dendrites of some motor neurons. Nerves that innervate proximal muscle groups are preferentially affected. Motor neurons throughout the brain stem and spinal cord are involved. In the intermediate form, neuronal chromatolysis and axonal swellings are less marked. Instead, a loss of motor neurons is the predominant pathologic change.

DEVELOPMENTAL DISORDERS CHARACTERIZED BY LOSS OF PERIPHERAL AXON

Giant Axonal Neuropathy in Alsatians (German Shepherds)

Giant axonal neuropathy is an autosomal recessive condition reported in Alsatian dogs in the United Kingdom.[34–37] Clinical signs of rear limb weakness, hyporeflexia, and hypotonia began shortly after 1 year of age and progressed slowly to include sensory deficits and fecal incontinence. Megaesophagus was also a common early feature of the disease. Electrophysiologically, spontaneous activity was first noted in the distal muscles of the pelvic limbs and progressed more proximally with time. Motor and sensory nerve conduction was reduced, and the evoked potentials were reduced and dispersed. Nerve conduction studies also became more abnormal as the disease progressed. Thoracic limbs were involved late in the disease.

Histologically, lesions were present in both the central and the peripheral nervous systems. Characteristically, distal myelinated and unmyelinated axons developed swellings that contained tightly packed, whorled neurofilaments. Swellings occurred throughout the nervous system but appeared to be concentrated in paranodal regions at the end of long motor and sensory tracts in the CNS and distally along peripheral nerves.[35] Based on the spatial-temporal spread of lesions, this disease has been classified as a central peripheral distal dying-back neuropathy.

Peripheral Neuropathy in Aged German Shepherd Dogs

Three German shepherd littermates, raised in separate environments, developed pelvic limb weakness at about 9 years of age that progressed to tetraparesis with marked muscle atrophy.[38] Both spinal and pupillary light reflexes were decreased. Histologically, endoneurial fibrosis resulted in gross thickening of the peripheral nerves. Wallerian degeneration, secondary demyelination, and regenerating fibers were present in between fibrous tissue. Muscle showed changes characteristic of denervation, with reinnervation by collateral sprouts from surviving axons. No lesions were described in the CNS.

Hereditary Polyneuropathy in Alaskan Malamutes

An autosomal recessive polyneuropathy has been described in Alaskan malamutes in Norway.[39] Clinical signs of posterior ataxia and exercise intolerance were first noticed between 7 and 18 months of age. Megaesophagus was a prominent feature of the disease. The clinical course was overall progressive; however, a remitting and relapsing course was described for some dogs. Muscle atrophy was prominent, especially in shoulder and thigh muscles. Patellar reflexes were diminished, but proprioception and pain sensation were preserved. Spontaneous activity was described in both proximal and distal limb muscles, and motor nerve conduction velocities were reduced. Degeneration of myelinated axons in all levels of peripheral nerves and nerve roots was reported, but recent reports suggest that the disease may have been associated with more demyelination than was originally described.[15] Scattered nerve fiber degeneration was also seen in white matter tracts in the brain stem and spinal cord. This disease was last reported in Norway in 1982.

Idiopathic Polyneuropathy in Alaskan Malamutes

A second familial polyneuropathy has recently been described in Alaskan malamutes in the United States.[40] Clinical signs of progressive parapareis with exercise intolerance, generalized hyperesthesia, hyporeflexia, and proprioceptive deficits began between 10 and 18 months of age. Megaesophagus was not observed. The disease is gradually progressive without remission. Electrophysiologically, spontaneous activity suggestive of denervation was noted in limb muscles, occasionally in a predominantly distal distribution. Motor nerve conduction was typically slowed, with a reduction in the amplitude of the evoked muscle action potential. Histologically, lesions were largely confined to the peripheral nervous system, with axonal degeneration of both myelinated and unmyelinated fibers predominating. Although increased degeneration was present in distal nerve segments of two dogs, more studies are necessary before the disease

CNS

can be classified as a distal axonopathy. There was no evidence of neurofilament accumulation or tubovesicular aggregates noted in other inherited neuropathies, and only occasional degenerating fibers were noted in the CNS. Although it is unusual for two separate genetic peripheral neuropathies to occur in the same breed, differences in clinical course and histologic appearance between this and hereditary polyneuropathy in Alaskan malamutes suggest that they may be separate entities.

Neuropathy in Birman Cats

Four Birman cats have been reported that developed plantigrade gait, posterior ataxia, and slight hypermetria in all limbs between 8 and 10 weeks of age.[41] Clinical signs were progressive. Histologically, there was a diffuse loss of myelinated fibers in the cerebral and cerebellar white matter and terminal ends of the fasciculi gracili and lateral pyramidal tracts. In the peripheral nervous system, a distal loss of myelinated fibers was observed in the sciatic nerves. Based on the distribution of lesions, this was classified as a central peripheral distal axonopathy of presumed inherited origin.

Polyneuropathy in Rottweiler Dogs

Several mature rottweilers between 1 and 4 years of age have been described with a distal sensorimotor polyneuropathy.[42] Clinical signs were characterized by paraparesis that progressed over 12 months to tetraparesis, hyporeflexia, and hypotonia, with muscle atrophy most prominent in distal limb muscles. In two dogs, the onset was more acute, and three dogs had a remitting and relapsing clinical course associated with corticosteroid therapy. EMG abnormalities of spontaneous activity were concentrated in distal limb muscles. Motor and sensory nerve conduction velocity was slowed in all dogs examined. No systemic diseases could be identified.

Histologically, degeneration of peripheral axons, both myelinated and unmyelinated, was noted in distal nerve segments. Morphometrically, medium to large diameter fibers were preferentially affected, with increased spread in the diameter and proximal distribution of affected nerves over time. Demyelination appeared secondary to axonal loss. The CNS has not been thoroughly evaluated, but only reactionary changes of central chromatolysis have been reported in motor neurons. The cause of the disease is unknown, but a genetic etiology is speculated.

Progressive Axonopathy in Boxer Dogs

Progressive axonopathy is an autosomal recessive condition of Boxer dogs. Clinical signs began between 2 and 3 months of age and slowly progressed until 12 to 18 months of age, when they appeared to stabilize.[43] Pelvic limb ataxia, hypotonia, and hyporeflexia were the initial complaints, with the forelimbs becoming involved later. Mild cerebellar signs may be evident late in the course of the disease.[44] Electrophysiologically, slowing of motor and sensory nerve conduction potentials could be detected as early as 4 months of age, but spontaneous activity suggestive of denervation developed only late in the course of the disease.

Histologically, mild axonal swellings developed in paranodal areas of dorsal and ventral nerve roots and proximal lumbar peripheral nerves.[45–47] These swellings contained accumulations of vesicles and vesiculotubular profiles in subaxolemmal areas and disorganized cytoskeletal elements,

especially neurofilaments. In distal nerve segments, large diameter axons did not appear to reach a normal caliper, and cervical nerve roots often contained regenerating clusters of nerve fibers. Axonal degeneration developed in distal peripheral nerves later in the disease. Myelin internodes appeared to be unusually shortened and thin, changes that suggested remyelination in areas of segmental myelin loss. In the CNS, axonal swellings and degeneration were prominent in lateral and ventral funiculi of the spinal cord. Axonal spheroids containing disorganized neurofilaments and branched vesiculotubular profiles were seen in nuclei and tracts of the caudal brain stem, cerebellum, and visual tracts. The pathophysiology of the disease process is not fully understood, but impaired transport of neurofilaments is theorized.

Laryngeal Paralysis-Polyneuropathy Complex in Young Dalmatians

A generalized polyneuropathy has been reported in both male and female Dalmatians.[48] Clinical signs typically began between 2 and 6 months of age. Acute respiratory distress accompanied by syncopal episodes, exercise intolerance, inspiratory stridor, and dysphonia indicated that laryngeal paralysis was a prominent feature of this disease. Dogs also developed megaesophagus, generalized weakness, hyporeflexia, and muscle atrophy. Facial and lingual muscles were also paralyzed in some dogs. Affected dogs usually died within a few months of diagnosis from aspiration pneumonia.

Electrophysiologically, spontaneous activity suggestive of denervation was observed in distal limb muscles. Motor and sensory nerve conduction velocity was variable but often slowed. Morphologically, neurons in the spinal cord, brain stem, and spinal ganglia were normal. However, distal segments of most peripheral nerves showed extensive axonal degeneration and loss of large and medium diameter myelinated fibers. Few degenerating fibers were found in distal spinal tracts. The disease is believed to be inherited in an autosomal recessive manner. No treatment is effective.

DEVELOPMENTAL DISORDERS CHARACTERIZED BY SCHWANN CELL DYSFUNCTION

Hypomyelinating Neuropathy in Golden Retrievers

Two golden retriever littermates that lacked the normal amount of myelin in peripheral nerves have been reported.[49, 50] The marked absence of myelin without evidence of onion bulb formation, inflammation, or other degenerative changes supported a disorder of synthesis rather than destruction of peripheral nerve myelin. The onset of clinical signs occurred between 5 and 7 weeks of age and was characterized by mild pelvic limb muscle atrophy, decreased spinal reflexes, and hind limb weakness and ataxia. Clinical signs were nonprogressive, but unlike similar disorders affecting myelination of the CNS, affected animals remained abnormal for life. Electrophysiologically, denervation potentials were rarely found. However, there was marked slowing of motor nerve conduction velocity in the sciatic-tibial and ulnar nerves. Nerve biopsy showed hypomyelination without evidence of demyelination or abortive attempts at remyelination. Schwann cell cytoplasm appeared increased and contained excessive amounts of endoplasmic reticulum and mitochondria. The etiology is unknown; however, an autosomal recessive condition is likely.

Hypertrophic Neuropathy in Tibetan Mastiffs

Hypertrophic neuropathy is an autosomal recessive trait in Tibetan mastiffs.[51] Clinically, affected pups were normal until between 7.5 and 10 weeks of age, when they developed rapidly progressive generalized weakness.[52, 53] The condition usually began in the rear limbs with an abnormal bunny-hopping gate but progressed to tetraparesis and areflexia within days. Muscle atrophy was minimal. Dysphonia was the only reported cranial nerve dysfunction. With supportive care, the animals regained the ability to stand within four to six weeks. However, recovered animals remained weak for the remainder of their lives. Electrophysiologically, there was marked reduction in motor and sensory nerve conduction velocities beginning with the onset of clinical signs and progressing throughout the animal's life. Using needle EMG, spontaneous activity suggestive of denervation was noted early in the course of the disease but diminished as the animals aged. A few animals exhibited increased protein in cerebrospinal fluid (CSF) without an increase in nucleated cells, but no other consistent clinical pathologic abnormalities were present.[53]

Histologically, extensive demyelination with remyelination was apparent in all levels of peripheral nerves. Characteristically, Schwann cells accumulated 6- to 7-nm neurofilaments in their adaxonal cytoplasm, which appeared to severely attenuate the underlying axon. Progressive axonal loss was seen in older animals and was believed to result from defective axonal transport secondary to axonal constriction.[53] Transplantation studies support the theory that there is an intrinsic Schwann cell defect with an associated inability to maintain myelin during rapid periods of growth, which explains the onset and subsequent stabilization of clinical signs.[54]

DEVELOPMENTAL DISORDERS CHARACTERIZED BY LOSS OF SENSORY NEURON OR AXON

Sensory Neuropathy in Longhaired Dachshunds

Three longhaired dachshunds with a primary sensory neuropathy have been described.[55] Clinical signs began around 8 to 10 weeks of age and consisted of abnormal rear limb abduction during sitting; rear limb weakness, especially during initial phases of ambulation; and urinary and fecal incontinence. Proprioception was reduced, but spinal reflexes were normal or exaggerated. There was a notable loss of pain sensation over the entire body, and one dog mutilated his genitals. Needle EMG was normal, and no abnormalities could be detected in motor nerve conduction velocity. Sensory nerve conduction was reduced in one affected animal.

Histologically, there was a distal loss of large myelinated and unmyelinated fibers in sensory nerves.[56] Mixed nerves were similarly affected, but to a lesser extent. Accumulations of degenerating cellular organelles were noted in myelinated axons, whereas unmyelinated fibers contained abundant neurotubules and vesiculotubular profiles often forming multilamellar whorls. Neurons in the CNS and dorsal root ganglion appeared normal, but degenerating axons were noted in distal areas of the fasciculus gracilis. These were thought to represent distal projections of primary sensory axons. The

cause of this neuropathy is unknown, but an inherited trait is considered likely. A similar neuropathy has also been reported in a Jack Russell terrier.[57]

Acral Mutilation in English Pointers and Shorthaired Pointers

Acral mutilation is an autosomal recessive trait in English Pointer dogs in the United States and shorthaired Pointer dogs in Europe.[58, 59] Clinical signs usually began between 3 and 8 months of age. The dogs started biting and licking their paws, with subsequent ulcerations and paronychia. More severe injury and painless fractures, osteomyelitis, and autoamputation developed in some animals as the disease progressed. The only detectable neurologic abnormality was loss of nociception, which was prominent only in the distal limbs. Pathologic lesions were concentrated in the dorsal root ganglia, where there was a significant decrease in the number of ganglionic cell bodies. The reduced number of primary sensory neurons was associated with a reduction in myelinated and unmyelinated fibers in the dorsolateral fasciculus of the spinal cord and a loss of sensory axons in peripheral nerves and dorsal root ganglion. Immunocytochemical reactivity of substance P, a neurotransmitter associated with nociceptive impulses in the central projections of primary sensory neurons, was also reduced.

DEGENERATIVE DISORDERS CONCENTRATED IN LARYNGEAL NERVES

Laryngeal Paralysis in Bouvier des Flandres

An autosomal dominant condition has been documented in Bouvier des Flandres dogs.[60, 61] Clinical signs began between 4 and 8 months of age and were characterized by exercise intolerance, inspiratory stridor, and dyspnea. The diagnosis of laryngeal paralysis was confirmed with laryngoscopy under light anesthesia. Denervation of intrinsic laryngeal muscles, especially the dorsal cricoarytenoid muscles, was identified electromyographically and confirmed on histopatholgy. Axonal degeneration was present in all levels of the recurrent laryngeal nerves, with neuronal loss evident in the nucleus ambiguus of the brain stem. Three affected dogs also had evidence of denervation of the anterior tibial nerves. Additional peripheral nerves were not evaluated, but the disease does not appear to progress clinically to involve other nerves.

Laryngeal Paralysis in Siberian Husky Dogs

A familial form of laryngeal paralysis has been reported in Siberian husky dogs and their crosses.[62, 63] Clinical signs of inspiratory dyspnea, stridor, and exercise intolerance began as early as 6 weeks of age. Intrinsic laryngeal muscles exhibited EMG and morphologic abnormalities compatible with denervation. Peripheral nerve histology was not reported. However, neuronal loss was documented in the vagal nuclei of one dog, suggesting that the disease may be similar to laryngeal paralysis reported in Bouviers.

DEGENERATIVE DISORDERS ASSOCIATED WITH INBORN ERRORS IN METABOLISM

Hyperchylomicronemia in Cats

Primary inherited disorders of lipoprotein metabolism have been reported in cats from New Zealand, the United

Kingdom, and the United States.[64] Affected cats have fasting hyperchylomicronemia and hypertriglyceridemia. Clinical signs occur secondary to lipid deposition and peripheral nerve compression in regions subject to trauma, such as bony prominences or vertebral foramina. Clinical signs vary with the nerves affected, but Horner's syndrome and tibial and radial nerve compression are most common. Clinical signs are reversible with reduction in plasma triglyceride concentrations.

Hyperoxaluria Type 2 in Domestic Shorthaired Cats

A series of domestic shorthaired cats from a single breeding colony with a condition analogous to primary hyperoxaluria type 2 in human beings was reported.[65] Affected cats developed acute renal failure between 5 and 9 months of age owing to deposition of calcium oxalate in the kidneys. Many of these cats also exhibited generalized weakness characterized by a crouching, cow-hocked stance. Spinal reflexes were depressed, and pain perception appeared diminished. Serology revealed changes compatible with primary renal failure, and urine samples contained increased concentrations of oxalate and L-glycerate. Enzymatic studies showed less than 5 per cent of the normal concentration of D-glycerate dehydrogenase in the livers of affected cats. Peripheral nerves showed evidence of wallerian degeneration. Axonal swellings containing accumulations of neurofilaments were present in proximal axons in spinal ventral horn cells, ventral roots, intramuscular nerves, and dorsal root ganglia. Oxalate crystals were not observed in tissues other than the kidneys. The metabolic defect is believed to be inherited as an autosomal recessive condition, but the pathogenesis of the peripheral nerve disorder is uncertain. A motor neuropathy has been observed in human patients with hyperoxaluria type 1, but axonal swellings were not apparent.

α-L-Fucosidosis in English Springer Spaniels

Deficiency of α-L-fucosidase results in accumulation of incompletely metabolized fucose-containing substrates in visceral organs and the nervous system.[66–69] This appears as an autosomal recessive condition in English springer spaniels in the United Kingdom, Australia, and Canada.[70] Neurologic signs became apparent between 12 and 18 months of age and progressed until the dogs were incapacitated around 4 years of age. The earliest changes consisted of behavioral changes and rapidly included generalized ataxia. Postural reactions were depressed, but tendon reflexes were maintained until late in the course of the disease. Both hearing and vision gradually declined as the disease progressed. Vacuolated lymphocytes were present in blood smears, and vacuolated mononuclear cells were present in CSF, contributing to the diagnosis. No changes were present electrophysiologically, even though the peripheral nerves were palpably thickened. Microscopic examination of peripheral nerves showed that nerve enlargement was caused by infiltration of foamy macrophages of loose fibroedematous tissue within the endoneurial spaces. Vacuolar distention occurred in neuronal cell bodies in peripheral ganglia, retinal ganglion cells, and CNS. Vacuolated mononuclear cells also accumulated beneath the leptomeninges and perivascular spaces in the CNS. Despite these lesions, there was little obvious axonal degeneration or demyelination in the central or peripheral nervous system. The diagnosis can be confirmed by demonstrating reduced α-L-fucosidase levels in serum and peripheral leukocytes.

Atypical GM₂ Gangliosidosis in Cats and a Mixed Breed Dog

Ganglioside storage diseases are a diverse group of inherited diseases caused by a deficiency of lysosomal hydrolases or cofactors necessary for the metabolism of gangliosides. Two major groupings, GM_1 and GM_2 gangliosidosis, are separated on the basis of the accumulated ganglioside. Hallmarks of all ganglioside storage disorders are widespread neuronal accumulation of finely granular material. Despite neuronal involvement, axonal necrosis is minimal. Clinical signs are typically restricted to dysfunction of CNS neurons. However, isolated cases of peripheral nerve involvement have been reported in cats and a mongrel dog with GM_2 gangliosidosis.[71, 72] In both species, there was wallerian degeneration of peripheral axons, with accumulation of lamellar inclusions in Schwann cells and endoneurial fibroblasts in cats.

Globoid Cell Leukodystrophy

Globoid cell leukodysrophy is a storage disease caused by deficiency of the lysosomal enzyme β-galactocerebrosidase.[73] Deficiency of this enzyme results in accumulations of galactocerebroside in macrophages within the central and peripheral nervous systems. The condition is an autosomal recessive condition in Cairn and West Highland white terriers but has been sporadically reported in other dogs, including beagles, poodles, Pomeranians, and basset and bluetick hounds, and in domestic shorthaired cats.[73–79] Clinical signs usually developed within the first 5 months of life. In some animals, signs of pelvic limb paresis predominated, while others had signs more typically associated with cerebellar dysfunction. Multifocal neurologic abnormalities, including behavioral changes, blindness, whole body tremors, and generalized ataxia, were usually apparent as the disease progressed. Lower motor neuron signs of hyporeflexia and hypotonia were rarely seen. Most animals were severely incapacitated by 1 year of age.

Histologically, there was a diffuse loss of myelin in both central and peripheral nervous systems. Globoid cells, macrophages distended with periodic acid–Schiff (PAS) positive material, were present in the regions of white matter destruction both perivascularly and in linear rows between myelinated fibers. Axonal degeneration and focal axonal swelling accompanied myelin loss. Ultrastructurally, two types of tubular shaped inclusions were found in globoid cells and occasionally Schwann cells, oligodendrocytes, and astrocytes. One inclusion type was straight or arched and polygonal in cross section. The other inclusion was small, twisted, round in cross section, and located within cytoplasmic sacs. Both were thought to be accumulations of galactocerebroside. Peripheral nerve biopsy may support the diagnosis.[80, 81] Measurement of enzyme activity in peripheral leukocytes can be used to identify animals both homozygous and heterozygous for the genetic defect.

Niemann-Pick Disease in Siamese Cats

Sphingomyelin lipidosis is an inherited defect that results in the visceral and neuronal accumulation of sphingomyelin. Five subtypes (A, B, C, D, and E) are recognized in humans that differ in age of onset, distribution of lesions, and levels of sphingomyelinase activity. Several animal models of Niemann-Pick disease have been recognized. Most present with cerebral and/or cerebellar signs. Three cats with chemical changes consistent with type A Niemann-Pick disease were described in which clinical signs were largely referable to peripheral nerve dysfunction.[82] Tetraparesis, hypotonia, and areflexia developed between 2 and 5 months of age. Spontaneous activity was detected with needle EMG, and motor and sensory conduction velocities were markedly slowed. Peripheral nerves showed marked demyelination and remyelination with vacuolated macrophages surrounding affected nerve fibers. Marked vacuolation and granular distention were seen in neurons, glial cells, endothelium, choroid plexus, and ependyma. Macrophages with accumulations or granular material were dispersed throughout the CNS and body organs. Diagnosis was based on clinical and pathologic changes and on biochemical evidence of reduced sphingomyelinase activity and accumulations of sphingomyelin, cholesterol, and glycosphingolipids in tissue.

Glycogen Storage Disease Type IV in Norwegian Forest Cats

A deficiency in glycogen branching enzyme has been reported as an autosomal recessive condition in Norwegian Forest cats.[83, 84] Clinical signs typically began around 5 months of age and progressed quickly. Hyperthermia was one of the initial clinical signs and was thought to be related to muscle injury secondary to glycogen accumulation. Evidence of multifocal peripheral and central nervous system dysfunction rapidly ensued. Generalized muscle atrophy, movement-associated whole body tremors, and ataxic gait were initial clinical signs. These progressed to tetraparesis with diminished myotactic and flexor reflexes, multiple cranial nerve dysfunction, seizures, and eventually death. Serum biochemical abnormalities included transient elevations in creatine kinase activity reflective of muscle lysis and increased alanine aminotransferase activity suggestive of liver disease. Electromyographically, spontaneous activity was present in all skeletal muscle. Nerve conduction studies showed minimal reduction in nerve conduction velocity but reductions in the amplitude and configuration of the evoked muscle action potential compatible with axonal loss. Other electrophysiologic studies such as electroencephalography and somatosensory evoked potentials reflected loss of central neurons as well. Histologically, PAS-positive material was present in multiple organs, including lymph nodes, lungs, gastrointestinal tract, liver, thymus, cardiac and skeletal muscle, and central and peripheral nervous systems. Accumulations of storage material in neuron cell bodies resulted in neuronal loss and axonal degeneration. These changes were present in motor, sensory, and autonomic nerves.

METABOLIC AND TOXIC DISORDERS

DIABETES MELLITUS

Diabetic neuropathy represents one of the most significant late complications of diabetes mellitus in human beings. The reported incidence in human diabetic populations varies with diagnostic criteria but ranges from 5 to 100 per cent.[85] Although no attempts have been made to identify the incidence, a causal relationship between diabetes mellitus and peripheral nerve disease has been identified in dogs and cats as well. In dogs, the neuropathy is usually subclinical.[86, 87]

Only rarely do diabetic dogs present with pelvic limb weakness, postural reaction deficits, and normal to depressed myotactic reflexes.[88–92] In cats, clinical signs are much more common.[93] Diabetic cats frequently present with a characteristic plantigrade stance, pelvic limb weakness, muscle wasting, and depressed myotactic reflexes. Electrodiagnostic abnormalities consist of spontaneous activity in skeletal muscle and slowed nerve conduction with smaller evoked muscle responses. In both species, better glycemic control results in resolution of clinical signs.

Peripheral nerves were carefully examined in a series of experimental dogs with subclinical neuropathy.[86] In teased fiber preparations, only 3 per cent of nerve fibers were abnormal. Nerve fibers with short intercalated internodes, or with uniformly and inappropriately short internodes for the diameter of the nerve fiber, had the most prominent changes. Paranodal and segmental demyelination or fibers with linear rows of myelin ovoids were much more rare. There was no evidence of active demyelination or nerve fiber degeneration in cross sections of peripheral nerves. In another study of biopsy material from a diabetic dog with clinically evident peripheral nerve disease, a much larger percentage of nerve fibers undergoing active wallerian degeneration were found.[88] These studies indicate that diabetic neuropathy in dogs consists of a mixture of demyelination and axonal degeneration. Similar findings have been reported in cats.[93]

The pathogenesis of diabetic neuropathy has been the subject of intensive study for years and is the subject of several recent reviews.[94, 95] Despite this fact, the mechanisms underlying diabetic neuropathy are still not understood. Current theories include nerve hypoxia subsequent to vascular changes and metabolic derangements associated with sorbitol accumulation. Altered protein synthesis and delayed axonal transport of molecules necessary to maintain distal axonal segments, together with immunologic mechanisms, may also play a role. Most authors agree that no single mechanism can explain the myriad clinical signs associated with diabetic neuropathy, and many of the proposed mechanisms are interrelated. The significance of this neuropathy in veterinary patients remains to be determined. It is interesting to note that both the incidence and the spectrum of clinical signs of diabetic neuropathy in dogs and cats are significantly lower than in the human counterpart. It has been clearly established that clinically detectable neuropathy in human beings is directly related to duration of diabetes.[85] One factor contributing to the differences may be that dogs and cats do not survive long enough after the diagnosis of diabetes to develop clinically significant neuropathy.

HYPOTHYROIDISM

The frequent association between hypothyroidism and a vast array of neurologic symptoms has led to a causal relationship between the two conditions. Despite hypothyroidism being one of the most widely recognized causes of neuromuscular disease in both humans and animals, it remains one of the least well characterized.

Early reports of dogs with neuromuscular disease and hypothyroidism were difficult to interpret because each animal had additional medical problems that could cause neuropathies.[96, 97] Four subsequent reports presented more convincing evidence.[98–101] In these reports, a total of 41 dogs were described. Each presented for neurologic disease, was diagnosed with hypothyroidism, and received thyroid supplementation. Either complete resolution or marked clinical improvement in neurologic signs was noted in each case within three days to three months after receiving thyroid replacement therapy. In two cases, clinical signs returned when treatment was discontinued and resolved once again with thyroid supplementation.[100]

The most common neurologic problem described is paresis. This varied from monoparesis to hemiparesis to quadriparesis, with an equally variable onset and rate of progression. Cranial neuropathies are the second most common presentation, with the facial, vestibulocochlear, and trigeminal nerves appearing most susceptible. Megaesophagus and laryngeal paralysis are also common clinical signs in dogs with hypothyroidism. Whether these are manifestations of a more generalized neuromuscular disorder or represent a unique form of the disease is presently unclear. Electrophysiologic evidence of a generalized neuropathy, including spontaneous activity in all limb muscles and slowed nerve conduction velocities, has been found in all cases examined. In addition, brain stem auditory evoked potentials are often reduced in amplitude and have prolonged latencies.[99, 101] Increased protein in CSF is a less consistent finding.

Unfortunately, the histologic changes of peripheral nerves have not been carefully examined in canine patients. Preliminary evidence suggests that both axonal necrosis and demyelination occur.[98, 101] In human and experimental animals, hypothyroidism has been associated with both Schwann cell and primary axonal injury, with glycogen aggregates occurring in the cytoplasm of both cells.[102] Remaining axons often appear to have shrunken axons with inappropriately thick myelin sheaths, suggesting that axonal atrophy may be a feature of the neuropathy in some cases. The pathogenesis is unclear. Thyroid hormones appear necessary for microtubule assembly, and slowed axonal transport has been identified in hypothyroid rats. Regardless of the pathogenesis, marked improvement in nerve function has been identified in all species examined after thyroid levels return to normal.

BOTULISM

Botulism in an acute, rapidly progressive, generalized lower motor neuron paralysis that results from ingestion of the exotoxin produced by *Clostridium botulinum*.[103] *C. botulinum* is a saprophytic soil organism with a worldwide distribution. Under anaerobic conditions, the toxin is elaborated from both vegetative cells and, to a lesser extent, spores. Although eight antigenically different types of botulinum neurotoxins have been identified, most cases of botulism in dogs are caused by type C.[104, 105] Naturally occurring cases of botulism in domestic cats have not been reported, even though the disease can be experimentally produced in this species. Clinical cases are usually attributable to ingestion of preformed toxin, usually in carrion.

Clinical signs may begin within hours of toxin ingestion or may be delayed up to six days. The severity of signs varies with both the amount and the potency of the toxin ingested, as well the susceptibility of the individual animal. Most often, clinical signs present as an ascending paralysis, with rear limb weakness preceding forelimb involvement. In severe cases, complete flaccid paralysis is accompanied by weakness of facial, pharyngeal, and esophageal musculature. Mydriasis, decreased tear production, and urinary and fecal retention are signs of cholinergic autonomic dysfunction. Hyperesthesia is not a prominent clinical feature, and interestingly, tail wag is preserved even in severe cases.

Electrophysiologic changes characteristic of botulism include a marked reduction in the amplitude of the muscle action potential evoked by electrical stimulation of a motor nerve, while motor conduction velocities are normal or only mildly reduced. EMG is usually normal. However, severe cases may have occasional spontaneous activity noted five to seven days after paralysis. The diagnosis of botulism is confirmed by identifying toxin in the food, serum, stomach contents, or feces. A mouse neutralization is available. By injecting toxin alone and in combination with specific antitoxins, both the type and the potency of the botulinum toxin can be identified. Radioimmunoassay, enzyme-linked immunosorbent assay (ELISA), and passive hemagglutination tests have been developed that evaluate the toxin and type but do not evaluate potency. Recovery of *C. botulinum* from fecal culture is also presumptive evidence of intoxication, as the organism rarely colonizes the normal canine intestine.

Pathophysiologically, ingested toxin is absorbed from the gastrointestinal tract and is transported to cholinergic nerve terminals. The toxin binds to presynaptic terminals, is internalized, and then blocks acetylcholine release, presumably by inhibiting calcium ion increases necessary for transmitter release. Recovery usually occurs in two to three weeks, following regrowth of terminal motor branches. Because most animals recover within weeks, treatment is largely supportive. Antibiotics should be used only to treat secondary infections, because they may facilitate intestinal colonization of *C. botulinum* by altering the normal gastrointestinal flora. An antitoxin is available and should be either a polyvalent antitoxin or specific for type C. Antitoxin is not effective after the toxin has entered nerve terminals, so it will only halt the progression of the disease and not reverse clinical signs. Recommended antitoxin dosage is 10,000 to 15,000 units intravenously (IV) or intramuscularly (IM) administered twice at four-hour intervals. Anaphylaxis is possible, so a test injection of 0.1 mL intradermally 20 minutes before antitoxin administration is advisable.

TICK PARALYSIS

Tick paralysis is an acute, rapidly progressive generalized lower motor neuron paralysis caused by a salivary neurotoxin produced by ticks.[106] Adult female *Dermacentor andersoni* (the Rocky Mountain wood tick) and *Dermacentor variabilis* (the American dog tick) are most often incriminated in North America, while *Ixodes holocyclus* is most often incriminated in Australia. Adult females, nymphs, and larvae of *Ixodes* ticks may produce the neurotoxin. Although additional sites of neuronal dysfunction may result from intoxication, the predominant clinical signs are produced by inhibition of acetylcholine release from motor nerve terminals.

In the United States, clinical signs are restricted to dogs. Cats are also susceptible to the effects of *Ixodes* neurotoxin in Australia and present with a similar set of clinical signs. In most cases, rear limb weakness begins five to seven days after tick attachment. This is rapidly followed by generalized weakness and eventually complete flaccid paralysis and areflexia within 24 to 72 hours. Cranial nerves, especially the facial nerve, may be mildly affected by the *Dermacentor* neurotoxin, but pain sensation is preserved, and the animals do not appear hyperpathic. In contrast, *Ixodes* neurotoxin causes more profound signs of facial paralysis, dysphagia, and megaesophagus. Autonomic signs include mydriasis with loss of pupillary light reflex, peripheral vasoconstriction and arterial hypertension, pulmonary hypertension and edema, and either tachycardia or bradycardia. Failure to diagnose tick paralysis in either country can result in death from respiratory paralysis within days.

Electrodiagnostic changes are similar in both forms of tick paralysis. EMG is usually normal. The evoked muscle action potential is reduced in amplitude or nonexistent, and there is mild slowing of both motor and sensory nerve conduction velocities.[107] The diagnosis is made by exclusion of other causes of rapidly progressive generalized lower motor neuron paralysis (e.g., botulism, acute polyradiculoneuritis, myasthenia gravis) and response to tick removal. Clinical signs improve within 24 hours after *Dermacentor* tick removal, and the animals are usually normal within 48 hours. In Australia, clinical signs may progress for 24 to 48 hours after tick removal. Administration of canine hyperimmune serum at 0.5 to 1 mL/kg IV has been recommended in these cases to bind circulating neurotoxin and prevent further progression. Because the only available hyperimmune serum is derived from dogs, cats should be pretreated with 30 mg/kg hydrocortisone, and epinephrine (1 mL of a 1:10,000 solution) should be available to counteract anaphylaxis. Autonomic dysfunction may be improved by administration of a combination of phenoxybenzamine hydrochloride 1 mg/kg as a 0.1 per cent solution administered IV over 15 minutes every 12 to 24 hours and acepromazine 0.05 to 0.10 mg/kg IV every 6 to 12 hours. Oxygen therapy and respiratory support may be necessary for severely affected cases. Dogs are susceptible to repeat bouts of tick paralysis. Even though an immune response develops against *Ixodes* neurotoxin, it has only a limited duration. Vaccines are currently unavailable, so minimizing tick infestation is the best method of prevention.

MISCELLANEOUS TOXINS

The nervous system is the target of a tremendous number of toxic compounds. The list of drugs, metals, and other environmental chemicals that have been associated with peripheral neuropathy in humans is lengthy and growing daily.[108] Unfortunately, the clinical significance of most of these agents in veterinary medicine is uncertain. There are far fewer documented toxic peripheral neuropathies in dogs and cats than in human beings. Potential explanations for this observation include difficulty in identifying toxin exposure without critical historical information, as well as difficulty in identifying subtle signs of sensory deficits and/or weakness in veterinary patients. Without overt clinical signs, a cause-and-effect relationship between chemical exposure and disease may be difficult to ascertain. Finally, there are clear differences in species susceptibility to recognized toxins. As an example, cats are much more susceptible to the distal dying-back neuropathy associated with organophosphate exposure than are dogs. Toxin exposure should be considered for any animal with an undiagnosed peripheral nerve disease. The national animal poison control center (1-900-680-0000) can provide valuable information regarding any suspicious exposure. Some of the recognized neurotoxicants that affect the peripheral nervous system in dogs and cats are listed in Table 108–3.

INFLAMMATORY AND IMMUNE-MEDIATED NEUROPATHIES

ACUTE POLYRADICULONEURITIS (COONHOUND PARALYSIS)

Acute polyradiculoneuritis is a common neuropathy affecting primarily dogs and occasionally cats.[128–132] The syndrome was first described in 1954 as an acute, rapidly progressive paralysis that occurred in dogs 7 to 10 days after contact with a raccoon.[133] An identical syndrome has subsequently been described in dogs and cats with no known exposure to raccoons.[134, 135] The syndrome was originally named coonhound paralysis to reflect the association between raccoons and paralysis. However, the recognition of additional cases suggests that the broader term acute polyradiculoneuritis better reflects the full spectrum of the disease.

Clinical signs of generalized weakness typically begin in the pelvic limbs and progress in an ascending fashion to involve thoracic limbs. In severe cases, cranial nerves and respiratory muscles may be affected as well. Even animals severely affected often retain voluntary tail movement and voluntary control of urination and defecation. Sensory function is likewise preserved, and many animals seem unusually sensitive to mild stimulation, indicating generalized hyperpathia. In rare cases, the thoracic limbs may be affected first or preferentially. Clinical signs may progressively worsen for up to 10 days after the onset of signs and then plateau. The severity of motor deficits once the plateau is reached varies from mild weakness to complete flaccid paralysis, areflexia, and respiratory paralysis. Spontaneous remission may begin as early as one week after the onset of clinical

TABLE 108–3. TOXIC NEUROPATHIES RECOGNIZED IN DOGS AND CATS

COMPOUND	SUSCEPTIBLE SPECIES	PATHOLOGY	REFERENCE
Vincristine	Dogs and cats	Distal axonopathy, loss of neurotubules with neurofilamentous accumulations in axons	109, 110
Pyridoxine	Dogs	Neuronal loss in sensory, dorsal root, and trigeminal ganglia	111
Mercury	Dogs and cats	Neuronal loss in sensory, dorsal root, and trigeminal ganglia	112–114
Thallium	Dogs and cats	Gastrointestinal irritation; skin lesions; neuronal loss in cerebrum, cerebellum, and sensory ganglia	115–117
Lead	Dogs and cats	Central nervous system signs predominate, rare megaesophagus; Schwann cell pathology in other species	118, 119
Organophosphates	Cats (experimental)	Distal axonopathy with tubovesicular profiles in axons	120–123
Acrylamide	Cats and dogs (experimental)	Distal axonopathy with neurofilament accumulation in axons	124, 125
Hexacarbons	Cats (experimental)	Distal axonopathy with giant neurofilamentous axonal swellings	126
Lasalocid	Dogs	Pathology not described, dogs recovered in 2–50 days	127

signs or may be delayed for several months. Recovery may take several months and is often incomplete. Some animals do not improve within the time frame during which supportive care is tenable. Unfortunately, there is no reliable prognostic criteria by which to gauge the probable speed or degree of functional recovery of individual cases.

Despite the fact that polyradiculoneuritis is a well-recognized syndrome, definitive diagnosis is not always straightforward. History of raccoon exposure shortly before the onset of clinical signs is helpful, but as previously mentioned, it is not present in all cases. Abnormal spontaneous activity is usually detected with needle EMG five to seven days after the onset of clinical signs. Motor nerve conduction is typically slowed at about the same time that EMG changes are present, and the muscle action potential is often dispersed, indicating both demyelination and axonal injury. Small motor potentials produced by orthodromic conduction of evoked motor action potentials to the cell body and then back to the muscle (F wave) are often delayed or absent, reflecting injury to ventral nerve roots.[136] Increased protein without an increase in white blood cells (albuminocytologic dissociation) is typically found in lumbar CSF but not in fluid collected from the cisterna magna.

Histologically, all regions of peripheral nerves have signs of injury, but lesions are usually concentrated in ventral roots. Demyelination and inflammatory cell infiltration are the predominant findings, with more variable degrees of axonal degeneration accompanying the inflammation. The pathogenesis of the disease is uncertain. However, an antigenic stimulus in raccoon saliva is thought to stimulate an immune reaction against peripheral nerve myelin. The source of antigenic stimulation in animals without raccoon exposure is unknown but may be viral, toxic, or infectious in origin. An immune theory is supported by several factors. Epidemiologic evidence indicates that not all dogs bitten by the same raccoon are affected. Once affected, repeated episodes can be precipitated in the same animal by raccoon exposure or injections of raccoon saliva. These two observations indicate that the disease is associated with an idiosyncratic response in some dogs. Dogs with an acute onset of clinical signs shortly after a known raccoon exposure have antibodies against an antigen in raccoon saliva.[136] Histologically, demyelination can occur in regions without inflammatory cells, suggesting antibody-mediated damage in some instances.[129] Finally, the disease shares many clinical and histopathologic features with human Guillain-Barré syndrome, an immune-mediated radiculoneuropathy in human beings.

Therapy for this disease is largely supportive. Despite the probable immune-mediated etiology, immune-suppressive therapy usually increases the incidence of secondary infections and muscle atrophy. Plasmapheresis has become standard in human beings with Guillain-Barré syndrome. Unfortunately, this is not widely available for veterinary patients. Recently, intravenous immunoglobulin therapy has shown promising results in humans with Guillain-Barré syndrome.[137] Although intravenous human immunoglobulin has shown efficacy in treating a number of immune-mediated diseases in veterinary patients, no one has reported its application in the treatment for acute polyradiculoneuritis.[138]

CHRONIC RELAPSING NEUROPATHY AND ACQUIRED DEMYELINATING NEUROPATHY

A generalized polyneuropathy that follows a remitting and relapsing clinical course has been identified in both dogs and cats of various breeds.[139–143] Clinical signs may be acute or chronic in onset and are often asymmetric in distribution. In most cases, an overall progressive course of generalized weakness, areflexia, and diffuse muscle atrophy is interrupted by spontaneous periods of partial remission. Cranial nerves may be affected as well. Electrophysiologic changes consist of variable degrees of spontaneous activity in limb muscles and marked slowing of nerve conduction velocities with more variable degrees of attenuation of the evoked response. These findings are most suggestive of a demyelinating neuropathy. CSF analysis in one dog with a year's duration of clinical signs showed increased protein concentrations without concomitant pleocytosis (albuminocytologic dissociation). Muscle biopsies contain changes characteristic of denervation, and primary demyelination with remyelination is seen in peripheral nerves. Variable degrees of mononuclear cell infiltrates are found in both peripheral nerves and nerve roots. The inflammatory response varies markedly between nerves and probably varies with stage of the disease process. Macrophages, monocytes, and lymphocytes are associated with prominent primary demyelination and remyelination. Redundant Schwann cell membranes forming concentric layers around nerve fibers (onion bulbs) are prominent in some cases, indicating repetitive cycles of demyelination and remyelination. Lesser degrees of axonal necrosis are also present in peripheral nerves, suggesting that axonal injury occurred as a consequence of the inflammatory reaction against peripheral nerve myelin. Immune-suppressive doses of prednisolone (2 mg/kg orally every 12 hours) resulted in reversal of clinical signs in two cats within weeks of therapy.[142, 143] Prednisolone was tapered after six or eight months, and both cats remained clinically normal. The pathogenesis of the neuropathy in all cases remains unknown. Based on the histologic appearance of an inflammatory response against peripheral nerve myelin and the response to immune-suppressive therapy, an immune-mediated etiology is likely. It is important to note that no other evidence of immune-mediated disease was present in any of the cases investigated.

Two similar cases, one in a 2-year-old rottweiler and one in a 4-year-old cat, have been reported.[144, 145] Both had similar histologic changes of an inflammatory demyelinating neuropathy, but neither followed a remitting and relapsing clinical course. Immune-suppressive doses of prednisolone were ineffective after 14 days in the dog but were not tried in the cat. It is uncertain whether these cases represent yet another disease process or a more severe form of chronic relapsing neuropathy.

BRACHIAL PLEXUS NEURITIS

Brachial plexus neuritis is an inflammatory neuritis involving primarily the ventral branches of spinal nerves that give rise to the brachial plexus. This rare condition has been reported in two unrelated dogs and in one cat.[146–148] Clinical signs consisted of an acute onset of flaccid paralysis in the thoracic limbs only, with diminished or absent spinal reflexes. Sensory nerves may be affected as well, causing anesthesia of the distal limb. Pelvic limb function remained unaffected in all reported cases. Electrophysiologic changes were confined to the affected limbs. Spontaneous activity suggested denervation in limb muscles, and nerve conduction studies were mildly slowed, with a reduced or small nerve action potential. CSF was evaluated only in the canine patients and was normal. Clinical recovery occurred spontaneously in the cat in four days and in one dog in four months.[147, 148] No improvement was noted in the other dog 45 days after the onset of clinical signs.[146] In the dog that was euthanized, axonal degeneration appeared concentrated in ventral branches of spinal nerves, with wallerian degeneration and mast cell infiltration present in most peripheral nerves in the thoracic limbs. More proximal portions of axons in ventral nerve roots were spared, and the disease process appeared mildly asymmetric between left and right brachial plexi. Retrograde sensory degeneration and chromatolysis in motor and sensory neurons were the only changes noted in the CNS. The cause of the condition is unknown but is thought to be associated with a hypersensitivity reaction. Both dogs experienced urticarial reactions before the onset of clinical signs, and clinical signs occurred shortly after ingestion of horse meat in one dog. A positive intradermal reaction to horse serum was subsequently found in that case. There are many similarities to an immunologic reaction in humans referred to as brachial plexus neuropathy. Antigenic differences in brachial plexus nerves from those elsewhere have not been identified, so many features of the disease remain unexplained.

SENSORY GANGLIONEURITIS

Sensory ganglioneuritis is a poorly defined sensory neuropathy that has been reported in young adult dogs of various breeds.[149–153] The onset of clinical signs may be subacute, acute, or chronic, with an equally variable rate of progression. Initial signs consist of rear limb ataxia that progresses over weeks or months to generalized ataxia. Facial hypalgesia, dysphagia, and regurgitation secondary to megaesophagus have been seen in some cases. A characteristic feature of the syndrome is preservation of limb muscle mass, strength, and tone, but diminished to absent proprioception and tendon reflexes. Withdrawal reflex is usually intact, and most have some preservation of nociception. Less frequent findings in some of these dogs include self-mutilation and masticatory muscle atrophy.

Electrophysiologically, needle EMG and motor conduction velocity are either normal or only mildly abnormal. However, sensory nerve conduction is usually not recordable. CSF is typically normal or may show mild increases in protein and white blood cell count. Axonal atrophy of large diameter fibers is found in biopsy material from a mixed or sensory nerve.

The pathology of this syndrome is characterized by a nonsuppurative inflammation of dorsal root ganglia and cranial sensory ganglia with loss of sensory neuronal cell bodies. There is a concomitant loss of larger diameter fibers corresponding to sensory axons involved in proprioception and stretch reflexes in both peripheral nerves and sensory tracts in the spinal cord. The masticatory muscle atrophy reported in a few dogs was attributed to the loss of motor fibers as they coursed through the trigeminal ganglion. The etiology is unknown, but immune-mediated, toxic, and viral causes have been considered. Similar clinical and pathologic changes can be produced by a number of toxins, including mercury intoxication, pyridoxine (vitamin B_6) excess, and doxorubicin. There is no treatment for the condition, and recovery has not been reported.

MYASTHENIA GRAVIS

Myasthenia gravis is a disorder characterized by inefficient neuromuscular transmission secondary to a reduction in acetylcholine receptors on the postsynaptic muscle membrane. Two forms of the disease are recognized in dogs and cats: congenital and acquired. In congenital myasthenia gravis, the deficiency in acetylcholine receptors has been attributed to reduced or imperfect synthesis, probably secondary to a genetic defect. In acquired myasthenia gravis, antibodies, usually IgG are generated against acetylcholine receptors. These autoantibodies block neuromuscular transmission by directly interfering with the actions of acetylcholine on receptors, accelerating the normal turnover rate of receptors, or activating complement-mediated lysis of the postsynaptic membrane.[154]

Acquired myasthenia gravis is the most common form of the disease. An increased risk has been identified in Akitas, various terriers, German shorthaired pointers, and Chihuahuas; rottweilers, Doberman pinschers, Dalmatians, and Jack Russell terriers have lower relative risks compared with mixed breed dogs. Despite these statistics, German shepherds and Labrador and golden retrievers are the breeds most commonly diagnosed with the disease.[155] Abyssinians and Somalis appear overrepresented among cats.[156–158] Two age groups appear most susceptible in dogs: those 2 to 3 years of age, and those older than 9 years of age. Intact male dogs are underrepresented, suggesting that testosterone may confer some protection from the disease.

Historically, clinical signs of myasthenia were described as generalized skeletal muscle weakness that worsens with exercise and improves with rest. It is now recognized that myasthenia presents with a spectrum of clinical signs that vary in both distribution and severity of muscle involvement. Three major categories have been identified in dogs: focal, chronic generalized, and acute fulminant generalized.[159] The focal form occurs in approximately 36 per cent of recognized cases and consists of variable degrees of facial, pharyngeal, laryngeal, and esophageal dysfunction. Subclinical evidence of appendicular muscle involvement has been demonstrated in some focal myasthenics. The two generalized forms are distinguished primarily by the rate at which clinical signs develop. Twenty-five per cent of dogs with generalized neuromuscular weakness have acute, fulminant clinical signs that result in nonambulatory tetraparesis and severe dyspnea within 72 hours. The remaining 39 per cent exhibit a more chronic onset and gradual progression of clinical signs. Recent studies indicate that not all dogs with generalized weakness worsen with exercise, and that weakness may be concentrated in pelvic limb muscles of some dogs. It is important to note that between 80 and 90 per cent of dogs with generalized myasthenia also have megaesophagus.[155] Cats appear to be similar in this regard. Chronic regurgitation and aspiration pneumonia are common complications of all three forms.

Currently the primary criterion for diagnosing all forms of acquired myasthenia in both dogs and cats is demonstrating serum antibodies that react with α-bungarotoxin extracted acetylcholine receptors.[160] This test is readily available and appears to be specific for myasthenia gravis. Sensitivity of this test is difficult to evaluate; however, approximately 15 per cent of suspected myasthenics are seronegative for acetylcholine receptor antibodies yet have immune complexes localized to end plates in their muscle biopsy samples, or have antibodies in the serum that bind the postsynaptic membrane of normal muscle.[161] Explanations for these apparent false-negative serum tests are speculative, but they may be caused by the production of high-affinity antibodies that are largely bound and not free in serum. Alternatively, antibodies may be directed to additional antigens on muscle membranes other than those recognized by α-bungarotoxin. Additional supportive evidence for the diagnosis of myasthenia can be obtained by demonstrating increased muscle strength following administration of the short-acting acetylcholinesterase agent edrophonium chloride (Tensilon) or by finding a decreasing evoked muscle response following repetitive nerve stimulation. Recommended dosages of Tensilon are 0.1 to 0.2 mg/kg IV and should cause temporary improvement in clinical signs within minutes. Esophageal musculature does not respond to Tensilon, limiting the usefulness of this test in focal myasthenics. Similarly, a large percentage of myasthenics have a decreasing response following repetitive motor nerve stimulation that will be blocked by Tensilon administration. Both false-positive and false-negative results occur with both of these tests, so they should be used for supportive evidence only.

Treatment is directed toward amelioration of generalized muscle weakness with longer-acting anticholinesterase agents that prolong the interaction of acetylcholine with any available receptors. Pyridostigmine bromide (Mestinon, Roche Laboratories) may be given 1 to 3 mg/kg every 8 to 12 hours in dogs and cats. Therapy should begin at the low end of the scale and gradually increase to desired effect. Alternatively, injectable neostigmine (Prostigmin, Roche Laboratories) has been recommended at a dosage of 0.04 mg/kg every 6 hours IM to bypass the problem of oral administration of medication in regurgitating animals. Esophageal motility is minimally affected by anticholinesterase therapy. Immune-suppressive therapy is controversial. Many cases can be adequately controlled with anticholinesterases, lessening the potential complications of immune suppression in animals with aspiration pneumonia. Corticosteroids may also exacerbate weakness in some cases.[162, 163] However, immune-suppressive therapy increased the probability of survival in one study and has been used successfully to shorten the course of disease in others.[159] The best advice is to tailor drug therapy to each individual animal while providing supportive care. Almost 50 per cent of myasthenics die within the first two weeks of diagnosis from aspiration pneumonia. The risk of aspiration pneumonia can be reduced by feeding in an upright position and holding the animal in an elevated position for 5 to 10 minutes after feeding. Percutaneous gastrostomy has been recommended for alimentary support but does not prevent aspiration pneumonia. Pneumonia may require additional therapy such as antibiotics and oxygen supplementation. Several drugs (e.g., aminoglycoside antibiotics, antiarrhythmic agents, phenothiazines, methoxyflurane, and magnesium) may reduce the efficiency of neuromuscular transmission and worsen clinical signs in myasthenic animals. Therefore, additional drugs should be used with caution.

A simple correlation between acetylcholine receptor antibody and severity and distribution of clinical signs does not exist in dogs with myasthenia gravis. However, the course of the disease may be monitored by evaluating serum acetylcholine receptor antibodies. Spontaneous remission occurs, and the antibody titer will decrease as the animal goes into remission. Duration of the disease varies from months to years, and recurrence is possible.[160] One of the most important yet unanswered questions about myasthenia is what initiates the immune response to acetylcholine receptors. An association has been made between the occurrence of thymomas and myasthenia in both dogs and cats.[164–167] This is probably related to antigenic similarity between neoplastic thymocytes and acetylcholine receptors. A less direct association has been made between myasthenia and other forms of neoplasia.[168, 169] A more recent association with immune-mediated endocrinopathies such as hypothyroidism and hypoadrenocorticism, myocarditis with third-degree atrioventricular block, myositis, and other immune-mediated diseases suggests that a generalized immune dysfunction may occur in many animals.[170, 171]

A congenital form has been reported as an autosomal recessive condition in Jack Russell terriers, smooth-haired fox terriers, and English springer spaniels.[172–175] It has also been reported in Siamese and domestic shorthaired cats.[157, 158] Clinical signs are similar to generalized acquired myasthenia gravis, with the exception that megaesophagus has been infrequently reported in smooth-haired fox terriers. Remissions have not been reported. Instead, clinical signs are chronically progressive, usually resulting in paralysis despite treatment with pyridostigmine bromide. Circulating autoantibodies are not present in congenital myasthenia gravis. Instead, the diagnosis is based on response to anticholinesterase agents, decreasing response on repetitive stimulation, and demonstration of reduced concentrations of acetylcholine receptors in skeletal muscle.

NEOPLASTIC NEUROPATHIES

The peripheral nervous system can be affected by neoplastic processes in at least three different ways. The most common clinical manifestation is the development of primary neural tumors that arise from the neoplastic transformation of cells intrinsic to the peripheral nervous system. Less commonly, secondary peripheral nerve tumors develop as peripheral nerves are invaded by neoplastic hemolymphatic cells or entrapped by nearby carcinomas or sarcomas. Finally, the peripheral nervous system can be the target of paraneoplastic processes. Both clinical and subclinical neuropathies have been attributed to the remote effects of a number of neoplastic processes.

PRIMARY PERIPHERAL NERVE TUMORS

The peripheral nervous system is composed of neurons and their cell processes surrounded by fibroblasts, Schwann cells, and perineural cells. Each of these cell types is capable of becoming neoplastically transformed.

Neuroblastomas, ganglioneuroblastomas, and ganglioneuromas are primary neural tumors that develop in the peripheral nervous system. These are rare tumors that arise from neural crest cells, usually in adrenal medulla or sympathetic ganglia, and are distinguished primarily by the degree of differentiation of the neoplastic cells. These tumors typically occur in young dogs in retroperitoneal or mediastinal locations.[176–180] Occasionally tumors are reported in the gastrointestinal tract, olfactory mucosa, and peripheral sympathetic ganglia.[179–182] A single case of a kitten with an intestinal ganglioneuroma has been reported.[183] Clinical signs vary with location of the tumor, with vomiting, diarrhea, and dyspnea being most common. Neurologic signs occur after metastasis to the brain or spinal cord.[176, 179, 184]

Primary tumors that develop from the neoplastic transformation of supporting cells in the peripheral nervous system are more common. Considerable controversy exists over the nomenclature of these tumors. They have been referred to as schwannomas, neurinomas, neurilemomas, neurofibromas, and neurofibrosarcomas. Much of the controversy stems from difficulty in determining the primary cell of origin.

Most canine primary nerve sheath tumors are poorly differentiated, pleomorphic neoplasms in which the cell of origin is difficult to identify.[15] Therefore, the term malignant nerve sheath tumor is preferred by most authors. Malignant nerve sheath tumors may arise along the course of any peripheral nerve, including cranial nerves and spinal nerve roots. They typically are slow-growing tumors that extend by local invasion along the peripheral nerve and its branches. They rarely invade surrounding tissue, and metastasis is rare.[185] Neurologic signs are created by compression of peripheral axons, spinal cord, or brain stem by the expanding neoplastic mass. Although any peripheral nerve may be affected, over 80 per cent of the reported cases have occurred in the brachial plexus or its nerve roots. The remaining 20 per cent of cases occur in the pelvic plexus, thoracolumbar nerve roots, and cranial nerves.[186-188] Of the cranial nerves, the trigeminal nerve is most commonly affected.

Clinical signs typically begin in mature dogs, with only rare examples of the disease in cats. No breed or sex predisposition has been identified. Clinical signs vary with the area affected, but these tumors typically present as a chronic, progressive forelimb lameness. Muscle atrophy, pain in the axillary area, and a palpable mass may be present. Horner's syndrome and loss of the ipsilateral panniculus response reflect loss of the first two thoracic nerve roots, which contain preganglionic sympathetic fibers that supply the face and give rise to the lateral thoracic nerve. Ipsilateral hemiparesis that progresses to paraparesis occurs with extension of neoplastic tissue and secondary spinal cord compression. In cases that involve the cranial nerves, multiple cranial nerve deficits are accompanied by ipsilateral hemiparesis as the tumor compresses the brain stem.

Diagnostically, EMG reveals denervation in muscles innervated by affected nerves. Survey radiographs may show enlarged intervertebral foramen, and myelography may show an intradural extramedullary mass if neoplastic cells have invaded nerve roots. Computed tomography has been helpful for identifying tumors in peripheral nerves.[189] Surgical exploration and biopsy of nerve or plexus may be necessary to confirm the diagnosis.

Surgical excision has been curative in a few isolated cases.[186, 187, 190] Unfortunately, inability to completely resect all neoplastic tissue usually results in tumor recurrence. In one study, median survival interval after diagnosis in dogs with tumors of the brachial plexus or nerve roots was 12 and 5 months, respectively.[186] Radiation therapy has been proposed as a potential treatment for malignant nerve sheath tumors, but results have not been reported.

SECONDARY PERIPHERAL NERVE TUMORS

Peripheral nerve involvement by non-neural tumors is rare. However, infiltration of cranial and spinal nerves by neoplastic lymphocytes has been reported in cats with lymphosarcoma.[191] More recently, two dogs with myelomonocytic neoplasia and infiltration of multiple cranial nerves and spinal nerve roots were reported.[192, 193] Both dogs had an acute onset of "dropped jaw" and facial hyperesthesia secondary to bilateral trigeminal neuropathy. One dog also had Horner's syndrome, and the other had clinical signs of optic nerve and hypoglossal nerve involvement. Antemortem diagnosis was made in one dog by identification of blast cells in lymph nodes and peripheral blood. In both cases, neoplastic myeloid cells were found infiltrating cranial nerves and spinal nerve roots on postmortem examination.

PARANEOPLASTIC NEUROPATHIES

The fact that cancer is a multisystem disease, affecting tissues well removed from the site of the tumor, is recognized in both human and veterinary medicine. Although paraneoplastic diseases can affect a variety of tissues, neurologic involvement can be quite disabling. In human medicine, several different paraneoplastic syndromes have been identified that affect all levels of the nervous system.[194] In veterinary medicine, peripheral nerves seem the most susceptible. The incidence of paraneoplastic peripheral neuropathy in veterinary patients is uncertain but probably varies with tumor type. Most cases with clinically significant neuropathies have been associated with insulinomas.[194-199] A total of six dogs with histologically confirmed insulinomas have been described that presented for tetraparesis. All had generalized muscle atrophy, diminished spinal reflexes, and electrophysiologic changes compatible with diffuse axonal degeneration. Angular atrophy of both type I and type II myofibers seen in muscle biopsy suggested denervation, and axonal degeneration was apparent in peripheral nerve sections. The association between clinically significant neuropathies and other tumor types in veterinary patients is more tenuous. Cardinet and Holliday reported denervation changes in skeletal muscle biopsies in two dogs with adenocarcinoma and clinical signs of muscular weakness.[199] Presthus and Teige described facial and pelvic limb weakness in a dog with gastric lymphosarcoma.[200] In the remaining cases, peripheral nerve changes were subclinical and were identified electrophysiologically or on postmortem examination.[201-204]

In an effort to identify the subclinical incidence of peripheral nerve changes in cancer patients, Braund et al. evaluated peripheral nerves from a series of 21 dogs with malignant tumors.[203] All the dogs examined with bronchogenic carcinoma, insulinoma, malignant melanoma, osteosarcoma, thyroid adenocarcinoma, and mammary adenocarcinoma and one dog with a mast cell tumor had significantly more degenerative changes than age-matched controls. A combination of demyelination, remyelination, and axonal necrosis was present in every case. However, the incidence of demyelination and remyelination was higher. Interestingly, lymphosarcoma had the least neuropathic effect in this study. The number of dogs with each tumor type was relatively small, and no correlation between duration of the tumor and degree of neuropathic change was attempted. Additional studies are needed to better define the true incidence of peripheral nerve changes in veterinary cancer patients. However, this study confirms that paraneoplastic neuropathies exist in animals and occur in a wide variety of neoplastic processes.

Several hypotheses have been proposed regarding the pathogenesis of paraneoplastic diseases. The most widely investigated include elaboration of a neurotoxic substance by the neoplastic cells, secondary nutritional deficiencies caused by competition between the tumor and the host for an essential metabolite, cancer-associated immune suppression predisposing affected individuals to opportunistic infections, and an immune-mediated disorder in which autoantibodies are produced against antigens shared by the tumor and the nervous system. To date, most evidence supports an immune-mediated disorder. Antibodies that recognize specific neuronal populations have been found in humans with a variety of paraneoplastic neurologic syndromes, including Eaton-Lambert myasthenic syndrome, cerebellar degeneration, subacute sensory neuropathy, and retinal degeneration.[194] Although they are probably responsible for the neurologic signs, identification of these antibodies has also proved useful as a serologic marker for neoplasia. In many instances, neurologic signs may antedate the diagnosis of cancer, and identification of these specific antibodies in serum provides presumptive evidence of occult neoplasia.

Treatment for paraneoplastic neuropathies has been unrewarding in veterinary patients. A single case with insulinoma-associated neuropathy improved with corticosteroid therapy.[198] Current therapy in humans takes two approaches: first, to treat the cancer, and second, to suppress the immune reaction. Successful treatment has been reported in individual cases. Unfortunately, the target of most human paraneoplastic neurologic syndromes is neurons, which do not regenerate, so the efficacy of treatment is often difficult to evaluate.

TRAUMATIC NEUROPATHIES

Research into peripheral nerve trauma suggests that there are at least five different classifications for the types of injury that can occur.[205] Class 1 is referred to as neurapraxia and describes the response to mild or moderate focal compression. Nerve conduction is reversibly blocked. Histologically there are either no lesions or mild segmental demyelination. Complete recovery may occur within hours or, with more severe compression, may be delayed up to six weeks. Class 2 injuries, or axonotmesis, usually occur with crush or percussion injuries. Axons are interrupted, but the supporting connective tissue remains intact. Wallerian degeneration usually occurs distal to the site of injury, but regeneration is usually effective, because regenerating axons can be guided back to the appropriate targets. Class 3, 4, and 5 injuries refer to varying degrees of neurotmesis. Class 3 injuries result in disruption of axons and endoneurium, but fascicular orientation is preserved by an intact perineurium. Class 4 injuries also disrupt the perineurium, and the entire peripheral nerve is severed in class 5 injuries. With increasing degrees of damage to supporting structures, the ability of regenerating axons to successfully bridge the gap and reinnervate original structures is lessened.

All five classes of injury are possible in veterinary patients, and more than one class can occur simultaneously. Unless the peripheral nerve is completely severed, most surgeons wait several weeks before attempting repair to assess how much functional return will occur. Surgical repair of transected nerves has been attempted using either direct end-to-end anastomosis or a nerve graft to bridge the defect. Autologous sensory nerves may be harvested to be used as a graft, or a non-neural conduit can be used. Experimentally, application of nerve growth factors to synthetic conduits has aided peripheral nerve regeneration after complete resection and may be clinically useful in the future.[206] Axonal regrowth occurs at a rate of approximately 1 to 2 mm/day. Therefore, the prognosis for functional return depends not only on class of injury or precision of surgical repair but also on the distance the axon must travel to reach its end organ.

Individual peripheral nerves can be injured in a number of ways. Injection injuries, trauma from bone fracture and repair, lacerations from fights, and automobile accidents are some of the more common sources in dogs and cats. Motor and sensory deficits associated with individual peripheral and cranial nerves are outlined in Tables 108–1 and 108–2. Diagnosis is usually based on clinical signs of motor and sensory deficits. EMG reveals denervation, and peripheral nerve conduction should fail five to seven days after the injury. Recently, ultrasonography has shown promise at imaging transected nerve stumps.[207]

BRACHIAL PLEXUS AVULSION

The brachial plexus is typically formed from the sixth cervical through the second thoracic spinal nerve roots. Because nerve roots lack a perineurium, traction of the forelimb or severe abduction of the scapula frequently results in avulsion of these nerve roots, usually within the dura. Depending on the direction and extent of forelimb traction, all or only part of the brachial plexus may be involved. The caudal portion of the plexus is more commonly involved in partial injuries.[208, 209]

Clinical signs are characterized by an acute, nonprogressive monoparesis, usually precipitated by an automobile accident or a fall. The resulting motor and sensory dysfunction in the limb varies with the extent of the avulsion. Avulsion of C8, T1, and T2 nerve roots injures the radial, median, and ulnar nerves. The limb may be carried in a flexed position because the musculocutaneous, axillary, and suprascapular nerves are intact, but weight bearing is impossible without the ability to extend the elbow and carpus. Injury to C8, T1, and T2 spinal nerve roots also results in Horner's syndrome and loss of the ipsilateral cutaneous trunci (panniculus) reflex owing to damage to the origins of the presynaptic sympathetic innervation to the face and lateral thoracic nerve, respectively. More rostral nerve root injuries also involve the musculocutaneous nerve and prevent flexion of the elbow. Any limb movement in this case is generated by advancement of the shoulder. Injury of only proximal portions of the brachial plexus is rare. Useful limb function depends on the radial nerve, and in a review of 30 cases, the radial nerve was involved in 92 per cent of dogs with brachial plexus avulsion.[210] Like motor function, sensory deficits depend on the number and distribution of nerve roots avulsed. In some instances, dorsal roots may be spared, resulting in some preservation of sensation even though motor function was lost with avulsion of the ventral roots. Despite the potential variability in sensory deficits, most cases are analgesic distal to the elbow.[211]

Diagnosis of brachial plexus avulsion depends on history, clinical signs, and electrophysiologic evidence of denervation in limb muscles. Motor nerve conduction is usually abolished in affected nerves. A sensory nerve evoked potential may be present even in the absence of conscious perception of pain if the dorsal nerve root is avulsed proximal to the dorsal root ganglion. Somatosensory evoked potentials produced by stimulation of a peripheral nerve and measuring the response of afferent neurons in the spinal cord and brain will be abolished if all nerve roots are avulsed. Unfortunately, somatosensory evoked potentials are less useful with partial lesions.[212]

Prognosis for functional return is hopeless if the radial nerve has been avulsed. Several salvage procedures have been described for distal radial nerve deficits, but triceps innervation is required for any useful limb movement. Neurapraxia is certainly a feature of any traumatic peripheral nerve injury. Therefore, a hopeless prognosis should not be given before a minimum of four to six weeks after the injury. Unfortunately, less than 12 per cent of reported cases regained radial nerve function.[210] Limb amputation should be considered if self-mutilation or other continuous trauma occurs in desensitized areas.

VASCULAR NEUROPATHIES

Acute obstruction of blood vessels supplying peripheral nerves is rare except in cats with aortic thromboembolism.

Occasional cases have been reported in dogs, especially in association with heartworm disease. Although thromboembolism of any major artery could produce clinical signs, the most common site is the terminal aorta obstructing the internal and external iliac arteries and the median sacral artery. Both physical restriction of blood flow by the embolus and the production of vasoactive substances, including serotonin and thromboxane, that limit collateral blood flow combine to produce ischemia of the sciatic nerve and adjacent muscles. Axonal necrosis occurs in the center of nerve fascicles in the distal sciatic nerve and its branches, and paranodal demyelination is evident in peripheral areas.[213] Muscle damage consists of focal necrosis, with inflammatory cell infiltrates and myophagia.

Clinical signs typically consist of an acute onset of pelvic limb paralysis. The femoral pulse is usually weak or absent, the rear limbs are cold, and the nail beds are ischemic and fail to bleed if cut. Rear limb musculature often feels stiff because of ischemic muscle contracture, and the cats often show signs of pain on muscle palpation. Evidence of cardiac disease is usually present in physical examination findings, thoracic radiographs, or echocardiography. Most cats have hypertrophic cardiomyopathy; however, other forms of cardiac disease are possible. Therapeutically, in addition to specific treatment for the cardiac disease, most cats benefit from warming of the limbs and administration of acepromazine 0.2 to 0.4 mg/kg subcutaneously every 8 hours to encourage vasodilatation and collateral blood flow. Heparin sodium (100 to 200 IU/kg IV initially, followed by 50 to 100 IU/kg subcutaneously every 6 to 8 hours) is recommended to prevent further thrombus formation, and analgesics such as butorphanol (0.2 to 0.4 mg/kg every 6 to 12 hours) should be used to control pain. Specific therapy to remove the clot has been attempted both surgically and medically using thrombolytic agents. The benefits versus risks of these measures, as well as specific treatment for feline cardiac diseases, are discussed in more detail in Chapter 117. If given enough time and supportive care, the clot will undergo spontaneous thrombolysis, and a significant number of cats will regain some limb function. In a recent review of 100 cases, 37 per cent survived the initial episode.[214] This percentage increased to 70 per cent if only cats with partial femoral arterial thrombosis were considered. However, the long-term prognosis for cats with aortic thromboembolism is poor, with average survival intervals ranging from 6 to 11.5 months.[214, 215]

IDIOPATHIC NEUROPATHIES

DISTAL DENERVATING DISEASE

Distal denervating disease is considered the most common neuropathy in dogs in the United Kingdom.[216] Dogs of all ages and breeds and both sexes are affected. The onset of clinical signs is variable, ranging from days to a month or more. Quadriparesis to quadriplegia is accompanied by neck weakness, loss of bark, diminished spinal reflexes, and muscle atrophy that is especially prominent in proximal limb muscles. Voluntary control of tail movement, urination, and defecation is maintained, and pain sensation is preserved. EMG reveals diffuse spontaneous activity in all muscles. Motor nerve conduction velocity is modestly reduced, but the evoked muscle action potential is usually small and dispersed. These electrophysiologic changes are most compatible with primary axonal loss with little demyelination.

Sensory nerve conduction is normal. Muscle and nerve biopsy confirms a distal axonopathy with denervation atrophy of muscle. Most cases spontaneously resolve without treatment, with complete recovery occurring four to six weeks after clinical signs plateau.[217] Pathologic changes are restricted to the distal motor axon. No changes have been reported in the CNS, nerve roots, or main portions of peripheral nerves. Intramuscular branches are reported to show extensive collateral axonal sprouting, with early cases also exhibiting modest degrees of terminal axonal degeneration. The etiology is unknown, but an unidentified toxin is considered likely.

DISTAL SYMMETRIC POLYNEUROPATHY

Numerous adult, large breed dogs have been described with distal sensorimotor polyneuropathies, which have been collectively referred to as distal symmetric polyneuropathy.[218, 219] There is a remarkable similarity to the polyneuropathy in rottweiler dogs described previously, but no breed association has been identified with this syndrome. Clinical signs are insidious in onset and gradually progressive over one to two months. Pelvic limb paresis is the initial presenting sign, but tetraparesis with atrophy of distal limb muscles and muscles of mastication eventually develops. Diffuse spontaneous activity is prominent with needle EMG. Motor nerve conduction velocities are usually normal or slightly slowed, but the amplitude and duration of the evoked muscle action potential are small and prolonged, suggesting axonal injury. Muscle and nerve biopsy confirms a distal axonopathy with denervation atrophy of skeletal muscles. No other abnormalities have been reported in peripheral blood or CSF. Histologically, lesions are confined to the distal regions of motor nerves. Degeneration of large diameter motor axons is prominent in distal limb nerves and the recurrent laryngeal nerve. Variable degrees of demyelination are also present but appear secondary to axonal loss. Sensory and autonomic nerves may be affected as well, but to a lesser degree. No lesions are found in the CNS. The etiology is obscure, but metabolic, toxic, and paraneoplastic neuropathies may appear similarly. Prognosis is poor, as the disease is chronic and progressive in nature, and no effective treatment has been described.

DANCING DOBERMAN DISEASE

Dancing Doberman disease is an unusual neuromuscular disorder that presently appears restricted to adult Doberman pinschers of both sexes.[220] Clinical signs begin between 6 months and 7 years of age and are gradually progressive over several years. Affected dogs have a characteristic habit of holding one or both pelvic limbs flexed while standing. The condition may begin in one limb and then spread to the other limb within three to six months. When both pelvic limbs are affected, the condition may appear as a shifting rear limb lameness, with an increased tendency for the dogs to sit rather than stand. Conscious proprioceptive deficits have been reported in two dogs five and six years after the disease was diagnosed. Exaggerated pelvic limb reflexes and atrophy of the gastrocnemius muscle are also common.

Electrophysiologic abnormalities suggest a mixture of myopathic and neuropathic changes. EMG shows spontaneous activity in affected muscles, but motor and sensory nerve conduction velocities are usually normal. Pathologic changes are confusing. Some dogs have multifocal pelvic limb muscular atrophy and hypertrophy, fiber type grouping, focal necrosis, and endomysial-perimysial fibrosis, suggestive of a form of myotonic myopathy.[219] Other dogs have peripheral nerve changes suggestive of a primary axonopathy. A single dog has been reported with neuronal degeneration and gliosis in the spinal cord and lumbosacral nerve roots.[220]

No treatment has proved beneficial to date. Although the syndrome is slowly progressive, affected animals remain functional pets for many years. Without definitive diagnostic criteria, the syndrome can be diagnosed only by ruling out other diseases such as lumbosacral stenosis, intervertebral disk disease, or nerve root tumors that might present initially with rear limb paresthesias without obvious motor impairment.

DYSAUTONOMIA

Dysautonomia is a general term for dysfunction of the autonomic nervous system. A syndrome characterized by diffuse autonomic dysfunction was first reported in cats in 1982 by Key and Gaskell.[221] Over the next two years, this previously undiagnosed disease was reported in epidemic proportions throughout the United Kingdom and later in Europe and the United States. The incidence of the disease has since markedly declined in cats. The first case of dysautonomia was reported in dogs in 1983, again in the United Kingdom.[222] Only sporadic reports of canine cases appeared until recently, when 11 dogs were identified in Missouri over a seven-year period.[223]

Animals between 6 weeks and 11 years of age have developed dysautonomia, but both dogs and cats younger than 3 years old appear to be more susceptible. Males and females are equally affected. The onset is acute in most cases, with clinical signs developing over two to three days. Rarely the onset is more insidious, lasting a week or more. Initial clinical signs are usually nonspecific and consist of lethargy, anorexia, and depression. Gastrointestinal signs, including regurgitation and vomiting, constipation, or diarrhea, follow. Dysuria with a distended urinary bladder, myiasis with depressed pupillary light reflexes, dry mucous membranes, prolapsed third eyelids, dysphagia, and weight loss are also commonly seen. More inconsistent features include loss of anal tone and mild postural reaction deficits. Many cats also have bradycardia, with heart rates less than 120 beats per minute.

No consistent abnormalities have been detected in peripheral blood or CSF. Radiographically, most animals have evidence of decreased peristaltic activity throughout the gastrointestinal tract, including megaesophagus, delayed gastric emptying, and generalized ileus. Electrodiagnostic testing is usually normal, with the exception of occasional spontaneous activity in limb muscles. Pharmacologic testing has been used to confirm parasympathetic and sympathetic nervous system dysfunction.

Histologically, sympathetic and parasympathetic ganglia are affected to an equal degree. Depletion of neuronal cell bodies is the more prominent change, with many remaining neurons containing atypical homogeneous cytoplasm, dissolution of Nissl substance, and an eccentric pyknotic nucleus. Axonal degeneration is present in autonomic nerves. Peripheral nerves are relatively spared, although occasionally smaller neurons in dorsal root ganglia and cranial nerve ganglia may show chromatolytic changes. A percentage of neurons in cranial nerve nuclei, ventral horn cells, and cells in the intermediolateral grey matter of the spinal cord may also show characteristic changes. Unusual ultrastructural changes consist of derangement of rough endoplasmic reticulum, with existing cisternae denuded of ribosomes and distended with electron-dense flocculent material.[224] No normal Golgi bodies are found, but instead there are stacks of smooth membranous profiles. Membranous dense bodies and autophagic vacuoles are common in some neurons.

Treatment is largely supportive. Pilocarpine (1 per cent) eye drops may improve mydriasis as well as stimulate lacrimation and salivation. Bethanechol (2.5 to 7.5 mg every 8 hours) should facilitate evacuation of the bladder at least temporarily. Metoclopramide enhances the actions of any available acetylcholine on muscarinic receptors in the gastrointestinal tract and enhances gastric emptying. Unfortunately, the prognosis is poor. Less than 25 per cent of affected cats survive, and recovery often takes over a year. The etiology of the disease remains a mystery, despite numerous attempts to identify an infectious or toxic agent. The clustering of cases in the United Kingdom and more recently Missouri suggests an environmental agent, but none has been identified. Based on histologic evidence, the agent disrupts protein synthesis in autonomic and some somatic neurons.

IDIOPATHIC TRIGEMINAL NEURITIS

The trigeminal nerve is most commonly injured by inflammatory or neoplastic intracranial diseases. Rarely, the trigeminal nerve is directly infiltrated by neoplastic cells, as described earlier for peripheral nerve neoplasia. The trigeminal nerve is also the target of an idiopathic, inflammatory condition referred to as trigeminal neuritis. Clinical signs are characterized by an acute onset of bilateral trigeminal motor paralysis, causing an inability to close the mouth ("jaw drop").[225] Facial sensation is usually preserved. Occasionally, Horner's syndrome may accompany trigeminal neuritis, presumably because the postganglionic sympathetic axons course with the ophthalmic branch of the trigeminal nerve.[226]

Biopsy of the muscles of mastication reveals denervation atrophy. Mild albuminocytologic dissociation may be seen in CSF. Histology is characterized by extensive nonsuppurative neuritis in all portions of the trigeminal nerve and ganglion, causing demyelination.[226] The brain stem is spared. Spontaneous recovery usually occurs in two to three weeks with only supportive care. Maintenance of hydration and alimentation is critical during this time. Percutaneous gastrostomy has been helpful in this regard.

IDIOPATHIC FACIAL NEURITIS

Because of its anatomic proximity to the inner and middle ear, the facial nerve is commonly injured in otitis media or interna. The facial nerve also has a superficial location after emerging from the stylomastoid foramen and is therefore susceptible to traumatic injury. The facial nerve is often affected in generalized peripheral nerve diseases, including polyradiculoneuritis, tick paralysis, and botulism. Less frequently, facial nerve paralysis results from no identifiable cause and has been referred to as idiopathic facial neuritis.[226]

Clinical signs of facial paralysis are characterized by an inability to move the lips, ears, and eyelids. Ptyalism and inability to blink are the most common admitting complaints. The facial nerve also provides parasympathetic innervation to lacrimal glands, and proximal injury may result in keratoconjunctivitis sicca. Xerostomia, focal hypalgesia to the pinna, and partial loss of taste may also occur with facial nerve paralysis, but these are difficult to appreciate clinically. Both dogs and cats have been reported with idiopathic facial neuritis.[227] The syndrome tends to occur in mature animals, and cocker spaniels have been identified in two studies as being predisposed.[227, 228] Clinical signs typically appear acutely and in the absence of any other systemic illness. One or both facial nerves may be initially affected. In cases with unilateral facial neuritis, the other side may become affected later. Electrophysiologically, spontaneous activity suggestive of denervation appears in superficial facial muscles. Stimulation of the facial nerve failed to evoke an action potential in one report.[228] Fascicular biopsy of the ventral buccal branch of the facial nerve in two dogs showed axonal degeneration.[228, 229]

The cause of this condition is unknown. A causal link has been made with hypothyroidism. Statistically, the relationship with hypothyroidism has been difficult to prove.[227] However, numerous cases have concurrent hypothyroidism and clinically improve with thyroid supplementation.[99, 10] Other theories that are also unproved include herpes viral neuritis or swelling of the facial nerve causing compression in the bony facial canal traversing the petrous temporal bone.[10]

The prognosis for idiopathic facial neuritis is poor. Steroid therapy has been recommended, but its efficacy is uncertain. Animals may improve within weeks or months. However, the facial nerve remains permanently paralyzed in a significant number of cases. Exposure keratitis, especially if compounded by decreased lacrimation, is the most significant complication.

IDIOPATHIC PERIPHERAL VESTIBULAR DISEASE

An idiopathic vestibular dysfunction has been identified in old dogs and in cats of all ages.[226] Clinical signs are acute in onset and consist of head tilt, nystagmus, falling, rolling, and ataxia. Postural reactions remain intact, and spinal reflexes are normal. Facial nerve deficits and Horner's syndrome, which are common features of otitis media or interna, are conspicuously absent in idiopathic vestibular disease. In cats, there is an unusually high frequency of cases in July and August.[230] The reason for this seasonal incidence is unknown. The diagnosis is based on clinical signs and failure to identify other causes of vestibular dysfunction, including trauma, otitis media or interna, or toxins. Aminoglycoside antibiotics, especially streptomycin in cats, can damage vestibular and auditory receptors and result in vestibular dysfunction. The prognosis for idiopathic vestibular dysfunction is excellent. Most cases spontaneously improve within weeks. Some animals have a residual head tilt. An association between idiopathic peripheral vestibular disease and hypothyroidism has been noted.[99, 101] Other inner and middle ear diseases are covered more thoroughly in Chapter 122.

REFERENCES

1. Gardner E, Bunge RP: Gross anatomy of the peripheral nervous system. In Dyck PJ, Thomas PK, Griffin JW, et al (eds): Peripheral Neuropathy, 3rd ed. Philadelphia, WB Saunders, 1993, p 8.
2. Thomas PK, et al: Microscopic anatomy of the peripheral nervous system. In Dyck PJ, Thomas PK, Griffin JW, et al (eds): Peripheral Neuropathy, 3rd ed. Philadelphia, WB Saunders, 1993, p 28.
3. Berthold C-H, Rydmark M: Morphology of normal peripheral axons. In Waxman SG, Kocsis JD, Stys PK (eds): The Axon, Structure, Function and Pathophysiology. New York, Oxford University Press, 1995, p 13.
4. Ritchie JM: Physiology of axons. In Waxman SG, Kocsis JD, Stys PK (eds): The Axon, Structure, Function and Pathophysiology. New York, Oxford University Press, 1995, p 68.
5. Bostock H: Impulse propagation in experimental neuropathy. In Dyck PJ, Thomas PK, Griffin JW, et al (eds): Peripheral Neuropathy, 3rd ed. Philadelphia, WB Saunders, 1993, p 109.
6. Gaber CE, et al: Laryngeal paralysis in dogs: A review of 23 cases. JAVMA 186:377, 1985.
7. Braund KG, et al: Laryngeal paralysis in immature and mature dogs as one sign of a more diffuse polyneuropathy. JAVMA 194:1735, 1989.
8. Gaynor AR, et al: Risk factors for acquired megaesophagus in dogs. JAVMA 211:1406, 1997.
9. Niederhauser UB, Holliday TA: Electrodiagnostic studies in disease of muscles and neuromuscular junctions. Semin Vet Med Surg 4:116, 1989.
10. Oliver JE, Lorenz MD, Kornegay JN: Handbook of Veterinary Neurology, 3rd ed. Philadelphia, WB Saunders, 1997.
11. Kimura J: Electrodiagnosis in Diseases of Nerve and Muscle: Principles and Practice. Philadelphia, FA Davis, 1983.
12. Braund KG: Nerve and muscle biopsy techniques. Prog Vet Neuro 2:35, 1991.
13. Braund KG, et al: Fascicular nerve biopsy in the dog. Am J Vet Res 40:1025, 1979.
14. Kreutzberg GW: Reaction of the neuronal cell body to axonal damage. In Waxman SG, Kocsis JD, Stys PK (eds): The Axon, Structure, Function and Pathophysiology. New York, Oxford University Press, 1995, p 355.
15. Summers BA, Cummings JF, de Lahunta A: Veterinary Neuropathology. St. Louis, Mosby, 1995.
16. Dyck PJ, et al: Pathologic alterations of nerves. In Dyck PJ, Thomas PK, Griffin JW, et al (eds): Peripheral Neuropathy, 3rd ed. Philadelphia, WB Saunders, 1993, p 514.
17. Verdon T, Suter U: Molecular biology of axon-glia interactions in the peripheral nervous system. Prog Nucleic Acid Res Molec Biol 56:225, 1997.
18. Scherer S: The biology and pathobiology of Schwann cells. Curr Opin Neurol 10:386, 1997.
19. Cummings JF, et al: Multisystemic chromatolytic neuronal degeneration in a Cairn terrier pup. Cornell Vet 78:301, 1988.
20. Palmer AC, Blakemore WF: A progressive neuronopathy in the young Cairn terrier. J Small Anim Pract 30:101, 1989.
21. Cummings JF, et al: Multisystemic chromatolytic neuronal degeneration in Cairn terriers. A case with generalized cataplectic episodes. J Vet Intern Med 5:91, 1991.
22. Cumming JF, et al: Focal spinal muscular atrophy in two German shepherd pups. Acta Neuropathol 79:113, 1989.
23. Inada S, et al: A clinical study on hereditary progressive neurogenic muscular atrophy in Pointer dogs. Jpn J Vet Sci 40:539, 1978.
24. Izumo S, et al: Morphological study on the hereditary neurogenic amyotrophic dogs: Accumulation of lipid compound–like structures in the lower motor neuron. Acta Neuropathol (Berl) 61:270, 1983.
25. Inada S, et al: Canine storage disease characterized by hereditary progressive neurogenic muscular atrophy: Breeding experiments and clinical manifestation. Am J Vet Res 47:2294, 1986.
26. Shell LG, et al: Familial lower motor neuron disease in rottweiler dogs: Neuropathological studies. Vet Pathol 24:139, 1987.
27. Shell LG, et al: Spinal muscular atrophy in two rottweiler littermates. JAVMA 190:878, 1987.
28. Sandefelt E, et al: Hereditary neuronal abiotrophy in the Swedish Lapland dog. Cornell Vet 63 (Suppl 3):7, 1973.
29. Sandefeldt E, et al: Infantile spinal muscular atrophy, Herdnig-Hoffmann disease. Animal model: Hereditary neuronal abiotrophy in Swedish Lapland dogs. Am J Pathol 82:649, 1976.
30. Sack GH, et al: Autosomal dominant inheritance of hereditary canine spinal muscular atrophy. Ann Neurol 15:369, 1984.
31. Lorenz MD, et al: Hereditary spinal muscular atrophy in Brittany spaniels: Clinical manifestations. JAVMA 175:833, 1979.
32. Cork LC, et al: Hereditary canine spinal muscular atrophy. Neuropathol Exp Neurol 37:209, 1979.
33. Cork LC, et al: Pathology of motor neurons in accelerated hereditary canine spinal muscular atrophy. Lab Invest 46:89, 1982.
34. Duncan ID, Griffiths IR: Peripheral nervous system in a case of canine giant axonal neuropathy. Neuropathol Appl Neurobiol 5:25, 1979.
35. Griffiths IR, et al: Further studies of the central nervous system in canine giant axonal neuropathy. Neuropathol Appl Neurobiol 6:421, 1980.
36. Duncan ID, Griffiths IR: Canine giant axonal neuropathy: Some aspects of its clinical, pathological and comparative features. J Small Anim Pract 22:491, 1981.
37. Duncan ID, et al: Inherited canine giant axonal neuropathy. Muscle Nerve 4:223, 1981.
38. Furuoka H, et al: Peripheral neuropathy in German shepherd dogs. J Comp Pathol 107:169, 1992.
39. Moe L: Hereditary polyneuropathy of Alaskan malamutes. In Kirk RW, Bonagura JD (eds): Current Veterinary Therapy XI Small Animal Practice. Philadelphia, WB Saunders, 1992, p 1038.
40. Braund KG, et al: Idiopathic polyneuropathy in Alaskan malamutes. J Vet Intern Med 11:243, 1997.
41. Moreau PM, et al: Peripheral and central distal axonopathy of suspected inherited origin in Birman cats. Acta Neuropathol 82:143, 1991.
42. Braund KG, et al: Distal sensorimotor polyneuropathy in mature rottweiler dogs. Vet Pathol 31:316, 1994.

43. Griffiths IR, Duncan ID, Barker J: A progressive axonopathy of Boxer dogs affecting the central and peripheral nervous system. J Small Anim Pract 21:29, 1980.

44. Griffiths IR: Progressive axonopathy: An inherited neuropathy of Boxer dogs. 1. Further studies of the clinical and electrophysiological features. J Small Anim Pract 26:381, 1985.

45. Griffiths IR, Kyriakides E, Scott J: Progressive axonopathy: An inherited neuropathy of Boxer dogs. Quantitative and morphometric analysis of the peripheral nerve lesion. J Neurol Sci 75:69, 1986.

46. Duncan ID, Griffiths IR: Peripheral neuropathies of domestic animals. In Dyck PJ, Thomas PK, Lambert EH, Bunge R (eds): Peripheral Neuropathy, 2nd ed. Philadelphia, WB Saunders, 1984, p 707.

47. Griffiths IR, et al: Progressive axonopathy: An inherited neuropathy of Boxer dogs. 4. Myelin sheath and Schwann cell changes in the nerve roots. J Neurocytol 16:145, 1987.

48. Braund KG, et al: Laryngeal paralysis-polyneuropathy complex in young Dalmatians. Am J Vet Res 55:534, 1994.

49. Matz ME, et al: Peripheral hypomyelinization in two golden retriever littermates. JAVMA 197:228, 1990.

50. Braund KG, et al: Congenital hypomyelinating polyneuropathy in two golden retriever littermates. Vet Pathol 26:202, 1989.

51. Sponenberg DP, de Lahunta A: Hereditary hypertrophic neuropathy in Tibetan mastiff dogs. J Hered 72:287, 1981.

52. Cumming JF, et al: Canine inherited hypertropic neuropathy. Acta Neuropathol (Berl) 53:137, 1981.

53. Cooper BJ, et al: Canine inherited hypertrophic neuropathy: Clinical and electrodiagnostic studies. Am J Vet Res 45:1172, 1984.

54. Cooper BJ, et al: Defective Schwann cell function in canine inherited hypertrophic neuropathy. Acta Neuropathol (Berl) 63:51, 1984.

55. Duncan ID, Griffiths IR: A sensory neuropathy affecting long-haired dachshund dogs. J Small Anim Pract 23:381, 1982.

56. Duncan ID, Griffiths IR, Munz M: The pathology of a sensory neuropathy affecting long haired dachshund dogs. Acta Neuropathol (Berl) 58:141, 1982.

57. Franklin RJM, et al: Sensory neuropathy in a Jack Russell terrier. J Small Anim Pract 33:402, 1992.

58. Cummings JF, et al: Acral mutilation and nociceptive loss in English Pointer dogs. A canine sensory neuropathy. Acta Neuropathol (Berl) 53:119, 1981.

59. Cummings JF, et al: Ganglioradiculoneuritis in the dog. A clinical, light and electronmicroscopic study. Acta Neuropathol 60:29, 1983.

60. Venker–van Haagen AJ, et al: Spontaneous laryngeal paralysis in young Bouviers. J Am Anim Hosp Assoc 14:714, 1978.

61. Venker–van Haagen AJ, et al: Hereditary transmission of laryngeal paralysis in Bouviers. J Am Anim Hosp Assoc 17:75, 1981.

62. Hendricks JC, O'Brien JA: Inherited laryngeal paralysis in Siberian husky crosses (abstract). Proceedings of the 3rd annual ACVIM Forum, 1985.

63. O'Brien JA, Hendricks H: Inherited laryngeal paralysis: Analysis in the husky cross. Vet Q 8:301, 1986.

64. Jones BR: Inherited hyperchylomicronaemia in the cat. J Small Anim Pract 34:493, 1993.

65. McKerrell RE, et al: Primary hyperoxaluria (L-glyceric aciduria) in the cat: A newly recognised inherited disease. Vet Rec 125:31, 1989.

66. Keller CB, Lamarre J: Inherited lysosomal storage disease in an English springer spaniel. JAVMA 200:194, 1992.

67. Hartley WJ, et al: A suspected new canine storage disease. Acta Neuropathol (Berl) 56:225, 1982.

68. Kelly WR, et al: Canine α-L-fucosidosis: A storage disease of springer spaniels. Acta Neuropathol (Berl) 60:9, 1983.

69. Taylor RM, et al: Canine fucosidosis: Clinical findings. J Small Anim Pract 28:291, 1987.

70. Barker CG, et al: Fucosidosis in English springer spaniels: Results of a trial screening programme. J Small Anim Pract 29:623, 1988.

71. Braund KG: Disorders of peripheral nerves. In Ettinger SJ, Feldman EC (eds): A Textbook of Veterinary Internal Medicine. Disease of the Dog and Cat, 4th ed. Philadelphia, WB Saunders, 1995, p 701.

72. Rotmistrovsky RA, et al: GM₂ gangliosidosis in a mixed-breed dog. Prog Vet Neurol 2:203, 1991.

73. Fletcher TF, Kurtz HJ: Animal model for human diseases: Globoid cell leukodystrophy, Krabbe's disease. Am J Pathol 66:375, 1972.

74. Fletcher TF, et al: Ultrastructural features of globoid-cell leukodystrophy in the dog. Am J Vet Res 32:177, 1971.

75. Johnson KH: Globoid leukodystrophy in a cat. JAVMA 157:2057, 1970.

76. Johnson GR, et al: Globoid cell leukodystrophy in a beagle. JAVMA 167:380, 1975.

77. Boysen BG, et al: Globoid cell leukodystrophy in the bluetick hound dog: 1. Clinical manifestations. Can Vet J 15:303, 1975.

78. Zaki FA, Kay WJ: Globoid cell leukodystrophy in a miniature poodle. JAVMA 163:248, 1973.

79. Luttgen PJ, et al: Globoid cell leukodystrophy in a basset hound. J Small Anim Pract 24:153, 1983.

80. Blakemore WF, et al: Value of a nerve biopsy in diagnosis of globoid cell leucodystrophy in the dog. Vet Rec 93:70, 1974.

81. Vicini DS, et al: Peripheral nerve biopsy for diagnosis of globoid cell leukodystrophy in a dog. JAVMA 192:1087, 1988.

82. Cuddon PA, et al: Polyneuropathy in feline Niemann-Pick disease. Brain 112:1429, 1989.

83. Fyfe JC, et al: Familial glycogen storage disease type IV in Norwegian Forest cats (abstract). Proceedings of the 8th annual ACVIM Forum, Washington, DC, 1990.

84. Coates JR, et al: A case presentation and discussion of type IV glycogen storage disease in a Norwegian Forest cat. Prog Vet Neurol 7:5, 1996.

85. Thomas PK, Tomlinson DR: Diabetic and hypoglycemic neuropathy. In Dyck PJ, Thomas PK, Griffin JW, et al (eds): Peripheral Neuropathy, 3rd ed. Philadelphia, WB Saunders, 1993, p 1219.

86. Braund KG, Steiss JE: Distal neuropathy in spontaneous diabetes mellitus in the dog. Acta Neuropathol (Berl) 57:263, 1982.

87. Steiss JE, et al: Electrodiagnostic analysis of peripheral neuropathy in dogs with diabetes mellitus. Am J Vet Res 42:2061, 1981.

88. Katherman AE, Braund KG: Polyneuropathy associated with diabetes mellitus in a dog. JAVMA 182:522, 1983.

89. Johnson CA, et al: Peripheral neuropathy and hypotension in a diabetic dog. JAVMA 9:1007, 1983.

90. Anderson PG, et al: Polyneuropathy and hormonal profiles in a chow puppy with hypoplasia of the islets of Langerhans. Vet Pathol 23:528, 1986.

91. Collyer JH, Gripper PL: Peripheral neuropathy in diabetic bitch (letter). Vet Rec 121:207, 1987.

92. Misselbrook NG: Peripheral neuropathy in diabetic bitch (letter). Vet Rec 121:287, 1987.

93. Kramek BA, et al: Neuropathy associated with diabetes mellitus in the cat. JAVMA 184:42, 1984.

94. Munana K: Long-term complications of diabetes mellitus. Part I: Retinopathy, nephropathy, and neuropathy. Vet Clin North Am Small Anim Pract 25:715, 1995.

95. Feldman EL, et al: Pathogenesis of diabetic neuropathy. Clin Neurosci 4:365, 1997.

96. Sims MH, et al: Depressed thyroid function in two tetraplegic dogs. JAVMA 171:178, 1977.

97. Dyer KR, et al: Peripheral neuropathy in two dogs: Correlation between clinical, electrophysiological and pathological findings. J Small Anim Pract 27:133, 1986.

98. Indrieri RJ, et al: Neuromuscular abnormalities associated with hypothyroidism and lymphocytic thyroiditis in three dogs. JAVMA 190:544, 1987.

99. Bichsel P, et al: Neurologic manifestations associated with hypothyroidism in four dogs. JAVMA 192:1745, 1988.

100. Budsberg SC, et al: Thyroid responsive unilateral forelimb lameness and generalized neuromuscular disease in four hypothyroid dogs. JAVMA 202:1859, 1993.

101. Jaggy A, et al: Neurological manifestations of hypothyroidism: A retrospective study of 29 dogs. J Vet Intern Med 8:328, 1994.

102. Pollard JD: Neuropathy in diseases of the thyroid and pituitary glands. In Dyck PJ, Thomas PK, Griffin JW, et al (eds): Peripheral Neuropathy, 3rd ed. Philadelphia, WB Saunders, 1993, p 1266.

103. Hatheway CL: Botulism: The present status of the disease. Curr Top Microbiol Immunol 195:55, 1995.

104. Cornelissen JM, et al: Type C botulism in five dogs. J Am Anim Hosp Assoc 21:401, 1985.

105. Barsanti JA: Botulism. In Greene CE (ed): Infectious Diseases of the Dog and Cat. Philadelphia, WB Saunders, 1990, p 515.

106. Malik R, Farrow BRH: Tick paralysis in North America and Australia. Vet Clin North Am Small Anim Pract 21:157, 1991.

107. Chrisman CL: Differentiation of tick paralysis and acute idiopathic polyradiculoneuritis in the dog using electromyography. J Am Anim Hosp Assoc 11:455, 1975.

108. Chang LW: Principles of Neurotoxicology. New York, Marcel Dekker, 1994.

109. Hamilton TA, et al: Vincristine-induced peripheral neuropathy in a dog. JAVMA 198:635, 1991.

110. Cho ES, et al: Neurotoxicity of vincristine in the cat: Morphological study. Arch Toxicol 52:83, 1983.

111. Krinke G, et al: Pyridoxine megavitaminosis produces degeneration of peripheral sensory neurons (sensory neuronopathy) in the dog. Neurotoxicology 2:13, 1980.

112. Gruber TA, et al: Chronic methyl mercurialism in the cat. Aust Vet J 54:115, 1978.

113. Charbonneau SM, et al: Subacute toxicity of methylmercury in the adult cat. Toxicol Appl Pharmacol 27:569, 1974.

114. Davies TS, et al: Pathology of chronic and subacute canine methylmercurialism. J Am Anim Hosp Assoc 13:369, 1977.

115. Ruhur LP, Andries J: Thallium intoxication in a dog. JAVMA 186:498, 1985.

116. Zook BC, et al: Thallium poisoning in cats. JAVMA 153:285, 1968.

117. Kennedy P, Cavanaugh JB: Sensory neuropathy produced in the cat with thallous acetate. Acta Neuropathol (Berl) 39:81, 1977.

118. Bratton GP, Kowalczyk DF: Lead poisoning. In Kirk RW, Bonagura JD (eds): Current Veterinary Therapy X. Philadelphia, WB Saunders, 1989, p 152.

119. Steiss JE, et al: Inability to experimentally produce a polyneuropathy in dogs given chronic oral low level lead. Can J Comp Med 49:401, 1985.

120. Prineas J: The pathogenesis of dying-back polyneuropathies. Part I. An ultrastructural study of experimental tri-ortho-cresyl phosphate intoxication in the cat. J Neuropathol Exp Neurol 28:571, 1969.

121. Bouldin TW, Cavanagh JB: Organophosphorous neuropathy. I. A teased-fiber study of the spatio-temporal spread of axonal degeneration. Am J Pathol 94:241, 1979.

122. Bouldin TW, Cavanagh JB: Organophosphorous neuropathy. II. A fine-structural study of the early stages of axonal degeneration. Am J Pathol 94:253, 1979.

123. Fikes JD, et al: Clinical, biochemical, electrophysiologic, and histologic assess-

ment of chlorpyrifos induced delayed neuropathy in the cat. Neurotoxicology 13:663, 1992.

124. Schaumburg HH, et al: Ultrastructural studies of the dying-back process. 1. Peripheral nerve terminal and axon degeneration in systemic acrylamide intoxication. J Neuropathol Exp Neurol 33:260, 1974.

125. Prineas J: The pathogenesis of dying-back polyneuropathies. Part II. An ultrastructural study of experimenta acrylamide intoxication in the cat. Neuropathol Exp Neurol 28:598, 1969.

126. Spencer PS, Schaumburg HH: Ultrastructural studies of the dying-back process. IV. Differential vulnerability of PNS and CNS fibers in experimental central-peripheral distal axonopathies. J Neuropathol Exp Neurol 36 300, 1977.

127. Safran N, et al: Paralytic syndrome attributed to lasalocid residues in a commercial ration fed to dogs. JAVMA 202:1273, 1993.

128. Cummings JF, Haas DC: Coonhound paralysis: An acute idiopathic polyradiculoneuritis in dogs resembling the Landry-Guillain-Barré syndrome. J Neurol Sci 4:51, 1967.

129. Cummings JF, de Lahunta A, Holmes DF, et al: Coonhound paralysis. Further clinical studies and electron microscopic observations. Acta Neuropathol (Berl) 56:167, 1982.

130. Holmes DF, et al: Experimental coonhound paralysis: Animal model of Guillain-Barré syndrome. Neurology 29: 186, 1979.

131. Luttgen PJ: Polyradiculoneuritis in a cat (abstract). Proceedings of the 5th annual ACVIM Forum, 1987.

132. Gerritsen RJ, et al: Acute idiopathic polyneuropathy in nine cats. Vet Q 18:63, 1996.

133. Kingma FJ, Catcott EJ: A paralytic syndrome in coonhounds. North Am Vet 35:115, 1954.

134. Northington JW, et al: Acute idiopathic polyneuropathy in the dog. JAVMA 179:375, 1981.

135. Northington JW, Brown MJ: Acute canine idiopathic polyneuropathy: A Guillain-Barré-like syndrome in dogs. J Neurol Sci 56:259, 1982.

136. Cuddon PA: Electrophysiological and immunological evaluation in coonhound paralysis. Proceedings of the 8th annual ACVIM Forum, Washington, DC 1990, p 1009.

137. Dalakas MC: Intravenous immune globulin therapy for neurologic diseases. Ann Intern Med 126:721, 1997.

138. Scott-Moncrieff JCR, Reagan WJ: Human intravenous immunoglobulin therapy. Semin Vet Med Surg 12:178, 1997.

139. Cummings JF, de Lahunta A: Hypertrophic neuropathy in a dog. Acta Neuropathol (Berl) 29:325, 1974.

140. Cummings JF, de Lahunta A: Chronic relapsing polyradiculoneuritis in a dog. A clinical, light- and electron-microscopic study. Acta Neuropathol (Berl) 28:191, 1974.

141. Flecknell PA, Lucke VM: Chronic relapsing polyradiculoneuritis in a cat. Acta Neuropathol (Berl) 41:81, 1978.

142. Shores A, et al: Chronic relapsing polyneuropathy in a cat. J Am Anim Hosp Assoc 23:569, 1987.

143. Malik R, et al: Prednisolone responsive neuropathy in a cat. J Small Anim Pract 32:529, 1991.

144. Bichsel P, Oliver JE, Tyler DE, et al: Chronic polyneuritis in a rottweiler. JAVMA 191:991, 1987.

145. Lane JR, de Lahunta A: Polyneuritis in a cat. J Am Anim Hosp Assoc 20:1006, 1984.

146. Cummings JF, Lorenz MD, de Lahunta A, et al: Canine brachial plexus neuritis: A syndrome resembling serum neuritis in man. Cornell Vet 63:589. 1973.

147. Alexander JW, et al: A case of brachial plexus neuropathy in a dog. J Am Anim Hosp Assoc 10:515, 1974.

148. Bright RM, Crabtree BJ, Knecht C: Brachial plexus neuropathy in the cat: a case report. J Am Anim Hosp Assoc 14:612, 1978.

149. Cummings JF, et al: Ganglioradiculoneuritis in the dog. A clinical, light and electronmicroscopic study. Acta Neuropathol 60:29, 1983.

150. Wouda W, et al: Sensory neuronopathy in dogs: A study of four cases. J Comp Pathol 183:437, 1983.

151. Steiss JE, et al: Sensory neuronopathy in a dog. JAVMA 190:205, 1987.

152. Wheeler SJ: Sensory neuropathy in a Border collie puppy. J Small Anim Pract 28:281, 1987.

153. Jeffery ND, et al: Sensory neuronopathy of possible toxic etiology in a dog. Prog Vet Neurol 4:145, 1993.

154. Shelton GD, Willard MD, Cardinet GH III, et al: Acquired myasthenia gravis: Selective involvement of esophageal, pharyngeal, and facial muscles. J Vet Intern Med 4:281, 1990.

155. Shelton GD, et al: Risk factors for acquired myasthenia gravis in dogs: 1,154 cases (1991-1995). JAVMA 211:1428, 1997.

156. Cuddon PA: Acquired immune-mediated myasthenia gravis in a cat. J Small Anim Pract 30:511, 1989.

157. Joseph RJ, et al: Myasthenia gravis in the cat. J Vet Intern Med 2:75, 1988.

158. Indrieri RJ, et al: Myasthenia gravis in two cats. JAVMA 182:57, 1983.

159. Dewey CW, et al: Clinical forms of acquired myasthenia gravis in dogs: 25 cases (1988-1995). J Vet Intern Med 11:50, 1997.

160. Shelton GD: Canine myasthenia gravis. In Kirk RW, Bonagura JD (eds): Current Veterinary Therapy XI. Philadelphia, WB Saunders, 1992, p 1039.

161. Shelton GD: Canine seronegative acquired myasthenia gravis. Proceedings of the 7th annual ACVIM Forum, San Diego, 1989, p 999.

162. Rusbridge C, et al: Treatment of acquired myasthenia gravis associated with thymoma in two dogs. J Small Anim Pract 37:376, 1996.

163. Shelton GD: Myasthenia gravis—1000 cases later. Proc Am Coll Vet Intern Med 14:658, 1996.

164. Aronsohn MG, et al: Clinical and pathological features of thymoma in 15 dogs. JAVMA 184:1355, 1984.

165. Lainesse MF, et al: Focal myasthenia gravis as a paraneoplastic syndrome of canine thymoma: Improvement following thymectomy. J Am Anim Hosp Assoc 32:111, 1996.

166. Rusbridge C, et al: Treatment of acquired myasthenia gravis associated with thymoma in two dogs. J Small Anim Pract 37:376, 1996.

167. Scott-Moncrieff JC, et al: Acquired myasthenia gravis in a cat with thymoma. JAVMA 196:1291, 1990.

168. Moore AS, et al: Osteogenic sarcoma and myasthenia gravis in a dog. JAVMA 197:226, 1990.

169. Krotje LJ, et al: Acquired myasthenia gravis and cholangiocellular carcinoma in a dog. JAVMA 197:488, 1990.

170. Dewey CW, et al: Neuromuscular dysfunction in five dogs with acquired myasthenia gravis and presumptive hypothyroidism. Prog Vet Neurol 6:117, 1995.

171. Hackett TB, et al: Third degree atrioventricular block and acquired myasthenia gravis in four dogs. JAVMA 206:1173, 1995.

172. Wallace WE, Palmer AC: Recessive mode of inheritance in myasthenia gravis in the Jack Russell terrier. Vet Rec 114:350, 1984.

173. Johnson RP, et al: Myasthenia in springer spaniel littermates. J Small Anim Pract 16:641, 1975.

174. Jenking WL, et al: Myasthenia gravis in a fox terrier litter. J S Afr Vet Assoc 47:59, 1976.

175. Miller LM, et al: Congenital myasthenia gravis in 13 smooth fox terriers. JAVMA 182:694, 1983.

176. Kelly DF: Neuroblastoma in the dog. J Pathol 116:209, 1975.

177. Hawkins KL, Summers BA: Mediastinal ganglioneuroma in a puppy. Vet Pathol 24:283, 1987.

178. Payne-Johnson CE, Brockman DJ: Neuroblastoma in the dog. J Small Anim Pract 33:395, 1992.

179. Louden C, et al: Peripheral neuroblastomas in two dogs. J Vet Diagn Invest 4:476, 1992.

180. Schultz KS, et al: Thoracic ganglioneuroblastoma in a dog. Vet Pathol 31:716, 1994.

181. Ribas JL, et al: Immunohistochemistry and ultrastructure of intestinal ganglioneuroma in a dog. Vet Pathol 27:376, 1990.

182. Mattix ME, et al: Olfactory ganglioneuroblastoma in a dog. A light, ultrastructural and immunohistochemical study. Vet Pathol 31:262, 1994.

183. Patnaik AK, et al: Intestinal ganglioneuroma in a kitten: A case report and review of the literature. J Small Anim Pract 19:735, 1978.

184. Schueler RO, et al: Spinal ganglioneuroma in a dog. JAVMA 203:539, 1993.

185. Uchida K, et al: Malignant schwannoma in the spinal root of a dog. J Vet Med Sci 54:809, 1992.

186. Brehm DM, et al: A retrospective study of 51 cases of peripheral nerve sheath tumors in the dog. J Am Anim Hosp Assoc 31:349, 1995.

187. Bradley RL, et al: Nerve sheath tumors in the dog. J Am Anim Hosp Assoc 18:915, 1982.

188. Zachary JF, et al: Multicentric nerve sheath fibrosarcomas of multiple cranial nerve roots in two dogs. JAVMA 188:723, 1986.

189. McCarthy RJ, et al: Preoperative diagnosis of tumors of the brachial plexus by use of computed tomography in three dogs. JAVMA 202:291, 1993.

190. Bailey CS: Long term survival after surgical excision of a schwannoma of the sixth cervical spinal nerve in a dog. JAVMA 196:754, 1990.

191. Zaki FA, Hurvitz A I: Spontaneous neoplasms of the central nervous system of the cat. J Small Anim Pract 17:773, 1976.

192. Christopher MM, et al: Acute myelomonocytic leukemia in neurologic manifestations in the dog. Vet Pathol 23:140, 1986.

193. Carpenter JL, et al: Bilateral trigeminal nerve paralysis and Horner's syndrome associated with myelomonocytic neoplasia in a dog. JAVMA 191:1594, 1987.

194. Dalmau JO, Posner JB: Paraneoplastic syndromes affecting the nervous system. Semin Oncol 24:318, 1977.

195. Shahar R, et al: Peripheral polyneuropathy in a dog with functional islet B-cell tumor and widespread metastasis. JAVMA 187:175, 1985.

196. Schrauwen E: Clinical peripheral neuropathy associated with canine insulinoma. Vet Rec 128:211, 1991.

197. Bergman PJ, et al: Canine clinical peripheral neuropathy associated with pancreatic islet cell carcinoma. Prog Vet Neurol 5:57, 1994.

198. Van Ham L, et al: Treatment of a dog with an insulinoma-related peripheral polyneuropathy with corticosteroids. Vet Rec 141:98, 1997.

199. Cardinet GH, Holliday TA: Neuromuscular diseases of domestic animals: A summary of muscle biopsies from 159 cases. Ann N Y Acad Sci 317:290, 1979.

200. Presthus J, Teige J: Peripheral neuromyopathy associated with lymphosarcoma in a dog. J Small Anim Pract 27:463, 1986.

201. Griffiths IR, et al: Peripheral polyneuropathies in dogs: A study of five cases. J Small Anim Pract 18:101, 1977.

202. Sorjonen DC, et al: Paraplegia and subclinical neuromyopathy associated with a primary lung tumor in a dog. JAVMA 180:1209, 1982.

203. Braund KG, McGuire JA, Amling KA, et al: Peripheral neuropathy associated with malignant neoplasms in dogs. Vet Pathol 24:16, 1987.

204. Braund KG, et al: Insulinoma and subclinical peripheral neuropathy in two dogs. J Vet Intern Med 1:86, 1987.

205. Terzis JK, Smith KL: The Peripheral Nerve: Structure, Function and Reconstruction. Norfolk, Hampton Press, 1990.

206. Fu SY, Gordon T: The cellular and molecular basis of peripheral nerve regeneration. Mol Neurobiol 14:67, 1997.

CNS

207. Hudson JA, et al: Ultrasonography of peripheral nerves during wallerian degeneration and regeneration following transection. Vet Radiol Utrasound 37:302, 1996.
208. Griffiths IR: Avulsion of the brachial plexus. 1. Neuropathology of the spinal cord and peripheral nerves. J Small Anim Pract 15:165, 1974.
209. Griffiths IR, et al: Avulsion of the brachial plexus. 2. Clinical aspects. J Small Anim Pract 15:177, 1974.
210. Steinberg HS: The use of electrodiagnostic techniques in evaluating traumatic brachial plexus root injuries. J Am Anim Hosp Assoc 15:621, 1979.
211. Bailey CS: Patterns of cutaneous aesthesia associated with brachial plexus avulsions in the dog. JAVMA 185:889, 1984.
212. Oliver JE, et al: Effect of lesions of spinal nerves on somatosensory evoked potentials from stimulation of thoracic limb nerves of the dog. Prog Vet Neurol 1:445, 1990.
213. Griffiths IR, Duncan ID: Ischaemic neuromyopathy in cats. Vet Rec 104:518, 1979.
214. Laste NJ, Harpster NK: A retrospective study of 100 cases of feline distal aortic thromboembolism: 1977–1993. J Am Anim Hosp Assoc 31:492, 1995.
215. Atkins CE, et al: Risk factors, clinical signs, and survival in cats with a clinical diagnosis of idiopathic hypertrophic cardiomyopathy: 74 cases (1985–1989). JAVMA 201:613, 1992.
216. Duncan ID, Griffiths IR: Peripheral neuropathies of domestic animals. In Dyck PJ, Thomas PK, Lambert EH, Bunge R (eds): Peripheral Neuropathy, 2nd ed. Philadelphia, WB Saunders, 1984, p 707.
217. Griffiths IR, Duncan I: Distal denervating disease: A degenerative neuropathy of the distal motor axon in dogs. J Small Anim Pract 20:579, 1979.
218. Braund KG, et al: Distal symmetrical polyneuropathy in a dog. Vet Pathol 17:422, 1980.
219. Braund KG: Disorders of peripheral nerves. In Ettinger SJ, Feldman EC (eds): A Textbook of Veterinary Internal Medicine. Disease of the Dog and Cat, 4th ed. Philadelphia, WB Saunders, 1995, p 701.
220. Chrisman CL: Dancing Doberman disease: Clinical findings and prognosis. Prog Vet Neurol 1:83, 1990.
221. Key TJA, Gaskell CJ: Puzzling syndrome in cats associated with pupillary dilation. Vet Rec 110:160, 1982.
222. Rochlitz I, Bennett AM: Key-Gaskell syndrome in a bitch. Vet Rec 112:614, 1983.
223. Longshore RC, et al: Dysautonomia in dogs: A retrospective study. J Vet Intern Med 10:103, 1996.
224. Pollin MM, Griffiths IR: Feline dysautonomia: An ultrastructural study of neurons in the XII nucleus. Acta Neuropathol (Berl) 73:275, 1987.
225. Powell AK: Idiopathic trigeminal neuritis in a dog. Can Vet J 32:265, 1991.
226. de Lahunta A: Veterinary Neuroanatomy and Clinical Neurology, 2nd ed. Philadelphia, WB Saunders, 1983.
227. Kren TJ, Erb HN: Facial neuropathy in dogs and cats: 95 cases (1975–1985). JAVMA 191:1604, 1987.
228. Braund KG, et al: Idiopathic facial paralysis in the dog. Vet Rec 105:297, 1979.
229. Wright JA: Ultrastructural findings in idiopathic facial paralysis in the dog. J Comp Pathol 98:111, 1988.
230. Burke EE, et al: Review of idiopathic feline vestibular syndrome in 75 cats. JAVMA 187:941, 1985.

CHAPTER 109

DISORDERS OF THE SKELETAL MUSCLES

Stephane Blot

Striated muscle, representing approximately 50 per cent of the body mass, is an intricate machine designed to convert chemical energy into mechanical energy. The component processes include excitation-contraction coupling, the contractile mechanism itself, various structural components, and the energy system that supports the activity and the integrity of the other systems. Proper function of striated muscle is therefore dependent on the integrity of all organs of the body. This chapter focuses on primary defects involved in skeletal muscle diseases (primary myopathies), but numerous secondary myopathies are encountered as a result of defects in other organs. For the understanding of the known mechanisms involved in myopathies, anatomic and physiologic features that underlie the various component processes of the striated muscle's complex function are presented before a discussion on specific myopathies. Disorders of the neuromuscular junction are discussed elsewhere.

ANATOMY AND PHYSIOLOGY

Skeletal muscles are composed of fusiform multinucleated cells called myofibers, connective tissue, vessels, and nerves.[1–3] During myogenesis, myofibers are produced by the fusion of myogenic cells, the myoblasts that stem from the same mesodermal embryonic tissue that provides bone, cartilage, and connective tissue. However, all muscles do not stem from the same origin, thus explaining immunologic differences between groups of muscles and therefore may account for specific topographic muscle lesions. Some multinucleated myogenic cells do not merge and lie beneath the basement membrane of mature muscle fibers. These are the satellite cells. When a muscle is damaged and necrosis occurs, the satellite cells develop and merge together to form new muscle fibers.

On transverse section of normal muscle, myofibers are all polygonal, roughly of equal size with peripheral nuclei; however, different types of myofibers are identified based upon physiologic and histochemical criteria (Table 109–1): the slow contraction fibers (type 1) withstand fatigue and use oxidative metabolism, whereas the fast contraction fibers extract their energy from the glycolytic pathway. Most skeletal muscles are made up with a mixture of these functional types, the proportion of each type being stable for a given muscle in each species.[4] In specific muscles, one type appears largely predominant. The functional type of each myofiber is actually determined by the neuronal cell body innervating the cell.[5, 6] All myofibers innervated by the same motor neuron define a motor unit whose size varies: muscles with fine movement are composed of small motor units (such as extraocular muscles), whereas antigravity muscles are composed of large units.

TABLE 109–1. CHARACTERISTICS OF MAMMALIAN MYOFIBER TYPES

Properties	Type 1	Type 2M*	Type 2A	Type 2B†	Type 2C‡
Histochemistry staining intensity					
ATPases pH 10,4/9,4	Low	Low	High	High	High
ATPases pH 4,63/4,53	High	Moderate	Low	Moderate	Moderate
ATPases pH 4,35	High	Low	Low	Low	Moderate
Oxydative					
NADH-TR, SDH	High		Moderate	Low	Moderate
Menadione	Low		Moderate	High	
Phosphorylase	Low		Moderate	High	
Periodic acid–Schiff	Low		High	Moderate	High
Physiologic/morphologic features					
Contraction speed	Slow		Intermediate/fast	Fast	—
Fatigue resistance	High		Intermediate	Low	—
Size	Small	—	Intermediate	Large	—
Myoglobin	High	—	High	Low	—
Energy metabolism	Oxidative	—	Oxi/glyccly	Glycolytic	—
Mitochondria	Many	—	Many	Few	—
Glycogen content	Low	—	High	Intermediate	—
Lipid content	High	—	Intermediate	Low	—

*Masticatory myofiber type.
†Type 2B does not exist in canine.[82]
‡Type 2C are primitive myofibers that may be precursors to types 2A and 2B.
From Guy PS, Snow DH: Skeletal muscle fibre composition in the dog and its relationship to athletic ability. Res Vet Sci 31 244, 1981.

Perimysial connective tissue defines fascicles that enclose several motor units. All motor units are closely intermingled with each other, producing a particular mosaic-like or checkerboard pattern. Each muscle fiber is surrounded by a thin layer of connective tissue (the endomysium), whereas the entire muscle is encased in epimysial connective tissue. Each myofiber is composed of hundreds of myofibrils made of thin and thick contractile filaments separated by an intermyofibrillar network containing aqueous sarcoplasm, mitochondria, glycogen, and the sarcoplasmic reticulum (calcium reservoir) with the associated transverse tubular system. The protein myosin is the main component of the thick filaments, whereas actin, troponin, and tropomyosin constitute the thin contractile filaments. Ultrastructurally, the regular spatial distribution of the contractile filaments exhibits a characteristic striated appearance that is due to the repetition of a transverse pattern. This repetitive pattern, called the sarcomere, contains an electron-dense area, or A band, produced by the overlapping of thick and thin filaments and an electron-lucent area the "I band," which contains thin filaments alone. In the middle of band A, the absence of thin filament produces an additional electron-lucent band, the H zone. The transverse line M in the H zone is composed of cross-linked thick filaments, whereas the transverse Z line in the I band is made of protein-anchoring adjacent thin filament. The sarcomere is thus the structural unit defined by two successive Z lines.

Molecular studies bring constant enlightenment about the components of the cytoskeletal, sarcolemmal, or contractile apparatus, thus leading to the discovery of molecular defects involved in degenerative myopathies. The muscle fiber converts a biochemical signal, the release of acetylcholine from the nerve terminal after arrival of a nerve action potential at the neuromuscular junction, into a mechanical force produced by the coordinated contraction of several thousands of sarcomeric units. In order to achieve this complex process, termed excitation-contraction coupling, several elementary phases are required: the depolarization of the sarcolemma, the transverse tubules, and the sarcoplasmic reticulum. Depolarization leads to the release of calcium into the sarcoplasm. At rest, tropomyosin (a regulating protein) blocks the active site of actin and prevents the myosin-actin interaction. Binding of the calcium to troponin moves tropomyosin, which then promotes formation of several cross-bridges between actin and myosin molecules. With the availability of energy (ATPase from myosin catalyzes hydrolysis of ATP, which comes from the phosphocreatine stock—the myofiber's battery—or from oxidative phosphorylation metabolism or from glycogenolysis), the thin filaments move on the thick myofilaments, leading to the shortening of the myofibrils. Dissociation of the cross-bridges, thus producing relaxation time, also requires energy.

GENERAL CLINICAL FEATURES

The main sign of a disease affecting appendicular musculature is weakness. Weakness induced by skeletal muscle disorders is usually persistent but may become more pronounced after exercise (increased fatigability). Rarely, weakness may disappear with exercise whereas the signs are exacerbated by rest (myotonia). Weakness may be discrete with a stiff gait, tremors, an abnormal posture such as neck ventroflexion (more pronounced in cats owing to the absence of a nuchal ligament), palmigrade or plantigrade stance, splaying digits, bunny hopping gait, or difficulty in negotiating simple motions (jumping over steps, climbing into the car ...). Weakness may also be extreme, mimicking a neurogenic disease. Muscle atrophy is frequent; however, hypertrophy can occur in some instances. In most cases, hypotony with normal tendon reflexes is encountered. However, hypertonic muscles are also observed (polymyositis, myotonia). Absent tendon reflexes are sometimes observed in congenital myopathies or later in the course of degenerative myopathies. Muscular fibrosis and contracture inducing reduced range of articular movement is a frequent feature in severe inflammatory or degenerative myopathies. Muscle pain (myalgia) can be occasionally identified in inflammatory conditions. The normal muscular response to percussion is a barely visible transient contraction of the myofibers. It disappears prematurely in primary muscle diseases, thus contrasting with the conservation of tendon reflexes. However,

CNS

mechanical excitability is exaggerated in neurogenic muscular atrophies. In the myotonic syndrome, the myotonic dimple persists for several seconds. Signs affect appendicular musculature and several other striated muscles such as masticatory, extraocular, cardiac, digestive, and respiratory musculature. Thus, disorders of striated muscle should be suspected as one cause of the condition in dogs and cats with regurgitation, vomiting, dysphagia, dysphonia, or ophthalmoplegia.

Weakness is a nonspecific sign that is frequently encountered in other nonmuscular diseases (see Chapter 3), thus requiring the use of ancillary tools to confirm a myopathy.

GENERAL DIAGNOSTIC FEATURES

Several serum enzymes, such as creatine kinase (CK), lactate dehydrogenase, aldolase, and aspartate aminotransferase, may be elevated in muscle diseases.[3] In particular, owing to its short half-life (around 6 hours), the level of serum CK is the best indication of a recent muscle lesion.[7] However, tremendous variability occurs with age (the younger the animal, the higher the value), the breed (the smaller the dog, the greater the value), with motor activity (increased with exercise), with recent intramuscular injections, and lastly with sampling methods. Although some myopathies are associated with dramatic persistent elevations (muscular dystrophies, polymyositis), numerous myopathies cause little, transient, or no elevation at all. Thus, a normal CK level should not exclude a muscle disease from the differential diagnosis.

Electrophysiologic testings (electromyography, nerve conduction studies, and repetitive stimulation) are more valuable in the evaluation of peripheral neuropathies than in myopathies.[8] If contractile activity is recorded, myopathies are classically associated with smaller, shorter, and sometimes polyphasic motor unit potentials. Spontaneous abnormal activity (fibrillation potentials, positive waves, high-frequency discharges, and complex repetitive discharges) may be recorded in numerous myopathies, but no activities are specific of certain myopathies except the myotonic burst that is pathognomonic of myotonia. If a muscle biopsy is planned, that muscle site should not be electrophysiologically tested, to avoid iatrogenic changes. When muscle disease is suspected, a muscle biopsy is indicated to confirm the diagnosis. The sampling is a relatively innocuous procedure, but certain guidelines must be followed if maximum information is to be gained.[9] Blood for serum muscle enzyme analysis should be collected before the biopsy is performed. Selection of the muscle for biopsy is guided by the electromyography, or, failing that, atrophic or hypertrophic muscles are chosen. Although a single muscle biopsy is usually satisfactory, chances of identifying characteristic lesions are considerably enhanced if several muscles are sampled (generally at least one muscle biopsy each from the pelvic and thoracic limbs). The biopsy specimen is taken at the center of the muscle belly by parallel incisions along the longitudinal axis of the myofibers. A section 4 to 5 mm wide and 2 cm long is satisfactory for routine light microscopic evaluation. Tools for reducing the shortening of the muscle sample may be used (muscle biopsy clamp or a sterile applicator stick). The muscle sample should then be divided into two fragments; one is fixed in 10 per cent buffered formalin and the other submitted prior to fixation, in a refrigerated gauze sponge, within 24 hours, in order to apply histochemical stains. Such stains are the only satisfactory method for analyzing degenerative myopathies. When muscle atrophy is of nervous origin, it is characterized by variability in fiber diameter, angular atrophied fibers, and by alteration of the normal checkerboard pattern.

Myopathies can be categorized as inflammatory or degenerative (Table 109–2). The inflammatory conditions are either infectious or immune mediated, whereas degenerative myopathies are acquired or inherited. The discussion will focus on the main myopathies in dogs and cats.

INFLAMMATORY MYOPATHIES

A classic separation is made between infectious myositis conditions and those that are immune mediated. In cases of infectious myositis, bacteria (*Leptospira* or *Clostridium*) or parasites (*Toxoplasma* or *Neospora*) are directly responsible. Some agents are capable of triggering noninfectious myositis by modifying muscle immunogenicity (leishmaniasis or ehrlichiosis).

INFECTIOUS BACTERIAL MYOSITIS

Bacterial myositis is a rare disorder in carnivores and occurs more frequently in food animals.[10] A distinction can be made between polymyositis and focal myositis. The manifestation of the latter is lameness accompanied by pain and muscle enlargement. This type of myopathy occurs with bacterial spread from a distant site of infection via the blood or after bacterial inoculation through external trauma such as a bite, a sting, or the contamination of surgical wounds.[11-14] Staphylococci and streptococci are often involved in canine traumatic infectious myositis. In cats, *Pasteurella multocida* is more frequently encountered. Clostridial myositis (*Clostridium perfringens*) is rarely found in domestic carnivores. *Leptospira icterohaemorrhagiae* is responsible for serious

TABLE 109–2. CLASSIFICATION OF MYOPATHIES

I. Inflammatory
  A. Infectious
    1. Bacterial
    2. Leptospirosis
    3. Toxoplasmosis/neosporosis
    4. Parasitic
  B. Immune-mediated
    1. Masticatory muscle myositis
    2. Polymyositis
    3. Dermatomyositis
II. Degenerative
  A. Acquired
    1. Endocrine
      a. Hyperadrenocorticism
      b. Hypothyroidism
      c. Hypokalemic polymyopathy in cats
    2. Fibrotic/ossifying myopathies
    3. Ischemic
    4. Nutritional
    5. Neoplastic
    6. Toxic
  B. Inherited
    1. Muscular dystrophy
      a. X-linked muscular dystrophy (dystrophin deficient)
      b. Other muscular dystrophies (dystrophin positive)
    2. Myotonia
    3. Metabolic
      a. Glycogen storage disease
      b. Mitochondrial myopathy
      c. Lipidic myopathy
      d. Malignant hyperthermia
    4. Centronuclear myopathy (Labrador retriever)
    5. Nemaline myopathy

myositis. However, the severe nature of the general signs masks the muscle damage. The treatment consists of lancing the wounds and draining any abscesses. In the case of secondary bacterial myositis, the first step consists of identifying the primary site. The antibiotic is selected by the results of sensitivity testing. Clindamycin (5 mg/lb orally, twice a day) is the antibiotic of choice for anaerobic bacterial myositis.[15–17]

PARASITIC MYOSITIS

Toxoplasmosis (Toxoplasma gondii). The disease develops clinically only in young animals (less than a year old) and often arises when another disease occurs. The muscular signs are characterized by abnormal gait, muscle pain, and muscle atrophy. Sometimes myositis with subsequent fibrosis evolves quickly.[18]

Neosporosis (Neospora caninum). Neurologic damage dominates the clinical presentation, and pups that are affected rapidly exhibit hyperextension of the hind limbs. The transplacental transmission mimics a hereditary disease. Clindamycin (5 mg/lb twice daily) or trimethoprim combined with sulfadiazine (7 mg/lb, twice per day) is the drug of choice; however, pelvic limb extensor rigidity does not respond to therapy.[19–21]

Other Parasites. *Trichinella spiralis, Ancylostoma caninum,* and *Sarcocystis* may be located in the muscle and only rarely produce clinical signs. Generally, they are discovered purely by chance.[18, 19, 22, 23]

IMMUNE-MEDIATED MYOSITIS

Myositis of the Masticatory Muscles

The muscle fibers of the masticator muscles have a distinct embryologic origin, thus explaining the presence of a particular type of fiber called 2M. These fibers enclose a specific myosin, which is specifically involved in this immune-mediated reaction. Type 1 fibers are spared. This myopathy affects all dogs of any age, sex, or breed, but the German shepherd seems to have a predisposition.[24–27]

In the acute form, hypertrophy of the temporal and masseter muscles is observed with myalgia. The animal is reluctant to open its mouth. It has difficulty eating and may dribble saliva. Sometimes the jaws remain open, as complete closing is impossible. Fever, inflammation of the tonsils, and local adenitis may also be found. In most cases, it is a chronic condition with severe progressive muscular atrophy accompanied by fibrosis that causes a reduced ability to open the mouth, and trismus or lockjaw.

The disorder is generally bilateral. Exophthalmos linked to enlargement of the temporal muscles can sometimes be the cause of an optic neuritis and produce vision disorders. Biochemical examinations are not specific, but the serum level of CK may be increased. Leukocytosis is sometimes found. EMG reveals abnormal spontaneous activity. Muscle biopsy shows sites of necrosis and phagocytosis of the 2M fibers with perivascular infiltration of mononucleate cells. In the serum of affected dogs, 2M anti-type antibodies are identified.

Administration of immunosuppressive doses of corticosteroids is the only advisable therapy. Clinical recovery is usually rapid and complete if the treatment is begun early. A dose of 0.5 to 1.0 mg/lb twice a day is maintained for 15 days, after which it is gradually reduced. Should a relapse

occur, the maximum dose should be administered again. Sometimes a prolonged course of treatment is required with small doses administered on alternate days. Therapy is ineffective when it is administered to an animal that has already experienced several inflammatory episodes which have resulted in extensive fibrosis.

Polymyositis

Polymyositis is an inflammatory polymyopathy with an immune-mediated etiology. It is sometimes associated with other immune-mediated diseases, such as systemic lupus erythematosus. Polymyositis may also be caused by parasitic disorders (toxoplasmosis and ehrlichiosis) or various forms of cancer (paraneoplastic syndrome).[27] In most cases, the etiology is unknown. Polymyositis affects all skeletal muscles of limbs, although there are occasionally reports of focal damage, such as the extraocular muscles.[28]

Large-sized adult dogs are most commonly affected. The signs include muscle weakness, which is sometimes exacerbated by exercise. Myalgia, pyrexia, amyotrophy, and muscle stiffness are sometimes noted. Dysphagia and regurgitation caused by megaesophagus are less common. Pneumonia is a frequent complication. Generally, an increase in the CK level is observed. Electromyographic abnormalities are similar to those seen in myopathy of the masticator muscles. The muscle biopsy reveals perivascular infiltrations of mononucleate cells. Necrosis and regeneration are also noted. The therapy is based on immunosuppressive doses of corticosteroids. Prognosis is guarded, especially when pneumonias arise. The combination of prednisolone and azathioprine is effective in certain cases that prove to be refractory to the administration of corticosteroids only.

Dermatomyositis is an inherited disorder in which myositis is associated with dermatitis. It has been reported in the collie, the Shetland sheepdog, and also in the Welsh corgi.[29–35] The manifestations of the nonpruritic cutaneous disorder are erythema, alopecia, and ulceration. The signs appear in 3- to 11-week-old pups, and the disease appears to wax and wane. The myopathic signs of weakness are usually observed within a few months. Myositis, especially involving the temporal muscles, is seen histologically.

DEGENERATIVE MYOPATHIES

ENDOCRINE MYOPATHY

Both myopathy and peripheral neuropathy have been associated with hypothyroidism.[36] They may occur simultaneously. The EMG examination may record high-frequency discharges. In most cases the muscle biopsy is normal, and if there are any lesions, they are not specific (glycogenic inclusions, type 2 atrophy, necrotic fibers, and centralized nuclei). Moderate signs can be resolved by administering a hormone supplementation. Abnormal serum electrolytes, in particular those that concern potassium, can cause a myopathic syndrome.[36]

There are reports of myopathy in spontaneous or iatrogenic hypercorticism in both dogs and cats.[46] Clinical forms vary from muscle weakness to a myotonic form. Myotonia causes limb stiffness and seems to affect the poodle in particular. In some cases, it is even associated with muscular hypertrophy. EMG shows bursts of pseudomyotonic potentials. Muscle biopsy demonstrates disorganized muscle fibers with an abnormal accumulation of mitochondria (ragged red fibers). Treatment of the underlying disease leads to improvement of the neuromuscular signs except for the pseudomyotonic form.

FELINE HYPOKALEMIC POLYMYOPATHY

Frequently clinical signs appear suddenly. They are dominated by a marked cervical ventroflexion, which indicates extreme muscle weakness.[36-40] There is occasionally muscular pain. Serum potassium concentrations are typically less than 3 mEq/L. The CK level increases and may rise to as much as 20,000 U/L. It should also be noted that there is an increase in the creatinine. Occasionally a metabolic acidosis appears. Therapy calls for supplementation, and parenteral administration of potassium for the most severe cases. An inherited disease associated with hypokalemia in Burmese cats is also described.[41]

HYPERKALEMIA

Hyperkalemic periodic paralysis is an inherited myopathy characterized by frequent episodes of weakness, during which serum potassium is elevated. A myotonic syndrome may often accompany this myopathy, and the fits of weakness can be triggered by oral administration of potassium. There is only one documented report of this in a female American pit bull aged 7 months. The administration of acetazolamide and fludrocortisone led to clinical improvement in the patient's condition.

FIBROTIC AND OSSIFYING MYOPATHIES

This myopathy is generally described as being a progressive ossifying myositis. It may occur in both localized and generalized forms. Clinically, the animal refuses to move. Upon radiographic investigation, intramuscular zones can be seen, and their density is close to that of bone. Histologically, there is a progressive ossification of the connecting intramuscular tissue where isolated patches of trabecular bone and cartilage are to be found, in addition to perivascular lymphocytic infiltrates, which are at the origin of the term of myositis used for this disorder. The term of fibrodysplasia is preferable, because neither the optical microscope nor the electron microscope shows any lesions to confirm that there is primary damage to the muscle fibers.[42, 43]

The appearance of a permanent focal contracture with muscle fibrosis (infraspinous, femoral quadriceps) causes lameness. The cause is often obscure: congenital malformation, *Neospora caninum* infection, or traumatic causes are proposed.[19, 44-47]

INHERITED MYOPATHIES

MUSCULAR DYSTROPHIES

Muscular dystrophies are a group of inherited myopathies clinically defined by a muscular weakness and histologically characterized by chronic degeneration and regeneration of muscle fibers accompanied by progressive fibrosis. Among them, the best known is X-linked muscular dystrophy.

X-LINKED MUSCULAR DYSTROPHY

X-linked muscular dystrophy results from an alteration of the gene dystrophin as is the case in Duchenne's muscular dystrophy in humans. The absence or the production of abnormal dystrophin leads to a degeneration of the muscle fibers. The gene is carried by the X chromosome, and in a natural environment only males are affected. The canine disease was initially identified in the golden retriever[48, 49] in which the mutation was cloned.[50] Since then, the disease has been detected in the rottweiler, Samoyed,[51] Groenendaeler shepherd,[52] and the miniature schnauzer.[53] The clinical signs appear at about 8 weeks of age and are manifested by muscular weakness, a stiffness in gait, and reduced opening of the mouth. Within a few weeks, exercise intolerance appears and the muscles become atrophic. Hypertrophy of the esophageal muscle, the tongue, and the diaphragm can lead to severe digestive signs. The gait of the dog becomes peculiar; abduction of the elbows, adduction of the hocks, and lordosis occurs in older animals. The signs usually stabilize by about 6 months of age and movement becomes restricted with the onset of muscular fibrosis. There is no neurologic deficiency. Life expectancy depends on the severity of the signs. Death may occur within the first few days, caused by severe diaphragmatic necrosis,[54] or the animal may survive for several years and die after the progressive deterioration of its general condition and difficulty eating. The onset of a dilated cardiomyopathy is gradual and is considered a major cause of mortality.[55] The CK levels vary (10,000 to 30,000 IU/L). Electromyography reveals high-frequency and pseudomyotonic discharges.

Muscle biopsy reveals necrosis with an influx of macrophages and phagocytosis, muscle regeneration, and sites of intracellular calcification.[56] Some muscles, such as the sartorius, the extensor carpi radialis, the deltoid, and the cranial tibial muscle, are affected earlier and more severely. Fiber size varies with the centralized nuclei.

In cats, the signs are discrete and there is no muscular weakness. At the age of 5 months, most muscles, including the tongue, with exception of the masticator and facial muscles, gradually become hypertrophied.[57-59] The neck is stiff, and the hocks are adducted. Because of the muscular stiffness, the animals cannot lie down normally and they have to let themselves drop onto one side. There is no difficulty in swallowing, though labored breathing may appear after moderate exercise. The CK values are very high, from 17,000 to more than 200,000. The EMG examination shows fibrillation potentials and bursts of high-frequency potentials similar to canine muscular dystrophy. Muscle histology shows a greater frequency of regeneration than in dogs, with increased muscle fiber size and progressive calcification. The fiber splitting is extremely important, producing a pseudo type-grouping. Numerous fibers have centralized nuclei. More moderate fibrosis of the endomysium is also observed. Lastly, cardiac mineralizations are noted.

OTHER MUSCULAR DYSTROPHIES

Several cases of canine muscular dystrophies without dystrophin deficiency are reported.[60, 61]

LABRADOR RETRIEVER MYOPATHY

This autosomal recessive myopathy, reported in the United States, Australia, Great Britain, and France, has been initially described as a dystrophic disease affecting type 2 muscle fibers.[29] The cause of the disease remains unknown; muscle biopsy specimens display a mixture of denervation and primary myopathies.

Clinical signs appear within 8 weeks to 11 months of age, the peak being around 4 months.[62, 63] General weakness is seen with muscle atrophy, most visible in the temporal muscles. Neck ventroflexion and a bunny hopping gait are also noted. Fatigability is variable. The animal exhibits a very slender profile contrasting with the muscular stature of a healthy Labrador. Tendon reflexes are absent or reduced. In some dogs, there is kyphosis or megaesophagus. Clinical signs stabilize after 8 months of age, and the disease is not lethal. The CK level is normal, and EMG reveals early fibrillation potentials, slow positive waves, and repetitive complex discharges that disappear in aged dogs. Muscle biopsy shows a marked diameter difference, with small-sized angular or round-shaped fibers and large fibers with centralized nuclei. Later in the course of the disease, most fibers display centrally placed nuclei.[64] Necrosis is visible on rare occasion.[29] A similar myopathy has been described in the Devon Rex cats.[65]

MYOTONIA

Non-dystrophic myotonia is caused by the dysfunction of one or several ionic sarcolemnal channels: mainly the chloride and the sodium channel. The myotonic or pseudomyotonic syndrome may be continuous or transient and can be drug-induced.

In the chow chow, myotonia is inherited with an autosomal recessive trait. Nonetheless, certain descendants may exhibit autosomal dominant transmission with incomplete penetrance. Clinical signs are visible at 10 to 12 weeks of age.[66, 67] These dogs have excess muscle mass. Immediately after rest, the gait is stiff and animals may frequently fall forward with the forelimbs spread out. Dyspnea and hypoxia are common because their respiratory muscles are unable to respond to the rise in metabolic requirements. A myotonic dimple persists several seconds after percussion on the surface of a muscle. Myopathy stabilizes after a few months, but because myotonia occurs in young animals, bone or articular deformations may appear. There is no satisfactory therapy. The disease itself is not life-threatening. The CK level is normal or only moderately increased. Myotonic discharges are seen on EMG. Muscle biopsy is not specific; it displays mild abnormalities, mainly hypertrophy of the muscle fibers with some centralized nuclei. Recent descriptions of congenital myotonia in cats[68] and of a possible dystrophic myotonia in boxer dogs[69] are available.

METABOLIC MYOPATHY

Glycogenoses are storage diseases due to an enzymatic deficiency in the glycolytic metabolism and lead to the accumulation of glycogen in cells. Signs are nonspecific. Muscular weakness, fatigability, syncope, rhabdomyolysis, and convulsions caused by hypoglycemia after a period of fasting or moderate exercise are clinical hallmarks. Among the seven types identified in human beings, only three types have been identified in dogs. Type II glycogenosis or Pompe's disease is caused by a deficiency in alpha-glucosidase (acid maltase). This disease is described in the spitz.[48] The mode of transmission is autosomal recessive. Clinical signs are usually observed by 6 months of age. The animals usually die in their second year.[70–72] Type III glycogenosis or Cori's disease is caused by a deficiency in amylo-1,6-glucosidase. In the German shepherd, clinical signs appear

during the second month and the disease is rapidly fatal.[73] Type VII glycogenosis is caused by a phosphofructokinase deficiency and has been identified in a colony of springer spaniels,[74] and in an American cocker spaniel.[75] The animals show exercise intolerance and suffer from muscle cramps and hemolytic anemia. Mitochondrial myopathies are characterized by a functional abnormality (an enzymatic deficiency) or a structural abnormality of the mitochondria (membrane transporter deficiency). An enzymatic deficiency in pyruvate dehydrogenase has been identified in the clumber spaniel and in the Sussex spaniel.[36] In these dogs, exercise leads to collapse and severe metabolic acidosis. Another mitochondrial myopathy is suspected in the Old English sheepdog, but the biochemical substrate remains unknown.[76]

Lipid storage has been noted in muscle in dogs with myopathies.[36, 77] Clinically, once the dogs reach adulthood, they exhibit muscle weakness and muscle pain. Tremors, stiffness, and fatigability may well be encountered.

NEMALINE MYOPATHY

In affected cats,[78] muscle weakness appears between the ages of 6 months and 1.5 years. Trembling may be noted. Movement becomes increasingly difficult, and gait becomes hypermetric. The femoral reflex is absent or diminished. EMG is normal, and the CK values are not increased. This disorder is characterized by the abundance of abnormal formations of long rows of twisted rods in the muscle fibers. Ultrastructurally, these formations appear to be related to the Z line of the myofibrils. A few cases of rod myopathy have been reported in dogs,[79] sometimes associated with hypothyroidism.[80]

REFERENCES

1. Engel AG, Franzini-Armstrong C: Myology, 2nd ed. New York, McGraw-Hill, 1994.
2. Fischbeck KH: Structure and function of striated muscle. In Asbury AK, et al (eds): Diseases of the Nervous System: Clinical Neurobiology, Philadelphia, WB Saunders, 1992, p 123.
3. Cardinet GH, III: Skeletal muscle function. In Kaneko JJ (ed): Clinical Biochemistry of Domestic Animals. San Diego, Academic Press, 1989, p 462.
4. Kuzon WM, Jr, et al: A comparative histochemical and morphometric study of canine skeletal muscle. Can J Vet Res 53:125, 1989.
5. Karpati G, Engel WK: Transformation of the histochemical profile of skeletal muscle by "foreign" innervation. Nature 215:1509, 1967.
6. Romanul FCA, Van Der Meulen JP: Reversal of the enzyme profiles of muscle fibres in fast and slow muscles by cross-innervation. Nature 215:1369, 1966.
7. Aktas M, et al: Creatine kinase in the dog: A review. Vet Res Commun 17:353, 1993.
8. Niederhauser UB, Holliday TA: Electrodiagnostic studies in diseases of muscles and neuromuscular junctions. Semin Vet Med Surg (Small Anim) 4:116, 1989.
9. Braund KG: Nerve and muscle biopsy techniques. Prog Vet Neurol 2:35, 1991.
10. Kornegay JN, Anson LW: Musculoskeletal infections. In Greene CE (ed): Infectious Diseases of the Dog and Cat. Philadelphia, WB Saunders, 1990, p 84.
11. Luttgen PJ: Miscellaneous myopathies. Semin Vet Med Surg (Small Anim) 4:168, 1989.
12. Mané MC, et al: A putative clostridial myositis in a dog. J Small Anim Pract 33:345, 1992.
13. Seddon ML, Barry SJ: Clostridial myositis in dogs. Vet Rec 131:84, 1992.
14. Thomson MJ, Eger CE: Management of a femoral fracture complicated by clostridial myositis. J Small Anim Pract 38:70, 1997.
15. Mané MC, et al: A putative clostridial myositis in a dog. J Small Anim Pract 33:345, 1992.
16. Poncelet L, et al: Polymyositis associated with Leptospira australis infection in a dog. Vet Rec 129:40, 1991.
17. Poonacha KB, et al: Clostridial myositis in a dog. JAVMA 194:69, 1989.
18. Craig TM: Parasitic myositis of dogs and cats. Semin Vet Med Surg (Small Anim) 4:161, 1989.
19. Braund KG: Idiopathic and exogenous causes of myopathies in dogs and cats. Vet Med 629, 1997.
20. Barber JS, Trees AJ: Clinical aspects of 27 cases of neosporosis in dogs. Vet Rec 139:439, 1996.

21. Ruehlmann D, et al: Canine neosporosis: A case report and literature review. J Am Anim Hosp Assoc 31:174, 1995.

22. Macintire DK. et al: Hepatozoonosis in dogs: 22 cases (1989–1994). JAVMA 210:916, 1997.

23. Vincent-Johnson NA, et al: A new *Hepatozoon* species from dogs: Description of the causative agent of canine hepatozoonosis in North America. J Parasitol 83:1165, 1997.

24. Anderson JG, Harvey CE: Masticatory muscle myositis. J Vet Dent 10:6, 1993.

25. Shelton GD, Cardinet GH, III: Canine masticatory muscle disorders. *In* Kirk RW (ed): Current Veterinary Therapy X. Philadelphia, WB Saunders, 1989, p 816.

26. Shelton GD, et al: Canine masticatory muscle disorders: A study of 29 cases. Muscle Nerve 10:753, 1987.

27. Smith MO: Idiopathic myositides in dogs. Semin Vet Med Surg (Small Anim) 4:156, 1989.

28. Carpenter JL, et al: Canine bilateral extraocular polymyositis. Vet Pathol 26:510, 1989.

29. Braund KG: Pediatric myopathies. Semin Vet Med Surg (Small Anim) 9:99, 1994.

30. Hargis AM, et al: Familial canine dermatomyositis. Am J Pathol 116:234, 1984.

31. Hargis AM, et al: A skin disorder in three shetland sheepdogs: comparison with familial canine dermatomyositis of collies. Compend Cont Educ Pract Vet 7:306, 1985.

32. Haupt KH, et al: Familial canine dermatomyositis: Clinicopathologic, immuno-logic, and serologic studies. Am J Vet Res 46:1870, 1985.

33. Haupt KH, et al: Familial canine dermatomyositis: Clinical, electrodiagnostic, and genetic studies. Am J Vet Res 46:1861, 1985.

34. Kunkle GA, et al: Dermatomyositis in Collie dogs. Compend Cont Educ Pract Vet 7:185, 1985.

35. White SD, et al: Dermatomyositis in an adult pembroke welsh corgi. J Am Anim Hosp Assoc 28:398, 1992.

36. LeCouteur RA, et al: Metabolic and endocrine myopathies of dogs and cats. Semin Vet Med Surg (Small Anim) 4:146, 1989.

37. Dow SW, Fettman MJ: Management of potassium-depleted cats. Compend Cont Educ Pract Vet 12:1612, 1990.

38. Dow SW, et al: Hypokalemia in cats: 186 cases (1984–1987). JAVMA 194:1604, 1989.

39. Dow SW, LeCouteur RA: Hypokalemic polymyopathy of cats. *In* Kirk RW (ed): Current Veterinary Therapy X. Philadelphia, WB Saunders, 1989, p 812.

40. Dow SW, et al: Potassium depletion in cats: Hypokalemic polymyopathy. JAVMA 191:1563, 1987.

41. Mason K: A hereditary disease in Burmese cats manifested as an episodic weak-ness with head nodding and neck ventroflexion. J Am Anim Hosp Assoc 24:147, 1988.

42. Cuddon PA: Feline neuromuscular diseases. *In* Kirk RW, Bonagura JD (eds): Kirk's Current Veterinary Therapy. Philadelphia, WB Saunders, 1992, p 1024.

43. Valentine BA, et al: Fibrodysplasia ossificans progressiva in the cat. A case report. J Vet Intern Med 6:335, 1992.

44. Capello V, et al: Myopathy of the gracilis-semitendinosus muscle complex in the dog. Eur J Comp Anim Prac 3:57, 1993.

45. Gomez-Villamandos R, et al: Tenotomy of the tibial insertion of the semitendino-sus muscle of two horses with fibrotic myopathy. Vet Rec 136:67, 1995.

46. Lewis DD: Fibrotic myopathy of the semitendinosus muscle in a cat. JAVMA 193:240, 1988.

47. Moore RW, et al: Fibrotic myopathy of the semitendinosus muscle in four dogs. Vet Surg 10:169, 1981.

48. Kornegay JN, et al: Muscular dystrophy in a litter of Golden Retriever Dogs. Muscle Nerve 11:1056, 1988.

49. Valentine BA, et al: Canine X-linked muscular dystrophy. An animal model of Duchenne muscular dystrophy: Clinical studies. J Neurol Sci 88:69, 1988.

50. Sharp NJH, et al: An error in dystrophin mRNA processing in golden retriever muscular dystrophy, an animal homologue of Duchenne muscular dystrophy. Genomics 13:115, 1992.

51. Presthus J, Nordstoga K: Congenital myopathy in a litter of samoyed dogs. Prog Vet Neurol 4:37, 1993.

52. Van Ham L, et al: Canine X-linked muscular dystrophy in belgian Groenendaeler Shepherds. J Am Anim Hosp Assoc 29:570, 1993.

53. Paola JP, et al: Muscular dystrophy in a miniature schnauzer. Prog Vet Neurol 4:14, 1993.

54. Valentine BA, Cooper BJ: Canine X-linked muscular dystrophy: Selective involve-ment of muscles in neonatal dogs. Neuromuscul Disord 1:31, 1991.

55. Valentine BA, et al: Development of Duchenne-type cardiomyopathy. Am J Pathol 135:671, 1989.

56. Valentine BA, et al: Intracellular calcium in canine muscle biopsies. J Comp Pathol 100:223, 1989.

57. Carpenter JL, et al: Feline muscular dystrophy with dystrophin deficiency. Am J Pathol 135:909, 1989.

58. Gaschen FP, et al: Dystrophin deficiency causes lethal muscle hypertrophy in cats. J Neurol Sci 110:149, 1992.

59. Gaschen FP, Burgunder JM: Clinical study of a breeding colony affected with hypertrophic feline muscular dystrophy. J Vet Intern Med 9:207, 1995 (abstract).

60. Braund KG, et al: Investigating a degenerative polymyopathy in four related Bouvier des Flandres dogs. Vet Med Small Anim Clin 85:558, 1990.

61. Hanson SM, et al: Juvenile-onset distal myopathy in rottweiler dogs. J Vet Intern Med 12:103, 1998.

62. McKerrel RE: Labrador myopathy: Clinical and pathological investigations. The-sis/dissertations University of Cambridge, 1989.

63. McKerrel RE, Braund KG: Hereditary myopathy in Labrador Retrievers: Clinical variations. J Small Anim Pract 28:479, 1987.

64. Blot S, et al: Canine inherited centronuclear myopathy. Neuropathol Appl Neuro-biol 22:111, 1996 (abstract).

65. Malik R, et al: Hereditary myopathy of Devon rex cats. J Small Anim Pract 34:539, 1993.

66. Farrow BRH, Malik R: Hereditary myotonia in the Chow-Chow. J Small Anim Pract 22:451, 1981.

67. Kortz G: Canine myotonia. Semin Vet Med Surg (Small Anim) 4:141, 1989.

68. Toll J, et al: Congenital myotonia in 2 domestic cats. J Vet Intern Med 12:116, 1998.

69. Smith BF, et al: Possible adult onset myotonic dystrophy in a boxer (letter). J Vet Intern Med 12:120, 1998.

70. Walvoort HC: Glycogen storage disease type II in the Lapland dog. Vet Q 7:187, 1985.

71. Walvoort HC, et al: Heterozygote detection in a family of Lapland dogs with a recessively inherited metabolic disease: Canine glycogen storage disease type II. Res Vet Sci 38:174, 1985.

72. Walvoort HC, et al: Canine glycogen storage disease type II: A clinical study of four affected Lapland Dogs. J Am Anim Hosp Assoc 20:279, 1984.

73. Ceh L, et al: Glycogenosis type III in the dog. Acta Vet Scand 17:210, 1976.

74. Harvey JW, et al: Polysaccharide storage myopathy in canine phosphofructokinase deficiency (Type VII glycogen storage disease). Vet Pathol 27:1, 1990.

75. Giger U, et al: Inherited phosphofructokinase deficiency in an American Cocker Spaniel. JAVMA 201:1569, 1992.

76. Breitschwerdt EB, et al: Episodic weakness associated with exertional lactic acidosis and myopathy in old English Sheepdog littermates. JAVMA 201:731, 1992.

77. Shelton GD: Canine lipid storage myopathies. Proceedings of the 11th Annual Veterinary Medical Forum, Washington, DC, 1993, p 707.

78. Cooper BJ, et al: Nemaline myopathy of cats. Muscle Nerve 9:618, 1986.

79. Huxtable CR, et al: Severe subacute progressive myopathy in a young silky terrier. Prog Vet Neurol 5:21, 1994.

80. Cardinet GH, III: Nemaline rods in neuromuscular disorders of the dog. Anat Histol Embryol 13:87, 1984 (abstract).

81. Guy PS, Snow DH: Skeletal muscle fibre composition in the dog and its relation-ship to athletic ability. Res Vet Sci 31:244, 1981.

82. Snow DH, et al: No classical type 2B fibres in dog skeletal muscle. Histochemistry 75:53, 1982.

SECTION VII

THE CARDIOVASCULAR SYSTEM

CHAPTER 110

PATHOPHYSIOLOGY OF HEART FAILURE AND CLINICAL EVALUATION OF CARDIAC FUNCTION

Helio Autran de Morais

The first indication of cardiac failure is to be found in diminished tolerance to exercise. Of the numerous tests of cardiac efficiency . . . there is none that approaches in delicacy the symptom breathlessness.

Sir Thomas Lewis, 1933

The cough is an early feature of left heart failure in dog and is usually the most distinctive and alarming feature of this condition.

Stephen J. Ettinger and Peter F. Suter, 1970

WHAT IS HEART FAILURE?

Heart failure is a clinical syndrome in which impaired pumping decreases ventricular ejection and impedes venous return. During heart failure, the heart cannot pump blood at a rate adequate to maintain metabolizing tissue requirements or can do so only with elevated filling pressures.[1] The hemodynamic abnormalities are in many cases complicated by depressed myocardial contractility and relaxation resulting from biochemical and biophysical disorders in the myocardial cells. The latter are due partly to molecular abnormalities that not only impair the heart's performance but also accelerate the deterioration of the myocardium and hasten myocardial cell death.[2] *Circulatory failure* is a decrease in cardiac output caused by abnormalities in one or more components of circulation (heart, blood volume, concentration of oxyhemoglobin, vasculature). Heart failure is therefore one of the many causes of circulatory failure (Fig. 110–1).

The heart, like any pump, has only two ways to fail. It either cannot pump enough blood into the aorta or pulmonary artery to maintain arterial pressure (low-output heart failure) or cannot adequately empty the venous reservoirs (congestive heart failure or CHF). Heart failure, therefore, can be recognized clinically by signs of low cardiac output (e.g., depression, lethargy, hypotension) or congestion (e.g.,

ascites, pleural effusion, pulmonary edema). Heart failure can also be classified according to the side that is failing in right, left, or bilateral heart failure. Right-sided heart failure is associated with signs of congestion in the systemic circulation (ascites, peripheral edema), whereas left-sided heart failure causes signs of congestion in the pulmonary circulation (pulmonary edema, dyspnea). Bilateral heart failure presents a combination of left- and right-sided signs and may cause pleural effusion. Either left- or right-sided heart failure can be associated with low-output signs.

WHY DO HEARTS FAIL?

Heart failure may be due to inability of the heart to eject blood properly (systolic failure), inadequate ventricular filling (diastolic failure), or a combination of the two. The final result in either case is a reduction in stroke volume leading to a decrease in cardiac output and a tendency to decrease arterial pressure. Patients with severe heart failure have reduced or inadequate cardiac output even at rest, whereas patients with mild heart failure or diastolic failure have inadequate increase in cardiac output with perturbation (e.g., exercise, stress).

SYSTOLIC FUNCTION AND DYSFUNCTION

Systemic arterial blood pressure (ABP) is a result of the interplay between the arterial system and the heart. Any pressure can be estimated as the product of flow times resistance. In the cardiovascular system, cardiac output (CO), or the amount of blood pumped at a given time, is the flow, whereas the aortic input impedance (Z), the opposition that the vasculature offers to the ejection of blood by the heart, is the resistance factor.

$$ABP \approx CO \times Z$$

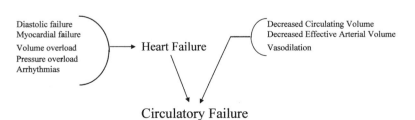

Figure 110–1. Causes of circulatory and heart failure.

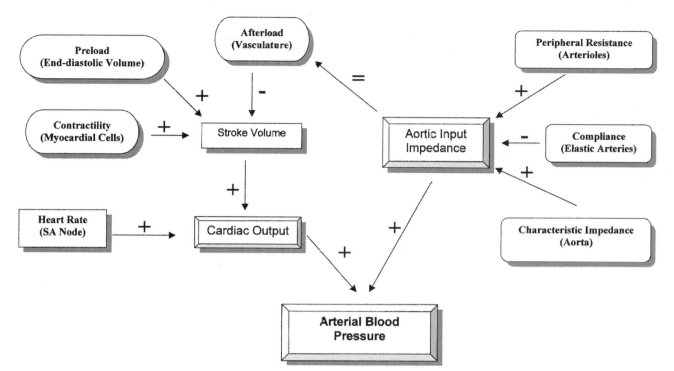

Figure 110–2. Determinants of arterial blood pressure. Arterial blood pressure is a function of the cardiac output and the arterial impedance. Contractility, preload, and afterload determine the stroke volume, which, mult plied by the heart rate, yields the cardiac output. Changes in arterioles, elastic arteries, and the aorta all influence the aortic input impedance (afterload). (+) increases in the parameter increase aortic input impedance, stroke volume, cardiac output, or arterial blood pressure; (−) increases in the parameter decrease aortic input impedance or stroke volume.

Cardiac output is a product of the left ventricular stroke volume (SV) and the heart rate (HR).

$$CO = SV \times HR$$

The higher the stroke volume, the higher the cardiac output. Increases in heart rate increase cardiac output linearly until a plateau is reached at which further increases in heart rate do not affect cardiac output. The latter effect occurs because there is less diastolic time for ventricular filling and increases in heart rate are balanced by decreases in stroke volume. With further increases in heart rate, cardiac output starts to fall. Stroke volume is primarily determined by an intrinsic property of the myocardial cell, contractility, and two coupling factors, preload and afterload. Preload and afterload are considered coupling factors because they are dependent on vascular changes. Stroke volume increases with increases in preload and contractility or decreases in afterload. *Preload* is the force acting to stretch the ventricular fibers at the end of diastole and to determine the maximal resting length of the sarcomeres.[3] Clinically, preload is estimated as the end-diastolic volume or, less precisely, the end-diastolic pressure. Substitution of pressure for volume in estimating preload is not accurate in all clinical situations (e.g., noncompliant or stiff ventricles). *Afterload* is the force opposing ventricular ejection. This opposition is presented by the vasculature to the ejecting ventricle and it is best described by the aortic input impedance.[4–6] An increase in afterload communicates itself to the ventricles during systole by increasing wall stress. The end-systolic wall stress, therefore, is used as an index of the afterload.[6] *Contractility* is a change in the ability of the heart to do work when preload, afterload, and heart rate are kept constant.[2, 6] Stroke volume is also affected by ventricular filling during diastole, ventricular wall motion abnormalities, space-occupying lesions, and arrhythmias.

The resistance factor in estimating blood pressure is best represented by the arterial impedance, which is the aortic pressure divided by aortic flow at a given time. The properties of the arterial system can be described by the total arterial compliance, the peripheral resistance, and the characteristic impedance.[7] Total arterial compliance is a property of elastic arteries and is the change in volume that results from a given change in pressure. The peripheral resistance is largely determined by small arteries and arterioles and represents the resistance to steady (nonpulsatile) flow. Aortic characteristic impedance, the opposition to pulsatile flow, is the quantity that accounts for the elastic wall properties and blood mass properties in the proximal aorta.[7] Increases in peripheral resistance and characteristic impedance and decreases in compliance increase left ventricular afterload. A decrease in compliance makes the ventricle eject into a stiff vasculature, increasing the energetic cost to maintain blood flow, increasing myocardial oxygen consumption (MVO_2), expending more energy to distend less compliant elastic arteries, and making less energy available for tissue perfusion.[8, 9] Characteristic impedance is a property of the proximal aorta and increases whenever the aorta becomes stiffer or its radius becomes smaller. Increases in peripheral resistance (by decreasing the cross-sectional area of the arterioles) increase mean aortic pressure and decrease left ventricular stroke work and stroke volume.[10–12] Peripheral resistance has a greater effect on ventricular performance than characteristic impedance or compliance.[9] One should bear in mind, however, that the left ventricle ejects blood into the proximal aorta and not into the arterioles. The principal factors involved in the determination of arterial pressure are shown in Figure 110–2.

Systolic failure is characterized by normal filling of the ventricle and a decrease in forward stroke volume. The

TABLE 110–1. MECHANISMS LEADING TO SYSTOLIC HEART FAILURE*

Myocardial failure
  Dilated cardiomyopathy
  Infective myocarditis
  Doxorubicin toxicity
  Cardiomyopathy of overload
  Myocardial infarct
  Right ventricular cardiomyopathy
Volume overload
  Valvular diseases
    Endocardiosis
    Endocarditis
    Rupture of mitral chordae tendineae
    Valvular dysplasia
  Patent ductus arteriosus
  Ventricular septal defect
  Atrial septal defect
  Thyrotoxicosis
  Chronic anemia
  Peripheral arteriovenous fistula
Pressure overload
  Subaortic stenosis
  Pulmonic stenosis
  Systemic hypertension
  Pulmonary hypertension
    Primary
    Pulmonary embolism
    Heartworm disease

*Many diseases are also associated with diastolic dysfunction.

decrease in forward stroke volume may result from a decrease in contractility (*myocardial failure*) or a primary increase in ventricular pressure (*pressure overload*) or ventricular volume (*volume overload*) (Table 110–1). Increases in volume are usually caused by a leaking valve or an abnormal communication between the systemic and the pulmonary circulation.

Myocardial Failure

Myocardial failure may be primary (e.g., dilated cardiomyopathy) or secondary to chronic volume or pressure overload. In patients with myocardial failure, a decrease in contractility lowers the stroke volume, cardiac output, and arterial blood pressure. Myocardial failure depresses the ability of the heart to compensate for the decrease in cardiac output (Fig. 110–3).

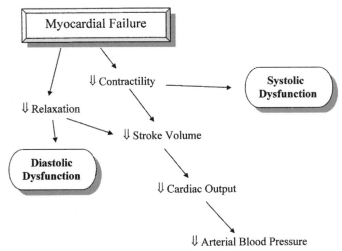

Figure 110–3. From myocardial failure to heart failure.

Pressure Overload

The most common reasons for pressure overload in small animal medicine are subaortic stenosis and systemic arterial hypertension on the left side and heartworm disease and pulmonic stenosis on the right side. The ventricle must overcome the increase in resistance to eject blood. The first response is to dilate, increasing the sarcomere length to the point at which overlap between myofilaments is optimal (approximately 2.2 μm). Dilation raises ventricular contractility and pressure by a length-dependent activation of contractility, helping to overcome the increase in resistance and to maintain stroke volume. This adaptation, however, increases ventricular wall stress and consequently MVo_2.

Left ventricular wall stress can be approximated by the product of intraventricular pressure by the left ventricular radius divided by the left ventricular wall thickness. During the initial dilatation, the ventricular radius increases and the wall thickness decreases, both of which raise ventricular wall stress. With a sustained pressure overload, the ventricular muscle adapts by undergoing concentric hypertrophy (Fig. 110–4). In this type of hypertrophy, there is an increase in wall thickness at the expense of a decrease in chamber size (decrease in ventricular radius), returning ventricular wall stress to normal and increasing contractility.

Myocardium that undergoes hypertrophy secondary to pressure overload is not normal.[13] There is a close link between hypertrophy and systolic dysfunction.[14] The hypertrophied ventricle is also prone to ischemia that leads to fibrosis and an increase in collagen content. The early increase in collagen helps to maintain systolic function but interferes with diastolic function. With progression of the myocardial hypertrophy, perimuscular fibrosis impairs both systolic and diastolic function.[15] As secondary myocardial failure settles in, the ventricle again dilates. The sequence of events in heart failure secondary to pressure overload is shown in Figure 110–5.

Volume Overload

Volume overload may occur with valve insufficiency, abnormal communications (e.g., patent ductus arteriosus, septal defects), and high-output states (e.g., hyperthyroidism). The initial event is an increase in chamber size because of the need to accommodate a large ventricular end-diastolic volume, raising the sarcomere length to the optimal level of 2.2 μm. Again, dilatation leads to an increase in wall stress, which in turn causes ventricular hypertrophy and normalizes wall stress. In a volume overload situation, there is eccentric hypertrophy, with a mild increase in wall thickness and increase in radius (see Fig. 110–4). The degree of hypertrophy is not as severe as in pressure overload states because the primary event now is an increase in volume, which causes only a mild increase in ventricular pressure. The performance of each functional unit of myocardium in a chronically volume-overloaded heart is normal or near normal, allowing a greater than normal stroke volume. The ventricle responds to a volume overload situation by increasing size and also by changing its geometry. Contrary to what happens in the pressure-overloaded myocardium, collagen formation is not a problem in the early stages of volume-overloaded hearts. There is a loss of myocardial collagen in volume-overloaded hearts. The loss of collagen causes the ventricle to dilate and increases ventricular compliance.[16] Left ventricular dilatation and increased compliance do not occur in volume-overloaded hearts when collagenase stimulation caused by mast cell degranulation is blocked.[17]

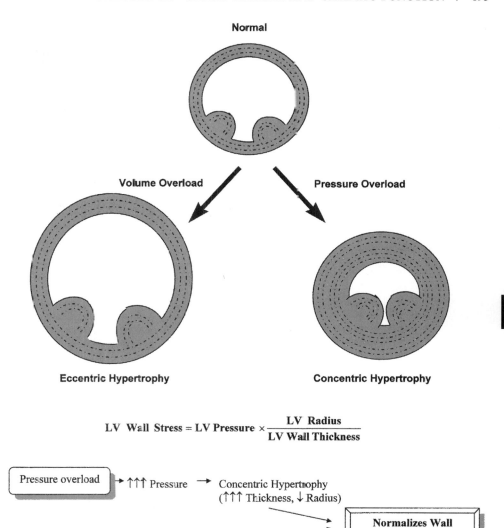

Figure 110–4. Types of ventricular hypertrophy. Increases in pressure lead to concentric hypertrophy, whereas increases in volume lead to eccentric hypertrophy.

CV

With progression of the disease, ventricular end-diastolic pressure again rises above the normal range, raising resting tension and compromising endocardial perfusion pressure.[13] The increase in tension that occurs in this setting is due to slippage of fibers with an excessive increase in chamber size. The mechanism for fiber slippage is poorly understood, but it is probably related to a disruption of normal collagen-myocyte interaction. If collagen fibers fail to support the myocytes, increases in intracavitary pressure may push the myocytes apart by means of fiber slippage.[13] Fiber slippage helps to maintain stroke volume by an unknown mechanism, probably by improving diastolic function. The stretched collagen and the longer fibers act in diastole in an opposite way to hypertrophied myocardium, therefore increasing diastolic compliance.[13] Fiber slippage, on the other hand, sets the stage for progressive disease. The increase in chamber size raises wall stress, increases $M\dot{V}O_2$, changes ventricular geometry, and may cause pressure hypertrophy and fibrosis. With progression of the disease secondary myocardial failure may ensue and the ventricle undergoes further dilatation. The sequence of events in heart failure secondary to volume overload is shown in Figure 110–6.

DIASTOLIC FUNCTION AND DYSFUNCTION

Diastolic dysfunction results from an impairment in ventricular filling. Diastolic heart failure exists when pulmonary venous congestion and resultant clinical signs occur in the presence of normal or near-normal left ventricular systolic function.[18] Approximately one third of human patients with heart failure have diastolic failure. Another third have systolic failure, and the remaining third have impairment of both systolic and diastolic function.[1] Mechanisms leading to diastolic heart failure are listed in Table 110–2.

If diastole is defined to start at the time of aortic valve closure (there are other definitions), diastole can be divided into four phases: (1) isovolumic relaxation (aortic valve closure to mitral valve opening), (2) rapid early mitral inflow (or rapid filling phase, in which the majority of ventricular filling occurs), (3) diastasis (or slow filling phase, in which there is little change in ventricular volume and pressure), and (4) atrial contraction (atrial systole and its contribution to ventricular filling). The latter three phases of diastole represent ventricular filling. Relaxation and chamber stiffness are two diastolic properties of the heart. Relaxation is

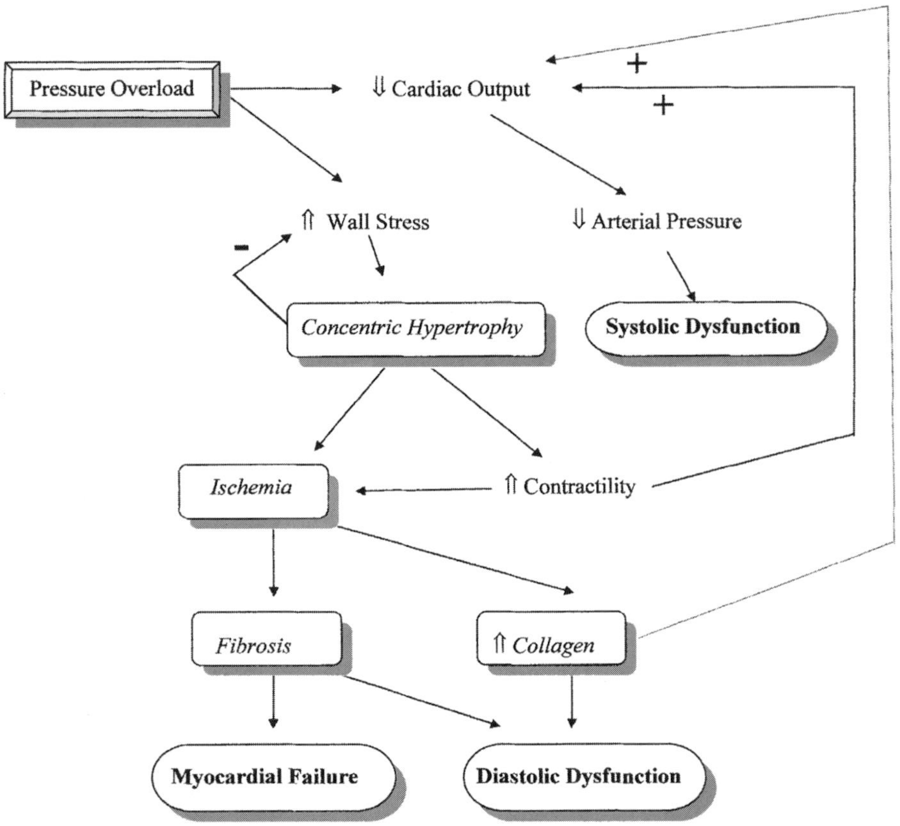

Figure 110–5. From pressure overload to heart failure. Pressure overload states increase wall stress, leading to concentric hypertrophy. Hypertrophy increases contractility and decreases wall stress. Unfortunately, pressure hypertrophy leads to ischemia, fibrosis, and increased collagen. The end result is myocardial failure and diastolic dysfunction leading to heart failure. (−) decreases wall stress; (+) increases cardiac output.

a dynamic, energy-dependent process that begins at the end of contraction and lasts throughout isovolumic relaxation and early ventricular filling. Relaxation is dependent on energy. Ischemia depletes ATP and delays relaxation, whereas beta-adrenergic stimulation improves relaxation. Asynchrony of relaxation, increase in afterload, ventricular hypertrophy, and abnormal calcium fluxes in the myocardial cells delay relaxation. Chamber stiffness or the change in pressure resulting from a given change in volume (e.g., how many millimeters of mercury left ventricular pressure increases for an increase of 1 mL in left ventricular volume) is measured at the end of diastole, after filling has ended. Chamber compliance, the inverse of chamber stiffness, is also measured at the end of diastole. Chamber stiffness increases as filling pressures increase, with increases in intrinsic myocardial stiffness (stiffness of a given unit of cardiac wall as occurs in infiltrative diseases, fibrosis, ischemia), with hypertrophy, and with cardiac tamponade. Lusitropy is a measure of global diastolic performance of the heart and encompasses relaxation and filling phases.[19]

Ventricular filling may be affected by several factors, including atrioventricular pressure gradient, isovolumic relaxation rate, synchronized atrial kick and ventricular relaxation, and compliance. The driving force for ventricular filling is the pressure gradient between left atrium and ventricle when the mitral valve opens. This gradient is affected mostly by the intravascular volume and the degree of vasodilatation of the patient. The isovolumic relaxation rate is also an important determinant of early ventricular filling. Adrenergic stimulation increases the rate of relaxation, improving relaxation to a greater extent than it improves contractility. Increases in heart rate decrease the duration of the diastasis. Incremental increases in heart rate up to 180 beats per minute in dogs progressively increase rate of relaxation,

improve left ventricular contractility, and decrease left ventricular end-diastolic pressure.[20, 21] These changes allow an increase in early filling in situations in which higher heart rates are needed (e.g., exercise). Patients with ventricular hypertrophy that are ischemic, however, show a decrease in left ventricular distensibility with increases in heart rate. Normal diastolic filling is also dependent on the synchronized contraction between the left ventricle and left atrium.[18]

Loss of atrial contraction is one of the reasons why dogs with dilated cardiomyopathy or mitral endocardiosis develop heart failure when their atria start to fibrillate. Asynchronous relaxation of the left ventricle may be observed in cats with

TABLE 110–2. MECHANISMS LEADING TO DIASTOLIC HEART FAILURE

Impaired energy-dependent ventricular relaxation or
    abnormal ventricular chamber or muscle properties
  Ventricular hypertrophy
    Hypertrophic cardiomyopathy
    Subaortic stenosis
    Pulmonic stenosis
    Heartworm disease
    Systemic hypertension
  Dilated cardiomyopathy
  Myocardial infarct
  Restrictive cardiomyopathy
Obstruction to ventricular filling at veins, atria, and
    atrioventricular valves
  Mitral stenosis
  Tricuspid stenosis
  Intracardiac neoplasia causing intracardiac obstruction
  Cor triatriatum
Pericardial abnormalities
  Constrictive disease
  Cardiac tamponade

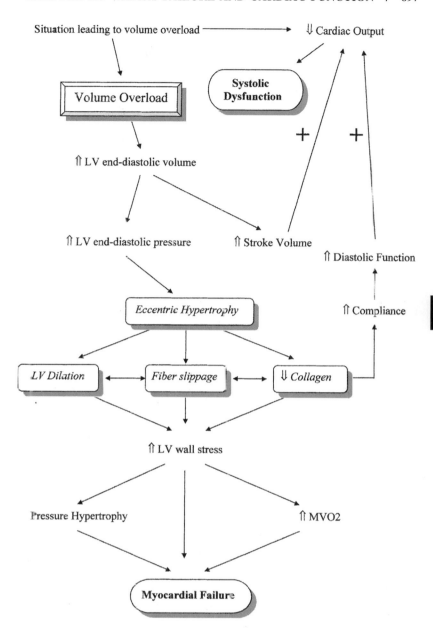

Figure 110–6. From volume overload to heart failure. Volume overload states decrease forward stroke volume, leading to systolic dysfunction, and increase end-diastolic volume. The increase in end-diastolic volume increases stroke volume but also increases end-diastolic pressure, leading to eccentric hypertrophy. Eccentric hypertrophy leads to a decrease in collagen that helps diastolic function, but it also causes fiber slippage, increasing wall stress and ultimately leading to myocardial failure. Patients with volume-overloaded hearts usually develop CHF secondary to a decrease in forward stroke volume, but some patients may have CHF secondary to myocardial failure. (+) increases cardiac output.

restrictive cardiomyopathy. A decrease in the uniformity of relaxation decreases ventricular filling[18] and may contribute to the development of heart failure in these patients. Left ventricular compliance also affects ventricular filling Patients with left ventricular hypertrophy have decreased left ventricular compliance and diastolic function caused by the increase in cardiomyocyte size, increase in collagen content, and increase in wall thickness.[18] The pericardium may also restrain ventricular filling in constrictive pericardial disease or cardiac tamponade. In the latter situations, ventricular filling is abruptly halted in mid-diastole by the abnormal pericardium, which imposes its mechanical properties on those of the ventricle during the final phases of diastole.[1] The mechanisms leading to development of CHF during diastolic dysfunction are shown schematically in Figure 110–7.

HOW DOES THE BODY REACT TO HEART FAILURE?

Regardless of the cause, a decrease in ventricular function causes CHF by decreasing cardiac output and arterial blood pressure. Maintenance of arterial blood pressure and maintenance of effective plasma volume are the main priorities of the cardiovascular system. As blood pressure falls, a series of neurohumoral responses are activated to bring blood pressure back to normal. The immediate response is to increase sympathetic drive, causing vasoconstriction (increasing arterial impedance) and tachycardia (increasing cardiac output). Decrease in renal blood flow causes renin release and activation of the renin-angiotensin-aldosterone system (RAS-aldosterone), contributing to vasoconstriction and causing sodium and water retention, which increases circulating volume. Compensatory mechanisms are acute responses that evolved to keep an animal alive during and right after bleeding. During heart failure, however, compensatory mechanisms are chronically activated (Fig. 110–8). In an effort to maintain blood pressure, the cardiovascular system allows the venous pressure to increase and redistributes cardiac output, maintaining blood flow mostly to essential organs (Fig. 110–9).

Compensation cannot be viewed as an isolated response of the circulation. The heart and the myocardial cells undergo changes to adapt to ventricular dysfunction. A common characteristic of all compensatory responses is that their

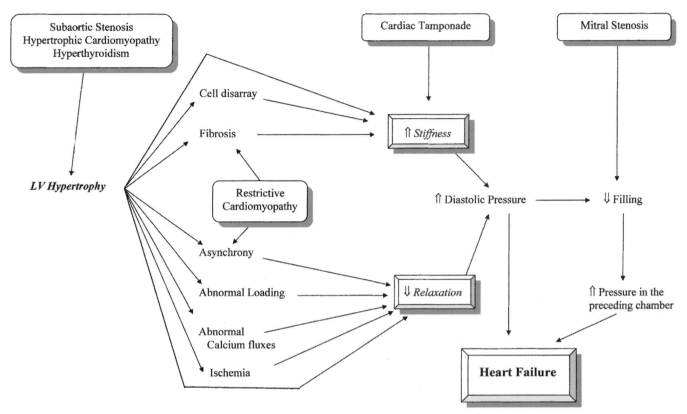

Figure 110–7. Sequence of events leading to diastolic heart failure. Most mechanisms leading to diastolic failure decrease lusitropy by increasing stiffness, decreasing relaxation, or both. Mitral stenosis leads to diastolic heart failure by interfering with left ventricular filling.

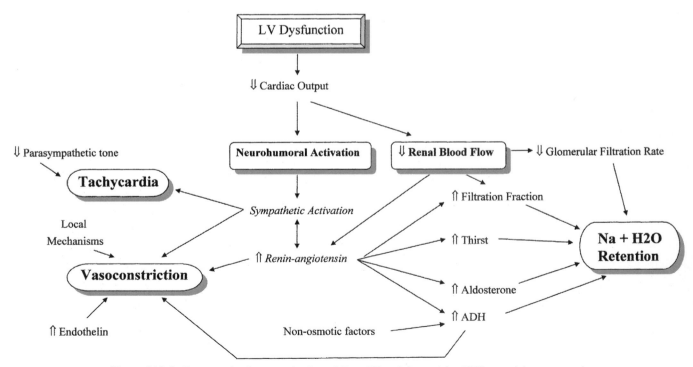

Figure 110–8. Compensation in congestive heart failure. LV = left ventricle; ADH = arginine vasopressin.

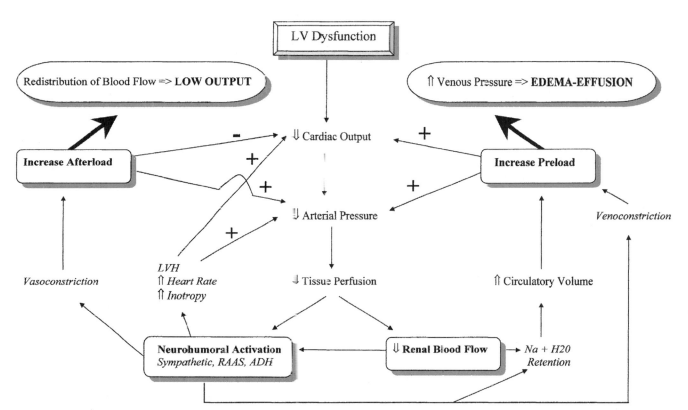

Figure 110–9. Compensation and clinical signs of congestive heart failure. (+) increases arterial pressure or cardiac output; (−) decreases cardiac output; LV = left ventricle; RAAS = renin-angiotensin-aldosterone system; LVH = left ventricular hypertrophy; ADH = arginine vasopressin.

short-term effects are helpful but the long-term effects are deleterious. In acute injuries to the heart, cardiac output decreases and acute heart failure may occur. This phase, known as "transient breakdown," initiates the activation of the compensatory mechanisms.[22] In small animals, heart failure is usually a chronic problem and the transient breakdown phase merges with the following phase. As compensation occurs, cardiac output and clinical signs steadily improve because extra work is being performed by the heart and the circulation. This compensated phase is known as "stable hyperfunction." Chronic hyperfunction leads to progression of left ventricular dysfunction, myocardial cell death, development of clinical signs, and death, the "exhaustion and

progressive cardiosclerosis" phase. The chronic effects of the compensatory mechanisms leading to progression of left ventricular dysfunction are shown in Figure 110–10.

NEUROHUMORAL ACTIVATION

Neurohumoral activation in CHF is a result of the decrease in cardiac output and atrial hypertension. Neurohumoral mechanisms include vasoconstrictive or sodium-retaining systems and vasodilator or natriuretic systems (Table 110–3). All neurohumoral mechanisms are fully operative during severe CHF. The exact time when activation of each particu-

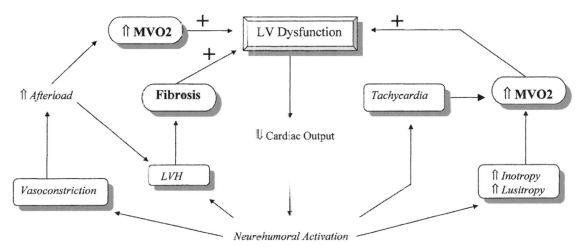

Figure 110–10. Compensation and progression of left ventricular (LV) dysfunction (+) causes further left ventricular dysfunction; LVH = left ventricular hypertrophy. MVo₂ = myocardial oxygen consumption.

TABLE 110–3. NEUROENDOCRINE FACTORS INCREASED IN HEART FAILURE

Vasoconstrictive or sodium retaining
↑ Sympathetic nervous system
↑ Renin-angiotensin II-aldosterone
↑ Arginine vasopressin
↑ Endothelin-1
↑ Tromboxane
↑ Neuropeptide Y
↑ Tumor necrosis factor
Vasodilators or natriuretic
↑ Atrial natriuretic factor
↑ NO (basal, decreased release upon stimulation)
↑ Prostaglandins (E_2, I_2)
↓ Kallikreins
↑ Dopamine
↓ Calcitonin gene–related peptide

lar neurohumoral mechanism starts is more controversial. Clinical data are still lacking for small animals with naturally occurring CHF. The underlying cause of ventricular dysfunction also plays a role in determining when the activation of a particular neurohumoral mechanism starts. The net effect of neuroendocrine activation is vasoconstriction, sodium and water retention, and left ventricular hypertrophy, leading to ventricular and peripheral vessel remodeling.

Autonomic Nervous System

CHF is accompanied by a generalized increase in sympathetic nerve activity and an attenuation of parasympathetic tone. Dogs with naturally occurring CHF caused by dilated cardiomyopathy and mitral regurgitation have increased norepinephrine concentrations that correlate positively with the clinical severity of CHF.[23] The increase in norepinephrine, however, does not correlate with the degree of myocardial dysfunction.[23] Norepinephrine concentration correlates with cardiac death in human patients with CHF. Increases in norepinephrine are due to increased release from adrenergic endings and its "spillover" into plasma and to a decrease in the uptake by adrenergic nerve endings. The decrease in left ventricular function leads to relative hypotension that stimulates the baroreceptors to activate the sympathetic nervous system.[24] The precise mechanisms responsible for the persistent sympathetic overactivity and blunted baroreflex control seen in CHF, however, remain obscure, and the effects cannot be solely explained by chronic withdrawal of baroreflex inhibition.[25] Augmented peripheral chemosensitivity has been demonstrated in CHF.[26] A link between increased peripheral chemosensitivity and impaired autonomic control, including baroreflex inhibition, has been demonstrated in human patients with CHF.[27] Overactivity of muscle metaboreceptors (ergoreceptors) may also contribute to the autonomic imbalance.[28]

Despite increases in plasma concentration of norepinephrine, patients with CHF have depletion of norepinephrine from atria and ventricles that blunts the IR response to sympathetic activation. Increased levels of norepinephrine in the vicinity of beta-adrenoreceptors lead to down-regulation of these receptors. Down-regulation of beta-adrenoreceptors occurs in patients with severe cardiomyopathy and correlates with severity of the heart disease. In patients with dilated cardiomyopathy, the down-regulation is consistently shown in beta$_1$-adrenoreceptors but not in the beta$_2$-adrenoreceptors, whereas in mitral disease and in ischemic cardiomyopathy both subsets of beta-adrenoreceptors are down-regulated.

The selective beta$_1$ down-regulation may occur because myocardial beta$_1$-adrenoreceptors are innervated and therefore exposed to the increased norepinephrine being released from the nerve endings, whereas myocardial beta$_2$-adrenoreceptors are not innervated. Postadrenoreceptor changes in the beta-adrenoreceptor–adenylate cyclase complex could contribute to changes in adrenergic responsiveness. In human patients with heart failure there is a subsensitivity of beta$_2$-adrenoreceptors even in patients with normal beta$_2$-adrenoreceptor numbers. The subsensitivity of the beta$_2$-adrenoreceptors is believed to be due to partial uncoupling of the beta$_2$-adrenoreceptors from the beta$_2$-adrenergic complex and not to down-regulation. The role of alpha-adrenoreceptors during heart failure is not as clear.

Increased sympathetic activity is partially responsible for vasoconstriction and sodium and water retention, whereas decreased norepinephrine stores and changes in adrenoreceptors lead to a decrease in contractile response of the myocardial cells and a decrease in chronotropic response of the sinoatrial node cells during exercise. Chronic adrenergic stimulation also leads to increased afterload, increased MVo_2, and ventricular arrhythmias and favors progression of the left ventricular dysfunction. Remodeling of the heart and peripheral vessels is also stimulated by the chronic sympathetic activation and also favors progression of left ventricular dysfunction.

Baroreflex control is altered during CHF, contributing to the increased sympathetic activity and blunted tachycardic response during exercise or hypotension. Abnormal baroreflexes also contribute to sodium and water retention. Normally, increases in atrial pressure stimulate atrial stretch receptors that inhibit antidiuretic hormone (ADH, arginine vasopressin) release, decrease sympathetic activity, and increase renal blood flow and glomerular filtration rate. During CHF, atrial and arterial receptors have a decreased response to stimulation. Decreased parasympathetic activity is present in CHF, decreasing the restraint of the sinoatrial node. The net result is a higher heart rate for a given arterial pressure and a decrease in heart rate variability. Decrease in parasympathetic tone in CHF carries a poor prognosis.

Renin-Angiotensin-Aldosterone System

Low cardiac output during CHF activates the renin-angiotensin system (RAS) by direct beta-adrenoreceptor stimulation and by the decrease in renal flow in the juxtaglomerular apparatus of the kidneys. Angiotensin II is a potent vasoconstrictor and also stimulates the release of aldosterone and ADH, increases sympathetic activity, constricts the efferent renal artery, and stimulates thirst.[29] Thus, activation of RAS contributes to the vasoconstriction and sodium water retention during CHF. Sympathetic activation usually precedes RAS activation, although some of the sympathetic activation during CHF is caused by RAS. Angiotensin stimulates vessel remodeling either by directly decreasing nitric oxide (NO) synthesis or by increasing local angiotensin-converting enzyme (ACE) breakdown of bradykinin, altering prostaglandin metabolism. Vascular remodeling causes structural changes that further decrease compliance of the arterial system. Angiotensin II can also stimulate smooth muscle cell growth, leading to cellular hyperplasia, hypertrophy, and apoptosis (programmed cell death).[29] Aldosterone increases total body water and may contribute to increased tissue water content, increasing the stiffness and decreasing the compliance of the arterial system.[29] Aldosterone may also have a direct vasoconstrictive action during CHF.[30] Aldosterone also increases potassium and magnesium excretion. Activation of RAS contributes to vasoconstriction, increasing afterload and MVo$_2$, and causes sodium and water retention by the kidneys. Remodeling of the heart and peripheral vessels is also stimulated by RAS, favoring progression of left ventricular dysfunction.

Other Vasoconstrictive Agents

Arginine vasopressin is increased in patients with heart failure, because of nonosmotic release, impairment of baroreceptor-mediated inhibition of brain stem centers, and increases in circulating angiotensin II. Arginine vasopressin may be increased even in patients with asymptomatic left ventricular dysfunction. Release of ADH leads to vasoconstriction and water reabsorption and favors the development of hyponatremia.

Endothelin is the most potent vasoconstrictor substance known for vascular smooth muscle cells. Endothelin was elevated in a canine pacing model of heart failure and the increase correlated well with right atrial or pulmonary capillary wedge pressure.[31] Endothelin plays an important role in maintaining blood pressure and blood flow during CHF and may be activated by angiotensin II.[32] Chronic blockage of endothelin receptors may prevent the progression of heart failure.[33]

Vasodilatory Agents

Atrial natriuretic peptide is stored in the right atrium and released by increases in atrial distending pressures. This peptide causes arterial dilatation, venodilatation, natriuresis, and water diuresis, counteracting the effects of vasoconstrictory agents. It also inhibits renin and aldosterone secretion and reduces sympathetic vasoconstriction.[34] Brain natriuretic peptide is stored in the ventricular myocardium and also causes vasodilatation and natriuresis. CHF is associated with an increase in atrial natriuretic peptide and the changes are related to the fall in ejection fraction and to the increase in cardiac filling pressures. Despite having beneficial effects during CHF, release of atrial natriuretic peptide is overridden by the release of agents that cause vasoconstriction as well as sodium and water retention.

Nitric oxide is the major physiologic regulator of basal blood vessel tone. There appears to be a dissociation of stimulated and basal release of NO in patients with heart failure. The stimulated endothelium-dependent dilatation exerted by acetylcholine in peripheral resistance vessels is blunted during heart failure, suggesting reduced release of NO on stimulation. This defective mechanism may be involved in the impaired vasodilator capacity in the peripheral circulation (e.g., during exercise).[35] In contrast, the basal release of NO from endothelium of resistance vessels appears to be preserved and may even be enhanced and may potentially play an important compensatory role in CHF during resting conditions by antagonizing neurohumoral vasoconstrictory forces.[35]

PERIPHERAL COMPENSATION

Peripheral compensation occurs outside the heart and is directed at normalizing arterial blood pressure. The main mechanisms involved in peripheral compensation are tachycardia, vasoconstriction, and sodium and water retention (Table 110–4).

Blood Vessels and Vasoconstriction

The mechanism responsible for the increased tone of the vascular smooth muscle in CHF is multifactorial, but it is basically a result of the neurohumoral activation and the interplay of local mechanisms. Decreased blood flow to muscles causes overactivity of muscle metaboreceptors (afferents sensitive to skeletal muscle work) and peripheral chemoreceptors, contributing to the autonomic imbalance. Increase in efferent sympathetic neuron discharge causes vasoconstriction. There is an increase in aortic stiffness (characteristic impedance), and a decrease in compliance of large arteries before the vasoconstriction of the small arterioles (increase in peripheral resistance) occurs in dogs with pacing-induced CHF.[36] Sympathetic activation occurs even in patients with asymptomatic left ventricular dysfunction. There appear to be further increases in plasma norepinephrine in these patients when signs of heart failure develop. The RAS is also activated by the decrease in cardiac output, further increasing vascular tone as a direct action of angiotensin II and indirectly via the facilitatory effect of angiotensin II in the alpha-adrenergic neurons. Unlike the sympathetic system, the RAS normalizes as compensation returns cardiac output to normal. It is still controversial whether dogs with asymptomatic mitral regurgitation or left ventricular dysfunction have activation of RAS.[37, 38] Arginine vasopressin may be increased even in patients with asymptomatic left ventricular dysfunction and contributes to the increase in peripheral vascular resistance in patients with heart failure.

Local vasoregulatory mechanisms are important in modulating vascular tone during heart failure. In normal dogs, shear stress related to pulsatile flow releases NO and prostacyclin and inhibits endothelin-1 leading to vasodilatation. During CHF, decreased shear stress secondary to decreased peripheral blood flow and neurohumoral activation decreases release of NO and increases endothelin-1, leading to vasoconstriction.[39] Endothelin is a potent vasoconstrictor that is elevated during CHF. Blocking of endothelin may prevent progression of CHF.

Vasoconstriction is primarily mediated by increased sympathetic tone, RAS activation, and increased endothelin concentration.[32, 40] Arginine vasopressin becomes an important vasoconstrictor agent only in hyponatremic patients.[40] These mechanisms also lead to venoconstriction, increasing venous pressure and increasing venous return to the heart. Vasoconstriction helps to maintain arterial pressure, but it also increases afterload, causing the stroke volume to fall. Failing ventricles are afterload dependent, and stroke volume falls with any given increase in afterload (Fig. 110–11). In this setting, the cardiovascular system redistributes cardiac output, decreasing blood perfusion to "less essential" organs. Increases in afterload also increase MVo$_2$ by increasing wall stress. In patients with severe mitral regurgitation the increase in opposition to ventricular ejection increases regurgitation, whereas in patients with left-to-right shunt it increases the shunting fraction.

Skeletal Muscles

Left ventricular dysfunction leads to a decrease in blood flow to the periphery, causing vasomotor changes and muscle alterations. Mechanisms not related to the decrease in blood flow (e.g., decreased activity, increased catabolic factors, insulin resistance) may also play a role in muscle changes during CHF. Patients with CHF have substantial skeletal

TABLE 110–4. COMPENSATORY MECHANISMS ACTING IN THE PERIPHERY

RESPONSE	MECHANISM	POTENTIAL BENEFIT	POTENTIAL HARM	MANIFESTATIONS	CORRELATES
Sympathetic activation	Decrease in arterial pressure RAS activation	Inotropic support Tachycardia Activates RAS Vasoconstriction Venoconstriction	Increases MVo$_2$ Increases afterload Sympathetic desensitization Excessive preload	Tachycardia Arrhythmias Pale mucous membranes	Norepinephrine concentration correlates with mortality Beta-adrenoreceptor blockade may increase survival
Vasoconstriction	Sympathetic activation RAS activation Increase in ADH Local blood vessel mechanisms	Maintains arterial pressure Maintains perfusion of "essential" organs	Increases MVo$_2$ Increases afterload Stimulates LVH Decreases cardiac output Potentiates mitral regurgitation Redirects blood flow	Pale mucous membranes	Modulation of excessive arterial tone with vasodilators is beneficial during heart failure
Activation of renin-angiotensin system	Sympathetic activation Decreased renal perfusion	Vasoconstriction Stimulates thirst Releases ADH Releases aldosterone Increases sympathetic tone	Increases MVo$_2$ Increases afterload Stimulates LVH Stimulates blood vessel remodeling Decreases cardiac output and tissue perfusion	Pale mucous membranes	Angiotensin-converting enzyme blockade increases survival time in patients with heart failure
Sodium and water retention	Poor renal perfusion Increases in thirst, ADH, and aldosterone	Increases preload Improves LV function	Congestion Excessive preload, increases wall stress Hypokalemia (aldosterone)	Edema and cavitary effusions Arrhythmias (hypokalemia)	Use of diuretics in CHF decreases sodium and water retention Aldosterone inhibition decreases chance of hypokalemia
Venoconstriction	Sympathetic activation	Increases preload and ventricular function	Congestion Excessive preload, increases wall stress	Edema and cavitary effusions Venous distention	Venodilators and nitrates can be used in the treatment of heart failure

ADH = antidiuretic hormone (vasopressin); CHF = congestive heart failure; LV = left ventricular; LVH = left ventricular hypertrophy; MVo$_2$ = myocardial oxygen consumption; RAS = renin–angiotensin system.

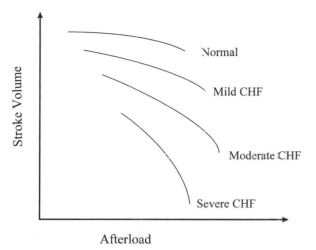

Figure 110–11. Effects of increasing afterload on left ventricular stroke volume in normal animals and in patients with congestive heart failure (CHF).

muscle atrophy, and the degree of atrophy correlates with muscle strength and peak oxygen consumption.[41] Skeletal muscles are morphologically and metabolically abnormal in CHF. Atrophy, changes in muscle fiber type and mitochondrial ultrastructure, and a decrease in oxidative enzymatic capacity leading to increased reliance on anaerobic metabolism and lactate production have all been demonstrated in patients with CHF. Increase in lactate during exercise stimulates (or serves as a marker for the presence of other stimulants) peripheral metaboreceptors. Patients with CHF, therefore, have greater metaboreceptor stimulation for a given degree of exercise than normal subjects.[25, 41] Metaboreceptor stimulation increases sympathetic outflow, adding to the vasoconstriction and reducing blood flow to exercising muscles, because alpha-adrenergically mediated vasoconstriction is not impaired during CHF.

Kidneys and Sodium and Water Retention

Several mechanisms are responsible for sodium and water retention in CHF. Competing vasodilator-natriuretic and vasoconstrictive–sodium-retaining mechanisms operate. Decrease in cardiac output decreases renal blood flow and increases sympathetic drive, which causes renal vasoconstriction and a further decrease in renal blood flow. Renin is released by activation of the juxtaglomerular apparatus by beta-adrenoreceptors stimulation and decreases in renal blood flow. The end result of renin release is an increase in angiotensin II and aldosterone. Angiotensin II stimulates thirst and release of ADH, leading to water retention. Aldosterone causes sodium and water retention and potassium wasting by the kidneys. Decreases in renal perfusion are countered by the release of prostaglandin E, which dilates the afferent renal arteriole and constricts the efferent renal arteriole, a response mediated by angiotensin II. These alterations combine to increase glomerular filtration pressure, increase filtration fraction (the ratio of glomerular filtration to renal plasma flow), and maintain glomerular filtration rate despite the reduction in renal blood flow. Sodium and water retention increases circulating volume and preload, helping to maintain cardiac filling pressures and increasing cardiac output. Retention of sodium and water, however, leads to an excessive increase in venous filling pressure, leading to the development of edema and cavitary effusions. It also increases afterload and favors progression of the left ventricular dysfunction.

CENTRAL COMPENSATION (HEART)

The heart participates actively in the compensation for the decrease in cardiac output. Sympathetic activation leads to an increase in heart rate, inotropy, and lusitropy, all of which increase cardiac output. In addition, hypertrophy helps to normalize cardiac output by increasing stroke volume. Compensatory mechanisms acting on the heart are shown in Table 110–5.

Tachycardia

During heart failure, the increase in sympathetic tone increases heart rate. Parasympathetic tone decreases, contributing to the tachycardia. It is usually believed that sinus rates above 160 beats per minute imply not only parasympathetic withdrawal but also sympathetic activation. The end result is an increase in heart rate and a decrease in heart rate variability. The increase in heart rate helps to normalize arterial pressure but at a high price, an increase in MVo$_2$. A decrease in heart rate variability is a negative prognostic factor for overall mortality in human patients with myocardial infarction. Decreased heart rate variability correlates with severity of CHF in dogs with chronic mitral valve disease.[42] Patients with decreased heart rate variability are also less likely to respond to vasodilator infusion. Increases in heart rate in patients with heart failure parallel the sympathetic activation, which in turn correlates with the severity of heart failure.

Increased Inotropy and Lusitropy

Beta-adrenergic stimulation by the increased sympathetic tone during heart failure increases calcium entry in the atrial and ventricular cells, increases calcium release from the sarcoplasmic reticulum, and increases interaction between contractile proteins. All of these actions increase contractility. Beta-adrenergic stimulation also increases lusitropy by increasing calcium efflux from the cell and calcium uptake by the sarcoplasmic reticulum.[2] The increase in calcium entry is largely responsible for the positive inotropic effect, whereas the facilitated dissociation from troponin and increased calcium uptake by the sarcoplasmic reticulum are the key factors in causing a positive lusitropic effect.[2] Beta-adrenergic stimulation increases cardiac output but also increases MVo$_2$ and may contribute to myocardial remodeling.

Myocardial Growth

An increase in afterload and neurohumoral activation leads to left ventricular hypertrophy. Hypertrophy decreases the load in individual cells and increases cardiac output. Hypertrophy causes growth of myocyte and nonmyocyte cells in the extracellular matrix of the myocardium. Growth of myocytes and growth of nonmyocyte cells are independent of each other. Chronic anemia and thyrotoxicosis cause myocyte growth without involvement of fibroblasts, whereas hypertrophy secondary to pressure overload is accompanied by reactive fibrosis that is not secondary to myocyte necrosis. Increases in preload, afterload, sympathetic activation, and growth hormone induce myocardial growth, whereas activation of RAS, prostaglandin E$_2$, transforming growth factor-

TABLE 110-5. COMPENSATORY MECHANISMS ACTING IN THE HEART

RESPONSE	MECHANISM	POTENTIAL BENEFIT	POTENTIAL HARM	MANIFESTATIONS	CORRELATES
Sympathetic desensitization	Down-regulation of beta$_1$-adrenoreceptors Uncoupling of beta$_2$-adrenoreceptors Myocardial norepinephrine depletion	Spares energy	Decreases contractility	Low-output signs	Beta-adrenoreceptor blockade may revert sympathetic desensitization
Tachycardia	Sympathetic activation Parasympathetic withdrawal	Increases cardiac output	Increases MVo$_2$	Tachycardia Decrease in heart rate variability	Decrease in heart rate variability correlates with mortality
Increased inotropy Increased relaxation	Sympathetic activation Sympathetic activation	Increases stroke volume Improves diastolic function (lusitropy)	Increases MVo$_2$ Increases MVo$_2$		
Appearance of slow myosin in the atria	Changes in isogene expression	Decreases cost to achieve normal tension Energy sparing Increases atrial kick	Atrial failure		Changes do not occur in the ventricles of dogs and cats
Myocardial ATPase activity reduction	Unknown (altered isoenzymes?)	Facilitates high-pressure, low-speed work Spares energy	Slows rate of contraction Decreases contractility	Low-output signs	Myocardial ATPase activity is increased in high-output CHF (e.g., thyrotoxicosis)
Pressure-overload (concentric hypertrophy)	Increase afterload Renin-angiotensin activation	Unloads individual muscle fibers Decreases wall stress Decreases MVo$_2$	Imbalance energy demand and supply Focal necrosis Fibrosis Increases collagen Diastolic dysfunction	Cardiomegaly Diastolic dysfunction increases venous congestion	Induces cardiomyopathy of overload Growth-inhibitory drugs (ACE inhibitors and nitrates) may delay the development of cardiomyopathy of overload
Volume overload (eccentric hypertrophy)	Fiber slippage Increase tension	Increases compliance? Increases stroke volume with same ejection fraction (dilatation)	Increases wall stress Increases MVo$_2$ Pressure hypertrophy	Cardiomegaly	Increase in wall stress leads to pressure hypertrophy

ACE = angiotensin-converting enzyme; ATPase = adenosinetriphosphatase; CHF = congestive heart failure; MVo$_2$ = myocardial oxygen consumption.

β1 (TGF-β$_1$), and insulin-like growth factor-1 induces remodeling of cardiac interstitium.[43] All these substances induce expression of proto-oncogenes and growth-regulating genes that play an important role in mediating hypertrophy.[44] Structural remodeling of myocardial collagen matrix contributes to progression of heart failure.

Hypertrophy in patients with CHF leads to a ventricle that is not normal. There are morphologic, biochemical, and genetic changes that cause ventricular remodeling leading to progression of the left ventricular dysfunction. Appearance of a "slow" myosin, a more efficient myosin that spares energy in the heart, has been detected in the atria[45] but not in the ventricle[46] of dogs with CHF. Pressure-induced hypertrophy unloads the individual myocardial cells and decreases wall stress and MVo$_2$. Hypertrophied ventricles have a capillary deficit and a decrease in the number of mitochondria, leading to a state of energy starvation.[47] The ischemia leads to necrosis, fibrosis, increase in collagen concentration, and diastolic dysfunction. Volume-induced hypertrophy decreases wall stress and MVo$_2$ and helps to maintain stroke volume, probably by increasing compliance. Fiber slippage, however, causes further dilatation of the heart, again increasing wall stress and MVo$_2$ and favoring progression of the left ventricular dysfunction.

WHAT ARE THE CLINICAL MANIFESTATIONS OF HEART FAILURE?

Clinical signs in heart failure may result from accumulation of fluids, low cardiac output, or changes in skeletal muscles (Table 110–6). Primary clinical manifestations of CHF differ among species. Dogs with CHF are usually brought to the clinic because of cough, dyspnea, exercise intolerance, abdominal enlargement, or syncope. Cats, on the other hand, are usually presented because they cannot breathe (pleural effusion or pulmonary edema) or cannot walk (aortic thromboembolism) properly.

Sodium and water retention increase circulating volume and venous pressure, an effect that is potentiated by venous constriction. Venous hypertension and microcirculatory congestion lead to transudation of fluids in body cavities (effusion) or interstitium (edema). These signs develop preferentially in the capillary beds drained by the failing ventricle. Thus, elevated pulmonary venous and capillary hydrostatic pressures in small animals lead to pulmonary edema and can be manifested as dyspnea, cough, pulmonary crackles, and exercise intolerance. Systemic venous hypertension causes jugular distention, hepatic congestion, ascites, and subcutaneous edema. In dogs, ascites always precedes subcutaneous edema in patients with right-sided CHF. Biventricular failure is characterized by a combination of left- and right-sided signs and is often associated with accumulation of pleural fluid. Pleural effusion in small animals is usually a sign of biventricular failure and not right-sided failure.[48] Although cats may occasionally develop pleural effusion during experimentally induced right-sided CHF,[49] almost all cat patients with pleural effusion from CHF have bilateral disease or a disease of the left side with pulmonary hypertension or atrial fibrillation. Dogs develop pleural effusion during experimentally induced right-sided CHF only when large volumes of crystalloid are infused, leading to severe hypoproteinemia.[50] In this setting, pleural effusion correlates better with pulmonary capillary wedge pressure than with right atrial pressure, suggesting that right-sided CHF was not the main cause of the development of pleural effusion.

Decrease in cardiac output may lead to exercise intolerance, tiring, and fatigue. Exercise intolerance can occur only in animals that exercise. Exercise intolerance, therefore, is not a prominent complaint of owners of cats and dogs that spend most of their life on the lap. Syncope may be due to low cardiac output of the failing heart or to concurrent arrhythmia. Low-output signs are nonspecific but, when related to CHF, tend to worsen with exercise.

Dyspnea may be caused by pulmonary edema or pleural effusion, but it may also occur before the patient develops severe fluid retention. Dyspnea and exercise intolerance may be related to skeletal muscle changes during CHF. Abnormal muscle function and increased fatigability during CHF have been linked to the decrease in muscle bulk, increased reliance on anaerobic metabolism, decreased muscle blood flow, and metaboreceptor activation.[25] Normal animals also became dyspneic during exercise in a manner similar to that in CHF. The main difference between a normal fit animal, an untrained animal, and a patient with CHF is the amount of exercise that leads to dyspnea and fatigue. Muscle fatigue is an important determinant of exercise intolerance and dyspnea (fatigue of respiratory muscle) during CHF. In human beings, the same patient may complain of fatigue or dyspnea, depending on the type of exercise being performed. It has been proposed that a sensation of fatigue during CHF is generated as a central mechanism to protect against hypoxic damage to essential organs.[51] Ergoreceptors may be responsible for mediating both dyspnea and sensation of fatigue.[25] The muscle hypothesis of CHF states that abnormalities in skeletal muscle blood flow, bulk, and function are major determinants of clinical signs leading to fatigue and increase ventilatory stimulus. Activation of ergoreceptors leads to persistent sympathetic activation increasing afterload and reducing blood flow. As cardiac function deteriorates, a catabolic state exacerbates muscle wasting (cardiac cachexia), whereas inactivity of the patient leads to further

TABLE 110–6. CLINICAL SIGNS IN CONGESTIVE HEART FAILURE

Low-output signs
    Complaints → exercise intolerance, syncope
    Clinical signs → weak arterial pulses, tachycardia, arrhythmias, cool extremities
Signs related to poor skeletal muscle function
    Complaints → loss of weight, exercise intolerance, dyspnea*
    Clinical signs → decreased muscle bulk
Signs related to fluid retention
    Left side (pulmonary edema)
        Complaints → dyspnea, orthopnea, exercise intolerance, cough†
        Clinical signs → pulmonary crackles, tachypnea, gallop rhythm, functional mitral regurgitation, cyanosis caused by ventilation-perfusion inequality
    Right side (systemic venous congestion)
        Complaints → abdominal enlargement (ascites), subcutaneous edema
        Clinical signs → jugular distention and pulsation, ascites, hepatomegaly, splenomegaly, hepatojugular reflux, gallop rhythm
    Bilateral
        Complaints → left side plus right side complaints, dyspnea caused by pleural effusion
        Clinical signs → left side plus right side clinical signs, muffled heart and lung sounds with fluid line in the chest (pleural effusion)
Other signs
    Arrhythmias
    Weight loss
    Cough

*Activation of metaboreceptors and peripheral chemoreceptors may contribute to dyspnea in patients without congestion.
†Cough may also occur in dogs without congestive heart failure because of left main stem bronchus compression.

deterioration of muscle function.[25] Such a progression of events leads to a vicious cycle wherein muscle abnormalities cause clinical signs and favor progression of left ventricular dysfunction, worsening muscle abnormalities and increasing clinical signs.[25]

Cardiac cachexia is a common finding during CHF. It is usually more prominent during right-sided CHF and in giant breeds with dilated cardiomyopathy. In one study, more than half of the dogs with CHF secondary to dilated cardiomyopathy were cachectic.[52] Is uncommon for an animal with overt CHF to be obese. Obesity is usually associated with respiratory problems. In situations in which CHF develops rapidly (e.g., rupture of one of the chordae tendineae, development of atrial fibrillation, a few Dobermans with dilated cardiomyopathy), time may not have been sufficient for to cardiac cachexia to develop and the animal may show a reasonably normal body condition. The cachectic state is a strong independent risk factor for mortality in patients with CHF.[53] Cachexia is more closely associated with hormonal changes in CHF than conventional hemodynamic measures of the severity of CHF.[54] Neurohumoral activation leading to increases in tumor necrosis factor-α (TNF-α), interleukin-1β, norepinephrine, and cortisol and to insulin resistance. All these factors appear to play a major role in the development of cardiac cachexia. There is an increase in TNF-α and its soluble receptors in chronic heart failure. This increase is associated with a rise in the cortisol/dehydroepiandrosterone (catabolic/anabolic) ratio, suggesting that an increase in TNF is a possible etiology for cardiac cachexia.[55] During right-sided failure, interference with normal absorption of nutrients in the gastrointestinal tract caused by intestinal and hepatic congestion may also contribute to cachexia.

Cough is common sign of heart disease in dogs but not in cats. Dogs with heart disease may cough because of left-sided CHF, compression of the left main stem bronchus without CHF, or a concomitant respiratory disease (e.g., collapsing trachea, chronic bronchitis). Dogs that cough because of pulmonary edema are frequently thin, with severe weight loss, and have a more subtle cough that tends to be worse at night and may be accompanied by pink nasal discharge or sputum. Dogs that cough because of left main stem bronchus compression or primary respiratory problem may be obese or have normal weight and tend to have dry, hacking coughs that are usually worse during the day. Dogs with left-sided CHF usually have fast heart rates caused by sympathetic activation, whereas dogs with left main stem bronchus compression or respiratory disease have normal heart rates with pronounced sinus arrhythmia resulting from high parasympathetic tone.

Arrhythmias in patients with heart failure may be caused by the underlying disease or by the CHF itself. In addition, chronic persistent tachycardia may cause left ventricular dysfunction and CHF. Enlargement, fibrosis, and hypertrophy that occur during left ventricular dysfunction lead to conduction abnormalities that predispose to arrhythmias. A rise in cytosolic calcium caused by sympathetic activation may also cause arrhythmias. The presence of arrhythmias is an important prognostic factor in patients with CHF.

Clinical signs suggestive of heart disease, not necessarily with CHF, include a diastolic, continuous or loud systolic murmur; arrhythmias with pulse deficit; gallop rhythms; and ascites with jugular distention and presence of hepatojugular reflux. The presence of an aortic thromboembolism (saddle thrombus) in cats also suggests the presence of a heart disease. Right-sided CHF is a clinical diagnosis in dogs. It is likely to be present in patients with ascites and jugular vein distention, hepatomegaly, and abnormal cardiac auscultation. Diagnosis of left-sided heart failure, however, requires a chest radiograph. Auscultatory pulmonary abnormalities during pulmonary edema are neither sensitive nor specific. A patient with dyspnea, cough, or pulmonary crackles, even with abnormal heart auscultation, may have respiratory signs caused by a primary respiratory disease. In cats, chest radiographs are useful in diagnosing both right- and left-sided CHF.

WHY DOES A PATIENT DEVELOP CLINICAL SIGNS OF CONGESTIVE HEART FAILURE?

CHF is a progressive disease, and systolic or diastolic function is eventually compromised to a degree that heart failure is inevitable. One should not conclude, however, that recent development or worsening of clinical signs is due to disease progression. In many patients, a precipitating factor for the CHF can be found and may not necessarily be related to the heart itself. Lack of client compliance is a common cause of treatment failure. Clients should be carefully questioned about the medications being used. Treatment of heart failure usually requires multiple drugs. Confusion about proper use of the medications is not uncommon. Doses employed, frequency and route of administration, and use of the proper formulation should be verified. Furthermore, the possibility that a person different from the owner (e.g., a dog sitter) may have been temporarily responsible for the dog should also be investigated. Inappropriate reduction of therapy is the most common reason for sudden worsening of the clinical condition in human patients with CHF. In small animal practice, inappropriate therapy is more likely when someone who is not completely familiar with the patient's clinical condition is caring for the dog or cat or when the patient goes through a long period without clinical signs and it is assumed to be "cured."

Development of complications is an important precipitating factor for CHF in small animal medicine. Extracardiac complications that pose an extra load on the cardiovascular system may induce CHF in patients with heart disease. Conditions that lead to a hyperdynamic circulation (e.g., anemia, hyperthyroidism, infections, fever) increase MVo_2 and sympathetic tone. Systemic arterial hypertension causes an increase in afterload that has a devastating effect in a failing myocardium. Systemic hypertension also increases regurgitant fraction in patients with aortic and mitral regurgitation. Physical, environmental, and emotional stress may also lead to CHF. A second unrelated disease may affect cardiac function indirectly. Renal failure potentially causes hypertension and may interfere with sodium excretion and exacerbate CHF.

A common cause of sudden decompensation of CHF is a cardiac complication. The two most common cardiac complications leading to CHF are development of mitral regurgitation and arrhythmias. Mitral regurgitation may suddenly develop because of dilatation of the mitral annulus in patients with dilated cardiomyopathy or because of the Venturi effect in cats with hypertrophic cardiomyopathy. The most devastating cause of acute worsening of mitral regurgitation leading to CHF, however, is the rupture of chordae tendineae that occurs in dogs with mitral endocardiosis. Sudden appearance of atrial fibrillation is a common cause of precipitation of CHF in dogs with dilated cardiomyopathy or mitral endocardiosis. Progression of the cardiac disease, usually with development of myocardial failure, eventually leads to the appearance of signs of CHF in patients with heart disease.

HOW CAN WE CLINICALLY EVALUATE HEART FUNCTION?

Is Heart Failure Present?

Heart disease is not synonymous with heart failure. A patient may be presented with a heart murmur or gallop or even have myocardial failure and may not necessarily be in CHF. To facilitate characterization of the severity of heart failure, functional classifications based on clinical signs at rest have been proposed (Table 110–7).[56] The presence of heart failure may be suspected during physical examination. Right-sided CHF is a clinical diagnosis based on jugular distention and pulsation, presence of ascites (dogs) and pleural effusion (cats, usually indicating bilateral failure), and peripheral edema. Diagnosis is confirmed by showing elevation of central venous pressure or more loosely by observing a large right heart on radiographs or echocardiography. Left-sided heart failure is a radiographic diagnosis that can be suspected in patients with dyspnea and abnormal respiratory sounds. It can be confirmed by showing elevation of the pulmonary capillary wedge pressure, but identifying pulmonary edema in association with left-heart enlargement would suffice from a clinical standpoint.

Some clinical findings may be helpful, providing indications of cardiovascular function. Gallop rhythms suggest the presence of ventricular dysfunction. The fourth heart sound (S_4 gallop) occurs during late diastole and represents atrial contraction. An S_4 gallop is associated with elevated ventricular end-diastolic pressure related to a decrease in ventricular compliance. An early diastolic filling sound (S_3 gallop) may occur during ventricular dysfunction of any cause and is a sensitive indication of ventricular dysfunction. Increased in loudness and splitting of the second heart sound suggest the presence of pulmonary hypertension. A distended and sometimes pulsating jugular vein suggests that right atrial pressure is elevated and the patient is in right-sided heart failure.

What Test Should Be Selected?

Laboratory examination is used to confirm the presence and cause of the heart disease, the presence and severity of the CHF and ventricular dysfunction, and presence of complications. Some tests are useful for diagnosing specific conditions and may offer no information regarding cardiovascular function, whereas others may assess only function or offer a combination of functional and diagnostic information. In addition to physical examination, confirmation of the exact cause of CHF by a combination of radiographic, electrocardiographic, echocardiographic, and laboratory examination is usually necessary. Echocardiography is helpful in determining the disease leading to CHF.

Electrocardiography can be used to evaluate heart rhythm but provides only indirect information regarding cardiovascular function. Arrhythmias may be due to heart disease but may also result from noncardiac causes. The electrocardiogram provides no definitive criteria for diagnosing heart failure. It may, however, contribute to the diagnosis (e.g., decreased QRS voltage and electrical alternans in pericardial effusion). One should bear in mind that a normal electrocardiogram does not rule out CHF or heart disease.

Chest radiographs are an important test in patients suspected to have heart disease. Changes in cardiac size and shape may show compensatory effects in the heart (cardiomegaly) and be helpful in determining the cause of CHF in dogs. Unfortunately, in cats, chest radiographs do not discriminate among the different myocardial diseases that may lead to heart failure and echocardiography is usually necessary. Chest radiographs are of paramount importance in determining the presence of left-sided CHF (pulmonary venous congestion, pulmonary interstitial or alveolar edema). They are also useful for visualizing pleural effusion in patients with CHF.

Echocardiographic examination is extremely helpful in determining the cause of CHF. There are no echocardiographic criteria for diagnosing CHF, but it is uncommon to see left-sided CHF without echocardiographic abnormalities such as left atrial enlargement in left-sided CHF and right-atrial enlargement or pericardial effusion in right-sided CHF.

Echocardiography, measurement of arterial blood pressure, and cardiac catheterization may all provide useful information about cardiovascular function. Cardiac catheterization has been used less and less, because most of the information provided by cardiac catheterization can now be obtained noninvasively and without the need to anesthetize the patient. Pressures behind the pumping chambers are useful for estimating ventricular filling pressures. Central venous pressure can be measured with a water- or saline-filled catheter placed in the cranial vena cava or right atrium. Central venous pressure provides an estimate of right ventricular end-diastolic pressure. Pulmonary capillary wedge pressure is obtained by placing a balloon-tipped (Swan-Ganz) catheter in the pulmonary artery and inflating the balloon to wedge the catheter tip and record the pressure. Pulmonary capillary wedge pressure provides an estimate of left ventricular end-diastolic pressure. Clinically speaking,

---

TABLE 110–7. FUNCTIONAL CLASSIFICATION OF HEART FAILURE

Modified from the New York Heart Association classification*
  I. Normal activity does not produce undue fatigue, dyspnea, or coughing.
 II. The dog or cat is comfortable at rest, but ordinary physical activity causes fatigue, dyspnea, or coughing.
III. The dog or cat is comfortable at rest, but minimal exercise may produce fatigue, dyspnea, or coughing. Signs may also develop while the patient is in a recumbent position (orthopnea).
 IV. Congestive heart failure, dyspnea, and coughing are present even when the dog or cat is at rest. Signs are exaggerated by any physical activity.
International Small Animal Cardiac Health Council†
  I. Asymptomatic patient
    Ia. Signs of heart disease but no cardiomegaly
    Ib. Signs of heart disease and evidence of compensation (cardiomegaly)
 II. Mild to moderate heart failure
    Clinical signs of heart failure are evident at rest or with mild exercise and adversely affect the quality of life.
III. Advanced heart failure
    Clinical signs of congestive heart failure are immediately obvious.
    III.a. Home care is possible.
    III.b. Hospitalization is recommended (cardiogenic shock, life-threatening edema, large pleural effusion, refractory ascites).

   * Adapted from Ettinger SJ, Suter PF: The recognition of cardiac disease and congestive heart failure. In Ettinger SJ, Suter PF (eds): Canine Cardiology. Philadelphia, WB Saunders, 1970, p 215.
   † Adapted from International Small Animal Cardiac Health Council: Recommendations for the diagnosis of heart disease and the treatment of heart failure in small animals. In Miller MS, Tilley LP (eds): Manual of Canine and Feline Cardiology. Philadelphia, WB Saunders, 1995, p 473.

CHF is evidenced by the presence of increased ventricular filling (end-diastolic) pressures.[57]

Several indices are available to evaluate systolic and diastolic function in intact animals. The plethora of indices (see Table 110–8 for a partial list) to evaluate systolic and diastolic function in intact animals probably reflects the fact that no index is really good. Only indices that are clinically useful are discussed here.

Systolic Function

Systolic function is assessed by evaluating the determinants of stroke volume (preload, afterload, and contractility) and indices of global ventricular systolic performance. To evaluate cardiac function, many indices require knowledge of the left ventricular volume or stroke volume. Left ventricular volume can be estimated echocardiographically or by angiography. The echocardiogram provides a good estimate of left ventricular volume noninvasively in dogs[58] and is economically feasible. Two-dimensional echocardiography

TABLE 110–8. SOME HEMODYNAMIC INDICES USED TO EVALUATE CARDIOVASCULAR FUNCTION

Pressure behind the pumping chamber
  Left or right ventricular end-diastolic pressure*
  Pulmonary capillary wedge pressure* (left side)
  Central venous pressure (right side)
Systolic function
  Preload
    LV volume
    LV end-diastolic pressure*
  Afterload
    Aortic input impedance*
    Effective arterial elastance
    Systemic vascular resistance
    Arterial blood pressure
  Contractility
    Isovolumic indices
      dP/dt_{MAX} and derived indices*
    Pressure-volume indices
      Preload recruitable stroke work*
      $dP/dt - EDV$ relation*
      End-systolic elastance*
  Integrated systolic function
    Systolic time intervals
    Ejection fraction
    Fractional shortening
    End-systolic volume index
    Mean normalized systolic ejection rate
    Mean velocity of circumferential fiber shortening
    Stroke work*
Diastolic function
  Diastolic time intervals
    Isovolumic relaxation period
  Flow and volume measurements
    Transmitral valve flow profile
    Transmitral filling fractions
    Filling fraction
    Peak filling rate
    dV/dt
  Other echocardiogram-derived indices
    Rate of change in wall thickness
    Rate of wall relaxation
    Relaxation half-time
  Pressure-derived isovolumic relaxation
    dP/dt_{MIN}*
    Time constant of relaxation* (τ)
  Pressure-volume indices
    End-diastolic pressure-volume relationship*
    Chamber stiffness*

*Require cardiac catheterization to be measured properly.
LV = left ventricular; EDV = end-diastolic volume.

is superior to M-mode echocardiography in estimating left ventricular volume in dogs.[59] Stroke volume can also be obtained by two-dimensional echocardiography (end-diastolic volume − end-systolic volume)[58] or preferentially by Doppler echocardiography. Using Doppler echocardiography, stroke volume can be determined from the average velocity of blood flow across the aorta or pulmonary artery multiplied by the cross-sectional area of the respective valve orifice.[60]

Preload

Left ventricular volume is the best clinical approximation of preload. M mode–based models for evaluating left ventricular volume are associated with unacceptably high variation, especially for end-diastolic volume. Whenever possible, left ventricular volume should be estimated with two-dimensional echocardiography, using Simpson's rule or the cylinder–truncated cone–cone method.[59] Alternatively, preload can be estimated as being equal to left ventricular end-diastolic pressure on the basis of the relationship between left ventricular pressure and volume. Pressure cannot be used instead of volume to estimate preload in stiff or noncompliant ventricles.

Afterload

Ideally, afterload should be measured as the aortic input impedance. Measurement of the impedance is not clinically feasible. An alternative is to use the effective arterial elastance (Ea). The Ea is a steady-state arterial parameter that incorporates the principal elements of vascular load including peripheral resistance, total vascular compliance, characteristic impedance, and systolic and diastolic time intervals. The Ea is obtained from the ratio end-systolic pressure to stroke volume.[8] To avoid the need for cardiac catheterization, mean femoral artery pressure can be used as an estimate of left ventricular end-systolic pressure.[61] Changes in Ea show a high correlation with changes in input impedance. Peripheral resistance is another option for estimating left ventricular afterload, but it accounts for only the opposition to steady flow and not the opposition to pulsatile flow. Peripheral vascular resistance can be calculated using cardiac output (CO), mean aortic pressure (MAP), and venous pressure (VP) as

$$SVR = 80 \times (MAP - VP)/CO$$

Arterial blood pressure can be used as a simple and noninvasive way to assess the opposition to left ventricular ejection. In CHF, however, there is an association between decreased cardiac output and increase in afterload. Because arterial blood pressure is dependent on both factors, it does not provide an adequate evaluation of left ventricular afterload.[62] Nevertheless, it is important to know whether a patient with CHF also has systemic hypertension. Arterial blood pressure may also be important in monitoring vasodilator therapy during CHF.

Contractility

Contractility is hard to define and even harder to measure without interference from preload and afterload. Ventricular contraction has an isovolumic phase and an ejection phase. Isovolumic indices evaluate only the isovolumic contraction phase but are less affected by load changes. Ejection phase indices are so affected by changes in afterload and preload that they reflect not the contractility but the integrated systolic function. Indices based on the pressure-volume relationship are relatively load independent and are probably the best indices for evaluating contractility in intact animals. However, they are not routinely used clinically and are beyond the scope of this chapter.

The most commonly used isovolumic index for evaluating cardiac contractility is the maximum rate of pressure rise (dP/dt_{MAX}). dP/dt_{MAX} is the tangent to the maximum slope of the ascending portion of the left ventricular pressure curve and therefore can be obtained only with left ventricular catheterization. dP/dt_{MAX} is influenced by preload (and to a lesser extent by afterload) and cannot be used in the presence of valvular regurgitation. It is a sensitive index of contractility but is not specific because of its load dependence. Many other indices based on dP/dt have been developed, but they have roughly the same limitations as dP/dt_{MAX}.

Integrated Left Ventricular Systolic Function

Indices of left ventricular function that evaluate global systolic function can be based on systolic time intervals, left ventricular volume, diameter, or flow characteristics.

Systolic time intervals can be used to evaluate integrated systolic function. The most commonly used systolic time intervals are the left ventricular ejection time (LVET) and the preejection period (PEP). The PEP corresponds to the electrical-mechanical interval plus the pressure rise time (onset of QRS to the opening of the aortic valve). It is influenced by changes in afterload, preload, and contractility. The LVET (opening to closing of the aortic valve) is affected by heart rate and contractility and only mildly affected by preload and afterload. The information necessary to determine PEP and LVET can be obtained with an electrocardiogram, phonocardiogram, and arterial pressure curve or M-mode echocardiogram of the aortic valve. The PEP/LVET ratio is independent of heart rate and inversely related to systolic function.[63]

Ejection fraction (stroke volume/end-diastolic volume) and fractional shortening ([end-diastolic dimension − end-systolic dimension]/end-diastolic dimension) are two indices of systolic function expressed as a percentage. They are sensitive and easy to measure using echocardiography but unfortunately they are influenced by changes in load. In addition, the low correlation between M mode–derived volumes and the true left ventricular end-diastolic volume[59] probably renders the ejection fraction obtained using M-mode echocardiography inaccurate. The left ventricle must also be contracting uniformly and the ultrasound beam must be parallel to the short axis of the ventricle for an M mode–derived volume to be representative of global ventricular function.

M-mode imaging of the left ventricle may be obtained using short- or long-axis views of the heart. When recording an M-mode image of the left ventricle, it is important to be in the center of the left ventricle, perpendicular to the left ventricular wall, and with the ultrasound beam just below the mitral valve. The short-axis view allows better centering of the beam in the heart, whereas the long-axis view is preferred to ensure that the beam is perpendicular to the wall. Either plan can be used to place the beam below the mitral valve. Choosing the view (short-axis versus long-axis or both) to obtain M-mode measurements of fractional shortening in dogs and cats remains a matter of personal preference.

Fractional shortening in dogs is also affected by body size, being smaller in giant-breed dogs. The end-systolic

volume index is the left ventricular volume obtained by M mode indexed to the body surface. It has been used in dogs,[64] but it is also dependent on afterload and M-mode estimation of left ventricular volume. The mean normalized systolic ejection rate (ejection fraction/duration of ejection) has theoretical advantages over the ejection fraction by relating ejection fraction to muscle shortening velocity. Mean normalized systolic ejection fraction has, however, proved less useful than the ejection fraction. The mean velocity of circumferential fiber shortening (fractional shortening/duration of ejection) is similar to the mean normalized systolic ejection rate except that it is calculated using fractional shortening instead of ejection fraction. It therefore has the same limitations as the mean normalized systolic ejection rate. Stroke work or the total mechanical energy expended during a cardiac cycle may also be used in assessing systolic function. Unfortunately, it is also affected by load conditions. Time to aortic peak velocity can be obtained by Doppler echocardiography and correlates well with global systolic function. It is, like all ejection indices, affected by changes in afterload.

Diastolic Function

Diastolic function is harder to evaluate noninvasively than systolic function. The information gathered is semiquantitative and is affected by many factors that affect ventricular filling. Some indices of diastolic function assess the ventricular function during a specific phase, whereas others evaluate "global" performance during diastole. Doppler echocardiography remains the primary technique for assessing diastolic function noninvasively.

Diastolic time intervals can be used to evaluate diastolic properties. The most commonly used diastolic time interval is the isovolumic relaxation period, which is the time from aortic valve closure to mitral valve opening when the left ventricular volume is constant. It is a relaxation index and can be obtained from phonocardiography (for aortic closure) and M-mode echocardiography (to mitral opening) or from Doppler echocardiography (time from cessation of aortic flow to commencement of transmitral flow). Unfortunately, the rate of decline in left ventricular pressure is only one of the several factors that determine this period. Aortic diastolic pressure and left atrial pressure affect the duration of this period. Isovolumic relaxation time cannot be used in patients with aortic or mitral regurgitation because there is no true isovolumic period.

Doppler echocardiogram–derived changes in blood flow can be used to evaluate diastolic function. Many indices have been proposed, but the ones based on the transmitral valve flow profile (E and A waves) are more commonly used. The E wave represents early ventricular filling and precedes the A wave (atrial filling wave). The E wave is normally larger than the A wave (E/A ratio usually greater than 1). During fast heart rates, especially in cats, E and A waves are often fused and the E/A ratio cannot be evaluated. Increase in size of the A wave and decrease in the E wave occur in patients with relaxation abnormalities. Unfortunately, with progression of the disease and increase in left ventricular end-diastolic pressure, presence of mitral regurgitation, and increase in left atrial pressure, there is a pseudonormalization of the E and A waves. Patients with restrictive diseases tend to have smaller A waves and larger E waves. Filling fractions can also be estimated with the transmitral flow by calculating the velocity time integral for both waves.

M-mode echocardiography can also be used to evaluate diastolic function. Rate of change in wall thickness, rate of wall relaxation, and relaxation half-time can be obtained with an M-mode echocardiogram (ideally digitized echocardiogram). The peak rate of posterior wall motion has also been used, but this measurement is susceptible to distortion because of translational motion.

Hemodynamic indices using pressure rather than volume have been used to evaluate the diastolic function. They all require cardiac catheterization. The peak negative dP/dt measures the maximal rate of decline of left ventricular pressure during relaxation and is usually taken as the lowest value of the first derivative of this pressure. It usually occurs around the time of aortic closure. It should be remembered that peak negative dP/dt occurs at one time point and does not represent the totality of events even during relaxation only. In addition, peak minimum dP/dt is highly dependent on left ventricular and aortic systolic pressure.

Integrated Function

Cardiac output is considered a measure of integrated cardiovascular performance. Cardiac output is usually measured by thermodilution, a technique based on the indicator dilution method.[65] Thermodilution offers advantages because it does not require arterial puncture or blood to be withdrawn, and an inert and inexpensive indicator, cold saline or 5% dextrose in water, is used with virtually no recirculation.[65] All indicator techniques, however, require a catheter placed in the pulmonary artery, making them impractical for routine use in clinical veterinary medicine outside critical care units. Doppler echocardiography can also be used to estimate cardiac output. Stroke volume can be determined from the average velocity of blood flow across the aorta or pulmonary artery multiplied by the cross-sectional area of the respective valve orifice.[60] Doppler determination of blood flow velocity is a noninvasive method that can be performed in awake, untrained, dogs.[66] It is useful for documenting beat-to-beat variations in stroke volume in dogs[67] and can be used to determine cardiac output when stroke volume is multiplied by the heart rate. As with thermodilution determination of cardiac output, Doppler-derived values for cardiac outputs are variable.[68] Cardiac outputs obtained by Doppler echocardiography and thermodilution show an excellent correlation,[69] but the technique for obtaining cardiac output by echocardiography appears to be quite operator dependent. It should be remembered that cardiac output at rest is not a sensitive indicator of heart function during CHF because all compensatory mechanisms act to increase cardiac output.

WHAT TESTS SHOULD I USE IN A CLINICAL PATIENT?

Of all the tests available for evaluating cardiovascular function, a few are routinely used. Chest radiography and echocardiography are performed in virtually all patients with CHF. Measurements of arterial blood pressure and central venous pressure can be easily performed and provide important information regarding cardiovascular status. Not surprisingly, the most commonly used tests of cardiovascular function are based on echocardiography, whereas chest radiographs are used to confirm left-sided CHF. In the majority of patients, systolic performance is assessed by either fractional shortening, ejection fraction, or end-systolic volume index. No clinical comparison of these indices in small animals has been performed. Choosing the index is a matter of personal preference. In selected patients, aortic velocity,

time to peak aortic velocity, and cardiac output can be measured using Doppler echocardiography. Diastolic performance is usually assessed by Doppler evaluation of transmitral flow. For patients undergoing cardiac catheterization, among other measurements, pressure traces, dP/dt$_{MAX}$, cardiac output, and estimated systemic vascular resistance can be obtained.

HOW DOES HEART FAILURE BECOME A PROGRESSIVE DISEASE?

THE VICIOUS CYCLES IN CONGESTIVE HEART FAILURE

Compensatory mechanisms activated during heart failure have the paradoxical role of serving simultaneously as adaptive, compensatory changes and as major contributing elements to the progression of CHF by causing myocardial cell death. Cell death in an overloaded heart adds further to the overload on surviving myocytes in a vicious cycle. There are three main interlocked vicious cycles that ultimately result in myocardial cell death (Fig. 110–12).

Increase in Left Ventricular Afterload and MVo₂ (Cycle 1)

Vasoconstriction and increases in cardiac contractility and heart rate help to maintain blood pressure but increase MVo₂. Increasing cardiac MVo₂ accelerates myocardial cell death. Wall stress (a function of afterload), contractility, and heart rate are the main determinants of MVo₂. Myocardial hypertrophy decreases the oxygen consumption by decreasing wall stress during ejection. Hypertrophy caused by increases in load, however, does not yield a normal heart. Load-induced hypertrophy sets the stage for myocardial death (see later). Increase in afterload leads to further left ventricular dysfunction, and the patient spirals down vicious cycle 1 until it reaches a new, decreased steady-state level, where the cardiac output is lower and vasoconstriction higher than is optimal for the patient.

Sodium and Water Retention and Increased Left Atrial Pressure (Cycle 2)

Sodium and water retention increase circulating volume, increasing preload and left atrial pressure. Increase in preload increases cardiac output, helps to maintain filling pressures, but also leads to signs of congestion and edema. Excessive preload increases ventricular pressures, volume, and wall stress, also adding to deterioration of left ventricular function.

Left Ventricular and Vascular Remodeling (Cycle 3)

Stretching of myocardium resulting from overload seems to be the initiating signal for an adaptive process in the myocardium to begin. This leads to hypertrophy through growth factor and proto-oncogene stimulation.[44, 47] Hypertrophy unloads the cells of the failing heart by adding new sarcomeres and also increases contractility and cardiac output. Unfortunately, hypertrophy ultimately leads to cellular abnormalities that result in mitochondrial DNA abnormalities and apoptosis (programmed cell death), hastening myocardial cell death.[47] Chronic neurohumoral activation, espe-

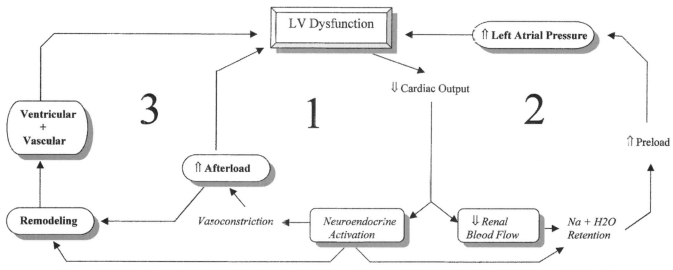

Figure 110–12. Interlocked vicious cycle in congestive heart failure: increased afterload (cycle 1), increased left atrial pressure (cycle 2), and ventricular and vascular remodeling (cycle 3). LV = left ventricle.

CV

cially increases in angiotensin II and norepinephrine, and increases in afterload lead to left ventricular and vascular remodeling (cycle 3). Globally, the remodeling process in the ventricle is characterized by progressive left ventricular enlargement and increased chamber sphericity. At the cellular level, the remodeling process is associated with myocyte slippage, hypertrophy, and accumulation of collagen in the interstitial compartment. The final result of this process is the so-called cardiomyopathy of overload. Angiotensin II also causes vascular remodeling leading to hypertrophy of smooth muscle cells of the vessel walls.[70] Vascular remodeling decreases vessel compliance and therefore increases ventricular afterload.

Cardiomyopathy of Overload

Long-term overload hypertrophy in the heart is accompanied by myocardial cell death and cardiac fibrosis. This abnormal, progressive, and eventually lethal growth abnormality has been called cardiomyopathy of overload.[22, -7, 71] In embryonic hearts, growth factors induce protein synthesis, leading to normal cell division. Early after the animal is born, cardiac myocytes withdraw from the cell cycle and can no longer divide, and protein synthesis is slowed to rates appropriate to maintain and repair the cells.[47] Stimulation of growth factors by chronic overload leads to an increase in protein synthesis. The cell cycle, however, remains blocked and the end result is not normal cell division but abnormal hypertrophy. Increases in angiotensin II, a peptide that is not only a vasoconstrictor but also a mitogen, appear to be an important mediator of reversal of inhibition of protein synthesis in the adult heart.

Overload-induced hypertrophy leads to an state of chronic energy starvation in the heart. The increase in cardiac mass is not accompanied by an increase in capillary vessels. The hypertrophied ventricle therefore outstrips its blood supply.[13] The cell volume occupied by sarcomeres increases, leading to an increased ratio of mitochondria to myofibrils, which can exacerbate the energy deficit. The net result is a decrease in capillary density and coronary reserve with the myocardium becoming prone to ischemia, especially in the subendocardium.[72] The relative decrease in oxygen delivery complicates the increased needs for oxygen of the failing heart,

which are already increased by vasoconstriction and sympathetic activation. There is a close link between hypertrophy and increasing systolic dysfunction.[14] The ischemia resulting from hypertrophy leads to development of focal fibrosis, which increases myocardial collagen content.[15] The early increase in collagen helps to maintain systolic function but interferes with diastolic function. With progression of the myocardial hypertrophy, the early interstitial fibrosis progresses to perimuscular fibrosis, impairing both systolic and diastolic function.[15] Myocardial cell necrosis occurs in overloaded hearts in the transition to heart failure. It has been suggested that myocyte cell death results not from necrosis (accidental cell death) but from apoptosis (programmed cell death).[47] Activation of proto-oncogenes and increased concentrations of TGF-β_1 that occur in CHF may induce apoptosis. Regardless of the cause, myocardial cell death occurs in overload hypertrophy, increasing the overload of the surviving myocytes in a vicious cycle (cycle 3). Cardiomyopathy of overload therefore represents an unnatural growth of the adult heart leading to myocardial cell death, progression of myocardial failure, and death.

SUMMARY

Heart failure is a state wherein the cardiac output is inadequate to meet the perfusion needs of the metabolizing tissues and exercise capacity is limited. It may result from inability of the heart to eject blood properly (systolic failure) or from inadequate ventricular filling (diastolic failure). Correct identification of the cause of heart disease and the mechanism leading to heart failure allows the clinician to choose the appropriate therapy, improving the prognosis.

Regardless of the mechanism, CHF is associated with a fall in blood pressure and activation of compensatory mechanisms that are aimed at restoring normal arterial blood pressure. These mechanisms include neurohumoral activation and renal retention of sodium and water. Vasoconstriction, tachycardia, and volume retention are the initial responses of circulation to the fall in blood pressure. An excessive compensatory response may lead to overcompensation, and compensatory mechanisms that are beneficial in the beginning become responsible for the development of clinical signs.

Therapy is aimed at modulation of the excessively activated compensatory mechanisms. The inciting cause of cardiac dysfunction and the neurohumoral activation also stimulate myocardial compensation leading to increased contractility and relaxation, sympathetic desensitization, and unnatural growth (hypertrophy). Modulation of the unnatural growth response with drugs that have growth inhibitory as well as vasodilatory properties (angiotensin-converting enzyme inhibitors and nitrates) may delay the appearance of cardiomyopathy of overload and improve the prognosis of patients with CHF. Myocyte changes determined by overload-induced hypertrophy ultimately lead to myocardial cell death, which further compromises myocardial function. Thus, once a certain point of myocardial dysfunction is reached, CHF becomes a progressive, irreversible disease.

REFERENCES

1. Colucci WS, Braunwald E: Pathophysiology of heart failure *In* Braunwald E (ed): Heart Disease. Philadelphia, WB Saunders, 1997, pp 394–420.
2. Katz AM: Physiology of the Heart, 2nd ed. New York, Raven Press, 1992.
3. Braunwald E, Ross J Jr: Control of cardiac performance. *In* Berne R, Sperelakis N, Geiser SR (eds): Handbook of Physiology, Section 2: The Cardiovascular System. Washington, DC, American Physiological Society, 1979, pp 533–580.
4. Nichols WW, Pepine CJ: Left ventricular afterload and aortic input impedance: Implications to pulsatile blood flow. Prog Cardiovasc Dis 24:293–306, 1982.
5. de Morais HSA: Resistance, impedance, compliance and reflectance or what is the load after the heart. Proceedings of the XIV Annual Forum of the American College of Veterinary Internal Medicine, 1996, pp 230–232.
6. Opie LH: The Heart: Physiology and Metabolism, 2nd ed. New York, Raven Press, 1991.
7. Westerhof N, Elzinga G, Sipkema P: An artificial arterial system for the pumping heart. J Appl Physiol 31:776–781, 1971.
8. Kelly RP, Ting CT, Yang TM, et al: Effective arterial elastance as index of arterial vascular load in humans. Circulation 86:513–521, 1992.
9. Fitchett DH: LV-arterial coupling: Interactive model to predict effect of wave reflections on LV energetics. Am J Physiol 261:H1026–H1033, 1991.
10. Elzinga G, Westerhof N: Pressure and flow generated by the left ventricle against different impedances. Circ Res 32:178–185, 1973.
11. O'Rourke MF, Avolio AP, Nichols WW: Coupling in health and disease. *In* Yin FCP (ed): Ventricular/Vascular Coupling. New York, Springer-Verlag, 1987, pp 1–19.
12. Sunagawa K, Maughan WL, Sagawa K: Optimal arterial resistance for the maximal stroke work studied in isolated canine left ventricle. Circ Res 56:586–595, 1985.
13. Opie LH: Compensation and overcompensation in congestive heart failure. Am Heart J 120:1552–1557, 1990.
14. Douglas PS, Berko B, Lesh M, et al: Alterations in diastolic function in response to progressive left ventricular hypertrophy. J Am Coll Cardiol 13:461–467, 1989.
15. Weber KT: Cardiac interstitium in health and disease: the fibrillar collagen network. J Am Coll Cardiol 13:1637–1652, 1989.
16. Caulfield JB, Norton P, Weager RD: Cardiac dilation associated with collagen alterations. Mol Cell Biochem 118:171–179, 1992.
17. Brower GL, Berry JRWD, Janicki JS: Pharmacological inhibition of mast cell degradation prevents ventricular remodeling secondary to chronic volume overload. Circulation 96(Suppl):I519–I521, 1997.
18. Lenihan JL, Gerson MC, Hoit BD, et al: Mechanisms, diagnosis, and treatment of diastolic heart failure. Am Heart J 130:153–166, 1995.
19. Katz AM: Influence of altered inotropy and lusitropy on ventricular pressure-volume loops. J Am Coll Cardiol 11:438–445, 1988.
20. Cheng CP, Freeman GL, Santamore WP, et al: Effect of loading conditions, contractile state, and heart rate on early diastolic filling in conscious dogs. Circ Res 66:814–823, 1990.
21. Miura T, Miyazaki S, Guth BD, et al: Heart rate and force-frequency effects on diastolic function of the left ventricle in exercising dogs. Circulation 89:2361–2368, 1994.
22. Katz AM: Cardiomyopathy of overload: A major determinant of prognosis in congestive heart failure. N Engl J Med 322:100–110, 1990.
23. Ware WA, Lund DD, Subieta AR, et al: Sympathetic activation in dogs with congestive heart failure caused by chronic mitral valve disease and dilated cardiomyopathy. JAVMA 197:1475–1481, 1990.
24. Harris P: Congestive cardiac failure: Central role of the arterial blood pressure. Br Heart J 58:190–203, 1987.
25. Clark AL, Poole-Wilson PA, Coats AJS: Exercise limitation in chronic heart failure: A central role for the periphery. J Am Coll Cardiol 28:1092–1102, 1996.
26. Chua TP, Ponikowski P, Webb-Peploe K, et al: Clinical characteristics of chronic heart failure patients with an augmented peripheral chemoreflex. Eur Heart J 18:480–486, 1997.
27. Ponikowski P, Chua TP, Piepoli M, et al: Augmented peripheral chemosensitivity as a potential input to baroreflex impairment and autonomic imbalance in chronic heart failure. Circulation 96:2586–2594, 1997.
28. Ponikowski P, Chua TP, Piepoli M, et al: Ventilatory response to exercise correlates with impaired heart rate variability in patients with chronic congestive heart failure. Am J Cardiol 82:338–344, 1998.
29. Teerlink JR: Neurohumoral mechanisms in heart failure: A central role for the renin-angiotensin system. J Cardiovasc Pharmacol 27(Suppl 2):S1–S8, 1996.
30. Zannad F: Aldosterone and heart failure. Eur Heart J 16(Suppl N):98–102, 1995.
31. Margulies KB, Hildebrand FL Jr, Lerman A, et al: Increased endothelin in experimental heart failure. Circulation 82:2226–2230, 1990.
32. Yazaki Y, Yamazaki T: Reversing congestive heart failure with endothelin receptor antagonists. Circulation 95:1752–1754, 1997.
33. Ohnishi M, Wada A, Tsutamoto T, et al: Chronic effects of a novel, orally active endothelin receptor antagonist, T-0201, in dogs with congestive heart failure. J Cardiovasc Pharmacol 31(Suppl 1):S236–S238, 1998.
34. Mancia G: Neurohumoral activation in congestive heart failure. Am Heart J 120:1532–1537, 1990.
35. Hornig B: Importance of endothelial function in chronic heart failure. J Cardiovasc Pharmacol 27(Suppl 2):S9–S11, 1996.
36. Eaton GE, Cody RJ, Binkley PF: Increase in aortic impedance precedes peripheral vasoconstriction at the early stage of ventricular failure in the paced canine model. Circulation 88:2714–2721, 1993.
37. Häggström J, Hansson K, Kvart C, et al: Effects of naturally acquired decompensated mitral valve regurgitation in the renin-angiotensin-aldosterone system and atrial natriuretic peptide concentration in dogs. Am J Vet Res 58:77–82, 1997.
38. Pedersen HD, Koch J, Poulsen K, et al: Activation of the renin-angiotensin system in dogs with asymptomatic and mildly symptomatic mitral valvular insufficiency. J Vet Intern Med 9:328–331, 1995.
39. Katz SD: The role of endothelium-derived vasoactive substances in the pathophysiology of exercise intolerance in patients with congestive heart failure. Prog Cardiovasc Dis 38:23–50, 1995.
40. Parmley W: Neuroendocrine changes in heart failure and their clinical relevance. Clin Cardiol 18:440–445, 1995.
41. Delehanty JM, Liang C: Metabolic control of the circulation: Implications for congestive heart failure. Prog Cardiovasc Dis 38:51–66, 1995.
42. Häggström J, Hamlin RL, Hansson K, et al: Heart rate variability in relation to severity of mitral regurgitation in Cavalier King Charles spaniels. J Small Anim Pract 37:69–75, 1996.
43. Wilke A, Funck R, Rupp H, et al: Effect of the renin-angiotensin-aldosterone system in the cardiac interstitium in heart failure. Basic Res Cardiol 91(Suppl 2):79–84, 1996.
44. Stys T, Stys A, Mallis G: Pathogenesis of congestive heart failure from compensation to decompensation. Coron Artery Dis 13:27–30, 1996.
45. Hoit BD, Shao Y, Gabel M, et al: Left atrial systolic and diastolic function after cessation of pacing in tachycardia-induced heart failure. Am J Physiol 273:H921–H927, 1997.
46. Williams RE, Kass DA, Kawagoe Y, et al: Endomyocardial gene expression during development of pacing tachycardia-induced heart failure in the dog. Circ Res 75:615–623, 1994.
47. Katz AM: The cardiomyopathy of overload: An unnatural growth response in the hypertrophied heart. Ann Intern Med 121:363–371, 1994.
48. Bonagura JD, Lemkuhl LB: Fluid and diuretic therapy in heart failure. *In* DiBartola SP (ed): Fluid Therapy in Small Animal Practice. Philadelphia, WB Saunders, 1992, pp 529–553.
49. Wisenbaugh T, O'Connor WN: Right ventricular hypertrophy long after reversal of severe pressure overload in cats. Am J Physiol 254:H1099–H1104, 1988.
50. Wiener-Kronish JP, Goldstein R, Matthay RA, et al: Lack of association of pleural effusion with chronic pulmonary arterial and right atrial hypertension. Chest 92:967–970, 1987.
51. Green HJ: Manifestations and sites of neuromuscular fatigue. Biochem Exerc 66:142–150, 1990.
52. Freeman LM, Rush JE, Kehayias JJ, et al: Nutritional alterations and the effects of fish oil supplementation in dogs with heart failure. J Vet Intern Med 12:440–448, 1998.
53. Anker SD, Ponikowski P, Varney S, et al: Wasting as independent risk factor for mortality in chronic heart failure. Lancet 349:1050–1053, 1997.
54. Anker SD, Chua TP, Ponikowski P, et al: Hormonal changes and catabolic/anabolic imbalance in chronic heart failure and their importance for cardiac cachexia. Circulation 96:526–534, 1997.
55. Anker SD, Clark AL, Kemp M, et al: Tumor necrosis factor and steroid metabolism in chronic heart failure: Possible relation to muscle wasting. J Am Coll Cardiol 30:997–1001, 1997.
56. International Small Animal Cardiac Health Council: Recommendations for the diagnosis of heart disease and the treatment of heart failure in small animals *In* Miller MS, Tilley LP (eds): Manual of Canine and Feline Cardiology. Philadelphia, WB Saunders, 1995, pp 469–502.
57. Ross J Jr: Assessment of cardiac function and myocardial contractility. *In* Schlant RC, Alexander RW (eds): Hurst's the Heart, 8th ed. New York, McGraw-Hill, 1994, pp 487–502.
58. Sisson DD, Daniel GB, Twardock AR: Comparison of left ventricular ejection fractions determined in healthy anesthetized dogs by echocardiography and gated equilibrium radionuclide ventriculography. Am J Vet Res 50:1840–1847, 1989.
59. de Morais HSA, Bonagura JD, Muir WW, et al: Left ventricular volumes obtained by echocardiography in intact dogs: Validation using the conductance catheter (abstract). J Vet Intern Med 11:140, 1997.

60. Gardin JM: Doppler echocardiography. *In* Talamo JV, Gardin JM (eds): Textbook of Two-Dimensional Echocardiography. New York, Grune & Stratton, 1983, pp 325–355.
61. de Morais HSA, Muir WW, Bonagura JD: Can we evaluate ventriculo-arterial coupling without cardiac catheterization in dogs? 15th Annual Veterinary Medical Forum ACVIM, 1997, pp 210–211.
62. Little WC, Braunwald E: Assessment of cardiac function. *In* Braunwald E (ed): Heart Disease: A Textbook of Cardiovascular Medicine. Philadelphia, WB Saunders, 1997, pp 421–444.
63. Atkins CE, Snyder PS: Systolic time intervals and their derivatives for evaluation of cardiac function. J Vet Intern Med 6:55–63, 1992.
64. Kittleson MD, Eyster GE, Knowlen GG, et al: Myocardial function in small dogs with chronic mitral regurgitation and severe congestive heart failure. JAVMA 184:455–459, 1984.
65. Grossman W: Cardiac catheterization. *In* Braunwald E (ed): Heart Disease, 4th ed. Philadelphia, WB Saunders, 1992, pp 180–203.
66. Brown DJ, Knight DH, King RR: Use of pulsed-wave Doppler echocardiography

to determine aortic and pulmonary velocity and flow variables in clinically normal dogs. Am J Vet Res 52:543–550, 1991.
67. Steingart RM, Miller J, Barovick J: Pulse-Doppler echocardiographic measurement of beat-to-beat changes in stroke volume in dogs. Circulation 62:542–548, 1980.
68. Marshall SE, Weyman AE: Doppler estimation of volumetric flow. *In* Weyman AE (ed): Principles and Practice of Echocardiography, 2nd ed. Philadelphia, Lea & Febiger, 1994, pp 955–978.
69. de Morais HSA, Bonagura JD, Muir WW, et al: Comparison of cardiac output obtained by Doppler echocardiography, thermodilution, and conductance catheter technique (abstract). J Vet Intern Med 11:140, 1997.
70. Geisterfer AA, Peach MJ, Owens GK: Angiotensin II induces hypertrophy, not hyperplasia, of cultured rat aortic smooth muscle cells. Circ Res 62:749–756, 1988.
71. Katz AM: The cardiomyopathy of overload: An unnatural growth response. Eur Heart J 16(Suppl O):110–114, 1995.
72. Braunwald E: Pathophysiology of heart failure. *In* Braunwald E (ed): Heart Disease, 4th ed. Philadelphia, WB Saunders, 1992, pp 393–418.

CHAPTER 111

THERAPY OF HEART FAILURE

Mark D. Kittleson

GENERAL PRINCIPLES

Cardiovascular Function. The primary functions of the cardiovascular system are to maintain a normal blood pressure and cardiac output at normal capillary pressures. When the heart fails, it loses its ability to maintain these functions sequentially, first losing its ability to maintain a normal capillary pressure, then its ability to maintain a normal cardiac output, and last its ability to maintain a normal blood pressure. Consequently, signs of congestion, edema, and effusion occur first in chronic heart failure and are generally the most severe. Congestion and edema are so common in animals with chronic heart failure that the terms heart failure and congestive heart failure are often used synonymously.

Primary Aims. The primary aim of treating chronic heart failure is to reduce the formation of edema and effusion. Most animals with clinical signs referable to heart failure and most of those that die of chronic heart failure do so because of severe edema or effusion. Consequently, drugs that reduce edema formation are generally more efficacious than drugs that primarily increase cardiac output. In human patients with severe chronic heart failure, inability to return pulmonary capillary pressure to normal with drug therapy is an independent predictor of mortality, whereas low cardiac output and blood pressure are not.[1] In general, the diuretics are the most efficacious of any drug class, and the loop diuretics are the most efficacious diuretic type, although no controlled studies have been performed to prove this. The angiotensin-converting enzyme (ACE) inhibitors are the next most efficacious drugs in the general heart failure population. A secondary goal in chronic heart failure patients is to increase cardiac output.

Almost all heart failure treatments are palliative rather than curative. Consequently, most animals that develop heart failure die from it, often within a relatively short time. No studies have been performed in veterinary medicine to determine whether any cardiovascular drug prolongs life. Certainly, diuretics prolong life, and without their administration, most animals with severe heart failure would die before leaving the hospital. ACE inhibitors have been shown to prolong life in humans with heart failure, but this prolongation is modest, usually being measured in months rather than years. Digoxin has recently been shown not to prolong life in humans with heart failure.[2] Often of more importance is the effect cardiovascular drugs have on the quality of life. Diuretics and ACE inhibitors definitely improve the quality of life in dogs and cats with heart failure. When animals become refractory to these drugs, other drugs may help reduce edema formation and improve perfusion, thus reducing clinical signs and increasing comfort.

Heart Failure Categories. For the purposes of deciding drug therapy and drug doses, animals are categorized into those that have mild, moderate, or severe disease and mild, moderate, severe, fulminant, or refractory heart failure. All animals with heart failure have severe disease. Heart failure can be further subdivided into acute and chronic heart failure. Most animals with acute heart failure present in severe or fulminant heart failure and require intensive therapy with intravenously administered agents such as furosemide or nitroprusside with or without dobutamine. Chronic left heart failure is graded based on the severity of pulmonary edema on thoracic radiographs, and chronic right heart failure is graded based on hepatic vein size on ultrasound examination and amount of ascites present clinically or ultrasonographically. Increasingly severe chronic heart failure is treated with escalating doses of furosemide, whereas an ACE inhibitor is administered at a fixed dose. Digoxin may also be used, depending on the underlying disease and the stage of heart failure. Refractory heart failure is treated by adding a thiazide diuretic, a vasodilator such as hydralazine, or a nitrate, depending on the underlying disease and monitoring capabilities.

Standard Therapy. Most canine and many feline patients with heart failure are treated with a diuretic and an ACE inhibitor. Digoxin is also commonly used. The use of digoxin is not always indicated and in some situations is contraindicated. The digitalis glycosides are contraindicated in animals with hypertrophic cardiomyopathy. There is no primary indication for the use of digitalis glycosides in small canine patients with primary mitral regurgitation, although there may be secondary indications. Although many animals are treated with these three standard drug classes, there are situations in which the addition of other drugs is beneficial.

It should be stressed that the efficacies of drugs used to treat heart failure vary considerably from drug class to drug class, from drug to drug, and from patient to patient. A drug's efficacy may be very different when used to treat acute heart failure and when used for chronic therapy.

DIURETICS

In most animals with chronic heart failure, edema is primarily the direct consequence of an increase in blood volume. Blood volume may be increased by as much as 30 per cent in animals with severe heart failure.[3] Diuretics decrease edema formation by decreasing this excess blood volume. The decrease in blood volume results in decreases in diastolic intraventricular, venous, and capillary pressures and hence a decrease in transudation of fluid across capillary membranes (i.e., edema formation).

Three classes of diuretics are used clinically in dogs to treat heart failure: thiazide, loop, and potassium-sparing diuretics. They differ in their ability to promote sodium and water excretion and in their mechanism of action. Thiazide diuretics are mildly to moderately potent agents.[4] They are most commonly used in conjunction with a loop diuretic in animals with severe congestive heart failure that is refractory to loop diuretics. The loop diuretics are the most potent and can be used in small doses in animals with mild to moderate heart failure and in higher doses in those with severe heart failure. They can be given orally for chronic administration or parenterally to animals with acute, severe heart failure. The use of potassium-sparing diuretics is reserved for those animals that become hypokalemic with other diuretics and for those refractory to other agents because of an elevated plasma aldosterone concentration. In the latter situation, potassium-sparing diuretics are administered in conjunction with another diuretic, usually a loop diuretic.

LOOP DIURETICS

The loop diuretics include furosemide, ethacrynic acid, and bumetanide. Furosemide is the most commonly used diuretic for treating heart failure in the dog and cat. Ethacrynic acid is rarely used. Bumetanide is a new agent that is 40 to 50 times as potent as furosemide and may offer some clinical advantages. Clinical experience with ethacrynic acid

and bumetanide is very limited. All loop diuretics inhibit sodium, potassium, and chloride reabsorption in the thick portion of the ascending loop of Henle.[5] In so doing, they inhibit sodium and obligatory water reabsorption in the nephron. The loop diuretics are capable of increasing the maximal fractional excretion of sodium from 1 per cent to 15 to 25 per cent of the filtered load, making them the most powerful natriuretic agents available.[6]

Furosemide

Furosemide is potent and will produce a response. It can be administered over a wide dose range, so the dose can be tailored to the individual animal's needs. It can be administered orally or parenterally and can be used for chronic administration or for emergency therapy. In dogs and cats, as long as the animal is eating and drinking normally and the drug is used judiciously, the side effects are few.[6]

Actions. Furosemide is a sulfonamide-type loop diuretic. It inhibits the reabsorption of electrolytes in the thick ascending loop of Henle and also decreases reabsorption of sodium and chloride in the distal renal tubule. Furosemide diuresis results in enhanced excretion of sodium, chloride, potassium, hydrogen, calcium, magnesium, and possibly phosphate ions. Chloride excretion is equal to or exceeds sodium excretion.[7, 8] A dose of 0.45 mg/lb to normal anesthetized dogs increases sodium excretion 17-fold.[8] This natriuretic effect is attenuated by aspirin administration in dogs.[9] Potassium excretion is much less affected than sodium excretion in dogs.[7, 10] In several studies, potassium excretion did not change or only doubled following administration of 0.45 mg/lb furosemide intravenously.[8, 11] Magnesium excretion increases by a factor of four.[8] Calcium excretion increases dramatically by as much as 50 times baseline. The effect on calcium excretion makes furosemide particularly useful in animals with hypercalcemia. Enhanced hydrogen ion excretion without a concomitant increase in bicarbonate excretion can result in metabolic alkalosis in normal dogs.[7] This effect is rarely clinically significant. The increase in net acid excretion produces a slight decrease in urinary pH after furosemide administration.[7] Urine specific gravity generally decreases to the 1.006 to 1.020 range.

In addition to its diuretic effects, furosemide acts as a venodilator, decreasing venous pressures before diuresis takes place (especially after intravenous administration).[12] The venodilatation requires the presence of the kidneys (it does not occur in anephric dogs or humans), meaning that this effect is probably an indirect one.[12, 13] Furosemide decreases renal vascular resistance; thus, it acutely increases renal blood flow (on the order of 50 per cent) without changing glomerular filtration rate (GFR).[14–16] Indomethacin and aspirin completely inhibit this increase in renal blood flow in dogs.[16]

Furosemide increases thoracic duct lymph flow in dogs, but only following high doses (4 to 5 mg/lb intravenously) and not after doses of 0.5 to 1 mg/lb.[17]

Furosemide acts as a bronchodilator in humans, horses, and guinea pigs.[18–20] It can be used as an inhalant in humans with asthma. Its effects in dogs and cats are unknown.[21]

Renin secretion is increased by furosemide administration.[22] This occurs via two mechanisms. There is an early and rapid increase in renin secretion following furosemide administration that is not prevented by beta blocker administration or ureterovenous anastomosis to prevent volume depletion. Consequently, this increase is a direct effect of the drug on the macula densa.[23] There is also a later (six hours) increase in renin secretion that is prevented by beta blocker administration and ureterovenous anastomosis. Consequently, this increase is due to volume depletion and secondary sympathetic stimulation. Renin secretion with subsequent aldosterone secretion should result in sodium and water retention. This effect is obviously easily overcome by furosemide's more potent actions on the nephron.

Pharmacokinetics. Furosemide is rapidly but incompletely absorbed after oral administration, with a bioavailability of 40 to 50 per cent.[24] The ratio of kidney to plasma concentration is 5:1.[25] After intravenous administration, furosemide has an elimination half-life of approximately one hour.[10] Intravenously, furosemide's onset of action is within five minutes, peak effects occur within 30 minutes, and duration of effect is two to three hours.[10] Also after intravenous administration, about 50 per cent of the drug is cleared from the body within the first 30 minutes, 90 per cent is eliminated within the first two hours, and almost all is eliminated within three hours.[26] The terminal half-life after oral administration is biexponential, with an initial phase that has a half-life of approximately 30 minutes and a second phase with a half-life of approximately seven hours.[24] The initial disposition phase has the most effect on plasma concentration, with plasma concentration decreasing from therapeutic to subtherapeutic range within the first four to six hours after oral administration. After oral administration, onset of action occurs within 60 minutes, peak effects occur within one to two hours, and duration of effect is approximately six hours.[24] In normal dogs, a dose of 1 mg/lb furosemide intramuscularly results in maximal natriuresis (beyond that dose there is no further increase in sodium excretion).[16] Because the diuretic effect of furosemide is dependent on its delivery to the kidney by blood flow, animals with decreased renal blood flow (e.g., those with heart failure) need a higher plasma concentration and higher doses to produce the same effect observed in normal dogs.

Experimentally induced renal failure (blood urea nitrogen [BUN] = 70 ± 26; creatinine = 2.4 ± 0.9 in one study) approximately doubles the serum half-life of furosemide in dogs and decreases renal clearance to 15 per cent of control.[27] Experimentally induced renal failure also markedly attenuates the diuretic effect of the drug to approximately one third of control. A higher concentration of furosemide is required to produce the same diuretic effect in dogs with renal failure. However, the relationship between the rate of urinary furosemide excretion and diuresis remains constant. Consequently, the decrease in diuresis in dogs with renal failure appears to be due to a decrease in delivery of furosemide to the nephron.

Very few studies have examined the effects of furosemide in cats. Cats may be more sensitive to furosemide than dogs. In one study, the increase in urine volume was comparable between normal cats and normal dogs in doses from 0.25 to 4.5 mg/lb intramuscularly.[28] However, sodium excretion was between 1.3 and 2.2 times (average, 1.7 times) that seen in dogs at each dosage. The slope and x-axis intercept of the regression equation between furosemide dose and sodium excretion (mmol/lb) for cats were both about twice that for dogs. In another study, fractional excretion of sodium increased from an average of 1.5 per cent at baseline to 23 per cent with a dose of 2.5 mg/lb furosemide intravenously.[29] Even with a dose of 0.45 mg/lb, fractional excretion of sodium was 18 per cent, indicating that the effect of furosemide starts to plateau somewhere between 0.5 and 2.5 mg/lb intravenously in cats. Clinically, cats commonly require no more than 1 mg/lb orally every 8 to 12 hours for the treatment of pulmonary edema.[30] However, higher doses may be needed in feline patients with severe heart failure because of the reduced renal blood flow.

Administration and Dosage. The canine oral dose of furosemide for the treatment of chronic heart failure ranges from 0.5 mg/lb every other day for very mild heart failure to 2 mg/lb every 8 hours for severe heart failure. The oral furosemide dose in cats ranges from 0.5 mg/lb every two to three days to 1 mg/lb every 8 to 12 hours in most cases.[30] The author, however, has used doses as high as 3 mg/lb every 12 hours and has administered up to 7 mg/lb once a day for months at a time to cats that are difficult to treat by pill. Owners must be warned that high-dose diuretic therapy can produce profound dehydration in animals that are not drinking or that stop drinking adequate quantities of water.

Severe pulmonary edema requires immediate intensive intravenous or intramuscular administration in dogs and cats (up to 3.5 mg/lb every one to two hours in dogs, and up to 2 mg/lb every one to two hours in cats). High-dose furosemide administration should be continued until the respiratory rate decreases and/or respiratory character improves. Such intensive dosing may result in mild hypokalemia (serum potassium concentration between 3 and 3.5 mEq/L), mild to moderate hyponatremia (serum sodium concentration between 135 and 145 mEq/L), and mild dehydration. These may need to be addressed after the life-threatening pulmonary edema has been controlled. However, in dogs, electrolyte disturbances and dehydration are usually corrected when the dog feels well enough to eat and drink once the pulmonary edema has resolved. In addition, the electrolyte abnormalities and dehydration are usually not clinically significant unless severe overdosing has occurred. Consequently, aggressive fluid therapy for these abnormalities is not required and is often contraindicated, because such fluid therapy can result in recrudescence of the heart failure. In cats, judicious administration of fluids may be required to rehydrate the animal after intensive diuresis, because cats often do not start to eat and drink as readily as do dogs. Clinically significant electrolyte disturbances (serum sodium concentration <135 mEq/L; serum potassium concentration <3.0 mEq/L) and moderate to severe dehydration are rare in dogs that are chronically administered furosemide unless maximal doses are employed and anorexia is present.[31] These abnormalities, especially dehydration, may be more common in cats.

An alternative to bolus injection of high doses of furosemide to animals with severe heart failure is continuous infusion. This method has been employed in human medicine. The same dose administered continuously over 24 hours produces greater natriuresis and diuresis than does bolus administration.[32]

Adverse Effects. Furosemide can produce adverse effects in dogs and cats. Those adverse effects shared with other diuretics are presented later. Furosemide has the potential for ototoxicity. However, when administered as the sole agent, doses in excess of approximately 10 mg/lb intravenously are required to produce any hearing loss in dogs.[33] Doses in the 25 to 50 mg/lb range produce profound loss of hearing. Furosemide can potentiate the ototoxic effects of other drugs such as the aminoglycosides. Furosemide also potentiates the nephrotoxic effects of the aminoglycosides in dogs.[34] This may occur because furosemide accelerates the accumulation of gentamicin in renal cells.[35] Furosemide does not have any nephrotoxic effects when administered by itself. Prerenal azotemia can occur if moderate to severe dehydration is produced in an animal with heart failure.

Theoretically, primary renal failure can occur if severe dehydration is produced in an animal with heart failure, resulting in a marked and prolonged decrease in renal perfusion.

THIAZIDE DIURETICS

Actions. The thiazides act primarily by reducing membrane permeability to sodium and chloride in the distal convoluted tubule.[4] They promote potassium loss at this site and produce large increases in the urine sodium concentration but only mild to moderate increases in urine volume. Consequently, only mild to moderate renal sodium loss is promoted. Thiazide diuretics increase renal sodium excretion from a normal value of about 1 per cent to 5 to 8 per cent of the filtered load, about one third that achieved with the loop diuretics. Thiazide diuretics also inhibit carbonic anhydrase in the proximal tubules, but this effect varies considerably among the various agents. The thiazides are ineffective when renal blood flow is low, which may explain their lack of efficacy in animals with severe heart failure.

Thiazide diuretics decrease GFR, which may explain their lack of efficacy in animals with renal failure. It is unknown whether this effect is due to a direct effect on renal vasculature or is secondary to the decrease in intravascular fluid volume.

In addition to their effects on sodium and chloride, the thiazides increase potassium excretion because of the increased sodium that reaches the distal tubular site of sodium-potassium exchange. Thiazides also increase bicarbonate excretion. Long-term thiazide administration can result in mild metabolic alkalosis associated with hypokalemia and hypochloremia in human patients. The effects in dogs and cats are less clear. Plasma renin concentration is increased by thiazide administration. This is probably due to the decrease in plasma volume.

Pharmacokinetics and Dosage. In dogs, the thiazides are well absorbed after oral administration. The action of chlorothiazide begins within one hour, peaks at four hours, and lasts six to 12 hours. The dosage is 9 to 18 mg/lb every 12 hours. Hydrochlorothiazide has an onset of action within two hours, peaks at four hours, and lasts 12 hours. The oral canine dose is 0.9 to 1.8 mg/lb every 12 hours; cats are administered 0.45 to 0.9 mg/lb every 12 hours. The newer, more lipid-soluble thiazides (trichlormethiazide, cyclothiazide) have not been studied in the dog or cat.

Indications. The most common use of the thiazide diuretics in veterinary patients is treatment of heart failure refractory to furosemide administration. Use of a thiazide diuretic in combination with furosemide in such animals commonly results in restoration of diuresis, decreased edema formation, and clinical improvement.

POTASSIUM-SPARING DIURETICS

Actions. This class of diuretics acts by inhibiting the action of aldosterone on distal tubular cells or blocking the entry of sodium in the latter regions of the distal tubule and collecting tubules.[36] In normal animals, plasma aldosterone concentration is relatively low, hence the effect of these diuretics is mild. In normal dogs, they can increase the maximal fractional excretion of sodium only from 1 to 2 per cent of the filtered load.[37] In dogs with heart failure and increased plasma aldosterone concentration, the effect of these diuretics may be greater. However, potassium-sparing diuretics are rarely used as sole agents in animals with heart failure. When potassium-sparing diuretics are administered with other diuretics, potassium loss is decreased. Consequently, they can be administered to animals that become hypokalemic because of the administration of other diuretic agents.

Spironolactone. Spironolactone is structurally similar to aldosterone and binds competitively to aldosterone's binding sites in the distal tubule. Its onset of action is slow in dogs, and peak effect does not occur until two to three days after administration commences.[38] The drug is extensively and rapidly metabolized to canrenone and other metabolites in plasma. These metabolites are pharmacologically active, but much less so than the parent compound. The duration of effect for spironolactone is two to three days after cessation of drug administration.[38] The dose of spironolactone for dogs is 0.9 to 1.8 mg/lb per day.

Triamterene. Triamterene is a potassium-sparing diuretic that is structurally related to folic acid. It acts directly on the distal tubule to depress the reabsorption of sodium and decrease the excretion of potassium and hydrogen.[39] It does not competitively inhibit aldosterone. Its action begins within two hours, peaks at six to eight hours, and lasts 12 to 16 hours.[38] The oral canine dose of triamterene is 0.9 to 1.8 mg/lb per day.

ADVERSE EFFECTS OF DIURETICS

Diuretic therapy has the potential of causing undesirable effects, primarily electrolyte disturbances and dehydration. These effects can occur in canine and feline patients, especially in those that are not eating and/or drinking or in animals being administered acute, high-dose therapy. Cats appear to be more susceptible than dogs to electrolyte depletion and dehydration while on diuretic therapy.

Electrolyte Abnormalities. Hypokalemia is one of the more common undesirable effects. However, the incidence of hypokalemia in dogs being administered furosemide chronically is low.[31, 40] In one study of 23 canine patients with heart failure being administered furosemide at doses of 1.3 to 9 mg/lb per day (mean, 4 mg/lb), serum potassium concentration ranged from 3.9 to 5.2 mEq/L (normal = 3.5 to 5.5 mEq/L). None of these dogs were being administered ACE inhibitors. All were outpatients that were eating and drinking normally. In another study, serum potassium concentration did not differ in control dogs and in dogs with heart failure treated with furosemide with or without digoxin and an ACE inhibitor.[41]

Hyponatremia may occur in animals on high-dose diuretic therapy. Animals with severe heart failure may also become hyponatremic owing to excess antidiuretic hormone (ADH) secretion and resultant water retention. It may be impossible to distinguish between these two causes in some heart failure patients.

Hypomagnesemia may be identified, but the incidence of clinically significant hypomagnesemia in dogs with heart failure that are administered diuretics is very low (see Chapter 63).[31, 41]

Dehydration. Dehydration is probably common in animals with severe heart failure that require maximal doses of diuretics. Usually the dehydration is subclinical. At times, however, animals appear mildly dehydrated on physical examination, and in some, prerenal azotemia is present. If the animal is clinically affected (e.g., not eating), the diuretic dose must be reduced, and in some cases, judicious fluid therapy must be employed. Animals that are not clinically affected by their dehydration and azotemia often need the dose of diuretic they are receiving. In those cases, the prerenal azotemia can be safely ignored as long as the azotemia is not severe (e.g., BUN not >60 mg/dL).

VASODILATORS: GENERAL PRINCIPLES

Actions. Vasodilators are drugs that relax arteriolar or venous smooth muscle to cause vasodilatation. Their effects depend on the vascular beds they influence, as well as relative drug potency. The effect of these drugs on the pulmonary vasculature is erratic or insignificant. This discussion is therefore limited to the systemic vascular beds.

In animals with heart disease, systemic arterioles are constricted so that a normal blood pressure can be maintained when cardiac output is reduced. In addition, systemic veins are constricted so that blood volume is shifted from the peripheral to the central compartment in order to increase ventricular preload, produce volume overload hypertrophy, and, in so doing, increase stroke volume and cardiac output. In animals with heart failure, these compensatory mechanisms become detrimental. Although systemic vasoconstriction is able to maintain a normal systemic blood pressure, it increases resistance to blood flow and contributes to producing an increased afterload. The normal systemic blood pressure and increased afterload decrease the effective transfer of mechanical energy into blood propulsion into the aorta.[42] The net result is a decrease in stroke volume and an increase in energy consumption by the heart. Systemic venoconstriction in heart failure patients contributes to the increase in central blood volume. In these animals, the ventricular chambers are unable to grow larger in response to this increase in volume. Consequently, the increase in central blood volume and venoconstriction contribute to the increase in ventricular diastolic pressures and hence to the increase in edema formation.

Vasodilators are generally classified as arteriolar dilators, venodilators, or combination (i.e., balanced) arteriolar and venodilators. Arteriolar dilators relax the smooth muscle of systemic arterioles, decreasing peripheral vascular resistance and impedance. This usually results in decreased systemic arterial blood pressure, systolic intraventricular pressure, and systolic myocardial wall stress (or afterload). Thus, the force that opposes myocardial fiber shortening is reduced. This allows the heart muscle to shorten further and increase stroke volume. Arteriolar dilators are especially useful in animals with mitral regurgitation, aortic regurgitation, ventricular septal defect, and patent ductus arteriosus. In mitral regurgitation, the left ventricle pumps blood in two directions—forward into the systemic circulation, and backward, either through a defect in the mitral or aortic valves or between the left and right circulations. In mitral regurgitation, the percentage of blood pumped into the systemic circulation versus the percentage pumped through the defect in the valve depends on the relative resistances to blood flow. If resistance to blood flow through the systemic circulation is reduced with drugs, systemic blood flow increases and the amount of blood flowing into the left atrium decreases (Fig. 111–1). Similarly, in aortic regurgitation, ventricular septal defect, and patent ductus arteriosus, a decrease in systemic vascular resistance results in increased forward flow and decreased flow through the aortic valve, the septal defect, or the patent ductus arteriosus.

Venodilators relax systemic venous smooth muscle, effec-

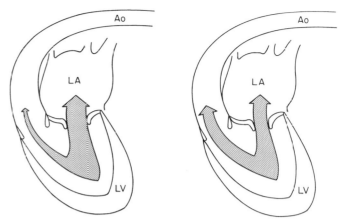

Figure 111–1. Schematic drawing of severe mitral regurgitation before (left) and after (right) the administration of a drug that dilates systemic arterioles. The relative amount of blood ejected into the systemic circulation versus into the left atrium is determined by the relative resistances to flow in each direction (forward vs. backward). The regurgitant fraction (percentage of stroke volume ejected backward into the left atrium) is approximately 80 per cent before drug administration. Following the administration of the arteriolar dilator, more blood is ejected forward into the systemic circulation and less is ejected backward into the left atrium.

tively redistributing some of the blood volume into the systemic venous reservoir (especially the splanchnic vasculature), decreasing cardiac blood volume, and reducing pulmonary congestion (Fig. 111–2). The net result is reduced ventricular diastolic pressures, decreased pulmonary and systemic capillary pressures, and diminished edema formation. Consequently, venodilators are used to reduce edema formation.

Vasodilators are also classified according to their mechanism of action. ACE inhibitors can be classified as vasodilators, but they also decrease plasma aldosterone concentration, which results in less sodium and water retention.

Therapeutic End Points. The therapeutic end point of vasodilator therapy is reduction in edema (reduced pulmonary capillary pressure and venous pressures) for venodilators and improved forward perfusion (elevation of cardiac output) for arteriolar dilators in patients with diseases such as dilated cardiomyopathy. When regurgitation or left-to-right shunting is present arteriolar dilators reduce edema

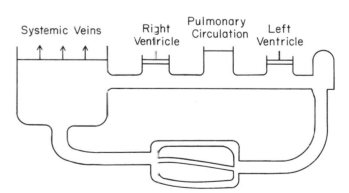

Figure 111–2. Schematic drawing of the circulation during the administration of a systemic venodilator. By increasing the capacitance of the systemic veins (*arrows pointed up*), blood is shifted from the central circulation (heart and lungs) into the peripheral circulation. The decrease in blood volume in the central circulation results in a decrease in diastolic intraventricular pressures. This results in a decrease in capillary hydrostatic pressure and thus a decrease in edema formation. By contrast, a diuretic decreases total blood volume to accomplish the same task.

formation and improve forward flow. Although it may not be feasible to measure these variables directly, close monitoring of the clinical signs referable to congestive heart failure and the radiographic appearance of the lungs is realistic. Blood lactate concentration and venous oxygen tension should improve following arteriolar dilator therapy if they were initially abnormal. Mean or systolic systemic arterial blood pressure is usually reduced by 10 to 30 mmHg. Mean pressure should be maintained at approximately 70 mmHg or above.

Adverse Effects. Although vasodilators enable one to achieve better therapeutic results, there is the potential for adverse effects. These drugs are often used in critically ill canine or feline patients or those with multiple problems that may be on several medications at the time of evaluation or during the course of treatment. These animals, in general, are at greater risk for experiencing adverse effects from a drug. To avoid adverse events and to use these drugs wisely, one must have a working knowledge of the mechanism of action, dosages, side effects, drug interactions, and patient risks. If adverse effects occur, one must be cognizant of what constitutes a life-threatening adverse event versus a relatively benign complication and how to deal with the more serious complications of drug therapy. One must have an accurate diagnosis before the institution of therapy. Complications can be expected to be more frequent if the animal is treated prior to establishing an accurate diagnosis. In cardiovascular medicine, thoracic radiographs, an electrocardiogram, and an echocardiogram are frequently required to establish the diagnosis.

The primary major adverse effect of vasodilator therapy is hypotension severe enough to cause clinical signs (usually weakness). This usually occurs as an isolated event following administration of the first doses of the drug or during titration of the dose and may warrant only a decrease in the dose rather than discontinuation of the drug. The additive effects of a diuretic and a vasodilator may be a factor in producing an adverse effect, especially if the animal is clinically dehydrated and severely volume depleted. Clinically significant hypotension is more common and often more severe when two arteriolar dilators are administered concurrently.

ACE INHIBITORS

Actions. The renin-angiotensin-aldosterone system plays an important role in regulating cardiovascular homeostasis in normal individuals and in those with heart failure. Renin is released from the juxtaglomerular apparatus in response to sympathetic stimulation and to decreased sodium flux by the macula densa. Renin is a protease that acts on the plasma glycoprotein angiotensinogen to form the polypeptide angiotensin I. ACE cleaves two amino acids from the decapeptide angiotensin I to form the octapeptide angiotensin II. This conversion occurs primarily in the vascular endothelium of the lung, although other vascular beds are involved.

ACE inhibitors bind to the same site on ACE as angiotensin I, effectively arresting its action.[43] This site contains a zinc ion, and ACE inhibitors contain a sulfhydryl, carboxyl, or phosphoryl group that interacts with this site. The relative potency of these compounds depends on the affinity of the compound for the active site. ACE inhibitors that are more tightly bound to the active site tend to be more potent. They also tend to have a longer duration of effect. The effects of ACE inhibitors occur as a result of the decreased concentra-

tion of circulating angiotensin II. Angiotensin II has several important effects in animals with heart failure: (1) it is a potent vasopressor, (2) it stimulates the release of aldosterone from the adrenal gland, (3) it stimulates vasopressin (ADH) release from the posterior pituitary gland, (4) it facilitates the central and peripheral effects of the sympathetic nervous system, and (5) it preserves glomerular filtration when renal blood flow is decreased. ACE inhibitors have several effects in animals with heart failure. Arteriolar and venous dilatation occurs as a direct result of the decreased concentration of angiotensin II. Consequently, ACE inhibitors are generally classified as vasodilators. One must remember, however, that ACE inhibitors also decrease plasma aldosterone concentration. This may, in fact, be their most important role. When the stimulus for aldosterone secretion is lessened, sodium and water excretion is enhanced, and edema is lessened.

The effects of ACE inhibitors become evident at different times following the onset of administration. Arteriolar dilatation is observed after the first dose is administered, whereas the lessening of sodium and water retention takes days to become clinically significant.[44] Because most dogs presenting with severe heart failure are dying from pulmonary edema, the ACE inhibitors are poor emergency heart failure drugs.

The ability of ACE inhibitors to decrease plasma aldosterone secretion may become attenuated or lost with time. In one study of Cavalier King Charles spaniels with severe mitral regurgitation, enalapril significantly decreased plasma aldosterone concentration after three weeks of administration.[45] However, six months later, the plasma aldosterone concentration was increased to an even higher level than at baseline. These dogs were also on furosemide at six months, which may have contributed to the increase.

ACE inhibitors act acutely and chronically as arteriolar dilators. In most canine patients, however, this effect is relatively mild when compared with the more potent arteriolar dilators such as hydralazine and nitroprusside. In general, ACE inhibitors can decrease systemic vascular resistance by 25 to 30 per cent, whereas hydralazine can decrease it by 50 per cent. This explains the reduced number of hypotensive events observed with ACE inhibitors. This also explains why the effect of ACE inhibitors on edema formation and cardiac output in dogs with mitral regurgitation is usually not as profound as that of hydralazine.

Benefits. The clinical benefits of ACE inhibitors in heart failure are reasonably good in human and canine studies. In general, ACE inhibitors improve clinical signs and improve quality of life in dogs with heart failure due to diverse causes.[46, 47] The improvement in clinical signs is primarily due to reduction in capillary pressure and edema formation and to increased perfusion of vascular beds. ACE inhibitors are one of the few drug types used to treat heart failure that have been proved to both improve symptoms and prolong life in humans.[48] Several large clinical trials have documented that captopril and enalapril significantly improve the quality of life and significantly increase survival time in human patients with heart failure.[49-51] A combination of hydralazine and isosorbide dinitrate has also been shown to prolong survival time in humans.[52] *One must be cognizant that vasodilator therapy is still palliative, however, and that even in people, death occurs at a relatively rapid pace despite intervention with ACE inhibitors.*

In veterinary medicine, the primary studies that have documented clinical benefit have been performed using enalapril. These benefits are outlined under the enalapril subsection.

Adverse Effects. The risks of interfering with angiotensin II formation lie in its role in preserving systemic blood pressure and GFR as renal flow decreases.[53] Blocking its action on peripheral arterioles can result in hypotension that leads to cerebral hypoperfusion and dizziness. The incidence of clinically significant hypotension in dogs appears to be much lower than in people, probably because dogs do not walk upright. The second risk is seen in patients that are very dependent on angiotensin II to maintain GFR. Glomerular efferent arteriolar constriction maintains normal GFR in mild to moderately severe heart failure when renal blood flow is reduced.[54] The primary stimulus for this vasoconstriction is increased plasma angiotensin II concentration, which is elaborated in response to the decrease in renal blood flow.[55] Glomerular capillary pressure provides the force for filtration, and glomerular capillary pressure is determined by renal plasma flow and efferent arteriolar resistance. When renal plasma flow is low (as in heart failure), angiotensin II causes efferent arterioles to vasoconstrict, bringing glomerular capillary pressure back to normal. GFR is preserved despite the decrease in flow, and normal BUN and serum creatinine concentrations are maintained. The filtration fraction (ratio of GFR to renal plasma flow) is increased. When an ACE inhibitor is administered, efferent arteriolar dilatation must occur. In some patients, this dilatation appears to be excessive, resulting in a moderate to marked reduction in GFR and subsequent azotemia. Those human patients at greatest risk for developing azotemia include patients with high plasma renin activity, low renal perfusion pressure, hyponatremia, and excessive volume depletion.[55–58] When angiotensin II concentration is decreased in at-risk patients, GFR becomes decreased and azotemia results. The azotemia is generally mild but occasionally can be severe in both human and canine patients. Functional azotemia can occur secondary to the administration of any ACE inhibitor. However, the longer-acting agents (e.g., enalapril, lisinopril, benazepril) may produce azotemia in human patients more frequently than do the shorter-acting agents (e.g., captopril).[59] Treatment consists of reducing the diuretic dose or stopping the administration of the ACE inhibitor.

A decrease in GFR and an increase in BUN and serum creatinine concentration are seen in 35 per cent of human patients receiving ACE inhibitors. In most cases, the increase in BUN is mild. In dogs, the incidence of clinically significant azotemia appears to be low. In fact, studies suggest that there are no differences between populations of dogs on placebo and furosemide and dogs on an ACE inhibitor.[46] However, the author's clinic and others have a number of documented cases in which severe azotemia (BUN >100 mg/dL) developed after initiating ACE inhibitor therapy in a canine patient that was on a stable dose of furosemide. This suggests that ACE inhibitor–induced functional renal insufficiency occurs frequently enough that any veterinarian using these drugs should be aware of the potential occurrence of azotemia. A rough estimate of animals that develop severe azotemia would be 1 in 50 animals treated. In the author's experience, mild to moderate increases in BUN (between 35 and 60 mg/dL) occur with some frequency. In these animals, BUN may increase without a concomitant increase in serum creatinine concentration, or the increase in creatinine may be milder. In such animals, an attempt should be made to reduce the diuretic dose, but in those that require the dose of diuretic they are on to treat their heart failure, the author's tendency is to ignore the change in BUN and

to maintain the administration of the ACE inhibitor as long as the animal continues to eat and act normally.

Because ACE inhibitors can reduce GFR and cause an increase in BUN and creatinine, clinicians (human and veterinary) are commonly reluctant to use these drugs in patients with mild to moderate azotemia. However, there is no evidence that there is any greater risk of exacerbating azotemia in patients with moderate renal failure than there is in patients with normal renal function. Human patients with moderate renal failure tolerate the administration of an ACE inhibitor without an increase in serum creatinine.[60] Some of the ACE inhibitors are excreted primarily via the kidneys. The dose of these drugs may need to be decreased in patients with renal failure, although the exact reduction in dosage is not known for dogs or cats.

Recommended veterinary guidelines (based on human studies and guidelines) for ACE inhibitor therapy with regard to azotemia are as follows: (1) identify high-risk animals (those with moderate to severe dehydration, hyponatremia) before therapy; (2) ensure that the animal is not clinically dehydrated, and ensure adequate oral fluid intake throughout therapy; (3) evaluate renal function at least once within one week after commencing therapy; and (4) decrease the dose of furosemide if moderate azotemia develops or discontinue the ACE inhibitor if the azotemia is severe or if a reduction in furosemide dose does not improve renal function.[56, 58, 61] The prescribing information for the veterinary formulation of enalapril states that if azotemia develops, the dose of diuretic should be reduced, and if azotemia continues, the dose should be reduced further or discontinued. This makes it sound as if diuretic administration should be discontinued permanently, but a recommendation to permanently discontinue furosemide therapy in an animal with a clear history of moderate to severe heart failure is not tenable. In human medicine, the recommendation is to discontinue diuretic therapy for 24 to 48 hours if needed, not permanently.[56] It should also be stressed that azotemia sometimes develops in a canine patient that appears to have no risk factors other than heart failure. Consequently, it is important to warn owners of the clinical signs of severe azotemia (usually anorexia and other gastrointestinal signs) and to measure serum creatinine concentration and BUN within the first week of initiating ACE inhibitor therapy. If an animal develops severe azotemia, the author generally discontinues use of the ACE inhibitor and makes sure that the animal is not dehydrated. If dehydration is moderate to severe, the author reduces the furosemide dose or discontinues its administration for one to two days and administers intravenous fluids cautiously. Once the dog is stable, the author reassesses the need for an ACE inhibitor. In many cases, the ACE inhibitor was being administered because of its potential benefits and the animal did not require it. If the animal is refractory to furosemide administration, other options are to lower the ACE inhibitor dose, use a short-acting ACE inhibitor such as captopril, add a thiazide diuretic, or use hydralazine in place of an ACE inhibitor.

Drug Interactions. It should be noted that the arteriolar dilating effect of enalapril, and probably other ACE inhibitors, is attenuated by the concomitant administration of aspirin in humans. In one study in humans, the usual decrease in systemic vascular resistance induced by an ACE inhibitor was blocked by aspirin.[62] However, aspirin did not attenuate the hemodynamic effects of enalaprilat in one study of experimental dogs with heart failure.[63]

Not all the effects of ACE inhibitors are beneficial in patients with heart failure. One study of human patients with acute heart failure documented that captopril acutely decreases the natriuretic and diuretic effects of furosemide.[64] This finding suggests that an ACE inhibitor should not be administered to a patient with severe, acute heart failure that needs the diuretic effect of furosemide to maintain life.

There are four ACE inhibitors that have been used in dogs and cats: captopril, enalapril, lisinopril, and benazepril. Enalapril is approved by the Food and Drug Administraton for use in dogs. Generally these drugs have similar effects. The primary difference is in duration of effect. Captopril is short-acting, lasting less than three to four hours. Enalapril's effects last 12 to 14 hours. Lisinopril is thought to be the longest acting and is advocated for once-a-day use in humans. In general, the ACE inhibitors have very similar effects on hemodynamics. The pharmacokinetics and dosages of the commonly used ACE inhibitors are listed in Table 111–1.

CAPTOPRIL

Actions. Captopril prevents the conversion of angiotensin I to angiotensin II by competing with angiotensin I for the active site of ACE.[65] As with all ACE inhibitors, administration of captopril results in arteriolar and venous dilatation and a decreased circulating plasma aldosterone concentration.[66]

The primary effect of captopril in the dog following its first dose is arteriolar dilatation.[44] Little change in pulmonary capillary pressure and thus edema formation is noted following the first dose. In addition, in human heart failure patients, acute captopril administration decreases the natriuretic and diuretic effects of furosemide.[64] Consequently, captopril is not a good emergency drug in dogs with severe pulmonary edema. The effect of reducing edema appears to take more than 48 hours to develop. After that time, clinically significant reductions in pulmonary capillary pressure can be noted.

Indications. Some dogs with acquired mitral regurgitation display marked improvement following captopril administration; others have no change or reduced cardiac output.[67] These variable effects may be explained by differences in baseline aldosterone concentration, but this remains to be studied. In dogs with dilated cardiomyopathy, clinical improvement is usually noted, although this improvement may be short-lived. In humans, captopril is thought to be an effective drug for treating all stages of heart failure in which therapy is required. The drug produces mild to moderate reductions in blood pressure, improves exercise tolerance, and prolongs life in human patients.[68] Improvement in survival time has not been documented in veterinary medicine.

A small study has been performed in large (45- to 70-lb) experimental dogs to examine the effects of captopril on mitral regurgitation before the onset of heart failure.[69] In this study, 10 dogs with induced mitral regurgitation were randomly assigned to placebo or captopril (0.9 mg/lb every eight hours). These dogs had moderate mitral regurgitation with an average regurgitant fraction of approximately 60 per cent. They were not in heart failure. The significant findings from this study were that forward ejection fraction (i.e., 1-regurgitant fraction) decreased significantly in the dogs administered placebo but did not change in the dogs administered captopril. This was accompanied by a significant decrease in total peripheral resistance. Unexpectedly, the significant increase in forward ejection fraction was not accompanied by a significant decrease in regurgitant fraction. However, this appeared to be due to the marked variability from dog to dog and the small number of dogs studied.

Administration and Dosage. The recommended dosage for captopril in dogs is 0.22 to 0.45 mg/lb orally every eight hours. Doses of 1.5 mg/lb every eight hours have been associated with glomerular lesions and renal failure in experimental dogs and in clinical canine patients. In a study performed by the author, the onset of activity of captopril was within one hour of the first dose.[44] Drug effect lasted less than four hours. A dose of 0.45 mg/lb produced slightly greater effects than a dose of 0.22 mg/lb. A dose of 0.9 mg/lb produced no additional benefit. Doses in excess of 3 mg/lb every eight hours can produce renal failure and should be avoided. The dose of captopril in cats with dilated, restrictive, or hypertrophic cardiomyopathy, determined from clinical experience, is 0.25 to 0.70 mg/lb every 8 to 12 hours.

Adverse Effects. Captopril is generally well tolerated in most animals. However, side effects can occur and include anorexia, vomiting, diarrhea, azotemia, and hypotension. Gastrointestinal side effects appear to be more common in dogs administered captopril than in dogs administered other ACE inhibitors.[70] In human patients, captopril produces fewer instances of azotemia and hypotension than do the longer-acting ACE inhibitors.[59]

ENALAPRIL

Actions. Enalapril is the ethyl ester of enalaprilat.[65] It has little pharmacologic activity until it is hydrolyzed in the liver to enalaprilat. Enalapril is available commercially as the maleate salt. In dogs, enalapril maleate is absorbed better from the gastrointestinal tract than is enalaprilat.[71] Enalapril is structurally and pharmacologically similar to captopril but contains a disubstituted nitrogen rather than the sulfhydryl group. The lack of the sulfhydryl group may result in a decreased risk of certain side effects in humans, such as taste disturbances and proteinuria. These adverse effects have not been documented in dogs or cats administered ACE inhibitors.[65]

Pharmacodynamics. The pharmacodynamics of enalapril have been examined in experimental dogs.[72] An oral dose of 0.14 mg/lb results in approximately 75 per cent

TABLE 111–1. PHARMACOLOGY OF ACE INHIBITORS IN DOGS

	CAPTOPRIL	ENALAPRIL	LISINOPRIL	BENAZEPRIL
Zinc ligand	Sulfhydryl	Carboxyl	Carboxyl	Carboxyl
Prodrug	No	Yes	No	Yes
Bioavailability	75% (40% if fed)	60%	25–50%	
Peak plasma concentration	1 h	3–4 h (enalaprilat)	4 h	1–3 h
Duration of effect	3–4 h	12–14 h	24 h	16 h
Route of elimination	Kidney	Kidney, liver	Kidney	Kidney, liver
Dosage range	0.22–0.45 mg/lb q8h	0.22 mg/lb q12–24h	0.22–0.45 mg/lb q24h	0.11–0.22 mg/lb q12–24h

inhibition of the pressor response to angiotensin I. This effect lasts for at least six hours and is completely dissipated by 24 hours after administration. A dose of 0.45 mg/lb produces only slightly better inhibition (approximately 30 per cent) for at least seven hours. About 15 per cent inhibition is still present 24 hours after oral administration.

Administration and Dosage. Dose ranging has been performed with enalapril in dogs with surgically induced mitral regurgitation and heart failure.[73] In these dogs, an oral dose of 0.22 mg/lb acutely produced a greater decrease in pulmonary capillary pressure than a dose of 0.12 mg/lb. A dose of 0.35 mg/lb produced no better response. After 21 days of administration, the dose of 0.22 mg/lb every 24 hours produced a significant decrease in heart rate, whereas the 0.12 mg/lb dose did not. Consequently, the enalapril dose is 0.22 mg/lb. Whether this dose should be administered once a day or twice a day is debatable. The package insert recommends starting with once-a-day dosing and increasing to twice-a-day dosing if the clinical response is inadequate. Based on the pharmacodynamics presented in the previous paragraph, the author generally starts with twice-a-day administration to dogs in heart failure, with the doses approximately 12 hours apart.

Efficacy and Safety. Studies of enalapril's efficacy in dogs with dilated cardiomyopathy and in dogs with primary mitral regurgitation with heart failure have been completed and reported. In one study, 58 dogs were enrolled for study at seven different centers.[47] This study was identified by the acronym IMPROVE (Invasive Multicenter Prospective Veterinary Evaluation of Enalapril Study). Of the 58 dogs, 35 had dilated cardiomyopathy, 22 had primary mitral regurgitation, and one had aortic regurgitation. Dogs were randomly assigned to be administered enalapril (n = 31) or a placebo (n = 27). The enalapril dose was 0.22 mg/lb every 12 hours. Physical examinations were performed and electrocardiograms, echocardiograms, and thoracic radiographs were obtained before and an average of 2 (range, 1 to 4) and 20 (range, 17 to 28) days after starting placebo or drug administration. In addition, a Swan-Ganz catheter was placed to monitor pulmonary capillary pressure, right atrial pressure, and cardiac output, and an arterial catheter was placed to measure systemic arterial blood pressure intermittently for the first 24 hours (baseline and 4, 8, 12, and 24 hours after drug administration). Forty-one dogs (19 placebo-treated and 22 enalapril-treated) completed the study. The acute (first 24 hours) hemodynamic effects of enalapril were not spectacular. Heart rate decreased significantly only at the four-hour period. Mean systemic arterial blood pressure decreased significantly only at the eight-hour period. Pulmonary capillary pressure decreased significantly at the eight-hour period. Cardiac output and right atrial pressure did not change at all. Clinical response over the 20 days was better. Overall, the dogs on enalapril improved clinically and had increased mobility when compared with dogs on the placebo (7 of 24 dogs on the placebo improved clinically, whereas 19 of 27 dogs on enalapril experienced an overall clinical improvement). Of the dogs administered enalapril, 26 per cent were classified as greatly improved, and 44 per cent were classified as improved. No dog that was administered the placebo was classified as greatly improved, but 29 per cent were classified as improved. This overall clinical improvement was significant only for dogs with dilated cardiomyopathy, not for dogs with primary mitral regurgitation. There were no significant changes in activity, attitude, cough, appetite, demeanor, respiratory effort, or murmur intensity. Radiographic evidence of pulmonary edema was decreased in 40

per cent of the dogs treated with enalapril on day 2, and 56 per cent were improved on day 20; this compares with 15 per cent of dogs treated with the placebo on day 2 and 17 per cent on day 20. There was no significant change in any echocardiographic variable. A significantly greater number of enalapril-treated dogs also improved clinically based on class of heart failure when compared with placebo-treated dogs.

A second study was performed and identified by the acronym COVE (Cooperative Veterinary Enalapril Study Group).[46] In this study, 211 dogs were studied at 19 centers. Of these, 141 dogs had primary mitral regurgitation and 70 had dilated cardiomyopathy as the primary diagnosis. All except one dog were being administered furosemide with (approximately 75 per cent) or without digoxin on entry into the study. Dogs were assigned to be administered either placebo or enalapril based on a randomized allocation schedule. The study was blinded so that neither the investigator nor the client knew which treatment the dog was receiving. Dogs with renal failure, other terminal disease, or uncorrected hypothyroidism were excluded from the study. Dogs that had been administered calcium antagonists or non-nitrate vasodilators within four days before entering the study were also excluded. Clinical evaluations of each dog were performed at baseline and at two and four weeks later. Dogs were evaluated by physical examination, electrocardiography, thoracic radiography, complete blood count (CBC), serum chemistry profile, urinalysis, and serum digoxin concentration at each time point. Echocardiography was performed at baseline to confirm the diagnosis. Fourteen subjective clinical variables were assessed by each investigator with the aid of the owner at each time point. The investigators had the option of removing a dog from the study at any point if they thought that continuation in a blinded study placed the dog at risk or if the dog was not improving adequately. Furosemide and digoxin doses did not change significantly during the study in either group. Significantly more enalapril-treated dogs (32 per cent) completed the study than placebo-treated dogs (15 per cent). More dogs in the placebo group died of heart failure (7 vs. 0) or were removed from the study because of progression of heart failure (16 vs. 7). In dogs with dilated cardiomyopathy, there was significant improvement in class of heart failure, overall evaluation, mobility, activity, and amount of pulmonary edema on both days 14 and 28. By day 28, there was further improvement, as evidenced by significant improvement in demeanor, cough, and appetite. In dogs with mitral regurgitation, there was no significant clinical improvement on day 14, but by day 28 there was significant improvement in activity, mobility, overall evaluation, and cough. Renal function tests were abnormal in approximately 45 per cent of the dogs in both groups at baseline. They did not change significantly in either group.

A long-term efficacy study has also been completed, known as the LIVE study (Long Term Investigation of Veterinary Enalapril Study).[74, 75] Dogs (n = 148) from the COVE and IMPROVE studies were continued on either the placebo (n = 71) or enalapril (n = 77) and studied in an identical manner to the COVE study for up to 15.5 months. Dogs remained in the study until they developed intractable heart failure (n = 48), died of heart failure (n = 17), died suddenly (n = 10), died of a noncardiac cause (n = 4), dropped out of the study for other reasons (n = 48), or the study ended (n = 21). Dogs administered enalapril remained in the study significantly longer (169 days) than dogs administered the placebo (90 days). Most of the benefit occurred in the first 60 days. After that, dogs in both groups either developed intractable heart failure or died at a similar rate. When divided into dogs with mitral regurgitation and those with dilated cardiomyopathy, the dogs with dilated cardiomyopathy that were administered enalapril remained in the study significantly longer (158 days) than did those that were administered the placebo (58 days). Dogs with mitral regurgitation that were administered enalapril did not remain in the study significantly longer (172 days) than those administered the placebo (110 days).

The three aforementioned studies are the result of one of the largest efforts ever put forth to document drug efficacy in small animal veterinary medicine. The results are quite clear. Enalapril, despite the fact that it produces minimal hemodynamic change, results in clinical improvement in dogs with heart failure due to mitral regurgitation or dilated cardiomyopathy. It appears to perform better in dogs with dilated cardiomyopathy but is clearly efficacious in many dogs with mitral regurgitation. However, in general and in both diseases, the clinical response is not profound. Rather, in most cases, the drug results in mild and gradual improvement that helps to stabilize the clinical course of the patient and improve the quality of life. As such, enalapril is a good adjunctive agent for treating animals with heart failure. It may be effective as the sole agent in some dogs with very mild heart failure, but in most cases it must be administered in conjunction with a more effective drug, usually furosemide. The drug's effects on survival are less clear. No true survival study has been performed, although the LIVE study determined the time to treatment failure or death. The data from this study may translate into increased survival, but this is not assured. The ability of enalapril to prolong the life of dogs with heart failure secondary to primary mitral regurgitation remains unanswered.

Enalapril has been shown to be beneficial in dogs with mitral regurgitation but of less benefit for the group as a whole than possibly expected. In the author's clinical experience, some dogs with mitral regurgitation have dramatic responses to an ACE inhibitor, many improve clinically, and a significant number have little response.

Early Intervention. Studies have been performed in humans to determine whether starting enalapril therapy in patients with left ventricular dysfunction but without evidence of heart failure is beneficial. Benefit has been defined as reduction in mortality, reduction in the incidence of heart failure, and reduction in the hospitalization rate. In a study of human patients with chronic cardiac disease, 4228 patients with ejection fractions less than 35 per cent (comparable to a shortening fraction <15 per cent) were randomized to receive either placebo or enalapril.[48] They were followed clinically for an average of 37 months. During that time, there was no reduction in mortality associated with enalapril administration, but there was a reduction in the incidence of heart failure and in hospitalizations for heart failure (the drug delayed the onset of heart failure).

Because of findings in humans, recommendations have been made to administer enalapril to canine patients with advanced cardiac disease but without heart failure.[74] Many veterinary cardiologists recommend that an ACE inhibitor be administered to dogs with mitral regurgitation when there is severe left atrial enlargement but no evidence of pulmonary edema. There certainly are theoretical grounds for doing this, but there is no proof that this tactic is beneficial. Presently, the author does not follow this approach and administers ACE inhibitors, usually in conjunction with furosemide, only when there is evidence of heart failure. Because

there is no proof that either approach is superior, each veterinarian must use his or her own judgment on how to approach this type of case. A few veterinary cardiologists recommend initiating ACE inhibitor therapy when mild to moderate mitral regurgitation is present. The author opposes this approach for several reasons. First and foremost, many dogs with mild to moderate mitral regurgitation will never develop heart failure. If these dogs are administered an ACE inhibitor, it condemns the owner to years of expensive treatment. Second, there is no clinical proof and no experimental evidence to suggest that administering an ACE inhibitor this early in the course of the disease is beneficial. Third, ACE inhibitors are not without side effects. Administering a drug that has the potential of producing side effects to a dog that does not need the drug (presuming the dog will never develop heart failure) is questionable medical practice. Currently, a second study is in progress to determine whether enalapril administration to dogs with severe mitral regurgitation but without heart failure is beneficial (in the first study, many dogs died of unrelated disease and the results were negative, so the study was aborted). Until the results of that study are known, recommendations to start enalapril before the onset of heart failure are premature. If the results of this trial show a true increase in survival time, there will be no doubt that administration of an ACE inhibitor to dogs with severe cardiac disease but without heart failure is warranted. If, however, it shows only that the onset of heart failure is delayed, early administration of such drugs should be undertaken only after detailed consultation with the client, primarily because of the cost of these drugs. If this scenario comes to pass, there undoubtedly will be clients who will opt for early therapy in order to delay the onset of their pets' respiratory distress, regardless of cost. There undoubtedly will be other clients who will choose not to spend several dollars a day just to delay the inevitable.

One study has examined the short- and long-term effects of enalapril on left ventricular size and function in Cavalier King Charles spaniels with myxomatous mitral valve degeneration and mild to moderate heart failure.[45] In this study, enalapril did not result in a decrease in left ventricular size after three weeks of drug administration. After this time, furosemide was administered in conjunction with enalapril. Six months later, the left ventricular size actually increased. In a comparable group administered hydralazine and furosemide, the left ventricular size remained the same. End-systolic diameter did not change at any time in either group, suggesting that afterload and myocardial function were not significantly altered.

LISINOPRIL

Actions. Lisinopril is a lysine derivative of enalaprilat. It does not require hydrolysis to become active. It has a higher affinity for ACE than either captopril or enalapril.

Pharmacodynamics. Lisinopril's effects last for 24 hours but are quite attenuated 24 hours after oral administration in dogs.[72] An oral dose of 0.15 mg/lb to dogs results in approximately 75 per cent inhibition of the pressor response to angiotensin I three hours after administration. This response decreases to about 60 per cent inhibition by six hours and to approximately 10 per cent at 24 hours. When an oral dose of 0.45 mg/lb is administered, greater than 90 per cent inhibition of the pressor response to angiotensin I is achieved four hours after drug administration. This response is still approximately 90 per cent inhibition at six hours after administration and is approximately 40 per cent 24 hours after administration.

Administration and Dosage. A clinically effective dose of lisinopril has not been identified in dogs or cats. The author and others generally use a dose of 0.22 mg/lb orally every 24 hours. From the pharmacodynamic data just presented, a dose of 0.12 to 0.22 mg/lb every 12 hours or a dose of 0.45 mg/lb every 24 hours may be more effective. The primary benefit of lisinopril is cost. Cost per day to treat a dog is often half that of other ACE inhibitors if a dose of 0.22 mg/lb every 24 hours is used. The major factor that retards its use is that studies to document its pharmacodynamics and efficacy have not been performed.

Indications and Adverse Effects. The indications for and the adverse effects of lisinopril are the same as for the other long-acting ACE inhibitors.

BENAZEPRIL

Actions. Benazepril is a nonsulfhydryl ACE inhibitor. Like enalapril, it is a prodrug that is converted to benazeprilat by esterases, mainly in the liver.[76]

Pharmacodynamics. The pharmacodynamics of benazepril have been studied in dogs by measuring plasma ACE activity before and after various doses of the drug.[77] A dose of 0.06 mg/lb every 24 hours appears to be too low. It inhibits plasma ACE activity to only about 80 per cent of baseline. A dose of 0.12 mg/lb decreases plasma ACE activity to less than 10 per cent of baseline within three hours of administration. This effect lasts for at least 12 hours. By 16 hours, plasma ACE activity is back to 20 per cent of baseline, and by 24 hours, it is approximately 30 per cent of baseline. Doses of 0.22 and 0.45 mg/lb cause the greater than 90 per cent suppression to last at least 16 hours. When benazepril is administered chronically, doses from 0.11 to 0.45 mg/lb produce indistinguishable effects at the time of peak effect, two hours after oral administration. The same can be said for dosage effects on plasma ACE activity 24 hours (trough) after oral administration. From these data, it can be concluded that the clinically effective dose of benazepril is probably between 0.11 and 0.22 mg/lb orally and that once-a-day administration will probably be clinically effective in dogs.

Indications and Adverse Effects. Benazepril, like other ACE inhibitors, can be used in dogs or cats with heart failure. However, no clinical studies have been performed to document safety and efficacy. Anticipated adverse effects would be the same as for other long-acting ACE inhibitors.

PURE VASODILATORS

HYDRALAZINE

Actions. Hydralazine directly relaxes the smooth muscle in systemic arterioles, probably by increasing the prostacyclin concentration in systemic arterioles.[78, 79] It also increases aortic compliance. Hydralazine has no effect on systemic venous tone.[80] Hydralazine decreases vascular resistance in renal, coronary, cerebral, and mesenteric vascular beds more than in skeletal muscle beds.[81]

Hydralazine is a very potent arteriolar dilator.[82] In dogs it is able to decrease systemic vascular resistance to less than 40 per cent of baseline, in comparison to captopril, which can decrease systemic vascular resistance only by about 25

per cent.[44, 83] Hydralazine's potency can be both beneficial and detrimental. Its potency is of benefit because it results in good to profound improvement in the majority of animals in which it is indicated. Its potency can be detrimental if it results in hypotension.

In small dogs with severe mitral regurgitation refractory to the administration of furosemide, regurgitant flow may constitute 80 to 85 per cent of stroke volume.[84] Left ventricular contractile function is usually normal or only mildly depressed.[85] Consequently, the major hemodynamic abnormalities are caused by marked regurgitant flow through an incompetent mitral valve. The ideal treatment would be mitral valve repair, but this is not technically feasible at this time. Consequently, the theoretical treatment of choice is arteriolar dilator administration (see Fig. 111–1). ACE inhibitors are usually the first choice for achieving mild arteriolar dilatation. Hydralazine is more potent and is reserved for cases that are refractory to ACE inhibitors or animals with acute heart failure secondary to mitral regurgitation. Hydralazine decreases regurgitant flow, increases forward aortic flow and venous oxygen tension, and decreases radiographic evidence of pulmonary edema.[86, 87] A therapeutic dosage decreases mean arterial blood pressure from 100 to 110 mmHg to 60 to 80 mmHg.

Indications. The primary indication for hydralazine administration in veterinary medicine is severe mitral regurgitation that is refractory to conventional therapy.[83, 86] The dose must be titrated, starting with a low dose and titrating upward to an effective end point. Hydralazine produces an all-or-nothing response. It is well absorbed from the gastrointestinal tract but undergoes first-pass hepatic metabolism by acetylation.[88] Presumably, dog-to-dog variation in the ability to acetylate hydralazine explains the wide dose range required to produce a response. Although hydralazine is not excreted by the kidneys, its biotransformation is affected by renal failure, which may increase serum concentration. The vasodilating effect of hydralazine occurs within 30 to 60 minutes after oral administration and peaks within three hours. The effect is then stable for the next 8 to 10 hours, after which it rapidly dissipates. The net duration of effect is about 12 hours.[83]

In dogs that are not being administered ACE inhibitors, the starting dose of hydralazine should be 0.45 mg/lb. This can then be titrated up to as high as 1.35 mg/lb if no response is observed at lower doses. Titration in these animals can be performed with or without blood pressure measurement. If blood pressure cannot be monitored, titration is performed more slowly, and clinical and radiographic signs are monitored. Baseline assessments of mucous membrane color, capillary refill time, murmur intensity, cardiac size on radiographs, and severity of pulmonary edema are made. A dose of 0.45 mg/lb is administered orally every 12 hours, and repeat assessments are made in 12 to 48 hours. If no response is identified, the dose is increased to 0.9 mg/lb and then to 1.35 mg/lb if no response is seen at the previous dose. Mucous membrane color and capillary refill time become noticeably improved in about 50 to 60 per cent of dogs. In most dogs with heart failure due to mitral regurgitation, the severity of the pulmonary edema improves within 24 hours. In many of these dogs, the size of the left ventricle and left atrium decreases. In some dogs, improvement is not great enough to identify with certainty. In those dogs, the titration may continue with the realization that some dogs will be mildly overdosed and clinical signs of hypotension may become evident. Owners should be warned to watch for signs of hypotension and notify the clinician if they are identified. If a dog becomes weak and lethargic following hydralazine administration, the dog should be rechecked by a veterinarian, but in almost all situations, the dog should be observed only until the drug effect wears off 11 to 13 hours later. The drug dose should then be reduced. In the rare event that signs of shock become evident, fluids and vasopressors may be administered. In human medicine, there has never been a death recorded that was secondary to the administration of hydralazine alone. The author has observed dogs become very weak following an overdose of hydralazine but has never observed a serious complication when the drug was not administered in conjunction with another vasodilator such as an ACE inhibitor.

More rapid titration can be performed if blood pressure monitoring is available. In this situation, baseline blood pressure is measured and 0.45 mg/lb hydralazine is administered. Blood pressure measurement should be repeated one to two hours later. If blood pressure (systolic, diastolic, or mean) has decreased by at least 15 mmHg, the dose (0.45 mg/lb) is effective and should be administered every 12 hours from then on. If no response is identified, another 0.45 mg/lb dose should be administered (cumulative dose of 0.9 mg/lb) and blood pressure measured again one to two hours later. This can continue until a cumulative dose of 1.35 mg/lb has been administered within a 12-hour period. The resultant cumulative dose then becomes the dose administered every 12 hours.

In dogs that are already being administered an ACE inhibitor, the addition of hydralazine must be performed with caution. ACE inhibition depletes the body's ability to produce angiotensin II in response to hydralazine-induced vasodilatation. Severe hypotension can occur if the hydralazine dose is not titrated carefully. In general, the dosage should start at 0.22 mg/lb and be titrated at 0.22 mg/lb increments until a response is identified. Blood pressure monitoring is strongly encouraged in this situation. Referral to a board-certified cardiologist or internist is also encouraged.

In dogs with acute, fulminant heart failure due to severe mitral regurgitation that are not already receiving an ACE inhibitor, hydralazine titration can be more aggressive. An initial dose of 0.9 mg/lb may be administered along with intravenous furosemide. This dose should produce a beneficial response in more than 75 per cent of dogs. This dose may produce clinically significant hypotension (i.e., signs of weakness), but the hypotension is rarely fatal, whereas fulminant pulmonary edema is commonly fatal.

Adverse Effects. Common side effects include first-dose hypotension and anorexia, vomiting, and diarrhea. Anorexia, vomiting, or both occur in approximately 20 to 30 per cent of animals. They are often intractable as long as the drug is being administered. Consequently, discontinuation of the drug may be necessary. Reducing the dose to 0.11 to 0.22 mg/lb every 12 hours for one to two weeks and then increasing the dose to its therapeutic range may be effective in some cases. The most serious adverse effect is hypotension, indicated by signs of weakness and depression. In most cases, this does not require treatment and will abate within 10 to 12 hours after the last dose of hydralazine. The dose should then be reduced. The author has observed dogs with clinical signs of hypotension or counseled owners over the telephone regarding dogs with clinical signs of hypotension, and only rarely have clinically significant sequelae occurred. The only time that clinically significant complications (e.g., renal failure) have occurred is in dogs that were also on an ACE inhibitor.

Reflex sympathetic tachycardia can occur in heart failure patients. In animals with heart failure, the sympathetic nervous system is already activated, and the heart's ability to respond to the sympathetic nervous system is blunted. However, in one study, heart rate in dogs with mild to moderate heart failure increased from an average of 136 beats per minute to 153 beats per minute following hydralazine administration.[45] Control of reflex tachycardia may require the addition of low doses of a beta-adrenergic blocking drug or of digoxin.

Rebound increases in renin and aldosterone secretion and decreased sodium excretion occur following hydralazine administration.[45] This is generally not a clinical problem, however. The beneficial effect on regurgitant fraction usually outweighs these effects.

Drug Interactions. Hydralazine administration may have beneficial effects on the pharmacokinetics and pharmacodynamics of other drugs. The increased renal blood flow produced by hydralazine administration can increase the GFR (if initially depressed) and thereby enhance digoxin excretion.[89] The increased renal blood flow also improves furosemide delivery to the nephron.[90] This increases furosemide's renal effects (increases natriuresis and diuresis), especially in animals that are refractory to furosemide administration because of decreased renal flow due to decreased cardiac output.

NITRATES

The organic nitrates, such as nitroglycerin, are esters of nitric oxide. Nitroprusside is a nitric oxide–containing compound without an ester bond. There are important differences in the biotransformation of these compounds, but it is generally accepted that they share a common final pathway of nitric oxide (endothelium-derived relaxing factor) production and a common therapeutic effect.[91]

Nitrates relax vascular smooth muscle. They do this through a complex series of events. Nitrates are denitrated in smooth muscle cells to form nitric oxide, which binds with the heme moiety on the enzyme guanylate cyclase.[91–93] This causes activation of guanylate cyclase, which enzymatically forms cyclic guanosine monophosphate (cGMP) from guanosine triphosphate (GTP). Cyclic GMP activates a serine/threonine protein kinase, which phosphorylates myosin light chains, resulting in smooth muscle relaxation.[91, 94]

Nitrates have been advocated as agents to produce systemic venodilatation in dogs and cats with heart failure.[95] Few studies have been performed to document the pharmacodynamics or establish the therapeutic dosage of nitrates in dogs or cats. Nitrates can be administered orally, intravenously, or transcutaneously to animals with heart failure. When administered transcutaneously or orally to humans, low plasma concentrations are achieved. Nitrates act primarily as venodilators at low plasma concentrations. When administered intravenously, higher concentrations are achieved, and arteriolar dilatation also occurs.

Nitrates are well absorbed from the gastrointestinal tract but are rapidly metabolized by hepatic organic nitrate reductase. Consequently, bioavailability of orally administered nitrates is very low, typically less than 10 per cent. In humans, the duration of effect after transcutaneous administration is three to eight hours.

Nitrate Tolerance. Tolerance to the organic nitrates is a common problem in human patients, occurring in up to 70 per cent of individuals exposed to intravenous infusions of nitroglycerin.[96] The exact mechanism is poorly understood.[97, 98]

Intermittent administration of nitrates prevents tolerance in human patients. However, this approach is limited by the fact that the hemodynamic benefit is interrupted. Concurrent administration of hydralazine with a nitrate appears to prevent nitrate tolerance in human heart failure patients.[99, 100]

NITROGLYCERIN

Nitroglycerin is an organic nitrovasodilator that possesses a nitrate ester bond. The biotransformation of nitroglycerin to nitric oxide is complex and not completely understood. Thiols (compounds containing sulfhydryl groups) appear to be important as intermediary structures.[91]

Pharmacokinetics. Nitroglycerin has a very short half-life of one to four minutes.[65] Transdermal systems are designed to provide continuous, controlled release of nitroglycerin to the skin, from which the drug is absorbed. The onset of action with the transdermal route of administration is delayed, and the duration of effect is prolonged. The rate of delivery and absorption of the drug vary in humans and probably do not translate into the actual rate of delivery for a dog or a cat.

Indications. In human patients with heart failure, transdermal administration of nitroglycerin results primarily in systemic venodilatation. This effect redistributes blood volume from the central to the peripheral vascular compartments, resulting in a decrease in diastolic intraventricular pressures and a reduction in the formation of edema fluid (see Fig. 111–2).[101, 102] Systemic vascular resistance is lowered to a lesser degree.[101] The dosage required to produce a beneficial effect is highly variable, and some patients are refractory to the drug. Tolerance develops quickly, within 18 to 24 hours.[101] A rebound increase in systemic vascular resistance is observed when nitroglycerin is withdrawn, which results in a decrease in cardiac output.[101] There is no rebound effect on ventricular diastolic and atrial pressures.

Transdermal administration of nitroglycerin has been advocated for use in dogs and cats with heart failure.[95] All references in the veterinary literature to the use of nitroglycerin in clinical patients, including dosing, are anecdotal. Nitroglycerin administered topically to the ears of experimental dogs has been shown to produce splenic venodilatation.[103] Nitroglycerin is most commonly administered in conjunction with furosemide to animals with severe heart failure. Beneficial effects in this situation cannot be directly ascribed to nitroglycerin, because it is well known that furosemide by itself can produce dramatically beneficial effects in these animals. Anecdotal reports of the skin in the region of administration turning red certainly suggest that there is local vasodilatation, but that does not directly translate into systemic vasodilatation. The author has on occasion observed beneficial effects in dogs that were not responding or had become unresponsive to other cardiovascular drugs, suggesting that there may be a limited role for this drug in veterinary patients. The author does not believe that nitroglycerin is a very effective drug and would never administer it as the sole agent to an animal with moderate to severe heart failure.

Nitroglycerin ointment is available in a 2 per cent formulation to be spread on the skin for absorption into the systemic circulation.[68] It is also supplied in a transcutaneous patch preparation by numerous manufacturers.[101] In dogs and cats, 2 per cent nitroglycerin cream has been used (half an inch per 5 lb body weight every 12 hours for dogs; one-eighth to one-quarter inch every 4 to 6 hours for cats),

but efficacy has not been documented.[95] If transcutaneous nitroglycerin cream is used, it should be applied on a hairless area (usually inside the ear flap) using gloves, because transcutaneous absorption will occur in the clinician or owner as well as in the animal. Cutaneous absorption in a human can cause a profound headache and a very unhappy client. Transdermal patches have been used successfully in large dogs with dilated cardiomyopathy.[104]

ISOSORBIDE DINITRATE

Isosorbide dinitrate is an organic nitrate that can be administered orally. Its efficacy in dogs and cats has not been studied. Isosorbide mononitrate has been studied in experimental dogs, and the dose of isosorbide dinitrate is probably similar to that of isosorbide mononitrate. In one study, a dose of 30 mg of isosorbide mononitrate orally every 12 hours to dogs weighing 33 ± 6.5 pounds (approximately 1 mg/lb) subjected to transmyocardial direct-current shock produced acute hemodynamic effects that lasted only two hours. When administered over days, however, this dose resulted in a chronic decrease in pulmonary capillary wedge pressure and a decrease in left ventricular volume and mass when compared with control dogs.[105]

NITROPRUSSIDE

Nitroprusside (sodium nitroferricyanide) produces nitric oxide in vascular smooth muscle. Unlike the organic nitrates, nitroprusside releases nitric oxide when it is nonenzymatically metabolized directly via one-electron reduction.[106] This may occur on exposure to numerous reducing agents and tissues such as vascular smooth muscle. The major difference between nitroprusside and the organic nitrates is that tolerance to nitroprusside does not develop.

Actions. Nitroprusside is a potent venodilator and a potent arteriolar dilator.[80] It may also increase left ventricular compliance.[107] It is administered intravenously and is used only for short-term treatment of dogs with severe or fulminant heart failure. In one study in normal dogs, nitroprusside (11 μg/lb per minute) decreased systemic arterial blood pressure by 23 per cent and increased cardiac output by 39 per cent.[108] This effect became attenuated over time. Because tolerance does not occur with nitroprusside, this attenuation of effect was probably due to reflex changes. The decrease in systemic blood pressure did result in a reflex increase in sympathetic discharge, as evidenced by increases in heart rate and myocardial contractility. As expected, left ventricular end-diastolic and end-systolic diameters decreased in this study, as did left ventricular end-diastolic pressure.

Pharmacokinetics. Nitroprusside is rapidly metabolized after intravenous administration, with a half-life of a few minutes. Consequently, no loading dose is required, and any untoward effects of the drug can be rapidly reversed by discontinuing drug administration. When nitroprusside is metabolized, cyanogen (cyanide radical) is produced. This is converted to thiocyanate in the liver by the enzyme thiosulfate sulfurtransferase (rhodanase).

Indications. Nitroprusside is beneficial in dogs with experimentally induced acute mitral regurgitation (comparable to a patient with a ruptured chorda tendinea). In one study, a dose of 2.2 μg/lb per minute reduced left ventricular systolic pressure 16 per cent and decreased left ventricular end-diastolic pressure from 23 mmHg to a normal value of

10 mmHg.[109] Left atrial pressure, left atrial diameter, and left ventricular diameter also decreased. The left atrial "v" wave decreased from 41 mmHg to 16 mmHg.

In humans with severe heart failure, nitroprusside can produce beneficial effects that are equal to or better than those achieved with the administration of intravenous furosemide.[110] In one study, nitroprusside reduced pulmonary capillary pressure from 31 to 16 mmHg while increasing the cardiac index from 2.33 to 3.62 L/min/M².[111] Furosemide (200 mg intravenously) in these same patients decreased pulmonary capillary pressure to 27 mmHg while the cardiac index did not change. Consequently, it appears that nitroprusside may be preferred for treating patients with acute, severe heart failure. Unfortunately, nitroprusside is often not a practical drug to use in clinical veterinary practice because blood pressure monitoring is required.

Administration and Dosage. The dose of nitroprusside is highly variable from patient to patient. In addition, the hemodynamic response can be varied, depending on the amount of change in filling pressures and cardiac output desired. Consequently, the dosage range is large. Doses from 1 to 12 µg/lb per minute reduce systemic arterial blood pressure in a dose-dependent manner in experimental dogs.[112] However, the decrease in blood pressure with 12 µg/lb per minute is only about 5 mmHg more than that observed with 5 µg/lb per minute. Consequently, it does not appear that doses greater than 5 µg/lb per minute provide much more benefit than lesser doses.[65]

Sodium nitroprusside is supplied as vials containing 50 mg of lyophilized dry powder for dilution in 5 per cent dextrose in water.[115] Sodium nitroprusside is sensitive to light, heat, and moisture. Exposure to light causes deterioration, which may be observed as a change in color from brown to blue, caused by reduction of the ferric ion to ferrous ion. If not protected from light, approximately 20 per cent of the drug in solution in glass bottles will deteriorate every four hours when exposed to fluorescent light. The drug deteriorates even faster in plastic containers. Consequently, sodium nitroprusside should be protected from light by wrapping the bottle with aluminum foil. When adequately protected from light, the solution is stable for 24 hours. Nitroprusside reacts with minute quantities of a variety of agents (including alcohol), forming blue, dark red, or green products. The solution should be discarded if this occurs.

Adverse Effects. Adverse effects of nitroprusside are hypotension and cyanide toxicity. Nitroprusside-induced hypotension can be rapidly (1 to 10 minutes) reversed by discontinuing drug administration. Sodium nitroprusside infusions in excess of 1 µg/lb per minute generate cyanogen in amounts greater than can be effectively buffered by the normal quantity of methemoglobin in the body. Deaths due to cyanogen toxicity can result when this buffering system is exhausted. In humans, this has been reported only in patients receiving infusion rates of 12 to 55 µg/lb per minute.[65] However, increased circulating cyanogen concentration, metabolic acidosis, and clinical deterioration have been observed at infusion rates within the therapeutic range. In humans, it has been recommended that an infusion rate of 5 µg/lb per minute should not last longer than 16 hours.[113, 114] In the presence of thiosulfate, cyanogen is converted to thiocyanate, which is excreted in the kidneys. Thiocyanate toxicity can occur, especially in patients that have a decreased GFR, are on prolonged infusions, or are receiving thiosulfate. Neurologic signs occur in humans at a serum concentration of 60 µg/mL, and death can occur at a concentration greater than 200 µg/mL.[65]

DIGITALIS GLYCOSIDES

The digitalis glycosides are used primarily to treat patients with heart failure due to systolic dysfunction. The means by which they improve cardiovascular function in heart failure patients is multifactorial. Digitalis glycosides act as positive inotropic agents. They also alter baroreceptor sensitivity and directly alter autonomic function. In so doing, they increase vagal efferent nerve traffic to the heart and tend to decrease sympathetic nervous tone when present in therapeutic concentrations. They may also directly produce diuresis and natriuresis and directly decrease renin release.[116]

Efficacy. Ever since the original clinical studies, the digitalis glycosides have been embroiled in controversy regarding their use, mechanisms of action, and efficacy. The human literature is replete with reports documenting the efficacy and lack of efficacy of digitalis in the treatment of heart failure patients.[117–124] More recent studies using blinded and placebo-controlled trials have more strongly suggested that digoxin is efficacious for treating human patients in sinus rhythm.[125–127] The issue of efficacy remains controversial, however. Recently, a large clinical trial designed to answer the question of digoxin's efficacy in human heart failure patients in sinus rhythm was completed.[2, 128] This trial enrolled 7788 human patients with heart failure. About 6800 of them had a low ejection fraction (<45 per cent). Most (80 to 90 per cent) were being treated with a diuretic and an ACE inhibitor at presentation. About 50 per cent of the patients were in class II (mild) heart failure, and about 30 per cent were in class III (moderate) heart failure. Patients were randomized to receive either placebo or digoxin. Patients were followed by measuring ejection fraction, measuring the cardiothoracic ratio on a chest radiograph, recording hospitalizations, and recording death. There was no difference in deaths from cardiovascular causes between the two groups. Consequently, it was concluded that digoxin has no impact on survival in human patients with heart failure. There was a trend toward a significant decrease in deaths due to heart failure, but this was offset by a higher incidence of other types of cardiac death (sudden death, acute myocardial infarction, bradyarrhythmias, low-output states, and surgery) in the digoxin group. The digoxin group had significantly fewer hospitalizations. However, for the average physician, only nine hospitalizations would be avoided for every 1000 patients treated each year.[129] In general, the effect of digoxin in this clinical trial can be described, for the average human patient, as underwhelming. As one editorial stated, "Digoxin's inability to substantially influence morbidity or mortality eliminates any ethical mandate for its use and effectively relegates it to be prescribed for the treatment of persistent symptoms after the administration of drugs that do reduce the risk of death and hospitalization."[129]

In small animal veterinary medicine, the question of digoxin's efficacy will probably never be answered. There is no reason to believe that results of studies examining digoxin's efficacy in human patients can be directly extrapolated to digoxin's efficacy in dogs or cats, and it is very unlikely that the funds for a large clinical trial to document efficacy in veterinary patients will ever become available. Consequently, controversy regarding the efficacy of digoxin in dogs and cats will probably continue until better means of dealing with severe cardiac disease are identified.

It is the author's opinion that, as with any cardiovascular drug, individual response to digoxin is highly variable. Although the majority of dogs and cats have no to minimal response to the drug, some animals have a mild to moderate response. The only way to identify such animals is to administer the drug and monitor the response. The author believes that digoxin should be administered to any animal that has severe myocardial failure, followed by careful monitoring for any signs of improvement both clinically and echocardiographically, if possible. If no response is identified, the drug can be either continued if there are no untoward effects identified or discontinued.

Efficacy could depend on dose. It is often thought that if a low dose of digoxin is ineffective, a larger dose may be beneficial. This is not necessarily true and may be false. A recent study in humans suggests that patients who receive a moderate dose of digoxin (0.25 mg every 24 hours) and have a moderate serum digoxin concentration (1.5 ng/mL) obtain no more benefit than patients who receive a low dose of digoxin (0.125 mg every 24 hours) and have a lower serum digoxin concentration (0.8 ng/mL).[130] In this study, increased contractility and decreased heart rate were the primary end points. Another human study suggested that a serum digoxin concentration greater than 1 ng/mL was associated with greater mortality than a serum concentration less than 1 ng/mL.[131]

Actions. The digitalis glycosides increase contractility in normal myocardium and may also do so in failing myocardium. However, their ability to increase contractility in normal myocardium is only about one third that of the sympathomimetics (e.g., dopamine, dobutamine) and bipyridine compounds (e.g., amrinone, milrinone).[132] This translates into a lesser inotropic response in clinical patients.[133]

The positive inotropic effect of digitalis is thought to be caused by the effect of digitalis on the Na^+,K^+-ATPase pumps located on myocardial cell membranes.[124] Digitalis competitively binds to the site at which potassium normally attaches and effectively stops pump activity.[134] A therapeutic concentration of digoxin "poisons" approximately 30 per cent of the Na^+,K^+-ATPase pumps in the myocardium. Thus, the cell loses some of its ability to extrude sodium from the intracellular space during diastole, resulting in an increase in intracellular sodium concentration. This leads to increased intracellular osmolality. The cell counters by exchanging the intracellular sodium for extracellular calcium via the Na^+/Ca^{++} cation exchanger or by reducing the exchange of intracellular calcium for extracellular sodium. The net result is an increase in the number of calcium ions within the cell. In a normal cell, these excess calcium ions are bound by the sarcoplasmic reticulum during diastole. They are subsequently released onto the contractile proteins during systole, causing increased contractility.[135] This mechanism also works in failing myocardium if the myocytes are able to bind the increased calcium. However, the effects of positive inotropic agents are usually reduced in the presence of myocardial failure. The author's clinical impression is that the positive inotropic effects of digoxin are severely reduced in most animals with severe myocardial failure.

Most investigators have focused on the positive inotropic effects of the digitalis glycosides in patients with heart failure. However, digitalis glycosides may have other beneficial effects that are unrelated to their positive inotropic effects. Only recently, investigators examined the renal effects of a digitalis glycoside (ouabain) and found it to have diuretic properties.[116] There are Na^+,K^+-ATPase pumps present on the basolateral aspect of renal tubular epithelial cells that may promote renal tubular reabsorption of sodium. There appears to be an up-regulation of pump activity in the proximal tubule in heart failure.[136] These pumps appear to be regulated by prostaglandins. Indomethacin decreases prostaglandin synthesis and increases Na^+,K^+-ATPase activity and renal sodium retention. Prostaglandin administration, in contrast, results in natriuresis. Digitalis had a similar effect in one study, increasing sodium excretion up to 284 per cent above the baseline in experimental dogs with rapid ventricular pacing–induced heart failure.[136] This would make digoxin a slightly better diuretic than spironolactone. This same study documented decreased renal renin release when digitalis was injected directly into the renal artery.

In addition to the aforementioned effects, the digitalis glycosides have effects on vascular baroreceptors. Baroreceptor function is reset to a lower value in human patients and experimental dogs with heart failure.[137, 138] This results in decreased vagal tone to the heart and increased sympathetic activity. This is clearly a compensatory mechanism, although it is commonly construed to be a primary abnormality.[138] This compensatory mechanism, however, can be detrimental in patients with heart failure. The digitalis glycosides clearly have the ability to increase baroreceptor function in normal cats, dogs, and humans.[139–141] The digitalis glycosides decrease plasma catecholamine concentrations, directly recorded sympathetic nerve activity, and plasma renin activity, which may all be related to increased baroreceptor activity.[142, 143] In addition, the increase in vagal tone observed with digitalis administration is in part due to this effect.

The digitalis glycosides are used as antiarrhythmic agents, mostly for controlling supraventricular tachyarrhythmias (see Chapter 114). These agents increase parasympathetic nerve activity to the sinus node, atria, and atrioventricular (AV) node when the digitalis serum concentration is within the therapeutic range.[144]

Indications. The digitalis glycosides are indicated for the treatment of myocardial failure and supraventricular tachyarrhythmias. Myocardial failure is always present in animals with dilated cardiomyopathy or a long-standing (>5 years) moderate-size patent ductus arteriosus. It is usually present in animals with heart failure secondary to chronic severe aortic regurgitation and in large dogs with severe mitral regurgitation. Myocardial function is usually not clinically significantly depressed in small dogs with heart failure secondary to severe mitral regurgitation, although it may become apparent (on an echocardiogram) by the time a dog has become refractory to conventional medical therapy. The use of digitalis in small dogs with mitral regurgitation and no myocardial failure is not contraindicated, but other drugs are more beneficial. Myocardial failure is never present in hypertrophic cardiomyopathy or pericardial disease. Digitalis is contraindicated in hypertrophic cardiomyopathy, because increased contractility can worsen systolic anterior motion of the mitral valve and increase the outflow tract gradient. It is not contraindicated in pericardial diseases, but beneficial effects should not be expected.

In dogs with myocardial failure, digitalis does not routinely result in a clinically significant increase in myocardial contractility. Of 22 dogs with dilated cardiomyopathy in one study, only five responded to digoxin.[145] All five dogs lived longer than six months after their response. Dogs with dilated cardiomyopathy that respond to digoxin live significantly longer than do those that do not respond.[67] Consequently, the author treats all animals with myocardial failure with digoxin but does not hesitate to take a dog off of digoxin if there has been no apparent response and complications of digoxin therapy have occurred.

The digitalis glycosides are used to treat supraventricular tachyarrhythmias. They are generally regarded as moderately effective in controlling supraventricular premature depolarizations, supraventricular tachycardia, and the ventricular rate in atrial fibrillation (see Chapter 114).

DIGOXIN

Pharmacokinetics. Digoxin is well absorbed after oral administration. Approximately 60 per cent of the tablet is absorbed, whereas about 75 per cent of the elixir is absorbed. There is very little hepatic metabolism, so almost all the drug that is absorbed reaches the serum. In the serum, an average of 27 per cent of digoxin is bound to albumin.[146] The volume of distribution is 5.5 to 7 L/lb.[147]

In the dog, the serum half-life of digoxin is 23 to 39 hours,[148] but much individual variability exists. Drug accumulation occurs until a steady-state serum concentration is reached. It takes one half-life to achieve 50 per cent of the steady-state serum concentration, two half-lives to reach 75 per cent, three half-lives to reach 87.5 per cent, and so forth. Theoretically, it takes about five half-lives to reach steady state, so it is commonly thought that five half-lives are required to achieve therapeutic serum concentrations. However, this is not the case. In one study of dogs given 0.01 mg/lb digoxin every 24 hours, the serum concentration was within therapeutic range by the second day.[149] Based on these data, maintenance doses of digoxin in dogs should be used to achieve therapeutic serum concentrations in almost all situations. Loading doses designed to achieve a therapeutic concentration within a shorter period should be used only for emergencies, and then with caution, because loading dose schedules can produce a toxic serum concentration.[150]

Most of a digoxin dose is excreted in the urine via glomerular filtration and renal secretion. About 15 per cent is metabolized in the liver. Renal failure reduces renal clearance, total body clearance, and volume of distribution, resulting in increased serum digoxin concentrations.[151] Digoxin should be avoided in dogs with renal failure, if possible. If a digitalis glycoside is required, tincture of digitoxin may be used instead, or a much lower dose of digoxin can be administered and the serum concentration monitored closely. Formulas have been devised to calculate the reduction in digoxin dosage needed to achieve therapeutic serum concentrations in humans with renal failure.[152] There is no correlation between the degree of azotemia and serum digoxin concentration in dogs or cats, so such formulas cannot be used.[153, 154] Digitoxin is not a viable option for cats owing to its long half-life in that species. Consequently, in cats with renal failure that are administered digoxin, the dosage should be markedly reduced and the serum concentration monitored.

The pharmacokinetics of digoxin in the cat are controversial. The half-life is extremely variable from cat to cat, ranging from 26 to 51 hours in one study (mean, 33 hours) and 39 to 78 hours in another report (mean, 58 hours).[148, 155] In a more recent study, the half-life in a group of six normal cats ranged from 30 to 173 hours, with a mean half-life of 82 hours.[154] The first study reported that the half-life of digoxin increased dramatically to an average of 73 hours after prolonged oral administration. When digoxin tablets are administered with food to cats, the serum concentration is reduced by about 50 per cent compared with the concentration without food.[156] The elixir form results in a serum concentration approximately 50 per cent higher than that obtained with the tablet.[156] However, cats generally dislike the taste of the alcohol-based elixir.

Administration and Dosage. Because of the variability in pharmacokinetics from animal to animal, digoxin administration to any animal should be viewed as a pharmacologic experiment. An initial dose should be chosen, that dose administered, and a serum concentration measured three to five days later to determine whether the chosen dose has resulted in a therapeutic serum concentration. The initial starting dose of digoxin in normal small dogs weighing less than 40 pounds can be based on body weight at 0.002 to 0.005 mg/lb administered orally every 12 hours. In dogs weighing more than 40 pounds, this dose cannot be safely used. Instead, the dosage should be based on body surface area (i.e., 0.25 mg/M² orally every 12 hours).[157]

Commonly, the initial starting dose of a digitalis glycoside needs to be modified because of factors that alter the pharmacokinetics of the drug. In a study in which digoxin dose (0.002 to 0.11 mg/lb per day) was plotted against serum concentration in dogs with heart failure, the correlation coefficient was only 0.39 (1.0 is a perfect correlation).[158] This weak correlation was statistically significant. The drug dosage is therefore a factor in determining serum concentration, but it is only one factor among a number of other variables to consider when administering digoxin.

Because most of a digitalis glycoside is bound to skeletal muscle, dogs or cats that have lost significant muscle mass (decreased volume of distribution) have an increased serum concentration for any given dose. Consequently, for animals that are cachectic, the dose must be reduced. Older dogs commonly have decreased muscle mass and impaired renal function, so digoxin dosing in these animals must be performed cautiously.

Digoxin is poorly lipid-soluble. Consequently, dosing should be based on a lean body weight estimate. Lean body weight is an estimate of what an obese animal should weigh. Conversely, digitoxin is lipid-soluble, so no change in the dosage is required for lean or obese dogs.

Digoxin does not distribute well into ascitic fluid. Consequently, the dose of digoxin must be reduced in animals with ascites if total body weight is used to calculate the dose.[159] In general, animals with mild ascites should have the dose reduced by 10 per cent. Animals with moderate ascites require a 20 per cent dose reduction, and those with severe ascites need a 30 per cent reduction.

The administration of other drugs along with digitalis may affect the serum concentration. Quinidine displaces digoxin from skeletal muscle binding sites and reduces its renal clearance, resulting in an increased serum digoxin concentration.[160] Quinidine probably also displaces digoxin from myocardial binding sites.[161, 162] This may lessen the direct cardiac toxicity of digoxin and decrease its positive inotropic effect. In general, the combination of digoxin and quinidine should be avoided. If both drugs must be used together, the rule of thumb in human medicine is to reduce the digoxin dosage by 50 per cent.[160] Because serum digoxin concentration approximately doubles following quinidine administration in dogs, this recommendation appears to be valid in veterinary patients.[161] No interaction between digitoxin and quinidine exists in the dog.[163] In humans, there are reports of numerous other drugs that increase the serum concentration of digoxin, including oral aminoglycosides (neomycin), amiodarone, anticholinergics, captopril, diltiazem, esmolol, flecainide, ibuprofen, indomethacin, nifedipine, tetracycline, and verapamil.[164, 165]

Drugs that alter hepatic microsomal enzymes may affect digoxin pharmacokinetics, because about 15 per cent of digoxin is metabolized in the liver.[166] Drugs that induce hepatic microsomal enzymes, such as phenylbutazone and the barbiturates, may have a tendency to increase digoxin clearance, whereas such drugs as chloramphenicol and tetracycline, which inhibit hepatic enzymes, should increase the serum digoxin concentration. However, one study documented that chloramphenicol decreases serum digoxin concentration in dogs.[167] The effects of these drugs on digitoxin elimination are unknown.

Hypokalemia predisposes to digitalis myocardial toxicity. Digitalis and potassium compete for the same binding site on the membrane Na^+,K^+-ATPase pumps.[168] Hypokalemia leaves more binding sites available for digitalis. Hyperkalemia displaces digitalis from the myocardium. Hypercalcemia and hypernatremia potentiate the positive inotropic and toxic effects of digitalis, whereas hypocalcemia and hyponatremia reduce these effects.

Hyperthyroidism increases the myocardial effects of digitalis.[151] The dose may need to be decreased in this situation. Although hypothyroidism has been reported to reduce renal clearance of digoxin in humans, this does not appear to be the case in dogs.[151] In one study, acute and chronic digoxin pharmacokinetics were measured in dogs before and after experimental induction of hypothyroidism.[169] There was no difference between the groups. Consequently, it is not necessary to adjust the digoxin dose in hypothyroid dogs.

Myocardial failure increases the sensitivity of the myocardium to the toxic effects of digitalis. Failing myocardial cells are usually thought to be overloaded with calcium. Digitalis may cause further calcium loading. Calcium-overloaded cells may become electrically unstable, resulting in tachyarrhythmias.[170] Digitalis should be administered cautiously in these animals, and loading doses should not be used.

Digoxin pharmacokinetics are not significantly altered in cats with compensated heart failure that are being administered furosemide and aspirin,[154] despite increases in serum urea and creatinine concentrations.

Strategy. In general, animals should be evaluated carefully before digoxin is administered. Factors that alter the dosage should be noted and an initial dose chosen. The animal should be monitored during the initial course of therapy for signs of toxicity or improvement. A decrease in heart rate or resolution of an arrhythmia is a documentable benefit in an animal with tachycardia or arrhythmia. Clinical responsiveness owing to improved hemodynamics in animals with heart failure is the desired end point of digitalis administration but can be difficult to identify for several reasons. First, other drugs are generally administered with digitalis, so it may be impossible to identify the beneficial drug. Second, many dogs do not respond to digoxin, so clinical resolution may never occur. The dosage in the latter case should not be increased unless the serum concentration has been measured and documented to be subtherapeutic (i.e., <0.5 to 1 ng/mL). In each case, serum digoxin concentration should be measured two to five days after initiating therapy. The serum sample should be acquired six to eight hours after the last dose and sent to a laboratory for analysis. Therapeutic range for serum digoxin concentration is somewhat controversial but can generally be considered to be between 0.5 and 2 ng/mL. A serum concentration greater than 2.5 ng/mL should be considered toxic. If such an elevation is identified in an animal and clinical signs are evident, digoxin administration should be discontinued until the serum concentration is less than 2.5 ng/mL. The dosage should be reduced accordingly.

Toxicity. Therapeutic end points for digitalis in animals with heart failure include clinical improvement or attainment of therapeutic serum concentration. Progressive dosing until signs of toxicity occur or until the PR interval on the electrocardiogram increases is not justified.[171] By the time gastrointestinal signs of toxicity are present in dogs with myocardial failure, myocardial toxicity may be present and may be fatal. Dogs without myocardial failure (e.g., small dogs with mitral regurgitation) tolerate digitalis toxicity better than do those with myocardial failure (i.e., myocardial toxicity occurs at a higher serum concentration) and generally show signs of anorexia and vomiting before exhibiting electrocardiographic evidence of myocardial toxicity.

In normal beagle dogs, a serum concentration of digoxin that exceeds 2.5 ng/mL generally produces clinical signs of toxicity.[172] However, dogs and cats may show clinical evidence of toxicity at a serum concentration less than 2.5 ng/mL, and occasionally a dog shows no clinical signs of toxicity at a serum concentration greater than 2.5 ng/mL.

The incidence of digoxin toxicity is unclear.[173] In the author's experience, clinically significant digitalis toxicity is rare if the drug is used judiciously and the serum concentration is monitored. Toxicity occurs most frequently when an owner becomes overzealous with drug administration when the animal is not responding, when the pet develops renal failure while on digoxin, and during the initial stages of digoxin administration. Owners should always be warned not to administer more of a digitalis glycoside if the pet does not appear to be improving on the medication.

Problems from digitalis intoxication fall into three general classes: those referable to the central nervous system, the gastrointestinal system, and the myocardium.[172] Most dogs that are intoxicated with digoxin appear depressed. Humans experience malaise and drowsiness and have headaches.[168] Anorexia and vomiting are common manifestations of digitalis intoxication and are probably due to the direct effect of the digitalis molecule on the chemoreceptor trigger zone located in the area postrema in the medulla.[174] In one study, normal dogs with a serum concentration of digoxin in the 2.5 to 6 ng/mL range decreased their food intake to about half of normal while maintaining a normal water intake; dogs with a serum concentration greater than 6 ng/mL stopped eating, decreased their water intake to less than a third of normal, and vomited.[175]

Autonomic tone to the heart is increased with digitalis toxicity. Increased vagal tone can result in a decrease in sinus node rate and altered AV nodal conduction and refractoriness. Increased sympathetic tone can counter these effects. Sinus node rate is variable in dogs with digitalis intoxication. In one study of normal dogs administered toxic doses of digoxin for two weeks, the heart rate initially decreased from baseline values of 90 to 130 beats per minute to 50 to 90 beats per minute after intravenous administration of digoxin but returned to baseline by 24 to 48 hours after dosing.[172] Despite continued administration of toxic doses, the heart rate remained at baseline values or was mildly decreased. During the periods of most severe toxicity, the heart rate increased to 130 to 190 beats per minute. Increased vagal tone predominates at the AV nodal level. First-degree AV block is a common finding in dogs with digoxin toxicity. Second-degree AV block may also occur, especially after prolonged intoxication.[176, 177] In dogs, blockade of the sympathetic nervous system increases the dose of digitalis required to produce arrhythmias.[168] However, in cats it has been shown that cardiac toxicity occurs at the same dosage with or without destruction of the area postrema.[178] Digitalis also slows conduction and alters the refractory period, making it easier for reentrant arrhythmias to develop. Triggered activity appears to be the most important reason for the development of arrhythmias in digitalis intoxication. The classic cellular event produced by digitalis intoxication is the formation of late afterdepolarizations in which the diastolic membrane potential oscillates, eventually reaches threshold potential, and depolarizes the cell.[170] The electrocardiographic counterpart of this depolarization would be a premature beat. Late afterdepolarizations are attributed to cellular calcium overload and are more easily induced in myocardium that has been stretched (analogous to a ventricle with an increased end-diastolic pressure) and is in a hypokalemic environment.[168]

Clinically, myocardial toxicity can take the form of almost every known rhythm disturbance. In the dog, ventricular tachyarrhythmias and bradyarrhythmias are most common. The ventricular tachyarrhythmias consist of ventricular premature depolarizations, ventricular bigeminy and trigeminy, and ventricular tachycardia. The common bradyarrhythmias are second-degree AV block, sinus bradycardia, and sinus arrest that occur because of increased vagal tone. Digitalis can also induce supraventricular premature depolarizations and tachycardia, junctional tachyarrhythmias, and other arrhythmias. At times it may be difficult or impossible to distinguish whether an arrhythmia is due to digitalis or to the underlying heart disease. Arrhythmias characterized by tachycardia with impaired conduction are highly suggestive of digitalis-induced problems. Ventricular tachyarrhythmias and AV nodal conduction disturbances that appear in a dog or cat being administered digitalis should generally be regarded as digitalis induced until proved otherwise.

Digoxin toxicity also causes renal damage. In one study, there was hydropic degeneration and epithelial necrosis in the proximal tubule and in the medullary collecting ducts.[172] This resulted in increases in serum concentrations of urea nitrogen and creatinine. There was a direct correlation between the degree of elevation in serum concentration and the severity of the tubular damage.

A digitalis overdose can produce hyperkalemia and hyponatremia.[179] In one study, moderate toxicity (serum digoxin concentration 2.5 to 6 ng/mL) resulted in serum concentrations of sodium between 130 and 145 mEq/L with a normal serum potassium concentration. Severe toxicity (serum digoxin concentration >6 ng/mL) produced serum sodium concentrations in the 110 to 130 mEq/L range and serum concentrations of potassium anywhere from 3.2 to 7.7 mEq/L. These electrolyte abnormalities are probably caused by digitalis inhibition of the Na^+,K^+-ATPase pumps throughout the body.

The mainstay of treating digitalis intoxication is discontinuing drug administration. Because the half-life of digoxin in a normal dog is between 24 and 36 hours, it should take one to one and a half days for the serum concentration to decrease to half the original concentration. Half-life is commonly prolonged in older animals and diseased animals. Consequently, the time to reach half the original concentration is prolonged.

Gastrointestinal signs related to a digitalis overdose are treated by drug withdrawal and correction of fluid and electrolyte abnormalities. Conduction disturbances and bradyarrhythmias usually require only digitalis withdrawal, although atropine administration is occasionally needed.[180] Ventricular tachyarrhythmias are generally treated aggressively, especially when ventricular tachycardia is present. It is estimated that two thirds of the human patients with ventricular tachycardia secondary to digitalis intoxication will not survive, despite therapy.[181]

Lidocaine is the drug of choice for treating ventricular

tachyarrhythmias due to digitalis intoxication.[180] It decreases sympathetic nerve traffic and can abolish reentrant arrhythmias and late afterdepolarizations.[182, 183] Lidocaine usually has little effect on sinus rate or AV nodal conduction, so it does not usually exacerbate these problems. It is safe in the dog, can readily be administered intravenously, and has a rapid onset of action. It may be administered as an initial bolus (1 to 2 mg/lb intravenously over one to three minutes) followed by continuous infusion of 14 to 45 μg/lb per minute for arrhythmia control.

Phenytoin (diphenylhydantoin) is the second drug of choice for the treatment of digitalis-induced toxicity in the dog. It has similar properties to lidocaine. When administered intravenously, the drug vehicle can produce hypotension and exert a depressant effect on the myocardium.[184] The total intravenous dose is 4.5 mg/lb, given in 1 mg/lb increments over three to five minutes.[185]

Serum potassium concentration should always be determined in animals intoxicated with digitalis. If serum potassium is less than 4 mEq/L, potassium supplements should be administered, preferably in intravenous fluids. Potassium competes with digitalis for binding sites on the Na^+,K^+-ATPase pumps and provides a more suitable environment for the antiarrhythmic agents to work.

Orally administered activated charcoal avidly binds digoxin and is useful after accidental ingestion or administration of a large oral dose. It decreases digoxin absorption up to 96 per cent.[186, 187] Cholestyramine, a steroid-binding resin, may also be useful early after digoxin ingestion but decreases absorption only 30 to 40 per cent.[186] Cholestyramine is more useful in digitoxin toxicity.[188] Cholestyramine binds digitalis in the intestinal tract. Digitoxin undergoes enterohepatic circulation and so can be bound by this resin. Digoxin undergoes minimal enterohepatic circulation, so cholestyramine administration is only useful soon after an accidental overdose of this drug.

A cardiac glycoside–specific antibody fragment is used in humans to bind digitalis glycosides in the bloodstream and thus remove them from myocardial binding sites.[189] This product (Digibind) is very expensive. There has been one report of its use in a dog.[190] It cost $1200 to treat this 50-pound Labrador retriever. Digibind binds with the antigenic epitope on the digoxin molecule. This complex cannot bind to Na^+,K^+-ATPase pumps and is cleared by glomerular filtration. These effects result in rapid resolution of clinical signs. In one report of its use in humans, the median time to initial response was 19 minutes, with 75 per cent of the patients having evidence of response within one hour.[191] In the same report, 80 to 90 per cent of patients had resolution of all clinical signs and symptoms of digitalis intoxication. The method of dosing Digibind can be found on the package insert.

DIGITOXIN

Pharmacokinetics. One formulation of digitoxin (Crystodigin) has superior pharmacokinetic properties in the dog as compared with digoxin.[173] Its half-life is only 8 to 12 hours. Therapeutic serum concentration can be achieved more rapidly than with digoxin, and serum concentration decreases more quickly if a dog becomes toxic; 95 to 100 per cent of tincture of digitoxin is absorbed. About 90 per cent of the drug is bound to serum protein, so a higher dose of digitoxin is needed relative to digoxin. Digitoxin is excreted by the liver and can therefore be used safely in dogs with renal failure. Bile duct ligation in experimental dogs increased the half-life of digitoxin from an average of 10 hours to 31 hours.[192]

In cats, the half-life of digitoxin is greater than 100 hours.[157] Consequently, this drug should be avoided in cats. Digoxin is the only recommended digitalis glycoside for this species.[30]

Administration and Dosage. The starting dose of digitoxin in dogs is 0.015 mg/lb administered orally every 8 to 12 hours.[173] In general, small dogs should receive the dose every 8 hours and large dogs every 12 hours. The cumulative daily dose in small dogs would be greater than that for large dogs on a per-weight basis but similar on a per–body surface area basis.

SYMPATHOMIMETICS

Sympathomimetic amines increase contractility, conduction velocity, and heart rate by binding to cardiac beta-adrenergic receptors. The increase in contractility is brought about by activation of adenyl cyclase within the cell. Adenyl cyclase cleaves adenosine triphosphate (ATP) to cyclic adenosine monophosphate (cAMP), which stimulates a cellular protein kinase system (Fig. 111–3). Protein kinases phosphorylate intracellular proteins, such as phospholamban on the sarcoplasmic reticulum, allowing it to bind more calcium during diastole and thereby release more calcium during systole.[193] Cyclic AMP also affects L-type calcium channels to increase calcium entry into the cell during systole.

Most sympathomimetics have the ability to increase contractility about 100 per cent above baseline, but many are unsuitable for treating heart failure because of other drug properties. Sympathomimetics can stimulate both alpha- and beta-adrenergic receptors. The degree to which each type of receptor is stimulated depends on the specific sympathomimetic and the dose administered.[194] Classic catecholamines, such as isoproterenol, norepinephrine, and epinephrine, produce too many untoward hemodynamic effects and are arrhythmogenic. All three of these drugs are therefore unsuitable for treating heart failure. Newer sympathomimetics, such as dopamine and dobutamine, are less arrhythmogenic, produce a smaller heart rate increase, and are more suitable for heart failure therapy.[195] The arrhythmogenic potential for all catecholamines is increased when dogs are anesthetized with drugs such as thiamylal and halothane. In this setting, the arrhythmogenic potential of epinephrine, dopamine, and dobutamine is similar.[196]

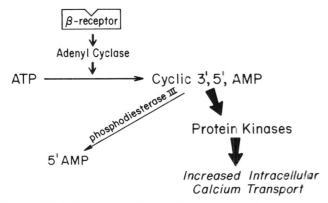

Figure 111–3. The cascade of events that occurs following beta-receptor stimulation by a sympathomimetic or phosphodiesterase inhibition by a bipyridine compound.

All currently available sympathomimetics have very short half-lives (one to two minutes). When administered orally they are metabolized extensively and rapidly by the liver before they reach the circulation.[197] Consequently, they must be administered intravenously, usually as a constant-rate infusion.

One of the major limitations of using sympathomimetics to treat animals with heart failure is the fact that the inotropic response to sympathomimetics decreases to approximately 50 per cent of baseline after a day or two of constant stimulation. This occurs because of a decrease in beta receptor number and sensitivity. As such, the efficacy of sympathomimetics decreases rapidly once therapy is initiated. Consequently, one should generally not consider using a sympathomimetic longer than two or three days for inotropic support.

DOPAMINE

Actions. Dopamine stimulates cardiac beta$_1$-adrenergic receptors as well as peripherally located dopaminergic receptors.[198] The latter appear to be located most prevalently in the renal and mesenteric vascular beds, where they produce vasodilatation. Dopamine administration to an animal with acute heart failure should improve contractility and thereby increase cardiac output. The renal and mesenteric vasodilatation should cause preferential blood flow to these areas. In humans, dopamine administration to patients with chronic heart failure can cause increased ventricular filling pressures and edema formation.[199] However, in one study of experimental heart failure in dogs induced by creating an aorta–left atrial shunt, dopamine decreased ventricular filling pressures.[200] Consequently, the effects of dopamine may be more advantageous in dogs than in humans. In one study, the hemodynamic effects of dopamine and dobutamine were indistinguishable, except for the increase in renal and mesenteric flow produced with dopamine, following a 15-minute infusion.[200] However, after a five-hour infusion, the mesenteric and renal vasodilatation was lost and the increase in contractility was attenuated.

Indications. In cardiovascular medicine, dopamine is recommended for short-term use in animals with myocardial failure. It has many other but similar indications in critical care and anesthetized animals.

Administration and Dosage. The dosage for dopamine in dogs is 0.5 to 5 μg/lb per minute intravenously. Doses higher than 5 μg/lb per minute can be used but result in norepinephrine release and increased peripheral vascular resistance and heart rate.[201] An initial dose of 1 μg/lb per minute may be started and titrated upward to obtain the desired clinical effect (improved hemodynamics).

Dopamine is supplied as a liquid in ampules, vials, and syringes. The liquid must be diluted in solutions suitable for intravenous administration. The solution is stable at room temperature for a minimum of 24 hours. Dopamine is inactivated when mixed with sodium bicarbonate or other alkaline intravenous solutions. The solution becomes pink or violet. The product should not be used if it is discolored.

DOBUTAMINE

Actions. Dobutamine is a synthetic catecholamine. It stimulates beta$_1$-adrenergic receptors, increasing myocardial contractility. In so doing, it decreases end-systolic volume, increases stroke volume, and increases cardiac output. It also weakly stimulates peripheral beta$_2$- and alpha$_1$-adrenergic receptors. As this response is balanced, systemic arterial blood pressure is usually unchanged after dobutamine administration.[202] Dobutamine is less arrhythmogenic than most of the other sympathomimetics in awake animals. In vagotomized experimental dogs under anesthesia, dobutamine is as arrhythmogenic as dopamine and epinephrine.[196] In one study of conscious dogs with experimental myocardial infarction, dobutamine did not increase the frequency of premature ventricular ectopic beats.[203]

Dobutamine's hemodynamic effects have been studied in normal conscious and normal anesthetized dogs.[201, 202] It has also been examined in conscious and anesthetized dogs following myocardial infarction.[204] In each situation, dobutamine produced dose-related increases in myocardial contractility, cardiac output, stroke volume, and coronary blood flow with no change in systemic arterial blood pressure. When administered to an animal with acute or chronic myocardial failure, it should increase contractility and cardiac output and decrease ventricular diastolic pressures, leading to a decrease in edema formation. This has been poorly documented in dogs and cats with chronic myocardial failure but has been well documented in human patients.[205, 206] In one canine study, dogs were placed on cardiopulmonary bypass with their aortas cross-clamped for one hour and studied after surgery.[207] Comparisons were made between a group treated with dobutamine (2 μg/lb per minute) and a group that received no treatment. Dobutamine administration resulted in an increased stroke volume, a decreased heart rate, an increase in blood pressure toward normal, and improved survival (75 vs. 37.5 per cent). There was no increase in arrhythmias.

Dobutamine's effects on heart rate are generally less than those of other catecholamines. When studied in normal dogs and in dogs with experimental myocardial infarction, the heart rate did not increase at infusion rates less than 9 μg/lb per minute.[202, 204] Dobutamine, however, does increase heart rate in a dose-dependent manner in dogs that are anesthetized.[201, 204]

Pharmacokinetics. Dobutamine must be administered as a constant-rate infusion. A plateau plasma concentration is achieved within approximately eight minutes of starting the infusion.[197] Upon cessation of the infusion, dobutamine rapidly clears from the plasma, with a terminal half-life of one to two minutes.

Indications. In clinical situations, dobutamine can be used to treat acute heart failure due to myocardial failure until inotropic support is no longer needed or until other longer-acting positive inotropic agents (e.g., digoxin) have taken effect. It can also be used to treat acute exacerbations of chronic heart failure requiring acute inotropic support.

Administration and Dosage. The dosage of dobutamine is 2 to 18 μg/lb per minute intravenously. Doses of 2 to 9 μg/lb per minute are generally adequate for dogs. Infusion rates of greater than 9 μg/lb per minute may produce tachycardia.[204] Cats may be administered 2 to 7 μg/lb per minute. The positive inotropic effect is dosage-dependent.

Adverse Effects. Dobutamine can exacerbate existing arrhythmias, especially ventricular arrhythmias. It can also produce new arrhythmias and increase heart rate.

BIPYRIDINE COMPOUNDS

Bipyridine compounds increase myocardial contractility and produce mild systemic arteriolar dilatation. Milrinone is about 30 to 40 times as potent as amrinone. Both compounds are active after oral administration, although only intravenous formulations are available commercially.

Actions. Bipyridine compounds primarily act as inhibitors of phosphodiesterase fraction III,[208] which is an intracellular enzyme that specifically breaks down cAMP in myocardial and vascular tissue (see Fig. 111–3). When phosphodiesterase III is inhibited, intracellular cAMP concentration increases. This increase results in the same type of inotropic effect in the myocardium produced by sympathomimetics. The major difference is that bipyridine compounds "bypass" the beta receptors, so there is no decrement in inotropic effect over time. Consequently, bipyridine compounds can be used to chronically increase contractility. Bipyridine compounds also produce arteriolar dilatation, probably also mediated by phosphodiesterase inhibition. Milrinone also increases left ventricular relaxation and distensibility in human heart failure patients.[209]

Cardiovascular effects of the bipyridine compounds are species-dependent. Myocardial contractility increases approximately 100 per cent above baseline in dogs and cats but increases only about 50 per cent above baseline in nonhuman primates and presumably humans.[210] When amrinone is administered to rats, contractility increases only about 25 per cent above baseline.[211] Because of this marked species difference, data obtained from other species cannot be extrapolated to dogs or cats.

AMRINONE

In normal anesthetized dogs, an intravenous bolus of amrinone (0.5 to 1.5 mg/lb) causes contractility to increase 60 to 100 per cent, systemic arterial blood pressure to decrease 10 to 30 per cent, and heart rate to increase 5 to 10 per cent.[212] The maximal contractility increase occurs within five minutes after injection and decreases 50 per cent by 10 minutes. Effects are dissipated within 20 to 30 minutes. This short duration of effect necessitates administering the drug by constant intravenous infusion following the initial bolus injection. Constant infusions in dogs take about 45 minutes to reach peak effect if a loading dose is not administered. Infusion rates of 5 to 45 μg/lb per minute in conscious experimental dogs increase contractility 10 to 80 per cent above baseline. In anesthetized dogs, an infusion of 5 μg/lb per minute does not decrease systemic blood pressure, whereas 14 μg/lb per minute decreases it 10 per cent and 45 μg/lb per minute decreases it 30 per cent. Heart rate does not increase at 5 μg/lb per minute but increases 15 per cent at 14 μg/lb per minute and 20 per cent at 45 μg/lb per minute. In anesthetized dogs with drug-induced myocardial failure, amrinone infusions increase contractility 40 to 200 per cent above baseline and increase cardiac output by 80 per cent. In experimental cats, amrinone infused at 14 μg/lb per minute causes contractility to increase 40 per cent above baseline. Peak effect occurs 90 minutes after starting an infusion.

Studies have not been performed to determine the hemodynamic changes brought about by amrinone administration in dogs or cats with naturally occurring heart failure. Based on the information from normal dogs, however, clinical recommendations can be made. The drug has a wide margin of safety, and the risk of toxicity is low. Amrinone is marketed only as a solution for intravenous administration and so is useful only for short-term administration. The initial dose should be 0.5 to 1.4 mg/lb administered as a slow intravenous bolus followed by a constant-rate infusion of 5 to 45 μg/lb per minute. One half the initial bolus may be administered 20 to 30 minutes after the first bolus. The same regimen may be effective in the cat.

MILRINONE

Milrinone is a bipyridine compound with pharmacologic effects that are almost identical to those of amrinone. Milrinone is currently marketed for intravenous administration only. No clinical studies of the effects of intravenous milrinone administration for acute myocardial failure in dogs or cats have been performed. Clinical studies of the effects of chronic oral administration have been performed, but this form of the drug has not been approved for veterinary use. The results of the veterinary clinical trials of chronic oral milrinone administration in dogs with heart failure have been reviewed.[213]

In normal anesthetized dogs, milrinone dosed at 14 to 140 μg/lb intravenously increases contractility 40 to 120 per cent while decreasing diastolic blood pressure 10 to 30 per cent.[214] Peak effect occurs within one to two minutes and is reduced to 50 per cent of maximum in 10 minutes; the effects are essentially gone in 30 minutes. Constant-rate intravenous infusions (0.5 to 4.5 μg/lb per minute) increase contractility 50 to 140 per cent, with peak effect in 10 to 30 minutes. In the normal unanesthetized dog, the oral administration of 0.05 mg/lb milrinone increases contractility 30 per cent above baseline, 0.14 mg/lb increases contractility 50 per cent above baseline, and 0.5 mg/lb increases contractility more than 80 per cent above baseline. Systemic arterial blood pressure is essentially unchanged at these doses, whereas heart rate increases up to 30 per cent at the 0.5 mg/lb dose. In the normal anesthetized cat, a constant-rate infusion of 0.5 μg/lb per minute increases contractility about 40 per cent, with peak effect occurring within 30 minutes.

Milrinone has been scrutinized by numerous investigators for chronic oral administration to human patients with heart failure. In 1991, the results of a large clinical trial (approximately 1100 patients were enrolled) were reported.[131] The investigators in this study found that chronic administration of milrinone to patients with heart failure resulted in an increased risk of sudden death. Consequently, the request for a new drug approval was removed from consideration with the Food and Drug Administration. Largely because of this event, the drug company that manufactures milrinone lost interest in pursuing approval for milrinone's chronic oral use in dogs, despite the fact that milrinone appears to be a better drug in dogs than it is in humans for the treatment of heart failure.

OXYGEN THERAPY

Dogs and cats with severe pulmonary edema develop life-threatening hypoxemia. The hypoxemia is primarily due to the decreased ability of oxygen to diffuse from the alveoli into the pulmonary capillaries.[215] Increasing the inspired concentration of oxygen increases the pressure gradient of oxygen from the alveoli to the capillaries, resulting in an increase in arterial oxygen tension. Consequently, dogs and cats with severe pulmonary edema and respiratory distress should have supplemental oxygen administered while they are treated for the pulmonary edema. In general, the percentage of inspired oxygen should be increased from the normal

21 per cent to 40 to 50 per cent. This can best be achieved by placing the animal in an oxygen cage or by administering oxygen via a nasal cannula (nasal insufflation). It can also be achieved with a tight-fitting mask. Masks should be used only if the animal will tolerate their placement without struggling. Oxygen cages must have a mechanism for removing carbon dioxide and for cooling the environment. Cages or enclosures contrived from plastic bags or boxes are dangerous and can cause death from hyperthermia or hypercarbia unless the flow rate of oxygen is very high to wash out the carbon dioxide and the temperature is controlled by some means. The oxygen must be humidified when supplied via nasal insufflation. Animals in extreme respiratory distress may benefit from sedation or anesthesia, endotracheal intubation, controlled ventilation, and 100 per cent oxygen administration. These animals usually have copious amounts of pulmonary edema fluid spew from the endotracheal tube. Postural drainage and suction must be used to remove this fluid.

THORACENTESIS AND ABDOMINOCENTESIS

Dyspneic animals with pleural effusion benefit from withdrawal of the fluid from the pleural space. Pleural effusion is a common cause of severe respiratory distress in cats. Any dyspneic cat suspected of having cardiac disease should undergo pleurocentesis to determine whether pleural effusion is the cause of the respiratory distress at the time of initial examination. This can usually be performed with the cat in sternal recumbency with a butterfly catheter. Fluid removal often results in prompt and dramatic improvement. Dogs with severe ascites benefit from fluid withdrawal. Although large quantities of protein are removed along with the fluid, this is rarely clinically significant unless hepatic failure or other complicating diseases are also present.

ANXIOLYTIC THERAPY

Dogs and cats with severe respiratory distress may become severely anxious and may benefit from sedation. However, most animals with respiratory distress in the author's hospital are not sedated.

Morphine is commonly recommended for its analgesic and antianxiety effects in humans with respiratory distress secondary to heart failure.[216] Morphine also has venodilating properties that may be beneficial. Morphine is generally not used in cats because they may become aggressive and agitated following its administration. In dogs, the dose is 0.05 to 0.12 mg/lb subcutaneously. The dose is repeated as necessary to achieve the desired effect. The primary adverse effect of morphine is respiratory depression. This can be a fatal complication in a hypoxemic animal, so this drug must be used carefully.

Phenothiazine tranquilizers may be used to produce similar effects. Acepromazine is the tranquilizer the author uses most commonly in heart failure patients with severe respiratory distress. It reduces the agitation in these animals and does not depress respiration. Acepromazine is also an alpha-adrenergic blocker that decreases peripheral vascular resistance, which may be beneficial, especially in animals with mitral regurgitation (see Chapter 19). The dose is 0.005 to 0.1 mg/lb intramuscularly or intravenously. This drug can cause severe hypotension and bradycardia in Boxers and probably should not be used in this breed.[217, 218] Acepromazine should not be used in combination with an opioid in animals with respiratory distress because of enhanced respiratory depression.[219]

BRONCHODILATOR THERAPY

Bronchodilators, such as theophylline and aminophylline, are occasionally prescribed for use in heart failure patients. However, attempting to produce bronchodilatation in patients with heart failure has been called into question in human medicine and is less likely to be of benefit in dogs. Aminophylline and theophylline are nonspecific phosphodiesterase inhibitors. Consequently, they have positive inotropic effects and may also act as diuretics. However, these effects are extremely mild and probably of little benefit. In general, these drugs are reserved for use in dogs with chronic airway disease.

COUGH SUPPRESSANTS

Cough suppressants are contraindicated in animals that have cough secondary to pulmonary edema. Consequently, pulmonary edema must be ruled out before initiating these drugs in a coughing animal. This can usually be done by obtaining a thoracic radiograph. In some dogs with mild edema, a trial of furosemide administration may be required to exclude pulmonary edema as a possible cause of a cough. In dogs with cough secondary to airway compression by an enlarged left atrium, hydrocodone bitartrate with homatropine (Hycodan, DuPont, Wilmington, DE) and butorphanol (Torbutrol, Fort Dodge Laboratories, Fort Dodge, IA) are generally the most effective drugs. Hycodan is supplied as 5-mg tablets. The oral dose in dogs is 2.5 to 10 mg every 6 to 12 hours or 0.12 mg/lb every 6 to 12 hours. Torbutrol is supplied as 1-, 5-, and 10-mg tablets. The dose in dogs is 0.25 to 0.5 mg/lb orally every 6 to 12 hours. Dextromethorphan (various preparations and manufacturers), as an over-the-counter drug, may also be effective in some situations. A dose has not been defined. The author generally bases the dose on a pediatric dose in comparison to the size of the dog.

REFERENCES

1. Saxon LA, Stevenson WG, Middlekauff HR, et al: Predicting death from progressive heart failure secondary to ischemic or idiopathic dilated cardiomyopathy. Am J Cardiol 72:62, 1993.
2. The Digitalis Investigation Group: The effect of digoxin on mortality and morbidity in patients with heart failure. N Engl J Med 336:525, 1997.
3. Vollmar AM, Montag C, Preusser U, et al: Atrial natriuretic peptide and plasma volume of dogs suffering from heart failure or dehydration. JAVMA 41:548, 1994.
4. Kunau RTJ, Weller DR, Webb HL: Clarification of the site of action of chlorothiazide in the rat nephron. J Clin Invest 56:401, 1975.
5. Puschett JB: Clinical pharmacologic implications in diuretic selection. Am J Cardiol 57:6A, 1986.
6. Puschett JB: Sites and mechanisms of action of diuretics in the kidney. J Clin Pharmacol 21:564, 1981.
7. Bosch JP, Goldstein MH, Levitt MF, Kahn T: Effect of chronic furosemide administration on hydrogen and sodium excretion in the dog. Am J Physiol 232:F397, 1977.
8. White MG, van Gelder J, Eastes G: The effect of loop diuretics on the excretion of Na$^+$, Ca^{2+}, Mg^{2+}, and Cl$^-$. J Clin Pharmacol 21:610, 1981.
9. Berg KJ, Loew D: Inhibition of furosemide-induced natriuresis by acetylsalicylic acid in dogs. Scand J Clin Lab Invest 37:125, 1977.
10. Hirai J, Miyazaki H, Taneike T: The pharmacokinetics and pharmacodynamics of furosemide in the anaesthetized dog. J Vet Pharmacol Ther 15:231, 1992.
11. Cohen MR, Hinsch E, Vergona R, et al: A comparative diuretic and tissue distribution study of bumetanide and furosemide in the dog. J Pharmacol Exp Ther 197:697, 1976.
12. Bayne EJ, Williamson HE: Effect of furosemide on peripheral venous compliance following ureteral ligation in the adult dog. Res Commun Chem Pathol Pharmacol 25:399, 1979.
13. Mukherjee SK, Katz MA, Michael UF, Ogden DA: Mechanisms of hemodynamic actions of furosemide: Differentiation of vascular and renal effects on blood pressure in functionally anephric hypertensive patients. Am Heart J 101:313, 1981.
14. Fernando ON, Newman SP, Hird VM, et al: Enhancement of renal blood flow in transplanted dog kidneys following perfusion with frusemide. Scott Med J 19(Suppl 1):50, 1974.
15. Ludens JH, Heitz DC, Brody MJ, Williamson HE: Differential effect of furosemide on renal and limb blood flows in the conscious dog. J Pharmacol Exp Ther 171:300, 1970.
16. Data JL, Rane A, Gerkens J, et al: The influence of indomethacin on the pharmacokinetics, diuretic response and hemodynamics of furosemide in the dog. J Pharmacol Exp Ther 206:431, 1978.
17. Szwed JJ, Kleit SA, Hamburger RJ: Effect of furosemide and chlorothiazide on the thoracic duct lymph flow in the dog. J Lab Clin Med 79:693, 1972.
18. Rubie S, Robinson NE, Stoll M, et al: Flunixin meglumine blocks frusemide-induced bronchodilation in horses with chronic obstructive pulmonary disease. Equine Vet J 25:138, 1993.
19. Stevens EL, Uyehara CF, Southgate WM, Nakamura KT: Furosemide differentially relaxes airway and vascular smooth muscle in fetal, newborn, and adult guinea pigs. Am Rev Respir Dis 146:1192, 1992.
20. Bianco S, Pieroni MG, Refini RM, et al: Inhaled loop diuretics as potential new anti-asthmatic drugs. Eur Respir J 6:130, 1993.
21. Padrid P: Chronic lower airway disease in the dog and cat. Probl Vet Med 4:320, 1992.
22. Imbs JL, Schmidt M, Velly J, Schwartz J: Comparison of the effect of two groups of diuretics on renin secretion in the anaesthetized dog. Clin Sci Mol Med 52:171, 1977.
23. Corsini WA, Hook JB, Bailie MD: Control of renin secretion in the dog. Effects of furosemide on the vascular and macula densa receptors. Circ Res 37:464, 1975.
24. Yakatan GJ, Maness DD, Scholler J, et al: Plasma and tissue levels of furosemide in dogs and monkeys following single and multiple oral doses. Res Commun Chem Pathol Pharmacol 24:465, 1979.
25. Cohen M: Pharmacology of bumetanide. J Clin Pharmacol 21:537, 1981.
26. Brown DJ, Knight DH, King RR: Use of pulsed-wave Doppler echocardiography to determine aortic and pulmonary velocity and flow variables in clinically normal dogs. Am J Vet Res 52:543, 1991.
27. Miyazaki H, Hirai J, Taneike T: The pharmacokinetics and pharmacodynamics of furosemide in anesthetized dogs with normal and experimentally decreased renal function. Jpn J Vet Sci 52:265, 1990.
28. Klatt P, Muschaweck R, Bossaller W, et al: Method of collecting urine and comparative investigation of quantities excreted by cats and dogs after administration of furosemide. Am J Vet Res 36:919, 1975.
29. Friedman PA, Roch-Ramel F: Hemodynamic and natriuretic effects of bumetanide and furosemide in the cat. J Pharmacol Exp Ther 203:82, 1977.
30. Fox PR: Feline myocardial diseases. In Kirk RW (ed): Current Veterinary Therapy VIII. Philadelphia, WB Saunders, 1983, p 387.
31. Edwards NJ: Serum potassium concentration in dogs administered furosemide. Personal communication, 1996.
32. Dormans TPJ, van Meyel JJM, Gerlag PGG, et al: Diuretic efficacy of high dose furosemide in severe heart failure: Bolus injection versus continuous infusion. J Am Coll Cardiol 28:376, 1996.
33. Brown RD: Comparative acute cochlear toxicity of intravenous bumetanide and furosemide in the purebred beagle. J Clin Pharmacol 21:620, 1981.
34. Raisbeck MF, Hewitt WR, McIntyre WB: Fatal nephrotoxicosis associated with furosemide and gentamicin therapy in a dog. JAVMA 183:892, 1983.
35. Nakahama H, Fukuhara Y, Orita Y, et al: Furosemide accelerates gentamicin accumulation in cultured renal cells (LLC-PK1 cells). Nephron 53:138, 1989.
36. Puschett JB: Pharmacological classification and renal actions of diuretics. Cardiology 84(Suppl 2):4, 1994.
37. Brater DC, Thier SO: Renal Disorders. New York, Macmillan, 1978.
38. Muir WW, Sams R: Pharmacodynamics of Cardiac Drugs. Columbus, Ohio State University, 1979.
39. Crosley AP, Ronquillo LM, Strickland WH, Alexander F: Triamterene, a new natriuretic agent. Ann Intern Med 56:241, 1962.
40. Edwards NJ: Magnesium and congestive heart failure. In Proceedings of the Ninth Annual Veterinary Medical Forum. Blacksburg, VA, American College of Veterinary Internal Medicine, 1990, pp 679–680.
41. O'Keefe D, Sisson DD: Serum electrolytes in dogs with congestive heart failure (abstract). J Vet Intern Med 7:118, 1993.
42. Asanoi H, Kameyama T, Ashizaka S, et al: Energetically optimal left ventricular pressure for the failing human heart. Circulation 93:67, 1996.
43. Brown NJ, Vaughan DE: Angiotensin-converting enzyme inhibitors. Circulation 97:1411, 1998.
44. Kittleson MD, Johnson LE, Pion PD, Mekhamer YE: The acute haemodynamic effects of captopril in dogs with heart failure. J Vet Pharmacol Ther 16:1, 1993.
45. Haggstrom J, Hansson K, Karlberg BE, et al: Effects of long-term treatment with enalapril or hydralazine on the renin-angiotensin-aldosterone system and fluid balance in dogs with naturally acquired mitral valve degeneration. Am J Vet Res 57:1645, 1996.
46. The COVE Study Group: Controlled clinical evaluation of enalapril in dogs with heart failure: Results of the Cooperative Veterinary Enalapril Study Group. J Vet Intern Med 9:243, 1995.

CV

47. The IMPROVE Study Group: Acute and short-term hemodynamic, echocardiographic, and clinical effects of enalapril maleate in dogs with naturally acquired heart failure: Results of the Invasive Multicenter Prospective Veterinary Evaluation of Enalapril Study. J Vet Intern Med 9:234, 1995.

48. The SOLVD Investigators: Effect of enalapril on mortality and the development of heart failure in asymptomatic patients with reduced left ventricular ejection fractions. N Engl J Med 327:685, 1992. (Published erratum appears in N Engl J Med 327:1763, 1992 [see comments])

49. Pfeffer MA, Braunwald E, Moye LA, et al: Effect of captopril on mortality and morbidity in patients with left ventricular dysfunction after myocardial infarction. Results of the survival and ventricular enlargement trial. The SAVE Investigators. N Engl J Med 327:669, 1992 (see comments).

50. The SOLVD Investigators: Effect of enalapril on survival in patients with reduced left ventricular ejection fractions and congestive heart failure. N Engl J Med 325:293, 1991 (see comments).

51. The CONSENSUS Trial Study Group: Effects of enalapril on mortality in severe congestive heart failure. Results of the Cooperative North Scandinavian Enalapril Survival Study (CONSENSUS). N Engl J Med 316:1429, 1987.

52. Cohn JN, Johnson G, Ziesche S, et al: A comparison of enalapril with hydralazine-isosorbide dinitrate in the treatment of chronic congestive heart failure. N Engl J Med 325:303, 1991 (see comments).

53. Packer M: Converting-enzyme inhibition in the management of severe chronic congestive heart failure: Physiologic concepts. J Cardiovasc Pharmacol 10(Suppl 7):S83, 1987.

54. Hollenberg NK: Control of renal perfusion and function in congestive heart failure. Am J Cardiol 62:72E, 1988.

55. Packer M, Lee WH, Kessler PD: Preservation of glomerular filtration rate in human heart failure by activation of the renin-angiotensin system. Circulation 74:766, 1986.

56. Packer M, Lee WH, Medina N, et al: Functional renal insufficiency during long-term therapy with captopril and enalapril in severe chronic heart failure. Ann Intern Med 106:346, 1987.

57. Lee WH, Packer M: Prognostic importance of serum sodium concentration and its modification by converting-enzyme inhibition in patients with severe chronic heart failure. Circulation 73:257, 1986.

58. Packer M, Lee WH, Kessler PD, et al: Identification of hyponatremia as a risk factor for the development of functional renal insufficiency during converting enzyme inhibition in severe chronic heart failure. J Am Coll Cardiol 10:837, 1987.

59. Packer M, Lee WH, Yushak M, Medina N: Comparison of captopril and enalapril in patients with severe chronic heart failure. N Engl J Med 315:847, 1986.(Published erratum appears in N Engl J Med 315:1105, 1986.)

60. Pitt B: ACE inhibitors in heart failure: Prospects and limitations. Cardiovasc Drugs Ther 11(Suppl 1):285, 1997.

61. Gottlieb SS, Robinson S, Weir MR, et al: Determinants of the renal response to ACE inhibition in patients with congestive heart failure. Am Heart J 124:131, 1992.

62. Hall D, Zeitler H, Rudolph W: Counteraction of the vasodilator effects of enalapril by aspirin in severe heart failure. J Am Coll Cardiol 20:1549, 1992.

63. Evans MA, Burnett JCJ, Redfield MM: Effect of low dose aspirin on cardiorenal function and acute hemodynamic response to enalaprilat in a canine model of severe heart failure. J Am Coll Cardiol 25:1445, 1995.

64. McLay JS, McMurray JJ, Bridges AB, et al: Acute effects of captopril on the renal actions of furosemide in patients with chronic heart failure. Am Heart J 126:879, 1993.

65. American Hospital Formulary Service: AHFS Drug Information. Bethesda, MD, American Society of Health-System Pharmacists, Inc., 1995.

66. Vidt DG, Bravo EL, Fouad FM: Captopril. N Engl J Med 306:214. 1982.

67. Kittleson MD: Positive inotropic agents and captopril. In Proceedings of the Ninth Annual Kal Kan Symposium. Vernon, CA, Kal Kan Foods, Inc., 1986, p 19.

68. Ader R, Chatterjee K, Ports T, et al: Immediate and sustained hemodynamic and clinical improvement in chronic heart failure by an oral angiotensin-converting enzyme inhibitor. Circulation 61:931, 1980.

69. Blackford LW, Golden AL, Bright JM, et al: Captopril provides sustained hemodynamic benefits in dogs with experimentally induced mitral regurgitation. Vet Surg 19:237, 1990.

70. Fox PR: Feline cardiomyopathy. In Bonagura JD (ed): Contemporary Issues in Small Animal Practice: Cardiology. New York, Churchill Livingstone, 1987, p 157.

71. Tocco DJ, deLuna FA, Duncan AE, et al: The physiological disposition and metabolism of enalapril maleate in laboratory animals. Drug Metab Dispos 10:15, 1982.

72. Sweet CS, Ulm EH: Lisinopril. Cardiovasc Drug Rev 6:181, 1988.

73. Benitz AM, Hamlin RL, Ericsson GF: Titration of enalapril dose for dogs with induced heart failure (abstract). In Proceedings of the Ninth Annual Veterinary Medical Forum. New Orleans, American College of Veterinary Internal Medicine, 1991, p 879.

74. Ettinger SJ, Benitz AM, Ericsson GF: Relationships of enalapril with other CHF treatment modalities In Proceedings of the Twelfth Veterinary Medical Forum. San Francisco, American College of Veterinary Internal Medicine, 1994. pp 251–253.

75. Fox PR: The effect of drug therapy on clinical characteristics and outcome in dogs with heart failure. In Proceedings of the Tenth Veterinary Medical Forum. San Diego, American College of Veterinary Internal Medicine, 1992, pp 592–593.

76. Waldmeier F, Schmid K: Disposition of [14C]-benazepril hydrochloride in rat, dog and baboon. Absorption, distribution, kinetics, biotransformation and excretion. Arzneimittelforschung 39:62, 1989.

77. King JN, Mauron C, Kaiser G: Pharmacokinetics of the active metabolite of benazepril, benazeprilat, and inhibition of plasma angiotensin-converting enzyme activity after single and repeated administration to dogs. Am J Vet Res 56:1620, 1995.

78. Greenwald JE, Wong LK, Alexander M, Bianchine JR: In vivo inhibition of thromboxane biosynthesis by hydralazine. Adv Prostaglandin Thromboxane Res 6:293, 1980.

79. Maekawa K, Liang CS, Tsui A, et al: Vasodilative effect of hydralazine in awake dogs: The roles of prostaglandins and the sympathetic nervous system. Circulation 70:908, 1984.

80. Tabrizchi R, Pang CC: Effects of drugs on body venous tone, as reflected by mean circulatory filling pressure. Cardiovasc Res 26:443, 1992.

81. Spokas EG, Wang HH: Regional blood flow and cardiac responses to hydralazine. J Pharmacol Exp Ther 212:294, 1980.

82. Yamamoto J, Trippodo NC, Ishise S, Frohlich ED: Total vascular pressure-volume relationship in the conscious rat. Am J Physiol 238:H823, 1980.

83. Kittleson MD, Hamlin RL: Hydralazine pharmacodynamics in the dog. Am J Vet Res 44:1501, 1983.

84. Brown WA, Kittleson MD: Color flow Doppler estimation of mitral regurgitation using the proximal flow convergence method in dogs with chronic degenerative valve disease (abstract). J Vet Intern Med 8:143, 1994.

85. Kittleson MD, Eyster GE, Knowlen GG, et al: Myocardial function in small dogs with chronic mitral regurgitation and severe congestive heart failure. JAVMA 184:455, 1984.

86. Kittleson MD, Johnson LE, Oliver NB: Acute hemodynamic effects of hydralazine in dogs with chronic mitral regurgitation. JAVMA 187:258, 1985.

87. Kittleson MD, Eyster GE, Olivier NB, Anderson LK: Oral hydralazine therapy for chronic mitral regurgitation in the dog. JAVMA 182:1205, 1983.

88. Koch-Weser J: Hydralazine. N Engl J Med 295:320, 1976.

89. Cogan JJ, Humphreys MH, Carlson CJ, et al: Acute vasodilator therapy increases renal clearance of digoxin in patients with congestive heart failure. Circulation 64:973, 1981.

90. Nomura A, Yasuda H, Katoh K, et al: Hydralazine and furosemide kinetics. Clin Pharmacol Ther 32:303, 1982.

91. Anderson TJ, Meredith IT, Ganz P, et al: Nitric oxide and nitrovasodilators: Similarities, differences and potential interactions. J Am Coll Cardiol 24:555, 1994.

92. Gruetter CA, Gruetter DY, Lyon JE, et al: Relationship between cyclic guanosine 3':5'-monophosphate formation and relaxation of coronary arterial smooth muscle by glyceryl trinitrate, nitroprusside, nitrite and nitric oxide: Effects of methylene blue and methemoglobin. J Pharmacol Exp Ther 219:181, 1981.

93. Ignarro LJ, Lippton H, Edwards JC, et al: Mechanism of vascular smooth muscle relaxation by organic nitrates, nitrites, nitroprusside and nitric oxide: Evidence for the involvement of S-nitrosothiols as active intermediates. J Pharmacol Exp Ther 218:739, 1981.

94. Tzeng TB, Fung HL: Pharmacodynamic modeling of the in vitro vasodilating effects of organic mononitrates. J Pharmacokinet Biopharm 20:227, 1992.

95. Hamlin RL: Evidence for or against clinical efficacy of preload reducers. Vet Clin North Am Small Anim Pract 21:931, 1991.

96. Abrams J: Tolerance to organic nitrates. Circulation 74:1181, 1986.

97. Fung HL: Solving the mystery of nitrate tolerance. A new scent on the trail? (editorial comment). Circulation 88:322, 1993.

98. Lis Y, Bennett D, Lambert G, Robson D: A preliminary double-blind study of intravenous nitroglycerin in acute myocardial infarction. Intensive Care Med 10:179, 1984.

99. Gogia H, Mehra A, Parikh S, et al: Prevention of tolerance to hemodynamic effects of nitrates with concomitant use of hydralazine in patients with chronic heart failure. J Am Coll Cardiol 26:1575, 1995.

100. Unger P, Berkenboom G, Fontaine J: Interaction between hydralazine and nitrovasodilators in vascular smooth muscle. J Cardiovasc Pharmacol 21:478, 1993.

101. Packer M, Medina N, Yushak M, Lee WH: Hemodynamic factors limiting the response to transdermal nitroglycerin in severe chronic congestive heart failure. Am J Cardiol 57:260, 1986.

102. Cohn JN, Franciosa JA: Vasodilator therapy of cardiac failure (first of two parts). N Engl J Med 297:27, 1977.

103. Hamlin RL: Increase in splenic size following transdermal nitroglycerin administration in experimental dogs. Personal communication, 1997.

104. Ware WA: Management of congestive heart failure. In Nelson RW, Couto CG (eds): Essentials of Small Animal Internal Medicine. St. Louis, Mosby, 1992, pp 42–58.

105. McDonald KM, Francis GS, Matthews J, et al: Long-term oral nitrate therapy prevents chronic ventricular remodeling in the dog. J Am Coll Cardiol 21:514, 1993.

106. Harrison DG, Bates JN: The nitrovasodilators. New ideas about old drugs. Circulation 87:1461, 1993.

107. Brodie BR, Grossman W, Mann T, McLaurin LP: Effects of sodium nitroprusside on left ventricular diastolic pressure-volume relations. J Clin Invest 59:59, 1977.

108. Pagani M, Vatner SF, Braunwald E: Hemodynamic effects of intravenous sodium nitroprusside in the conscious dog. Circulation 57:144, 1978.

109. Sasayama S, Takahashi M, Osakada G, et al: Dynamic geometry of the left atrium and left ventricle in acute mitral regurgitation. Circulation 60:177, 1979.

110. Guiha NH, Cohn JN, Mikulic E, et al: Treatment of refractory heart failure with infusion of nitroprusside. N Engl J Med 291:587, 1974.
111. Franciosa JA, Silverstein SR: Hemodynamic effects of nitroprusside and furosemide in left ventricular failure. Clin Pharmacol Ther 32:62, 1982.
112. Finegan BA, Chen HJ, Singh YN, Clanachan AS: Comparison of hemodynamic changes induced by adenosine monophosphate and sodium nitroprusside alone and during dopamine infusion in the anesthetized dog. Anesth Analg 70:44, 1990.
113. Spinale FG, Crawford FAJ, Hewett KW, Carabello BA: Ventricular failure and cellular remodeling with chronic supraventricular tachycardia. J Thorac Cardiovasc Surg 102:874, 1991.
114. Cottrell JE, Casthely P, Brodie JD, et al: Prevention of nitroprusside-induced cyanide toxicity with hydroxocobalamin. N Engl J Med 298:809, 1978.
115. Palmer RF, Lasseter KC: Drug therapy. Sodium nitroprusside. N Engl J Med 292:294, 1975.
116. Lloyd MA, Sandberg SM, Edwards BS: Role of renal Na$^+$,K$^{(+)}$-ATPase in the regulation of sodium excretion under normal conditions and in acute congestive heart failure. Circulation 85:1912, 1992.
117. Brandt RB, Laux JE, Spainhour SE, Kline ES: Lactate dehydrogenase in rat mitochondria. Arch Biochem Biophys 259:412, 1987.
118. Kleiman JH, Ingels NB, Daughters G 2nd, et al: Left ventricular dynamics during long-term digoxin treatment in patients with stable coronary artery disease. Am J Cardiol 41:937, 1978.
119. Arnold SB, Byrd RC, Meister W, et al: Long-term digitalis therapy improves left ventricular function in heart failure. N Engl J Med 303:1443, 1980.
120. Mulrow CD, Feussner JR, Velez R: Reevaluation of digitalis efficacy. New light on an old leaf. Ann Intern Med 101:113, 1984.
121. Gheorghiade M, Beller GA: Effects of discontinuing maintenance digoxin therapy in patients with ischemic heart disease and congestive heart failure in sinus rhythm. Am J Cardiol 51:1243, 1983.
122. Taggart AJ, Johnston GD, McDevitt DG: Digoxin withdrawal after cardiac failure in patients with sinus rhythm. J Cardiovasc Pharmacol 5:229, 1983.
123. McHaffie D, Purcell H, Mitchell-Heggs P, Guz A: The clinical value of digoxin in patients with heart failure and sinus rhythm. Q J Med 47:401, 1978.
124. Hougen TJ, Smith TW: Inhibition of myocardial monovalent cation active transport by subtoxic doses of ouabain in the dog. Circ Res 42:856, 1978.
125. Gheorghiade M, Zarowitz BJ: Review of randomized trials of digoxin therapy in patients with chronic heart failure. Am J Cardiol 69:48G, 1992 (discussion on p 62G).
126. Uretsky BF, Young JB, Shahidi FE, et al: Randomized study assessing the effect of digoxin withdrawal in patients with mild to moderate chronic congestive heart failure: Results of the PROVED trial. PROVED Investigative Group. J Am Coll Cardiol 22:955, 1993 (see comments).
127. Packer M, Gheorghiade M, Young JB, et al: Withdrawal of digoxin from patients with chronic heart failure treated with angiotensin-converting-enzyme inhibitors. RADIANCE Study. N Engl J Med 329:1, 1993 (see comments).
128. Ruskin JN, Goldstein S, Bittl JA, Grines CL: The Major Clinical Trials: Bringing Results to Practice. Orlando, FL, AVW/Sound Images, 1996.
129. Packer M: End of the oldest controversy in medicine. Are we ready to conclude the debate on digitalis? (editorial comment). N Engl J Med 336:575, 1997.
130. Slatton ML, Irani WN, Hall SA, et al: Does digoxin provide additional hemodynamic and autonomic benefit at higher doses in patients with mild to moderate heart failure and normal sinus rhythm? J Am Coll Cardiol 29:1206, 1997.
131. Packer M, Carver JR, Rodeheffer RJ, et al: Effect of oral milrinone on mortality in severe chronic heart failure. The PROMISE Study Research Group. N Engl J Med 325:1468, 1991 (see comments).
132. Mahler F, Karliner JS, O'Rourke RA: Effects of chronic digoxin administration on left ventricular performance in the normal conscious dog. Circulation 50:720, 1974.
133. Goldstein RA, Passamani ER, Roberts R: A comparison of digoxin and dobutamine in patients with acute infarction and cardiac failure. N Engl J Med 303:846, 1980.
134. Caprio A, Farah A: The effect of the ionic milieu on the response of rabbit cardiac muscle to ouabain. J Pharmacol Exp Ther 155:403, 1967.
135. Mason DT, Zelia R, Amsterdam EA: Unified concept of the mechanism of action of digitalis: Influence of ventricular function and cardiac disease on hemodynamic response to fundamental contractile effect. In Marks BH, Weissler AM (eds): Basic and Clinical Pharmacology of Digitalis. Springfield, IL, CV Mosby, 1972, p 283.
136. Wald H, Scherzer P, Popovtzer MM: Na,K-ATPase in isolated nephron segments in rats with experimental heart failure. Circ Res 68:1051, 1991.
137. Higgins CB, Vatner SF, Eckberg DL, Braunwald E: Alterations in the baroreceptor reflex in conscious dogs with heart failure. J Clin Invest 51:715, 1972.
138. Creager MA, Creager SJ: Arterial baroreflex regulation of blood pressure in patients with congestive heart failure. J Am Coll Cardiol 23:401, 1994.
139. Ferrari A, Gregorini L, Ferrari MC, et al: Digitalis and baroreceptor reflexes in man. Circulation 63:279, 1981.
140. Spotnitz HM, Sonnenblick EH: Structural conditions in the hypertrophied and failing heart. Am J Cardiol 32:398, 1974.
141. McLain PL: Effects of ouabain on spontaneous afferent activity in the aortic and carotid sinus nerves of cats. Neuropharmacology 9:399, 1970.
142. Ferguson DW, Berg WJ, Sanders JS, et al: Sympathoinhibitory responses to digitalis glycosides in heart failure patients. Direct evidence from sympathetic neural recordings. Circulation 80:65, 1989.
143. Covit AB, Schaer GL, Sealey JE, et al: Suppression of the renin-angiotensin system by intravenous digoxin in chronic congestive heart failure. Am J Med 75:445, 1983.
144. Moe GK, Farah AE: Digitalis and allied cardiac glycosides. In Goodman LS, Gilman A (eds): Pharmacological Basis of Therapeutics, 4th ed. New York, Macmillan, 1970, p 677.
145. Kittleson MD, Eyster GE, Knowlen GG, et al: Efficacy of digoxin administration in dogs with idiopathic congestive cardiomyopathy. JAVMA 186:162, 1985.
146. Baggot JD, Davis LE: Plasma protein binding of digitoxin and digoxin in several mammalian species. Res Vet Sci 15:81, 1973.
147. Button C, Gross DR, Johnston JT, Yakatan GJ: Pharmacokinetics, bioavailability, and dosage regimens of digoxin in dogs. Am J Vet Res 41:1230, 1980.
148. Weidler DFJ, Jallad NS, Movahhed HS: Pharmacokinetics of digoxin in the cat and comparisons with man and the dog. Res Commun Chem Pathol Pharmacol 19:57, 1987.
149. Pedersoli WM: Serum digoxin concentrations in healthy dogs treated without a loading dose. J Vet Pharmacol Ther 1:279, 1978.
150. DeMots H, McAnulty JH, Porter GA: Effects of rapid and slow infusion of ouabain on systemic and coronary vascular resistance in patients not in clinical heart failure (abstract). Circulation 52:II-77, 1975.
151. Smith TW, Haber E: Digitalis (third of four parts). N Engl J Med 289:1063, 1973.
152. Doherty JE: Digitalis glycosides. Pharmacokinetics and their clinical implications. Ann Intern Med 79:229, 1973.
153. Gierke KD, Perrier D, Mayersohn M, Marcus FI: Digoxin disposition kinetics in dogs before and during azotemia. J Pharmacol Exp Ther 205:459, 1978.
154. Atkins CE, Snyder PS, Keene BW, Rush JE: Effects of compensated heart failure on digoxin pharmacokinetics in cats. JAVMA 195:945, 1989.
155. Bolton GRP: Pharmacokinetics of Digoxin in the Cat. Snowbird, UT, Academy of Veterinary Cardiology, 1985.
156. Erichsen DF, Harris SG, Upson DW: Plasma levels of digoxin in the cat: Some clinical applications. J Am Anim Hosp Assoc 14:734, 1978.
157. Kittleson MD: Drugs used in the management of heart failure. In Kirk RW (ed): Current Veterinary Therapy VIII. Philadelphia, WB Saunders, 1983, p 285.
158. Bonagura JD, Ware WA: Atrial fibrillation in the dog: Clinical findings in 81 cases. J Am Anim Hosp Assoc 22:111, 1986.
159. Button C, Gross DR, Allert JA: Application of individualized digoxin dosage regimens to canine therapeutic digitalization. Am J Vet Res 41:1238, 1980.
160. Bigger JTJ: The quinidine-digoxin interaction. Mod Concepts Cardiovasc Dis 51:73, 1982.
161. Warner NJ, Barnard JT, Leahey EBJ, et al: Myocardial monovalent cation transport during the quinidine-digoxin interaction in dogs. Circ Res 54:453, 1984.
162. Warner NJ, Leahey EBJ, Hougen TJ, et al: Tissue digoxin concentrations during the quinidine-digoxin interaction. Am J Cardiol 51:1717, 1983.
163. Peters DN, Hamlin RL, Powers JD: Absence of pharmacokinetic interaction between digitoxin and quinidine in the dog. J Vet Pharmacol Ther 4:271, 1981.
164. Cardiology Drug Facts. New York, JB Lippincott, 1989.
165. Lesko LJ: Pharmacokinetic drug interactions with amiodarone. Clin Pharmacokinet 17:130, 1989.
166. Breznock EM: Effects of phenobarbital on digitoxin and digoxin elimination in the dog. Am J Vet Res 36:371, 1975.
167. Pedersoli WM: Serum digoxin concentration in dogs before and after concomitant treatment with chloramphenicol. J Am Anim Hosp Assoc 16:839, 1980.
168. Akera T, Brody TM: Pharmacology of cardiac glycosides. In Sperelakis N (ed): Physiology and Pathophysiology of the Heart, 3rd ed. Boston, Kluwer Academic Publishers, 1995, pp 495–510.
169. Snyder PS, Panciera DL, Volk L: Digoxin pharmacokinetics in dogs with experimental hypothyroidism (abstract). In Proceedings of the Eleventh Annual Veterinary Medical Forum. Washington, DC, American College of Veterinary Internal Medicine, 1993, p 950.
170. Karagueuzian HS, Katzung BG: Relative inotropic and arrhythmogenic effects of five cardiac steroids in ventricular myocardium: Oscillatory afterpotentials and the role of endogenous catecholamines. J Pharmacol Exp Ther 218:348, 1981.
171. Gross DR, Hamlin RL, Pipers FS: Response of P-Q intervals to digitalis glycosides in the dog. JAVMA 162:888, 1973.
172. Teske RH, Bishop SP, Righter HF, Detweiler DK: Subacute digoxin toxicosis in the beagle dog. Toxicol Appl Pharmacol 35:283, 1976.
173. Hamlin RL: Basis for selection of a cardiac glycoside for dogs. In Proceedings of the First Symposium on Veterinary Pharmacology and Therapeutics. Baton Rouge, American Academy of Veterinary Pharmacology and Therapeutics, 1978.
174. Borison HL, Borison R, McCarthy LE: Role of the area postrema in vomiting and related functions. Fed Proc 43:2955, 1984.
175. Kaplinsky E, Ogawa S, Balke CW, Dreifus LS: Two periods of early ventricular arrhythmia in the canine acute myocardial infarction model. Circulation 60:397, 1979.
176. Singh BN: Controlling cardiac arrhythmias by lengthening repolarization: Historical overview. Am J Cardiol 72:18F, 1993.
177. Somberg JC, Smith TW: Localization of the neurally mediated arrhythmogenic properties of digitalis. Science 204:321, 1979.
178. Thron CD, Riancho JA, Borison HL: Lack of protection against ouabain cardiotoxicity after chronic ablation of the area postrema in cats. Exp Neurol 85:574, 1984.
179. Citrin D, Stevenson IH, O'Malley K: Massive digoxin overdose: Observations on hyperkalaemia and plasma digoxin levels. Scott Med J 17:275, 1972.
180. Smith TW, Willerson JT: Suicidal and accidental digoxin ingestion. Report of five cases with serum digoxin level correlations. Circulation 44:29, 1971.
181. Dreifus LS, McKnight EH, Katz M, Likoff W: Digitalis intolerance. Geriatrics 18:494, 1963.

182. Hoffman BF, Rosen MR: Cellular mechanisms for cardiac arrhythmias. Circ Res 49:1, 1981.
183. Peon J, Ferrier GR, Moe GK: The relationship of excitability to conduction velocity in canine Purkinje tissue. Circ Res 43:125, 1978.
184. Rall TW, Schleifer LS: Drugs effective in the therapy of the epilepsies. In Gilman AG, Goodman LS, Gilman A (eds): The Pharmacological Basis of Therapeutics, 6th ed. New York, Macmillan, 1980, p 539.
185. Fogoros RN, Elson JJ, Bonnet CA, et al: Long-term outcome of survivors of cardiac arrest whose therapy is guided by electrophysiologic testing. J Am Coll Cardiol 19:780, 1992 (see comments).
186. Neuvonen PJ, Kivisto K, Hirvisalo EL: Effects of resins and activated charcoal on the absorption of digoxin, carbamazepine and frusemide. Br J Clin Pharmacol 25:229, 1988.
187. Eyster GE, Anderson LK, Sawyer DC, et al: Beta adrenergic blockade for management of tetralogy of Fallot in a dog. Circulation 87:1954, 1993.
188. Caldwell JH, Greenberger NJ: Interruption of the enterohepatic circulation of digitoxin by cholestyramine. I. Protection against lethal digitoxin intoxication. J Clin Invest 50:2626, 1971.
189. Smith TW, Butler VPJ, Haber E, et al: Treatment of life-threatening digitalis intoxication with digoxin-specific Fab antibody fragments: Experience in 26 cases. N Engl J Med 307:1357, 1982.
190. Senior DF, Feist EH, Stuart LB, Lombard CW: Treatment of acute digoxin toxicosis with digoxin immune Fab (Ovine). J Vet Intern Med 5:302, 1991.
191. Antman EM, Wenger TL, Butler VPJ, et al: Treatment of 150 cases of life-threatening digitalis intoxication with digoxin-specific Fab antibody fragments. Final report of a multicenter study. Circulation 81:1744, 1990.
192. Miyazawa Y, Sato T, Kobayashi K, et al: Influence of induced cholestasis on pharmacokinetics of digoxin and digitoxin in dogs. Am J Vet Res 51:605, 1990.
193. Katz AM: Congestive heart failure: Role of altered myocardial cellular control. N Engl J Med 293:1184, 1975.
194. Adams HR: New perspectives in cardiopulmonary therapeutics: Receptor-selective adrenergic drugs. JAVMA 185:966, 1984.
195. Maekawa K, Liang CS, Hood WBJ: Comparison of dobutamine and dopamine in acute myocardial infarction. Effects of systemic hemodynamics, plasma catecholamines, blood flows and infarct size. Circulation 67:750, 1983.
196. Bednarski RM, Muir WW: Catecholamine infusion in vagotomized dogs during thiamylal-halothane and pentobarbital anesthesia. Cornell Vet 75:512, 1985.
197. Murphy PJ, Williams TL, Kau DL: Disposition of dobutamine in the dog. J Pharmacol Exp Ther 199:423, 1976.
198. McNay JL, McDonald RH, Goldgern LI: Direct renal vasodilation produced by dopamine in the dog. Circ Res 16:510, 1965.
199. Loeb HS, Bredakis J, Gunner RM: Superiority of dobutamine over dopamine for augmentation of cardiac output in patients with chronic low output cardiac failure. Circulation 55:375, 1977.
200. MacCannell KL, Giraud GD, Hamilton PL, Groves G: Haemodynamic responses to dopamine and dobutamine infusions as a function of duration of infusion. Pharmacology 26:29, 1983.
201. Robie NW, Goldberg LI: Comparative systemic and regional hemodynamic effects of dopamine and dobutamine. Am Heart J 90:340, 1975.
202. Vatner SF, McRitchie RJ, Braunwald E: Effects of dobutamine on left ventricular performance, coronary dynamics, and distribution of cardiac output in conscious dogs. J Clin Invest 53:1265, 1974.
203. Tuttle RR, Mills J: Dobutamine: Development of a new catecholamine to selectively increase cardiac contractility. Circ Res 36:185, 1975.
204. Willerson JT, Hutton I, Watson JT, et al: Influence of dobutamine on regional myocardial blood flow and ventricular performance during acute and chronic myocardial ischemia in dogs. Circulation 53:828, 1976.
205. Akhtar N, Mikulic E, Cohn JN, Chaudhry MH: Hemodynamic effect of dobutamine in patients with severe heart failure. Am J Cardiol 36:202, 1975.
206. Andy JJ, Curry CL, Ali N, Mehrotra PP: Cardiovascular effects of dobutamine in severe congestive heart failure. Am Heart J 94:175, 1977.
207. Eyster GE, Anderson LK, Bender G, et al: Effect of dobutamine in postperfusion cardiac failure in the dog. Am J Vet Res 36:1285, 1975.
208. Braunwald E: A symposium: Amrinone. Introduction. Am J Cardiol 56:1B, 1985.
209. Piscione F, Jaski BE, Wenting GJ, Serruys PW: Effect of a single oral dose of milrinone on left ventricular diastolic performance in the failing human heart. J Am Coll Cardiol 10:1294, 1987.
210. Keister DM: A Summary of Phase IV Clinical Data on Milrinone (Wincardin), a Canine Cardiotonic. Protocol H. Rensselaer, NY, Sterling-Winthrop Research Institute, 1988
211. Emmert SE, Stabilito II, Sweet CS: Acute and subacute hemodynamic effects of enalaprilat, milrinone and combination therapy in rats with chronic left ventricular dysfunction. Clin Exp Hypertens 9:297, 1987.
212. A Summary of Laboratory and Clinical Data on Inocor (brand of amrinone). Rensselaer, NY, Sterling-Winthrop Research Institute, 1980.
213. Kittleson MD: The efficacy and safety of milrinone for treating heart failure in dogs. Vet Clin North Am Small Anim Pract 21:905, 1991.
214. Alousi AA, Canter JM, Montenaro MJ, et al: Cardiotonic activity of milrinone, a new and potent cardiac bipyridine, on the normal and failing heart of experimental animals. J Cardiovasc Pharmacol 5:792, 1983.
215. Puri S, Baker BL, Dutka DP, et al: Reduced alveolar-capillary membrane diffusing capacity in chronic heart failure. Its pathophysiological relevance and relationship to exercise performance. Circulation 91:2769, 1995.
216. Guidelines for the evaluation and management of heart failure. Report of the American College of Cardiology/American Heart Association Task Force on Practice Guidelines (Committee on Evaluation and Management of Heart Failure). J Am Coll Cardiol 26:1376, 1995.
217. Plumb DC: Acepromazine maleate. In Plumb DC (ed): Veterinary Drug Handbook, 2nd ed. Ames, Iowa State University Press, 1995, pp 1–3.
218. Hall LW, Clarke KW: Anaesthesia of the dog. In Hall LW, Clarke KW (eds): Veterinary Anaesthesia, 9th ed. London, Bailliere Tindall, 1991, pp 290–323.
219. Jacobson JD, McGrath CJ, Smith EP: Cardiorespiratory effects of four opioid-tranquilizer combinations in dogs. Vet Surg 23:299, 1994.(Published erratum appears in Vet Surg 23:434, 1994.)

CV

CHAPTER 112

CONGENITAL HEART DISEASE

D. David Sisson, William P. Thomas, and John D. Bonagura

CLINICAL APPROACH TO CONGENITAL HEART DISEASE

Malformations of the heart and adjacent great vessels constitute a small but clinically significant percentage of cardiovascular disorders in dogs and cats.[1a–14a] The etiologies, pathogenesis, and types of defects in animals parallel those in humans.[15a, 16a, 1b] There are also similar clinical findings in animals and humans with similar cardiac defects, and most of the diagnostic and therapeutic methods used in veterinary cardiology have been adapted from those used in the management of children and adults with congenital heart disease.

Examination for congenital heart defects and other con-

References superscripted with [a] are from the third edition of *Textbook of Veterinary Internal Medicine*; references superscripted with [b] are from the fourth edition.

genital disorders is important in the evaluation of newly acquired pets and purebred dogs and cats intended for breeding. Although precise identification and evaluation of congenital heart disease may require referral for echocardiography or cardiac catheterization, every veterinarian should be aware of the most common cardiac defects in small animals and should be able to distinguish between murmurs caused by these defects and the innocent murmurs that are often heard in neonates. Clinicians should also have a general understanding of the proven or suspected genetic/etiologic basis of congenital heart disease in order to counsel breeders properly.[17a–21a]

HISTORY AND PHYSICAL EXAMINATION

The diagnostic approach to the pet with suspected congenital heart disease is similar to that used in the evaluation of acquired cardiac disorders.[1a, 9a, 15a, 22a–36a, 2b] The breed is important to note because some cardiac malformations have a proven genetic basis, and most have breed predilections. The noninvasive evaluation always includes the patient history and physical examination, and this is often supplemented by thoracic radiography, electrocardiography, routine hematologic tests, and two-dimensional echocardiography. Based on these evaluations, an anatomic diagnosis can often be made. Definitive diagnosis and determination of severity often requires Doppler echocardiography and may necessitate cardiac catheterization and angiocardiography. The extent of the evaluation is influenced by client expectations, the nature and severity of the disorder and any clinical signs, and surgical considerations.

HISTORY

The age, sex, and breed should be considered when evaluating animals with suspected congenital heart disease. Table 112–1 lists the breed predilections reported for canine cardiac defects in North America and Europe.[1–6] These associations provide support for a suspected genetic basis of many malformations. Sex predispositions are weak or poorly established in dogs, except for the higher prevalence of patent ductus arteriosus in females.[1a, 4a, 8a] In cats, the Siamese, Burmese, and Oriental shorthair breeds may be predisposed to some defects, and male kittens seem to be affected more often than females.[2 [36a]] However, sex predilection has little influence on the evaluation of an individual patient. Age may be an important factor when interpreting the results of initial examinations. Most defects are detectable shortly after birth, but the severity of the hemodynamic abnormalities may change significantly during the first 6 to 12 months of life. For example, the lesion of congenital discrete subaortic stenosis may not be present at birth but will develop during the first 2 months of life,[2a, 9a] and the severity of the obstruction and associated physical findings often increase progressively during the first year of life. Similarly, left-to-right shunting defects may not be fully manifest until pulmonary vascular resistance and right heart pressures, which are high in the fetus and remain increased immediately after birth, decrease to normal low levels several weeks after birth.

Most animals with congenital heart defects are asymptomatic when first examined; these defects are initially recognized when a heart murmur is detected, often during a routine examination. Even dogs and cats with hemodynamically severe valvular, obstructive, or shunting defects may appear asymptomatic and well to the owner during the first 6 to 12 months. Dogs with severe subaortic stenosis may look well and act normally to the owner, yet they can collapse and die suddenly with or without exercise provocation. Similarly, young animals with patent ductus arteriosus (PDA) and imminent cardiac failure often appear normal to the owner until pulmonary edema becomes life-threatening and causes acute dyspnea. Therefore, the veterinarian should not necessarily conclude from an unremarkable history that the underlying defect is mild. Clinical signs that may develop with severe defects include small stature, exertional fatigue, dyspnea/tachypnea, abdominal swelling, cyanosis, episodic weakness or syncope, seizures, or sudden death.

PHYSICAL EXAMINATION

With occasional exceptions, dogs and cats with congenital heart defects are so identified when a heart murmur is discovered. The typical characteristics of the heart murmurs associated with the most common heart defects are listed in Table 112–2. When a murmur is first detected, the examiner must decide whether it is pathologic or innocent, because normal pups and kittens can exhibit innocent systolic cardiac murmurs. Innocent murmurs are typically soft (grade 1–3/6), are best heard over the left mid- or cranial precordium, are short and confined to the first half of systole, and often vary with heart rate and changing body position. The first and second heart sounds are clearly preserved, and the re-

TABLE 112–1. CANINE BREED PREDILECTIONS FOR CONGENITAL HEART DISEASE

BREED	DEFECT(S)
Basset hound	PS
Beagle	PS
Bichon frisé	PDA
Boxer	SAS, PS, ASD
Boykin spaniel	PS
Bull terrier	MVD, AS
Chihuahua	PDA, PS
Chow chow	PS, CTD
Cocker spaniel	PDA, PS
Collie	PDA
Doberman pinscher	ASD
English bulldog	PS, VSD, TOF
English springer spaniel	PDA, VSD
German shepherd	SAS, PDA, TVD, MVD
German shorthair pointer	SAS
Golden retriever	SAS, TVD, MVD
Great Dane	TVD, MVD, SAS
Keeshond	TOF, PDA
Labrador retriever	TVD, PDA, PS
Maltese	PDA
Mastiff	PS, MVD
Newfoundland	SAS, MVD, PS
Pomeranian	PDA
Poodle	PDA
Rottweiler	SAS
Samoyed	PS, SAS, ASD
Schnauzer	PS
Shetland sheepdog	PDA
Terrier breeds	PS
Weimaraner	TVD, PPDH
Welsh corgi	PDA
West Highland white terrier	PS, VSD
Yorkshire terrier	PDA

AS = aortic stenosis, ASD = atrial septal defect, CTD = cor triatriatum dexter, MVD = mitral valve dysplasia, PDA = patent ductus arteriosus, PPDH = peritoneopericardial diaphragmatic hernia, PS = pulmonic stenosis, SAS = subaortic stenosis, TOF = tetralogy of Fallot, TVD = tricuspid valve dysplasia, VSD = ventricular septal defect.

TABLE 112–2. AUSCULTATORY FINDINGS IN CONGENITAL HEART DISEASE

LESION	TIMING	FEATURES	LOCATION (PMI)	COMMENTS
Atrial septal defect	Systolic (diastolic)	Ejection (diastolic rumble)	Left base	Systolic murmur ends prior to S_2, which is usually split; murmur(s) due to relative pulmonic (tricuspid) stenosis
(Sub)aortic stenosis	Systolic*	Ejection (crescendo-decrescendo)	Left base	Often nearly as loud at the right base; diastolic murmur of aortic regurgitation may also occur
Mitral valve dysplasia†	Systolic	Regurgitant (holosystolic)	Left apex	May radiate widely
Patent ductus arteriosus	Continuous	Machinery	Left base	Murmur peaks at S_2, often radiates to right base and thoracic inlet
Pulmonary hypertension (Eisenmenger's syndrome)	None (systolic)	Split S_2 (ejection)	Left base	Accentuated and split S_2; systolic murmur of tricuspid regurgitation or blowing decrescendo diastolic murmur of pulmonic regurgitation may also occur
Pulmonic stenosis	Systolic	Ejection (crescendo-decrescendo)	Left base	Occasional systolic ejection sound; blowing, decrescendo diastolic murmur of pulmonic regurgitation may occur
Tetralogy of Fallot	Systolic	Ejection (crescendo-decrescendo)	Left base	Murmur is due to pulmonic stenosis; murmur may be soft or absent with pulmonary artery hypoplasia
Tricuspid valve dysplasia†	Systolic	Regurgitant (holosystolic)	Right midprecordium	Often low-pitched and rumbling
Ventricular septal defect	Systolic*	Regurgitant (holosystolic)	Right base	Often higher pitched and more cranially located than tricuspid regurgitation; may also be loud at left base

* = At times a diastolic murmur of aortic regurgitation may also be present.
† = Mitral stenosis and tricuspid stenosis are rare but may cause diastolic murmurs over the affected valve and ventricle.

mainder of the examination is usually normal. Innocent murmurs usually, but not invariably, diminish in intensity or resolve by the time the animal is 4 to 5 months of age, but short, early systolic innocent murmurs may occasionally be heard in mature animals.

Cardiac murmurs of congenital heart disease are more often louder (grade 3–5/6), are of longer duration, may obscure the normal heart sounds, and may be accompanied by a precordial thrill. However, the intensity of the murmur should *not* be relied upon by itself to speculate about the severity of the underlying defect. A murmur may occasionally be soft or even inaudible with certain large septal defects, atrioventricular (AV) valve stenosis, or even in some cases of severe cyanotic heart disease. In addition, mild subaortic stenosis may generate only a soft, variable systolic murmur that can easily be confused with an innocent murmur. Thus, any grade of cardiac murmur may represent potential congenital heart disease. Additional auscultatory abnormalities, such as an accentuated or split-second heart sound, may offer further evidence of congenital heart disease.

Abnormalities of the arterial pulse, mucous membranes, jugular venous pulse, or precordial impulse may support a suspicion of congenital heart disease. Hyperkinetic, bounding ("waterhammer") arterial pulses are characteristic of lesions that cause abnormal diastolic run-off of aortic blood and low arterial diastolic pressure, such as PDA or aortic regurgitation. Hypokinetic pulses are typical of moderate-to-severe left ventricular outflow obstruction (aortic stenosis) or other severe defects accompanied by low left ventricular output. Peripheral cyanosis suggests a possible systemic-to-pulmonary (right-to-left) shunt but may also develop in animals with severe congestive failure and secondary pulmonary dysfunction. Increased jugular pulsations indicate an abnormality of the right side of the heart, such as pulmonic stenosis and/or tricuspid regurgitation. A precordial impulse of increased strength or area often indicates enlargement of the underlying ventricle(s). Precordial thrills accompany the loudest cardiac murmurs (grade 5–6/6), and the focus of this vibration is the point of maximal murmur intensity, which is characteristic of the associated defect (see Table 112–2).

Laboratory Tests

In most cases, hematologic tests are not an important part of the congenital heart disease work-up. Although serum biochemical tests may be abnormal when there is congestive heart failure (especially right) or intercurrent organ disease (e.g., portosystemic shunting), the complete blood count, biochemical profile, and urinalysis are typically normal. Distinctive abnormalities may occur in animals with right-to-left shunting defects such as tetralogy of Fallot, PDA with pulmonary hypertension, and other complex cyanotic heart disease. These include arterial hypoxemia, hypocarbia, metabolic acidosis and, eventually, polycythemia. Any animal with absolute polycythemia should be evaluated for a right-to-left shunting cardiovascular defect.

Despite a strong clinical suspicion of congenital heart disease based on history and physical examination, definitive diagnosis of the animal with a cardiac murmur generally requires additional studies. In this regard, an electrocardiogram (ECG), thoracic radiographs, and two-dimensional and Doppler echocardiograms are required.

ELECTROCARDIOGRAPHY
(see also Chapter 114)

The ECG can provide helpful information in dogs and cats with congenital heart disease.[7b] Whereas a normal ECG does not rule out a cardiac malformation, an abnormal ECG often indicates at least the side of the heart that is affected and may suggest one or more specific defects.[5a, 9a, 15a] For example, a normal frontal plane QRS axis with increased QRS voltages is typical of PDA but very unlikely in pulmonic stenosis or tricuspid dysplasia. Left axis deviation (more common in cats, rare in dogs) may indicate left ventricular hypertrophy or a partial left bundle branch block. Persistence of a right ventricular hypertrophy-type pattern after the first few weeks of age in the dog is abnormal[31a] and is most commonly associated with simple or complicated pulmonic stenosis, tricuspid valve dysplasia, atrial septal defect, large ventricular septal defect, or a shunting defect with pulmonary hypertension. Right heart defects with right ventricular enlargement can also result in conduction delay with right axis deviation and widening of the QRS complex (partial or complete right bundle branch block).[5a, 32a] These must be distinguished from congenital right bundle branch block, an uncommon conduction disorder that may occur with or without an underlying congenital heart defect.

CARDIAC IMAGING

RADIOGRAPHY

Survey radiographs of the thorax are important for the determination of cardiac size, initial identification of chamber enlargement and size of the great vessels, pulmonary circulatory dynamics, and congestive heart failure.[5a, 22a–24a, 3b] While typical radiographic features are discussed later for each defect, some general comments about radiographic interpretation can be offered. Subjective or objective detection of cardiomegaly is relatively easy; however, distinguishing between right heart, left heart, and bilateral enlargement may be difficult or impossible without echocardiography. There is a tendency to overinterpret the size of the right heart in neonates, in which some right ventricular prominence is normal. This may lead to an erroneous diagnosis of pulmonic stenosis in a pup with a functional (innocent) left base murmur. The frequent occurrence of apex shifting may also confuse an inexperienced clinician, resulting in an erroneous diagnosis. Thus, the radiographic evaluation is best conducted in conjunction with an ECG and, when possible, an echocardiogram. Thoracic radiographs provide a good general indicator of the severity of congenital heart disease when the underlying condition is characterized by volume overload from left-to-right shunting or valvular insufficiency. This is not the case, however, for outflow obstruction, pulmonary hypertension, or right-to-left shunts, in which ventricular hypertrophy is concentric and better appreciated by echocardiography.

Dilatation of the great vessels may provide clues to the underlying cardiac malformation. Ascending aortic dilatation in the cranial mediastinum may represent the post-stenotic dilatation of subaortic stenosis or the aortic anomaly sometimes noted with tetralogy of Fallot. Aneurysmal dilatation of the proximal descending aorta is common with PDA. Dilatation of the main pulmonary artery may occur with turbulent post-stenotic flow from pulmonic stenosis, increased pulmonary flow caused by a left-to-right shunt, or pulmonary hypertension.

Because of its variability, pulmonary vascularity must be assessed with caution, but it may be used to help identify pulmonary overcirculation, undercirculation, and pulmonary venous congestion. Central cranial and caudal lobar arteries and veins, as well as peripheral pulmonary vascular markings, should be examined. Right-to-left shunts cause decreased pulmonary blood flow, with diminished peripheral perfusion and normal-to-small lobar arteries and veins. Vascularity can also appear to be decreased with pulmonic stenosis and severe tricuspid dysplasia. Pulmonary hypertension with bidirectional or right-to-left shunting causes an enlarged main pulmonary artery, variable prominence of the central lobar arteries, and variable diminished peripheral lung vasculature. Conversely, left-to-right shunts cause increased size of the main pulmonary artery, lobar arteries and veins, and increased peripheral vascular markings that may be misinterpreted as interstitial lung densities. Increased right or left atrial pressure and impending right or left heart failure usually cause visible widening of the caudal vena cava or pulmonary veins, respectively.

ECHOCARDIOGRAPHY (see also Chapter 115)

In recent years, the development of echocardiography, which permits detailed imaging of internal cardiac anatomy, has markedly reduced the necessity for invasive cardiac catheterization and angiocardiography to establish a definitive diagnosis of congenital heart disease.[27a, 28a, 4b–6b] When combined with basic two-dimensional anatomic imaging, Doppler echocardiography, which can identify normal and abnormal blood flow patterns and estimate intravascular pressures, greatly increases the value of ultrasound studies.[7, 8, 29a] Contrast echocardiography, in which microbubbles created by the rapid intravenous injection of agitated saline or indocyanine-green dye provide the intravascular echo contrast targets,[27a, 28a, 30a] is another method that can detect intracardiac blood shunting (especially right-to-left shunting) when Doppler technology is unavailable.

Doppler echocardiography, which uses the principle of sound frequency shifting of ultrasound as it reflects from moving structures, is used to measure the velocity and flow direction of blood cells. Because the magnitude and direction of the frequency shift is directly proportional to the velocity and direction of the flowing cells, the technique permits the recognition of normal laminar and abnormal turbulent blood flow, detection and measurement of abnormal high-velocity flow jets in the heart and blood vessels, and estimation of intracardiac and vascular blood pressures.[8, 29a (b–d)] A careful "echo-Doppler" study can usually provide a detailed diagnosis and eliminate the need for cardiac catheterization and angiocardiography in most animals. The velocity and direction of flow can be displayed as a "spectral" tracing. Range-gated or *pulsed-wave Doppler* allows interrogation of blood cell velocities in specific locations by having the operator direct a depth-range "gate" that is superimposed over a two-dimensional (2D) image to the region of interest. This mode provides accurate information about the exact anatomic site of the abnormal flow and relative direction of flow. It is limited to the measurement of relatively low velocities because of a sampling phenomenon called "aliasing" (related mainly to the sampling rate), in which velocities greater than a known limit (the "Nyquist limit") appear to reverse direction and cause an ambiguous display. *Continuous-wave Doppler* uses two crystals (a constant transmitter and constant receiver) to achieve very high sampling rates and allow recording and measurement of very high velocities along the directed ultrasound beam. The velocities of all cells along the beam line are recorded and displayed, allowing the high-flow velocities across stenotic or insufficient valves to be displayed and measured, but preventing precise localization of the abnormal flow. The two modes are therefore complementary, with pulsed-wave being used to identify and localize a lesion and continuous-wave being used to measure any high velocities.

2D color-flow Doppler imaging is a special form of pulsed-wave Doppler in which Doppler shift signals from multiple points in a two-dimensional area are collected, color coded, and then displayed as an overlay on the two-dimensional anatomic image. The Doppler shift or velocity is color-coded to indicate velocity, direction, and the presence of disturbed, turbulent flow. The current standard scheme codes flow toward the transducer in shades of red and flow away from the transducer in shades of blue. Turbulent blood flow is indicated by special "turbulence" or "variance" maps, which add an additional color (usually green or white) to the display. This complex imaging method, which combines 2D anatomy, pulsed-wave Doppler, and color designation of red blood cell direction and velocity, is often called *color-flow* or *color-Doppler* imaging. The technique is very sensitive and provides detailed images of blood flow through the heart and adjacent great vessels throughout the cardiac cycle. It greatly facilitates the identification and localization of flow abnormalities associated with most congenital heart defects.

A typical echo-Doppler study usually proceeds as follows: (1) detailed anatomic evaluation, cardiac function, and cardiac dimensions are determined by 2D and M mode imaging; (2) color-flow imaging and/or contrast 2D studies are used to identify areas of abnormal blood flow; (3) pulsed-wave spectral Doppler may be used as a supplement to the color-flow examination to locate areas of abnormal or high-velocity blood flow; (4) any high-velocity flow jets are confirmed and measured using continuous-wave spectral Doppler. Although details of the methods and calculations used in these studies are beyond the scope of this chapter, one important calculation that is routinely used in evaluation of congenital heart disease is the modified Bernoulli equation. This equation, a much simplified version of the original Bernoulli principle, provides a good estimate of the instantaneous peak pressure difference (gradient) across a stenosis, septal defect, or regurgitant valve, using the peak velocity of blood in the jet by continuous-wave Doppler (pressure gradient in mmHg = 4 × [peak velocity in m/s]^2). The peak velocity of flow is thereby converted to a pressure gradient across the lesion. This gradient is useful in grading the severity of obstructive lesions and in determining the advisability of surgical intervention. In addition, by estimating the pressure on one side of a lesion, the Doppler pressure gradient may be used to estimate the pressure on the other side of the lesion. Details of these principles are in Chapter 115 and in the references.[8, [29a, (b)]]

OTHER IMAGING FORMATS

Single-pass or blood-pool radionuclide scanning studies may be used to detect cardiac shunting and measure ventricular volumes, but the resolution of these studies is not high enough to evaluate details of cardiac and vascular anatomy. Computerized tomography and magnetic resonance imaging are newer techniques that may be applicable to evaluation of congenital heart diseases. Magnetic resonance imaging, in particular, is an effective method of evaluating the aortic arch and related vascular anomalies in humans. Because of their expense and limited availability to veterinarians, there are currently no reports of the clinical application of these techniques to animals with congenital heart disease.

ANGIOCARDIOGRAPHY AND CARDIAC CATHETERIZATION

Cardiac catheterization is an invasive procedure used to diagnose structural malformations of the heart and to evaluate the physiologic derangements caused by these anatomic lesions.[9 [5a, 15a, 24a–26a, 33a–35a]] To many older cardiologists who were trained before the ultrasound era, selective catheterization with angiocardiography remains the "gold standard" by which to diagnose and evaluate congenital heart disease. During the 1990s, the combination of 2D anatomic echocardiography with color and spectral Doppler imaging has rapidly become the primary method for the clinical identification and assessment of anatomic cardiac defects in animals. Ultrasound imaging is less expensive, less invasive, safer, and often superior to angiography in examining the dynamic, detailed three-dimensional anatomy of the heart and central great vessels. However, determination of intracardiac and vascular pressures, cardiac output, oximetry, and the anatomy of the pulmonary or systemic vasculature may be necessary for determining prognosis and recommending treatment choices for some patients.

ANGIOCARDIOGRAPHY

Selective angiocardiography[5a, 24a–26a] has been used to identify most of the common congenital heart defects reported in dogs and cats. To achieve the best contrast outline of the defect and affected chambers, contrast injections should be made as close to the lesion(s) as possible. For shunting and obstructive lesions, the contrast should be injected into the chamber *proximal to* (upstream from) the defect. For valvular insufficiencies, the contrast should be injected in the chamber *distal to* (downstream from) the defect. For animals with congenital heart disease, it is common to perform both right ventricular and left ventricular injections. Additional injections are selected based on the specific defect(s) known or suspected to be present. The right ventriculogram is used to identify defects such as tricuspid regurgitation, pulmonic stenosis, right-to-left shunting ventricular septal defect, tetralogy of Fallot, transposition of the great vessels, (pseudo)truncus arteriosus, aorticopulmonary window, and right-to-left PDA and to distinguish abnormal pulmonary vascularity from pulmonary vascular disease/pulmonary hypertension. The left ventriculogram is used to identify defects such as mitral regurgitation, left-to-right shunting ventricular septal defect, subaortic and aortic valve stenosis, (pseudo)truncus arteriosus, and supravalvular aortic lesions. Pulmonary artery injection is useful for identifying defects such as anomalous pulmonary venous return (to the right atrium), left-to-right shunting atrial septal defect, and mitral valve stenosis. Aortic root injection is useful for identifying aortic valve regurgitation, left-to-right shunting aorticopulmonary window, anomalous coronary arteries, anomalous branching from the aortic arch, coarctation or interruption of the aorta, left-to-right shunting PDA, and bronchoesophageal or other collateral pulmonary circulation. Angiograms are recorded on videotape, multiple or continuous x-ray films, 16 or 35 mm film, or digitally on magnetic media. With modern ultrasound technology, most of the same lesions listed above can also be imaged and the abnormal blood flow clearly demonstrated by a good echo-Doppler examination.

Additional injections of contrast media may be indicated for identification of specific lesions. For example, injection of contrast into the left jugular vein identifies persistent left cranial vena cava. A right atrial or vena caval injection is used to demonstrate a right-to-left shunting atrial septal defect or tricuspid valve stenosis/hypoplasia/atresia. A caudal vena caval injection is used to visualize a partitioned right atrium from cor triatriatum dexter.

CARDIAC CATHETERIZATION

Insertion of catheters into peripheral arteries or veins and guidance into the heart allows the clinician to record the pressures in cardiac chambers, measure cardiac output, obtain blood samples for oxygen content or saturation (oximetry), and perform indicator dilution studies. More complete details of these techniques and their interpretation are in the references.[9] [5a, 15a, 33a]

The variable most commonly measured during catheterization is intravascular hydrostatic pressure. Normal pressure tracings from the right and left heart chambers are shown in Figure 112–1. As the tracings show, the peak systolic pressure in the left ventricle and aorta (100 to 120 mmHg) is much higher than in the right ventricle and pulmonary artery (20 to 25 mmHg).[5a] Because right and left ventricular outputs are nearly the same, pulmonary vascular resistance is normally much lower than systemic vascular resistance. Blood is normally propelled through the heart by generation of small instantaneous pressure gradients; however, peak pressures on either side of a normal open valve are nearly equal. The large systolic pressure difference between the ventricles and corresponding atria are because of the intervening atrioventricular valve. When a valve or other structure becomes stenotic, a pressure gradient (increased pressure proximal to the obstruction, relative to the pressure distal to the obstruction) is required to maintain normal flow. Intracardiac obstruction is proven by demonstration of the pressure gradient, and its magnitude is commonly used to classify the severity of obstruction. A systolic pressure gradient across a semilunar valve indicates the presence of pulmonic or aortic stenosis (Fig. 112–2). A diastolic pressure gradient across an atrioventricular valve is indicative of mitral or tricuspid stenosis. Gradients across fixed obstructions vary with the rate of flow through the region and can be diminished by heart failure, anesthesia, or hypovolemia and increased by exercise, anemia, or other causes of increased cardiac output. A mild systolic pressure gradient (5 to 15 mmHg) may also occur across a normal pulmonary valve when the right ventricular stroke volume is markedly increased, most often due to a large left-to-right shunt proximal to the valve. Such a physiologic flow-related gradient is termed "relative" pulmonic stenosis.

Because of the differences in pressure between the two sides of the heart, anatomically small (*restrictive*) communications between the atria (atrial septal defect [ASD]), ventri-

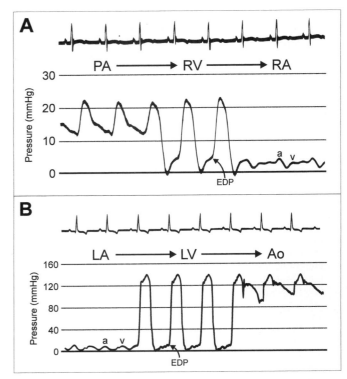

Figure 112–1. Normal intracardiac pressures in the dog. *A,* Right heart pressure recording during withdrawal of a catheter from the pulmonary artery (PA) to the right ventricle (RV) and right atrium (RA). Of note is the normal low PA and RV systolic pressure (<25 mmHg) and the low mean RA pressure (<6 mmHg). *B,* Left heart pressure recording during withdrawal of a catheter from the left atrium (LA) to the left ventricle (LV) and aorta (Ao). Note the higher pressure scale on the left heart compared with that for the right heart. The configurations of the tracings in each area are similar for both sides of the heart. Notice that when the cardiac valve regions are normal, the peak systolic pressure in the PA and RV are almost identical, and the diastolic pressures in the RV and RA are very similar.

cles (ventricular septal defect [VSD]), or great vessels (PDA) cause left-to-right shunting of blood. Uncomplicated shunting defects result in significant pulmonary overperfusion and dilatation of all chambers and vessels along the shunt circuit. However, large (*unrestrictive*) communications between the ventricles or great vessels cause the pressures on both sides of the defect to equilibrate at left heart pressure levels and the ventricles to behave as a common chamber. Flow direction and magnitude across the defect then depend on the relative resistance downstream from each side. Because the systemic vascular resistance is usually normal, the shunt becomes dependent mainly on the resistance to outflow from the right ventricle. If pulmonary vascular resistance is near normal, a very large left-to-right shunt may result. If pulmonary vascular resistance is increased or pulmonic stenosis is also present, the shunt may be left-to-right but reduced, bidirectional (usually right-to-left during systole, left-to-right during diastole), or mainly right-to-left. Pulmonary vascular resistance may increase secondary to left heart failure (with elevated pulmonary venous and capillary pressure) or due to pulmonary arteriolar vasoconstriction or pathologic narrowing.

The systemic arterial pressure configuration may also be altered by congenital heart defects. In the presence of decreased left ventricular stroke volume (hypovolemia, heart failure), the mean arterial pressure may be maintained by peripheral vasoconstriction, but the arterial pulse pressure (systolic minus diastolic) narrows, and the palpable pulse is

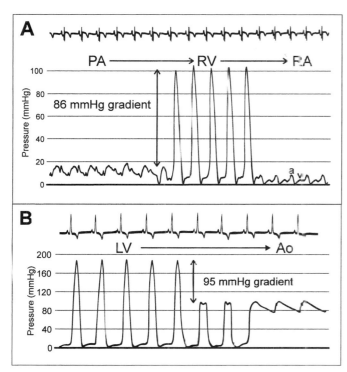

Figure 112–2. Intracardiac pressure tracings from two dogs with obstructive congenital heart defects. *A*, Right heart pressure tracing from a dog with valvular pulmonic stenosis. The pulmonary artery (PA) pressure is normal. As the catheter is withdrawn across the pulmonic valve into the right ventricle (RV), there is a sudden increase in systolic pressure to near systemic levels. The peak-to-peak systolic pressure gradient between the RV and PA is 86 mmHg. The mean right atrial (RA) pressure is normal, but the atrial (a) wave component is increased due to RV hypertrophy and reduced compliance. *B*, Left heart pressure tracing from a dog with subaortic stenosis. The pressure in the body of the left ventricle (LV) is increased (190 mmHg). As the catheter is withdrawn, there is a sudden decrease in systolic pressure while the recording tip is still within the ventricle. The peak-to-peak systolic pressure gradient is 95 mmHg. Further withdrawal across the aortic valve into the aorta (Ao) shows no pressure gradient at the valve level and therefore no valvular component to the stenosis.

weak. In cases of severe aortic stenosis, the arterial pressure systolic upstroke is slow-rising, the systolic pressure is decreased, and the pulse feels weak or sluggish, with a weak early systolic wave. Diastolic arterial pressure is normally determined mainly by the resistance to peripheral arterial diastolic run-off. In the presence of PDA or aortic regurgitation, the arterial systolic pressure is increased by the increased left ventricular stroke volume, and the arterial diastolic pressure is decreased by increased diastolic run-off into the pulmonary artery or left ventricle. The result is a wide arterial pulse pressure and an exaggerated (bounding, hyperkinetic, waterhammer) pulse.

The other abnormality that may be identified by pressure recording is elevation of ventricular end-diastolic (filling) pressure. This may be caused by increased diastolic ventricular stiffness (decreased compliance) from ventricular hypertrophy or fibrosis, volume overloading from valvular regurgitation or a left-to-right shunt, ventricular myocardial failure, or pericardial disease. When ventricular end-diastolic pressure and corresponding atrial and venous pressure exceed 15 to 20 mmHg, signs of overt congestive heart failure with edema are usually present or imminent.

Cardiac output may be measured at catheterization by the indicator (thermal or indocyanine green dye) dilution technique or by combining measurements of oxygen content of arterial and mixed-venous blood (oximetry) and oxygen

consumption in respiratory gases.[9] Blood hemoglobin oxygen saturation (per cent) or blood oxygen content (mL O$_2$/dL blood) are determined by the partial pressure of oxygen in the blood, characteristics of the hemoglobin-oxygen dissociation curve, and the blood hemoglobin concentration.[15a, 33a] Oximetry and selective indicator dilution may also be used to detect and quantify intracardiac shunts. On each side of the heart, oxygen content or saturation should be very similar within the atrium, ventricle, and great artery (see caution below). When oxygen saturations are recorded sequentially from the right and left heart chambers, a significant increase or step-up (≥ 5 per cent) in oxygen saturation within the right heart indicates the presence of a left-to-right shunt proximal to the site of the step-up. A significant decrease in oxygen saturation within the left heart indicates the presence of a right-to-left shunt proximal to the site of the decrease. For example, a marked increase in oxygen saturation in the right ventricular outflow tract occurs with a left-to-right shunting ventricular septal defect. Formulas may be used to estimate the degree of cardiac shunting, using either oxygen saturation or indicator dilution techniques.[9] [33a, 35a] Caution must be exercised when interpreting oxygen measurements in the right heart. Whereas oxygen saturations from the left atrium, left ventricle, ascending aorta, and descending aorta are normally within 1 to 2 per cent of each other, the right atrium receives blood from several sources with different oxygen saturations (up to 3 to 4 per cent differences), and there is incomplete mixing of blood in this chamber. Typically, the lowest oxygen saturation is measured in the coronary sinus, and saturation in the caudal vena cava may be slightly higher than in the cranial vena cava. These differences make it more difficult to diagnose atrial septal defects by comparing single right atrial samples with those from the right ventricle. Differences of 5 to 6 per cent saturation are suggestive of an atrial level shunt but not definitive. Differences greater than 8 per cent are almost always indicative of a shunt.

CAUSES, PREVALENCE, AND CLASSIFICATION OF CONGENITAL HEART DISEASE

CAUSES OF CARDIAC MALFORMATIONS

Congenital cardiac defects may be caused by genetic, toxicologic, nutritional, infectious, environmental, and pharmacologic factors.[17a–21a] Although most of these factors have been studied in the laboratory, little is known about the role of nongenetic factors in the occurrence of spontaneous congenital heart defects in dogs and cats. Although breed predispositions have been suggested for certain malformations in cats,[2] the evidence for a genetic basis of congenital heart disease is stronger in dogs, in which the heritable basis of several defects in certain breeds have been proved.

The pioneering studies of Patterson et al have clearly demonstrated a genetic basis for several specific congenital heart defects in certain dog breeds.[2a–4a, 17a–19a] Most of these studies indicated a probable polygenic basis for transmission of each defect, although data from Newfoundland dogs with subaortic stenosis have suggested that this defect may be inherited as an autosomal dominant with modifiers. As stated by Patterson, "these genetic factors have specific effects on cardiac morphogenesis, resulting in specific types of cardiovascular malformations."[20a] Multiple genes with additive effects may produce a discrete phenotypic trait once a

CV

genetic threshold has been attained. Polygenic inheritance helps to explain the spectrum of subclinical-to-severe malformations found in families of keeshond dogs with conotruncal septal defects and tetralogy of Fallot.[2a] Unfortunately, the absence of a simple mendelian mode of inheritance makes it difficult to counsel breeders about the breeding of individual dogs. Although there have been recent attempts to screen dogs for congenital heart disease before breeding, morphologic normalcy does not equal genetic normalcy. Even with careful attention to pedigree and results of breeding trials, it may be impossible to eliminate or markedly reduce the prevalence of cardiac defects until genetic testing for specific defects becomes a reality. The interested reader is referred to Patterson's studies for more detail.[1a–4a]

PREVALENCE OF CONGENITAL HEART DISEASE

Both prevalence and breed associations reported for congenital heart defects in the dog and cat exhibit national and regional variations.[1–6 2a, 12a, 14a, 36a] Most surveys have reported that PDA is the most common malformation in the dog, and either ASD or atrioventricular valve dysplasia is most common among cats; however, over the past 2 decades subaortic stenosis has gradually increased to become the most commonly diagnosed defect in dogs in many regions of the world. Hospital surveys of congenital heart defects in the United States have been reported by Patterson and Detweiler in dogs and by Liu and by Harpster in cats.[2a, 12a, 14a, 36a] In the largest survey of dogs from the 1960s, 325 malformations were detected in 290 dogs, and the overall prevalence in a university hospital population was 6.8 per 1000 dogs.[1a, 2a, 14a] The frequency of diagnoses was approximately 28 per cent for PDA, 20 per cent for pulmonic stenosis, 14 per cent for aortic stenosis, 8 per cent for persistent right aortic arch, 7 per cent for ventricular septal defect, and less than 5 per cent for tetralogy of Fallot, persistent left cranial vena cava, and atrial septal defects. In a 1989 survey of 339 cases of congenital cardiac defects in dogs in the United Kingdom, the most common diagnoses were subaortic stenosis (32 per cent), PDA (20 per cent), mitral valve dysplasia (14 per cent), pulmonic stenosis (12 per cent), and ventricular septal defect (8 per cent). A more recent report by Buchanan,[1 9b] which includes prevalence information from a North American database of over 1300 cases, indicates that PDA is still most frequently reported (31.7 per cent of cases), but that subaortic stenosis (22.1 per cent) now exceeds pulmonic stenosis (18.3 per cent) in prevalence. The overall prevalence of congenital heart disease in dogs has been reported to range from 0.46 to 0.85 per cent of hospital admissions.[9b]

Harpster's review[36a] of congenital heart disease in cats summarizes data from the literature, the Angell Memorial Animal Hospital (Boston), and the Animal Medical Center (New York City). The prevalence of congenital heart disease was between 2 and 10 cats per 1000 admissions (0.2 to 1 per cent) and included a total of 287 reported anomalies. The most common defects reported were ASD 24 per cent (including ventricular septal defect, atrial septal defect, and endocardial cushion defect), atrioventricular valve dysplasia 17 per cent, endocardial fibroelastosis 11.5 per cent, PDA 11 per cent, aortic stenosis 6 per cent, and tetralogy of Fallot 6 per cent of the reported diagnoses. Males were affected nearly twice as often as females in the series reported by Harpster.

Table 112–3 lists the reported common and uncommon

TABLE 112–3. CONGENITAL CARDIOVASCULAR DEFECTS IN THE DOG AND CAT

CANINE

Most Common Defects

Patent ductus arteriosus
Subaortic stenosis
Pulmonic stenosis
Tricuspid valve dysplasia
Mitral valve dysplasia
Ventricular septal defect
Tetralogy of Fallot
Persistent right aortic arch
Persistent left cranial vena cava
Peritoneopericardial diaphragmatic hernia

Uncommon Defects

Aortic hypoplasia/interruption
Aortic stenosis (valvular)
Aorticopulmonary window
Anomalous pulmonary venous return
Arteriovenous fistula
Atrial septal defect
Coarctation of the aorta
Cor triatriatum dexter
Double aortic arch
Double outlet right ventricle
Ebstein's anomaly of the tricuspid valve
Endocardial cushion defect
Endocardial fibroelastosis
Retroesophageal left subclavian artery
Situs inversus
Vascular anomalies
ECG conduction disorders
    Right bundle branch block
    Ventricular pre-excitation

FELINE

Most Common Defects

Atrioventricular (AV) septal defects
    Ventricular septal defect
    Atrial septal defect
    AV canal (endocardial cushion) defect
Tricuspid valve dysplasia
Mitral valve dysplasia
Patent ductus arteriosus
Aortic stenosis
Endocardial fibroelastosis
Tetralogy of Fallot
Pulmonic stenosis
Persistent right aortic arch
Peritoneopericardial diaphragmatic hernia

Uncommon Defects

Anomalous right atrium
Cor triatriatum
Double outlet right ventricle
Taussig-Bing complex
Truncus arteriosus
Vascular anomalies
    Anomaly of vena cava
    Pulmonary vein stenosis

congenital cardiac defects in dogs and cats. Table 112–1 summarizes the breed predispositions reported for dogs with congenital heart disease.

CLASSIFICATION OF CONGENITAL HEART DISEASE

Although a number of classification systems can be used to classify congenital heart defects, the following system emphasizes both the anatomy and physiology of the primary malformations.

Systemic to pulmonary shunting
Patent ductus arteriosus
Aorticopulmonary window (see Vascular Anomalies)
Atrial septal defect
Anomalous pulmonary venous return
Ventricular septal defect
Endocardial cushion defect/atrioventricular septal defect
Ventricular outflow obstruction
Pulmonic stenosis
Aortic stenosis
Coarctation and interruption of the aorta (see Vascular Lesions)
Malformations of atrioventricular valves
Dysplasia of the mitral valve
Dysplasia of the tricuspid valve
Cyanotic heart disease (pulmonary to systemic shunting)
Eisenmenger's syndrome (pulmonary hypertension with right-to-left shunting)
Tricuspid atresia/right ventricular hypoplasia
Tetralogy of Fallot
Double outlet right ventricle
Transposition of the great vessels
Miscellaneous cardiac defects
Endocardial fibroelastosis
Anomalous development of the atria: cor triatriatum
Multiple cardiac anomalies
Pericardial defect
Peritoneopericardial hernia
Vascular anomalies
Persistent right aortic arch
Other vascular ring anomalies
Coarctation of the aorta
Interruption of the aortic arch
Persistent left cranial vena cava
Other venous anomalies

This system emphasizes the pathophysiologic rather than the embryologic basis for maldevelopment and resulting clinical signs. Some lesions fit into more than one pathophysiologic category, and others are very rare or have been reported only in combination with other defects. The reader is encouraged to review the hemodynamic principles in the previous section on cardiac catheterization when considering individual defects.

CARDIAC MALFORMATIONS CAUSING SYSTEMIC TO PULMONARY (LEFT-TO-RIGHT) SHUNTING

PATENT DUCTUS ARTERIOSUS

The fetal ductus arteriosus is derived from the left sixth embryonic aortic arch. It connects the main pulmonary artery to the proximal descending aorta, allowing the shunting of fetal blood from the pulmonary artery to the systemic circulation.[37a–42a] This function diverts blood away from the nonfunctional fetal lung into the descending aorta and back toward the placenta where fetal oxygenation occurs. Following parturition and the onset of breathing, the rapid increase in arterial oxygen tension inhibits local prostaglandins and causes constriction of ductal smooth muscle and functional closure of the ductus. Anatomic obliteration occurs by necrosis and fibrosis during the first few weeks of life. The ductus may be probe-patent in pups less than 4 days of age, and it is usually closed securely by about 7 to 10 days after birth.[4a, 41a, 42a] Abnormal postnatal patency of the ductus (PDA) is

the first or second most commonly diagnosed congenital cardiac defect in the dog, in which it has been extensively studied.[37a–61a] It is much less common but well recognized in the cat.

Pathogenesis

Failure of ductal closure in dogs appears to be the result of histologic abnormalities within the ductal wall. The normal fetal ductal wall contains a loose branching pattern of circumferential smooth muscle throughout its length. In prenatal pups bred to have a high probability of PDA, varying portions of the ductal wall resemble the wall of the aorta, lacking constricting smooth muscle. According to the seminal work of Patterson and Buchanan et al,[4a] increasing genetic liability to PDA results in "extension of the non-contractile wall structure of the aorta to an increasing segment of the ductus arteriosus, progressively impairing its capacity to undergo physiologic closure." In its mildest form, the ductus closes at the pulmonary arterial end only, and there is a blind, funnel-shaped outpouching of the ventral aspect of the aorta, called a *ductus diverticulum*. This hidden form (*forme fruste*) of PDA can be diagnosed only by angiography or necropsy, but it indicates that the dog possesses genes for this defect.[4a, 39a–40a] Increasing genetic liability results in a moderate form, the typical tapering, funnel-shaped PDA (Fig. 112–3A and B) with left-to-right shunting. The most severe, but least common, form is the cylindrical, nontapering PDA with persistent, postnatal pulmonary hypertension (Eisenmenger's syndrome) and bidirectional or predominantly right-to-left shunting (Fig. 112–3C and D). Based on the breeding studies of poodle-type dogs by Patterson et al, the mode of transmission of PDA in dogs is polygenic.

Pathophysiology

In the typical left-to-right shunting PDA, aortic pressure is higher than pulmonary artery pressure throughout the cardiac cycle, and blood shunts continuously from the aorta to the pulmonary artery. This results in a continuous cardiac murmur, increased pulmonary flow, and volume overloading and diastolic dilatation of the left atrium and left ventricle. The left ventricle also undergoes eccentric hypertrophy and, in moderate-to-severe cases, increased left ventricular end-diastolic pressure. If the defect is wide enough to allow a large shunt and pulmonary vascular resistance remains low, the end result may be left ventricular failure with pulmonary edema. Left ventricular stroke volume is increased (Frank-Starling principle) and is reflected in an increased arterial systolic pressure. In addition, rapid run-off of blood from the aorta via the ductus causes a decreased aortic and arterial diastolic pressure. The wide arterial pulse pressure is felt as a bounding, hyperkinetic (waterhammer, Corrigan's) arterial pulse. Increased volume flow in the aortic arch and pulmonary artery causes dilatation of the aorta and main pulmonary artery. The right ventricle never handles the shunted blood and remains normal unless there are increases in pulmonary vascular resistance and pulmonary arterial pressure.

In a small percentage of cases, the lumen of the post-natal PDA remains cylindrical and wide enough to prevent the normal postnatal decline in pulmonary vascular resistance. In these cases, the aortic and pulmonary artery pressures are the same at systemic pressure levels, and the right ventricle remains concentrically hypertrophied after birth. In Patterson's colony of dogs, this type of ductus was the most severe, and the pattern of pulmonary hypertension and bidi-

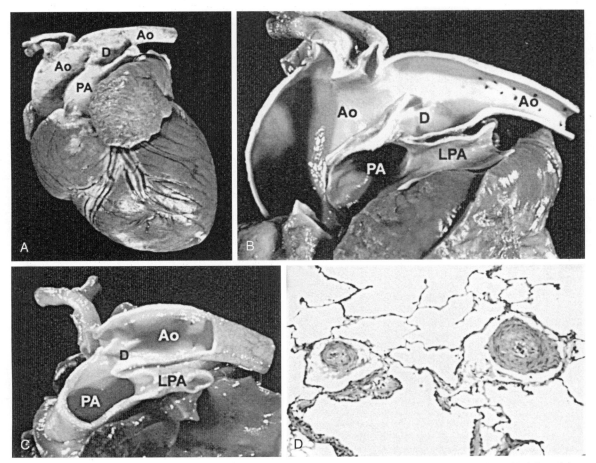

Figure 112–3. Pathology of patent ductus arteriosus (PDA). *A,* Left view of the heart from a young dog with left-to-right shunting PDA, showing the anatomic location of the ductus (D) between the aorta (Ao) and main pulmonary artery (PA). The left auricle appears enlarged. *B,* Cutaway view of the great vessels from the heart in *A.* The ductus (D) is funnel-shaped, with its narrowest orifice at the pulmonary arterial end, and the wall of the pulmonary artery (PA) is thinner than that of the adjacent aorta (Ao). LPA = left pulmonary artery. *C,* Cutaway view of the great vessels from a young dog with right-to-left shunting PDA. The ductus (D) is short, wide, and nontapering, and the thickness of the main PA is similar to that of the aorta (Ao). *D,* Histologic section of lung from a dog with right-to-left PDA and marked pulmonary hypertension. Two small PAs are visible, showing very narrow lumina and walls thickened by intimal proliferation and medial hypertrophy.

rectional or reversed (right-to-left) shunting developed within the first few weeks of life.[39a] This pattern also fits the clinical picture of most dogs with "reversed" PDA, in which there is usually no evidence of a continuous murmur or large left-to-right shunt earlier in life. Dogs and cats with reversed PDA exhibit diminished pulmonary flow, a comparatively small left ventricle, and marked hypertrophy of the right ventricle. The exact mechanism by which the pulmonary vascular resistance increases is not completely understood, but anatomic descriptions of the pulmonary microvasculature are similar for both humans and animals. Histologic changes within small pulmonary arteries include hypertrophy of the media, thickening of the intima and reduction of lumen dimensions, and plexiform lesions of the vessel wall (Fig. 112–3*D*).[60a, 61a] Most of these changes are considered to be irreversible.

Clinical Findings

The clinical features of PDA have been defined in both a breeding colony and in clinic populations.[10] [1a–4a, 37a–53a] Females developed PDA at a rate of 2.49 per 1000 versus 1.45 per 1000 for males.[2a] The chihuahua, collie, maltese, poodle, pomeranian, English springer spaniel, keeshond, bichon frisé, and Shetland sheepdog are most frequently affected,

although other breeds such as the Cavalier King Charles spaniel may also be predisposed (see Table 112–1). Many other breeds, including larger dogs such as German shepherds, Newfoundlands, and Labrador retrievers, may also be prone to PDA in some regions. Pups may appear thin or tachypneic from left heart failure. However, the majority of dogs and cats with PDA are reported to be asymptomatic and developing normally at the time of their initial recognition. Clinical signs rarely develop within the first week of life, and many diagnoses are made at the time of initial examination at 6 to 8 weeks of age or later.

Left-to-Right Shunting PDA

In all but the mildest cases with very small shunts, arterial pulses are hyperkinetic (bounding). Mucous membranes are pink in the absence of heart failure. The precordial impulse is often exaggerated and more diffuse than normal due to cardiac enlargement. A continuous thrill may be palpated at the heart base, and a continuous murmur is audible at the same point(s) (Fig. 112–4). The focus (point of maximal intensity [PMI]) of the murmur is the main pulmonary artery at the dorsal left base, and it may radiate cranially to the thoracic inlet and to the right base, where it is almost always softer.[5a, 39a, 47a] Often, only a systolic murmur is audible over

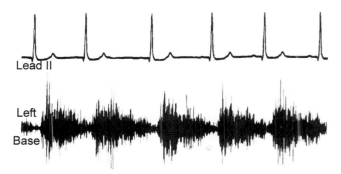

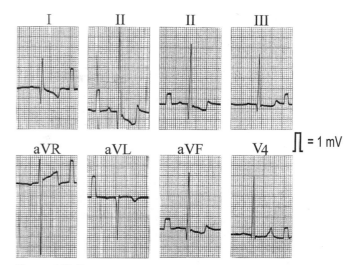

Figure 112–4. Phonocardiogram recorded at the left heart base from a dog with left-to-right patent ductus arteriosus. The lead II ECG is recorded simultaneously for timing purposes (ventricular mechanical systole is approximately the period from the middle of the QRS complex to the end of the T wave; the remainder of the time is diastole). The recorded murmur is continuous, increasing in intensity during systole, peaking near the end of systole, and decreasing in intensity during diastole.

Figure 112–5. Electrocardiogram from a dog with left-to-right patent ductus arteriosus. The mean QRS axis is normal (+80°), but the QRS voltage (amplitude) is increased in several leads, including leads II, III, aVF, and V_4, consistent with left ventricular enlargement. (The square waves in each lead are 1 mV standardization impulses). Paper speed = 50 mm/s.

the mitral area. This murmur may simply reflect the greater intensity and radiation of the systolic component of the continuous murmur, but the murmur may also be contributed to by secondary mitral regurgitation, which usually develops in cases with severe left ventricular dilatation. In the cat, the murmur may be heard best somewhat more caudoventrally than in the dog, even sounding shorter or holosystolic.

Noninvasive studies are usually diagnostic. Electrocardiography usually indicates left ventricular enlargement by a normal frontal plane QRS axis and increased R-wave voltages in craniocaudal leads II, III, and aV_F and in the left chest leads V_2 and V_4 (Fig. 112–5). Left atrial enlargement may also be indicated by widening of P waves. Radiography demonstrates cardiomegaly and pulmonary hypervascularity in proportion to the magnitude of the left-to-right shunt and left atrial and left ventricular enlargement (Fig. 112–6). On the dorsoventral view, there may be prominence to the left auricle and main pulmonary artery. The most specific finding is the appearance of an aortic bulge near the origin of the

ductus, which is caused by the widened aortic arch and abrupt tapering of the descending aorta just caudal to the ductus origin (Fig. 112–6B). In cats, the left apex may be displaced into the right hemithorax. The diagnosis can be proved by echocardiography in almost all cases. The 2D and M-mode studies demonstrate dilatation of the left atrium, left ventricle, aorta, and pulmonary artery (Fig. 112–7A to D).[11] The left ventricular shortening fraction is often in the "normal" range and not elevated in proportion to the degree of left ventricle dilatation. The ductus can be imaged from the left cranial position in most cases (Fig. 112–7D), and Doppler studies show the continuous retrograde ductal flow jet in the pulmonary artery (Fig. 112–7E and F). If the pulmonary artery pressure is near normal, the peak velocity

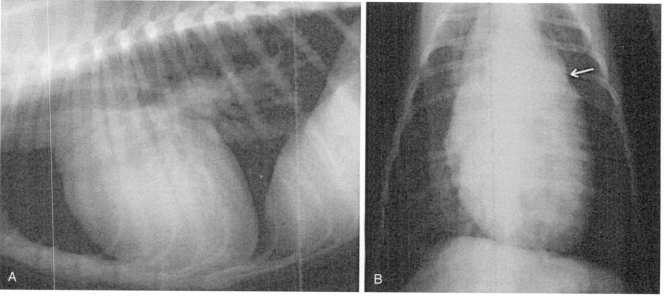

Figure 112–6. Thoracic radiographs from a dog with left-to-right PDA. A, Lateral view shows moderate cardiomegaly with prominence to the left atrium, pulmonary vasculature, and aortic arch. B, Dorsoventral view shows moderate cardiomegaly, a normal shape to the cardiac silhouette, prominence of the pulmonary vasculature (especially the arteries), and a lateral protrusion of the aorta (arrow) near the origin of the ductus.

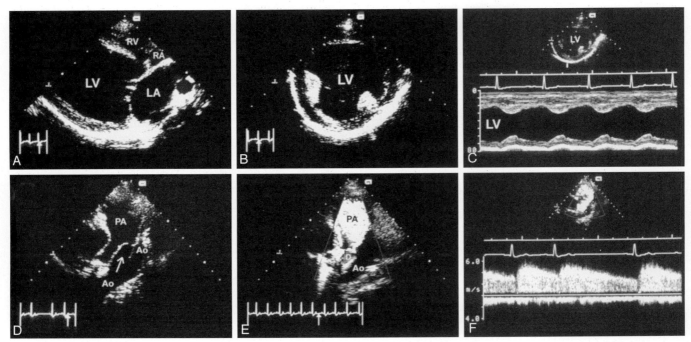

Figure 112–7. Echocardiography in left-to-right patent ductus arteriosus (PDA). *A,* The right long-axis view shows dilatation of the left atrium (LA) and left ventricle (LV). The right atrium (RA) and right ventricle (RV) are normal. *B,* The right short-axis view from the same dog shows dilatation of the left ventricle (LV). *C,* The M-mode tracing from the same dog shows dilatation of the left ventricle (LV) and increased septal motion consistent with LV volume overload. The LV shortening fraction is 34 per cent. *D,* Left cranial view of the ductus (D) between the aorta (Ao) and pulmonary artery (PA). *E,* View similar to *D.* The grey-scale depiction of a two-dimensional color Doppler image shows retrograde flow from the ductus (D) into the pulmonary artery (PA) during ventricular diastole. *F,* Continuous-wave Doppler recording of the PDA jet in the PA, obtained from the left heart base. There is continuous retrograde flow toward the transducer. The peak velocity (5.3 m/s) occurs near the end of ventricular systole.

of this jet is about 4.5 to 5.0 m/s. Other findings may include mildly increased left ventricle outflow velocity (1.8 to 2.3 m/s) and modest secondary mitral valve and pulmonary valve insufficiency.

Cardiac catheterization and angiocardiography are unnecessary to confirm a diagnosis of PDA unless the Doppler echocardiographic study is ambiguous or additional malformations are suspected.[12, 13] In dogs with PDA, associated cardiac defects are uncommon,[4a, 44a] and catheterization is not justified if noninvasive data support the diagnosis and indicate no complications. With large shunts, catheterization data may show elevated left ventricle diastolic, left atrial, pulmonary capillary wedge, and pulmonary artery pressures.[39a, 58a] The aortic pulse pressure is wide, and pulmonary artery and right ventricular pressures are normal to mildly elevated in cases uncomplicated by heart failure or pulmonary vascular disease (Fig. 112–8). Oxygen saturation in the pulmonary artery is higher than the right ventricle. When contrast material is injected into the left ventricle or ascending aorta, the PDA is seen, and both aorta and pulmonary artery are opacified (Fig. 112–9A and B). Modest mitral valve and pulmonary valve regurgitation may be present due to dilatation of the valve annuli.

PDA With Pulmonary Hypertension

When a PDA is complicated by high pulmonary vascular resistance and right-to-left shunting, a diagnosis of "reversed PDA" is made.[14, 5a, 8a, 9a, 39a, 46a, 59a-61a] Although unproven, there may be an increased incidence of this type of PDA in dogs living at altitudes above 5000 to 6000 feet.[16] Many owners do not recognize obvious clinical signs in their pet during the first 6 to 12 months of life. Because of the lack

of a loud heart murmur, cursory physical examination may not detect the more subtle signs of this defect (see below). Clinical signs invariably develop, although some animals are not diagnosed until 3 to 4 years of age or even later. The symptomatic patient may exhibit exertional fatigue and shortness of breath, hyperpnea, hind limb weakness or collapse, or seizures.

Clinical examination is very different from the more common left-to-right PDA. Physical examination reveals either no murmur or only a soft, early systolic murmur at the left heart base. The most common finding is an accentuated and split-second heart sound over the left heart base. Differential cyanosis (cyanosis of the caudal mucous membranes with pink cranial membranes) may be observed, but recognition may require examination after exercise. Differential cyanosis is caused by the location of the PDA, which shunts right-to-left from the pulmonary artery into the descending aorta (see Fig. 112–3C). Perfusion of the kidneys with hypoxemic blood leads to secondary polycythemia and hyperviscosity, with the PCV gradually increasing to 65 per cent or greater.[59a] Polycythemia may occur during the first year but often does not become severe until 18 to 24 months of age. The electrocardiogram shows changes of right ventricular hypertrophy (right axis deviation, $S_I S_{II} S_{III}$). Thoracic radiographs show right heart enlargement, dilatation of the main pulmonary artery, and variable appearance of the lobar and peripheral arteries. Echocardiography demonstrates right ventricular hypertrophy and a dilated main pulmonary artery, and the ductus may be imaged in some cases (Fig. 112–10A and B). The most sensitive way to demonstrate the right-to-left shunt is by means of contrast echocardiography. Injection of agitated saline into a cephalic or saphenous vein results in opacification of the right heart and pulmonary

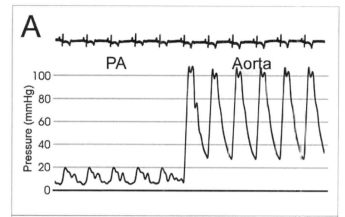

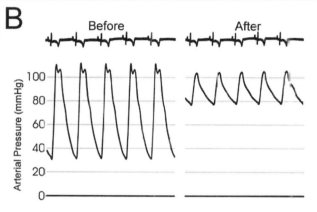

Figure 112–8. Vascular pressures from a dog with left-to-right patent ductus arteriosus (PDA). *A*, Pressure tracing obtained by retrograde catheterization of the PDA from the femoral artery. The pulmonary arterial (PA) pressure is normal. As the catheter is withdrawn into the ductus and aorta (Ao), the pressure increases abruptly. The aortic systolic pressure is normal, but the diastolic pressure is markedly reduced, resulting in a very wide arterial pulse pressure. *B*, The same aortic pressure recorded just before and immediately after closure of the PDA by coil occlusion. There is a marked increase in diastolic pressure and decreased width of the pulse pressure after occlusion.

artery and the descending aorta (best observed by abdominal imaging of the aorta dorsal to the bladder), but not the left heart or ascending aorta (Fig. 112–10C).

Cardiac catheterization shows pulmonary artery hypertension with elevation of right ventricular systolic pressure to equal left ventricular or aortic pressure. Right ventricular contrast injection demonstrates right ventricular hypertrophy and usually outlines a wide PDA that appears to continue distally as the descending aorta (Fig. 112–9C and D). The lobar pulmonary arteries may appear nearly normal, especially during the first year of life (Fig. 112–9C), or show increased tortuosity (Fig. 112–9D), and bronchoesophageal collateral vessels may be outlined.

Natural History of PDA

Eyster reported that approximately 64 per cent of dogs diagnosed with left-to-right shunting PDA will be dead from complications within 1 year of diagnosis without surgical correction.[53a] Complications include left heart failure with pulmonary edema, atrial fibrillation, mild pulmonary hypertension secondary to left heart failure, and mitral regurgitation secondary to left ventricular dilatation.[53a, 58a] Some dogs

and cats with PDA and modest shunts will survive to maturity, and a few may live to 10 years of age or greater.[10] In humans, gradual development of pulmonary hypertension and shunt reversal is a significant risk in uncorrected PDA. However, rapid or gradual development of pulmonary hypertension appears to be extremely rare in dogs and probably in cats with left-to-right PDA after 6 months of age.

When persistent pulmonary hypertension in the neonate leads to reversed shunting, congestive heart failure almost never develops. Clinical signs result from hypoxemia and polycythemia/hyperviscosity, and cardiac arrhythmias and sudden death may occur. Animals with reversed PDA often live at least 3 to 5 years, and a few survive beyond 7 years if the PCV is kept below 65 per cent.

Clinical Management

Surgical correction is recommended in all cases of left-to-right shunting PDA in animals younger than 2 years of age. When this condition is diagnosed in older pets, a cardiologist should be consulted. Recommended preoperative studies include an ECG and chest radiographs to help assess the severity of the shunt and resulting cardiomegaly and echocardiography to verify the diagnosis and rule out additional defects. The timing of surgery is debatable, but the authors usually recommend PDA correction at an early age or as soon as the diagnosis is made, especially if cardiac failure is imminent. If congestive heart failure has developed, the patient is treated medically for heart failure (furosemide, digoxin, etc.) before surgery. Treatment with prostaglandin inhibitors such as indomethacin, often used in premature human infants to assist closure of a structurally normal but functionally immature PDA, has been unsuccessful in dogs and cats, most likely because of the histologic nature of the lesion (absence of smooth muscle in the ductal wall).

Two approaches to PDA correction are currently available. For many years, left thoracotomy and PDA ligation has been the recommended surgical treatment.[15] This technique and its results have been described in detail in several reports, indicating a high surgical success rate and excellent prognosis after successful surgery.[48a–54a, 10b–12b] Surgical mortality should be less than 3 per cent in uncomplicated cases.[53a, 10b–12b] Postoperative ductal recanalization has been reported but is very uncommon, occurring in less than 2 per cent of cases, most commonly associated with infection.[16] Postoperative fever and pulmonary infiltrates may indicate infection at the surgical site and hematogenous pneumonia.[57a] Depending on the animal's age and severity of cardiomegaly, most pets become clinically normal following surgery, and overall cardiac size decreases toward normal, although the heart and great vessels often continue to be misshapen in outline.[44a] A soft, left apical systolic murmur, usually from residual secondary mitral regurgitation, is often heard for a variable period after ductus ligation.[47a] Left ventricular systolic function, as assessed echocardiographically by left ventricle shortening fraction and left ventricle end-systolic volume, appears to decline sharply immediately after surgery, indicative of secondary myocardial failure from volume overload. When atrial fibrillation or advanced congestive heart failure are present, the anesthetic and operative risks are high, and the postoperative prognosis is much more guarded. Postoperative Doppler examination may indicate a small residual shunt, although the continuous murmur is usually absent, and the clinical outcomes are good. The owner should be informed of the suspected heritable nature

CV

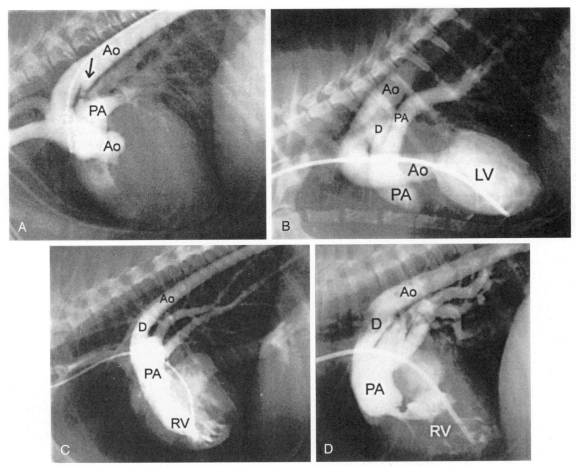

Figure 112–9. Angiographic diagnosis of patent ductus arteriosus (PDA). *A,* Aortic root injection from a dog with small left-to-right PDA. The contrast outlines the aortic arch (Ao), a thin conical PDA (arrow), and part of the main pulmonary artery (PA). *B,* Left ventricular injection from a cat with large left-to-right PDA. Contrast outlines the dilated left ventricle (LV), aortic arch (Ao), wide conical ductus (D), and pulmonary artery (PA). *C,* Right ventricular injection from a dog with a reversed (right-to-left) PDA. Contrast outlines the right ventricle (RV); PA and its main branches; the wide, cylindrical PDA (D), and the descending aorta (Ao). *D,* Right ventricular injection from another dog with right-to-left PDA. Contrast outlines the hypertrophied RV, the main PA and its tortuous branches, the wide PDA (D), and the descending aorta (Ao). The appearance of narrowing of the RV outflow region below the pulmonary valve is caused by the excessive ventricular hypertrophy.

of the defect and that the animal should not be used for breeding.

Within the past few years, less invasive minor surgical alternative techniques for PDA occlusion have been reported in dogs.[17–21] Development of thin metal coils imbedded with thrombogenic dacron strands, which can be delivered through relatively small catheters, has made coil embolization of PDA possible in small animals. Although details of the technique continue to evolve, one or more coils are delivered to the ductus through a catheter via the femoral artery or other peripheral vessel. The coil(s) lies in the funnel-shaped ductus and stimulate thrombosis, which occludes the PDA. Following PDA coil embolization, chest radiographs show the coil(s) at the site of the ductus (Fig. 112–11). The advantages of PDA coil embolization over thoracotomy and ligation include lower morbidity and mortality rates, shorter hospitalization, and faster recovery. To date, the success rate of this technique has been good, and the major complication rate has been low, consisting mainly of pulmonary embolization of a coil.[17–21] Further study will define the limitations of and contraindications to coil embolization as well as refine the technique to maximize success rate and minimize complications.

Animals with *reversed PDA* have irreversible obstructive pulmonary vascular disease. Ligation of the PDA is strongly contraindicated as it invariably leads to late operative or early postoperative acute right heart failure and death. Management of these patients consists of limitation of exercise, avoidance of stress, and maintenance of the PCV between 58 and 65 per cent by periodic phlebotomy.[22] In four dogs, periodic phlebotomy without intravenous fluid replacement was subjectively associated with clinical improvement and few or no adverse effects.[22a] Bleeding should be performed cautiously to avoid weakness or collapse, and intravascular volume may be supported during phlebotomy by infusing crystalloid solutions, if needed. Attempts to reduce the red blood cell volume of reversed PDA cases using drug therapy (e.g., hydroxyurea) have not been reported.

ATRIAL AND VENTRICULAR SEPTAL DEFECTS

During cardiac embryonic development, the atria and ventricles begin as a common chamber. The heart becomes partitioned into the normal four-chambered heart by growth of cardiac septa.[15a] The atria are partitioned by a wall formed mainly from two septa: the septum primum, which forms first, and the septum secundum, which develops to the right of the septum primum. The foramen ovale, a slit-like passageway that persists between these septa, permits right-

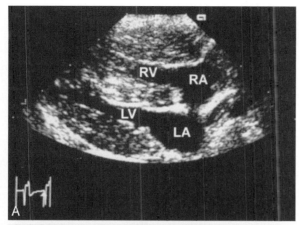

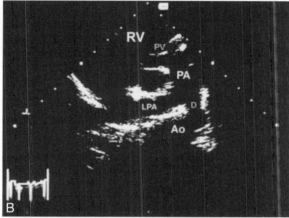

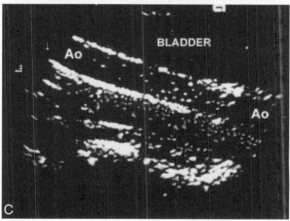

Figure 112–10. Echocardiography in reversed (right-to-left) patent ductus arteriosus (PDA) in the dog. *A,* The right long-axis view shows marked concentric hypertrophy of the right ventricle (RV). *B,* The left base short-axis view shows wide, nontapering PDA (D) between the main pulmonary artery (PA) and descending aorta (Ao). RV = right ventricle; PV = pulmonary valve; LPA = left pulmonary artery. *C,* Image of the abdominal aorta (Ao) dorsal to the bladder following cephalic vein injection of agitated saline. Microbubbles are seen as bright white dots in the aorta, confirming the presence of a right-to-left shunt.

to-left atrial shunting in the fetus but functionally and anatomically closes in the neonate when left atrial pressure rises. Most of the ventricular septum forms by inward growth from the ventricular walls. The area of atrioventricular confluence, including the upper ventricular septum, lower atrial septum, and atrioventricular valves, is formed primarily by growth and differentiation of the endocardial cushions. Defects in the development of the embryonic ventricular septum, the primum or secundum atrial septa, or the endocardial cushions may result in postnatal atrial and/or ventricular

septal defects. Congenital septal defects are common in both dogs and cats as isolated lesions and as components of more complex combination lesions such as tetralogy of Fallot.[4a–13a, 62a–79a]

Pathogenesis

Except for the proven genetic basis of ventricular septal defect in keeshond dogs with conotruncal malformation,[124a] there are no data on the cause(s) of spontaneous septal defects in dogs or cats.[-a] ASDs are usually classified based on the region of the malformation.[15a, 16a] Defects at or near the foramen ovale are called ostium (or septum) secundum defects, and defects of the lower atrial septum are called ostium primum defects (Fig. 112–12). Rare sinus venosus atrial septal defects are found dorsocranial to the fossa ovalis near the entrance of the cranial vena cava.[13a, 62a–67a] Because the endocardial cushions are responsible for partitioning the lowermost atrial septum and because they also contribute to the development of the atrioventricular (AV) valves, septum primum defects found in association with AV valve malformations are often referred to as "endocardial cushion defects." A defect in this area may include anomalous development of the atrioventricular valves and a "cleft" in the septal leaflet of the mitral valve (see Fig. 112–12). A complete endocardial cushion defect is a large defect of the lower atrial septum and upper ventricular septum with fusion of the septal leaflets of both AV valves. This malformation is sometimes referred to as a (complete or incomplete) AV canal defect, since the embryonic atrioventricular canal area never partitions and there is communication between all four cardiac chambers. Patent foramen ovale is not a true ASD inasmuch as the atrial septum forms normally but the walls of the foramen may be pushed apart, usually by conditions which increase right atrial pressure.[62a] A patent foramen ovale achieves clinical significance when it allows right-to-left shunting, as may occur with severe pulmonic stenosis or tricuspid valve dysplasia.

Most ventricular septal defects (VSD) are located in the upper ventricular septum (Fig. 112–13).[68a] Muscular apical or midventricular septal defects are uncommon in small animals. On the left side, the typical location of a VSD is just below the aortic valve, most often centered between the right coronary and noncoronary cusps. On the right side, the opening is often described by its position relative to the crista supraventricularis muscular ridge.[15a] An infracristal (subcristal) VSD is located proximal to the crista supraventricularis near the cranial aspect of the septal leaflet of the tricuspid valve, which may partially cover it. A supracristal VSD is located distal to the crista supraventricularis just below the pulmonic valve. Large defects may obliterate the crista and are usually associated with additional defects, as in tetralogy of Fallot (see Fig. 112–13).[2a, 4a] The right side of the root of the aorta, including the right coronary and noncoronary cusps, may be displaced to the right so that the aorta straddles the defect. The altered geometry of the aortic root that accompanies many VSDs often results in aortic valve regurgitation.

Pathophysiology

The magnitude and direction of blood shunting across septal defects are affected by the size of the orifice, the pressure difference across the defect, and/or the relative resistances in the systemic and pulmonary circulations.[15a, 62a, 68a, 72a, 73a] Shunting across small (restrictive) defects depends primarily on the pressure difference, whereas shunting across

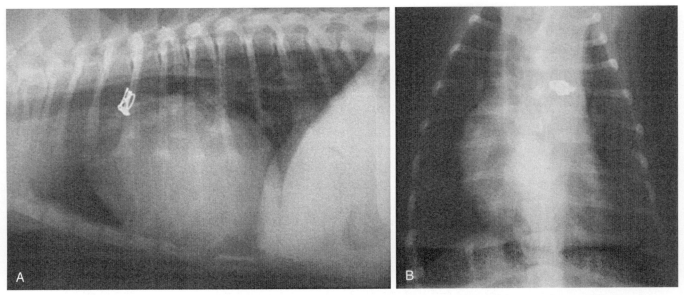

Figure 112–11. Lateral (A) and dorsoventral (B) thoracic radiographs from a dog with left-to-right patent ductus arteriosus (PDA) following closure of the defect by coil embolization. Two metallic coils are lodged in the PDA at the base of the heart. The coils were delivered to the site through a femoral artery catheter.

large (nonrestrictive) defects depends primarily on relative resistance. When left and right heart pressures and arterial resistances are near normal, the direction of shunting is left-to-right, and all of the cardiac chambers and vessels that handle the shunted blood dilate and enlarge. If pressure on the right side of the defect is increased by complications or additional defects, left-to-right shunting decreases and, ultimately, right-to-left shunting may develop. The most common conditions that complicate septal defects and result in reversed shunting are pulmonic stenosis, tricuspid regurgitation, and pulmonary hypertension.

Atrial Septal Defect

When an ASD is present, flow across the defect occurs primarily during diastole, the pressure difference across the defect is low, and the resulting shunt is determined mainly by the relative diastolic resistance to inflow for each ventricle.[15a, 65a] Normally, the right ventricle is thinner and more compliant than the left, and blood preferentially shunts left to right into the right atrium and ventricle. The result is volume overload of the right atrium, right ventricle, pulmonary artery, and pulmonary veins. The left atrium receives the shunted blood, but most of the increased pulmonary venous return is shunted immediately into the right atrium, resulting in minimal left atrial dilatation. If significant left atrial enlargement is observed in an animal with an ASD, an additional defect, such as an endocardial cushion defect with mitral regurgitation, should be suspected.

Left-to-right shunting increases oxygen saturation in the right atrium, right ventricle, and pulmonary artery. The shunt flow across an ASD does not generate a heart murmur (because of the very low pressure gradient between the atria); the increased flow volume and velocity across the tricuspid and pulmonic valves, which can be measured by Doppler echocardiography, can cause murmurs of relative pulmonic stenosis (common) or tricuspid stenosis (rare). In addition, delayed closure of the pulmonic valve (and early closure of the aortic valve) causes splitting of the second heart sound.[62a, 63a] Because the volume overload affects the right ventricle and not the left, right heart failure occurs in

severe cases. Complete endocardial cushion (AV canal) defects may cause left-sided or bilateral congestive heart failure.

Ventricular Septal Defect

When a VSD is present, flow across the defect occurs primarily during ventricular systole. As with ASDs, the magnitude of left-to-right shunting with small (restrictive) defects is mainly determined by the diameter of the defect and the systolic pressure difference (gradient) between the ventricles. Since the normal left ventricle systolic pressure is four to five times that of the right ventricle, a left-to-right shunt occurs, and oxygen saturation in the right ventricular outflow tract and pulmonary artery is higher than in the right atrium. The peak pressure difference across the defect can be measured by catheters inserted into each ventricle, or it may be estimated noninvasively by Doppler echocardiography. Using the peak flow velocity (m/s) in the jet passing through the defect, the pressure gradient is calculated using the simplified Bernoulli equation ($\Delta P = 4V^2$). A restrictive defect with normal right ventricle pressure is expected to have a peak jet velocity of ≥ 4.5 m/s, corresponding to a peak pressure gradient across the defect of ≥ 80 mmHg. If the peak velocity is lower than predicted, right ventricle systolic pressure is increased, usually due to the presence of pulmonic stenosis or increased pulmonary vascular resistance (pulmonary hypertension).

Because most of the VSD shunt flow occurs during ventricular systole, flow across restrictive defects in the upper septum is pumped mainly into the right ventricular outflow tract and directly into the pulmonary artery, with only limited volume going into the body of the right ventricle.[72a, 73a] As a result, the pulmonary vasculature, left atrium, and left ventricle become volume overloaded, while the right ventricle may be only mildly affected, unless the defect and shunt are relatively large. Large shunts (e.g., greater than 3:1 pulmonary-to-systemic flow ratio) may overload the left and/or right heart enough to increase ventricular diastolic pressure and cause signs of left, right, or biventricular failure.

The degree of right ventricular dilatation and hypertrophy depends on the diameter of the VSD, the state of the pul-

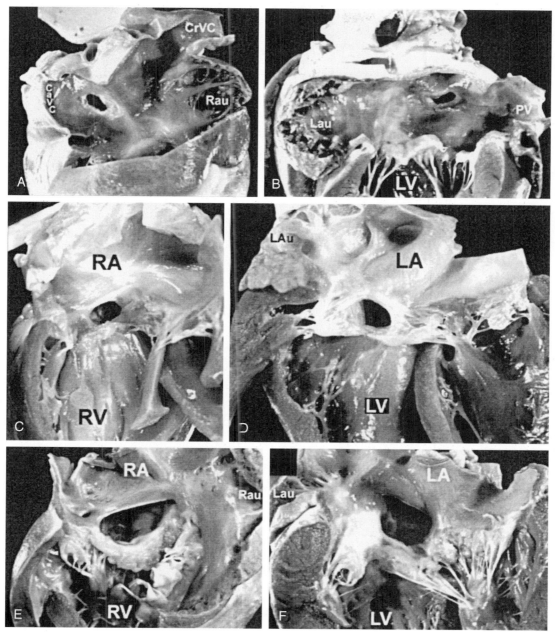

Figure 112–12. Pathology of atrial septal defect (ASD). *A* and *B*, Small septum secundum ASD in an 18-year-old dachshund, viewed from the right atrium and left atrium, respectively. The defect is located at the site of the fetal foramen ovale. It was an incidental finding at autopsy. Note the severe degenerative mitral valve disease and ruptured chorda tendineae in *B*. *C* and *D*, Septum primum ASD (partial AV canal defect) in a young Abyssinian cat, viewed from the right atrium and left atrium, respectively. In the right atrium, the defect is located just above the septal leaflet of the tricuspid valve. In the left atrium, the defect extends ventrally into the upper ventricular septum and has split the septal leaflet of the mitral valve into two parts. *E* and *F*, Large septum primum ASD in a 12-year-old Brittany spaniel dog, viewed from the right atrium and left atrium, respectively. In the right atrium, the defect is located in the lower septum just above the septal leaflet of the tricuspid valve. In the left atrium, the defect is located just above the mitral valve. The middle of the septal leaflet of the mitral valve has a prominent cleft and is affixed to the septum beneath it, but the defect does not extend ventrally into the ventricular septum. The dog also has moderately severe degenerative mitral and tricuspid valve disease. LA = left atrium; Lau = left auricle; LV = left ventricle; RA = right atrium; Rau = right auricle; RV = right ventricle; CaVC = caudal vena cava; CrVC = cranial vena cava; PV = pulmonary vein.

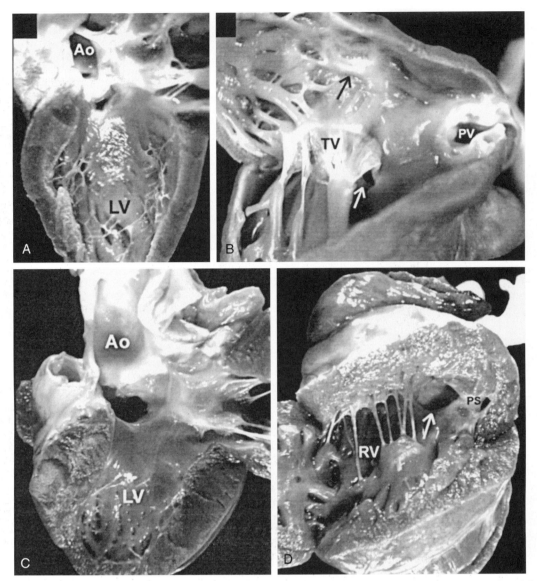

Figure 112–13. Pathology of ventricular septal defect (VSD). *A* and *B,* Small, restrictive VSD in a young cat, viewed from the left ventricle and right ventricle, respectively. In the left ventricle, the defect is located in the upper septum just beneath the aortic valve. In the right ventricle, the defect is located near the cranial part of the septal leaflet of the tricuspid valve (white arrow). The pale area of endocardial fibrosis on the right ventricular lateral wall (black arrow) is a jet lesion from the high-velocity VSD jet. *C* and *D,* Large, unrestricted VSD in a young dog with tetralogy of Fallot, viewed from the left ventricle and right ventricle, respectively. In the left ventricle, the defect is located just below the aortic valve, which is partially obscured by the rightward displacement of the root of the aorta toward the right ventricle. In the right ventricle, the large defect is located just cranial to the tricuspid valve (arrow). The right ventricle (RV) is markedly thickened, and there is a narrow fibrous ring of subvalvular pulmonic stenosis (PS) in the area where the pulmonic valve should be seen. Ao = aorta; LV = left ventricle; PV = pulmonic valve; TV = tricuspid valve.

monic valve, and the pulmonary vascular resistance. Very large, nonrestrictive VSDs cause the pressures in both ventricles to equalize and the two ventricles to behave as a common chamber. The ratio of blood ejected into the aorta versus into the pulmonary artery becomes inversely proportional to the ratio of left ventricle versus right ventricle outflow resistance. If the pulmonary valve and the pulmonary vascular resistance are normal, a very large left-to-right shunt will occur, and left heart failure may develop. If pulmonic stenosis or increased pulmonary vascular resistance are present, left-to-right shunting is proportionally decreased, and bidirectional or mainly right-to-left shunting may occur.

Eisenmenger's Syndrome

As with PDA, a newborn animal with a large VSD may maintain or develop high pulmonary vascular resistance and

pulmonary hypertension.[13b, 14b] Because of the size of the defect, right ventricular systolic and diastolic pressures equilibrate at systemic (left ventricle) levels, and bidirectional or reversed shunting may occur. Pulmonary hypertension associated with a shunting cardiac defect is known as Eisenmenger's physiology or syndrome. When the defect is a VSD, it is known as Eisenmenger's complex. The high pulmonary vascular resistance is caused by proliferative changes in the pulmonary arteries similar to those mentioned in the section on reversed PDA. As with PDA, the altered physiology and shunt reversal with VSD usually become established shortly after birth. Although humans with uncorrected left-to-right shunts may develop gradual pulmonary vascular disease and progressive pulmonary hypertension over several to many years, similar cases in dogs and cats with typical left-to-right shunting ASD or VSD appear to be very rare. Eisenmenger's syndrome is a permanent condition

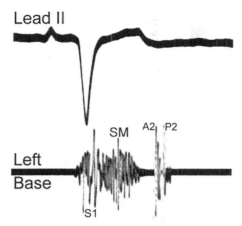

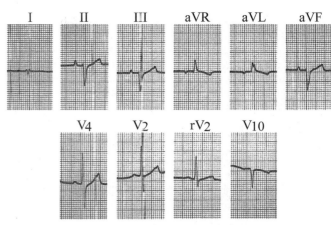

Figure 112–14. Phonocardiogram recorded at the left heart base from a dog with a primum atrial septal defect (ASD). The lead II ECG has a negative, slightly prolonged QRS complex indicative of a right ventricular conduction disorder (partial or incomplete right bundle branch block). The phonocardiogram shows a systolic ejection murmur (SM) that ends well before the second heart sound, which is widely split. S1 = first heart sound; A2 = aortic component of the second heart sound; P2 = pulmonic component of the second heart sound.

Figure 112–15. Electrocardiogram from a dog with a primum atrial septal defect. The QRS axis is shifted to the right and cranially (+265°), and the last two-thirds of the complex is prolonged, as shown by widened and notched S waves in leads III and aVF. There is also a prominent S wave in lead V$_4$. These changes are consistent with a right ventricular conduction disorder that is often referred to as partial or incomplete right bundle branch block. Paper speed = 50 mm/s, 10 mm = 1 mV.

caused by irreversible obliterative pulmonary arterial disorder. Afflicted animals become hypoxemic and cyanotic, especially with exertion, and eventually develop polycythemia and hyperviscosity.

Clinical Findings

Breed predispositions for atrial and ventricular septal defects are indicated in Table 112–1. Clinical findings of the typical left-to-right ASD include a grade 2–3/6 systolic ejection murmur over the left heart base and splitting of the second heart sound (Fig. 112–14).[23–25] The murmur is often misinterpreted initially as pulmonic stenosis. A low-pitched, right-sided diastolic murmur of relative tricuspid stenosis may occur, but it is usually not audible, especially in smaller patients. Cyanosis is rare unless there is an additional defect such as pulmonic stenosis or tricuspid valve dysplasia[15b] or

a complication such as pulmonary hypertension.[26] Heart failure may develop in advanced cases. Differential diagnosis includes anomalous pulmonary venous return, an extremely rate anomaly in dogs and cats.[80a]

The main cardiac structural change caused by an ASD is volume overload and dilatation of the right atrium and ventricle. The ECG may suggest right ventricular enlargement, but intraventricular conduction disturbances, especially partial or complete right bundle branch block (Fig. 112–15), are also common, especially with primum atrial or atrioventricular septal defects.[4a, 64a, 66a] Thoracic radiographs show cardiomegaly, enlargement of the right heart and main pulmonary artery, and pulmonary hypervascularity proportional to the magnitude of the shunt (Fig. 112–16). The left atrium is usually minimally enlarged unless there is also mitral regurgitation from a cleft mitral valve. Echocardiography usually allows direct imaging of the atrial defect, and Doppler exam-

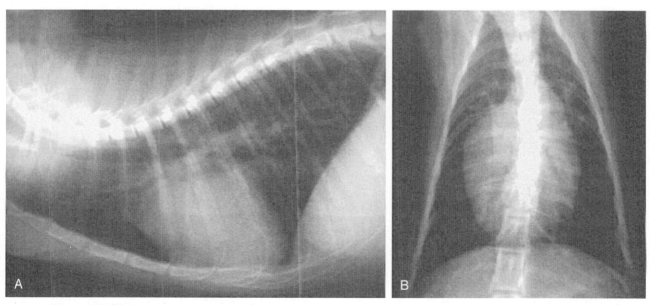

Figure 112–16. Lateral (A) and dorsoventral (B) thoracic radiographs from a 9-month-old cat with a large primum atrial septal defect. The cardiac silhouette is moderately enlarged, and the enlargement appears to be bilateral. The left atrium is moderately enlarged, and the pulmonary vasculature is prominent.

ination shows laminar or mildly turbulent diastolic flow through the ASD (Fig. 112–17), increased right ventricle outflow and pulmonary artery velocity, and associated problems such as mitral regurgitation.[16b] Contrast echocardiography may also be useful in some cases to demonstrate right-to-left passage of bubbles through the defect when an ASD is complicated and right atrial pressure is increased.

Cardiac catheterization of animals with ASD may be used to evaluate the magnitude of a left-to-right shunt as well as to document complications. Using oximetry and sampling from the venae cavae, cardiac chambers, and great vessels, the step-up in oxygen saturation in the right ventricle can be detected, and the magnitude of systemic-to-pulmonary shunting can be estimated (subject to the limitations discussed earlier for cardiac catheterization).[9] If congestive heart failure is present or imminent, central venous and right ventricular diastolic pressures will be elevated. Increased systolic flow across the pulmonic valve may result in "relative" pulmonic stenosis, identified by a mild systolic pressure gradient (5 and 15 mmHg) between the right ventricle and pulmonary artery.[63a] Although echocardiography is superior for imaging ASDs, angiocardiography may also be used. Contrast injection into the pulmonary artery will outline left-to-right shunting defects during the left-sided phase of the study. Following pulmonary venous return, the atrial septum can usually be seen between the left atrium and aorta on the lateral projection. Passage of dye from the left atrium into the right atrium and vena cavae confirms the presence

of the defect. In addition, a catheter can often be passed from the right atrium through the defect into the left atrium for confirmation. With more extensive endocardial cushion (AV canal) defects, a left ventriculogram may outline a VSD, mitral regurgitation, and occasionally left ventricular to right atrial shunting.

The clinical features of a VSD also depend on the magnitude of the shunt and presence of complications or other defects. In a typical small, infracristal VSD, a harsh, holosystolic murmur is heard best over the right mid- to cranial precordium.[23, 27, 28 [5a–10a, 68a]] In rare cases of supracristal VSD, the defect opens just under the pulmonic valve, and the systolic murmur may be best heard at the left base. Splitting of the second heart sound may occur but is often not recognized because of the inclusion of S_2 in the end of the murmur. If distortion of the aortic root causes significant aortic regurgitation, a blowing, decrescendo diastolic murmur will be audible over the left ventricular outflow area. Occasionally, the aortic regurgitation flows into the right ventricle, and the diastolic murmur may be heard on the right side.[17b] Mitral regurgitation may also occur if the defect is part of a more extensive endocardial cushion defect.

As with ASD, electrocardiography in animals with VSD is also variable. With moderate or large left-to-right shunts there may be changes of left atrial or left ventricular enlargement, and right ventricular conduction defects may also occur. The frontal plane leads may demonstrate a subtle

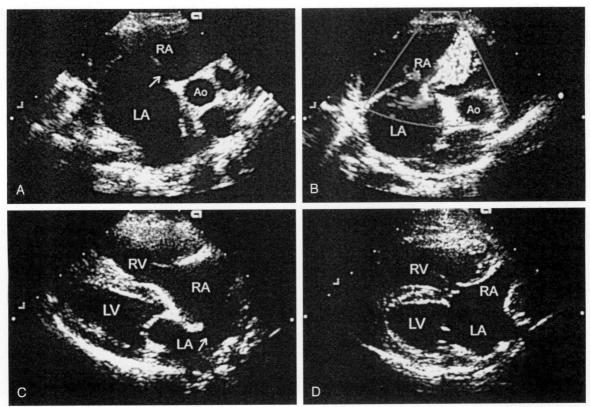

Figure 112–17. Echocardiography of atrial septal defect (ASD). *A,* Right short-axis view from a 3-year-old cat with other defects shows dilatation of both the left atrium (LA) and right atrium (RA). There is a small defect in the atrial septum (arrow). In this view, it is difficult to distinguish the ASD from simple echo dropout because of beam alignment. *B,* View similar to A from the same cat. The grey-scale depiction of a two-dimensional color Doppler image shows a flow jet from the LA into the right atrium RA during ventricular diastole. *C,* Right long-axis view from an 18-month-old miniature pinscher dog. The RA and right ventricle (RV) are both dilated. There is a moderately large secundum defect in the upper portion of the atrial septum (arrow). *D,* Right long-axis view from a 6-year-old cat. The RV is markedly dilated. There is a very large ASD involving most of the atrial septum, giving the appearance of a single large atrial chamber. Ao = aorta; LA = left atrium; LV = left ventricle.

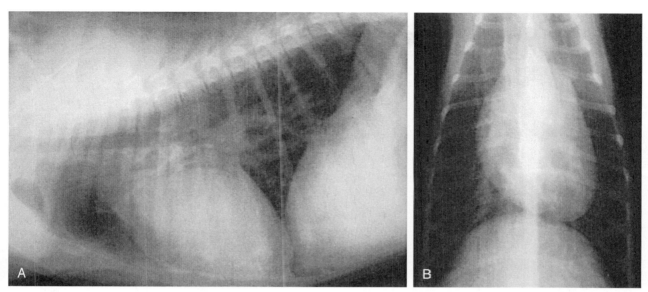

Figure 112–18. Lateral *(A)* and dorsoventral *(B)* thoracic radiographs from a 1-year-old Siberian husky dog with a small ventricular septal defect and a small left-to-right shunt. The cardiac silhouette is only very mildly enlarged. The left atrium is slightly enlarged on the lateral view, and the pulmonary vasculature is mildly prominent in both views.

abnormality in early ventricular septal activation, characterized by a Q-wave that is wide or contains high-frequency notching.[69a] Right axis deviation and a narrow QRS complex in a dog with VSD usually indicate right ventricular hypertrophy and a more complex lesion, such as VSD with pulmonic stenosis or pulmonary hypertension. Thoracic radiographs are very useful in assessing the magnitude of the shunt. In animals with very small defects, radiographs may appear entirely normal. In most uncomplicated left-to-right VSDs, however, pulmonary hypervascularity and left atrial and left ventricular enlargement are observed in proportion to the shunt magnitude (Figs. 112–18 and 112–19).[21a–24a] With larger defects and shunts, the right ventricle may also enlarge. The main, lobar, and peripheral pulmonary arteries are usually prominent. Cases of VSD complicated by pul-

monic stenosis or pulmonary hypertension may have hypovascular lungs with small peripheral pulmonary vasculature despite the prominence of the main pulmonary artery. 2D echocardiography usually identifies all but the smallest VSDs, although confirmation of patency of the defect may require Doppler study (Figs. 112–20 and 112–21). Color 2D Doppler imaging allows identification of jets through uncomplicated VSDs in almost every case (Fig. 112–20B). Spectral Doppler studies can also localize and quantify the high-velocity jet through a small, restrictive VSD. As explained previously, the peak pressure gradient across the defect can be measured from the peak jet velocity using the formula $\Delta P = 4V^2$ (Fig. 112–20C). From this value and an estimate of LV systolic pressure (100 to 120 mmHg), peak right ventricle systolic pressure can be estimated. Contrast

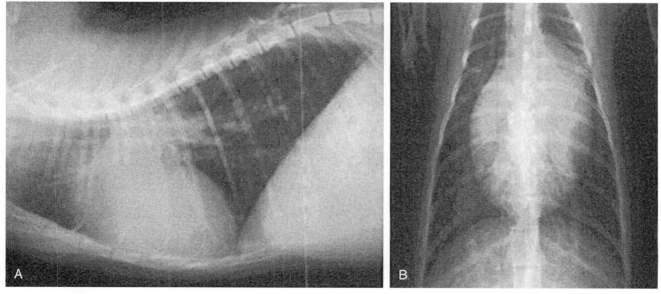

Figure 112–19. Lateral *(A)* and dorsoventral *(B)* radiographs from an 18-month-old domestic cat with a ventricular septal defect and a large left-to-right shunt. The cardiac silhouette is markedly enlarged, and the enlargement appears to be bilateral. There is moderate enlargement of the left atrium (lateral) and marked enlargement of the main pulmonary artery (DV), and the pulmonary vasculature is prominent in both views.

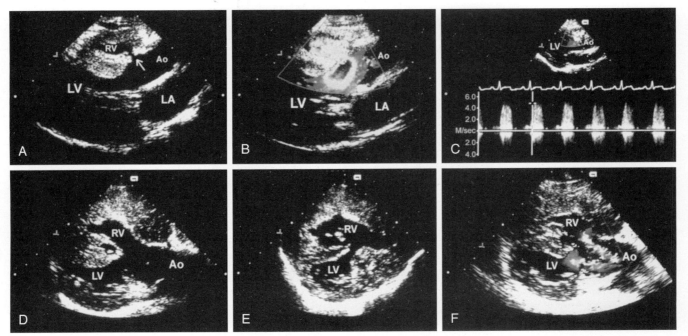

Figure 112–20. Echocardiography of ventricular septal defect (VSD). *A* to *C,* 6-month-old husky dog with a small VSD. *A,* Right long-axis view shows a small defect (arrow) in the upper ventricular septum just below the root of the aorta (Ao). *B,* The grey-scale depiction of a two-dimensional color Doppler image shows a flow jet from the left ventricular (LV) outflow tract into the right ventricle (RV) during ventricular systole. *C,* Continuous-wave Doppler recording of the VSD jet in the pulmonary artery, obtained from the same view as in *A* and *B.* The jet is oriented toward the transducer, and the peak systolic velocity is 4.8 m/s (calculated peak pressure gradient 92 mmHg). *D* to *F,* 2-year-old Rottweiler dog with a large VSD as part of tetralogy of Fallot. *D,* Right long-axis view shows marked thickening of the RV, a large septal defect between the upper portions of the ventricles, and displacement of the aortic root toward the RV (overriding aorta). *E,* Right short-axis view shows severe RV hypertrophy and a portion of the septal defect. *F,* The grey-scale depiction of a two-dimensional color Doppler image shows simultaneous laminar flow from both ventricles into the aorta during ventricular systole. LA = left atrium.

echocardiography may also be used to identify flow through the defect, but it is clearly inferior to Doppler imaging for this purpose.

Cardiac catheterization and angiocardiography in animals with VSD allow identification of the anatomic defects and estimation of the degree of shunting.[27] [65a] Oximetry demonstrating an oxygen step-up is recorded in the right ventricular outflow tract and pulmonary artery. With small defects, all intracardiac pressures may be normal. With larger shunts and ventricular volume overload, end-diastolic ventricular pressure becomes elevated. As with ASD, a mild systolic pressure gradient of 5 to 15 mmHg, indicating relative pulmonic stenosis, may be measured in some animals with a left-to-right shunting VSD. If the defect is complicated by pulmonary hypertension or pulmonic stenosis, increased right ventricle systolic pressure will be found, and right-to-left shunting may be present in the most severe cases. In uncomplicated VSD, a left ventricular angiocardiogram outlines the defect and shunt and may also demonstrate any geometric alterations of the great vessels, especially the aortic root (Fig. 112–22). Aortic root contrast injection can also be used to demonstrate the presence of aortic regurgitation.[17b]

Natural History

The longevity and quality of life of dogs and cats with atrioventricular septal defects depend on the defect size and magnitude of any shunt and the presence of complications or additional lesions. Animals with uncomplicated small defects and modest shunts may live a normal lifespan without ever developing recognizable clinical signs. Although spontaneous closure of small VSDs often occurs in humans and has been reported in dogs,[71a] the authors' experience is that this is very rare in dogs and cats. Larger defects and shunts with moderate or severe cardiomegaly may eventually lead to congestive heart failure. In addition, complication by moderate or severe aortic regurgitation may substantially shorten survival.[17b] It may initially be difficult to predict the prognosis of a very young animal with a septal defect and modest cardiomegaly until the animal grows closer to its adult size at 6 to 12 months of age. Any septal defect complicated by pulmonary hypertension (Eisenmenger's syndrome) has a guarded short-term and a very guarded to poor long-term prognosis, although survival beyond 7 years is possible. Cats with severe endocardial cushion defects often have marked cardiomegaly and may develop biventricular congestive heart failure at a relatively early age (<2 years), warranting a very guarded to poor prognosis.

Clinical Management

Open heart correction of atrial or ventricular septal defects is uncommon for animals because of the usual requirement for cardiopulmonary bypass or other techniques to arrest the heart.[29–31] [76a, 77a] Palliative treatment of VSD may be accomplished without bypass using pulmonary artery banding to create supravalvular pulmonic stenosis and reduce the magnitude of left-to-right shunting (Fig. 112–23).[75a] This procedure is recommended for dogs and cats showing signs of marked or progressive cardiomegaly and overt or impending congestive heart failure. Other conditions that may increase resting cardiac output and shunting, such as anemia, should be treated.[78a] In animals with large left-to-right shunts and increased risk of congestive heart failure, arterial vasodilators may be prescribed to try to reduce both systemic vascular resistance and the left-to-right shunt.[79a] As noted for reversed PDA, septal defects with Eisenmenger's syndrome cannot be corrected and usually require medical management, primarily by periodic phlebotomy. Maintenance of the PCV at 58 to 65 per cent is recommended.

VENTRICULAR OUTFLOW OBSTRUCTIONS

PULMONIC STENOSIS

Pulmonic stenosis (PS) is one of the three most common congenital heart defects occurring in dogs, and it is occasionally recognized in cats.[1–5, 32, 33 [81a–89a]] Pulmonic stenosis often occurs as an isolated heart defect, but it is sometimes accompanied by additional cardiac anomalies. Congenital obstructions of the right ventricular outflow tract (RVOT) can develop in the infundibulum, subvalvular region, and above the pulmonic valve, but primary malformation of the pulmonary valve (dysplasia) is the most frequently observed defect in dogs. Patterson and associates,[86a] who studied the heritability and pathology of pulmonic valve dysplasia in the beagle,

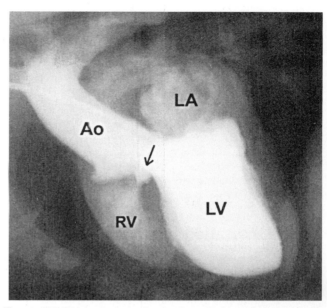

Figure 112–22. Angiography from a 6-month-old Australian heeler dog with a small ventricular septal defect (VSD). The catheter has been inserted into a carotid artery and advanced retrograde into the ascending aorta (Ao) and left ventricle (LV). Left ventricular injection of contrast outlines the LV and Ao and shows a narrow jet passing from the left to the right ventricle (RV) through a small defect in the ventricular septum just below the area of the aortic valve (arrow). The right coronary sinus at the aortic root just distal to the septal defect is distorted and bulges toward the RV. There is very slight artifactual mitral regurgitation of contrast into the left atrium

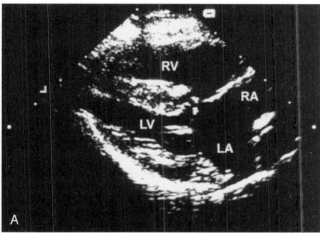

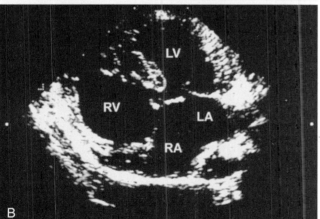

Figure 112–21. Echocardiogram from a 6-year-old miniature poodle with a large AV canal–type septal defect and pulmonary hypertension. *A,* Right long-axis view shows dilatation and hypertrophy of the right ventricle (RV). The large septal defect involves most of the atrial septum and the upper portion of the ventricular septum. *B,* The left-apical four-chamber view shows the markedly dilated RV and the large septal defect. This view more clearly shows the ventricular septal portion of the defect and the joining of the septal leaflets of the mitral and tricuspid valves.

initially suggested a polygenic mode of transmission for this defect. These breeding studies did not, however, exclude the possibility of a single-gene mechanism with variable penetrance. This latter hypothesis is imbued with the virtue of simplicity, and future studies should clarify which hypothesis is correct. The pattern of inheritance of PS has not been studied in other predisposed dog breeds (see Table 112–1), in dogs with other forms of RVOT obstruction, or in cats.

Pathology

Valvular lesions consist of varying degrees of valve thickening, fusion of the leaflets, and/or hypoplasia of the annulus. Whereas some dogs manifest a thin dome-shaped valve with a central orifice (Fig. 112–24A), most dogs have more complicated lesions resembling atypical PS in children (Fig. 112–24B).[15a, 86a, 88a] The valve leaflets are often very thick and misshaped, and the leaflets are often fused. The annulus of the pulmonic valve is hypoplastic in some dogs. Histologic abnormalities include thickening of the valve spongiosa and the presence of bands of fusiform cells in a dense collagen network. These changes are thought to represent overproduction of normal valve elements or a failure of conversion of the cushion-like embryonic valve primordia. Blood-filled spaces and endothelium-lined spaces are also found in one or more cusps of affected dogs.[86a] Some affected dogs have a fibrous ring just below the valve leaflets accompanying the valvular changes (Fig. 112–24C). In other dogs, the obstructive lesion occurs in the infundibular region of the RVOT (Fig 112–24D). On occasion, the RVOT is partitioned from the body (inflow region) of the right ventricle by a well-developed, fibromuscular ridge, resulting in an anomaly referred to as double- or dual-chambered right ventricle. Supravalvular PS is a very uncommon defect in

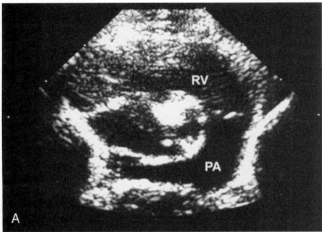

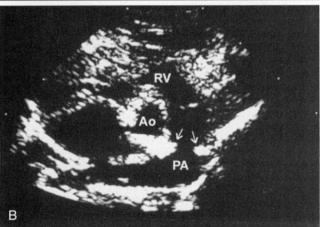

Figure 112–23. Echocardiogram from a 6-month-old domestic cat with a ventricular septal defect and large left-to-right shunt, before *(A)* and after *(B)* creation of pulmonic stenosis by surgical placement of a pulmonary artery band. *A,* Preoperative right short-axis view at the base of the heart shows the dilated main pulmonary artery. The pulmonic valve is seen in the 3 o'clock position. *B,* Similar view obtained postoperatively shows the constricting pulmonary artery band (arrows) 1 cm above the pulmonic valve. RV = right ventricle, Ao = aorta.

dogs. In the authors' experience, it is most often observed in giant schnauzers. In some English bulldogs and boxers, subvalvular PS is accompanied by anomalous development of the coronary arteries.[18] In this anomaly, the left and right coronary arteries branch from a single large coronary artery that originates from the right aortic sinus of Valsalva (Fig. 112–25A). From this location, the left coronary artery encircles the RV outflow tract just below the pulmonary valve, thereby contributing to the subvalvular component of this complex malformation (Fig. 112–25B to D). The precise relationship between the coronary artery anomaly and PS is uncertain as RVOT obstruction occurs in bulldogs and boxers with normally developed coronary arteries.

Increased resistance to systolic ejection results in concentric right ventricular hypertrophy, which generally develops in proportion to the severity of the obstructing defect. Although this compensatory response serves to normalize wall stress, it can have deleterious consequences. In some dogs with PS, secondary hypertrophy of the infundibular region of the RVOT contributes to outflow obstruction, particularly during exercise or stress (dynamic RVOT obstruction). The operation of this secondary mechanism of obstruction can complicate the clinical outcome of otherwise successful repair of valvular pulmonic stenosis. Although rare, extreme

hypertrophy of the interventricular septum resulting from PS can narrow the left ventricular outflow tract and cause a dynamic LVOT obstruction similar to that observed in the obstructive form of hypertrophic cardiomyopathy.

Other cardiac defects can complicate the physiology and alter the clinical presentation of dogs or cats with PS. In the authors' experience, mild (subclinical) deformities of the tricuspid valve often accompany pulmonic stenosis, particularly in the larger breeds of dogs. Many of these defects are inconsequential, but severe malformations of the tricuspid valve are sometimes observed (Fig. 112–26A and B). Pulmonic stenosis and tricuspid valve dysplasia can be a particularly lethal combination; such malformations often cause intractable right heart failure. Inasmuch as the volume of tricuspid regurgitation is a function of the size of the regurgitant orifice (severity of tricuspid valve dysplasia) and the systolic pressure gradient (severity of PS), massive tricuspid regurgitation develops in affected dogs.

Patent connections between the right and left heart occur in a substantial percentage of dogs with PS. Some dogs with severe PS become cyanotic as a result of right-to-left shunting through an atrial septal defect or patent foramen ovale. VSDs are also fairly common in dogs with PS. Many of these malformations result from maldevelopment of the conotruncal septum. Left-to-right or reversed shunting may occur, depending on the location and severity of the outflow obstruction. These types of defects are discussed more thoroughly in the section on tetralogy of Fallot.

Pathophysiology

Obstruction to right ventricular outflow causes increased resistance to ejection and a proportional increase in ventricular systolic pressure. Concentric hypertrophy of the right ventricle serves to normalize wall stress. During systole, blood ejected from the right ventricle accelerates as it traverses the obstructing orifice. Flow velocity and turbulence become maximal just beyond this point. A post-stenotic dilatation develops in the main pulmonary artery as the turbulent jet of blood decelerates and expends some of its kinetic energy against the vessel wall. Increased stiffness of the right ventricle is responsible for the vigorous contractions of the hypertrophied right atrium and the resulting giant a waves that are sometimes evident in the external jugular veins.

Heart failure develops as a consequence of systolic and diastolic right ventricular dysfunction and, in many cases, from concurrent tricuspid regurgitation. Tricuspid regurgitation results from progressive dilatation of the right ventricle, from valvular dysplasia, or from a combination of these factors.[85a] Sodium and water retention causes further dilatation of the right heart, increasing the severity of tricuspid valve insufficiency and, thereby, establishing a vicious cycle of deteriorating right heart function. As right atrial pressure approaches 15 mmHg, jugular distension, ascites, and other signs of right-sided congestive heart failure develop.

The physiologic mechanisms responsible for syncope in dogs with PS have not been evaluated extensively. Hypotension is presumed to develop as a consequence of reduced cardiac output (bradycardia, or worsening of a dynamic obstruction) in combination with peripheral arteriolar vasodilatation (with or in anticipation of exercise). Pronounced bradycardia and hypotension may result from stimulation of pressure receptors in the right ventricle. Reduced right coronary blood flow has been documented in some dogs with

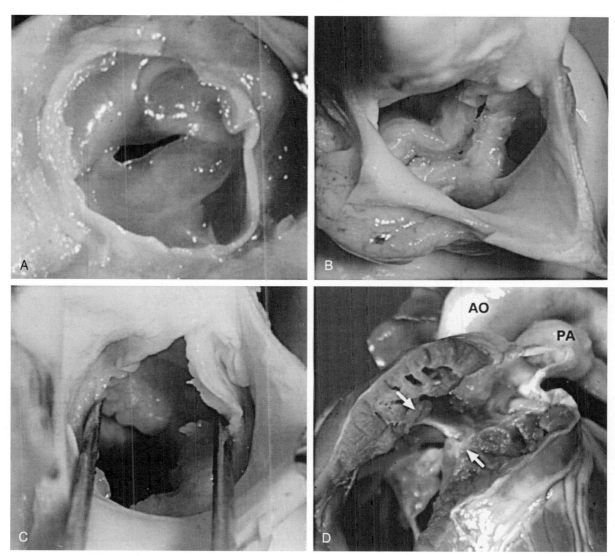

Figure 112–24. Pathology specimens from dogs with pulmonic stenosis (PS). *A,* The pulmonic valve leaflets are thin but fused with a central orifice in this 1-year-old Labrador retriever; they are similar to the domed valves of children with PS. *B,* A very thick (dysplastic) and bicuspid pulmonic valve is shown (Staffordshire terrier). *C.* Same dog as in *(B)*; the leaflets have been distracted to show a small subvalvular ridge. *D,* A fibromuscular ring (arrows) is shown in the right ventricular infundibulum several centimeters below the pulmonic valve.

pulmonic stenosis and may contribute to the development of syncope, exercise intolerance, and myocardial failure.

Clinical Findings

Pulmonic stenosis is common in certain breeds, including the beagle, Samoyed, Chihuahua, English bulldog, miniature schnauzer, cocker spaniel, Boykin spaniel, Labrador retriever, mastiff, Samoyed, chow-chow, Newfoundland, Basset hound, and other terrier and spaniel breeds.[8a, 9a, 9b 19b] Miniature pinschers also seem predisposed. Most dogs with PS are asymptomatic during the first year of life when the condition is usually first discovered. Severely affected dogs may evidence exertional fatigue or syncope at a young age. Signs of congestive right heart failure, such as ascites, are most often reported in dogs that are older.[88a] Cyanosis may be noted when PS is complicated by right-to-left shunting across a patent foramen ovale or coexisting ASD or VSD.

The most prominent physical examination finding is a left basilar ejection murmur that is best heard over the pulmonic valve area and that often radiates dorsally. In some cases the

murmur is heard equally well on the right cranial thorax, possibly due to tricuspid regurgitation. In dogs with concurrent valvular insufficiency, the systolic murmur is accompanied by a soft diastolic murmur best heard just ventral to the pulmonic valve region. A holosystolic murmur of tricuspid regurgitation may be noted over the right hemithorax in dogs with this complication. Large-amplitude jugular pulses may be noted in the lower third of the neck either from a giant a wave or a regurgitant c–v wave even in the absence of heart failure. Jugular venous distention and prominent jugular pulses are evident in most dogs with right heart failure and ascites.

Right ventricular enlargement is usually evident on the electrocardiogram unless the lesion is very mild.[31a, 32a, 90a] Right axis deviation, an $S_{I}S_{II}S_{III}$ pattern, and deep S waves on the left precordial chest leads are reliable indicators of right heart enlargement. Thoracic radiographs typically show a prominent right heart and post-stenotic dilatation of the main pulmonary artery (Fig. 112–27).[8a, 22a–24a, 88a] These changes are usually most evident on the dorsoventral view. Additional and more variable findings include dilatation of the proximal left pulmonary artery, diminished size of the

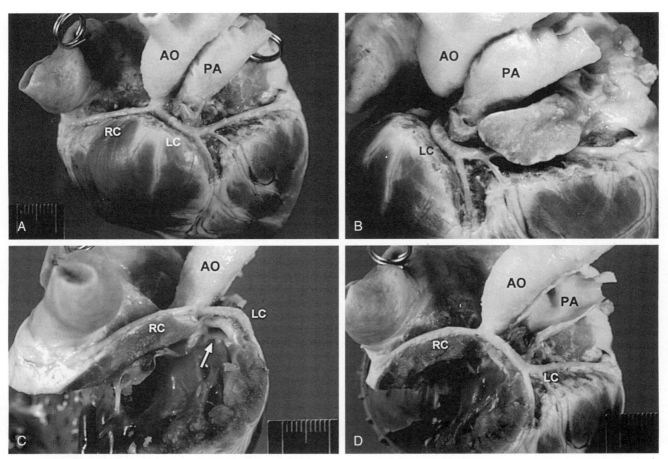

Figure 112–25. The coronary artery anomaly seen in some English bulldogs with pulmonic stenosis is shown in *A* to *D*. In *(A)* the left and right coronary arteries are seen to branch from a single large coronary artery that originates from the right aortic sinus of Valsalva. From this location, the left coronary artery encircles the right ventricle (RV) outflow tract just below the pulmonary valve *(B)*, thereby contributing to the subvalvular component of this complex malformation *(C* and *D)*. *C,* The left coronary artery is seen to course over the RV outflow tract just below the annulus of the pulmonic valve (arrow). *D,* The anterior wall of the pulmonary artery (PA) has been removed to show the hypoplastic pulmonic annulus, diminutive proximal PA, and the crowded and thickened valve leaflets.

pulmonary vasculature, and enlargement of the caudal vena cava.

Angiocardiography is most often performed at the time of balloon valvuloplasty or in anticipation of surgery. Such studies clearly demonstrate the anatomic location of the obstruction, the degree of right ventricular hypertrophy, and post-stenotic dilation of the pulmonary artery. The angiographic features of pulmonic valve dysplasia (Fig. 112–28) consist of any combination of the following: narrowing at the immediate base of the valve sinuses, asymmetrical valve sinuses, hypoplasia of the annulus or a valve sinus, thickening of individual valve leaflets producing a lucent filling defect, narrowing of the dye column with a central or asymmetric jet of contrast observed within a narrowed valve orifice, or systolic doming of the valve (indicating fusion of the commissures).[86a, 88a] Dynamic muscular obstruction of the right ventricular infundibulum (Fig. 112–29) is often visible in dogs with PS. The term "double-chambered right ventricle" (Fig. 112–30) is applied when the right ventricle is divided into a low-pressure region (the infundibulum) and a region of high pressure (the apex and inlet portion of the right ventricle) by a muscular or fibromuscular ridge deep in the infundibulum. Left ventricular angiography or coronary arteriography are performed to demonstrate any suspected abnormalities of the left heart or coronary circulation (Fig. 112–31A to D). Such studies should be performed whenever

surgery or balloon valvuloplasty is contemplated in an English bulldog or boxer dog. Enlargement of the right coronary artery is an expected finding in dogs with PS and right ventricular hypertrophy.

Hemodynamic confirmation of outflow tract obstruction is accomplished by measuring a systolic pressure difference across the lesion. Characteristic pressure tracings obtained from a dog with valvular pulmonic stenosis are shown in Figure 112–2. Pulmonary artery pressure is usually normal. As the catheter is withdrawn into the right ventricle, a sudden increase in systolic pressure is observed. The severity of the obstruction is often defined as the difference in peak systolic pressures measured above and below the obstruction (peak-to-peak pressure gradient). Inasmuch as the recorded gradient varies with the rate of flow across the obstruction, this measurement is greatly affected by myocardial contractility and the anesthetic regimen selected. Despite these limitations, the systolic pressure gradient has been used to divide patients with pulmonic stenosis into mild (<50 mmHg), moderate (50 to 80 mmHg), and severe (>80 mmHg) categories.[87a, 88a, 93a]

Echocardiography is the most commonly used method for confirming a diagnosis of PS. M-mode and 2D imaging typically show concentric hypertrophy of the right ventricle, increased prominence of the papillary muscles, deformity in the region of the obstruction(s), narrowing of the right ventri-

CV

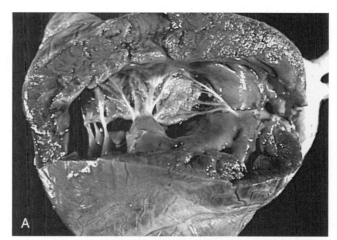

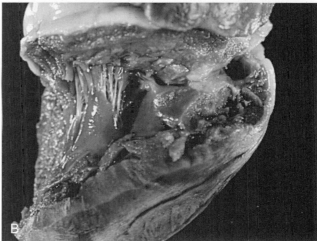

Figure 112–26. Pathology specimens from a dog *(A)* and a cat *(B)* with severe pulmonic stenosis and tricuspid dysplasia. Marked right ventricle (RV) hypertrophy is evident in both specimens. *A,* A curtain-like deformity of the tricuspid valve shows leaflet tissue attaching directly to the RV papillary muscles. *B,* The tricuspid valve of this is very unusual, with one very large papillary muscle receiving most of the chordae tendineae.

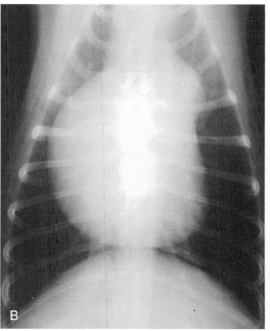

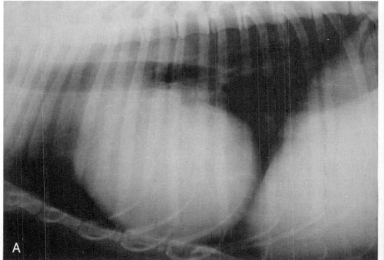

Figure 112–27. These radiographs from a young dog with severe pulmonic stenosis (PS) show marked right ventricle enlargement with dorsal displacement of the heart's apex on the lateral view *(A)* and a reverse D and enlarged pulmonary artery segment (post-stenotic dilation) on the dorsoventral view *(B)*. As shown here, the pulmonary vessels often appear small and the lung fields appear hypolucent in dogs with severe PS, even in the absence of a right-to-left shunt.

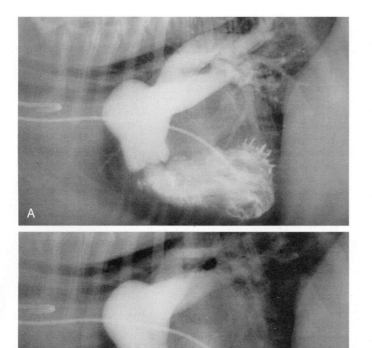

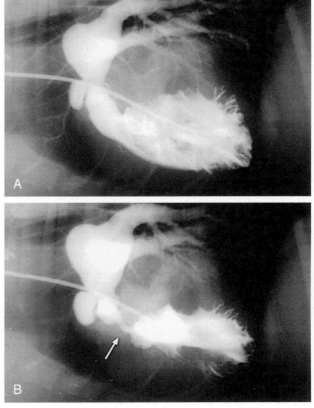

Figure 112–28. Diastolic *(A)* and systolic *(B)* frames of a right ventricle (RV) angiogram in a dog with pulmonic stenosis. Note the narrow jet of contrast as it passes through the pulmonic orifice. Post-stenotic dilatation of the pulmonary artery is visible on both frames as is hypertrophy of the RV wall and papillary muscles.

Figure 112–29. Right ventricular angiocardiogram from a dog with severe pulmonic stenosis. Comparison of the diastolic *(A)* and systolic *(B)* frames shows complete obliteration of the outflow tract due to vigorous contraction of the hypertrophied infundibulum. Compare with Figure 112–28. Also note the distortion of the pulmonic valve sinuses (arrow).

cle outflow tract, varying degrees of right atrial enlargement, and post-stenotic dilation of the main pulmonary artery (Fig. 112–32). In some cases, the images are sufficiently clear to reveal the exact location and nature of the obstruction, but in many dogs the details of the deformity are not discernable. It is often particularly difficult to identify a discrete subval-

vular obstruction close to the pulmonary valve. The pulmonic valve leaflets are typically thickened and often fused and sometimes appear to dome upwards during systole. Hypoplasia of the pulmonic valve annulus can often be appreciated, and recognition of this finding can influence the approach to treatment. Obstructions that occur deeper in the infundibulum of the right ventricle are usually accompanied

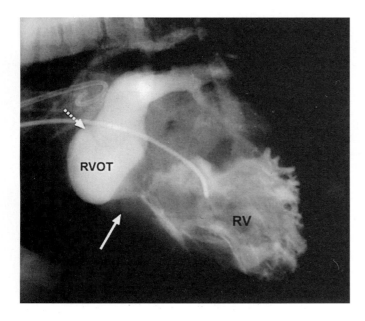

Figure 112–30. Right ventricular angiocardiogram recorded from a Rottweiler dog with an unusual form of subvalvular muscular pulmonic stenosis. Some refer to this lesion as a "double-chambered right ventricle" to distinguish it from dynamic collapse of the hypertrophied infundibulum (Fig. 112–28). Others use the term only when the lesion is deeper within the right ventricle, and some avoid the term altogether. Solid arrow indicates the muscular obstructing lesion in the right ventricular outflow tract. The dashed arrow indicates the location of the pulmonic valve.

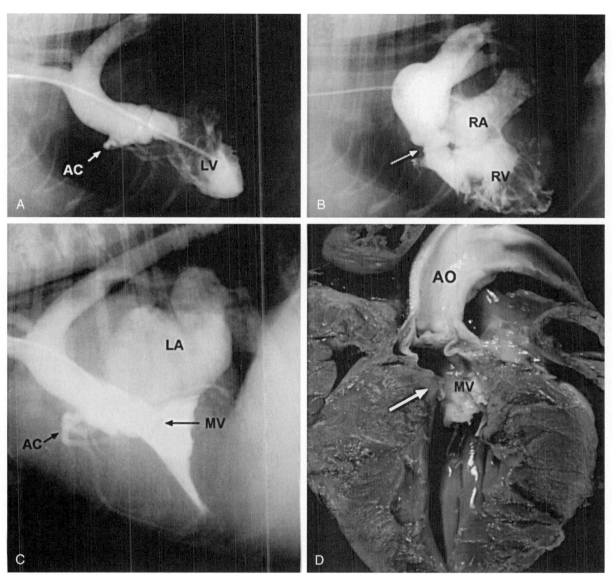

Figure 112–31. Angiographic studies in a bulldog. *A* This left ventricular angiogram shows a large, single aberrant coronary artery (AC, arrow) leaving the right coronary sinus on the anterior aspect of the aorta and giving rise to both the left and right coronary arteries. *B*, A right ventricular injection in this same dog shows a notch-like deformity (arrow) just below the pulmonic valve that is caused by the encircling left coronary artery. Tricuspid regurgitation and post-stenotic dilation of the main pulmonary artery is also seen. *C*, Also from a bulldog, this left ventricular angiogram shows aberrant coronary artery development, marked left ventricle (LV) hypertrophy, and dynamic left ventricular outflow tract obstruction accompanied by mitral regurgitation. *D*, Pathology from the same dog as in *(C)* demonstrates marked hypertrophy of the interventricular septum and LV free wall. An impact lesion was present on the interventricular septum (arrow), presumably from systolic anterior motion of the thickened mitral valve.

by post-stenotic dilation of the distal part of the right ventricle infundibulum.

Color flow Doppler echocardiography is useful in establishing the anatomic type of the obstruction, as the turbulent, high-velocity jet can usually be seen emerging from the obstructive orifice (Fig. 112–32C). Mild-to-moderate pulmonic valve insufficiency is also apparent in most affected dogs. To quantify the severity of the obstruction accurately, the peak velocity of the jet must be recorded on a spectral Doppler tracing acquired with the continuous-wave Doppler beam precisely in alignment with the direction of flow (Fig. 112–32D). This is usually accomplished from either the right or left cranial parasternal locations. The modified Bernoulli equation, $\Delta P = 4V^2$, is applied to relate the instantaneous pressure gradient across an obstruction (ΔP, in mmHg) to the peak velocity of jet distal to the obstruction (V, in m/s).

As a general rule, Doppler-derived gradients are 40 to 50 per cent higher than the catheterization gradient measured in an individual dog.[20b] There are several reasons for this apparent discrepancy. Doppler studies are performed in awake or lightly-sedated animals, and transvalvular flow is considerably higher in these circumstances than in dogs that have been anesthetized for a cardiac catheterization. In addition, hemodynamic studies indicate the severity of obstruction as a peak-to-peak pressure gradient, and such measures are almost always lower than the instantaneous peak pressure gradient that is calculated from Doppler measures of peak flow velocity.

Doppler interrogation of the tricuspid valves is particularly helpful for identifying and assessing the severity of coexisting tricuspid valve insufficiency. In some dogs, the severity of the obstruction is most accurately assessed by measuring

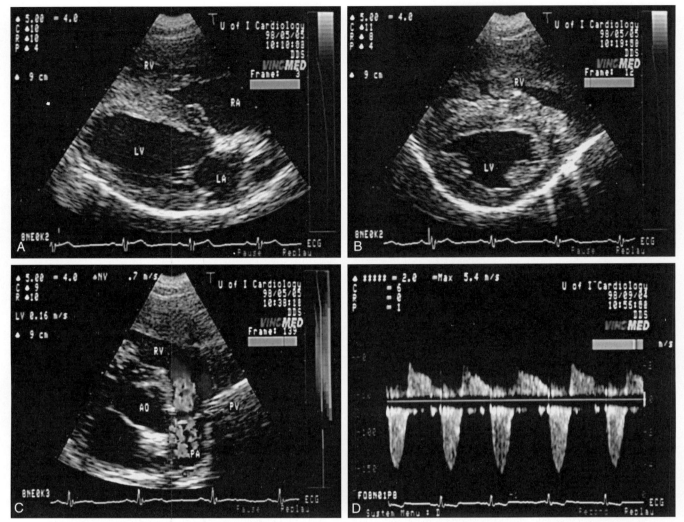

Figure 112–32. Echocardiographic findings in a dog with pulmonic stenosis (PS) are shown. *A,* Long axis two-dimensional echocardiogram showing a hypertrophy of the interventricular septum and the right ventricle (RV) wall. The thick papillary muscle and shortened chordae tendineae suggest some degree of tricuspid valve dysplasia. *B,* This short, right parasternal short-axis view, recorded at the level of the papillary muscles, shows marked RV hypertrophy. *C,* This color Doppler recording shows the blood beginning to accelerate in the RV outflow tract, but the highest velocities and greatest turbulence occur in the proximal pulmonary artery. *D,* This continuous-wave Doppler recording from another dog with more mild PS shows a peak velocity of about 4.0 m/s, indicating an instantaneous pressure gradient of 64 mmHg.

the velocity of this regurgitant jet. A complete Doppler examination includes measurement of aortic velocities to detect concurrent aortic stenosis and careful inspection of the atria and ventricle for evidence of shunting defects in these locations.

Natural History

Precise criteria for establishing an accurate prognosis have not been developed for dogs and cats with PS. There is general agreement that most dogs with mild and even moderate PS (Doppler-derived gradient <80 mmHg) usually live normal or nearly normal lives. This generalization does not encompass those dogs with other complicating defects. The problem of concurrent tricuspid valve dysplasia and its relation to developing heart failure has already been discussed. Although systolic pressure gradients are not always predictive of clinical outcome, the authors have found a general correlation between pressure gradient and survival. Dogs with Doppler-derived gradients greater than 125 mmHg frequently develop one or more debilitating problems, including

secondary tricuspid regurgitation, heart failure, exertional syncope, or a serious cardiac arrhythmia (atrial fibrillation). When an ASD, patent foramen ovale, or VSD coexists with PS, there is the potential for right-to-left shunting, hypoxemia, polycythemia, and serious debilitation. Sudden death occurs in some dogs with severe PS, but this outcome is uncommon.

Clinical Management

Following noninvasive studies, the attending clinician can generally determine if the stenosis is likely to be mild to moderate or moderate to severe. When radiographic, electrocardiographic, and echocardiographic changes are evident, or if the patient has clinical signs of disease, the pressure gradient should be determined by Doppler echocardiography. It cannot be stated with certainty at what pressure gradient an operation should be recommended. However, a dog with a Doppler gradient of greater than 100 to 125 mmHg should be considered a candidate for balloon valvuloplasty or surgery. Dogs with less severe gradients are also candidates for these procedures if they exhibit compatible clinical signs: syncope or exertional fatigue. If the clinician elects to delay surgery in a dog with moderate to severe stenosis, then the dog should be reevaluated in 6 to 12 months. Over time, progressive infundibular hypertrophy can substantially worsen the severity of the obstruction. Tricuspid regurgitation may also worsen. Moreover, right ventricle hypertrophy and fibrosis can lead to diastolic or systolic dysfunction that can induce elevated right atrial pressures and right-sided congestive heart failure. The development of overt congestive heart failure substantially lessens the chance for a successful outcome. Even mildly affected dogs should not be bred.

The goal of treatment for dogs with PS is to abolish or to reduce the systolic pressure gradient to the mild range before signs of heart failure develop. Until the last decade, surgery was the only available option for treating PS. A number of surgical techniques have been advocated.[34, 35 [21b, 22b, 37a, 91a–94a]] Closed procedures include valve dilation, patch grafting, or the placement of a conduit from the right ventricle to the pulmonary artery. Open valvotomy or valvectomy, performed with direct examination of the defect under total venous inflow occlusion or with complete cardiac bypass, allows more extensive revision of the obstructing lesion. The open patch-graft technique is a particularly versatile and cost-effective method for treating dogs with PS, particularly when there is a substantial subvalvular obstruction.[34, 35 [22b]] This technique is well-suited to the treatment of some situations not amenable to balloon valvuloplasty: e.g., dogs with muscular RVOT obstructions, double-chambered right ventricle, or severe hypoplasia of the pulmonic anulus.

An alternative to surgery that has been increasingly utilized over the last decade is catheter balloon valvuloplasty.[35–39 [20b, 23b, 24b, 94a,b,c]] This procedure uses a dilation catheter with an inflatable balloon to expand the obstructing orifice (Fig. 112–33). Successful reduction of the obstructive gradient by 50 per cent or more has been reported in 75 to 80 per cent of the dogs treated with this technique. Improvements in balloon catheter design and refinements in technique have expanded the application of this procedure to dogs weighing as little as 4 pounds.[40] Delayed re-stenosis can occur, but this is not thought to be an important problem. Balloon valvuloplasty is most successful when the pulmonary anulus is normally developed and the valves are thin and fused. More variable results are obtained in dogs with complex lesions and hypoplasia of the pulmonary annulus.[38, 41] In the authors' experience, balloon dilation is of little value in dogs with muscular RVOT obstructions or double-chambered right ventricle–type defects. While balloon valvuloplasty is generally regarded as a safe procedure with a low complication rate, life-threatening problems do occur. Dogs with hypoplasia of pulmonary annulus or anomalous development of the coronary arteries are at particular risk for serious complications.[36]

When congestive heart failure or atrial fibrillation develops secondary to PS, the prognosis is poor. If medical stabilization can be achieved, balloon valvuloplasty or surgery can be attempted.

CV

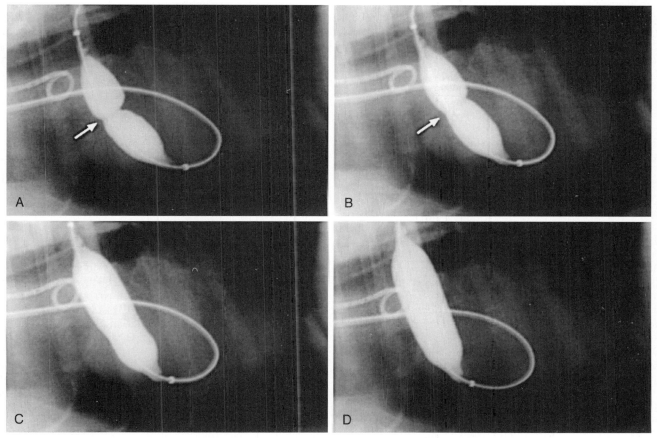

Figure 112–33. This sequence of radiographs was taken during balloon dilation in a dog with valvular pulmonic stenosis. The balloon catheter is seen to traverse the cranial vena cava, right atrium and ventricle, and pulmonary artery. Radio-opaque markers on the catheter are used to help position the balloon across the valve. A prominent stenotic lesion (arrow) is seen on inflation of the balloon (A); it becomes less obvious as the lesion is stretched or torn open in (B) and (C); and it is no longer evident at the time the balloon is fully inflated (D).

SUBAORTIC STENOSIS

Subaortic stenosis (SAS) is the most common congenital cardiac malformation in large-breed dogs.[1–5, 42 [97a–109a]] It is a troublesome disorder because it is very difficult to diagnose in mildly affected dogs, and it is difficult to treat when it is severe. The phenomenon of dynamic LVOT obstruction is also being recognized with increasing frequency in dogs and cats with a variety of cardiac disorders, including SAS, mitral valve dysplasia, hypertrophic cardiomyopathy, and other conditions causing hypertrophy of the interventricular septum (PS, tetralogy of Fallot).[43, [26b]] Isolated valvular aortic stenosis is much less common than fixed or dynamic SAS. Many dogs with SAS have a thickened aortic valve, and aortic valve opening is impaired in many dogs when the stenotic ring involves the base of the valves. Other dogs with aortic stenosis, such as bull terriers, have a small LVOT and thickened aortic leaflets, and it is difficult to tell which lesion is mainly responsible for the obstruction. The authors have recognized an increased number of dogs with aortic valvular stenosis since the introduction of color-flow Doppler echocardiography. Aortic stenosis has been described in a small number of cats,[44, [12a, 13a, 36a, 25b]] including one case of supravalvular stenosis.[101a]

Pathology and Pathogenesis

Subvalvular aortic stenosis has been extensively studied, particularly in the Newfoundland dog. Breeding studies of the Newfoundland dog have established a genetic basis for the perpetuation of SAS in this breed.[4a, 100a] The inheritance of SAS in the Newfoundland dog is most compatible with an autosomal dominant mode of transmission with modifying genes, but a polygenic mechanism cannot be excluded. The breeding colony studies of Pyle and Patterson[4a, 99a, 100a, 103a, 104a] further indicate that the obstruction may not be present at birth but instead develops during the first 4 to 8 weeks of life. This progression has particular significance relative to the identification of cardiac murmurs in pups of breeds known to be at risk for SAS.

The lesions of SAS in Newfoundland dogs have been described in postmortem studies as mild (grade 1), consisting of "small, whitish, slightly raised nodules on the endocardial surface of the ventricular septum immediately below the aortic valve"; moderate (grade 2), consisting of a "narrow ridge of whitish, thickened endocardium" extending partially about the LVOT; and severe (grade 3), consisting of "a fibrous band, ridge, or collar completely encircling the left ventricular outflow tract just below the aortic valve."[4a, 100a] This ring is raised above the endocardium and extends to and may involve the cranioventral leaflet of the mitral valve and the base of the aortic valves (Fig. 112–34A and B). The stenotic ring consists of loosely arranged reticular fibers, mucopolysaccharide ground substance, and elastic fibers. Discrete bundles of collagen and even cartilage are found in advanced lesions.[100a] Cardiac catheterization of dogs with grade 1 lesions failed to reliably detect the postmortem lesion, whereas grade 2 lesions were often associated with soft cardiac murmurs and only minimal systolic pressure gradients. From these studies it is clear that clinical detection of SAS may be quite difficult in mild cases and that genetic counseling may be fraught with error. A number of cardiac abnormalities can accompany SAS, most notably mitral valve dysplasia, PDA, and a variety of aortic arch abnormalities.

In many dogs with SAS, including some golden retrievers,

the pathologic findings diverge from the classical description in the preceding paragraph. Many dogs do not manifest a discrete subvalvular membrane. Instead, a broad fibromuscular ridge, arising from the base of the interventricular septum, protrudes into the LVOT (Fig. 112–34C and D). Large muscular ridges, resembling an accessory papillary muscle when viewed in cross section, traverse the long axis of the LVOT, eventually fusing into the interventricular septum. Malformed and misaligned papillary muscles, thickened chordae tendineae, and elongated or distorted mitral leaflets are found in many affected dogs. Pathologic and clinical evidence of dynamic LVOT obstruction and mitral regurgitation is obvious in many affected dogs. Bull terrier dogs also have an unusual form of aortic stenosis, often occurring together with a malformation of the mitral valve. The nature of the LVOT obstruction is not well characterized, but the outflow tract appears smaller than normal, and the aortic valve leaflets are thickened and rigid.

Concentric hypertrophy of the left ventricle develops in dogs with SAS more or less in proportion to the severity of the outflow obstruction, albeit that the correlation between wall thickness and the magnitude of the measured gradient is often poor.[45] Structural and functional abnormalities of the coronary circulation have been documented in dogs with SAS.[103a, 104a] Abnormal coronary flow has also been measured in the larger, extramural arteries with diminished baseline diastolic flow and reversal of coronary flow during systole.[8a, 104a] Focal areas of myocardial infarction and fibrosis are commonly observed in the papillary muscles and subendocardium of dogs with severe SAS, often in association with abnormal intramural coronary arteries. Histologic changes of the intramural coronary arteries in these locations include intimal proliferation of connective tissue and smooth muscle as well as medial degeneration. These changes are presumably related to the high wall tension found in this condition, and their genesis may be related to the elaboration of angiotensin II or other biochemical mediators. Moreover, these lesions may be important in the genesis of sudden death.

Pathophysiology

Obstruction to LV outflow causes an increase in left ventricular systolic pressure and concentric hypertrophy of the left ventricle. As a consequence of fixed obstruction, left ventricular ejection is delayed, causing a small and late rising arterial pulse (parvus et tardus). High-velocity and turbulent flow across the stenotic area causes the systolic cardiac murmur and results in post-stenotic dilatation of the ascending aorta, aortic arch, and brachiocephalic trunk. Left atrial hypertrophy develops as a consequence of the reduced compliance of the hypertrophied left ventricle. Mild aortic regurgitation is presumably due to thickening of the valve leaflets or dilatation of the ascending aorta. Damage to the valvular endothelium (jet lesions) predisposes dogs with SAS to bacterial endocarditis, leaflet destruction, and rapidly progressing aortic regurgitation. Left ventricular hypertrophy and myocardial ischemia are responsible for the changes in the QRS complex and ST-T segment. Critical SAS can lead to left-sided congestive heart failure from myocardial failure, increased ventricular stiffness, mitral regurgitation, atrial fibrillation, or a combination of these factors. More often, exertional syncope or sudden death is reported, presumably as a consequence of myocardial ischemia and the development of malignant ventricular arrhythmias. In some dogs, exertional collapse results from hypotension precipitated by

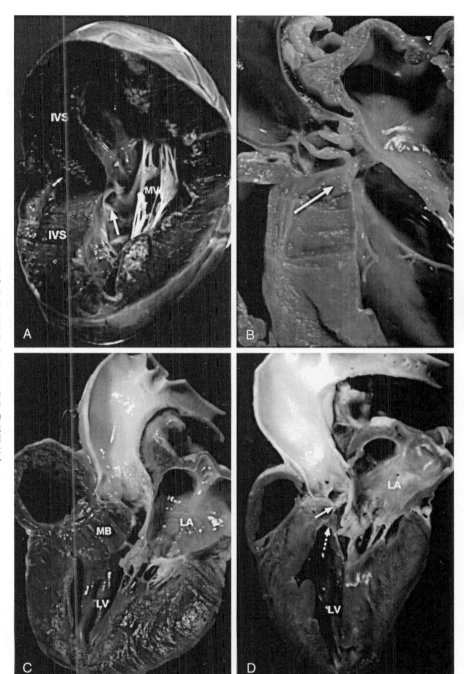

Figure 112–34. The gross pathology of subvalvular aortic stenosis is shown. *A,* Viewed from the left apex, a fibrous collar is shown completely encircling the left ventricular outflow tract (LVOT) just below the aortic valve. This ring was also adherent to the cranioventral (anterior) leaflet of the mitral valve. *B,* In this dog, a fibromuscular ridge protrudes into the LVOT. A fibrous ring is seen extending from the base of the aortic valve leaflet to the base of the mitral valve. The valve leaflets are thickened and unable to open completely as a result. *C,* In this specimen from a young golden retriever, the LVOT is obstructed by a large protruding bundle of muscle and a malpositioned and malformed mitral valve. *D,* The heart of this golden retriever has lesions somewhere in between those shown in *(B)* and *(C).* The base of the septum protrudes into the LVOT; there is an encircling fibrous ring (arrow) at the base of the aortic and mitral valves; and there is evidence of an impact lesion on the septum caused by systolic anterior motion of the dysplastic mitral valve.

exercise-induced increases in left ventricular pressure, activation of ventricular mechanoreceptors, and inappropriate bradycardia or vasodilation.

Clinical Findings

Congenital SAS is most common in the Newfoundland, boxer, Rottweiler, golden retriever, and German shepherd breeds.[8a, 9b] The clinical findings of SAS vary with the severity of the obstruction and the presence of concurrent cardiac defects. Clinical findings in pups with mild SAS are often subtle and easily overlooked.[5a–9a, 98a–100a] Asymptomatic dogs have a soft to moderately intense ejection murmur that can easily be confused with an innocent or functional heart murmur. Inasmuch as the lesions of SAS can develop during the postnatal period, the murmur may become increasingly prominent during the first 6 months of life. Severely affected dogs may also be asymptomatic. Alternatively, they may present with exertional tiring, syncope, or left-sided congestive heart failure. Sudden death, without premonitory signs, is common.

Recognition of severe SAS is not difficult, as the murmur generally becomes louder and longer when the obstruction is more severe.[46] The murmur of severe SAS is usually best heard at the left heart base. In some dogs, the systolic murmur is equally loud or louder at the right cardiac base, presumably from radiation into the ascending aorta. The murmur of aortic stenosis also tends to radiate up the carotid arteries and even to the calvarium. In some affected dogs, the systolic murmur is accompanied by a soft diastolic murmur secondary to aortic valve insufficiency. A number of dogs exhibit both SAS and mitral regurgitation, but these murmurs

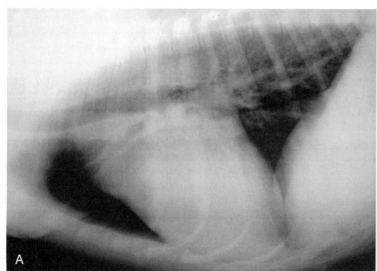

Figure 112–35. Electrocardiogram from a dog with congenital subaortic stenosis. There is a single interpolated ventricular premature complex and significant ST segment depression (arrow). This may indicate ischemia in this dog. Paper speed = 50 mm per second; calibration: 5 mm = 1 mV.

are usually difficult to identify specifically given their similar timing and overlapping areas of maximal intensity. Other physical abnormalities detected in moderate to severely affected dogs include a diminished and late rising arterial pulse and a prominent left ventricular heave arising from the hypertrophied left ventricle.

The electrocardiogram is often normal but may, in severe cases, indicate left ventricular hypertrophy as reflected by increased R-wave amplitudes or left-axis deviation. Depression of the ST segment and T-wave changes suggest myocardial ischemia, particularly when these alterations are precipitated by exercise or occur in the company of ventricular ectopia (Fig. 112–35). Compared with the resting electrocardiogram, 24-hour Holter ECG studies offer a more sensitive method of detecting ventricular arrhythmia and ST segment changes, particularly when such changes are only precipitated by exercise. The severity of arrhythmias detected in this fashion are often, but not always, related to the severity of disease.

Thoracic radiographs can be normal or may indicate left ventricular hypertrophy (Fig. 112–36A and B).[8a, 22a–24a] Post-

stenotic dilation of the often horizontally inclined aorta causes loss of the cranial waist on the lateral radiograph and widening of the mediastinum on the dorsoventral radiograph. Mild left atrial enlargement is common in dogs with moderate or severe SAS, but marked left atrial enlargement suggests concurrent mitral regurgitation. Angiocardiography is useful for delineating the site of obstruction, which is usually most evident in the ventral aspect of the outflow tract when viewed on the lateral projection (Fig. 112–37A). Other changes include post-stenotic dilation of the ascending aorta, enlargement of the left coronary artery and its extramural branches, a small left ventricular cavity, hypertrophy of the papillary muscles, and thickening of the left ventricle wall. Other abnormalities, such as mitral regurgitation (Fig. 112–37B) or dynamic LVOT obstruction, are observed in some dogs. The latter phenomenon is more likely to be visualized when a post-extrasystolic beat is captured on the angiocardiogram (see Fig. 112–31D). Supravalvular aortic injections are sometimes performed to identify insufficiency of the aortic valve, but Doppler echocardiography is a more sensitive technique. Hemodynamic recordings are made to docu-

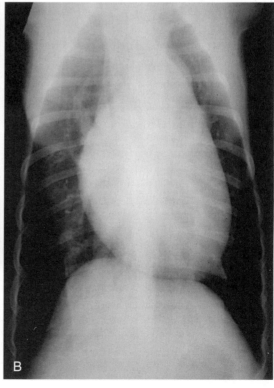

Figure 112–36. These radiographs from a 1-year-old golden retriever show moderate left ventricle enlargement. On the lateral view (A), the post-stenotic dilatation of the horizontally inclined aorta (see Fig. 112–37) has abolished the cranial waist of the cardiac silhouette. On the dorsoventral view (B), the post-stenotic dilatation is seen protruding into the cranial mediastinum at 12 o'clock.

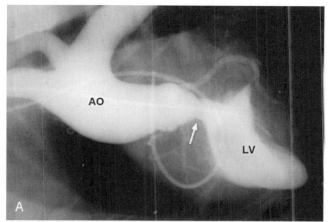

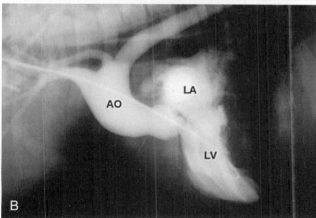

Figure 112–37. Angiocardiograms from two dogs with subvalvular aortic stenosis. *A,* The arrow points to a narrow portion of a funnel-shaped subvalvular obstruction. Note the prominent post-stenotic dilatation of the aorta that extends to the brachiocephalic trunk and left subclavian artery. With some effort, the reader should be able to distinguish the enlarged left circumflex coronary artery from the NIH catheter that loops through the right heart. *B,* This angiocardiogram from a young golden retriever shows a subvalvular obstruction located just below the aortic valve. Concurrent mitral valve dysplasia resulted in considerable mitral regurgitation.

ment the presence of a systolic pressure gradient across the obstruction and to document its severity (see Fig. 112–2B). Such recordings are also useful for detecting elevated left ventricular diastolic pressure.[8a, 105a] As a result of diminished flow, pressure gradients recorded from dogs with SAS are depressed by general anesthesia to approximately 40 to 50 per cent of that measured in the unanesthetized state.[47]

Moderate to severe SAS is easily confirmed by 2D echocardiography. Typical findings include concentric left ventricular hypertrophy, a subvalvular fibrous or fibromuscular obstructing lesion, and post-stenotic dilatation of the aorta (Fig. 112–38A).[27a, 106a] The tips of the papillary muscles and various segments of the ventricular myocardium often appear hyperechoic, presumably reflecting the fibrotic changes induced by chronic ischemia. Structural changes in the mitral valve can often be appreciated, and abnormal motion of the mitral valve (systolic anterior motion) can be detected in those dogs with coexisting mitral valve dysplasia and/or dynamic obstruction. All of these changes are often lacking in dogs with mild SAS. Doppler interrogation of the LVOT appears to be the most sensitive means of verifying a mild obstructing lesion, and disease severity is frequently estimated by measuring peak velocity of flow in the LVOT (Fig. 112–38B).[48] Doppler-derived gradients show excellent correlation with invasive measures.[49] Doppler measurements

from recordings made with the transducer in a subcostal location are generally higher than those made from the left apical window or the suprasternal notch.[27b] However, several windows are routinely evaluated because the best location for optimal alignment varies from patient to patient. Doppler-estimated pressure gradients between 75 and 100 mmHg (peak flow velocities ranging from 4.3 to 5.0 m/s) indicate moderate LVOT obstruction, and higher gradients indicate severe obstruction. As in dogs with PS, these designations are somewhat arbitrary. Color-flow Doppler recordings are also valuable for detecting and estimating the severity of coexisting aortic or mitral valve insufficiency.

Detection of mild SAS by Doppler echocardiography remains somewhat controversial. The upper limit for aortic velocity in normal dogs is not well established, and conditions other than mild SAS can cause slight elevation in aortic velocities. The maximum aortic velocity in the authors' laboratories is 1.7 m/s. Values above 2.2 m/s are regarded as indicative of mild SAS, and values from 1.7 to 2.2 m/s are regarded as equivocal. A diagnosis of mild SAS is more secure when mildly elevated velocity measures are accompanied by disturbed flow or when velocity flow suddenly accelerates over a discrete region in the LVOT.

Natural History

Severe SAS is a discouraging condition because many dogs either die suddenly or develop congestive heart failure. The natural history of SAS was reported in a retrospective survey of 96 affected dogs examined between 1967 and 1991.[50] Of these dogs, 21 died suddenly, usually within the first 3 years of life. Eleven dogs developed endocarditis (6 dogs) or heart failure (7 dogs), and 32 dogs evidenced exercise intolerance or syncope. Doppler echocardiography or cardiac catheterization is usually required to confirm the severity of SAS and to formulate an accurate prognosis. Dogs with higher pressure gradients are more likely to die suddenly, and they tend to die at a younger age than more mildly affected dogs. Dogs with minimal ventricular hypertrophy, mild ventricular outflow obstruction, and a maximal Doppler pressure gradient of less than 50 mmHg are likely to be near-normal pets. Dogs with Doppler gradients in excess of 125 mmHg are likely to develop serious complications or to experience sudden death. Complicating factors that may lead to an adverse outcome include mitral regurgitation, aortic regurgitation, aortic valve endocarditis, and atrial fibrillation.[51–53]

Clinical Management

Dogs with mild SAS are not treated. Given the established and substantial risk of bacterial endocarditis,[53] prophylactic antibiotics can be considered for dogs with open skin wounds or that will undergo dental procedures or surgery, but the efficacy of this approach has not been proved. A number of treatment options can be considered for dogs with moderate to severe SAS, but many (most) are of questionable or unproven value. As sudden death often occurs during or shortly after vigorous exercise, such activity should be avoided.

Open resection of the obstructing lesion during cardiopulmonary bypass clearly offers the best opportunity to substantially and permanently reduce the systolic pressure gradient.[54, 55] Unfortunately, an otherwise successful procedure does not preclude the later occurrence of sudden death.[55] Other surgical procedures employed to dilate or

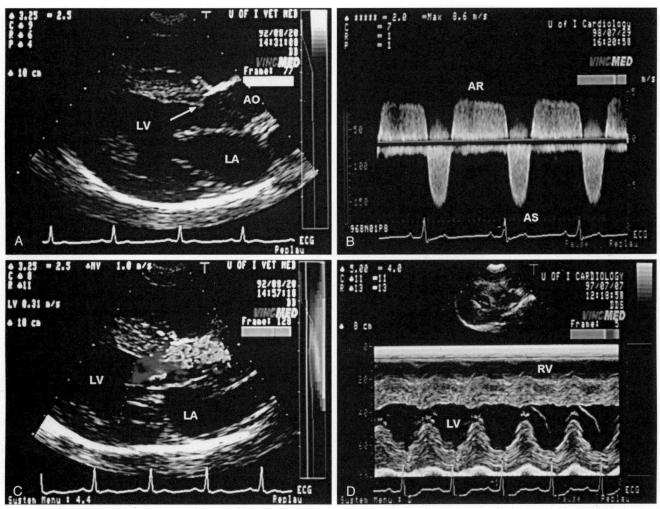

Figure 112–38. Representative echocardiographic findings in dogs with aortic stenosis. *A*, A visible ridge of tissue extending into the left ventricular outflow tract (LVOT) below the aortic valve (arrow), LV hypertrophy (modest in this dog), and post-stenotic dilatation of the aorta (not shown). *B*, High-velocity flow out of the LVOT, recorded with a continuous-wave Doppler transducer, in this case from the left apex. High-velocity flow away from the transducer is shown below the line (AS), and flow from coexisting aortic regurgitation is shown above the line. *C*, This black-and-white representation of a color flow echocardiogram is from the same dog as *(A)*. Note the disturbed blood flow in the proximal aorta. *D*, M-mode echocardiography is helpful for measuring wall thickness (very thick in this example from a dog with subaortic stenosis) and assessing contractility.

bypass the obstruction have either failed to achieve a sustained reduction of the systolic pressure gradient or they entail an unacceptable risk of complications.[56, 57] Moreover, these remedies are too limited in their availability and too expensive to be considered practical options.

Balloon catheter dilatation has also been effectively used to reduce the severity of obstruction in dogs with SAS, at least in the short term. On average, an immediate 50 per cent decrease in the gradient can be accomplished in dogs with SAS.[29b] However, this benefit attenuates in some (and perhaps a majority) over time.[48] Balloon dilatation in dogs with SAS is more difficult and more risky than balloon valvuloplasty in dogs with PS. Life-threatening complications of SAS include fatal arrhythmia during inflation, avulsion of the brachiocephalic artery during balloon withdrawal, and development of aortic endocarditis within a week or two of the procedure. The long-term results of balloon dilatation should soon be available, but the results of surgical dilatation cast a shadow of skepticism over this once promising remedy. Given the expense and limitations of surgery, balloon

dilatation of SAS will remain an option for at least some of the more severely affected dogs.

The authors often prescribe beta-adrenergic receptor blocking drugs empirically to dogs with high gradients (>75 to 100 mmHg) and to those dogs with a history of syncope or near-syncope (and without chronic heart failure). The observation of significant ST-T changes or frequent ventricular extrasystoles on a post-exercise or Holter ECG provides an additional impetus to recommend treatment. Atenolol is the drug most often used by the authors; but other beta blockers can also be used. Beta blockers reduce maximal heart rate and decrease myocardial oxygen consumption, thereby reducing ST segment changes and decreasing the frequency of ventricular extrasystoles. Moreover, dogs on high doses of beta blockers seem less willing (or are less able) to indulge in prolonged vigorous exercise. From a theoretical viewpoint, treatment with calcium channel blockers or angiotensin-converting enzyme may also be of value in dogs with SAS. None of these strategies has been proved effective in a controlled clinical trial.

PULMONIC AND AORTIC VALVE INSUFFICIENCY

Pulmonic Insufficiency

Primary congenital pulmonic insufficiency (PI) is an uncommon abnormality resulting from abnormal development of valve leaflets or dilation of the pulmonary artery annulus.[95a, 96a] Pulmonic valve insufficiency causes volume overload and eccentric hypertrophy of the right ventricle. The main and proximal branches of the right and left pulmonary arteries enlarge to accommodate the concomitant increase in stroke volume. Isolated pulmonic valve insufficiency is often well tolerated, but heart failure can develop when severe PI is induced experimentally in dogs. Congenital PI is more likely to cause heart failure if pulmonary vascular resistance subsequently increases as a result of severe pulmonary parenchymal or vascular disease. Mild PI occurs in most dogs with pulmonic valve stenosis, but occasionally PI is severe. Trivial PI is often observed in dogs with a PDA, presumably from dilation of the main pulmonary artery. PI can also develop solely as a consequence of pulmonary hypertension or as a result of surgery or balloon dilation to relieve PS.

Clinical features of PI include variable systolic (due to increased flow) and diastolic murmurs best heard at the left heart base. This to-and-fro murmur should not be confused with the continuous murmur of PDA. Fortunately, the supporting electrocardiographic and radiographic findings of these two conditions are quite dissimilar.[95a] Electrocardiograms from dogs with congenital PI may be normal or reflective of right ventricular hypertrophy. Thoracic radiographs show enlargement of the main pulmonary artery and right ventricle (Fig. 112–39), giving the erroneous impression of pulmonic stenosis to the uninitiated. Angiography (Fig. 112–40A and B) documents regurgitation of blood from the dilated pulmonary arteries (in excess of that expected from the catheter) and slow clearance of contrast from the

dilated and thin-walled right ventricle. Doppler echocardiography can demonstrate these same features without the expense or risks of anesthesia and cardiac catheterization (Fig. 112–40C). Doppler studies can also clarify the pathogenesis of PI. When the velocity of the regurgitant jet exceeds 3 m/s, pulmonary hypertension is the likely cause of the pulmonary artery dilatation and valvular insufficiency.

Treatment for PI has not been described in companion animals. Some dogs tolerate the lesion well, and medical therapy is not indicated unless signs of heart failure are observed.

Aortic Regurgitation

Isolated congenital aortic regurgitation (AR) is a rare disorder. It is occasionally detected in young or older dogs with idiopathic dilation of the aorta. One of the authors (Sisson) has documented mild to moderate aortic insufficiency in a Boxer dog and a hound with a quadricuspid aortic valve. AR is also being recognized with increasing frequency as a complication of other cardiac malformations.[108a, 109a] Aortic insufficiency often complicates subaortic stenosis and has been observed with ventricular septal defects, tetralogy of Fallot, and following balloon catheter dilation. The potential mechanisms for aortic valvular insufficiency in these conditions have been reviewed by Eyster et al.[108a] The to-and-fro systolic and diastolic murmurs resulting from AR are best heard over the left hemithorax, but many dogs with mild AR do not evidence an audible murmur. The diagnosis of AR is supported by palpation of a hyperkinetic arterial pulse. Left ventricular dilatation and hypertrophy develop in proportion to the severity of the leak. Severe AR often leads to left ventricular failure. Documentation of AR and estimation of its severity requires angiocardiography or Doppler echocardiography.

Definitive repair of AR requires cardiac bypass surgery and valve replacement. Arterial vasodilators reduce the re-

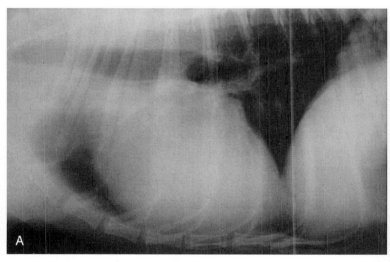

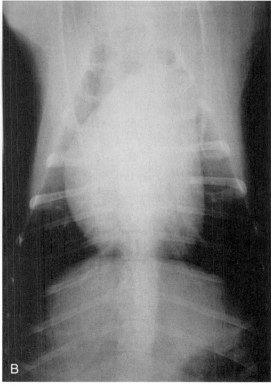

Figure 112–39. These radiographs from a Cavalier King Charles spaniel with congenital pulmonic valve insufficiency show convincing evidence of right ventricle enlargement in the lateral (A) and dorsoventral (B) projections. The pulmonary artery segment is markedly enlarged (see text for discussion).

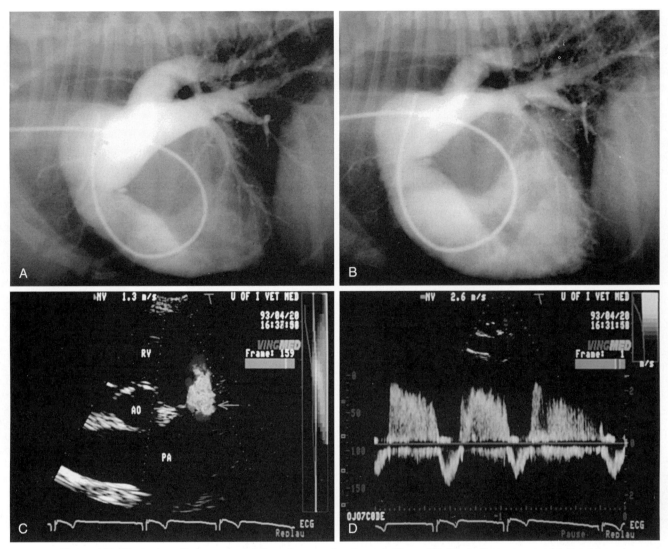

Figure 112–40. Angiocardiogram recorded from the same dog shown in Figure 112–39. *A,* Contrast material injected into the pulmonary artery leaks immediately back into the right ventricle (RV) through the incompetent tricuspid valve. *B,* Several frames later, the RV has filled with contrast, establishing substantial pulmonic valve incompetence. A dysplastic valve remnant is also visible. *C,* Color Doppler was performed several years later in the same dog. Disturbed flow entering the RV from the pulmonary artery is shown on this black-and-white rendition of a color study. Note the very dilated main pulmonary artery. *D,* Pulsed-wave Doppler shows that the diastolic flow is moving at a relatively low velocity (just over 2.0 m/s), excluding the possibility of pulmonary hypertension.

gurgitant volume and may delay the onset of heart failure. Treatment with angiotensin-converting enzyme inhibitors may also be beneficial.

DYSPLASIA OF THE ATRIOVENTRICULAR VALVES

Congenital malformations of the mitral and tricuspid valves are being reported with increasing frequency in both cats and dogs.[1–5, 58–62] [12a, 110a–121a] Functional sequelae to these malformations include mitral and tricuspid regurgitation, inflow obstruction, mitral or tricuspid valve stenosis, and dynamic obstruction of the LVOT. Mitral valve dysplasia is one of the most important congenital heart defects in cats. Malformed atrioventricular valves, as a general rule, are incompetent. In many ways, the pathophysiology and clinical course of congenital valvular insufficiency is similar to acquired degenerative valvular disease in the dog. For this reason, only the salient features of these conditions will be reviewed, and the reader is directed to Chapter 113 for

greater detail. Congenital stenosis of the atrioventricular valves is being recognized more frequently, clearly due to the increased utilization of Doppler echocardiography. The importance of mitral valve malformations in cats with dynamic outflow tract obstruction is unknown. The phenomenon of systolic excursion of the mitral apparatus into the outflow tract in cats has been largely associated with and attributed to hypertrophic cardiomyopathy (see Chapter 117). This traditional view is being challenged by the opposing notion that some dogs and cats develop LV hypertrophy secondary to primary mitral valve dysplasia and the dynamic obstruction.

Pathology and Pathogenesis

The causes of mitral and tricuspid valve dysplasia are unknown. Undoubtedly, a genetic basis exists in certain breeds (see Table 112–1); however, detailed breeding trials have not been reported. A wide spectrum of lesions has been identified in dogs and cats with atrioventricular valve malformations, including shortening, rolling, notching, and thickening of the valve leaflets; incomplete separation of valve components from the ventricular wall; elongation, shortening, fusion, and thickening of the chordae tendineae; direct insertion of the valve cusp into a papillary muscle; and atrophy, hypertrophy, fusion, and malpositioning of the papillary muscles and chordae tendineae.[113a–120a] The usual functional consequence of these changes is valvular insufficiency. Examples of mitral and tricuspid dysplasia in dogs and cats are shown in Figure 112–41A–F. Mitral valve dysplasia is particularly common in bull terriers, often occurring together with valvular or subvalvular aortic stenosis. Mitral stenosis is a unique form of mitral valve dysplasia in dogs, and it occurs most often in this breed (Fig. 112–42A and B).[40b] A rare and previously unreported parachute deformity of the mitral valve is shown in Figure 112–42C and D.

Whether some cases of tricuspid dysplasia represent Ebstein's anomaly is unresolved.[63] [120a, 121a] In the latter condition, the anomalous tricuspid valve is displaced down into the ventricle (Fig. 112–41C). Simultaneous intracardiac pressure and electrode studies are needed to document a ventricular electrogram in the lowermost portion of the downwardly displaced right atrium.[15a] Dogs and cats with mitral or tricuspid dysplasia can also have patency of the foramen ovale or a concurrent ASD, resulting in left-to-right or right-to-left shunting.

Pathophysiology

The essential pathophysiologic abnormalities of the various types of atrioventricular valve malformations are briefly summarized here. Valve regurgitation causes volume overloading, atrial dilation, and eccentric hypertrophy on the affected side. Congestive heart failure often develops at a very young age. Valve stenosis obstructs ventricular filling, thereby limiting cardiac output. Syncope or collapse with exertion may occur. The atrium behind the stenotic valve is hypertrophied and dilated, and increased left or right atrial pressure results in pulmonary edema or ascites, respectively. Pulmonary hypertension and right heart failure can develop secondary to mitral stenosis when left atrial pressures are chronically elevated. Dogs and cats with congenital valvular stenosis or regurgitation are predisposed to cardiac arrhythmia, particularly atrial fibrillation. The consequences of atrial fibrillation are devastating in both circumstances. The potential for right to left shunting through the foramen ovale or an ASD is fully realized in some cases of tricuspid dysplasia.

Clinical Findings

Cats, great Danes, German shepherds, bull terriers, golden retrievers, Newfoundlands, Dalmations, and mastiffs are predisposed to mitral dysplasia.[30b, 111a–114a] Tricuspid dysplasia

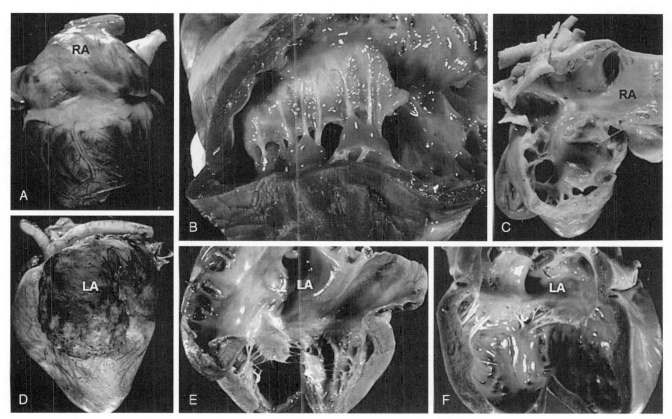

Figure 112–41. Pathology specimens of tricuspid valve dysplasia *(A, B, C)* and mitral valve dysplasia *(D, E, F)* obtained from dogs *(A, B, F)* and cats *(C, D, E)*. Animals with atrioventricular valve dysplasia often have a tremendously enlarged atrium. *A,* The large right atrium seen in *(B)* resulted from the malformation shown in *(B)*. *B,* Note the similarity of this curtain-like deformity of the tricuspid valve to that shown in Figure 112–25. *C,* This example of tricuspid valve dysplasia shows some of the pathologic features of Ebstein's anomaly, as the tricuspid valve is displaced into the right ventricle. The papillary muscles also form a peculiar pattern. *D,* Marked left atrial dilatation in a cat with mitral valve dysplasia. *E,* The mitral valve in this cat shows a bizarre malformation of the anterior (cranioventral) leaflet. Also, the posterior (caudodorsal) papillary muscle is abnormally located, and it attaches directly to the leaflet with no intervening chordae. *F,* This puppy with mitral valve dysplasia died from congestive heart failure. The papillary muscles are small and dorsally displaced. The chordae tendineae are short and thickened. The chambers of the left heart are markedly dilated.

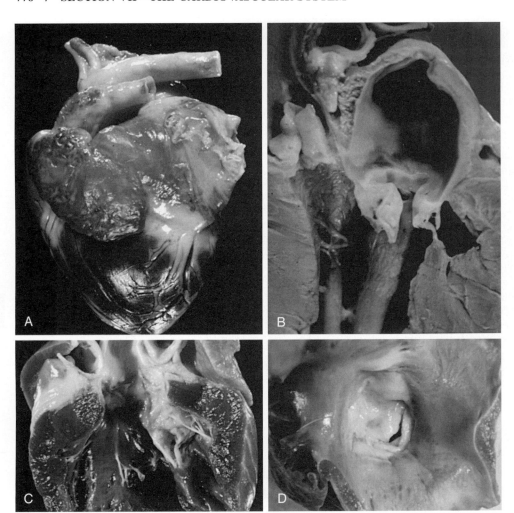

Figure 112–42. Pathology specimens from dogs with congenital mitral valve stenosis. *A,* Marked dilatation of the left atrium is seen as a result of obstructed flow into the left ventricle. *B,* This grossly distorted mitral valve was from a bull terrier with concurrent stenosis and insufficiency of the mitral valve. A thickened aortic valve, causing mild aortic stenosis, is just visible on the left side of the picture. *C,* Parachute deformity of the mitral valve results when all or most of the chordae tendineae insert on a single papillary muscle. *D,* This skyline view of a stenotic mitral valve is from the same dog shown in *(A)* and *(C)*. This dog suffered from intermittent left and right heart failure as it also developed pulmonary hypertension, presumably as a result of the parachute mitral valve deformity.

occurs in cats but seems to be most common in large male dogs.[9a] Old English sheepdogs, German shepherds, Weimaraners, and Labrador retrievers are at increased risk. Presenting signs, if any, are referable to exercise intolerance or to right, left, or biventricular congestive heart failure. The hallmark of valvular insufficiency is a holosystolic murmur heard best over the affected valve area. A loud gallop may also be detected.[111a] A soft diastolic murmur is sometimes auscultated in dogs or cats with valvular stenosis (Fig. 112–43), but this finding is often absent or missed.

Left or right atrial enlargement is seen with mitral dysplasia or tricuspid dysplasia, respectively. Evidence of ventricular enlargement is common in animals with valvular insufficiency but is not present with isolated valvular stenosis. Splintered QRS complexes (Rr', RR', rR', rr') are a distinctive and common finding in dogs and cats with tricuspid dysplasia (Fig. 112–44).[64] Atrial arrhythmias, especially atrial fibrillation, are recorded in some affected animals. The patterns of chamber enlargement on the thoracic radiographs (Fig. 112–45) generally reflect the involvement of the tricuspid or mitral valve and the functional consequences of the offending defect. The possibility of valvular stenosis should be considered whenever the atrium is markedly dilated without enlargement of the ipsilateral ventricle. Both chambers will be enlarged when the valve is insufficient.

Definitive diagnosis of atrioventricular valve malformation requires echocardiography or cardiac catheterization and angiocardiography. Abnormal location, shape, motion, or attachment of the valve apparatus is observed by echocardi-

ography (Fig. 112–46).[62] [39b, 40b] In case of valve stenosis, a diastolic jet is seen traversing the stenotic orifice during the color Doppler examination (Fig. 112–46C and D). Transvalvular flow velocities are increased, and the EF slope is reduced, compared with the normal Doppler measures, reflecting the presence and severity of the diastolic pressure. Doppler echocardiography can also document the regurgitant jet in cases of valvular insufficiency and increased outflow tract velocities in animals with dynamic LVOT obstruction.

Left Apex
log-log

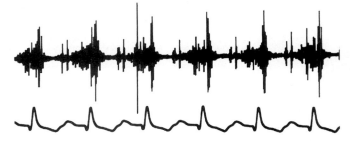

Figure 112–43. This phonocardiogram was recorded from a bull terrier with mitral valve stenosis. Note that the murmur occurs during the diastolic interval. The extra heart sound near S_2 was not specifically identified but could be an opening snap of a stenotic mobile valve. Feel free to speculate.

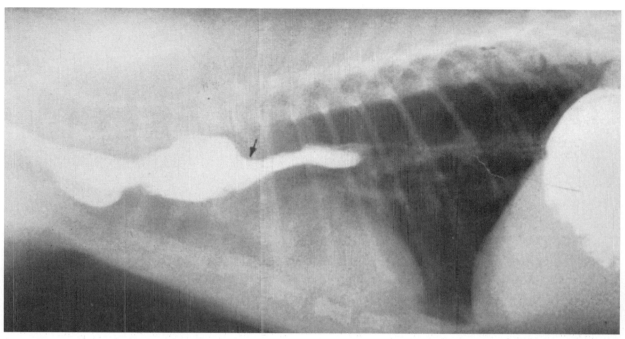

Figure 112–44. Persistent right aortic arch in a cat. The barium swallow indicates constriction of the esophagus at the base of the heart (arrow).

In dogs or cats with valvular insufficiency, the ventricular injection of contrast material outlines a dilated ventricle, regurgitant valve orifice, and a dilated atrium (Fig. 112–47). Demonstration of tricuspid valve stenosis is easily demonstrated by recording the diastolic pressure gradient across the tricuspid valve and by injecting contrast material into the right atrium. Demonstration of mitral valve stenosis can be accomplished by trans-septal catheterization of the left atrium or by injecting contrast material into the pulmonary arteries and allowing it to pass into the left heart.

Clinical Management

The natural history of atrioventricular valve dysplasia has not been reported. In the authors' experience, some animals tolerate what appears to be a serious defect for many years. In other cases there is rapid progression to heart failure and death. Only the most severely affected animals are likely to be described in clinical reports. These papers have emphasized that heart failure and atrial arrhythmias often develop within the first year of life.[114a, 119a] Surgical replacement of the dysplastic valve has been successfully accomplished in a small number of animals.[65–67] Partially successful balloon valvuloplasty has also been described in one dog with tricuspid stenosis.[68]

In most affected animals, medical treatment is instituted only when heart failure develops. Treatment of valvular insufficiency consists largely of diuretics, an ACE inhibitor and/or vasodilators, and digoxin. Diuretics are also used to control edema in animals with stenotic valves. Tachycardia

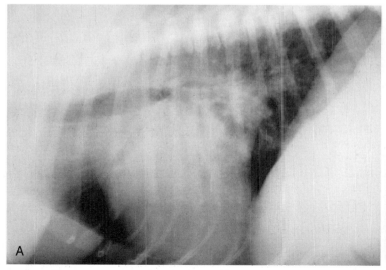
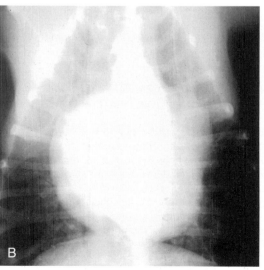

Figure 112–45. These chest radiographs were recorded from a bull terrier with mitral valve stenosis. Note the marked left atrial enlargement visible on the lateral (A) and dorsoventral (B) projections. The pulmonary veins are distended, and there is mild pulmonary congestion. The right heart also appears enlarged.

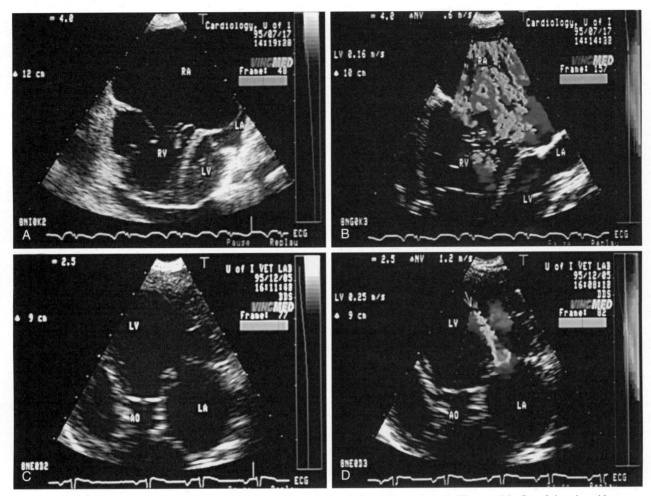

Figure 112–46. Echocardiograms from two dogs with atrioventricular malformations. *A*, The septal leaflet of the tricuspid valve is tethered to the interventricular septum, resulting in severe tricuspid valve dysplasia. The right heart chambers are very dilated. *B*, This color-flow echocardiogram shows a huge turbulent jet filling the right atrium. *C*, Incomplete opening of the mitral valve recorded at the point of maximal diastolic excursion in a bull terrier. The left atrium is moderately dilated. Also note the thick (hyperechoic) aortic valve leaflet on this diastolic frame. *D*, Color Doppler recordings (black-and-white rendition) confirmed mitral valve stenosis as a narrow diastolic jet streamed into the left ventricle during diastole.

is poorly tolerated in these patients, and every effort should be made to avoid stress and exercise. Administration of beta blockers, calcium channel blockers, and/or digoxin are helpful in some cases. The same drugs are useful for the management of atrial fibrillation, the onset of which is typically characterized by sudden and severe congestive heart failure (see Chapter 114).

ANOMALOUS DEVELOPMENT OF THE ATRIA, COR TRIATRIATUM, AND COR TRIATRIATUM DEXTER

Cor triatriatum has been reported in cats,[69] [156a] and cor triatriatum dexter and other saccular anomalies of the caudal right atrium have been seen in dogs and cats.[70–72] [33b, 156a–158a] In cor triatriatum the venous drainage enters an additional, accessory atrial chamber, which is separated from the true atrium by a membrane. When the membrane is obstructive, dilation of the venous chamber and the entering veins is evident, and congestion develops in the lungs. In contrast to mitral stenosis, blood flows through the stenotic orifice during both systole and diastole. This aside, the functional consequences of these defects are very similar. One of the authors (Thomas) has evaluated several cats that appear to have supravalvular mitral stenosis. The distinction between

this defect and cor triatriatum is the location of the obstructing membrane. With supravalvular mitral stenosis, the membrane is located ventral to the foramen ovale, whereas the membrane is located dorsally with true cor triatriatum. If the foramen ovale is closed, there is no functional difference between these defects. Affected cats typically present with signs of pulmonary congestion.

Cor triatriatum dexter results from persistence of the embryologic right sinus venosus valve.[71] In dogs with this malformation, the right atrium is partitioned by a diaphragm located caudal to the tricuspid valve and foramen ovale. Affected dogs present with ascites but without jugular distention or an audible murmur. Other clinical findings include diarrhea and prominence of the cutaneous abdominal veins. Congenital obstructions of the caudal vena cava can present with similar clinical findings. Electrocardiography is normal in most affected dogs, and thoracic radiographs are unremarkable with the notable exception of caudal vena cava enlargement. Diagnosis can be accomplished by echocardiography or angiography. One of the authors (Bonagura) has examined cats with saccular dilations of the caudal right atrium. These protruded into the left hemithorax but did not cause clinical signs.

Treatment for cor triatriatum and its right-sided counterpart generally requires surgical resection or bypass of the

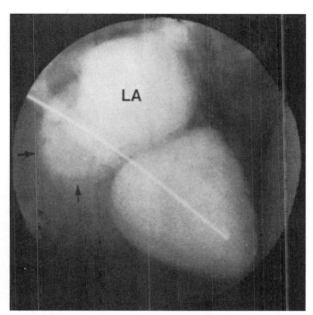

Figure 112–47. Angiocardiogram from a cat with mitral valve dysplasia. Following injection of contrast into the left ventricle, there is opacification of the dilated left atrium (LA) and the left auricular appendage (arrows). The left ventricle is significantly enlarged.

obstruction.[73, 74] Balloon dilation of the obstructing membrane can also be attempted.

LESIONS CAUSING RIGHT-TO-LEFT SHUNTING

CYANOTIC HEART DISEASE

The term "cyanotic congenital heart disease" is both useful and misleading. Whereas most clinicians immediately think of lesions that cause pulmonary to systemic shunting, such as the tetralogy of Fallot, a wide variety of malformations can induce arterial hypoxemia and cyanosis. Moreover, when congenital heart malformations of any type lead to congestive heart failure with pulmonary dysfunction, cyanosis can develop. Thus, the pup or kitten with left-to-right shunting PDA, left ventricular overload, pulmonary edema, and ventilation/perfusion inequality is as likely to be blue as the pup with the tetralogy of Fallot. Still, cyanotic heart disease is a useful designation for classifying a variety of conditions that result in systemic arterial desaturation.[122a–147a] Because the pathophysiology and clinical signs of these conditions are similar, they will be considered as a group. Only the most important defects are discussed to illustrate the clinical syndrome common to these conditions.

Pathophysiology of Cyanotic Heart Disease

Mechanisms of Right-to-Left Shunting

In order for desaturated venous blood to shunt into the systemic arteries, there must be either a transposition of the great vessels (or systemic veins) or a defect between pulmonary and systemic circulations and a mechanism to raise pressure on the right side of the circulation. A septal defect between the atria, ventricles, or aorticopulmonary trunk causes blood to flow from the path of greatest to least resistance and pressure. Accordingly, right-to-left shunting generally will not develop unless there is an obstruction to

blood flow on the right side of the circulation or there is a substantial increase in pulmonary vascular resistance. Tricuspid stenosis (or atresia) and pulmonic stenosis (or atresia) are examples of obstructive right heart lesions. The term Eisenmenger's physiology (or syndrome) refers to that situation wherein a left-to-right shunt reverses to right to left in response to marked increases in pulmonary vascular resistance.[148a–150a] The factors underlying the development of pulmonary hypertension are incompletely understood in children and in animals.[15a, 49a, 60a, 148a, 150a] Cardiologists are aware of the association between large-bore defects and pulmonary vascular disease. Reversed shunting has been observed with PDA, aorticopulmonary communication, VSD, and ASD. Although the number of exceptions is growing, Eisenmenger's syndrome usually develops rapidly in small animals and almost always before 6 months of age.

The anatomic changes in the muscular and small pulmonary arteries observed in dogs and cats with Eisenmenger's physiology are similar to those of humans as described by Edwards and Heath and amended by Roberts.[15a, 148a] Intimal thickening, medial hypertrophy, and plexiform lesions are the salient abnormalities in most cases. The plexiform lesion is considered irreversible consequently, neither medical therapy nor closure of the shunt will effectively improve the condition once these lesions have developed. In fact, surgical closure of the shunt pathway forces the right ventricle to work against a tremendous resistance, because the systemic circulation, which acts as a "pop-off" valve, can no longer be accessed. Such closure usually causes a marked decline in cardiac output, right ventricular failure, and death. Thus, a reversed PDA should not be closed surgically.

Effects of Hypoxemia

Systemic hypoxemia is best detected by measuring the oxygen content (and partial pressure) in an arterial blood sample obtained while the animal breathes room air. Providing 100 per cent oxygen does not significantly improve the hypoxemia caused by right-to-left shunting.[15a] Clinical signs of cyanotic heart disease are a result of tissue hypoxia and include stunting, weakness, anxiety, syncope, and seizures.[5a–9a, 15a, 59a, 137a–139a] Because systemic hypoxemia increases plasma erythropoietin concentrations, secondary polycythemia develops in most dogs and cats with cyanotic heart disease. When the PCV exceeds the 65 to 68 per cent range, hyperviscosity can predispose to thrombosis and microvascular complications.[15a, 148a] Metabolic acidosis is another potential complication of protracted hypoxemia.[15a, 59a]

Systemic Pulmonary Resistance

The magnitude of right-to-left shunting fluctuates with the systemic vascular resistance or the ratio of pulmonary to systemic resistance.[15a] Exercise promotes peripheral arteriolar vasodilation and decreases the systemic/pulmonary resistance ratio, thereby increasing the magnitude of right-to-left shunting. Tachycardia or elevated sympathetic tone can increase the magnitude of right-to-left shunting in dogs and cats with right ventricular hypertrophy and a VSD. This phenomenon is explained by the development or exacerbation of dynamic right ventricular outflow tract obstruction, increased resistance to ejection, and a corresponding reduction in pulmonary blood flow.[15a] Beta-adrenergic blocking drugs are used to blunt or prevent this phenomenon in some forms of cyanotic heart disease.[139a, 140a] These drugs also

CV

tend to limit exercise, offering another explanation for their efficacy in some patients. Anemia or even relative anemia (normal hematocrit level in a hypoxemic patient) reduces the ratio of systemic to pulmonary resistance when the pulmonary resistance is fixed.[138a] By this mechanism, overzealous phlebotomy can increase the severity of arterial hypoxemia just as it decreases the oxygen-carrying capacity of blood. The effects of phlebotomy on systemic/pulmonary resistance has not been studied in animals with pulmonary hypertension.

Additional Circulatory Factors

Right-to-left shunting leads to compensatory increases in nutritive blood flow to the lung via the bronchial arteries. These tortuous systemic collateral vessels are easily recognized at angiography. Blood from these vessels may return via the pulmonary veins and increase venous admixture. While uncommon, it is possible for these vessels to rupture, leading to hemoptysis. Another potential problem in right-to-left shunting is paradoxical embolization. This is defined as a venous-to-systemic embolus. Normally, the pulmonary vasculature filters systemic venous emboli before they can reach the left side of the circulation. With reversed shunting, the possibility of coronary, cerebral, or other systemic emboli must always be considered, particularly when intravenous catheters are used. Clots, bacteria, or air may gain access to vital organs by this mechanism.

Clinical Evaluation of the Cyanotic Heart Disease Patient

History and Physical Examination

Most cases of cyanotic congenital heart disease encountered in veterinary medicine are associated with pulmonic stenosis, pulmonary hypertension, or tricuspid valve disease. In the last case, shunting is invariably across an ASD or patent foramen ovale. Presenting signs include failure to grow, cyanosis, shortness of breath, exercise intolerance, weakness, syncope, and seizures. Affected animals often gasp when stressed. Arterial P_{O_2}, and P_{CO_2} are decreased. These animals may develop adverse reactions (particularly bradycardia) to sedatives and tranquilizers and may not improve appreciably following administration of supplemental oxygen. Most cases are polycythemic, but the hemoglobin concentration must be compared with that in age-matched normal animals.[128a] Clinical features of Eisenmenger's syndrome tend to be similar, regardless of the underlying lesions, whereas reversed shunting associated with tetralogy of Fallot differs in some important ways.[8a, 9a, 128a] One important auscultatory feature of Eisenmenger's syndrome is the loud or split-second heart sound of pulmonary hypertension. This may be the only audible abnormality, and it is lacking in tetralogy of Fallot. An ejection sound with a soft, short, systolic murmur also may be evident at the left heart base in dogs with Eisenmenger's syndrome. Diastolic murmurs of pulmonic insufficiency are rare in the authors' experience.

Cyanotic heart disease, with rare exception (tricuspid atresia and anomalous systemic venous return), is characterized by right ventricular hypertrophy, which is usually evident on an echocardiogram, ECG, and the thoracic radiograph. However, marked cardiomegaly is atypical of most cyanotic cardiac conditions, and the heart often does not appear enlarged on survey films. As a general rule, the lungs appear underperfused in cyanotic heart diseases.[24a] The main pulmonary artery and proximal lobar arteries are dilated when Eisenmenger's syndrome is the basis for reversed shunting, but they are not enlarged in tetralogy of Fallot or pulmonary or tricuspid atresia.

Echocardiography

The echocardiogram is very helpful in assessing the cyanotic patient because most large defects can be easily visualized, the right ventricular inflow and outflow tracts can be evaluated, and the site of right-to-left shunting can be identified through echocontrast or by color-flow imaging.[15b] Detailed ultrasound studies often make cardiac catheterization unnecessary, unless surgery is contemplated and pulmonary hypertension (as opposed to pulmonic stenosis) cannot otherwise be ruled out. Estimation of pulmonary vascular pressures can be easily accomplished by measuring the peak velocity of even a small jet of pulmonic valve insufficiency. A peak velocity of <2.2 m/s (corresponding to a pulmonary artery–right ventricular diastolic gradient of 10 mmHg) precludes a diagnosis of pulmonary hypertension. The same conclusion is reached when the velocity of a tricuspid insufficiency jet velocity is <3.3 m/s in the absence of right heart failure.

Cardiac Catheterization

Cardiac catheterization and angiocardiography are invaluable for the evaluation of cyanotic patients, particularly when an uncommon or complex defect is suspected. In addition to showing the location and severity of the shunt, angiography outlines the anatomy of the defect (pulmonic stenosis, tricuspid dysplasia) and permits visualization of the pulmonary vasculature. Direct measurements of intravascular pressure are invaluable for assessing pulmonic stenosis severity and for confirming the presence of pulmonary hypertension or tricuspid valve stenosis. Measurement of pulmonary artery pressure is essential when cardiac or vascular surgery is contemplated in a patient with cyanotic heart disease. When pulmonary vascular resistance is normal, pulmonary flow can be augmented and systemic hypoxemia improved by creation of the shunt between a systemic and a pulmonary artery.[15a, 128a, 136a, 141a] Elevated pulmonary vascular resistance negates the usefulness of such surgery as left-to-right shunting cannot be successfully produced. Angiocardiograms in complicated cyanotic heart disease can be very confusing. For this reason, it is helpful to include a vena caval and possibly a right atrial injection of contrast material in the angiographic series. The operator must also watch for abnormal catheter positions as a clue to large septal defects and vessel transpositions.

Tetralogy of Fallot

The four salient anatomic features of the tetralogy of Fallot include right ventricular outflow obstruction (pulmonic stenosis), secondary right ventricular hypertrophy, a subaortic VSD, and an overriding aorta (see Fig. 112–13D). Pulmonic stenosis can occur in combination with an isolated VSD, producing similar but not identical findings. In these defects the infundibular septum is not malaligned, the aorta is normal sized, and the infundibulum of the right ventricle not narrowed.[75] These distinctions are commonly ignored in veterinary patients because corrective surgery is rarely performed.

Pathogenesis

Patterson and colleagues studied this malformation in keeshond breeding colonies and observed a spectrum of lesions, ranging from the subclinical to the clinically complicated.[31b, 124a–127a] Patterson graded the conotruncal defects pathologically as follows. Grade 1: persistence of the conus septum fusion line, aneurysm of the ventricular septum, and absence of the papillary muscle of the conus (these represent the subclinical malformations). Grade 2: pulmonic stenosis or VSD, plus the grade 1 lesions. Grade 3: tetralogy of Fallot: pulmonic stenosis, VSD, and dextropositioned aorta (with secondary right ventricular hypertrophy), plus the grade 1 lesions. Additional abnormalities found in some dogs included dilated and tortuous ascending aorta, pulmonary atresia, hypoplasia of the supraventricular crest, and anomalies of the aortic arch system. Early studies suggested that the transmission of conotruncal defects best fit a polygenic model with multiple thresholds. Based on more recent studies, Patterson et al[76] has concluded that conotruncal defects are inherited in an autosomal recessive trait with variable expression. According to Patterson: "the mutant CTD allele causes conotruncal malformations in homozygous animals by interfering with myocardial growth in the conotruncus during the critical window of conotruncal septation." The reader is referred to the excellent studies of Patterson et al for further detail.[76 [4a, 124a–127a]]

Pathophysiology

As with other right-to-left shunts, the essential components are the increased right-sided resistance and pressure and the communication between pulmonary and systemic circulations. As a result of the outflow obstruction and elevated right ventricular pressure, desaturated blood shunts through the septal defect to mix with blood coming from the left ventricle.[122a–123a] Pulmonary arterial flow and venous return are scant, and the left atrium and left ventricular cavity remain small as a result. The addition of unoxygenated blood from the right ventricle to the systemic side of the circulation causes arterial hypoxemia, decreased hemoglobin oxygen saturation, cyanosis, and secondary polycythemia. Systemic collateral circulation increases via the bronchial arterial system. These vessels supply blood to the capillaries of the pulmonary parenchyma either directly or via anastomosing connections with a larger pulmonary artery. A substantial portion of this blood can participate in pulmonary gas exchange. Other aspects of clinical pathophysiology have been previously described (see Clinical Manifestations of Cyanotic Heart Disease).

Clinical Findings

Tetralogy of Fallot is common in the keeshond and English bulldog and in some families of other breeds. It has also been recognized in the cat.[9a] Presenting complaints and clinical complications are similar to those previously described for cyanotic heart disease. In cyanotic patients, the murmur of the tetralogy of Fallot is produced by blood flowing through the stenotic defect.[75] Murmurs in dogs with severe pulmonic stenosis and a small restrictive VSD also sound like isolated pulmonic stenosis. The murmur of the VSD predominates only when pulmonic stenosis is mild and left-to-right shunting occurs across the VSD, i.e., such as in an acyanotic defect. Some dogs have no obvious murmur. This phenomenon is related to pulmonary atresia and/or polycythemia with hyperviscosity (which decreases turbulence) and ejection across a large, nonrestrictive VSD. Cyanosis occurs in the classic, fully manifested form of tetralogy of Fallot, but acyanotic cases are not uncommon. Exercise or excitement may induce or exacerbate cyanosis by accentuating right-to-left shunting

Radiography usually shows a small or normal-sized heart with rounding of the right ventricular border (Fig. 112–48).

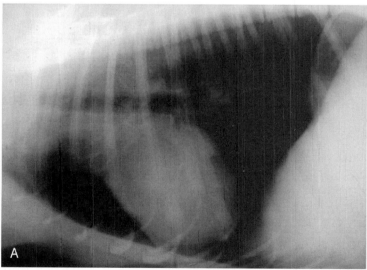
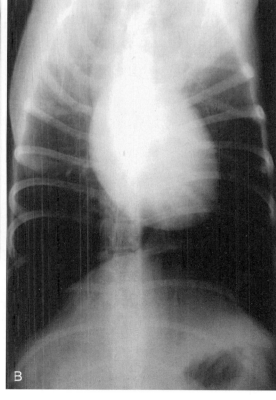

Figure 112–48. These radiographs are from a keeshond dog with tetralogy of Fallot. *A,* The heart appears small, and the pulmonary vessels are difficult to identify. In the dorsoventral projection *(B)* the heart assumes the shape of a golf club (wood). This appearance is due to enlargement of the right ventricle, a small left heart, and hypoplasia of the pulmonary artery.

CV

The main pulmonary artery is not enlarged, in contrast to the usual finding in cases of pulmonic stenosis with an intact ventricular septum. The pulmonary circulation is diminished, and the left auricle may be inconspicuous subsequent to decreased venous return. While the ECG usually exhibits a right-axis deviation, a left or cranial axis may be found in some cases.[129a] Echocardiography reveals right ventricular hypertrophy, small left chamber dimensions, a large subaortic VSD, and right ventricular outflow obstruction (see Fig. 112–20D and E). Doppler studies document right-to-left shunting at the ventricular outflow level (see Fig. 112–20F).[130a]

Cardiac catheterization demonstrates virtual equilibration of left and right ventricular systolic pressures in most cases, compatible with a large VSD.[128a] An oxygen step-down is recorded at the left ventricular outflow level, and the aortic blood is relatively desaturated. Angiocardiography reveals right ventricular hypertrophy; narrowing of the right ventricle infundibulum; pulmonic stenosis with minimal post-stenotic dilatation; a large subaortic VSD; a small, dorsally displaced left ventricle; an enlarged and overriding aorta; and prominent bronchial circulation (Fig. 112–49).[124a–128a] Either valvular or subvalvular pulmonic stenosis, or both, may be found. Bidirectional shunting across the VSD is common in the anesthetized animal. Anticoagulation therapy (e.g., heparin) should be considered to prevent cerebral embolization during and immediately after cardiac catheterization.

Clinical Management

The *natural history* of tetralogy of Fallot in dogs and cats is not well characterized. Many affected animals are severely limited in their activities. Like other cyanotic heart diseases, this defect can be tolerated for years, provided pulmonary blood flow is maintained and hyperviscosity is controlled. In cases of pulmonary atresia, pulmonary blood flow must be derived from a PDA, a bronchial artery, or an elaborate network of systemic collaterals. Sudden death is common, related to complications of hypoxia, hyperviscosity, or cardiac arrhythmia. Unlike pulmonic stenosis with an intact ventricular septum, congestive heart failure is extremely unlikely.

Both medical and surgical *therapy* can be employed in the management of tetralogy of Fallot. Although definitive correction of the defect (closing the VSD and removing or bypassing the pulmonic stenosis) can be done as part of cardiopulmonary bypass, such surgery is rarely performed in animals.[77] The pulmonic stenosis should not be relieved if the VSD cannot be closed because marked left-to-right shunting with subsequent left ventricular failure may develop.[128a] Surgical palliation through the creation of a systemic-to-pulmonary shunt can be quite rewarding.[78, 79 [128a, 141a] Subclavian to pulmonary artery (Blalock-Taussig), ascending aorta to pulmonary artery (Potts), and aorta to right pulmonary artery (Waterston-Cooley) connections have been made in dogs and cats. By increasing pulmonary venous return, left heart size increases, and there is a greater contribution of oxygenated blood to the systemic circulation. The size of the shunt must be controlled to prevent overloading of the diminutive left ventricle and subsequent pulmonary edema. The extent to which these shunts remain patent postoperatively has not been reported.

Periodic phlebotomy, performed to maintain the PCV between 62 and 68 percent, produces a satisfactory result in most cases. Excessive bleeding should be avoided, and the blood that is withdrawn should be replaced with crystalloid

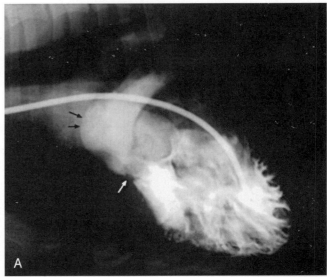

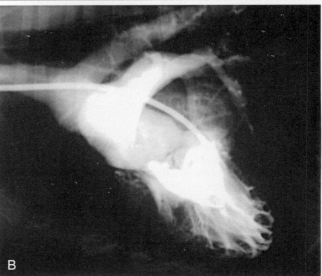

Figure 112–49. Right heart angiocardiogram in a keeshond with tetralogy of Fallot; same dog shown in Figure 112–48. *A,* The presence of a large, nonrestrictive, ventricular septal defect (VSD) allowed filling of both the right ventricle (RV) and left ventricle. The outflow region of the RV appears narrowed (white arrow), and the suspicion of pulmonic stenosis is supported by identification of a post-stenotic dilatation of the main pulmonary artery (black arrows). *B,* The contrast agent that first appeared in the pulmonary artery and aorta in *(A)* is more obvious, confirming the presence of a right-to-left shunt. The location of a large VSD is more obvious, and an enlarged aorta is seen overriding this defect (dextropositioning of the aorta).

fluids to maintain cardiac output and tissue oxygen delivery.[138a] Some children with tetralogy of Fallot benefit from beta blockade with propranolol; however, controlled studies of the clinical efficacy of this treatment in animals have not been reported.[139a, 140a] Severe hypoxic spells should be treated with cage rest, oxygen, and sodium bicarbonate (if metabolic acidosis is evident). Drugs with marked systemic vasodilating properties should be avoided.

Other Causes of Cyanotic Congenital Heart Disease

Pulmonary Atresia

Pulmonary atresia with a VSD is essentially an exaggerated form of tetralogy of Fallot. All of the blood ejected from the right heart is shunted right to left across a large

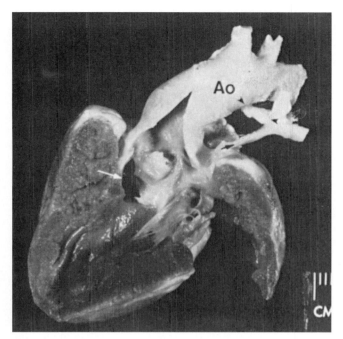

Figure 112–50. Tetralogy of Fallot. From a cat with tetralogy of Fallot and pulmonary artery atresia (pseudotruncus arteriosus). The left ventricle has been opened to expose the large ventricular septal defect (white arrow), the hypoplastic pulmonary artery (small arrow), and the dilated aorta (Ao). Pulmonary flow was through the ductus arteriosus, the origin and termination of which are shown by arrowheads. While the lobar pulmonary arteries were patent almost no blood was found in the main pulmonary artery.

VSD and into a much enlarged aorta (often referred to as a pseudotruncus arteriosus). The term "pseudotruncus arteriosus" has been used to describe this defect because a superficial inspection of the heart shows a single vessel arising from both ventricles (Fig. 112–50). Careful dissection reveals an imperforate pulmonic valve and a vestigial cord representing the main pulmonary trunk.

Aortic Atresia

Aortic atresia with a hypoplastic left heart is a rare form of cyanotic heart disease in dogs. The aortic orifice is often imperforate, the ascending aorta is hypoplastic, and the mitral valve is usually atretic or hypoplastic (Fig. 112–51). In the absence of a VSD, the left ventricle is very small; when a VSD is present, the left ventricle is better developed. The right heart supplies the entire pulmonary and systemic circulations, resulting in profound cyanosis and, in most cases, early death.

Tricuspid Valve Atresia

Tricuspid valve dysplasia, particularly atresia or stenosis of the valve, can cause cyanosis because the elevated right atrial pressure behind the obstruction may maintain patency of the foramen ovale or shunt through an ASD.[117a] In some cases, the pulmonic valve is also atretic (Fig. 112–52). The right ventricle is small or hypoplastic unless there is an associated VSD, in which case there may be a functional remnant of the ventricular outflow tract. The combination of severe pulmonic stenosis with an ASD can also cause cyanosis through increased diastolic pressures in the right heart.

Double Outlet Right Ventricle

Double outlet right ventricle, wherein both great vessels exit from the right ventricle, has been reported in dogs and cats.[146a, 147a] A VSD provides the left ventricle with an avenue for outflow into the great vessels. Pulmonary overcirculation is present unless there is pulmonic stenosis or pulmonary hypertension develops. Cyanosis is likely based on the origin of the aorta and is most severe if there is pulmonic stenosis or pulmonary hypertension.

Transposition of the Great Arteries

In dextro-transposition of the great arteries, the aorta originates from the right ventricle and the pulmonary trunk from the left ventricle.[15a, 145a] In the pure and fatal case, two independent circulations exist, and the systemic arteries never receive oxygenated blood. Survival of an animal with dextro-transposition depends on the presence (or production)

Figure 112–51. This specimen is from a dog that exhibited severe cyanosis from birth. *A,* The proximal aorta is hypoplastic, and an aortic opening (valve) could not be identified. A huge pulmonary artery gives origin to the right and left pulmonary branches, and a large patent ductal segment connects to the aortic arch, supplying the brachiocephalic vessels, the descending aorta, and the hypoplastic aorta. *B,* Note the marked hypertrophy of the opened right ventricle and the ventricular septal defect that received blood from the underdeveloped left heart.

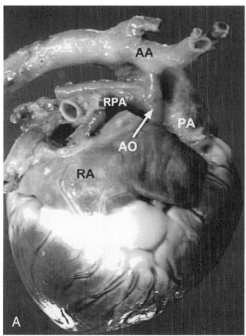

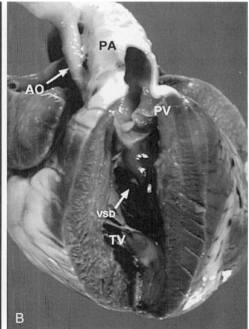

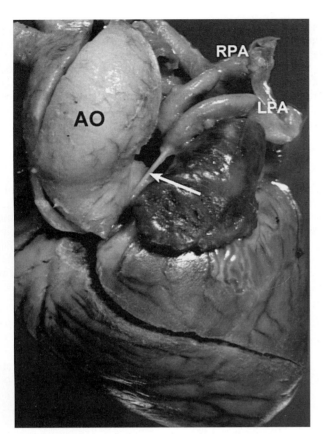

Figure 112–52. This specimen of pulmonary atresia (arrow) superficially resembles that shown in Figure 112–50. In this instance, there was no ventricular septal defect, excluding the possibility of a conotruncal defect. Instead, there was a large atrial septal defect. The lungs were supplied entirely by the brachial artery and systemic collateral vessels.

of shunts between the two circulations to allow for mixing of blood to prevent fatal hypoxemia. These defects are complex, generally lethal, and probably underdiagnosed in animals, relative to children, because neonatal care is rarely supervised by veterinarians.

MISCELLANEOUS CARDIAC DEFECTS

The potential for different anatomic forms and physiologic variants of congenital heart disease is tremendous, and it is beyond the scope of this chapter to discuss rare malformations. The following section summarizes clinically relevant aspects of cardiac and pericardial defects not yet discussed.

Endocardial fibroelastosis has been reported in dogs and cats and is probably familial in some lines of Burmese and Siamese cats.[79] [12a, 13a, 36a, 151a–155a] The gross anatomic findings include left ventricular and left atrial dilatation, with severe endocardial thickening grossly characterized by diffuse, white, opaque thickening of the luminal lining. Histologic lesions in the cat include diffuse hypocellular, fibroelastic thickening of the endocardium with layering of thin, randomly organized collagen and elastic fibers.[151a, 153a] Edema of the endocardium with dilatation of lymphatics is prominent, and there is no evidence of myocardial inflammation or necrosis.

The clinical features of endocardial fibroelastosis include early development of left or biventricular failure, generally before six months of age. Mitral regurgitation may be detected. Left ventricular and atrial dilatation are evident on radiographs and on the ECG. Limited echocardiographic

studies performed to date suggest reduction of left ventricular myocardial function, as opposed to pure valvular disease in which shortening fraction tends to be normal or increased.[155a] Left ventricular diastolic pressures are elevated at catheterization, compatible with ventricular stiffness, ventricular failure, or volume overload from mitral regurgitation.[155a]

The diagnosis of primary endocardial fibroelastosis is, at times, tenuous, inasmuch as chronic left ventricular dilatation may lead to similar changes, particularly in the setting of mitral dysplasia, aortic stenosis, dilated cardiomyopathy, or myocarditis. Dogs with endocardial fibroelastosis often have thickening of the mitral valve leaflets and mitral regurgitation.[154a, 155a] Similar difficulties in diagnosis exist in children with this disorder.[15a] Affected animals fail to thrive. Medical treatment of congestive heart failure may be effective in prolonging life, but recovery is unlikely in actual cases of endocardial fibroelastosis.

Multiple cardiac anomalies have been described in kittens and in pups by a number of authors.[34b, 159a–162a] Pyle and Patterson studied a family of Boxer dogs with multiple defects in which secundum-type atrial septal defects were prominent.[161a] Other abnormalities included RVOT and LVOT obstruction and persistent fetal elements of the right atrium. Ogburn et al[162a] described multiple defects in a family of Saluki dogs that included PDA, tricuspid and pulmonic abnormalities, and mitral insufficiency. *Cordis ectopia,* ectopic location of the heart, has been reported in pups.[35b]

Peritoneopericardial diaphragmatic hernia is a relatively common developmental anomaly of dogs and cats.[163a–170a] This condition is not a true cardiac anomaly, but it can be confused with other congenital and acquired conditions. The reader is referred to Pericardial Disease (Chapter 118).

VASCULAR ANOMALIES

Vascular anomalies can be classified based on their location within the vascular system. A number of vascular malformations have been reported.[49a, 50a, 171a–196a] PDA represents the most important of the vascular malformations. Peripheral vascular disorders, including abnormal abdominal and hepatic venous drainage and arteriovenous fistulas,[37b] are detailed in their respective chapters. Unilateral atresia of a pulmonary artery has been described in a cat with respiratory difficulty.[185a] Coronary arteries can develop anomalously, but they rarely cause documented clinical disease except when associated with pulmonic stenosis.[18b] Other major vascular defects center about the aorta and the systemic venous drainage, and these will be briefly addressed.

AORTIC ANOMALIES

Persistent Right Aortic Arch

Persistence of the right, as opposed to the left, fourth aortic arch causes regurgitation in weanlings.[49a, 50a, 171a–183a] Vascular ring anomalies include this common malformation and other total or partial ring anomalies such as those formed by retroesophageal subclavian arteries, double aortic arch, or left aortic arch with right-sided ligamentum arteriosum.[177a, 179a, 180a, 184a] The cardinal feature of these defects is regurgitation of solid food due to obstruction of the esophagus rather than circulatory dysfunction. The condition is quite common in German shepherd dogs and has been recognized in many other canine breeds, including Irish

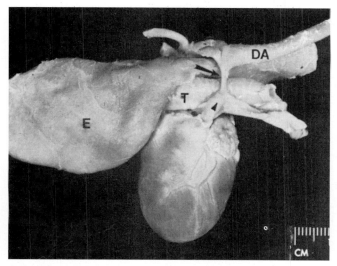

Figure 112–53. Left lateral view of the heart, the esophagus, and trachea of a cat with patent ductus arteriosus, right aortic arch, and vascular ring anomaly. The esophagus (E) is dilated proximal to the vascular ring. The trachea (T), ductus arteriosus (large arrow), and the aorta form the vascular ring. In the normal situation, the aortic arch would have formed to the left of the trachea and esophagus and there would not have been entrapment. DA = descending aorta; the junction of the pulmonary artery and the ductus is indicated by the arrowhead.

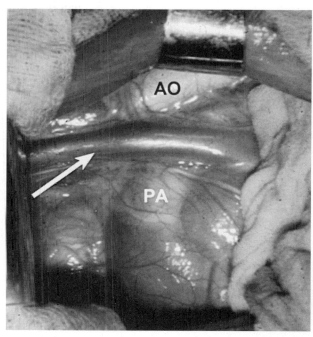

Figure 112–54. A surgeon's view of a persistent left cranial vena cava. This venous anomaly is often encountered during the approach to a patent ductus arteriosus. No hemodynamic consequences result from this anomaly.

setters and great Danes. The condition is uncommon in cats. Occasionally, other cardiac defects are present, including PDA (Fig. 112–53). This condition is described more fully in Chapter 135.

Aorticopulmonary Septal Defect (Window)

As opposed to PDA, this persistent aorticopulmonary communication is caused by failure of the truncus arteriosus

to differentiate.[188a–191a] Subsequently, shunting develops between the ascending aorta and pulmonary artery. Although a clinical condition similar to that of PDA can develop, the authors' experience and reports in the literature suggest that in most cases pulmonary hypertension develops during the first year of life and that clinical signs are similar to those in dogs that develop Eisenmenger's syndrome due to other defects. Management is similar to that for a reversed PDA.

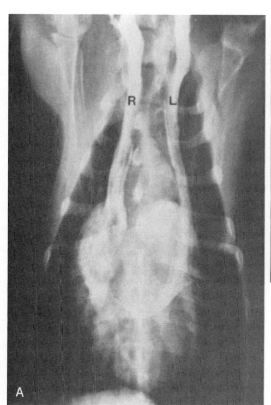

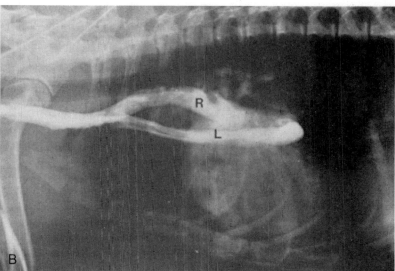

Figure 112–55. Persistent left cranial vena cava in a dog. Contrast was injected simultaneously into both the right and left jugular veins. The normal right cranial vena cava is evident (R) as well as a persistent left vena cava (L). Notice that the left vena cava empties in the caudal portion of the right atrium into the coronary sinus.

Surgery is difficult without cardiopulmonary bypass and should not be attempted if pulmonary vascular resistance is markedly elevated. This defect is not synonymous with a short, wide PDA that is sometimes referred to as a "window."

Coarctation and Interruption of the Aorta

This is a rare defect in dogs that is characterized by narrowing of the aorta distal to the subclavian artery, adjacent to the ductus arteriosus. A case reported by Eyster had systolic and diastolic murmurs and left ventricular failure.[193a] The clinical features of coarctation in children are well described and in many ways are similar to this case.[15a] Aortic interruption has been reported in two dogs,[80][193a] and a case of tubular hypoplasia of the ascending aorta in a dog has been described.[194a] Although these lesions differ from coarctation, they are additional examples of malformation of the aorta in small animals. Definitive diagnosis usually requires angiography, although magnetic resonance imaging and computed tomographic scanning are effective methods for evaluating lesions of the aortic arch. Surgical correction has been successful in affected dogs.

VENOUS ANOMALIES

Thoracic venous anomalies rarely cause cardiac problems in small animals. Total or partial anomalous pulmonary venous return has been reported in a dog and behaves functionally as a left-to-right shunt at the atrial level.[80a] Abnormalities of abdominal venous drainage, such as patent ductus venosus, can induce hepatic encephalopathy. A relatively common venous abnormality of clinical significance during thoracic surgery is the persistent left cranial vena cava (Fig. 112–54).[81][195a] This vessel, normally present in the fetus as part of the left cardinal venous system, may persist and drain into the embryologically related coronary sinus in the caudal aspect of the right atrium (Fig. 112–55). Persistent left cranial vena cava may interfere with surgical exposure, particularly during surgical treatment of persistent right fourth aortic arch, but otherwise it is of no known functional significance. As with right fourth aortic arch, this vascular anomaly is common in German shepherds and has been reported in other canine breeds as well as in cats.[133a, 195a] Division of this vessel generally poses no clinical problem, provided the normal right cranial vena cava is also present. Venous aneurysms or related anomalies are rare.[38b]

REFERENCES

1. Buchanan JW: Changing breed predispositions in canine heart disease. Canine Pract 18:12, 1993.
2. Stur I, et al: Investigation into a familial accumulated occurrence of congenital cardiac anomalies in Siamese and Oriental shorthaired cats. Kleintierpraxis 36:85, 1991.
3. Kvart C, Westmoreland H: Congenital heart diseases in dogs. Svensk Veterinar 48:549, 1996.
4. Westmoreland H: Congenital heart diseases in dogs at the animals hospitals in Uppsala and Stromsholm. Svensk Veterinar 48:12, 559, 1996.
5. Tidholm A: Retrospective study of congenital heart defects in 151 dogs. J Small Anim Pract 38:94, 1997.
6. Bohn FK: Eradication of congenital defects of the heart and the large blood vessels in the dog. Praktische Tierarzt 76:339, 1995.
7. Wakao Y: Echocardiography in cases of hereditary heart disease in small animals. J Vet Med Japan 46:417, 1993.
8. Darke PGG, et al: Transducer orientation for Doppler echocardiography in dogs. J Small Anim Pract 34:2, 1993.
9. Thomas WP: Sisson D: Cardiac catheterization. In Fox PR, Sisson DD, Moise NS (eds): Textbook of Canine and Feline Cardiology. Principles and Clinical Practice, 2nd ed. Philadelphia, WB Saunders, in press.
10. Goodwin JK, Lombard CW: Patent ductus arteriosus in adult dogs: Clinical features of 14 cases. J Amer Anim Hosp Assoc 28:349, 1992.
11. Pouchelon JL, et al: An ultrasonography classification system for patent ductus arteriosus in the dog using 24 case studies. Recueil Med Vet 172:623, 1996.
12. McEntee K, et al: Clinical vignette [Tetralogy of Fallot associated with a patent ductus arteriosus in a German Shepherd dog]. J Vet Intern Med 12:53, 1998.
13. Malik R, et al: Aberrant branch of the bronchoesophageal artery mimicking patent ductus arteriosus in a dog. J Am Anim Hosp Assoc 30:162, 1994.
14. Oswald GP, Orton EC: Patent ductus arteriosus and pulmonary hypertension in related Pembroke Welsh Corgis. JAVMA 202:761, 1993.
15. Buchanan JW: Patent ductus arteriosus. Sem Vet Med Surg Small Anim 9:168, 1994.
16. Peeters D, et al: Bacterial endocarditis and third degree atrio-ventricular block associated with a patent ductus arteriosus in a young dog. Ann Med Vet 141:225, 1997.
17. Miller MM, et al: Percutaneous catheter occlusion of patent ductus arteriosus. Proc 13th Ann Forum, Am Coll Vet Int Med, 1995, pp 308–310.
18. Snaps FR, et al: Treatment of patent ductus arteriosus by placement of intravascular coils in a pup. JAVMA 207:724, 1995.
19. Grifka RG, et al: Transcatheter occlusion of a patent ductus arteriosus in a Newfoundland puppy using the Gianturco-Grifka vascular occlusion device. J Vet Intern Med 10:42, 1996.
20. Schneider M, et al: Transvenous coil embolization for closure of persistent arterial duct in a dog. Kleintierpraxis 41:685, 1996.
21. Fox PR, et al: Nonsurgical transcatheter coil occlusion of patent ductus arteriosus in two dogs using a preformed nitinol snare delivery technique. J Vet Intern Med 12:182, 1998.
22. Goodwin JK: The medical management of pets with congenital heart defects. Vet Med 87:670, 1992.
22a. Côté E, Ettinger SJ, Sisson DD: Long-term treatment of reversed patent ductus arteriosus (rPDA) in four dogs using phlebotomy alone (abstract). J Vet Int Med 11:139, 1997.
23. Eyster GE: Atrial septal defect and ventricular septal defect. Sem Vet Med Surg Small Anim 9:227, 1994.
24. Glardon OJ, Amberger CN: Atrial septum defect in a dog. Schweizer Archiv Tierheilkunde 140:321, 1998.
25. Kosztolich A, et al: Diagnosis of an atrial septum defect in a cat: A case report. Kleintierpraxis 43:207, 1998.
26. Church DB, Allan GS: Atrial septal defect and Eisenmenger's syndrome in a mature cat. Aust Vet J 67:380, 1990.
27. Hagen A, Keene B: Presentation of a ventricular septum defect in a dog by colour-doppler-echocardiography, by angiography and by selective oxymetry. Schweizer Archiv Tierheilkunde 135:208, 1993.
28. Doiguchi O, et al: Echocardiographic study of the long-term development of a case of ventricular septal defect in a dog. J Vet Med Japan 49:728, 1996.
29. Hunt GB, et al: Ventricular septal defect repair in a small dog using cross-circulation. Aust Vet J 72:10, 379, 1995.
30. Monnet E, et al: Diagnosis and surgical repair of partial atrioventricular septal defects in two dogs. JAVMA 211:569, 1997.
31. Nakayama T, et al: A case report of surgical treatment of a dog with atrioventricular septal defect (incomplete form of endocardial cushion defect). J Vet Med Sci 56:981, 1994.
32. McEwan J, Dukes-McEwan J: Pulmonic stenosis in the cat. Veterinary Pract 27:12, 1995.
33. Malik R, et al: Valvular pulmonic stenosis in bullmastiffs. J Small Anim Pract 34:288, 1993.
34. Orton EC, Monnet E: Pulmonic stenosis and subvalvular aortic stenosis: Surgical options. Semin Vet Med Surg 9:221, 1994.
35. Hunt GB, et al: Use of a modified open patch-graft technique and valvulectomy for correction of severe pulmonic stenosis in dogs: Eight consecutive cases. Aust Vet J 70:244, 1993.
36. Thomas WP: Therapy of congenital pulmonic stenosis. In Kirk RW, Bonagura JD (eds): Current Veterinary Therapy XII. Philadelphia, WB Saunders, 1995, p 817.
37. de Madron E, et al: Five cases of valvuloplasty with a balloon catheter for stenotic pulmonary valves in dogs. Pratique Medicale and Chirurgicale de l'Animal de Compagnie 29:383, 1994.
38. de Madron E, Bussadori C: Valvuloplasty in valvular pulmonic stenosis: The European experience. Proc 13th Ann Forum, Am Coll Vet Ind Med, 1995, p 327.
39. Gerlach KF, et al: Balloon valvuloplasty for the treatment of pulmonary stenosis in dogs. Tierarztl Prax Ausg K Klientiere Heimtiere 25:643, 1997.
40. Miller M, Sisson DD: Balloon valvuloplasty in small dogs. Proc 16th Ann Forum, Am Coll Vet Ind Med, 1998, p 87.
41. Bussadori C: Breed-related echocardiographic prognostic indicators in pulmonic and subaortic stenosis. Proc 16th Ann Forum, Am Coll Vet Ind Med, 1998.
42. Fuentes VL, Luis-Fuentes V: Aortic stenosis in Boxers. Vet Annu 33:220, 1993.
43. Buoscio DA, et al: Clinical and pathological characterization of an unusual form of subvalvular aortic stenosis in four Golden Retriever puppies. J Am Anim Hosp Assoc 30:100, 1994.
44. King JM: Subaortic stenotic ring in a cat. Vet Med 92:236, 1997.
45. Oyama M, Thomas WP: Echocardiographic predictors of congenital subaortic stenosis severity in dogs (abstract). J Vet Int Med 11:140, 1997.
46. Kvart C, et al: Analysis of murmur intensity, duration and frequency components in dogs with aortic stenosis. J Small Anim Pract 39:318, 1998.
47. Burwash IG, et al: Dependence of the Gorlin formula and continuity equation valve areas on transvalvular flow rate in valvular aortic stenosis. Circulation 89:827, 1994.

48. Lehmkuhl LB, Bonagura JD: CVT update: Canine subvalvular aortic stenosis. In Kirk RW, Bonagura JD (eds): Current Veterinary Therapy XII. Philadelphia, WB Saunders, 1995, p 822.

49. Lehmkuhl LB, et al: Comparison of catherization and Doppler-derived pressure gradients in a canine model of subaortic stenosis. J Am Soc Echocardiogr 8:611, 1995.

50. Kienle RD, et al: The natural clinical history of canine congenital subaortic stenosis. J Vet Int Med 8:423, 1994.

51. Nakayama T, et al: Progression of subaortic stenosis detected by continuous-wave Doppler echocardiography in a dog. J Vet Intern Med 10:97, 1996.

52. Bussadori C, Mingardi M: Congestive heart failure in a Boxer with subaortic stenosis. Veterinaria Cremona 12:89, 1998.

53. Roth L: Bacterial aortic valvular endocarditis associated with subaortic stenosis. J Small Anim Pract 35:169, 1994.

54. Komtebedde J, et al: Resection of subvalvular aortic stenosis: Surgical and perioperative management in seven dogs. Vet Surg 22:419, 1993.

55. Monnet E, et al: Open resection for subvalvular aortic stenosis in dogs. J Am Vet Med Assoc 209:1255, 1996.

56. Linn K, Orton EC: Closed transventricular dilation of discrete subvalvular aortic stenosis in dogs. Vet Surg 21:441, 1992.

57. Dhokarikar P, et al: Closed aortic valvotomy: A retrospective study in 15 dogs. J Am Anim Hosp Assoc 31:402, 1995.

58. Moise NS: Tricuspid valve dysplasia in the dog. In Kirk RW, Bonagura JD (eds): Current Veterinary Therapy XII. Philadelphia, WB Saunders, 1995, p 813

59. Mai W, et al: Tricuspid valve dysplasia in a Labrador retriever. Summa 15:63, 1998.

60. Atwell RB, Sutton RH: Atrioventricular valve dysplasia in Dalmations. Aust Vet J 76:249, 1998.

61. Bussadori C, Mingardi M: Dysplasia of the mitral valve in a golden retriever. Veterinaria Cremona 12:129, 1998.

62. Fox PR, et al: Clinical, echocardiographic, and Doppler imaging characteristics of mitral valve stenosis in two dogs. J Am Vet Med Assoc 10:1575, 1992.

63. Larsson MH, et al: Tricuspid dysplasia associated with Ebstein's anomaly in a dog: A case report. Braz J Vet Res Anim Sci 33:302, 1996.

64. Kornreich BG, Moise NS: Right atrioventricular valve malformation in dogs and cats: An electrocardiographic survey with emphasis on splintered QRS complexes. J Vet Int Med 11:226, 1997.

65. Breznock EM: Tricuspid and mitral valvular disease: Valve replacement. Semin Vet Med Surg 9:234, 1994.

66. White RN, et al: Mitral valve replacement for the treatment of congenital mitral valve dysplasia in a bull terrier. J Small Anim Pract 36:407, 1995.

67. White RN, et al: Surgical management of subvalvular aortic stenosis and mitral dysplasia in a golden retriever. J Small Anim Pract 38:251, 1997.

68. Brown WA, Thomas WP: Balloon valvuloplasty of tricuspid stenosis in a Labrador retriever J Vet Int Med 9:419, 1995.

69. Braz-Ruivo L, O'Grady M: Echocardiographic diagnosis of cor triatriatum sinistrum in cats (abstract). J Vet Int Med 9:199, 1995.

70. Tobias AH, et al: Cor triatriatum dexter in two dogs. J Am Vet Med Assoc 202:285, 1993.

71. Brayley KA, et al: Cor triatriatum dexter in a dog. J Am Anim Hosp Assoc 30:153, 1994.

72. Fossum TW, Miller MW: Cor triatriatum and caval anomalies. Semin Vet Med Surg 9:177, 1994.

73. Kaufman AC, et al: Surgical correction of cor triatriatum dexter in a puppy. J Am Anim Hosp Assoc 30:157, 1994.

74. Wander KW, et al: Surgical correction of cor triatriatum sinister in a kitten. J Am Anim Hosp Assoc 34:383, 1998.

75 Perloff JK: Ventricular septal defect with pulmonic stenosis. In Perloff JK: The Clinical Recognition of Congenital Heart Disease. 3rd ed. Philadelphia, WB Saunders, 1987, p 404.

76. Patterson DF, et al: A single gene defect underlying cardiotruncal malformations interferes with myocardial growth during embryonic development: Studies in the CTD line of keeshond dogs. Am J Hum Genet 52:388, 1993.

77. Lew LJ, et al: Open-heart correction of tetralogy of Fallot in an acyanotic dog. J Am Vet Med Assoc 213:652, 1998.

78. Weber UT, et al: Palliative treatment of tetralogy of Fallot in a dog using a PTFE (polytetrafluorethylene) vascular graft. Schweizer Archiv für Tierheilkunde. 137:430, 1995.

79. Rozengurt N: Endocardial fibroelastosis in common domestic cats in the UK. J Comp Path 110:295, 1994.

80. Schulz K, et al: What is your diagnosis? [Interruption of aortic arch and subaortic stenosis in a dog]. J Am Vet Med Assoc 203:645, 1993.

81. Fernandez del Palacio MJ: Dilated coronary sinus in a dog with persistent left cranial vena cava. Vet Radiol Ultrasound 38:376, 1997.

CV

CHAPTER 113

ACQUIRED VALVULAR HEART DISEASE

Clarence Kvart and Jens Häggström

CHRONIC MITRAL VALVE INSUFFICIENCY

OCCURRENCE

Chronic mitral valve insufficiency (CMVI) is the most common heart disease in dogs and is estimated to account for 75 to 80 per cent of cardiac diseases.[1–3] The prevalence of CMVI is age-dependent: 1 to 5 per cent of cases occur in dogs younger than 1 year of age, and 75 per cent in dogs older than 16 years.[1–3] CMVI is encountered in all breeds, but the prevalence of the disease varies greatly: dogs of small- to medium-size breeds, such as the Papillon, poodle, dachshund, and Cavalier King Charles spaniel, are most commonly affected.[4–7] CMVI is more prevalent in males than in females.[8] The prevalence of CMVI in cats without primary myocardial disease is unknown but is presumed to be low.

SIGNIFICANCE

CMVI is characterized by chronic progression. Many affected dogs need therapy for heart failure and will die or be euthanized owing to refractory cardiac failure (Fig. 113–1). CMVI has been reported to account for 75 per cent of the cases of congestive heart failure in dogs[1, 2] and a considerably higher proportion in affected breeds.[5, 9, 10] Furthermore, the presence of CMVI and ongoing medical treatment for heart failure may negatively interact with other drugs, decisions for surgical procedures, or anesthesia.

PATHOLOGY

The lesions characteristic of CMVI are caused by an acquired chronic structural degeneration of the atrioventricu-

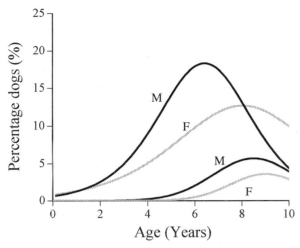

Figure 113–1. Proposed model for progression of chronic mitral valve insufficiency (CMVI) in the Cavalier King Charles spaniel population. Shown is the effect of age on the annual percentage of new cases of heart murmurs attributable to CMVI out of the total population in male dogs *(upper black line)* and female dogs *(upper grey line)* and on the annual percentage of deaths and euthanasias caused by heart failure *(lower black or grey line)*. Note that both curves resemble a distribution of a random variable, with means of approximately 6 to 7 years (heart murmurs) and 9 to 10 years (deaths and euthanasias). The male and female populations differ in their epidemiology concerning age of onset of mitral regurgitation (MR) and mortality attributable to CMVI. Initiated breeding programs aim at pushing the curve of new cases of CMVI to a higher age in order to reduce the number of cases of congestive heart failure. (From Häggström J: Chronic valvular disease in Cavalier King Charles spaniels—epidemiology, inheritance and pathophysiology. Thesis, Swedish University of Agricultural Sciences, 1996.)

lar valves defined as endocardiosis or myxomatous degeneration. Initial findings are small nodules along the free margin of the leaflets. With progression, the nodules coalesce into larger nodules, areas of opacity appear on the valve surface, and the free edge of the leaflet becomes thickened and irregular (Fig. 113–2A).[1] The chordae tendineae become thickened at the valve attachment, elongate, and may rupture,[11] leading to an unattached free edge or a flail leaflet.[12] Ultrastructurally, there is myxomatous proliferation of the valve, in which the spongiosa component of the valve is unusually prominent and the quantity of acid-staining glucosaminoglycans (GAGs) is increased.[1–3, 11] There is haphazard arrangement, disruption, and fragmentation of the collagen fibrils (Fig. 113–2B). Inflammation is not an apparent part of the degenerative changes. The valvular regurgitation leads to secondary changes, including left atrial and ventricular dilatation (eccentric hypertrophy), atrial endocardial lesions (fibrosis) opposite the mitral orifice (i.e., "jet lesions"), and varying degrees of atrial rupture, such as endomyocardial splits, ruptured pectinate muscles in the atrial appendage, acquired atrial septal defects, and hemopericardium. Myxomatous degeneration is not restricted to the mitral valve, and it may be detected in any of the four intracardiac valves. The incidence of valve involvement in dogs was reported as follows: mitral valve alone, 62 per cent; mitral and tricuspid valves, 32.5 per cent; and tricuspid valve alone, 1.3 per cent.[1] The pulmonary and aortic valves were rarely affected. Other findings in dogs with advanced stages of CMVI include arteriosclerosis and multiple intramural myocardial infarcts.[13]

ETIOLOGY AND INHERITANCE

The etiology of CMVI has not been ascertained. However, the localization and the nature of the lesions associated with

CMVI suggest that the condition may be caused by an inherently determined weakness of connective tissue. Heredity has long been suspected to play a role in CMVI, owing to the strong association of this disease with certain small to medium-size breeds. Recent research suggests that CMVI is a multifactorial, polygenic threshold trait[8]; multiple genes influence the trait, and certain thresholds have to be reached before CMVI develops.[8] This means that a combination of a sire and a dam that both have an early onset of CMVI will produce offspring that have, on average, an early onset of CMVI (and heart failure). A combination of dogs with late onset will produce offspring that manifest the disease at old age or never. Breeding programs accounting for age at manifestation and ancestral background have subsequently been initiated.[14]

PATHOPHYSIOLOGY

Proper mitral closure requires an anatomically and functionally intact valve apparatus. Mitral regurgitation (MR) can be due to alterations of the valve leaflet, dilatation of the atrioventricular annulus, rupture of chordae tendineae, or inappropriate contraction of the papillary muscles. More than one of these factors can usually be identified when CMVI is present. The consequences of CMVI depend on several factors[15]: the reduction in forward flow, the regurgitant volume, the size and compliance of the left atrium, the compliance of the pulmonary arterial tree, the development of atrial or ventricular tachyarrhythmias, and the rupture of the left atrial wall.

Primary MR of lesser degree does not induce any apparent changes in indices of cardiac size or function. The forward stroke volume is maintained, and the small regurgitant volume is easily accepted by the left atrium. With progression of the valve lesions, the regurgitant part of the total left ventricular stroke volume increases, but several cardiac and noncardiac (e.g., renal, neurohumoral, and vascular) compensatory mechanisms contribute to maintain the forward stroke volume.[9, 15] The left ventricle compensates for the loss of forward stroke volume by increasing the end diastolic volume (preload), but the heart rate is usually not affected until advanced stages of CMVI, when it increases.[9, 15] The increased preload causes an increased force of contraction according to the Frank-Starling mechanism.[16] The resistance to ventricular emptying is reduced because the blood is ejected into both the aorta and the left atrium. These mechanisms lead to exaggerated motion of the left ventricle (i.e., hyperkinesia). Myocardial systolic function is relatively well preserved, and animals may be sustained for years even with severe CMVI.[1, 15] Nevertheless, because of chronic volume overload, myocardial contractility decreases slowly but progressively and inexorably,[1] and arteriosclerosis may complicate the condition by causing multiple myocardial infarctions.[13]

The left atrium has an important function in allowing the regurgitant volume to be absorbed within the atrial cavity, and it protects the pulmonary vascular bed from hypertension.[17] Increased left atrial pressure results in pulmonary venous congestion and edema. The effect of regurgitant volume on left atrial pressure and volume depends on the left atrial size, as well as on the compliance of the left atrial wall. Consequently, left atrial compliance is determined by the rate of increase in regurgitant volume, which itself is determined by the rate of progression of CMVI, and by left ventricular compliance. In cases of slowly progressing CMVI, there is often a drastic enlargement of the left atrium,

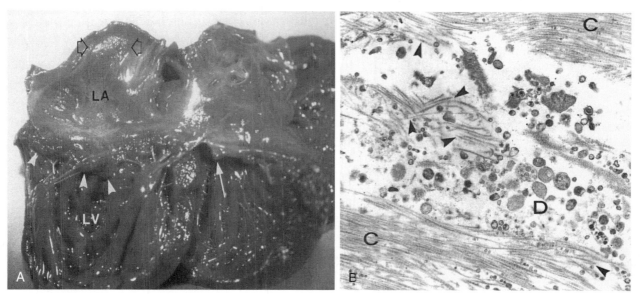

Figure 113–2. *A,* Postmortem specimen of an opened left ventricle (LV) and left atrium (LA) from a dog suffering from chronic mitral valve insufficiency. The left ventricle and atrium are dilated, and the mitral valve leaflets are thickened and contracted, with nodules rolling in the free edges *(arrowheads).* There is evidence of chordal involvement in the form of a missing, presumably ruptured, chorda on the septal leaflet *(arrow).* Jet lesions present on the atrial wall *(between open arrows)* result when the regurgitant streams of blood from the left ventricle strike the atrial wall. *B,* Electron micrograph of the same mitral valve. Collagen fibers (C) are fragmented and have a spiraling appearance in longitudinal section *(arrowheads).* There is aggregation of cellular debris (D) in between the collagen bundles. (Magnification: 3500×.) (From Häggström J: Chronic valvular disease in Cavalier King Charles spaniels—epidemiology, inheritance and pathophysiology. Thesis, Swedish University of Agricultural Sciences, 1996.)

whereas pulmonary congestion and pulmonary edema develop late. The enlarged left atrium may induce coughing by compressing the left main stem bronchus that lies dorsal to the left atrium. In cases of acutely increased MR, as in rupture of a tendinous cord, the left atrium is unable to adapt, resulting in a rapid elevation of left atrial pressure. Pulmonary capillary pressure subsequently increases, leading to pulmonary congestion and edema.

Advanced cases of CMVI may be complicated by processes that are related to increased left atrial size and pressure.[1, 2] The left atrium may rupture, causing cardiac tamponade; right-sided heart failure may develop as a consequence of pulmonary artery hypertension; and tachyarrhythmias may develop as a consequence of ultrastructural changes in the myocardium. These complications are discussed later.

CLINICAL SIGNS

The progress of CMVI from the detection of a soft heart murmur to the end stage is often a matter of years. The first clinical signs of decompensation are usually mild but may aggravate within days or sometimes weeks. Because these signs are vague and not specific for decompensated heart failure, the differential diagnostic challenge in CMVI is often not whether the disease is present but whether CMVI is responsible for the clinical signs. The signs relate to the presence and degree of one or more of the following pathophysiologic events, listed in order of relative importance: (1) elevated left atrial and pulmonary venous pressure, resulting in respiratory distress and cough due to pulmonary edema and main stem bronchial compression; (2) reduced left ventricular or right ventricular forward flow, resulting in weakness and reduced stamina; (3) right-sided heart failure, resulting in pleural effusion and ascites; and (4) acute fulminant pulmonary edema or ventricular fibrillation causing sudden death.

Mild to moderate CMVI is usually not associated with any signs of disease. Most dogs with CMVI are free from clinical signs for most of their lives, although exercise intolerance might be noted. Cough is the most common presenting complaint in CMVI. Although this sign is not specific for heart disease or heart failure, it merits further evaluation. In the case of advanced CMVI, the cough may be caused by pressure of the left atrium on the left main stem bronchus, by pulmonary congestion and edema, or, most commonly, by a combination.[2] With the presence of pulmonary edema, other common complaints are tachypnea and dyspnea. The dogs are often anxious and restless during the night while lying in lateral recumbency (orthopnea) and prefer sternal positioning. In more advanced cases, respiratory sounds, often wheezes, may be audible. These dogs are often inactive and have differing degrees of inappetence. Varying degrees of cardiac cachexia may develop, although a loss of body weight may be masked by a concurrent edema. Dogs with left main stem bronchial compression may have coughing spells at any time during the day, especially during physical exercise or excitement. Otherwise, they do not demonstrate tachypnea, dyspnea, orthopnea, exercise intolerance, or reduced alertness or appetite.

Syncope is encountered in some dogs with CMVI. Syncope may be associated with a tachyarrhythmia, but the course of events often resembles that described in vasovagal syncope.[18] The episodes vary from occasional spells to several attacks per day. Other causes of syncope include tussive fainting, which may occur in conjunction with paroxysms of coughing, or exercise in the presence of pulmonary hypertension.

PHYSICAL EXAMINATION

A midsystolic click is frequently encountered in early stages of CMVI.[19] The presence of this sound depends on heart rate and body position.[19] A systolic click may be accompanied by a low-intensity systolic murmur of variable duration. With progression, the most prominent clinical finding is a systolic heart murmur. The sound begins as a soft apical systolic murmur on the left side of the thorax; it may be intermittent and is sometimes audible only during inspiration. In the early stages of CMVI, the murmur can often be augmented by physical maneuvers, such as a short run.[19] With further progression, the sound becomes holosystolic and more intense[9, 19–21] and may radiate to the right side of the thorax. A thrill may be palpated over the left thoracic wall (cardiac apical area). Musical murmurs (whoop sounds) of high intensity occur less frequently. This type of murmur does not indicate the severity of CMVI. There is usually a shift in the relative intensity of S_1 and S_2.[20] In the absence of significant myocardial failure, the first heart sound is usually enhanced, whereas the second heart sound becomes less intense.[2, 20] A low-intensity third heart sound is often present, but this sound is often difficult to detect by auscultation. The presence of a clearly audible third (gallop) sound is a strong indicator of myocardial failure.[20] Finally, the heart sounds and murmurs may be muffled by pleural effusion or cardiac tamponade. Thus, even though auscultatory findings may be suggestive, the clinician must rely on the supporting historical, clinical, echocardiographic, and radiographic data to determine the hemodynamic significance of the insufficiency.

The presence of sinus arrhythmia in advanced CMVI indicates that heart failure is absent.[22] The heart rate increases as decompensation develops, in response to decreased forward cardiac output. A rapid and irregular heart rate is indicative of arrhythmia. The most common form of ectopy is atrial premature contractions. In progressed CMVI, supraventricular tachycardia, atrial fibrillation, and ventricular premature contractions may be encountered.

With sinus rhythm, the femoral arterial pulse is usually normal. Weak pulses may be noted in heart failure. Weak and variable pulses with deficits can also be observed with rhythm disturbances. If tamponade occurs, owing to a tear in the left atrium and pericardial hemorrhage, the femoral pulse will be weak. Jugular venous distention may be present in severe heart failure, pulmonary hypertension, or pericardial effusion.

In cases of CMVI without signs of heart failure, the lung sounds are expected to be normal. Crackles, snaps, and popping sounds, best heard at the end of inspiration, may be detected in advanced CMVI with pulmonary interstitial edema. Similar findings are common in dogs with small airway disease[23]; if this occurs along with CMVI, it may be a diagnostic challenge to determine the cause of the clinical signs. In more severe cases with alveolar edema, the pulmonary sounds are usually more pronounced and may be auscultated even without a stethoscope.

Mucous membranes are usually normal, even in animals with pulmonary edema, but may be cyanotic, greyish, or ashen in advanced cases of heart failure. Ascites in isolated CMVI is uncommon, but progressed CMVI often tends to involve the right side of the heart as a consequence of pulmonary hypertension. In these dogs, ascites and hepatic and splenic enlargement are common findings.

RADIOGRAPHIC FINDINGS

It is not possible to establish the precise etiology of mitral insufficiency radiographically. The value of radiographs is in assessing the hemodynamic consequences of CMVI, and they can help exclude other possible causes for the clinical signs, which is of particular interest in geriatric dogs. At least two orthogonal projections should be obtained: lateral and dorsoventral or ventrodorsal.

In dogs with CMVI, the most important structures to evaluate are the left atrium, left ventricle, main stem bronchi, pulmonary vessels, and lung field. Dogs with a low degree of CMVI usually have a normal heart size, normal lung fields, and normal vascular markings. Left atrial enlargement is one of the earliest and most consistent radiologic features of CMVI. With progression, the left atrium and left ventricle continue to enlarge. Signs of left atrial and left ventricular enlargement in lateral projection include dorsal elevation of the distal portion of the trachea and carina; dorsal displacement of the main stem bronchi (the left bronchus appears more dorsal than the right); and visible prominence of the left atrium, causing the caudal border of the heart to appear straight (Fig. 113–3). In the dorsoventral (or ventrodorsal) projection, the enlarged left atrium may be identified as a bulge in the left cranial part of the cardiac border (between the two and three o'clock positions). The border of the enlarged left ventricle appears rounded, and there is a shift of the cardiac apex to the left. In advanced cases of CMVI, pleural effusion, ascites, and enlargement of the liver and spleen are commonly encountered as a consequence of congestive heart failure.

During the progression of CMVI, radiologic signs of pulmonary congestion and edema usually develop. The degree of cardiac enlargement is poorly related to the severity of pulmonary congestion and edema (see Pathophysiology). Thus, therapy should be based primarily on the presence of pulmonary edema and congestion, not the degree of cardiac enlargement. Venous distention is an early indication of pulmonary congestion; the diameter of the veins is greater than that of the corresponding pulmonary arteries, and they often become tortuous (especially in cats). With progression, interstitial and, in severe cases, alveolar edema develops. In dogs, alveolar edema is often first detected in the perihilar region and the caudal lung lobe—sometimes more prominent on the right side—but an acute edema may also spread to the cranial lobes. In cats, the alveolar edema develops in the periphery of the lung fields and has a patchy distribution.

Pulmonary findings may be inconclusive, because early radiographic changes of pulmonary interstitial edema and the bronchial pattern resemble the radiographic appearance of chronic airway disease. The tendency is to overdiagnose pulmonary edema of heart failure. It is therefore important to have a series of radiographs, if possible, and to evaluate other evidence of left-sided heart failure that should be present by the time pulmonary edema has developed (e.g., venous distention) before deciding on a diagnosis.

ELECTROCARDIOGRAPHIC FINDINGS

Electrocardiographic findings in CMVI vary from normal tracings to marked abnormalities in rate, rhythm, or configuration of complexes. With the exception of documenting and classifying a certain arrhythmia, the electrocardiogram (ECG) is of limited use in the diagnosis or management of CMVI. ECG is an insensitive indicator of cardiac enlargement and cannot detect heart failure or pulmonary edema.

Sinus arrhythmia is usually preserved during the early course of CMVI. In heart failure, sinus tachycardia and a loss of sinus arrhythmia are common.[22] Thus, heart failure from CMVI should be questioned in a coughing animal with sinus arrhythmia. Cats with MR usually maintain sinus

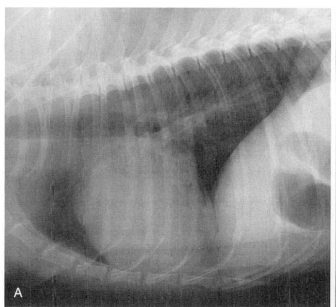

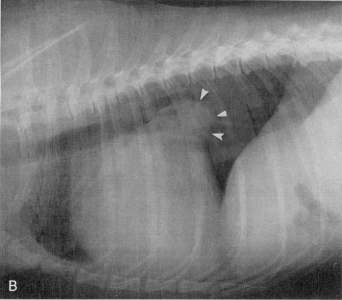

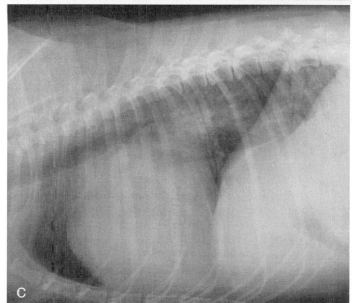

Figure 113–3. Radiographs in left lateral projection of a dog with chronic mitral valve insufficiency. *A,* The dog was asymptomatic at this time, and the radiograph shows a slight left atrial enlargement and normal vascular perfusion. *B,* Radiograph of the same dog four years later. The dog had developed exercise intolerance and persistent cough. Visible are marked left atrial *(white arrowheads)* and left ventricular enlargement and elevation and slight compression of the left main stem bronchus, whereas the vascular markings are within normal limits. *C,* Six months later, the dog had also developed dyspnea and had suffered episodes of syncope. In addition to the findings in the previous radiograph *(B),* there is a more obvious compression of the left main stem bronchus and evidence of pulmonary congestion and interstitial edema. (Courtesy of Dr. Kerstin Hansson, Department of Clinical Radiology, Faculty of Veterinary Medicine, Uppsala, Sweden.)

CV

rhythm, although atrial fibrillation and/or ventricular ectopy may develop.

Most ECG abnormalities associated with CMVI are the result of accentuations of the normal ECG. The mean electrical axis in the frontal plane often remains within the normal range throughout the progression of the disease. In cases of significant left atrial enlargement, the P wave may be prolonged. In cases of significant left ventricular enlargement, the QRS complex may be prolonged and the R wave amplitude in lead II may be increased,[24] but the former is generally a more reliable criterion to detect left ventricular enlargement.

Supraventricular premature beats are common in CMVI. In most cases, this finding is of little hemodynamic significance. Atrial fibrillation, paroxysmal supraventricular tachycardia, atrioventricular disassociation, ventricular premature beats, and ventricular tachycardia are less common. These arrhythmias are most often encountered in advanced cases and often indicate a poor prognosis.

ECHOCARDIOGRAPHIC FINDINGS

Echocardiography is used to obtain a definite diagnosis of CMVI and, thereafter, to study the progression of the condition, although it cannot diagnose heart failure. A systolic bulging of one or both leaflets to the atrial side of the mitral annulus is an early indication of affected valves.[25] At later stages with insufficient valves, the degree of displacement is reported to relate well to the severity of MR.[25] Early cases of CMVI with a low degree of MR have no echocardiographic signs of left atrial or left ventricular enlargement. Apart from a possible systolic displacement, the mitral leaflets usually have a normal appearance. It is rare, even in severe cases of CMVI, to detect incomplete closure of the leaflets as a means of confirming the presence of MR. Instead, the valvular insufficiency may be detected and quantified by spectral or color-flow Doppler.[19] With progression, the degenerative changes become more prominent, most commonly on the anterior leaflet of the mitral valve (Fig.

113–4*B*). Chordal thickening may be identified, and in some cases, a partial prolapse of the leaflet may be evident (Fig. 113–4*C*). The finding of a flail leaflet leads to the suspicion of chordal rupture.[12] Mild pericardial effusion may be present in heart failure, whereas severe pericardial effusion should raise the suspicion of left atrial rupture.

CMVI causes a volume overload of the left atrium and ventricle. Echocardiography reveals an increased left ventricular end-diastolic minor-axis dimension and exaggerated motion of the left ventricular and septal walls (hyperkinesia). Thus, the values of ejection phase indices (e.g., left ventricular fractional shortening, ejection fraction, and mean velocity of circumferential shortening) are often normal or greater than normal owing to the ability of the left ventricle to decompress rapidly into the low-pressure left atrium.[1, 26] Therefore, in the setting of moderate or severe MR, a normal fractional shortening represents a significant reduction of myocardial contractility. End-systolic volume indices (e.g., left ventricular end-systolic minor dimension or end-systolic volume index) more accurately estimate myocardial contractility in MR.[1, 26] However, when heart failure is present and the sympathetic nervous system is activated, even these measurements overestimate intrinsic myocardial contractility.

DIFFERENTIAL DIAGNOSIS

The signalement, clinical signs, and physical examination findings often strongly suggest CMVI. Although the usual cause for MR is myxomatous degeneration, other causes are noteworthy: dilated and hypertrophic cardiomyopathy; widespread arteriosclerosis with myocardial infarcts; bacterial endocarditis of the mitral valve; and undiscovered congenital heart disease, such as mitral valve dysplasia and patent ductus arteriosus (PDA). Although bilateral regurgitation is commonly encountered, isolated tricuspid regurgitation does occur. In these cases, the heart murmur may radiate to the left side of the thorax. Although CMVI may readily be diagnosed, the true diagnostic challenge lies in determining the underlying cause of clinical signs. Unfortunately, the hallmarks of left-side heart failure—coughing and dyspnea—may be caused by several conditions such as small airway disease, tracheal collapse, pulmonary fibrosis, neoplasia, heartworm disease, and pneumonia. Many of these differential diagnoses can be excluded by different clinical tests, but in some cases, the results may be inclusive. In these cases, a 48- to 72-hour trial of diuretic therapy with repeat radiographs might help distinguish the underlying etiology.

MANAGEMENT

Ideally, the therapy of CMVI should cease the progress of the valvular degeneration or involve the improvement of valvular function by surgical repair or valve replacement. However, no therapy is currently available for inhibiting or preventing the valvular degeneration, and surgery is seldom ethically, economically, or technically possible in dogs and cats. The management of CMVI is therefore concerned with improving quality of life by ameliorating the clinical signs and with improving survival. This usually means that therapy is tailored for the individual animal, owner, and practitioner and often involves concurrent treatment with two or more drugs. Medical treatment of CMVI is controversial. The key question is at what stage of CMVI medical therapy should commence. At present, there is no solid evidence that any medication given to an animal with asymptomatic CMVI has a preventive effect on the development and progression of clinical signs of heart failure or improves survival. In advanced CMVI with heart failure, angiotensin converting enzyme (ACE) inhibitors in combination with diuretics alleviate clinical signs and increase exercise tolerance.[27–29] In addition, there are indications that ACE inhibitors in combination with diuretics prolong life in dogs with CMVI and heart failure.[27–29] Management of CMVI is discussed in three groups of animals: those with left main stem bronchial compression, those with pulmonary edema, and those with severe or refractory heart failure. Possible complications are discussed separately.

Animals With Left Main Stem Bronchial Compression Without Pulmonary Congestion. With significant coughing, therapy is aimed at suppressing the cough reflex or reducing the influence of the underlying cause for the compression—the left atrial enlargement. Cough suppressants such as butorphanol, hydrocodone, or dextromethorphan may alleviate the coughing in some cases. Many dogs have evidence of concurrent tracheal collapse or chronic small airway disease. Some of these animals may be improved by administering a bronchodilator or a brief course of glucocorticoids. Different xanthine derivatives, such as aminophylline and theophylline, are commonly used bronchodilators.

Reduction of left atrial size may be effected either by reducing the regurgitation over the mitral valve or by reduc-

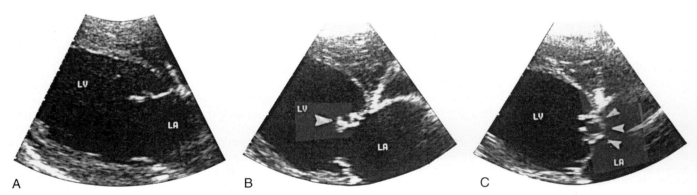

Figure 113–4. Echocardiographic long-axis views of the left atrium (LA) and left ventricle (LV) during diastole (*A* and *B*) and systole *(C)* in a normal dog *(A)* and in the same dog with chronic mitral valve insufficiency (*B* and *C*). The mitral valve appears thickened *(B, arrowhead)*, and there is systolic displacement of both leaflets to the atrial side of the mitral annulus *(C)*.

ing pulmonary venous pressure. Diminished regurgitation can be achieved by reducing aortic impedance with an arterial dilator or by contracting blood volume with a diuretic. The place of a positive inotrope in the management of CMVI is controversial, because signs of left-side heart failure usually precede overt myocardial failure. It is difficult to predict the individual response to drugs with significant positive inotropic effect. These drugs may reduce MR by decreasing the size of the left ventricle and the mitral valve annulus through a more complete emptying of the left ventricle. To the contrary, the increased contractility leads to increased pressure gradient over the mitral valve, which may generate increased regurgitation in some cases with high peripheral vascular resistance. Furthermore, with the exception of digoxin, a comparably weak positive inotrope, many of the positive inotropes have been shown to increase mortality when administered chronically to people in heart failure.[30] Reductions in systemic arterial resistance may be achieved by ACE inhibitors and nitrovasodilators, such as hydralazine.[31] The ACE inhibitors are substantially weaker arterial vasodilators than the nitrovasodilators.[31] Side effects are infrequent, but monitoring of renal function and serum electrolytes, particularly potassium, may be indicated. Hydralazine, a direct-acting arterial vasodilator, has been used widely in animals with CMVI. Hydralazine therapy is often initiated at a dosage of 0.25 mg/lb orally every 12 hours, and the dosage is increased at daily to weekly intervals to an appropriate maintenance dose of 0.5 to 1 mg/lb every 12 hours, or until hypotension develops, detected either by blood pressure measurements or by clinical signs. Reflex tachycardia may develop in response to hypotension, and gastrointestinal problems are sometimes observed. In tachycardia, digoxin may be considered to limit the resting heart rate. As a consequence of hypotension, hydralazine may induce fluid retention, thereby necessitating concurrent diuretic therapy.[32] Animals receiving hydralazine should routinely be monitored, including having the owner check the heart rate at home and having renal function assessed periodically. Diuretic monotherapy may be considered to decrease MR by contracting the extracellular fluid compartment, blood volume, and left ventricular size. However, diuretics activate the renin-angiotensin-aldosterone system (RAAS).[32] Accordingly, these drugs are often reserved for animals with signs of pulmonary congestion and edema or those in which cough suppressants and vasodilators have failed to alleviate clinical signs.

Animals With Pulmonary Edema Secondary to CMVI. Considering the pathophysiology of CMVI, therapy should be directed toward (1) reducing the venous pressures to alleviate edema and effusions; (2) maintaining adequate cardiac output to prevent signs of weakness, lethargy, and prerenal azotemia; (3) reducing the cardiac workload and MR; and (4) protecting the heart from negative long-term effects of neurohumoral influence. Animals with less pronounced pulmonary interstitial edema may be managed on an outpatient basis, but with regular reexaminations. Animals with more pronounced pulmonary edema need intensive care, including cage rest and sometimes oxygen supplementation.

Diuretics. Diuretics relieve the pulmonary congestion and evacuate the edema by decreasing the left atrial and pulmonary venous pressures. As a consequence of contracting the blood volume, diuretics reduce the left ventricular dilatation and, thereby, the mitral valve annulus. However, overzealous use of diuretics may lead to weakness, hypotension, syncope, aggravation of prerenal azotemia, and acid-base and electro-

lyte imbalances. Consequently, it is important to use the appropriate dosage of the diuretic to relieve clinical signs but to avoid unnecessarily high maintenance dosing. This medication should preferably be based on clinical signs rather than radiographic findings. An animal may breathe with ease even in the presence of radiologic signs of peribronchial and interstitial edema, or vice versa. The usual course is an initial intensive treatment with furosemide (1 to 2 mg/lb every 8 to 12 hours) for two to three days, followed by a decrease to a maintenance dose of furosemide (0.5 to 1 mg/lb every 12 to 48 hours or lower). Thereafter, the dosage often has to be gradually increased, often over weeks or years. When the dose of furosemide has reached a level of approximately 2 to 2.5 mg/lb every 8 to 12 hours, sequential blocking of the nephron should be considered by adding another oral diuretic such as spironolactone (2 to 5 mg/lb every 12 to 24 hours) or a thiazide such as hydrochlorothiazide (1 to 2 mg/lb every 12 hours), triamterene (0.5 to 1 mg/lb every 12 hours), or amiloride (0.05 to 0.15 mg/lb every 24 hours). The documentation of triamterene and amiloride in veterinary medicine is limited. Because the furosemide treatment precedes and is used concomitantly with these drugs, the risk of hyperkalemia is low, even when they are added to ongoing treatment with an ACE inhibitor and furosemide. It should be noted that the chance of inducing prerenal azotemia, hypotension, and acid-base and electrolyte imbalances increases with the intensity of the diuretic treatment. However, the practitioner usually has to accept some degree of such risk when treating an animal with heart failure.

ACE Inhibitors. ACE inhibitors, such as enalapril, benazepril, and lisinopril, are considered to be first-line adjuncts to diuretic therapy when managing animals with heart failure and pulmonary edema. These drugs are likely to result in comparable benefits, but enalapril is the one best documented in veterinary medicine. In the case of enalapril, full effect is observed in two to three weeks,[28, 33] and the frequency of side effects is low, regardless of the type of ACE inhibitor used.[28, 29] In the dose range that is recommended for use in dogs and cats, the vasodilating actions of the drug are not prominent, and side effects associated with hypotension, such as fainting and syncope, are rare.[28, 29, 31] The major reason for this observation is believed to be that the effects of ACE inhibitors are dependent on the activity of RAAS before administration of the drug; the higher the activity, the more pronounced the effect of the drug.[34] In combination with diuretics, such as furosemide, the ACE inhibitors have a synergistic effect with the diuretic by counteracting the reflective stimulation of RAAS that occurs in diuretic therapy. Thus, it decreases the tendency for fluid retention and counteracts peripheral vasoconstriction and other negative effects on the heart. ACE inhibitors may be combined with most of the drugs commonly used in heart disease, but they should be avoided in combination with spironolactone without concurrent furosemide treatment, to avoid hyperkalemia.

Cardiac Glycosides. The use of digoxin is controversial in this setting (see the previous section). Many cardiologists initiate digoxin therapy when the signs of heart failure first appear. Although myocardial failure may not be a prominent feature of CMVI until later stages of the disease, digoxin has a place in this scenario by reducing reflex tachycardia, normalizing baroreceptor activity, and reducing central sympathetic activity.[35] Thus, digoxin may be useful to reduce the heart rate (especially when hydralazine is administered

CV

or in atrial fibrillation) and to abolish or limit the frequency of syncope.

Nitrovasodilators. If the animal does not respond with appropriate diuretic, ACE inhibitor, and digoxin treatment, adding another vasodilator, such as hydralazine, may be considered. The potential risk for hypotension is increased with the use of a second arterial vasodilator.[31] Therefore, it is especially important to start with a low dose of hydralazine, such as 0.1 mg/lb orally every 12 hours, and slowly increase to the eventual maintenance level, such as 0.25 to 0.75 mg/lb orally every 12 hours. In cases of severe heart failure and venous congestion, a direct-acting venodilator, such as nitroglycerine ointment topically or isosorbide dinitrate,[1] may also be considered.

Low-Sodium Diet. The use of a low-sodium diet as complementary therapy in heart failure is controversial, and there are currently no clinical studies to support its beneficial use in managing heart failure in dogs and cats. However, excessive intake of sodium should be avoided in the management of animals with symptomatic CMVI (see Chapter 69).

Other Therapies. Some cases of CMVI with evidence of myocardial failure also have evidence of disseminated myocardial infarctions, most commonly as a consequence of widespread arteriosclerosis.[13] Some of these animals may benefit from prophylactic antithrombotic and antiplatelelet therapy, although this has not been evaluated in veterinary medicine.

Animals With Severe or Refractory Heart Failure.

Intravenous agents are generally reserved for dogs with acute severe heart failure or chronic heart failure that is nonresponsive to maximal oral doses of digoxin, diuretics, ACE inhibitors, and vasodilators. In severe acute MR, such as in the case of a ruptured tendinous chord, large doses of diuretics such as furosemide (3 to 4 mg/lb intravenously every two to eight hours) may by required over the first 24 hours. In these cases, dobutamine may also be used in combination with an intravenous vasodilator such as nitroprusside (1.25 to 7 μg/lb/minute) to stabilize animals with otherwise intractable heart failure. Both drugs are administered by constant infusions. Hypotension is the most serious side effect of nitroprusside, but it can be reversed by discontinuing the infusion. Usually the animal must be weaned from intravenous to oral therapy within one to two days.

COMPLICATIONS

Acute Exacerbation of Pulmonary Congestion and Edema due to Ruptured Chordae Tendineae. Ruptured chordae tendineae (RCT) may be suspected in all dogs suffering from CMVI with a drastic aggravation of pulmonary congestion and edema, whereas RCT is a rare finding in cats. The most important ruptures involve those of first-order chordae that are attached to the septal leaflet, and these animals are expected to die rapidly from acute volume overload and fulminant pulmonary edema. Ruptures of lesser-order chordae or perhaps first-order chordae that are attached to the free wall leaflet may result in minor clinical signs or none at all. Significant RCT causes acutely increased MR, and the clinical findings may differ from those encountered in chronic MR. Owing to the acute increase in MR, there may be a marked increase in left atrial and pulmonary venous pressures, leading to acute pulmonary edema, pulmonary artery hypertension, and right heart failure.[3, 15, 17] The physical examination of these animals often reveals a heart murmur of lower intensity than that of chronic

MR, an S_3 gallop is more likely to be present, and jugular venous distention is more likely to be present with pulsations. The radiographic and echocardiographic findings of cardiac size vary, depending on how far the CMVI had progressed before the onset of RCT. Doppler echocardiography shows severe MR, and various degrees of mitral valve prolapse may be detected using two-dimensional views. Thoracic radiographs show a marked increased interstitial and alveolar pattern with distention of the pulmonary veins. These animals require intensive care to stabilize the condition and then maintenance therapy for CMVI (see under Management). As long as a first-order chorda attaching to the septal leaflet has not occurred, many of these animals can be sustained with the aid of appropriate medication.

Right-Sided Heart Failure due to Pulmonary Hypertension. Many animals with a long-standing history of CMVI develop pulmonary hypertension and right-sided heart failure. In CMVI, the condition occurs presumably secondary to the persistent elevation of the left atrial and pulmonary venous pressures, but concurrent chronic airway disease may also contribute. Because the right ventricle is thinner and more compliant than the left ventricle, it can accept relatively large increases in volume but not in pressure.[36] Even small increases in pulmonary artery pressure cause sharp decreases in right ventricular stroke volume.[36] Individuals with pulmonary hypertension are sensitive to exercise, with signs of weakness or collapse even with mild exercise. A physical examination may reveal evidence of right heart failure, such as ascites, hepatic and splenic congestion, distention of the jugular veins with abnormal pulsations, and pleural effusion. The presence and degree of pulmonary hypertension may be indirectly quantitated by Doppler echocardiography.[3]

Individuals with pulmonary hypertension may be difficult to manage. The goal of therapy is to eliminate contributing factors and to restrict even mild exercise. Oxygen supplementation is indicated in cases of acute collapse. Because persistently increased left atrial and pulmonary venous pressures are in large part responsible for the condition, therapy should be as for CMVI with pulmonary congestion (see Management). At present, there is no vasodilator available that specifically acts on the pulmonary artery, but hydralazine may be one of the better drugs in this respect.[3] Bronchodilator therapy may also be indicated, and methylxanthines and β-2-selective agonists may be considered in these cases. Particularly aggressive diuretic treatment may be required to resolve ascites.

Acute Exacerbation of Pulmonary Congestion due to Tachyarrhythmia. An enlarged left atrium predisposes to supraventricular premature beats, atrial fibrillation, and supraventricular tachycardia. Ventricular arrhythmias are less common but may occur in cases that have progressed. A tachycardia with a ventricular rate greater than 180 beats per minute is of hemodynamic significance. These animals often have a long-standing history of CMVI, with an acute onset of pulmonary edema. In addition to other findings characteristic of CMVI, these animals have a change in cardiac rhythm. The goal of therapy is to relieve the pulmonary edema, as described earlier, and to reduce heart rate to an acceptable rate for improving cardiac output. Digoxin is the drug of choice in cases of supraventricular tachycardia. Should this fail to control heart rate, diltiazem (0.22 to 0.68 mg/lb orally every 8 hours) or a β-1-receptor antagonist such as atenolol (3 to 5.5 mg/lb orally every 12 hours) or metoprolol (0.25 to 0.45 mg/lb orally every 8 to 12 hours) could be added. It should be noted that some individuals with CMVI are highly dependent on sympathetic drive, so these drugs may not be well tolerated in the recommended dose range. Therefore, both types of drugs should be initiated at the lowest possible dose and then gradually increased with careful monitoring.

Left Atrial Rupture and Cardiac Tamponade. As a consequence of the left atrial dilatation in CMVI, the left atrium becomes thin walled and more vulnerable to increases in pressure, such as in the case of a ruptured chorda or trauma. Endocardial splitting is a frequent postmortem finding in dogs with a history of long-standing CMVI.[1] The significance of this finding is that it may progress to rupture of the left atrium with the sudden development of hemoperi-cardium, cardiac tamponade, and sudden death. In most cases of atrial rupture and cardiac tamponade, the animals die suddenly. There is often a history of trauma, excitement, or physical exercise preceding the atrial rupture and sudden death. For those surviving the initial event, clinical signs of cardiac tamponade along with evidence of CMVI can be expected. Thus, acute development of ascites, collapse, or marked exercise intolerance is usual. The physical examination may reveal signs of pericardial effusion (see Chapter 118), together with evidence of CMVI. Echocardiography is often required for definite diagnosis by identifying the presence of significant pericardial effusion, whereas the left atrial tear is often difficult to detect. Treatment of atrial rupture with hemopericardium and cardiac tamponade is usually futile. Immediate pericardiocentesis is indicated, and pericardial fluid should be removed to alleviate the tamponade without removing so much that further bleeding is stimulated. If the bleeding continues after pericardiocentesis, the final option is emergency thoracotomy with pericardiectomy and closure of the tear, but the prognosis for this procedure is grim.

TRICUSPID VALVE INSUFFICIENCY

Since the advent of Doppler echocardiography, tricuspid valve insufficiency (TVI) has been recognized as a common incidental finding in dogs and cats.[37] TVI of clinical significance most often occurs concomitant with chronic CMVI as a consequence of primary valvular changes, secondary right ventricular enlargement, or both.[1] In these circumstances, the degenerative changes of the tricuspid valve apparatus are identical to those found in CMVI (see the previous section under Pathology).[1] Other processes that may affect the tricuspid valve apparatus itself include infective endocarditis and, more seldom, chordal rupture.[1-3] Secondary or functional TVI may occur as a consequence of right ventricular dilatation in all conditions associated with increased right ventricular pressure. These include heartworm disease, pulmonary thromboembolism, pulmonary hypertension secondary to left heart disease, and idiopathic hypertension. In addition, secondary TVI occurs in biventricular dilated cardiomyopathy and in congenital pulmonic stenosis. TVI occurs in cats with cardiomyopathy and hyperthyroidism.[38]

PATHOPHYSIOLOGY

TVI, in the absence of concurrent obstruction of the pulmonary valve or pulmonary artery hypertension, is comparably well tolerated.[39] However, because the right ventricle is designed to contract against a low-pressure artery, it is vulnerable to increases in pressure. It responds poorly to the increased work; even relatively small acute increases in

pulmonary artery pressure cause sharp decreases in right ventricular stroke volume.[36] Thus, TVI is of significance if pulmonary hypertension is present. In addition to the right ventricular dilatation, right atrial enlargement develops and adds to the tricuspid annular dilatation and TVI. Enlargement of this chamber may result in atrial tachyarrhytmias, such as atrial fibrillation and supraventricular tachycardia. As a consequence of increased right atrial pressure, ascites, pleural effusion, pericardial effusion, hepatomegaly, and spleno-megaly may develop.

CLINICAL SIGNS

Isolated TVI is not expected to result in clinical signs of disease.[1-3] Evidence of reduced exercise tolerance, weakness, or syncope occurs mainly in instances of pulmonary hypertension secondary to CMVI or tachyarrhythmia. It is common for these animals to show signs of right heart failure as well, including respiratory distress due to pleural effusion; abdominal distention due to ascites, hepatomegaly, or spleno-megaly; or gastrointestinal signs such as diarrhea, vomiting, and anorexia.

PHYSICAL EXAMINATION

Significant TVI is characterized by a holosystolic murmur with varying intensity and with the point of maximal intensity over the tricuspid area, and by the presence of venous distention and pulsations in the jugular veins. The heart sounds may be muffled in cases of pleural effusion. Abdominal distention may be present with ascites, hepatomegaly, or splenomegaly. A rapid irregular heart rhythm and femoral artery pulse are observed in the presence of tachyarrhythmia, and pulse deficits may be detected. A weak femoral artery pulse may be found in cases of pulmonary hypertension or left-side heart failure.

ELECTROCARDIOGRAPHIC FINDINGS

ECG has a low sensitivity in detecting right atrial and right ventricular enlargement secondary to primary TVI.[1] In significant TVI with pulmonary hypertension, the ECG changes may include evidence of right atrial enlargement (tall P wave) and right ventricular enlargement.[24] However, even in severe cases of TVI and pulmonary hypertension secondary to CMVI, these signs may not be obvious because of the concurrent changes to the left cardiac side. In these cases, the recording may show evidence of only left-side involvement.[1-3] Arrhythmias, such as supraventricular premature beats, atrial fibrillation, and ventricular premature beats, may be noted.

RADIOGRAPHIC FINDINGS

Mild right atrial and ventricular enlargement is usually not associated with detectable radiologic signs. Signs of moderate to severe right atrial enlargement in lateral projection include bulging of the right atrium in the craniodorsal direction. This causes the cranial border of the heart to appear straight rather than convex and elevates the trachea as it courses dorsally over the right atrium. In addition to elevations of the trachea and caudal vena cava, signs of right ventricular enlargement include increased sternal contact and rounding of the right heart border. In the dorsoventral (or ventrodorsal) projection, the enlarged right atrium may be identified as a bulge in the right cranial part of the cardiac border (in the 9 to 12 o'clock position). The border of the enlarged right ventricle appears rounded and, in severe enlargement, may resemble an inverted *D* sign. There is a shift of the cardiac apex to the left. Signs of right heart failure may be observed, including pleural effusion, abdominal effusion, hepatomegaly, and splenomegaly. If biventricular failure occurs, the global cardiac size is increased, and signs of left heart failure may be present.

ECHOCARDIOGRAPHIC FINDINGS

Echocardiography is useful to detect increased right atrial and right ventricular size and for the evaluation of tricuspid valve morphology. Thus, it is an important tool to rule out other differential diagnoses, such as undiscovered congenital heart defect. With the use of spectral or color-flow Doppler, TVI may be detected and semiquantified, and right ventricular stroke volume and degree of pulmonary hypertension may be indirectly estimated.[3]

MANAGEMENT

Because primary TVI is usually benign, animals with clinical signs of right-sided heart failure with suspected TVI must be thoroughly evaluated for other concurrent conditions that may mimic or exaggerate TVI. Examples of these include congenital heart defects, heartworm disease, CMVI, pulmonary hypertension, pericardial effusion, restrictive pericarditis, and mitral valve stenosis. The signs of right heart failure (i.e., abdominal and pleural effusions) may be alleviated with diuretic treatment involving two or more drugs to obtain sequential blocking of the nephron (see CMVI under Management), but abdominocentesis is likely to be required. If tachyarrhythmias are present, successful management depends on controlling the increased heart rate or preferably abolishing the tachyarrhythmia.

SEMILUNAR VALVE INSUFFICIENCY

With the advent of color-flow echocardiography, a low degree of aortic and, more commonly, pulmonic valve insufficiency is frequently detected.[37] In many cases, this finding is of no clinical significance, but in others, it occurs with different types of congenital heart disease. Aortic valve insufficiency (AVI) occurs most often in dogs as a consequence of subaortic stenosis, and pulmonic valve insufficiency (PVI) as a consequence of pulmonic valve stenosis.[1-3] Acquired AVI of clinical significance, except in association with bacterial endocarditis (see Infective Endocarditis), is a rare disorder in dogs and cats. PVI is observed in the majority of cases with pulmonary artery hypertension and in cases of pulmonary artery dilatation, such as in PDA and heartworm disease. Isolated PVI as cause of clinical signs is extremely rare. Although myxomatous degeneration of one or both semilunar valves is sometimes evident at postmortem,[1-3] it is not expected to lead to significant insufficiency associated with clinical signs.

INFECTIVE ENDOCARDITIS

Infective endocarditis (IE) is a life-threatening disorder resulting from microorganisms colonizing the cardiac endo-

cardium, commonly destroying valves or other structures within the heart. Bacteremia is by far the most common etiology, with the mitral and aortic valve most frequently affected.[40] Vegetation may cause thromboembolism or metastatic infections involving multiple body organs, producing a large variety of clinical signs and making diagnosis difficult. The incidence of IE in necropsied animals has been reported to range from 0.06 to 6.6 per cent in dogs[3, 41] and 2 to 5 per cent in cats.[42] Medium to large breed middle-aged male dogs are reported to be predisposed.[40] Animals with congenital heart disease have a low incidence of IE,[3] but associations have been reported with subaortic stenosis[43] and occasionally with PDA.[44] IE has not been found to have any association with CMVI in dogs.[3, 9, 41]

PATHOLOGY

Vegetation caused by IE affects mainly the left heart, with the highest incidence involving the mitral valve.[45] Involvement of the right heart or mural endocardium is uncommon.[45] Pathologic findings vary and depend on the virulence of the infecting organism, the duration of infection, and the immunologic response. Necrosis and destruction of the valve stroma or chordae tendineae proceed rapidly in peracute or acute IE, causing valvular insufficiency and cardiac failure. Intracardiac vegetation consists of different layers of fibrin, platelets, bacteria, and red and white cells, often covered by an intact endothelium. Bacteria may continue to grow despite antibiotic therapy, owing to the location deep within the vegetation and a slow metabolic rate (Fig. 113–5).[46]

ETIOLOGY AND PATHOGENESIS

Transient or persistent bacteremia is a prerequisite for the development of IE. A large number of bacteria have been associated with bacteremia[47] (see the section on blood culture), and some are known to cause IE.[45, 47] Most bacteria require predisposing factors to cause IE, such as depression of the immune system or endothelial damage, sometimes with depositions of platelet-fibrin complexes, to adhere and create IE.[46] The origin of the bacteremia may be active infections, with localization varying within the body.[47] In many cases of IE, there is no clinically detectable source of infection.[45, 47] Possible routes for bacteria to reach and infect the endocardium are by direct contact with the surface endothelium via the bloodstream or from capillaries within the valve (vasculitis).[48] The consequences of IE depend on several factors: virulence of the infective agent, site of infection, degree of valvular destruction, influence of vegetation on valvular function, production of exo- or endotoxins, interaction with the immune system and the formation of immune complexes,[49] and development of thromboembolism and metastatic infections. Gram-negative bacteremia results more often in a peracute or acute clinical manifestation, whereas gram-positive bacteremia results in a subacute or chronic condition. The vegetation may cause valvular insufficiency or obstruction. The destruction of valvular tissue is caused by the action of bacteria or the cellular response from the immune system. Deposition of immune complexes in different organs may cause glomerulonephritis, myositis, or polyarthritis.[49] Septic embolization that produces clinical signs is uncommon, but postmortem findings of glomerulonephritis were reported in 16 percent of 44 dogs with IE.[40]

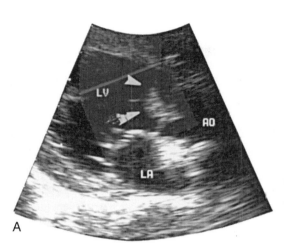

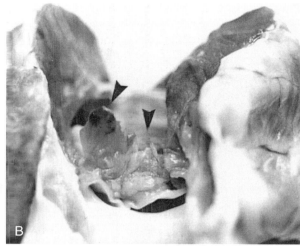

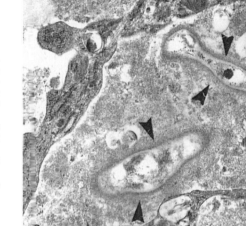

CV

Figure 113–5. *A*, Echocardiographic long-axis view from a 3-year-old male Boxer. The dog had previously been diagnosed with slight aortic stenosis but had recently suffered recurrent episodes of fever and lethargy. An irregular-shaped echogenic mass was attached to the aortic valve *(arrowheads)*. *B*, A valvular vegetation *(arrowheads)* localized to the base of the aortic valve leaflet was evident at postmortem examination. *C*, Electron micrograph showing two rod-shaped bacteria *(arrowheads)* about 1 μm in diameter located intracellularly in a phagocytic cell found within the vegetation. (Magnification: 35,000x.) (Courtesy of Profs. L. Jönsson and T. Nikkile, Department of Pathology, Faculty of Veterinary Medicine, Uppsala, Sweden.)

CASE HISTORY AND CLINICAL SIGNS

The diagnosis of IE can easily be overlooked because the case history and clinical signs are not specific, and there may be an absence of predisposing factors to raise the suspicion of IE. Clinical signs are variable and occur in different combinations. Commonly reported signs include lethargy, weakness, fever (sometimes recurrent), anorexia, weight loss, gastrointestinal disturbances, and lameness.[46, 49] Stiffness and pain originating from joints or muscles may be caused by immune-mediated responses, and abdominal pain may be caused by secondary renal or splenic infarction, septic embolization, or abscess formation. If the condition leads to severe valvular damage, especially of the aortic valve, signs of cardiac failure and syncope from arrhythmias may occur. Predisposing factors that in combination with clinical signs should raise the suspicion of IE are immune-suppressive drug therapy, such as corticosteroids[47, 50]; aortic stenosis;[43] recent surgery, especially in conjunction with trauma to mucosal surfaces in the oral or genital tract; or infections in these body regions, especially prostatitis, indwelling catheters, infected wounds, abscesses, or pyoderma.[47]

PHYSICAL EXAMINATION

Most clinical signs lack specificity for IE. However, fever, heart murmur (particularly if newly developed), and lame-

ness are considered classic signs. Fever is reported to occur in 80 to 90 percent of dogs with IE.[40] Absence of fever is reported to be more common in cases of aortic valve involvement[45] but may also be attributed to treatment with antibiotics or corticosteroids. Because aortic insufficiency is otherwise uncommon in dogs, the finding of a diastolic murmur and bounding peripheral pulse should raise the suspicion of IE. Systolic murmurs may be caused by destruction of the mitral valve, resulting in MR or vegetations obstructing the aortic outflow tract, leading to stenosis.[40] These forms of murmurs are poor indicators of IE, because they frequently occur in dogs with other problems, such as CMVI and aortic stenosis. It should be noted that 26 percent of dogs with IE are reported to lack audible murmurs.[40] Lameness is also an inconsistent finding in IE, with an incidence of 34 percent in one study.[41] A range of other physical findings may occur, depending on which organs are affected by circulating immune complexes or septic embolization. Possible findings are pain reactions from muscles or abdomen (spleen, intestines, or kidneys), cold extremities, cyanosis and skin necrosis from severe embolization, and a variety of neurologic disturbances if the central nervous system is affected.

BLOOD CULTURES

Positive blood cultures are crucial evidence of IE. The theory that bacteremia from IE is intermittent has changed in recent years to the opinion that if it exists, it is continuous.[46] Thus, negative or intermittent positive cultures are unusual when collection and handling of samples are conducted properly.[46] The time for sampling is probably not critical, but a constant finding through repeat samplings is valuable to exclude sample contamination. The technique for obtaining samples aseptically and anaerobically is important and is described in detail later. In cases of positive blood culture, it is important to evaluate whether the microorganism is compatible with the diagnosis of IE. Microorganisms known to commonly cause IE in dogs are beta-hemolytic *Streptococcus, Staphylococcus aureus, Escherichia coli, Pseudomonas aeruginosa, Erysipelothrix rhusiopathiae, Corynebacterium* spp.,[45] and *Bartonella vinsonii.*[51] Dog or cat bites have been reported to occasionally cause IE in humans, with a high mortality (30 percent) due to infection with *Capnocytophaga canimorsus,* a commensal in the saliva of dogs and cats.[52] Negative cultures may be due to antibiotic therapy, chronic situations with "encapsulated" infections, noninfective IE (only platelets and fibrin in vegetation), or failure to grow organisms from samples. Some bacteria may grow slowly, and samples should not be regarded as definitely negative until they have been incubated for 10 days. More common is a rapid growth of microorganisms, with 90 percent of cultures positive within 72 hours of incubation.[53]

Obtaining Blood Cultures. Contact the referral laboratory for the preferred type of prepared vials before obtaining a sample; special additives are available if the animal has been on antibiotics. Pediatric vials are useful, because less blood is required. To avoid contamination, strictly aseptic sampling should be observed, including thorough shaving and disinfection of the sampling site (sampling through indwelling catheters should be avoided) and strict use of sterile gloves. Try to obtain three samples with adequately filled vials from different puncture sites. If samples are collected with a syringe, suction should cease before withdrawal of the needle, to avoid contamination with skin bacteria, and a new sterile needle should be used to transfer blood into the bottles; the bottles should be prewarmed to 37°C and, after sampling, incubated at the same temperature. The former recommendation to draw samples over 24 hours has changed, because multiple samples drawn simultaneously have been shown to be equally sensitive.[46]

ELECTROCARDIOGRAPHIC FINDINGS

Arrhythmia is reported to occur in 50 to 75 per cent of dogs with IE.[40, 45] Ventricular premature beats and tachyarrhythmias are the most commonly encountered arrhythmias, but they are usually not life-threatening. Deviations in the ST segment suggest myocardial hypoxia and may indicate coronary artery embolism or ischemia from heart failure. Evidence of chamber enlargement may occur in chronic IE. All these ECG abnormalities are, however, nonspecific.

RADIOGRAPHIC FINDINGS

Radiography often does not add any information specific for IE. In cases of chronic IE with aortic or mitral insufficiency, left-sided cardiac enlargement may be detected.

ECHOCARDIOGRAPHIC FINDINGS

The development and increasing use of echocardiography have significantly improved the possibilities for diagnosing and monitoring animals with IE.[47] Valvular vegetations may be detected using two-dimensional echocardiography, although minor lesions may be difficult to distinguish from CMVI. M-mode can be used to measure secondary changes in cardiac size and to detect mitral valve motions as fluttering from aortic regurgitation. Mitral or aortic regurgitation may be detected using continuous or color-flow Doppler echocardiography.

OTHER LABORATORY FINDINGS

Mild anemia is found in 50 to 60 percent of animals with IE.[40, 45] The anemia is similar to that from other infections, usually being normocytic and normochromic. Leukocytosis is found in about 80 per cent of dogs with IE, usually owing to neutrophilia and monocytosis (left shift). Other findings that may be encountered include elevated blood urea nitrogen (BUN) due to embolization, metastatic infection, heart failure, or immune-mediated disease. Urinalysis may reveal pyuria, bacteriuria, or proteinuria. Elevated serum alkaline phosphatase may be found, probably caused by circulating endotoxins,[47] and reduced hepatic function may cause hypoalbuminemia.[41] Serum glucose may be decreased, and serologic tests for immune-mediated disease, such as Coombs' test, may be positive.[47]

DIAGNOSIS

Because the clinical signs of IE are often a result of complications rather than a reflection of intracardiac infection, the diagnosis may easily be overlooked. Major criteria for IE are positive blood cultures with typical microorganisms for IE from two separate samples plus evidence of cardiac involvement.[46] Cardiac involvement needs confirmation from echocardiographic visualization of vegetations. In the absence of positive cultures, a tentative diagnosis of IE can be made if there is clinical and laboratory evidence of systemic infection, such as fever and leukocytosis, plus cardiac involvement and eventually signs of embolization.

MANAGEMENT

The goal of therapy is to eradicate the infective microorganism and to treat all secondary complications. A successful outcome is based on early diagnosis and immediate and aggressive treatment. Only bactericidal antibiotics or a combination of agents capable of penetrating fibrin should be considered. The antibiotic concentration in serum and deep within vegetations should exceed the organism's minimal inhibitory concentration, and preferably the minimal bactericidal concentration, continuously or throughout most of the interval between doses. Treatment should continue for at least six weeks to eradicate dormant microorganisms.[46]

Management of Cases With a Tentative Diagnosis of IE. Obtain blood cultures (see earlier) and an antibiotic sensitivity profile. Initiate immediate intravenous treatment with a high dosage of bactericidal antibiotic, such as cephalosporin, while waiting for results from cultures and sensitivity tests. Alternatives to cephalosporin are combinations of penicillin G or ampicillin with gentamicin, depending on the suspected source of infection and possible resistance pattern. Identify the source of infection and treat it as aggressively as possible, including surgical drainage or debridement.[54] Identify possible secondary problems, such as heart or renal failure, that need therapy or may impair the prognosis. When results are available from blood cultures, select appropriate antibiotics and continue aggressive intravenous treatment for 5 to 10 days while monitoring renal function. If results from cultures are negative, the decision to continue antibiotic therapy should be based on clinical improvement. Depending on the early outcome of therapy, after 5 to 10 days, subcutaneous administration may substitute for intravenous treatment, followed by the use of oral preparations. The duration of therapy should be at least six weeks on the effective antibiotic. Perform frequent clinical examination, blood screening, and urinalysis.

PROGNOSIS

Factors that indicate a poor prognosis include late diagnosis and late start of therapy; vegetations on valves (especially the aortic)[45]; gram-negative infection or heart or renal failure that does not respond to therapy; septic embolization or metastatic infection; elevation of serum alkaline phosphatase and hypoalbuminemia (70 percent mortality is reported if this is found in cases of IE)[41]; ongoing treatment with corticosteroids, regardless of whether antibiotics are given simultaneously[40, 50]; and treatment with bacteriostatic antibiotics or premature termination of antibiotic therapy. Factors that indicate a more favorable prognosis include only mitral valve involvement (47 percent of dogs are reported to survive)[40]; gram-positive infections; and origin of infection being the skin, abscess, cellulitis, or wound infection.[47]

PREVENTION

Prophylactic antibiotics may be indicated 1 to 2 hours before and 12 to 24 hours after diagnostic or surgical procedures in cases in which turbulent blood flow is suspected to have damaged the endocardium (e.g., aortic stenosis, PDA, or ventricular septal defect). In these cases, it is also important to institute early treatment of all manifest infections to avoid bacteremia and reduce the risk for IE, and caution should be observed when bleeding or infection is anticipated or evident in the oral, urogenital, intestinal, or respiratory tract. Amoxicillin may be the first choice, but other antibiotics, such as clindamycin or cephalosporins, may also be considered, depending on the organ system involved and the site of infection.[46]

REFERENCES

1. Sisson D, et al: Acquired valvular heart disease in dogs and cats. In Fox P (ed): Canine and Feline Cardiology, 2nd ed. Philadelphia, WB Saunders, in press.
2. Ettinger SJ: Valvular heart disease. In Ettinger S (ed): Textbook of Veterinary Internal Medicine, 3rd ed. Philadelphia, WB Saunders, 1989, pp 1031–1050.
3. O'Grady M: Acquired valvular heart disease. In Ettinger SJ, Feldman E (eds): Textbook of Veterinary Internal Medicine, 4th ed. Philadelphia, WB Saunders, 1995, pp 945–959.
4. Thrusfield MV, et al: Observations on breed and sex in relation to canine heart valve incompetence. J Small Anim Pract 26:709, 1985.
5. Häggström J, et al: Chronic valvular disease in the Cavalier King Charles spaniel in Sweden. Vet Rec 131:549, 1992.
6. Darke PGG: Valvular incompetence in Cavalier King Charles spaniels. Vet Rec 120:365, 1987.
7. Beardow A, et al: Chronic mitral valve disease in Cavalier King Charles spaniels: 95 cases (1987–1991). JAVMA 203:1023, 1993.
8. Swenson L, et al: Relationship between parental cardiac status in Cavalier King Charles spaniels and prevalence and severity of chronic valvular disease in offspring. JAVMA 208:2009, 1996.
9. Häggström J: Chronic valvular disease in Cavalier King Charles spaniels—epidemiology, inheritance, and pathophysiology. Thesis, Swedish University of Agricultural Sciences, 1996.
10. Bonnett B, et al: Mortality in insured Swedish dogs: Rates and causes of death in various breeds. Vet Rec 141:40, 1997.
11. Kogure K: Pathology of chronic mitral valve disease in the dog. Jpn Vet Sci 42:323, 1980
12. Jacobs G, et al: Echocardiographic detection of flail left atrioventricular valve cusp from ruptured chordae tendineae in 4 dogs. J Vet Intern Med 9:341, 1995.
13. Tidholm A, et al: Histopathologic and echocardiographic diagnosis of dilated cardiomyopathy in dogs. JAVMA 212:1732–1734, 1998.
14. Häggström J, et al: Update on mitral valve disease in dogs. Proc 15th ACVIM Forum, Orlando, FL, 1997, pp 202–204.
15. Braunwald E: Valvular heart disease. In Braunwald E (ed): Heart Disease, 5th ed. Philadelphia, WB Saunders, 1997, pp 1017–1035.
16. Komamura K, et al: Exhaustion of Frank-Starling mechanism in conscious dogs with heart failure. Am J Physiol 265:H1119, 1993.
17. Kihara Y, et al: Role of left atrium in adaptation of the heart to chronic mitral regurgitation in conscious dogs. Circ Res 62:543, 1988.
18. Kapoor W: Syncope and hypotension. In Braunwald E (ed): Heart Disease, 5th ed. Philadelphia, WB Saunders, 1997, p 863.
19. Pedersen H, et al: Auscultation in mild mitral regurgitation in dogs: Observer variation, effects of physical maneuvers, and agreement with color Doppler echocardiography and phonocardiography. J Vet Intern Med 1998, in press.
20. Häggström J, et al: Heart sounds and murmurs: Changes related to severity of mitral regurgitation in Cavalier King Charles spaniels. J Vet Intern Med 9:75, 1995.
21. Pedersen H, et al: Echocardiographic mitral valve prolapse in Cavalier King Charles spaniels: Epidemiology and role in development of regurgitation. Vet Rec 1998, in press.
22. Häggström J, et al: Heart-rate variability in relation to severity of mitral regurgitation in the Cavalier King Charles spaniel. J Small Anim Pract 37:69, 1996.
23. Bonagura JD, et al: Chronic respiratory disease in the dog. In Kirk R, Bonagura JD (eds): Current Veterinary Therapy X. Philadelphia, WB Saunders, 1989, pp 351–368.
24. Tilley L: Essentials of Canine and Feline Electrocardiography, 3rd ed. Philadelphia, Lea & Febinger, 1992, pp 62–74, 104–109.
25. Pedersen HD, et al: Mitral valve prolapse in 3-year old healthy Cavalier King Charles spaniels. An echocardiographic study. Can J Vet Res 59:294, 1995.
26. Kittleson M, et al: Myocardial function in small dogs with chronic mitral regurgitation and severe congestive heart failure. JAVMA 184:455, 1984.
27. The Consensus Trial Study Group: Effect of enalapril on mortality in severe congestive heart failure. N Engl J Med 316:1429, 1987.
28. The COVE Study Group: Controlled clinical evaluation of enalapril in dogs with heart failure: Results of the Cooperative Veterinary Enalapril Study Group. J Vet Intern Med 9:243, 1995.
29. The Benazepril Veterinary Investigator Groups: Treatment of heart failure in dogs with benazepril—results of European double-blind placebo controlled study. Proc 14th ACVIM Forum, San Antonio, TX, 1996, p 745.
30. The PROMISE Study Research Group: Effect of oral milrinone on mortality in severe chronic heart failure. N Engl J Med 325:1468, 1991.
31. DeLellis L, et al: Current uses and and hazards of vasodilator therapy in heart failure. In Kirk R, Bonagura JD (eds): Current Veterinary Therapy XI. Philadelphia, WB Saunders, 1992, pp 700–708.
32. Häggström J, et al: Effects of long-term treatment with enalapril or hydralazine on the renin-angiotensin-aldosterone system and fluid balance in dogs with naturally acquired mitral valve regurgitation. Am J Vet Res 57:1645, 1996.
33. The IMPROVE Study Group: Acute and short-term hemodynamic, echocardiographic, and clinical effects of enalapril maleate in dogs with naturally acquired heart failure: Results of the invasive multicenter prospective veterinary evaluation of enalapril study. J Vet Intern Med 9:234, 1995.
34. Häggström J, et al: Effects of naturally acquired decompensated mitral valve regurgitation on the renin-angiotensin-aldosterone system and atrial natriuretic peptide concentration in dogs. Am J Vet Res 58:77, 1997.
35. Packer M, et al: Withdrawal of digoxin from patients with chronic heart failure treated with angiotensin-converting enzyme inhibitors. N Engl J Med 329:1, 1993.
36. Wiedeman H, et al: Cor pulmonale. In Braunwald E (ed): Heart Disease, 5th ed. Philadelphia, WB Saunders, 1997, pp 1604–1625.
37. Yuill C, et al: Doppler-derived velocity of blood flow across the cardiac valves in the normal dog. Can J Vet Res 55:185, 1991.
38. Jacobs G, et al: Congestive heart failure associated with hyperthyroidism in cats. JAVMA 188:52, 1986.
39. Barbour D, et al: Valve excision only versus valve excision plus replacement for active infective endocarditis involving the tricuspid valve. Am J Cardiol 57:475, 1986.
40. Calvert CA: Valvular bacterial endocarditis in the dog. JAVMA 180:1080, 1982.
41. Calvert CA, et al: Cardiovascular infections in dogs: Epizootiology, clinical manifestations, and prognosis. JAVMA 187:612, 1985.
42. Stalis IH, et al: Feline endomyocarditis and left ventricular endocardial fibrosis. Vet Pathol 32:122, 1995.
43. Kienle RD, et al: The natural clinical history of canine congenital subaortic stenosis. J Vet Intern Med 8:423, 1994.
44. Goodwin JK, et al: Patent ductus arteriosus in adult dogs: Clinical features of 14 cases. JAVMA 28:349, 1992.
45. Sisson D: Acquired valvular heart disease in dogs and cats. In Bonagura J (ed): Contemporary Issues in Small Animal Practice. New York, Churchill Livingstone, 1987, pp 59–116.
46. Karchmer A: Infective endocarditis. In Braunwald E (ed): Heart Disease, 5th ed. Philadelphia, WB Saunders, 1997, p 1077.

CV

47. Calvert CA: Endocarditis and bacteremia. *In* Fox PR (ed): Canine and Feline Cardiology. New York, Churchill Livingstone, 1988, pp 419–434.
48. Järplid B, et al: Observations of apparent early valvular endocarditis in swine. J Vet Diagn Invest 9:449, 1997.
49. Bennett D, et al: Bacterial endocarditis and inflammatory joint disease in the dog. J Small Anim Pract 29:347, 1988.
50. Cornelius LM, et al: Four case studies in the use and misuse of corticosteroid therapy. Vet Med 86:1186, 1991.
51. Breitschwerdt E, et al: Endocarditis in a dog due to infection with a novel *Bartonella* subspecies. J Clin Microbiol 33:154, 1995.
52. Lion C, et al: *Capnocytophaga canimorsus* infections in human: Review of the literature and cases report. Eur J Epidemiol 12:521, 1996.
53. Julander IG, et al: Detection times for blood culture isolates using a biphasic medium. Eur J Clin Microbiol 2:54, 1983.
54. Ellison GW, et al: Medical and surgical management of multiple organ infarctions secondary to bacterial endocarditis in a dog. JAVMA 193:1289, 1988.

CHAPTER 114

ELECTROCARDIOGRAPHY

Stephen J. Ettinger, Gérard Le Bobinnec, and Etienne Côté

The criteria for the normal electrocardiogram (ECG) serve as a rough guide for evaluating heart diseases. These criteria are not based on controlled studies identifying sensitivity or specificity. Electrocardiographic parameters for dogs or cats by breed, body type, age, and sex are not established. An abnormal heart may have a normal ECG and vice versa. The ECG, like a blood count, is not an absolute indicator of normalcy or disease. Deviations from normal suggest but do not identify structural heart disease. ECGs best demonstrate cardiac rhythm abnormalities. The ECG of the dog received major attention first in 1949, later in the decades of the 1960s and 1970s, and is once again being revisited.[1–3, 5, 24]

CRITERIA FOR THE NORMAL CANINE ELECTROCARDIOGRAM*

Heart rate: 70 to 160 beats/min in adult dogs; 60 to 140 beats/min in giant breeds; to 180 beats/min in toy breeds; 220 beats/min in puppies.

Heart rhythm: Normal sinus rhythm; sinus arrhythmia; wandering sinoatrial pacemaker. Cyclic changes in the R-R interval are associated with cyclic alterations in amplitudes.

P wave: To 0.4 mv in amplitude; to 0.04 second in duration (0.05 second in large breeds); positive in leads II and aV_F; positive or isoelectric in lead I.

PR interval: 0.06 to 0.13 second (inversely related to heart rate).

QRS complex: Positive in leads II and aVF, negative in lead V_{10}; mean electrical axis, frontal plane: 40 to 100 degrees; amplitude—maximum R wave 2.5 to 3.0 mv leads II, III, and aVF (dogs older than 2 years); R in V_1 or V_{10} less than 3 mv; V_2 and V_4 less than 5.0 mv. Minimum amplitude for R-wave leads II, III, and aVF is 0.5 mv.

    Duration—to 0.05 second (0.06 second in large breeds).

    S in V_4 not deeper than 0.7 mv.

    QRS negative in V_{10}.

QT segment: 0.15 to 0.25 second; varies with heart rate.

ST segment and T wave:

ST segment free of marked coving (repolarization changes).

ST segment depression not greater than 0.2 mv in limb leads and not greater than 0.25 mv in chest leads.

ST segment elevation not greater than 0.15 mv in leads II and III.

T wave positive in lead V_1 (rV_2) and negative in V_{10} (except in the Chihuahua).

T-wave amplitude not greater than 25 per cent of amplitude of the R wave.

T waves may be positive, negative, or biphasic.

CRITERIA FOR THE NORMAL FELINE ELECTROCARDIOGRAM*

Heart rate: To 240 beats/min (usually 140 to 180 bpm)

Heart rhythm: Normal sinus rhythm or physiologic supraventricular tachycardia

P wave: Positive to 0.2 mv in leads II and aVF; may be positive or isoelectric in lead I; duration should not exceed 0.04 second (rate dependent).

PR interval: duration 0.04 to 0.09 second (inversely related to heart rate)

QRS complex:

    More variable than in the canine; the mean electrical axis in the frontal plane is often irrelevant and may be isoelectric in all frontal plane limb leads; mean electrical axis from 0 to +160 degrees (frontal plane).

    Amplitude of the R wave is usually low; maximum is 0.9 mv.

    Duration: Under 0.04 second.

QT segment: duration 0.12 to 0.18 second; varies inversely with heart rate.

ST segment and T wave: ST segment and T wave should be small and free of repolarization changes, marked

---

*These criteria represent commonly encountered numbers for dogs and cats. The ECG is extremely variable; serial ECGs are recommended. Measurements outside these ranges suggest but do not identify cardiac disease. Values are from references and personal experience.[1–4]

depression, or elevation. T waves positive, negative, or biphasic; up to 0.3 mv in height.

There are few established rules for the V leads in cats. R in V_4 should not exceed 1.0 mv.

BASIC ELECTROCARDIOGRAPHIC CONCEPTS

ELECTROPHYSIOLOGY

The ECG is a graphic record of the voltage produced by cardiac muscle cells during depolarization and repolarization plotted against time (Fig. 114–1). The resting heart muscle cell has an electrical potential of −90 mv across the cell membrane. The inside of the cell is negative with respect to the exterior. When the cell is stimulated to depolarize, positively charged sodium and calcium ions flow into the cell across the semipermeable cell membrane, reversing the polarity of the stimulated portion of the cell membrane. The electrical gradient across the cell wall becomes +30 mv. The electrical gradient across the cell membrane is thus reversed and is registered as a voltage deflection on the ECG. The stimulated muscle cell contracts as calcium catalyzes excitation-contraction coupling. Potassium begins to diffuse to the outside of the cell during depolarization. When diffusion of potassium ions to the exterior exceeds the influx of sodium, repolarization begins, resulting in higher concentrations of extracellular potassium and intracellular sodium. Repolarization of the heart muscle produces another series of voltage deflections. During the diastolic (resting) phase, sodium returns slowly to the exterior of the cell and potassium returns to the interior. Whereas random electrical activity is characteristic of other tissue, the electrical activity in the heart muscle is more highly organized, creating a "functional syncytium" of cardiac muscle that permits excitation of the entire atrial and/or ventricular mass when one fiber is properly stimulated.

MONOPHASIC ACTION POTENTIAL AND SPONTANEOUS DISCHARGE CYCLE

Muscle fibers incapable of pacemaker ability have a monophasic action potential when stimulated. When a stimulus strong enough to raise the resting transmembrane potential to a critical or threshold potential is applied to a cell, a monophasic action potential representing cellular depolarization is produced. The rapidly induced action potential of depolarization (phase 0) is followed by slower cellular repolarization (phases 1 to 3), which returns the resting transmembrane potential to its constant −90 mv (phase 4). During phase 0, cellular depolarization occurs, represented by the QRS complex. Repolarization, recognized by the ST segment and T wave on the ECG, is associated with cellular phases 2 and 3.

Whereas all cardiac tissue has the ultimate capability of spontaneous discharge, the sinoatrial (SA) node, some atrial fibers, the bundle of His and its branches, and the Purkinje fibers demonstrate spontaneous or automatic discharge. Other atrial and ventricular muscle cells are capable of automaticity only in unusual circumstances. There are no automatic fibers in the atrioventricular (AV) node and conduction through the AV node is slow. Cells within the heart capable of spontaneous discharge are called pacemaker cells. These cells either act directly as the cardiac pacemaker or have the potential for this action. The fibers with the highest rate of spontaneous depolarization of the cell membrane (normally the SA node) assume the function of the cardiac pacemaker. After repolarization is complete (phase 3) in the cells, there is spontaneous, gradual decay of the transmembrane potential of pacemaker tissue (phase 4) as electrolytes leak across the semipermeable cell membrane. An action potential representing cellular depolarization (phase 0) occurs when slow, spontaneous depolarization (phase 4) reaches the threshold potential.

THE CARDIAC VECTOR

The measurable properties of a cardiac electrical force or potential are magnitude (size) and direction (vector), represented by an arrow. The cardiac vector represents an electrical force of known magnitude and direction determined by resolution of all the cardiac forces into one. An ECG lead is a hypothetical line drawn between two sites on the body surface where electrodes are placed. The ECG deflection for any lead is a measure of the projection of the

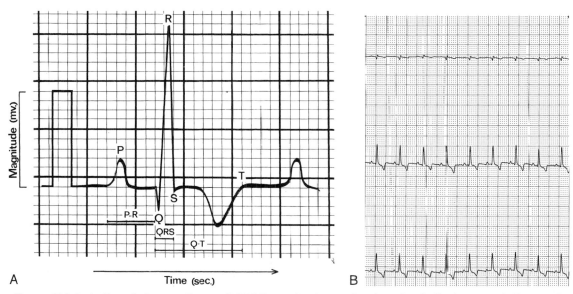

Figure 114–1. *A,* Normal electrocardiogram, P-QRS-T complex from a dog. 1mv. Standardization precedes P wave. *B,* Normal sinus rhythm in a dog. Leads I, I, and III recorded simultaneously at 25 mm/s. The heart rate is 136 beats/min in this dog. (From Ettinger SJ, Suter PM: Canine Cardiology. Philadelphia, WB Saunders, 1970.)

cardiac vector on that lead. The length of the projection of the cardiac vector on any lead depends on the degree to which the vector is parallel to the lead (Fig. 114–2).

The electrocardiographic galvanometer records a positive deflection when the cardiac vector is directed toward the positive electrode but a small or isoelectric deflection (nil) when the vector is perpendicular to the lead being recorded.

TECHNIQUES OF ELECTROCARDIOGRAPHY

ECG tracings record the cardiac vector from the limb leads (I, II, III), the augmented unipolar leads (aVR, aVL, aVF), and the precordial or V leads (exploring thoracic lead). Adhesive patch electrodes or, better yet, alligator clips (with the jaws bent slightly open) are used as electrodes.

For standardization, where feasible, dogs are held in right lateral recumbency, the right forearm of the handler over the dog's neck and right hand holding the forelimbs perpendicular to the torso. The handler's left arm is placed over the hindquarters, and the left hand holds the hindlimbs extended perpendicular to the body. Contact between the electrodes is avoided. The position of the forelimbs should not differ, as

slight positional changes cause significant ECG variations. Feline ECGs are preferably recorded with the cat in a sternal position and held gently by the scruff of the neck.

The electrodes are attached to the skin; right fore (RA) and left fore (LA) are just proximal to the right and left olecranon, right hind (RL) and left hind (LL) proximal to the right and left patella. Leads too close to the thorax are influenced by precordial potentials. The V (C) lead is the exploring chest lead. Alcohol is a contact agent. It is not necessary to clip the hair. In thin-skinned pets, pain is alleviated by attaching the clips over a gauze pad. The moistened electrodes must not come in contact with each other or the handler. Cable tips and electrodes should be clean. Anesthesia or tranquilization is almost never necessary. Anxious or excited animals are muzzled. The table surface is insulated from the ground; metal tables can be used if covered with a large piece of rubber sheeting or a woolen blanket.

LEADS USED IN ELECTROCARDIOGRAPHY

Bipolar Leads (I, II, III)

Using Einthoven's three-lead system[6] as modified for the dog, electrodes are placed on four limbs.[5] The electrical

A

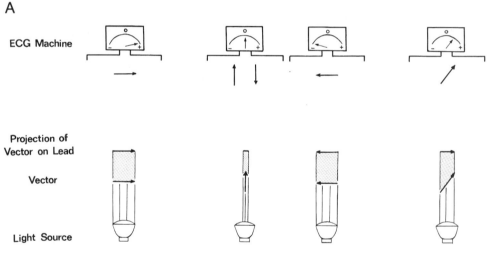

B

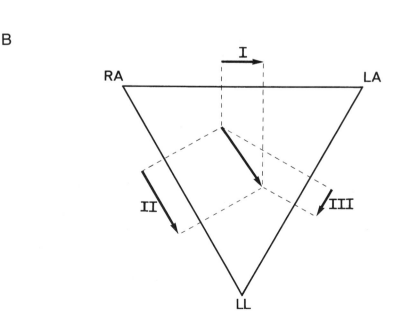

Figure 114–2. Cardiac vector. (From Ettinger SJ, Suter PM: Canine Cardiology. Philadelphia, WB Saunders, 1970.)

ground wire (RL) connects the patient to the ground. In lead I, LA is the positive terminal and RA is the negative terminal; in lead II, LL is the positive terminal and RA the negative; and in lead III, LL is the positive terminal and LA the negative. Because the limbs act as wire extensions of the electrical field, each electrode is considered to measure the electrical field at the site of attachment of the limb to the torso. The electrodes are considered to be relatively equidistant electrically from the heart and from each other. In theory, the bipolar limb leads form an equilateral triangle (Einthoven's triangle) with the origin of the cardiac vector, the zero point of the electrical field, at the center point of the triangle. The three limb lead axes can be redrawn with exactly the same direction, length, and polarity but all passing through the zero point at the electrical center of the heart, because parallel sides of a parallelogram are of equal length.

Augmented Unipolar Leads (aVR, aVL, aVF)

The unipolar limb leads compare the voltage detected by an exploring electrode placed on one limb with that of the center of the electrical field, which is electrically equivalent to zero. The system, modified and augmented, compares the electrical activity at one limb with the sum of that at the other two (i.e., LL with RA + LA) rather than with the entire field (lead I + [−lead II] + lead III). For each augmented unipolar lead, the voltage at one limb electrode (the positive terminal) is compared with the average voltage across the other two electrodes, which are connected to the negative terminal. A triaxial unipolar reference system similar to that drawn for leads I, II, and III may be drawn from these relationships. Thus, six lead axes, I, II, III, aVR, aVL, and aVF, are recorded at different orientations in the frontal plane (head to tail and right to left) (Fig. 114–3).

Unipolar Precordial Leads (V Leads)

The positive terminal is the exploring electrode (C or V) and is placed on the thorax, and the voltage is compared with the average voltage across the three standard limb leads (theoretically equivalent to zero) at the negative terminal.[23] In human beings, leads V_1 through V_6 record the electrical activity as measured on the chest at the fourth and fifth intercostal spaces from the sternum to the left midaxillary line. With these leads, the horizontal or transverse vector (right-to-left and dorsoventral planes) is explored. The exploring V leads used in the dog[5, 7] are

- V_1 ($CV_5RL;rV_2$)—fifth right intercostal space near the edge of the sternum at the most rounded part of the costal cartilage
- V_2 (CV_6LL)—sixth left intercostal space near the edge of the sternum at the most curved part of the costal cartilage
- V_4 (CV_6LU)—sixth left intercostal space at the costochondral junction
- V_{10}—Over the dorsal spinous process of the sixth to seventh thoracic vertebra and vertical to the V_4 position

Unipolar precordial leads provide data for diagnosis of right and left heart enlargement, bundle branch blocks (BBBs), arrhythmias, and ischemic changes.

Other Leads and Electrocardiographic Systems

More accurate, corrected lead systems were devised to minimize variations such as electrode placement, position of the heart within the thorax, and the heterogeneous nature of the body as a conducting medium.[1] An uncorrected distorted orthogonal lead system might be designed:

Lead I: the sinistrodextral axis (X)
Lead aVF: craniocaudal axis (Y)
Lead V_{10}: dorsoventral axis (Z)

Signal-Averaged Electrocardiography. Low-amplitude, high-frequency signals occur in some patients with delayed (10 to 40 ms) ventricular activation into the ST segment. They imply the substrate for reentry and life-threatening ventricular arrhythmias and are more likely to occur in abnormal hearts. These signals are not appreciated in the scalar ECG because of skeletal muscle noise. In signal-averaged ECG (SAECG) the noise is decreased through filtering, amplification, and signal averaging of the last 40 ms of the QRS complex. With signal averaging of large numbers of QRS complexes, high-frequency, low-amplitude (75 to 90 ms; less than 40 μv) signals in the terminal position of the QRS (10 to 40 ms) can be observed. Such late potentials were observed in a group of Doberman pinschers[8, 9] and other dogs,[9] many of whom later died suddenly of a presumed cardiac arrhythmia. Late potentials plus other trigger mechanisms set the stage for fatal tachyarrhythmias. SAECG is a method used for detection late after depolarizations and thus can identify arrhythmia candidates before they develop problems.

THE MEAN ELECTRICAL AXIS

A single determination of the mean ventricular electrical axis (MEA), or average vector, is made for the frontal plane. It may be abnormal with cardiac enlargement or an intraventricular conduction disturbance. In the cat, it is often erroneous, not supported clinically, and often disregarded. The MEA is only a rough calculation, the number being less important than the trend.

Choose a complete QRS complex from any two limb lead recordings. Determine the positive and negative deflections and measure the overall amplitude of the QRS complex.

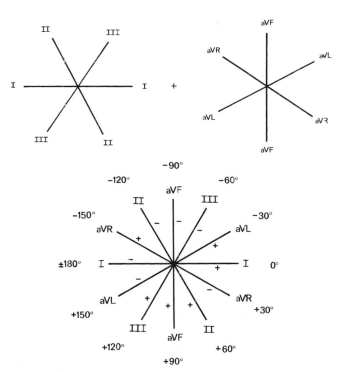

Figure 114–3. Bailey six-axis reference system. (From Ettinger SJ, Suter PM: Canine Cardiology. Philadelphia, WB Saunders, 1970.)

Identify the two leads on the six-axis reference (see Fig. 114–3) system. Draw a perpendicular line from each, extending until the lines intersect at the calculated MEA. The same method may be used to determine the MEA of atrial depolarization (P wave).

The MEA of ventricular depolarization in the frontal plane in most normal dogs is between +40 and +100 degrees. An axis less than +40 degrees is called left axis deviation, and an axis over +100 degrees is right axis deviation. In the dog, deviations from normal warrant further investigation. The MEA need not correspond to the physical axis as observed on radiography. It has been observed that in dogs with a narrow thorax (collies) the MEA in the frontal plane is usually closer to 90 degrees, whereas in dogs with a wide thorax the axis is usually less than 90 degrees. The electrical axis changes artifactually with position of the limbs and torso. Variations within normal are not significant, whereas major shifts to the right (> +90 degrees) or the left (< +40 degrees) are relevant.

THE CARDIAC CONDUCTION SYSTEM AND THE ELECTROCARDIOGRAM

The cardiac conduction system is composed of specialized tissue that conducts electrical impulses through the heart. This system consists of the SA node, the interatrial bundles, the AV node, the common bundle of His, the right and left branches of the bundle of His, and the Purkinje fibers. With the exception of the AV node, the cardiac conduction system consists entirely of specialized muscle tissue, which spreads the wave of excitation more rapidly than can the myocardium. Conduction is slow through the AV node, permitting completion of atrial excitation and enabling the ventricle to fill with blood before contracting.

The *P wave* represents atrial depolarization. The SA node is located at the junction of the right atrium and the cranial vena cava. The *PR segment* of the ECG is the isoelectric or zero potential period that follows the P wave, reflecting the delay of the cardiac impulse in the AV node. The AV node lies above the septal leaflet of the tricuspid valve just anterior to the ostium of the coronary sinus. The period from the beginning of the P wave to the end of the PR segment, that is, the beginning of the QRS complex, is called the *PR interval.*

After a delay in the AV node, the impulse is transmitted through the common bundle of His, the right and left branches of the bundle of His, and the Purkinje fibers, resulting in activation of all fibers within the ventricles. When the impulse reaches the ventricular myocardium, depolarization of the cardiac muscle occurs, the *QRS complex.*

The *ST segment* and the *T wave* represent ventricular repolarization. The ST segment represents the period of slow repolarization of the ventricles when calcium slowly reenters the cells, and the T wave indicates the period of more rapid repolarization as potassium leaks profusely out of the cell. Repolarization of the atria occurs during the QRS complex, so it is not seen on the ECG because the small electrical potential is obliterated by that of ventricular depolarization.

THE NORMAL ELECTROCARDIOGRAM

Highly trained animals, such as Alaskan sled dogs with athletic hearts, deviate significantly from the heart rate numbers established at the beginning of the chapter.[10] In the feline, the normal heart rate extends up to 240 beats/min. The low end varies at home, resting, or in the hospital. Generally, 70 to 80 beats/min would be considered low normal for a cat. In most normal dogs, heart rates range between 60 and 160 beats/min. Rates above these limits are classified as tachycardias and those below 70 bpm are bradycardias. Bursts of sinus tachycardia of up to 300 bpm have been identified for brief periods in normal dogs observed under monitored conditions.[2] Ambulatory electrocardiographic (Holter) testing provides an excellent opportunity to evaluate the real heart rate and identifies a higher prevalence of arrhythmias than seen with conventional monitoring.[16] Heart rate variability in disease has been studied.[17]

The P wave is the first deflection on the ECG after isoelectric diastole. It should be positive in leads II and aVF, isoelectric or positive in lead I. It may be negative in leads III, aVR, aVL, V_2, and V_{10}. The first half of the P wave represents right atrial activation, the second half left atrial activation. The spread of atrial excitation begins in the upper portion of the right atrium at the SA node and spreads across the atrium, depolarizing the left atrium. The maximum normal amplitude of the P wave in any limb lead is 0.4 mv in the dog and 0.2 mv in the cat. The amplitude of the P wave may increase during inspiration and with increased heart rate. Vagal influences within the SA node account for variations in the amplitude of the P wave from beat to beat. The amplitude of the P wave may vary between tracings. These variations are probably the result of changes in the pacemaking site, with higher centers for early activation and lower rates and lower amplitude P waves being associated with lower centers of activation closer to the AV node.[2]

The duration of the P wave should not exceed 0.04 second in the dog (0.05 second in larger breeds) and 0.04 second in the cat. Notching of the P wave is not significant unless the duration of the wave exceeds stated limits, in which case it is associated with left atrial enlargement. Conversely, P waves of increased amplitude are most often associated with right atrial strain, enlargement, or hypoxia.

The form and amplitude of the P wave in dogs are more variable than in other animals, more so in the limb leads than in the thoracic leads. The mean P-wave axis in all normal dogs is within 90 degrees of the maximal QRS vector in the frontal plane.[2]

The PR segment is the isoelectric period that follows the P wave on the ECG. It is measured from the end of the P wave to the beginning of the first deflection away from the baseline, indicating ventricular activity. During the PR segment, the electrical impulse is being conducted slowly through the AV node. Atrial repolarization is occurring during this period and into the QRS but is often too low in amplitude to detect on surface recordings. Abnormalities related to large P waves with increased atrial repolarization result in t_a waves within the PR segment.

The period from the onset of the P wave to the onset of the QRS complex is the PR interval. The duration of the PR interval varies inversely with the heart rate. With rapid heart rates it may be 0.04 second, but it usually varies from 0.06 to 0.14 second (dog) and from 0.04 to 0.09 second (cat). Normal dogs vary considerably. Prolongation represents first-degree heart block—an electrocardiographic, not a pathologic term. Common causes of prolongation of the PR interval are digitalis intoxication and abnormalities of the atrial conduction system. Short PR intervals suggest rapid rates or accessory pathways that bypass normal AV conduction.

The QRS complex is the ECG representation of ventricular depolarization. It occurs immediately after the PR interval. The Q wave is the first negative deflection occurring before a positive wave after the isoelectric PR segment. The R wave is the first positive deflection after the PR segment, regardless of whether a Q wave precedes it. The S wave is a negative deflection occurring after a Q and/or R deflection. If no positive waves are present, the negative deflection is called a QS complex. Positive or negative deflections that occur after the R or S wave has returned to the baseline are called prime (R', S') waves. Any of the following ventricular patterns may arise: QR, QS, RS, R, and QRS plus prime deflections. If the wave amplitude is small (e.g., less than 0.5 mv), a lower case letter is used (e.g., q); if it is greater than 0.5 mv, a capital letter is used (i.e., Q).[2] Significant feline QRS voltage attenuation was identified when commercial ECG machine filtering frequencies (less than 150 Hz) were turned on.[11]

Left ventricular (LV) muscle mass normally exceeds right ventricular (RV) mass. Depolarization of the left ventricle overwhelmingly controls the magnitude and direction of the forces of the QRS complex in the dog and the cat. The interventricular septum, except for the basilar region, is depolarized first, followed by bilateral apical and central endocardial to epicardial activation until a single cone of depolarized muscle surrounds each cavity. Terminal electrical activity proceeds from apex to base, exciting the basal septum and basal and lateral left ventricle. Ventricular activation occurs in three smooth, transitional phases: initial, main, and terminal. The vector is directed from left to right in the interventricular septum; then from the endocardium to the epicardium, depolarizing the free (lateral) ventricular walls; and finally basally in the upper walls and septum (ventricular outflow tracts).[24] These phases are normally 0.01, 0.025 to 0.035, and 0.01 second in duration, respectively, in the dog.[12, 13]

The initial ventricular vector is oriented rightward, craniad, and ventrad. Leads I and V_{10} should each have a Q wave, indicating a rightward (lead I) and ventrad (lead V_{10}) force. The Q wave in canine leads II and aVF represents cranially directed initial forces (duration less than 0.01 second). The initial vector is directed cranially for only a short period before turning caudad. If a Q wave is present in older dogs in leads I, II, III, and aVF and if its amplitude is greater than -0.5 mv in lead II, it is probably abnormal and specifically suggests right heart enlargement or BBB.

The main portion of the QRS complex reflects depolarization of the left and right ventricular free walls. The main ECG deflection is depolarization of the LV wall directed to the left, caudad, and ventrad, producing an R wave in leads I, II, III, and aVF (leftward and caudad) and a Q wave in lead V_{10} (ventrad).

The terminal force of the QRS complex represents dorsal basal (apicobasilar) depolarization. The force is either rightward or leftward, depending on the extent to which the basal region of the left ventricle lies to the right of the midline. If part of the dorsal basal region lies electrically to the right side of the thorax, there is a small S wave in leads I, II, III, and aVF. There is normally no S wave in lead I, and it may also be absent in lead II. Lead V_{10} should always have a Qr complex, the small r wave representing the terminal dorsal basal depolarization of the heart.

The mean direction of the QRS complex (i.e., the sum of electrical forces depolarizing the ventricles) in the dog is leftward, caudad, and ventrad. The mean frontal plane electrical axis of the QRS complex is considered normal between $+40$ and $+100$ degrees. Prolongation of the QRS complex

beyond 0.05 second (0.06 second in large breeds) indicates delayed ventricular depolarization. In cats, durations exceeding 0.04 second are unusual. Ventricular hypertrophy, BBB, electrolyte disorders, formation of premature ventricular ectopic beats, and aberrantly conducted beats could result in prolonged complexes.

The upper normal amplitude of the canine R wave is 2.5 mv; above 3.0 mv is abnormal. Abnormally tall R waves suggest ventricular enlargement. R waves of amplitude less than 0.5 mv in leads I, II, and III are small.[2] Cyclic changes in heart rate may cause cyclic variations in QRS complex size. Diminished amplitudes of the electrocardiographic complexes suggest pericardial and/or pleural effusion, intrathoracic mass, hypovolemia, hypothyroidism, hypothermia, or obesity. This abnormality is true only if ventricular complexes are diminished in all leads, including the V leads.

Occasionally the QRS complex is nearly isoelectric in all six limb leads, referred to as a *horizontal heart*. The electrical axis is indeterminate in the frontal plane. In this case, normal values for mean frontal plane electrical axis and wave amplitudes cannot be applied. Interval durations are not altered. Detweiler[2] referred to this as a "butterfly" QRS loop condition because the resulting vector loop resembles butterfly wings. Such loops result from the position of the heart directing the QRS mostly craniad and ventrad.

The QT interval varies with the preceding R-R interval. Despite wide variations in heart rate in the dog, the QT interval does not vary during respiratory sinus arrhythmia.[15] The QT interval encompasses the time from the earliest activation to the latest repolarization of the ventricular myocardium, and the T wave proper is the result of repolarization gradients within the ventricles of the heart.[25]

The ST segment and T wave represent ventricular repolarization. The ST segment, which represents the slower phase of repolarization and slow channel calcium activity, begins with the end of the ventricular complex (J or junctional point) and ends with the first deflection of the T wave. The T wave represents the most rapid period of ventricular repolarization while potassium continues to leak out of the cell. It ends when the wave returns to the isoelectric baseline. The ST segment and T wave should be examined for depression or elevation from the baseline. The ST segment is isoelectric or slightly concave or convex. Polarity of the T wave need not be the same as that of the QRS complex, as is usually the case in humans. The degree of ST deviation appears to vary cyclically with the R-R interval and deviation increases with shorter preceding R-R intervals.[2] Criteria established for changes of the ST segment and T wave in humans should not be transferred empirically. If the amplitude of the T wave is greater than 25 per cent of that of the R wave (Q wave if it is deeper), LV enlargement may be suspected. ST and T-wave changes are usually reported as being associated with hypoxia, nonspecific electrolyte changes, or cardiac hypertrophy.

Normally, the T wave is positive in lead V_2 and negative in V_{10} or RV hypertrophy is suggested (exception: Chihuahua). Suspect myocardial hypoxia if depression or elevation of the ST segment is excessive. Abnormal deviations of the ST segment are depression of 0.2 mv or elevation of 0.15 mv in leads II and III and depression or elevation of 0.3 mv in lead V_4. ST segment elevation associated with pericardial effusion is thought to represent an epicardial injury current.

Evolution of the Electrocardiogram. At birth the normal canine ECG is directed rightward, cranially, and ventrally. Over the first 3 months of life this slowly changes in the normal dog to leftward, caudal, and ventrad. The criteria used to establish a "normal" ECG are not the same for a dog younger than 12 weeks of age as for an older dog.[14]

VAGAL MANEUVERS

Vagal maneuvers involve stimulation (by carotid sinus compression) or inhibition (by atropine injection) of the parasympathetic system. They are helpful in the electrocardiographic differentiation and diagnosis of arrhythmias.[20, 21] The autonomic nervous system includes the sympathetic cardiostimulating system and the parasympathetic inhibitory system. The cardiac anatomic division of the nerve fibers of these two antagonistic systems is quite different. The vagal parasympathetic innervation is primarily at the supraventricular level (sinus node, atrial tissue, and AV node), whereas the sympathetic innervation involves the ventricular level as well. Physiologic responses identified on the surface ECG include, for the sympathetic system, a positive chronotropic effect (increased rate), positive dromotropic effect (increased speed of conduction), and positive ventricular bathmotropic effect (increased ventricular excitability). For the parasympathetic system there are a negative chronotropic effect (decreased rate), negative dromotropic effect (decreased speed of conduction), and positive atrial bathmotropic effect (increased atrial excitability).[20]

CAROTID SINUS COMPRESSION

Carotid sinus compression (CSC) involves noninvasive stimulation of the vagal nerve to enhance vagal tone. The technique consists of gently squeezing the thumb and index fingers progressively along the neck in the anatomic natural depression located between the atlas, the angle of the mandible, and the larynx. This direct manual stimulation of vagal baroreceptors located at the bifurcation of the carotid arteries triggers the cardioinhibitory center of the medulla in the brain.

The cholinergic effects recorded on the ECG are negative chronotropism, dromotropism, and shortening of the atrial refractory period. The consequent parasympathetic cardiac effects are reduced heart rate, possible second-degree AV block, and cardiac standstill with escape complexes (Fig. 114–4A). When pressure is slackened, a short reflex sinus tachycardia appears because of the feedback release of epinephrine (may reveal concealed ventricular excitability).

CSC is helpful in differentiating tachycardias and ventricular ectopy.[21, 22] For example, a false interpretation of ventricular tachycardia arises from the combination of atrial fibrillation and right BBB. This classic pitfall in ECG analysis is avoided by CSC, which may transiently slow the tachycardia and yet would have no effect on a true ventricular tachycardia (Fig. 114–4B).

CSC can help to differentiate ventricular reentry from parasystole.[21] After CSC with ventricular reentry, there is a negative dromotropic effect that breaks the reentrant loop. In parasystole the frequency of ventricular premature beats increases because the sinus rhythm is slowed.

For latent arrhythmias, CSC can sometimes replace a Holter recording by revealing concealed excitability. Concealed excitability may be revealed by a direct effect of CSC on increasing supraventricular sensitivity (Fig. 114–4C) and also indirectly by the triggering of the sympathetic reflex that occurs after cessation of CSC.

CSC is safe in dogs.[20] In human cardiology, a danger has been described with digitalized patients, but we have not experienced any difficulties even in animals who are digitalized. Although CSC has been useful in our hands, others have reported relatively limited beneficial diagnostic effects of CSC.[19]

ATROPINE INJECTION

Vagal inhibition is induced by atropine injected intravenously (IV)[21] at 0.02 mg/lb.[18] This maneuver is complementary to that of CSC. It should be undertaken after the CSC maneuver because the vagolysis induced by atropine persists for 20 to 30 minutes. Indications include all conduction disturbances (bradycardias and blocks). The only contraindication is that of a preexistent tachycardia. Atropine injection promotes a parasympatholytic effect and is used principally to demonstrate that a bradycardia was of sinus origin or to identify concealed conduction (Fig. 114–4D). It may also help to identify conduction irregularities by explaining the mechanism. Atropine analogues are used therapeutically in treating the bradycardia of sick sinus syndrome.

CLASSIFICATION OF CARDIAC RHYTHM DISTURBANCES

A classification scheme useful in a practical setting is one that separates cardiac arrhythmias into three groups: disturbances of impulse formation (cardiac excitability), disturbances of impulse transmission (cardiac conduction), and complex disturbances involving abnormalities of both excitation and conduction. Some rhythm disturbances fit poorly into any category. Some disturbances of cardiac excitability are secondary to conduction disturbances (e.g., junctional or ventricular escape rhythms). Disturbances are listed according to the anatomic level of their origin (atrial, junctional, or ventricular).

Excitation disturbances can cause either excessive or inadequate contraction of the heart or its parts. Increased excitability produces extrasystoles if intermittent, tachycardia if sustained. Decreased excitability leads to loss of impulse formation with electrical quiescence, resulting in bradycardia or asystole.

Conduction disturbances within the heart are all called blocks. Their categorization depends on the anatomic location of the block and its extent or degree. First-degree block refers to slowing of conduction, second-degree block implies complete but intermittent interruption, and third-degree block involves complete and permanent interruption of conduction. Block can occur at the SA node (rare), the AV node, or in branches of the His bundle (BBBs).

Finally, two disturbances combining excitability and conduction abnormalities are discussed. Preexcitation is a syndrome in which accessory conduction pathways bypass part of the normal AV conduction pathway. Sick sinus syndrome generally involves periods of bradycardia and tachycardia caused by dysfunction of the sinus node and supraventricular conductive tissues.

INCIDENCE OF RHYTHM DISTURBANCES

The rhythm disturbances just mentioned do not all have the same clinical importance. Some are commonly encountered, whereas others are extremely rare (Table 114–1). Fur-

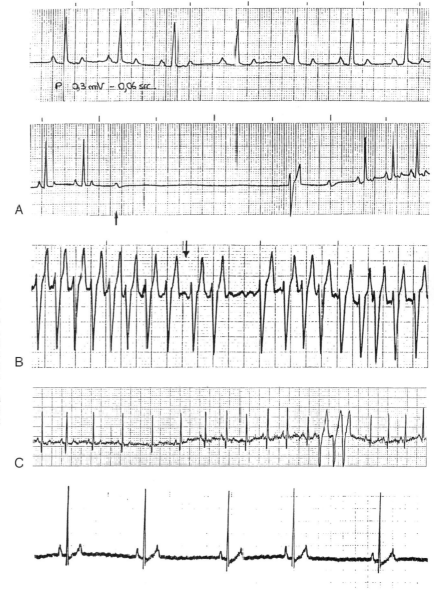

Figure 114–4. Carotid sinus compression (CSC). *A,* This single-channel, lead II tracing demonstrates second-degree AV block, sinus pause, and ventricular escape as a result of CSC (first arrow). *B,* CSC slows a tachycardia, demonstrating that this is atrial fibrillation (following second complex after the arrow) with right bundle branch block and not ventricular tachycardia. *C,* Upon releasing CSC, a brief sinus tachycardia occurs, followed by a cluster of three ventricular premature complexes, revealing concealed ventricular excitability in this dog with thoracic trauma. *D,* Atropine injection (second tracing) identifies the vagal origin of the bradycardia in the first tracing.

thermore, interspecies differences are marked. In cats, preexcitation and isorhythmic AV dissociation have been associated with feline cardiomyopathies. In the dog, disturbances of excitability, especially extrasystoles and atrial fibrillation, are more common than are disturbances of conduction, the majority of which are AV blocks.[1–4]

The hemodynamic consequences of cardiac arrhythmias depend on at least 10 factors: (1) the ventricular rate, (2) the duration of the abnormal rate, (3) the temporal relationship between the atria and ventricles, (4) the sequence of ventricular activation, (5) the functional cardiac status, (6) cycle length irregularity, (7) drug therapy, (8) other disease, (9) preservation of the functional state of the extracardiac system, and (10) the anxiety associated with the irregularity.[31] Ultimately, the sum of these factors—not just the rhythm—determines the impact of the arrhythmia on the patient. This is why some animals with ventricular tachycardia are asymptomatic whereas others are moribund.

CLINICAL ASPECTS OF RHYTHM DISTURBANCES

Before considering the symptoms caused by rhythm disturbances, it is important to place them in their clinical

TABLE 114–1. INCIDENCE OF MAJOR RHYTHM DISTURBANCES THROUGH DIFFERENT STATISTICAL SURVEYS*

ARRHYTHMIAS	PATTERSON (1961) 95 ARRHYTHMIAS DETECTED IN 3000 DOGS		KERSTEN (1969) 215 ARRHYTHMIAS		TILLEY (1985) 396 ARRHYTHMIAS IN 2000 TRANSTELEPHONIC ECGs	
	Number	*%*	*Number*	*%†*	*Number*	*%†*
Extrasystoles						
all	60	63	139	65	214	54
ventricular	43	45	66	31	101	26
atrial	14	15	48	22	113	28
junctional	3	3	25	12	113	28
Atrial fibrillation	13	14	26	12	63	16
First-degree AV block	12	13	50	23	30	8
Second-degree AV block	12	13	32	15	35	9
Sinus tachycardia, sinus bradycardia	—	—	23	11	—	—
Third-degree AV block	2	2	6	3	5	1
Atrial tachycardia, paroxysmal atrial tachycardia	3	3	—	—	13	3
Ventricular tachycardia, paroxysmal ventricular tachycardia	8	8	2	1	11	3
Junctional tachycardia, paroxysmal junctional tachycardia	—	—	1	1	—	—
Wolff-Parkinson-White	1	1	0	0	1	0.25
Junctional rhythm	—	—	—	—	2	0.5

*The incidence of rhythm disturbances indicated in the text is the mean (average) of these three statistical analyses.
†The total exceeds 100 per cent when multiple rhythm disturbances occur on one ECG.

context. If the rhythm disturbance is a result of primary heart disease, the arrhythmia typically increases the severity of clinical signs of the primary heart problem. In some cases, the arrhythmia may be responsible for the first clinical manifestations of a heart problem in an animal with latent or subclinical cardiac disease (e.g., the occurrence of atrial fibrillation in dilated cardiomyopathy). Finally, if the rhythm disturbance is not caused by a primary cardiac problem, it may bring on the first manifestation of a systemic disorder, as seen in electrolyte disturbances.

Simultaneous palpation (or auscultation) of the precordium and femoral pulse reveals the heart rate and the regularity or irregularity of the rhythm and allows detection of pulse deficits. Other complementary studies more precisely define the clinical picture. Echocardiography has the substantial advantage of simultaneously displaying the ECG tracing and its associated effect on cardiac motion, especially in M mode. Spectral Doppler echocardiography can evaluate the influence of this arrhythmia on the cardiac output. The combination of Doppler echocardiography and ECG provides diagnostic, prognostic, and often therapeutic information. Clinicopathologic and radiographic analyses help to evaluate concurrent, primary, or underlying disorders.

IDENTIFICATION OF RHYTHM DISTURBANCES

Although the "gold standard" for assessing arrhythmias, clinical ambulatory ECG or "Holter monitoring," is increasingly popular, most clinical electrocardiography in veterinary medicine today relies on in-hospital ECGs. Rhythm disturbances are identified on the ECG using a methodic four-point examination. First, the rapid, cursory evaluation from left to right of the entire tracing gives a general idea of the cardiac rhythm and an initial diagnostic orientation. This step reveals whether a single rhythm or many rhythms are present. (Are all QRS complexes of the same morphology? Are the R-R intervals the same?) One grossly assesses the heart rate (slow, normal, or fast), determines whether the rhythm is regular or irregular, and detects premature or delayed complexes.

Second, the R-R intervals are evaluated in representative sections of the entire tracing (Table 114–2). In cats, variability of the R-R interval is not consistent with normal sinus rhythm and is considered pathologic.[18] In dogs, cyclic (i.e., rhythmic, patterned) variation of the R-R interval is normal. Irregularly irregular R-R variations are always abnormal in both species (see Table 114–2).

Third, the examination of individual QRS complexes consists of determining whether they are narrow or wide. Narrow QRS complexes generally identify ventricular depolarization of supraventricular origin. Wide QRSs represent asynchronous depolarization of the two ventricles, which may be due either to the ventricular origin of a depolarization or to preexcitation or block.

Fourth, examination of the P waves (present, absent; positive, negative) provides information on the depolarization of the atria. The PR interval is examined to determine whether a P wave exists for every QRS complex and a QRS complex for every P wave, to assess AV synchrony, and measured to assess AV nodal conduction.

Finally, the basic underlying rhythm and any additional or secondary rhythms that are superimposed are identified. Normally, there is a P wave for every QRS complex (an atrial depolarization for every ventricular depolarization). Abnormalities causing more than one P wave for each QRS complex include second- and third-degree AV blocks, and abnormalities causing more than one QRS for every P include ventricular arrhythmias in which the ventricular rate is greater than the atrial rate.

DISTURBANCES OF EXCITABILITY

Disturbances of Sinus Excitability

These arrhythmias are variations of the sinus rhythm (Fig. 114–5) and are most commonly linked to normal, autonomic inputs in a healthy individual. They may also be abnormal and then are potentially detrimental. For example, sinus tachycardia is a normal and appropriate physiologic phenomenon during exercise, but it is commonly encountered in heart failure, in which, pathologically, it occurs even at rest.

TABLE 114–2. DETERMINING THE HEART RHYTHM ON THE BASIS OF R-R INTERVAL VARIATION

REGULAR (R-R INTERVAL CONSTANT THROUGHOUT THE TRACING)	REGULARLY IRREGULAR (CYCLIC, METHODICAL VARIATION IN R-R INTERVAL)	IRREGULARLY IRREGULAR (ERRATIC, PATTERNLESS VARIATION IN R-R INTERVAL)
Sinus tachycardia (HR>180)	Respiratory sinus arrhythmia	Atrial fibrillation
Supraventricular tachycardia (HR>180)	Supraventricular premature complexes	Atrial tachycardia with block
Sustained ventricular tachycardia (HR>180)	Ventricular premature complexes	Multifocal ventricular tachycardia
Normal sinus rhythm (HR = 70–80)	(e.g., bigeminy, trigeminy)	Advanced second-degree AV block
Sinus bradycardia (HR<70)		Sick sinus syndrome
Second- and third-degree AV block (HR<70)		Supraventricular premature complexes
		Ventricular premature complexes

AV = atrioventricular; HR = heart rate (beats per minute).

Sinus Tachycardia

Sinus tachycardia is a sinus rhythm occurring at an elevated rate (see Fig. 114–5). The wide range of resting heart rates in normal cats and dogs makes the cutoff between normal sinus rhythm and sinus tachycardia unclear. In dogs, sinus tachycardia exists when the increase in heart rate (P-QRS-T complexes of normal sinus origin) gives rise to loss of respiratory sinus arrhythmia, the latter being a normal physiologic phenomenon in the dog (see next section). Diagnosing this arrhythmia on the ECG is difficult only when the heart rate is extremely elevated, causing T and P waves to blend together. Carotid sinus massage, which temporarily slows the heart rate, separates the P and T waves and clarifies that the tachycardia is of sinus origin.

The causes of sinus tachycardia are diverse and are all marked by sympathetic predominance over parasympathetic inputs. Treatment of this arrhythmia is therefore aimed at the underlying cause when one exists. To slow a sinus tachycardia is indicated only if the tachycardia itself is producing clinical signs and is poorly controlled with treatment of the underlying disorder. For example, in hyperthyroidism, a beta blocker may be given concurrently with antithyroid treatment. (**Antiarrhythmic drugs to consider: class II.**)

Sinus Bradycardia

Sinus bradycardia is a sinus rhythm in which the heart rate is abnormally low (Fig. 114–6). There is a 1:1 ratio of normal-appearing QRS complexes and P waves. As with sinus tachycardia, the notion of bradycardia varies according to species, breed, and body weight.

Sinus bradycardia generally indicates the physiologic (e.g., brachycephalic, athletic individual) or pathologic (e.g., toxicity) predominance of the parasympathetic system. A diagnostic aid is the response to an injection of atropine (0.02 mg/lb IV; evaluate response 15 minutes after injection[18]), which helps differentiate between bradycardias of purely vagal origin (atropine increases the rate) and bradycardias caused by conduction disturbances (atropine has no effect). Only severe, symptomatic bradycardias (syncope, malaise) warrant specific treatment with drugs or pacemaker implantation. (**Antiarrhythmic drugs to consider: parasympatholytics, sympathomimetics; pacemaker.**)

Respiratory (Normal) Sinus Arrhythmia

In the dog, the balance between the sympathetic and parasympathetic inputs to the heart tilts mainly in favor of the parasympathetic system. This characteristic is in contrast to the adult human and the cat. The vagal predominance in the dog produces two particular features of sinus rhythm on the canine ECG: respiratory sinus arrhythmia (RSA) and wandering pacemaker.

RSA is the result of vagal effects that occur within the thorax during each respiratory cycle (Fig. 114–7). In dogs, it is a normal physiologic phenomenon requiring no treatment. The result is a correlation between heart rate and respiratory rate, with slowing of the heart rate during expiration and acceleration of the heart rate during inspiration. The cyclic nature of this arrhythmia is its hallmark. RSA is first noted in the puppy after 4 weeks of age,[2] generally disappears when the heart rate exceeds 150 beats/min,[1, 2] and is often enhanced when severe dyspnea is present (pneumothorax, fibrosis, emphysema) caused by increased intrathoracic pressure.[2, 3] Interestingly, the presence of RSA may be a valuable diagnostic clue in a common clinical situation, namely in the chronically coughing small breed dog. It is common for these dogs to have concurrent mitral valvular disease (typical murmur is auscultated) and collapsing trachea. It may therefore be difficult to pinpoint which of the two diseases is responsible for the animal's cough. The presence of RSA makes decompensated mitral valvular dis-

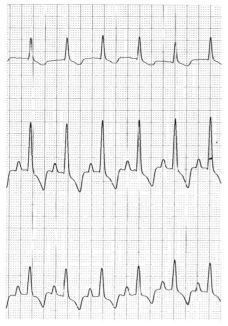

Figure 114–5. Sinus tachycardia. Leads I, II, and III recorded simultaneously at 50 mm/s. This dog with congestive heart failure has a heart rate of 190 beats/min at rest with regular R-R intervals that are 15.5 boxes apart.

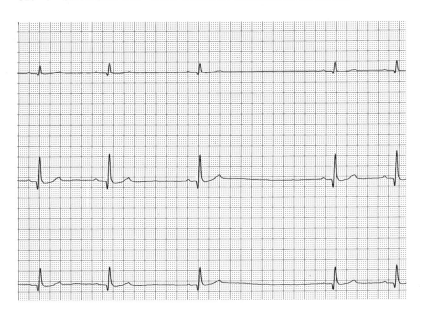

Figure 114–6. Sinus bradycardia. Leads I, II, and III recorded simultaneously at 50 mm/s. Note the normal PQRST waves in this dog with sinus bradycardia and sinus arrhythmia. The heart rate is approximately 65 beats/min.

ease as the sole cause of the cough highly unlikely, because heart failure would bring on increased sympathetic tone and loss of RSA.

In the treatment of congestive heart failure (CHF) with tachycardia (sinus or other supraventricular), successful digitalization may cause the reappearance of RSA. This return of RSA is due to the reactivation of baroreceptors, which had been "worn out" by the ongoing sympathetic stimulation of heart failure. In cats, RSA is unusual and is typically associated with underlying disease.[71]

Wandering Pacemaker

Wandering pacemaker (WP) is a normal, physiologic phenomenon in dogs that is not associated with pathologic conditions and requires no treatment (Fig. 114–8).

In the dog, the origin of depolarization in the heart is not fixed but may move within the right atrium, by an unknown mechanism, between the SA node and the AV node. On the ECG, the result is variation in the P-wave amplitude, with QRS complexes that retain a normal, supraventricular appearance. This variability in the P wave is often cyclic, and often associated with RSA. In this situation, the amplitude of the P wave increases with increased heart rate (inspiration) and decreases with decreased heart rate (expiration),

sometimes to the point of disappearance (isoelectric P wave) or, rarely, negativity in leads II, III, and aVF.[1, 2] The ECG differential diagnosis for WP includes morphologic abnormalities (e.g., P pulmonale) and supraventricular extrasystoles.

Disturbances of Atrial Excitability

Disturbances of atrial excitability are common, especially in the dog. Indeed, in the most common forms of heart disease in dogs (endocardiosis and cardiomyopathy), atrial distention leads to pathologic disorganization of the atrial tissue, which can then generate atrial hyperexcitability and conduction disturbances.

Atrial Extrasystoles

Atrial extrasystoles (atrial premature complexes or contractions [APCs], atrial premature depolarizations [APDs]) are premature depolarizations that originate in an ectopic atrial focus (Fig. 114–9). Identification of atrial extrasystoles is based on a combination of one or more of the following five abnormalities but must always include the first point: (1) prematurity of the P-QRS-T sequence; (2) a P wave of

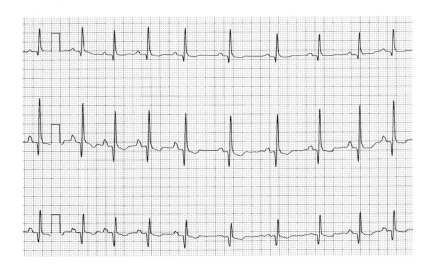

Figure 114–7. Respiratory sinus arrhythmia. Leads I, II, and III recorded simultaneously at 50 mm/s. Cyclic variations in the R-R interval identify normal sinus arrhythmia and a heart rate of approximately 140 beats/min. P waves vary in height, being taller when the rate is higher and lower when the rate is lower. The ECG characterizes P mitrale and signs of left-sided cardiac enlargement. The first P-QRS-T complex is followed by a 1-mv standardization marker.

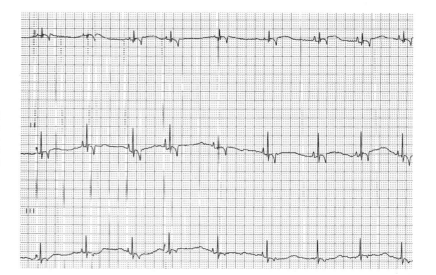

Figure 114–8. Wandering pacemaker. Leads I, II, and III recorded simultaneously. This tracing identifies a regularly varying heart rate affected by respiration (normal sinus arrhythmia). Notice the variation in the P waves from shorter to taller during the respiratory and cardiac cycle in this normal dog; 25 mm/s.

CV

different amplitude than sinus P waves, including negative, biphasic, or positive P waves, but always preceding the QRS complexes; (3) a PR interval that is often different from the sinus PR interval, either shorter or longer[1]; (4) QRS complexes that have a supraventricular appearance in that they are narrow and comparable in shape to the sinus QRS complexes but may, rarely, be absent or widened in cases of atrial extrasystoles that are exceptionally early and thus occur during the total or partial refractory period; and (5) a post-extrasystolic pause that is most often noncompensatory. The pathogenesis of atrial extrasystoles is most commonly related to a structural cardiac lesion. Distention of the atria is the main cause of ectopic foci, but atrial tumors (hemangiosarcoma), hyperthyroidism in the cat, and digitalis toxicity are also recognized causes.[31] Clinical repercussions of atrial extrasystoles are minor, except in cases of multiple repeated bursts, and the main interest in identifying atrial extrasystoles is to add weight to a suspicion of atrial disease. Treatment is therefore first aimed at addressing the underlying cause rather than resorting to antiarrhythmic drugs specifically.

Atrial Tachycardias

An atrial tachycardia is a series of atrial extrasystoles occurring at a rate greater than the sinus rhythm (Fig. 114–10). It may be continuous (sustained atrial tachycardia) or intermittent (paroxysmal atrial tachycardia), the latter being the more common of the two in the dog, the former in the cat. Identifying paroxysmal atrial tachycardia is usually straightforward: the ECG shows a burst of atrial extrasystoles. Establishing a diagnosis of sustained atrial tachycardia is, however, more difficult because P waves may be difficult or impossible to identify, each being buried within the previous QRS complex. Differentiation between sustained atrial tachycardia and "high" ventricular tachycardia (i.e., originating near the AV node) can therefore be accomplished only by exteriorizing the P waves, which occurs after carotid sinus massage and subsequent slowing of the tachycardia or even sinus capture (resumption of sinus rhythm). Causes of atrial tachycardias include the causes listed earlier for atrial extrasystoles as well as the Wolff-Parkinson-White (WPW) syndrome.[5, 6, 7] The clinical impact of an atrial tachycardia depends on its duration, rate, and underlying cardiac lesions.

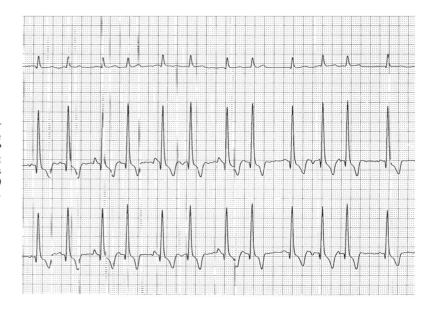

Figure 114–9. Atrial extrasystoles. Note the irregular rhythm and premature beats (beats 4, 6, 8, 10, and 11). The premature beats are associated with early and abnormal P waves that are either positive or negative in deflection. Left atrial and left ventricular enlargement are suggested by this ECG. Leads I, II, and III simultaneously recorded at 50 mm/s in this older poodle with chronic valvular heart disease.

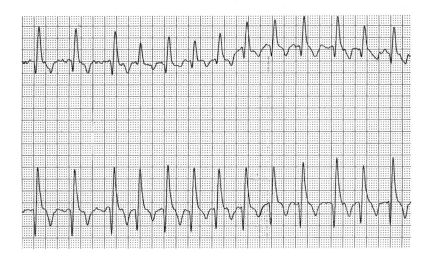

Figure 114–10. Atrial tachycardia. Notice the burst of premature supraventricular tachycardia that begins with the fourth beat. The ECG suggests left-sided cardiac enlargement. Leads I and II were recorded at 50 mm/s simultaneously.

As with atrial extrasystoles, atrial tachycardias often precede the development of atrial fibrillation. Treatment of the underlying disease is an essential part of managing these arrhythmias. (**Antiarrhythmic drugs to consider: digoxin, class II, IV.**)

Atrial Flutter

Atrial flutter is characterized by a rapid, sustained, and regular series of atrial depolarizations without a rest phase between P waves (Fig. 114–11). Identification of this arrhythmia is therefore based on the occurrence of regular P waves, usually at a high rate (often greater than 300 per minute), without returning to baseline ("sawtooth" appearance), and with QRS complexes of a supraventricular appearance with a variable R-R interval. Atrial flutter is different from other atrial tachycardias in that there is no return to the isoelectric baseline after each P wave in atrial flutter. The causes and the treatment of atrial flutter are the same as those of atrial fibrillation.

Atrial Fibrillation

Atrial fibrillation is particularly important in small animal cardiology; it is a common arrhythmia (14 per cent of all canine arrhythmias, including a 50 per cent incidence in cases of dilated cardiomyopathy) (see Table 114–1) and it can bring on clinically overt hemodynamic changes requiring specific treatment. Atrial fibrillation is characterized by complete electrical disorganization at the atrial level, leading to a chaotic, rapid series of depolarizations (300 to 600 per minute) (Fig. 114–12). In atrial fibrillation, the AV node acts as a "gatekeeper" for this chaotic electrical activity, allowing only the electrical depolarizations whose intensity and orientation are optimal to pass through to the ventricles, thus controlling the ventricular rate.[20]

There are four ECG characteristics of atrial fibrillation: (1) a high ventricular rate (often at or above 180 to 200 beats/min), (2) supraventricular-appearing QRS complexes (narrow, upright, and of only slightly variable amplitude in lead II, unless ventricular aberration or BBBs are concurrent), (3) an irregularly irregular rhythm, and (4) no visible P waves (often replaced by fine undulations of the isoelectric line, termed "f waves"). The absence of organized atrial depolarizations has major hemodynamic, and therefore clinical, consequences. During diastole, active filling is associated with the P wave (i.e., atrial contraction), which accounts for 30 per cent of total ventricular filling. Its absence therefore can reduce ventricular volume to suboptimal levels. Furthermore, the rapid heart rate, as well as the prematurity of some QRS complexes, brings about poor diastolic filling. For these reasons, some contractions may be ineffective and therefore without a corresponding palpable arterial pulse ("pulse deficit"). Atrial fibrillation is one of the few arrhythmias that may be suspected from the moment of palpation during the physical examination on the basis of the irregularity of the heartbeat in the chest, together with pulse deficits; ventricular tachycardia and frequent ventricular premature complexes or contractions (VPCs), however, should be included in the differential diagnosis.

A major diagnostic impostor on the ECG is the combination of atrial fibrillation and BBB, which produces wide QRS complexes and therefore mimics ventricular tachycardia, but without P waves to indicate AV association (BBB) or dissociation (ventricular tachycardia). In such a delicate situation, the mild irregularity in QRS complex shape or amplitude may suggest that the rhythm is not ventricular tachycardia, and that suspicion may be reinforced if carotid sinus massage briefly reduces the heart rate. Also, sustained, monomorphic ventricular tachycardia is often characterized by regular R-R intervals, whereas atrial fibrillation with BBB is not.

Atrial fibrillation is most often caused by a primary, underlying cardiac disease. However, A fib may also be noncardiogenic in origin (e.g., anesthesia, hypothyroidism, cardiac tamponade) or idiopathic in certain large breeds (Irish wolfhound). There are two goals of treatment: managing the

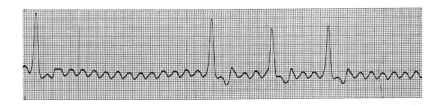

Figure 114–11. Atrial flutter. Sawtooth P waves occurring at the rate of 214 per minute identify the atrial flutter along the baseline. Wide, irregularly occurring, and aberrantly shaped QRS complexes are seen as well throughout the ECG. Recorded at 50 mm/s, lead II.

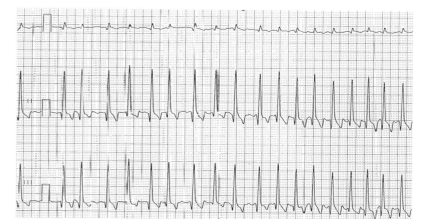

Figure 114–12. Atrial fibrillation. Leads I, II, and III recorded simultaneously at 50 mm/s in an older Labrador dog with dilated cardiomyopathy. Rapid, irregularly irregular ventricular beats are present in all leads. P waves are absent, with an undulating irregular baseline instead. The QRS complexes vary modestly from beat to beat but are generally similar in appearance.

underlying problem(s) and maximizing cardiac output by controlling (slowing) the rate of conduction through the AV node. Conversion to sinus rhythm is not usually undertaken. (**Antiarrhythmic drugs to consider: digoxin; class II or class IV agents +/− in association with positive inotropes.**)

Disorders of Junctional Excitability

Some parts of the junctional AV node possess automaticity (the middle and distal portions). Therefore, it is possible for disturbances in excitability to affect these areas and give rise to a supraventricular arrhythmia. Characteristics include a supraventricular-appearing QRS complex, a regular R-R interval, and no evidence of ventricular preexcitation. The arrhythmias are referred to as paroxysmal or sustained supraventricular tachycardias[70] (Fig. 114–13A and B).

Disturbances of Ventricular Excitability

Disturbances of ventricular excitability are important because they involve the main element in the cardiac pump and may therefore have severe hemodynamic and clinical repercussions. However, it must be recognized that ventricular arrhythmias have diverse mechanisms and etiologies (es-

pecially noncardiac), so that severity, treatment, and prognosis depend on more than ECG findings alone.

Ventricular Extrasystoles

Ventricular extrasystoles (premature ventricular complexes or contractions, beats, or depolarizations) are premature depolarizations generated by an ectopic focus located in the ventricular tissue (Fig. 114–14A and B). These arrhythmias are the most commonly recognized of all rhythm disturbances at present (34 per cent of cases) (see Table 114–1). Their identification is often simplified by the wide QRS complex they generate, which differs in morphology (shape) from a normal sinus QRS complex. Most ventricular extrasystoles have a wide, often bizarre-appearing QRS complex (greater than 0.07 second), without an associated P wave, and a large associated T wave. It is important to differentiate the other major causes of widened QRS complexes: morphologic changes related to cardiomegaly, intraventricular conduction disturbances within the bundle branches, and wide but nonpremature QRS complexes in ventricular escape beats (these three causes of wide QRSs are not ventricular arrhythmias, do not involve a pathologic focus in the ventricle, do not carry a risk of degeneration to ventricular tachycardia or ventricular fibrillation, and therefore are not treated

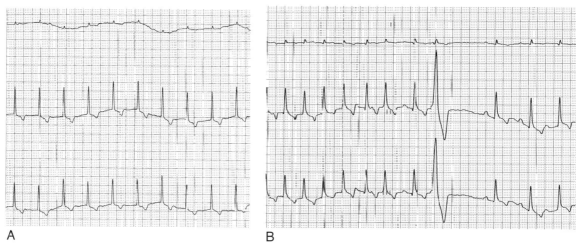

A   B

Figure 114–13. A, A junctional-type rhythm with regularly spaced R-to-R intervals in this three-lead (I, II, III) simultaneous ECG taken at 25 mm/s in a dog. Atrial fibrillation would be associated with a more irregular baseline and an irregularly irregular R-to-R interval in contrast to this rhythm. A differential diagnosis for this tracing is sinoventricular rhythm. B, Junctional rhythm. Note the initial junctional tachycardia followed by ventricular premature contraction and spontaneous resetting to the normal rhythm in a three-lead (I, II, III) simultaneous recording at 50 mm/s.

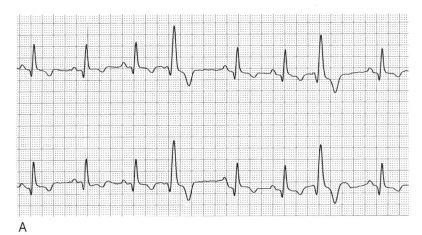

A

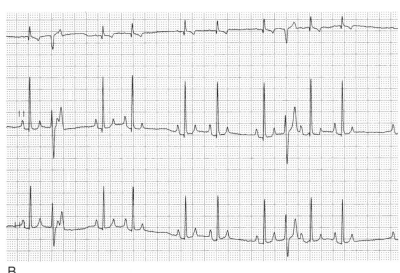

B

Figure 114–14. *A,* Ventricular extrasystoles. Ventricular premature contractions are seen in this taurine-deficient collie with dilated cardiomyopathy in leads II and III recorded simultaneously at 50 mm/s and at one-half amplitude. Beats 4 and 7 are premature with aberrant QRS-T complexes. The R-R interval for the two beats preceding the ventricular premature complex (VPC) equal two R-R intervals from the beat before the VPC to the beat after the VPC, indicating a compensatory pause. This type of pause is also characteristic of a VPC. *B,* This three-lead simultaneous recording at 25 mm/s in a middle-aged German shepherd dog with myocarditis identifies single VPCs (numbers 2 and 8) occurring intermittently. Beat number 8 occurs in between two normal beats and is an example of a true extrasystole (interpolated beat).

with antiarrhythmic drugs). The most challenging aspect of managing ventricular extrasystoles remains the evaluation of their severity and therefore assessment of the need for treatment (see Therapy of Arrhythmias).

There are only two goals of treatment of ventricular tachycardias: to reduce the ventricular rate so as to optimize cardiac output and to reduce the risk of progression to a lethal arrhythmia. Some (ECG) features that have been claimed to indicate severity (and perhaps to warrant antiarrhythmic treatment) are etiology, clinical manifestations, frequency (e.g., if more than 10 per cent of QRSs are ventricular extrasystoles), rate of occurrence (single versus pairs or bursts), morphology (polymorphic: multiple ectopic foci), and R-on-T phenomenon or degree of prematurity. None of these parameters has yet been shown to affect an animal's prognosis, and these "criteria" remain anecdotal in veterinary medicine. (**Antiarrhythmic drugs to consider: class I, II, III.**) "Prophylactic" treatment of asymptomatic ventricular arrhythmias is detrimental and therefore not recommended in human medicine.

Ventricular Tachycardia

Ventricular tachycardia is a series of three or more ventricular extrasystoles occurring at a high rate (Fig. 114–15). It may be continuous (sustained) or intermittent (paroxysmal). Ventricular tachycardias are much less common than ventric-

ular extrasystoles, constituting approximately 4 per cent of rhythm disturbances (see Table 114–1), but their causes are just as diverse. Clinical manifestations are frequent (weakness, syncope) but their occurrence depends directly on the hemodynamic consequences of the rhythm. The greater the rate, the greater the likelihood that cardiac output is decreased, resulting in overt signs. Doppler echocardiography has shown that ventricular tachycardia may be asymptomatic because it has been demonstrated in conjunction with an adequate cardiac output. This situation is particularly true in cases of accelerated idioventricular rhythms (see later), in which case the need to treat with antiarrhythmics becomes highly questionable.

The identification of ventricular tachycardia is easier when it is paroxysmal: the typical appearance is one or several series of QRS complexes that are widened (greater than 0.07 second), do not resemble the sinus QRS complexes, are associated with giant T waves, are not linked to P waves, and may include capture beats (sinus QRS complexes) and fusion beats (QRS complexes whose morphology is intermediate between that of sinus QRS complexes and that of ectopic QRS complexes) (see Fig. 114–15). The ECG diagnosis can become more challenging when ventricular tachycardia is continuous, particularly when it is of septal origin and thus produces QRS complexes that are fairly narrow and resemble supraventricular complexes. Wide QRS complexes caused by other factors (see earlier) must not be mistaken

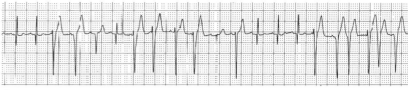

Figure 114-15. *A,* Ventricular tachycardia. A lead II electrocardiogram taken at 25 mm/s initially has two normal beats followed by two VPCs, then two fusion beats (numbers 5 and 6) followed thereafter by a burst of ventricular tachycardia (7 to 12). A series of three capture beats then occurs, followed again by a burst of ventricular tachycardia. Note the R-on-T phenomenon in the next to last abnormal beat. *B,* This full lead tracing demonstrates two episodes of paroxysmal ventricular tachycardia. In the initial portion of the ECG, note three capture beats that precede the initial burst of ventricular tachycardia. Leads V_1, V_2, and V_3 are actually V_2, V_4, and V_{10}. The tracing is at 25 mm/s.

for ventricular tachycardia. (**Antiarrhythmic drugs to consider: class I, II, and III antiarrhythmics.**)

Ventricular Flutter

Ventricular flutter is a rapid and prefibrillatory stage of ventricular tachycardia. The ECG appearance of this rhythm is a tight, tall sinusoidal wave in which it is impossible to separate QRS complexes and T waves and in which neither capture nor fusion beats are seen. This intermediate stage between ventricular tachycardia and ventricular fibrillation is rare, brief, and precedes cardiac arrest. It must be considered a severe ventricular arrhythmia and warrants immediate intravenous antiarrhythmic treatment or possibly electrical defibrillation.

Ventricular Fibrillation

Ventricular fibrillation is a disorganized, chaotic sequence of ventricular depolarizations involving complete desynchronization of ventricular electrical activity. Hemodynamically, it produces circulatory collapse and arrest. It is therefore a preagonal state leading to death within minutes. The ECG appearance consists of erratic, patternless waves of variable morphology, amplitude, and frequency (Fig. 114-16). The underlying cause is generally a severe disorder, such as myocardial trauma, anoxia, severe electrolyte disturbance, or advanced state of shock. Ventricular fibrillation is often preceded, and therefore heralded, by ventricular extrasystoles demonstrating the R-on-T phenomenon, then sustained ventricular tachycardia, then ventricular flutter.[1] When the rhythm has reached ventricular fibrillation, treatment (cardiopulmonary resuscitation), although often unrewarding, must be instituted immediately and generally involves electrical defibrillation if available. (**Antiarrhythmic treatments to consider: electrical defibrillation, KCl and CaCl$_2$, class III.**)

Torsades de Pointes

Torsades de pointes is an intermediate ventricular arrhythmia that arises from prolongation of the QT interval.[69] The rotation of the peaks of the QRS complexes on the horizontal axis of the ECG is due to the ever-changing geometry of the reentry circuit, which finds no stable position. The diagnosis of torsades de pointes is based on the following criteria: (1) the rhythm immediately before the onset of torsades is slow and the QT interval is prolonged (greater than 0.25 second); (2) the onset of torsades involves an R-on-T ventricular extrasystole (e.g., depolarization [R wave] occurs during the vulnerable part of the T wave); (3) the ensuing rapid (greater than 180 beats/min) ventricular rhythm has QRS complexes that are more regular than in ventricular fibrillation but are continuously changing in amplitude and polarity (Fig. 114-17). The total duration is usually brief (5 to 10 seconds) but torsades may also evolve lethally into ventricular fibrillation. Torsades de pointes is rare in the dog but may be caused by any disorder that prolongs the QT interval: congenital long-QT syndrome (Dalmatian), hypokalemia, hypocalcemia, and overdosage or toxicity of antiarrhythmic drugs, particularly class IA antiarrhythmics such as quinidine. The treatment is highly specific and requires discontinuation of all antiarrhythmic drugs and institution of intravenous magnesium sulfate (10 to 30 mg/lb slowly IV).[20, 26, 69]

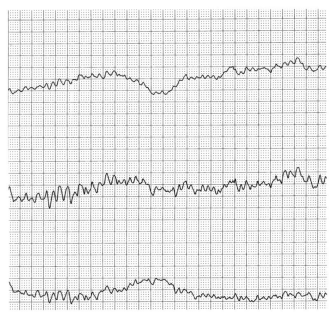

Figure 114–16. Ventricular fibrillation. This three-channel (leads I, II, and III) ECG shows chaotic ventricular activity as erratic, patternless waves varying in morphology. The erratic electrical activity is associated with a nonfunctional ventricle equivalent to cardiac arrest hemodynamically.

Accelerated Idioventricular Rhythms

Identified as a specific subset of ventricular tachycardia for the past 30 years and paradoxically named "slow ventricular tachycardia" at first, accelerated idioventricular rhythms (AIVRs) have several of the same ECG characteristics as ventricular tachycardia, including AV dissociation; wide, bizarre QRS complexes; and the possibility of capture beats and fusion beats. However, the rate of accelerated idioventricular rhythms is between 70 and 160 beats/min, which places it between idioventricular rhythm (less than 70 beats/min) and true ventricular tachycardia in terms of rate. The slower AIVRs (70 to 100 beats/min) occur as a response to bradycardia and are a type of ventricular escape that is faster than the usual 20 to 70 beats/min.[31] The more rapid AIVRs (100 to 160 beats/min) are rare but may be seen with cardiomyopathy (particularly Boxer type), shock (gastric dilatation and volvulus syndrome), digitalis intoxication, and general anesthesia.[26] In general, AIVRs are well tolerated. Treatment is directed at the underlying cause.

Ventricular Parasystole

Ventricular parasystole ("one heart beats as two") is a complex arrhythmia that results from the concurrent and independent activity of two pacemakers, one being a normal supraventricular pacemaker and the other existing in a protected site in a ventricle. By definition, parasystole has (1) a ventricular focus with independent, abnormal automaticity and a rate greater than that of an escape focus and (2) a unidirectional (entry) block that shields this focus from sinus

depolarizations. The rate of sinus depolarizations is normal for parasystole versus escape rhythms, in which it is slow or absent. Parasystole therefore has several ECG characteristics: (1) unlike the situation in reentry, coupling intervals (R-R intervals between normal beat and ectopic beat) are variable; (2) intervals that separate ectopic complexes are related to one another in a simple arithmetic relationship (which is a multiple of the duration of the ectopic cycle); (3) fusion complexes occur; and (4) parasystolic complexes appear when the heart is excitable, such as during pauses or during slowing of the sinus node, and therefore the frequency of ventricular extrasystoles increases during carotid sinus massage with parasystole (Fig. 114–18). In the dog, parasystole is most commonly associated with Boxer cardiomyopathy and hypothyroidism.[20] Parasystole is most often benign, does not warrant antiarrhythmic treatment, and is usually refractory to therapy.

DISORDERS OF CONDUCTION

Disorders arising from faulty intracardiac conduction are simply referred to as blocks. Blocks are grouped according to anatomic and functional criteria. Anatomic criteria separate them on the basis of their anatomic location: SA blocks, AV blocks, and BBBs.

Functional criteria characterize blocks according to their degree of severity: first degree, delay in conduction; second degree, complete intermittent block; and third degree, complete permanent block. In addition to conduction blocks, there are disturbances of excess conduction. Although rare, the more common of these are due to rapid accessory pathways that short-circuit the normal, slow AV route of conduction between the atria and the ventricles (preexcitation syndromes).

Sinoatrial Blocks

SA block is a rarely detected conduction disturbance that occurs between the SA node and the atrial tissue. It should not be mistaken for the much more common AV blocks ("heart blocks") (see later). In SA block, the impulse is properly generated by the sinus node but is not transmitted to the atria or beyond them. SA blocks may be of first degree (slowing of the impulse from the SA node to the atria), second degree (intermittent block), and third degree (permanent block). The only form of SA block that is detectable with routine ECG is second-degree SA block, in which a sinus pause occurs whose duration is, in theory, an exact multiple of the P-P interval in the basic rhythm. This type of block occurs in brachycephalic dogs secondary to intoxication (e.g., iatrogenic digitalis overdose). Treatment naturally revolves around etiology, namely reducing the dose of digitalis to appropriate levels in cases of toxicity. This rhythm may be difficult to detect, given some normal dogs' propensity for marked sinus arrhythmia.

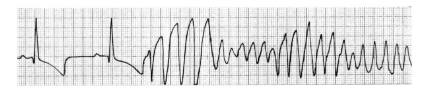

Figure 114–17. Torsades de pointes. This single-channel recording from a dog at 50 mm/s identifies an initial slow heart rate, prolongation of the QT interval, followed by a run of rotating QRS complexes constantly changing in amplitude and polarity.

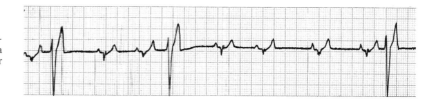

Figure 114–18. Parasystole. This hypothyroid dog demonstrates two independent rhythms; a sinus rhythm with a normal P-QRS-T complex and an independent idioventricular rhythm. Lead II tracing at 25 mm/s.

Atrioventricular Block

AV blocks are defined as delays or stoppages of conduction, transient or permanent, between the atria and the ventricles (specifically, between the upper part of the AV node and the common trunk of the His bundle). AV blocks are common conduction disturbances in small animal cardiology. First- and second-degree AV blocks occur frequently (15 and 12 per cent, respectively) (see Table 114–1) but are often barely, or not at all, symptomatic. Third-degree AV blocks are much less common (2 per cent) (see Table 114–1) but usually have much more apparent clinical effects (exercise intolerance, syncope).

First-degree AV block is a simple delay in AV conduction (Fig. 114–19). It may be permanent or transient and may arise from a structural lesion or be simply functional. The ECG diagnosis is based on normal, sinus-appearing QRS complexes and a prolonged PR interval. The clinical manifestations are nil; first-degree AV block is an ECG finding only and does not warrant treatment. Its importance is essentially diagnostic, drawing the clinician's attention to possible causes of delayed conduction, which include AV nodal damage in the major forms of heart disease, and functional abnormalities in iatrogenic AV blocks such as excessive digitalis or antiarrhythmic therapy.

Second-degree AV blocks involve complete, but not permanent, interruption of AV conduction. There are two important subtypes of second-degree AV block. Mobitz's type I second-degree AV block is characterized by a progressive lengthening of the PR interval until ultimately a P wave is blocked (P wave without QRS complex), known as the Wenckebach phenomenon. Anatomically, Mobitz's type I second-degree AV block originates high in the AV node and has a good prognosis because it is closely related to first-degree AV block (and is almost always asymptomatic). Mobitz's type II second-degree AV block demonstrates perfectly regular PR intervals until one or more P waves are blocked (Fig. 114–20). In simple Mobitz's type II second-degree AV block, there are more conducted P waves than blocked P waves, whereas in advanced Mobitz's type II second-degree AV block there are more blocked P waves than conducted P waves. Mobitz's type II second-degree AV block arises from the AV bundle and carries a more guarded to poor prognosis because it more closely resembles third-degree AV block. Simple Mobitz's type II second-degree AV blocks may on occasion produce clinical manifestations such as exercise intolerance, whereas the more advanced Mobitz's type II second-degree AV blocks commonly produce clinical signs that are similar to those of third-degree AV block: weakness and syncope, even at rest.

Third-degree AV block is a complete and permanent interruption of AV conduction. The ventricles depolarize according to an autonomic rhythm, called an escape rhythm (junctional or ventricular; see later) (Fig. 114–21). Therefore, communication between the atria and ventricles is abolished (complete AV dissociation). The ECG diagnosis is based on the complete absence of P-wave conduction (frequent Ps without QRSs, no consistent PR interval) and on slow ventricular QRS complexes (20 to 70 beats/min), which are often regular. Symptomatic, third-degree AV blocks produce marked exercise intolerance, weakness, and syncope. Even so, it is possible to encounter older animals, not active by nature, who have "asymptomatic" third-degree AV blocks.[2, 3]

The causes of AV blocks are diverse. First-degree AV and Mobitz's type I second-degree AV blocks are frequently functional (high vagal tone in healthy individuals, negative dromotropic effects of digitalis, antiarrhythmics, or alpha$_2$-stimulating anesthetics). Less commonly, cardiac disease with atrial dilatation and AV nodal pathology may be present. Mobitz's type II second-degree AV block and third-degree AV block are sometimes functional (hyperkalemia, digitalis toxicity, alpha$_2$-stimulating anesthetics) but are more commonly associated with a structural lesion or inflammatory (endocarditis, Lyme disease, traumatic myocarditis) or degenerative (physical disruption arising from cardiomyopathy, endocardiosis, or fibrosis) condition. Treatment is therefore aimed at the underlying cause. In advanced Mobitz's type II second-degree AV blocks or third-degree AV blocks, the response to parasympatholytic or sympathomimetic drugs tends to be fairly disappointing and potentially dangerous. Pacemaker implantation is a better choice (see Fig. 114–21B).

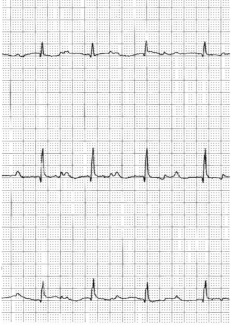

Figure 114–19. First-degree heart block. This tracing demonstrates prolongation of the PR interval to 0.20 second. Three-channel (leads I, II, III) simultaneous tracings at 50 mm/s.

Bundle Branch Blocks

BBBs are slowings or interruptions of conduction involving one or more of the ventricular branches of the His

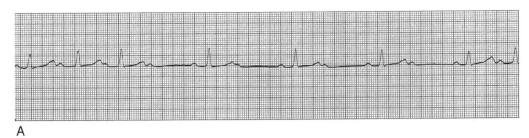

A

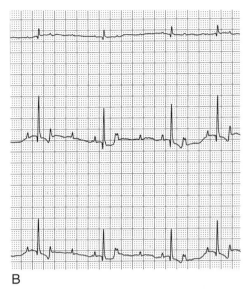

B

Figure 114–20. Second-degree AV block. *A*, Type I (Wenckebach) second-degree AV block is seen. The P-R interval progressively lengthens until the QRS is dropped. *B*, Second-degree AV block, Mobitz type II. This is a triple-channel tracing (leads I, II, and III) of a dog experiencing weakness. Extra heart sounds were ausculted. The P waves occur regularly every 10 boxes, resulting in a 2:1 and 3:1 atrial-to-ventricular rhythm. Recording at 25 mm/s.

bundle. Blocks may be functional (functional interruptions caused by the depolarizations occurring during the refractory period) or structural (permanent interruptions caused by a physical disturbance).

The ECG diagnosis of bundle branch block is based on the change in shape of the QRS complexes, which become widened because of the desynchronization of the two ventricles. The duration of the QRS complexes is greater than 0.07 second, and the polarity is positive in lead II for left bundle branch blocks and negative in lead II for right bundle branch blocks (Figs. 114–22 and 114–23). If bundle branch block occurs with a sinus rhythm, the ECG diagnosis is straightforward, because other than the abnormal appearance of the QRS complexes, the P-QRS-T sequence throughout the ECG is normal: there is a P wave before each QRS and the PR interval is fixed and normal.

Establishing a diagnosis of bundle branch block can become much more challenging if the block occurs concurrently with a nonsinus rhythm, such as atrial fibrillation. A BBB together with atrial fibrillation imitates ventricular extrasystoles or ventricular tachycardia, which may misdirect therapeutic decisions, especially with regard to digitalis (see Atrial Fibrillation, earlier). Cats with heart disease (especially cardiomyopathy) are prone to develop block in a subdivision of the left bundle branch known as the left anterior fascicle (LAF).[26] LAF block produces a tall R wave in leads I and aVL and a deep S wave in leads II, III, and aVF (Fig. 114–24).

The causes of BBB are many; they may be due to all types of ventricular abnormality including hypertrophy, as in feline hypertrophic cardiomyopathy; dilatation, as seen in dilated cardiomyopathy (especially in Boxer and Doberman dogs); and inflammation (endocarditis, traumatic myocarditis). In the dog, right bundle branch block is often a completely normal, if potentially disturbing-looking, ECG finding. Clinical manifestations of bundle branch blocks alone generally do not occur. These disturbances therefore do not warrant specific treatment beyond treatment of their underlying cause. It is important to recognize BBBs because they could be the first indicators of underlying cardiac disease that itself warrants further diagnosis and treatment.

Escape Rhythms

Escape rhythms arise from a physiologic (as opposed to pathologic) ectopic focus when a superior focus (pacemaker) fails to fire. For example, a ventricular escape rhythm and ventricular tachycardia could have identically shaped QRS complexes, but escape complexes, occurring at 40 beats/min in an otherwise electrically silent heart, are rescuing the heart from asystole and must not be suppressed. They arise from pacemaker cells whose rate is slower than that of the SA node. Therefore, they occur only when there is a failure to generate (sinus pause or arrest) or to conduct (third-degree SA or AV block) the sinus impulse, and thus they rescue the cardiac rhythm. The "rescue" ectopic foci that generate escape rhythms generally exist at one of two levels: supraventricular or ventricular.

For junctional supraventricular escape rhythms, the QRS complexes are narrow and the P wave may not be seen if it occurs within the QRS complex. The heart rate is typically 40 to 70 beats/min.

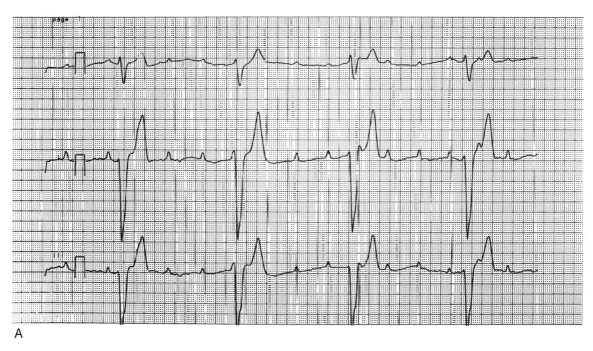

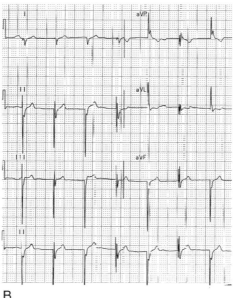

Figure 114–21. Third-degree AV block. *A,* Leads I, II and III simultaneously recorded at 50 mm/s. Note the regularly occurring P waves, unrelated to the QRS complexes (varying PR intervals) and the slow, aberrant-appearing QRS complexes. *B,* A simultaneous recording from a cat with an implanted pacemaker. Note the regular pacemaking spikes on each QRS complex occurring exactly 16 boxes apart. Recording taken at 25 mm/s.

In ventricular escape rhythms, the QRS complexes are wide, with a rate generally between 20 and 40 beats/min (see Fig. 114–21). Any serious condition depressing sinus excitability (sinus arrest) or affecting supraventricular conduction should lead to a junctional rhythm or an idioventricular (ventricular escape) rhythm. For example, animals do not develop asystole and die when they have third-degree AV block because of the emergence of an escape rhythm.

Other than the escape beats, which are generally highly regular, the remainder of the tracing depends on the rhythm disturbance that led to the appearance of the escape rhythm in the first place. For example, in cases of failure to generate a sinus impulse, there is no physical P wave (except the retrograde, negative P waves between the QRS complex and the T wave that arise from lower junctional rhythms). In such cases, termed "sinus arrest," differentiating the rhythm from a sinoventricular rhythm or atrial standstill may be difficult. In cases of AV block, P waves exist but they have no connection to the QRS complexes (AV dissociation).

In isorhythmic AV dissociation (IAVD) the atria and ventricles beat independently (e.g., third-degree AV block, ventricular tachycardia), yet the ventricular rhythm happens to occur at the same rate as the sinus (P wave) rate. Thus, Ps and QRSs occur at the same rate even though there is no correlation between the two (AV dissociation). To establish this diagnosis on the basis of an ECG can be a delicate task, because it may appear that the P waves are related to the QRS complexes, when in fact there is no AV conduction.

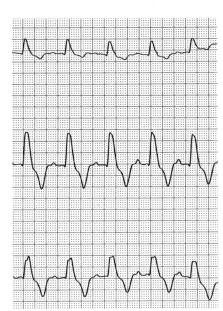

Figure 114–22. Left bundle branch block. Three simultaneously recorded leads (I, II, III) at 50 mm/s characterize this condition by regular appearing P-QRS-T complexes with wide QRS complexes, greater than 0.07 second. This 13-year old Vizsla dog had asymptomatic chronic mitral valvular disease.

Careful examination of the PR interval demonstrates not only that it varies but also that there are P-QRS-T sequences that are incoherent (e.g., sequences in which positive P waves occur between the QRS complex and the T wave), showing that there must be complete dissociation between the atria and ventricles. Performing a vagal maneuver slows the P waves but not the QRSs, strengthening the diagnosis of IAVD. Isorhythmic AV dissociation, which is unusual in the dog, is seen in cats with hypertrophic cardiomyopathy.[20, 26] This arrhythmia is rarely symptomatic, given the nearly normal rate of ventricular depolarization. There-fore, it does not warrant therapy beyond treatment of the underlying problem.

Atrial Standstill (or Silent Atrium or Sinoventricular Rhythm)

This rhythm disturbance does not strictly fall into the category of blocks. It is an arrhythmia characterized by total absence of atrial depolarization despite normal impulse formation in the SA node (Fig. 114–25). Without depolarizing the atria, the sinus impulse is nevertheless properly conducted to the AV node, and the ventricular depolarization is normal. Therefore, the rhythm is referred to as sinoventricular. This type of atrial standstill is rare in the dog, somewhat less so in the cat, and may arise from two etiologies. First, it may be a structural anatomic lesion, consisting of atrial parenchymal hypoplasia, occasionally associated with a dystrophic form of neuromyopathy, particularly in the springer spaniel dog breed. Second, it may be functional, caused by severe hyperkalemia (K^+ usually greater than 7.5 mEq/L), because the atrial myocardium is particularly sensitive to the potassium ion. Either way, the ECG appearance is therefore of a supraventricular rhythm with a normal rate but without detectable P waves. Differentiating between the two causes of this rhythm using the ECG alone is difficult, and measurement of serum electrolytes is warranted.

DISORDERS OF BOTH EXCITABILITY AND CONDUCTION

Of the multiple rhythm disturbances that have been described, many can occur jointly on the same ECG tracing, producing mixed disturbances of excitability and of conduction. This section discusses examples of disturbances of excitability and of conduction that produce specific clinical syndromes.

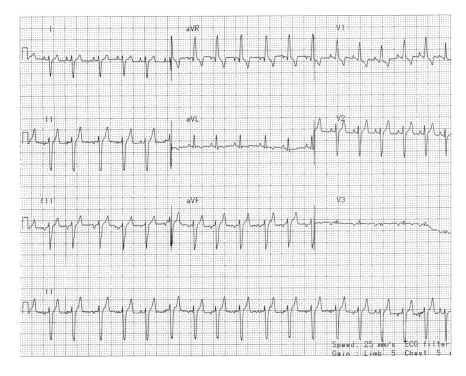

Figure 114–23. Right bundle branch block. Note wide QRS complexes with deep, prolonged S waves in leads I, II, and III, a positive large R wave in V, and normal P-QRS-T progression. V_1, V_2, V_3 represent leads V_1, V_4, and V_{10}. Simultaneously recorded 9-lead strip @ 25 mm/s with a lead II rhythm strip at the bottom.

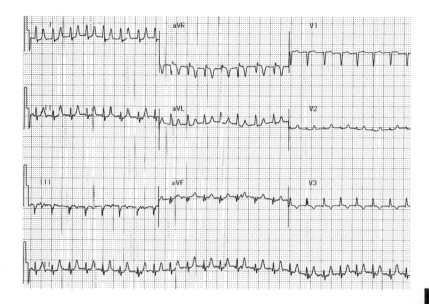

Figure 114–24. Left hemibranch block. Left axis deviation with positive leads I and aVL is seen in this cat with hypertrophic cardiomyopathy and probable atrial fibrillation (resulting in a loss of P waves and irregularly irregular and rapid QRS complexes). V_1, V_2, and V_3 as identified were recorded as V_1, V_4, and V_{10}. The tracing at 25 mm/s and $2\times$ standardization suggests left axis deviation and left ventricular enlargement. However, the conduction disturbance makes these diagnoses suspect and warrants further evaluation of the clinical state. The predominant QRS direction is leftward in this cat.

Preexcitation Syndromes

These syndromes link a conduction disturbance (conduction that is accelerated by passage through an accessory conduction pathway that short-circuits the normal AV nodal–His pathway) to a disturbance of excitability (supraventricular tachycardia related to reentry via macro circuits involving the accessory pathways). Classically, three types of bundles of abnormal, highly conductive tissue ("accessory pathways") have been identified pathologically.[24] The Kent bundle directly connects the atria to the ventricles. On the ECG, the anterograde passage of the sinus impulse through the Kent bundle produces a shortened PR interval (less than 0.08 second) and a notching of the QRS complex by a delta wave, which indicates the premature depolarization of part of the ventricles (Fig. 114–26A and B). However, a sinus impulse passing first in an anterograde direction through the AV node, then in retrograde fashion (often more conductive

than the anterograde direction) through the Kent bundle, may lead to a circuit referred to as a macro reentry circuit, or circus rhythm, that produces a potentially rapid and symptomatic supraventricular tachycardia. This type of condition is termed the Wolff-Parkinson-White syndrome. It is a rare condition in the dog and slightly less so in the cat, in which it is occasionally associated with hypertrophic forms of cardiomyopathy.[1, 2, 20, 26, 31] Initial treatment can involve carotid sinus massage, which, through its slowing of AV conduction (i.e., negative dromotropic action), breaks the cycle of reentry. Amiodarone, an excellent supraventricular antiarrhythmic with few negative inotropic effects, can be used in the management of such tachyarrhythmias. Conversely, digoxin is contraindicated because of its powerful negative dromotropic effect on the AV node, which then redirects passage of the depolarization through the accessory pathway.

A second type of accessory pathway, the James bundle, directly connects the atria to the upper part of the His bundle. The ECG outcome is a tracing in which the PR interval is short (the AV node is bypassed) with no widening of the QRS complex (the two ventricles are activated synchronously) and no delta wave. This type of rhythm is occasionally encountered in dogs with CHF and in humans causes the Lown-Ganong-Levine syndrome.

The third type of accessory pathway, the Mahaim fibers, directly connects the AV node to the ventricles, thus bypassing the common trunk of the bundle of His. The ECG appearance of this rhythm involves a normal PR interval with a QRS complex that is more widened than that in a Kent bundle aberration. At present, this third type of preexcitation has not been described in small animals.

Sick Sinus Syndrome (Bradycardia-Tachycardia Syndrome)

This syndrome involves a complex disturbance of the cardiac conductive tissues, producing simultaneous defects in sinus activity (sinus bradycardia and SA block), AV conduction disturbances (first-degree and second-degree AV blocks), and disturbances in supraventricular and ventricular excitability (Fig. 114–27). Therefore, the disturbance is not a problem involving only the SA node, as the name "sick sinus syndrome" suggests, but rather an illness that affects cardiac tissue at all levels.

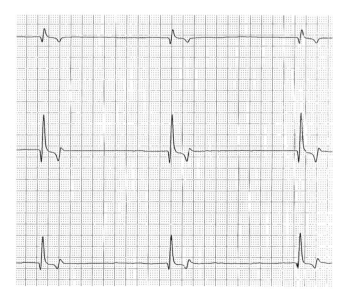

Figure 114–25. Atrial standstill. Six-year-old male retriever-cross dog with hypoadrenocorticism. Chronic vomiting, weight loss, and hyperkalemia were present. The ECG identifies a slow heart rate, absence of P waves (atrial standstill), and wide but normal QRS complexes. Three-channel simultaneous recording (leads I, II, III) at 50 mm/s.

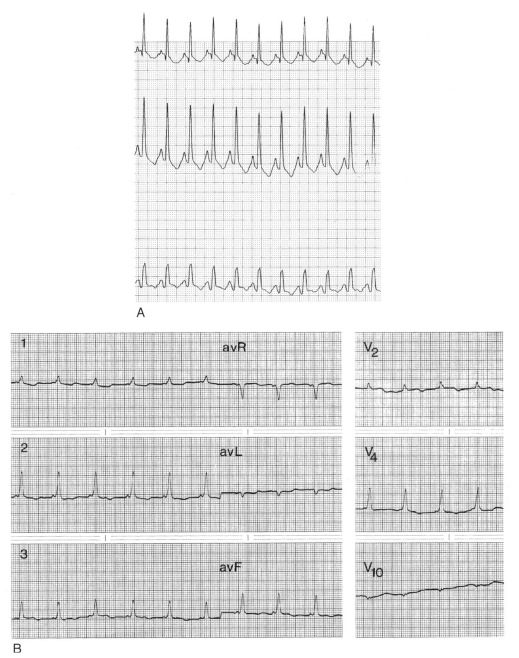

Figure 114–26. *A,* Ventricular preexcitation. A three-channel, simultaneously recorded ECG (leads I, II, III at 50 mm/s) suggests a preexcitation tracing in this cat. This disorder is identified by an increased heart rate and shortened PR segment. *B,* This tracing identifies a very short PR interval with notching of the upstroke of the R wave in some of the leads.

The etiology of sick sinus syndrome is unknown, but certain features stand out from cases reported in the literature. Female small breed dogs are more commonly affected, with a clear predilection for the miniature schnauzer breed. The age of onset is middle to late years (6 to 10 years), and the association with chronic mitral valvular disease is common but not obligatory. Histopathologically, nodal tissue fibrosis is seen, associated with vascular disturbances (microcoronary arteritis). The ECG diagnosis requires repeated and sufficiently long (2- to 3-minute) tracings in order to demonstrate properly all of the aspects of sick sinus syndrome: sinus bradycardia (often with first- or second-degree AV block), prolonged sinus pauses with variable escape beats, and bursts of supraventricular tachycardia (see Fig. 114–27). In some cases, especially in miniature schnauzer dogs, only sinus bradycardia occurs. The most common overt clinical manifestation of this arrhythmia is syncope induced by bradycardia. Vagolytic drugs may acutely improve the situation by reducing the impact of bradycardia episodes and pauses, but definitive treatment may require the implantation of a pacemaker. Digitalis glycosides are usually contraindicated.

THERAPY OF ARRHYTHMIAS

Underlying and predisposing factors involved in the precipitation of arrhythmias should be identified and resolved when possible. A practical approach to choosing antiarrhythmic therapy incorporates known clinical efficacy, adverse

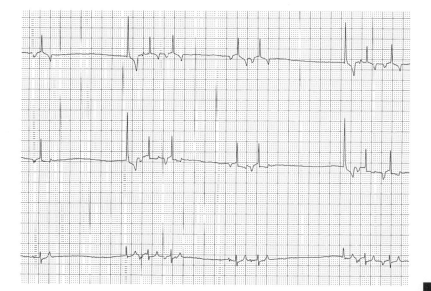

Figure 114–27. Sick sinus syndrome. A 9-year-old female schnauzer with lethargy, panting, and malaise and a 3/6 systolic murmur. The ECG shows an irregular rhythm, ventricular escape beats. negative P waves, sinus pauses, and a bradyarrhythmia. These and other irregularities, often supraventricular in nature, are characteristic of sick sinus syndrome. Periods of both tachycardia and bradycardia are common and alternating in this condition. Leads I, II, III recorded simultaneously at 25 mm/s.

drug reactions, pharmacokinetic effects, and results of administration.

During the past decade, significant changes in the approach to antiarrhythmic therapy have evolved. This, in large part, is the result of the 1991 Cardiac Arrhythmia Suppression Trial in human beings after myocardial infarction. In this multigroup placebo-controlled double-blind study, researchers unexpectedly found an increased rather than decreased risk of death when certain type IC antiarrhythmic agents were administered. Although ambient arrhythmias are still regarded as a risk factor, the rush to treat asymptomatic VPCs has been markedly reduced.[27]

The decision to treat ventricular arrhythmias in veterinary medicine should be based on the functional effects of the rhythm and not the frequency or morphologic complexity of the abnormal beats.[27] Whereas arrhythmias are still considered a marker of risk for arrhythmia progression, asymptomatic complex arrhythmias without signs do not necessarily represent an increased risk of sudden death.

The veterinary experience may or may not be significantly different from the human. Long-term outcome studies of arrhythmic conditions have not been completed. We do not know what happens to dogs or cats with arrhythmias of different etiologies, nor are we able to compare arrhythmias of different etiologies regarding outcome or specific drug therapies. In general, dogs with mitral regurgitation are not likely to die suddenly of arrhythmic causes, whereas some cardiomyopathic Doberman pinschers and Boxers and dogs with advanced subaortic stenosis are at risk of sudden death if they have an arrhythmic condition.

"When to treat?" probably remains the single most important and unresolved question in veterinary cardiology. Therapy based on human medical recommendations may be inappropriate because of the principal differences in disease etiology between the species. Survival and efficacy studies of complex arrhythmias in veterinary medicine are few. Of these, none were double blind or placebo controlled. Mortality studies have not been completed, and it is impossible to verify the actual benefits of antiarrhythmics that have been administered. When symptoms are present, it is difficult to argue with therapeutic efforts to contain the arrhythmia. When clinical signs are absent, it is relevant to compare the potential side effects of therapy, including proarrhythmia, with the potential benefit of a stabilized or normalized rhythm. Proarrhythmia aside, Calvert et al.[29] have shown the adverse effects of routine anesthesia and surgery in Doberman pinschers with occult cardiomyopathy, thereby reminding the clinician to consider the dangers of medical procedures that may exacerbate uncontrolled arrhythmias.[29]

CLASSIFICATION SYSTEMS FOR ANTIARRHYTHMIC AGENTS

Antiarrhythmic drugs have traditionally been classified in four groups according to their predominant effect on the action potential. Dissatisfaction with the shortcomings of the Vaughn-Williams (V-W) classification scheme for antiarrhythmic drugs (Table 114–3) resulted in the creation of a competing classification system[30] correlating antiarrhythmic drugs with the mechanism of the arrhythmia and vulnerable parameters as well as actions of the drug (Tables 114–4 and 114–5).[72] The scheme, known as the Sicilian gambit (SG), is based on the actions of drugs on arrhythmogenic mechanisms and is another attempt at providing a rational basis for therapy.

Limitations of the traditional V-W system include its incomplete classification, crossover within the system among specific drugs, and discussion principally of blocking mechanisms while activation of channels and/or receptors is not considered. Antiarrhythmic agents may be effective in a number of ways: slowing tachycardias, terminating arrhythmias, making them tolerable, or preventing their initiation.[30] The V-W classification is based only on the electrophysiologic drug effects on isolated, normal cardiac tissue (except for class II agents), which differ from those in the disease state. The classification excludes compounds such as digitalis, adenosine, and alpha-adrenergic blocking agents. The V-W classification system assumes that we know more than we really do. Not all drugs within a class have the same physiologic or clinical effects. The danger in using only the simplified scheme is that most drugs have more than one mode of action and not all the drugs within a category are always the same.

The SG first tries to identify the mechanism of the arrhythmia. A vulnerable parameter, that is, the electrophysiologic property of the arrhythmia most susceptible to modification, is identified; a target likely to influence that parameter is

TABLE 114–3. VAUGHAN-WILLIAMS CLASSIFICATION OF ANTIARRHYTHMIC DRUGS

ELECTROPHYSIOLOGIC EFFECTS	EXPECTED ELECTROCARDIOGRAPHIC EFFECTS	DRUGS USED IN VETERINARY MEDICINE
Class I		
Drugs with direct action (Na$^+$ channel blockade)		
Ia Depress phase 0	Widen QRS interval	Quinidine
Slow conduction	Prolong QT interval	Procainamide
Prolong repolarization		
Lengthen refractory periods		
Ib Little effect on phase 0 in normal tissue	Limited effect on QRS and conduction	Lidocaine
Depress phase 0 in abnormal fibers	Shorten QT interval	Tocainide
Shorten repolarization		Mexiletine
Elevate fibrillation thresholds		
Ic Markedly depress phase 0	Widen QRS interval	Encainide
Markedly slow conduction		Lorcainide
Limited effect on repolarization		Flecainide
		Propafenone
Class II		
Sympatholytic drugs	No effect on ECG except slowing of sinus rhythm	Propranolol
		Metoprolol
		Atenolol
		Esmolol
Class III		
Drugs that prolong repolarization	Prolong Q-T interval	Amiodarone
		Sotalol
		Bretylium
Class IV		
Calcium channel blocking drugs	Slowing of the sinus rate	Diltiazem
	Possible P-R prolongation (mild)	Verapamil
		Amlodipine

selected; and a drug known to modify the target is chosen. Although this is academically reasonable, there are few instances in small animal medicine in which these parameters can be accurately assessed.

Veterinarians seldom have access to electrophysiologic monitoring, and we rely on past experience as well as trial and error. We are required to rely more on ECG and Holter monitoring than detailed electrophysiologic (EPH) testing. In human beings, there is little or no difference in drug efficacy when arrhythmias are identified by electrophysiologic testing or Holter monitoring.[38] Physicians usually cannot match drug to mechanism and must instead rely on empirical drug selection.[38] Despite the known actions of the agents and the recognized mechanisms of arrhythmia induction, clinical correlation is difficult as the cellular mechanism is often not deducible from the surface ECG.

Antiarrhythmic therapy is described in this textbook for the practicing veterinarian with access to ECG monitoring, possibly telemetry, and echocardiography. EPH monitoring and terminology, although desirable, are with few exceptions not used in practice. Therefore, the discussion of these techniques is limited to what is required to make knowledgeable medical decisions. Most veterinarians should find our approach practical and reasonable. There are excellent specialty textbooks and cardiology journals for additional information. Only commonly used and available drugs or those likely to be useful for canine or feline heart disease are discussed. New drugs are identified, as are new uses for older drugs. In general, drug dosages are omitted in the text and may be found in Table 114–6. Where new drugs or dosages are recommended, brief discussions of dosage, route of administration, or other specifics are included in the text.

Class I Antiarrhythmics

Class I drugs selectively block the fast sodium channels, decreasing sodium influx during phase 0. A reduced slope of phase 0 leads to decreased conduction velocity. Slowed conduction velocity can interrupt a reentrant pattern.[31] These drugs work best in cells dependent on the fast sodium channel for their action potential, such as normal and ischemic Purkinje cells and myocardial cells. Within this class are three subgroups, distinguished by their electrophysiologic and antiarrhythmic differences (see Table 114–3). Most of the compounds in this class fail to perform adequately in the presence of hypokalemia.

Class Ia Drugs

Class Ia antiarrhythmic drugs markedly depress the phase 0 action potential, depress conduction of electrical impulses through the heart, and slow cardiac repolarization by lengthening the effective refractory period.[31] By depressing the conduction velocity and prolonging the refractory period, arrhythmias dependent on reentry may be interrupted. Drugs in this class include quinidine (prototype Ia drug), procainamide, and disopyramide. Quinidine decreases the rate of spontaneous depolarization in pacemaker fibers, prolongs antegrade refractoriness in the accessory pathway, and can suppress or trigger delayed afterdepolarizations. Quinidine may prolong the PR interval, widen the QRS complex, and lengthen the QT interval and is indicated for the control of supraventricular and ventricular arrhythmias.

An anticholinergic property of quinidine can lead to increased AV conduction; therefore, caution is warranted if supraventricular tachycardia is present. Intravenous use can induce hypotension by alpha blockade and is not recommended. The rare dog benefits from high doses of quinidine by permanent conversion of recent-onset (e.g., postanesthetic) atrial fibrillation to sinus rhythm. Quinidine is contraindicated in third-degree AV block, digitalis intoxication, ventricular tachycardia associated with long QT intervals, myasthenia gravis, and severe hepatic failure. Relative con-

TABLE 114–4. CLASSIFICATION OF DRUG ACTIONS ON ARRHYTHMIAS BASED ON MODIFICATION OF VULNERABLE PARAMETER

ARRHYTHMIA	MECHANISMS	VULNERABLE PARAMETER	DRUGS
	Automaticity (a) Enhanced normal		
Inappropriate sinus tachycardia Some idiopathic ventricular tachycardias		Phase 4 depolarization (decrease)	Beta-adrenergic blocking agents Na^+ channel blocking agents
	(b) Abnormal		
Atrial tachycardia		Maximal diastolic potential (hyperpolarization) or	M_2 agonist
		Phase 4 depolarization (decrease)	Ca^{2+} or Na^+ channel blocking agents M_2 agonists
Accelerated idioventricular rhythms		Phase 4 depolarization (decrease)	Ca^{2+} or Na^+ channel blocking agents
	Triggered activity (a) EAD		
Torsades de pointes		Action potential duration (shorten) or	Beta agonists; vagolytic agents (increase rate)
		EAD (suppress)	Ca^{2+} channel blocking agents; Mg^{2+}; beta-adrenergic blockers
	(b) DAD		
Digitalis-induced arrhythmias		Calcium overload (unload) or	Ca^{2+} channel blocking agents
		DAD (suppress)	Na^+ channel blocking agents
Certain autonomically mediated ventricular tachycardias		Calcium overload (unload) or	Beta-adrenergic blocking agents
		DAD (suppress)	Ca^{2+} channel blocking agents, adenosine
	Reentry (Na^+ channel dependent) (a) Long excitable gap		
Atrial flutter type I		Conduction and excitability (depress)	Na^+ channel blocking agents (except lidocaine, mexiletine, tocainide)
Circus movement tachycardia in WPW		Conduction and excitability (depress)	Na^+ channel blocking agents (except lidocaine, mexiletine, tocainide)
Sustained monomorphic ventricular tachycardia		Conduction and excitability (depress)	Na^+ channel blocking agents
	(b) Short excitable gap		
Atrial flutter type II		Refractory period (prolong)	K^+ channel blockers
Atrial fibrillation		Refractory period (prolong)	K^+ channel blockers
Circus movement tachycardia in WPW		Refractory period (prolong)	Amiodarone, sotalol
Polymorphic and sustained monomorphic ventricular tachycardia		Refractory period (prolong)	Quinidine, procainamide, disopyramide
Bundle branch reentry		Refractory period (prolong)	Quinidine, procainamide, disopyramide, bretylium
Ventricular fibrillation		Refractory period (prolong)	
	Reentry (Ca^{2+} channel dependent)		
AV nodal reentrant tachycardia		Conduction and excitability (depress)	Ca^{2+} channel blocking agents
Circus movement tachycardia in WPW		Conduction and excitability (depress)	Ca^{2+} channel blocking agents
Verapamil-sensitive ventricular tachycardia		Conduction and excitability (depress)	Ca^{2+} channel blocking agents

AV = atrioventricular; DAD = delayed afterdepolarization; EAD = early afterdepolarization; WPW = Wolff-Parkinson-White.
Reproduced with permission from Task Force of the Working Group on Arrhythmias of the European Society of Cardiology: The Sicilian gambit. A new approach to the classification of antiarrhythmic drugs based on their actions on arrhythmogenic mechanisms. Circulation 84:1831, 1991. Copyright 1991. American Heart Association.

traindications exist for patients with milder forms of AV block. Hypokalemia may predispose to torsades de pointes. Quinidine increases serum digoxin, verapamil, and amiodarone levels; cimetidine decreases the metabolism of quinidine. Combined with verapamil or a beta blocker, quinidine may induce negative inotrope and hypotension. Sodium bicarbonate administration and metabolic alkalosis transiently increase protein binding of quinidine.[32, 33] Proarrhythmic effects necessitate discontinuation of the drug.

Quinidine is well absorbed orally, is metabolized by the liver, and is eliminated by the kidneys. It is widely bound to plasma and tissue proteins.[33]

Principal side effects include anorexia, nausea, vomiting, diarrhea, intestinal cramping, confusion, skeletal muscle weakness, ataxia, and seizures. Thrombocytopenia, dermatopathies, and fever are possible.[33]

Procainamide has cardiac effects similar to those of quini-

dine. The propensity for IV-induced hypotension or increased ventricular rates caused by increased AV conduction is diminished. Like quinidine, procainamide is used for control of APCs, VPCs, atrial fibrillation, accessory pathway slowing, and atrial and ventricular tachycardias. Procainamide has been demonstrated to prolong the effective refractory period and slow conduction in the accessory pathway of dogs with orthodromic AV reciprocating tachycardia.[35]

Procainamide is metabolized by the liver and eliminated by the kidney. The sustained-release formulations may be poorly absorbed and even eliminated as intact tablets in the feces of dogs.

Procainamide may be used in conjunction with other class I agents and beta blockers for refractory arrhythmias. Oral administration of the drug at higher than usually recommended dosages to achieve trough serum concentrations of 10 to 12 μg/mL was successful in controlling some

TABLE 114–5. ACTIONS OF ANTIARRHYTHMIC DRUGS*

DRUG	CHANNELS — NA Fast	Medium	Slow	Ca	K	I_f	RECEPTORS α	β	M₂	P	PUMPS Na⁺, K⁺-ATPase	CLINICAL EFFECTS Left Ventricular Function	Sinus Rate	Extra-cardiac	ECG EFFECTS PR Interval	QRS Width	JT Interval
Lidocaine	○											→	→	Ⓐ			↓
Mexiletine	○											→	→	Ⓐ			↓
Tocainide	○											→	→	●			↓
Moricizine	●I											↓	→	○		↑	
Procainamide		●A			Ⓐ							↓	→	●	↑	↑	↑
Disopyramide		●A			Ⓐ				○			↓	→	Ⓐ	↑↓	↑	↑
Quinidine		●A			Ⓐ		○		○			→	↑	Ⓐ	↑↓	↑	↑
Propafenone		●A						Ⓐ				↓	→	○	↑	↑	
Flecainide			●A		○							↓	→	○	↑	↑	
Encainide			●A									↓	→→	○		↑	↑
Bepridil	○			●	Ⓐ							?	↓	○			↑
Verapamil	○			●			Ⓐ					↓	↓	○	↑		↑
Diltiazem				Ⓐ								↓	↓	○	↑		↑
Bretylium					●		▣	▣				→	↓	○			↑
Sotalol					●			●				↓	↓	○	↑		↑
Amiodarone	○			○	●		Ⓐ	Ⓐ				→	↓	●	↑		↑
Alinidine					Ⓐ	●						?	↓	●			
Nadolol								●				↓	↓	○	↑		
Propranolol	○							●				↓	↓	○	↑		
Atropine									●			→	→	Ⓐ	↓		
Adenosine										□		?	↓	○	↓		
Digoxin										□	●	↑	↓	●	↑		↓

*Relative potency of block: ○ = low; Ⓐ = moderate; ● = high; □ = agonist; ▣ = agonist/antagonist. A = activated state blocker; I = inactivated state blocker.
From Schwartz PJ, Zaza A: The Sicilian gambit revisited—Theory and practice. Eur Heart J *13*:23, 1992. Copyright © 1992 reproduced by permission of the publisher W.B. Saunders Company Limited.

supraventricular tachyarrhythmias.[34, 35] Procainamide is contraindicated in the presence of third-degree AV block. Side effects are anorexia, nausea, vomiting, fever, proarrhythmia, and agranulocytosis but are infrequent.

Disopyramide is similar to quinidine and procainamide. Excretion is primarily renal with some hepatic metabolism. It is rarely used in veterinary medicine, and there is little clinical experience in dogs and less in cats. Side effects are principally anticholinergic and negative inotrope. It is contraindicated in the presence of CHF, pulmonary edema, glaucoma, urine retention, advanced AV block, and sinus node dysfunction. Hyperkalemia accentuates its myocardial depressant effect.[31]

Class Ib Drugs

Class Ib agents shorten repolarization, decrease the slope of phase 0, depress automaticity, and increase the threshold for ventricular fibrillation. These drugs have an affinity for binding with inactivated sodium channels, thereby acting selectively on diseased or ischemic tissue. There are minimal effects on the sinus node, AV node, and atrial muscle or on inotrope. Lidocaine, phenytoin, tocainide, and mexiletine are examples of drugs in this class.

Lidocaine is used for acute control of life-threatening ventricular arrhythmias. It is not likely to affect myocardial contractility, systemic arterial blood pressure, the QRS complex, or AV conduction time.[31] Lidocaine significantly suppresses automaticity and conduction velocity and prolongs refractoriness in diseased (ischemic) cardiac cells.

Lidocaine is effective only when used IV owing to first-pass hepatic metabolism. It is less than 10 per cent protein bound. Hepatic disease, chloramphenicol, propranolol, halothane, cimetidine, and norepinephrine may all delay hepatic metabolism of lidocaine. Hepatic microenzyme inducers enhance degradation.[32]

Lidocaine intoxication results in seizures. These usually subside within minutes after lidocaine is discontinued. Diazepam or a short-acting barbiturate may be necessary to control the seizure. Sudden death and bradyarrhythmia may be complications with its IV use in the cat. Lidocaine may be administered by slow (2- to 5-minute) IV loading bolus (2 to 4 mg/lb) followed by a continuous-rate infusion (CRI) of 10 to 30 μg/lb/min in dogs. Alternatively, after the initial bolus, an additional amount can be given at half the dosage every 10 minutes to maintain the rhythm. Cats are more sensitive to lidocaine and require lower bolus dosages of 0.25 to 0.5 mg/lb slowly over 5 minutes followed by 5 to 20 μg/lb/min CRI. Intramuscular lidocaine is rarely utilized and is less efficacious. It may be administered in emergency situations when IV access is not possible at a dosage of 2 to 4 mg/lb intramuscularly in the dog.

Tocainide and mexiletine are structurally analogous to lidocaine but have oral bioavailability. Response to lidocaine may not be a predictor of response to these oral agents.

Tocainide is orally absorbed and undergoes hepatic metabolism and renal excretion. It may be used after lidocaine or as initial treatment in a hemodynamically stable patient. At 6.8 to 11.4 mg/lb orally every 8 hours, peak levels were reached in cardiomyopathic Doberman pinscher dogs after 2 hours and began to diminish by 8 hours. Fifteen of 23 dogs experienced a 90 per cent diminution of their ventricular tachycardias and there was a 70 per cent reduction of all VPCs in 80 per cent of the cardiomyopathic dogs. Although there was no relationship between dosage and serum concentration, nontoxic dogs had serum levels less than 11 mg/L and all those with toxic signs had levels greater than 14 mg/L.[36]

Side effects observed within 8 days are weakness, head tremor, ataxia, and head bobbing. In the long term, corneal dystrophy, corneal edema, or renal failure was observed in more than 50 per cent of dogs.[36, 37]

Mexiletine is absorbed orally and undergoes less than 10 per cent first-pass hepatic elimination. It is 70 per cent protein bound. The half-life varies depending on the urine pH. The drug is eliminated by renal excretion. Side effects are infrequent in the dog but can include nausea, inappetence, and tremor.[40] Sinus bradycardia, ataxia, dizziness, and thrombocytopenia are potential problems. There are no data regarding its use in cats. Twenty-two dogs with frequent VPCs and multiform VPCs related to DCM (7), myocarditis (11), and unknown causes (4) were studied and received mexiletine at 2 to 5 mg/lb every 8 hours. Sixty-four per cent had effective control of their arrhythmia for 2 weeks to 8 months as determined by brief, in-hospital ECGs. Four of seven incomplete responders improved when quinidine was added to the schedule. No dog experienced more serious arrhythmias or morphologic P or QRS alterations.[40] This was an open label study without conclusions about mortality or clinical benefits. Mexilitine is available only in the oral formulation in North America.

Intravenous mexiletine antagonized the prolongation effect on the QT interval of sotalol and its proarrhythmic effect in a canine model of torsades de pointes.[41] Both mexiletine and tocainide appear to have synergistic properties when combined with class Ia or class II agents.

Class IC Drugs

Class IC drugs profoundly depress phase 0 and conduction velocity. They exert a minimal effect on refractoriness or action potential duration. They may be indicated for supraventricular and ventricular tachyarrhythmias and arrhythmias involving accessory pathways. They are notorious in humans for their proarrhythmic tendencies. They depress contractility, cardiac output, and systemic blood pressure. These drugs are contraindicated in the presence of AV block, BBB, and myocardial depression. Flecainide and propafenone are class IC agents.

Flecainide is indicated for paroxysmal supraventricular tachycardia and paroxysmal atrial fibrillation but not for chronic atrial fibrillation or patients with ventricular dysfunction, ventricular hypertrophy, ischemic heart disease, or valvular heart disease. Its use has not been reported in clinical small animal medicine. This drug may induce or aggravate CHF.

Propafenone has local anesthetic effects and a direct stabilizing action on myocardial tissue as well as weak beta-adrenergic blocking activity. It prolongs AV nodal conduction (A-H and H-V) and has negative inotropic action. It is effective against many SVT, accessory pathway arrhythmias as well as ventricular arrhythmias. Proarrhythmia is unlikely in humans with structurally normal hearts. Propafenone is available only in the oral form in North America.

Class II Antiarrhythmics

Class II antiarrhythmics reverse or nullify the electrophysiologic and arrhythmogenic effects of beta-adrenergic sympathetic stimulation.[48] The magnitude of the beta-blockade effect is dependent on the prevailing level of sympathetic tone. Sympathetic stimulation increases the likelihood of slow calcium channels opening and the rate of pacemaker discharge. Overall, beta blockers depress the slope of phase 4 depolarization and minimally raise the threshold for activation in sinus and AV nodal cells, thereby suppressing automaticity. The effect of beta blockers on normal cell refractoriness and conduction is modest and it is unlikely that they influence cardiac repolarization. As a result of the negative inotropic, chronotropic, and dromotropic effects, cardiac output is reduced and myocardial oxygen requirements and LV work are decreased.

Beta blockade is indicated for supraventricular tachycardias, including atrial flutter, atrial fibrillation, and preexcitation tachyarrhythmias. It may be even more effective in controlling the ventricular rate response to atrial fibrillation in combination with digitalis. Beta blockade should be helpful in ventricular arrhythmias induced by sympathetic stimulation.[44] It may be used in combination with a class I agent for refractory ventricular tachyarrhythmias in the dog or alone as the primary agent in the cat. Beta blockade has traditionally been useful in the treatment of hypertension, obstructive heart disease, thyrotoxicosis, and digitalis toxicity. In addition, a role in the management of pheochromocytoma, theobromine intoxication, dilated cardiomyopathy, and portal hypertension is possible.[48]

Contraindications include AV block and sick sinus syndrome. Many beta blockers are not cardioselective; that is, they exert their effects on both beta$_1$ and beta$_2$ receptors, resulting in bronchial smooth muscle constriction. Nonselective beta blockers are contraindicated in patients with dynamic bronchial disease. Relative contraindications for use include concurrent myocardial depression, CHF, hypotension, and peripheral vascular disease. Beta blockers, especially nonselective types, may interfere with the compensatory response to hypoglycemia and exercise.[48]

Because of the potential for adverse effects of excess beta blockade, the dosage rate must be individually titrated. Side effects include lethargy, fatigue, depression, anorexia, vomiting, and diarrhea. Thrombocytopenia and agranulocytosis are unlikely. Adverse reactions such as hypotension, CHF, sinus bradycardia, AV block, bronchospasm, and hypoglycemia can occur. If adverse reactions occur, myocardial depression may be addressed with careful infusion of isoproterenol or dobutamine. Sinus bradycardia responds to atropine or glycopyrrolate administration. Serum glucose levels should be monitored. After chronic oral use, drug withdrawal should be gradual to prevent acute arrhythmia induction or hypertension.

Cardioselective (beta$_1$-blocking) agents exert their primary effect on cardiac beta$_1$ receptors, especially at lower doses. This property is helpful in patients with asthma, chronic obstructive pulmonary disease, hypoglycemia, peripheral vascular disease, or thrombosis. Atenolol, esmolol, and metoprolol are examples. Other beta blockers have mild intrinsic sympathomimetic activity (ISA) that provides some protection for patients with underlying myocardial failure or those dependent on high sympathetic tone to maintain cardiac output. Some beta-blocking agents such as carvedilol, bucindolol, and labetalol have alpha$_1$-blocking activity, providing vasodilatation.[48] These drugs reduce peripheral vascular resistance and may be useful in hypertension, dilated cardiomyopathy, and arrhythmias.

Propranolol has been the standard beta blocker used in veterinary medicine for years. It blocks both beta$_1$ and beta$_2$ receptors. It is well absorbed orally, experiences large and variable first-pass hepatic and portal elimination, and has variable plasma protein binding. The half-life is 3 to 6 hours in dogs, but effects may persist long enough to require only twice-daily dosing. Lethargy in cats is a prominent side effect. Beta-blocking agents with longer durations of action are often used in place of propranolol.

TABLE 114–6. DRUGS USED FOR THE TREATMENT OF CARDIAC ARRHYTHMIAS

GENERIC NAME	TRADE NAME	ADMINISTRATION ROUTE	COMMON INDICATIONS	DOSAGE	COMMENTS
Adenosine	Adenocard	IV	Terminates acute paroxysmal supraventricular tachycardia	1.5–3.0 mg/dose; repeat in 1 min to maximum of 6–12 mg	Side effects: sinus arrest, sinus bradycardia, and atrioventricular block
Amiodarone	Cordarone	Oral	Recurrent ventricular fibrillation; recurrent hemodynamically unstable ventricular tachycardia	2–4 mg/lb q12h	Side effects include proarrhythmias, pulmonary fibrosis, hypothyroidism, liver necrosis, photosensitivity and others; minimum use in veterinary medicine at this time.
Atenolol	Tenormin	Oral	Same as propranolol	0.2–0.5 mg/lb bid in the dog; 1.4 mg/lb sid to bid in the cat	Weakness; depression; hypotension; bradycardia; inappetence.
Atropine Tablets Injectable		Oral; IV, IM, SQ	1. Test responsiveness of sinus node 2. Hyperactive carotid sinus reflex (SA arrest) 3. AV block (second and third degree)	0.01–0.03 mg/lb IV, IM, SQ	1. Do not use in states of heart failure. 2. Do not administer when bronchial tree secretions are a problem. 3. Used infrequently in heart block.
Digoxin Tablets Elixir Injectable	Lanoxin Cardoxin	Oral Oral IV	1. Supraventricular premature contractions and tachyarrhythmias 2. Right heart failure 3. Pump dysfunction	0.22 mg/m² bid PO as maintenance dosage; double dosage initially first 24 h for rapid effect; lower dosage in large (>30 lb) and giant breeds of dogs 0.0312 mg eod PO in cats	1. Digitalize cautiously. 2. Monitor with ECG. 3. All doses are approximate and the patient must be monitored frequently. 4. Side effects—malaise, anorexia, vomiting, diarrhea.
Diltiazem	Cardizem	Oral IV	Supraventricular tachyarrhythmias; feline hypertrophic cardiomyopathy	0.2–0.7 mg/lb q8h PO in dogs 0.7 mg/lb q8h PO in cats IV: 0.05–0.1 mg/lb; repeat every 2 min to effect	Side effects include bradycardia, hypotension, collapse and severe weakness; sudden death may occur.
Disopyramide	Norpace	Oral	Ventricular arrhythmias	5–10 mg/lb q8h (q12h using long-acting product)	May be used in conjunction with quinidine or procainamide.
Esmolol	Brevibloc	IV	Supraventricular tachycardia	25–100 µg/lb/min 0.22 mg/lb IV Effects occur within 2 min	Short-term IV agent; used to control ventricular rate while agents are given for long-term effects; used for atrial fibrillation, atrial flutter, supraventricular tachycardia; side effect is rapid, severe hypotension; do not use in congestive heart failure–compromised patient.
Isoproterenol Injectable	Isuprel Injectable	IM, IV, SC	1. Advanced second-degree and third-degree heart block 2. SA arrest 3. Sinus bradycardia(?)	For bradyarrhythmias: 1 mg/500 mL D5W IV to increase heart rate, use to effect (0.5–1 mL/min) 0.1–0.2 mg SQ or IM q4h for heart block. (Variable efficacy by these routes.)	May be used on temporary basis parenterally until conduction improves or a pacemaker is implanted. Do not use when hypotension is present.
Lidocaine 2% without epinephrine	Xylocaine	IV only	1. Ventricular tachyarrhythmias	1. 2–4 mg/lb IV slow bolus over 2 min or until arrhythmia controlled. 2. 1 mg/lb IV slowly, then 10–30 µg/lb/min continuous infusion or 1 mg up to 4 times over 5 minutes to effect. 3. For cats, 0.25–0.5 mg/lb IV bolus, then 5–20 µg/lb/min CRI	1. Reserve for serious arrhythmias. 2. Toxicity includes convulsions and respiratory arrest. 3. Single IV dose lasts 15–20 min only. 4. Excretion is hepatic.
Metoprolol	Lopressor Toprol XL	Oral	Hypertension, beta blockade	0.2–0.5 mg/lb sid or divided in multiple doses bid-tid depending on product used	Used for hypertension, beta blockade; ?arrhythmias.
Mexiletine	Mexitil	Oral	Ventricular tachyarrhythmias	2–5 mg/lb q8-12h (dogs)	Few side effects; may be used with digoxin and class I antiarrhythmic agents; hepatic excretion.

Drug	Brand	Route	Indications	Dosage	Comments
Phenytoin Capsules Injectable	Dilantin	Oral IV	1. Some ventricular tachyarrhythmias 2. May be useful in treating arrhythmias caused by digitalis overdose	7–14 mg/lb q8h orally 2.24–4.5 mg/lb IV	Infrequently used as an antiarrhythmic drug; hepatic excretion.
Pindolol	Visken	Oral	Hypertension	1–3 mg bid-tid orally	Do not discontinue abruptly; often used with thiazide; not commonly used in veterinary medicine.
Procainamide Capsules Tablets Injectable	Pronestyl Pronestyl-SR Procan SR	Oral IV	1. Ventricular premature contractions 2. Ventricular tachycardia	1. 3–10 mg/lb q2–6h (to 8h sustained-release form) 2. Dogs: 1–10 mg/lb IV over 30 min, then infuse 10–20 µg/lb/min CRI 3. Cats: 0.5–1.0 mg/lb IV bolus, then 5–10 µg/lb/min CRI	1. IV effect is brief, and oral maintenance dose must be given q4h 2. Oral forms available in sustained-release tablets may not be absorbed 3. Hepatic excretion
Propafenone	Rhythmol	Oral IV (?)	(a) Supraventricular tachyarrhythmias (b) Accessory conduction arrhythmias (c) Ventricular tachycardia	Unknown. Begin in medium to large size dogs with 75–125 mg orally tid	May be proarrhythmic in structural heart disease
Propranolol Tablets Injectable	Inderal	Oral IV	1. Supraventricular tachyarrhythmias 2. To slow ventricular rate in atrial fibrillation or to distinguish the latter from ventricular tachycardia 3. Arrhythmias of digitalis intoxication 4. Preexcitation syndromes 5. Some ventricular arrhythmias, when other agents fail	Oral: general 0.2–0.5 mg/lb q8h: 2.5–20 mg/lb q8-12h small dogs; 10–40 mg q8-12h medium and large dogs; 40–80 mg q8-12h large and giant dogs; 2.5 mg q12–24h cats; 0.25–0.5 mg IV no more frequently than q1–3 min to 5 mg maximum; administer until rate slows or toxicity occurs. Cats: 0.25–0.5 mg IV bolus, then 2.5 5 mg/cat PO sid-bid	1. Use with caution: as a negative inotropic agent it may induce congestive heart failure 2. Excessive dosage causes reduction in cardiac rate and prolongation of PR and QT intervals
Quinidine gluconate Injectable Tablets	Quinidine gluconate Quinaglute Qinidex	IM Oral	Same as quinidine sulfate	3–10 mg/lb (of base) q2–4h IM, PO; delayed-release forms are same dosage but given q8 12h orally	Same as quinidine sulfate Injectable product is not used IV—only IM (epaxial)
Quinidine sulfate Tablets	Quinidne sulfate	Oral	1. Ventricular premature contractions 2. Ventricular tachycardia	3–10 mg/lb (of base) IM or PO q6–8h; may be given q2h until loading dose controls arrhythmia or induces toxicity	1. Do not use in presence of congestive heart failure unless this is being treated simultaneously 2. Toxicity results in increased heart rate and prolongation of the PR, QRS, and QT intervals 3. Often effective in lower doses when used with procainamide, mexiletine, or a beta-blocking agent 4. Hepatic excretion 5. IV use may cause hypotension
Sotalol	Betapace	Oral	Class II and III for ventricular arrhythmias	Canine: 2.2–3.6 mg/lb bid-tid Feline: 10–20 mg/lb bid-tid	May need to use with other class Ia antiarrhythmic agents for better effect; hepatic excretion
Tocainide	Tonocard	Oral	Ventricular tachyarrhythmias	/–11 mg/lb q8–12h (dogs)	Side effects are weakness, collapse, bradycardia; contraindicated in shock, heart block, sick sinus syndrome, congestive heart failure, ventricular tachycardia
Verapamil	Isoptin	Oral IV	Supraventricular tachycardia	Oral: 0.2–1.0 mg/lb bid-tid IV: 0.02 mg IV to maximum of 0.07 mg/lb	

As with all beta blockers, dosage must be titrated individually. It is rare to need 80 mg per dose of propranolol even in giant breed dogs. Retitration is required when switching to the sustained-release formulation. Intravenous therapy is reserved for acute arrhythmias, especially anesthetic- or pre-excitation-related supraventricular tachycardias.

Atenolol is a beta$_1$-selective agent with the advantage of requiring once- or twice-daily dosing in cats. In nine normal cats, atenolol reduced heart rates for up to 12 hours and thus should perhaps be given on a twice-daily schedule. Beta blockade was not evident at 24 hours with an oral dosage of 1.4 mg/lb.[46] Another longer acting drug, metoprolol, is effective in dogs requiring beta blockade as well as in those with congestive heart failure associated with mitral valve disease or dilated cardiomyopathy. Studies (human) in heart failure suggest a possible beneficial increase in ejection fraction when beta-blocking agents are added.

Esmolol is an ultrashort-acting (9 minutes), rapid-onset (2 minutes), cardioselective beta blocker. It has been used as a trial agent (450 µg/lb infusion over 6 minutes) to reduce LV outflow tract gradients in cats with obstructive hypertrophic cardiomyopathy.[45]

Class III Antiarrhythmics

Each drug in this class frequently displays properties of other antiarrhythmic classes. Class III drugs specifically prolong the action potential duration and the refractory period, principally by inhibiting the repolarizing potassium channel (I_K). They are antiarrhythmic by reducing the initiation of an arrhythmia. Tissue cannot generate a new action potential before repolarizing, which slows or terminates a tachycardia. They should have few effects at normal heart rates but lengthen the action potential duration in a tachycardia.[47] They are noted for increasing the threshold for atrial and ventricular fibrillation. This drug group includes amiodarone, sotalol, ibutilide, and bretylium.

Amiodarone has had moderate success in controlling supraventricular and ventricular tachyarrhythmias in humans. It exhibits class I, II, and IV properties as well. Amiodarone has not been shown to be associated with increased mortality, nor is there evidence that it favorably affects survival except for a trend toward reduced mortality in human nonischemic cardiomyopathy.[49] It may be useful in dogs with LV systolic dysfunction to offer rate control as well as for converting acute atrial fibrillation to sinus rhythm.[20] Amiodarone is also able to relax vascular smooth muscle, resulting in decreased afterload. Side effects reported in humans include pulmonary fibrosis, liver damage, photosensitization, thyroid derangements, and ocular lesions. Amiodarone increases serum digoxin levels, so the dose of digoxin should be halved. Quinidine and procainamide levels are also elevated.[38]

Sotalol provides both class III (higher dose) and class II (l isomer, lower dose) effects.[59] It is not a negative inotrope and does not decrease LV ejection fraction. It induces systolic and diastolic hypotension and is considered to have approximately 30 per cent beta-blocking potency compared with propranolol. Considered to be protective against proarrhythmia, it is effective particularly for life-threatening ventricular arrhythmias.

Sotalol was shown to be more effective than six other antiarrhythmics in the human ESVEM trial.[49] The sotalol group had a lower 2-year mortality than groups receiving other antiarrhythmics. However, there was not a placebo control group with which to compare these results. The addition of IV mexiletine antagonized the proarrhythmic effects of sotalol on QT duration in a canine study, reducing torsades de pointes.[41]

In the only reported veterinary study utilizing sotalol, three classes of cardiomyopathic Boxer dogs were identified with ventricular arrhythmia: asymptomatic, syncopal, and CHF. Slowing of the heart rate and first-degree AV block were the only side effects observed, but proarrhythmic effects were seen in other dilated cardiomyopathy dogs with sotalol. The dosage of sotalol administered was 0.44 to 2.8 mg/lb/day given once a day, orally titrated to effect. The dogs with heart failure received less medication, up to 104 mg/day on average, compared with the syncopal group at 183 mg/day. Syncopal symptoms were diminished by sotalol therapy, and dogs with markedly diminished shortening fraction did not appear to exhibit untoward drug effects.[59] Oral dosages as high as 2.3 to 3.6 mg/lb increased the action potential duration in experimental dogs.[50] Sotalol has been effectively administered to cats with severe ventricular arrhythmias at 10 to 20 mg orally every 8 to 12 hours.[51] It is thought that class III effects are predominant at lower dosages and class II effects are predominant only at higher dosages (greater than 160 mg in humans).

Sotalol's good oral absorption is reduced when it is given with food. Steady state is reached within 2 to 3 days. It is indicated for life-threatening ventricular arrhythmias, may be used with caution in CHF, and should not be abruptly discontinued. Sotalol is used cautiously with other drugs that decrease blood pressure as well as other antiarrhythmics, specifically those that prolong the QT interval. It is contraindicated for patients with bronchospastic disease, second- or third-degree heart block, sinus bradycardia, and uncontrolled CHF.

Ibutilide is another (I_K) type III agent, particularly effective in humans for terminating recent-onset atrial fibrillation or atrial flutter.[52]

Bretylium produces a state resembling chemical sympathectomy after initial catecholamine release. Its principal use is to suppress ventricular fibrillation or prevent its recurrence. A canine dose of 2 to 5 mg/lb IV over 10 minutes is repeated every 4 to 6 hours.

Class IV Antiarrhythmics

Class IV drugs, known as calcium channel blockers, selectively inhibit slow inward calcium current channels (L type) during the action potential. Reentry can thus be interrupted. Calcium channel blockers interrupt arrhythmias resulting from abnormal automaticity and triggered mechanisms. They slow the sinus rate and, more profoundly, AV conduction by blocking the inward calcium current carried by the L-type (and probably T-type) channels.[53] By decreasing release of Ca^{2+} from the sarcoplasmic reticulum, they also decrease the force of contraction. Decreasing the amount of calcium into the myocyte may help to decrease myocardial protein synthesis and thus attenuate the pathologic process of hypertrophy. They are indicated for the control of most supraventricular tachycardias. Contraindications include sinus bradycardia, AV block, myocardial failure, sick sinus syndrome, and digoxin toxicity. Calcium channel blockers are classified as either dihydropyridines, which do not affect conduction and act principally on the vasculature (nifedipine and amlodipine), or nondihydropyridines, which have SA and AV nodal but minimal vascular effects (verapamil, diltiazem).

Verapamil has potent negative inotropic effects, moderate rate control, and minimal peripheral vascular effects. It is used in dogs to slow the sinus rate, increase AV conduction time, or decrease the ventricular response. In acute supraventricular tachycardias, it is given in 0.02 mg/lb IV increments to a maximum of 0.07 mg/lb. Acute hypotension, AV block, collapse, or hypocalcemia may result. Judicious calcium chloride administration may correct these iatrogenic disturbances.

Diltiazem is the favored drug of this class. Its effective antiarrhythmic properties combined with minimal inotropic depressive action, make it a popular drug for the veterinary patient. Its frequency-dependent channel blockade in the AV node makes it effective in slowing supraventricular arrhythmias. It is usually used in combination with digoxin to slow the rate in atrial fibrillation, although studies comparing it with beta blockade and digoxin in dogs are not available. Diltiazem-induced vasodilatation may create a reduction in afterload that is beneficial to the patient with heart failure.[53] Diltiazem has been administered to cats with hypertrophic cardiomyopathy in a non–placebo-controlled study. Over 6 months, there was a reduction in LV and septal wall thickness as well as left atrial size. Left atrial size was significantly improved.[54] The dosage of diltiazem for dogs and cats is 0.2 to 0.7 mg/lb every 8 hours. Using diltiazem CD, a sustained-release formulation, similar plasma concentrations were obtained in normal cats receiving 0.44 mg/lb oral diltiazem three times a day and 4.4 mg/lb oral diltiazem CD once a day.[55] For IV treatment of supraventricular tachyarrhythmias, diltiazem is recommended at 0.05–0.1 mg/lb repeating every 2 minutes until conversion or a safe maximal dosage has been reached. Continuous ECG and blood pressure monitoring is important.

Amlodipine and nifedipine are potent vasodilators and produce a marked decline in arterial blood pressure. They have a minimal effect on AV nodal tissue and are not used as antiarrhythmic agents but are used instead for treating isolated hypertension (see Chapter 50).

DIGITALIS GLYCOSIDES

Digitalis glycosides have multiple effects on cardiac muscle and conductive tissues. Their predominant antiarrhythmic properties result from a parasympathomimetic action on the SA and AV nodes and atrial muscle. AV nodal conduction is slowed, AV nodal refractoriness is increased, and vagal tone to ventricular muscle is increased. Of the antiarrhythmic agents, digitalis glycosides are among the few to produce a positive inotropic effect. Their primary indications for use are treatment of supraventricular tachycardias, which they accomplish by modifying the ventricular rate response. Often a second agent in combination, such as a beta blocker or calcium channel blocker, is needed to attain adequate rate control.

They are contraindicated in patients with accessory pathway preexcitation as they may speed conduction through the accessory pathway, promoting ventricular fibrillation. Concern exists about the use of digoxin in the presence of ventricular arrhythmias. If existent CHF is not due to the ventricular arrhythmia, digoxin may improve the arrhythmia by improving cardiac output. However, if the myocardium is diseased, the increased oxygen demands made by digoxin may worsen the arrhythmia. Dosing and pharmacokinetics are discussed in Chapter 111.

Digitalis intoxication is a serious, potentially life-threatening event. Gastrointestinal signs such as anorexia, nausea, vomiting, and diarrhea may be the first symptoms observed. Myocardial poisoning may take one of several forms. In-

creased sympathetic tone may result in increased automaticity. Slowed conduction and altered refractoriness may precipitate reentry. Increased intracellular calcium levels predispose the cell to delayed afterdepolarizations. Any of these changes can be the source of arrhythmogenesis. Electrocardiographically, ventricular tachycardia, supraventricular tachycardia, junctional escape complexes, SA arrest, Wenckebach's or other forms of AV block, and tachycardias with aberrant conduction may be seen. Stop the drug; provide supportive fluid and electrolyte therapy as necessary. Hypokalemia exacerbates digitalis intoxication. Specific treatment for ventricular tachycardias may be needed. Lidocaine decreases sympathetic tone and abolishes reentry and delayed afterdepolarizations. Phenytoin and propranolol are alternatives but should be used only if more traditional options have been exhausted. Atropine may help patients that are symptomatic because of bradyarrhythmias. Acute ingestion may be treated with cholestyramine or activated charcoal to reduce absorption. Digitalis Fab fragments bind serum digitalis molecules, preventing the myocardial effects. This treatment is prohibitively expensive.

There are numerous potential drug interactions of which one must be aware when using digitalis glycosides. Kaolin-pectin, metoclopramide, neomycin, antacids, and bran decrease oral absorption. Decreased digoxin clearance occurs with quinidine and, in cats, with concurrent furosemide, aspirin, and low-sodium diets. In humans, increased excretion is seen with hydralazine and nitroprusside. Decreased excretion may result with captopril, verapamil, and spironolactone.[31]

ADENOSINE, EDROPHONIUM, PHENYLEPHRINE

Adenosine is an endogenous nucleoside occurring in all cells of the body. Therapeutically, it slows AV nodal conduction and restores sinus rhythm in patients with paroxysmal supraventricular tachycardia. Electrophysiologically, it produces effects similar to those of acetylcholine by activating K+ channels. This shortens the atrial action potential duration, hyperpolarizes membrane potentials, and decreases atrial contractility. After IV injection, adenosine is taken up rapidly by red blood cells and vascular endothelial cells with an elimination half-life of less than 10 seconds. It is competitively antagonized by methylxanthines (caffeine and theophylline).

Adenosine is the drug of choice for terminating acute paroxysmal supraventricular tachyarrhythmias including accessory pathway (WPW) arrhythmias. It does not correct atrial flutter, atrial fibrillation, or ventricular tachycardia. It may help to differentiate wide QRS tachycardias by terminating supraventricular tachycardia but not ventricular tachycardia. It does not have adverse consequences in these arrhythmias.

Adenosine is preferred to verapamil unless the patient is receiving high-dose theophylline. This is principally due to its effectiveness and ultrashort duration of action and the ability to use the drug in the presence of uncontrolled CHF. It may be used in patients receiving digoxin, angiotensin-converting enzyme inhibitors, beta blockers, and calcium channel blocking agents. Side effects include transient AV block, sinus bradycardia, and sinus arrest. These occur commonly but are transient and of brief duration.

Human beings receiving this drug often experience transient (up to 1 minute) dyspnea, chest pain, and flushing. Adenosine is available in 2-mL vials (3 mg/mL). It is administered IV, followed by a rapid saline flush. The dosage is repeated after 1 minute if ECG changes have not occurred. Reports on clinical experience with adenosine in dogs and cats are not available. Suggested dosages are 1.5 to 3.0 mg initially repeated to a maximum of 6 to 12 mg.[19]

Edrophonium is an anticholinesterase agent with both nicotinic and muscarinic side effects. This drug has been used to treat supraventricular tachycardia and is often available in veterinary clinics (Tensilon, used for diagnosis of myasthenia gravis). The drug is administered at 0.05 mg/lb IV. Side effects are vomiting and muscular twitching.[57]

Phenylephrine, an alpha-adrenergic agonist, slows AV nodal conduction and induces vasoconstriction and hypertension. Reflex baroreceptor tone is thought to be the mode of slowing supraventricular tachycardia. It is given at 0.002 to 0.004 mg/lb IV.[56]

RADIOFREQUENCY ABLATION

In human medicine, electrophysiologic evaluation followed by radiofrequency catheter ablation of supraventricular circuits has become the treatment of choice for AV nodal reentry or AV reciprocating tachycardia. This permanently interrupts the pathways that allow the tachyarrhythmia to self-propagate.

The high rate of success, low mortality and morbidity, and cost-effectiveness of this technique have resulted in an entirely new subspecialty of human medicine often associated with pacemaker specialists who study and treat specific electrophysiologic dysfunctions of the heart. In veterinary medicine, pacemakers (see next section) are occasionally implanted and radiofrequency ablation has received limited attention.[57, 58] Although radiofrequency ablation will clearly become a more utilized procedure with time, costs and specialized requirements along with limited need will probably restrict its use to specialized cardiac institutions.

PACEMAKER THERAPY

Implantable cardiac pacemakers were first placed in human beings in 1958.[61] During the intervening period, there has been a revolution in the understanding and treatment of bradyarrhythmias as well as pacemaker and electrode technology.[60] Whereas over one-half million pacemakers are now placed annually by physicians, only several thousand have been implanted clinically in dogs and cats during the past four decades.

Pacemakers are utilized predominantly for bradyarrhythmia therapy, including sinus node dysfunction, AV block, and fascicular block. In human beings, implantable electrical devices are used for pacing and cardioversion, defibrillation, and specific forms of heart failure.[62] Historical reports of pacing are summarized from the human[61, 62] and veterinary[63–66] literature.

Costs, availability of pacemaker generators and electrode leads, the age and debilitated state of the dog or cat, and concerns regarding complications, aftercare, and general philosophy continue to restrict the availability of this technique to a limited number of our patients. The human literature is replete with articles and current recommendations such as for dual-chamber versus single-chamber ventricular pacing.[67] The balance of this section identifies current veterinary techniques and experiences with pacemaker implantation in North America. Although we are not up to human standards, it identifies what we presently do.

Reported methodology, problems, side effects, and expectations are limited to several refereed articles on dogs[63, 65] and one on cats.[64] Pacemakers were originally implanted transdiaphragmatically using epicardial leads. Most are now implanted in the dog transvenously through the jugular vein and attached to the RV wall. This is accomplished with either a "tined" lead or a lead that is screwed into the ventricular wall. Adverse reactions to transvenous leads have been observed in cats, and the trend today is to implant epicardial leads in cats requiring such treatment. Anesthesia has been performed with a balanced formula avoiding barbiturates. The generator is usually buried in a subcutaneous pocket of the neck or cranial abdomen and is connected to the electrode wire through a subcutaneous tunnel.

Pacemakers are usually identified by a three-letter code. The first letters identify the chamber(s) paced and sensed and the response to sensing. Whereas the DDD mode is the preferred pacemaker mode for most humans, the VVI mode is used most often for dogs and cats. Some electrophysiologists use two additional descriptive letters (Table 114–7).

Most veterinary cardiologists and internists secure their pacemakers from private sources, morgues, or the ACVIM Cardiology Specialty group. With limited availability of equipment, especially lead wires, we must be gracious about the gifts we receive. New pacemakers and wires would otherwise run into the tens of thousands of dollars for each unit. One additional word of caution: always ascertain in advance that the pacemaker is functional, that the lead wire is effective and compatible with the pacemaker, and that the pacemaker is single or dual programmed to the compatible lead wire.

In the largest and most recent pacemaker survey in dogs, Lehumkuhl and Sisson[66] reviewed pacemaker implantation in over 120 dogs at seven referral centers. Most dogs were paced for syncope or exercise intolerance secondary to AV block or sick sinus syndrome. Pacemaker rates were arbi-

TABLE 114–7. THE NASPE-BPEG GENERIC (NBG) PACEMAKER CODE*

POSITION: CATEGORY:	I CHAMBER(S) PACED	II CHAMBER(S) SENSED	III RESPONSE TO SENSING	IV PROGRAMMABILITY, RATE MODULATION	V ANTITACHYARRHYTHMIA FUNCTION(S)
Letters:	0 = none A = atrium V = ventricle D = dual (A + V)	0 = none A = atrium V = ventricle D = dual (A + V)	0 = none T = triggered I = inhibited D = dual (T + I)	0 = none P = simple programmable M = multiprogrammable C = communicating R = rate modulation	0 = none P = pacing (antitachyarrhythmia) S = shock D = dual (P + S)
Manufacturers' designation only:	S = single (A or V)	S = single (A or V)			

*Positions I through III are used exclusively for antibradyarrhythmia function. NASPE = North American Society of Pacing and Electrophysiology; BPEG = British Pacing and Electrophysiology Group.
Modified from Bernstein AD, Camm AJ, Fletcher RD, et al: The NASPE/BPEG Generic Pacemaker Code for antibradyarrhythmia and adaptive-rate pacing and antitachyarrhythmia devices. Pace 10:794, 1987. From Braunwald E (ed): Heart Disease: A Textbook of Cardiovascular Medicine, 5th ed. Philadelphia, WB Saunders, 1997, p 706.

trarily set at 100 beats/min. Whether long-term damage results from chronic pacing at this rate is not yet established. Major complications included cardiac arrest, perforation of the right ventricle, acute renal failure, CHF, lead or generator displacement, and pacemaker malfunction. Minor complications included seroma formation, arrhythmias, and twitching of the skin and subcutaneous muscle. Mean survival after pacing was 16 months for this group of dogs, and owner satisfaction after the procedure was usually high.[66]

REFERENCES

1. Ettinger SJ, Suter PF: Canine Cardiology. Philadelphia, WB Saunders, 1970.
2. Detweiler DK: The dog electrocardiogram: A critical review. In MacFarlane PW, Veitch Laurie TD (eds): Comprehensive Electrocardiology. New York, Pergamon, 1989, pp 1267–1329.
3. Detweiler DK: Electrocardiography in toxicological studies. In Sipes G, McQueen C, Gandolfi A (eds): Comprehensive Toxicology. New York, Pergamon, 1997, pp 95–115.
4. Miller MS, et al: Electrocardiography. In Fox PR, Sisson D, Moise NS (eds): Small Animal Cardiology, 2nd ed. Philadelphia, WB Saunders, 1999, Chap 6.
5. Lannek N: A Clinical and Experimental Study on the Electrocardiogram in Dogs. Thesis, Stockholm, 1949.
6. Einthoven W: The galvanometric registration of the human electrocardiogram, likewise a review of the use of the capillary electronometer in physiology. Translated in Willium F, Keys T (eds): Classics of Cardiology, Vol 2. New York, M Schuman, 1941, p 722.
7. Hahn AW, et al: Standards for canine electrocardiography. Academy of Veterinary Cardiology Committee Report, 1977.
8. Jacobs GJ: Signal averaged electrocardiography. Proceedings 16th Annual ACVIM Forum, San Diego, 1998, pp 121–122.
9. Calvert CA, et al: Possible late potentials in 4 dogs with sustained ventricular tachycardia. J Vet Intern Med 12:96, 1998.
10. Hinchcliff KW, et al: Electrocardiographic characteristics of endurance-trained Alaskan sled dogs. JAVMA 211:1138, 1997.
11. Schrope DP, et al: Effects of electrocardiograph frequency filters on P-QRS-T amplitudes of the feline electrocardiogram. Am J Vet Res 56:1534, 1995.
12. Hellerstein HK, Hamlin RL: QRS component of the spatial vectorcardiogram and of the spatial magnitude and velocity electrocardiograms of the normal dog. Am J Cardiol 6:1049, 1960.
13. Hamlin RL: Electrocardiographic detection of ventricular enlargement in the dog. JAVMA 153:1461, 1968.
14. Trautvetter E, et al: Evolution of the electrocardiogram in young dogs during the first twelve weeks of life. J Electrocardiol 14:267, 1981.
15. Oguchi Y, Hamlin R: Rate of change of QT interval in response to sudden change in the heart rate in dogs. Am J Vet Res 55:1618, 1994.
16. Ulloa H, et al: Arrhythmia prevalence during ambulatory electrocardiographic monitoring of beagles. Am J Vet Res 56:275, 1995.
17. Haggstrom J, et al: Heart rate variability in relation to severity of mitral regurgitation in Cavalier King Charles spaniels. J Small Anim Pract 37:69, 1996.
18. Rishniw M, et al: Characterization of chronotropic and dysrhythmogenic effects of atropine in dogs with bradycardia. Am J Vet Res 57:337, 1996.
19. Moise NS: Diagnosis and management of cardiac arrhythmias. In Fox PR, Sisson SD, Moise NS (eds): Canine and Feline Cardiology, 2nd ed. Philadelphia, WB Saunders, 1999.
20. Collet M, Le Bobinnec G: Électrocardiographie et Rhythmologie Canine. Paris, Point Veterinarire, 1990.
21. Le Bobinnec G: Vagal maneuvers. Proceedings 10th ACVIM Forum, San Diego, 1992.
22. Miller M: Diagnostic maneuvers used in the differential diagnosis of cardiac arrhythmias. Proceedings 9th ACVIM Forum, New Orleans, 1991, pp 177–180.
23. Wilson FN, et al: Electrocardiograms that present the potential variations of a single electrode. Am Heart J 9:477, 1934.
24. Hurst JW: Naming of the waves in the ECG, with a brief account of their genesis. Circulation 98:1937, 1998.
25. Yan G, Antzelevitch C: Cellular basis for the normal T wave and the electrocardiographic manifestations of the long-QT syndrome. Circulation 98:1928, 1998.
26. Tilley LP: Essentials of Canine and Feline Electrocardiography. Interpretation and Treatment, 2nd ed. Philadelphia, Lea & Febiger, 1985.
27. Myerburg RJ, et al: Interpretation of outcomes of antiarrhythmic clinical trials. Circulation 97:1514, 1998.
28. Knight DH, Allen CL: Ventricular arrhythmias in ICU patients: Prevalence, management, and outcome assessment. Proceedings 15th ACVIM Forum, Orlando, FL, 1997, pp 205–207.
29. Calvert CA, et al: Unfavorable influence of anesthesia and surgery on Doberman pinschers with occult cardiomyopathy. J Am Anim Hosp Assoc 32:57, 1996.
30. Rosen MR, et al: The Sicilian gambit. Circulation 84:1831, 1991.
31. Lunney J, Ettinger SJ: Cardiac arrhythmias. In Ettinger SJ, Feldman EC (eds): Textbook of Veterinary Internal Medicine, 4th ed. Philadelphia, WB Saunders, 1995, pp 959–994.
32. Muir WW: Antiarrhythmic drugs. Vet Clin North Am Small Anim Pract 21:957, 1991.
33. Muir WW, Sams RA: Pharmacology and pharmacokinetics of antiarrhythmic drugs. In Fox PR (ed): Canine and Feline Cardiology. New York, Churchill Livingstone, 1988, pp 309–333.
34. Wright KN, et al: Supraventricular tachycardia in four young dogs. JAVMA 208:75, 1996.
35. Atkins CE: Orthodromic reciprocating tachycardia and heart failure in a dog with a concealed posteroseptal accessory pathway. J Vet Intern Med 9:43, 1995.
36. Calvert CA, et al: Efficacy and toxicity of tocainide for the treatment of tachyarrhythmias in Doberman pinschers with occult cardiomyopathy. J Vet Intern Med 10:235, 1996.
37. Jacobs G: Tocainide in ventricular arrhythmias. Proceedings 13th ACVIM Forum, Orlando, FL, 1995.
38. Mason JW, et al: A comparison of electrophysiologic testing with Holter monitoring to predict antiarrhythmic drug efficacy for ventricular tachyarrhythmias. N Engl J Med 329:445, 1993.
39. Gratzek AT, et al: Corneal edema in dogs treated with tocainide. Prog Vet Comp Ophthalmol 3:47, 1993.
40. Lunney J, Ettinger SJ: Mexiletine administration for management of ventricular arrhythmia in 22 dogs. J Am Anim Hosp Assoc 27:597, 1991.
41. Chezalviel-Guilbert F, et al: Mexiletine antagonizes effects of sotalol on Q-T interval duration and its proarrhythmic effects in a canine model of torsades de pointes. J Am Coll Cardiol 26:787, 1995.
42. Singh SN, et al: Amiodarone in patients with congestive heart failure and asymptomatic ventricular arrhythmia. N Engl J Med 333:77, 1995.
43. Calvert CA, et al: Bradycardia-associated episodic weakness, syncope, and aborted sudden death in cardiomyopathic Doberman pinschers. J Vet Intern Med 10:38, 1996.
44. Moise NS: Treatment of supraventricular arrhythmias. Proceedings 15th ACVIM Forum, Orlando, FL, 1997, pp 123–125.
45. Bonagura JD, et al: Acute effects of esmolol in left ventricular outflow obstruction in cats with hypertrophic cardiomyopathy: A Doppler-echocardiographic study. J Vet Intern Med 5:123, 1991.
46. Quincnes M, et al: Pharmacokinetics of atenolol in clinically normal cats. Am J Vet Res 57:1050, 1996.
47. Hondegum LM: Class III agents: Amiodarone, bretylium, and sotalol. In Zipes D, Jalife J (eds): Cardiac Electrophysiology, 2nd ed. Philadelphia, WB Saunders, 1995, Chap 114.
48. Singh BN: Beta-blockers and calcium channel blockers as antiarrhythmic drugs. In Zipes D, Jalife J (eds): Cardiac Electrophysiology, 2nd ed. Philadelphia, WB Saunders, 1995, Chap 113.
49. Mason JW, et al: A comparison of seven antiarrhythmic drugs in patients with ventricular tachyarrhythmias. N Engl J Med 329:452, 1993.
50. Gomoll AW, et al: Comparability of the electrophysiologic responses and plasma and myocardial tissue concentrations of sotalol and its d stereoisomer in the dog. J Cardiovasc Pharmacol 16:204, 1990.
51. Fox PR, Liu SK: Arrhythmic right ventricular cardiomyopathy/dysplasia. Proceedings ACVIM 15th Annual Forum, San Diego, 1998, p 89.
52. Murray KT: Ibutilide. Circulation 97:493, 1998.
53. Cooke KL, Synder PS: Calcium channel blockers in veterinary medicine. J Vet Intern Med 12:123, 1998.
54. Bright JM, et al: Evaluation of the calcium channel blocking agents diltiazem and verapamil for treatment of feline hypertrophic cardiomyopathy. J Vet Intern Med 5:272, 1991.
55. Johnson LM, et al: Pharmacokinetic and pharmacodynamic properties of conventional and CD-formulated diltiazem in cats. J Vet Intern Med 10:316, 1996.
56. Moise NS, et al: Diagnosis of inherited ventricular tachycardia in German shepherd dogs. JAVMA 210:403, 1997.
57. Scherlag B, et al: Radiofrequency ablation of a concealed accessory pathway as treatment for incessant supraventricular tachycardia in a dog. JAVMA 203:1147, 1993.
58. Wright KN, et al: Transcatheter modification of the atrioventricular node in dogs, using radiofrequency energy. Am J Vet Res 57:229, 1996.
59. Meurs KM, Brown WA: Update on Boxer cardiomyopathy. Proceedings 16th ACVIM Forum, San Diego, 1998, pp 119–120.
60. Ellenbogen KA: Cardiac Pacing, 2nd ed. Cambridge, Blackwell Science, 1996.
61. Jeffrey K, Parsonnet V: Cardiac pacing. Circulation 97:1978, 1998.
62. Gregoratos G, et al: ACC/AHA guidelines for implantation of cardiac pacemakers and antiarrhythmia devices: Executive summary. Circulation 97:1325, 1998.
63. Darke PG, et al: Transvenous cardiac pacing in 19 dogs and one cat. J Small Anim Pract 30:491, 1989.
64. Fox PR, et al: Techniques and complications of pacemaker implantation in four cats. JAVMA 199:1742, 1991.
65. Sisson D, et al: Permanent transvenous pacemaker implantation in forty dogs. J Vet Intern Med 5:322, 1991.
66. Lehmkuhl LB, Sisson DD: Pacing practices and outcomes in the 1990s. Proceedings 16th ACVIM Forum, San Diego, 1998, pp 123–124.
67. Ovsyschner IE, et al: Dual chamber pacing is superior to ventricular pacing. Circulation 97:2368, 1998.
68. Mason JW, et al: A comparison of electrophysiologic testing with Holter monitoring to predict antiarrhythmic-drug efficacy for ventricular tachyarrhythmias. N Engl J Med 329:445, 1993.
69. Baty CJ, et al: Torsades de pointes–like polymorphic ventricular tachycardia in a dog. J Vet Intern Med 8:439, 1994.
70. Zipes DP: Specific arrhythmias: Diagnosis and treatment. In Braunwald E (ed): Heart Disease, 5th ed. Philadelphia, WB Saunders, 1997, pp 640–704.
71. Rishniw M, Bruskiewicz K: ECG of the month. JAVMA 208:1811, 1996.
72. Zipes DP: Management of specific arrhythmias: Pharmacological, electrical, and surgical techniques. In Braunwald E (ed): Heart Disease, 5th ed. Philadelphia, WB Saunders, 1997, pp 593–639.

CV

CHAPTER 115

ECHOCARDIOGRAPHY

John D. Bonagura and Virginia Luis Fuentes

Echocardiography is widely used for the diagnosis and management of congenital and acquired cardiac diseases. Although a number of different echocardiographic formats are used in clinical practice (Table 115–1), each involves reflection of ultrasound from cardiovascular tissues, specialized processing of returned (echoed) signals, and the ultimate display of this information in some recognizable visual or auditory format. Echocardiography has become increasingly sophisticated, and the combined modalities have largely replaced cardiac catheterization and angiocardiography for diagnosis and assessment of cardiac lesions. Although the newest technologies are expensive and limited to referral hospitals and clinics, many practicing veterinarians use, or will soon acquire, echocardiographs. Furthermore, veterinarians who are not yet performing echocardiographic studies often find referral for echocardiography helpful or even essential for establishing a cardiac diagnosis, assessing ventricular function, determining a prognosis, and guiding medical or surgical therapy.

The echocardiographic examination must be placed within a proper clinical perspective. Foremost, echocardiography is not a substitute for a careful clinical examination. Cardiac auscultation is still a most cost-effective and expedient examination for identifying serious heart diseases. Echocardiography should be performed, and echocardiograms are best interpreted by clinicians who understand the pertinent issues and questions regarding specific cardiovascular diseases. Furthermore, the clinical assessment and treatment plan prescribed should be directed by an individual capable of integrating information from all sources, including the history and physical examination. These decisions should not be abdicated to a sonographer unless that individual has a full understanding of the entire clinical situation and has physically examined the patient. The echocardiographer must appreciate ultrasound physics and instrumentation so that artifacts are not overinterpreted and important information is not suppressed. Echocardiographic studies are repeatable in experienced hands, but results can be highly operator and equipment dependent.

The veterinarian should appreciate the advantages and limitations of an echocardiographic study. A complete echocardiographic study should (1) reveal the pertinent congenital or acquired anatomic lesions (morphologic diagnosis), (2) estimate hemodynamic burden through quantitation of cardiac chamber size (dilatation and hypertrophy), (3) quantify ventricular systolic function, (4) estimate ventricular diastolic function, and (5) evaluate valvular function. Properly gathered and interpreted, this information should lead to a definitive cardiac diagnosis and illustrate the hemodynamic consequences of structural and functional cardiac lesions. Such detailed information can be obtained through complementary echocardiographic modalities; however, limited echo studies can also be useful in selected situations, as with rapid screening for pericardial effusion or when an expedient estimate of left ventricular ejection fraction is needed.

This chapter begins by reviewing the types of echocardiographic studies currently used and briefly examines the clinical utility of each modality. The authors then consider the results of the echocardiographic study in terms of five main issues: anatomic diagnosis, cardiac chamber size, systolic function, diastolic function, and valvular function. Our goal is illustration of important principles of echocardiography, although we also refer the reader to other sources for details of ultrasound physics and instrumentation.[1–4] Specific examples of these echocardiographic abnormalities can be found here, in veterinary textbooks[5–8] and in many other chapters in this section.

IMAGING FORMATS

TWO-DIMENSIONAL ECHOCARDIOGRAPHY

The most often performed and easiest to understand study produces a two-dimensional echocardiogram (2DE), which is also called a B-mode (for brightness mode) study or sector scan. These images are the consequence of numerous adjacent lines of B-mode ultrasound. These lines are composed at extraordinary speed to form a slice-of-pie-shaped image displayed within hundreds of "dots" of varying shades of gray and subsequently displayed in the pixels of the video screen. By updating the image frame—usually at rates between 30 and 60 frames per second—cardiac motion can be appreciated. Newer digital echocardiographs can generate extraordinary frame rates exceeding 150 frames per second. These 2D studies are typically viewed in "real time" and are simultaneously recorded on a videotape or optical disk for subsequent slow-motion replay.

The 2DE provides substantial anatomic information and serves as the anatomic template for guiding M-mode and Doppler studies. The 2DE examination is also useful for quantitation of cardiac size and function. Various imaging planes are generally recorded to provide sufficient anatomic detail in three dimensions (Table 115–2). Image planes can be categorized as long axis (sagittal), short axis (coronal), apical (transducer positioned near the left apex), or angled (specialized or hybrid imaging planes). The specific tomograms used for any given study depend in part on the clinical situation, but most echocardiography laboratories develop standards for specific examinations. A few centers are performing transesophageal echocardiography[9]; however, because of the limited availability of this equipment and the requirement for general anesthesia to perform the study, we do not consider these imaging planes further. Examples of typical transthoracic image planes are illustrated (Figs. 115–1 to 115–3).

M-MODE ECHOCARDIOGRAPHY

The M-mode echocardiogram is generated by a single line of B-mode ultrasound (Figs. 115–4 and 115–5). The

TABLE 115–1. ECHOCARDIOGRAPHIC MODALITIES*

STUDY	MORPHOLOGIC DETAIL	ASSESSMENT OF CHAMBER SIZE AND HEMODYNAMIC BURDEN†	MEASUREMENTS OF VENTRICULAR FUNCTION	ABNORMAL BLOOD FLOW	VALVULAR FUNCTION
M-mode	Limited	Indirect estimates from detection of chamber enlargement, hypertrophy, abnormal valve movements, or altered ventricular septal motion	Left ventricular shortening fraction; velocity of circumferential fiber shortening, systolic time intervals; mitral valve E-point to septal separation‡	Does not detect	Poor Indirect assessment from imaging and valve motion
Two-dimensional	Excellent	As per M-mode echo; dilatation of the great vessels can also be detected readily	Ventricular ejection fraction from volume estimates or shortening areas from short-axis tomograms	Does not detect	Limited Indirect assessment from imaging and valve motion
Contrast echo	Limited to imaging of the blood pool	Indirect—inferred from abnormal blood flow patterns	None	Sensitive, especially for right-to-left shunting	Limited unless performed during cardiac catheterization
Pulsed-wave Doppler	None	Indirect—inferred from abnormal blood flow patterns Limited by inability to quantify high-velocity signals§	Systolic estimates include aortic and pulmonary artery maximal velocity, velocity time integral, and acceleration time; diastolic estimates are based on analysis and measurements of mitral valve inflow velocity profiles and analysis of flow in pulmonary veins	Sensitive	Sensitive measure of valvular stenosis or insufficiency
Color-coded Doppler	Limited to color coding of the blood pool	Indirect—inferred from abnormal blood flow patterns Quantitation by analysis of the flow convergence region	Tissue Doppler imaging can be used to assess diastolic ventricular function	Sensitive	Sensitive measure of valvular insufficiency; stenosis can be detected but must be verified by other modalities
Continuous-wave Doppler	None	Indirect—inferred from abnormal blood flow patterns Quantitation through calculation of pressure gradients across lesions	Similar to pulsed-wave Doppler	Sensitive	Sensitive measure of valvular stenosis or insufficiency

*Major points are emphasized; this table does not consider experimental or developing technologies.

†Hemodynamic load refers to the increase in volume pumped or pressure generated by the ventricle during each cardiac cycle. In general, the more severe the cardiac lesion, the greater the hemodynamic burden.

‡For M-mode indices of ventricular function, left ventricular shortening fraction = (ventricular diastolic dimension − ventricular systolic dimension)/diastolic dimension; velocity of circumferential fiber shortening = shortening fraction/ejection time; systolic time intervals include pre-ejection period (onset of QRS to aortic opening) and ejection time; mitral valve E-point to septal separation = distance in centimeters from mitral valve opening to the ventricular septum.

Ejection fraction = ventricular stroke volume/ventricular end-diastolic volume.

§A special form of pulsed-wave Doppler—high pulse repetition frequency Doppler—can measure high-velocity flow signals; this is a hybrid of pulsed and continuous-wave Doppler.

transducer emits a pulse of ultrasound and then processes echoes reflected from moving cardiac tissues using a high sampling rate. The echocardiograph continually updates the depth of the tissues along the line of the ultrasound pulses and displays the structures as grey-scale "dots" that are spaced relative to the static transducer. By sweeping paper (or videotape) along this continuously updated output, a graph of cardiac motion is displayed, showing time (seconds; x axis) and depth (centimeters; y axis).

Standard M-mode studies of the left ventricle include those recorded between the tips of the ventricular papillary muscles, at the level of the chordae tendineae, across the peak diastolic excursion of the cranioventral (anterior) mitral valve leaflet, and through the aortic valves and left atrium. M-mode studies must be recorded with care to avoid angula-

tion errors and erroneous measures. Recordings should be guided by the 2DE long- and short-axis images.

Interpretation of the M-mode study requires knowledge of normal M-mode echocardiogram images and of cardiac motion at different levels of the heart. Although it is not difficult to comprehend, the graphic nature of this format and the lack of easily recognizable anatomic landmarks have diminished its importance. The M-mode study of the left ventricle and the calculation of left ventricular (LV) shortening fraction (see Fig. 115–5 and later) remain a standard for assessing global LV systolic function. However, the clinician should not rely on a single dimensional measure or function index without considering qualifying conditions such as species, breed, body weight, use of tranquilizers, heart rhythm, volume status, mitral valve competence, and global function

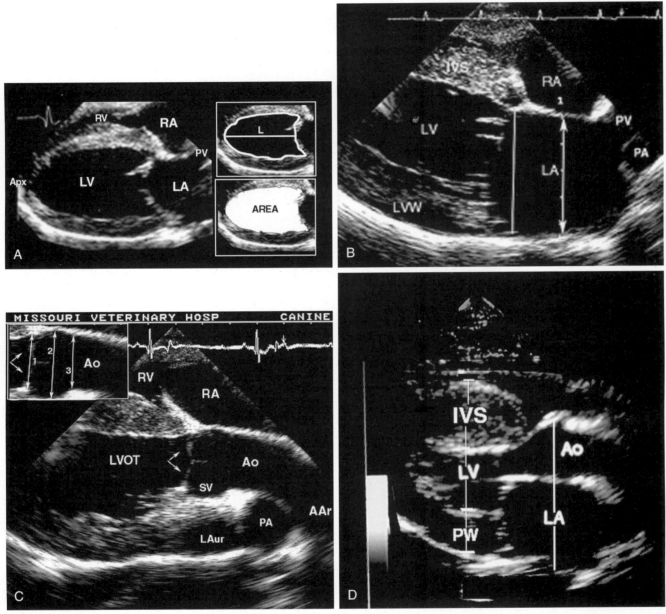

Figure 115–1. *A,* Right parasternal (intercostal) long-axis image of the heart recorded from a dog. The right atrium (RA), left atrium (LA), right ventricle (RV), and left ventricle (LV) are labeled. Although the "true" left apex (apx) may be difficult to visualize, this approach provides the best length measurement of the LV. Both area-length methods and other approaches to volumetric analysis of the left ventricle can be used with this image plane (insets). *B,* Right parasternal long-axis image of the heart recorded from a dog. The image is optimized for left atrial size and is frozen in systole. A reference line is drawn across the mitral anulus. Measurement of the left atrial diameter can be made as shown *(arrows).* Abbreviations as in *A.* Pulmonary vein (PV), pulmonary artery (PA), interventricular septum (IVS), and left ventricular free wall (LVW) are also labeled. *C,* Right parasternal long-axis image of the left ventricular outflow tract (LVOT) and ascending aorta (Ao) and is frozen in diastole. Abbreviations as in *B.* Left auricle (LAur), aortic arch (AAr), pulmonary vein (PV), pulmonary artery (PA), interventricular septum (IVS), and one aortic sinus of Valsalva (SV) are also labeled. Inset: methods of measuring the aorta at the valve hinge points (1), across the sinuses (2), and at the sinotubular junction (3). *D,* Right parasternal long-axis image of the heart recorded from a cat with hypertrophic cardiomyopathy and asymmetric septal hypertrophy (IVS). The end-diastolic image is optimized for the left ventricle and shows both the left atrium and aorta. This image is slightly different from that in dogs, in which only a small portion of the left atrium–auricle is evident when the aorta is in the long-axis imaging plane.

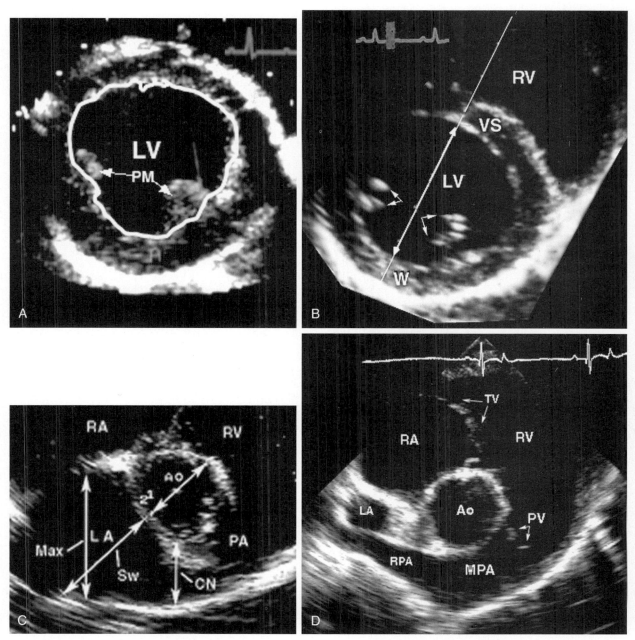

Figure 115–2. Right parasternal (intercostal) short-axis images of the side of the heart recorded from different dogs. *A,* Diastolic image across the "high" papillary muscle level of the left ventricle (LV). A method for measuring left ventricular short-axis area is depicted. The papillary muscles (PM) are disregarded in the area measurement. *B,* Diastolic image of the left ventricle (LV) recorded at the level of the chordae tendineae *(arrows)* and demonstrating placement of the M-mode cursor for measurement of the ventricular diameter *(arrows)*. The cursor bisects the chamber crossing the ventricular septum (VS), the lumen, and the posterior ventricular wall (W). Note that the image was "moved" to the edge of the sector to obtain this view. *C,* Frozen systolic image at the base of the heart showing the left atrium (LA) and methods used in measuring this chamber. The conventional (CN) method of M-mode measurement in dogs crosses the junction of the left atrium–auricle. The maximum diameter (Max) is obtained by disregarding the auricle and roughly bisecting the atrium with the measurement extending from the atrial septum to the right of the pulmonary vein The "Swedish" method first reported by Hansson (SW) would be measured in *diastole* and compares the aortic diameter (Ao) with the left atrial diameter along a line to the closure line of the noncoronary and left coronary cusps of the aortic valve. (The approximate path is shown here for comparative purposes.) RA = right atrium; RV = right ventricle; PA = proximal pulmonary artery. *D,* Diastolic image at the base of the heart demonstrating the right ventricular inlet and outlet. The aorta (Ao) is in short-axis and right heart structures are in angled or long-axis planes. RA = right atrium; RV = right ventricle; PA = pulmonary valve; MPA = main pulmonary artery; RPA = right pulmonary artery; LA = small portion of the left atrium.

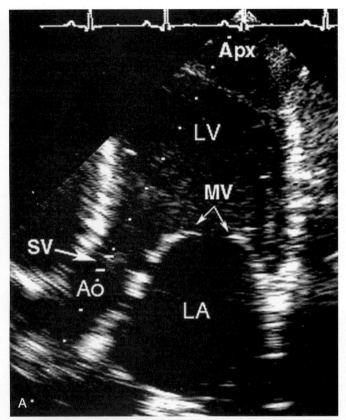

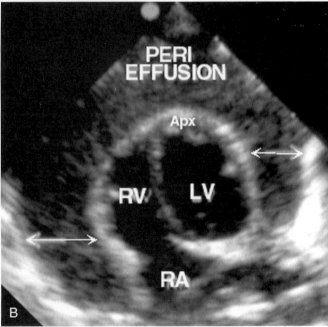

Figure 115–3. *A,* Left apical three-chamber image of a normal dog. Ventricular wall resolution is suboptimal, in part because of the parallel alignment of the ultrasound beam and the wall targets. However, excellent alignment with left ventricular inflow and outflow flow can be obtained from these planes as demonstrated by the cursor and pulsed-wave sample volume (SV) aligned parallel to and within the left ventricular outflow tract. MV = mitral valve; Apx = left apex. *B,* Left apical image from a cat with septic pericardial effusion. The pericardial space is distended with a mixed echoic fluid typical of an exudative or cellular process. The arrows show the span between epicardium and parietal pericardium. Apx = apex; RA = right atrium; RV = right ventricle; LV = left ventricle.

of the ventricles as seen on the 2DE. These factors must be studied and appreciated to prevent misinterpretation of M-mode–derived values.

Despite limitations, which are further considered later in this chapter, the M-mode echocardiogram is useful for quantifying cardiac wall thickness, ventricular luminal size, and LV function. M-mode studies can be combined with contrast echocardiography or color-coded Doppler imaging for accurate detection and timing of flow events. This modality is also capable of recording high-frequency motion,

as with a fluttering valve, which might be missed by the slower sampling of a 2D echocardiographic study.

CONTRAST ECHOCARDIOGRAPHY

Two-dimensional or M-mode contrast echocardiography is performed to identify abnormal blood flow. The contrast echocardiogram is produced by altering the sonographic appearance of a small portion of the blood pool through the

TABLE 115–2. IMAGING PLANES USED IN ECHOCARDIOGRAPHY

Right hemithorax
  Long-axis intercostal (parasternal) images of the left ventricle
    Four-chamber view*
    Optimized for the left ventricular inlet and atrial septum
    Optimized for the left ventricular outlet and ascending aorta
    Optimized for the right atrium and tricuspid valve
    Left ventricular inlet–left ventricular outlet view
  Short-axis intercostal (parasternal) images at the level of the
    Left ventricular apex
    Left ventricular papillary muscles
    Left ventricular chordae tendineae
    Mitral valve
    Aorta and left atrium
  Angled image optimized for the right ventricular inlet and outlet, pulmonary valve, and pulmonary artery
  Angled image optimized for the aortic arch
Left hemithorax
  Apical (caudal intercostal) images
    Four-chamber view optimized for the left ventricular inlet, mitral valve, and pulmonary veins
    Five-chamber view† optimized for the left ventricular outflow tract and proximal aorta
    Two-chamber view optimized for the left ventricular inlet
    Three-chamber view‡ optimized for the left ventricular outlet and ascending aorta
    Four-chamber view optimized for the right ventricular inlet
    Angled image of the caudal vena cava
  Angled view of the left auricle
  Cranial long-axis views
    Optimized for the left ventricular inlet and mitral valve
    Optimized for the left ventricular outlet, aortic valve, and ascending aorta
    Optimized for a long-axis image of the pulmonary artery
    Optimized for the cranial vena cava
  Cranial short-axis and angled image planes
    Short-axis image of the aorta, atrial septum, and atria
    Angled image of the right atrium, right ventricular inlet and outlet, and pulmonary artery (± descending aorta)
    Cranial angled views optimized for the right auricle and right ventricular inlet
  Other imaging locations
    Subcostal image of the left ventricular outlet
    Subcostal image of the aortic arch and pulmonary artery
    Subcostal images of the atrioventricular valves
    Suprasternal notch images of the great vessels, cranial mediastinal vessels

*Four chamber refers to left atrium, left ventricle, right atrium, and right ventricle.
†Five chamber refers to left atrium, left ventricle, ascending aorta, right atrium, and right ventricle.
‡Three chamber refers to left atrium, left ventricle, and aorta.

injection of agitated (sonicated) saline or dextrose solution, iodinated contrast medium indocyanine green dye, albumin solution, or carbon dioxide. After injection of the contrast agents into a peripheral vein, the acoustic impedance of the blood changes as microcavitations develop and act as powerful ultrasonic reflectors. The commonly used contrast agents do not pass through the pulmonary capillaries; therefore, finding echo-dense contrast within the left side of the heart indicates a right-to-left shunt (Fig. 115–6). For example, with the tetralogy of Fallot, echo-dense blood can be traced along its path from the right ventricle to the LV outlet.

Although Doppler studies have largely replaced contrast echocardiography, the technique is useful and sensitive and results are often less ambiguous than results of color-coded Doppler studies. Contrast echocardiography is used especially for identification of right-to-left shunts at the atrial septal level or with reversed patent ductus arteriosus (with imaging over the abdominal aorta to detect the presence of contrast agent).

DOPPLER ECHOCARDIOGRAPHY—PRINCIPLES

Doppler echocardiography represents a special processing of cardiac ultrasound that is characterized by a continuously updated display of blood velocity during the cardiac cycle.[2, 4] Doppler examinations, pulsed-wave (PW) examination, continuous-wave (CW) studies, and color-coded Doppler echocardiography, are applicable to veterinary patients.[10-12] The sonographer can obtain the following information from the Doppler examination: (1) the instantaneous direction of blood flow relative to the stationary transducer, (2) the instantaneous *velocity* of blood flow within the sample volume (PW) or along the line of interrogation (CW), and (3) the absence or presence of disturbed flow or "turbulence" in the heart or blood vessels. This information, when interpreted in conjunction with other echocardiographic findings, can be used to identify abnormal patterns of blood flow such as shunting, valvular regurgitation, or stenosis. Doppler examinations are also used to assess systolic and diastolic cardiac function and to quantify the severity of a lesion.

Doppler studies are based on the principle described by Johann Christian Doppler, who first described the frequency shift that occurs when light (or ultrasound) waves are reflected back by a moving object.[3, 4] This principle is embod-

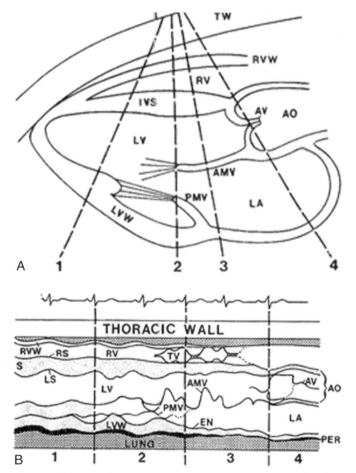

Figure 115–4. *A,* Cartoon demonstrating the approximate path of an ultrasound beam across the heart when recording "standard" M-mode echocardiograms. *B,* The resultant M-mode study. RVW = right ventricular wall; RS/LS = right/left side of the ventricular septum (S); LVW = left ventricular wall; EN = endocardium; PER = pericardium; PMV = posterior leaflet of mitral valve; AMV = anterior leaflet of mitral valve; AV = aortic valve; AO = aortic root.

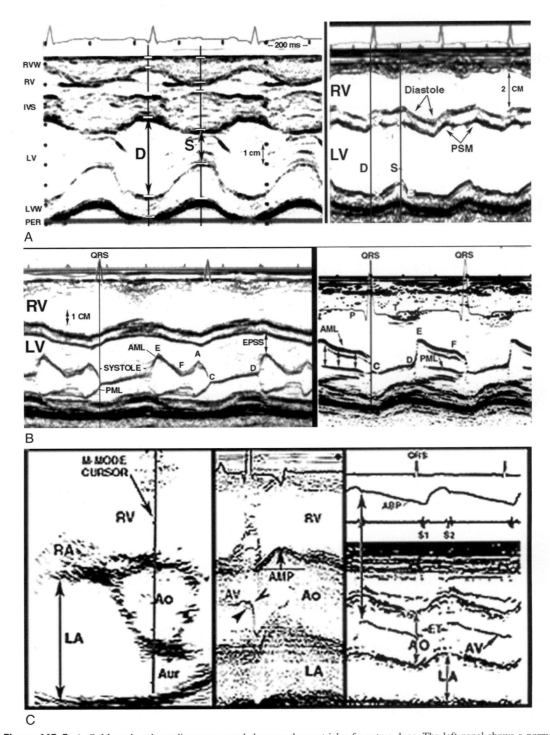

Figure 115–5. *A–C,* M-mode echocardiograms recorded across the ventricles from two dogs. The left panel shows a normal dog under isoproterenol stimulation. The fractional shortening (D − S/D) is high. Note the prominent thickening of the ventricular walls during systole. The right panel demonstrates a dilated heart in a dog with biventricular heart failure. The right ventricle is dilated, the left ventricular shortening fraction (D − S/D) is reduced, and there is paradoxical septal motion (PSM) related to right-sided volume overload, which depresses the septum down into the left ventricle during diastole. There is some ventilation-related variation on right ventricular filling as well. RVW = right ventricular wall; RV = right ventricle; IVS = interventricular septum (S); LV = left ventricle; LVW = left ventricular wall; D = diastolic LV dimension; S = systolic LV dimension. *B,* M-mode echocardiograms recorded across the mitral level from two dogs. The left panel represents a dog with dilated cardiomyopathy. Mitral movements are labeled: C is the closure point in early systole; D-E represents initial transmitral filling; E-F represents the rate of mid-diastolic closure; A indicates the atrial contraction. The E-point to septal separation (EPSS) is slightly increased in this dog, indicating dilation and decreased ventricular ejection fraction. The tracing on the right is from a dog with congenital mitral valve stenosis. There is reduced diastolic separation between the leaflets and the posterior leaflet follows the anterior leaflet, typical of a mobile but stenotic valve. The EF slope is also decreased, indicating maintenance of a diastolic pressure gradient during mid-diastole. PMV = posterior leaflet of mitral valve; AMV = anterior leaflet of mitral valve; ECG waveforms are also labeled (P, QRS). *C,* M-mode examination across the aortic root–left atrium. The left and middle panels are from a healthy greyhound. The M-mode cursor is evident (highlighted). Note the course taken in dogs by the cursor compared with a maximum LA diameter in this plane *(arrows).* The derived M-mode study is shown to the right of this in the middle panel. The amplitude of the aortic root during systole (AMP) is a general marker of systolic performance. The aortic valve closure is illustrated *(arrowheads).* The recording at the right is from another dog and shows hemodynamic correlates of the aortic valve (AV) motion within the aortic root (AO), relative to the electrocardiogram, arterial blood pressure (ABP), and phonocardiogram with recorded heart sounds (1 and 2). Measurements of the aortic root in end diastole and left atrium in systole are shown *(arrows).* Note that the aortic valve closes coincident with the incisura of the ABP curve and the second heart sound.

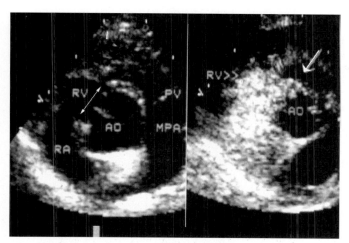

Figure 115–6. Contrast echocardiogram from a dog with tetralogy of Fallot. A large ventricular septal defect is seen in the left panel *(arrows)* at the root of the aorta (AO). After injection of agitated saline into a peripheral vein, there is opacification of the right atrium (RA) and right ventricle (RV) proximal to the outflow obstruction *(arrow)*, with spilling of echo-dense blood across the defect and into the aortic root. PV = pulmonary valve; MPA = main pulmonary artery.

ied in the Doppler equation, solved for velocity as $V = F_d$ (C) / $2F_0 \cos \Theta$, where F_d is the frequency shift (change in wavelength) caused by the reflection of ultrasound by a mass moving at a given velocity (V); F_0 is the initial transmitted frequency; the constant, C, is the speed of ultrasound in tissue; and Θ is the angle of incidence (or intercept angle) formed by the reflector and the interrogating ultrasonic beam. For Doppler studies, the initial or carrier frequency (F_0) is that emitted by the ultrasound transducer (generally between 1.9 and 7.5 megahertz). Also known are the speed of ultrasound in tissue (about 1540 m/s) and the angle of incidence of the ultrasound beam to blood flow. The latter is generally maintained by the examiner at less than 20 degrees to flow. The reflector is represented by the red blood cell (RBC) pool, which is moving either toward (causing a positive Doppler frequency shift) or away from (causing a negative Doppler frequency shift) the stationary handheld transducer (Fig. 115–7). The Doppler echocardiograph continuously measures returning Doppler frequency shifts, calculates the Doppler equation (assuming an angle of 0 or 180 degrees and a cosine function of 1), and displays the output of interest, namely the direction and velocity of blood flow (Figs. 115–8 and 115–9). If ultrasound reflects from targets moving at right angles to the emitted beam, no signal is returned (as the cosine of 90 degrees is zero). Reflections of ultrasound associated with larger beam-intercept angles (greater than 20 degrees) underestimate the true RBC velocity. Because Doppler frequency shifts are quite small—measured in kilohertz—they fall within the audible frequency range. Accordingly, Doppler instruments contain an audio channel that permits the operator to listen to the pitch of returning Doppler frequency shifts.

The major differences between PW and CW Doppler studies can be understood by considering briefly the concepts of sample volume, range gating, pulse repetition frequency, signal aliasing, and range ambiguity.[3, 4, 12] PW studies define Doppler shifts within a narrowly defined anatomic area of interest or *sample volume*. After each ultrasound pulse is emitted, the echocardiograph sampling ceases until the precise moment at which ultrasound returns to the transducer from the focal area of interest. This process is called *range*

gating and is the basis for the precise anatomic localization that characterizes the PW Doppler format. The actual sample volume size and location are operator controlled, and the region of interest is generally directed across the 2D echocardiograph image used as an anatomic template. Any time-velocity spectra recorded by this method represent flow within this narrow sample volume. However, the maximum velocity of RBC flow that can be recorded by this method is limited by a number of factors, including the *pulse repetition frequency*. Because high emitted ultrasound pulse rates cannot be achieved with standard PW Doppler, high-velocity flow patterns may not be faithfully recorded. When the returning RBC Doppler frequency shift is greater than twice the pulse repetition frequency (the *Nyquist limit*), the velocity spectrum becomes "wrapped" around the graph, displaced to the opposite side of the zero baseline, and displayed as if flow were in the opposite direction. This phenomenon, called *signal aliasing*, is common in both PW and color-coded Doppler studies (Fig. 115–10A; see Fig. 115–8B). It is analogous to the situation in a motion picture in which the spokes of a wagon wheel appear to be moving backward because the sampling rate of the film is too slow to record the direction of movement accurately. The principal way to overcome this limitation is to employ techniques capable of higher pulse repetition frequencies, including CW Doppler or *high pulse repetition frequency* PW Doppler (a hybrid of PW and CW methods) as shown in Figures 115–10B and 115–11.

The CW Doppler examination is used to quantify high-velocity blood flow (see Fig. 115–11). This format uses two ultrasound crystals that independently emit and receive ultrasound. Extremely high pulse repetition frequencies are possible with CW Doppler, although there is one significant limitation. All returning ultrasound is sampled and processed along the line of interrogation causing the various Doppler

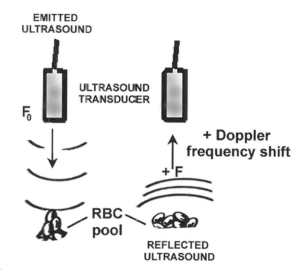

Figure 115–7. Drawing illustrating Doppler frequency shifts. The handheld transducer is oriented to interrogate blood flow with a small (less than 20 degrees) angle of incidence. As the ultrasound signal is transmitted across the heart, some waves are reflected back from the *(moving)* blood pool to the transducer, leading to a frequency shift (+F) between the emitted (F_0) and received signals. This small difference in ultrasound wavelength frequency is termed the Doppler shift and is directly proportional to the velocity of the moving red blood cell targets. Flow moving toward the transducer, as in this example, results in a higher returning frequency (shorter wavelength of ultrasound) or positive Doppler shift. The instantaneous Doppler shifts are displayed above the zero-velocity baseline. Flow moving away from the transducer (not shown) would yield a lower returning frequency with velocity spectra displayed below the baseline.

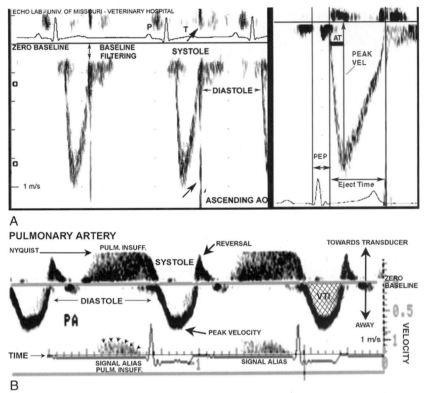

Figure 115–8. *A,* Aortic velocity spectra recorded from two dogs. At the left is a pulsed-wave Doppler recording across the aortic valve (50 mm/s). The normal triangular appearance of the systolic flow signal is evident. Peak velocity is about 1 m/s. The acceleration limb is compact with greater spectral dispersion observed at the peak and along the deceleration limb. The baseline is filtered using a low-velocity reject filter in order to limit the valve noise artifact. Such filtering results in a band of unrecorded Doppler shifts immediately adjacent to the baseline. Prominent aortic valve closure artifacts are evident *(arrows)*. At the right, a single velocity signal is recorded at higher paper speed (100 mm/s). Systolic time intervals are indicated as PEP (pre-ejection period) and ejection (Eject) time. The PEP/ET ratio is inversely related to myocardial contractility. The time from baseline to peak velocity can be used to calculate average aortic acceleration (dv/dt), a measure of ventricular performance. Similarly, the area under the triangular velocity curve (velocity-time integral) is directly related to ventricular stroke volume. *B,* Pulsed-wave Doppler recording across the pulmonary valve (canine study). Note the more rounded velocity peak. The area under the systolic flow spectrum (velocity-time integral or VTI) is proportional to the ventricular stroke volume. A brief, normal flow reversal is observed at the end of systole and into early diastole. This reversal can be extremely prominent in cats. Physiologic pulmonary insufficiency is evident as a broad band of flow disturbance. The peak velocity of the regurgitant signal attains the Nyquist limit for this recording, "wraps around" the top of the record, and generates a signal alias appearing at the bottom of the recording and representing the continuation of flow toward the transducer. Aliasing in this case could have been avoided by shifting the zero baseline down.

frequency shifts to superimpose. Thus, although it is capable of measuring extremely high velocity flow, the CW study is hampered by *range ambiguity*: the operator does not know the precise location of the returning signals. This limitation is managed by using the PW and CW examinations as complementary studies. When an area of high velocity or disturbed flow is localized by a signal alias in the PW examination, the CW mode is activated to record the peak velocity within the flow disturbance.

The PW and CW studies are processed to produce a constantly updated graph of instantaneous blood flow direction (positive or negative) and velocity (displayed along the y axis) relative to time, which is correlated with the electrocardiogram and displayed along the x axis (see Figs. 115–8 to 115–11). The RBCs do not travel at exactly the same velocity; thus, the Doppler display is not of a thin line but of a wider velocity spectrum. The outputs of PW and CW studies are referred to as *spectral Doppler* displays. Most Doppler processors generate spectral displays with shades of contrast (grey scale) with the brightest zones within the spectra representing the greatest numbers of RBCs. Normal flow is characterized by relatively tight spectra exhibiting small velocity variations around a modal

(brightest) time-velocity curve. A flow disturbance, as might develop with RBC movement across an incompetent or stenotic valve, is characterized by marked spectral broadening of the time-velocity curve (see Figs. 115–8B and 115–11). Such patterns are generally considered to indicate disturbed or turbulent flow.[5, 13]

PULSED-WAVE DOPPLER ECHOCARDIOGRAPHY

The principles of PW studies have been described in the preceding section. The PW Doppler examination is a component of a complete echocardiographic study. The typical PW Doppler examination is generally preceded by 2D and M-mode examination and by color Doppler imaging if that format is available. Color Doppler images (see later) represent essentially hundreds of PW sample volumes, so an efficient "screening" of the heart can be done that can be further refined by spectral Doppler techniques. The Doppler examination should include routine recordings of transvalvular flows[5, 14, 15] and also be guided by clinical findings and identification of lesions during 2D echo imaging. Reference values from canine and feline studies obtained without angle

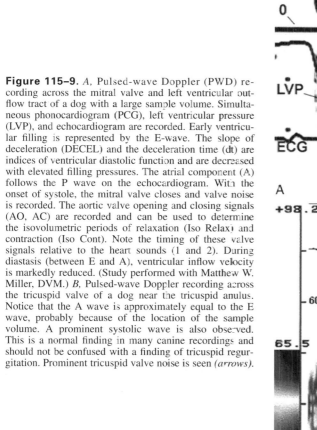
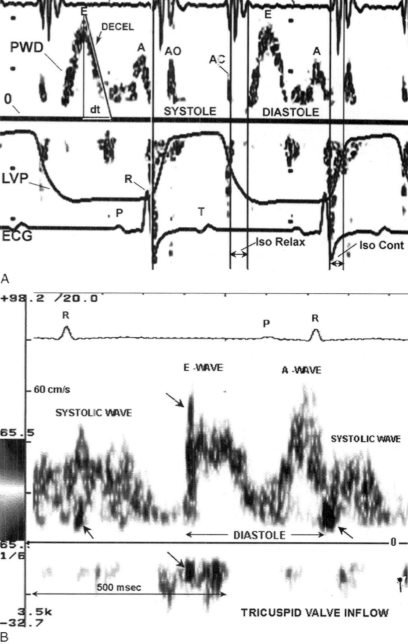

Figure 115–9. *A,* Pulsed-wave Doppler (PWD) recording across the mitral valve and left ventricular outflow tract of a dog with a large sample volume. Simultaneous phonocardiogram (PCG), left ventricular pressure (LVP), and echocardiogram are recorded. Early ventricular filling is represented by the E-wave. The slope of deceleration (DECEL) and the deceleration time (dt) are indices of ventricular diastolic function and are decreased with elevated filling pressures. The atrial component (A) follows the P wave on the echocardiogram. With the onset of systole, the mitral valve closes and valve noise is recorded. The aortic valve opening and closing signals (AO, AC) are recorded and can be used to determine the isovolumetric periods of relaxation (Iso Relax) and contraction (Iso Cont). Note the timing of these valve signals relative to the heart sounds (1 and 2). During diastasis (between E and A), ventricular inflow velocity is markedly reduced. (Study performed with Matthew W. Miller, DVM.) *B,* Pulsed-wave Doppler recording across the tricuspid valve of a dog near the tricuspid anulus. Notice that the A wave is approximately equal to the E wave, probably because of the location of the sample volume. A prominent systolic wave is also observed. This is a normal finding in many canine recordings and should not be confused with a finding of tricuspid regurgitation. Prominent tricuspid valve noise is seen *(arrows).*

Ventricular Outflow Tracts

Normal Doppler shifts in the ventricular outflow tracts yield spectra that are roughly triangular in profile (see Fig. 115–8) and produce a smooth, high-pitched, whistling sound in the audio channels of the echocardiograph. The *aortic* velocity signal has rapid acceleration, with a thin acceleration envelope and relatively sharp peak. Systolic RBC velocities increase substantially, roughly doubling from approximately 70 to 150 cm/s, as the sample volume is mapped from the proximal outflow tract (at the level of the open mitral valve) and across the subaortic zone to the aortic valve. The peak velocities then increase further as flow crosses the aortic valve, reaching a peak just distal to the valve. The peak aortic velocity is highly dependent on ventricular stroke volume and cross-sectional outlet area. Peak velocity recorded using PW Doppler from the left apex in the dog is generally between 0.9 and 1.6 m/s (see Tables 115–3 and 115–4), varying with sympathetic activity (enhances), sedation (depresses), variable cardiac cycle length (greater after long pauses), or the presence of obstructive lesions. Variation is also observed in peak velocity during ventilation, especially with translational movement of the heart relative to the stationary sample volume. In our experience, the aortic peak velocity can approach 2.8 m/s in healthy dogs subjected to catecholamine infusions and in high-flow states such as with patent ductus arteriosus even

correction,[14, 16, 17] as well as results for healthy and sedated dogs, are summarized in Tables 115–3 and 115–4.

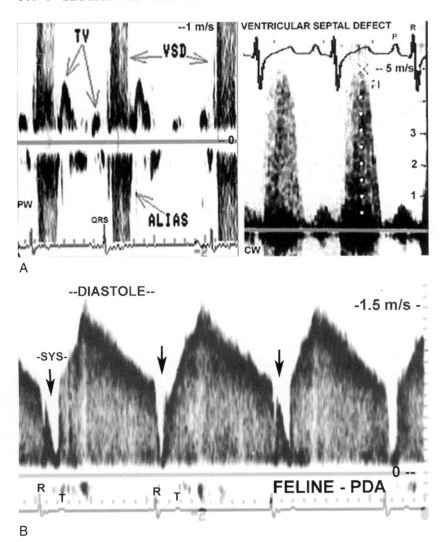

A

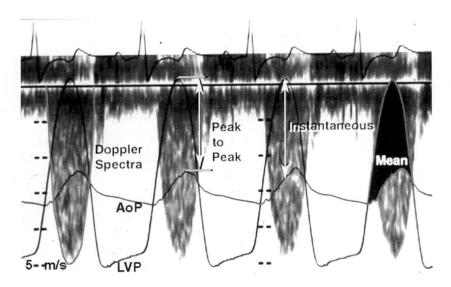

B

Figure 115–10. *A,* Doppler recordings of ventricular septal defect in two dogs. The left panel is a pulsed-wave Doppler recording of flow across the defect. A high-velocity, turbulent, systolic signal with aliasing is noted. Normal diastolic trans-tricuspid velocity profile is also observed (TV). The right panel, recorded from the right hemithorax, shows a continuous-wave Doppler recording of high velocity (about 5 m/s), indicating a restrictive defect. *B,* Patent ductus arteriosus in a cat. There is continuous turbulent flow throughout the cardiac cycle with a brief interruption during early systole. The peak velocity is not high, indicating either poor alignment with flow or (as in this case) substantial pulmonary hypertension.

in the absence of aortic stenosis (AS). The deceleration limb in healthy dogs is approximately twice the thickness of the acceleration limb and the slope is less steep. Aortic regurgitation in not common in healthy, unanesthetized dogs[12, 14, 17, 18] and should be regarded with suspicion.

The *pulmonary* artery signal is slower to accelerate, more rounded at the peak, and slightly lower in maximum velocity than flow in the ascending aorta (see Fig. 115–8B).[14, 17, 18] Pulmonary hypertension can alter the appearance of the pulmonary artery signal, producing a sharp, pointed spec-

Figure 115–11. Continuous-wave Doppler recording obtained from the subcostal position in a dog with congenital subvalvular aortic stenosis. Simultaneous aortic (Ao) and left ventricular (LV) pressures are recorded. Peak outflow velocity is markedly increased (approximately 5 m/s). The Doppler study can identify two types of gradients. Tracing the envelope (first cycle) yields a mean pressure gradient. This is analogous to the mean gradient measured by tracing the systolic area between the LV and aorta (see last cycle). The instantaneous gradient *(arrows)* can be measured by using the modified Bernoulli equation (gradient = $4V^2$ as described in the text). There is no Doppler correlate of the peak-to-peak gradient *(arrows)* typically measured at cardiac catheterization. (Study performed with Linda B. Lehmkuhl, DVM.)

TABLE 115–3. REFERENCE VALUES FOR CANINE AND FELINE PULSED-WAVE DOPPLER VARIABLES*

CARDIAC VALVE	GABER[18]	YUILL AND O'GRADY[17]	BROWN ET AL[14]	BONAGURA AND MILLER[33]	DOMANJKO AND THOMAS[16]
Species	Canine	Canine	Canine	Canine	Feline
Aortic (cm/s)	118.9 (17.8)	118.1 (10.8)	106.0 (21.0)	115.4 (15.3)	104 (14)
Pulmonary (cm/s)	99.8 (15.3)	98.1 (9.4) right side	84.0 (17.0)	106.0 (13.8) right side	95 (13) right side
		95.5 (10.3) left side		106.8 (10.2) left side	96 (13) left side
Mitral E wave (cm/s)	75.0 (11.8)	86.2 (9.5)		73.9 (8.9)	69 (12)
Mitral A wave (cm/s)	53.8 (8.7)	Not measured		45.9 (10.6)	54 (8)
Tricuspid E wave (cm/s)	56.2 (16.1)	68.9 (8.4)		59.7 (8.8)	60 (10)
					Combined E and A waves
Tricuspid A wave (cm/s)	Not measured			45.4 (5.8)	
Comments	Averaged six signals over respiratory cycle, n = 28	Averaged peak velocities, n = 20	Averaged five cycles over respiratory cycle, pooled heart rate = 96/min, n = 28	Averaged peak velocities; pooled heart rate = 108.9/min, n = 15	Unsedated cats, values obtained represent 32 to 53 determinations

*Values represent mean (and standard deviation); data reported have *not* been angle corrected; see references for further details.

trum, often with a notched peak, and altering the duration and acceleration time to peak pulmonary velocity. In one study, the acceleration time–ejection period was inversely correlated with the degree of pulmonary hypertension in dogs with dirofilariasis (r = −0.84).[19] It is common to observe physiologic pulmonary insufficiency of low peak velocity (usually less than 2.2 m/s in early diastole) in healthy dogs.[12, 14, 17, 18] In the setting of pulmonary hypertension, pulmonary insufficiency becomes associated with higher velocity spectra because the RBCs are driven into the right ventricle under higher pulmonary arterial pressure.

Outflow tract velocity profiles of cats are generally similar to those of dogs, but peak velocities have been similar to slightly lower in the aorta in the limited data reported thus far.[16] It is quite difficult to align the cursor with blood flow in the aorta of cats, especially in animals with outflow tract obstruction or with dilatation of the ascending aorta. In these cases, peak aortic velocity is certainly underestimated.

Ventricular Inlets

The velocity profiles related to ventricular filling are more complicated.[3, 4] Filling patterns in the left ventricle are related to numerous factors including ventricular relaxation and distensibility, atrial pressure and atrioventricular pressure gradient, heart rate, loading conditions,[20] ventilation, and presence of cardiac lesions (e.g., mitral valve disease, ischemia, left-to-right shunt, pericardial diseases). Inspection of the transmitral and pulmonary venous waveforms and measurements of filling times, wave amplitude, and wave duration can be used to evaluate ventricular diastolic function, particularly on the left side of the heart.

The typical appearance of *transmitral* flow recorded at the tips of the opened mitral valve is an "M-shaped" waveform consisting of two triangles, one representing early ventricular filling and the second atrial contraction (see Fig. 115–9A). An accompanying audio produces a variably pitched, bipha-

TABLE 115–4. EFFECTS OF SEDATION ON PULSED-WAVE DOPPLER VARIABLES

SITE	MEAN	MINIMUM	MAXIMUM	STANDARD DEVIATION	CV* (%)
Healthy dogs tranquilized with acepromazine†					
Aorta (cm/s)	112.4	96.5	141.0	15.17	13.9
PA—right parasternal (cm/s)	104.6	91.4	125.0	9.64	9.4
PA—left parasternal (cm/s)	99.9‡	76.1	118.0	9.99	10.0
Mitral valve E (cm/s)	70.4	42.5	86.2	11.23	16.3
Mitral valve A (cm/s)	38.3‡	25.7	51.7	6.74	17.6
Tricuspid valve E (cm/s)	58.2	41.0	72.8	8.79	15.3
Tricuspid valve A (cm/s)	41.5‡	27.4	55.3	7.47	17.3
Heart rate§ (beats per minute)	97.5‡	60.0	150.0	17.28	15.3
Healthy dogs sedated with acepromazine and buprenorphine¶					
Aorta (cm/s)	116.9	95.3	169.0	22.6	19.3
PA—right parasternal (cm/s)	87.6**	73.8	107.0	10.0	11.4
PA—left parasternal (cm/s)	82.7**	68.4	97.1	8.6	10.1
Mitral valve E (cm/s)	71.2	53.2	85.0	9.9	13.7
Mitral valve A (cm/s)	37.6††	25.9	58.0	10.8	28.8
Tricuspid valve E (cm/s)	65.8	38.7	79.1	11.5	17.5
Tricuspid valve A (cm/s)	33.0**	20.5	41.3	7.1	21.4
Heart rate (beats per minute)	83.3**	47.2	117	22.7	27.3

*CV = coefficient of variation, a measure of relative variation among variables = standard deviation/mean.
†Sedated with acepromazine, 3 mg/m², subcutaneously. Dogs were selected from the same population as in Table 115–3[33]; n = 10. Values were obtained by averaging three to five maximum velocity measures per variable per dog.
‡Indicates that mean value is significantly lower than the value without sedation; $P < .05$.
§Heart rate is the pooled average of all measured heart rates over the study.
¶Data for young, healthy, purpose-bred research dogs that could not be examined without sedation; n = 12.[33] Sedated with acepromazine (0.03 mg/kg) mixed with buprenorphine (0.0075 mg/kg) and administered intravenously. Values were obtained by averaging three to five maximum velocity measures per variable per dog.
**Indicates mean value is significantly lower ($P < .05$) than the value for a comparison group of young, unsedated dogs (n = 15).
††$P < .053$.
PA = pulmonary artery.

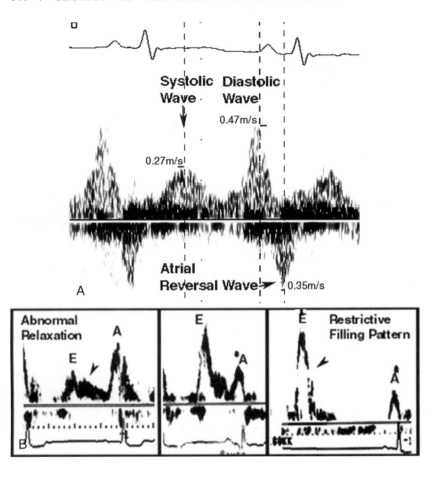

Figure 115–12. *A,* Pulmonary venous velocity profile of a cat with cardiomyopathy and left ventricular hypertrophy. Pulmonary venous signals are useful for assessing diastolic function and filling pressures. The systolic, diastolic, and atrial reversal waves are illustrated (see text for details). *B,* Pulsed-wave Doppler recordings from three different dogs. The left panel shows impaired relaxation in a dog with dilated cardiomyopathy. There are prolonged early deceleration *(arrow)* and E/A wave reversal. The center panel represents a normal dog, although this pattern can also be observed in the transition from abnormal relaxation to restrictive filling when atrial pressures are increased. In that case, the pattern is termed pseudonormal. The tracing on the far right demonstrates a "restrictive" filling pattern, with a large abbreviated E wave and small A wave, indicating that most ventricular filling was confined to early diastole. This pattern can be seen with elevated filling pressures and reduced left ventricular compliance, as well as in normal animals with enhanced ventricular relaxation.

sic, diastolic signal. Initial LV filling is rapid, usually achieving a maximal E-wave velocity of about 75 cm/s (see Tables 115–3 and 115–4). After this comes a less steep but brisk deceleration of inflow. During diastasis that is recorded at lower heart rates, there is minimal flow velocity in the ventricular inlet. Atrial contraction follows the P wave, producing a second inflow pattern with a distinct peak (the A wave, averaging about 55 cm/s). The mitral velocity spectra are relatively "tight" with little dispersion. The signals become stronger, of greater amplitude, and more dispersed with increased transmitral flow and often exceed 1 m/s with high-cardiac-output states, left-to-right shunts, anemia, severe mitral regurgitation (MR), and some tachycardias. At lower heart rates, the areas under the two inflow triangles can be measured to estimate relative filling fraction (early versus atrial contribution). In addition, the clinician can measure acceleration and deceleration times to and from the E wave. These variables have been used to estimate ventricular diastolic function, although the issue is complicated and requires further clarification (see later).

The normal relationship between the mitral filling waves changes as one moves the sample volume closer to the mitral anulus and into the left atrium. This yields a time-velocity spectrum with a larger atrial (A wave) than E wave and may be useful if one is timing the duration of early and late cardiac filling. This must be appreciated as normal variation because E/A reversal is considered abnormal when recorded from the tips of the mitral valve. The E/A ratio may decrease in older dogs as it does in older people[21] Rapid heart rates, which are common in the dog and typical of most cats, can lead to progressive increases in the amplitude of the A wave

relative to the E wave. As heart rate increases further, there is fusion of the terminal portion of the E wave with the A wave, a finding that impedes Doppler analysis of diastolic function. Most feline studies demonstrate a single, peaked inflow wave, unless the cat is heavily sedated or receives a beta-adrenergic blocker.

As the sample volume is retracted further into the left atrium, *pulmonary venous* flow patterns can be recorded. These velocity spectra have been measured in healthy dogs under a variety of conditions using both transthoracic[22] and transesophageal techniques and in dogs with experimentally induced perturbations in ventricular function and left atrial pressure.[23–30] Flow across the pulmonary veins is driven by pressure gradients between the pulmonary veins and the left atrium, which are in turn influenced by ventricular diastolic and systolic function. In transthoracic Doppler studies of dogs, pulmonary venous flow profiles are polyphasic, consisting of either one or two systolic (S) forward flow waves, a reversal wave after systolic flow, a prominent early diastolic forward flow wave (D), and a reversal wave (R) related to atrial contraction (Fig. 115–12). Maximal pulmonary flow velocity in transthoracic canine studies was approximately 40 cm/s during systole and 55 cm/s in early diastole.[22, 31] The initial systolic wave is related to atrial relaxation (after the P wave). The second systolic wave depends on either the suction created by the descent of the mitral anulus during ventricular contraction or the retrograde right ventricular (RV) stroke volume.[32] The prominent diastolic wave reflects the veno-ventricular pressure gradient established during early ventricular filling. The reversal wave represents atrial contraction. Resistance to ventricular filling, elevated ventricular pressure, or increased atrial pressure may increase the size of the Rwave. Severe MR can cause retrograde systolic flow extending into the pulmonary veins.

The *tricuspid* valve recording is qualitatively similar to that of the mitral valve with some important differences (see Fig. 115–9B). The peak inlet velocities are usually lower than for the left heart. There is often greater spectral dispersion of the inlet signal, which may indicate difficulties in aligning to inflow in all planes. In many studies, a distinct systolic wave is observed, which can be confusing if a simultaneous ECG is not recorded. Physiologic tricuspid regurgitation is also common in dogs, evident in at least 50 per cent of dogs studied[12, 18, 33, 34]

CONTINUOUS-WAVE DOPPLER ECHOCARDIOGRAPHY

CW Doppler studies use two independent crystals to emit ultrasound and receive reflected waves. Sampling is rapid and extremely high velocity flow patterns can be faithfully recorded. This is important inasmuch as flow patterns associated with MR, AS, and ventricular septal defect often exceed 5 m/s.

There are important quantitative clinical uses for CW Doppler–derived measurements. Foremost is the estimation of pressure gradients (Table 115–5). In the normal heart, the peak systolic and peak diastolic pressures measured at either side of a cardiac valve are equal, although they do not occur at precisely the same time. Although the normal peak-to-peak pressure gradient is zero, an instantaneous pressure gradient can be detected. These so-called impulse gradients drive blood through the circulation, but they are typically small, usually between 2 and 10 mmHg. These normal gradients generate RBC velocities between 0.25 and 1.7 m/s. Abnormal, high-velocity flow develops in many cardiac conditions, including AS, pulmonary stenosis, dynamic ventricular outflow stenosis (hypertrophic cardiomyopathy), mitral or tricuspid valve stenosis, ventricular septal defect, valvular regurgitation, and patent ductus arteriosus. In each of these conditions, a pressure gradient drives blood across a restrictive orifice. Most of these gradients are either reflections of the normal intravascular pressures or consequences of increased intracardiac pressures needed to move blood across a stenosis. Pressure gradients can be estimated using Doppler echocardiography by employing the simplified Ber-

CV

TABLE 115–5. ESTIMATING PRESSURE WITH DOPPLER ECHOCARDIOGRAPHY

General approach
  Record flow velocities across all valves in systole and diastole using PW and CW Doppler techniques; interrogate the ventricular septum in cases of ventricular septal defect or ductal flow in the case of patent ductus arteriosus.
  When abnormal flow is detected, quantify peak and mean velocities during the duration of the abnormal flow period using CW Doppler.
  Use the simplified Bernoulli equation (gradient = $4V^2$) to determine the maximum and mean pressure gradients using software in the echocardiograph.
  Measure systolic arterial blood pressure noninvasively with a Doppler flowmeter and appropriate cuff.
  Estimate right atrial pressure from the jugular veins or the hepatic veins in cases of right heart disease.
Aortic stenosis
  Record the peak velocity profile in meters per second across the stenosis.
  Use the simplified Bernoulli equation (gradient = $4V^2$) to determine the maximum and mean pressure gradients across the outlet.
  Peak left ventricular systolic pressure = peak gradient + systolic arterial blood pressure.
Pulmonic stenosis
  Record the peak velocity profile in meters per second across the stenosis.
  Use the simplified Bernoulli equation (gradient = $4V^2$) to determine the maximum and mean pressure gradients.
  If a dynamic subvalvular component is identified, identify both jets; calculate the gradient for the proximal dynamic obstruction (V_1) as gradient = $(4V_1)^2$ and for the distal valvular obstruction as gradient = $4(V_2 - V_1)^2$.
  Right ventricular systolic pressure = peak gradient + 22 (where 22 is an estimate of pulmonary artery systolic pressure based on catheterization experience).
Pulmonary hypertension
  Measure the peak velocity of any tricuspid regurgitation present (high-velocity tricuspid regurgitation correlates with elevated right ventricular systolic pressure (abnormal velocity is usually >2.6 m/s).
  In the absence of right ventricular outflow obstruction, high-velocity TR generally indicates systolic pulmonary hypertension. The PA systolic pressure equals right ventricular systolic pressure; this equals the calculated RV-to-RA instantaneous pressure gradient plus right atrial pressure.
  To estimate diastolic pulmonary artery pressure, record the maximal velocity of any pulmonary insufficiency and calculate the PA pressure in early and late diastole using the simplified Bernoulli equation. The PA diastolic pressure = right ventricular diastolic pressure + Doppler-derived PA-to-RV diastolic pressure gradient (the RV diastolic pressure is assumed to be zero or is estimated by measuring the venous pressure from inspection of the jugular veins or from a CVP recording).
Ventricular septal defect
  Determine the peak velocity across the aortic valve. If the aortic velocity is less than 2 meters/sec. assume LV systolic pressure = the systemic arterial systolic pressure measured simultaneously by noninvasive means. (If the velocity is >2 meters/sec, calculate the gradient; see aortic stenosis).
  Measure the peak velocity across the septal defect. *Assuming close parallel alignment with flow,* one can use the simplifed Bernoulli equation to estimate the peak instantaneous left ventricular to right ventricular pressure gradient.
  RV systolic pressure equals systolic arterial blood pressure minus the pressure gradient between the left and right ventricles.
  Interpretation is difficult if there is concurrent right ventricular obstruction or subaortic stenosis, or if the angle of Doppler interrogation is greater than 20 degrees.
Patent ductus arteriosus
  Use the simplified Bernoulli equation to estimate the peak aortic to pulmonary artery pressure gradient and pulmonary artery systolic pressure.
  PA systolic pressure equals systolic arterial blood pressure minus the pressure gradient between the aorta and pulmonary artery.
  The peak aortic to pulmonary artery systolic gradient should be approximately 80 to 100 mm Hg in normotensive animals with left to right shunting PDA. Poor alignment with flow, or a long, narrow ductus may produce a low gradient despite normal pulmonary arterial pressure.
Mitral or tricuspid valve stenosis
  Estimate the transvalvular diastolic gradients from the modified Bernoulli equation (maximal and mean gradients)
  Also calculate the pressure half-time, the time (in seconds) required for the instantaneous pressure gradient to decrease by ½ as calculated from the Bernoulli equation (see text).
  Results can be impacted by a high heart rate (which shortens diastolic flow time), increased transvalvular flow (from a concurrent shunt, atrioventricular valvular regurgitation), or general high cardiac output states (sympathetic activity, fever, or anemia).

CVP = central venous pressure; CW = continuous wave; LV = left ventricular; PA = pulmonary artery; PDA = patent ductus arteriosus; PW = pulsed wave; RA = right atrial; RV = right ventricular; TR = tricuspid regurgitation.

noulli equation,[1] where gradient (mmHg) = maximal velocity[2] × 4 and where maximal velocity is in meters per second. The Bernoulli relationship works well for this clinical application and often obviates the need for cardiac catheterization (see Fig. 115–11).

COLOR DOPPLER IMAGING

Color Doppler Imaging (CDI) is a sophisticated form of ultrasound technology in which blood flow and velocity information is overlaid on a B-mode, 2D, grey-scale image. This imaging technique—also called color Doppler echocardiography, color-coded Doppler, Doppler color flow imaging, and color flow imaging—is a type of PW Doppler echocardiography. Because the anatomic site of received Doppler shift information can be readily determined, CDI is useful for documenting normal blood flow patterns and for screening the heart and great vessels for areas of abnormal flow. Color Doppler technology can also be combined with M-mode echocardiography to generate a precise temporal resolution of flow events[4, 6] and assess ventricular diastolic function.[35] Newer technologies, such as color-coded tissue Doppler imaging, may prove useful for assessment of wall motion and ventricular diastolic function.[36]

The basic principles of PW Doppler echocardiography are quite applicable to CDI. Relevant aspects of Doppler physics still apply, including the concepts of the Doppler equation, the Nyquist limit, signal aliasing, angle of incidence relative to flow, and signal filtering and processing. Many of these points were addressed earlier. There are also major instrumentation issues to be mastered before one can become proficient with this technology.[2, 4–6, 37, 38]

Major differences between spectral PW Doppler echocardiography and CDI include the number of sample volumes used, the angle of incidence of beam interrogation to flow (the beam-flow intercept), the approach to temporal (time) analysis, the methods of displaying flow direction, quantitation of RBC velocity, and display of disturbed flow or turbulence. Traditional PW Doppler echocardiography records frequency shifts within a single operator-guided sample volume. With CDI, the Doppler shifts are received from scores of individual, adjacent sample volumes confined to a

defined region of interest. The sample volume data are computer averaged and filtered to generate a smooth transition of color and hues. In PW Doppler studies, only a single line of interrogation intercepts RBC flow, whereas CDI represents dozens of individual lines, each projecting spokelike from the apex of the sector scan, to record from a different beam-flow intercept angle. In the PW Doppler study is plotted time along the horizontal axis, but in CDI each 2D image must be quickly processed, displayed, and then updated within milliseconds so that flow over time can be shown. Blood flow direction and velocity are demonstrated in PW Doppler studies using a graphical display in which velocity and direction are plotted on the vertical axis and time along the abscissa. In CDI, the direction and relative velocities of blood cells within the region of interest are determined by inspecting each color image frame and comparing the color signals with a reference map (Fig. 115–13). Flow "toward" the transducer is coded in one color (generally red) and flow "away from" the transducer is displayed in another color (typically blue). These colors do not correspond to arterial and venous blood flow but indicate the direction within the sample volumes along the line of interrogation.

The reference color map is qualitatively similar to the vertical axis of the PW Doppler spectral display.[4, 38, 39] In standard color flow mapping, zero-velocity flow—which is analogous to the zero baseline of a spectral Doppler trace—is coded in black. Positive Doppler shifts (flow toward the transducer) are color coded in red and negative Doppler shifts (flow away from the transducer) are coded in blue. As with spectral Doppler, the zero baseline can be shifted up or down to increase the maximal velocity scale in one direction, although this is not particularly helpful except for estimation of mitral regurgitant volume (see later). Color maps vary, although most instruments use red toward, blue away (RTBA) maps. Enhanced velocity maps display higher velocities as increasingly bright hues (e.g., a color change from black to dark blue to light blue to cyan). Such color maps are largely semiquantitative. The Nyquist limits, displayed at each end of the color map, are generally quite low, promoting signal aliasing of even normal flow patterns. Flow rates exceeding the displayed maximal velocity "wrap around" the color bars and become an aliased signal with

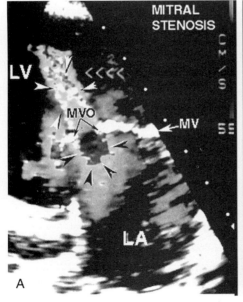
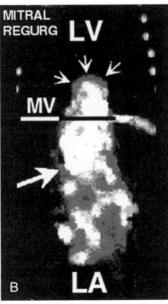

Figure 115–13. Black-and-white reproductions of color Doppler imaging in mitral disease. *A,* Congenital mitral stenosis in a dog. As red cells converge toward the stenotic mitral valve orifice (MVO), there is a prominent hemisphere of flow convergence represented by the aliased signal *(black arrowheads).* Flow in the ventricle is disturbed *(white arrowheads),* indicating rapid and turbulent flow across the narrowed area. *B,* Focused image of a mitral regurgitant jet in a dog. Flow converges proximal to the mitral valve (MV) orifice that is identified by the line. A hemisphere of aliased flow is evident on the left ventricular (LV) side of the valve *(small arrows).* A relatively wide band of regurgitation is observed in the left atrium (LA, *arrow*).

involved sample volumes coded to the color opposite to that of the true direction of flow. Extremely fast flows can actually wrap two or three times, presenting a challenging image analysis. Aliased signals are easier to identify with enhanced maps because the surreptitious flow is surrounded by a brightly coded flow pattern of the direction opposite to that of the aliased core (e.g., cyan surrounded by bright orange).

The principal use of CDI is to detection of abnormal flow, and specialized maps have been developed for this purpose. Turbulence, variance, high-velocity, and hot-white maps are useful for identifying areas of abnormal flow and function. The most common of these function by adding green or yellow to pixels representing sample volumes with "disturbed" flow. In some systems, disturbed flow appears almost completely as yellow-green, whereas in other systems a mosaic of color is generated. Because the algorithms for determining variance or turbulence are not uniform in the industry, disturbed flow coding may be inconsistent among instruments and even with different transducers on the same Doppler echocardiograph. The finding of turbulence by CDI can be normal and any suspicious flow pattern detected by CDI—be it an aliased signal, high-velocity signal, or turbulence—must be qualified and quantified using a spectral Doppler technique.

There are a number of advantages of CDI. Because large areas of the heart can be examined with each frame, screening for valvular regurgitation and other abnormal flow patterns is easier to perform than with the tedious mapping required with conventional, PW Doppler studies. Small shunts, muscular ventricular septal defects, small regurgitant jets, and other subtle lesions are more readily diagnosed with CDI than with spectral Doppler methods. Furthermore, the color flow study is useful for guiding placement of sample volumes and steerable CW Doppler cursors through regions of suspicious flow.

ASSESSMENT OF CARDIAC CHAMBER SIZE

One of the questions most often directed to the sonographer pertains to cardiac mensuration: is the heart dilated or hypertrophied? Furthermore, the clinician wants to know whether the enlargement is mild, moderate, or severe. This would seem to be a simple question inasmuch as the 2D and M-mode studies are ideal for imaging the chambers and walls. There are, in fact, numerous reports of ventricular and atrial measurements in dogs and cats (Tables 115–6 through 115–8).[7] Nevertheless, a number of complicated issues confound assessment of ventricular volume and mass estimates. These are discussed here and in the subsequent section that details estimation of systolic function.

TABLE 115–6. NORMAL CANINE LEFT VENTRICULAR CHAMBER DIMENSIONS*

BREED	N	BODY WEIGHT (kg)	LVDd (mm)	LVDdI (mm)	LVDs (mm)	LVDsI (mm/m²)	LVFWd (mm)	LVFWdI (mm/m²)	LVFWs (mm)	IVSd (mm)	IVSs (mm)	SF (%)
Miniature poodles[56]	20	3	20 (16–28)	100	10 (8–16)	50	5 (4–6)	25	8 (6–10)	—	—	47 (35–57)
Beagles[102]	20	8.9 ± 1.5	26.3 19.5–33.1	61.2	15.7 8.9–22.5	36.5	8.2 4.4–12	19.1	11.4 7.6–15.2	6.7 4.5–8.9	9.6 6.6–12.6	40 22–58
West Highland white terriers[136]	24	10.3 ± 0.9	28.8 17.4–40.2	61.3	20 12.6–27.4	42.6	6.4 4–8.8	13.6	9.8 7.2–12.4	6.9 4.1–9.7	10.2 5.2–15.2	35 21–49
English cocker spaniels[137]	12	12.2 ± 2.25	33.8 27.2–40.4	63.8	22.2 16.6–27.8	41.9	7.9 5.7–10.1	14.9	—	—	—	34.3 25.3–43.3
Corgis[56]	20	15 (8–19)	32 (28–40)	53.3	19 (12–23)	31.7	8 (6–10)	13.3	12 (8–13)	—	—	44 (33–57)
Pointers[61]	16	19.2 ± 2.8	39.2 34.4–44	54.4	25.3 20.5–30.1	35.1	7.1 5.7–8.5	9.9	11.5 8.9–14.1	6.9 4.7–9.1	10.6 8.6–12.6	35.5 27.5–43.5
Afghan[56]	20	23 (17–36)	42 (33–52)	51.9	28 (20–37)	34.6	9 (7–11)	11.1	12 (9–18)	—	—	33 (24–48)
Greyhounds[97]	16	26.6 ± 3.5	44.1 28.1–50.1	49.6	32.5 25.5–39.5	36.5	12.1 8.7–15.5	13.6	15.3 10.9–19.7	10.6 7.2–14	13.4 8.2–18.6	25.3 12.7–37.9
Boxers[138]	30	28 ± 7.1	40 30–50	43.5	26.8	29.1	10 6–14	10.9	15 11–19	9 5–13	13 9–17	33 17–49
Greyhounds[159]	11	29.1 ± 3.7	46.9 40.7–53.1	49.9	33.3 28.1–38.5	35.4	11.6 8.2–15	12.3	—	13.4 10–16.8	—	28.8 20.4–37.2
Golden retrievers[56]	20	32 (23–41)	45 (37–51)	44.6	27 (1.8–3.5)	26.7	10 (8–12)	9.9	15 (10–19)	—	—	39 (27–55)
Dobermans[98]	23	—	40.1 34.7–45.5	—	31.4 25.9–36.9	—	8 5.6–10.4	—	11.2 8.3–14.1	—	—	21.7 14.4–29
Dobermans[41]	21	36	46.8 38.5–55.1	42.9	30.8 24.2–37.4	28.3	9.6 3.4–10.8	8.8	14.1	9.6 8.4–10.8	14.3 13–15.6	34.2 30.6–37.8
Spanish mastiffs[140]	12	52.4 ± 3.3	47.7 44.9–50.5	33.8	29 26.8–31.2	20.6	9.7 8.9–10.5	6.9	15.2 14.4–16	9.8 9–10.6	15.6 14.6–16.6	39.2
Newfoundlands[62]	27	61 47–69.5	50 44–60	32.1	35.5 29–44	22.8	10 8–13	6.4	15 11–15	11.5 7–15	15 11–20	30 22–37
Great Danes[62]	15	62 52–75	53 44–59	32.3	39.5 34–45	24.1	12.5 10–16	7.6	16 11–19	14.5 12–16	16.5 14–19	25 18–36
Irish wolfhounds[52]	20	68.5 50–80	50 46–59	28.6	36 33–45	20.6	10 9–13	5.7	14 11–17	12 9–14.5	15 11–17	28 20–34

*All values expressed as mean, ±2 standard deviations or (range). Values indexed to body surface area are of group mean divided by mean group body surface area.
LVDd = left ventricular diameter in diastole; LVDdI = left ventricular diastolic diameter index; LVDs = left ventricular diameter in systole; LVDsI = left ventricular systolic diameter index; LVFWd = left ventricular free wall thickness in diastole; LVFWs = left ventricular free wall thickness in systole; IVSd = interventricular septal thickness in diastole; IVSs = interventricular septal thickness in systole; SF = left ventricular shortening fraction.

TABLE 115–7. NORMAL CANINE LEFT ATRIAL DIMENSIONS

BREED	N	BODY WEIGHT (kg)	M-MODE LA (mm)	M-MODE Ao (mm)	M-MODE LA/Ao
Poodles[56]	20	3	12	10	1.2
Mixed[141]	27	11.1 ± 8.8	22.6	22.9	0.99
			7.7–37.6	8.7–37.1	
Corgis[56]	20	15	21	18	1.17
Pointers[61]	16	19.2	22.6	24.1	0.94
			18.6–22.6	20.7–27.5	0.8–1.08
Mixed[40]	20	19.3	—	—	0.95
					0.88–1.02
Mixed	20	22.1 ± 6.2	22.4	22.4	0.93
			9.4–35.4	12–37.4	0.53–1.33
Afghans[56]	20	23	26	26	1.0
Mixed	40	24 ± 10	22	23	0.99
			12–32	15–31	0.79–1.19
German shorthaired pointers†	13	26.9 ± 3.8	23.2	22.1	1.05
			20.4–25.9	19.4–24.8	0.9–1.2
Boxers[138]	30	28 ± 7.1	23	22	1.06
			19–27	18–26	1.04–1.08
Golden retrievers[56]	20	32	27	24	1.13
Dobermans[41]	21	36	26.6	29.9	0.89
			23.6–29.6	25.3–34.5	
Spanish mastiffs[140]	12	52.4	28.5	27.6	1.03
			26.7–30.3	26–29.2	
Newfoundlands[62]	27	61	30	29	1.0
			24–33	26–33	0.8–1.25
Great Danes[62]	15	62	33	29.5	1.1
			28–46	28–34	0.9–1.5
Irish wolfhounds[62]	20	68.5	31	30	1.0
			22–35	29–31	0.9–1.5

All values expressed as mean ± 2 standard deviations (or as a range).
†Unpublished data.
M-mode LA = M-mode left atrial diameter in systole; M-mode Ao = M-mode aortic diameter in diastole; M-mode LA/Ao = ratio of M-mode left atrium to aortic diameter.

TABLE 115–8. NORMAL FELINE M-MODE VALUES

VARIABLE	PIPERS ET AL (1979)[143]	JACOBS AND KNIGHT (1985)[60]	FOX ET AL (1985)[143]	MOISE ET AL (1986)[144]	SISSON ET AL (1991)[145]
Sedation	None	None	Ketamine	None	None
Number of cats	25	30	30	11	79
Body weight (kg)	4.7 ± 1.2	4.1 ± 1.1	3.9 ± 1.2	4.3 ± 0.5	4.7 ± 1.2
HR (beats per minute)	167 ± 29	194 ± 23	245 ± 36	182 ± 22	—
LVDd (mm)	14.8	15.9	14	15.1	15
	9.6–20	12.1–19.7	11.4–16.6	11–19	11–19
LVDs (mm)	8.8	8	8.1	6.9	7.2
	4–13.6	5.2–10.8	4.9–11.3	2.5–11	4.2–10.2
IVSd (mm)	4.5	3.1	3.6	5	4.2
	2.7–6.3	2.3–3.9	2–5.2	3.6–5.6	2.8–5.6
IVSs (mm)	NR	5.8	NR	7.6	6.7
		4.6–7		5.2–10	4.3–9.1
LVPWd (mm)	3.7	3.3	3.5	4.6	4.1
	2.1–5.3	2.1–4.5	2.5–4.5	3.6–5.6	2.7–5.5
LVPWs (mm)	NR	6.8	NR	7.8	6.8
		5.4–8.2		5.8–9.8	4.6–9
LA (mm)	7.4	12.3	10.3	12.2	11.7
	4–10.8	9.5–15.1	7.5–13.1	8.6–16	8.3–15.1
Ao (mm)	7.5	9.5	9.4	9.5	9.5
	3.9–11.1	7.3–11.7	7.2–11.6	6.5–13	6.7–12.3
LA/Ao	0.99	1.3	1.1	1.29	1.25
		0.96–1.64	0.74–1.46	0.83–1.75	0.89–1.61
RVd (mm)	NR	6	5	5.4	4.6
		3–9	0.8–9.2	3.4–7.4	1.2–8
SF (%)	41	49.8	42.7	55	52.1
	26.4–55.6	39.3–60.3	26.5–58.9	35–75	37.9–66.3

All values expressed as mean ± 2 standard deviations (or as a range).
LVDd = left ventricular diameter in diastole; LVDdI = left ventricular diastolic diameter index; LVDs = left ventricular diameter in systole; LVDsI = left ventricular systolic diameter index; LVFWd = left ventricular free wall thickness in diastole; LVFWs = left ventricular free wall thickness in systole; IVSd = interventricular septal thickness in diastole; IVSs = interventricular septal thickness in systole; LA = left atrial diameter in systole; Ao = aortic diameter in diastole; LA/Ao = left atrial/aortic ratio; RVD = right ventricular diastolic diameter; SF = left ventricular shortening fraction.

LEFT ATRIAL SIZE

Dilatation of the left atrium develops in association with left-to-right shunts, mitral valve disease, cardiomyopathies, and virtually any cause of significant systolic or diastolic dysfunction of the left ventricle. High-output states, including hyperthyroidism and anemia, can lead to left atrial dilation. The atrium may dilate in primary atrial cardiomyopathies or consequent to chronic bradyarrhythmias or tachyarrhythmias. The magnitude of left atrial dilation is often taken to represent the severity and hemodynamic burden of a lesion. Certainly, a normal left atrial size portends a better short-term prognosis for most cardiac lesions involving the left side of the heart. One notable exception occurs with the setting of peracute MR (ruptured chordae tendineae, bacterial endocarditis), wherein left atrial dilation may be minimal but heart failure severe. Assessment of left atrial mass is problematic because atrial wall thickness is more difficult to resolve.

M-Mode Estimates

The M-mode measurement of left atrial size in dogs markedly underestimates maximal atrial dimensions as recorded by 2D studies (see Figs. 115–1 to 115–4). The method used generally crosses the center of the aorta but only the junction of the left atrium or auricle. The image plane can determine the left atrial dimension obtained. Careless cursor placement can lead to erroneous results or even sampling of the pulmonary artery in lieu of the left atrium. Furthermore, the cursor often crosses extracardiac fat located between the two structures, which is eventually included in the measurements. Many M-mode reference values for left atrial size in dogs and cats are relatively old and were obtained without benefit of 2D guidance.[40–43] Many authors index the atrial dimension to the aorta to accommodate the marked differences in atrial size across the various canine breeds (see Tables 115–7 and 115–8). Certainly, when the left atrial/aortic ratio exceeds 1.2 to 1.3, left atrial dilatation is likely; however, a normal M-mode atrial/aortic ratio does not rule out atrial enlargement.

The M-mode cursor tends to cross a more representative portion of the left atrium in cats. A left atrial/aortic ratio greater than 1.3 is highly suggestive of atrial dilatation. 2D measures may still be useful. Internal atrial diameter measurements exceeding 19 mm in cats indicate a risk for atrial thrombosis and systemic thromboembolism.

Two-Dimensional Echocardiographic Estimates

The authors have used three general 2D echo approaches for measuring internal left atrial diameters (see Figs. 115–1 to 115–3). One method is to measure an internal right-to-left cranial-to-caudal diameter from the right parasternal long-axis view recorded at end systole.[44] Absolute values cannot be compared among dogs of different sizes; however, the left atrial measurement can be indexed to body surface area and then related to body weight. Even when these calculations are accomplished, the left atrial index is much higher in dogs weighing less than 10 kg and demonstrates a curvilinear relationship across all body weights. When the left systolic atrial dimension is divided by the 2D aortic diastolic diameter, measured across the sinuses of Valsalva, a left atrial/aortic ratio can be constructed. This value is somewhat less affected by body size and is typically between 1.6 (larger dogs) and 1.8 (smaller dogs). The left atrial dimension in

healthy cats should be less than 16 mm in this view and the left atrial/aortic ratio less then 1.3.

Another approach to left atrial quantitation uses a diastolic short-axis image of both the aorta and left atrium and measures aortic and left atrial diameters across the line of closure of the left and noncoronary cusps of the aortic valve.[45] A normal diastolic left atrial/aortic ratio is 0.88 to 1.12. Although this method does not evaluate peak left atrial size, it has been useful for following the severity of MR in small-breed dogs.[46]

A third method involves measuring the left atrium in systole across its maximal right-to-left, cranial-to-caudal aspect with the line placed right and caudal to the aortic root and left and cranial to the right pulmonary venous ostium. Either a 2D or M-mode measurement can be made. This view often provides the greatest atrial diameter measurement; however, the usefulness of this and all other atrial measurement approaches is limited by a lack of large studies across breeds of varying body size. Nevertheless, each of these methods can at least be used to follow the progression of left atrial size.

A fourth approach involves measurement of the left atrium or left atrial area from the left-sided, apical four-chamber plane. Area measures can also be made from right-sided, long-axis images.[44] These approaches are uncommonly used in veterinary practice.

ESTIMATION OF LEFT VENTRICULAR CHAMBER SIZE

The diseased left ventricle can undergo simple dilatation, dilate, and hypertrophy while maintaining a normal wall thickness (eccentric hypertrophy), thicken at the expense of the ventricular lumen (concentric hypertrophy), or develop a mixed pattern of concentric hypertrophy with chamber dilatation. Severe dilatation is seen in the worst cases of dilated cardiomyopathy or myocarditis. Eccentric hypertrophy is typical of volume overload (valvular regurgitation, left-to-right shunts) and compensated dilated cardiomyopathy. Concentric hypertrophy is most often seen with AS, idiopathic hypertrophic cardiomyopathy, systemic hypertension, and some cases of hyperthyroidism. Mixed hypertrophy is observed in combined aortic stenosis-insufficiency, with aortic stenosis or hypertrophic cardiomyopathy combined with myocardial failure, or in some cats with hyperthyroidism.

Identification of LV chamber size, cardiac dilatation, and ventricular hypertrophy is an important goal of an echocardiographic study. These changes are indirect measures of the severity of many cardiac lesions. The sonographer must appreciate that accuracy in assessment of ventricular diameter or volume or in estimates of ventricular mass may depend on the approach, the type of heart disease, the species, and even the breed of dog undergoing examination. Linear, area, and volumetric approaches can be taken to analysis of the left ventricle.[4]

Models of the Left Ventricle

The simplest approaches to the left ventricle consider the chamber a sphere or a prolate ellipse. In the latter model, the chamber has two equal minor axes and one long axis equal to twice the minor axis.[4] Assuming that this model is representative of the ventricular lumen, one can simply measure the minor dimension to identify cardiomegaly or cube the minor axis to estimate ventricular volume. This approach, or modifications (e.g., Teicholtz's method[2, 47]), is used routinely in measuring LV size, volume, and systolic function by M-mode echocardiography (see later). Of course, the ventricle is not a prolate ellipse, and in conditions of cardiac dilatation or concentric hypertrophy, this approach may not be suitable. Moreover, systolic dimensions or volume estimates may be depicted inaccurately because minor-axis approaches neglect shortening in the apical-basilar dimension, along the major axis of the ventricle. More accurate methods of estimating ventricular luminal size consider the short-axis area of the ventricle as well as the length of the ventricle.[48] Various area-length models can be used for more accurate assessment of ventricular volume and estimatation of ventricular systolic function; however, these models require additional measurements and an image of the left ventricle that includes length (see Fig. 115–1A). The method of disks or Simpson's rule is an example of an advanced area-length method that can be calculated by many echocardiographic software packages and yields a reasonable estimate of LV diastolic and systolic volumes.[48, 49] These methods may also be more accurate for estimating ventricular systolic function (see later).

LV wall mass can be estimated by both M-mode and 2D echo methods (see Figs. 115–1 to 115–4). Linear measures of LV and ventricular septal wall thickness recorded by M-mode studies are best related to body surface area as an index. M-mode measurements can be misleading, however, if the cursor crosses a papillary muscle or fails to sample the thickest portion of the LV wall or septum. In some situations, as with feline hypertrophic cardiomyopathy, other wall segments must be measured in order to detect ventricular hypertrophy.[50] 2D echocardiographic measures of LV wall thickness can be made in a variety of ways. Both linear and area measures of wall segments can be made and ventricular mass calculated. The general approach involves measuring the internal endocardial area and the external epicardial area and calculating the difference. Myocardial tissue volume is then calculated using a mathematical model of the ventricle and multiplied by 1.05 (the specific gravity of myocardial tissue) to obtain ventricular mass. These methods are beyond the scope of this chapter but are well described elsewhere.[51–54]

Great care must be taken in diagnosing ventricular hypertrophy in volume-depleted patients. Loss of plasma volume reduces ventricular cavity size and the lack of intraluminal distending pressure increases the wall thickness. This ventricular *pseudohypertrophy* can mimic hypertrophic cardiomyopathy or other causes of concentric hypertrophy.[55]

Indexing Measurements to Body Surface Area or Mass

It seem logical that chamber dimensions and wall thickness should be related to body size. In fact, most studies do demonstrate a general relationship of chamber size and wall thickness to body size when compared across breeds of markedly different sizes, as summarized by Boon.[7] However, this issue is not simple, and in some breeds there is little variation in dimensions over a range of body weights.[56] Reference data also suffer from relatively small sample sizes and a lack of data points at the extreme ends of low and high body weights. Accordingly, the 95 per cent confidence limits that define "normal" tend to diverge widely at the extremes, making it difficult to diagnose dilatation or wall hypertrophy in larger breed dogs. It seems evident that breed-specific normal values are needed in many instances.

For example, it has been suggested that maximal LV, diastolic dimensions in Doberman pinschers should be no greater than 45 to 49 mm.[41, 57–59] Values for other breeds have been reported (see Tables 115–6 and 115–7). It seems conceivable that a sonographer may need a number of different reference normal values to diagnose cardiomegaly accurately. One solution is to use dimensions that have been indexed to body surface area. These relationships are approximately linear over the range of medium to large dog sizes. However, the relationships demonstrated in Figure 115–14 become curvilinear when smaller breed dogs (less than 8 kg) are included (not shown), and the values increase almost exponentially so that quite small dogs have larger dimension/body surface area indices.

Left Ventricular Measures in Cats

Reference values reported for cats have been slightly more uniform, probably related to the smaller dispersion in body size; however, some variables demonstrate a statistical correlation with body size.[60] Table 115–8 is a summary of various feline studies. In our laboratory, we generally consider a few key measurements. The most important measurements in cats include the diastolic thickness of the LV wall and the ventricular septum because values exceeding 5.5 mm (sensitive) to 6 mm (specific) are assumed to indicate hypertrophy. It should be noted that many older cats have focal hypertrophy in the dorsal portion of the ventricular septum that may have minimal clinical significance. As already discussed, volume depletion can lead to pseudohypertrophy and an erroneous diagnosis of hypertrophic cardiomyopathy. The LV diastolic internal dimension in healthy cats averages about 15 mm and is generally less than 19 mm. The LV systolic dimensions in cats average between 7 and 8 mm in most studies.

QUANTITATION OF RIGHT-SIDED HEART CHAMBERS

The right atrial and right ventricular cavities are more complex geometrically and are therefore more difficult to quantify. The acoustic windows available for imaging of right heart structures are also limited. The RV free wall diastolic and systolic thickness can be measured with a high-frequency transducer from the right parasternal windows. Diastolic thickness is typically about one third that of the LV wall and should be less than 50 per cent of the LV measurement. The RV cavity is difficult to measure because it is a rapidly tapering triangle when viewed from the right parasternal long-axis view and forms an arc around the left ventricle when viewed in the short-axis planes. Reported values indicate a smaller internal dimension than for the left ventricle when measured by M-mode from the right hemithorax.[42, 61, 62] The size of the right atrium from the right parasternal windows depends largely on how dorsally one can place or angulate the transducer. The left apical four-chamber view is better for identifying moderate to severe right atrial enlargement, as both atria are relatively circular in this plane and the left atrium normally appears larger than the right atrium. There are no definitive studies of internal right atrial or RV measurements and the clinician is frequently forced to use experience and multiple image planes to identify right-sided cardiomegaly.

MEASUREMENT OF THE GREAT VESSELS

Cardiomegaly may be accompanied by dilatation of the aorta or the pulmonary artery. Dilatation of the pulmonary

LV end-diastolic diameter index

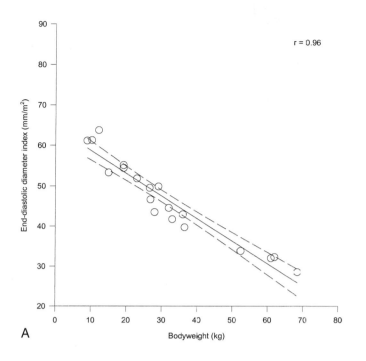

r = 0.96

LV end-systolic diameter index

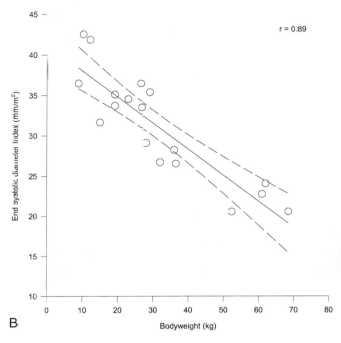

r = 0.89

LV free wall diastolic index

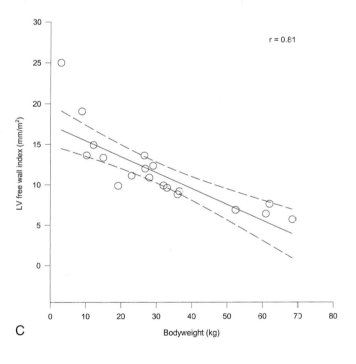

r = 0.81

Figure 115–14. *A*, Plot of end-diastolic left ventricular diameter index (mm diameter per square meter of body surface area) against body weight (kg). Notice the relatively linear relationship with larger dogs having smaller diameter indices. The same relationship is also true for the end-systolic diameter index (*B*) and ventricular wall index (*C*). It should be emphasized that values for smaller breeds do not fall along these lines and when present alter the line to a curvilinear relationship. Each point represents data from an individual study of a single breed (see text and tables for details and study sources).

artery is usually associated with three major abnormalities: left-to-right shunts, pulmonary hypertension (including dirofilariasis), and pulmonic stenosis. Dilatation of the aorta can develop in a number of situations: AS, patent ductus arteriosus, malformations of the conotruncal septum (tetralogy of Fallot, pulmonary atresia), systemic hypertension, and some cases of feline hypertrophic cardiomyopathy. Older cats often develop dilatation and tortuosity of the aorta.

These findings are often quite evident from subjective evaluation of the great vessels when an experienced exam-

iner performs a study. Normal values for aortic root dimension (at the level of the aortic valves), aortic sinuses, and the ascending aorta have been reported.[44] Dimensions across the aortic sinuses are wider than those measured at the attachment points of the aortic valve or the sinotubular junction. As a general rule, the normal main pulmonary artery appears no larger than the aorta in image planes that include both structures. Assuming normal aortic dimensions, this rule of thumb can be used to identify a dilated or attenuated pulmonary artery.

PRINCIPLES OF ANATOMIC DIAGNOSIS

The most important part of any echocardiographic examination is high-quality imaging that permits evaluation of morphology and cardiac motion. This aim is accomplished primarily by the 2D examination and is supported by M-mode studies; Doppler examinations are more useful for identification of abnormal blood flow and for estimation of pressure gradients and aspects of diastolic cardiac function.

The anatomic echocardiographic diagnosis can be categorized in a number of ways. One approach is simply to divide morphologic abnormalities into congenital and acquired heart diseases. This approach is summarized in Tables 115–9 and 115–10. However, when performing and interpreting an echocardiographic study, a more general anatomic approach, as advanced by Weyman,[4] may be preferable because many aspects of congenital and acquired diseases overlap. Furthermore, a systematic approach fosters an open mind with respect to anatomic and functional abnormalties. This type of approach is illustrated in the following and in Table 115–11.

LEFT ATRIUM

The left atrial cavity may be normal, small, or volume loaded. The atrial intraluminal dimension can be measured readily by 2D methods.[63, 64] Estimation of atrial wall thick-

TABLE 115–9. USUAL ECHOCARDIOGRAPHIC FINDINGS IN CONGENITAL HEART DISEASE*

CARDIAC DISORDER	TWO-DIMENSIONAL ECHOCARDIOGRAPHY	M-MODE ECHOCARDIOGRAPHY	DOPPLER STUDIES
Atrial septal defect	"Dropout" of atrial septal echoes (ASD); dilatation of the RA, RV, PA, ± LA	Paradoxical ventricular septal motion and right ventricular volume overload	Low-velocity shunt across the defect§
Patent foramen ovale	Separation of septum primum and septum secundum in place of a normal fossa ovalis; contrast echocardiography demonstrates right-to-left shunting	Evidence of right ventricular volume or pressure overload	Low-velocity right-to-left shunt across the foramen ovale; other findings indicating a right-sided cardiac lesion(s)
Ventricular septal defect	"Dropout" of ventricular septal echoes (VSD); dilatation of the LA, LV, ± RV, ± PA; ± evidence of RV outlet obstruction; rarely prolapse of aortic valve into VSD	Evidence of volume overload; normal LV shortening fraction	Turbulent, high-velocity systolic jet crossing the defect; possibly aortic regurgitation†,‡
Patent ductus arteriosus	Dilation of the LA, LV, Ao, PA; can generally image ductal ampulla	Normal to reduced shortening fraction	Continuous, high-velocity, turbulent flow traversing the ductus and entering the pulmonary artery†,‡
Tetralogy of Fallot	Large subaortic ventricular septal defect; RV hypertrophy; RA dilation; right ventricular outflow obstruction; aortic malalignment (override); contrast echocardiography demonstrates right-to-left shunting	RV hypertrophy; malalignment of the aorta; flat ventricular septal motion; relatively small left heart chambers	Turbulent, high-velocity systolic signal in the RV outlet and pulmonary artery; low-velocity shunt from right to left across the VSD
Mitral valve dysplasia (congenital mitral regurgitation)	Valve thickening, abnormal chordae tendineae or papillary muscles, possible leaflet fusion; dilated LA and LV	Thick mitral valve; abnormal valve motion; dilated LA and LV; increased LV shortening fraction	Turbulent, high-velocity, systolic signal of mitral regurgitation in the LA; possible increase in diastolic mitral valve velocities¶
Tricuspid valve dysplasia (congenital tricuspid regurgitation)	Valve thickening, abnormal chordae tendineae or papillary muscles, possible leaflet fusion; dilated RA and RV	Thick tricuspid valve; abnormal valve motion; dilated RA and RV; paradoxical ventricular septal motion	Turbulent, high-velocity systolic signal in the RA; possible increase in diastolic tricuspid valve velocities¶
Pulmonic stenosis	Thick, hypoplastic, or fused pulmonary valve leaflets; less often a subvalvular or supravalvular obstruction; dilated main pulmonary artery; RV hypertrophy; ± dynamic RV outlet obstruction, ± RA dilation	RV hypertrophy; RA dilation; flat ventricular septal motion	Turbulent and high-velocity systolic signal in the RV outlet and PA; pulmonary insufficiency is also typical A concurrent, high-velocity signal of tricuspid regurgitation is commonly recorded in the RA
Subaortic stenosis	Subaortic ridge, collar, or hyperechoic tissue; narrowed left ventricular outlet; LV hypertrophy; dilated ascending aorta; ± hyperechoic LV subendocardium (indicates myocardial fibrosis)	LV hypertrophy; normal to increased shortening fraction	Turbulent, high-velocity systolic signal in the left ventricular outlet and Ao A diastolic signal of aortic regurgitation is also recorded in most cases

*Major points are emphasized; this table is not comprehensive.

†Mild increases in diastolic mitral (PDA, VSD) and systolic aortic velocities (PDA) will usually be recorded owing to increased volume flow.

‡The velocity depends on the relative pressure between the systemic and pulmonary circulations; generally the velocity is directly related to pressure differences and inversely related to the diameter of the defect.

§Mild increases in diastolic tricuspid and systolic pulmonary artery velocities will usually be recorded owing to increased transvalvular flow.

¶Congenital atrioventricular valve stenosis is relatively rare, but would be associated with other findings including a narrowed valve orifice or tethered valve leaflets, dilated atrium, increased transvalvular diastolic velocities (E and A waves), prolonged pressure half-time, and often concurrent valvular regurgitation.

LA = left atrium; RA = right atrium; LV = left ventricle; RV = right ventricle; Ao = aorta; PA = pulmonary artery; PDA = patent ductus arteriosus; VSD = ventricular septal defect; ASD = atrial septal defect.

TABLE 115–10. ECHOCARDIOGRAPHIC FINDINGS IN COMMON ACQUIRED HEART DISEASES*

CARDIAC DISORDER	TWO-DIMENSIONAL ECHOCARDIOGRAPHY	M-MODE ECHOCARDIOGRAPHY	DOPPLER STUDIES
Pericardial effusion†	Fluid-filled, sonolucent or mixed-echoic pericardial space; possible cardiac or heart base tumor; collapse of the RA and RV in cardiac tamponade; may observe pleural effusion as well	Sonolucent pericardial space evident; abnormal cardiac motion; RA and RV collapse if tamponade; respiratory variation in cardiac filling	Exaggerated respiratory variation in the transvalvular tricuspid and mitral valve velocity signals with constrictive disease
Feline hypertrophic cardiomyopathy	LA dilatation; LV hypertrophy: hypertrophy may be symmetric and involving the entire ventricle, asymmetric with predominant hypertrophy of the septum or free wall, or focal hypertrophy of the ventricle	Normal to decreased LV dimensions; LV hypertrophy; LA dilatation; normal to increased shortening fraction; possible systolic anterior motion of the septal mitral valve leaflet	Turbulent, high-velocity systolic signal of mitral regurgitation often recorded in the LA; turbulent, high-velocity systolic signal recorded in the left ventricular outlet in cats with obstructive form of hypertrophic cardiomyopathy; ± abnormal isovolumetric relaxation time
Feline restrictive (intermediate) cardiomyopathy	LA dilatation, RA dilatation, ± RV dilatation; mild LV dilatation with variable hypertrophy; hyperechoic subendocardium; regional ventricular wall dysfunction is possible	Normal to mildly decreased LV shortening fraction, LA dilatation; possible regional wall motion abnormalities	Variable; turbulent high-velocity systolic signals of mitral or tricuspid regurgitation may be recorded; restrictive ventricular filling pattern
Dilated cardiomyopathy	LA and LV or generalized cardiac dilatation; global ventricular hypokinesis or marked depression of systolic ventricular free wall contraction and thickening	Ventricular and atrial dilatation; decreased LV shortening fraction is required to establish the diagnosis; increases E-point to septal separation, ± delayed mitral valve closure (B-shoulder) indicates elevated atrial and ventricular diastolic pressures	Turbulent, high-velocity systolic signals of mitral and tricuspid regurgitation are common; decreased aortic velocity and acceleration time; abnormal indices of diastolic ventricular function
Feline hyperthyroidism	Mild to moderate LA and LV dilatation; LV hypertrophy; variable RA and RV dilatation; if heart failure, all chambers dilated and pleural effusion	LV hypertrophy; mild to moderate LV and LA dilatation; increased LV shortening fraction in most cases; normal to decreased shortening fraction if heart failure	Variable: may observe turbulent jets of mitral regurgitation or tricuspid regurgitation; increased aortic velocity may be recorded
Mitral regurgitation (degenerative)	Valvular thickening—diffuse or focal; may observe prolapse of a valve (or rarely a flail leaflet) related to stretching or rupture of chorda tendineae; LA and LV dilatation; hyperdynamic left ventricle in primary mitral degeneration in small breed dogs	LV and LA dilatation; valvular thickening; variable LV shortening fraction depending on etiology, duration, and severity of valvular regurgitation; fractional shortening can be high in cases of mitral regurgitation when myocardial contractility is preserved	Turbulent, high-velocity systolic signal of mitral regurgitation in LA; increased diastolic mitral valve inflow velocities‡
Aortic regurgitation	Valvular thickening—diffuse or focal, if severe and irregular consider bacterial endocarditis (± flail leaflet); ± aortic root dilatation (cats); LV dilatation with severe aortic regurgitation	Possible LV dilation and hypertrophy; aorta may be dilated; thickened aortic valve may be observed; ± diastolic fluttering of aortic or mitral valves	Turbulent, high-velocity diastolic signal of aortic regurgitation in the LV outflow tract; ± increased systolic outflow velocity‡
Tricuspid regurgitation	Valvular thickening—diffuse or focal; may observe prolapse of a valve; RA and RV dilatation; if dilated PA consider pulmonary hypertension as cause of tricuspid regurgitation.	RV and RA dilatation; possible valvular thickening	Turbulent, high-velocity systolic signal of tricuspid regurgitation in RA; the peak velocity of the regurgitant jet is variable and depends on RV systolic pressure; increased diastolic tricuspid inflow velocities may be observed‡
Bacterial endocarditis	Valvular thickening—irregular or oscillating echo densities on aortic or mitral valves; long-standing cases may appear calcified; dilation of the left atrium and left ventricle if volume overload is severe	Highly thickened valve; echo-dense material moves in association with the cardiac cycle; cardiomegaly related to volume or pressure overload; premature closure of the mitral valve in peracute, severe aortic regurgitation	Evidence of valvular regurgitation and increased transvalvular flow velocities‡ across the affected heart valve; in cases of chronic endocarditis the valve may become stenotic with Doppler evidence of aortic or mitral valve stenosis
Heartworm disease	Dilated PA, RV, RA; may observe echogenic densities (double, parallel lines) in the main or branch PA; in caval syndrome heartworms create echogenic masses within the tricuspid valve orifice; in cats adult filaria may be evident in the right ventricle and right atrium	If severe, RV dilatation and flat or paradoxical ventricular septal motion	Possibly a high-velocity diastolic signal of pulmonary insufficiency in the RV outlet; possibly high-velocity tricuspid regurgitation

*Major points are emphasized; this table is not comprehensive.

†Constrictive pericardial diseases may be associated with small pericardial effusions (constrictive-effusive disease) or no demonstrable fluid; marked diastolic flutter of the ventricular septum may be observed because of disparate rates of ventricular filling; marked respiratory variation in ventricular filling is observed.

‡Mild increases in velocities owing to increased transvalvular flow.

LA = left atrium; RA = right atrium; LV = left ventricle; RV = right ventricle; Ao = aorta; PA = pulmonary artery; PDA = patent ductus arteriosus; VSD = ventricular septal defect; ASD = atrial septal defect.

TABLE 115–11. APPROACH TO ECHOCARDIOGRAPHIC DIAGNOSIS

General principles
    Evaluate the ECG relative to cardiac motion and cardiac rhythm disturbances.
    Determine image planes needed on the basis of clinical situation and laboratory standards.
    Identify structures including the atria, ventricles, cardiac septa, great vessels, and cardiac valves.
    Note dilatation, attenuation, or absence of the aorta or pulmonary artery.
    Note presence or absence of anticipated structures.
    Identify extracardiac or cardiac mass lesions.
    Identify abnormal external structures such as dilated coronary sinus.
    Identify pleural effusion.
Left atrium and pulmonary veins
    Identify pulmonary veins and pulmonary venous ostia.
    Examine left atrium for attenuation: if small, rule out volume depletion, right-to-left shunt, or low cardiac output.
    Examine left atrium for enlargement: if enlarged, rule out left-to-right shunt, mitral valve disease, left ventricular systolic or diastolic failure, primary atrial disease.
    Identify mass lesions or thrombi.
    Measure left atrial diameter.
    Examine the atrial septum for abnormal bowing into the left or right atrium (high atrial pressure).
    Examine the atrial septum for septal defects or patent foramen ovale.
    Examine the blood pool for spontaneous contrast.
    Examine the atrioventricular groove for dilated vascular structure: rule out dilated coronary sinus and left cranial vena cava.
Mitral valve
    Identify valve leaflets and cusps.
    Identify support apparatus (chordae tendineae, papillary muscles).
    Increased valve echogenicity: rule out vegetation, degenerative thickening, malformation, thrombus.
    Cleft or common septal leaflet: rule out endocardial cushion defect or primum atrial septal defect.
    Observe motion during cardiac cycle.
        Reduced diastolic (E-F) slope: rule out stenosis, decreased transvalvular flow.
        Lack of diastolic separation or increased mitral E point to septal distance: rule out LV dilation with left ventricular failure, mitral stenosis, or aortic regurgitation.
        Prolapse of leaflet into atrium: rule out degenerative disease, elongated or ruptured chordae tendineae.
        Flail leaflet: rule out ruptured chordae tendineae or avulsion of papillary muscle.
        Diastolic mitral valve fluttering: rule out aortic regurgitation.
        Systolic mitral or tricuspid valve fluttering: rule out AV insufficiency.
        Chaotic valve motion: rule out arrhythmia, ruptured chordae tendineae.
        Premature (diastolic) closure of the AV valve: rule out severe semilunar valve insufficiency, long PR interval, or atrioventricular block.
        Delayed (systolic) closure (B-shoulder): rule out LV failure and elevated atrial pressure.
Left ventricle
    Hypertrophy: rule out hypertension, aortic or subaortic stenosis, hyperthyroidism, hypertrophic cardiomyopathy, coarctation of the aorta.
    Dilation: rule out causes of volume overload, dilated cardiomyopathy, myocarditis, mitral or aortic valvular disease, left-to-right shunts, AV fistula, anemia, persistent tachyarrhythmia or bradyarrhythmia.
    Hyperkinesis: rule out mitral or aortic insufficiency, compensated aortic stenosis, volume overload with preserved myocardial function, bradycardia, hyperthyroidism, sympathetic tone stimulation, hypertrophic cardiomyopathy.
    Dyskinesis: rule out cardiomyopathy, ischemia, infarct, arrhythmia.
    Aneurysm: rule out congenital lesion or prior myocarditis or infarct.
    Giant or thickened papillary muscle: rule out ventricular hypertrophy, AV valve dysplasia.
Left ventricular outlet and aorta
    Examine for subvalvular aortic stenosis—congenital or acquired.
    Identify aortic valve leaflets and motion during cardiac cycle.
        Thickened leaflets: rule out malformation, degeneration, endocarditis.
        Diastolic fluttering of the aortic valve: rule out aortic insufficiency.
        Systolic fluttering or the aortic valve: normal or high-flow state.
        Prolapse into ventricle: rule out ventricular septal defect or bacterial endocarditis.
        Lack of systolic separation: rule out low cardiac output, arrhythmia, stenosis.
        Premature (midsystolic) closure: rule out outflow tract obstruction, ventricular septal defect.
        Systolic doming: rule out congenital valve stenosis.
    Decreased aortic diameter: rule out low cardiac output; hypotension.
    Dilation of the aorta: rule out subaortic or aortic stenosis, tetralogy of Fallot, pulmonary artery atresia, patent ductus arteriosus, systemic hypertension, or idiopathic dilatation.
Ventricular septum
    Hypertrophy: rule out causes of left or right ventricular hypertrophy (above); rule out idiopathic hypertrophic cardiomyopathy.
    Hyperkinesis: as per left ventricle.
    Hypokinesis: as perlet ventricle; also rule out RV pressure or volume overload.
    Paradoxic motion: rule out moderate to severe RV pressure or volume overload such as atrial septal defect, tricuspid regurgitation.
    Examine for ventricular septal defects.
    Discontinuity of septum and anterior aortic root: rule out simple ventricular septal defect (peri- or paramembranous; inlet septal VSD; muscular VSD; outlet septal VSD), tetralogy of Fallot, pulmonary artery atresia, truncus arteriosus, or a false defect caused by angle of the ascending aorta or aortic dilatation.
Right atrium
    Examine right atrium for attenuation: if small, rule out volume depletion.
    Examine right atrium for enlargement: if enlarged, rule out tricuspid regurgitation, tricuspid stenosis or atresia, cardiomyopathy, primary atrial myocardial diseases, right heart failure, atrial septal defect, hyperthyroidism, moderate to severe anemia, or arteriovenous fistula.
    Identify mass lesions such as tumor or thrombus.
    Examine the atrial septum for abnormal bowing into the left or right atrium (high atrial pressure).
    Examine the atrial septum for septal defects or patent foramen ovale.
    Obstructive partitioning of right atrium: rule out cor triatriatum dexter.

TABLE 115–11. APPROACH TO ECHOCARDIOGRAPHIC DIAGNOSIS *Continued*

Tricuspid valve
  Identify valve leaflets and cusps.
  Identify support apparatus (chordae tendineae, papillary muscles).
  Increased valve echogenicity: rule out vegetation, degenerative thickening, malformation, thrombus.
  Cleft or common septal leaflet: rule out endocardial cushion defect/primum atrial septal defect.
  Motion during cardiac cycle.
    Reduced diastolic (E-F) slope or separation: rule out stenosis, decreased transvalvular flow.
    Prolapse of leaflet into atrium: rule out degenerative disease, elongated or ruptured chordae tendineae.
    Flail leaflet: rule out ruptured chordae tendineae or avulsion of papillary muscle.
    Chaotic valve motion: rule out arrhythmia, ruptured chordae tendineae.
    Premature (diastolic) closure of the AV valve: rule out severe semilunar valve insufficiency, long PR interval, or atrioventricular block.
  Echogenic parasites in the right atrium and right ventricular inlet: caval syndrome of heartworm disease.
Right ventricle
  Hypertrophy: rule out pulmonic stenosis, tetralogy of Fallot, large ventricular septal defect, pulmonary hypertension.
  Dilation: rule out tricuspid insufficiency, chronic right ventricular pressure overload, atrial septal defect, large ventricular septal defect, severe
    pulmonary insufficiency, Chagas' disease, myocarditis, right ventricular cardiomyopathy, persistent tachyarrhythmia or bradyarrhythmia, or
    arteriovenous fistula.
  Aneurysm: rule out congenital lesion or prior myocardial (traumatic) rupture.
Right ventricular outlet and pulmonary artery
  Narrowing of the outflow tract: rule out valvular stenosis with secondary hypertrophy; rule out VSD with secondary hypertrophy.
  Examine outlet for subvalvular pulmonic stenosis.
  Identify valve leaflets and motion during cardiac cycle.
    Thick leaflets or fused leaflets: rule out congenital stenosis or dysplasia.
    Diastolic fluttering: rule out valvar insufficiency.
    Systolic fluttering: normal or high-flow state.
    Lack of systolic separation: rule out low cardiac output, arrhythmia, stenosis.
    Systolic doming: rule out valve stenosis.
  Pulmonary artery, absence or attenuation of: rule out atresia or hypoplasia.
  Pulmonary artery, dilation of: rule out pulmonic stenosis, left-to-right shunt, pulmonary hypertension, dirofilariasis.
  Examine the main pulmonary artery and branches for *Dirofilaria immitis* or large pulmonary thrombi.
Other vascular structures
  Identify cranial vena cava.
  Identify caudal vena cava.
  Identify hepatic veins.
Pericardium and pericardial space
  Rule out peritoneopericardial diaphragmatic hernia, pericardial effusion, pericardial constriction, or mass lesion.
  Diastolic collapse of the right atrium or right ventricle: rule out cardiac tamponade or large bilateral pleural effusion.
  Rule out extrapericardial mass lesion of the lung, mediastinum, or pleural space.
  Rule out pleural effusion.

ECG = electrocardiogram; LV = left ventricular; AV = atrioventricular; RV = right ventricular; VSD = ventricular septal defect.

ness is much more difficult and requires a system with fine resolution. General reasons for left atrial dilatation include left-to-right shunt, mitral valvular disease, and LV diastolic or systolic failure. Primary atrial muscle disease is a rare cause of dilatation. Issues of quantitation were discussed in the previous section. The most common congenital lesions of the atria recognized by echocardiography are atrial septal defects. Lesions can be located in the fossa ovalis (secundum septal defects or patent foramen ovale associated with a right-sided heart lesion) or the ventral atrial septum (primum atrial septal defect) or dorsally in the case of the sinus venosus defect.[65–67] Rare lesions include cor triatriatum (partitioning of the left atrium) and near absence of the atrial septum. Acquired mass lesions include left atrial thrombi, which are most common in cats, and intracardiac or extrinsic mass lesions including tumors and granulomas. Cats with a propensity for atrial thrombosis may demonstrate spontaneous echogenic contrast or "smoke" within the atrial cavity. Identification of a dilated structure in the atrioventricular groove is suggestive of a dilated coronary sinus as might be seen with persistent left cranial vena cava.

MITRAL VALVE

Mitral valvular lesions commonly encountered in practice include congenital malformations, degenerative diseases, infective endocarditis, chordal ruptures, and dysfunction secondary to myocardial disease. Dysplasia of the atrioventricular valves refers to a spectrum of lesions that includes thick or shortened valve cusps, either long or stout chordae tendineae, and anomalies of the papillary muscles. Less frequently, there is stenosis or even atresia of the atrioventricular valve.[68, 69] Acquired mitral disorders typically lead to valve thickening. Abnormal valve motion, including valve prolapse[70–74] or flail leaflet,[75] may be observed with loss of valvular support as with chordae tendineae stretch or rupture. Reduced opening of the valve is most often due to low cardiac output, although it can also be seen with aortic regurgitation or congenital valvular stenosis. Diastolic fluttering of the mitral valve, impaired opening of the septal leaflet, and premature mitral valve closure are indicators of aortic regurgitation with the regurgitant jet directed toward the mitral valve.[76] Systolic mitral valve fluttering has been observed with myxomatous disease in dogs with musical murmurs. Delayed mitral closure may be a sign of high left atrial pressure and is best observed by M-mode study.[77] Systolic anterior motion of the valve (toward the septum) is typical of dynamic ventricular outflow obstruction.

LEFT VENTRICLE

The general anatomic responses of the left ventricle have already been discussed, and Table 115–11 indicates many of the abnormalities potentially affecting the left ventricle. The clinician should determine whether morphologic abnormalities such as dilatation or hypertrophy are primary (e.g., cardiomyopathy) or secondary to increased workloads such as hypertension, AS, anemia, or primary mitral valve disease. Endocrinopathies such as hyperthyroidism can affect the left ventricle (see Chapter 150).[78, 79] Abnormalities of the papillary muscles may be observed in some cases of mitral valve malformation (especially in cats) or associated with concentric hypertrophy or idiopathic hypertrophic cardiomyopathy. The overall systolic motion of the left ventricle generally reflects contractility and loading conditions (see later). Wall motion abnormalities may be evident with arrhythmias, in feline restrictive cardiomyopathy, and in the rare cases of myocardial infarction or myocarditis.

LEFT VENTRICULAR OUTLET AND AORTA

The LV outlet extends from the tips of the open anterior mitral valve leaflet, along the ventricular septum, across the aortic valve, and into the ascending aorta. Obstruction to outflow may occur in the subaortic, aortic valvular, or supravalvular zone. The most common lesions observed by echocardiography are congenital subaortic stenosis in dogs[5] and dynamic LV outflow tract obstruction associated with hypertrophic obstructive cardiomyopathy in cats.[80] The latter is characterized by mitral valve–septal contact during systole. Thickening of the aortic valve is observed occasionally in congenital AS. Some older dogs and aged cats also develop aortic valve thickening that predisposes to varying degrees of aortic regurgitation. Marked thickening of the valve, an irregular oscillating appearance, or evidence of valve calcification are highly suggestive of infective endocarditis.

A number of motion patterns of the aortic valve may be observed. Normal aortic valve motion involves opening in early systole and often systolic fluttering of the leaflets. This fluttering can be pronounced in high-output states or with aortic stenosis. Incomplete opening may suggest stenosis or simply low cardiac output. Premature, midsystolic closure is typical of dynamic obstruction in the outflow tract. Diastolic fluttering of the aortic valve is observed in some cases of aortic insufficiency. Prolapse of the valve is observed in some cases of ventricular septal defect and with avulsion of a leaflet as with severe endocarditis.

The ascending aortic diameter may appear reduced in hypotension or as a variant in some breeds (some Boxer dogs). Dilatation of the ascending aorta is common with hypertension, with hyperthyroidism,[81] as an incidental finding in many older cats (without the aforementioned conditions), and associated with some congenital defects including aortic stenosis (see Table 115–9). Aortic dilatation is observed sporadically as an incidental finding in dogs.

VENTRICULAR SEPTUM

The ventricular septum is generally considered part of the left ventricle but can thicken in concert with an LV or RV hypertrophic process. Isolated septal hypertrophy is occasionally observed in cats with hypertrophic cardiomyopathy. In older cats, isolated hypertrophy of the dorsal septum is not uncommon. Dynamic obstruction between the ventricular septum and the mitral outlet is common in cats with hypertrophic cardiomyopathy and can be observed with high-frame-rate 2D studies or by M-mode methods.

Ventricular septal defects are typically classified by location within the right ventricle. The most common defects can be observed using short-axis or angled tomograms of the aortic root and the U-shaped RV inlet and outlet. The typical peri- or paramembranous defects are evident ventral to the aortic root and enter adjacent to the tricuspid valve. Large defects associated with the outlet or tetralogy of Fallot may be evident at the opposite extreme of the ventricle just below the pulmonary valve. Rare muscular defects are ventral and require multiple views to identify. Inlet ventricular septal defects, such as develop with endocardial cushion defects, are often best observed with a left apical four-chamber view (also see Congenital Heart Disease). Discontinuity of the septum and anterior aortic root is observed with so-called malalignment septal defects, including those seen with tetralogy of Fallot, pulmonary artery atresia, or truncus arteriosus. In some cases, the defect is partially closed by a prolapsing aortic valve leaflet.[82]

It can be useful to inspect the shape and motion of the ventricular septum in animals with heart disease.[83, 84] Ventricular septal motion is a reflection of overall LV shape but responds to the relative pressure and volume loads of the ventricles and is a factor in ventricular interdependence. Abnormalities in septal motion and in the radius of ventricular septal curvature are often noted in animals with spontaneous pressure or volume overload of the right ventricle. The normal septal arc is circular throughout the cardiac cycle on short-axis images of the left ventricle (see Fig. 115–2A and B). Normal ventricular septal motion on the M-mode echocardiogram is toward the contracting ventricular free wall in systole (see Figs. 115–4 and 115–5). The septal nadir occurs just before or during the free wall apogee in most studies. With significant RV volume overload, the septum is deviated and may actually invert into the left ventricle. After the QRS complex, as intracardiac pressures increase, the higher LV pressure suddenly forces the septum back into the right ventricle, recreating a circular septal arc. The M-mode correlate of this is paradoxical ventricular septal motion in which the septum moves away from the contracting LV free wall. In RV pressure overload (as with pulmonic stenosis), the ventricular septum is either circular or flat in diastole. During ventricular systole, septal motion may be minimal or initially paradoxical on the M-mode study, and on the short-axis 2D echo, cardiogram the septum may appear quite flattened, especially if RV and LV systolic pressures are nearly equal.

RIGHT ATRIUM

Compared with the left atrium, the right atrium is more difficult to examine because of its more complex and less circular geometry (see Fig. 115–1). Changes in right atrial size are reflections of plasma volume status and right atrial pressure. Disorders that change atrial size are summarized in Table 115–11. Atrial septal defects, tricuspid valve disease, and pulmonary hypertension are important causes of right atrial enlargement. High-output states, including hyperthyroidism, anemia, and arteriovenous fistula, can also lead to right atrial enlargement. Normally, the atrial septum is relatively straight (with a slight concavity into the left atrium) when viewed from the right using a parasternal long-axis image. Marked bowing of the septum into either the left or the right atrium generally suggests increased volume or pressure in the contralateral chamber. The congenital defect cor triatriatum dexter is characterized echocardiographically by a persistent intra-atrial membrane that partitions the right atrium into two chambers.[85, 86] The right atrium is also a common location for atrial tumors in dogs, most often hemangiosarcoma of the right auricle.[87] The mass lesion can vary from subtle (just filling the auricle) to massive with invasion of the atrioventricular free wall or encroachment of the atrial lumen. Extracardiac masses can also impinge on the atria, impairing venous return (Fig. 115–15).

TRICUSPID VALVE

Many of the points made previously concerning the mitral valve are pertinent to echocardiographic examination of the tricuspid valve; however, there are some differences that should be addressed. The tricuspid valve in the dog is actually composed of two leaflets, a small septal leaflet that adheres closely to the septum and an expansive lateral leaflet. Tricuspid valve malformation is probably more common in dogs than mitral dysplasia, and the most common features involve long leaflets and chordae tendineae with an abnormal papillary muscle in the RV apex. Thrombi are more likely to adhere to the tricuspid than the mitral valve. The tricuspid valve can develop incompetence with minimal morphologic abnormality, particularly when there is pulmonary hypertension or pulmonic stenosis. Endocarditis of the tricuspid valve and chordal rupture are both rare conditions in dogs and cats. In the caval syndrome of dirofilariasis, adult heartworms span the tricuspid orifice, moving into the atrium and caudal vena cava during systole and into the right ventricle during diastole.[88]

RIGHT VENTRICLE

The right ventricle is a complicated structure anatomically and echocardiographically. The chamber is difficult to measure accurately, and consistently useful echocardiographic indices of RV performance are still lacking. The overall cavity is crescent shaped, extending around the left ventricle and the aortic root. The right ventricle is roughly partitioned into an inlet and outlet by a ridge of muscle, the supraventricular crest (see Figs. 115–2D and 115–6). This muscle can become a prominent echocardiographic structure in condi-

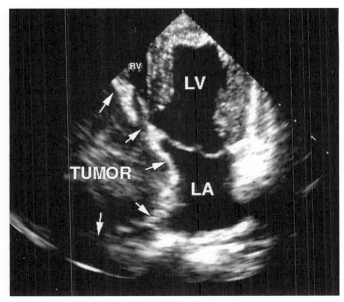

Figure 115–15. Large extracardiac tumor impinging on the right atrium, right ventricle (RV), and left atrium (LA). Left apical image plane recorded from an Afghan hound.

tions of RV hypertrophy subsequent to pulmonic stenosis, tetralogy of Fallot, ventricular septal defect, or pulmonary hypertension. It is not uncommon to observe dynamic, infundibular, outflow obstruction in these situations. Even normal cats appear prone to narrowing of the lumen in this area when they are subjected to high sympathetic drive.

Causes of RV hypertrophy, dilatation, and other morphologic lesions are indicated in Table 115–11. It should be appreciated that concentric hypertrophy is less common in acquired conditions, but pressure overload in congenital heart disease often results in marked hypertrophy of the entire chamber, including the papillary muscles. Cardiomyopathies may lead to RV dilatation consequent to pulmonary hypertension, arrhythmia, or generalized myocardial involvement. An unusual isolated RV cardiomyopathy is occasionally diagnosed in cats and dogs. In some but not all cases, there is concurrent right atrial disease.

RIGHT VENTRICULAR OUTLET AND PULMONARY ARTERY

Distal to the supraventricular crest are the RV outflow tract, pulmonary valve, and pulmonary artery. Congenital valvular dysplasia and stenosis represent common congenital defects in dogs. A variety of valvular malformations may be evident, ranging from fused mobile valves to marked thickening with a hypoplastic anulus. Subvalvular stenosis is more typical of tetralogy of Fallot or secondary to acquired stenosis from a ventricular septal defect. Supravalvular stenosis is uncommon.

Dilation of the pulmonary artery is a relatively common 2D echocardiographic finding and generally indicates either pulmonary hypertension, pulmonic stenosis, or a left-to-right shunt. Atresia and hypoplasia of the pulmonary artery represent rare congenital defects. Imaging of the pulmonary artery, along with the main branches, may be the most sensitive study with which to diagnose feline dirofilariasis.[89–91] However, in our experience echocardiography is not as useful for routine diagnosis of canine heartworm infections, except in dogs with caval syndrome.[92, 93]

OTHER VASCULAR STRUCTURES

Depending on the clinical circumstances, it may be useful to image vascular structures extending out from the heart. The cranial vena cava can be examined from left cranial intercostal positions and appears as a vascular structure running parallel to the aorta in the far field. The cranial vena cava may be obstructed or dilated by masses in the cranial mediastinum. Similarly, the caudal vena cava can be imaged from an angled view in the left apical image planes[94] or from the right with the transducer placed over the caudal, dorsal intercostal spaces. Dilation of the caudal vena cava and hepatic veins is typical in right-sided congestive heart failure. Precise values that define this vascular enlargement are lacking.

VENTRICULAR SYSTOLIC FUNCTION

Quantification of myocardial function is an important role of echocardiography. Deterioration in systolic performance often has prognostic repercussions, and the ability to identify myocardial failure in a noninvasive way has enormous benefits. There are limitations, however; and it is important to be aware of the effects of preload, afterload, and heart rate on most functional indices measured by echocardiography. Drug intervention may also affect these indices, either by directly influencing contractility or by altering loading conditions. It is often not possible to separate changes in echocardiographic indices produced by altered inotropic state versus altered loading conditions.

LV ejection fraction has traditionally been the standard index of LV systolic function and is defined as the fraction of end-diastolic volume ejected from the left ventricle during systole (Tables 115–12 and 115–13). As with most systolic indices, ejection fraction is affected by both contractility and loading conditions, so it provides a measurement of overall cardiac performance rather than a specific assessment of ventricular contractility. Nevertheless, it is still considered the "gold standard" clinical measurement for the assessment of global ventricular systolic function. Many other ejection phase indices derived from echocardiography are simpler measurements intended to approximate ejection fraction.

LINEAR INDICES

Linear estimates of ejection fraction include the LV shortening fraction (SF), which is measured from the M-mode echocardiogram. The SF is defined as the percentage reduction in LV diameter in systole and therefore represents shortening in one minor-axis dimension. As it is readily derived from M-mode studies, it has been widely used in veterinary medicine.[95, 96] The clinician should be wary, however, in placing undue emphasis on a single measurement of LV function, such as SF. SF is difficult to measure accurately when the septum and free wall do not contract synchronously; SF may be reduced despite active wall motion in this setting. Other potential problems with relying on SF include masking of myocardial failure by increased preload or decreased afterload. Small dogs with MR and normal myocardial function generally have supranormal values for SF, as they have both enhanced preload and reduced afterload. In the context of severe MR, a normal value for SF might indicate myocardial failure. Dogs with aortic stenosis may also have normal or increased values of SF. Conversely, apparently healthy dogs may have SF values between 20 and 25 per cent,[97] which might otherwise be considered abnormal in terms of many published reference values. In breeds that are predisposed to dilated cardiomyopathy, the problem becomes still more difficult. Values as different as 34.2 per cent[41] and 21.7 per cent[98] have been published for asymptomatic Doberman pinschers. Low values of SF in asymptomatic animals may represent normality or occult dilated cardiomyopathy. Clearly, it is better to use a wide range of echocardiographic variables and to interpret them carefully within their clinical context.

The situation in cats is far less confusing. Normal feline values are higher, generally exceeding 35 per cent in most situations. Occult dilated cardiomyopathy is not considered a significant problem at this time.

Other reported indices derived from M-mode include percentage systolic free wall thickening and the amplitude of LV free wall excursion. Both indices are unaffected by the presence of paradoxical or asynchronous septal motion. The mitral valve E-point to septal separation (EPSS) is also a linear measure, based on M-mode recordings at the mitral valve level.[41] It is increased with myocardial failure but can also be increased when affected by a jet of aortic regurgita-

tion (impinging on the valve) or rare cases of mitral valve stenosis. A combination of LV dilatation with reduced SF and increased EPSS is more likely to indicate myocardial failure than abnormality of only one of these variables. Mitral anular motion is a linear measure in the long-axis dimension.[99] Whereas SF is measured from an M-mode recording in the short-axis dimension, mitral anular motion is measured from an M-mode recording with a cursor placed parallel to the long-axis of the ventricle in a left apical view. This allows assessment of shortening of the ventricle in an apicobasilar direction, which is not assessed by conventional M-mode linear estimates.

AREA INDICES

Area-based measurements of systolic function include left ventricular shortening area. This measurement is derived from the 2DE short-axis image of the left ventricle and is the percentage reduction in LV cross-sectional area in systole. It has advantages over SF in that it represents wall motion over the entire short-axis area and is therefore less sensitive to asynchronous wall motion. Nevertheless, it does not address shortening in the apicobasilar direction. Preliminary data from our laboratory suggest that values between 50 and 72 per cent are normal in dogs.

VOLUMETRIC INDICES

Volume-based measurements of systolic function have generally been based on M-mode minor-axis measurements and used variations of the diameter-cubed formula or Teichholz formula (see Table 115–12).[47, 100] As discussed earlier, there are inherent limitations in using volume estimates based on a single minor-axis dimension, and there are many reports of the inferiority of M-mode volume estimates for dogs to those obtained with 2DE formulas.[48, 101] Many different 2DE formulas have been used for calculation of LV volumes, although it is generally acknowledged that calculations based on a modified Simpson's rule are likely to be the most accurate and the least affected by abnormal chamber geometry.[49] Although left apical views are usually used for 2DE volume measurements in humans, these views often result in a truncated view of the apex in dogs.[94] Right parasternal long-axis views have been validated for LV volume estimation in dogs.[51, 52] Despite the inclusion of measurement software to allow 2DE volume calculations in most current echocardiography machines, there are still few reports of normal canine 2DE volume measurements.[44] Normal values for ejection fraction obtained using an M-mode–derived diameter have been reported for dogs,[62, 102, 103] although this is reported less as an index of systolic function than in the human literature. Ejection fractions calculated from 2DE take into account asynchronous wall motion as well as shortening in an apicobasilar direction and should be much more reliable than calculations based on M-mode studies.

An end-systolic volume index calculated from M-mode studies has been used to identify myocardial failure in dogs with MR.[104] Care should be taken in extrapolating from values used in human studies, as in our experience the normal values are different for dogs of different sizes, even though the measurement is indexed to body surface area.

SYSTOLIC TIME INTERVALS

Systolic time intervals include the pre-ejection period (PEP; onset of the QRS to onset of ejection) and the ejection period. Systolic time intervals can be recorded with either M-mode or Doppler echocardiography.[105–107] Although systolic time intervals are also influenced by loading conditions, they provide an alternative means of assessing global systolic function. Mean velocity of circumferential fiber shortening is an extension of SF and is calculated by dividing the SF by the LV ejection time. It is therefore subject to many of the same limitations as the SF. PEP and LV ejection time (LVET) are affected by heart rate and loading conditions, although the ratio (PEP/LVET) may be less heart rate independent.[105] As myocardial dysfunction tends to increase PEP and decrease LVET, their ratio may be more sensitive than either variable alone. RV systolic time intervals may be applicable to the assessment of pulmonary hypertension.[19]

BLOOD FLOW INDICES

A variety of quantitative Doppler echocardiographic variables can be used to assess aortic flow indices. The area under the aortic or pulmonic flow signal (the velocity-time integral) is directly related to stroke volume, which can be calculated by multiplying the velocity-time integral by the cross-sectional area of the vessel. Measurement of stroke volume and cardiac output has been related to invasive techniques such as thermodilution in dogs. Correlations between traditional invasive indices (such as the rate of LV pressure rise: LV dP/dt) have been shown with other Doppler variables, such as aortic peak acceleration (dV/dt_{max}) and peak aortic velocity.[108] Although these variables may be useful in assessing acute changes in LV function, they are less useful in documenting chronic changes and have little role in guiding cardiac therapy. Peak aortic velocity has been found to be abnormal in dogs with dilated cardiomyopathy,[106] but generally myocardial dysfunction must be severe for blood flow indices to be affected. Neurohormonal activation and Starling's law of the heart generally help to maintain cardiac output in the failing heart until these compensatory mechanisms are overcome, so a detectable fall in cardiac output is a late change in most clinical cases with myocardial failure, although stroke volume index is more likely to decrease. The rate of acceleration (dV/dt) of MR has shown a more direct relationship with LV contractility or at least with LV dP/dt.[109]

VENTRICULAR DIASTOLIC FUNCTION

Diastolic function is more complex than systolic function, and there is no single index of diastolic function that can incorporate all the factors that contribute to ventricular filling. These factors include active ventricular relaxation, ventricular fiber restoring forces, myocardial and chamber stiffness, pericardial restraint, RV-LV interaction, and left atrial contractility and compliance. Interplay among these factors is dynamic and complex. For example, chamber stiffness increases as the ventricle fills, so that ventricular compliance changes throughout the cardiac cycle. In addition, preload, afterload, and systolic function influence ventricular filling. Although invasive indices of diastolic function have been used to assess diastolic function and ventricular relaxation in particular (peak negative dP/dt, time constant of isovolumic

pressure decline), echocardiography has assumed increasing importance as a noninvasive means of evaluating overall diastolic performance (Table 115–14). Conditions such as feline hypertrophic cardiomyopathy may lead to congestive heart failure as a result of primary diastolic dysfunction (see Chapter 117), and echocardiography can offer functional information in addition to a simple measure of LV wall thickness. Diastolic abnormalities may also be present in other conditions such as dilated cardiomyopathy, in which the functional disturbances are overshadowed by the more obviously recognized systolic dysfunction.

PEAK RATE OF LEFT VENTRICULAR WALL THINNING

The rate of wall thinning is related to the rate of ventricular relaxation and can be obtained by digitizing M-mode recordings.[110] This must often be carried out off-line, so it has not found much favor.

ISOVOLUMIC RELAXATION TIME

The isovolumic relaxation time is the time from aortic valve closure to mitral valve opening. It can be recorded with an M-mode study of the mitral valve and aortic valve concurrently or with a mitral valve M-mode study and a phonocardiogram. It can also be recorded using spectral Doppler, with a large sample volume placed to record mitral inflow and aortic outflow simultaneously.[27, 111] It is affected by ventricular relaxation and aortic end-systolic pressure, as well as by intrinsic myocardial factors and atrial loading conditions. Doppler-derived measures of isovolumetric relaxation time have been reported in healthy, unsedated cats,[111] with a mean reported value of 55.4 ± 13.2 ms.

MITRAL INFLOW PATTERNS

Mitral inflow is determined by the left atrial–left ventricular pressure gradient, which in turn is subject to the whole array of forces influencing ventricular filling described earlier. The normal pattern of mitral inflow consists of early rapid filling (mitral E wave), a period of little or no transmitral flow (diastasis), and then another wave of filling after atrial contraction (mitral A wave). In a normal ventricle under normal loading conditions and at low heart rates, most filling occurs early in diastole, resulting in a large E wave and smaller A wave.[113] When ventricular relaxation is impaired, the early left atrial–left ventricular pressure gradient is reduced so that the early filling component is diminished (and a greater proportion of total filling occurs after atrial contraction). This results in a reduced mitral E/A ratio. Conversely, factors increasing chamber stiffness cause the ventricular pressure to rise disproportionately as the ventricle fills, thus reducing the left atrial–left ventricular pressure gradient in late diastole. This reduces the proportion of filling in late diastole and increases the mitral E/A ratio. This has been termed "restrictive" physiology. It should be noted that an increased mitral E/A ratio is also seen with enhanced relaxation (increased suction forces early in diastole) and with elevated mean atrial pressures, both of which increase the left atrial–left ventricular pressure gradient early in diastole. An apparently normal (or pseudonormal) mitral E/A ratio may be seen when impaired relaxation coexists with elevated atrial pressures or increased chamber stiffness,

TABLE 115–12. ECHOCARDIOGRAPHIC MEASURES OF VENTRICULAR SYSTOLIC FUNCTION

METHOD	ECHO MODE(S) USED	MEASUREMENTS REQUIRED	CALCULATION	EFFECT OF LV FAILURE	COMMENTS
LV shortening fraction (SF%)	M-mode at chordal level	LV diameter in diastole (LVDd); LV diameter in systole (LVDs)	$\dfrac{\text{LVDd} - \text{LVDs}}{\text{LVDd}} \times 100$	↓	Contractility, preload, and afterload dependent; Affected by asynchronous wall motion; Measures only shortening in minor-axis dimension
LV free wall thickening (%FWth)	M-mode at chordal level	LV free wall thickness in diastole (LVFWd); LV free wall thickness in systole (LVFWs)	$\dfrac{\text{LVFWs} - \text{LVFWd}}{\text{LVFWd}} \times 100$	↓	Contractility, preload, and afterload dependent; Can be used in presence of paradoxical septal motion; Less reproducible than SF%
Amplitude of LV free wall motion (FWamp)	M-mode at chordal level	Distance between endocardial surface of LV free wall in diastole and systole	—	↓	Contractility, preload, and afterload dependent; Few advantages over SF% or %FWth; Limited normal reference values
Mitral valve E-point to septal separation (EPSS)	M-mode at mitral valve level	Distance between maximum opening of mitral valve in early diastole (E-point) and endocardial surface of interventricular septum	—	↑	Contractility, preload, afterload dependent; Not valid in mitral stenosis
Velocity of circumferential fiber shortening	M-mode at chordal level + (a) M-mode at aortic valve level OR (b) Doppler aortic flow signal	LVDd, LVDs + (a) Time from aortic valve opening to aortic valve closure (LVET) (b) Duration of aortic flow signal (LVET)	$\dfrac{(\text{LVDd} - \text{LVDs})}{(\text{LVDd} \times \text{LVET})} = \dfrac{\text{SF\%}}{\text{LVET}}$ To normalize for heart rate: $\dfrac{(\text{LVDd} - \text{LVDs}) \times 100}{(\text{LVDd} \times \text{LVET} \times \text{HR})}$ OR Rate-corrected Vcf$_c$: Vcf $\times \sqrt{\text{preceding RR interval}}$ on ECG	↓	Contractility, afterload, and heart rate dependent; Reflects global LV function better than SF% alone; Can be corrected for heart rate
Ratio of pre-ejection period to LV ejection time (PEP/LVET)	(a) M-mode at aortic valve level OR (b) Doppler aortic flow signal	PEP: (a) Time from onset of QRS on ECG to opening of aortic valve (b) Time from onset of QRS on ECG to start of aortic flow LVET: (a) Time from aortic valve opening to aortic valve closure (b) Duration of aortic flow signal	$\dfrac{\text{PEP}}{\text{LVET}}$	↑	Contractility, preload, and afterload dependent; More sensitive than PEP or LVET alone; ↑ with mitral regurgitation; ↓ with aortic stenosis
LV shortening area (%SA)	2DE right parasternal short axis	2DE short-axis area in diastole (LVAd) and systole (LVAs)	$\dfrac{\text{LVAd} - \text{LVAs}}{\text{LVAd}} \times 100$	↓	Contractility, preload, and afterload dependent; Less affected by asynchronous wall motion than SF%

Parameter	Method/View	Measurements	Formula	Change	Comments
End-systolic volume index (ESVI)	(a) M-mode at chordal level OR (b) 2DE right parasternal long axis view ± 2DE short axis view at chordal level (b) is preferred	(a) LVDs (b) (i) LV chamber area in systole + LV long-axis length in systole OR (ii) LV long-axis length in systole + LV short-axis area in systole	$ESVI = \dfrac{ESV}{BSA}$ ESV Cube formula $= (LVDs)^3$ $Teichholz = \dfrac{7 \times (LVDs)^3}{2.4 + LVDs}$ Short-axis area-length $= \dfrac{5AL}{6}$ Long-axis area-length $= \dfrac{8A^2}{3\pi L}$ Modified Simpson's $= \dfrac{\pi}{4} \sum\limits_{i=1}^{20} \dfrac{A^2 L}{20}$	↑	Contractility, preload, and afterload dependent Measurements based on M-mode (cube, Teichholz formulas) are relatively inaccurate 2DE measurements that include LV length preferred Lack of normal reference values—may differ for dogs of different size, as well as with formula used
LV ejection fraction (EF%)	(a) M-mode at chordal level OR (b) 2DE right parasternal long-axis view ± 2DE short-axis view at chordal level (b) is preferred	(a) LVDd, LVDs (b) (i) LV chamber area in systole and diastole + LV long-axis length in systole and diastole OR (ii) LV long-axis length in systole and diastole + LV short-axis area in systole and diastole	$EF\% = \dfrac{EDV-ESV}{EDV} \times 100$ For LV volumes, see ESVI above	→	Traditional estimate of LV global systolic function Contractility, preload, and afterload dependent Measurements based on M-mode (cube, Teichholz formulas) are relatively inaccurate 2DE measurements that include LV length are preferred Lack of normal reference values— may differ according to formula used
Mitral annular motion (MAM)	M-mode from left apical view, with cursor through mitral annulus	Distance between mitral annulus in systole and diastole		→	Contractility, preload, and afterload dependent Reflects shortening in the long-axis dimension, which is not measured with SF%
Aortic blood flow acceleration (dV/dt)	Doppler aortic blood flow	Acceleration of aortic spectral signal	—	→	Contractility, preload, afterload, and heart rate dependent Relatively insensitive marker of myocardial failure
Cardiac output (CO)	PW Doppler aortic blood flow at sinotubular junction + 2DE image of aorta	Velocity time integral of aortic spectral signal (VTI) + diameter of aorta at sinotubular junction (d) + heart rate (HR)	Stroke volume (SV) $= VTI \times (d/2)^2 \times \pi$ $CO = SV \times HR$	↓ (unless compensated)	Contractility, preload, afterload, and heart rate dependent Requires accurate measurement of aortic diameter Normal output often maintained in chronic disease
LV dP/dt	CW Doppler of mitral regurgitation flow signal	Time (dt) taken for mitral regurgitation blood flow signal to accelerate from 1 to 3 m/s	$\dfrac{dP}{dt} = \dfrac{32\ mmHg}{dt\ (seconds)}$	→	Less affected by preload and afterload than most systolic indices Requires mitral regurgitation signal

2DE = two-dimensional echocardiography; LV = left ventricle; L = LV length; A = LV area; HR = heart rate; ESV = LV end-systolic volume; EDV = LV end-diastolic volume; dP/dt = rate of rise of LV pressure.

TABLE 115–13. SYSTOLIC ECHOCARDIOGRAPHIC INDICES IN CONSCIOUS DOGS*

BREED	N	MEAN BODY WEIGHT (kg)	SF (%)	FWth (%)	FWamp (mm)	EPSS (mm)	VcF (circs/s)	PEP/LVET	ESVI (mL/m²)	EF (%)
Beagles[102]	50	8.9	40 22–58	39	—	—	—	—	—	77 57–97
Mixed[141]	27	11.1	30.1 15.5–45.9	56 17.2–94.8	—	6.4 0.1–12.8	1.96 1.2–2.8	—	—	—
Mixed[146]	16	17.6	30.8	—	—	—	—	—	27	66.6 55.6–77.6
Mixed[44]	17	18.5	25 15–35	31 7–55	—	—	—	—	—	50 34–66
English pointers[61]	16	19.2	35.5 27.5–43.5	62	—	—	—	—	—	—
Mixed[40]	20	19.3	36.3 33.6–38.9	61.7 55.2–68.3	—	—	2.07 1.58–2.79	—	—	—
Mixed[22]	14	23	31 23–39	—	—	—	1.56†,‡ 0.86–2.26	0.35†,‡ 0.25–0.45	—	58† 44–72
Mixed[42]	40	24	39 27–51	—	10 4–16	—	—	—	—	—
Mixed[147]	31	24	—	36 16–56	—	—	—	—	—	—
Greyhounds[97]	16	26.6	25.3 12.7–37.9	26.5	—	—	—	—	—	49.9 34.5–65.3
Greyhounds[139]	11	29.1	28.8 20.4–37.2	—	—	—	1.6 1.02–2.18	0.38 0.26–0.5	—	—
Dobermans[98]	23	—	21.7 14.4–29	42.4 11.7–73.1	6.5 4–9	—	1.27	0.44 0.41–0.46	—	—
Dobermans[41]	21	36	34.2 30.5–37.8	32.1 25.9–38.3	—	4.8 1.8–7.8	2.07 1.75–2.39	0.41	—	—
Spanish mastiffs[140]	12	52.4	39.2	—	—	6.7 6.1–7.3	—	—	—	—
Newfoundlands[62]	27	61	30 22–37	31 11–40	—	6 3–14	1.7 1.1–2.5	—	38 22–56	57 44–66
Great Danes[62]	15	62	25 18–36	18 –9–29	—	8 5–12	1.7 1.0–2.3	—	42 26–55	48 33–65
Irish wolfhounds[62]	20	68.5	28 20–34	24 10–38	—	7 1–10	1.7 1.0–2.2	—	33 26–69	54 38–61

*All values expressed as mean ± 2 standard deviations or (range). Unless otherwise stated, volumes and ejection fractions are obtained from M-mode and the cube or Teichholz formula.
†Volumes measured from 2DE.
‡Systolic time intervals obtained from Doppler studies.
SF = left ventricular shortening fraction; FWth = left ventricular free wall thickening; FWamp = amplitude of left ventricular free wall motion; EPSS = mitral valve E-point to septal separation; Vcf = velocity of circumferential fiber shortening; PEP/ET = ratio of pre-ejection period to left ventricular ejection time; ESVI = end-systolic volume index; EF = left ventricular ejection fraction.

TABLE 115–14. ECHOCARDIOGRAPHIC MEASURES OF DIASTOLIC FUNCTION

METHOD	ECHO MODE(S) USED	MEASUREMENTS REQUIRED	COMMENTS
Rate of LV wall thinning	M-mode at chordal level	Digitized rate of wall thinning	Most machines lack digitizing software Affected by LV relaxation, LA pressures, preload, afterload, contractility, and heart rate
Isovolumic relaxation time	(a) M-mode at aortic valve with concurrent mitral valve M-mode (b) M-mode at mitral valve level with concurrent phonocardiogram (c) Spectral Doppler signals of aortic flow and concurrent mitral inflow	(a) Time from aortic valve closure to mitral valve opening (b) Time from S2 on phonocardiogram to mitral valve opening on M-mode (c) Time from end of aortic flow signal (or valve closure noise) to onset of mitral E wave	Influenced by LV relaxation, LA filling pressures, aortic end-systolic pressure Normal 0.06 second $\pm$ 0.02[22] (dogs) Normal 0.055 second $\pm$ 0.013[109] (cats)
Mitral E/A ratio	Spectral Doppler with sample volume at tips of mitral valve leaflets	Maximum velocity of early mitral filling (E) wave, maximum velocity of mitral filling after atrial contraction (A wave)	Cannot use with fused E and A waves (i.e., at fast heart rates) Sensitive to sample volume position Influenced by filling pressures, rate of LV relaxation, LV compliance, and heart rate
Mitral E deceleration time	Spectral Doppler with sample volume at tips of mitral valve leaflets	Time from maximum mitral E wave velocity to end of mitral E wave	Cannot use with fused E and A waves Influenced by filling pressures, rate of LV relaxation, LV compliance, and heart rate ↓ with vigorous relaxation or ↓ chamber compliance Normal 0.08 second $\pm$ 0.02[22]
Pulmonary venous flow systolic fraction	Spectral Doppler with sample volume in right or left cranial lobar pulmonary vein	$$\frac{\text{Systolic velocity-time integral (VTI)} \times 100}{\text{Systolic VTI} + \text{diastolic VTI}}$$	↓ with ↑ filling pressures (or in vigorous normal filling) Normal 42.3% $\pm$ 9.8[22]
Mitral A wave duration (A_{dur})/ pulmonary venous flow atrial reversal duration (AR_{dur})	Spectral Doppler of mitral inflow at mitral inflow at mitral anulus and in right or left cranial lobar pulmonary vein	$$\frac{A_{dur}}{AR_{dur}}$$	↓ ratio suggests ↑ LV end-diastolic pressure Normal ratio > 1.0[22]
Doppler tissue imaging of LV free wall ($LVFW_{DTI}$)	Pulsed-wave Doppler tissue imaging (DTI) with sample volume in LV free wall (short-axis view at papillary muscle level)	Peak diastolic velocity of LV free wall (PDV)	Limited availability and few normal reference values reported Influenced by relaxation and loading conditions Normal cats PDV = 12.1 $\pm$ 2.3 cm/s (Gavaghan et al, 1998)

LA = left atrial; PW = pulsed wave.

thus reducing the usefulness of mitral E/A ratios.[114] Mitral E/A ratios are also sensitive to sample volume position, decreasing as the sample volume is moved from the leaflet tips to the mitral anulus. Further limitations include the dependence on heart rate—at high heart rates, diastasis is obliterated and the E and A waves frequently fuse. This is commonly the case with cats. The absence of A waves in arrhythmias such as atrial fibrillation also limits the use of this index.

The mitral deceleration time is another transmitral flow index that has been used to assess ventricular filling forces. Rapid mitral deceleration may be a sensitive predictor of elevated pulmonary capillary wedge pressures,[115] as well a poor prognostic sign in human patients with dilated cardiomyopathy.

PULMONARY VENOUS FLOW

Including the assessment of pulmonary venous flow may circumvent some of the problems associated with transmitral flow analysis. A pulsed-wave sample volume is placed in the right or left pulmonary vein. Pulmonary venous flow normally consists of a forward flow wave in diastole and a forward flow wave in systole (sometimes with two components), with a reverse flow wave after atrial contraction.[22, 116] In human cardiology there has been a tendency to move away from the goal of assessing "diastolic function" with Doppler echocardiography in favor of obtaining some insight into filling pressures. Studies in human patients have shown that pulmonary venous flow analysis can yield information that correlates with mean left atrial and LV end-diastolic pressures.[1-7]

COLOR M-MODE

Studies have shown that the rate of LV filling can be assessed with color M-mode analysis.[35, 118] The M-mode cursor is placed across the mitral anulus in a left apical view, parallel to the direction of LV filling. The slope of the early filling flow pattern appears to be related to the rate of LV relaxation.

DOPPLER TISSUE IMAGING

Doppler tissue imaging is a relatively new echocardiographic mode that may prove useful in the assessment of diastolic function. Doppler tissue imaging is used to interrogate the velocity and direction of the LV wall or mitral valve anulus instead of the movement and direction of blood flow, as in conventional Doppler echocardiography.

VALVULAR FUNCTION

GENERAL APPROACH TO ASSESSING VALVULAR FUNCTION

Valvular regurgitation and stenosis can be recognized using a number of echocardiographic modalities. The simplest approach combines information from the clinical examination, including auscultation of a murmur, with 2D and M-mode imaging of the cardiac valves. This approach is often sufficient to generate a reliable diagnosis when the morphologic lesions are clear and are congruous with the clinical findings. Analysis of cardiac chamber sizes by 2D and M-mode echocardiography provides additional insight into the hemodynamic significance of the flow disturbance (see earlier)

A more sensitive method for evaluation of valvular function involves interrogation of the valves using Doppler methods.[5, 7, 10, 39] (Fig. 115–16; see Figs. 115–8, 115–9, 115–11, and 115–13). The main PW Doppler and CDI finding of valvular dysfunction is either increased flow velocity or abnormal direction of transvalvular flow. These flow disturbances should be observed consistently during a particular phase of the cardiac cycle. In most instances, abnormal transvalvular flow recorded by PW Doppler produces signal aliasing and a broadly disturbed velocity band. Abnormal transvalvular flow is coded in CDI by signal aliasing and activation of turbulence algorithms.[38] A number of imaging planes may be required for accurate identification of the origin and extent of the abnormal flow event. The examiner should quantify the velocity profile and pressure gradient with CW (or high pulse rate repetition) Doppler, aiming to record velocity spectra with well-defined envelopes and clear peak velocities. It is also crucial to time the duration of the event relative to the ECG and cardiac cycle using either spectral Doppler or color M-mode techniques. The examiner must also remember that Doppler displays of blood flow indicate RBC direction and velocity, as predicted by instantaneous pressure gradients, not absolute volumetric flow.

Doppler studies are sensitive to detection of abnormal flow; however, estimating the severity of valvular regurgitation is far more difficult. Commonly used methods for semiquantitation of regurgitation include mapping the length or area of the regurgitant jet using PW Doppler or CDI, evaluating the signal strength of the PW regurgitant signal, and measuring the area of the regurgitation at the valve orifice. The last approach, although difficult, is accurate provided orthogonal planes are evaluated and the true regurgitant orifice can be measured. Overall signal strength depends in part on instrumentation factors. Regurgitant flow patterns in the receiving chamber are influenced strongly by forces that

are better explained by fluid mechanics; these include driving pressure, orifice size and shape, concurrent flow, and characteristics of the receiving chamber.[4, 39] For a simple analogy, consider a garden hose nozzle that can be adjusted to control flow rate and spray area. One can adjust the nozzle orifice to produce a diffuse spray that covers a large area with a fine mist but actually involves little volumetric flow through the orifice. Conversely, a wide orifice conducts a large volume of fluid that is confined to a relatively small area. For similar reasons, analyzing the receiving chamber flow pattern in valvular regurgitation is fraught with difficulties.

Doppler diagnosis of valvular and outflow tract stenosis is also quite sensitive. Rapid acceleration, increased peak velocity, and flow disturbances distal to the obstruction are typical findings.[3] Identifying and quantifying the severity of moderate to severe valvular stenosis is relatively straightforward; however, precise identification of mild stenosis can be problematic. One must understand first that normal transvalvular flows can alias and activate turbulence mapping in CDI; thus, spectral Doppler studies must be used to confirm an abnormality recorded by color-coded techniques. Next, it should be appreciated that the absolute limit of normal flow velocity in various breeds under different hemodynamic conditions is unresolved. In our experience, most ejection murmurs are associated with peak flow velocities that exceed 1.6 to 1.7 m/s and most studies suggest that values exceeding this range represent abnormal flow (see Tables 115–3 and 115–4). However, these limits can be exceeded in normal dogs subjected to sympathetic stimulation or in situations in which stroke volume is increased. Finally, one must consider other pitfalls of Doppler diagnosis. Some of these are summarized in Table 115–15 and explained in the following sections.

AORTIC STENOSIS

Subvalvular AS is the most common congenital heart defect of dogs. Anatomic lesions are evident in moderate to severe cases of AS (see Table 115–9) but may not be obvious in mild disease. Flow abnormalities that develop in this condition are best understood by considering the *continuity equation* and the *Bernoulli relationship*.[1–4, 13, 119, 120] The product of flow velocity and cross-sectional area is maintained across a stenotic zone (s) such that as the cross-sectional area (CSA) decreases abruptly from the normal, proximal flow region (p) there is an acceleration of flow across the narrowed zone:

$$\text{Velocity}_p \times \text{CSA}_p = \text{velocity}_s \times \text{CSA}_s \text{ (the continuity relationship)}$$

This acceleration of flow is generated in the hypertrophied ventricle by an increased ventricular systolic pressure that increases the kinetic energy of RBCs as they are propelled across the stenosis. Immediately distal to the obstruction (vena contracta), flow reaches a peak velocity that is directly proportional to the pressure gradient across the stenosis (as defined by the Bernoulli relationship). Distal to the obstruction there is flow disturbance characterized by loss of kinetic energy in the form of heat and friction.

PW Doppler studies are ideal for detecting the proximal acceleration of flow and the flow disturbance distal to the stenosis. In moderate to severe AS, the peak velocity signal is generally aliased requiring CW Doppler (or techniques

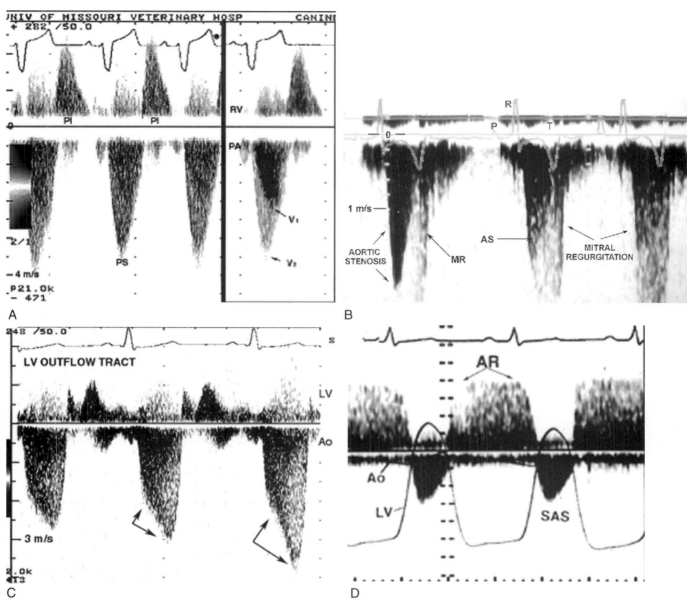

Figure 115–16. *A,* Continuous-wave recording from a dog with congenital pulmonary stenosis (PS) and concurrent dynamic ventricular outflow obstruction caused by marked right ventricular hypertrophy. A high-velocity systolic signal is recorded indicating PS. There is also a strong signal of pulmonary insufficiency (PI). The velocity spectra on the right have been postprocessed to reveal the relative contributions of proximal dynamic obstruction (V_1) to the velocity peak, V_2, which is related to flow across the stenotic pulmonic valve. In this case, a simplified Bernoulli equation would not be adequate to assess the severity of valvar stenosis (see text for details). *B,* Contamination of an aortic stenosis (AS) flow signal by a concurrent jet of mitral regurgitation (MR) in a dog with mild subvalvular AS. The three beats demonstrate progressive migration of the cursor from the left ventricular outflow tract to the mitral valve orifice. Note that the peak velocity of the MR jet on the right is much greater. The beat in the middle could be easily mistaken for a high-velocity jet of AS, although the width of turbulent signal is probably too long to represent an ejection phenomenon. (Study performed with Linda B. Lehmkuhl, DVM.) *C,* Continuous-wave Doppler recording obtained from the left apical position of a pup with both fixed and dynamic subvalvular aortic stenosis. Peak velocities increase across the three beats, exceeding 3 m/s. Note the typical "dagger" shape of the velocity spectra *(arrows)* related to the development of an early to midsystolic obstruction and pressure gradient from left ventricle to aorta as the dog becomes excited *(arrows).* The peak velocity when the dog was quiet and after β-adrenergic blockade was less than 2 m/s. *D,* Continuous-wave Doppler recording from the subcostal position of a dog with aortic stenosis and aortic regurgitation (AR). There is a well-defined, high-velocity, envelope of AR *(arrows),* indicating good alignment to both jets. The flat appearance of the AR jet indicates maintenance of the diastolic pressure gradient from aortia to left ventricle and argues against severe AR. Left ventricular pressure and aortic pressure tracings (obscured by the Doppler signal) are also recorded. (Study performed with Linda B. Lehmkuhl DVM.)

with high pulse repetition frequency) to record faithfully the high velocity of the vena contracta (see Figs. 115–11 and 115–16*B*). By using the simplified Bernoulli equation (pressure gradient = $V^2 \times 4$, where V is velocity in m/s), one can accurately predict the peak and the mean pressure gradients in mmHg.[121] Such gradients are considered key determinants of severity. For example, a peak velocity of 4 m/s would indicate a peak gradient of 64 mmHg ($4^2 \times 4$) or an obstruction of "moderate" severity. Peak gradients greater than 75 to 100 mmHg are generally considered "severe." The examiner should also obtain recordings in the subcostal position because this provides the best alignment

TABLE 115–15. COMMON SOURCES OF ERROR IN DOPPLER ECHOCARDIOGRAPHIC STUDIES

PITFALL	POSSIBLE CONSEQUENCE
Instrumentation and examination errors	
Failure to use lower frequency transducer crystals for optimal Doppler sensitivity	Underestimation of abnormal flow signal strength and spatial resolution
Not setting power, gain, and compression appropriately	Inability to visualize flow signals in spectral display
	Creation of color flow artifacts
Excess pulse-wave Doppler gain	Expansion and elongation of the flow "envelope" causing overestimation of velocity and lesion severity
Excessive color flow Doppler gain	Expansion of the color signal causing overestimation of flow patterns and color "bleeding" into areas without flow
Excessive tissue gain during color flow studies	Pixel cannot be occupied by color coding; poor color flow characterization
Inadequate filtering of low velocity, strong reflectors (including cardiac valves, chamber walls, and lungs)	Spectral and color flow artifacts
	False color Doppler diagnosis of valvular regurgitation
Excessive filtering of low velocity signals	Failure to identify low-velocity flow patterns or normal signals interrogated at a wide angle
Excessive angle of interrogation (greater than 20 degrees to flow)	Underestimation of maximum velocity
	Increased spectral dispersion in the PW Doppler mode
Activating angle correction features for evaluation of cardiac flow disturbances	Overestimation of true velocity and lesion severity
Failure to use the visual and audio displays to obtain optimal Doppler signals	Inability to record peak velocities in the azimuthal plane
Lack of familiarity with cardiac disorders	Not understanding the issues that must be addressed during the echocardiographic and Doppler study; incomplete assessment
	Missed flow disturbance(s)
Failure to obtain appropriate and complementary images of the heart for Doppler studies	
Failure to use appropriate transducer placement sites (e.g., subcostal position to measure aortic velocity; left apex to record mitral or tricuspid regurgitation) and sufficient tomographic planes	Underestimation of maximal velocity or spatial distribution
Failure to recognize the simultaneous interrogation of multiple jets during CW Doppler studies (e.g., crossing subaortic stenosis and mitral regurgitation)	Erroneous conclusions about lesion severity; overestimating the severity of valvular stenosis
Failure to time flow events, relative to the ECG, with spectral Doppler tracings or through color M-code recordings	Duration of flow events is uncertain; normal backflow or diastolic regurgitation may be misinterpreted
Inability to maintain the PW Doppler sample volume or CW Doppler line of interrogation within the abnormal flow throughout its duration	Limits the faithful recording of the peak Doppler spectrum during the cardiac cycle
Errors of Interpretation	
Assuming one can reliably image all minor lesions or definitively identify the source of all murmurs using Doppler methods	Overinterpretation of normal variation or trivial lesions
	False-positive diagnoses
Failure to appreciate normal variation	Misdiagnosis of normal backflow, physiologic regurgitation, or diastolic regurgitation as clinically significant valve regurgitation
Lack of familiarity with cardiac lesions	Misdiagnoses or incomplete assessment
Over-reliance on qualitative information such as spectral dispersion in pulsed wave studies, "acceleration" of flow, or "turbulence" maps in color coded studies	Misdiagnoses such as "aortic stenosis"
Overinterpreting color "bleeding"	False-positive diagnosis, including septal defects and aorticopulmonary communications
Relying on a single frame of 2D-color information or the position of a color frame relative to the ECG (without reviewing complementary spectral Doppler or color M-mode studies)	Inadequate temporal resolution of events
	Misdiagnosis of early systolic backflow as significant regurgitation
Failure to appreciate the effects of cardiac output and stroke volume on Doppler derived velocities and estimated pressure gradients	False-positive diagnosis of valvular stenosis
	Over- or underestimation of lesion severity
Quantifying valvular regurgitation from only color Doppler studies	Analysis of receiving chamber flow patterns may lead to misinterpretation of severity (see text)

PW = pulsed wave; CW = continuous wave; ECG = electrocardiogram; 2D = two-dimensional.

with flow in most cases.[122] Experience with subvalvular AS has indicated that general anesthesia depresses the pressure gradient by approximately 50 per cent; however, when both pressure gradients are recorded simultaneously there is little difference between the methods.[121] Variable stroke volume also affects the gradient. An important pitfall of accurate diagnosis arises in the presence of AS with concurrent MR. In this situation, both jets may be crossed by the CW cursor, leading to contamination of the AS jet and potential overestimation of the pressure gradient (as the LV-to-atrial gradient is always much higher than the ventricular-to-aortic gradient).

The CDI study in AS demonstrates acceleration of flow as blood is propelled at increasing velocities toward and across the stenosis.[5, 6, 13, 123] The velocity signal is aliased more proximal to the valve than is normal, but this is not sufficient evidence to make a diagnosis. Turbulent signals develop at the obstruction and continue into the great vessel, where a prominent post-stenotic flow disturbance is recorded. Concurrent semilunar valve incompetence is almost always present. Each of these findings should be supported by spectral Doppler studies.

Although the diagnosis of moderate to severe AS is straightforward, difficulties are encountered in the Doppler diagnosis of mild AS. Findings such as "mild spectral disturbance" or acceleration of peak flow across the ventricular outlet are relatively subjective, and in our experience 2D imaging lesions are not consistently evident in mild or trivial obstruction. It is also normal for the peak velocity to increase (at least double) when velocities are mapped from the apical portion of the outflow tract to the ascending aorta. A fundamental problem is identification of the point at which flow in the LV outflow tract becomes abnormal. Peak velocities greater than 1.7 m/s, recorded by PW Doppler with the transducer placed near the left apex, fall outside the normal range established for most laboratories (see Tables 115–3 and 115–4) and are usually associated with an ejection murmur. However, this value may be too conservative for recordings made in the subcostal position, when the more sensitive CW transducer is used, when cardiac cycle lengths are variable (as with sinus arrhythmia), or when sympathetic tone is high. Thus, we view a peak PW Doppler ejection velocity between 1.7 and 2.0 m/s as raising suspicion of AS (or equivocal) in our laboratory and values greater than 2.0 m/s are considered abnormal. For dogs with marked variation related to sinus arrhythmia, it may be reasonable to average 5 to 10 aortic velocity signals. The presence of concurrent holodiastolic aortic regurgitation generally supports the diagnosis because it is not a usual finding in young, unanesthetized dogs. Establishing a diagnosis of mild AS by Doppler methods alone is difficult, if not impossible, in cases of uncorrected patent ductus arteriosus because outflow velocities are generally increased and often range between 2 and 2.8 m/s.

The special situation of dynamic LV outflow obstruction associated with hypertrophic obstructive cardiomyopathy, certain mitral valve malformations, or fixed subvalvular AS is characterized by high-velocity systolic flow in the LV outflow tract. The peak outflow tract velocity and flow disturbance are labile, increasing with heart rate and sympathetic drive but attenuated by beta-blockers. A typical "dagger-shaped" signal is expected, with sudden acceleration of velocity beginning in early to midsystole, coincident with the onset of dynamic ventricular obstruction (see Fig. 115–16C).[50]

PULMONIC STENOSIS

The diagnosis of pulmonic stenosis can generally be made by a combination of 2D imaging (see Table 115–9) and PW Doppler findings.[124, 125] The typical PW examination findings include marked acceleration of RBC velocity across the subpulmonic outflow tract, increased peak pulmonary artery velocity (greater than 1.6 m/s), flow disturbance distal to the valve, and often prominent pulmonary insufficiency. CDI also demonstrates many of these qualitative abnormalities. Peak ejection velocity can be used to quantify the severity of obstruction using the Bernoulli equation. Frequently, the velocity proximal to the valvular stenosis is substantially augmented because of dynamic, muscular outflow tract obstruction. This leads to a prominent, high-velocity subvalvular profile (V_1), superimposed on the increased peak velocity (V_2), on CW Doppler recordings (Fig. 115–16C). In such cases, the simplified Bernoulli equation cannot be used to estimate the pressure drop across the stenotic valve without additional consideration of the proximal obstruction and velocity (V_1). The equation used to calculate the valvular obstruction then becomes.[1]

$$\text{Transvalvular gradient} = 4(V_2^2 - V_1^2)$$

Inasmuch as pulmonary insufficiency is normal in dogs, this finding is not specific for a dysplastic valve, although subjectively, the signal strength of the pulmonary incompetence is usually greater than that associated with physiologic backflow. It is emphasized that Doppler gradients recorded in awake dogs can be substantially higher than those recorded by cardiac catheterization. This is explained by the negative impact of inhalation anesthetics on ventricular stroke volume.[125]

MITRAL REGURGITATION

MR is the most common and clinically important valvular disorder in small animals. Causes of MR include malformation, degeneration (endocardiosis), ruptured chordae tendineae, virtually any cause of LV dilation or hypertrophy, dynamic outflow obstruction with systolic anterior motion of the mitral valve, and bacterial endocarditis. The precise cause of MR can be identified from clinical findings and 2D imaging (see Tables 115–9 and 115–10). Overall ventricular systolic function depends on the underlying cause and whether or not systolic function is preserved.[104] In general, any Doppler evidence of MR is taken to indicate disease of the mitral apparatus. Exceptions are brief (less than 50 ms) periods of early systolic backflow, which are often seen in dogs; diastolic MR associated with bradyarrhythmias; and MR consequent to premature ventricular complexes. As most dogs develop some degree of progressive mitral degeneration with age, it is not uncommon to observed trivial MR, silent to auscultation, using Doppler studies. In cats, MR is generally caused by valve malformation or a form of myocardial disease that either distorts the mitral apparatus or causes systolic anterior motion of the mitral valve leading to valvular incompetence.

Examination with CDI is an effective method to screening for one or more jets of MR.[6, 8, 10, 126–128] If the color map zero baseline is shifted down (to produce a negative Nyquist limit of 18 to 30 cm/s), one can observe that abnormal regurgitant flow begins proximal to the valve. As the regurgitant mass accelerates toward the valve orifice, the signal is aliased and a roughly hemispheric zone of color change is identified. This proximal flow field is called the zone of flow convergence and can be likened to isovelocity shells of fluid accelerating toward the regurgitant orifice (see Fig. 115–13B). A number of studies have demonstrated the value of this proximal isovelocity field analysis for predicting the actual flow rate across the regurgitant orifice.[4, 129, 130] If the distance between the aliased signal and the orifice is measured, the radius of the hemisphere is known. The velocity at the hemisphere can be read from the Nyquist limit of the color bar. From these variables, the peak mitral regurgitant flow rate can be calculated.

The regurgitant flow field continues to narrow and forms a high-velocity jet that is coded as turbulent flow. The regurgitant jet(s) can be single or multiple, central or eccentric. The typical mitral regurgitant jet originates from the center of the mitral orifice, especially when the cause is LV dilatation. In primary valvular diseases—including mitral dysplasia, valvular endocardiosis, bacterial endocarditis, or rupture of the chordae tendineae—the regurgitant jet may be central or arise from eccentric locations. The regurgitant jet in cats with hypertrophic obstructive cardiomyopathy originates from the septally displaced anterior mitral leaflet and is usually directed parallel to the posterior (mural) leaflet.[50] Distal to the vena contracta, the flow field in the left atrium is quite variable but is typically displayed in CDI as turbulent. The jet may entrain venous return within the atrium, expanding the zone of turbulence. Alternatively, the regurgitant fluid mass may be directed eccentrically along the atrial walls or atrial septum. The duration of MR varies,

CV

although typical cases are holosystolic, preceding ejection and extending into isovolumetric relaxation. Protomesosystolic regurgitation is often observed in mild MR. Delayed onset of regurgitation is typical of MR caused by systolic anterior motion of the mitral valve.

PW and CW studies of MR are characterized by high-velocity, turbulent, systolic jets recorded at the valve orifice and within the left atrium (see Fig. 115–16B).[3, 4, 11] The audio channel concurrently emits a harsh, mixed-frequency, signal. The peak CW velocity of MR in normotensive animals should range between 5 and 6 m/s provided parallel alignment to flow is obtained during the examination. In cases of systemic hypertension, AS, or dynamic LV outflow obstruction, the peak velocity may exceed 6 m/s owing to elevated ventricular systolic pressure. Conversely, in severe dilated cardiomyopathy or with atrial fibrillation, both peak velocity and rate of velocity change are often lower, reflecting reductions in systolic pressure and vigor of LV contraction as well as a higher left atrial pressure that further reduces the gradient for regurgitant flow.

Doppler echocardiographic grading of MR severity as mild, moderate, or severe is not straightforward. Traditional methods of analysis have considered signal intensity and the jet width, length, and area as measures of severity.[1, 2, 127, 128] Assuming proper flow alignment and correct instrumentation, the finding of a narrow central jet that extends no more than half of the distance into the atrium would be typical of trivial or mild MR. In contrast, a wide-origin, regurgitant jet that extends to the pulmonary veins generally indicates moderate to severe MR. As discussed earlier, the area of jet "spray" can be misleading, and a wide distribution of turbulence need not indicate severe MR. Similarly, a long narrow jet may simply indicate a high ventricular driving pressure. The size of a jet that is carried along an atrial wall usually underestimates the severity of the condition producing it. These semiquantitative aspects are generalizations but are useful when combined with other imaging and clinical criteria of severity.

Transmitral flow during diastole should also be evaluated in patients with MR. Significant MR is often associated with increased diastolic filling velocities, with E waves often exceeding 1.25 m/s. In addition, abnormalities of diastolic ventricular function may be uncovered in cases of severe volume overload. It is also essential to distinguish diastolic mitral (and tricuspid) regurgitation from that which occurs during systole. Diastolic regurgitation is common with bradycardia and with arrhythmias and probably indicates small reversed pressure gradients during cardiac filling.[131, 132] Failure to time the events can lead to a false-positive diagnosis of clinically significant valvular regurgitation.

TRICUSPID REGURGITATION

The Doppler echocardiographic features of systolic and diastolic tricuspid regurgitation (TR) are similar to those of MR with a few exceptions (also see Tables 115–9 and 115–10). Foremost is the common occurrence of physiologic TR that is silent to auscultation in many healthy dogs (50 per cent or more).[12, 33, 34] The distinction between physiologic and pathologic regurgitation in dogs without tricuspid murmurs becomes an issue in breeds such as Labrador retrievers, which are prone to tricuspid valve malformations. Pathologic tricuspid regurgitant jets may stem from valve malformation, tricuspid endocardiosis, cardiomyopathy, RV hypertrophy, dirofilariasis, and pulmonary hypertension.

The diagnostic features of TR include detection of retrograde flow converging toward the tricuspid orifice, a high-velocity regurgitant jet across the valve, and a holosystolic flow disturbance in the right atrium. The right atrium is more complicated to map than the circular left atrium and orientation of TR jets is not consistent. Regurgitant velocity is affected by peak ventricular pressure and varies with arrhythmias and erratic cardiac filling (Fig. 115–17). The velocity of the regurgitant flow generally peaks at less than 2.6 m/s unless there is an elevation in RV pressure that forces RBCs into the atrium at a higher velocity. Usual causes of high-velocity TR (above 3 m/s) are pulmonary hypertension and pulmonic stenosis. Infrequently, florid TR is associated with an increased peak regurgitant velocity for uncertain reasons.

The CDI patterns observed in tricuspid valve regurgitation are qualitatively similar to those described before for MR. It is likely that TR jets are under-recognized because transthoracic imaging planes are less effective for examining the normal-sized right atrium and the tricuspid orifice is wider and more complicated to interrogate.

ATRIOVENTRICULAR VALVE STENOSIS

Stenoses of the atrioventricular valves are rare conditions in small animals, usually caused by valve malformation.[133–135] Echocardiographic findings are compatible with anatomic obstruction to ventricular diastolic filling. The salient features are imaging lesions of the valve with atrial dilatation (see Table 115–9), acceleration of the diastolic flow signal (flow convergence) at the atrial side of the atrioventricular orifice, increased filling velocities with high-velocity E and A waves, and prolongation of the pressure half-time (Fig. 115–18; see Fig. 115–13A). A classic CDI appearance of an aliased inflow core with a bright, turbulent rim likened to a candle flame has been observed in people and in animals. Some cases of atrioventricular valve stenosis are associated with very high-velocity A waves (often above 1.5 m/s), presumably representing atrial hypertrophy with a vigorous atrial contraction. Frequently there is concurrent evidence of valvular regurgitation. The pressure half time represents the time (seconds) needed for the peak Bernoulli-calculated transmitral pressure gradient to decrease by 50 per cent.[1, 3, 134] This prolonged decline in inflow velocity distinguishes mitral or tricuspid stenosis from other causes of high inflow velocity such as severe atrioventricular valve regurgitation or left-to-right shunts.

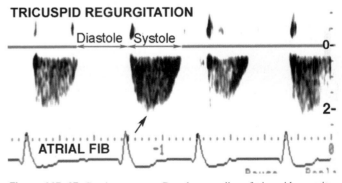

Figure 115–17. Continuous-wave Doppler recording of tricuspid regurgitation in a dog with atrial fibrillation and dilated cardiomyopathy. Note the beat-to-beat variation in signal. The peak velocity recorded (arrow) is about 2 m/s, predicting a normal right ventricular and pulmonary artery systolic pressure.

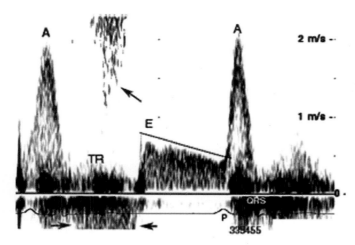

Figure 115–18. Continuous-wave Doppler recording from a dog with congenital tricuspid stenosis. The trans-tricuspid flow signals are increased in velocity. The deceleration time for flow after the E-point is markedly prolonged, with an abnormal pressure half-time (note slope of the line). There is marked elevation of the atrial signal (A) related to a vigorous atrial contraction and high instantaneous atrial-to-ventricular pressure gradient. A weak jet of tricuspid regurgitation (TR) is also recorded, with signal aliasing at the top of the recording (arrow).

AORTIC REGURGITATION

Aortic regurgitation is encountered in association with subvalvular aortic stenosis, in some cases of ventricular septal defect, and as a complication of bacterial endocarditis. Trivial aortic regurgitation, silent to auscultation, is often observed in older dogs during Doppler studies. Presumably this is a consequence of age-related valve thickening. Similarly, older cats may develop aortic regurgitation, possibly related to dilatation of the aorta (a common finding in aged cats).

Imaging lesions in aortic regurgitation vary (see Tables 115–10 and 115–11), but the Doppler diagnosis is straightforward. Placement of the sample volume below the closed aortic valve demonstrates a broad, turbulent, diastolic signal that ends abruptly with ventricular ejection (see Fig. 115–16D). The regurgitant jet is often quite eccentric and may mix with transmitral flow in the LV inlet while causing diastolic fluttering of the mitral valve on the M-mode study. Thin regurgitant jets that extend minimally from the valve orifice are rarely significant. Longer or wider jets may indicate significant aortic regurgitation; however, the length and area of the jet correlate poorly with regurgitant volume. In contrast, the width of the aortic regurgitant jet in two orthogonal planes or the cross-sectional area of the regurgitant orifice is related to regurgitant flow volume.[4] The orifice area may be appreciated in a short-axis image planes. Assuming the sample volume can be maintained within—and well aligned to—the regurgitant jet throughout diastole, the severity of aortic regurgitation can also be evaluated using CW Doppler by calculating the pressure drop at the beginning and end of diastole using the simplified Bernoulli equation. Severe aortic regurgitation increases LV diastolic pressure, reducing the pressure gradient and leading to a sudden drop in velocity of regurgitation (indicating near-equal aortic and ventricular end-diastolic pressures).

PULMONARY INSUFFICIENCY

Pulmonary insufficiency, silent to auscultation, is normal and is encountered in 80 per cent or more of normal dogs examined by PW Doppler (see Fig. 115–8B). Pulmonary insufficiency is rarely a clinical problem, even when severe or associated with pulmonary valve dysplasia, pulmonary hypertension, or patent ductus arteriosus. The main value of identifying pulmonary insufficiency during a Doppler examination is in the information gained about pulmonary arterial pressure.[3] Increasing pulmonary arterial pressure is associated with progressively higher regurgitant velocities as predicted by the Bernoulli relationship.

REFERENCES

1. Hatle LK, Angelsen B: Doppler Ultrasound in Cardiology, 2nd ed. Philadelphia, Lea & Febiger, 1985.
2. Feigenbaum H: Echocardiography, 5th ed. Philadelphia, Lea & Febiger, 1994.
3. Goldberg SJ, Allen HD, Marx GR, et al: Doppler Echocardiography, 2nd ed. Philadelphia, Lea & Febiger, 1988.
4. Weyman AE: Principles and Practice of Echocardiography, 1st ed. Philadelphia, Lea & Febiger. 1994.
5. Kienle RD, Thomas WP: Echocardiography. In Nyland TG, Mattoon JS (eds): Veterinary Diagnostic Ultrasound. Philadelphia, WB Saunders, 1995, pp 198–256.
6. Darke PGG, Bonagura JD, Kelly DF: Colour Atlas of Veterinary Cardiology. London, CV Mosby, 1996.
7. Boon JA: Manual of Echocardiography. Philadelphia, Lea & Febiger, 1998.
8. Kittleson MD, Kienle RD: Small Animal Cardiovascular Medicine. St. Louis, CV Mosby, 1998.
9. Loyer C, Thomas WP: Biplane transesophageal echocardiography in the dog—Technique, anatomy and imaging planes. Vet Radiol Ultrasound 36:212–226, 1995.
10. Bonagura JD, Miller MW: Veterinary echocardiography. Echocardiography 6:229–264, 1989.
11. Darke PGG: Doppler echocardiography. J Small Anim Pract 33:104–112, 1992.
12. Gaber CE: Doppler echocardiography. Probl Vet Med 3:479–499, 1991.
13. Moise NS: Doppler echocardiographic evaluation of congenital cardiac disease. J Vet Intern Med 3:195–207, 1989.
14. Brown DJ, Knight DH, King RR: Use of pulsed-wave Doppler echocardiography to determine aortic and pulmonary velocity and flow variables in clinically normal dogs. Am J Vet Res 52:543–550, 1991.
15. Darke PGG, Bonagura JD, Miller MW: Transducer orientation for Doppler echocardiography in dogs. J Small Anim Pract 34:2–8, 1993.
16. Domanjko A, Thomas WP: Pulsed wave Doppler echocardiography in normal cats (abstract). Proceedings of the 6th European Society of Veterinary Cardiology Meeting. Veldhoven Free Communications, 1996.
17. Yuill CDM, O'Grady MR: Doppler-derived velocity of blood flow across the cardiac valves in the normal dog. Can J Vet Res 55 185–192, 1991.
18. Gaber CE: Normal pulsed Doppler flow velocities in adult dogs (abstract). Proceedings of the Fifth Annual Veterinary Internal Medicine Forum, 1987, p 923
19. Uehara Y: An attempt to estimate the pulmonary-artery pressure in dogs by means of pulsed Doppler echocardiography. J Vet Med Sci 55:307–312, 1993.
20. Nishimura RA, Abel MD, Hatle LK, et al: Significance of Doppler indices of diastolic filling of the left ventricle: Comparison with invasive hemodynamics in a canine model Am Heart J 118:1248–1258, 1989.
21. Vandenberg BF, Kieso RA, Fox Eastham K, et al: Effect of age on diastolic left ventricular filling at rest and during inotropic stimulation and acute systemic hypertension: Experimental studies in conscious beagles. Am Heart J 120:73–81, 1990.
22. Schober KE, Fuentes VL, McEwan JD, French AT: Pulmonary venous flow characteristics as assessed by transthoracic pulsed Doppler-echocardiography in normal dogs. Vet Radiol Ultrasound 39:33–41, 1998.
23. Choong CY, Abascal VM, Thomas JD, et al: Combined influence of ventricular loading and relaxation on the transmitral flow velocity profile in dogs measured by Doppler echocardiography. Circulation 78:672–683, 1988.
24. Courtois M, Mechem CJ, Barzilai B, et al: Delineation of determinants of left ventricular early filling Saline versus blood infusion. Circulation 90:2041–2050, 1994.
25. Courtois M, Kovacs SJ Jr, Ludbrook PA: Transmitral pressure-flow velocity relation. Importance of regional pressure gradients in the left ventricle during diastole Circulation 78:661–671, 1988.
26. Little WC, Ohno M, Kitzman DW, et al: Determination of left ventricular chamber stiffness from the time for deceleration of early left ventricular filling. Circulation 92:1933–1939, 1995.
27. Myreng Y, Smiseth CA, Risoe C: Left ventricular filling at elevated diastolic pressures: Relationship between transmitral Doppler flow velocities and atrial contribution. Am Heart J 119:620–626, 1990.
28. Nakatani S, Beppu S, Miyatake K, et al: Left ventricular function and the relationship between left atrial pressure and peak early diastolic filling velocity in dog. Cardiovasc Res 26: 109–114, 1992.
29. Yamamoto K, Masuyama T, Tanouchi J, et al: Effects of heart rate on left ventricular filling dynamics: Assessment from simultaneous recordings of

CV

pulsed Doppler transmitral flow velocity pattern and haemodynamic variables. Cardiovasc Res 27:935–941, 1993.

30. Yamamoto K, Masuyama T, Tanouchi J, et al: Peak early diastolic filling velocity may decrease with preload augmentation: Effect of concomitant increase in the rate of left atrial pressure drop in early diastole. J Am Soc Echocardiogr 6:245–254, 1993.

31. Chiang CH, Hagio M, Yoshida H, Okano S: Pulmonary venous flow in normal dogs recorded by transthoracic echocardiography—Techniques, anatomic validations and flow characteristics. J Vet Med Sci 60:333–339, 1998.

32. Appleton CP: Hemodynamic determinants of Doppler pulmonary venous flow velocity components: New insights from studies in lightly sedated normal dogs. J Am Coll Cardiol 30:1562–1574, 1997.

33. Bonagura JD, Miller MW: Doppler echocardiography I: Pulsed and continuous wave studies. Vet Clin North Am Small Anim Pract, in press.

34. Bonagura JD, Miller MW: Doppler echocardiography II: Color Doppler imaging. Vet Clin North Am Small Anim Pract, in press.

35. Stugaard M, Risoe C, Ihlen H, et al: Intracavitary filling pattern in the failing left ventricle assessed by color M-mode Doppler echocardiography. J Am Coll Cardiol 24:663–670, 1994.

36. Gorcsan J 3rd, Strum DP, Mandarino WA, et al: Quantitative assessment of alterations in regional left ventricular contractility with color-coded tissue Doppler echocardiography. Comparison with sonomicrometry and pressure-volume relations. Circulation 95:2423–2433, 1997.

37. Omoto R: Color Atlas of Real-Time Two-Dimensional Doppler Echocardiography. Tokyo, Shindan-To-Chiryyosha, 1987.

38. Kisslo JA, Adams DB, Belkin RN: Doppler Color Flow Imaging. New York, Churchill Livingstone, 1998.

39. Sahn DJ: Instrumententation and physical factors related to visualization of stenotic and regurgitant jets by Doppler color flow mapping. J Am Coll Cardiol 12:1234, 1998.

40. Boon J, Wingfield WE, Miller CW: Echocardiographic indices in the normal dog. Vet Radiol 24:214–221, 1983.

41. Calvert CA, Brown J: Use of M-mode echocardiography in the diagnosis of congestive cardiomyopathy in Doberman pinschers. JAVMA 189:293–297, 1986.

42. Lombard CW: Normal values of the canine M-mode echocardiogram. Am J Vet Res 45:2015–2018, 1984.

43. Bonagura JD, O'Grady MR, Herring DS: Echocardiography. Principles of interpretation. Vet Clin North Am Small Anim Prac 15:1177–1194, 1985.

44. O'Grady MR, Bonagura JD, Powers JD, et al: Quantitative cross-sectional echocardiography in the normal dog. Vet Radiol 27:34–49, 1986.

45. Haggstrom J, Hansson K, Karlberg BE, et al: Plasma concentration of atrial natriuretic peptide in relation to severity of mitral regurgitation in Cavalier King Charles spaniels. Am J Vet Res 55:698–703, 1994.

46. Haggstrom J, Hansson K, Kvart C, et al: Effects of naturally acquired decompensated mitral valve regurgitation on the renin-angiotensin-aldosterone system and atrial natriuretic peptide concentration in dogs. Am J Vet Res 58:77–82, 1997.

47. Teichholz LE, Kreulen T, Herman MV, et al: Problems in echocardiographic volume determinations: Echocardiographic-angiographic correlations in the presence or absence of asynergy. Am J Cardiol 37:7–11, 1976.

48. Wyatt HL, Heng MK, Meerbaum S, et al: Cross-sectional echocardiography. II. Analysis of mathematic models for quantifying volume of the formalin-fixed left ventricle. Circulation 61:1119–1125, 1980.

49. Schiller NB, Shah PM, Crawford M, et al: Recommendations for quantitation of the left ventricle by two-dimensional echocardiography. J Am Soc Echocardiogr. 2:358–367, 1989.

50. Fox PR, Liu SK, Maron BJ: Echocardiographic assessment of spontaneously occurring feline hypertrophic cardiomyopathy. An animal model of human disease. Circulation 92:2645–2651, 1995.

51. Wyatt HL, Heng MK, Meerbaum S, et al: Cross-sectional echocardiography. I. Analysis of mathematic models for quantifying mass of the left ventricle in dogs. Circulation 60:1104–1113, 1979.

52. Schiller NB, Skioldebrand CG, Schiller EJ, et al: Canine left ventricular mass estimation by two-dimensional echocardiography. Circulation 68:210–216, 1983.

53. Coleman B, Cothran LN, Ison-Franklin EL, et al: Estimation of left ventricular mass in conscious dogs. Am J Physiol 251:H1149–H1157, 1986.

54. Stack RS, Ramage JE, Bauman RP, et al: Validation of in vivo two-dimensional echocardiographic dimension measurements using myocardial mass estimates in dogs. Am Heart J 113:725–731, 1987.

55. Di SE, Preisman S, Ohad DG, et al: Echocardiographic left ventricular remodeling and pseudohypertrophy as markers of hypovolemia. An experimental study on bleeding and volume repletion. J Am Soc Echocardiogr 10:926–936 1997.

56. Morrison SA, Moise NS, Scarlett J, et al: Effect of breed and body weight on echocardiographic values in four breeds of dogs of differing somatotype. J Vet Intern Med 6:220–224, 1992.

57. Calvert CA: Cardiomyopathy in the Doberman pinscher dog. Calif Vet 38:7–12, 1984.

58. Calvert CA: Dilated congestive cardiomyopathy in Doberman pinschers. Compend Contin Educ Pract Vet 8:430–417, 1986.

59. Calvert CA, Hall G, Jacobs G, Pickus C: Clinical and pathological findings in Doberman pinschers with occult cardiomyopathy that died suddenly or developed congestive heart failure—54 cases (1984–1991). JAVMA 210:505–505, 1997.

60. Jacobs G, Knight DH: M-mode echocardiographic measurements in nonanesthe-

tized healthy cats: Effects of body weight, heart rate, and other variables. Am J Vet Res 46:1705–1711, 1985.

61. Sisson DD, Schaeffer D: Changes in linear dimensions of the heart, relative to body weight, as measured by M-mode echocardiography in growing dogs. Am J Vet Res 52:1591–1596, 1991.

62. Koch J, Pedersen HD, Jensen AL, et al: M-mode echocardiographic diagnosis of dilated cardiomyopathy in giant breed dogs. Zentralbl Veterinarmed A 43:297–304, 1996.

63. O'Grady MR, Bonagura JD, Powers JD, et al: Quantitative cross-sectional echocardiography in the normal dog. Vet Radiol 27:34–49, 1986.

64. DeMadron E, Bonagura JD, Herring DS: Two-dimensional echocardiography in the normal cat. Vet Radiol 26:149–158, 1985.

65. Kirberger RM, Berry WL: Atrial septal defect in a dog: The value of Doppler echocardiography. J S Afr Vet Assoc 63:43–48, 1992.

66. Monnet E, Orton EC, Gaynor J, et al: Diagnosis and surgical repair of partial atrioventricular septal defects in 2 dogs. JAVMA 211:569–569, 1997.

67. Nakayama T, Wakao Y, Uechi M, et al: A case-report of surgical-treatment of a dog with atrioventricular septal-defect (incomplete form of endocardial cushion defect). J Vet Med Sci 56:981–984, 1994.

68. Stamoulis ME, Fox PR: Mitral valve stenosis in three cats. J Small Anim Pract 34:452–456, 1993.

69. Lehmkuhl LB, Ware WA, Bonagura JD: Mitral stenosis in 15 dogs. J Vet Intern Med 8:2–17, 1994.

70. Beardow AW, Buchanan JW: Chronic mitral valve disease in Cavalier King Charles spaniels: 95 cases (1987–1991). JAVMA 203:1023–1029, 1993.

71. Nakayama T, Wakao Y, Uechi M, et al: Relationship between degree of mitral protrusion assessed by use of B-mode echocardiography and degree of mitral regurgitation using an experimental model in dogs. J Vet Med Sci 59:551–555, 1997.

72. Pedersen HD, Kristensen BO, Lorentzen KA, et al: Mitral valve prolapse in 3-year-old healthy Cavalier King Charles spaniels. An echocardiographic study. Can J Vet Res 59:294–298, 1995.

73. Pedersen HD, Kristensen BO, Norby B, Lorentzen KA: Echocardiographic study of mitral-valve prolapse in dachshunds. Zentralbl Veterinarmed A 43:103–110, 1996.

74. Pedersen HD, Lorentzen KA, Kristensen BO: Observer variation in the 2-dimensional echocardiographic evaluation of mitral-valve prolapse in dogs. Vet Radiol Ultrasound 37:367–372, 1996.

75. Jacobs GJ, Calvert CA, Mahaffey MB, et al: Echocardiographic detection of flail left atrioventricular valve cusp from ruptured chordae tendineae in 4 dogs. J Vet Intern Med 9:341–346, 1995.

76. Sisson DD, Thomas WP: Endocarditis of the aortic valve in the dog. JAVMA 184:570–577, 1984.

77. Pipers FS, Bonagura JD, Hamlin RL, et al: Echocardiographic abnormalities of the mitral valve associated with left sided heart diseases in the dog. JAVMA 179:580–586, 1981.

78. Bond BR, Fox PR, Peterson ME, et al: Echocardiographic findings in 103 cats with hyperthyroidism. JAVMA 192:1546–1549, 1988.

79. Jacobs G, Hutson C, Dougherty J, et al: Congestive heart failure associated with hyperthyroidism in cats. JAVMA 188:52–56, 1986.

80. Fox PR, Liu SK, Maron BJ: Echocardiographic assessment of spontaneously occurring feline hypertrophic cardiomyopathy. An animal model of human disease. Circulation 92:2645–2651, 1995.

81. Bond BR, Fox PR, Peterson ME, et al: Echocardiographic findings in 103 cats with hyperthyroidism. JAVMA 192:1546–1549, 1988.

82. Sisson DD, Luethy M, Thomas WP: Ventricular septal defect accompanied by aortic regurgitation in five dogs. J Am Anim Hosp Assoc 27:441–448, 1991.

83. DeMadron E, Bonagura JD, O'Grady MR: Normal and paradoxical ventricular septal motion in the dog. Am J Vet Res 46:1832–1841, 1985.

84. Tanaka H, Tei C, Nakao S, et al: Diastolic bulging of the interventricular septum toward the left ventricle. An echocardiographic manifestation of negative interventricular pressure gradient between left and right ventricles during diastole. Circulation 62:558–563, 1980.

85. Brayley KA, Lunney J, Ettinger SJ: Cor striatriatum dexter in a dog. J Am Anim Hosp Assoc 30:153–156, 1994.

86. Tobias AH, Thomas WP, Kittleson MD, et al: Cor triatriatum dexter in two dogs. JAVMA 202:285–290, 1993.

87. Thomas WP, Sisson DD, Bauer TG, et al: Detection of cardiac masses in dogs by two-dimensional echocardiography. Vet Radiol 25:65–72, 1984.

88. Atkins CE: Caval syndrome in the dog. Sem Vet Med Surg (Small Anim) 2:64–71, 1987.

89. Borgarelli M, Venco L, Piga PM, et al: Surgical removal of heartworms from the right atrium of a cat. JAVMA 211:68–69, 1997.

90. Prieto C, Venco L, Simon F. Genchi C: Feline heartworm (Dirofilaria immitis) infection—Detection of specific IgG for the diagnosis of occult infections. Vet Parasitol 70:209–217, 1997.

91. Selcer BA, Newell SM, Mansour AE, McCall JW: Radiographic and 2-D echocardiographic findings in 18 cats experimentally exposed to D. immitis via mosquito bites. Vet Radiol Ultrasound 37:37–44, 1996.

92. Atkins CE, Keene BW, McGuirk SM: Pathophysiologic mechanism of cardiac dysfunction in experimentally induced heartworm caval syndrome in dogs: An echocardiographic study. Am J Vet Res 49:403–410, 1988. [Published erratum appears in Am J Vet Res, 49:964, 1988.]

93. Kitagawa H, Sasaki Y, Ishihara K: Clinical studies on canine dirofilarial hemoglobinuria: Relationship between the presence of heartworm mass at the tricuspid valve orifice and plasma hemoglobin concentration. Jpn J Vet Sci 48:99–103, 1986.

94. Thomas WP: Two-dimensional, real-time echocardiography in the dog. Vet Radiol 25:50–64, 1984.

95. Monnet E, Orton EC, Salman M. et al: Idiopathic dilated cardiomyopathy in dogs—survival and prognostic indicators. J Vet Intern Med 9:12–17, 1995.

96. Koch J, Pedersen HD, Jensen AL, et al: Activation of the renin-angiotensin system in dogs with asymptomatic and symptomatic dilated cardiomyopathy. Res Vet Sci 59:172–175, 1995.

97. Page A, Edmunds G, Atwell RB: Echocardiographic values in the greyhound. Aust Vet J 70:361–364, 1993.

98. Minors SL, O'Grady MR: Resting and dobutamine stress echocardiographic factors associated with the development of occult dilated cardiomyopathy in healthy Doberman pinscher dogs. J Vet Intern Med 12:369–380, 1998.

99. Schober KE, Luis Fuentes V, Dukes McEwan J, et al: Atrioventricular annular displacement in healthy dogs and dogs with heart disease: Relation to left ventricular systolic function (abstract). British Small Animal Veterinary Association Congress Proceedings, 1997, p 312.

100. Sisson DD, Daniel GB, Twardock AR: Comparison of left ventricular ejection fractions determined in healthy anesthetized dogs by echocardiography and gated equilibrium radionuclide ventriculography. Am J Vet Res 50:1840–1847, 1989.

101. Schapira JN, Kohn MS, Beaver WL, et al: In vitro quantitation of canine left ventricular volume by phased-array sector scan. Cardiology 67:1–11, 1981.

102. Crippa L, Ferro E, Melloni E, et al: Echocardiographic parameters and indices in the normal beagle dog. Lab Anim 26:190–195, 1992.

103. Mashiro I, Nelson RR, Cohn JN, et al: Ventricular dimensions measured noninvasively by echocardiography in the awake dog. J Appl Physiol 41:953–959, 1976.

104. Kittleson MD, Eyster GE, Knowlen GG, et al: Myocardial function in small dogs with chronic mitral regurgitation and severe congestive heart failure. JAVMA 184:455–459, 1984.

105. Atkins CE, Snyder PS: Systolic time intervals and their derivatives for evaluation of cardiac function. J Vet Intern Med 6:55–63, 1992.

106. Darke PGG, Fuentes VL, Champion SR: Doppler-echocardiography in canine congestive cardiomyopathy. In Denovo R (ed): Proceedings of the Eleventh Annual Veterinary Medical Forum. Blacksburg, American College Veterinary, 1993, pp 531–534.

107. Kittleson MD, Pipers FS, Knauer KW, et al: Echocardiographic and clinical effects of milrinone in dogs with myocardial failure. Am J Vet Res 46:1659–1664, 1985.

108. Wallmeyer K, Wann LS, Sagar KB, et al: The influence of preload and heart rate on Doppler echocardiographic indexes of left ventricular performance: Comparison with invasive indexes in an experimental preparation. Circulation 74:181–186, 1986.

109. Chen C, Rodriguez L, Guerrero JL, et al: Noninvasive estimation of the instantaneous first derivative of left ventricular pressure using continuous-wave Doppler echocardiography. Circulation 83:2101–2110, 1991.

110. Lee CH, Hogan JC, Gibson DG: Diastolic disease in left ventricular hypertrophy: Comparison of M mode and Doppler echocardiography for the assessment of rapid ventricular filling. Br Heart J 65:194–200, 1991.

111. Santilli RA, Bussadori C, Bigliardi E, Borgarelli M: Systemic hypertension in (the) cat: A Doppler echocardiographic study. Eur Soc Vet Cardiol (Newslett) September–December, 1997.

112. Picard MH: M-mode echocardiography: Principles and examination techniques. In Weyman AE (ed): Principles and Practice of Echocardiography, 2nd ed. Philadelphia, Lea & Febiger, 1994, pp 282–301.

113. Appleton CP, Hatle LK, Popp RL: Relation of transmitral flow velocity patterns to left ventricular diastolic function: New insights from a combined hemodynamic and Doppler echocardiographic study. J Am Coll Cardiol 12:426–440, 1988.

114. Appleton CP, Hatle LK: The natural history of left ventricular filling abnormalities: Assessment by two-dimensional and Doppler echocardiography. Echocardiography 9:437–457, 1992.

115. Giannuzzi P, Imparato A, Temporelli PL, et al: Doppler-derived mitral deceleration time of early filling as a strong predictor of pulmonary capillary wedge pressure in postinfarction patients with left ventricular systolic dysfunction. J Am Coll Cardiol 23:1630–1637, 1994.

116. Santilli RA, Bussadori C: Hemodynamic assessment of diastolic function by echo-Doppler in feline cardiopathies (abstract). Proceedings of the 5th ESVIM Congress, 1995, p 55.

117. Rossvoll O, Hatle LK: Pulmonary venous flow velocities recorded by transthoracic Doppler ultrasound: Relation to left ventricular diastolic pressures. J Am Coll Cardiol 21:1687–1696, 1993.

118. Brun P, Tribouilloy C, Duval AM: Left ventricular flow propagation during early filling is related to wall relaxation: A color M-mode Doppler analysis. J Am Coll Cardiol 20:420–432, 1992.

119. Burwash IG, Thomas DD, Sadahiro M, et al: Dependence of Gorlin formula and continuity equation valve areas on transvalvular volume flow rate in valvular aortic stenosis. Circulation 89:827–835, 1994.

120. Lehmkuhl LB, Bonagura JD: Comparing transducer placement for quantifying outflow gradients in subaortic stenosis. In Denovo R (ed): Proceedings of the Eleventh Annual Veterinary Medical Forum. Blacksburg, American College Veterinary, 1993, pp 528–529.

121. Lehmkuhl LB, Bonagura JD, Jones DE, et al: Comparison of catheterization and Doppler-derived pressure gradients in a canine model of subaortic stenosis. J Am Soc Echocardiogr 3:611–620, 1995.

122. Lehmkuhl LB, Bonagura JD: Comparison of transducer placement sites for Doppler-echocardiography in dogs with subaortic stenosis. Am J Vet Res 55:192–198, 1994.

123. Bonagura JD, Darke PGG: Congenital heart disease. In Ettinger SJ, Feldman EC (eds): Textbook of Veterinary Internal Medicine, 4th ed. Philadelphia, WB Saunders, 1995, pp 892–943.

124. Thomas WP: Doppler echocardiographic estimation of pressure gradients in dogs with congenital pulmonic and subaortic stenosis. Proceedings of the 8th ACVIM Forum, 1990, pp 867–869.

125. Martin MWS, Godman M, Fuentes VL, et al: Assessment of balloon pulmonary valvuloplasty in six dogs. J Small Anim Pract 33:443–449, 1992.

126. Chetboul V, Pouchelon JL, Bonhoeffer P: Cardiac examination by Doppler ultrasonography in domestic carnivores. Rec Med Vet 171:799–818, 1995.

127. Uehara Y, Takahashi M: Hemodynamic changes during administration of drugs for mitral regurgitation in dogs. J Vet Med Sci 60:213–218, 1998.

128. Uehara Y, Takahashi M: Quantitative evaluation of the severity of mitral-insufficiency in dogs by the color Doppler method. J Vet Med Sci 58:249–253, 1996.

129. Schwammenthal E, Chen C, Giesler M, et al: New method for accurate calculation of regurgitant flow rate based on analysis of Doppler color flow maps of the proximal flow field. Validation in a canine model of mitral regurgitation with initial application in patients. J Am Coll Cardiol 27:161–172, 1996.

130. Brown WA, Kittleson MD: Color flow Doppler estimation of mitral regurgitation using the proximal flow convergence method in dogs with chronic degenerative mitral valve disease (CDMVD) (abstract). Proceedings of the 12th ACVIM Forum, 1994, p 974.

131. Appleton CP, Basnight MA, Gonzalez MS: Diastolic mitral regurgitation with atrioventricular conduction abnormalities: Relation of mitral flow velocity to transmitral pressure gradients in conscious dogs. J Am Coll Cardiol 18:843–849, 1991.

132. Rosenthal SL, Fox PR: Diastolic mitral regurgitation detected by pulsed wave Doppler-echocardiography and color-flow Doppler mapping in 5 dogs and 2 cats with 2nd-degree and 3rd-degree atrioventricular block. Vet Radiol Ultrasound 36:152–156, 1995.

133. Fox PR, Miller MW, Liu SK: Clinical, echocardiographic, and Doppler imaging characteristics of mitral valve stenosis in two dogs. JAVMA 201:1575–1579, 1992.

134. Lehmkuhl LB, Ware WA, Bonagura JD: Mitral stenosis in 15 dogs. J Vet Intern Med 8:2–17, 1994.

135. Stamoulis ME, Fox PR: Mitral valve stenosis in three cats. J Small Anim Pract 34:452–456, 1993.

136. Baade H, Schober K, Oechtering G: Echokardiographische Normwerte bei West Highland White Terriern und Boxern unter besonderer Beruecksichtigung der Rechtsherzfunktion. Proceedings of the 7th Annual Congress of the German Society of Veterinary Internal Medicine and Laboratory Diagnostics, in press.

137. Gooding JP, Robinson WF, Mews GC: Echocardiographic assessment of left ventricular dimensions in clinically normal English cocker spaniels. Am J Vet Res 47:296–300, 1986.

138. Herrtage ME: Echocardiographic measurements in the normal boxer (abstract). Proceedings of the 4th European Society of Veterinary Internal Medicine Congress, 1994, p 172.

139. Snyder PS, Sato T, Atkins CE: A comparison of echocardiographic indices of the nonracing, healthy greyhound to reference values from other breeds. Vet Radiol Ultrasound 36:387–392, 1995.

140. Bayon A, Delpalacio MJF, Montes AM, et al: M-mode echocardiography study in growing Spanish mastiffs. J Small Anim Pract 35:473–479, 1994.

141. DeMadron E: Update on normal TM (M-mode) echocardiographic values in the dog. Prat Med Chir Anim Cie (Fr) 30:647–657, 1995.

142. Pipers FS, Reef V, Hamlin RL: Echocardiography in the domestic cat. Am J Vet Res 40:882–886, 1979.

143. Fox PR, Bond BR, Peterson ME: Echocardiographic reference values in healthy cats sedated with ketamine hydrochloride. Am J Vet Res 46:1479–1484, 1985.

144. Moise NS, Dietze AE, Mezza LE, et al: Echocardiography, electrocardiography, and radiography of cats with dilatation cardiomyopathy, hypertrophic cardiomyopathy, and hyperthyroidism. Am J Vet Res 47:1476–1486, 1986.

145. Sisson DD, Knight DH, Helinski C, et al: Plasma taurine concentrations and M-mode echocardiographic measures in healthy cats and in cats with dilated cardiomyopathy. J Vet Intern Med 5:232–238, 1991.

146. Mashiro I, Nelson RR, Cohn JN, Franciosa JA: Ventricular dimensions measured noninvasively by echocardiography in the awake dog. J Appl Physiol 41:953–959, 1976.

147. Smucker ML, Kaul S, Woodfield JA, et al: Naturally occurring cardiomyopathy in the Doberman pinscher: A possible large animal model of human cardiomyopathy? J Am Coll Cardiol 16:200–206, 1990.

148. Jacobs G, Knight DH: Change in M-mode echocardiographic values in cats given ketamine. Am J Vet Res 46:1712–1713, 1985.

CV

CHAPTER 116

PRIMARY MYOCARDIAL DISEASE IN THE DOG

D. David Sisson, William P. Thomas, and Bruce W. Keene

Myocardial diseases are those in which the heart muscle itself is affected by a pathologic process. As with other organs, myocardial diseases may result from degenerative, infectious, immune-mediated, genetic, metabolic, ischemic, toxic, or a combination of these common disease-producing processes. Primary myocardial diseases are called cardiomyopathies. These are diseases in which the pathologic changes in the heart muscle cannot be explained by the effects of congenital or acquired diseases of the heart valves, coronary vessels, pericardium, or other organs whose altered function affects the health of the myocardium (such as the thyroid, lung, or kidney). The most recent World Health Organization (WHO) classification system for primary myocardial diseases or cardiomyopathies divides them into three broad groups—dilated, hypertrophic, and restrictive.[1] The WHO classification system is based on the fundamental morphologic (echocardiographic or necropsy) and physiologic (echocardiographic or hemodynamic) characteristics of the diseased heart, rather than on etiologic considerations. Because the myocardium responds in limited ways to a variety of injuries, each of the clinically recognized forms of cardiomyopathy actually represents an etiologically heterogeneous group of myocardial diseases that at the time of diagnosis share a common morphologic, physiologic, and often (but not always, because their causes and subsequent natural history might be different) clinical result.

Myocardial diseases caused by well-defined conditions that profoundly affect the morphology and function of the myocardium in concert with or secondary to their effects on other organ systems (e.g., hyperthyroidism) are often classified as secondary myocardial diseases. Secondary myocardial diseases are generally named by the specific cause of the disease, such as hyperthyroid heart disease, although terms such as hyperthyroid cardiomyopathy are also common.[2]

CANINE DILATED CARDIOMYOPATHY

Dilated cardiomyopathy (DCM) describes any primary myocardial disease that is characterized by cardiac chamber dilatation (usually all four chambers to some degree, but sometimes predominantly left or more rarely predominantly right ventricular) and systolic ventricular dysfunction caused by impaired myocardial contractility.[1] Diastolic dysfunction also occurs in DCM, but it is less notable than the characteristically severe systolic dysfunction and is more difficult to document.[3, 4]

PREVALENCE AND DEMOGRAPHICS

Few estimates of the prevalence of DCM in the overall population of dogs have been reported in the veterinary literature.[5] In a study conducted in Italy, Fioretti and Delli Carri identified DCM in 1.1 per cent of 7148 dogs.[6] Based on a search of the Veterinary Medical Data Base (VMDB) at Purdue University for visits recorded from January 1986 through December 1991 (Fig. 116–1), DCM (coded as acquired, congestive, or right-sided cardiomyopathy) was diagnosed in 1681 (approximately 0.5 per cent) of the 342,142 dogs presented for veterinary services at participating (primarily referral) institutions.[7] Although these estimates are subject to referral and other biases (because they are not truly population-based studies),[8] they demonstrate that DCM is one of the most common acquired heart diseases of dogs. Only degenerative valvular disease and, in some regions of the world, heartworm infection are more common causes of cardiac morbidity and mortality in dogs.

Although DCM appears to be occurring with increasing frequency in medium-size breeds such as English and American cocker spaniels and Dalmatians, it is still recognized most commonly in large and giant purebred dogs.[5–15] According to the VMDB information cited earlier, the prevalence rate of DCM in mixed breed dogs was approximately 0.16 per cent, compared with 0.65 per cent in purebred dogs. Breeds most commonly affected according to the VMDB include Scottish deerhounds, Doberman pinschers, Irish wolfhounds, Great Danes, Boxer dogs, Saint Bernards, Afghan hounds, Newfoundlands, and Old English sheepdogs. In comparing breed prevalence data from different sources, it becomes obvious that a few breeds in some geographic locations are at greater risk for development of DCM than the same breed in other locations. In a recent study of dogs with DCM from Sweden, Tidholm and Jonsson found that Airedale terriers, English cocker spaniels, and standard poodles were at increased risk, and although some of the same breeds frequently seen with DCM in North America were also at increased risk in Sweden (Boxers, Doberman pinschers, Newfoundlands, and Saint Bernards), Great Danes and Old English sheepdogs were not at increased risk in the Swedish population, and Irish wolfhounds showed only a statistically nonsignificant trend toward increased risk.[14] Whether these differences reflect genetic or environmental differences is not known, and with the data currently available, it is not possible to compare absolute population prevalence rates between geographic locations. In all studies, DCM is rare in dogs less than 12 kg, although it has been reported in dogs as small as a Papillon.[14]

In several retrospective studies of various breeds, the median age of dogs with DCM is between 4 and 8 years, a generally younger population of dogs than those afflicted with degenerative valvular disease.[9–16] Also in contrast to acquired valvular disease, there are significant numbers of puppies younger than 1 year of age afflicted with DCM.[14] In retrospective studies performed on populations of dogs with

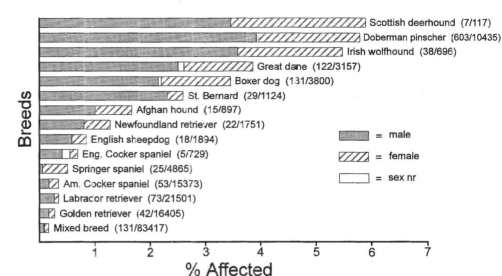

Figure 116–1. The prevalence of dilated cardiomyopathy (DCM), displayed as a percentage of new hospital admissions, is highest in large and giant purebred dogs. Male predominance is observed in most but not all affected breeds. (From the Veterinary Medical Data Base, Purdue University.)

Scottish deerhound (7/117)
Doberman pinscher (603/10435)
Irish wolfhound (38/696)
Great dane (122/3157)
Boxer dog (131/3800)
St. Bernard (29/1124)
Afghan hound (15/897)
Newfoundland retriever (22/1751)
English sheepdog (18/1894)
Eng. Cocker spaniel (5/729)
Springer spaniel (25/4865)
Am. Cocker spaniel (53/15373)
Labrador retriever (73/21501)
Golden retriever (42/16405)
Mixed breed (131/83417)

= male
= female
= sex nr

Breeds

% Affected

heart failure or sudden death attributed to DCM, males are affected nearly twice as often as females.[7, 14, 15] This male predominance has been questioned in asymptomatic Doberman pinschers or Boxers with clinical signs due to ventricular arrhythmia only,[17, 18] but males are significantly overrepresented in almost all other studies, including recent investigations of Doberman pinschers with occult cardiomyopathy that died suddenly or developed congestive heart failure.[19]

PATHOLOGY

Gross necropsy findings in dogs with DCM typically disclose marked dilatation of all cardiac chambers (Fig. 116–2).[8, 20–22] The myocardium often appears pale, soft, and flabby, and the ratio of ventricular wall thickness to chamber diameter is decreased. The eccentric myocardial hypertrophy typical of DCM is best noted on gross necropsy by measurement and calculation of the total heart weight to body weight ratio, which should always be increased. The thickness of the ventricular walls and interventricular septum may be decreased or normal despite the increased mass of the myocardium, a reflection of the fact that the eccentrically hypertrophied cardiac myocytes surround a larger chamber volume. The papillary muscles usually appear grossly flattened and atrophied. The circumferences of the mitral tricuspid valve annuli are generally increased in proportion to the magnitude of the chamber dilatation. The valves themselves should be reasonably normal in appearance, although incidental, modest degenerative changes (mild to moderate thickening of the valves and/or chordae) may be seen in older animals. If present, valvular changes in DCM are modest and in stark contrast to those observed in dogs that die from chronic valvular heart disease.

The endocardium of the left ventricle and sometimes the left atrium is often mildly to moderately thickened and may present a translucent, whitish sheen when examined under strong light. In the past, this endocardial thickening attending congenital DCM was sometimes termed primary endocardial fibroelastosis.[23] It is now generally thought that these changes are not pathognomonic for endocardial fibroelastosis or DCM, but rather represent subendocardial fibrosis that attends chronic left ventricular or atrial dilatation from any cause.[24]

In general, histologic and ultrastructural changes are moderate, unexciting, and usually etiologically unenlightening in the face of the devastating nature of the functional myocardial defect in DCM. On histopathologic examination, small scattered areas of myocyte degeneration, necrosis, and fibrosis are often observed, but these lesions are neither extensive nor pathognomonic for DCM.[21, 22] These histopathologic lesions are usually most pronounced in the subendocardial regions of the left ventricular free wall and papillary muscles (Fig. 116–3). In a relatively large retrospective case series, histopathologic examination of 67 cases showed diffuse subendocardial fibrosis in 67 per cent, with 99 per cent of the cases displaying at least some so-called attenuated wavy fibers, which represent degenerating or atrophied cardiac myocytes.[14] In evaluating the presence of these fibers in a randomized, blind fashion in conjunction with myocardial specimens from dogs that died of heart diseases other than DCM, the presence of attenuated wavy fibers appeared to be specific for the diagnosis of DCM.[25] Occasional mononuclear cells (lymphocytes, plasma cells, or macrophages) may be observed in histologic sections of myocardium from dogs with DCM, but active myocarditis (meeting the Dallas criteria for lymphocytic infiltration and myocyte necrosis)[26] appears to be relatively rare in the absence of clinically apparent infectious disease.[14, 24, 25, 27]

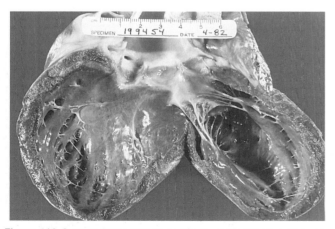

Figure 116–2. Heart from a Doberman pinscher with dilated cardiomyopathy. The left ventricle is markedly dilated, but grossly, the myocardium appears normal.

CV

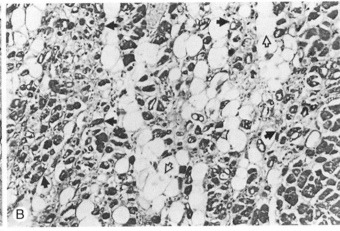

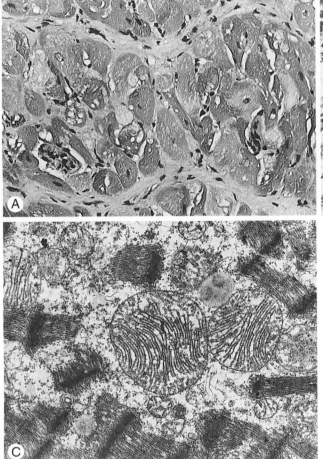

Figure 116–3. *A,* Nonspecific vacuolization of left ventricular myocytes and myocardial fibrosis in a dog dying from dilated cardiomyopathy. *B,* Large areas of ventricular myocardium are replaced by fatty infiltration *(open arrows)* in a Boxer dog with dilated cardiomyopathy. Solid arrows indicate areas of myofiber atrophy, myocyte degeneration, and myocardial fibrosis. *C,* Electron micrograph of cardiac muscle illustrating loss of myofilaments, disorientation of remaining myofibers, and increased size of abnormal mitochondria (Magnification: 15,000×) (*A* and *C* from Sandusky GE, et al: Histologic and ultrastructural evaluation of cardiac lesions in idiopathic cardiomyopathy in dogs. Can J Comp Med 48:81, 1984; *B* from Harpster NK: Boxer cardiomyopathy—a review of the long-term benefits of antiarrhythmic therapy. Vet Clin North Am 21:989, 1991).

Boxers in New England have been reported to have a pathologically distinct form of DCM, in which the right ventricular wall is the earliest and most severely affected region of the heart, coinciding clinically with the early onset of ventricular arrhythmias with typical left bundle branch block morphology, suggesting that the premature depolarizations have their origin in the diseased right ventricle.[18, 28] In advanced cases, widespread areas of myocardial fibrosis and fatty infiltration are observed (see Fig. 116–3). The pathology of cardiomyopathy in Boxer dogs is similar in some ways to right ventricular cardiomyopathy in humans, a condition often causing sudden death that has also been termed arrhythmogenic right ventricular dysplasia.[29–32] In general, however, the pathologic changes of myocyte loss and replacement with either adipose tissue or fibrous connective tissue appear to be less severe in Boxers than is typical for the human disease. Like Boxers, however, most humans with so-called right ventricular cardiomyopathy have been shown to have at least some involvement of the left ventricle, and the disease in humans is no longer generally considered an isolated disease of the right ventricle.[33] A syndrome of predominantly right ventricular cardiomyopathy has been reported separately in a dachshund and a bull mastiff, both of which had pathologic findings of more extensive myocyte loss and replacement of right ventricular myocardium with adipose tissue and fibrous connective tissue than is typically seen in Boxers, and closely mimicking right ventricular cardiomyopathy in humans.[34, 35]

Ultrastructural abnormalities described in dogs with DCM include scattered foci of degenerated myocardial cells exhibiting varying degrees of myocytolysis; mild to marked sarcoplasmic vacuolization; increased intracytoplasmic collections of large, dense lipofuscin granules; increased numbers of mitochondria with mild to moderate internal degenerative changes; and evidence of individual myocyte hypertrophy.[22, 36, 37] In more severely affected myocardial cells, the myofibrils are disrupted, disoriented, and loosely arranged in the cytoplasm, together with scattered deposits of what appears to be glycogen (see Fig. 116–3). These ultrastructural changes are generally regarded as nonspecific markers of myocyte damage. Histopathologic and ultrastructural studies to date have failed to illuminate the mechanisms responsible for reduced myocardial function in dogs with DCM.

ETIOLOGY AND PATHOGENESIS

The cause of most individual cases of DCM in dogs (as well as in most other species, including humans) remains unknown. Canine DCM has been associated with a variety of different potential insults to the myocardium, including (but probably not limited to) those caused by genetic mutations,[38–44] infectious agents,[45–63] mitochondrial and protein biochemical defects,[64–72] toxins,[73–83] nutritional deficiencies,[84, 85] rapid pacing (tachyarrhythmias),[86–90] immunologic mechanisms,[91–93] and even pregnancy.[94] The plethora of apparent potential causes and the wide variety of myocardial biochemical defects associated with DCM pose a difficult problem for clinicians, pathologists, and researchers seeking a unifying etiologic theory that might yield effective prevention or treatment strategies. The relative morphologic, histologic, ultrastructural, and functional homogeneity of patients with clinical DCM suggests that there are probably important similarities in the response of the myocardium to a variety of different types of injuries, and that some common cellular pathways that respond to those injuries cause and/or exacerbate the structural and functional changes typical of DCM. The familial nature, male predominance, and geographic variation in breed prevalence rates all suggest that genetic characteristics (apparently sometimes inherited in an autosomal dominant pattern)[95] play an important role in the pathogenesis of DCM in dogs. Recent molecular genetic investigations in humans, mice, hamsters, and dogs with DCM have yielded exciting results, identifying genes that may initiate inherited DCM and/or influence the progression of DCM caused by environmental (i.e., nongenetic) injuries.[38, 39, 40, 96, 97]

Defects (mutations) in two kinds of genes have been implicated in the etiology of DCM in some humans and dogs. The first group of implicated genes encodes structural proteins, including dystrophin. Dystrophin is part of a multiprotein complex (the dystrophin-associated glycoprotein complex) that is believed to link the muscle cytoskeleton to the extracellular matrix, anchoring the cardiac myocytes in their extracellular environment. These cytoskeletal anchors maintain the structural integrity of the muscle, allowing effective contraction and muscle shortening to occur. The health of the cytoskeleton also appears to be critical for myocyte viability, because mutations in cytoskeletal proteins lead to the death of cardiac myocytes.[4, 38] Mutations in the dystrophin gene have been shown to cause a relatively rare X-linked form of DCM in dogs (golden retrievers) and humans in association with Duchenne's muscular dystrophy.[41, 43, 44] Mutations in other cytoskeletal genes, including those that encode muscle LIM protein and cardiac actin, have also been shown to cause DCM in mice and humans.[96, 98] Recent prospective work indicates that many cases of DCM that were presumed to be sporadic are in fact familial,[99] further magnifying the importance of basic genetic findings. As suspected in many cases of familial DCM in dogs, these defects also appear to be inherited in an autosomal dominant pattern. Viewed as a whole, the mounting numbers of molecular cytoskeletal abnormalities that cause DCM suggest that defective force transmission may be the cause of myocardial failure and ventricular dilatation in some cases of the disease.

The second kind of gene implicated in the etiology of DCM encodes nuclear transcription factors (factors that control which specific parts of the DNA in a cell's nucleus get transcribed into messenger RNA to direct subsequent protein synthesis) specifically in the cardiac myocyte. One such gene, encoding the cyclic AMP response-element binding protein (a transcription factor that regulates the expression of genes in response to a wide variety of extracellular signals), has been manipulated in a mouse model to produce DCM clinically similar to that seen in dogs and humans.[38] It is hoped that further work will determine the molecular mechanism that couples extracellular signals to cardiac gene expression, potentially revealing how the interpretation of extracellular signals is modified by mutations in the genes that control transcription factors and detailing which extracellular signals are affected by such mutations. Basic research in this area has enormous potential clinical relevance, because understanding the complete mechanism by which extracellular signals trigger the expression of a typical DCM phenotype might logically enable the design of pharmaceutical or other interventions to prevent or interrupt the initiation or progression of the disease.

In addition to genetic contributions to the initiation or progression of DCM, several other kinds of myocardial injuries or defects have been associated with the pathogenesis of DCM. Although current evidence suggests that active myocarditis is an infrequent finding in dogs with clinical DCM, it is possible that viral or other infections may "smolder" in the myocardium, possibly triggering genetic or immunologic responses that could result in DCM months or years after the infection was acquired. For this reason, interest has grown in the potential application of molecular genetic techniques such as the polymerase chain reaction to amplify and identify segments of viral genes that might be present in fixed or frozen myocardial specimens if there is an association between past viral infection and DCM.[100]

A wide variety of biochemical abnormalities have been associated with DCM in dogs, including altered activity and concentrations of mitochondrial enzyme systems, abnormal calcium regulation, and altered membrane receptors.[64–72, 101–103] Specific biochemical abnormalities that have been reported in the hearts of dogs with DCM include reduced myocardial myoglobin content,[69, 70] myocardial calcium cycling and mitochondrial respiratory chain defects,[71b, 71c] reduced concentrations of myocardial troponin-T and creatine kinase MB isoenzyme,[72] and decreased beta receptor–mediated adenylate cyclase activity.[67] Reported alterations in dogs with experimentally induced heart failure and humans with DCM include selective down-regulation of beta-receptors,[122] increased G_i and decreased G_s regulatory proteins,[102, 123, 124] altered gating mechanism of the Ca^{++} release channel of the sarcoplasmic reticulum,[125] alterations in the proteins of the sarcoplasmic reticulum,[126] decreased contractile performance with increasing heart rate (inverse of the normal force-frequency relationship),[127] and reduced content of the regulatory light chain protein LC2, related to the presence of increased concentration of an active protease.[128] Because few animals (or humans) undergo myocardial biochemical investigation before the onset of DCM, it has been difficult to sort out the "chicken or egg" question regarding the presence of most of these biochemical defects in association with heart failure and DCM (i.e., does an identified defect cause DCM, is the defect caused by DCM, or is the defect simply associated with heart failure?). Uncertainty regarding their pathogenetic significance, combined with potential methodologic and technical problems[104] associated with some of these demanding studies, has limited the clinical impact of much of the literature in this area. Identification of potentially treatable biochemical abnormalities (e.g., carnitine or taurine deficiency) has, however, sometimes been shown to have significant therapeutic impact on the clinical course of DCM in affected individuals or families of individuals with those specific defects.[68, 105]

Myocardial L-carnitine deficiency has received considerable attention in recent years as a possible cause of or contributor to cardiomyopathy in dogs and humans.[64, 66, 68, 130–138] Carnitine plays several essential roles in mitochondrial metabolism, including transporting long-chain free fatty acids into the inner mitochondrial membrane where beta oxidation occurs. Because fatty acids are the heart's major metabolic fuel, it is theorized that inadequate amounts of free L-carnitine to transport fatty acids cause myocardial dysfunction as a result of altered energy metabolism.[134–139] Reduced concentrations of myocardial L-carnitine have been measured in several breeds of dogs with DCM, including Boxers, Doberman pinschers, and American cocker spaniels.[105, 130–132] Dogs with low myocardial L-carnitine concentrations often have normal plasma concentrations, suggesting the possibility of a membrane transport defect,[140, 141] and rendering plasma carnitine concentrations an insensitive test for myocardial carnitine deficiency. The response of dogs with DCM to oral L-carnitine supplementation is variable. A few dogs treated with large doses (50 mg/kg every eight hours) of oral L-carnitine have experienced dramatic objective improvement.[68] Others improve by subjective measures, but improved cardiac function, as assessed by echocardiographic evaluation, occurs in only a small percentage of treated dogs.[131, 132] Still others (including two Boxers with proven myocardial L-carnitine deficiency) experience no documentable benefit from carnitine supplementation.[133] Preexisting cardiac arrhythmias are not abolished, and sudden death does not appear to be prevented by L-carnitine supplementation. The available evidence suggests that L-carnitine deficiency is not the primary cause of most cases of canine or human DCM, but that it occurs secondary to some other genetic or acquired abnormality, such as a mitochondrial defect, in approximately 40 per cent of canine cases.[130, 136–139]

Decreased plasma concentrations of both carnitine and taurine have been reported in American cocker spaniels with DCM, and supplementation with a combination of taurine and carnitine proved in a blinded, placebo-controlled trial to be beneficial in these animals.[105] At the outset of this trial, some dogs had failed to improve on individual supplementation of either taurine or carnitine, and the efficacy of taurine or carnitine supplementation alone has not been rigorously examined. There are anecdotal reports that supplementation with one or the other may be efficacious, and there is one case report of a cocker spaniel that appeared to respond to taurine supplementation alone.[142] With the exception of American cocker spaniels and possibly some other "unusual" breeds with DCM, and in marked contrast to cats with DCM, taurine deficiency appears to be uncommon in dogs with DCM.[143]

Various toxic insults, ranging from doxorubicin (Adriamycin, an anthracycline antibiotic used for its antineoplastic properties) to avocados to ionizing radiation, have been associated with DCM in dogs.[73–83] Of these toxins, only the widely used cancer chemotherapeutic agent doxorubicin is known to be a relatively frequent cause of cardiotoxicity mimicking primary DCM in companion animals. Acute toxicosis following intravenous administration of doxorubicin includes anaphylaxis and cardiac arrhythmias, and administration of cumulative doses greater than 180 mg/M^2 can result in progressive cardiomyopathy characterized histologically and ultrastructurally by severe vacuolar degeneration, myocytolysis, myofibril atrophy, and interstitial fibrosis.[73, 74, 106] Clinical findings may include cardiomegaly, cardiac arrhythmias and conduction disturbances (especially atrioventricular block and bundle branch blocks), congestive heart failure, and sudden death. Severe doxorubicin cardiac toxicity is generally progressive and fatal, even if the drug is stopped, and prevention depends primarily on limiting the cumulative dose. As medical treatment of cancer in dogs has become increasingly aggressive and these animals are living longer after therapy, several centers have reported the development of DCM in dogs treated for neoplasms with doxorubicin alone or in combination with other drugs.[107–110]

The immunology of DCM is another area of active research in dogs as well as in humans. Several studies have found the presence of autoantibodies to various critical components of the heart to be present in some cases of DCM, and there is speculation that these antibodies may play an important etiologic role in the development and/or progression of the disease.[91–93] Preliminary evidence in humans suggests that immunoadsorption, a commercially available technique used in Germany to remove immunoglobulins from the circulation (including autoantibodies directed against beta$_1$ adrenoceptor), may result in substantial therapeutic benefit in some advanced cases of human DCM.[111] This technique might conceivably be useful in treating *Trypanosoma cruzi* infections in dogs, an infectious cardiomyopathy also shown to generate anti–heart tissue antibodies in association with down-regulation of the beta-adrenergic receptor complex.[112, 113]

Sustained tachycardia, usually induced by rapid electronic ventricular pacing, is a commonly used research method for creating experimental heart failure in dogs.[144–146] Depending on the protocol used, tachycardia-induced cardiomyopathy evokes neurohormonal responses similar to those observed in spontaneously occurring heart failure, including activation of the renin-angiotensin-aldosterone system and sympathetic nervous system.[147, 149] Beta-receptor desensitization has recently been shown to precede heart failure in this model.[150] Although rapid pacing of the ventricles is modestly more efficient in producing heart failure than induction of a sustained supraventricular tachyarrhythmia, supraventricular tachyarrhythmias can also produce a syndrome of heart failure and DCM in dogs, a fact with important implications for clinical patients with sustained supraventricular tachycardias either with or without preexisting structural heart disease.[152, 153] Rapid pacing also causes remodeling of the coronary vasculature with a reduction in the volume fraction of capillaries and increased capillary diffusion distance,[148] and some protocols can cause morphologic, structural, and functional changes in the ventricle and cardiac myocytes that mimic those of DCM.[151] Interestingly, the rapid pacing model has also provided a potential explanation for the widely held clinical impression that dogs with DCM are difficult to resuscitate from ventricular fibrillation, in that the defibrillation threshold is significantly elevated after the induction of heart failure.[154] Some important preliminary evidence for drug efficacy in the treatment of heart failure and DCM has also been generated in this model.[155]

PATHOPHYSIOLOGY

The variety of potential causes of DCM, coupled with the shared morphologic, functional, and clinical features of the disease that result from these various causes, supports a three-phase conceptual pathophysiologic model of heart failure caused by DCM. In this model, popularized by Bristow,[97] the myocardial injury inflicted by any of the genetic, infectious, metabolic, nutritional, toxic, or immunologic causes of DCM serves as an initiating or index event (phase I). In DCM, these defects or injuries primarily impair the systolic function of the myocardium. If this event is of sufficient severity, the initiating event triggers a physiologic (including activation of various cytokine, sympathetic nervous, and renin-angiotensin-aldosterone systems)[156, 157] and genetic cascade of events (phase II) that leads to further loss of cardiac myocytes, pathologic hypertrophy of the remaining myocytes, ongoing loss of contractile and pump function, and dilatation of the cardiac chambers. This progressive damage eventually results in the hemodynamic and clinical syndrome of heart failure (phase III), at which time the disease is most commonly recognized clinically in dogs. Typical hemodynamic findings in canine DCM at this stage include elevated ventricular end-diastolic, atrial, and venous pressures. Ultimately, clinical signs of right- or left-sided congestive heart failure appear, and markedly reduced cardiac output may be manifested as weakness, exercise intolerance, syncope, or cardiogenic shock.

Other factors that can contribute to ventricular dysfunction and the hemodynamics of cardiac failure in DCM include atrioventricular valvular insufficiency secondary to atrial and ventricular dilatation and the presence of cardiac arrhythmias. Based on color-flow Doppler studies in our laboratories, mitral and tricuspid insufficiency is observed in most dogs with DCM, but the magnitude of regurgitation is usually mild. Moderate to severe mitral regurgitation is observed occasionally in a dog with concurrent myxomatous degeneration of the mitral valve. Cardiac arrhythmias, such as atrial fibrillation or ventricular ectopia, are frequently detected in dogs with DCM. The frequency and severity of ventricular arrhythmia are believed to be important determinants of the risk of sudden death in Boxers and Doberman pinschers with DCM.[16, 18, 19, 28, 118–121] Specifically, sustained (>30 second) bouts of ventricular tachycardia observed on Holter studies appear to predict sudden death in Doberman pinschers.[19]

The development of atrial fibrillation has important immediate and chronic consequences for dogs with DCM. Cardiac output declines by as much as 25 per cent in healthy dogs with induced atrial fibrillation as a result of decreased and irregular diastolic filling times and the loss of atrial and ventricular synchronization.[158, 159] Darke has shown that stroke volume is severely reduced in dogs with DCM and atrial fibrillation when the R-R interval is less than 0.30 seconds.[160] Thus, signs of rapidly decompensated heart failure may occur when dogs with DCM develop atrial fibrillation, particularly if the heart rate is greater than 200 beats per minute. Chronic atrial fibrillation with a rapid ventricular response may also contribute to progressively deteriorating myocardial contractility by the mechanisms discussed earlier.

CLINICAL MANIFESTATIONS

The spectrum of clinical signs exhibited by dogs with DCM is similar in all breeds, but the observed frequency of these signs varies with breed, geographic location, family, and, to some extent, lifestyle of the animal. In a recent retrospective summary of 189 DCM cases from Sweden, cough, depression, inappetence, dyspnea, weight loss, panting, syncope, and polydipsia were all noted as presenting complaints.[14] In U.S. referral institutions, clinical manifestations of right heart or biventricular failure, including abdominal distention, anorexia, weight loss, and fatigue, often predominate in giant breeds, whereas signs of left heart failure (dyspnea caused by pulmonary edema), episodic weakness, or syncope are more common in Doberman pinschers and Boxers.[114–121] Working dogs are often presented because of a gradual onset of exercise intolerance that the owner has noted over several months. Dogs with a more leisurely lifestyle are often presented with rapidly progressing clinical signs that the owner has been aware of for only a few days or weeks.

Recognition of DCM in dogs without evidence of overt heart failure is becoming increasingly common, spurred by the widespread availability of diagnostic ultrasonography and commercially available Holter (24-hour electrocardiogram) monitoring combined with increased breeder interest in screening programs. About one third of Boxers in the northeastern United States with idiopathic myocardial disease are asymptomatic at the time of diagnosis. Only one third of Boxers are reported to exhibit signs of heart failure at the time of diagnosis, with the remaining one third presenting for syncope or episodic weakness associated with ventricular arrhythmias. Most asymptomatic or syncopal Boxers with ventricular arrhythmias are reported to have normal echocardiographic contractile indices.[18] In contrast, most asymptomatic Doberman pinschers with "occult" DCM exhibit ventricular arrhythmias in association with significantly impaired myocardial function and ventricular dilatation.[19] Some giant breed dogs, without signs of heart failure and regarded as healthy by their owners, exhibit atrial fibrillation with or without soft regurgitant-quality murmurs and mildly or moderately decreased myocardial function. Although most asymptomatic dogs with proven myocardial dysfunction (and especially those with atrial fibrillation or serious ventricular ectopy) eventually develop DCM with signs of heart failure or sudden death,[19] careful comparison of normal animals of various breeds to those with DCM reveals a sizable "grey area" of potential overlap between normal cardiac dimensions, function, and rhythm and parameters that clearly indicate that a diagnosis of "occult" DCM is justified.[129] The fate of individual asymptomatic dogs with these kinds of abnormalities is not known with certainty at this time.

Physical Examination. In dogs with clinical signs of DCM, a careful physical examination almost always reveals evidence of underlying heart disease. A protodiastolic (S_3) or presystolic (S_4) gallop is an important clinical finding that is most easily appreciated by using the bell of the stethoscope on dogs in sinus rhythm (although S_3 is often present in atrial fibrillation, recognition is complicated by the variable intensity of the heart sounds and the chaotic nature of the rhythm). Soft and often variable-intensity regurgitant systolic murmurs, typically grades 1–3 of 6, may be heard over the left and/or right atrioventricular valve regions in about one half of dogs with DCM. Soft murmurs and gallop sounds may be easily overlooked in dogs with atrial fibrillation or other rhythm disturbances. A variety of ventricular and supraventricular arrhythmias and conduction disturbances are observed in dogs with DCM, underscoring the importance of electrocardiogram (ECG) evaluation of all affected dogs.[7, 114–116, 153]

Rales or crackles and increased lung sounds may be auscultated in dogs with left heart failure and pulmonary edema. Jugular venous distention, jugular pulses, hepatomegaly, and ascites are easily detected in most dogs with right-sided heart failure. Equivocal findings of right heart failure may be clarified by measurement of central venous pressure (generally > 9 cm H_2O in untreated animals with right heart failure). In dogs with biventricular failure, the heart and lung sounds may be muffled as a result of pleural effusion. The arterial pulses are typically weak and are often irregular, with a pulse deficit due to accompanying atrial or ventricular tachyarrhythmias. Pulsus alternans, an alternating arterial pulse amplitude in the absence of cardiac arrhythmia, is an uncommon finding that usually signifies severe myocardial failure. Weight loss and muscle wasting are common but variable findings in dogs with DCM, and peripheral edema is unusual.

Electrocardiographic Changes. Most dogs with DCM have an abnormal ECG, although the changes may be subtle. High-amplitude or widened QRS complexes, indicating left ventricular enlargement, and widened P waves, indicating left atrial enlargement, are commonly observed in dogs with

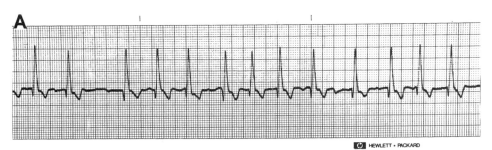

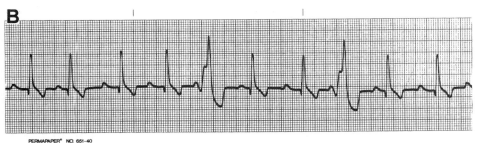

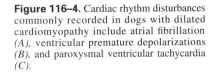

Figure 116–4. Cardiac rhythm disturbances commonly recorded in dogs with dilated cardiomyopathy include atrial fibrillation (A), ventricular premature depolarizations (B), and paroxysmal ventricular tachycardia (C).

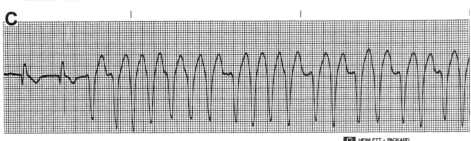

overt heart failure. Of greater clinical importance is the high prevalence of cardiac rhythm disturbances in dogs with DCM. Atrial fibrillation is a common rhythm disturbance reported to be present in as many as 75 to 80 per cent of some giant breed dogs with DCM[7, 114–116, 158] (Fig. 116–4). Other common rhythm disturbances include ventricular premature depolarizations (VPDs) and ventricular tachycardia. Ventricular rhythm disturbances are of particular concern in Boxers and Doberman pinschers, both of which suffer a high rate of sudden death associated with the development of DCM.[16–19] As many as 80 per cent of Dobermans with congestive heart failure manifest ventricular arrhythmias, especially VPDs, on resting ECGs.[16, 19] Using 24-hour ambulatory ECG (Holter) recordings, 81 per cent of asymptomatic Doberman pinschers with DCM had complex ventricular arrhythmias, and almost 30 per cent had sustained or nonsustained ventricular tachycardia.[19, 19a] The prevalence of ventricular tachycardia and VPDs in Boxers is similar to or greater than that observed in Dobermans, and they are often observed to have a left bundle branch block configuration on the ECG[18, 28] (Table 116–1). Although other arrhythmias and conduction disturbances occur in dogs with DCM, they are less common.

Radiographic Changes. The radiographic appearance of the heart often fails to reflect the severity of the underlying myocardial impairment. In breeds such as Doberman pinschers and Boxers, left atrial and left ventricular enlargement is usually present but may be overlooked unless radiographs are compared directly with those of known normals of the breed or cardiomegaly is accompanied by pulmonary venous enlargement or pulmonary edema (Fig. 116–5). Greater and more generalized cardiomegaly is typical in cocker spaniels and the other large and giant breed dogs

(Fig. 116–6). In these breeds, there is often evidence of right-sided or biventricular heart failure, including an enlarged caudal vena cava, hepatomegaly, ascites, or a large pleural effusion.

Hemodynamic and Angiographic Studies. Left heart catheterization and angiocardiography, though rarely performed in clinical practice, are helpful for illustrating the anatomic and functional changes resulting from DCM. Typical findings include increased left atrial and left ventricular

TABLE 116–1. PREVALENCE OF CARDIAC ARRHYTHMIAS AND CONDUCTION DISORDERS IN BOXER DOGS AND DOBERMAN PINSCHERS WITH DILATED CARDIOMYOPATHY

	PREVALENCE (% AFFECTED)	
	Boxer (n = 112)	Doberman (n = 39)
Supraventricular arrhythmias		
Premature depolarizations	18.8	7.7
Atrial tachycardia	8.0	N.R.
Atrial fibrillation	10.7	17.9
Ventricular arrhythmias		
Premature depolarizations	45.5	92.3
Ventricular tachycardia	38.4	40.0
Conduction disturbances		
Left bundle branch block	2.7	N.R.
Complete atrioventricular block	2.7	N.R.

N.R. = none recorded.
Modified from Harpster NK: Boxer cardiomyopathy: A review of the long-term benefits of antiarrhythmic therapy. Vet Clin North Am: Small Anim Pract 21:989, 1991; and Calvert CA: Dilated congestive cardiomyopathy in Doberman pinschers. Comp Contin Ed 8:417, 1986.

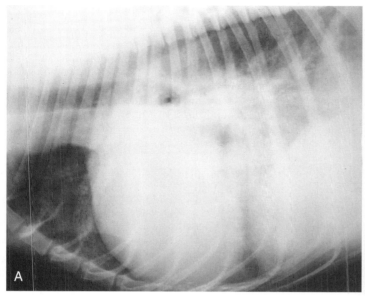

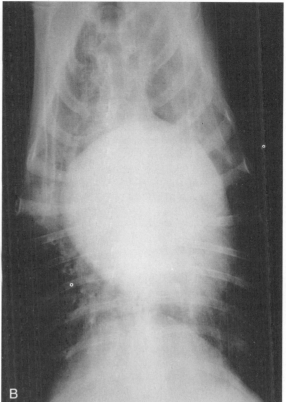

Figure 116–5. Lateral *(A)* and dorsoventral *(B)* radiographs from a Doberman pinscher with dilated cardiomyopathy. Cardiac enlargement is predominantly left-sided, and perihilar pulmonary edema is evident.

volumes, markedly diminished left ventricular ejection fraction, mild to moderate mitral regurgitation, decreased ventricular compliance, and elevated left atrial and left ventricular end-diastolic pressures.[116] Hemodynamic studies using a balloon-tipped Swan-Ganz thermodilution catheter positioned in the pulmonary artery, together with direct or indirect measures of systemic arterial pressure, are more clinically applicable and have been reported in a much larger number of dogs with DCM. Reported findings include decreased cardiac output and stroke volume, moderate to severe increases in pulmonary capillary wedge pressure, and modest proportional increase in pulmonary artery systolic and diastolic pressures.[161–154] Right atrial pressure is variable and dependent on the severity of right heart involvement, while arterial pressure is usually normal. Invasive hemodynamic monitoring is particularly useful to avoid serious hypotension when potent vasodilators are administered and to avoid excessive reductions in preload in dogs treated aggressively with diuretics.

Echocardiography. In dogs with DCM, echocardiogra-

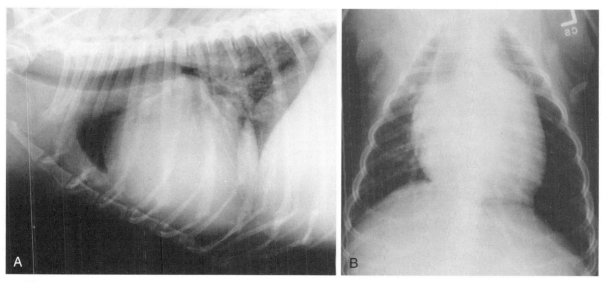

Figure 116–6. Lateral *(A)* and dorsoventral *(B)* radiographs from an American cocker spaniel with dilated cardiomyopathy show biventricular and biatrial enlargement.

phy is used to document and quantify myocardial dysfunction and to exclude other causes of heart disease such as primary acquired valvular or pericardial disease.[19, 129, 165–168] In humans, the clinical and echocardiographic diagnosis of DCM is presumably subject to greater error than in veterinary medicine, primarily because of the much higher prevalence of ischemic heart disease and possibly myocarditis, which can mimic DCM in humans.[186] The astute veterinarian should also keep these differential diagnoses for cardiac chamber dilatation and/or loss of systolic function in mind before rendering a definitive diagnosis of DCM, especially in small or otherwise atypical breeds. Chamber dilatation is easily recognized and quantified by either M-mode or two-dimensional measurements (Fig. 116–7). Short-axis end-systolic and end-diastolic dimensions of the left ventricle (LV), indexed for body weight, are usually much larger in dogs with DCM than in normal dogs. The walls of the LV are usually normal in thickness or slightly thinner than normal during diastole, but there is markedly decreased inward motion and thickening during systole. Generalized and symmetric LV hypokinesis is observed in most dogs with DCM, but dogs with concurrent moderate mitral regurgitation may show asymmetric contraction of the LV with greater septal than LV posterior wall motion. Excursions of the mitral valve leaflets are often diminished, and mitral valve closure may be delayed. An increased left atrial–aortic ratio results primarily from left atrial dilatation and, to a lesser extent, from reduced aortic diameter due to the reduced stroke volume. Right atrial and ventricular dimensions are increased in giant breeds and other dogs with biventricular failure but may be normal in dogs with predominant left heart involvement, especially Boxers and Doberman pinschers.

Echocardiography allows excellent noninvasive evaluation of LV systolic performance in dogs with DCM. Systolic ejection phase indices, such as LV fractional shortening, ejection fraction, and velocity of circumferential fiber shortening, are decreased in proportion to the severity of systolic dysfunction. The distance between the mitral valve at its maximal opening (E) point in early diastole and the interventricular septum (E point septal separation) is also increased as a result of a low ejection fraction. Mildly to moderately diminished ejection phase indices (fractional shortening 15 to 25 per cent) have been identified by Calvert in up to 46 per cent of asymptomatic Doberman pinschers, suggesting

the existence of occult myocardial disease and possibly a prolonged preclinical phase of DCM in this breed.[19] It is important to remember, however, that there may be significant overlap between the chamber dimensions and indices of systolic ventricular function in normal dogs and in dogs with "occult" cardiomyopathy, making indiscriminate echocardiographic "screening" hazardous until more is known regarding the natural history of these animals.[129]

Changes in ejection phase indices are frequently used to try to demonstrate the efficacy of drug therapy in groups of dogs or humans with DCM.[169, 170] However, it is important to understand the limitations of echocardiography and the low reliability of observed changes in ejection phase indices for determining prognosis or treatment response in an individual patient.[171, 172] Because of these limitations, therapeutic decisions are rarely based solely on echocardiographic measurements. Absence of echocardiographic changes with therapy does not preclude a beneficial therapeutic response, and improved echocardiographic measures are of little consolation to patients that are dying of pulmonary congestion or low-output heart failure. Echocardiographic findings may be more useful for prognostic purposes, as patient survival has been shown to correlate with the ejection phase indices in humans and dogs with DCM in some studies,[19, 173, 174] though not in all.[175] Systolic time intervals, including LV ejection time and pre-ejection period, can also be obtained noninvasively using echocardiography.[176, 177] Though rarely used in clinical practice, systolic time intervals have been effectively used to detect LV dysfunction in dogs and cats with DCM and to evaluate response to therapy.[176]

Spectral and color-flow Doppler echocardiography is also helpful in assessing cardiac function in dogs with DCM.[177] With these techniques, the presence and severity of valvular insufficiency can be quickly and noninvasively determined. Doppler indices of systolic performance derived from aortic flow velocity profiles, such as peak acceleration rate and time to peak acceleration, are reduced in humans and dogs with DCM.[178, 179] The value of these measurements relative to other ejection phase indices is uncertain, and the technology is not as widely available as two-dimensional imaging. Diastolic cardiac performance, which is cumbersome to assess by traditional M-mode and two-dimensional echocardiography, can be crudely assessed by evaluation of spectral Doppler mitral inflow velocity profiles. Preliminary studies

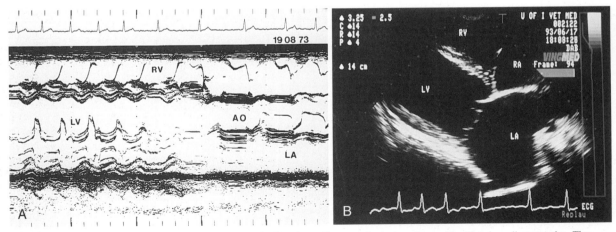

Figure 116–7. M-mode (A) and two-dimensional (B) echocardiograms from two dogs with dilated cardiomyopathy. The M-mode recording was obtained from a Great Dane with biventricular heart failure and shows a dilated right ventricle (RV), left ventricle (LV), and left atrium (LA). Fractional shortening is markedly decreased, and the amplitudes of LV, septal, and aortic (Ao) wall motion are diminished. The two-dimensional echocardiogram was obtained at end-systole and demonstrates dilated atria and increased end-systolic dimensions of the left and right ventricles.

in humans with DCM suggest that certain abnormalities of diastolic function, such as a prolonged relaxation time and increased early diastolic to atrial wave ratio, are associated with markedly reduced exercise tolerance and an adverse outcome (poor survival) in patients with DCM.[189]

Laboratory Findings. Clinical pathologic changes in dogs with DCM reflect the effects of low cardiac output, organ congestion, and neurohormonal activation.[14, 71, 156, 181] Serum electrolyte and protein concentrations are often in the normal range, but there may be mild hypoproteinemia, hyponatremia, hyperkalemia, and a decreased anion gap.[71] Other laboratory abnormalities include modestly elevated serum liver enzymes and bile acids, reduced bromosulphthalein clearance, and increased serum urea and creatinine concentrations in a small percentage of cases.[14, 71, 182-184] Serum thyroid concentrations are often depressed due to nonthyroidal systemic illness or altered protein binding.[71, 185] As a result of neurohormonal activation, increased serum norepinephrine concentrations and urine catecholamines are reported in dogs with advanced heart failure.[71, 156]

TREATMENT

Therapy for DCM can be considered in the context of the three-phase pathophysiologic model discussed earlier. Currently, with the exception of a small minority of cases in which carnitine or taurine deficiency appears to play a central role in the cause or progression of DCM, the apparent initiating or index event or injury (phase I) that causes DCM can rarely be identified, much less treated or prevented. Because identification of the cause of DCM offers the best hope of rational and effective treatment to eliminate the cause or reverse the myocardial damage caused by the event, highly motivated clients who wish to pursue every diagnostic and treatment avenue are best referred to one of the many centers researching the disease and offering state-of-the-art diagnostic testing to rule out known treatable causes of DCM.

If, as will be true in the vast majority of cases, no specific cause for the disease can be identified, some progress in prolonging survival and improving the quality of life of DCM patients (both dogs and humans) has been made by implementing therapy directed at minimizing the activation of the neurohormonal and genetic cascade of events (phase II) that contributes to the progression of systolic myocardial dysfunction and chamber dilatation in DCM (e.g., activation of the renin-angiotensin-aldosterone and sympathetic nervous systems).[164, 188-192] This pharmacologic "deactivation" of the physiologic responses to reduced cardiac output has been shown over time to improve not only the hemodynamics of heart failure but also the biologic properties of the myocardium itself to varying degrees.[97] Phase II therapy in canine DCM currently begins with an optimal dose of an angiotensin-converting enzyme (ACE) inhibitor (in the United States, enalapril is the only one approved by the Food and Drug Administration for use in dogs; in European Union countries, benazepril is also approved) to reduce the activation of the renin-angiotensin-aldosterone system. There are no placebo-controlled clinical trials in dogs with spontaneous DCM to document the benefits or define the hazards of beta blockers, digitalis glycosides, angiotensin II receptor blockers, neutral endopeptidase inhibitors, or calcium channel blockers—all classes of drugs known to potentially modify the neurohormonal imbalances that contribute to the pathophysiology of heart failure in DCM. Because there are

no definitive clinical studies of these important treatments in veterinary medicine, veterinarians must make informed judgments based on logical extrapolation from what is known about the pathophysiology of the disease and its treatment in humans or experimental canine models.[193-204]

Therapy for the hemodynamic manifestations (clinical signs) of heart failure (phase III) may include a potentially staggering (and sometimes confusing) array of pharmacologic interventions aimed at optimizing preload, afterload, heart rate, and rhythm and improving myocardial contractility to a degree that will allow comfortable routine existence. Keeping the pathophysiology of DCM in mind, it is important to remember that some drugs that favorably modify the hemodynamics of heart failure (e.g., ACE inhibitors causing modest acute reductions in preload and afterload)[163, 164, 193, 198, 205] also reduce the activity or effects of neurohormonal activation. Other drugs (e.g., furosemide causing dramatic preload reduction) that are strongly indicated for their lifesaving hemodynamic effects in acute, symptomatic heart failure (e.g., cardiogenic pulmonary edema) further activate the renin-angiotensin-aldosterone system,[206] making it desirable to limit their chronic use to the minimum needed to maintain the animal's quality of life. Treatment for heart failure must be tailored to the individual dog and owner, because no single drug or combination of drugs is effective or even feasible for every dog with DCM. Further discussion of congestive heart failure and its therapy can be found in Chapter 111.

Most dogs diagnosed in practice with DCM present because of signs of congestive heart failure (dyspnea and soft cough secondary to pulmonary edema and/or ascites or pleural effusion, or low-output signs such as weakness and lethargy). Parenteral or oral furosemide is used to reduce plasma volume and control congestive signs (pulmonary edema, pleural effusion, ascites) in dogs with DCM.[207] Intravenous administration (1 to 2 mg/lb) is indicated to relieve acute, life-threatening pulmonary edema, and oral therapy (0.5 to 1 mg/lb every 8 to 12 hours) is usually needed to control and prevent congestive signs in most dogs with chronic heart failure. Furosemide is a safe and effective drug for treating heart failure, but aggressive use of this drug can have adverse effects. The most common side effects are excessive reduction of preload, dehydration, decreased cardiac output, and azotemia. Electrolyte disorders, especially hypokalemia, are not common but can occur. Many of these problems can be minimized by using a lower dose of furosemide in combination with modest dietary sodium restriction and ACE inhibitors.[187] There is ample evidence in human medicine of the benefits of lower doses of furosemide combined with venodilators, or of lower doses given by continuous intravenous infusion—methods that have not been clinically investigated in dogs.[208-211] There is also intriguing evidence in people that long-term furosemide therapy may result in myocardial depression that may be reversed by thiamine supplementation.[212] Some dogs with DCM develop ascites or pleural effusion refractory to high doses of oral furosemide (2 to 4 mg/lb every eight hours). Furosemide absorption may be reduced in dogs with right heart failure. In this circumstance, furosemide should be administered parenterally (in combination with cage rest) or replaced by a better absorbed loop diuretic such as bumetanide.[213] Alternatively, fluid accumulations or edema that is refractory to furosemide alone can often be effectively managed by the addition of spironolactone,[214] a venodilator, or an increased dose (if possible without compromising renal function) of an ACE inhibitor.[215]

Digoxin is indicated in dogs with DCM and signs of heart failure.[216, 217] Although its effects are variable and difficult to quantify, digoxin has been shown to exert a significant positive inotropic effect in some dogs with DCM.[169] Digoxin is also moderately effective for slowing the ventricular rate in dogs with atrial fibrillation.[218] Digoxin reduces activation of the sympathetic nervous system and the renin-angiotensin-aldosterone system.[219] In several large clinical trials in humans, digoxin therapy reduced symptoms, improved exercise capacity, and decreased the risk of clinical deterioration of heart failure.[220–223] Studies of this magnitude are not likely to be duplicated in dogs.

Two other classes of positive inotropic drugs, beta-adrenergic agonists and phosphodiesterase inhibitors, both of which lack digoxin's ability to reduce the activity of the sympathetic nervous system, have been used effectively in the acute treatment of dogs with DCM.[224–228] However, none of these drugs is specifically approved for use in dogs. Both groups of drugs improve myocardial contractility by increasing the concentration of intracellular cyclic AMP. Beta-agonist drugs must be administered intravenously, and their use is limited to the short-term management of severe, refractory congestive heart failure. In this circumstance, dobutamine (1 to 5 μg/lb per minute) may be lifesaving, particularly when used in combination with vasodilators. Higher dosages often result in unacceptably high heart rates or ventricular arrhythmias. Treatment with dobutamine is usually limited to a few days owing to the rapid development of tolerance induced by down-regulation of cardiac beta-adrenergic receptors.

Two phosphodiesterase inhibitors, amrinone and milrinone, are approved for short-term intravenous therapy of heart failure in humans. Both drugs (sometimes referred to as "inodilators") are more potent inotropes than digoxin, and both possess substantial vasodilating properties. These agents do not act via the beta$_1$ receptor and therefore may be more effective than the beta agonists in replenishing depleted cyclic AMP levels and improving contractility in dogs with DCM. Kittleson et al. demonstrated that oral milrinone improves cardiac contractility, hemodynamic function, and clinical signs in dogs with DCM.[228] Based on these studies, milrinone appears to be an effective drug for short-term use in dogs with DCM. The suitability of milrinone for long-term therapy is controversial. Evidence of increased mortality in human patients receiving milrinone has generated concern that the same may be true in dogs.[229] Proponents of milrinone argue that this concern may not be relevant because dogs, unlike humans, rarely have coronary artery disease. Other promising (but commercially unavailable) positive inotropic drugs, such as pimobendan, increase the sensitivity of the myofilaments to calcium.[230, 231] A recent report of a relatively small clinical trial in Europe suggests that pimobendan has beneficial hemodynamic and possibly survival effects in refractory heart failure secondary to DCM in dogs.[232]

Placebo-controlled clinical trials have shown that dogs with DCM treated with diuretics and digoxin gain both a hemodynamic and a survival benefit from the additional use of the ACE inhibitor enalapril.[163, 164, 189] As reported in the Invasive Multicenter Prospective Veterinary Enalapril (IMPROVE) trial, the hemodynamic effects of enalapril (0.22 mg/lb [0.5 mg/kg] every 12 hours) in dogs with heart failure caused by DCM or chronic mitral regurgitation include small decreases in heart rate and pulmonary capillary wedge pressure.[163, 164] In a study of short duration (four weeks), investigators in the Cooperative Veterinary Enalapril (COVE) study group reported that enalapril, used in combination with conventional drugs (digoxin and furosemide), significantly reduced the clinical signs of heart failure and improved exercise tolerance in dogs with congestive heart failure due to DCM or mitral regurgitation.[189] In dogs, as in humans, these benefits appear to be sustained with chronic therapy.[188, 233–236] Lisinopril, ramipril, and benazepril have similar pharmacodynamic properties with minor pharmacokinetic differences from enalapril, whereas captopril has a much shorter pharmacodynamic half-life.[237] None of these alternative ACE inhibitors has been tested as extensively as enalapril in dogs with heart failure.

The use of direct-acting arterial vasodilators, such as hydralazine, in dogs with DCM is limited by their inability to decrease ventricular filling pressures and, with chronic administration, their tendency to activate neurohormonal reflexes.[162] By activating the sympathetic nervous system and stimulating the release of renin, these agents cause sodium and water retention and often a reflex tachycardia. In addition, hypotension is more likely to occur if myocardial failure is severe and the heart cannot increase its stroke output in response to arterial vasodilatation. However, combination therapy with hydralazine and a nitrate is an acceptable alternative for animals that do not tolerate ACE inhibitors.[188, 238] Hydralazine may also be useful adjunct therapy for dogs with persistent signs of heart failure following treatment with digoxin, furosemide, and ACE inhibitors. Other vasodilating drugs that do not trigger adverse neurohormonal responses, such as flosequinan, have been developed (but not approved) for use in humans but have not yet been evaluated in dogs.[239, 240] Unfortunately, flosequinan (like milrinone) was associated with excess mortality in the treatment versus placebo group, and a further study (PROFILE, the Prospective Randomized Flosequinan Longevity Evaluation) was also halted owing to excess mortality in the flosequinan group.[241]

Nitroprusside is an ultra-short-acting but extremely potent vasodilator that is primarily used to treat dogs with severe, life-threatening left heart failure and pulmonary edema. Beneficial hemodynamic effects of nitroprusside, including increased cardiac output and decreased pulmonary capillary wedge pressures, have been documented in dogs with spontaneous congestive heart failure due to DCM.[162] Nitroprusside must be administered by continuous intravenous infusion (0.5 to 5 μg/lb per minute) titrated to effect by monitoring arterial blood pressure and pulmonary capillary wedge pressure.

Calcium channel and beta-adrenergic receptor blocking drugs are frequently used in dogs with DCM and atrial fibrillation, because digoxin alone generally fails to adequately control the heart rate. Both drugs effectively reduce heart rate in this circumstance. Calcium antagonists and beta-adrenergic blocking drugs have also been advocated for treating heart failure patients, especially those with DCM, in sinus rhythm.[190–192, 242] Chronic treatment with beta-adrenergic blocking agents improves survival, exercise tolerance, quality of life, and hemodynamic parameters in humans with DCM and chronic heart failure.[190–192, 243–246] Despite efforts to predict which patients will respond best to beta-adrenergic blockade (those with the highest systolic arterial blood pressure and worst diastolic function),[247] this medical strategy has not yet been widely embraced in general human or veterinary practice, in part because of the potential acute detrimental hemodynamic and clinical effects of traditional (nonselective or beta$_1$ selective) beta blockade in some patients with severe heart failure. Nonetheless, evidence continues to mount that beta-adrenergic blocking drugs improve exercise capacity and prolong life in patients with DCM. Carvedilol has combined alpha$_1$ and nonselective beta-adrenergic blocking properties that give it a more favorable hemodynamic profile than standard beta-adrenergic blocking drugs for the chronic treatment of congestive heart failure.[244–246] Although not approved for use in dogs, the pharmacodynamics of carvedilol have been investigated in dogs,[248] and the hemodynamic effects are similar to those observed in humans (reductions in heart rate are accompanied by reductions in peripheral vascular resistance, in contrast to propranolol, which raises peripheral resistance, jeopardizing cardiac output). Convincing evidence exists that carvedilol improves both hemodynamics and survival in humans with DCM and mild, moderate, or severe heart failure.[192, 249] A small number of dogs with DCM in the authors' practices have been treated with carvedilol (starting at 1.5 mg every 12 hours) in addition to an ACE inhibitor, digoxin, and furosemide. The dosage is gradually titrated (doubled weekly) up to a maximal dose of 0.5 mg/lb every 12 hours. There is insufficient data or experience with carvedilol to make a general recommendation for its use in canine DCM at this time. It is also unknown whether its long-term effects on survival are actually superior to those of other beta-adrenergic receptor blockers.

The use of calcium antagonists in humans with heart failure is also controversial. Most of the calcium channel blocking drugs do not produce long-term symptomatic benefit, nor do they enhance exercise capacity.[250] Some of the calcium channel blocking drugs, notably verapamil and nifedipine, exacerbate signs of heart failure in humans owing to their inherent negative inotropic and chronotropic effects or increase the risk of sudden death as a result of reflex neurohormonal activation. Results using diltiazem are more encouraging.[242] Other calcium channel blockers such as amlodipine, which decreases sympathetic nervous activity, increase exercise capacity in humans with heart failure and appear to have beneficial acute hemodynamic (primarily afterload reducing) and potentially long-term survival benefits, at least in canine models of heart failure and in humans with nonischemic DCM (no survival benefit was demonstrated overall in the PRAISE [Prospective Randomized Amlodipine Survival Evaluation] study, but subgroup analysis of nonischemic DCM patients showed significant benefit).[204, 257, 259]

The use of antiarrhythmic drugs to treat dogs or humans with ventricular arrhythmias secondary to DCM is also controversial. There is no evidence that any Class I antiarrhythmic drug, including procainamide, quinidine, tocainide, or mexiletine, actually reduces the risk of sudden death in humans or dogs with heart failure. In humans, significant proarrhythmic effects and increased rates of sudden death have been reported with the use of some antiarrhythmic drugs.[251, 252] No controlled trials evaluating the safety or efficacy of antiarrhythmic drug therapy in dogs have been performed. Preliminary studies indicate the presence of proarrhythmic effects of some antiarrhythmic drugs in dogs,[253] but the prevalence of these effects and their impact on survival of dogs with heart disease are unknown. Tocainide was more effective in suppressing ventricular arrhythmias in Doberman pinschers than other Class I drugs tested, but there was no evidence of increased survival.[254] Preliminary data suggest improved survival of Boxers with DCM with the use of procainamide, usually in combination with propranolol.[18] Calvert et al. also reported in depth on their experience with tocainide, documenting apparently positive

clinical responses, with substantial adverse effects of long-term therapy.[255]

The authors' current philosophy is to recommend Holter monitoring when DCM is diagnosed in Doberman pinschers and Boxers (breeds with known high risk for sudden death). The authors treat dogs with DCM and symptomatic arrhythmias (syncope or episodic weakness associated with arrhythmia), sustained ($>$30 second) episodes of ventricular tachycardia, or other serious complex ventricular ectopy thought to pose a serious risk of sudden death (frequent, rapid, polymorphic nonsustained ventricular tachycardia, frequent R on T phenomenon, and so forth)[255, 256] on Holter examination. In otherwise asymptomatic dogs, atenolol (or another beta-adrenergic receptor blocker) is started. Holter monitoring is repeated, and the owner is asked to keep a diary (similar to a seizure diary) and note any episodes of weakness or syncope. If the arrhythmia persists, a Class I drug, usually procainamide, is administered (see Chapter 49). Refractory arrhythmias are treated by discontinuing the Class I drug and administering sotalol.[258] Mexiletine and tocainide may also be effective for treating some otherwise resistant ventricular arrhythmias.[255] Noncomplex and infrequent VPDs on a resting ECG are not treated or are further evaluated by 24-hour ambulatory ECG recordings. Several clinical trials of amiodarone as well as implantable defibrillators are ongoing. The applicability of all these trials to DCM in dogs is unknown, because many of the human patients studied have a presumably different arrhythmogenic substrate (ischemic heart disease and previous myocardial infarction).

In addition to the traditional pharmacologic therapy of heart failure secondary to DCM discussed earlier, two surgical approaches to therapy have been published in the veterinary literature. Dynamic cardiomyoplasty transposes the right latissimus dorsi muscle into the thoracic cavity, where an electronic myostimulator is implanted into the muscle, and the muscle is wrapped around the failing heart. The muscle is then "trained" over a period of approximately two months, after which cardiosynchronous stimulation provides the heart with a muscular assist approximately every third beat. In the single case reported by Orton and colleagues at Colorado State University, the cardiomyoplasty was successful, and the dog (a 5-year-old Rhodesian ridgeback with severe DCM) recovered nearly completely and was alive 22 months after the report.[260, 261]

The second surgical method involved the use by White and colleagues in Great Britain of the left latissimus dorsi muscle, which was similarly transposed and stimulated but wrapped instead around the descending aorta and pulsed counter to the heartbeat instead of synchronously with it. This method met with some significant technical difficulty and perioperative mortality but also showed promise in the four dogs (of seven) in which it worked.[262] Although these novel approaches have no practical application at this time in general practice, their refinement over the coming years could represent a serious new form of therapy for canine DCM.

A variety of "alternative" or neutraceutical therapies for DCM have also been advocated or are commercially available. There are no clinical trials to support any of these products. Coenzyme Q-10 is being marketed for use in canine DCM and heart failure in general. The results of small clinical trials of coenzyme Q-10 in humans are inconclusive, with some trials showing benefit[263, 264] and other well-controlled small trials failing to show benefit or showing very modest benefit.[265, 266] There are few hard data in the literature regarding vitamin E and cardiomyopathy.[267]

CV

PROGNOSIS

The diagnosis of DCM can be devastating to clients, because there is currently no cure available for the vast majority of dogs with DCM, and spontaneous recovery from this disorder has not been reported, although a few asymptomatic (or minimally symptomatic) animals may survive for years with the disease. Death most commonly results from progressive, intractable heart failure or malignant arrhythmia. The overall probability of one-year survival from recent multibreed retrospective analyses varied from 17.5 to 37.5 per cent, and at two years from 7.5 to 28 per cent.[175, 268] Median survival varied from 27 to 65 days between the two analyses, presumably at least in part owing to a higher incidence of euthanasia at the time of diagnosis in Sweden. The prognosis of any individual is difficult to predict, because some very ill dogs (requiring intravenous inotropic and vasodilator support) improve to a remarkable degree with treatment and live comfortably for many months or even years. Other dogs do not survive the initial 48 hours of hospitalization. The prognosis appears to be much better for American cocker spaniels, especially those treated with a combination of carnitine and taurine, than for most dogs with DCM.[105] Various retrospective studies have examined the prognosis of dogs with DCM, and the dramatic differences in their findings highlight the cultural differences in the treatment of dogs, as well as potential differences in the actual progression or severity of the disease and/or the success with which it is treated.[15–18, 175, 268] Prognosis estimates vary with breed, severity of disease, and presence and severity of some signs of heart failure, including dyspnea (pulmonary edema) and ascites, or biventricular failure. In some studies, younger age is a poor prognostic indicator.[175] Statistically significant indicators of poor prognosis in both of the two largest multibreed studies (one from Colorado[268] and one from Sweden[175]) were the presence of pulmonary edema, pleural effusion, or ascites. Common echocardiographic indices of systolic ventricular function, such as fractional shortening, were not good predictors of survival in either study. Some dogs with echocardiographic evidence of decreased myocardial contractility, but with no clinical signs of congestive heart failure, may live for a very long time. Data from a recent study by Koch et al. in Denmark emphasize that there is an echocardiographic overlap between individual normal dogs (followed in this study for at least four years) and those that go on to develop cardiomyopathy, necessitating caution when diagnosing "occult" DCM.[129]

Studies in humans have identified a number of risk factors for reduced survival in DCM, including increased heart size, decreased ejection fraction, increased norepinephrine levels, decreased exercise capacity, and evidence of restricted diastolic filling.[269–275] Four independent predictors of sudden death identified in humans with DCM include LV ejection fraction, cardiac output, number of paired VPDs per 24 hours, and presence of atrial fibrillation.[275]

A worse average prognosis has been reported for Doberman pinschers with symptomatic DCM.[16] Recent retrospective studies showed that survival after diagnosis is shorter in Doberman pinschers with DCM than in other breeds in some locations (Canada),[276] although breed differences in survival were not documented in Sweden and did not reach significance in the Colorado study.[175, 268] At initial examination, the average LV shortening fraction measured in Doberman pinschers is significantly lower than in other breeds. Survival of Doberman pinschers with DCM has been reported to correlate inversely with the severity of myocardial failure as measured by LV end-systolic dimension.[277] This dependence of survival on shortening fraction or chamber dimensions has not been found in all studies,[175] and the response to medical therapy and the subsequent clinical course of DCM in any individual dog is extremely variable and difficult to predict from any single finding. In dogs with severe heart failure at the time of presentation, a prudent approach is to recommend medical therapy and evaluate the initial response before rendering a tentative prognosis.[278]

CANINE HYPERTROPHIC CARDIOMYOPATHY

Hypertrophic cardiomyopathy (HCM) describes primary myocardial disorders characterized by the presence of a nondilated, hypertrophied left ventricle in the absence of a perivalvular or systemic illness that could cause LV hypertrophy.[1, 2] Human patients with HCM are further classified into two categories: those with dynamic left ventricular outflow tract (LVOT) obstruction, and those without. This definition of HCM is intended to exclude individuals with fixed LVOT obstruction, severe systemic hypertension, or one of the many metabolic disorders or endocrinopathies capable of inducing LV hypertrophy.[318]

INCIDENCE AND DEMOGRAPHICS

In stark contrast to the situation in cats, HCM appears to be a rare disease in dogs.[116, 279–287] The number of reported cases is too low to draw conclusions regarding age, sex, and breed predispositions. Of 10 dogs reported by Liu et al. to have HCM at necropsy, eight were males and four were German shepherd dogs.[279, 280] Most of the dogs identified by the authors (unpublished observations) have been rottweilers or Dalmatians, but a number of other breeds have been recognized, including a Walker hound, a cocker spaniel, a Pointer, several Boston terriers, a Rhodesian ridgeback, and a Shih Tzu. Most of these dogs were males, and most were identified before reaching 3 years of age.

PATHOLOGY

The most consistent feature of HCM is marked idiopathic concentric LV hypertrophy, usually with a small LV cavity (Fig. 116–8). As a result, the heart weight to body weight ratio is usually increased. The hypertrophy may be symmetric or asymmetric.[288–290] Asymmetric septal hypertrophy, wherein septal thickness greatly exceeds LV wall thickness, was once the only recognized form of HCM in humans. This pattern of hypertrophy is still observed in most human cases, but it is now well established that the distribution of hypertrophy in the left ventricle can be extremely variable.[288–292] Some recurring patterns of hypertrophy recognized as part of the HCM complex in humans include symmetric LV hypertrophy, apical hypertrophy, and focal hypertrophy of the base or middle region of the interventricular septum.[292, 293] One of the most prominent pathologic features of HCM in humans is disarray or malalignment of myofibers in the hypertrophied septum or LV free wall (see Fig. 116–8). Myocardial fiber disarray is now cited as the most consistent feature of HCM in humans, lending credence to the hypothesis that this disease is primarily a disease of the sarcomere.[290]

Obstructive and nonobstructive forms of HCM are also

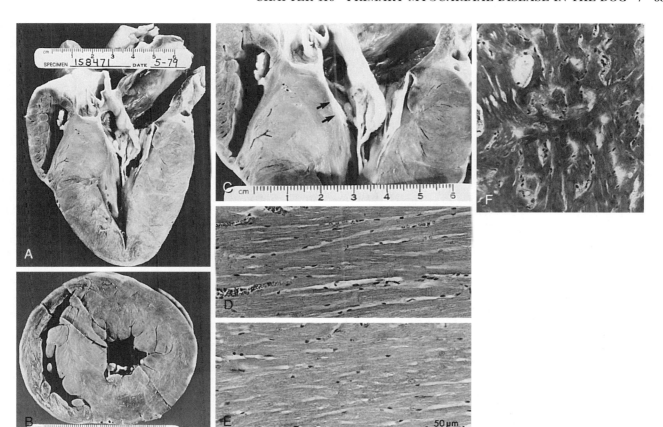

Figure 116–8. Pathology of the obstructive form of hypertrophic cardiomyopathy in a Walker hound. Gross photographs (A–C) show marked left ventricular hypertrophy, a small left ventricular cavity, and a fibrous plaque on the septal endocardium opposite a thickened and fibrotic mitral valve. Normally arranged myocardial fibers were found in sections from the septum and left ventricular free wall (D and E, respectively) (H&E; magnification 125×). F, Disorganized myofibers are shown in a section of myocardium from the septum of another dog with hypertrophic cardiomyopathy (H&E; magnification: 100×). D and E from Thomas WP, et al: Hypertrophic obstructive cardiomyopathy in a dog: Clinical, angiographic, and pathologic studies. J Am Anim Heart Assoc 20:253, 1984; F from Liu S-K, et al: Canine hypertrophic cardiomyopathy. JAVMA 174:708, 1979.)

recognized. In the obstructive form of the disease, abnormal systolic anterior motion (SAM) of the mitral valve toward the interventricular septum narrows and obstructs the outflow tract.[283, 290] As a result, a fibrous endocardial plaque develops on the septum directly opposite a thickened anterior mitral valve leaflet (see Fig. 116–8). Although this abnormality of LV ejection is now recognized to occur occasionally in other diseases and circumstances, it remains highly suggestive of HCM.[294, 295] Development of SAM was once attributed solely to narrowing of the LVOT from septal hypertrophy, but it now appears that malpositioning or malformation of the mitral valve apparatus also contributes to LVOT obstruction. A variety of structural mitral valve alterations have been documented in humans with HCM, suggesting that HCM is not simply a disease of the myocardium.[296, 297]

Based on the authors' observations and the pathologic findings reported in a small number of dogs, HCM in dogs appears to differ from the human disease in several important respects. In contrast to humans, disproportionate hypertrophy of the septum and myocardial fiber disarray are observed infrequently in dogs with HCM.[279–283] Dynamic LVOT obstruction has been observed in most of the dogs with HCM examined by the authors. Intramural coronary arteries in the LV wall, septum, and papillary muscles are often abnormal, with proliferative and degenerative changes of the intima and media. Similar changes are observed in the intramural coronary arteries of humans with HCM and dogs with sub-

aortic stenosis (SAS).[290, 294, 298] Focal areas of myocardial necrosis, fibrosis, and dystrophic calcification may be observed in the papillary muscles, the septum, and the LV wall. It must be emphasized that a reliable diagnosis of HCM in dogs requires more than the finding of LV hypertrophy at necropsy. Pathologic findings must be interpreted in association with clinical studies to exclude other causes of LV hypertrophy.

The relationship between HCM and fixed SAS in dogs is uncertain.[294, 299] It is of interest that approximately half of the HCM cases reported in dogs involved breeds (rottweiler, German shepherd, and Boxer) predisposed to congenital fixed subvalvular aortic stenosis.[5, 294, 299, 300] SAS in dogs was described in early reports as a discrete fibrous obstruction encircling the LVOT a variable distance below the aortic valve.[293] More recent observations suggest that the morphology of SAS in dogs is more diverse.[301] In some dogs, the obstructing subvalvular lesion is a less distinct fibromuscular bulge occupying the base of the interventricular septum (Fig. 116–9). Also, some dogs with fixed SAS show dynamic LVOT obstruction. Further complicating the distinctions between SAS and HCM is the observation that mitral valve dysplasia commonly coexists with SAS in dogs, offering a plausible explanation for the dynamic LVOT obstruction observed in some dogs with SAS.[288, 294, 301] Clearly, consideration must be given to the possibility that some cases of suspected HCM in dogs represent a muscular variant of

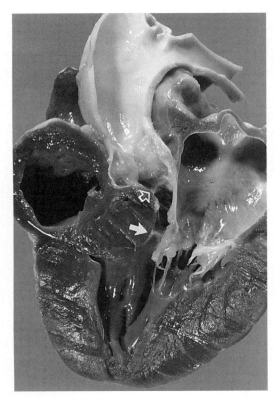

Figure 116–9. Dynamic obstruction of the left ventricular outflow tract in a golden retriever dog with mild fixed subvalvular aortic stenosis *(open arrow)*. Dynamic obstruction due to systolic apposition of the mitral valve with the malformed muscular base of the interventricular septum is evidenced by a linear fibrous plaque on the endocardium *(solid arrow)*. (From Buoscio D, et al: An unusual form of subvalvular aortic stenosis in golden retriever dogs. J Am Anim Hosp Assoc, in press.)

congenital SAS or an unusual consequence of a malformed mitral valve.

PATHOGENESIS AND ETIOLOGY

The cause of HCM in dogs is uncertain, although a heritable basis is suspected in most cases. Breeding studies performed by one of the authors demonstrated the heritability of dynamic LVOT obstruction and LV hypertrophy in Pointer dogs.[285] A polygenic or autosomal recessive pattern of inheritance best explained the observed pattern of occurrence in this study. Neither the propositus nor any of the offspring had evidence of fixed SAS. Approximately 60 per cent of human HCM cases are familial (usually autosomal dominant inheritance), and the remainder are sporadic.[302, 303] A variety of different mutations on seven different genes, all encoding sarcomeric proteins, have been associated with human familial HCM.[303–305] Geisterfer-Lowrance et al. working at Harvard Medical School have documented the fact that these mutations actually cause the clinical HCM phenotype by introducing one such mutation into a mouse model of beta-myosin heavy chain–induced HCM.[306]

PATHOPHYSIOLOGY

The two main functional abnormalities in humans with HCM are impaired diastolic filling and dynamic LVOT obstruction.[289, 290, 302] Diastolic dysfunction results from the combined influences of decreased chamber size, increased wall thickness, intrinsic changes in wall stiffness, and reduced rate and uniformity of ventricular relaxation in early diastole.[289, 302] These abnormalities are accentuated at rapid heart rates. Altered diastolic filling is the most pervasive hemodynamic change in patients with HCM because it is abnormal in patients with and without LVOT obstruction. The consequences of diastolic dysfunction include an impaired ability to increase cardiac output during stress or exercise, and pulmonary congestion and edema owing to increased left atrial and pulmonary venous pressures.

In dogs with the obstructive form of HCM, LV ejection is abnormal.[283] Although exceptions have been noted, obstruction typically occurs in early to mid-systole from systolic apposition of the mitral valve to the septum. This abnormality of mitral motion usually also causes mild to moderate mitral regurgitation. The cardinal features of this form of obstruction are the variability and lability of the resulting systolic pressure gradient. Physiologic changes or interventions that tend to reduce LV end-systolic volume, including increased contractility or reduced preload or afterload, tend to augment the severity of the obstruction. The consequences of LVOT obstruction are increased wall stress, increased myocardial oxygen consumption, reduced coronary blood flow, and myocardial ischemia, all of which are also worsened at rapid heart rates.[302] The extent to which dynamic LVOT obstruction acts as a stimulus to myocardial hypertrophy is unknown. It remains a topic for lively debate whether the dynamic obstruction is the primary disorder and the LV hypertrophy is secondary, or vice versa.

CLINICAL MANIFESTATIONS

The clinical signs reported in dogs with HCM are variable. Some dogs show no signs, and others exhibit exertional fatigue, tachypnea, cough, syncope, or sudden death. The clinical diagnosis of HCM is usually made during evaluation of a heart murmur or arrhythmia detected during physical examination. Systolic murmurs of variable intensity are heard over the left heart base or the apex (mitral area). Murmurs may be absent at rest but may be provoked by exercise, excitement, or short-acting pharmacologic agents that increase contractility or reduce afterload (isoproterenol, amyl nitrate). In the absence of these physical findings, a diagnosis of HCM may be easily overlooked.

Electrocardiographic and Radiographic Changes. Evidence of left atrial and ventricular enlargement may be present on a standard 10-lead ECG, but the prevalence of this observation is unknown. Arrhythmias reported in a small number of dogs with HCM include ventricular premature beats, paroxysmal ventricular tachycardia, and first-degree and third-degree atrioventricular block.[279–283] Thoracic radiographs usually show modest to moderate left atrial and ventricular enlargement and may show enlargement of the pulmonary veins and pulmonary edema (Fig. 116–10).

Echocardiography. The principal echocardiographic feature of HCM is concentric LV hypertrophy. The extent and distribution of hypertrophy are variable, but it is usually global, and asymmetric septal hypertrophy (septal–free wall thickness ratio >1.3) is not pronounced in dogs. Other findings include normal or reduced LV chamber dimensions, increased left atrial size, systolic anterior motion (SAM) of the mitral valve and narrowing of the LVOT, and partial systolic closure and coarse fluttering of the aortic valve (Fig. 116–11). Spectral Doppler echocardiography and two-dimensional color-flow mapping are useful for confirming

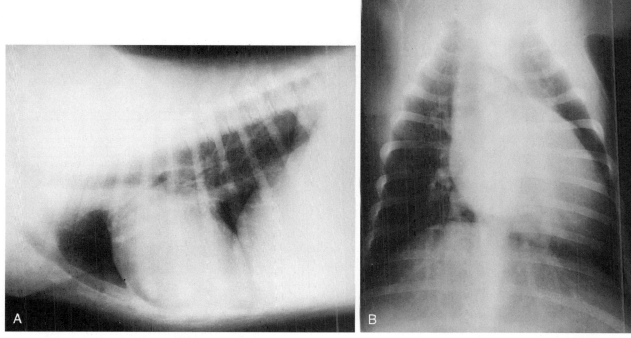

Figure 116–10. Lateral *(A)* and dorsoventral *(B)* radiographs of a dog with hypertrophic cardiomyopathy, showing moderate left heart enlargement. (From Thomas WP, et al: Hypertrophic obstructive cardiomyopathy in a dog: Clinical, angiographic, and pathologic studies. J Am Anim Heart Assoc 20:253, 1984.)

the presence and severity of LVOT obstruction and mitral regurgitation. In humans, diastolic LV function is evaluated by measurement of the isovolumetric relaxation time, peak filling rate, time to peak filling rate, and absolute and relative amplitudes of early diastolic and atrial peak flow velocities at the mitral valve orifice.[289, 302] Studies of these diastolic parameters have not been reported in dogs with HCM.

Hemodynamic and Angiographic Studies. Left ventricular angiography is useful for demonstrating the pattern and severity of LV hypertrophy, the presence of dynamic obstruction, and the severity of mitral regurgitation (Fig. 116–12).[116, 302] Obstruction is often absent in anesthetized dogs but can be provoked by drugs or physical maneuvers

(see Fig. 116–12). Diastolic dysfunction causes increased LV diastolic pressure and prominence of the atrial "a" wave.

TREATMENT AND PROGNOSIS

Too few dogs have been evaluated to define the natural history of this disease, but sudden death and congestive heart failure have been reported at a variety of ages.[171–173] Survival to at least middle age without clinical signs has also been documented. Treatment of HCM in dogs has not been reported.[285, 285, 294] The goals of treatment in humans with HCM are to improve diastolic filling, alleviate congestive signs,

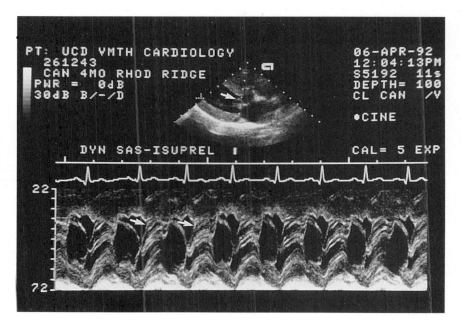

Figure 116–11. Two-dimensionally guided M-mode echocardiogram from a dog with the obstructive form of hypertrophic cardiomyopathy recorded during the infusion of isoproterenol. Systolic anterior motion of the mitral valve with systolic apposition with the septum (S) is apparent *(arrows)* on the M-mode recording.

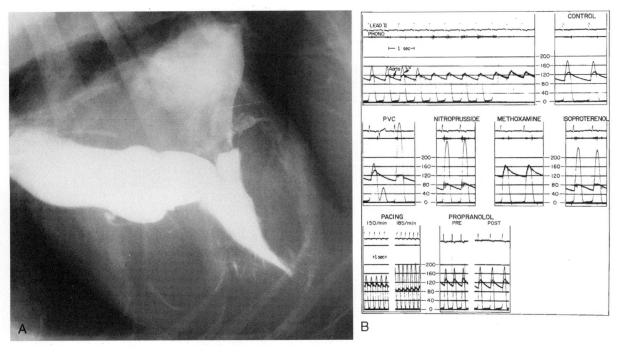

Figure 116–12. *A,* Left ventricular angiogram recorded at end-systole from a dog with hypertrophic cardiomyopathy. The walls of the left ventricle are thick, the left ventricular cavity is small, and systolic anterior motion of the mitral valve causes obstruction of the left ventricular outflow tract and mitral regurgitation. *B,* Hemodynamics of obstructive hypertrophic cardiomyopathy in a dog. The upper left panel demonstrates a mild initial obstructive gradient (40 mmHg). Remaining panels show the augmentation of the gradient and decreased aortic pulse pressure following a premature ventricular contraction, infusion of nitroprusside and isoproterenol, and rapid pacing. The gradient is abolished by infusion of methoxamine but is unaffected by infusion of propranolol. (From Thomas WP, et al: Hypertrophic obstructive cardiomyopathy in a dog: Clinical, angiographic, and pathologic studies. J Am Anim Heart Assoc 20:253, 1984.)

reduce or abolish obstructive gradients, control arrhythmias, and prevent sudden death. Beta-adrenoreceptor blocking drugs, such as propranolol, are used to reduce dynamic LVOT obstruction, slow the heart rate, and improve diastolic filling.[307, 308] The calcium channel blocker verapamil also reduces dynamic obstruction by its negative inotropic effects.[309] More importantly, verapamil improves diastolic filling by improving ventricular relaxation and reducing heart rate.[310] Diastolic dysfunction also improves with diltiazem, but this drug is less effective for reducing outflow obstruction because it causes less myocardial depression.[310, 311] Calcium channel blockers are preferred by some for treating the nonobstructive form of HCM because of their effects on ventricular relaxation and diastolic filling. In addition, diuretics are often used to control pulmonary edema. The value of antiarrhythmic drug therapy in humans with HCM is controversial.[312, 313] There is no conclusive evidence that antiarrhythmic drugs improve survival. In recent years, Class III antiarrhythmic drugs, such as amiodarone, have been advocated for treating symptomatic and life-threatening arrhythmias in affected humans.[314]

Surgical myectomy of the asymmetrically hypertrophied region of the upper interventricular septum is an effective treatment in humans with obstructive HCM.[315] This operation often eliminates the LVOT pressure gradient and abolishes coexisting mitral regurgitation. Surgery is reported to reduce symptoms, improve exercise capacity, and possibly prolong life in such patients.[316] Dual-chamber artificial pacing has also been shown to reduce LVOT obstruction and reduce symptoms in humans.[317] These effects are dependent in part on the programmed atrioventricular interval and appear to result from paradoxic septal motion induced by the altered sequence of ventricular activation.[316] In some pa-

tients, this beneficial effect persists after pacing is discontinued.[317]

CANINE RESTRICTIVE CARDIOMYOPATHY

Restrictive-infiltrative myocardial disease is the third major category of idiopathic myocardial disease. The pathologic features of this group of diseases in humans are diverse, but the primary functional consequence is diminished myocardial compliance and impaired diastolic filling. Specific diseases reported to cause restrictive myocardial disease in humans, such as amyloidosis, sarcoidosis, hemochromatosis, and eosinophilic or fibrosing endomyocardial disease, have not been reported in dogs.

CANINE ATRIOVENTRICULAR MYOPATHY

Atrioventricular myopathy (AVM) is a progressive idiopathic myocardial disease of dogs that may or may not be associated with a poorly characterized form of shoulder girdle skeletal muscular dystrophy. Miller et al. divided animals with AVM into two clinical groups—one associated with skeletal muscular dystrophy, and the other associated with long-standing cardiac disease of many types.[319] Tilley and Liu listed a third category for cases without evidence of other pathology.[320] The distinguishing features of these various groups are not clearly defined, and pathologic findings may vary with the stage of the disease. The unique features of this disorder include the marked degree of myocardial destruction and fibrosis and the characteristic bradyarrhythmias that result. Pathologic studies often reveal dilated, thin, almost transparent atria with little or no visible muscle.[319, 320] Involvement of the ventricles, especially the right ventricle, occurs somewhat later and is more variable. Histologic findings include variable amounts of mononuclear infiltration, myofiber necrosis and disappearance, and extensive replacement fibrosis. In dogs with muscular dystrophy, changes in skeletal muscle include muscle atrophy, hyalinized degenerated muscle fibers, and mild to moderate steatosis. A similar cardiac disorder has been observed in human patients with Emery-Dreyfuss (scapulohumeral) muscular dystrophy.[322-325]

The most commonly affected dogs are English springer spaniels and Old English sheepdogs. Affected dogs are usually presented for weakness, collapse, or syncope caused by severe bradycardia.[319, 321] Less commonly, dogs present with signs of right or biventricular congestive heart failure. Soft murmurs of atrioventricular valve insufficiency are audible in many cases. The most common ECG abnormality is persistent atrial standstill, but complete heart block and other rhythm and conduction disturbances may occur. Atrial enlargement is often found on thoracic radiographs, and generalized cardiomegaly is present in some dogs. Dilated, immobile atria can be identified by echocardiography or fluoroscopy. The clinical course is usually characterized by declining contractility, progressive ventricular dilatation, and eventually heart failure. Treatment of the bradyarrhythmia by artificial pacemaker implantation usually results in immediate improvement in clinical signs, but most dogs eventually develop refractory myocardial failure.

REFERENCES

1. Richardson P, et al: Report of the 1995 World Health Organization/International Society and Federation of Cardiology Task Force on the Definition and Classification of Cardiomyopathies. Circulation 93:841, 1996.
2. Goodwin JF: Cardiomyopathies and specific heart muscle diseases. Definitions, terminology, classifications, and new and old approaches. Postgrad Med J 68(suppl 1): s3, 1992.
3. Lord PF: Left ventricular diastolic stiffness in dogs with congestive cardiomyopathy and volume overload. Am J Vet Res 37:953, 1976.
4. Towbin JA: The role of cytoskeletal proteins in cardiomyopathies. Curr Opin Cell Biol 10:131, 1998.
5. Buchanan JW: Causes and prevalence of cardiovascular disease. In Kirk RW, Bonagura JD (eds): Kirk's Current Veterinary Therapy XI. Philadelphia, WB Saunders, 1992, pp 647–655.
6. Fioretti M, Delli Carri E: Epidemiological survey of dilatative cardiomyopathy in dogs (abstract). Veterinaria 2:81, 1988.
7. Sisson D, Thomas WP: Myocardial diseases of dogs and cats. In Ettinger S (ed): Textbook of Veterinary Internal Medicine, 4th ed. Philadelphia, WB Saunders, 1995, pp 995–1032.
8. Redfield MM, et al: Natural history of idiopathic dilated cardiomyopathy: Effect of referral bias and secular trend. J Am Coll Cardiol 22:1921, 1993.
8a. Thomas RE: Congestive cardiac failure in young cocker spaniels (a form of cardiomyopathy?): Details of eight cases. J Small Anim Pract 28:265, 1987.
9. Gooding JP, et al: Echocardiographic characterization of dilatation cardiomyopathy in the English cocker spaniel. Am J Vet Res 47:1936, 1986.
10. Miller MW, et al: ECG of the month. JAVMA 192:336, 1988.
11. Gooding JP, et al: A cardiomyopathy in the English cocker spaniel: A clinicopathological investigation. J Small Anim Pract 23:133, 1982.
12. Staaden RV: Cardiomyopathy of English cocker spaniels. JAVMA 178:1289, 1981.
13. Freeman LM, et al: Idiopathic dilated cardiomyopathy in dalmatians: Nine cases (1990–1995). JAVMA 209:1592, 1996.
14. Tidholm A, Jonsson L: A retrospective study of canine dilated cardiomyopathy (189 cases). J Am Anim Hosp Assoc 33:544, 1997.
15. Tidholm A, Jonsson L: Dilated cardiomyopathy in the Newfoundland: A study of 37 cases (1983–1994). J Am Anim Hosp Assoc 32:465, 1996.
16. Calvert CA, et al: Signalment, survival, and prognostic factors in Doberman pinschers with end-stage cardiomyopathy. J Vet Intern Med 11:323, 1997.
17. O'Grady MJ, et al: Occult dilated cardiomyopathy: An echocardiographic and electrocardiographic study of 193 asymptomatic Doberman pinschers (abstract). J Vet Intern Med 6:112, 1992.
18. Harpster NK: Boxer cardiomyopathy: A review of the long-term benefits of antiarrhythmic therapy. Vet Clin North Am Small Anim Pract 21:989, 1991.
19. Calvert CA, et al: Clinical and pathological findings in Doberman pinschers with occult cardiomyopathy that died suddenly or developed congestive heart failure: 54 cases (1984–1991). JAVMA 210:505, 1997.
19a. Calvert C: Long-term electrocardiographic (Holter) monitoring as an aid in the diagnosis of occult cardiomyopathy in Doberman pinschers. Proceedings of the Ninth Annual Veterinary Medical Forum, 1991, pp 691–692.
20. Tilley LP, Liu SK: Cardiomyopathy in the dog. Recent Adv Stud Cardiac Struct Metab 10:641, 1975.
21. Van Vleet JF, et al: Pathologic alterations in congestive cardiomyopathy of dogs. Am J Vet Res 42:416, 1981.
22. Sandusky GE Jr, et al: Histological and ultrastructural evaluation of cardiac lesions in idiopathic cardiomyopathy in dogs. Can J Comp Med 48:81, 1984.
23. Lombard CW, Buergelt CD: Endocardial fibroelastosis in four dogs. J Am Anim Hosp Assoc 20:271, 1984.
24. Robinson WS, Maxie MG: The cardiovascular system. In Jubb KVF, Kennedy PC, Palmer N (eds): Pathology of Domestic Animals. New York, Academic Press, 1993, pp 37–38.
25. Tidholm A, et al: Prevalence of attenuated wavy fibers in myocardium of dogs with dilated cardiomyopathy. JAVMA 212:1732, 1998.
26. Aretz HT: Myocarditis: The Dallas criteria. Hum Pathol 18:619, 1987.
27. Keene BW, et al: Myocarditis in canine dilated cardiomyopathy (abstract). J Vet Intern Med 7:118, 1993.
28. Harpster NK: Boxer cardiomyopathy. In Kirk RW (ed): Kirk's Current Veterinary Therapy VIII. Philadelphia, WB Saunders, 1983, pp 329–337.
29. Marcus IF, et al: Right ventricular dysplasia: A report of 24 adult cases. Circulation 65:384, 1982.
30. Nava A, et al: Familial occurrence of right ventricular dysplasia: A study involving nine families. J Am Coll Cardiol 12:1222, 1988.
31. Thiene G, et al: Right ventricular cardiomyopathy and sudden death in young people. N Engl J Med 318:129, 1988.
32. Corrado D, et al: Spectrum of clinicopathologic manifestations of arrhythmogenic right ventricular cardiomyopathy/dysplasia: A multicenter study. J Am Coll Cardiol 30:1512, 1997.
33. Pinamonti B, et al: Left ventricular involvement in right ventricular cardiomyopathy. Eur Heart J 10(suppl D):20, 1989.
34. Simpson KW, et al: Right ventricular cardiomyopathy in a dog. J Vet Intern Med 8:306, 1994.
35. Bright JM, McEntee M: Isolated right ventricular cardiomyopathy in a dog. JAVMA 207:64, 1995.
36. Van Fleet J, Ferrans VJ: Myocardial diseases of animals. Am J Pathol 124:98, 1986.
37. Bishop L: Ultrastructural investigations of cardiomyopathy in the dog. J Comp Pathol 96:685, 1986.
38. Leiden JM: The genetics of dilated cardiomyopathy—emerging clues to the puzzle. N Engl J Med 337:1080, 1997.
39. Beggs AH: Dystrophinopathy, the expanding phenotype. Dystrophin abnormalities in X-linked dilated cardiomyopathy. Circulation 95:2344, 1997.
40. Muntoni F, et al: Deletion of the dystrophin muscle-promoter region associated with X-linked dilated cardiomyopathy. N Engl J Med 329:921, 1993.
41. Valentine BA, et al: Development of Duchenne-type cardiomyopathy. Morphologic studies in a canine model. Am J Pathol 135:671, 1989.
42. Beggs AH: Dystrophinopathy, the expanding phenotype. Dystrophin abnormalities in X-linked dilated cardiomyopathy. Circulation 95:2344, 1997.
43. Moise NS, et al: Duchenne's cardiomyopathy in a canine model: Electrocardiographic and echocardiographic studies. J Am Coll Cardiol 17:812, 1991.
44. Moise NS: Duchenne cardiomyopathy in a canine model. Proceedings of the Eighth Annual Veterinary Medical Forum, 1990, pp 897–905.
45. Liu SK: Myocarditis and cardiomyopathy in the dog and cat. Heart Vessels Suppl 1:122, 1985.
46. Hayes MA, et al: Sudden death in young dogs with myocarditis caused by parvovirus. JAVMA 174:1197, 1979.
47. Carpenter JL, et al: Intestinal and cardiopulmonary forms of parvovirus infection in a litter of pups. JAVMA 175:1269, 1980.
48. Gagnon AN, et al: Myocarditis in puppies: Clinical, pathological and virological findings. Can Vet J 21:195, 1980.
49. Lenghaus C, Studdert MJ: Generalized parvovirus disease in neonatal pups. JAVMA 181:41, 1982.
50. Cimprich RE, et al: Degenerative cardiomyopathy in experimental beagles following parvovirus exposure. Toxicol Pathol 9:19, 1981.
51. Meunier PC, et al: Experimental viral myocarditis: Parvoviral infection of neonatal pups. Vet Pathol 21:509, 1984.
52. Lenghaus C, Studdert MJ: Animal model of human disease: Acute and chronic viral myocarditis; acute diffuse suppurative myocarditis and residual myocardial scarring following infection with canine parvovirus. Am J Pathol 115:316, 1984.
53. Barr SC, et al: Clinical, clinicopathologic, and parasitologic observations of trypanosomiasis in dogs infected with North American Trypanosoma cruzi isolates. Am J Vet Res 52:954, 1991.
54. Barr SC, et al: Pathologic features of dogs inoculated with North American Trypanosoma cruzi isolates. Am J Vet Res 52:2033, 1991.
55. Andrade ZA, et al: Damage and healing in the conducting system of the heart (an experimental study of dogs infected with Trypanosoma cruzi). J Pathol 143:93, 1984.
56. Barr SC, et al: Chronic dilatative myocarditis caused by Trypanosoma cruzi in two dogs. JAVMA 195:1237, 1989.
57. Dubey JP, et al: Newly recognized fatal protozoan disease of dogs. JAVMA 192:1269, 1988.
58. Dubey JP, et al: Neonatal Neospora caninum infection in dogs: Isolation of the causative agent and experimental transmission. JAVMA 193:1259, 1988.

CV

59. Hay WH, et al: Diagnosis and treatment of *Neospora caninum* infection in a dog. JAVMA 197:87, 1990.
60. Cohen ND, et al: Clinical and epizootiologic characteristics of dogs seropositive for *Borrelia burgdorferi* in Texas: 110 cases (1988). JAVMA 197:893, 1990.
61. Levy SA, Duray PH: Complete heart block in a dog seropositive for *Borrelia burgdorferi*—similarity to human Lyme carditis. J Vet Intern Med 2:138, 1988.
62. Greene RT: An update on the serodiagnosis of canine Lyme borreliosis. J Vet Intern Med 4:167, 1990.
63. Oden M, Dubey JP: Sudden death associated with *Neospora caninum* myocarditis in a dog. JAVMA 203:831, 1993.
64. Keene BW, et al: Carnitine-linked defects of myocardial metabolism in canine dilated cardiomyopathy. Proceedings of the Fourth Annual Veterinary Medical Forum, 1986, pp 14–54.
65. Bishop LM: Biochemical investigations of cardiomyopathy in the dog. Res Vet Sci 43:1, 1987.
66. Keene BW, et al: Myocardial carnitine deficiency associated with dilated cardiomyopathy in Doberman pinschers (abstract). J Vet Intern Med 3:126, 1989.
67. Hoey A, et al: Canine dilated cardiomyopathy—are there defects at the receptor level? (abstract). Proc British Small Anim Vet Med Assoc, 1991, p 142.
68. Keene BW, et al: Myocardial L-carnitine deficiency in a family of dogs with dilated cardiomyopathy. JAVMA 198:647, 1991.
69. O'Grady MJ, et al: Myocardial myoglobin deficiency: An etiology for Doberman dilated cardiomyopathy (abstract). J Vet Intern Med 6:113, 1992.
70. O'Brien PJ, et al: Myocardial myoglobin deficiency in various animal models of congestive heart failure. J Mol Cell Cardiol 24:721, 1992.
71. O'Brien PJ, et al: Clinical pathologic profiles of dogs and turkeys with congestive heart failure, either noninduced or induced by rapid ventricular pacing, and turkeys with furazolidone toxicosis. Am J Vet Res 54:60, 1993.
71a. Cory CR, et al: Compensatory asymmetry in down-regulation and inhibition of the myocardial Ca^{2+} cycle in congestive heart failure produced in dogs by idiopathic dilated cardiomyopathy and rapid ventricular pacing. J Mol Cell Cardiol 26:173, 1994.
71b. O'Brien, et al: Myocardial mRNA content and stability, and enzyme activities of Ca-cycling and aerobic metabolism in canine dilated cardiomyopathies. Mol Cell Biochem 142:139, 1995.
71c. McCutcheon LJ, et al: Respiratory chain defect of myocardial mitochondria in idiopathic dilated cardiomyopathy of Doberman pinscher dogs. Can J Physiol Phrmacol 70:1529, 1992.
72. O'Brien PJ: Deficiencies of myocardial troponin-T and creatine kinase MB isoenzyme in dogs with idiopathic dilated cardiomyopathy. Am J Vet Res 58:11, 1997.
73. Bristow MR, et al: Acute and chronic cardiovascular effects of doxorubicin in the dog: The cardiovascular pharmacology of drug-induced histamine release. J Cardiovasc Pharmacol 2:487, 1980.
74. Susaneck SJ: Doxorubicin therapy in the dog. JAVMA 182:70, 1983.
75. Tomlinson CW, et al: Adriamycin cardiomyopathy: Pathological and membrane functional changes in a canine model with mild impairment of left ventricular function. Can J Cardiol 2:368, 1986.
76. Unverferth DV, et al: Canine cobalt cardiomyopathy: A model for the study of heart failure. Am J Vet Res 44:989, 1983.
77. Rona G: Catecholamine cardiotoxicity. J Mol Cell Cardiol 17:291, 1985.
78. Gillette EL, et al: Isoeffect curves for radiation induced cardiomyopathy in the dog. Int J Radiat Oncol Biol Phys 11:2091, 1985.
79. McChesney SL, et al: Canine cardiomyopathy after whole heart and partial lung irradiation. Int J Radiat Oncol Biol Phys 14:1169, 1988.
80. Sandusky GE, et al: Experimental cobalt cardiomyopathy in the dog: A model for cardiomyopathy in dogs and man. Toxicol Appl Pharmacol 60:263, 1981.
81. Unverferth DV, et al: Canine cobalt cardiomyopathy: A model for the study of heart failure. Am J Vet Res 44:989, 1983.
82. Unverferth DV, et al: The evolution of beta-adrenergic dysfunction during the induction of canine cobalt cardiomyopathy. Cardiovasc Res 18:44, 1984.
83. Buoro IB: Putative avocado toxicity in two dogs. Onderstepoort J Vet Res 61:107, 1994.
84. VanVleet JF: Experimentally induced vitamin E/selenium deficiency in the growing dog. JAVMA 166:769, 1975.
85. Green PD, Lemckert JWH: Vitamin E and selenium responsive myocardial degeneration in dogs. Can Vet J 18:290, 1977.
86. Armstrong PW, et al: Rapid ventricular pacing in the dog: Pathophysiological studies of heart failure. Circulation 74:1075, 1986.
87. O'Brien PJ, et al: Rapid ventricular pacing of dogs to heart failure: Biochemical and physiological studies. Can J Physiol Pharmacol 68:34, 1990.
88. O'Brien PJ, et al: Clinical pathologic profiles of dogs and turkeys with congestive heart failure, either noninduced or induced by rapid ventricular pacing, and turkeys with furazolidone toxicosis. Am J Vet Res 54:60, 1993.
89. Liu Yu, et al: Myocyte nuclear mitotic division and programmed myocyte cell death characterize the cardiac myopathy induced by rapid ventricular pacing dogs. Lab Invest 73:771, 1995.
90. Kajstura J, et al: The cellular basis of pacing-induced dilated cardiomyopathy. Myocyte cell loss and myocyte cellular reactive hypertrophy. Circulation 92:2306, 1995.
91. Cobb MA, et al: Use of indirect immunofluorescence and Western blotting to assess the role of circulating antimyocardial antibodies in dogs with dilated cardiomyopathy. Res Vet Sci 56:245, 1994.
92. Goldman JH, McKenna WJ: Immunopathogenesis of dilated cardiomyopathies. Curr Opin Cardiol 10:306, 1995.
93. Bertrand F, et al: A clinical case of myocarditis associated with a high titer of antinuclear antibodies in a dog. Pratique médicale et chirurgicale de l'Anim de Cie 25:271, 1990.
94. Sandusky GE, Cho DY: Congestive cardiomyopathy in a dog associated with pregnancy. Cornell Vet 74:60, 1984.
95. Meurs KM, et al: Familial dysrhythmias in Boxer dogs appear to be inherited as an autosomal dominant trait (abstract). J Vet Intern Med, in press.
96. Arber S, et al: MLP-deficient mice exhibit a disruption of cardiac cytoarchitectural organization, dilated cardiomyopathy, and heart failure. Cell 88:393, 1997.
97. Bristow MR, Gilbert EM: Improvement in cardiac myocyte function by biological effects of medical therapy: A new concept in the treatment of heart failure. Eur Heart J 16(suppl F):20, 1995.
98. Olson TM, et al: Actin mutations in dilated cardiomyopathy, a heritable form of heart failure. Science 280:750, 1998.
99. Grunig E, et al: Frequency and phenotypes of familial dilated cardiomyopathy. J Am Coll Cardiol 31:186, 1998.
100. Why HJF, Meny BT, Richardson PJ, et al: Clinical and prognostic significance of detection of enteroviral RNA in the myocardium of patients with myocarditis or dilated cardiomyopathy. Circulation 89:2582, 1994.
101. Gilbert SJ, et al: Increased expression of promatrix metalloproteinase-9 and neutrophil elastase in canine dilated cardiomyopathy. Cardiovasc Res 34:377, 1997.
102. Lai LP: Differential changes of myocardial beta-adrenoceptor subtypes and G-proteins in dogs with right-sided congestive heart failure. Eur J Pharmacol 309:201, 1996.
103. Colbatzky F, et al: Synthesis and distribution of atrial natriuretic peptide (ANP) in hearts from normal dogs and those with cardiac abnormalities. J Comp Pathol 108:149, 1993.
104. Dos Remedios CG, et al: Different electrophoretic techniques produce conflicting data in the analysis of myocardial samples from dilated cardiomyopathy patients: Protein levels do not necessarily reflect mRNA levels. Electrophoresis 17:235, 1996.
105. Kittleson MD, et al: Results of the multicenter spaniel trial (MUST): Taurine- and carnitine-responsive dilated cardiomyopathy in American cocker spaniels with decreased plasma taurine concentration. J Vet Intern Med 11:204, 1997.
106. Page RL, Keene BW: Doxorubicin cardiomyopathy. In Kirk RW, Bonagura JD (eds): Kirk's Current Veterinary Therapy XI. Philadelphia, WB Saunders, 1992, pp 783–785.
107. Loar AS, Susaneck SJ: Doxorubicin-induced cardiotoxicity in five dogs. Semin Vet Med Surg 1:68, 1986.
108. Mauldin GE, et al: Doxorubicin-induced cardiotoxicosis—clinical features in 32 dogs. J Vet Intern Med 6:82, 1992.
109. Price GS, et al: Efficacy and toxicity of doxorubicin/cyclophosphamide maintenance therapy in dogs with multicentric lymphosarcoma. J Vet Intern Med 5:259, 1991.
110. Hammer AS, et al: Efficacy and toxicity of VAC chemotherapy (vincristine, doxorubicin, and cyclophosphamide) in dogs with hemangiosarcoma. J Vet Intern Med 5:160, 1991.
111. Wallukat G, et al: Removal of autoantibodies in dilated cardiomyopathy by immunoabsorption. Int J Cardiol 54:191, 1996.
112. Barr SC: Anti-heart tissue antibodies during experimental infections with pathogenic and non-pathogenic *Trypanosoma cruzi* isolates in dog. Int J Parasitol 23:961, 1993.
113. Morris SA, et al: Myocardial beta-adrenergic adenylate cyclase complex in a canine model of chagasic cardiomyopathy. Circ Res 69:185, 1991.
114. Fox PR: Myocardial diseases. In Ettinger SJ (ed): Textbook of Veterinary Internal Medicine, 3rd ed. Philadelphia, WB Saunders, 1989, p 1097.
115. Fox PR: Canine myocardial disease. In Fox PR (ed): Canine and Feline Cardiology. New York, Churchill Livingstone, 1988, p 467.
116. Thomas WP: Myocardial diseases of the dog. In Bonagura JD (ed): Contemporary Issues in Small Animal Practice: Cardiology. New York, Churchill Livingstone, 1987, p 117.
117. Harpster NK: Boxer cardiomyopathy. A review of the long-term benefits of antiarrhythmic therapy. Vet Clin North Am Small Anim Pract 21(5):989–1004, 1991.
118. Calvert CA, Chapman WL, Toal RL: Congestive cardiomyopathy in Doberman pinscher dogs. JAVMA 181:598, 1982.
119. Calvert CA, Brown J: Use of M-mode echocardiography in the diagnosis of congestive cardiomyopathy in Doberman pinschers. JAVMA 189:293, 1986.
120. Calvert CA, et al: Congestive cardiomyopathy in Doberman pinscher dogs. JAVMA 181:598, 1982.
121. Calvert CA, et al: Signalment, survival, and prognostic factors in Doberman pinschers with end-stage cardiomyopathy. J Vet Intern Med 11:323, 1997.
122. Anderson FL, et al: Myocardial catecholamine and neuropeptide Y depletion in failing ventricles of patients with idiopathic dilated cardiomyopathy. Circulation 85:46, 1992.
123. Feldman AM, et al: Increase of the 40,000 mol wt pertussin toxin substrate (G protein) in the failing human heart. J Clin Invest 82:189, 1988.
124. Lau C-P, et al: Reduced stimulatory guanine nucleotide binding regulatory protein in idiopathic dilated cardiomyopathy. Am Heart J 122:1787, 1991.
125. D'Agnolo A, et al: Contractile properties and Ca^{2+} release activity of the sarcoplasmic reticulum in dilated cardiomyopathy. Circulation 85:518, 1992.
126. Meyer M, et al: Alterations of sarcoplasmic reticulum proteins in failing human dilated cardiomyopathy. Circulation 92:778, 1995.
127. Pieske B, et al: Alterations in intracellular calcium handling associated with the inverse force-frequency relation in human dilated cardiomyopathy. Circulation 92:1169, 1995

128. Margossian SS, et al: Light chain 2 profile and activity of human ventricular myosin during dilated cardiomyopathy: Identification of a causal agent for impaired myocardial function. Circulation 85:1720, 1992.

129. Koch J, Pedersen HD, Jensen AL, Flagstad A: M-mode echocardiographic diagnosis of dilated cardiomyopathy in giant breed dogs. Zentralbl Veterinarmed A 43:297, 1996.

130. Keene BW, et al: Frequency of myocardial carnitine deficiency associated with spontaneous canine dilated cardiomyopathy (abstract). Proceedings of the Sixth Annual Veterinary Medical Forum, 1988, p 757.

131. Keene BW: L-carnitine supplementation in the therapy of canine dilated cardiomyopathy. Vet Clin North Am Small Anim Pract 21:1005, 1991.

132. Keene BW: L-carnitine deficiency in canine dilated cardiomyopathy. In Kirk RW, Bonagura JD (eds): Kirk's Current Veterinary Therapy XI. Philadelphia, WB Saunders, 1992, pp 780–783.

133. Costa ND, Labuc RH: Case report: Efficacy of oral carnitine therapy for dilated cardiomyopathy in Boxer dogs. J Nutr 124:2687S, 1994.

134. Gilbert EF: Carnitine deficiency. Pathology 17:161, 1985.

135. Ino T, et al: Cardiac manifestations in disorders of fat and carnitine metabolism in infancy. J Am Coll Cardiol 11:1301, 1988.

136. Winter SC, et al: Plasma carnitine deficiency. Clinical observations in 51 pediatric patients. Am J Dis Child 141:660, 1987.

137. Angelini C, et al: Clinical varieties of carnitine and carnitine palmitoyltransferase deficiency. Clin Biochem 20:1, 1987.

138. Winter SC, et al: The role of L-carnitine in pediatric cardiomyopathy. J Child Neurol 10(suppl 2):S45, 1995.

139. Scholte HR, et al: The role of the carnitine system in myocardial fatty acid oxidation: Carnitine deficiency, failing mitochondria and cardiomyopathy. Basic Res Cardiol 82(suppl1):63, 1987.

140. Tein I, et al: Impaired skin fibroblast carnitine uptake in primary systemic carnitine deficiency manifested by childhood carnitine-responsive cardiomyopathy. Pediatr Res 28:247, 1990.

141. York CM, et al: Cardiac carnitine deficiency and altered carnitine transport in cardiomyopathic hamsters. Arch Biochem Biophys 221:526, 1983.

142. Gavaghan BJ, Kittleson MD: Dilated cardiomyopathy in an American cocker spaniel with taurine deficiency. Aust Vet J 75:862, 1997.

143. Kramer GA, Kittleson MD, Fox PR, et al: Plasma taurine concentrations in normal dogs and in dogs with heart disease. J Vet Intern Med 9:253, 1995.

144. Armstrong PW, et al: Rapid ventricular pacing in the dog: Pathophysiological studies of heart failure. Circulation 74:1075, 1986.

145. O'Brien PJ, et al: Rapid ventricular pacing of dogs to heart failure: Biochemical and physiological studies. Can J Physiol Pharmacol 68:34, 1990.

146. O'Brien PJ, et al: Clinical pathologic profiles of dogs and turkeys with congestive heart failure, either noninduced or induced by rapid ventricular pacing, and turkeys with furazolidone toxicosis. Am J Vet Res 54:60, 1993.

147. Redfield MM, et al: Cardiorenal and neurohumoral function in a canine model of early left ventricular dysfunction. Circulation 87:2016, 1993.

148. Spinale FG, et al: Alterations in the myocardial capillary vasculature accompany tachycardia-induced cardiomyopathy. Basic Res Cardiol 87:65, 1992.

149. Spinale FG, et al: Angiotensin-converting enzyme inhibition and the progression of congestive cardiomyopathy. Effects on left ventricular and myocyte structure and function. Circulation 92:562, 1995.

150. Vatner DE, et al: Beta-adrenoceptor desensitization during the development of canine pacing-induced heart failure. Clin Exp Pharmacol Physiol 23:688, 1996.

151. Yamamoto K, et al: Ventricular remodeling during development and recovery from modified tachycardia-induced cardiomyopathy model. Am J Physiol 271:R1529, 1996.

152. Zupan I, et al: Tachycardia induced cardiomyopathy in dogs: Relation between chronic supraventricular and chronic ventricular tachycardia. Int J Cardiol 56:75, 1996.

153. Atkins CE: Orthodromic reciprocating tachycardia and heart failure in a dog with a concealed posteroseptal accessory pathway. J Vet Intern Med 9:43, 1995.

154. Lucy SD, et al: Pronounced increase in defibrillation threshold associated with pacing-induced cardiomyopathy in the dog. Am Heart J 127:366, 1994.

155. Allworth MS, et al: Effect of enalapril in dogs with pacing-induced heart failure. Am J Vet Res 56:85, 1995.

156. Ware WA, et al: Sympathetic activation in dogs with congestive heart failure caused by chronic mitral valve disease and dilated cardiomyopathy. JAVMA 197:1475, 1990.

157. Koch J, Pedersen HD, Jensen L, Flagstad A: Activation of the renin-angiotensin system in dogs with asymptomatic and symptomatic dilated cardiomyopathy. Res Vet Sci 59:172, 1995.

158. Bonagura JD, Ware WA: Atrial fibrillation in the dog: Clinical findings in 81 cases. J Am Anim Hosp Assoc 22:111, 1986.

159. Naito M, et al: The hemodynamic consequences of cardiac arrhythmias: Evaluation of the relative roles of abnormal atrioventricular sequencing, irregularity of ventricular rhythm, and atrial fibrillation in a canine model. Am Heart J 106:284, 1983.

160. Darke PGG: An evaluation of cardiac dysrhythmias by Doppler echocardiography. Proceedings of the Tenth Annual Veterinary Medical Forum, 1992, pp 602–603.

161. Kittleson MD, et al: The acute hemodynamic effects of milrinone in dogs with severe idiopathic myocardial failure. J Vet Intern Med 1:121, 1987.

162. Sisson D: Evidence for or against the efficacy of afterload reducers for management of heart failure in dogs. Vet Clin North Am Small Anim Pract 21:945, 1991.

163. Sisson D (for the IMPROVE Study Group): Efficacy of enalapril with chronic heart failure (abstract). J Vet Intern Med 6:139, 1992.

164. The IMPROVE Study Group: Acute and short-term hemodynamic, echocardiographic, and clinical effects of enalapril maleate in dogs with naturally acquired heart failure: Results of the invasive multicenter prospective veterinary evaluation of enalapril study. J Vet Intern Med 9:234, 1995.

165. Bonagura JD, Herring DS: Echocardiography: Acquired heart disease. Vet Clin North Am Small Anim Pract 15:1209, 1985.

166. Moise NS: Echocardiography: Therapeutic implications. In Kirk RW (ed): Kirk's Current Veterinary Therapy X. Philadelphia, WB Saunders, 1989, pp 201–218.

167. Moise NS: Echocardiography. In Fox PR (ed): Canine and Feline Cardiology. New York, Churchill Livingston, 1988, pp 113–154.

168. Lombard CW: Echocardiographic and clinical signs of canine dilated cardiomyopathy. J Small Anim Pract 25:59, 1984.

169. Kittleson MD, et al: Efficacy of digoxin administration in dogs with idiopathic congestive cardiomyopathy. JAVMA 186:162, 1985.

170. Kittleson MD, et al: Echocardiographic and clinical effects of milrinone in dogs with myocardial failure. Am J Vet Res 46:1659, 1985.

171. Sisson D: Myocardial diseases. In Ettinger SJ (ed): Textbook of Veterinary Internal Medicine, 3rd ed. Philadelphia, WB Saunders, 1989, pp 923–938.

172. Clark RD, et al: Serial echocardiographic evaluation of left ventricular function in valvular disease, including reproducibility guidelines for serial studies. Circulation 62:564, 1980.

173. Douglas PS, et al: Left ventricular shape, afterload and survival in idiopathic dilated cardiomyopathy. J Am Coll Cardiol 13:311, 1989.

174. Shah PM: Echocardiography in congestive or dilated cardiomyopathy. J Am Soc Echocardiogr 1:20, 1988.

175. Tidholm A, et al: Surviva and prognostic factors in 189 dogs with dilated cardiomyopathy. J Am Anim Hosp Assoc 33:364, 1997.

176. Atkins CE, Snyder PS: Systolic time intervals and their derivatives for evaluation of cardiac function. J Vet Intern Med 6:55, 1992.

177. Darke GG, et al: Doppler echocardiography in canine congestive cardiomyopathy. Proceedings of the Eleventh Annual Veterinary Medical Forum, 1993, p 531.

178. Bennet ED, et al: Ascending aortic blood velocity and acceleration using Doppler ultrasound in the assessment of left ventricular function. Cardiovasc Res 18:632, 1984.

179. Brown KK: Noninvasive evaluation of ventricular ejection dynamics in dogs. Proceedings of the Tenth Annual Veterinary Medical Forum, 1992, pp 613–615.

180. Werner GS, et al: Clinical and prognostic implications of left ventricular filling abnormalities in idiopathic dilated cardiomyopathy (abstract). Circulation 86 (suppl I):I, 1992.

181. Knowlen GG, et al: Comparison of plasma aldosterone concentration among clinical status groups of dogs with chronic heart failure. JAVMA 183:991, 1983.

182. O'Keefe D, Sisson DD: Serum electrolytes in dogs with congestive heart failure (abstract). J Vet Intern Med 7:115, 1993.

183. Longhofer SL, et al: Renal function in heart failure dogs receiving furosemide and enalapril maleate (abstract). J Vet Intern Med 7:123, 1993.

184. Longhofer SL, et al: Renal effects of two starting dosages of enalapril maleate in dogs with heart failure (abstract). J Vet Intern Med 7:124, 1993.

185. Lumsden JH, et al: Prevalence of hypothyroidism and von Willebrand's disease in Doberman pinschers and the observed relationship between thyroid, von Willebrand and cardiac status (abstract). J Vet Intern Med 7:115, 1993.

186. Kasper EK, et al: The causes of dilated cardiomyopathy: A clinicopathologic review of 673 consecutive patients. J Am Coll Cardiol 23:586, 1994.

187. Roudebush P, et al: The effect of combined therapy with captopril, furosemide and a sodium-restricted diet on serum electrolyte concentrations and renal function in normal dogs and dogs with congestive heart failure. J Vet Intern Med 8:337, 1994.

188. Cohn JN, et al: A comparison of enalapril with hydralazine-isosorbide dinitrate in the treatment of chronic congestive heart failure. N Engl J Med 325:303, 1991.

189. The COVE Study Group: Controlled clinical evaluation of enalapril in dogs with heart failure: Results of the cooperative veterinary enalapril study group. J Vet Intern Med 9:243, 1995.

190. Waagstein F: Efficacy of beta blockers in idiopathic dilated cardiomyopathy and ischemic cardiomyopathy. Am J Cardiol 80:45J, 1997.

191. Zarembski DG, et al: Meta-analysis of the use of low-dose beta-adrenergic blocking therapy in idiopathic or ischemic dilated cardiomyopathy. Am J Cardiol 77:1247, 1996.

192. The PRECISE Trial. Prospective Randomized Evaluation of Carvedilol on Symptoms and Exercise: Double-blind, placebo-controlled study of the effects of carvedilol in patients with moderate to severe heart failure. Circulation 94:2793, 1996.

193. Allworth MS, et al: Effect of enalapril in dogs with pacing-induced heart failure. Am J Vet Res 56:85, 1995.

194. Persson PB, et al: Modulation of natriuresis by sympathetic nerves and angiotensin II in conscious dogs. Am J Physiol 256:F485, 1989.

195. Shimoyama H, et al: Effect of beta-blockade on left atrial contribution to ventricular filling in dogs with moderate heart failure. Am Heart J 13:772, 1996.

196. Sabbah HN, et al: Effects of ACE inhibition and beta-blockade on skeletal muscle fiber types in dogs with moderate heart failure. Am J Physiol 270:H115, 1996.

197. Liang CS, et al: Chronic beta-adrenoceptor blockade prevents the development of beta-adrenergic subsensitivity in experimental right-sided congestive heart failure in dogs. Circulation 84:254, 1991.

CV

198. Nakazawa M, et al: Hemodynamic effects of benazeprilat in the anesthetized dog with acute left ventricular failure. Jpn J Pharmacol 56:369, 1991.

199. Andersson B, et al: Improved exercise hemodynamic status in dilated cardiomyopathy after beta-adrenergic blockade treatment. J Am Coll Cardiol 23:1397, 1994.

200. Zhang X, et al: Neutral endopeptidase and angiotensin converting enzyme inhibitors increase nitric oxide production in isolated canine coronary microvessels by a kinin-dependent mechanism. J Cardiovasc Pharmacol 31:623, 1998.

201. Seymour AA, et al: Systemic hemodynamics, renal function and hormonal levels during inhibition of neutral endopeptidase 3.4.24.11 and angiotensin-converting enzyme in conscious dogs with pacing-induced heart failure. J Pharmacol Exp Ther 266:872, 1993.

202. Seymour AA, et al: Inhibition of neutral endopeptidase 3.4.24.11 in conscious dogs with pacing induced heart failure. Cardiovasc Res 27:1015, 1993.

203. Cavero PG, et al: Cardiorenal actions of neutral endopeptidase inhibition in experimental congestive heart failure. Circulation 82:196, 1990.

204. Kloner RA, et al: Absence of hemodynamic deterioration in the presence of amlodipine following experimental myocardial infarction. J Cardiovasc Pharmacol 20:837, 1992.

205. Kittleson MD, et al: The acute hemodynamic effects of captopril in dogs with heart failure. J Vet Pharmacol Ther 16:1, 1993.

206. Broqvist M, et al: Neuroendocrine response in acute heart failure and the influence of treatment. Eur Heart J 10:1075, 1989.

207. Hamlin RL: Evidence for or against clinical efficacy of preload reducers. Vet Clin North Am Small Anim Pract 21:931, 1991.

208. Cotter G, et al: Randomised trial of high-dose isosorbide dinitrate plus low-dose furosemide versus high-dose furosemide plus low-dose isosorbide dinitrate in severe pulmonary oedema. Lancet 351:389, 1998.

209. Cotter G, et al: Increased toxicity of high-dose furosemide versus low-dose dopamine in the treatment of refractory congestive heart failure. Clin Pharmacol Ther 62:187, 1997.

210. van Meyel JJ, et al: Continuous infusion of furosemide in the treatment of patients with congestive heart failure and diuretic resistance. J Intern Med 235:329, 1994.

211. Dormans TP, et al: Diuretic efficacy of high dose furosemide in severe heart failure: Bolus injection versus continuous infusion. J Am Coll Cardiol 28:376, 1996.

212. Shimon I, et al: Improved left ventricular function after thiamine supplementation in patients with congestive heart failure receiving long-term furosemide therapy. Am J Med 98:485, 1995.

213. Smith TW, et al: The management of heart failure. In Braunwald E (ed): Heart Disease: A Textbook of Cardiovascular Medicine, 4th ed. Philadelphia, WB Saunders, 1992, pp 464–519.

214. Pacher R, et al: Effects of two different enalapril dosages on clinical, haemodynamic and neurohumoral response of patients with severe congestive heart failure. Eur Heart J 17:1223, 1996.

215. The Randomized Aldactone Evaluation Study Group: Effectiveness of spironolactone added to an angiotensin-converting enzyme inhibitor and a loop diuretic for severe chronic congestive heart failure (the Randomized Aldactone Evaluation Study [RALES]). Am J Cardiol 78:902, 1996.

216. Knight DH: Efficacy of inotropic support of the failing heart. Vet Clin North Am Small Anim Pract 21:879, 1991.

217. Snyder PS, Atkins CE: Current uses and hazards of the digitalis glycosides. In Kirk RW, Bonagura JD (eds): Kirk's Current Veterinary Therapy XI. Philadelphia, WB Saunders, 1992, pp 689–693.

218. Hamlin RL: Therapy of supraventricular tachycardia and atrial fibrillation. In Kirk RW, Bonagura JD (eds): Kirk's Current Veterinary Therapy XI. Philadelphia, WB Saunders, 1992, pp 745–749.

219. Ferguson DW, et al: Sympathoinhibitory responses to digitalis glycosides in heart failure patients: Direct evidence from sympathetic neural recordings. Circulation 80:65, 1989.

220. Young JB, et al (PROVED study investigators): Multicenter, double-blind, placebo-controlled randomized withdrawal trial of the efficacy and safety of digoxin in patients with mild to moderate chronic heart failure not treated with converting enzyme inhibitors (abstract). J Am Coll Cardiol 19:259A, 1992.

221. Packer M, et al: Withdrawal of digoxin from patients with chronic heart failure treated with angiotensin-converting-enzyme inhibitors. N Engl J Med 329:1, 1993.

222. DiBianco R, et al for the Milrinone Multicenter Trial Group: A comparison of oral milrinone, digoxin, and their combinations in the treatment of patients with chronic heart failure. N Engl J Med 320:677, 1989.

223. The Digitalis Investigation Group: The effect of digoxin on mortality and morbidity in patients with heart failure. N Engl J Med 336:525, 1997.

224. Kittleson MD: Dobutamine. JAVMA 177:642, 1980.

225. Keene BW, Rush JE: Therapy of heart failure. In Ettinger SJ (ed): Textbook of Veterinary Internal Medicine, 3rd ed. Philadelphia, WB Saunders, 1989, pp 939–975.

226. Keister DM, et al: Milrinone: A clinical trial in 29 dogs with moderate to severe congestive heart failure. J Vet Intern Med 4:79, 1990.

227. Cobb MA: Idiopathic dilated cardiomyopathy: Advances in aetiology, pathogenesis and management. J Small Anim Pract 33:113, 1992.

228. Kittleson MD: The efficacy and safety of milrinone for treating heart failure in dogs. Vet Clin North Am Small Anim Pract 21:905, 1991.

229. Packer M, et al for PROMISE study research group: Effect of oral milrinone on mortality in severe chronic congestive heart failure. N Engl J Med 325:1468, 1991.

230. Hagemeijer F: Intractable heart failure despite angiotensin-converting enzyme inhibitors, digoxin, and diuretics: Long-term effectiveness of add-on therapy with pimobendan. Am Heart J 122:517, 1991.

231. Le Bobinnec G: The place of inodilators in the treatment of congestive heart failure (CHF): Clinical trial of pimobendan in dogs. Proceedings of the Eleventh Annual Veterinary Medical Forum, 1993, pp 550–552.

232. Luis-Fuentes, V, et al: Placebo-controlled evaluation of pimobendan in the therapy of heart failure secondary to dilated cardiomyopathy (abstract). J Vet Intern Med, in press.

233. The CONSENSUS Trial Study Group: Effects of enalapril on mortality in severe congestive heart failure: Results of the Cooperative North Scandinavian Enalapril Survival Study (CONSENSUS). N Engl J Med 316:1429, 1987.

234. The SOLVD Investigators: Effect of enalapril on survival in patients with reduced left ventricular ejection fraction and congestive heart failure. N Engl J Med 325:293, 1991.

235. Captopril Multicenter Research Group: A placebo-controlled trial of captopril in refractory congestive heart failure. J Am Coll Cardiol 2:755, 1983.

236. Pfeffer MA, et al: Effect of captopril on mortality and morbidity in patients with left ventricular dysfunction after myocardial infarction. N Engl J Med 327:669, 1992.

237. Hamlin RL, Nakayama T: Comparison of some pharmacokinetic parameters of 5 angiotensin converting enzyme inhibitors in normal beagles. J Vet Intern Med 12:93, 1998.

238. Cohn JN, et al: Effect of vasodilator therapy on mortality in chronic congestive heart failure: Results of a Veterans Administration cooperative study. N Engl J Med 314:1547, 1986.

239. Gilbert EM, et al: Flosequinan selectively lowers cardiac adrenergic drive in the failing human heart (abstract). Circulation 86(suppl I):I-644, 1992.

240. Packer M, et al (for the REFLECT I and REFLECT II study groups): Efficacy of flosequinan in patients with heart failure who are withdrawn from therapy with converting-enzyme inhibitors (abstract). Circulation 86(suppl I):I-644, 1992.

241. Packer M, et al: Double blind placebo controlled study of the efficacy of flosequinan in patients with chronic heart failure. J Am Coll Cardiol 22:65, 1993.

242. Figulla HR, et al: Beneficial effects of long-term diltiazem treatment in dilated cardiomyopathy. J Am Coll Cardiol 13:653, 1989.

243. Andersson B, et al: Changes in early and late diastolic filling patterns induced by long-term adrenergic beta-blockade in patients with idiopathic dilated cardiomyopathy. Circulation 94:673, 1996.

244. Bristow MR, et al: Second- and third-generation beta-blocking drugs in chronic heart failure. Cardiovasc Drugs Ther 11(suppl1):291, 1997.

245. Gilbert EM, et al: Comparative hemodynamic, left ventricular functional, and antiadrenergic effects of chronic treatment with metoprolol versus carvedilol in the failing heart. Circulation 94:2817, 1996.

246. Demopoulos L, et al: Nonselective beta-adrenergic blockade with carvedilol does not hinder the benefits of exercise training in patients with congestive heart failure. Circulation 95:1764, 1997.

247. Eichhorn EJ, et al: 154 predictors of systolic and diastolic improvement in patients with dilated cardiomyopathy treated with metoprolol. J Am Coll Cardiol 25:763, 1995.

248. Abshagen U: A new molecule with vasodilating and beta adrenoceptor blocking properties. J Cardiovasc Pharmacol 10(suppl 11):S23, 1987.

249. Colucci WS, et al: Carvedilol inhibits clinical progression in patients with mild symptoms of heart failure. Circulation 94:2800, 1996.

250. Packer M: Pathophysiological mechanisms underlying the adverse effects of calcium channel-blocking drugs in patients with chronic heart failure. Circulation 80(suppl IV):IV-59, 1989.

251. Akhtar M, et al: CAST and beyond. Implications of the Cardiac Arrhythmia Suppression Trial. Circulation 81:1123, 1990.

252. Koga Y, et al: Sudden death in hypertrophic and dilated cardiomyopathy. Jpn Circ J 53:1546, 1989.

253. Hamlin RL: Antiarrhythmic (Anti) and proarrhythmic (Pro) effects of antiarrhythmics (A) on spontaneous ventricular premature beats in dogs (abstract). Proceedings of the Fifth Annual Veterinary Medical Forum, 1987, p 924.

254. Calvert CA: Effect of medical therapy on survival of patients with dilated cardiomyopathy. Vet Clin North Am Small Anim Pract 21:919, 1991.

255. Calvert CA, et al: Efficacy and toxicity of tocainide for the treatment of ventricular tachyarrhythmias in Doberman pinschers with occult cardiomyopathy. J Vet Intern Med 10:235, 1996.

256. Rush JE, Keene BW: ECG of the month. The sudden death of a dog with dilatative cardiomyopathy. JAVMA 194:52, 1989.

257. Lazzara R: A comparison of seven antiarrhythmic drugs in patients with ventricular tachyarrhythmias. N Engl J Med 329:452, 1993.

258. Waldo AL, et al: Effect of d-sotalol on mortality in patients with left ventricular dysfunction after recent and remote myocardial infarction. Lancet 348:7, 1996.

259. Packer M, et al: Effect of amlodipine on morbidity and mortality in severe chronic heart failure. N Engl J Med 335:1107, 1996.

260. Orton EC, et al: Dynamic cardiomyoplasty for treatment of idiopathic dilatative cardiomyopathy in a dog. JAVMA 205:1415, 1994.

261. Monnet E, Orton EC: Dynamic cardiomyoplasty for dilated cardiomyopathy in dogs. Semin Vet Med Surg (Small Anim) 9:240, 1994.

262. White RN, et al: Skeletal muscle extra-aortic counterpulsation in dogs with dilated cardiomyopathy. J Small Anim Pract 38:554, 1997.

263. Morisco C, et al: Effect of coenzyme Q10 therapy in patients with congestive heart failure: A long-term multicenter randomized study. Clin Investig 71(suppl 8):S134, 1993.

264. Langsjoen PH, et al: Long-term efficacy and safety of coenzyme Q10 therapy for idiopathic dilated cardiomyopathy. Am J Cardiol 65:521, 1990.
265. Permanetter B, et al: Ubiquinone (coenzyme Q10) in the long-term treatment of idiopathic dilated cardiomyopathy. Eur Heart J 13:1528, 1992.
266. Hofman-Bang C, et al: Coenzyme Q10 as an adjunctive in the treatment of chronic congestive heart failure. The Q10 Study Group. J Card Fail 1:101, 1995.
267. Li RK, et al: Vitamine E and oxidative stress in the heart of the cardiomyopathic Syrian hamster. Free Radic Biol Med 24:252, 1998.
268. Monnet E, Orton EC, Salman M, Boon J: Idiopathic dilated cardiomyopathy in dogs: Survival and prognostic indicators. J Vet Intern Med 9:12, 1995.
269. Arola A, Tuominen J, Ruuskanen O. Jokinen E: Idiopathic dilated cardiomyopathy in children: Prognostic indicators and outcome. Pediatrics 101:369, 1998.
270. Douglas PS, et al: Left ventricular shape, afterload and survival in idiopathic dilated cardiomyopathy. J Am Coll Cardiol 13:311, 1989.
271. Olshausen KV, et al: Long-term prognostic significance of ventricular arrhythmias in idiopathic dilated cardiomyopathy. Am J Cardiol 61:146, 1988.
272. Cohn JN, Rector TS: Prognosis of congestive heart failure and predictors of mortality. Am J Cardiol 62:25A, 1988.
273. Keren A, et al: Mildly dilated congestive cardiomyopathy: Use of prospective diagnostic criteria and description of the clinical course without heart transplantation. Circulation 81:506, 1990.
274. Romeo F, et al: Predictors of sudden death in idiopathic dilated cardiomyopathy. Am J Cardiol 63:138, 1989.
275. Franciosa JA, et al: Survival in men with severe chronic left ventricular failure due to either coronary heart disease or idiopathic dilated cardiomyopathy. Am J Cardiol 51:831, 1983.
276. Lamontagne J, DiFruscia R: Cardiomyopathie dilatée canine: La survie après le diagnostic. Le Médecin Vétérinaire Du Quebec 21:141, 1991.
277. Calvert CA: Update: Canine dilated cardiomyopathy. In Kirk RW, Bonagura JD (eds): Kirk's Current Veterinary Therapy XI. Philadelphia, WB Saunders, 1992, pp 773–779.
278. Stevenson LW, et al: Importance of hemodynamic response to therapy in predicting survival with ejection fraction <20% secondary to ischemic or nonischemic dilated cardiomyopathy. Am J Cardiol 66:1348, 1990.
279. Liu S-K, et al: Canine hypertrophic cardiomyopathy. JAVMA 174:708, 1979.
280. Liu S-K, et al: Hypertrophic cardiomyopathy in the dog. Am J Pathol 94:497, 1979.
281. Maron BJ, et al: Spontaneously occurring hypertrophic cardiomyopathy in dogs and cats: A potential animal model of a human disease. In Kaltenbach M, Epstein SE (eds): Hypertrophic Cardiomyopathy. New York, Springer-Verlag, 1982, pp 73–87.
282. Yamada E: A canine case of hypertrophic cardiomyopathy. J Jpn Vet Med Assoc 36:12, 1983.
283. Thomas WP, et al: Hypertrophic obstructive cardiomyopathy in a dog: Clinical, hemodynamic, angiographic, and pathologic studies. J Am Anim Hosp Assoc 20:253, 1984.
284. Swindle MM, et al: Mitral valve prolapse and hypertrophic cardiomyopathy in a pup. JAVMA 184:1515, 1984.
285. Sisson DD: Heritability of idiopathic myocardial hypertrophy and dynamic subaortic stenosis in pointer dogs (abstract). J Vet Intern Med 4:118, 1990.
286. Liu SK, et al: Comparison of morphologic findings in spontaneously occurring hypertrophic cardiomyopathy in humans, cats and dogs. Am J Cardiol 72:944, 1993.
287. Marks CA: Hypertrophic cardiomyopathy in a dog. JAVMA 203:1020, 1993.
288. Braunwald E: Hypertrophic cardiomyopathy—continued progress. N Engl J Med 320:800, 1989.
289. Maron BJ, et al: Hypertrophic cardiomyopathy: Interrelations of clinical manifestations, pathophysiology, and therapy. N Engl J Med 316:780, 844, 1987.
290. Maron BJ: Asymmetry in hypertrophic cardiomyopathy: The septal to free wall thickness ratio revisited. Am J Cardiol 55:835, 1985.
291. Webb JG, et al: Apical hypertrophic cardiomyopathy: Clinical follow-up and diagnostic correlates. J Am Coll Cardiol 15:83, 1990.
292. Lewis JF, Maron BJ: Elderly patients with hypertrophic cardiomyopathy: A subset with distinctive left ventricular morphology and progressive clinical course late in life. J Am Coll Cardiol 13:36, 1989.
293. Sisson DD: Fixed and dynamic subvalvular aortic stenosis in dogs. In Kirk RW, Bonagura JD (eds): Kirk's Current Veterinary Therapy XI. Philadelphia, WB Saunders, 1992, pp 760–765.
294. Panza JA, et al: Utility of continuous wave Doppler echocardiography in the noninvasive assessment of left ventricular outflow tract pressure gradient in patients with hypertrophic cardiomyopathy. J Am Coll Cardiol 19:91, 1992.
295. Sisson D, Thomas WP: Dynamic subaortic stenosis in a dog with congenital heart disease. J Am Anim Hosp Assoc 20:657, 1984.
296. Klues HG, et al: Diversity of structural mitral valve alterations in hypertrophic cardiomyopathy. Circulation 85:1651, 1992.
297. Mikami T, et al: Mitral valve and its ring in hypertrophic cardiomyopathy—a mechanism creating surplus mitral leaflet involved in systolic anterior motion. Jpn Circ J 52:597, 1988.
298. Muna FT, et al: Discrete subaortic stenosis in Newfoundland dogs: Association of infective endocarditis. Am J Cardiol 41:746, 1978.
299. Jones CL: Inheritable left ventricular outflow tract obstruction in the golden retriever. Proceedings of the Seventh Annual Veterinary Medical Forum, 1989, pp 851–853.
300. O'Grady MR: The occurrence and breed distribution of subaortic stenosis in the dog (abstract). J Vet Intern Med 5:145, 1991.
301. Buoscio DA, et al: Clinical and pathologic characterization of an unusual form of subvalvular aortic stenosis in four golden retriever dogs. J Am Anim Hosp Assoc, in press.
302. Wynne J, Braunwald E: The cardiomyopathies and myocarditides: Toxic, chemical, and physical damage to the heart. In Braunwald E (ed): Heart Disease: A Textbook of Cardiovascular Medicine, 4th ed. Philadelphia, WB Saunders, 1992, pp 1394–1450.
303. Maron BJ, et al: Hypertrophic cardiomyopathy. Lancet 350:127, 1997.
304. Kimura A, et al: Mutations in the cardiac troponin I gene associated with hypertrophic cardiomyopathy. Nat Genet 16:379, 1997.
305. Poetter K, et al: Mutations in either the essential or regulatory light chains of myosin are associated with a rare myopathy in human heart and skeletal muscle. Nat Genet 13:63, 1996.
306. Geisterfer-Lowrance A, et al: A mouse model of familial hypertrophic cardiomyopathy. Science 272:731, 1996.
307. Bonow RO, et al: Medical and surgical therapy of hypertrophic cardiomyopathy. Cardiovasc Clin 19:221, 1988.
308. Fox PR: Evidence for or against efficacy of beta-blockers and aspirin for management of feline cardiomyopathies. Vet Clin North Am Small Anim Pract 21:1011, 1991.
309. Chatterjee K: Calcium antagonist agents in hypertrophic cardiomyopathy. Am J Cardiol 59:146B, 1987.
310. Bright JM, Golden AL: Evidence for or against efficacy of calcium channel blockers for management of hypertrophic cardiomyopathy in cats. Vet Clin North Am Small Anim Pract 21:1023, 1991.
311. Fananapazir L, et al: Sudden death during empiric amiodarone therapy in symptomatic hypertrophic cardiomyopathy. Am J Cardiol 67:169, 1991.
312. Fananapazir L, et al: Prognostic determinants in hypertrophic cardiomyopathy. Prospective evaluation of therapeutic strategy based on clinical, Holter, hemodynamic, and electrophysiologic findings. Circulation 86:730, 1992.
313. McKenna WJ, et al: Improved survival with amiodarone in patients with hypertrophic cardiomyopathy. Br Heart J 53:412, 1985.
314. Seiler C, et al: Long-term follow-up of medical versus surgical therapy for hypertrophic cardiomyopathy: A retrospective study. J Am Coll Cardiol 17:634, 1991.
315. Cohn LH, et al: Long-term follow-up of patients undergoing myotomy/myectomy for obstructive hypertrophic cardiomyopathy. Am J Cardiol 70:657, 1992.
316. McAreavey D, Fananapazir L: Altered cardiac hemodynamic and electrical state in normal sinus rhythm after chronic dual-chamber pacing for relief of left ventricular outflow obstruction in hypertrophic cardiomyopathy. Am J Cardiol 70:651, 1992.
317. Jeanrenaud X, et al: Effects of dual-chambered pacing in hypertrophic obstructive cardiomyopathy. Lancet 339:1318, 1992.
318. Walvoort HC, et al: Canine glycogen storage disease type II: A clinical study of four affected Lapland dogs. J Am Anim Hosp Assoc 20:279, 1984.
319. Miller MS, et al: Persistent atrial standstill (atrioventricular muscular dystrophy). In Kirk RW, Bonagura JD (eds): Kirk's Current Veterinary Therapy XI. Philadelphia, WB Saunders, 1992, pp 786–791.
320. Tilley LP, Liu SK: Persistent atrial standstill in the dog and cat (abstract). Am Coll Vet Int Med Scientific Proceedings, 1983, p 43.
321. Jeraj K, et al: Atrial standstill, myocarditis and destruction of cardiac conduction system: Clinicopathologic correlation in a dog. Am Heart J 99:185, 1980.
322. de Visser M, et al: The heart in Becker muscular dystrophy, facioscapulohumeral dystrophy, and Bethlem myopathy. Muscle Nerve 15:591, 1992.
323. Emery AE: Emery-Dreifus syndrome. J Med Genet 26:637, 1989.
324. Perloff JK: Neurological disorders and heart disease. In Braunwald E (ed): Heart Disease: A Textbook of Cardiovascular Medicine, 4th ed. Philadelphia, WB Saunders, 1992, pp 1810–1826.
325. Yates JRW, et al: Emery-Dreyfus muscular dystrophy: Linkage to markers in distal Xq28. J Med Genet 30:108, 1993.

CHAPTER 117

FELINE CARDIOMYOPATHIES

Philip R. Fox

DEFINITIONS AND CLASSIFICATION

Cardiomyopathy describes a heterogeneous class of disorders whose dominant feature relates to structural abnormality or functional impairment of the heart muscle (*cardio*—heart, *myopathy*—muscle). Cardiomyopathies exclude conditions resulting from valvular, hypertensive, vascular, pericardial, pulmonary, or congenital derangements. A variety of schemes have been proposed to define myocardial diseases.[1-8] In cats, classification is facilitated by clinical, pathologic, or physiologic information corresponding to (1) morphologic phenotype (e.g., hypertrophic or dilated cardiomyopathy); (2) etiology (e.g., taurine deficiency myocardial failure; thyrotoxic heart disease); (3) myocardial function (e.g., systolic or diastolic dysfunction); (4) pathology (e.g., infiltrative cardiomyopathy); and (5) pathophysiology (e.g., restrictive cardiomyopathy). In addition, *idiopathic* (primary) cardiomyopathy describes the myocardium as the sole source of heart disease when a cause cannot be identified, whereas *secondary* cardiomyopathy denotes heart muscle disease resulting from an identifiable systemic, metabolic, or nutritional disorder (Table 117–1). Four types of idiopathic myocardial disease are recognized—hypertrophic, dilated, restrictive, and arrhythmogenic right ventricular (RV) cardiomyopathy.[3] Unfortunately, any scheme is self-limiting, and many cases have overlapping features or do not fit readily into a particular category. This has given rise to an increasingly acknowledged designation, unclassified cardiomyopathy.[1, 3, 9]

HEART FAILURE DUE TO DIASTOLIC DYSFUNCTION: HYPERTROPHIC AND RESTRICTIVE CARDIOMYOPATHY

DIASTOLIC FUNCTION

Chamber compliance can be reduced by increased myocardial stiffness, pericardial constraint, or increased chamber volume. Relaxation abnormalities may occur with myocardial ischemia, hypoxia, and hypertrophy. These abnormalities can increase left ventricular (LV) filling pressure and mean left atrial (LA) pressure and can result in pulmonary edema.[10, 11] Doppler echocardiography provides a non-invasive technique to assess diastolic function. Trans-mitral Doppler velocity curves can be interpreted as a representation of the overall diastolic cardiac filling characteristics (Fig. 117–1). These have aided diagnosis, prognosis, and treatment of diastolic function in humans,[10, 12, 15, 16] but mitral flow velocities vary (loading conditions, age, heart rate)[10, 17, 18] and rapid feline heart rates often cause E and A velocity waves to summate, confounding interpretation.

HYPERTROPHIC CARDIOMYOPATHY

Definitions and Nomenclature

Hypertrophic cardiomyopathy (HCM) is characterized by a hypertrophied, non-dilated left ventricle in absence of other cardiac disease or systemic or metabolic abnormalities (e.g., aortic stenosis, arterial hypertension, hyperthyroidism) capable of producing hypertrophy. The hallmark histopathologic feature is myocyte disarray.[3, 19–24] A distinctive clinical feature in some affected cats is a dynamic LV outflow tract obstruction and related subaortic pressure gradient (obstructive form of HCM).

Prevalence and Demographics

Liu recorded a 5.2 per cent incidence of HCM based on 4933 consecutive feline necropsies at The Animal Medical Center (1962–1976) in New York City.[19] A 1.6 per cent prevalence of HCM was reported from a retrospective clinical study at the Veterinary Teaching Hospital of North Carolina State University from 1985 to 1998.[25] Between 1985 and 1997, LV hypertrophy (predominantly idiopathic HCM) was diagnosed in 27 to 64 per cent of the cats examined by echocardiography for suspected heart disease at The Animal Medical Center (Fig. 117–2). Recorded ages range from 3 months to 17 years,[4–7, 22, 23, 25–31] with a mean age of 4.8[30] to 7 years.[22] Domestic short-hair cats are most frequently reported. Heritable transmission is suspected in Maine coon cats,[31, 32] American shorthairs,[33] and Persians.[19, 21, 30] A male predominance (up to 87 per cent) has been widely reported.[4–8, 19, 22, 23, 25, 27, 29]

Etiology

In humans, HCM is a familial disorder with an autosomal dominant pattern of transmission caused by genes that encode cardiac sarcomere protein. Mutations in the genes encoding cardiac beta-myosin heavy chain, cardiac troponin T, and alpha-tropomyosin account for up to 70 per cent of human familial HCM.[34–36] A heritable form of HCM has been identified in a highly interrelated colony of Maine coon cats compatible with autosomal dominance with 100 per cent penetrance.[31, 32] Familial transmission suggestive of an autosomal dominant pattern has also been reported in related American short-hair cats with systolic anterior motion of the mitral valve and/or HCM[33] and in an inbred colony of Persian cats with LV hypertrophy.[30]

Pathophysiology

Diastolic Dysfunction. Diastolic dysfunction has been documented in feline HCM with congestive heart failure (CHF).[22, 37–39] As a consequence of delayed LV relaxation and abnormal distensibility (stiffness), left-sided heart filling

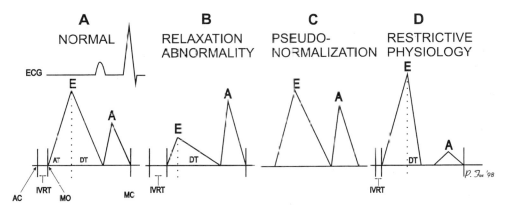

Figure 117–1. Diagram depicting trans-mitral inflow velocity patterns obtained by pulsed-wave Doppler echocardiography in normal states and with diastolic dysfunction. Optimal recordings are made at the left apical parasternal transducer location in this four-chamber inflow view with the pulsed-wave Doppler echo sample volume gate positioned at the mitral valve leaflet tips in diastole. Alterations in velocity profiles occur in myocardial diseases that share similar diastolic properties, and there is overlap in Doppler patterns between disease states. Documentation of these classic filling patterns in cats is often frustrated by rapid feline heart rates and attendant summation of E and A waves. *A, Normal*—In healthy cats with normal left-sided pressures, a high velocity, early diastolic filling wave (E wave) is followed by a smaller (lower velocity), late diastolic wave caused by atrial contraction (A wave). The isovolumic relaxation time (IVRT) is an index of LV relaxation. It represents the time from aortic valve closure (AC) (approximated from the Doppler spectral trace as the time from cessation of aortic blood flow) to mitral valve opening (MO). MC = mitral valve closure. *B, Relaxation abnormality*—Impaired LV relaxation may be indicated by a low, early peak velocity (E wave) and very high, atrial velocity (A wave). The IVRT is prolonged, the acceleration time (AT) is reduced, and the deceleration time (DT) is prolonged. Left ventricular diastolic pressures may be increased. *C, Pseudonormal*—"Pseudonormalization" describes an apparently normal pattern that is actually a transition between impaired relaxation and restrictive physiology. *D, Restrictive physiology*—Typical features include a high early velocity (E wave) and a very low atrial velocity (A wave). Both the IVRT and DT are shortened. This pattern may accompany markedly elevated LV filling pressures. (From Fox PR: Feline cardiomyopathies. *In* Fox PR, Sisson DD, Moïse NS [eds]: A Textbook of Canine and Feline Cardiology: Principles and Clinical Practice, 2nd ed. Philadelphia, WB Saunders, 1999.)

pressures increase.[40, 41] The LA dilates in response to increased end-diastolic pressures, and pulmonary venous pressures may eventually become elevated. Pulmonary congestion may result from this and other associated neurohormonal changes.

Myocardial Ischemia. Intrinsic diastolic function becomes abnormal with myocardial ischemia.[24, 42] Cats with HCM have coronary remodeling (arteriosclerosis or "small vessel disease") similar to humans,[23, 24, 43, 44] which reduces the lumen diameters.[21–24, 45] The severity of coronary changes is linearly related to the degree of myocardial hypertrophy.[46] Other causes of myocardial ischemia include elevated LV filling pressures[47] and prolonged diastolic relaxation,[37] resulting in increased myocardial wall tension and LV outflow tract gradients and tachyarrhythmias,[22] which can increase myocardial oxygen demand.[48, 49]

Figure 117–2. Prevalence of feline cardiomyopathy based on 6522 consecutive echocardiographic examinations performed between 1985–1998 at The Animal Medical Center in New York City. All cats were presented for cardiovascular examination based on a clinical suspicion of heart disease. The annual incidence does not add up to 100 per cent because only those cats that had myocardial disease compatible with a diagnosis of dilated cardiomyopathy (DCM), restrictive cardiomyopathy (RCM), or pathologic left ventricular hypertrophy (LVH) are listed. Known cases of hyperthyroidism or systemic hypertension were excluded and the LVH category represents predominantly idiopathic hypertrophic cardiomyopathy. Data for 1998 are limited to the first trimester. (From Fox PR: Feline cardiomyopathies. *In* Fox PR, Sisson DD, Moïse NS [eds]: A Textbook of Canine and Feline Cardiology: Principles and Clinical Practice, 2nd ed. Philadelphia, WB Saunders, 1999.)

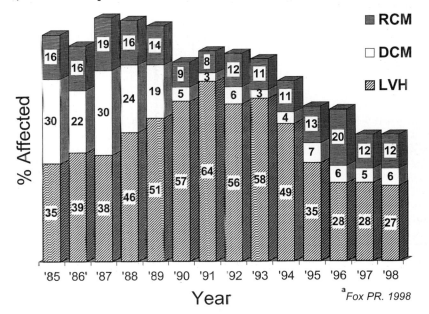

Feline Cardiomyopathy Prevalence Survey 6,522 Sequential Echos: 1985-1998, AMC[a]

[a]Fox PR. 1998

TABLE 117–1. CAUSES OF FELINE MYOCARDIAL DISEASE

Idiopathic

Hypertrophic cardiomyopathy
Restrictive cardiomyopathy
Dilated cardiomyopathy
Arrhythmogenic right ventricular cardiomyopathy

Secondary (Including Specific Cardiomyopathies)

Inflammatory
  Viral (panleukopenia?)
  Bacterial
  Protozoal
  Fungal
  Algal
  Parasitic
Metabolic
  Nutritional
    Taurine deficiency
    Obesity
  Endocrine
    Thyrotoxicosis
    Acromegaly
    Diabetes mellitus
    Uremia
    Cushing's syndrome
  Toxic
    Anthracyclines (doxorubicin)
Infiltrative
  Neoplastic
  Glycogen storage disorders
  Mucopolysaccharidosis
Fibroplastic
  Endomyocardial fibrosis
  Endocardial fibroelastosis
Genetic
  Hypertrophic cardiomyopathy
Neuromuscular
  Facioscapulohumeral muscular dystrophy
Physical agents
  Heat stroke
Unclassified cardiomyopathies
  Idiopathic unclassified cardiomyopathy
  Persistent atrial standstill
Miscellaneous
  Ischemia
  Excessive left ventricular moderator bands

Ventricular and Supraventricular Tachyarrhythmias. Elevated heart rates diminish systolic and diastolic function,[50] reduce diastolic filling, which can increase outflow gradients, and reduce forward cardiac output.[10, 51] Excessive myocardial oxygen utilization and ischemia may result,[49] increasing myocardial stiffness and reducing ventricular filling. Myocardial fibrosis may contribute to the arrhythmogenesis by enhancing re-entrant excitation in ischemic heart disease.[52]

Dynamic LV Outflow Tract Obstruction. Hypertrophic obstructive cardiomyopathy (HOCM), an entity of HCM, is associated with several characteristic abnormalities[22, 24, 53–68]: (1) narrowing of the LV outflow tract; (2) systolic anterior motion of the mitral valve; and (3) production of an LV outflow tract pressure gradient (Figs. 117–3 and 117–4). The LV outflow tract is formed by the hypertrophied interventricular septum anteriorly and the anterior mitral valve leaflet posteriorly. Dynamic LV outflow tract obstruction is commonly associated with systolic apposition of the mitral apparatus with the hypertrophied interventricular septum.[22, 53, 54, 56, 57, 65, 66] A number of mechanisms have been proposed, including narrowing of the subaortic outlet; longer anterior and posterior mitral leaflets and anteriorly displaced papillary muscles that poorly support leaflet tissue; increased LV outflow velocities; a Venturi effect that sucks the mitral leaflet toward the septum; and a high-velocity turbulent flow in the ascending aorta as a consequence of systolic anterior motion of the mitral valve. One study reported systolic apposition and dynamic LV outflow obstruction in 42 per cent of HCM cats. The magnitude of LV outflow tract obstruction varied from trivial to severe (25 to 110 mmHg).[22] LV outflow tract gradients may be present at rest, can be provoked with stress and excitement, and are increased by reduced LV volume (i.e., preload), decreased afterload, and increased contractility.[1, 51, 54, 55, 66–68] Obstructions can potentially increase systolic intraventricular pressure, increase myocardial wall stress, exacerbate subendocardial ischemia, increase myocardial oxygen demand, and stimulate ventricular hypertrophy.[1] Dynamic mitral regurgitation frequently accompanies HCM with obstruction.[22] Mitral regurgitation results from systolic anterior malposition of the mitral valve and increased tension on leaflets caused by papillary muscle displacement.[53] The related cardiac murmur in cats generally becomes louder as the pressure gradient (and degree of systolic apposition) increases. Negative inotropes can eliminate mid-ventricular septal contact and LV outflow obstruction.[54, 69] When the gradient and systolic apposition are markedly reduced or eliminated by these therapies (particularly beta-blocking drugs), both the degree of mitral regurgitation and the loudness of the murmur may decrease (Fox PR, unpublished data, 1998).

Right Ventricular Outflow Tract Obstruction and Pressure Gradients. Systolic abnormalities are not limited to the left ventricle. RV outflow tract gradients have been recorded from cats with HCM. The etiology is undetermined, and most gradients are relatively mild (<25 mmHg).

End-Stage Myocardial Failure. Occasionally, HCM progresses to a stage of chamber dilatation and systolic dysfunction. In humans, this structural and functional evolution is due to severe myocyte death and massive replacement fibrosis, probably associated with impaired coronary vasodilator reserve and myocardial ischemia produced by an abnormal coronary microcirculation.[70] Similar coronary and myocardial lesions are observed in cats with suspected end-stage HCM (Fox PR, Liu SK, unpublished data, 1998). This phase resembling dilated cardiomyopathy is usually associated with refractory heart failure and poor prognosis.

Pathology

The principal pathologic feature of idiopathic HCM is a hypertrophied, non-dilated left ventricle in absence of causative cardiac, systemic, or metabolic disease (Fig. 117–5).[1–3] LV hypertrophy exhibits a broad morphologic spectrum.[5–7, 19–23, 31, 33, 71–74] Biatrial enlargement is common. Mild to moderate RV hypertrophy is often present. The hallmark histopathologic lesion is LV myofiber disarray (cellular disorientation in more than 5 per cent of the tissue section) (Fig. 117–6).[19, 21–23, 71, 75, 76] Other common findings include coronary microcirculation remodeling (arteriosclerosis or "small vessel" disease) and matrix changes characterized by myocyte necrosis and fibrous connective tissue changes (see Fig. 117–6).[21–23, 43–46, 71, 75, 76] Myocardial infarction is frequently present.[77] The LV free (posterior) wall or LV apex is usually affected, although the RV free wall is occasionally involved. Pulmonary congestion or edema may occur, and, less commonly, pericardial, pleural, or abdominal effusions are present. Thromboembolism is common.

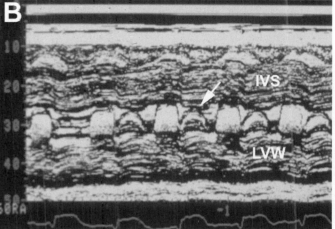

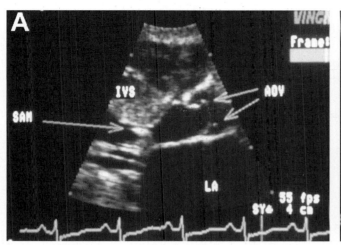

Figure 117–3. Dynamic LV outflow tract obstruction in feline hypertrophic cardiomyopathy defined with echocardiography. *A,* Two-dimensional recording (right parasternal long-axis view). During systole, systolic anterior motion (SAM) with mitral valve/septal contact is present (arrow). Note the aortic valve leaflets (AOV), which are open during ejection. The left atrium (LA) is enlarged. IVS = interventricular septum. (From Fox PR, Liu SK, Maron BJ Echocardiographic assessment of spontaneously occurring feline hypertrophic cardiomyopathy: An animal model of human disease. Circulation 92:2645–2651, 1992.) *B,* M-mode tracing showing marked SAM and prolonged contact between anterior mitral leaflet and thickened interventricular septum (IVS), producing an outflow gradient of 90 mm Hg. LVW = left ventricular posterior wall. (From Fox PR: Feline cardiomyopathies. *In* Fox PR, Sisson DD, Moïse NS [eds]: A Textbook of Canine and Feline Cardiology: Principles and Clinical Practice, 2nd ed. Philadelphia, WB Saunders, 1999.)

Clinical Manifestations

History. A broad range of clinical abnormalities have been described.[4–7, 21, 22, 25–29, 31–33, 38, 73, 74, 78] Many cats are asymptomatic. In others, peracute signs (<24 hours) associated with pulmonary edema are heralded by severe dyspnea and orthopnea. Anorexia and vomiting may precede respiratory signs by 1 or 2 days. Coughing is rarely observed. Acute paresis is the second most common clinical sign and is associated with arterial thromboembolism. Syncope occurs less commonly and may result from tachyarrhythmia or dynamic LV outflow tract obstruction. Sudden death without CHF is uncommon but has been documented by the author to occur in HCM cats with stress, sudden activity, or Valsalva maneuvers (defecation or urination).

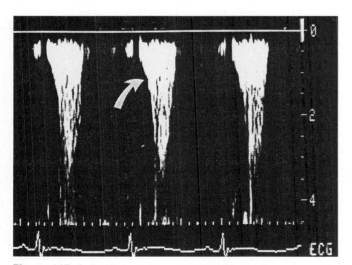

Figure 117–4. Continuous-wave Doppler echocardiogram recorded through the LV outflow tract from a cat with the obstructive form of hypertrophic cardiomyopathy. The maximal velocity was 3.6 m/s (normal, <1.3 m/s), which corresponded to an estimated outflow gradient of 52 mm Hg by the modified Bernoulli equation (i.e., pressure gradient = 4 × velocity²). Note the characteristic mid-systolic velocity acceleration (arrow) and "dagger-shaped" spectral waveform.

Physical Examination. The left precordial apex beat is usually palpably normal or hyperdynamic. Auscultation may reveal a soft, systolic murmur (I to III/VI) heard loudest over the mitral and/or tricuspid valve areas or over the sternum. A diastolic gallop rhythm is common and usually represents a fourth heart sound, S₄. Rales, arrhythmias, and femoral arterial pulse deficits occur commonly with CHF. Heart and lung sounds will be muffled if a large pleural or pericardial effusion is present. Paresis and absence of femoral arterial pulses accompany distal aortic thromboembolism. Abnormal jugular venous pulses may be present with severe right-sided heart failure. Ascites and cachexia may occur in chronic, end-stage disease.[4–7, 20, 21, 25–29, 38]

Electrocardiography. ECG changes are highly variable, generally non-specific, and frequently unremarkable.[4–7, 27, 29, 38, 73, 79, 80] A left-axis deviation compatible with left anterior fascicular block has been reported in 11 per cent (Table 117–2), 30 per cent,[29] and 33 per cent[73] of cats with HCM. In contrast, it has been detected in 3 to 6 per cent of cats with hyperthyroidism[81] and is infrequently recorded in other forms of myocardial disease. Other changes include LA and LV enlargement and ventricular and supraventricular arrhythmias.

Radiography. The ventrodorsal or dorsoventral view is the most sensitive radiographic position to disclose auricular enlargement. Radiographic changes include interstitial and/or alveolar pulmonary densities; pulmonary venous distention (congestion) with or without pulmonary arterial congestion; and, occasionally, mild pleural effusion (Fig. 117–7). Pulmonary edema may be diffuse, patchy, or focal and often involves the right caudal lung lobe. With chronic or advanced HCM, generalized cardiomegaly and severe biventricular failure can occur.[4–7, 27, 29, 38, 47, 73, 74, 78, 79]

Angiocardiography. Largely replaced by echocardiography, non-selective angiocardiographic features include (1) LV free wall hypertrophy; (2) pronounced LV chamber reduction (which often appears slit like); (3) extremely hypertrophied papillary muscles; (4) moderate to severe LA and sometimes RA enlargement; (5) distended pulmonary veins;

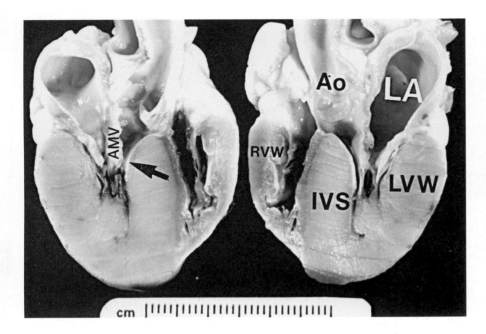

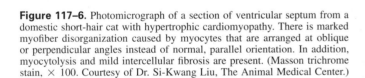

Figure 117–5. Gross heart from a cat with idiopathic hypertrophic cardiomyopathy. This specimen was sectioned in a long-axis plane to demonstrate the LV outflow tract and mitral inflow tract. Severe, generalized, concentric hypertrophy involving the interventricular septum (IVS) and LV posterior wall (LVW) reduces the LV cavity. The left atrium (LA) is moderately enlarged, the RV wall (RVW) is hypertrophied, and the anterior mitral valve leaflet (AMV) is thickened. Ventricular septal hypertrophy is maximal at the basilar region where it bulges into, and narrows, the LV outflow tract. At this point, a fibrous contact plaque (arrow) lies in close proximity to the anterior mitral valve leaflet (AMV), presumably a result of systolic apposition of the AMV and the ventricular septum (see Fig. 117–3).

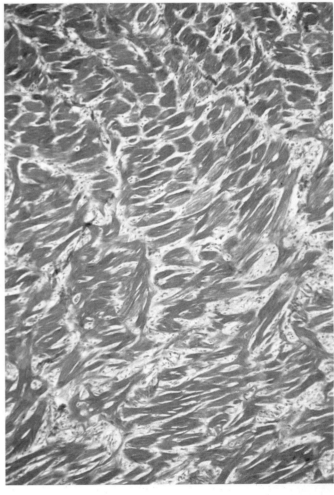

Figure 117–6. Photomicrograph of a section of ventricular septum from a domestic short-hair cat with hypertrophic cardiomyopathy. There is marked myofiber disorganization caused by myocytes that are arranged at oblique or perpendicular angles instead of normal, parallel orientation. In addition, myocytolysis and mild intercellular fibrosis are present. (Masson trichrome stain, × 100. Courtesy of Dr. Si-Kwang Liu, The Animal Medical Center.)

TABLE 117–2. FREQUENCY (PER CENT) OF SELECTED ARRHYTHMIAS RECORDED FROM CATS WITH CARDIOMYOPATHY

	HYPER-TROPHIC CARDIO-MYOPATHY (n = 46)*	RESTRICTIVE CARDIO-MYOPATHY (n = 37)†	MYO-CARDIAL FAILURE (n = 49)[282],‡
First-degree AV block	0	7	37
LAFB	10	7	3
APCs	10	22	15
PAT/Atrial Fib.	10	2	2
VPCs	41	53	43
VT	10	7	23

*Unpublished data from cats in reference 25.
†Fox PR: Unpublished data, 1998.
‡Five cats had severe taurine depletion.
LAFB = left-axis deviation compatible with left anterior fascicular block; APCs = atrial premature complexes; PAT = paroxysmal atrial tachycardia Atrial Fib = atrial fibrillation; VPCs = ventricular premature complexes; VT = ventricular tachycardia.

(6) normal to accelerated circulatory transit time; and (7) ball thrombi in the LA or LV (Fig. 117–8).[4–7, 27, 47, 82–84]

Echocardiography. Echocardiography (see Fig. 117–3) is used to (1) verify and assess severity of LV hypertrophy and cardiac chamber dimensions, (2) detect dynamic LV outflow tract obstruction, (3) evaluate myocardial function, (4) detect intracavitary ball thrombi or pre-thrombotic conditions (e.g., spontaneous echo contrast formation), and (5) diagnose other cardiac conditions. Diagnosis of pathologic hypertrophy requires that the thickness of the ventricular septum or LV posterior (free) wall measured at end-diastole is 6 mm or greater.[22]

Hypertrophic cardiomyopathy is characterized by a broad range of phenotypic patterns of LV hypertrophy ranging from localized and relatively mild wall thickening involving any one particular wall segment to diffuse and pronounced hypertrophy of all portions of the left ventricle.[22, 55, 71–74] No single pattern can be considered characteristic of the disease. In a study assessing the distribution of LV hypertrophy in 46 HCM cats, four patterns of LV hypertrophy were identified[22]: When viewed from the short axis, most often (in 31 cats) hypertrophy was diffuse and substantial, involving portions of ventricular septum as well as contiguous anterolateral and posterior free wall. Fifteen of the 31 cats showed a concentric distribution of hypertrophy of all segments, and 16 had involvement of the anterior portion of the septum as well as anterolateral and posterior free wall (but not posterior septum). Less often (in the remaining 15 cats), segmental patterns of hypertrophy were recorded. In 13 of these 15 cats, wall thickness was confined to only one LV segment (anterior septum in 12 cats and posterior free wall in 1 cat). In 2 of the 15 cats, wall thickening involved non-contiguous segments of LV (i.e., anterior septum or posterior free wall). When viewed from the longitudinal axis, 26 of the 46 cats showed greater wall thickening of the basal rather than apical portion of the left ventricle. Some had proximal septal thickening that protrudes into the LV outflow tract. The other 20 cats had diffuse thickening involving the basal and apical left ventricle. Additional findings include LA and often RA enlargement, decreased LV internal dimensions with hypertrophied papillary muscles, normal to elevated LV fractional shortening, mild hypertrophy of the RV wall and mild to moderate hypertrophy of the RV outflow tract, RV dilation (late in the disease course of some cases), and pericardial effusion. In cases of dynamic LV outflow tract obstruction, there is systolic anterior motion of the mitral apparatus and mid-systolic aortic valve closure (see Fig. 117–3), narrowed LV outflow tract, a fibrous plaque on the basal ventricular

CV

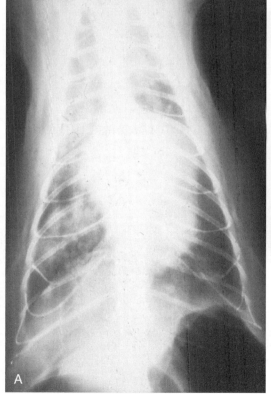
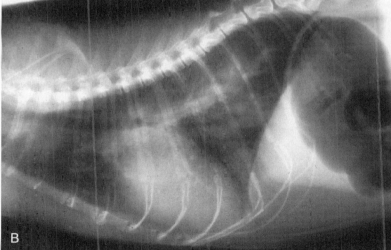

Figure 117–7. Ventrodorsal *(A)* and right lateral *(B)* thoracic radiographs of a cat with acute dyspnea and hypertrophic cardiomyopathy. The left atrium, left ventricle, and right atrium are moderately enlarged. Diffuse, patchy, interstitial and alveolar infiltrates with air bronchograms are present, particularly in the right caudal lung lobe. These changes are compatible with pulmonary edema. After furosemide therapy, these infiltrates cleared.

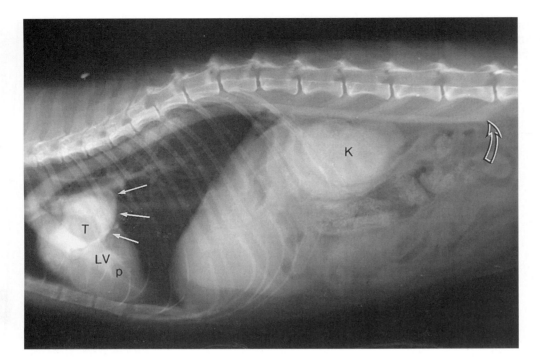

Figure 117–8. Non-selective angiocardiogram of a 7-year-old domestic short-hair cat with hypertrophic cardiomyopathy that had acute posterior paresis. Within the severely dilated left atrium (arrows) is a filling defect caused by a large ball thrombus (T). The LV cavity (LV) is markedly reduced owing to concentric hypertrophy. Note the thickened LV posterior wall and the finger-like apical filling defect caused by papillary muscle (p) hypertrophy. Radiocontrast dye opacifies the aorta but stops abruptly near its terminus owing to complete occlusion (arrow) by a "saddle" embolus. The kidneys (K) are opacified.

septum corresponding to a point of systolic anterior mitral valve contact, and thickening of the anterior mitral valve leaflet.[4–6, 22, 33, 51, 53–58, 65, 73, 74]

Doppler Echocardiography. Mitral regurgitation is common. In 46 cats with HCM, mild to moderate mitral regurgitation was detected in 96 per cent, regardless of whether the obstructive or non-obstructive form was present.[22] Cats with systolic anterior motion usually have eccentric mitral regurgitation jets oriented toward the posterolateral wall. These jets result from systolic disruption of the mitral valve apparatus. Tricuspid regurgitation is less common. With dynamic LV outflow tract obstruction, the maximal LV outflow tract velocity is increased. Waveforms display a characteristic concave and asymmetrically shaped pattern (see Fig. 117–4) because they increase relatively slowly in early systole but then rise abruptly and peak in mid systole. Mitral inflow Doppler waveforms may be normal or indicate a relaxation abnormality indicative of diastolic dysfunction (see Fig. 117–1).[16, 39, 51, 85] Occasionally, a mid LV gradient may be present.

Clinical Pathology. Effusions, when present, are obstructive transudate or modified transudate.[86] Mild prerenal azotemia may result from anorexia and vomiting. Anorectic cats are usually hypokalemic. These changes may be exacerbated by overzealous diuretic administration.[4–7, 87] Thromboembolism will cause elevations of serum muscle and hepatic enzymes and, occasionally, hyperkalemia.[4–8, 29, 79] Hypersomatotropism has been reported in hypertrophic cats,[88] but its significance, if any, is uncertain.

Differential Diagnosis

Conditions that cause LV hypertrophy must be excluded before idiopathic HCM can be diagnosed. Thus, the two most common differential diagnoses are hyperthyroidism and systemic hypertension. Rarely, valvular or subvalvular aortic stenosis is encountered. Because right-sided CHF may occur with HCM, non-cardiac causes of pleural effusions must be excluded. Pericardial diseases must be considered when pericardial effusion is present.

Natural History and Prognosis

Predicting the clinical course and outcome is difficult because of the wide variation in complexity of disease expression. No particular clinical finding has been reliably associated with subsequent sudden death or early recrudescence of CHF. Many cats with HCM achieve adulthood without clinical signs and appear to have a normal life expectancy, often without major therapeutic interventions. Some cats will be presented with severe CHF, become compensated with or without drug administration, and then remain asymptomatic. Others experience recurrent CHF and ultimately die. In a series of 46 HCM cats in which 43 were observed for up to 49 months,[22] non-survivors showed a significantly greater magnitude and extent of LV hypertrophy (maximum wall thickness, 8.1 ± 1.5 mm) than survivors (7.3 ± 0.9 mm); non-survivors also had significantly larger LA dimension (20.1 ± 4.6 mm) compared with survivors (16.8 ± 3.4 mm). In addition, systolic anterior motion was more common in survivors (16 of 18 cats [89 per cent]) than non-survivors (10 of 21 cats [48 per cent]), suggesting that the non-obstructive form of feline HCM without systolic anterior motion had a more unfavorable prognosis. In another series of 61 HCM cats for which follow-up evaluation was possible,[25] median survival time was 732 days. Longevity was not affected by age, breed, gender, or body weight. Cats without clinical signs lived longer (median survival > 1830 days) than those with clinical signs (cats in heart failure survived a median of 92 days and cats with arterial embolism survived a median of 61 days). At 6 months after diagnosis, all cats with embolism and 60 per cent of cats with heart failure were dead. Cats with heart rates less than 200 beats per minute at initial examination survived significantly longer than those with heart rates greater than 200 beats per minute. In a series of 15 HCM cats that had CHF, a mean survival time of 1147 days was recorded, although treatments varied and no controls were included.[89]

A disease pattern of HCM has been reported in a highly interrelated colony of Maine coon cats with familial HCM. When individuals with phenotypic LV hypertrophy were mated to cats without hypertrophy, HCM was not evident before 1 year of age, usually became apparent during adolescence, and usually progressed to severe disease by 2 to 4 years of age. In cats from affected to affected matings, HCM became apparent as early as 3 months of age and progressed to severe disease between 6 to 18 months of age. [31]

RESTRICTIVE CARDIOMYOPATHY

Definitions and Nomenclature

Restrictive cardiomyopathy (RCM) is defined as heart muscle disease that results in impaired diastolic ventricular filling, normal or decreased ventricular diastolic volume, generally normal systolic function, and normal to increased ventricular wall thickness.[3] In humans, it represents a spectrum of conditions that includes idiopathic RCM and RCM that occurs secondary to systemic or metabolic disorders. These different causes result in a variety of clinical and morphologic phenotypes, pathophysiologic derangements, and diastolic dysfunction.[1-3, 19, 51, 90-108] Thus, the only justification to use the term *restrictive cardiomyopathy* is that the case should be characterized by a cardiomyopathic process that restricts diastolic ventricular filling and excludes HCM. Accordingly, RCM is a specific pathophysiologic entity characterized within a broader group of conditions that cause diastolic dysfunction or diastolic heart failure.[105] Two basic categories of RCM are recognized in humans[1-3, 8, 9, 51, 91-93, 103, 105] and appear to be valid for cats as well[4-7, 19, 94-98]: (1) *myocardial RCM* (most prevalent) and (2) *endomyocardial RCM*.

Prevalence and Demographics

Prevalence data have been complicated by controversies in clinical diagnosis and antemortem recognition. The incidence of RCM diagnosed by echocardiography relative to other cardiomyopathies is illustrated in Figure 117–1. There are no known gender or breed predilections. Ages of affected cats are variable, but middle-aged or older animals are most commonly affected.[94, 98]

Etiology

Both myocardial and endomyocardial forms of feline RCM are idiopathic. The myocardial form is poorly characterized in cats but is generally a non-infiltrative disease. In humans, this form of RCM most commonly results from amyloid infiltration,[1, 2, 8, 9, 90, 92] although other causes have been reported.[8] A familial form of idiopathic myocardial RCM has also been documented, both with[08, 109] and without[110] skeletal myopathy in humans but, currently, not in cats. Endomyocardial feline RCM has been associated with endomyocarditis of undetermined origin in a small number of cases.[98] The ability of many viruses to infect and potentially injure myocardial tissue and activate the immune system has been suggested.[111-115] Isolation of parvoviral genomic material from feline hearts with idiopathic cardiomyopathy including RCM gives credence to a similar mechanism.[116] The endomyocardial form of human RCM and eosinophilic cardiomyopathy (Löffler's endocarditis) are thought to be different manifestations of restrictive obliterative cardiomyopathy associated with eosinophilia.[117] In cats, eosinophilic cardiomyopathy has not been described per se, although hypereosinophilic syndrome with multi-organ eosinophilic infiltration including the heart has been reported.[99, 101] Thus, a possible pathogenic relationship between direct eosinophilic involvement or indirect immune-mediated injury is speculated for some cases. Causes of the myocardial form of feline RCM have not been proposed.

Pathophysiology

The hallmark of RCM is diastolic dysfunction. Early LV filling is rapid but is then suddenly restrained, impeded by rigid ventricular walls or endocardium that impairs myocardial elasticity.[1, 51, 118] This results in elevated filling pressures with resultant pulmonary and systemic congestion. Contractility (systolic function) is generally normal or only mildly impaired.

Pathology

Myocardial (Non-infiltrative) Form of Idiopathic RCM. In humans, RCM most often results from systemic or metabolic processes that infiltrate the interstitial matrix.[1, 8, 92] Although RCM is poorly characterized in cats, neither amyloid infiltration nor deposition of abnormal metabolic material within myocytes has been identified. Thus, the feline condition represents a non-infiltrative, idiopathic RCM. Gross pathologic features include mild to moderate increase in heart weight and heart weight/body weight ratio, biatrial enlargement with particularly severe LA dilation, relatively normal LV internal cavity size, and normal to mildly increased LV wall thickness. Patchy endocardial fibrosis is common. Ball thrombi may be present in the LA or LV. Histopathologic findings include diffuse or patchy interstitial fibrosis and myocyte necrosis.

Endomyocardial Form of Idiopathic RCM. Two forms of endomyocardial RCM, hypereosinophilic syndrome (Löffler's endocarditis) and endomyocardial fibrosis, have received the most attention in humans and may represent different manifestations of the same disease. Activated eosinophils cause myocardial toxicity,[119] a theory supported by animal models of hypereosinophilic syndromes (HES).[98, 99, 120, 121] In a single cat with HES, the echocardiogram was unremarkable but focal mononuclear cell infiltration was present within the myocardium.[99] In another report of three cats with HES, two were necropsied and had subendocardial eosinophilic infiltration without fibrosis or gross cardiac lesions.[101] In the endomyocardial form of feline RCM, endomyocarditis and LV endomyocardial fibrosis have been reported, occurring both separately and together.[19, 98, 122, 123] Gross pathologic findings include greater than normal heart weight and heart weight to body weight ratio; severe LV endocardial scar (typically in the mid to apical cavity), often obliterating the distal chamber, causing mid-ventricular stenosis, or fusing and distorting the mitral apparatus; normal to hypertrophied LV wall; severe LA and often RA enlargement; myocardial infarction; variable RV hypertrophy; and LA or LV mural ball thrombi (Fig. 117–9). Histologic findings include marked LV endocardial thickening and scar; intramural coronary arteriosclerosis; endomyocardial necrosis and fibrosis; and, in cases of LV endomyocarditis, variable endomyocardial infiltrates (predominantly neutrophils and macrophages but occasionally lymphocytes and plasma cells).

Clinical Manifestations

History. Tachypnea and dyspnea may be acute or subacute with pulmonary edema. In chronic stages of the dis-

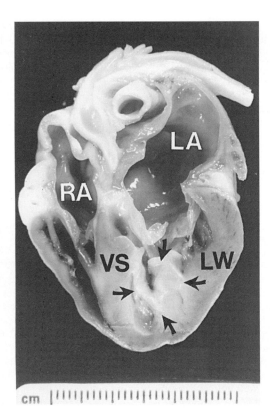

Figure 117–9. Gross heart from a cat with the endomyocardial form of idiopathic restrictive cardiomyopathy. The specimen was sectioned in a modified four-chamber long-axis plane to reveal the left ventricular inflow tract. The LV chamber is deformed by a massive, endocardial scar (arrows). This fibrous plaque bridges the interventricular septum (VS) and LV posterior wall (LW), nearly obliterating the mid and apical LV cavity. The left atrium (LA) is severely enlarged, and the right atrium is moderately dilated.

ease, effusions may predominate and cause gradual signs of dyspnea and weight loss associated with cachexia. Aortic thromboembolism is common and results in paresis.[92]

Physical Examination. Dyspnea and tachypnea may be present. Thoracic auscultation may reveal dull heart and lung sounds in the presence of marked pericardial or pleural effusion, or respiratory crackles may be associated with severe pulmonary edema. Soft, systolic heart murmurs may be detected over the mitral or tricuspid valve area or between the mitral valve area and sternum. Gallop heart rhythms are sometimes present. Distended jugular veins and elevated jugular venous pressures may accompany right-sided CHF. Irregular heart rates and arterial pulse deficits may be detected. Paresis is associated with thromboembolic complications.

Electrocardiography. Arrhythmias are common (see Table 117–2), and a variety of ECG changes may be recorded. Low voltage QRS complexes may be noted when severe pericardial and pleural effusions are present. Evidence of LA enlargement (P wave duration > 40 ms) or LV enlargement ($R_{II} > 0.8$ mV or QRS duration > 40 ms) is common.

Radiography. Classic radiographic changes include moderate to severe LA enlargement and, often, RA enlargement. Pulmonary edema and pleural effusion are common. Generalized cardiomegaly may be evident if pericardial effusion is present. Ascites may be detected, especially in chronic cases.

Angiocardiography. Findings include severe LA enlargement; an irregular LV cavity, often with partial mid-

ventricular constriction or striking obliteration of the apical cavity caused by severe endocardial scar formation; and LA or LV filling defects suggesting intracavitary ball thrombi (Fig. 117–10). The non-infiltrative myocardial form of RCM is characterized by severe LA enlargement with a relatively normal-appearing LV cavity. Ball thrombi may also be present. Right-sided changes are variable.

Echocardiography. Cardinal features of endomyocardial RCM include (1) pronounced endocardial scar, most commonly at the level of the mid-left ventricle, bridging the free wall and ventricular septum, which may cause mild to severe mid-ventricular constriction, resulting in a diastolic and systolic pressure gradient identifiable by Doppler echocardiography; and (2) severe LA enlargement with pronounced left auricular dilation. Additionally, the ventricular septum or LV posterior (free) wall may be mildly hypertrophied (e.g., end-diastolic thickness 5.5 to 6 mm) or normal. The LV posterior wall may appear non-homogeneous owing to focal hyperechoic areas or diffuse speckling. LV cavity dimensions may be normal or reduced, or severe endocardial fibrosis may result in obliteration of the apical LV cavity. The RA is usually enlarged, and RV changes vary from mild hypertrophy to dilation. Intracavitary ball thrombi (LA or LV) are common. Mitral and tricuspid valvular insufficiency are often present, but regurgitation is usually mild. Contractility is generally normal.

In contrast, the myocardial form of RCM is characterized by (1) marked LA or biatrial enlargement, (2) a relatively normal LV chamber, (3) normal ventricular septum or LV free wall thickness or mild hypertrophy (end-diastolic wall dimensions 5.5 to 6 mm), and (4) lack of severe left heart volume overload. Valvular insufficiency, if present, is mild.

Differential Diagnosis

From a pathophysiologic perspective, diagnosis of the myocardial form of RCM requires either Doppler echocardi-

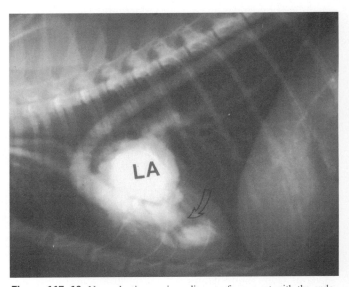

Figure 117–10. Non-selective angiocardiogram from a cat with the endomyocardial form of restrictive cardiomyopathy. This animal had acute pulmonary edema 2 days earlier. The left atrium (LA) is severely enlarged; pulmonary veins are prominent and tortuous, suggesting elevated left-sided heart filling pressures. A mid LV filling defect is indicated by lack of radiocontrast dye (arrow), and the apical cavity is irregular. These changes were caused by a large endocardial scar bridging the ventricular septum and left ventricular free wall, which nearly obliterated the mid left ventricular cavity.

ographic evidence of LV restrictive physiology or LV relaxation abnormality, in the absence of severe idiopathic LV hypertrophy. When Doppler echocardiographic evidence of diastolic dysfunction is lacking, a presumptive diagnosis of RCM is based on cardiac morphology that closely conforms to classic phenotypes of RCM (see Echocardiography, earlier) and excludes HCM, myocardial infarction, and other cardiomyopathies. Thus, RCM is diagnosed from the presence of a number of structural and physiologic features and by the absence of others. A diagnosis of RCM is not tenable in the presence of significant LV dilation or with severe LV hypertrophy without an LV endocardial scar. Accordingly, a diagnosis of RCM is often somewhat uncertain. In many cases, myocardial diseases may be more appropriately labeled *unclassified cardiomyopathy* when echocardiographic findings are equivocal, when mitral regurgitation is severe, when LA enlargement is mild, or when Doppler trans-mitral filling patterns are normal. RCM causes a syndrome that is hemodynamically similar to constrictive pericarditis, an exceedingly rare condition in cats.

Natural History and Prognosis

The true natural history of RCM is unknown. The rate of progression of diastolic dysfunction has not been determined. Frequently, RCM has an insidious onset with development of progressive right-sided CHF. Prognosis is generally poor when marked right-sided CHF is present, especially when accompanied with tachyarrhythmias such as atrial fibrillation.

THERAPY FOR HEART FAILURE ASSOCIATED WITH DIASTOLIC DYSFUNCTION

Optimal strategies for treating asymptomatic or mildly symptomatic cases is unclear. There is currently no consensus among cardiologists regarding therapeutic approaches for asymptomatic cases or even for chronic management, and there is little evidence-based data on which treatment strategies can be based.

HYPERTROPHIC CARDIOMYOPATHY

Therapies in Asymptomatic but Potentially High-Risk Patients

There are several important features of HCM that may increase risks of morbidity and mortality. Accordingly, prophylactic therapy may be warranted in these circumstances based on certain pathophysiologic considerations.

Myocardial Infarction. Myocardial infarction (MI) may be more prevalent than once believed.[77, 124] Clinical suspicion of MI is based on echocardiographic evidence of regional LV hypokinesis or dyskinesis, LV free wall thinning (end-diastolic measurement < 2 mm), or ECG evidence of marked (>0.2 mV) ST segment elevation or depression. In cats and humans with HCM, MI causes significant morbidity and may be related to intramural arteriosclerosis.[21–25, 45, 46] Myocardial ischemia is commonly associated with MI and myocardial fibrosis in human HCM[23, 50, 76, 124] and, presumably, in feline HCM as well, given their similar histopathologic lesions.[19, 20, 21–24, 31, 45, 71, 77] Ischemia may be associated with severe and potentially lethal arrhythmias.[125] Several drug therapies may be considered for treating MI.

Beta-adrenergic Blocker Therapy. Compelling evidence for beta-blocker therapy is based on human trials. These agents decreased mortality in patients with acute MI and cardiac arrhythmias.[125, 127] With chronic MI, beta-blockers reduced long-term mortality by their anti-arrhythmic effects and by prevention of re-infarction, particularly when decreased contractility and ventricular arrhythmias were present.[128, 129] Because LV diastolic function is very sensitive to increases in sympathetic tone,[130] sympathetic nervous system antagonists may indirectly improve ventricular compliance by reducing heart rate and myocardial ischemia. In cats with suspected ischemic myocardial injury, propranolol (2.5 to 5 mg q8–12h PO) or atenolol (6.25–12.5 mg per cat q12–24h PO) can be administered. Beta-blockers may occasionally cause bradycardia, hypotension, or lethargy.

Angiotensin-Converting Enzyme (ACE) Inhibitor Therapy. ACE inhibitors have been advocated in human post-MI trials based on their role in reducing cardiovascular remodeling and improving hemodynamics and survival.[131–134] There is clear evidence that ACE inhibitors decrease mortality in acute MI[135] and that chronic therapy reduces ischemic events in humans.[136] Enalapril (0.23 mg/lb q24h PO), benazepril (0.23 mg/lb q24h PO), and lisinopril (0.11 to 0.23 mg/lb q24h PO) have been used safely in cats. Because ACE inhibitors may reduce blood pressure, they can be contraindicated in cats with hypotension and with overzealous diuretic therapy.

Calcium Channel Blocker Therapy. Based on extrapolation from human studies, one might exercise caution when considering these agents in cats with MI. Calcium channel blockers have not been efficacious (i.e., no reduction of subsequent cardiovascular events) in treating human MI.[137, 138] Furthermore, diltiazem and other calcium-blocking agents were harmful when MI and LV dysfunction were present,[139–141] possibly because of activation of the neuroendocrine system.[142] Accordingly, calcium antagonists are not recommended for routine secondary prevention after infarction in humans.[143] Whether these data are relevant to treatment strategies for feline myocardial diseases remains to be determined.

Tachyarrhythmias. Tachycardia diminishes systolic and diastolic function[50]; reduces diastolic filling, which can increase outflow gradients and reduce forward cardiac output[10, 51]; and can result in excessive myocardial oxygen utilization and ischemia.[49] In some cases, tachycardia precipitates weakness or syncope. Beta-adrenergic blockers (propranolol, 5–10 mg q8–12h PO; atenolol, 6.25–12.5 mg q12–24h PO) antagonize the sympathetic nervous system and may therefore be useful for treating paroxysmal ventricular tachycardia or frequent multi-form ventricular arrhythmias. Digoxin (0.031 mg [i.e., one fourth of a 0.125-mg tablet] per 10-lb cat q48h PO) or diltiazem may be administered for atrial tachyarrhythmias. However, heart rate control often requires the addition of a beta-blocker that is titrated to effect.

Massive Left Ventricular Hypertrophy. Although the severity of hypertrophy is not a recognized risk factor for sudden death in human HCM,[55, 144–146] unfavorable prognosis may be associated with severe LV hypertrophy in cats.[22, 31] Marked hypertrophy is present when the maximal LV free wall or interventricular septal thickness measured at end-diastole exceeds 8 mm. Several drugs are available for pharmacotherapy, but clinical efficacy data are scant.

Beta-Blocker Therapy. These agents may be selected for the following reasons[55, 63, 147–150]: (1) heart rate control (negative chronotropism) and associated indirect improvement of diastolic filling; (2) reduction of dynamic LV outflow tract obstruction; (3) reduction in myocardial oxygen utilization; (4) antiarrhythmic effects; (5) ability to blunt sympathetic myocardial stimulation; or (6) improved survival. Clinical reduction of resting heart rate to 120 to 160 beats per minute is usually attainable with atenolol (6.25–12.5 mg q12–24h PO) or propranolol (5–10 mg q8–12h PO) for an average size (10 lb) cat.

Calcium Channel Blocker Therapy. These drugs are often advocated based on their action to promote positive lusiotropy (i.e., to directly improve ventricular diastolic relaxation and filling).[37–39] Diltiazem may slow the heart rate in some cats but not in others, and heart rate reduction is much weaker than results from beta-blocker therapy. Several preparations of diltiazem are available: diltiazem (Cardizem; 7.5 mg q8–12h); Cardizem CD capsules (a long-acting formulation; 4.5 mg/lb q24h); and extended-release diltiazem. In extended-release diltiazem each 240-mg capsule contains four controlled-released 60-mg tablets and the starting dosage is 30 mg every 12 to 24 hours. (Some cats may tolerate 60 mg once to twice daily, although vomiting is a common side effect.)

ACE Inhibitor Therapy. ACE inhibitors may blunt neuroendocrine activation and prevent deleterious cardiovascular remodeling. The merits of ACE inhibitors for treating feline HCM have a scientific basis,[148, 151–154] and ACE inhibitors have been used safely, most commonly added to other therapies.[89] Enalapril (0.23 mg/lb q24h PO) and benazepril (0.23 mg/lb q24h PO) are well tolerated.

Syncope. Recurrent syncope is a risk factor for sudden death in humans with HCM[155–158] and can be associated with tachyarrhythmias and bradyarrhythmias,[157] dynamic LV outflow obstruction,[159] altered baroreflexes,[160] and ischemia.[161] In cats, syncope is most often clinically associated with physical activity or exertion and obstructive HCM. Symptoms can often be managed successfully with beta-blockers, which alleviate or abolish dynamic LV outflow tract obstruction.

Spontaneous Echo Contrast ("Smoke") and Stasis. An echo phenomenon called *spontaneous echo contrast* is frequently observed in the LA or LV of cardiomyopathic cats and is associated with LA blood stasis. It is considered to presage thrombosis and is associated with increased thromboembolic risk.[162–164] "Smoke" has been attributed to erythrocyte aggregation at a low shear rate[165, 166] or to platelet aggregates.[167, 168] Many interrelated factors are involved in thrombogenesis, including blood stasis.[169, 170] Given the many pathologic and hemodynamic derangements common to feline and human heart disease, spontaneous echo contrast and stasis should be considered a clinical marker for incipient thromboembolism and invoke a more aggressive therapeutic strategy.

"Malignant" Family History (High-Risk Genotype). Pedigrees are occasionally identified in which a heritable pattern of HCM with severe morbidity and mortality is documented. For example, LV hypertrophy, heart failure, thromboembolism, and death have been reported in multiple generations of Maine coon cats,[31, 32] and other examples of familial transmission have been documented.[33] Thus, echocardiographic surveillance is warranted to evaluate disease progression, direct therapy, and assist prognosis. In such animals, early intervention with calcium channel blockers or beta-adrenergic receptor blockers may be contemplated. This unproven strategy is based on experimental and theoretical considerations, which hold that a pathway to the phenotypic expression of LV hypertrophy is influenced by triggers such as higher LV pressure and workload.[124, 171]

Myocardial Failure. In some HCM cats, LV contractility is mildly to moderately reduced (e.g., fractional shortening, 23–29 per cent; LV end-systolic dimension, 12–15 mm). This can result from acute or chronic myocardial infarction, particularly involving the LV posterior wall. Global LV failure has been observed with diffuse LV necrosis and fibrosis. Occasionally, HCM progresses to a stage of chamber dilatation and systolic dysfunction resembling dilated cardiomyopathy. This is usually associated with refractory heart failure and poor prognosis. Oral taurine supplementation (250 mg q12–24h) is initiated whenever myocardial failure is detected. An ACE inhibitor may be added for its beneficial effect to counteract neurohormonal activation and reduce deleterious remodeling. Digoxin may be administered (0.031 mg q48h) if contractility deteriorates or if supraventricular tachyarrhythmias (particularly atrial tachycardia or atrial fibrillation) develop. Beta-blocker therapy might be beneficial if myocardial infarction is suspected or if a tachyarrhythmia warrants control of ventricular heart rate despite other therapies.

Treatment of Symptomatic Cats

Acute Pulmonary Edema. Acute pulmonary edema is rapidly progressive and life threatening. Furosemide is the most commonly used agent to rapidly reduce cardiogenic pulmonary edema. It inhibits renal tubular reabsorption of sodium or its accompanying anions, promotes diuresis, and reduces vascular volume, thereby decreasing LV filling pressures (i.e., cardiac preload) and pulmonary congestion.[172] Initially, furosemide is administered intravenously (0.5–1.0 mg/lb) every 1 to 2 hours until the congestive state is substantially reduced. Then, the dosage frequency is decreased, typically to every 8 to 12 hours, and the drug is given intramuscularly or subcutaneously. Peak diuresis usually occurs within 30 minutes of intravenous administration. Resolution of edema may be enhanced in the first 24 to 36 hours of therapy by adding the preload reducer 2 per cent nitroglycerin ointment (1/8 to 1/4 inch q6h cutaneously; alternate 12 hours with and 12 hours without nitroglycerin therapy to reduce development of tolerance). Supplemental oxygen (40 to 60 per cent oxygen-enriched inspired gas) may be beneficial to improve pulmonary gas exchange. Clinical resolution is indicated by reduced respiratory rate and work of breathing, resolved auscultatory lung crackles, and radiographic clearing of alveolar infiltrates (usually complete by 24 to 36 hours).[4, 5, 7] The end point of diuretic therapy is relief of clinical signs or progressive increase in blood urea nitrogen (BUN) and creatinine levels. Cardiac responses to diuresis include decreased LA diameter and reduced Doppler echocardiographic trans-mitral E wave velocity.[173, 174] Dehydration and hypokalemia can result from overzealous diuresis, especially in the anorectic cat.[87]

Chronic Maintenance Therapy. Chronic therapies are individualized to maintain cardiac compensation; prevent arterial thromboembolism; halt, slow, or reverse myocardial dysfunction (theoretically); promote enhanced quality of life; and prolong survival. Underlying conditions and risk factors (e.g., arterial hypertension, taurine-deficient diets, hyperthyroidism, anemia) are treated when identified. There are currently no data to indicate which are the most effective drugs, whether combined therapy is more advantageous than monotherapy alone, or, for that matter, whether therapy is significantly better than no therapy. Because drugs are administered on an empirical basis, relying on clinical experiences, preferences, and theoretical benefits, advantages and disadvantages of current therapies are discussed next.

Diuretics. As soon as congestion is resolved and breathing improves, furosemide is changed to oral administration (typically, 6.25 mg q12–24h) and then gradually decreased to the lowest effective dosage. Some cats remain stable on daily therapy, whereas in others, diuretics may be largely unnecessary and can be safely discontinued. In contrast, upward titration is necessary with recurrent CHF, although diuretic resistance may occur as heart failure progresses.[175, 176] Cats with chronic CHF that have acute exacerbations of congestion are likely to benefit from intravenous furosemide, which has higher bioavailability, or from administration of two diuretics (see Recurrent and Refractory Congestive Heart Failure, later). It is prudent to assess BUN, creatinine, and electrolytes in anorectic or decompensated cats receiving diuretics.[87]

Beta-adrenergic Blockers. Prolonged activation of the sympathetic nervous system may lead to cardiovascular injury that exacerbates disease progression,[177, 178] causes arrhythmias,[179] or stimulates vasoconstriction and secondary tissue anoxia.[180] Sustained vasoconstriction, elevated ventricular afterload, and other mechanisms contribute to abnormal cardiovascular remodeling and progression to CHF.[181–183] Because LV diastolic function is very sensitive to increases in sympathetic tone,[184] by decreasing heart rate with beta-blockers, diastole is prolonged and passive ventricular filling and compliance are improved. Prolonged diastolic filling also allows more time for coronary blood flow and reduces myocardial ischemia.[184–186] Beta-blockers decrease myocardial oxygen requirements by reducing cardiac sympathetic stimulation, heart rate, LV contractility, systolic myocardial wall stress, and systemic blood pressure.[185, 187] Dynamic LV outflow tract obstruction and related pressure gradient are often reduced or abolished with beta-blocker therapy.[54, 188] Propranolol (5–10 mg q8–12h PO) has been recommended for more than 25 years.[4–7, 26, 27, 189, 190] It improves clinical signs, reduces heart rate, decreases severity of dynamic LV outflow tract obstruction, and is safe.[188, 190] Disadvantages include its need for frequent (thrice daily) dosing in some cats (half-life, 0.49 hour)[191] and its poor and variable oral bioavailability owing to extensive first-pass hepatic metabolism.[192] Atenolol (6.25–12.5 mg q12–24h PO) has become popular for several reasons. Its high oral bioavailability (90 ± 9 per cent) results in small inter-individual kinetic variability. Atenolol has a longer half-life (3.66 = 0.39 hours) than propranolol, and the heart rate attenuation after oral administration persists for at least 12 hours in normal cats.[193] Adverse reactions to beta-blockers are uncommon but include lethargy or hypotension, typically within an hour of first administration.[5, 6, 188]

Calcium Channel Blockers. These agents are used to enhance diastolic performance.[16, 24, 37, 38, 40] Diltiazem appears to improve LV diastolic function in human HCM.[194–196] In general, calcium antagonists may reduce heart rate (verapamil much more so than diltiazem) and blood pressure; exert a mild negative inotropic effect (reducing myocardial oxygen consumption); and improve rapid diastolic ventricular filling.[37, 38, 197–202] Diltiazem is less effective than verapamil with LV outflow obstruction.[54, 55, 149, 203] In a small clinical trial in which furosemide was combined with either diltiazem or propranolol to treat HCM cats with pulmonary edema, the diltiazem group (12 cats) had congestion resolved and indices of LV relaxation and filling improved. However, too few patients (5 cats) were allocated to the propranolol group to make comparative assessment meaningful.[38]

Whereas regression of LV wall thickness was a reported sequela of diltiazem therapy, this phenomenon is generally regarded to occur uncommonly.

Pharmacokinetic data have been reported in healthy cats given diltiazem. For diltiazem (Cardizem, 0.8 to 1.1 mg/lb tid PO), the half life was 113 ± 24 minutes; peak concentration after oral administration was achieved in ≤5 ± 36 minutes; and bioavailability was 50 to 80 per cent. Clinically, this drug is given orally at 7.5 mg three times a day. For a long-acting diltiazem formulation (Cardizem CD, 4.5 mg/lb PO q24h), the half-life was 411 ± 59 minutes; peak concentration after oral administration was achieved in 340 ± 140 minutes; and bioavailability was 22 to 59 per cent.[204] A disadvantage of the Cardizem CD preparation is that it is currently available only in capsules. Another diltiazem preparation, Dilacor XR, is available in an extended-release formulation. Although feline pharmacokinetic data are lacking, this preparation has become popular. Each 240-mg capsule contains four controlled-released 60-mg tablets. Starting dose for a 10-lb cat is 30 mg every 24 hours, and titration to 60 mg daily is tolerated in some patients, although vomiting is a side effect.

Because myocardial infarction is relatively common in feline myocardial diseases, and because there is no relevant treatment data for cats,[124] the results of human myocardial infarction trials may be informative.[205–207] Whether these negative data are relevant to treatment strategies for feline myocardial diseases remains to be determined.

ACE Inhibitors. Because neurohormonal activation plays an important role in heart failure,[208] disruption of neurohormonal activation should provide therapeutic rationale for using ACE inhibitors.[209, 210] Pathologic features of HCM are related to systolic and/or diastolic dysfunction associated with LV hypertrophy and derangements of myocardial extracellular matrix.[22, 23, 37, 38, 43, 45, 211–213] The renin-angiotensin-aldosterone system (RAS) plays a prominent role in human HCM patients by influencing or regulating the expression of myocardial hypertrophy.[214] There is some evidence that the RAS is activated in cats with HCM.[215] Inhibition of the RAS has a beneficial effect on extracellular remodeling in CHF,[216] and ACE inhibitors reduce ventricular remodeling by blocking the tropic effects of angiotensin II on myocytes.[217, 218] Given the clear survival value provided by early use of ACE inhibitors in acute human myocardial infarction,[219] background therapy with these agents might theoretically confer beneficial effects in similar circumstances. Recently, ACE inhibitors have been used to treat HCM in humans[220] and cats.[89]

Many clinicians combine an ACE inhibitor (usually enalapril) with furosemide, with or without a beta-blocker or calcium channel blocker, particularly when recurrent right-sided heart failure is present, if pulmonary edema recurs, or if progressive atrial enlargement is detected.[89] Enalapril and benazepril are clinically well tolerated.[89, 188, 221, 222] After oral administration of enalapril dosed at 0.1 and 0.23 mg/lb, a 95 per cent reduction in ACE occurred between 2 and 4 hours after either dose, and it remained depressed to less than 50 per cent of control for 2 to 3 days.[221] After single doses of benazepril (0.23 mg/lb), peak plasma benazepril levels were achieved 2 hours after oral administration and more than 90 per cent of plasma ACE inhibition persisted at 24 hours.[222] Other ACE inhibitors are also available. The optimal timing for ACE inhibitor administration, the most effective dosage, and the effects of these agents on morbidity and mortality in feline cardiomyopathy remain to be determined.

Reduction/Elimination of LV Outflow Tract Gradient. Negative inotropic drugs that reduce or eliminate obstruction have been widely used in humans with the obstructive form of HCM.[54, 223, 224] In cats, reduction of outflow gradient is usually best accomplished with beta-blocker therapy. Stimuli that provoke or intensify LV outflow tract gradients should be avoided, including positive inotropes, reduction of LV volume, or decreased afterload. The clinical importance of decreasing obstruction, particularly in asymptomatic cats, has not been established.

Recurrent and Refractory CHF. When pulmonary edema or biventricular failure recurs, emergency treatment may be required to increase the diuretic dose, increase the "primary" drug dose, change to a different class of primary drugs, or add a second or even third primary agent. For recurrent congestion in spite of these manipulations, particularly with severe, chronic effusions, further upward dose titration of furosemide (to 2 mg/lb q8–12h PO) may be required. Alternatively, the addition of a second diuretic agent that acts at a different site in the nephron (and, thus, synergistically with furosemide) may be helpful in some cases. Hydrochlorothiazide (1–2 mg/lb PO q12–24h) and hydrochlorothiazide-spironolactone (1 mg/lb q24h PO) have proven to be useful "second" diuretic agents.[87] Close monitoring for dehydration, azotemia, hyponatremia, and hypokalemia is advised. Digitalization may be prescribed when right-sided heart failure is unresponsive to diuretics, ACE inhibitors, or other therapy or if myocardial (systolic) failure occurs.

RESTRICTIVE CARDIOMYOPATHY

Acute therapy for pulmonary edema is similar to that described for HCM (see earlier). When moderate to severe pleural effusion is present, therapeutic thoracocentesis may be helpful. There are currently no clinical data indicating optimal chronic management of RCM. Consideration may be given to ACE inhibitors with the rationale for blunting neurohormonal activation and reducing ventricular remodeling; for beta-blockers, particularly when myocardial infarction is suspected or tachyarrhythmias are present; or for aspirin when LA enlargement is severe. Digoxin is added for severe or refractory right-sided CHF or to help reduce the ventricular rate with atrial fibrillation.

SYSTOLIC (MYOCARDIAL) DYSFUNCTION

TAURINE DEFICIENCY DILATED CARDIOMYOPATHY AND IDIOPATHIC MYOCARDIAL FAILURE

Definitions and Nomenclature. When the ventricles fail to generate normal systolic contractile force to maintain forward cardiac output, *systolic dysfunction* is said to be present. Synonymous terminology includes *myocardial failure, pump failure, systolic failure, contractile dysfunction,* and *reduced contractility.* Dilated cardiomyopathy (DCM) is the prototypical example of systolic dysfunction and is characterized by LV or biventricular dilatation and impaired contractility.[3]

Prevalence and Demographics. DCM represented the second most common form of feline myocardial disease before 1990 and was associated with the highest cardiac mortality. Ages of cats with DCM varied from 5 months to 16 years (mean, 7.5 years), and there was a male predisposi-

tion.[27, 122] Although all breeds were affected, a high incidence was observed in the Siamese, Abyssinian, and Burmese breeds.[5, 7] In 1987, an association between taurine deficiency and reversible myocardial failure (DCM) was reported[225] and subsequently corroborated.[226–237] In response, pet food manufacturers re-formulated their feline diets to include more taurine, which resulted in a dramatic reduction of feline taurine deficiency DCM by 1990 (see Fig. 117–2). More recently, 49 cats with myocardial failure were evaluated between 1990 and 1995. Ages ranged from 2 to 20 years (mean, 9.8 ± 4.4 years; median, 9.5 years); 69 per cent were male. Five cats (10 per cent) had markedly reduced taurine concentrations, and their clinical condition was compatible with taurine deficiency DCM. Ten additional cats (20 per cent) had somewhat reduced whole blood taurine concentrations compared with normal levels.[238] Currently, idiopathic myocardial failure represents 3 to 7 per cent of the cardiomyopathic cats evaluated at The Animal Medical Center for suspected heart disease. There is wide variation in degree of systolic impairment and LV morphology.

Etiology. A clear causal relationship has been demonstrated between deficiency of the amino acid taurine and reversible feline myocardial failure.[225, 232–235] Before 1987, most DCM was apparently related to consumption of commercial cat foods that either contained inadequate amounts of taurine[232] or whose taurine was rendered unavailable owing to processing and canning.[234] Although taurine deficiency alone was probably not the only factor responsible for the development of myocardial failure,[226, 228] the incidence of DCM became dramatically reduced after commercial feline diets were fortified with taurine. Although taurine deficiency DCM is still encountered,[238] it has remained a relatively rare cause of feline heart failure. Currently, most cats diagnosed with myocardial failure are idiopathic. Human idiopathic DCM represents a common expression of myocardial injury caused by a number of poorly understood myocardial insults.[1] Three basic mechanisms of myocardial damage include genetic and familial causes,[239, 240] viral myocarditis and other cytotoxic factors,[241–243] and abnormalities of cellular and humeral immunity.[244, 245] Other causes including energetic, metabolic, and contractile abnormalities have been proposed.[1, 2, 244] Some cats with idiopathic myocardial failure have had prominent myocardial fibrosis and infarction.[238] A heritable form of feline DCM has been reported.[246] The possibility that myocarditis is associated with at least some cases of feline DCM is suggested by the isolation of parvoviral genomic DNA from myocardial tissues of cats with DCM.[116]

Pathophysiology. When the LV fails to generate normal contractile force and ejection fraction is severely reduced, end-systolic and end-diastolic ventricular volumes increase, and myocardial wall tension becomes elevated. Alterations in LV relaxation and diastolic compliance co-exist with impaired contractile function and contribute to elevated filling pressure.[247, 248] Activation of the sympathetic and renin-angiotensin-aldosterone systems further increases cardiac preload and afterload. End-systolic volume increases as a result of impaired LV contractility. Pulmonary congestion, effusions, and signs of low cardiac output can result. Urinary acidification combined with potassium depletion may reduce tissue stores of taurine.[249] Taurine deficiency can also result when inappropriate diets are fed.[117, 225, 250, 251] Taurine is an essential dietary amino acid for cats because of their limited ability to synthesize taurine from cysteine and methionine. This is associated with a low concentration of cysteine-sulfinic acid decarboxylase, an enzyme required in taurine

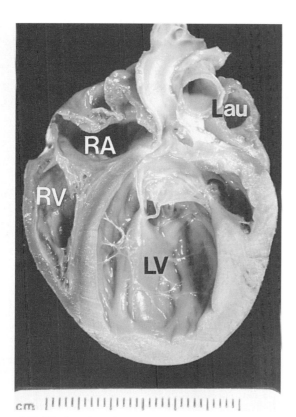

Figure 117–11. Gross heart from a cat with idiopathic dilated cardiomyopathy. The specimen was sectioned in a modified four-chamber long-axis plane. The left ventricle is severely dilated (note the rounded, convex apex). The right atrium (RA), right ventricle (RV), and left atrium (the left auricular appendage [Lau] is visualized) were moderately dilated.

biosynthesis.[252, 253] Cats are unable to conjugate significant amounts of bile acids with glycine and, therefore, must utilize taurine for conjugation. When taurine depleted, cats lose taurine in the bile, which creates severe whole-body taurine loss.[254, 255] Taurine is essential for normal structural and functional integrity of the heart.[225, 256, 257]

Pathology. In classic taurine deficiency DCM there is severe dilation of all four cardiac chambers. Gross features of idiopathic myocardial failure are more variable (Fig. 117–11). There is generally biatrial enlargement with or without hypertrophy. The LV is dilated, and the apex may be thinned. The ventricular septum may be thin or normal, and thinning of the LV free wall is common, typically occurring in the posterior segment of free wall as viewed in cross section. The RV may be dilated, and the RV free wall may be thickened or thinned. Myocytolysis and necrosis, fibrosis, and intramural coronary artery remodeling (arteriosclerosis) are common. Ball thrombi may occur in the LA or LV.

Clinical Manifestations

History. Clinical signs are usually vague and most commonly include anorexia, dyspnea, and lethargy. Vomiting is commonly reported from 1 to 3 days before presentation. Paresis of a front or rear leg results from acute arterial embolization[4–7, 238] in approximately one fifth of cats with idiopathic myocardial failure.

Physical Examination. Lethargy, depression, dehydration, and hypothermia are frequently present. Gallop rhythms (presumably S_3) are often reported; a 2–3/6, systolic, heart murmur heard over the left apex, sternum, or right apex may occur.[4–7, 26, 27, 29, 248] CHF was detected in 94 per cent of

cats with idiopathic myocardial failure.[238] Lung sounds of pulmonary edema or muffled heart and lung sounds with pericardial or pleural effusion are auscultated. Jugular veins may be distended or pulsatile. Hydroperitoneum, hepatomegaly, and pericardial and pleural effusion may accompany right-sided CHF. Persistent central retinal degeneration results from taurine deficiency.[225, 258]

Electrocardiography. ECG changes may include widened P waves (P-mitrale), tall R waves or widened QRS voltages, or various arrhythmias (see Table 117–2). Low-voltage R waves may indicate severe pericardial or pleural effusion.[4–7, 27, 29] First-degree atrioventricular block[26, 80, 82] was recorded in 35 per cent of cats with idiopathic myocardial failure.[228]

Radiography. Characteristic changes include generalized cardiomegaly and pleural effusion (Fig. 117–12). The latter may silhouette the cardiac shadow. Pulmonary venous congestion or mild, patchy, pulmonary edema may be present concurrently but is often obscured by effusion.[4–7, 26, 27] In 49 cats with myocardial failure, pleural effusion was present in 71 per cent and pulmonary edema in 22 per cent.[238]

Echocardiography. Myocardial failure is present if the %FS is less than 30 per cent and LV end-systolic dimension exceeds 12 mm (Fig. 117–13). Several patterns of cardiac dilation and degrees of myocardial failure have been identified. In classic taurine deficiency DCM, generalized enlargement of all four heart chambers, increased LV and RV end-diastolic and end-systolic dimensions, severely depressed global fractional shortening and ejection fraction, and pericardial and pleural effusion were often present. [4–7, 225, 229] Current cases of idiopathic myocardial failure[238] generally display either LV dilation with focal segmental LV hypertro-

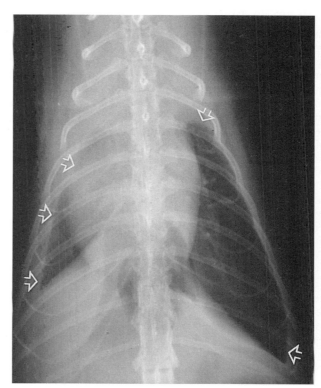

Figure 117–12. Ventrodorsal radiograph from a cat with dilated cardiomyopathy and right-sided congestive heart failure. Pleural effusion is present, causing the lung lobes to retract (arrows), filling the anterior mediastinum, and silhouetting the heart. There is generalized, moderate cardiomegaly. (From Fox PR: Feline myocardial diseases. *In* Fox PR [ed]: Textbook of Canine and Feline Cardiology. New York, Churchill Livingstone, 1998, p 435.)

CV

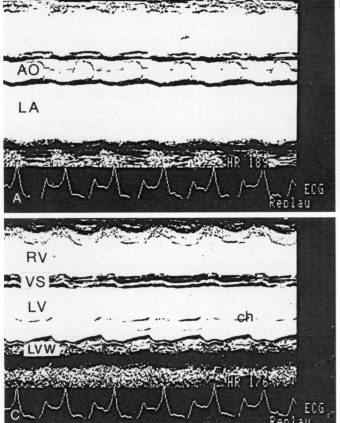

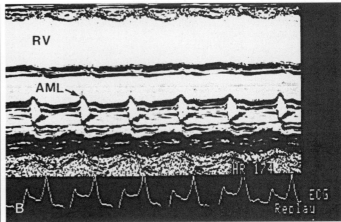

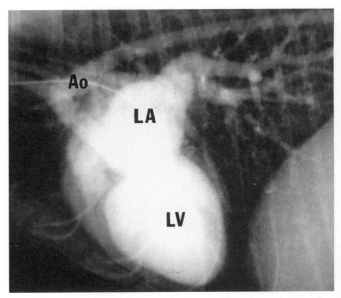

Figure 117–13. M-mode echocardiograms recorded at the three standard imaging planes from a cat with idiopathic dilated cardiomyopathy. *A,* Level of aortic root (AO) and left atrium (LA). The LA is moderately dilated. Poor (hypokinetic) aortic root motion is compatible with myocardial failure. Aortic valves are evident within the AO. *B,* Mitral valve level. Both the right ventricle (RV) and left ventricle are extremely dilated. There is wide separation between the anterior mitral valve leaflet (AML) and the ventricular septum due to left ventricular dilation. *C,* Chordae tendineae (ch) level. Biventricular dilation is evident. LV contractility is markedly decreased, as indicated by reduced systolic excursions of the LV posterior wall (LVW) and, especially, the interventricular septum (VS), which appears almost flat.

phy or LV dilation with ventricular septal or LV free wall hypokinesis, coupled with hyperdynamic motion of the opposite wall. Biatrial enlargement and variable right-sided enlargement are present. Indices of LV contractility may be mildly to severely compromised, that is, decreased LV ejection time and prolonged pre-ejection period; decreased fractional shortening or circumferential fiber shortening; aortic root, interventricular septal, and LV free wall hypokinesis; and reduced velocity-time integral. Mild mitral and/or tricuspid insufficiency are commonly detected. Mural LA or LV thrombi may be present.

Angiocardiography. Salient angiocardiographic features include generalized heart chamber dilation, enlarged and torturous pulmonary veins (and occasionally, pulmonary arteries), reduced cardiac output suggested by increased circulatory transit time of injected radiocontrast dye, and LA or LV intracavitary thrombi (Fig. 117–14)[5–8, 29, 83]

Clinical Pathology. Most cats are azotemic from reduced cardiac output, anorexia, and fluid sequestration (effusions). Effusions are usually obstructive transudate or modified transudate.[4–7, 26, 27, 29, 86] Normal plasma taurine concentration is more than 60 nmol/mL; in cats at risk it is less than 30 nmol/mL. However, plasma taurine concentration is very labile. Even 24 hours of fasting or anorexia can cause plasma levels to fall below 30 nmol/mL. In contrast, whole-blood taurine concentrations are less labile and fasting does not significantly affect values. Normal whole-blood taurine is more than 200 nmol/mL; in cats at risk it is less than 100 nmol/mL.[225, 227, 230, 232, 233, 259, 260]

Differential Diagnosis. Idiopathic myocardial failure is diagnosed on the basis of severe LV dilation and impaired contractile performance. Other known etiologic factors must

be excluded, including severe volume overloads (mitral regurgitation, patent ductus arteriosus, aortic regurgitation), atrioventricular fistulas, left-to-right shunting congenital anomalies, high output states such as severe anemia, and taurine deficiency.

Figure 117–14. Non-selective angiocardiogram from a cat with dilated cardiomyopathy. The left atrium (LA) is moderately enlarged, and the left ventricle (LV) is severely dilated. Papillary muscles (p) are thin and atrophic. The aorta (Ao) is thin and poorly opacified, suggesting diminished forward stroke volume.

Initial Therapy (First 24 to 48 Hours)

Treatment Goals. Initial therapy is directed to reduce or eliminate pulmonary and systemic venous congestion, promote increased forward cardiac output, control serious tachyarrhythmias or bradyarrhythmias, and improve myocardial contractility. General supportive measures such as external heating to combat hypothermia, oxygen administration, and minimization of stress are important.

Thoracocentesis. If breathing is compromised by severe pleural effusion, thoracocentesis is advised. In the severely dyspneic cat, this should be performed even before radiographs are taken.

Acute Pulmonary Edema. Life-threatening pulmonary edema is uncommon with myocardial failure. When edema is severe, refer to HCM, acute pulmonary edema.

Intravenous Inotropic Support. Synthetic sympathomimetic amines possess greater inotropic activity, provide quicker onset of action, and allow finer control than digoxin. Dobutamine (1 to 2.5 µg/lb/min) is the preferred agent for hemodynamic support of the failing heart. It exerts its positive inotropic effects through direct stimulation of myocardial beta-adrenergic receptors.[261-263] Dobutamine exerts a lesser effect on the sinoatrial node (and therefore heart rate) than on myocardial tissue and does not stimulate renal dopaminergic receptors (like dopamine).[261, 264, 265] A common adverse side effect is seizures,[4, 7] typically focal-facial but occasionally generalized. Seizures have been observed at infusion rates as low as 1.1 mg/lb/min but abate as soon as the dobutamine infusion is discontinued. Often, they do not recur when the dose is reduced by 50 per cent. Dopamine is a norepinephrine precursor that preferentially reduces renal vascular resistance and increases glomerular filtration rate, renal blood flow, urine flow, and solute excretion.[256] It is a second-line parenteral inotropic agent. Dopamine is dosed at 1 to 2.5 mg/lb/min (constant-rate infusion).

Taurine Supplementation. The only known cause of reversible myocardial failure is taurine deficiency. Because taurine supplementation is effective in such cases,[225] it is empirically administered (250 mg q12h to 24h PO). Analysis of blood taurine concentration should ideally be determined from a blood sample drawn and frozen before taurine administration. However, because this assay is not widely available, and because oral taurine supplementation is safe and inexpensive, oral taurine administration is endorsed for any case of myocardial failure.

General Supportive Measures. In absence of pulmonary edema, judicious fluid therapy (10 to 15 mL/lb/day by constant-rate infusion) is occasionally beneficial to combat the effect of cardiogenic shock and circulatory failure. Potassium chloride must often be supplemented (e.g., 5 to 7 mEq for each 250 mL of fluids, or according to serum potassium concentration) and serum electrolytes monitored. The infusion rate and dose varies with each patient and must be balanced to optimize clinical response without exacerbating pulmonary edema or effusions.[4-7] Central venous pressure monitoring may help guide infusion rate. Symptomatic or hemodynamically significant tachyarrhythmias are uncommon. For life-threatening ventricular tachycardia, lidocaine can be judiciously administered (0.1 to 0.45 mg/lb IV bolus over 5 minutes, or 1 mg boluses up to 4 mg maximum over 5 minutes; 5–20 µg/lb/min IV constant-rate infusion).

Chronic Maintenance Therapy

Diuretics. Furosemide is tapered to the lowest effective dose and interrupted or temporarily discontinued if anorexia, dehydration, or marked azotemia occurs. To manage chronic effusions, upward dose titration (1–2 mg/lb q8–12h PO) may be effective.[4-7, 29] Refractory cases may require periodic thoracocentesis and additional diuretic agents such as hydrochlorothiazide and spironolactone,[87, 267] although thiazides may be ineffective in the presence of renal failure.

ACE Inhibitors. ACE inhibitors blunt neurohormonal alterations, limit cardiac chamber remodeling (dilation), and prevent or delay clinical deterioration.[268, 269] Enalapril monotherapy (0.23 mg/lb PO daily) has been used to successfully manage some cases of mild idiopathic myocardial failure (%FS 23–29 per cent; LVDs 12–14 mm). Systolic failure often requires the addition of diuretics and digoxin.

Digitalis (Digoxin). Although digitalis is the traditional agent for chronic management of myocardial failure, there are little clinical data for its use in cardiomyopathic cats, and digoxin's low therapeutic index makes its role controversial.[233, 270] Although higher plasma levels and more accurate dosing can be achieved with the elixir form,[271, 272] it is less palatable to cats than tablets. Males may develop higher serum levels than females of the same body weight, and food administered in conjunction with digoxin may decrease drug absorption.[271, 272] The mean half-life after chronic oral administration of elixir (0.022 mg/lb bid) was 79 hours (range, 33 to 22 hours).[273] In DCM cats given oral digoxin in tablet form (0.003–0.006 mg/lb q48h), mean half-life was about 64 hours and steady state was reached after about 10 days.[270] Renal insufficiency will reduce digoxin clearance and increase serum concentration.

Digoxin therapy should be initiated when the cat is hydrated and eating. Based on a calculated dose of 0.0022 to 0.0045 mg/lb lean body weight and relatively normal BUN/creatinine, the following guidelines are suggested[7]: for cats weighing 4 to 12 lbs, one fourth of a 0.125-mg digoxin tablet (0.031 mg) every 2 to 3 days; and for cats weighing more than 13 lbs, one fourth of a tablet daily (occasionally, twice daily). Blood concentration should be evaluated 10 to 14 days after initiating therapy. When blood is drawn 10 to 12 hours after administration, a serum digoxin concentration of 1 to 2 ng/mL is presumed to be therapeutic. Anorexia and depression are early signs of toxicity.[4-7] The most striking ECG changes reported with digoxin toxicosis in one study was ST segment elevation, and PR interval prolongation may be noted at non-toxic concentrations.[273] Clinical illness in normal cats given toxic doses may last up to 96 hours.[271, 272]

Beta-adrenergic Blockers. Advocated for managing human DCM,[244, 274-279] beta-blockers may reduce myocardial oxygen demand owing to negative inotropic effect; protect against catecholamine-induced myonecrosis; improve diastolic relaxation; upregulate (increase) myocardial beta-adrenergic receptor density; and improve myocardial calcium handling.[278-280] Clinical benefits have not been evaluated in cats with myocardial failure. In cases of severe myocardial infarction or symptomatic or electrically unstable tachyarrhythmia, addition of a beta-blocker to conventional therapy may be warranted. A low oral test dose can be given and patient response observed, followed by judicious administration (propranolol, 2.5 mg q8–12h or atenolol, one eighth of a 25-mg tablet q24h).

Dietary Modifications. Causes of low body taurine (e.g., urinary acidification combined with potassium depletion, or inappropriate diets) should be eliminated.[117, 225, 249-251] Oral taurine supplementation should continue if concern exists about dietary taurine deficiency or when taurine depletion is confirmed. Sodium-reduced diets should be advocated in advanced heart failure.

Natural History and Prognosis. Echocardiographic improvements become noticeable between 3 and 16 weeks after beginning taurine supplementation, but time to recovery is extremely variable. In severely affected cats, mortality is significant within the first 30 days of treatment. Cats surviving more than 1 month remain clinically stable after adequate taurine intake was ensured, and discontinuation of all drugs is usually possible.[225, 229, 232, 233] Cats with idiopathic myocardial failure do not respond to taurine administration. Their clinical course is unpredictable, but symptomatic cats generally have poor prognosis with a median survival of approximately 13 days.[238] A minority of cats may have a prolonged period of clinical stability.

ARRHYTHMOGENIC RIGHT VENTRICULAR CARDIOMYOPATHY

DEFINITIONS AND NOMENCLATURE

Arrhythmogenic RV cardiomyopathy (ARVC) is characterized by progressive fibrofatty infiltration of the RV myocardium. Initially a regional phenomenon, it progresses to global RV and some LV involvement, with relative sparing of the ventricular septum.[3, 281, 282] Some authors have used the term *dysplasia* (i.e., ARVD)[283]; however, because this morbid entity is considered a progressive heart muscle disease of unknown etiology, the term *cardiomyopathy* (i.e., ARVC) is preferred.[3, 284] In humans, ARVC is classified as isolated RV dysplasia (includes the pure form of ARVC, RV outflow tract tachycardia, Uhl's anomaly, non-arrhythmogenic ARVC, and others) and dysplasia with major LV involvement.[285] ARVC characterized by fibrofatty replacement of RV myocardium with or without changes in wall thickness should be differentiated from Uhl's anomaly, which is distinguished by partial or total absence of RV myocardium with marked RV wall thinning.[286]

PREVALENCE AND DEMOGRAPHICS

Many cases of ARVC are misdiagnosed as tricuspid valve dysplasia, but recognition of this distinctive cardiomyopathy should increase as its clinicopathologic features become more widely published. The prevalence of ARVC in cats represents 2 to 4 per cent of feline myocardial diseases diagnosed at The Animal Medical Center. Cats from 2 to 20 years of age and several breeds have been identified with ARVC.

ETIOLOGY

The wide polymorphism of ARVC may be related to consecutive stages of cardiomyopathic disease progression.[287] The majority of humans (80 per cent)[287–289] and cats[290] with fibrofatty ARVC have lymphocytic infiltrates and fat interspersed within the myocardium. Inflammation leads to fibrosis and scarring, transforming the fatty form of ARVC to the fibrofatty form, the latter representing an end stage of a remote inflammatory process or superimposed condition.[291] Suggested causes include recurrent episodes of myocarditis,[292] autoimmune disease,[285] apoptotic cell death,[290, 293, 294] and a familial basis.[295–298]

PATHOPHYSIOLOGY

ARVC is a primary heart muscle disorder (cardiomyopathy). It involves a dynamic injury-repair process with a tendency to progress from RV to LV involvement. It is characterized by a progressive loss of myocardium and fibrofatty replacement, which causes cardiac electrical instability. Cell death and fibrofatty replacement constitutes a pathologic substrate for arrhythmias, including supraventricular tachyarrhythmias and life-threatening ventricular tachycardia.[299, 300] Severe RV failure results from loss of functional myocytes.

PATHOLOGY

Characteristic gross changes include marked RV and RA chamber enlargement (Fig. 117–15). The RV wall thickness may be normal or severely thinned. Thinning may be focally aneurysmal (i.e., external bulging of a thinned ventricular region) or diffuse and facilitate trans-illumination of light. There is trabecular disarrangement with loss of some trabecular structure. The tricuspid valve apparatus is distorted owing to severe RV dilation and papillary muscle derangement. Histopathologic lesions are pathognomonic and represent two types: fibrofatty (the predominant form) and fatty myocardial replacement. Myocarditis (inflammatory infiltrates associated with myocyte damage or necrosis) is common, particularly with the fibrofatty variety.

CLINICAL MANIFESTATIONS

The history may be vague and reveal only lethargy, anorexia, or dyspnea. Some cats are asymptomatic or have

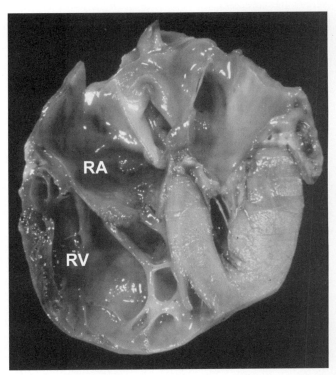

Figure 117–15. Gross transverse heart section from a cat with arrhythmogenic RV cardiomyopathy. Characteristic findings include severe dilation of the right atrium (RA) and ventricle (RV), segmental RV wall thinning, and RV trabecular disruption and disorientation. (From Fox PR: Feline cardiomyopathies. *In* Fox PR, Sisson DD, Moïse NS [eds]: A Textbook of Canine and Feline Cardiology: Principles and Clinical Practice, 2nd ed. Philadelphia, WB Saunders, 1999.)

syncope due to sustained ventricular tachycardia. Physical examination may reflect right-sided CHF, including tachypnea, dyspnea, distended abdomen, and jugular venous distention. Thoracic auscultation may reveal muffled heart and lung sounds if pericardial or pleural effusion is present. A holosystolic, regurgitant, soft to medium intensity murmur of tricuspid regurgitation may be detected. Femoral arterial pulse deficits are associated with arrhythmias. ECG abnormalities include supraventricular tachycardias, conduction abnormalities, and ventricular ectopia (frequently with a left bundle-branch type pattern). Some cats may have no recorded changes on short rhythm strips. Dramatic radiographic enlargement of the RA and RV is characteristic. Moderate to severe LA enlargement may also be present. Pleural, pericardial, or abdominal effusions are common. Echocardiography discloses severe, segmental, or diffuse RV dilatation; localized RV aneurysms (akinetic or dyskinetic areas with diastolic bulging); severe RA enlargement; abnormal trabecular muscle morphology (especially in the apical RV cavity); and, often, LA enlargement with a normal LV or mild LV impairment. Color flow Doppler may reveal mild to moderate tricuspid regurgitation.

DIFFERENTIAL DIAGNOSIS

Tricuspid dysplasia is commonly misdiagnosed when ARVC is present. Tricuspid insufficiency may result from derangement of the tricuspid valve apparatus secondary to myocardial diseases, but the valves are not dysplastic. Biventricular involvement can make diagnosis of ARVC challenging. Pure myocarditis may be arrhythmogenic but would not include characteristic right-sided heart enlargement.

NATURAL HISTORY AND PROGNOSIS

This disorder is not limited just to the right side of the heart. The natural history is not known in felines, although an arrhythmic phase and a right-sided or biventricular CHF phase have been observed. Treatment of right-sided CHF is unrewarding, although management of severe ventricular tachyarrhythmias for more than 1 year has been possible.

THERAPY

Right-sided CHF is treated with furosemide, digoxin, and an ACE inhibitor. For atrial fibrillation or atrial tachycardia, digoxin combined with diltiazem or atenolol is used to maintain the resting heart rate between 140 and 160 beats per minute. Symptomatic ventricular tachycardia has been successfully managed acutely with lidocaine (5–20 μg/lb/min constant-rate infusion) and chronically with sotalol (1–2 mg/lb q12h PO).

UNCLASSIFIED CARDIOMYOPATHIES

Some myocardial diseases have features that do not fit into a discrete category of HCM, RCM, DCM, or ARVC or display characteristics of more than one type of cardiomyopathy. These cases are more appropriately labeled "unclassified cardiomyopathies."[3] Their description can be enhanced by adding a qualifier describing the status of systolic function (i.e., normal vs. myocardial failure), as the case may be.

INCREASED LEFT VENTRICULAR MODERATOR BANDS

A pathologic condition associated with abnormal networks of LV moderator bands has been reported in some cats with cardiomyopathy and heart failure (Fig. 117–16).[4, 5, 7, 123, 301] The significance of these bands and their relationship to the presence of concurrent heart disease is uncertain because many healthy cats also have networks of LV moderator bands. In a study of 21 cats with increased moderator bands, 11 older cats (mean age, 8.7 years) had dilation of the LV and 8 younger cats (mean age, 4 years) had LV or septal hypertrophy.[301] Many of the clinical and pathologic findings described were typical of feline DCM or HCM. Mean heart weight in cats with increased moderator bands was less than that in cats with HCM or DCM. Also, conduction disturbances and bradycardia were more common. It was hypothesized that extensive networks of LV moderator bands may cause or contribute to cardiac dysfunction in some cats but that, in many instances, they are an incidental congenital anomaly.

SECONDARY MYOCARDIAL DISEASES

HYPERTHYROIDISM

Hyperthyroidism is the most common feline endocrine disorder (see Chapter 150). Cardiovascular abnormalities are detected in most affected animals, some of which develop arrhythmias and signs of CHF. Early studies reported CHF

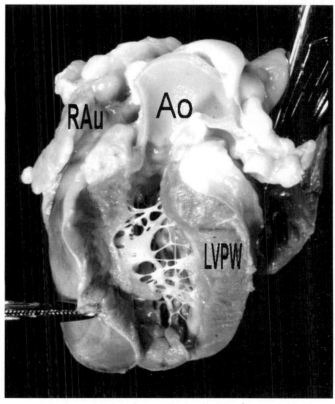

Figure 117–16. Feline heart incised from the apex through the LV outflow tract revealing abnormal, extensive, LV moderator bands. The left ventricle is also hypertrophied. This cat had acute, severe dyspnea and pulmonary edema. RAu = right auricle; Ao = aortic arch; LVPW = left ventricular posterior wall.

CV

in as many as 20 per cent of affected cats, but the prevalence of this complication appears to have declined with increased awareness and earlier diagnosis.[301a] Furosemide will effectively resolve acute pulmonary edema, but the key to continued compensation is maintenance of a euthyroid state. Initial heart failure therapy is continued until hyperthyroid management is under way.

ACROMEGALY (HYPERSOMATOTROPISM)

A syndrome resembling acromegaly in humans was reported in middle-aged and older cats, with a predisposition for neutered males. These animals had growth hormone–secreting tumors of the pituitary gland.[302, 303] In one study of 14 cats, systolic murmurs (9/14), radiographic evidence of cardiomegaly (12/14), and echocardiographic evidence of septal (7/8) and LV wall (5/8) hypertrophy were reported. None had ECG abnormalities, and 6 cats developed CHF. Necropsy of 10 cats revealed LV dilation in 1 cat and LV hypertrophy in 7 others. Myocardial histologic lesions included myofiber hypertrophy, multi-focal myocytolysis, interstitial fibrosis, and intramural arteriosclerosis.[302] Hypersomatotropism with LV hypertrophy and heart failure has also been identified in a glucose-intolerant, non-diabetic, 12-year-old male cat.[303] Increased plasma growth hormone concentration has been reported in some cats with HCM,[88] although the significance of this finding is unclear.

HYPERTENSIVE CARDIOMYOPATHY

The incidence of clinically significant feline systemic hypertension is unknown (see Chapter 50). Pathologic features have not been detailed, but cardiac changes in some cases may resemble feline HCM.

MISCELLANEOUS DISORDERS

INFILTRATIVE MYOCARDIAL DISEASE

Neoplastic cardiac infiltration is rare, and most cases involve lymphosarcoma. Diagnosis can sometimes be confirmed by echocardiography. Other feline cardiac tumors include chemodectoma, metastatic hemangiosarcoma, pulmonary carcinoma, and mammary gland carcinoma.[4–7, 304–306] Reported cardiac abnormalities include arrhythmias and pericardial and pleural effusion. Regression of neoplastic infiltration was observed in one cat with lymphoma.[304]

DRUGS, TOXINS, AND PHYSICAL INJURY

Many agents can injure the heart, but very few are identified in feline practice. Doxorubicin can cause cardiac injury.[307, 308] Decreased fractional shortening and increased LV end-systolic dimensions were recorded in 4 of 6 experimental cats given cumulative doses of 170 to 240 mg/m.[308] In cats with malignancies treated with doxorubicin, none developed overt heart failure and arrhythmias were rare.[307]

MYOCARDITIS

Although myocarditis is infrequently recognized, it may play an important role in certain myocardial diseases.[98, 100,] [112–115, 233, 285–292, 309, 310] A syndrome of idiopathic, acute, non-suppurative myocarditis and acute, unexpected death was described in 25 young cats (mean age, 2.6 years).[309] Pathologic lesions included diffuse or focal endomyocardial infiltration with mononuclear cells and occasional neutrophils. Other reported causes of myocarditis in cats include toxoplasmosis[311] and metastatic infection from sepsis or bacterial endocarditis.[4–7, 27, 29, 312, 313] Endocardial fibroelastosis, a rare disease characterized by diffuse thickening of LV endocardium due to proliferation of fibrous and elastic tissue, has chiefly been reported in Siamese[19, 314, 315] and Burmese breeds.[316–318] Recent evidence suggests that fibroelastosis may be a sequela of viral myocarditis.[318a]

PERSISTENT ATRIAL STANDSTILL AND OTHER UNCOMMON DISORDERS

Persistent atrial standstill has been reported in 11 cats (8 Siamese, 1 Burmese, 2 mixed-breed cats).[123, 319] Seven cats were necropsied, and all had DCM with severe atrial myocardial atrophy. In contrast to dogs with atrial standstill, none of the cats had evidence of skeletal muscular dystrophy. Cardiac involvement has been described in several cats with a Duchenne-like muscular dystrophy.[320] Genetic mucopolysaccharidosis has been reported in cats—Hurler's syndrome (MPS I) in domestic short-hair cats,[321] and Maroteaux-Lamy syndrome (MPS VI) in Siamese cats,[322] but cardiac involvement has not been significant. Bundle branch fibrosis, infiltration and degeneration, and atrioventricular node degeneration have been reported.[19, 323]

ARTERIAL THROMBOEMBOLISM

DEFINITIONS AND NOMENCLATURE

Thrombotic and thromboembolic complications of feline cardiomyopathy have long been recognized.[324] *Thrombosis* represents clot formation within a cardiac chamber or vascular lumen. Thrombi may be found in the body of the LA, in the atrial appendage, or in the LV. *Embolization* occurs when a clot or other foreign material lodges within a vessel.[325, 326] The systemic arterial system is almost exclusively involved because right-sided heart and deep venous thrombosis is rare in cats.

PREVALENCE AND DEMOGRAPHICS

Cardiogenic emboli cause significant morbidity and mortality with myocardial disease. Clinical studies have reported significant incidences of arterial thromboembolism in feline heart disease.[22, 25, 74, 229, 233, 238] Most cats with systemic arterial thromboembolism have CHF concurrently at the time of clinical embolism.[4–7, 22] Thromboembolism is uncommon with hyperthyroidism, and a 3 per cent incidence of thyrotoxicosis was recorded in 100 cats with saddle embolism.[327] The site of cardiogenic embolism is variable, but distal aortic ("saddle") embolization occurs in more than 90 per cent of cases (Fig. 117–17). The right brachial artery is occasionally occluded (the left brachial artery is only rarely embolized). Left-sided mural thrombi are sometimes present, particularly in the left auricle and less often in the left ventricle. Other organs may become embolized as a consequence of systemic embolic "showers," especially the kidneys.[4–7]

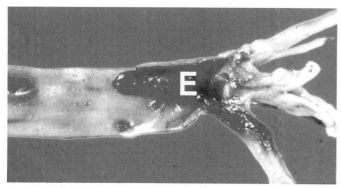

Figure 117–17. "Saddle" embolus (E) occluding the distal aorta at its trifurcation in a cat with restrictive cardiomyopathy.

PATHOPHYSIOLOGY

Thrombosis requires one or more of three essential conditions, known as *Virchow's triad,* to be present[328]:

1. *Local vessel or tissue injury*—Endomyocardial injury is common in all forms of feline cardiomyopathy.[9–23, 28, 71, 77, 123, 325] Such lesions may present reactive substrates to circulating blood and trigger a thrombotic process by inducing platelet adhesion and aggregation, with subsequent activation of the intrinsic clotting cascade.

2. *Circulatory stasis*—Cardiac chamber dilation, particularly when associated with reduced contractility, results in large end-systolic volumes and blood stasis.[163, 164, 170, 326, 329, 330] Impaired blood flow decreases clearance of activated clotting factors, which sets up clot formation in areas of tissue injury.

3. *Altered blood coagulability*—Disseminated intravascular coagulation associated with consumptive coagulopathy, liver-mediated coagulopathy, or thromboembolism was present in more than 75 per cent of cardiomyopathic cats in one study.[331, 332] In addition, feline platelets are very reactive and responsive to ADP and other agonists of platelet aggregation.[333, 334]

The influence of hypercoagulable states in human thrombogenesis has become the focus of great interest, particularly resistance to factor V Leiden (APC), proteins C and S deficiency, antithrombin III (AT III) deficiency, antiphospholipid syndrome, and hyperhomocysteinemia.[335] Hyperhomocysteinemia is present in some cardiomyopathic cats with thrombosis (Hohenhaus AE, Simantov R, Fox PR, unpublished data, 1998). Collateral circulation plays a critical role in progression and resolution of clinical thromboembolic disease and is modulated by vasoactive substances (e.g., serotonin and others) released by the clot and other substrates.[336, 337] Chemicals such as thromboxane A_2 also cause vasoconstriction.[338] Synthesis of thromboxane A_2 can be reduced by anti-prostaglandin drugs such as aspirin. Sudden arterial occlusion with almost instantaneous and complete interruption, coupled with decreased collateral circulation, causes substantial tissue injury. Ischemic neuromyopathy is a predictable consequence of arterial occlusion and, in particular, of clot associated with inhibition of collateral circulation.[339] Distal limbs below the stifle are most severely injured. Cranial tibial muscles are more effected than gastrocnemius muscles, inhibiting hock flexion more than extension. Hip flexion and extension is maintained. This results in a dragging motion of the hind legs.[340]

CLINICAL MANIFESTATIONS

The clinical consequences of arterial thromboembolism depend on the site of embolization, the severity and duration of occlusion, the degree of functional collateral circulation, and the development of serious complications (e.g., hyperkalemia, limb necrosis, self-mutilation).

History. Distal arterial embolism characteristically results in peracute clinical signs of lateralizing paresis, vocalization, and pain. Occasionally, intermittent claudication or right front paresis is reported. Signs of CHF are often present concurrently and include dyspnea, tachypnea, anorexia, and syncope.

Physical Examination. Clinical signs are attributable to CHF and specific tissues or organs that are embolized (e.g., azotemia from renal infarction, bloody diarrhea from mesenteric infarction, posterior paresis from saddle embolus). Thoracic auscultation may reveal heart murmurs, gallop rhythms, pulmonary crackles, or muffled heart and lung sounds. Most affected cats are clinically dehydrated, and many are hypothermic. More than 90 per cent of affected cats present with a lateralizing posterior paresis caused by a "saddle clot" at the distal aortic trifurcation. Clinical signs are characterized by the 4 *Ps,* which relate to the extremities: *paralysis, pain, pulselessness* (lack of palpable femoral arterial pulses), and *polar* (cold distal limbs and pads). Anterior tibial and gastrocnemius muscles are often firm or become so from ischemic myopathy by 10 to 12 hours after embolization. In most cases they become softer 24 to 72 hours later. Acutely affected cats can move their back legs by flexing and extending the hip in a "dragging" manner, but they cannot flex and extend the hock. Nail beds are cyanotic and distal limbs are commonly swollen. Intermittent claudication may be observed. In such cases, arterial pulses may be palpated, foot pads feel warm (normal), and nail beds are not cyanotic. This frequently precedes a more severe thromboembolic event. Occasionally, a single brachial artery is embolized, causing monoparesis (usually right front leg).

Thoracic Radiography. Cardiomegaly is usually evident. In most cases, biatrial enlargement is present and the left auricular appendage is often prominent in the ventrodorsal or dorsoventral view. The majority of affected cats have concurrent extracardiac signs of CHF (e.g., pulmonary edema, pleural effusion).[4–7, 22, 327, 341] Normal cardiac silhouettes were reported in only 11 per cent of cats with thromboembolism.[327]

Electrocardiography. ECG changes were reported in 85 per cent of cats with thromboembolism. Sinus rhythm was present in 60 per cent. 7 per cent had supraventricular tachycardia including atrial fibrillation; 3 per cent had ventricular tachycardia; and 28 per cent had sinus tachycardia. Isolated supraventricular (19 per cent) and ventricular extrasystoles (19 per cent) were also recorded.[327] Development of atrial standstill and a sinoventricular rhythm indicates hyperkalemia, a catastrophic consequence of re-perfusion muscle injury.[342]

Clinical Pathology. Most cats have clinical pathologic abnormalities.[327, 331, 332] Elevated BUN and creatinine levels were recorded in a little over half of cats at presentation.[327] Pre-renal azotemia may result from dehydration, although renal infarction may play a role in some cases.[4, 5, 8, 123, 331] Serum concentrations of alanine aminotransferase and aspartate aminotransferase are elevated by about 12 hours and peak by 36 hours after embolization, indicating hepatic and skeletal muscle inflammation and necrosis. Lactate dehydrogenase and creatine phosphokinase enzymes are greatly in-

CV

creased shortly after embolization, indicating widespread cellular injury. Hyperglycemia, mature leukocytosis, lymphopenia, and hypocalcemia may be present. Acute hyperkalemia can result from re-perfusion injury of skeletal muscles downstream from the embolus. Hypokalemia is a common consequence of anorexia and diuretic therapy.[5, 7, 87] Coagulation abnormalities may be detected,[332] including hyperhomocysteinemia.

Echocardiography. Echocardiography provides rapid, non-invasive assessment of cardiac structure and function, detects intracardiac thrombi (Fig. 117–18), and assists in formulating therapy and prognosis. *Spontaneous echo contrast* ("smoke") present in the LA or LV is associated with blood stasis and is considered a harbinger and marker for increased thromboembolic risk.[162–164] LA enlargement (LAE) is usually, but not invariably, present. In a retrospective study of cats with saddle emboli, severe LAE (LA:Ao ratio $\geq$ 2.0) was recorded in 57 per cent and moderate LAE (LA:Ao 1.63–1.99) or mild LAE (LA:Ao, 1.25–1.629) in 22 per cent; and 5 per cent of cats had normal LA measurements (LA:Ao < 1.25).[327]

Angiocardiography. Non-selective angiocardiography can be considered in the stabilized patient if echocardiography is not available. It is occasionally used to determine the anatomic location or extent of systemic thromboembolism and assess collateral flow (Fig. 117–19). Severe myocardial failure and hemodynamically or electrically unstable arrhythmias constitute relative contraindications.

DIFFERENTIAL DIAGNOSES

Trauma, intervertebral disk extrusion, spinal lymphosarcoma and other neoplasia, and fibrocartilaginous infarction may cause posterior paresis. Thromboembolism uncommonly occurs in the setting of a structurally normal or mildly abnormal heart. Neoplasia is sometimes discovered in the thorax or abdomen (although the mechanistic relationship, if

any, is unclear), or systemic inflammation or endocarditis can represent cardiovascular sources of emboli.

NATURAL HISTORY AND PROGNOSIS

Short-term prognosis depends on the nature and responsiveness of the cardiomyopathic disorder and heart failure state. In cases of saddle embolism, motor ability may begin to return in one or both legs within 10 to 14 days. By 3 weeks, significant motor function (i.e., hock extension and flexion) has often returned, typically better in one leg than in the other. Motor function may be completely normal by 4 to 6 weeks, although a conscious proprioceptive deficit or conformational abnormality (e.g., extreme hock flexion) may persist in one leg. Unfortunately, most cats experience additional thromboembolic episodes within days to months of the initial event, although survival of several years including repeat embolic episodes have been observed.[4, 5, 7, 331] In one study, 34 of 92 cats (37 per cent) survived an initial event of saddle embolism and the mean long-term survival was 11.5 months.[327] A more favorable prognosis may be suggested by resolution of CHF and/or control of serious arrhythmias, lack of LA/LV thrombi or spontaneous echo contrast, re-establishment of appetite, maintenance of relatively normal BUN/creatinine and electrolytes, return of limb viability and function (e.g., loss of swelling; return of normal limb temperature; return of motor ability), return of femoral arterial pulses and pink nail beds, lack of self-mutilation, and a committed owner. A grave prognosis is suggested by refractory CHF or development of malignant arrhythmias; acute hyperkalemia (from re-perfusion of injured muscles); declining limb viability (e.g., progressive hardening of the gastrocnemius and anterior tibial muscle group; failure of these muscles to become soft 48–72 hours after presentation; development of distal limb necrosis); clinical evidence of multi-organ or multi-systemic embolization; history of previous embolic episodes; presence or development of LA/LV thrombus or spontaneous echo contrast; rising BUN/creatinine; disseminated intravascular coagulation; unresponsive hypothermia; severe LA enlargement with tachyarrhythmia and myocardial failure; and an uncommitted owner with limited financial resources.

THERAPY FOR THROMBOEMBOLISM

Treatment Goals. Therapy is directed toward managing concomitant CHF or serious arrhythmias when present; general patient support, including nutritional supplementation, correction of hypothermia, and prevention of self-mutilation; adjunctive therapies to limit thrombus growth or formation; close patient monitoring; and prevention. Limb and/or organ viability is enhanced by rapid resolution of arterial occlusion. Embolectomy or surgery is generally contraindicated.

Supportive Therapies. Various medical treatments have been proposed, although most are empirical and efficacy is unsubstantiated. Aspirin is administered for myalgia associated with ischemic myopathy, in addition to antiplatelet effects. It is important to maintain hydration, electrolyte balance, and nutritional support. Placement of a nasoesophageal feeding tube is advocated for anorectic cats. Self-mutilation is common after a saddle embolus and is characterized by excessive licking or chewing of the toes or lateral hock. Application of a loose-fitting bandage, stockinette, or other barrier is usually effective. Placement of indwelling venous

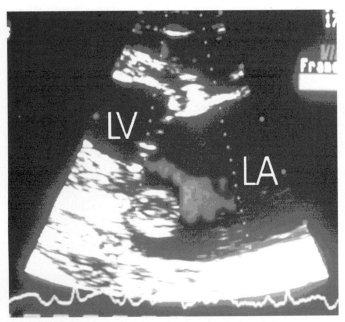

Figure 117–18. Color flow Doppler echocardiogram recorded at the right parasternal long-axis view recorded from a cat with restrictive cardiomyopathy that had acute posterior paresis. The left atrium (LA) is severely enlarged and contains a ball thrombus. A small jet of mitral regurgitation is evident (shown here in black and white). LV = left ventricle.

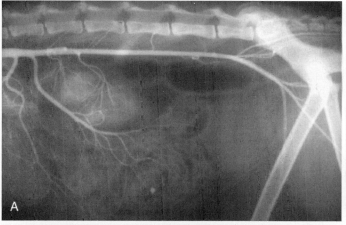

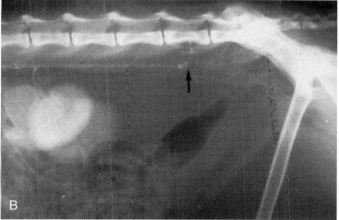

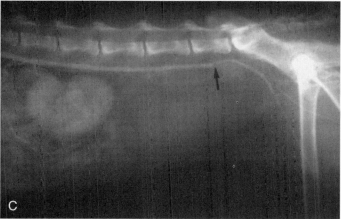

Figure 117–19. Arteriograms from two different cats. *A*, Normal cat. *B*, Cat with hypertrophic cardiomyopathy 24 hours after embolization. A large "saddle" embolus causes complete distal aortic occlusion (arrow), and femoral arterial pulses were absent. Note lack of collateral circulation (compare with *A*). In *C*, 4 days after embolization a small filling defect (arrow) is visible, indicating the saddle embolus; flow occurs past the block. Femoral arterial circulation (and palpable pulses) were re-established. However, collateral circulation, although improved, was still reduced (compare with *A*).

catheters into veins of legs devitalized by occlusive embolus should always be avoided.

Thrombolytic Therapy. Streptokinase and urokinase generate the non-specific proteolytic enzyme plasmin through conversion of the proenzyme plasminogen. This causes a generalized lytic state with the incipient hazard of bleeding complications.[343] Experimentally,[344] when streptokinase was administered as an IV loading dose (90,000 IU/cat over 20–30 minutes) followed by a constant-rate infusion (45,000 IU/h) for 3 hours, it produced systemic fibrinolysis with no detectable adverse effects. However, it failed to produce significant improvement, as measured by venous angiograms, thermal circulatory indices, or statistically significant reduction in mean thrombus weight. Clinical studies are lacking. Recombinant tissue-type plasminogen activator (t-PA) has a lower affinity for circulating plasminogen and does not induce a systemic fibrinolytic state. It binds to fibrin within the thrombus and converts the entrapped plasminogen to plasmin. This initiates a local fibrinolysis with limited systemic proteolysis.[345] When t-PA was administered (0.11 to 0.45 mg/lb/h IV for a total dose of 0.45 to 4.4 mg/lb) to cats with thromboembolism,[346] successful thrombolysis was reported in 50 per cent; 43 per cent of the cats survived therapy and ambulated within 48 hours of presentation. Fifty per cent of the cats died during therapy, which raised major concerns regarding rapid thrombolysis. Complications resulted from hyperkalemia (70 per cent) or heart failure (15 per cent), or sudden death occurred (15 per cent). Bleeding into and around the kidney was also observed in several cats.

Anticoagulation Therapy. Heparin and warfarin (Coumadin) have no effects on established thrombi. Their use has been based on the premise that, by retarding clotting factor synthesis or accelerating their inactivation, thrombosis from activated blood clotting pathways can be prevented. Heparin binds to lysine sites on plasma antithrombin III, enhancing its ability to neutralize thrombin and activated factors XII, XI, X, and IX; this prevents activation of the coagulation process.[347] Efficacy in treating cats with thromboembolism has not been established, and reported dosages vary widely. It may be administered at the time of admission as an initial intravenous dose (45–100 IU/lb), then 22–45 IU/lb subcutaneously every 6 to 8 hours.[327] The dose is then adjusted to prolong activated partial thromboplastin time one and one-half to two times pre-treatment values. Bleeding is a major complication, and clotting profiles must be closely monitored. Warfarin impairs hepatic vitamin K metabolism, a vitamin necessary for synthesis of procoagulants (factors II or prothrombin and factors VII, IX, and X).[348] The initial oral daily dosage (0.10 to 0.22 mg/cat) is adjusted to prolong the prothrombin time to twice the normal value; alternatively, it is adjusted by the international normalization ratio (INR) to maintain a value of 2.0 to 3.0 as follows[349, 350]:

$$INR = [Cat\ Prothrombin\ Time \div Control\ Prothrombin\ Time]^{ISI}$$

Hemorrhage is a potential complication (see Chapter 181).

Anti-Platelet Drugs. Exposure of blood to subendothelial connective tissue leads to rapid platelet activation, formation of platelet plugs, and subsequent thrombus. Pharmacologic measures are directed to modify platelet aggregation. Aspirin can be used based on its theoretic benefit during and after a thromboembolic episode to prevent further thromboembolism. Aspirin induces a functional defect in platelets by irreversibly inactivating (through acetylation) cyclooxygenase. This enzyme is critical for converting arachidonic acid to thromboxane A_2[351–353] and in the vascular wall is responsible for converting arachidonic acid to prostacyclin.[353, 354] Thromboxane A_2 induces platelet activation (through release of platelet adenosine diphosphate) and vasoconstriction (as does serotonin), whereas prostacyclin inhibits platelet aggregation and induces vasodilation.[355, 356] The aspirin-induced acetylation of the cyclooxygenase enzyme is irreversible and persists for the life of the platelet (7 to 10 days), as does platelet aggregation and release response to various agonists. In cats, aspirin (one fourth of a 5-grain tablet q48–72h PO) effectively inhibits platelet function for 3 to 5 days and is relatively safe.[357–360] The optimal aspirin dose that will inhibit thromboxane A_2 production but spare vascular endothelial prostacyclin synthesis has not yet been established for cats. Side effects of aspirin are mainly gastrointestinal and can be severe with overdosage.

PRIMARY PREVENTION OF THROMBOEMBOLISM

Although aspirin has been demonstrated to exert antiplatelet aggregating properties to feline platelets in vitro, there are no data to support routine prophylactic administration to cats with cardiomyopathy unless countervailing risk factors (see earlier) have been identified. Multi-center clinical trials have not been performed to evaluate optimal preventative strategies.

REFERENCES

1. Wynne JW, Braunwald E: The cardiomyopathies and myocarditides. In Braunwald E (ed): Heart Disease: A Textbook of Cardiovascular Medicine, 5th ed. Philadelphia, WB Saunders, 1997, p 1404.
2. Goodwin JF: Cardiomyopathies and specific heart muscle diseases. Definitions, terminology, classifications and new and old approaches. Postgrad Med J 68:S3, 1992.
3. Richardson P, McKenna W, Bristow M, et al: Report of the 1995 World Health Organization/international society and federation of cardiology task force on the definition and classification of cardiomyopathies. Circulation 93:841, 1996.
4. Fox PR: Feline myocardial diseases. In Fox PR, Sisson DD, Moise NS (eds): Textbook of Canine and Feline Cardiology: Principles and Practice, 2nd ed. Philadelphia, WB Saunders, 1999.
5. Fox PR: Feline myocardial disease. In Fox PR (ed): Canine and Feline Cardiology. New York, Churchill Livingstone, 1988, p 435.
6. Sisson DD, Thomas W: Myocardial diseases. In Ettinger SJ, Feldman EC (eds): Textbook of Veterinary Internal Medicine, 4th ed. Philadelphia, WB Saunders, 1995, p 995.
7. Fox PR: Feline myocardial diseases. In Kirk RW (ed): Current Veterinary Therapy VIII. Philadelphia, WB Saunders, 1983, p 337.
8. Kushwaha SS, Fallon JT, Fuster V: Restrictive cardiomyopathy. N Engl J Med 336:267, 1997.
9. Keren A, Popp RL: Assignment of patients into the classification of cardiomyopathies. Circulation 86:1622, 1992.
10. Choong CY: Left ventricle: V. Diastolic function—its principles and evaluation. In Weyman AE (ed): Principles and Practice of Echocardiography, 2nd ed. Philadelphia, Lea & Febiger, 1994, p 721.
11. Little WC, Downes TR: Clinical evaluation of left ventricular diastolic performance. Prog Cardiovasc Dis 32:273, 1990.
12. Nishimura RA, Tajik AJ: Evaluation of diastolic filling of left ventricle in health and disease: Doppler echocardiography is the clinician's Rosetta stone. J Am Coll Cardiol 30:8, 1997.
13. Gilbert JC, Glantz SA: Determinants of left ventricular filling and the diastolic pressure-volume relation. Circ Res 64:827, 1989.
14. Brutsaert DL, Rademakers FE, Sus SU: Triple control of relaxation: Implication in cardiac disease. Circulation 69:190, 1984.
15. Nishimura RA, Housmans PR, Hatle LK, et al: Assessment of diastolic function of the heart: Background and current applications of Doppler echocardiography. Mayo Clin Proc 64:71, 1989.
16. Maron BJ, Spirito P, Green KJ, et al: Noninvasive assessment of left ventricular diastolic function by pulsed Doppler echocardiography in patients with hypertrophic cardiomyopathy. J Am Coll Cardiol 10:733, 1987.
17. Pozzoli M, Traversi E, Cioffi G, et al: Loading manipulations improve the prognostic value of Doppler evaluation of mitral flow in patients with chronic heart failure. Circulation 95:1222, 1997.
18. Harrison MR, Clifton GD, Pennell AT, et al: Effect of heart rate on left ventricular diastolic transmitral flow velocity patterns assessed by Doppler echocardiography in normal subjects. Am J Cardiol 67:622, 1991.
19. Liu SK: Pathology of feline heart disease. Vet Clin North Am 7:323, 1977.
20. Van Vleet JF, Ferrans V: Myocardial diseases of animals. Am J Pathol 124:97, 1986.
21. Tilley LP, Liu SK, Gilbertson SR, et al: Primary myocardial disease in the cat: A model for human cardiomyopathy. Am J Pathol 87:493, 1977.
22. Fox PR, Liu SK, Maron BJ: Echocardiographic assessment of spontaneously occurring feline hypertrophic cardiomyopathy: An animal model of human disease. Circulation 92:2645, 1995.
23. Liu SK, Roberts WC, Maron BJ: Comparison of morphologic findings in spontaneously occurring hypertrophic cardiomyopathy in humans, cats and dogs. Am J Cardiol 72:944, 1993.
24. Maron BJ, Bonow RO, Cannon RO III, et al: Hypertrophic cardiomyopathy: Interrelations of clinical manifestations, pathophysiology, and therapy (first of two parts). N Engl J Med 316:844, 1987.
25. Atkins CE, Gallo AM, Kurzman ID, et al: Risk factors, clinical signs, and survival in cats with a clinical diagnosis of idiopathic hypertrophic cardiomyopathy: 74 cases (1985–1989). JAVMA 201:603, 1992.
26. Fox PR, Tilley LP, Liu SK: The cardiovascular system. In Pratt PW (ed): Feline Medicine. Santa Barbara, CA, American Veterinary Publications, 1983, p 249.
27. Harpster NK: The cardiovascular system. In Holzworth J (ed): Diseases of the Cat, Vol I. Philadelphia, WB Saunders, 1986, p 820.
28. Van Vleet J, Ferrans VJ, Weirich WE: Pathologic alterations in hypertrophic and congestive cardiomyopathy of cats. Am J Vet Res 41:2037, 1980.
29. Harpster NK: Feline myocardial diseases. In Kirk RW (ed): Current Veterinary Therapy IX. Philadelphia, WB Saunders, 1986, p 380.
30. Martin L, VandeWoude S, Boon J, et al: Left ventricular hypertrophy in a closed colony of Persian cats (abstract). J Vet Intern Med 8:143, 1994.
31. Kittleson MD, Meurs KM, Kittleson J, et al: Heritable characteristics, phenotypic expression, and natural history of hypertrophic cardiomyopathy in Maine coon cats (abstract). J Vet Intern Med 12:198, 1998.
32. Kittleson MD, Kittleson JA, Mekhamer Y: Development and progression of inherited hypertrophic cardiomyopathy in Maine coon cats (abstract). J Vet Intern Med 10:165, 1996.
33. Meurs K, Kittleson MD, Towbin J, et al: Familial systolic anterior motion of the mitral valve and/or hypertrophic cardiomyopathy is apparently inherited as an autosomal dominant trait in a family of American shorthair cats (abstract). J Vet Intern Med 11:138, 1997.
34. Seidman CE, Seidman JG: Gene mutations that cause familial hypertrophic cardiomyopathy. In Hager E (ed): Scientific American Molecular Cardiovascular Medicine. New York, Scientific American, 1995, p 193.
35. Marian AJ, Roberts R: Recent advances in the molecular genetics of hypertrophic cardiomyopathy. Circulation 92:1336, 1995.
36. Marian AJ, Yu Q-T, Mann FL, Roberts GR: Expression of a mutation causing hypertrophic cardiomyopathy disrupts sarcomere assembly in adult feline cardiac myocytes. Circ Res 77:98, 1995.
37. Golden AL, Bright JM: Use of relaxation half-time as an index of ventricular relaxation in clinically normal cats and cats with hypertrophic cardiomyopathy. Am J Vet Res 51:1352, 1990.
38. Bright JM, Golden L, Gompf R, et al: Evaluation of the calcium channel–blocking agents diltiazem and verapamil for treatment of feline hypertrophic cardiomyopathy. J Vet Intern Med 5:272, 1991.
39. Bright JM, Hertage ME: Pulsed Doppler assessment of left ventricular diastolic function in normal and cardiomyopathic cats. In: Proceedings of the 15th Annual Veterinary Medicine Forum, 1997, p 212.
40. Wiggle ED: Impaired left ventricular relaxation in hypertrophic cardiomyopathy: Relation to extent of hypertrophy. J Am Coll Cardiol 15:814, 1990.
41. Gwathmey JK, Warren SE, Briggs GM, et al: Diastolic dysfunction in hypertrophic cardiomyopathy: Effect on active force generation during systole. J Clin Invest 87:1023, 1991.
42. Grossman W, McLaurin LP: Diastolic properties of the left ventricle. Ann Intern Med 84:316, 1974.
43. Maron BJ, Wolfson JK, Epstein SE, et al: Intramural ("small vessel") coronary artery disease in hypertrophic cardiomyopathy. J Am Cardiol 8:545, 1986.
44. Tanaka M, Fuijiwara H, Onodera T, et al: Quantitative analysis of narrowing of intramyocardial small arteries in normal heart, hypertensive hearts, and hearts with hypertrophic cardiomyopathy. Circulation 75:1130, 1987.
45. Liu SK: The intramural coronary arterial lesions in 102 cats with hypertrophic cardiomyopathy (abstract). In: Scientific Proceedings of the International Academy of Pathology, 1989, p 54.
46. Krams R, Kofflard MJM, Duncker DJ, et al: Decreased coronary flow reserve in hypertrophic cardiomyopathy is related to remodeling of the coronary microcirculation. Circulation 97:230, 1998.
47. Lord PF, Wood A, Tilley LP: Radiographic and hemodynamic evaluation of cardiomyopathy and thromboembolism in the cat. JAVMA 164:154, 1974.
48. Sarnoff SJ, Braunwald E, Welch GH Jr, et al: Hemodynamic determinants of oxygen consumption of the heart with special reference to the tension-time index. Am J Physiol 192:148, 1958.
49. Boerth RC, Covell JW, Pool PE, et al: Increased myocardial oxygen consumption and contractile state associated with increased heart rate in dogs. Circ Res 24:725, 1958.
50. Cannon RO III, Rosing DR, Maron BJ, et al: Myocardial ischemia in patients with hypertrophic cardiomyopathy: Contribution of inadequate vasodilator reserve and elevated left ventricular filling pressures. Circulation 71:234, 1985.

51. Levine RA: Echocardiographic assessment of the cardiomyopathies. *In* Weyman AE (ed): Principles and Practice of Echocardiography, 2nd ed. Philadelphia, Lea & Febiger, 1994, p 781

52. Peters NS, Wit AL: Myocardial architecture and ventricular arrhythmogenesis. Circulation 97:1746, 1998.

53. Levine RA, Lefebvre X, Guerrero JL, et al: Unifying concepts of mitral valve function and disease: SAM, prolapse and ischemic mitral regurgitation. J Cardiol 24(Suppl 38):15, 1994.

54. Sherrid MV, Pearle G, Gunsburg DZ: Mechanism of benefit of negative inotropes in obstructive hypertrophic cardiomyopathy. Circulation 97:41, 1998.

55. Wigle ED, Rakowski H, Kimball BP, et al: Hypertrophic cardiomyopathy: Clinical spectrum and treatment. Circulation 92:1680, 1995.

56. Nakatani S, Schwammenthal E, Lever HM, et al: New insights into the reduction of mitral valve systolic anterior motion after ventricular septal myectomy in hypertrophic obstructive cardiomyopathy. Am Heart J 131:294, 1996.

57. Lin C-S, Chen K-S, Lin M-C, et al: The relationship between systolic anterior motion of the mitral valve and the left ventricular outflow tract Doppler in hypertrophic cardiomyopathy. Am Heart J 122:1671, 1991.

58. Spirito P, Maron BJ, Rosing DR: Morphologic determinants of hemodynamic state after ventricular septal myotomy-myectomy in patients with obstructive hypertrophic cardiomyopathy: M-mode and two-dimensional echocardiographic assessment. Circulation 70:84, 1984.

59. Jiang L, Levine RA, King ME, et al: An integrated mechanism to explain the systolic anterior motion of the mitral valve in hypertrophic cardiomyopathy based on echocardiographic observations. Am Heart J 113:633, 1987.

60. Murgo JP: The hemodynamic evaluation in hypertrophic cardiomyopathy: Systolic and diastolic dysfunction. Cardiovasc Clin 19:193, 1988.

61. Knight C, Kurbaan AS, Seggewiss H, et al: Nonsurgical septal reduction for hypertrophic obstructive cardiomyopathy: Outcome in the first series of patients. Circulation 95:2075, 1997.

62. Sasson Z, Yock PG, Hatle LK, et al: Doppler echocardiographic determination of the pressure gradient in hypertrophic cardiomyopathy. J Am Coll Cardiol 11:752, 1988.

63. Spirito P, Seidman CE, McKenna WJ, et al: The management of hypertrophic cardiomyopathy. N Engl J Med 336:775, 1997.

64. Pai RG, Jintapakorn W, Tanimoto M, et al: Role of papillary muscle position and mitral valve structure in systolic anterior motion of the mitral leaflets in hyperdynamic left ventricular function. Am J Cardiol 76:623, 1995.

65. Klues HG, Schiffers A, Maron BJ: Phenotypic spectrum and patterns of left ventricular hypertrophy in hypertrophic cardiomyopathy: Morphologic observations and significance as assessed by two-dimensional echocardiography in 600 patients. J Am Coll Cardiol 26:1699, 1995.

66. Klues HG, Roberts WC, Maron BJ: Morphological determinants of echocardiographic patterns of mitral valve systolic anterior motion in obstructive hypertrophic cardiomyopathy. Circulation 87:1570, 1993.

67. Gilligan DM, et al: Cardiac responses assessed by echocardiography to changes in preload in hypertrophic cardiomyopathy. Am J Cardiol 73:312, 1994.

68. McCully RB, Nishimura RA, Tajik AJ, et al: Extent of clinical improvement after surgical treatment of hypertrophic obstructive cardiomyopathy. Circulation 94:467, 1996.

69. Bonagura JD, Stepien RL, Lehmkuhl LB: Acute effects of esmolol on left ventricular outflow obstruction in cats with hypertrophic cardiomyopathy: A Doppler-echocardiographic study (abstract). J Vet Intern Med 5:123, 1991.

70. Maron BJ, Spirito P: Implications of left ventricular remodeling in hypertrophic cardiomyopathy. Am J Cardiol 81:1339, 1998.

71. Liu SK, Maron BJ, Tilley LP: Feline hypertrophic cardiomyopathy: Gross anatomic and quantitative histologic features. Am J Pathol 102:388, 1981.

72. Maron BJ, Gottdiener JS, Epstein SE: Patterns and significance of distribution of left ventricular hypertrophy in hypertrophic cardiomyopathy: A wide-angle, two-dimensional echocardiographic study of 125 patients. Am J Cardiol 48:418, 1981.

73. Bright JM, Golden AL, Daniel GB: Feline hypertrophic cardiomyopathy: Variations on a theme. J Small Anim Pract 33:66, 1992.

74. Peterson EN, Moise NS, Brown CA, et al: Heterogeneity of hypertrophic cardiomyopathy in feline hypertrophic heart disease. J Vet Intern Med 7:183, 1993.

75. Maron BJ, Roberts WC: Quantitative analysis of cardiac muscle cell disorganization in the ventricular septum of patients with hypertrophic cardiomyopathy. Circulation 59:689, 1979.

76. St. Johns, Lie JT, Anderson KR, et al: Histopathological specificity of hypertrophic obstructive cardiomyopathy: Myocardial fibre disarray and myocardial fibrosis. Br Heart J 44:433, 1980.

77. Liu SK, Fox PR: Myocardial ischemia and infarction. *In* Kirk RW, Bonagura JD (eds): Current Veterinary Therapy XI. Philadelphia, WB Saunders, 1992, p 791.

78. Bonagura JD: Cardiovascular diseases. *In* Sherding RG (ed): The Cat: Diseases and Clinical Management, 2nd ed. New York, Churchill Livingstone, 1994, p 819.

79. Kittleson ME: Feline hypertrophic cardiomyopathy. *In* Bonagura JD (ed): Current Veterinary Therapy XII. Philadelphia, WB Saunders, 1995, p 854.

80. Fox PR, Kaplan P: Feline arrhythmias. *In* Bonagura JD (ed): Contemp Issues Small Anim Pract, Vol 7. New York, Churchill Livingstone, 1987, p 251.

81. Fox PR, Broussard JD, Peterson ME: Electrocardiographic and radiographic changes in cats with hyperthyroidism: Comparison of populations evaluated during 1979–1982 vs. 1992–1993 (abstract). J Vet Intern Med 7:118, 1993.

82. Bond BR, Fox PR: Advances in feline cardiomyopathy. Vet Clin North Am 14:1021, 1984.

83. Fox PR, Bond BR: Nonselective and selective angiocardiography. Vet Clin North Am 13:259, 1983.

84. Fox PR: Feline cardiomyopathy. *In* Bonagura JD (ed): Contemp Issues Small Anim Pract, Vol 7. New York, Churchill Livingstone, 1987, p 157.

85. Appleton CP, Hatle LK: The natural history of left ventricular filling abnormalities: Assessment of two-dimensional and Doppler echocardiography. Echocardiography 9:437, 1992.

86. Wilkins RJ: Clinical pathology of feline cardiac disease. Vet Clin North Am 7:285, 1977.

87. Fox PR: Current usage and hazards of diuretic therapy. *In* Kirk RW, Bonagura JD (eds): Current Veterinary Therapy XI. Philadelphia, WB Saunders, 1992, p 668.

88. Kittleson MD, Pion PD, DeLellis LA, et al: Increased serum growth hormone concentration in feline hypertrophic cardiomyopathy. J Vet Intern Med 6:320, 1992.

89. Rush JE, Freeman LM, Brown DJ, et al: The use of enalapril in the treatment of feline hypertrophic cardiomyopathy. Am Anim Hosp Assoc 34:88, 1998.

90. Angelini A, Calzolari V, Thiene G, et al: Morphologic spectrum of primary restrictive cardiomyopathy. Am J Cardiol 80:1046, 1997.

91. Hirota Y, Shimizu G, Kita Y, et al: Spectrum of restrictive cardiomyopathy: Report of the national survey in Japan. Am Heart J 120:188, 1990.

92. Reisinger J, Dubrey SW, Falk RH: Cardiac amyloidosis. Cardiol Rev 5:317, 1997.

93. Lewis AB: Clinical profile and outcome of restrictive cardiomyopathy in children. Am Heart J 123:1539, 1992.

94. Fox PR: Restrictive cardiomyopathy. *In:* Proceedings of the 14th Annual Veterinary Medicine Forum, 1996, pp 235–236.

95. Bonagura JB, Fox PR: Restrictive cardiomyopathy. *In* Bonagura JD (ed): Current Veterinary Therapy XII. Philadelphia, WB Saunders, 1995, p 863.

96. Liu SK, Fox PR: Restrictive cardiomyopathy in the cat (abstract). Lab Invest 68:25A, 1993.

97. Saxon B, Hendrick M, Waddle JR: Restrictive cardiomyopathy in a cat with hypereosinophilic syndrome. Can Vet J 32:367, 1991.

98. Stalis IH, Bossbaly MJ, Van Winkle TJ: Feline endomyocarditis and left ventricular endocardial fibrosis. Vet Pathol 32:122, 1995.

99. Scott DW, Randolph JF, Walsh KM: Hypereosinophilic syndrome in a cat. Feline Pract 14:22, 1985.

100. Pedersen NC, Giffey S, Graham R, et al: A transmissible myocarditis/diaphragmitis of cats manifested by transient fever and depression. Feline Pract 21:13, 1993.

101. McEwen SA, Valli VEO, Hilland TJ: Hypereosinophilic syndrome in cats: A report of three cases. Can J Comp Med 49:248, 1985.

102. Zientek DM, King DL, Dewan SJ, et al: Hypereosinophilic syndrome with rapid progression of cardiac involvement and early echocardiographic abnormalities. Am Heart J 130:1295, 1995.

103. Arbustini E, Morbini P, Grasso M, et al: Restrictive cardiomyopathy, atrioventricular block and mild to subclinical myopathy in patients with desmin-immunoreactive material deposits. Am Coll Cardiol 31:645, 1998.

104. Gottdiener JS, Maron BJ, Schooley RT, et al: Two-dimensional echocardiographic assessment of the idiopathic hypereosinophilic syndrome: Anatomic basis of mitral regurgitation and peripheral embolization. Circulation 67:572, 1983.

105. Shabetai R: Controversial issues in restrictive cardiomyopathy. Postgrad Med J 68:S47, 1992.

106. Child JS, Perloff JK: The restrictive cardiomyopathies. Cardiol Clin 6:289, 1988.

107. Spyrou N, Foale R: Restrictive cardiomyopathies. Curr Opin Cardiol 9:344, 1994.

108. Katritsis D, Wilmshurst PT, Wendon JA, et al: Primary restrictive cardiomyopathy: Clinical and pathologic characteristics. J Am Coll Cardiol 18:1230, 1991.

109. Fitzpatrick AP, Shapiro LM, Rickards AF, et al: Familial restrictive cardiomyopathy with atrioventricular block and skeletal myopathy. Br Heart J 63:114, 1990.

110. Aroney C, Bett N, Radford D: Familial restrictive cardiomyopathy. N Z J Med 18:877, 1988.

111. Mady C, Barretto AC, Oliveira SA, et al: Evolution of the endocardial fibrotic process in endomyocardial fibrosis. Am J Cardiol 68:402, 1991.

112. Fujioka S, Koide H, Kitaura Y: Molecular detection and differentiation of enteroviruses in endomyocardial biopsies and pericardial effusions from dilated cardiomyopathy and myocarditis. Am Heart J 131:760, 1996.

113. Martin A, Webber S, Fricker F, et al: Acute myocarditis: Rapid diagnosis by PCR in children. Circulation 90:330, 1994.

114. Schowengerdt KO, Ni J, Denfield SW, et al: Association of parvovirus B19 genome in children with myocarditis and cardiac allograft rejection. Circulation 96:3549, 1997.

115. Ni J, Bowles N, Kim Y, et al: Viral infection of the myocardium in endocardial fibroelastosis: Molecular evidence for the role of mumps virus as an etiologic agent. Circulation 95:133, 1997.

116. Meurs KM, Fox PR, Magnon A, et al: Polymerase chain reaction (PCR) analysis for feline viruses in formalin-fixed cardiomyopathic hearts identifies panleukopenia (abstract). J Vet Intern Med 12:201, 1998.

117. Fauci AS, Harley JB, Roberts WC, et al: The idiopathic hypereosinophilic syndrome: Clinical, pathophysiologic, and therapeutic considerations. Ann Intern Med 97:79, 1982.

118. Appleton CP, Hatle LK, Popp RL: Demonstration of restrictive ventricular physiology by Doppler echocardiography. J Am Coll Cardiol 11:757, 1988.

119. Tai PC, Ackerman SJ, Spry CJ, et al: Deposits of eosinophil granule proteins in cardiac tissues of patients with eosinophilic endomyocardial disease. Lancet 1:643, 1987.

120. Schaffer SW, Dimayuga ER, Kayes SG: Development and characterization of a

model of eosinophil-mediated cardiomyopathy in rats infected with *Toxocara canis.* Am J Physiol 262:H1428, 1992.

121. Berger PB, Duffy J, Reeder GS, et al: Restrictive cardiomyopathy associated with the eosinophilia-myalgia syndrome. Mayo Clin Proc 69:162, 1994.

122. Liu SK, Tilley LP: Animal models of primary myocardial diseases. Yale J Biol Med 53:191, 1980.

123. Liu SK: Cardiovascular pathology. *In* Fox PR (ed): Canine and Feline Cardiology. New York, Churchill Livingstone, 1988, p 625.

124. Maron BJ, Epstein SE, Roberts WC: Hypertrophic cardiomyopathy and transmural myocardial infarction without significant atherosclerosis of the extramural coronary arteries. Am J Cardiol 43:1086, 1979.

125. von Dohlen TW, Prisant LM, Frank MJ: Significance of positive or negative thallium-201 scintigraphy in hypertrophic cardiomyopathy. Am J Cardiol 64:498, 1989.

126. Teo KK, Yusuf S, Furberg CD: Effects of prophylactic antiarrhythmic drug therapy in acute myocardial infarction. JAMA 270:1589, 1993.

127. Kennedy HL, Brooks MM, Barker AH, et al: Beta-blocker therapy in the Cardiac Arrhythmia Suppression Trial. Am J Cardiol 74:674, 1994.

128. ISIS-1 (First International Study of Infarct Survival) Collaborative Group: Mechanisms for the early mortality reduction produced by beta blockade started early in acute myocardial infarction: ISIS-1. Lancet 1:921, 1988.

129. Yusuf S, Peto R, Lewis J, et al: Beta blockade during and after myocardial infarction: An overview of the randomized trials. Prog Cardiovasc Dis 27:335, 1985.

130. Clarkson PBM, Wheeldon NM, Macleod C, et al: Systolic and diastolic effects of beta-adrenergic stimulation in normal humans. Am J Cardiol 75:206, 1997.

131. Foy SG, Crozier IG, Turner JG, et al: Comparison of enalapril vs captopril on left ventricular function and survival three months after acute myocardial infarction (the "PRACTICAL" Study). Am J Cardiol 73:1180, 1994.

132. Køber L, Torp-Pedersen C, on behalf of the TRACE Study Group: Clinical characteristics and mortality of patients screened for entry into the transolapril cardiac evaluation (TRACE) study. Am J Cardiol 76:1, 1995.

133. Greenberg B, Quinones MA, Koilpillai C, et al: Effects of long-term enalapril therapy on cardiac structure and function in patients with left ventricular dysfunction. Results of the SOLVD Echocardiographic Substudy. Circulation 91:2573, 1995.

134. Torp-Pedersen C, Køber L, Burchardt H: The place of angiotensin-converting enzyme inhibition after acute myocardial infarction. Am Heart J 134:S25, 1997.

135. Latini R, Maggioni AP, Flather M, et al: ACE-inhibitor use in patients with myocardial infarction: Summary of evidence from clinical trials. Circulation 32:3232, 1995.

136. Rutherford JD, Pfeffer MA, Moye LA, et al: Effects of captopril on ischemic events after myocardial infarction: Results of the Survival and Ventricular Enlargement Trial. Circulation 90:1731, 1994.

137. Skolnick AE, Frishman WH: Calcium channel blockers in myocardial infarction. Arch Intern Med 149:1669, 1989.

138. Hager WD, Davis BR, Riba A, et al: Absence of a deleterious effect of calcium channel blockers in patients with left ventricular dysfunction after myocardial infarction: The SAVE study experience. Am Heart J 135:406, 1998.

139. The Multicenter Postinfarction Trial Research Group (MDPIT): The effect of diltiazem on mortality and reinfarction after myocardial infarction. N Engl J Med 319:385, 1988.

140. Ishikawa K, Nakai S, Takenaka T, et al: Short-acting nifedipine and diltiazem do not reduce the incidence of cardiac events in patients with healed myocardial infarction. Circulation 95:2368, 1997.

141. Kostis JV, Lacy CR, Cosgrove RN, et al: Association of calcium channel blocker use with increased rate of acute myocardial infarction in patients with left ventricular dysfunction. Am Heart J 133:550, 1997.

142. Packer M: Calcium channel blockers in chronic heart failure: The risk of "physiological rationale" therapy. Circulation 82:2254, 1990.

143. ACC/AHA guidelines for the management of patients with acute myocardial infarction. J Am Call Cardiol 78:153, 1996.

144. Maron B, Shirani J, Poliac LC, et al: Sudden death in young competitive athletes, clinical, demographic, and pathological profiles. JAMA 276:199, 1996.

145. Wigle ED: Novel insights into the clinical manifestations and treatment of hypertrophic cardiomyopathy. Curr Opin Cardiol 10:29, 1995.

146. Maron B, Shirani J, Poliac LC, et al: Sudden death in young competitive athletes, clinical, demographic, and pathological profiles. JAMA 276:199, 1996.

147. Bristow MR: Mechanism of action of beta-blocking agents in heart failure. Am J Cardiol 80:26L, 1997.

148. Cody RJ: The sympathetic nervous system and the renin-angiotensin-aldosterone system in cardiovascular diseases. Am J Cardiol 80:9J, 1997.

149. Maron BJ, Bonow RO, Cannon RO III, et al: Hypertrophic cardiomyopathy: Interrelations of clinical manifestations, pathophysiology and therapy (second of two parts). N Engl J Med 316:780, 1987.

150. Heidenreich PA, Lee TT, Massie BM: Effect of beta-blockade on mortality in patients with heart failure: A meta-analysis of randomized clinical trials. J Am Coll Cardiol 30:27, 1997.

151. Rials SJ, Wu Y, Pauletto FJ, et al: Effect of an intravenous angiotensin-converting enzyme inhibitor on the electrophysiologic features of normal and hypertrophied feline ventricles. Am Heart J 132:989, 1996.

152. Pfeffer MA, Pfeffer JM: Pharmacologic regression of cardiac hypertrophy in experimental hypertension. J Cardiovasc Pharmacol 6:S865, 1989.

153. Dell'Itallia LJ, Oparil S: Cardiac renin angiotensin system in hypertrophy and the progression to heart failure. Heart Failure Rev 1:63, 1966.

154. Oshikawa T, Handa S, Anzai T, et al: Early reduction of neurohumoral factors plays a key role in mediating the efficacy of β-blocker therapy for congestive heart failure. Am Heart J 131:329, 1996.

155. Maron BJ, Roberts WC, Epstein SE: Sudden cardiac death in hypertrophic cardiomyopathy: A profile in 78 patients. Circulation 65:1388, 1982.

156. Maron BJ, Cecchi F, McKenna WJ: Risk factors and stratification for sudden death in patients with hypertrophic cardiomyopathy. Br Heart J 72:S13, 1994.

157. Schiavone WA, Malone JD, Lever HD, et al: Electrophysiologic studies of patients with hypertrophic cardiomyopathy with syncope of undetermined etiology. PACE Pacing Clin Electrophysiol 9:476, 1989.

158. Nienaber CA, Hiller S, Spielmann RP, et al: Syncope in hypertrophic cardiomyopathy: Multivariate analysis of prognostic determinants. J Am Coll Cardiol 15:948, 1990.

159. McAreavey D, Dilsizian V, Panza J, et al: Favorable prognosis in 88 young hypertrophic cardiomyopathy patients during therapy based on hemodynamic electrophysiologic and thallium scintigraphy findings (abstract). Circulation 88(Suppl I):I-209, 1993.

160. Gilligan DM, Nihoyannopoulos P, Chan WL, et al: Investigation of a hemodynamic basis for syncope in hypertrophic cardiomyopathy: Use of a head-up tilt test. Circulation 85:140, 1992.

161. Dilsizian V, Bonow RO, Epstein SE, et al: Myocardial ischemia detected by thallium scintigraphy is frequently related to cardiac arrest and syncope in young patients with hypertrophic cardiomyopathy. J Am Coll Cardiol 22:796, 1993.

162. Black IW, Hopkins AP, Lee LCL, et al: Left atrial spontaneous echo contrast: A clinical and echocardiographic analysis. J Am Coll Cardiol 18:398, 1991.

163. Leung DYC, Black IW, Cranney GB, et al: Prognostic implications of left atrial spontaneous echo contrast in nonvalvular atrial fibrillation. J Am Coll Cardiol 24:755, 1994.

164. Tsai LM, Chen JH, Fang CJ, et al: Clinical implications of left atrial spontaneous echo contrast in nonrheumatic atrial fibrillation. Am J Cardiol 70:327, 1992.

165. Black IW, Chesterman CN, Hopkins AP, et al: Hematologic correlates of left atrial spontaneous echo contrast and thromboembolism in nonvalvular atrial fibrillation. J Am Coll Cardiol 21:451, 1993.

166. Fatkin D, Herbert E, Feneley MP: Hematologic correlates of spontaneous echo contrast in patients with atrial fibrillation and implications for thromboembolic risk. Am J Cardiol 73:672, 1994.

167. Mahoney C, Ferguson J: The effect of heparin versus citrate on blood echogenicity in vitro: The role of platelet and platelet-neutrophil aggregates. Ultrasound Med Biol 18:851, 1992.

168. Kearney K, Mahoney C: Effect of aspirin on spontaneous contrast in the brachial veins of normal subjects. Am J Cardiol 75:924, 1995.

169. Karalis DG, Ross JJ, Neri JL: Left ventricular thromboembolism. Circulation 97:498, 1998.

170. Tsai L-M, Chen J-H, Tsao C-J: Relation of left atrial spontaneous echo contrast with prethrombotic state in atrial fibrillation associated with systemic hypertension, idiopathic dilated cardiomyopathy, or no identifiable cause (lone). Am J Cardiol 81:1249, 1998.

171. Marian AJ, Roberts R: Recent advances in the molecular genetics of hypertrophic cardiomyopathy. Circulation 92:1336, 1995.

172. Brater DC: Diuretic therapy. N Engl J Med 339:387, 1998.

173. Appleton CP, Hatle LK, Popp RL: Relation of transmitral flow velocity patterns to left ventricular diastolic function: New insights from a combined hemodynamic and Doppler echocardiographic study. J Am Coll Cardiol 12:426, 1988.

174. Gilligan DM, Chan WL, Stewart R, et al: Cardiac responses assessed by echocardiograph to changes in preload in hypertrophic cardiomyopathy. Am J Cardiol 73:312, 1994.

175. Vasko MR, Cartwright DB, Knochel JP, et al: Furosemide absorption altered in decompensated congestive heart failure. Ann Intern Med 102:314, 1985.

176. Ellison DH: The physiologic basis of diuretic synergism: Its role in treating diuretic resistance. Ann Intern Med 114:886, 1991.

177. Mann DL, Kent RL, Parsons B, et al: Adrenergic effects on the biology of the adult mammalian cardiocyte. Circulation 85:790, 1992.

178. Cohn JN: Plasma norepinephrine and mortality. Clin Cardiol 18(Suppl I):I-9, 1995.

179. Bigger JT: Why patients with congestive heart failure die: Arrhythmias and sudden cardiac death. Circulation 75(Suppl IV):IV28, 1987.

180. Mancia G: Sympathetic activation in congestive heart failure. Eur Heart J 11(Suppl A):3, 1990.

181. Collucci WS: Molecular and cellular mechanisms of myocardial failure. Am J Cardiol 80:15L, 1997.

182. Francis GS, Cohn JN: Heart failure: Mechanisms of cardiac and vascular dysfunction and the rationale for pharmacologic intervention. FASEB J 4:3068, 1990.

183. Eaton GM, Cody RL, Nunziata E, et al: Early left ventricular dysfunction elicits activation of sympathetic drive and attenuation of parasympathetic tone in the paced canine model of congestive heart failure. Circulation 92:555, 1995.

184. Clarkson PBM, Wheeldon NM, Macleod C, et al: Systolic and diastolic effects of beta-adrenergic stimulation in normal humans. Am J Cardiol 75:206, 1997.

185. Thompson DS, Naqvi N, Juul SM, et al: Effects of propranolol on myocardial oxygen consumption, substrate extraction, and haemodynamics in hypertrophic obstructive cardiomyopathy. Br Heart J 44:488, 1980.

186. Harrison DC, Braunwald E, Glick G, et al: Effects of beta adrenergic blockade on the circulation, with particular reference to observations in patients with hypertrophic subaortic stenosis. Circulation 29:84, 1964.

187. Newton GE, Parker JD. Acute effects of β₁-selective and nonselective β-adrener-

gic receptor blockade on cardiac sympathetic activity in congestive heart failure. Circulation 94:353, 1996.

188. Fox PR: Therapy for feline myocardial diseases. *In* Bonagura JD (ed): Current Veterinary Therapy XIII. Philadelphia, WB Saunders, 1999.

189. Tilley LP, Weitz J: Pharmacologic and other forms of medical therapy in feline cardiac disease. Vet Clin North Am 7:415, 1977.

190. Fox PR: Evidence for and against beta-blockers and aspirin for management of feline cardiomyopathies. Vet Clin North Am 21:1011, 1991.

191. Muir WW: Clinical pharmacodynamics of beta-adrenoceptor blocking drugs in veterinary medicine. Compend Contin Ed Pract Vet 6:156, 1939.

192. Frishman WH: β-adrenergic blockers. Med Clin North Am 72:37, 1988.

193. Quiñones M, Dyer DC, Ware WA, et al: Pharmacokinetics of atenolol in clinically normal cats. Am J Vet Res 57:1050, 1996.

194. Iwase M, Sotobata I, Takagi S, et al: Effects of diltiazem on left ventricular diastolic behavior in patients with hypertrophic cardiomyopathy: Evaluation with exercise pulsed Doppler echocardiography. J Am Coll Cardiol 2:143, 1987.

195. Suwa M, Hiroto Y, Kawamura K: Improvement in left ventricular diastolic function during intravenous and oral diltiazem therapy in patients with hypertrophic cardiomyopathy: An echocardiographic study. Am J Cardiol 54:1047, 1984.

196. Betocchi S, Piscione F, Losi MA, et al: Effects of diltiazem on left ventricular systolic and diastolic function in hypertrophic cardiomyopathy. Am J Cardiol 78:451, 1996.

197. Henry PD: Comparative pharmacology of calcium antagonists: Nifedipine, verapamil, and diltiazem. Am J Cardiol 46:1047, 1980.

198. Walsh RA: The effects of calcium-entry blockade of left ventricular systolic and diastolic function. Circulation 75(Suppl V):V43, 1997.

199. Rosing DR, Idänpään-Heikkilä U, Maron BJ, et al: Use of calcium-channel blocking drugs in hypertrophic cardiomyopathy. Am J Cardiol 55(Suppl):185B, 1985.

200. Bonow RO, Rosing DR, Bacharach SL, et al: Effects of verapamil on left ventricular systolic function and diastolic filling in patients with hypertrophic cardiomyopathy. Circulation 64:787, 1981.

201. Hess OM, Grimm J, Krayenbuehl HP: Diastolic function in hypertrophic cardiomyopathy: Effects of propranolol and verapamil on diastolic stiffness. Eur Heart J 4(Suppl F):47, 1983.

202. Udelson JE, Bonow RO, O'Gara PT, et al: Verapamil prevents silent myocardial perfusion abnormalities during exercise in asymptomatic patients with hypertrophic cardiomyopathy. Circulation 79:1052, 1989.

203. Natarajan D, Sharma SC, Sharma VP: Pulmonary edema with diltiazem in hypertrophic obstructive cardiomyopathy. Am Heart J 120:229, 1990.

204. Johnson LM, Atkins CE, Keene BW, et al: Pharmacokinetic and pharmacodynamic properties of conventional and CD-formulated diltiazem in cats. J Vet Intern Med 10:316, 1996.

205. Hager WD, Davis BR, Riba A, et al: Absence of a deleterious effect of calcium channel blockers in patients with left ventricular dysfunction after myocardial infarction: The SAVE study experience. Am Heart J 135:406, 1998.

206. Ishikawa K, Nakai S, Takenaka T, et al: Short-acting nifedipine and diltiazem do not reduce the incidence of cardiac events in patients with healed myocardial infarction. Circulation 95:2368, 1997.

207. Messerli FH, Michalewicz L: Safety of heart rate-lowering calcium antagonists: Lessons from controlled trials. Am Heart J 134(Suppl):S21, 1997.

208. Packer M: The neurohormonal hypothesis: A theory to explain the mechanism of disease progression in heart failure. J Am Coll Cardiol 20:248, 1992.

209. Chatterjee K: Heart failure therapy in evolution. Circulation 94:2689, 1996.

210. Consensus Trial Study Group: Effects of enalapril on mortality in severe congestive heart failure: Results of the cooperative North Scandinavian Enalapril Survival Study (CONSENSUS). N Engl J Med 316:1429, 1987.

211. Sun Y, Weber KT: Fibrosis and myocardial ACE: Possible substrate and independence from circulating angiotensin II. J Cardiac Failure 1:81, 1994.

212. Weber KT, Brilla CG: Pathological hypertrophy and cardiac interstitium: Fibrosis and renin-angiotensin-aldosterone system. Circulation 83:1849, 1991.

213. Factor SM, Butany J, Sole MK, et al: Pathologic fibrosis and matrix connective tissue in the subaortic myocardium of patients with hypertrophic cardiomyopathy. J Am Coll Cardiol 17:1343, 1991.

214. Lechin MM, Quiñones MA, Omran A, et al: Angiotensin-I converting enzyme genotypes and left ventricular hypertrophy in patients with hypertrophic cardiomyopathy. Circulation 92:1808, 1995.

215. Hodges RD, Lothrop CD Jr: Atrial natriuretic factor concentration in the cat (abstract). J Vet Intern Med 5:129, 1991.

216. Weber KT: Extracellular matrix remodeling in heart failure: A role for de novo angiotensin II generation. Circulation 96:4065, 1997.

217. Vaughn DE, Pfeffer MA: Angiotensin converting enzyme inhibitors and cardiovascular remodeling. Cardiovasc Res 28:159, 1994.

218. Dahlof B: Effect of angiotensin II blockade on cardiac hypertrophy and remodeling: A review. J Hum Hypertens 9(Suppl):S37, 1995.

219. ACE Inhibitor Myocardial Infarction Collaborative Group: Indications for ACE inhibitors in the early treatment of acute myocardial infarction: Systematic overview of individual data from 100,000 patients in randomized trials Circulation 97:2202, 1998.

220. Hartmann A, Puetz A, Hopf R: Effects of long term ACE-inhibitor therapy in hypertrophic cardiomyopathy (HCM). J Am Coll Cardiol Suppl A:234A, 1995.

221. Sanders N, Hamlin R, Buffington T, et al: Effects of enalapril on healthy cats (abstract). J Vet Intern Med 6:139, 1992.

222. King JN, Humbert-Droz, Maurer M: Pharmacokinetics of benazepril and inhibition of plasma ACE activity in cats (abstract). J Vet Intern Med 10:163, 1996.

223. Pollick C: Disopyramide in hypertrophic cardiomyopathy: Noninvasive assessment after oral administration. Am J Cardiol 62:1252, 1988.

224. Rosing DR, Kent KM, Maron BJ, et al: Verapamil therapy: A new approach to the pharmacologic treatment of hypertrophic cardiomyopathy: II. Effects on exercise capacity and symptomatic status. Circulation 60:1208, 1979.

225. Pion PD, Kittleson MD, Rogers QR, et al: Myocardial failure in cats associated with low plasma taurine: A reversible cardiomyopathy. Science 237:764, 1987.

226. Pion PD, Kittleson MD, Rogers QR, et al: Taurine deficiency myocardial failure in the domestic cat. *In* Fasante-Morales H (ed): Functional Neurochemistry of Taurine. New York, Alan R Liss, 1990, p 423.

227. Pion PD, Lewis J, Greene K, et al: Effect of meal-feeding and food deprivation on plasma and whole-blood taurine concentrations in cats. J Nutr 121:S177, 1991.

228. Pion PD, Kittleson MD, Lewis J, et al: Taurine deficiency myocardial failure: Incidence and relation to tissue taurine concentration (abstract). J Vet Intern Med 5:123, 1991.

229. Sisson DD, Knight DH, Helinski C, et al: Plasma taurine concentrations and M-mode echocardiographic measures in healthy cats and cats with dilated cardiomyopathy. J Vet Intern Med 5:232, 1991.

230. Skrodzki M, Trautvetter E, Monch E: Plasma taurine levels in healthy cats and cats with cardiac disorders. J Nutr 121:S171, 1991.

231. Pion PD, Kittleson MD, Stiles ML, et al: Dilated cardiomyopathy associated with taurine deficiency in the domestic cat: Relationship to diet and myocardial taurine content. *In* Lombardini JB, Schaffer SW, Azuma J (eds): Taurine. New York, Plenum Press, 1992 p 63.

232. Pion PD, Kittleson MD, Thomas WP, et al: Clinical findings in cats with dilated cardiomyopathy and relationship of findings to taurine deficiency. JAVMA 201:267, 1992.

233. Pion PD, Kittleson MD, Thomas WP, et al: Response of cats with dilated cardiomyopathy to taurine supplementation. JAVMA 201:275, 1992.

234. Morris JG, Rogers QR: The metabolic basis for the taurine requirement of cats. *In* Lombardini JB, Schaffer SW, Azuma J (eds): Taurine: New Dimensions on Nutrition and Mechanisms of Action. New York, Plenum Press, 1992.

235. Fox PR, Sturman JA: Myocardial taurine concentrations in cats with cardiac disease and in healthy cats fed taurine-modified diets. Am J Vet Res 53:237, 1992.

236. Novotny MJ, Hogan PM, Paley DM, et al: Systolic and diastolic dysfunction of the left ventricle induced by dietary taurine deficiency in cats. Am J Physiol 261:H121, 1991.

237. Fox PR, Trautwein EA, Hayes KC, et al: Comparison of taurine, α-tocopherol, retinol, selenium, and total triglycerides and cholesterol concentrations in cats with cardiac disease and in healthy cats. Am J Vet Res 54:563, 1993

238. Fox PR, Petrie JP, Liu SK, et al: Clinical and pathologic features of cardiomyopathy characterized by myocardial failure in 49 cats: 1990–1995 (abstract). J Vet Intern Med 11:139, 1997.

239. Grünig E, Tasman JA, Kücherer H, et al: Frequency and phenotypes of familial dilated cardiomyopathy. J Am Coll Cardiol 31:186, 1998.

240. Baig MK, Goldman JH, Caforio ALP, et al: Familial dilated cardiomyopathy: Cardiac abnormalities are common in asymptomatic relatives and may represent early disease. J Am Coll Cardiol 31:195, 1998.

241. Martino TA, Liu P, Sole MJ: Viral infection and the pathogenesis of dilated cardiomyopathy. Circ Res 74:182, 1994.

242. Rose NR, Neumann DA, Herskowitz A: Coxsackievirus myocarditis. Adv Intern Med 37:411, 1992.

243. Latham RD, Mulrow JP, Virmani R, et al: Recently diagnosed idiopathic dilated cardiomyopathy: Incidence of myocarditis and efficacy of prednisone therapy. Am Heart J 117:876, 1989.

244. Dec GW, Fuster V: Medical progress: Idiopathic dilated cardiomyopathy. N Engl J Med 331:1564, 1994.

245. Neumann DA: Autoimmunity and idiopathic dilated cardiomyopathy. Mayo Clin Proc 69:193, 1994.

246. Lawler DF, Templeton AJ, Monti KL: Evidence for genetic involvement in feline dilated cardiomyopathy. J Vet Intern Med 7:383, 1993.

247. Grossman W, McLaurin LP, Rolett EL: Alterations in left ventricular relaxation and diastolic compliance in congestive cardiomyopathy. Cardiovasc Res 13:514, 1979.

248. Lord PF: Left ventricular diastolic stiffness in dogs with congestive cardiomyopathy and volume overload. Am J Vet Res 37:953, 1976.

249. Dow SW, Fettman MJ, Smith KR, et al: Taurine depletion and cardiovascular disease in adult cats fed a potassium-depleted acidified diet. Am J Vet Res 53:402, 1992.

250. Ballèvre O, Piguet-Welsh C, Staempfli A, et al: Taurine kinetics in cats fed processed diets. Vet Int 1:17, 1993.

251. Morris JG, Rogers QR, Kim SW, et al: Dietary taurine requirement of cats is determined by microbial degradation of taurine in the gut. Vet Clin Nutr 1:118, 1994.

252. Huxtable RJ, Sebring LA: Cardiovascular actions of taurine. *In* Kuriyama K, Huxtable RJ, Iwata H (eds): Sulfur Amino Acids: Biochemical and Clinical Aspects. New York, Alan R Liss, 1983, p 5.

253. Sturman JA: Nutritional taurine and central nervous system development. Ann NY Acad Sci 477:196, 1986.

254. Hayes KC: A review of the biological function of taurine. Nutr Rev 34: 61, 1976.

255. Rabin B, Nicolosi RJ, Hayes KC: Dietary influences on bile acid conjugation in the cat. J Nutr 106:1241, 1976.

256. Knopf K, Sturman JA, Armstrong M, et al: Taurine: An essential nutrient for the cat. J Nutr 108:773, 1978.

CV

257. Sturman JA: Taurine in development. Physiol Rev 73:119, 1993.

258. Wen GY, Sturman JA, Wisniewski HM, et al: Tapetum disorganization in taurine-depleted cats. Invest Ophthalmol Visual Sci 18:1201, 1979.

259. Trautwein EA, Hayes KC: Gender and dietary amino acid supplementation influence the plasma and whole blood taurine status of taurine depleted cats. J Nutr 121:3170, 1991.

260. Trautwein EA, Hayes KC: Taurine concentrations in human plasma and whole blood: Estimation of error from intra- and inter-individual variation and sampling technique. Am J Clin Nutr 52:758, 1990.

261. Colucci WS, Wright RF, Braunwald E: New positive inotropic agents in the treatment of congestive heart failure: Mechanisms of action and recent clinical developments (first of two parts). N Engl J Med 314:290, 1986.

262. Kenakin TP: An in vitro quantitative analysis of the alpha adrenoceptor partial agonist activity of dobutamine and its relevance to inotropic selectivity. J Pharmacol Exp Ther 216:210, 1981.

263. Ruffolo RR Jr, Spradlin TA, Pollock GD, et al: Alpha and beta adrenergic effects of the stereoisomers of dobutamine. J Pharmacol Exp Ther 219:447, 1981.

264. Maskin CS, Le Jemtel MD, Sonnenblick EH: Inotropic drugs for treatment of the failing heart. Cardiovasc Clin 14:1, 1984.

265. Kittleson MD: Dobutamine. JAVMA 177:642, 1980.

266. McDonald RH Jr, Goldberg LI, McNay JL, et al: Effects of dopamine in man: Augmentation of sodium excretion, glomerular filtration rate, and renal plasma flow. J Clin Invest 43:1116, 1964.

267. Brest AN: Clinical pharmacology of diuretic drugs. Cardiovasc Clin 14:31, 1984.

268. Regitz-Zagrosek V, Leuchs B, Krulls-Munch J, et al: Angiotensin-converting enzyme inhibitors and β-blockers in long-term treatment of dilated cardiomyopathy. Am Heart J 129:754, 1995.

269. Sabbah HN, Shimoyama H, Kono T, et al: Effects of long-term monotherapy with enalapril, metoprolol, and digoxin on the progression of left ventricular dysfunction and dilation in dogs with reduced ejection fraction. Circulation 89:2852, 1994.

270. Atkins CE, Snyder PS, Keene BW, et al: Efficacy of digoxin for treatment of cats with DCM. JAVMA 196:1463, 1990.

271. Erichsen DF, Harris SG, Upson DW: Therapeutic and toxic plasma concentrations of digoxin in the cat. Am Anim Hosp Assoc 14:734, 1978.

272. Erichsen DF, Harris SG, Upson DW: Plasma levels of digoxin in the cat: Some clinical applications. Am Anim Hosp Assoc 14:734:1994, 1982.

273. Bolton GR, Powell AA. Plasma kinetics of digoxin in the cat. Am J Vet Res 43:1994, 1982.

274. Andersson B, Hamm C, Persson S, et al: Improved exercise hemodynamic status in dilated cardiomyopathy after beta-adrenergic blockade treatment. J Am Coll Cardiol 23:1397, 1994.

275. Eichhorn EJ, Heesch CM, Barnett JH, et al: Effect of metoprolol on myocardial function and energetics in patients with nonischemic dilated cardiomyopathy: A randomized, double-blinded, placebo-controlled study. J Am Coll Cardiol 24:1310. 1994.

276. Waagstien F: Adrenergic beta-blocking agents in congestive heart failure due to idiopathic dilated cardiomyopathy. Eur Heart J 16(Suppl O):128, 1996.

277. Regitz-Zagrosek V, Leuchs B, Krulls-Munch J, et al: Angiotensin-converting enzyme inhibitors and β-blockers in long-term treatment of dilated cardiomyopathy. Am Heart J 129:754, 1995.

278. Asseman P, McFadden E, Bauchart JJ, et al: Why do beta-blockers help in idiopathic dilated cardiomyopathy-frequency mismatch? Lancet 344:803, 1994.

279. Sato H, Hori M, Ozaki H, et al: Exercise-induced upward shift of diastolic left ventricular pressure-volume relation in patients with dilated cardiomyopathy. Effects of beta-adrenergic blockade. Circulation 88:2215, 1993.

280. Ishida S, Makino N, Masumoto K, et al: Effect of metoprolol on the beta-adrenoceptor density of lymphocytes in patients with dilated cardiomyopathy. Am Heart J 125:1311, 1993.

281. McKenna WJ, Thiene G, Nava A, et al: Diagnosis of arrhythmogenic right ventricular dysplasia/cardiomyopathy. Task Force of the Working Group Myocardial and Pericardial Disease of the European Society of Cardiology and of the Scientific Council on Cardiomyopathies of the International Society and Federation of Cardiology. Br Heart J 71:215, 1994.

282. Giles TD: New WHO/ISFC Classification of a task not completed (letter). Circulation 96:2081, 1996.

283. Frank R, Fontaine G, Vedel J, et al: Electrocardiologie de quatre cas de dysplasie ventriculaire droite arythmogene. Arch Mal Coeur Vaiss 71:963, 1978.

284. Thiene G, Basso C, Nava A: About the histology of arrhythmogenic right ventricular dysplasia (letter). Circulation 96:2089, 1997.

285. Fontaine G, Fontaliran F, Frank R: Arrhythmogenic right ventricular cardiomyopathies: Clinical forms and main differential diagnoses. Circulation 97:1532, 1998.

286. Gerlis LM, Schmidt-Ott SC, Ho SY, et al: Dysplastic conditions of the right ventricular myocardium: Uhl's anomaly versus arrhythmogenic right ventricular dysplasia. Br Heart J 69:142, 1993.

287. Burke AP, Farb A, Tashko G, et al: Arrhythmogenic right ventricular cardiomyopathy and fatty replacement of the right ventricular myocardium: Are they different? Circulation 97:1571, 1998.

288. Corrado D, Basso C, Thiene G, et al: Spectrum of clinicopathologic manifestations of arrhythmogenic right ventricular cardiomyopathy/dysplasia: A multicenter study. J Am Coll Cardiol 30:1512, 1997.

289. Basso C, Thiene G, Corrado D, et al: Arrhythmogenic right ventricular cardiomyopathy: Dysplasia, dystrophy, or myocarditis? Circulation 94:983, 1996.

290. Fox PR, Basso C, Maron BJ, et al: Spontaneous occurrence of arrhythmogenic right ventricular cardiomyopathy in the domestic cat: A new animal model of human disease. Circulation 98(Suppl I):297, 1998.

291. Fontaine G, Fontaliran F, Rosas Andrade F, et al: The arrhythmogenic right ventricle: Dysplasia versus cardiomyopathy. Heart Vessels 10:227, 1995.

292. Pinamonti B, Sinagra G, Salvi A, et al: Left ventricular involvement in right ventricular dysplasia. Am Heart J 123:711, 1992.

293. Mallat Z, Tedgui A, Fontaliran F, et al: Evidence of apoptosis in arrhythmogenic right ventricular dysplasia. N Engl J Med 335:1190, 1996.

294. James TN, Nichols MM, Sapire DW, et al: Complete heart block and fatal right ventricular failure in an infant. Circulation 93:1588, 1996.

295. Rakover C, Rossi L, Fontaine G, et al: Familial arrhythmogenic right ventricular disease. Am J Cardiol 58:377, 1986.

296. Nava A, Scognamiglio R, Thiene G, et al: A polymorphic form of familial arrhythmogenic right ventricular dysplasia. Am J Cardiol 59:1405, 1987.

297. Nava A, Thiene G, Canciani B, et al: Familial occurrence of right ventricular dysplasia: A study involving nine families. J Am Coll Cardiol 12:1222, 1988.

298. Canciani B, Nava A, Toso V, et al: A casual spontaneous mutation as possible cause of the familial form of arrhythmogenic right ventricular cardiomyopathy (arrhythmogenic right ventricular dysplasia). Clin Cardiol 15:217, 1992.

299. Dungan NT, Garson A Jr, Gillette PC: Arrhythmogenic right ventricular dysplasia: A cause of ventricular tachycardia in children with apparent normal hearts. Am Heart J 102:745, 1981.

300. Brembilla-Perrot B, Jacquemin L, Houplon P, et al: Increased atrial vulnerability in arrhythmogenic right ventricular disease. Am Heart J 135:748, 1998.

301. Liu SK, Fox PR, Tilley LP: Excessive moderator bands in the left ventricle of 21 cats. JAVMA 180:1215, 1982.

301a. Fox PR, Peterson ME, Broussard JD: Electrocardiographic and radiographic changes in cats with hyperthyroidism: Comparison of populations evaluated during 1992–1993 vs. 1979–1982. Am Anim Hosp Assoc 35:27, 1999.

302. Peterson ME, Taylor RS, Greco DS, et al: Acromegaly in 14 cats. J Vet Intern Med 4:192, 1990.

303. Morrison SA, Randolph J, Lothrop CD Jr: Hypersomatotropism and insulin-resistant diabetes mellitus in a cat. JAVMA 194:91, 1989.

304. Brummer DG, Moise NS: Infiltrative cardiomyopathy responsive to chemotherapy in a cat with lymphoma. JAVMA 195:1116, 1989.

305. Tilley LP, Bond B, Patnaik A, et al: Cardiovascular tumors in the cat. J Am Anim Hosp Assoc 17:1009, 1981.

306. Patnaik AK, Liu SK: Angiosarcomas in cats. J Small Anim Pract 18:191, 1977.

307. Mauldin GN, Matus RE, Patnaik AK, et al: Efficacy and toxicity of doxorubicin and cyclophosphamide used in the treatment of selected malignant tumors in cats. J Vet Intern Med 2:60, 1988.

308. O'Keefe DA, Sisson DD, Gelberg HB, et al: Systemic toxicity associated with doxorubicin administration in cats. J Vet Intern Med 7:309, 1993.

309. Liu S-K: Myocarditis and cardiomyopathy in the dog and cat. Heart Vessels 1(Suppl 1):122, 1985.

310. Liu S-K: Myocarditis and cardiomyopathy in the dog and cat. In Sekiguchi M, Olsen EGJ, Goodwin JF (eds): Myocarditis and Related Disorders. Tokyo, Springer-Verlag, 1985, p 122.

311. Dubey JP, Johnstone I: Fatal neonatal toxoplasmosis in cats. J Am Anim Hosp Assoc 18:461, 1982.

312. Yamaguchi RA, Pipers FS, Gamble DA: Echocardiographic evaluation of a cat with bacterial vegetative endocarditis. JAVMA 183:118, 1983.

313. Shousse CL, Meier H: Acute vegetative endocarditis in the dog and cat. JAVMA 129:278, 1956.

314. Harpster NK: Cardiovascular diseases of the domestic cat. Adv Vet Sci Comp Med 21:39, 1977.

315. van der Linde-Sipman JS, van den Ingh TSGAM, Koeman JP: Congenital heart abnormalities in the cat: A description of sixteen cases. Zentralbl Veterinärmed A 20:419, 1973.

316. Paasch LH: The comparative pathology of endocardial fibroelastosis in Burmese cats. PhD dissertation, George Washington University, 1979.

317. Paasch LH, Zook BC: The pathogenesis of endocardial fibroelastosis in Burmese cats. Lab Invest 42:197, 1980.

318. Zook BC, Chandra RS, Casey HW: The comparative pathology of endocardial fibroelastosis in Burmese cats. Virchows Arch [Pathol Anat] 390:211, 1981.

318a. Ni J, Bowles N, Kim Y, et al: Viral infection of the myocardium in endocardial fibroelastosis: Molecular evidence for the role of mumps virus as an etiologic agent. Circulation 96:3549, 1997.

319. Tilley LP, Liu SK: Persistent atrial standstill in the dog and cat (abstract). In: Scientific Proceedings of the American College of Veterinary Internal Medicine, 1983, p 43.

320. Carpenter JL, Hoffman EP, Ramanul FC, et al: Feline muscular dystrophy with dystrophin deficiency. Am J Pathol 135:909, 1989.

321. Haskins ME, Aguirre GD, Jezyk PF, Desnick RJ: Mucopolysaccharidosis in a domestic short-haired cat: A disease distinct from that seen in the Siamese cat. JAVMA 175:384, 1979.

322. Haskins ME, Aguirre GD, Jezyk PF, et al: The pathology of feline arylsulfatase B deficient mucopolysaccharidosis. Am J Pathol 101:657, 1980.

323. Liu SK, Tilley LP, Tashijian RJ: Lesions of the conduction system in the cat with cardiomyopathy. Recent Adv Card Struct Metab 10:681, 1975.

324. Collet P: Thrombose de l'aorte posterieur chez un chat. Bul Soc Sci Vet Lyon 33:136, 1930.

325. Liu SK, Hsu FS, Lee RCT: An Atlas of Cardiovascular Pathology. Taiwan, Republic of China, Pig Res Inst Taiwan, Wonder Enterprise Co, Ltd, and Shin Chan Color Printing Inc, 1989, p 311.

326. Waller BF: Anatomic basis of cardiac emboli: A morphologic review. In Daniel

WG, Kronzon I, Mügge A (eds): Cardiogenic Embolism. Baltimore, Williams & Wilkins, 1996, p 7.

327. Laste NJ, Harpster NK: A retrospective study of 100 cases of feline distal aortic thromboembolism: 1977–1993. J Am Anim Hosp Assoc 31:492, 1995.

328. Virchow R: Neuer Fall von Todlicher: Embolie der Lungenarterien. Arch Pathol Anat 10:225, 1856.

329. Roussell L, Biller J, Hajduczok Z, et al: Ischemic cerebrovascular complications and risk factors in idiopathic hypertrophic subaortic stenosis. Stroke 22:1143, 1991.

330. Fatkin D, Kelly R, Feneley MO: Relations between left atrial appendage blood flow velocity, spontaneous echocardiographic contrast and thromboembolic risk in vivo. J Am Coll Cardiol 23:961, 1994.

331. Fox PR: Feline thromboembolism associated with cardiomyopathy. In: Scientific Proceedings of the Fifth Annual Veterinary Medicine Forum, American College of Veterinary Internal Medicine, 1987, p 714.

332. Fox PR, Dodds WJ: Coagulopathies observed with spontaneous aortic thromboembolism in cardiomyopathic cats (abstract). In: Scientific Proceedings of the American College of Veterinary Internal Medicine, 1982, p 83

333. Weiser MG, Kociba GJ: Platelet concentration and platelet volume distribution in healthy cats. Am J Vet Res 45:518, 1984.

334. Helinski CA, Ross JN: Platelet aggregation in feline cardiomyopathy. J Vet Intern Med 1:24, 1987.

335. Jones MP, Alving BM: Evaluation of the hypercoagulable patient. Intern Med 18:37, 1997.

336. Schaub RG, Meyers KM, Sande RD: Serotonin as a factor in depression of collateral blood flow following experimental arterial thrombosis. J Lab Clin Med 90:645, 1977.

337. Golino P, Ashton JH, Buja LM, et al: Local platelet activation causes vasoconstriction of large epicardial canine coronary arteries in vivo: Thromboxane A$_2$ and serotonin are possible mediators. Circulation 79:154, 1989.

338. Grygleski RJ: Prostaglandins, platelets and atherosclerosis. CRC Crit Rev Biochem 7:291, 1980.

339. Griffith IR, Duncan ID: Ischaemic neuromyopathy in cats. Vet Rec 104:518, 1979.

340. Imhoff RK: Production of aortic occlusion resembling acute aortic embolism syndrome in cats. Nature (Lond) 192:979, 1961.

341. Flanders JA: Feline aortic thromboembolism. Compend Contin Ed 8:473, 1986.

342. Fox PR, Moïse NS, Price RA, et al: Analysis of continuous ECG (Holter) monitoring in normal cats and cardiomyopathic cats in congestive heart failure (abstract). J Vet Intern Med 12:199, 1998.

343. Kaplan AP, Castellino FJ, Collen D, et al: Molecular mechanisms of fibrinolysis in man. Thromb Haemost 39:263, 1978.

344. Killingsworth CR, Eyster GE, Adams T, et al: Streptokinase treatment of cats with experimentally induced aortic thrombosis. Am J Vet Res 47:1351, 1986.

345. Sherry S: Tissue plasminogen activator (t-PA). N Engl J Med 313:1014, 1985.

346. Pion PD, Kittleson MD: Therapy for feline aortic thromboembolism. In Kirk RW (ed): Current Veterinary Therapy X. Philadelphia, WB Saunders, 1989, p 295.

347. Rosenberg RD, Lam, L: Correlation between structure and function of heparin. Proc Natl Acad Sci U S A 76:1218, 1979.

348. Bell RW: Metabolism of vitamin K and prothrombin synthesis: Anticoagulants and the vitamin K–epoxide cycle. Fed Proc 37:2599, 1978.

349. Goldhaber SZ, Sors H: Treatment of venous thrombus and pulmonary embolism. In Fuster V, Verstraete M (eds): Thrombosis in Cardiovascular Disorders. Philadelphia, WB Saunders, 1992, p 465.

350. Baty CJ: Warfarin prophylaxis in feline aortic thromboembolism. In: Scientific Proceedings of the 11th Annual Veterinary Medicine Forum, 1993, p 519.

351. Roth GJ, Stanford N, Majerus PW: Acetylation of prostaglandin synthesis by aspirin. Proc Natl Acad Sci U S A 72:3073, 1975.

352. Burch JW, Stanford PW: Inactivation of platelet prostaglandin synthetase by oral aspirin. J Clin Invest 61:314, 1979.

353. Majerus PW: Arachidonate metabolism in vascular disorder. J Clin Invest 72:1521, 1983.

354. Preston FE, Whipps, Jackson CA, et al: Inhibition of prostacyclin and platelet thromboxane A$_2$ after low dose aspirin. N Engl J Med 304:76, 1981.

355. Hirsch J: Hypercoagulability. Semin Hematol 14:409, 1977.

356. Moncada S, Vane JR: Pharmacology and endogenous roles of prostaglandin endoperoxides, thromboxane A$_2$ and prostacyclin. Pharmacol Rev 30:293, 1978.

357. Schaub RG, Gates KA, Roberts RE: Effect of aspirin on collateral blood flow after experimental thrombosis of the feline aorta. Am J Vet Res 43:1647, 1982.

358. Allen DG, Johnstone IB, Crane S: Effects of aspirin and propranolol alone and in combination on hemostatic determinants in the healthy cat. Am J Vet Res 46:660, 1985.

359. Greene CE: Aspirin and feline platelet aggregation. JAVMA 188:1820, 1985.

360. Yeary RA, Swanson W: Aspirin dosages for the cat. JAVMA 163:1177, 1973.

CV

CHAPTER 118

PERICARDIAL DISORDERS

Matthew W. Miller and D. David Sisson

Diseases affecting the pericardium account for approximately 1 per cent of all animals with cardiovascular disease.[1] Although primary pericardial disease represents a small percentage of the total number of cardiac diseases in small animals, it is an important cause of right heart failure in the dog. Pericardial diseases of all types are uncommon in the cat.[2, 3] Several types of primary and secondary pericardial diseases occur, the most common of which are those resulting in the accumulation of pericardial effusion. Reported causes of pericardial disease in dogs[4–6] and cats[2, 3] are listed in Table 118–1.

ANATOMY

The pericardium envelopes the heart in a strong, flask-shaped sac with extensions that enclose the origins of the ascending aorta at the level of the aortic arch, the pulmonary artery at its bifurcation, the proximal pulmonary veins, and the vena cavae. The adventitia of the great arteries blends with fibrous tissues of the pericardium to form strong attachments. The pericardium is firmly attached to the diaphragm via the pericardiophrenic ligament. The pericardium is composed of two layers: a fibrous outer layer, and an inner serous membrane composed of a single layer of mesothelial cells. The inner serous layer is intimately attached to the epicardium to form the visceral pericardium, and this inner serous membrane reflects back on itself to line the outer fibrous layer to form the parietal pericardium.

"The pericardium is furnished with a liquid like to serum or urine lest the heart grow overheated by its perpetual movement" (Sir William Harvey, 1616).

The pericardial cavity is filled with a variable amount of pericardial fluid. This fluid is an ultrafiltrate of serum containing between 1.7 and 3.5 g/dL of protein and having a colloid osmotic pressure approximately 25 per cent that of serum. The volume of pericardial fluid present in normal

TABLE 118–1. PERICARDIAL DISEASES OF THE DOG AND CAT

Congenital disorders
  Pericardial defects
  Peritoneopericardial hernia
  Pericardial cyst (?)
Acquired disorders
  Pericardial effusion
    Transudate (hydropericardium)
      Congestive heart failure
      Hypoalbuminemia
      Peritoneopericardial hernia
    Exudate (pericarditis)
      Infection—bacterial, fungal
      Sterile—idiopathic, uremia, other infectious diseases (FIP), other
      (?)
    Hemorrhage (hemopericardium)
      Neoplasia—hemangiosarcoma, heart base tumor, mesothelioma,
        lymphosarcoma, other
      Trauma—iatrogenic, external
      Cardiac rupture, especially left atrium
      Idiopathic (pericarditis)
Constrictive pericarditis
  Idiopathic pericarditis
  Infection—bacterial (actinomycosis, nocardiosis, tuberculosis), fungal
    (coccidioidomycosis)
  Pericardial foreign body (metal)
  Neoplasia—heart base tumor, mesothelioma
Intrapericardiac masses (± effusion/fibrosis)
  Pericardial cyst
  Neoplasm
  Granuloma—actinomycosis, coccidioidomycosis
  Pericardial abscess

From Thomas WP: Pericardial disorders. *In* Ettinger SJ (ed): Textbook of Veterinary Internal Medicine, 3rd ed. Philadelphia, WB Saunders, 1989.

dogs ranges from 1 to 15 mL. The pericardial fluid contains phospholipids, which purportedly serve to lubricate the heart so that it can undergo motion without friction or damage to the epicardium.[7] The lymphatic drainage of the pericardium is similar to that of the myocardium, with most drainage via subendocardial lymphatics rather than from the parietal pericardium.

PERICARDIAL FUNCTION

Accepted functions of the pericardium include its ability to fix the heart anatomically and prevent excessive motion associated with changes in body position. Reducing friction between the heart and surrounding structures and preventing extension of infection or malignancy from contiguous organs are other functions commonly ascribed to the pericardium.[7] Because congenital absence of the pericardium is not associated with significant disturbances in cardiac function, the role of the pericardium in the regulation of the circulation is controversial. Studies have demonstrated that the pericardium may play a role in limiting acute cardiac dilatation and hemodynamic interaction between the left and right ventricles.[8–10]

It has been suggested that the pericardium plays an important role in limiting cardiac dilatation in acute mitral regurgitation (MR).[11] Although hemodynamic patterns in acute MR are similar to those observed in constrictive pericardial disease, evidence suggests that the role of the pericardium in the immediate hemodynamic response to acute, severe MR is minor.[12] The restraining effects of the pericardium have been observed early in the course of chronic overload caused by formation of an arteriovenous fistula in dogs. This restraining effect is no longer apparent following enlargement of the pericardium by stretch or hypertrophy late in the course of the volume overload.[13]

The pericardium contributes to the diastolic coupling between the two ventricles. The distention of one ventricle diminishes the distensibility of the other.[14, 15] When the pericardium is intact, right and left ventricular filling pressures are closely correlated, and the left ventricular lumen is smaller than in the absence of the pericardium. In the absence of the pericardium, cardiac distensibility is determined primarily by properties of the myocardium.[14] The effect of the pericardium on the interaction between the two ventricles is accentuated in experimental constrictive pericarditis.[16] This effect of the pericardium is present at normal filling pressures and becomes more important as right ventricular filling pressures increase. It has been suggested that the pericardium couples diastolic function of the ventricles primarily via its effects on right ventricular filling and distensibility.[17, 18]

The role of the pericardium in the pathogenesis of chronic heart failure has received increased attention.[19] Although chronic cardiac enlargement frequently results in pericardial enlargement and hypertrophy, it is possible that acute increases in venous return in patients with heart failure could increase the effects of the pericardium on both diastolic and systolic ventricular function. The effects of exercise in human patients with chronic heart failure showed that pericardial constraint became evident when stroke volume abruptly became invariant. In addition, a similar increment of elevation in right and left heart filling pressures occurred during increased venous return associated with exercise.[19] It appears that the pericardium can be an important determinant of the limits of systolic pump function and result in coupling of the right and left ventricular diastolic pressures in patients with chronic heart failure.

PATHOPHYSIOLOGY

PERICARDIAL EFFUSION

Pericarditis is often associated with the accumulation of an abnormal amount of pericardial fluid (pericardial effusion). The hemodynamic effects of pericardial effusion are primarily dependent on the rate and volume of fluid accumulation and the distensibility or compliance of the pericardium. If the effusion accumulates slowly, the pericardium will expand and hypertrophy to accommodate the fluid, intrapericardiac pressure will not increase significantly, and cardiac filling will not be compromised. In contrast, acute tamponade occurs when fluid accumulates rapidly in the pericardial space, compressing the ventricles, restricting ventricular filling, and reducing cardiac output.

Rapid accumulation of fluid within the pericardial sac increases pericardial pressure, and the slope of the pericardial pressure-volume curve increases as fluid is added. Although a significant volume of fluid may be required to raise pericardial pressure initially, when the steep portion of the curve is reached, an additional small accumulation of fluid may markedly increase intrapericardial pressure, significantly impeding ventricular filling. Because of their thin walls and low pressures, the right atrium and ventricle are much more vulnerable than the left to the effects of cardiac compression. The right ventricle is affected earlier and more severely than the left as tamponade begins to develop.

Acute tamponade is characterized by rapidly rising intracardiac and jugular venous pressures, falling cardiac output, and decreasing arterial pressures. In part, systemic venous pressure rises because of the diminution of right ventricular end-diastolic and stroke volumes and the resulting rise in end-diastolic and right atrial pressures. In addition, early in the course of tamponade, left ventricular output is maintained, shifting some of the blood out of the pulmonary circuit and into the systemic circuit. This further contributes to the rise in systemic venous pressures, a potentially beneficial compensatory response that would tend to overcome the rise in pericardial pressure.

During tamponade, blood flows from the vena cavae to the heart during atrial diastole (the x descent), but virtually no blood flow occurs during ventricular diastole (the y descent) (Fig. 118–1). This is because as the ventricles try to expand, rising pressure in the pericardial sac is transmitted to the atria, keeping atrial pressure elevated and impeding caval flow. The y descent of the atrial pressure wave is markedly diminished. Absence of the y descent is dependent on the ability of the fluid-filled pericardial sac to instantaneously transmit changing pressure; therefore, this sign is specific for cardiac tamponade rather than for pericardial constriction.

In tamponade, the right ventricle is usually the first to be compromised by cardiac compression. Once pericardial pressure exceeds left ventricular end-diastolic pressure, the pressures in both ventricles are determined primarily by intrapericardiac pressure. Diastolic pressures on both sides of the heart are not simply elevated; they become identical: the pulmonary wedge pressure (reflecting mean left atrial and left ventricular end-diastolic pressures), diastolic pulmonary arterial pressure, right ventricular end-diastolic pressure, and mean right atrial pressure (see Fig. 118–1).

Cardiac tamponade refers to the decompensated phase of cardiac compression resulting from an unchecked rise in the intrapericardiac fluid pressure. Cardiac tamponade develops when intrapericardiac pressure becomes elevated and compresses the heart. Tamponade is the mechanism by which low cardiac output and congestive heart failure (CHF) develop. Important features include increased (positive) intrapericardiac pressure, diastolic collapse of the right atrium (and right ventricle in some cases), reduction of ventricular filling, decreased cardiac output, and arterial hypotension. Compensatory measures are activated to maintain cardiac output; these include activation of the sympathetic nervous system and the renin-angiotensin-aldosterone system. Signs of right heart failure predominate, because this thinner chamber is more influenced by high intrapericardiac pressures. Myocardial systolic function is usually unaffected.

CONSTRICTIVE PERICARDIAL DISEASE

Pericardial constriction occurs when the visceral and parietal pericardial layers become fused or thickened, densely fibrotic, or inelastic, forming a rigid case around the heart. The pericardial space may become totally obliterated or may contain a small amount of fluid. Constrictive pericardial disease may develop asymmetrically so that one ventricle is more affected than the other, a situation that can be very confusing diagnostically.[20] In most cases, however, both ventricles are affected nearly equally.

Because early ventricular relaxation is usually normal in constrictive pericarditis, ventricular pressure decreases rapidly during early diastole. However, rapid ventricular filling occurs during a shortened interval that terminates as the limit of ventricular distensibility is reached. As filling continues, the ventricular pressure tracing displays an abrupt rise to an elevated diastolic plateau, commonly referred to clinically as the "square root sign" because of its appearance on the hemodynamic tracing (see Fig. 118–1). An audible "pericardial knock" may accompany early diastolic filling and is attributed to vibrations produced by the sudden deceleration of blood as it strikes the encased, nondistensible ventricular wall. In contrast to cardiac tamponade, in which the y descent of the atrial pressure tracing is obliterated, the y descent is prominent in constriction, reflecting appropriate pressure changes in the atrium and ventricle during early ventricular diastole. Because the atrioventricular valves are open, the atrial y descent also shows an abrupt termination, rising to a plateau as rapid ventricular filling terminates abruptly (see Fig. 118–1).

The pulmonary wedge pressure, pulmonary diastolic pressure, right ventricular end-diastolic pressure, and mean right atrial pressure all tend to be elevated and equal in constrictive pericarditis, because all the chambers of the heart are encased in the same rigid pericardial sac. Because the obliterated pericardial sac can no longer undergo pressure changes associated with respiration, the decrease in caval pressure normally associated with inspiration may be absent. In severe cases, there may be an actual increase in systemic venous pressure during inspiration (Kussmaul's sign).[21]

As constriction worsens, cardiac output declines, even though myocardial systolic function may be maintained. Fluid retention initiated by chronically reduced cardiac output further contributes to venous congestion, which is most commonly manifested as hepatomegaly and ascites accumulation. Peripheral edema is uncommon. As in chronic heart failure, chronic elevation in venous pressures commonly results in deleterious changes in abdominal viscera (e.g., hepatic dysfunction, malabsorption, protein-losing enteropathy, and splenic dysfunction).[22]

INTRAPERICARDIAC MASS LESIONS

The hemodynamic effects of intrapericardiac mass lesions that do not cause pericardial effusion are caused primarily by physical compression of cardiac structures by the mass. Signs of venous congestion may be detected if the mass lesion impinges on venous return. Compression of the outflow tract of one or both of the ventricles may cause signs of reduced cardiac output or syncope.

CONGENITAL DISEASES

There are several congenital diseases of the pericardium recognized in small animal species. While peritoneopericardial diaphragmatic hernia (PPDH) is the most common type of congenital abnormality encountered,[1] sporadic reports of partial pericardial defects[5, 8] and intrapericardiac cysts[4] have been published. Congenital complete absence of the pericardium is quite rare.[5]

PERICARDIAL DEFECTS

Congenital pericardial defects can be classified embryologically as those due to deficiency in the development of the pleuropericardium (which include partial defects and complete absence of the pericardium) and those due to deficiency in the development of the pericardioperitoneal communication. Evidence suggests that partial pericardial

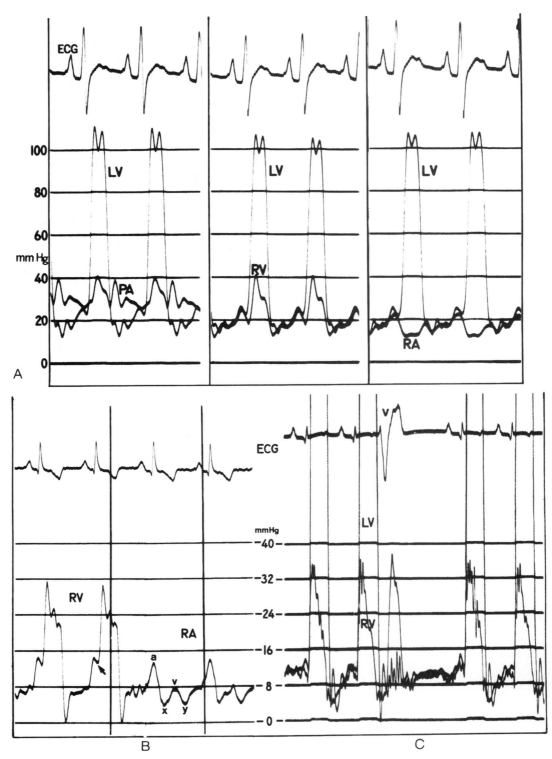

Figure 118–1. Hemodynamics of pericardial disease. *A*, Intracardiac pressures from a dog with pericardial effusion and cardiac tamponade. There is elevation (20 to 25 mmHg) and equilibration of end-diastolic pressures and superimposition of diastolic tracing in the left ventricle (LV), pulmonary artery (PA), right ventricle (RV), and right atrium (RA). Early diastolic (y) descent on the atrial and ventricular tracings is not prominent. *B*, Right ventricular (RV) and right atrial (RA) pressures from a dog with constrictive pericarditis. There is an early diastolic dip and mid-diastolic plateau on the ventricular tracing, the RV end-diastolic pressure is elevated to 14 mmHg *(arrow)*, and the RA, a wave, and x and y descents are prominent. *C*, Right (RV) and left (LV) ventricular pressures from a dog with constrictive pericarditis show mild elevation (12 mmHg) of end-diastolic pressures, a prominent early diastolic descent, and mid-diastolic plateau, seen best during the pause following a premature ventricular beat (V). (From Thomas WP, et al: Constrictive pericardial disease in the dog. JAVMA 184:546, 1984.)

defects and complete absence of the pericardium result from premature atrophy of the left duct of Cuvier, resulting in a compromised vascular circulation to the pleuropericardial membrane that would ultimately become the left pericardium. In the case of PPDH, it is probable that the embryologic abnormality is in the septum transversum because of the ventral position of the hernia and the position of the septum transversum as the shared diaphragmatic and pericardial anlage.

Most partial pericardial defects are clinically silent. Clinical signs may occur if a portion of the heart herniates through the defect and becomes incarcerated. Constriction of a portion of the heart can cause partial stasis within the herniated portion and predispose to embolic disease. Radiographically, herniated portions of the heart may be difficult to differentiate from specific cardiac chamber enlargements or pulmonary mass lesions (Fig. 118–2).

PPDH is commonly reported in dogs and cats.[23–25] Several studies have reported the occurrence of other abnormalities of midline closure (cranial abdominal hernia, sternal deformities) and congenital cardiac defects (e.g., ventricular septal defect) associated with PPDH.[24, 25] PPDHs have been reported in littermates, but there is no reported evidence that the lesion is hereditary. It has been suggested that Weimaraners are predisposed to PPDH.[6]

A large portion (48 per cent) of dogs and cats with PPDH are diagnosed prior to 1 year of age, and another 36 per cent are diagnosed between 1 and 4 years of age.[6] Clinical signs are most commonly gastrointestinal (anorexia, vomiting, discomfort following a meal) or respiratory (cough, dyspnea). Signs of cardiac compromise (abdominal distention and acute collapse) may occur, but are uncommon.

Physical examination may reveal an apical impulse that is displaced or decreased in intensity. Cardiac murmurs may be detected if concurrent cardiac malformations are present. If the hernia is large and a significant amount of abdominal viscera has herniated, the abdomen may seem empty on palpation. Signs of CHF (ascites, jugular venous distention) may be present but are uncommon. Concurrent defects (sternal malformations, cranial abdominal hernias) may be detected.

Thoracic radiographs are extremely helpful in establishing a definitive diagnosis of PPDH. Radiographic abnormalities

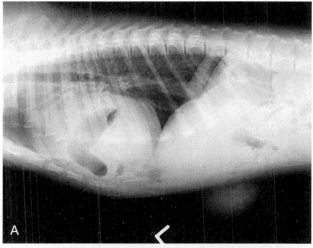
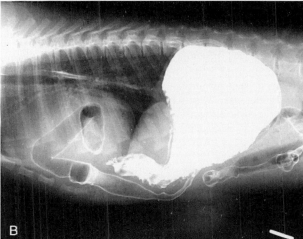

Figure 118–3. A, Lateral thoracic radiograph obtained from a dog with a peritoneopericardial diaphragmatic hernia. Notice the variability in radiographic densities detected within the cardiac silhouette and the cranial abdominal hernia. B, Lateral thoracic radiograph obtained following oral administration of barium sulfate. Notice that the barium-filled bowel loops that cross the diaphragm are located within the pericardial sac.

may include overlap of the caudal cardiac silhouette and cranial diaphragm, variable radiographic densities within the cardiac silhouette, gas-filled bowel loops crossing the diaphragm, and sternal malformations (Fig. 118–3). Oral administration of barium may help outline bowel loops present within the pericardial sac (see Fig. 118–3). Ultrasonography can readily identify the presence of abdominal viscera within the pericardial sac and help establish a definitive diagnosis.[23] Abnormalities on the electrocardiogram may include reductions in QRS amplitude from the presence of viscera within the pericardial sac or fluid accumulation. Axis shifts may be either due to cardiac displacement or associated with concurrent cardiac malformations.

Surgical correction of the hernia with replacement of viable herniated viscera is the recommended therapy. The severity of concurrent congenital malformations should be considered before surgical intervention. In uncomplicated cases (no concurrent malformations), the prognosis following surgical repair is excellent.

PERICARDIAL CYSTS

Pericardial cysts are very uncommon. The exact embryologic cause for the formation of these cysts is unknown. The

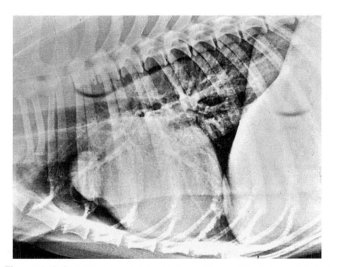

Figure 118–2. Lateral radiograph of a dog with a partial pericardial defect. Notice the well-circumscribed density located just cranial to the cardiac silhouette. Necropsy documented that the right auricle was herniated through the defect. This dog showed no signs associated with this defect.

clinical and echocardiographic features of six young dogs with intrapericardiac cysts have been reported.[4] Some of the cysts developed as a result of congenital herniation and entrapment of the omentum or a portion of the falciform ligament within the pericardial sac. The dogs were all 3 years of age or younger (range 6 months to 3 years) and were presented for signs associated with right heart failure (ascites). Definitive diagnosis was made with pneumopericardiography in two dogs and with echocardiography in the remaining dogs. Surgical removal of the cyst and subtotal pericardiectomy were curative in all five dogs in which they were attempted.[4]

ACQUIRED PERICARDIAL DISEASES

PERICARDIAL EFFUSION

Diseases causing pericardial effusion are the most common causes of clinically significant pericardial disease in the dog.[1] Pericardial effusions are commonly categorized by the characteristics of the fluid that accumulates. Transudation into the pericardial space usually occurs secondary to CHF, PPDH, cyst, hypoalbuminemia, infection, toxemia, or other causes of increased vascular permeability. Exudation caused by infective or noninfective pericarditis can develop. Pericarditis has been associated with feline cardiomyopathy and feline infectious peritonitis (FIP) virus infection.[2, 3] Intrapericardial hemorrhage with or without pericardial reaction is the most common cause of pericardial effusion in dogs. Neoplasia of the heart, heart base, or pericardium is the most common cause of hemorrhagic effusion in dogs.[1] Clinically important tumor types in dogs include hemangiosarcoma of the right atrium (especially common in German shepherds and golden retrievers).[26, 27] This tumor may be multicentric, and it is common to find splenic or hepatic involvement at the time the cardiac lesion is first identified.[26, 27] Aortic body tumors (chemodectoma, nonchromaffin paraganglioma) with invasion of the heart base are most commonly seen in aged brachycephalic breed dogs, ectopic (heart base) thyroid carcinoma, mesothelioma of the pericardium, and metastatic carcinoma to the heart. Another frequent situation is idiopathic pericardial hemorrhage in dogs, with golden retrievers being overrepresented.[28–30] A well-recognized but uncommon cause of intrapericardial hemorrhage in small breed dogs is left atrial tear secondary to severe chronic endocardiosis of the mitral valve.

Diagnosis

Signalment and History

Special breed predilections have been noted previously. Most frequently, animals with pericardial disease are presented with vague signs. Clients frequently describe lethargy, exercise intolerance, and anorexia. Occasionally, animals are presented for signs of compromise of right heart function: abdominal distention, respiratory difficulty, or syncope.

Physical Examination

Signs of increased right heart pressures are consistently present in animals with clinically significant pericardial disease. Jugular venous distention or a positive hepatojugular reflux is invariably present but commonly overlooked. Measurement of central venous pressure documents systemic venous hypertension and frequently exceeds 10 to 12 mmHg (normal = < 6 mmHg) if tamponade is present. Heart sound intensity is frequently diminished. Lung sounds may be diminished if pleural effusion is present. Other auscultatory abnormalities (gallop rhythms, cardiac murmurs, arrhythmias) are uncommon. Dogs with left atrial tears secondary to chronic degenerative valvular disease have systolic murmurs that may be decreased in intensity when compared with previous examinations. Hepatomegaly and free abdominal fluid are common findings. If the disease is chronic, significant weight loss may be observed.

Systemic arterial hypotension is common when tamponade has developed, and alterations in pulse quality (i.e., pulsus paradoxus) may be detected. Pulsus paradoxus is a valuable clinical sign that may be seen in cardiac tamponade. It is defined as an inspiratory fall in systemic arterial pressure exceeding 10 mmHg (Fig. 118–4). In tamponade, when the systemic veins are distended and ventricular enlargement is limited by pericardial effusion, an inspiratory increase in venous return to the right side of the heart further raises intrapericardial pressure, reducing left ventricular distensibility. Moreover, because the increased venous return cannot be accommodated by expansion of the right ventricular freewall, the interventricular septum is displaced toward the left ventricle, causing a significant reduction in left ventricular filling, stroke volume, and systemic cardiac output.

Radiography

Thoracic radiography usually demonstrates abnormalities when there is significant accumulation of pericardial fluid. The cardiac silhouette loses its angles and waists and becomes globe shaped (Fig. 118–5). Most cases are not classic and require integration with the other data. Pulmonary vascularity is often reduced as a result of low cardiac output, in contrast to CHF from cardiomyopathy or valvular disease, in which the pulmonary vascularity may be increased (especially the pulmonary veins). If CHF has developed, distention of the caudal vena cava, hepatomegaly, and pleural effusion are usually evident. Less commonly, distention of the pulmonary veins and increased pulmonary interstitial densities (edema) may be detected.[31] Heart base tumors may deviate the trachea and produce a mass effect.

Fluoroscopy may demonstrate reduced cardiac motion. Pneumopericardiography is useful for identifying intrapericardial mass lesions (Fig. 118–6).[32] Angiography usually shows filling defects or tumor vascularity ("blush") (see Fig. 118–6) if neoplasia is the cause of the effusion; furthermore, angiography shows increased endocardial-pericardial distance typical of pericardial effusion. Although these modalities have been shown to be very reliable when properly used,[32, 33] in most situations, echocardiography has supplanted most indications for their use.[29, 34, 35]

Laboratory Evaluation

The complete blood count may indicate inflammation or infection; increased numbers of circulating nucleated red blood cells are suggestive of hemangiosarcoma of the heart and spleen. Cardiac enzymes may be elevated owing to ischemia or myocardial invasion; other abnormalities may be associated with the primary disease or with CHF. Analysis of pleural or peritoneal effusions generally indicates that they are obstructive (transudate or modified transudate). Bacterial cultures of the effusion, serum fungal titer (coccidioidomycosis), or enzyme-linked immunosorbent assay

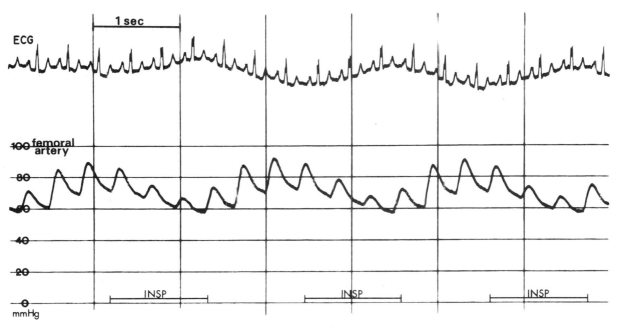

Figure 118–4. Pulsus paradoxus in a dog with cardiac tamponade. This direct femoral artery pressure tracing shows an exaggerated fall in arterial systolic and mean pressures (15 to 20 mmHg) and a markedly decreased pulse pressure during inspiration.

(ELISA) tests for feline leukemiavirus or FIP (cats) may be positive when pericarditis is related to these infections. (The pH value appears to be an effective discriminator between benign and neoplastic causes of pericardial effusion. High correlation exists, and pH values of fresh sampled effusates are often 7.5 or greater when neoplasia exists—The Editors.)[58]

Electrocardiography

Although there are no pathognomonic electrocardiographic findings for pericardial disease, several abnormalities are commonly seen.[36] Electrical alternans (Fig. 118–7) is a beat-to-beat voltage variation of the QRS or ST-T complexes. It may be recorded in as many as 50 per cent of patients with pericardial effusion. It is caused by swinging of the heart within large pericardial effusions rather than alterations in conduction within the heart. Even in the presence of large pericardial effusions, electrical alternans is not always present. A recent study using a nonlinear heart model showed that electrical alternans is rate-dependent and most likely to occur at heart rates between 90 and 144 beats per minute.[37]

Elevation of the ST segment is commonly recorded in patients with pericardial disease, representing an epicardial injury.[36] Reductions in QRS voltage (R < 1 mV in lead II) are commonly recorded in dogs with pericardial effusion.

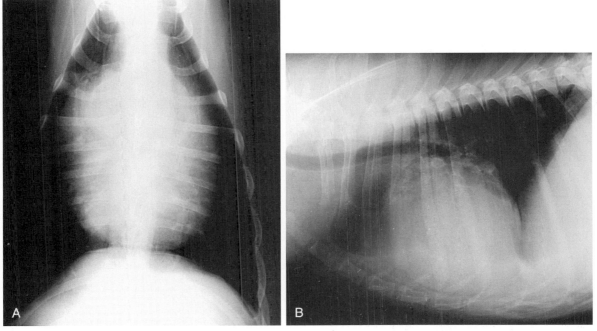

Figure 118–5. Radiographic features of pericardial effusion in the dog. Dorsoventral *(A)* and lateral *(B)* radiographs show a moderately enlarged, round cardiac silhouette in a dog with a moderate pericardial effusion.

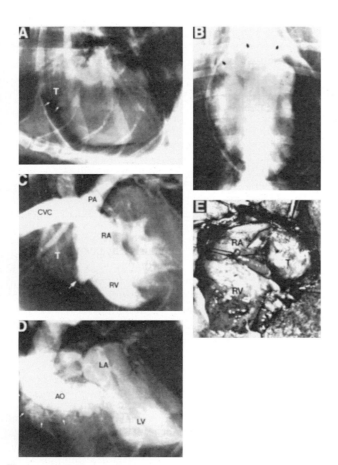

Figure 118–6. Heart base tumor (chemodectoma) in an 11-year-old Samoyed. *A,* Right lateral pneumopericardiogram shows a tumor mass (T) preventing gas from outlining the cranial heart base region above the right auricle *(arrows). B,* Dorsoventral pneumopericardiogram also shows failure of gas to reach the cranial heart base *(arrows). C,* Nonselective angiogram shows a nonopacified soft tissue mass (T) cranial to the right atrium (RA) and right auricle *(arrow).* CVC = cranial vena cava; RV = right ventricle; PA = pulmonary artery. *D,* Later in the series, during left heart opacification, the circular tumor mass *(arrows)* causes a vascular blush adjacent to the ascending aorta (AO). LA = left atrium; LV = left ventricle. *E,* At surgery, the tumor (T) was adherent to the ascending aorta medial to the right auricle (retracted by suture). (From Thomas WP, et al: Diagnostic pneumopericardiography in dogs with spontaneous pericardial effusion. Vet Radiol 25:2, 1984.)

Low electrocardiographic QRS voltage is considered a weak predictor of the presence of pericardial effusion.[38] Other causes of reduced complex size include hypovolemia, hypothyroidism, pleural effusion, obesity, and intrathoracic mass lesions.[36] In the authors' experience, arrhythmias other than sinus tachycardia are uncommon in primary pericardial disease.[39, 40] Others have suggested that up to 40 per cent of dogs with pericardial disease have ventricular or supraventricular arrhythmias.[41]

Echocardiography

Echocardiography is the most sensitive and specific noninvasive method of detecting pericardial effusion currently available. The hemodynamic consequences of pericardial effusion depend not only on the amount of pericardial effusion present but also on the rapidity with which the effusion has accumulated. A small or moderate amount of fluid accumulating rapidly (left atrial rupture) may produce significant hemodynamic compromise, whereas a large amount of effusion accumulating over months may have little hemody-

namic effect. These principles should be remembered when assessing the significance of an echocardiographically detected pericardial effusion. Echocardiography can detect as little as 15 mL of intrapericardial fluid. An anechoic space between the epicardium and pericardium is the classic echocardiographic finding in pericardial effusion. Cardiac motion is commonly abnormal, often with dramatic side-to-side movement (Fig. 118–8). Overall cardiac chamber size is usually diminished owing to impaired cardiac filling.[34] Intrapericardiac or cardiac mass lesions may be visualized (Fig. 118–9 and 118–10). If it does not compromise patient care, echocardiography should be performed before pericardiocentesis, as the pericardial fluid greatly enhances the ability to visualize heart base masses.[35, 42]

There are echocardiographic findings (diastolic right atrial and right ventricular collapse) that strongly suggest the presence of cardiac tamponade.[34] An experimental study has challenged the specificity of these findings in the presence of large pleural effusions. In a canine study, it was shown that large-volume pleural effusion can result in right atrial and ventricular collapse similar to that seen with pericardial effusion and cardiac tamponade.[43] If right ventricular filling pressures are elevated before the development of pericardial effusion, pericardial pressure can be markedly increased, with significant hemodynamic effects on right heart function, but diastolic cardiac collapse may not be seen.[44] Conversely, in the presence of hypovolemia, significant collapse of the right atrium and right ventricle may occur with only minor elevations in intrapericardial pressure.[44]

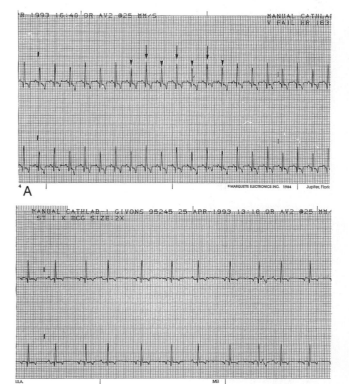

Figure 118–7. Electrocardiographic features of pericardial effusion in the dog. *A,* Before pericardiocentesis, a decrease in QRS voltages (<1.0 mV) is present in lead I. Electrical alternans of the QRS complexes can be seen *(arrows vs. arrowheads).* Paper speed = 25 mm/sec; 1 cm = 0.5 mV. *B,* Following pericardiocentesis, the electrical alternans is no longer evident, the heart rate has decreased, and the QRS size has increased. Paper speed = 25 mm/sec; 1 cm = 1.0 mV.

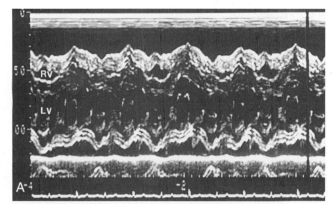

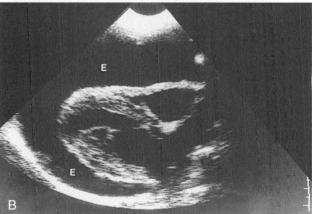

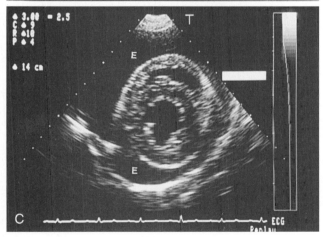

Figure 118–8. Echocardiographic features of pericardial effusion in the dog. *A,* M-mode echocardiogram recorded in a dog with a large pericardial effusion. The effusion is recognized as an echo-free space between the chest wall and right ventricle (RV) proximally and between the pericardium and the left ventricle (LV) distally. The left ventricular chamber dimension is decreased. *B,* Long-axis and *C,* short-axis two-dimensional echocardiograms from dogs with moderate idiopathic pericardial effusion. The anechoic effusion (E) surrounds the heart within the pericardium.

Magnetic Resonance Imaging and Computed Tomography

Little has been reported regarding the clinical use of either magnetic resonance imaging (MRI) or computed tomography (CT) in the evaluation of veterinary patients with pericardial disease.[6] Motion artifact, which has posed a significant problem in the past, has largely been eliminated with the use of physiologic gating, and the use of CT and MRI will most likely increase in the future.[45, 46] MRI can readily identify normal pericardium and thickening of the pericardium asso-

ciated with constrictive pericardial disease.[47] The ability to differentiate among intrapericardial fat, pericardial cysts, and intrapericardiac tumors with MRI has been documented.[48]

Therapy and Prognosis

Pericardiocentesis

The first use of therapeutic pericardiocentesis is commonly credited to Romero, who performed it in 1819. There is, however, a reference to pericardiocentesis in *Parzival*, a medieval German heroic poem written around 1200 by Wolfram von Eschenbach. In this poem, Lord Gawain comes upon a knight who has apparently been mortally wounded during a jousting match. Lord Gawain says to the knight's lady, "I could keep this knight from dying and I feel sure I could save him if I had a reed. You would soon see and hear him in health, because he is not mortally wounded. The blood is only pressing on his heart." The poem goes on to describe the procedure, as well as the fallen knight's dramatic recovery. It is hypothesized that the obsession of medieval court society with the sport of jousting probably made traumatic hemopericardium with cardiac tamponade a common ailment.

Pericardiocentesis is the treatment of choice for initial stabilization of dogs and cats with pericardial effusion and cardiac tamponade (Fig. 118–11).[49, 50] When performed properly, pericardiocentesis is associated with minimal complications. Before performing pericardiocentesis, it is necessary to shave and surgically prepare a large area of the right hemithorax (sternum to mid-thorax, third to eighth rib). Local anesthesia is usually adequate; however, mild sedation is sometimes necessary. It is important to ensure that the pleura has been infiltrated, as pleural penetration seems to cause significant discomfort. The animal is placed in sternal or lateral recumbency, depending on demeanor. Occasionally, pericardiocentesis can be accomplished in the standing animal, but adequate restraint is essential to prevent cardiac puncture or pulmonary laceration. Electrocardiographic monitoring during the procedure is helpful, because epicardial contact often causes ventricular arrhythmias (see Fig. 118–11).

The puncture site is usually determined based on the location of the heart on thoracic radiographs. This is most commonly between the fourth and sixth rib spaces at the costochondral junction. Ultrasound guidance is infrequently necessary unless the volume of effusion is very small or the effusion is compartmentalized.[51] The size of the needle or catheter used is dependent on the size of the animal. In cats, a 19- to 21-gauge butterfly catheter may be adequate, whereas in large dogs, a 16-gauge over-the-needle catheter (usually with additional side holes) may be needed. The needle or catheter should be attached to a three-way stopcock, extension tubing, and syringe to allow constant negative pressure to be applied during insertion and drainage. Care should be taken to avoid the large vessels that run along the caudal border of the ribs. Once the catheter has been inserted through the skin, negative pressure should be applied. If pleural effusion is present, it will be obtained immediately upon entering the thoracic cavity. It is most commonly a clear to pale yellow color. As the catheter is advanced and contacts the pericardium, a scratching sensation will be noticed. Minimal advancement will result in penetration of the pericardium.

Most pericardial effusions are hemorrhagic and have a "port wine" appearance. Once effusion of this character is

CV

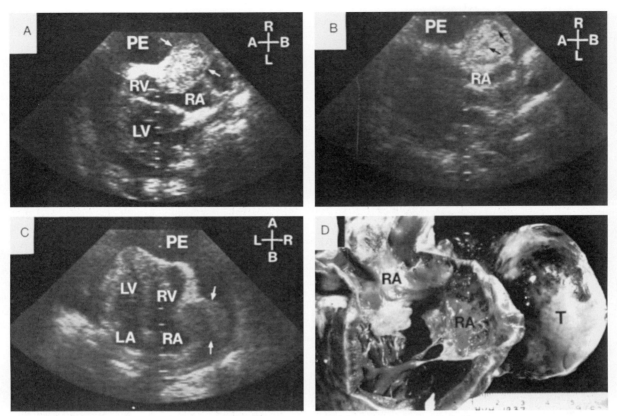

Figure 118–9. Right atrial hemangiosarcoma and pericardial effusion in a dog. *A,* Right intercostal long-axis view shows ovoid tumor mass *(arrows)* arising from right atrial wall. *B,* Similar view shows small hypoechoic areas within the tumor *(arrows). C,* Left intercostal four-chamber view shows the tumor *(arrows)* indenting the right heart near the atrioventricular junction. *D,* Necropsy specimen one month later shows the tumor (T) protruding from the epicardial surface of the right atrium. A = apex; B = base; R = right; L = left; PE = pericardial effusion; RV = right ventricle; RA = right atrium; LV = left ventricle; LA left atrium. (From Thomas WP, et al.: Detection of cardiac masses in dogs by two-dimensional echocardiography. Vet Radiol 25:65, 1984.)

obtained, the catheter should be advanced over the needle, and the needle removed. The remainder of the drainage should be performed using the catheter. Advancing the needle too far will result in contact with the epicardium. This is often felt as a tapping or more intense scratching sensation and commonly results in ventricular arrhythmias (see Fig. 118–11). These arrhythmias are usually self-limited following retraction of the needle or catheter.

Pericardial effusion can be differentiated from peripheral blood in that it rarely clots unless it is from very recent hemorrhage. The packed cell volume (PCV) is typically significantly lower than that of peripheral blood.[28–30] Every attempt should be made to drain the pericardial space as completely as possible. Drainage of the pericardium is often associated with an increase in the complex size on the electrocardiogram, a reduction in heart rate, and an improvement in arterial pulse quality. Potential complications include cardiac puncture (with resultant hemorrhage or arrhythmias), coronary artery laceration, lung puncture or laceration, and dissemination of infection or neoplasia throughout the thoracic cavity. Diagnostic evaluations of fluid obtained should include PCV and cytologic evaluation. Bacterial culture and sensitivity should be performed if indicated by cytologic evaluation. Caution should be exercised when evaluating the cellular component of pericardial effusion.[52] Clinically important neoplasia of the heart and pericardium (hemangiosarcoma, chemodectoma) commonly does not exfoliate, resulting in frequent false-negative evaluations. Reactive mesothelial cells within the pericardial sac are commonly overinterpreted as being neoplastic, causing false-positive results.

The long-term prognosis for dogs with hemorrhagic effusion is dependent on the underlying etiology. With idiopathic hemorrhagic pericardial effusion, the first pericardiocentesis may be curative. In most cases, repeat centesis is necessary to control clinical signs. Fluid may reaccumulate rapidly (within several days) or may not recur for months to years. In animals requiring more than two centeses, the authors recommend subtotal pericardiectomy. There are no controlled studies to confirm the efficacy of anti-inflammatory therapy for pericardial effusions. Subtotal pericardiectomy is usually curative in dogs with idiopathic pericardial effusion.

Pericardiectomy

If cardiac or pericardial neoplasia is the cause of the pericardial effusion, the recommended therapy is subtotal pericardiectomy. The prognosis is again dependent on the nature of the underlying etiology. Aortic body tumors are commonly associated with slow growth and are late to metastasize. Subtotal pericardiectomy may afford palliation for up to three years.[5] Hemangiosarcoma of the right atrium is associated with a poor long-term prognosis. Most mass lesions involving the right atrium or right ventricle are not amenable to surgical removal. The tumor has commonly spread to the lungs at the time of diagnosis, and these animals may have neoplastic lesions in the spleen or liver

CV

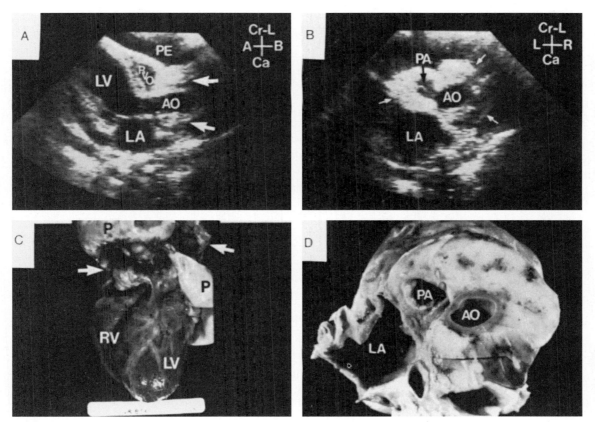

Figure 118–10. Heart base tumor (chemodectoma) and pericardial effusion in a dog. *A*, Left intercostal long-axis view shows a soft tissue mass on both sides of the ascending aorta *(arrows)*. *B*, Left intercostal short-axis view shows tumor *(white arrows)* surrounding the aorta and pulmonary artery. *C* and *D*, Necropsy specimen shows intra- and extrapericardial portions of the tumor *(arrows)* and infiltration around both great vessels as seen in *B*. (From Thomas WP, et al.: Detection of cardiac masses in dogs by two-dimensional echocardiography. Vet Radiol 25:65, 1984.)

as well. In these animals, subtotal pericardiectomy should be considered palliative.

Reports have suggested that percutaneous pericardial balloon dilatation may be a reasonable alternative to subtotal pericardiectomy in both neoplastic and benign effusions.[53, 54] Following pericardiocentesis, a balloon catheter is placed into the pericardial sac, and a window is formed with the balloon catheter. This allows the pericardial fluid to drain into the pleural space to be reabsorbed. This may provide significant palliation for animals with pericardial effusion and the resultant cardiac tamponade, without necessitating a thoracotomy. This therapy warrants further evaluation in canine patients.

CONSTRICTIVE PERICARDIAL DISEASE

History and Signalment

Medium to large breed dogs are most commonly affected with constrictive pericardial disease. In the largest series of

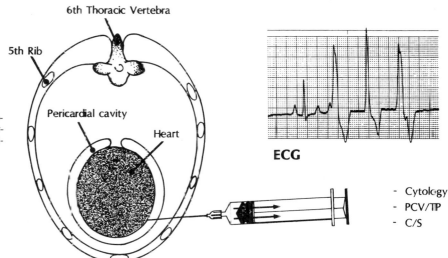

Figure 118–11. Graphic representation of the procedure of pericardiocentesis. Notice the typical morphology of the ventricular arrhythmia when the epicardium of the right ventricle is contacted.

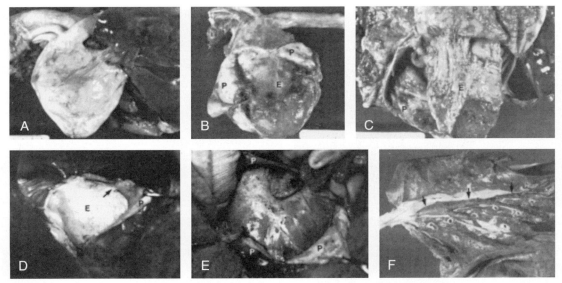

Figure 118–12. Pathology of constrictive pericardial disease in the dog. *A* and *B*, Heart showing thickened opaque pericardium surrounding the heart. The parietal pericardium (P) is thickened, there is epicardial fibrosis (E) over the lateral left ventricle, and epicardial adhesions are present. *C*, Actinomycotic pericarditis. A layer of fibrin coats the epicardium (E) and reflected pericardium (P). The dark area at the apex is an area of pericardial adhesion. *D*, Heart viewed during surgery. The parietal pericardium (P) has been partially resected, revealing marked epicardial fibrosis (E) and an area of pericardial adhesion *(arrow)*. *E*, Similar surgical view in another dog shows thickening of the reflected parietal pericardium (P), but minimal epicardial involvement and no adhesions. *F*, Left caudal lung lobe from a dog that died several days after pericardiectomy. A large thrombus is present in the lobar pulmonary artery and its branches *(arrows)*. (From Thomas WP, et al: Constrictive pericardial disease in the dog. JAVMA 184:546, 1984.)

cases reported, the average age was 6.6 years. The most common owner observation was abdominal enlargement. Less frequently, owners reported dyspnea or tachypnea, weakness or syncope, and weight loss. The duration of illness is variable, from weeks to months. Occasionally, there is a medical history that includes idiopathic pericardial effusion.

Diagnosis

The most common physical examination findings in dogs with constrictive pericardial disease are ascites and jugular venous distention. The femoral artery pulses may be diminished, and the heart sound intensity may be decreased as well. Systolic murmurs may occasionally be detected. A prominent pericardial knock (frequently described in human patients) is uncommonly detected in dogs.

Electrocardiographic abnormalities that may be detected include prolongation of the P wave, reductions in QRS voltage amplitude, and sinus tachycardia. In one dog reported with a coccidioidomycosis granuloma, a right ventricular hypertrophy pattern was described. Right ventricular hypertrophy patterns have also been described in human patients with constrictive pericardial disease. Sinus rhythm or sinus tachycardia is the most common rhythm detected.

Pleural effusion may be evident on thoracic radiographs. The cardiac silhouette may be rounded but is typically not as dramatically enlarged as in pericardial effusion. Dilatation of the caudal vena cava is common. Fluoroscopic examination may reveal diminished motion of the cardiac silhouette.

Central venous pressure is elevated in dogs with evidence of right heart failure. Classically, high mean atrial and ventricular diastolic pressures are detected. Simultaneous recording of atrial and ventricular pressures commonly shows equilibration of diastolic pressures. The classic finding of a prominent wide descent on atrial tracing and a prominent early diastolic dip and midsystolic plateau is infrequently

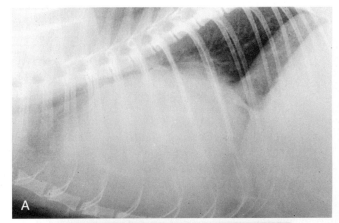

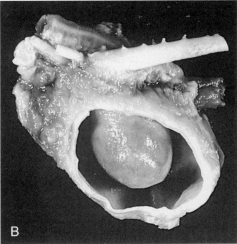

Figure 118–13. *A*, Lateral radiograph showing massive enlargement of the cardiac silhouette secondary to pericardial effusion associated with feline pericardial disease (FIP). *B*, Necropsy specimen demonstrating the pericardial dilatation and thickening secondary to FIP.

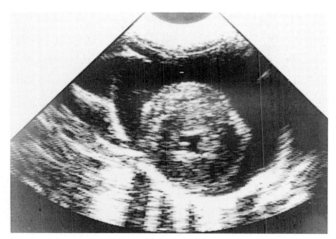

Figure 118–14. Right parasternal short-axis view obtained from a cat with hypertrophic cardiomyopathy and pericardial effusion. Notice the dramatic concentric hypertrophy of the left ventricle and the large anechoic space surrounding the heart.

detected. This again may reflect the fact that many dogs with constrictive pericardial disease have a small amount of fluid accumulation within the pericardial space and minimal epicardial involvement (constrictive-effusive physiology).

There are echocardiographic findings suggestive of constrictive pericardial disease. Differentiation between constrictive pericardial disease and restrictive myopathy may be quite difficult, however. Flattening of the left ventricular endocardium during diastole and abnormal diastole (early notch) and systolic septal motion are some of the more consistent findings in patients with constrictive pericarditis.[55] Doppler echocardiography has been shown to be helpful in the definitive diagnosis of constrictive pericarditis in human patients. Pulse Doppler echocardiographic evaluation of the hepatic vein and transesophageal Doppler echocardiographic evaluation of pulmonary venous flow have been helpful in

making a definitive diagnosis of constrictive pericarditis.[56, 57] The use of these diagnostic modalities in the evaluation of constrictive pericardial disease has not been reported.

Therapy and Prognosis

The therapy of choice for constrictive pericarditis is surgical removal of the pericardium. Complications associated with surgery include development of arrhythmias (most notably atrial fibrillation) and/or ventricular tachycardia. The success of surgical therapy is dependent on the severity of the underlying disease. If the visceral pericardium and epicardium are significantly involved (Fig. 118–12), the surgical outcome is less favorable. Although removal of the parietal pericardium is associated with significant improvement if epicardial involvement is severe, epicardial stripping may be necessary. A high degree of morbidity and mortality is associated with this challenging procedure. Reported complications following surgery in canine patients have included massive pulmonary embolic disease in the immediate postoperative period.[39] The cause of this complication is unknown. Chronic right heart failure can cause splenic dysfunction (functional hyposplenism) and protein-losing enteropathy. Hyposplenism can result in increased numbers of circulating activated platelets, and protein-losing enteropathy may exacerbate the splenic dysfunction and cause reductions in circulating antithrombin III levels.[22] Both conditions promote a hypercoaguable state and may help explain this complication.

FELINE PERICARDIAL DISEASE

Pericardial diseases appear to be quite uncommon in cats.[2, 3] Reports addressing the topic suggest that the most common single cause of pericardial disease in the cat is FIP.[2, 3] FIP infection can cause massive accumulations of intrapericardial fluid and resultant cardiac compromise (Fig. 118–13). Peri-

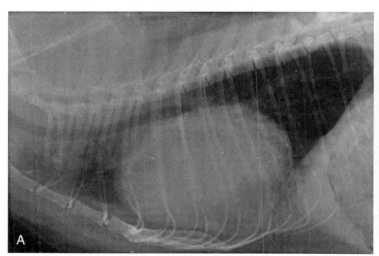

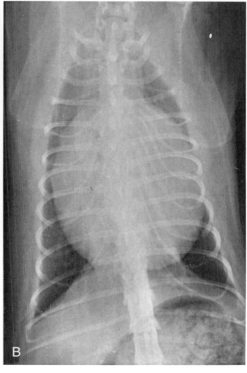

Figure 118–15. *A,* Lateral radiograph of a cat with a PPDH. Notice the variable radiographic densities within the cardiac silhouette, the contact between the cardiac silhouette and the diaphragm, and the sternal deformity. *B,* Ventrodorsal view from the same cat showing massive enlargement of the cardiac silhouette.

cardial effusion is common secondary to cardiomyopathy. Echocardiography can readily detect pericardial effusion and determine the nature of concurrent myocardial disease (Fig. 118–14). PPDHs may go undiagnosed for years in cats. Sternal abnormalities are commonly observed along with the PPDH (Fig. 118–15). Frequently, only falciform fat and liver are present within the pericardial sac, making barium contrast studies less informative in cats than they are in dogs.

REFERENCES

1. Buchanan JW: Causes and prevalence of cardiovascular disease. *In* Kirk RW, Bonagura JD (eds): Kirk's Current Veterinary Therapy XI: Small Animal Practice. Philadelphia, WB Saunders, 1992, pp 647–655.
2. Rush JE, Keene BW, Fox PR: Pericardial disease in the cat: A retrospective evaluation of 66 cases. J Am Anim Hosp Assoc 26:39, 1990.
3. Harpster NK: The cardiovascular system. *In* Holzworth J (ed): Diseases of the Cat. Medicine and Surgery. Philadelphia, WB Saunders, 1987, pp 820–887.
4. Sisson D, Thomas WP, Reed J, et al: Intrapericardial cysts in the dog. J Vet Intern Med 7:364, 1993.
5. Thomas WP: Pericardial disorders. *In* Ettinger SJ (ed): Textbook of Veterinary Internal Medicine, 3rd ed. Philadelphia, WB Saunders, 1989, pp 1132–1150.
6. Reed HRL: Pericardial diseases. *In* Fox PR (ed): Canine and Feline Cardiology. New York, Churchill Livingstone, 1988, pp 495–518.
7. Hills BA, Butler BD: Phospholipids identified on the pericardium and their ability to impart boundary lubrication. Ann Biomed Eng 13:573, 1985.
8. Santamore WP, Bartlett R, Van Buren SJ, et al: Ventricular coupling in constrictive pericarditis. Circulation 74:597, 1986.
9. Smiseth OA, Frais MA, Kingma I: Assessment of pericardial constraint in dogs. Circulation 71:158, 1985.
10. Smiseth OA, Frais MA, Kingma I: Assessment of pericardial constraint: The relation between right ventricular filling pressure and pericardial pressure measured after pericardiocentesis. J Am Coll Cardiol 7:307, 1986.
11. Tyson GS, Maier GW, Olsen CO, et al: Pericardial influences on ventricular filling in the conscious dog. Circ Res 54:173, 1984.
12. Freeman GL, LeWinter MM: Role of parietal pericardium in acute, severe mitral regurgitation in dogs. Am J Cardiol 54:217, 1984.
13. Freeman GL, LeWinter MM: Pericardial adaptations during chronic cardiac dilation in dogs. Circ Res 54:294, 1984.
14. Lorell BH, Palacios I, Daggett WM: Right ventricular distention and left ventricular compliance. Am J Physiol 240:H87, 1981.
15. Hoit BD, Dalton N, Bhargava V, Shabetai R: Pericardial influences on right and left ventricular filling dynamics. Circ Res 68:197, 1991.
16. Santamore WP, Bartlett R, Van Buren SJ: Ventricular coupling in constrictive pericarditis. Circulation 74:597, 1986.
17. Shabetai R: Pericardial and cardiac pressure. Circulation 77:1, 1988.
18. Tyson GS Jr, Maier GW, Olsen CO: Pericardial influences on ventricular filling in the conscious dog. Circ Res 54:173, 1984.
19. Janicki JS: Influence of the pericardium and ventricular interdependence on left ventricular diastolic and systolic function in patients with heart failure. Circulation 81:15, 1990.
20. Chuttani K, Pandian NG, Mohanty PK: Left ventricular diastolic collapse: An echocardiographic sign of regional cardiac tamponade. Circulation 83:1999, 1991.
21. Meyer TE, Sareli P, Marcus RH, et al: Mechanisms underlying Kussmaul's sign in chronic constrictive pericarditis. Am J Cardiol 64:1069, 1989.
22. Bonagura JD, Darke PGG: Congenital heart disease. *In* Ettinger SJ, Feldman EC (eds): Textbook of Veterinary Internal Medicine, 4th ed. Philadelphia, WB Saunders, 1995, p 892.
23. Lunney J: Congenital peritoneal pericardial diaphragmatic hernia and portocaval shunt in a cat. J Am Anim Hosp Assoc 28:163, 1992.
24. Bellah JR, Whitton DL, Ellison GW, Phillips L: Surgical correction of concomitant cranioventral abdominal wall, caudal sternal, diaphragmatic, and pericardial defects in young dogs. JAVMA 195:1722, 1989.
25. Bellah JR, Spencer CP, Brown DJ, Whitton DL: Congenital cranioventral abdominal wall, caudal sternal, diaphragmatic, pericardial, and intracardiac defects in cocker spaniel littermates. JAVMA 194:1741, 1989.
26. Keene BW, Rush JE, Cooley AJ, Subramanian R: Primary left ventricular hemangiosarcoma diagnosed by endomyocardial biopsy in a dog. JAVMA 197:1501, 1990.
27. Aronsohn M: Cardiac hemangiosarcoma in the dog: A review of 38 cases. JAVMA 187:922, 1985.
28. Berg RJ, Wingfield W: Pericardial effusion in the dog: A review of 42 cases. J Am Anim Hosp Assoc 20:721, 1984.
29. Berg RJ, Wingfield WE, Hoopes PJ: Idiopathic hemorrhagic pericardial effusion with organized thrombi in a dog. JAVMA 185:998, 1984.
30. de Madron E, Prymak C, Hendricks J: Idiopathic hemorrhagic pericardial effusion with organized thrombi in a dog. JAVMA 191:324, 1987.
31. Sznajder JI, Evander E, Pollak ER: Pericardial effusion causes interstitial pulmonary edema in dogs. Circulation 76:843, 1987.
32. Thomas WP, Reed JR, Gomez JA: Diagnostic pneumopericardiography in dogs with spontaneous pericardial effusion. Vet Radiol 25:2, 1984.
33. Reed JR, Thomas WP, Suter PF: Pneumopericardiography in the normal dog. Vet Radiol 24:112, 1983.
34. Berry CR, Lombard CW, Hager DA, et al: Echocardiographic evaluation of cardiac tamponade in dogs before and after pericardiocentesis: Four cases (1984–1986). JAVMA 192:1597, 1988.
35. Thomas WP, Sisson D, Bauer TG, Reed JR: Detection of cardiac masses in dogs by two-dimensional echocardiography. Vet Radiol 25:65, 1984.
36. Tilley LP: Essentials of Canine and Feline Electrocardiography, 3rd ed. Philadelphia, Lea & Febiger, 1992.
37. Sacks E, Widman LE: Nonlinear heart model predicts range of heart rates for 2:1 swinging in pericardial effusion. Heart Circ Physiol 33:h1716, 1993.
38. Casale PN, Devereux RB, Kligfield P, et al: Pericardial effusion: Relation of clinical echocardiographic and electrocardiographic findings. J Electrocardiol 17:115, 1984.
39. Thomas WP, Reed JR, Bauer TG, Breznock EM: Constrictive pericardial disease in the dog. JAVMA 184:546, 1984.
40. Spodick DH: Frequency of arrhythmias in acute pericarditis determined by Holter monitoring. Am J Cardiol 53:842, 1984.
41. Harpster NK: The pericardium. *In* Gourley IM, Vasseur PB (eds): General Small Animal Surgery. Philadelphia, JB Lippincott, 1985, pp 837–847.
42. Tominaga K, Shinkai T, Eguchi K, et al: The value of two-dimensional echocardiography in detecting malignant tumors in the heart. Cancer 58:1641, 1986.
43. Vaska K, Wann LS, Sagar K, Klopfenstein HS: Pleural effusion as a cause of right ventricular diastolic collapse. Circulation 86:609, 1992.
44. Labib SB, Udelson JE, Pandian NG: Echocardiography in low pressure cardiac tamponade. Am J Cardiol 63:1156, 1989.
45. Gouliamos A, Andreou J, Steriotis J, et al: Detection of pericardial heart disease by computed tomography. Clin Radiol 35:397, 1984.
46. Hackney D, Slutsky RA, Mattrey R, et al: Experimental pericardial inflammation evaluated by computed tomography. Radiology 151:145, 1984.
47. Sechtem U, Tscholakoff D, Higgins CB: MRI of the abnormal pericardium. AJR Am J Roentgenol 147:245, 1986.
48. Stark DD, Higgins CB, Lanzer P, et al: Magnetic resonance imaging of the pericardium: Normal and pathologic findings. Radiology 150:469, 1984.
49. Kopecky SL, Calahan JA, Tajik AF, Seward JB: Percutaneous pericardial catheter drainage: Report of 42 consecutive cases. Am J Cardiol 58:633, 1986.
50. Patel AK, Koosolcharoen PK, Nallasivan M, Kronke GM: Catheter drainage of the pericardium: Practical method to maintain long term patency. Chest 92:1018, 1987.
51. Callahan JA, Seward JB, Tajik AJ: Cardiac tamponade: Pericardiocentesis directed by two-dimensional echocardiography. Mayo Clin Proc 60:344, 1985.
52. Sisson D, Thomas WP, Ruehl WW: Diagnostic value of pericardial fluid analysis in the dog. JAVMA 51:184, 1984.
53. Ziskind AA, Pearce AC, Lemmon CC, Burstein S: Percutaneous balloon pericardiotomy for the treatment of cardiac tamponade and large pericardial effusions: Description of technique and report of the first 50 cases. J Am Coll Cardiol 21:1, 1993.
54. Palacios IF, Tuzcu EM, Ziskind AA, Younger J: Percutaneous balloon pericardial window for patients with malignant pericardial effusion and tamponade. Cathet Cardiovasc Diagn 22:244, 1991.
55. Engel PJ, Fowler NO, Tei C, et al: M-mode echocardiography in constrictive pericarditis. J Am Coll Cardiol 6:471, 1985.
56. Hatle LK, Appleton CP, Popp RL: Differentiation of constrictive pericarditis and restrictive cardiomyopathy by Doppler echocardiography. Circulation 79:357, 1989.
57. Schiavone WA, Calafiore PA, Currie PJ, Lytle BW: Doppler echocardiographic demonstration of pulmonary venous flow velocity in three patients with constrictive pericarditis before and after pericardiectomy. Am J Cardiol 63:145, 1989.
58. Edwards NJ: The diagnostic value of pericardial fluid pH determination. JAAMA 32:63, 1996.

CHAPTER 119

DIROFILARIASIS IN DOGS AND CATS

Ray Dillon

Infection with *Dirofilaria immitis*, first described in 1921,[1] has a worldwide distribution and has been reported to infect a wide variety of species of animals (dog, cat, ferret, fox, wolf, sea lion, horse). The distribution is influenced by the population of animals (usually dogs) that complete the life cycle and have microfilaremia and a mosquito vector that will complete the early larval stages. Different mosquito feeding patterns influence the areas and species of animal infected. For a cat (or alternate host) to develop heartworm disease, the mosquito must feed on a dog and then, after adequate warm environmental exposure, feed on a cat.[2–4]

LIFE CYCLE OF *DIROFILARIA* AND PATHOGENESIS

Adult *Dirofilaria* females (27 cm long) and males (17 cm long) normally reside in the pulmonary arteries and right ventricles without causing major occlusion of the blood supply (Fig. 119–1). Microfilariae (315 μm long and 6–7 μm wide) are discharged into the bloodstream and survive 1 to 3 years. The number of circulating microfilariae in dogs is increased in warm ambient temperature, after eating, and late at night. The microfilariae are ingested by a mosquito during feeding. The infective larvae (L1) migrate to the stomach and then the mouth parts (L3) during development (Fig. 119–2). The rate of development can be as short as 8 days at 30°C or as long as 28 days at 18°C. After a mosquito acquires the microfilariae (L1), adequate exposure to warm temperatures must occur during the relatively short life span (1 month) of that mosquito. The infective larvae are deposited on the skin of an animal when the mosquito feeds again and the L3 larvae enter through the bite wound. A maximum of 10 to 12 L3 larvae can be transmitted by a single mosquito.[2, 3]

The L3 larvae molt and migrate to the pulmonary arteries, arriving as L5 larvae (1–2 cm in length) (Fig. 119–3) approximately 100 days after infection (Table 119–1). These small L5 larvae are distributed mainly to the caudal distal pulmonary arteries, and over the next 2 to 3 months they develop to sexually mature adults and migrate back toward the right ventricle. If both sexes are present, microfilariae are produced 6 to 7 months after L3 larval exposure. The common detection methods for adult antigen are positive 1 month before or at the time of the production of the initial microfilaremia.[5] The initial arrival of L5 larvae in the small vessels of the lungs is associated with an intense eosinophilic reaction (Fig. 119–4), and a diffuse radiographic pattern and clinical signs of coughing may be present, preceding the production of microfilariae and circulating antigen by 2 to 3 months.[6, 7] Clinical diagnosis of early disease is difficult at this stage, especially in the cat and ferret. No pathologic process has been associated with circulating live microfilariae.

Adult heartworms can live 3 to 5 years. Although an endarteritis is produced, embolization and total vascular occlusion are rare when the worms are alive. The severity of the pathology is influenced by the number of parasites but also exacerbated by the shear stress of high blood flow associated with exercise.[8] Severe pathology can be induced by low worm burdens in athletic dogs. The classically described cor pulmonale syndrome is only induced in dogs

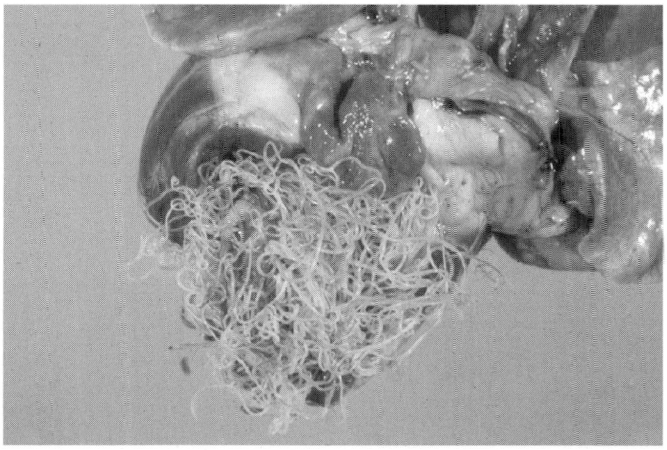

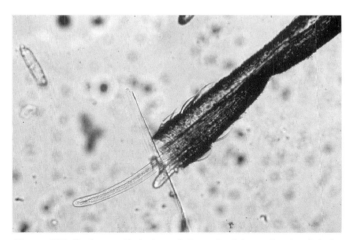

Figure 119–1. More than 150 adult heartworms were present in this asymptomatic dog presented for a traumatic death. Even in endemic areas, large worm burdens are unusual, with the average infection being 14 adult heartworms.

Figure 119–2. A magnified view of the end of the proboscis of *Aedes vexans* with two L3 larvae emerging.

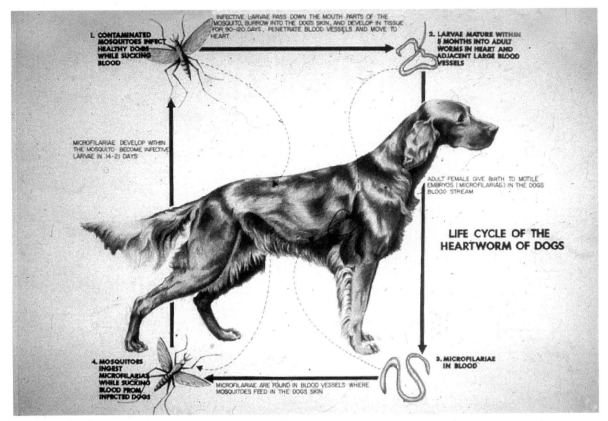

Figure 119–3. The life cycle of the heartworm is typically described as a 6-month cycle from mosquito bite to the production of microfilariae in the dog. However, the arrival of the immature L5 larvae at 100 days is the initiation of the pathology associated with the pulmonary parenchyma.

with an exercise pattern, forcing right ventricular hypertrophy from increased cardiac outputs and increased pulmonary vascular resistance. In endemic areas, the average worm burden in the dog is about 15 worms, and in the cat it is 1 to 3 worms. High worm burdens can be found in dogs with minimal cardiac changes if the dog is sedentary. The death of worms, either spontaneous or induced, is associated with severe pulmonary parenchymal disease. Respiratory failure may result and in the cat and ferret can be associated with a single worm infection.

RELATIVE RESISTANCE TO INFECTION

If dogs not previously exposed to heartworms are infected with 100 L3 larvae, between 60 to 75 adult worms develop in about 90 per cent of dogs.[2, 3] The cat is a resistant, but susceptible, host. Cats develop adult *D. immitis* infection, but it takes a greater exposure than in dogs[9–11] (see Table 119–1). If cats not previously exposed to heartworms are infected with 100 L3 larvae, 3 to 10 adult worms develop

in about 75 per cent of these cats.[10–13] The frequency of heartworm infection in the cat is generally accepted to correlate with the dog population of the area, but at a lower incidence[13] (Fig. 119–5).

Experimentally, the percentage of infective larvae (L3) developing into adult worms is less in cats (1 to 25 per cent) than in dogs (40 to 90 per cent).[10–12] Cats are at greatest risk in endemic areas where repeated bites by infected mosquitoes would occur over a short period of time (2 to 3 months).

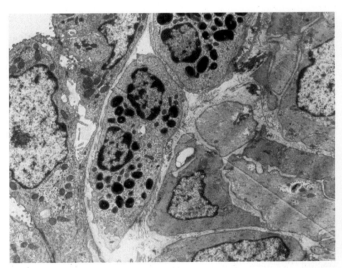

Figure 119–4. Transmission electron microscopy of a section of lung shows the initial eosinophilic (cells with "slashed football" granules) reaction associated with the early L5 stages.

TABLE 119–1. COMPARISON OF THE HOST SUITABILITY OF THREE ANIMAL SPECIES TO *D. IMMITIS* AFTER SUBCUTANEOUS INOCULATION OF L3

HOST	MICROFILARIAE (NO./DURATION)	INFECTION RATE (%)	WORM RECOVERY (%)
Ferret	Few/transient	100	34–54
Dog	Many/extended	100	56
Cat	Few/transient	56–90	6

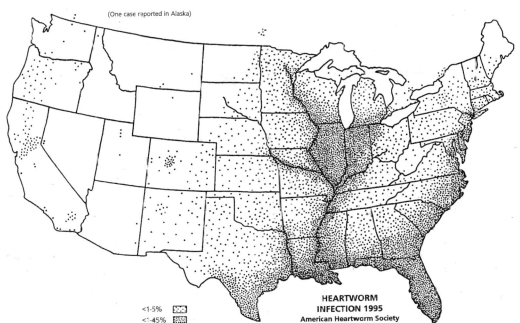

Figure 119–5. Incidence map demonstrating the endemic areas for heartworm disease in the United States.

Depending on the species, the average mosquito can transmit a maximum of 10 infective larvae; therefore, an experimental infection with 100 L3 larvae would represent 10 to 15 mosquitoes all feeding at the same time.[2, 11] Infective larvae in the cat are poorly oriented; therefore, ectopic sites for the L5 larvae (brain, subcutaneous tissue, abdomen) are more common than in the dog. Experimentally, up to 30 adult worms have been induced in a cat and 300 adult worms in dogs.[2, 3, 9] If immature L5 larvae are removed from the pulmonary arteries and are placed subcutaneous, 68 per cent of worms in cats and 58 per cent of worms in dogs will be found in the pulmonary arteries 1 to 2 months later.[14]

REACTION TO INFECTION

Microfilariae live for up to 2 years and are present in about 60 per cent of dogs with heartworms (Table 119–2). Once infected by adult heartworms by means of either infective larvae (L3) or transplantation (from experimentally superinfected dogs), the natural resistance of the cat induces a shortened period of patency and a lower concentration or absent circulating microfilaremia. Because microfilariae are rarely observed in the blood, the cat is not considered to be a reservoir host that can provide mosquitoes with a site to acquire potential larvae.[2, 15] The life cycle would then dictate that for a cat to become infected, a mosquito must feed on a species of animal with a patent infection (usually a dog) and then, after proper climate conditions, feed on a cat.[16] The feeding pattern of the mosquito determines which cat or dog acquires the infective larvae. Some species of mosquitoes will readily feed on both dogs and cats; others prefer only one species.[17, 18] The incidence of heartworms in cats is very high in some areas (25 per cent) and may reflect the willingness of a species of mosquito in the area to feed on both dogs and cats. Thus, as noted on incidence maps, there is no consistent ratio between the percentage of mongrel dogs with heartworms and the percentage of cats in the same area with heartworms. Based on necropsy data, some areas with moderate canine infections (e.g., Tennessee, Kentucky) have a greater percentage of cats with heartworms than areas with higher canine heartworm infections (e.g., Florida)[13, 19] (Fig. 119–5).

Of the L5 larvae that arrive in the distal pulmonary arteries as 1- to 2-cm immature adults, there is a higher mortality of the L5 larvae in the cat compared with the dog.[11, 20] The acute reaction often noted 3 to 4 months after infection may be the result of the arrival and death of immature L5 larvae.[2, 3, 21–23] Based on limited long-term studies, adult heartworms in the cat have a relatively short life span (probably less than 2 years) compared with the dog (approximately 5 years).[2, 7]

PATHOLOGY IN THE DOG

Although heartworms are frequently explained to owners as a "spaghetti size worm that lives in the pulmonary outflow tract and blocks blood going to the lungs," the pathogenesis is complex. The emphasis on the physical changes to the endothelium and intima of the main pulmonary arteries has demonstrated villous myointimal proliferation with endothelial cell swelling, widening intercellular junctions, and increased permeability. With endothelial sloughing, platelets and leukocytes are activated, resulting in thrombosis. The

TABLE 119–2. MORPHOLOGIC DIFFERENTIATION OF MICROFILARIAE

SMEAR	DIROFILARIA	DIPETALONEMA RECONDITUM
Fresh smear	Few to large numbers	Usually small numbers
	Undulate in one place	Move across field
Stained smear*	Straight body	Curved body
	Straight tail	Posterior extremity hook ("button-hook" tail); inconsistent finding
	Tapered head	Blunt head
	>290 μm long	<275–280 μm long
	>6 μm wide	<6 μm wide

*Size criteria given for lysate prepared using 2 per cent formalin (modified Knott's test); microfilariae tend to be smaller with lysate of filter tests. Width and morphology are the best discriminating factors.

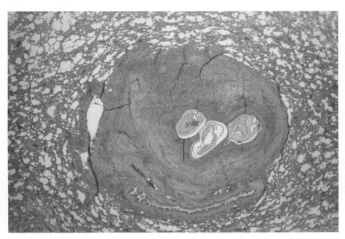

Figure 119–6. Periarteritis in a dog with heartworms demonstrates the intense inflammatory reaction adjacent to small pulmonary arteries and extending into the pulmonary parenchyma. Some of the arterial enlargement noted on radiographs is associated with this perivascular inflammation.

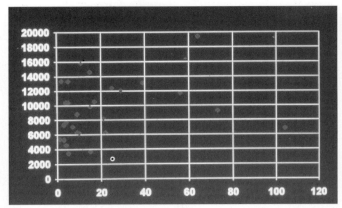

Figure 119–7. No correlation has been noted in naturally infected asymptomatic dogs between heartworm number and the degree of pulmonary vascular disease as measured by pulmonary vascular resistance (PVR). PVR takes into consideration cardiac output and pulmonary arterial pressure and body weight, being more sensitive than pulmonary arterial pressure alone. Some dogs with 10 worms have a higher PVR than dogs with 100 worms. Severely affected dogs may have a PVR of over 5 times normal.

endothelial cell damage and/or other trophic factors stimulate the proliferation of smooth muscle and thickening of the media. This villous proliferation is most severe in the caudal lung lobes, and the arteries lose their taper and become blunted or pruned. The proximal vessels become dilated and may have aneurysms, resulting in a tortuous appearance. This lesion blocks flow, and vascular bed and pulmonary hypertension develops, resulting in right ventricular strain and cor pulmonale.[3, 24]

Lesions are more severe when associated with the physical location of the parasite, but cardiovascular alterations develop at other levels[8, 25] (Figs. 119–6 to 119–8). The host-parasite reaction is more important than worm number in development of clinical signs. No correlation is noted between worm number and severity of pulmonary vascular resistance. High flow rates through the lung exacerbate pathology. Vessel responsiveness is altered in dogs with heartworm disease, not just in the pulmonary vasculature but also as blunting of femoral arterial vasodilation.[26] The heartworm represents an intravascular chemical factory releasing immune modulators and products that affect vascular tone

systemically.[27, 28] The airway may be compromised further by bronchoconstriction. Cyclooxygenase products from heartworms cause marked constriction of tracheal rings in vitro.[29] Heartworms release foreign proteins that, depending on the vascular bed, leak into the periarterial and parenchymal areas.[25, 30] This inflammatory response outside the vessel and separate from the physical presence of the heartworm can further dictate the severity of pathology and the resulting clinical signs.

With the initial arrival of L5 larvae as 1.5-cm worms in the right and left caudal arteries, small vessel disease and lung parenchymal pathologic processes are initial insults. The host response is locally eosinophilic. As the worms increase in size and grow back up the pulmonary arteries, the arterial lesions become more evident. The periarteritis allows additional leakage, and inflammation may extend into the lung parenchyma. At the distal capillary bed level, even the alveolar septa will develop edema and injury. High flow at critical times of early lesions will promote fibrosis rather than normal repair. Demonstration of heartworm antigen in interstitial areas distal to the physical presence of heart-

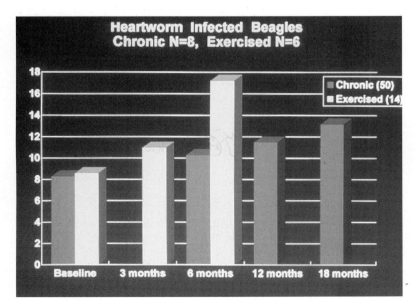

Figure 119–8. In experimental beagles, a group with only 14 heartworms for 6 months, which were exercised for 0.25 mile 5 days a week, had a higher PVR than a group with 50 heartworms for 2 years, which were confined.

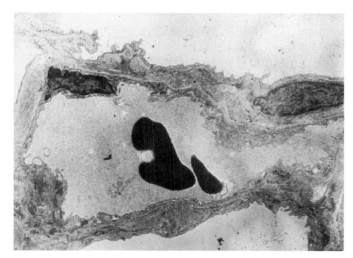

Figure 119–9. Transmission electron microscopy of canine lung at the capillary beds demonstrates the fibrosis and thickening of the alveolar gas exchange areas typical of severe heartworm disease.

worms emphasizes that the inflammatory response is throughout the pulmonary parenchyma. The microvascular lesions are severe when worms are alive but become exaggerated associated with worm death.[31] Type 1 pneumocytes are disrupted from the endothelial cells, leaving the alveolar sacs denuded. Although more severe in lobes where heartworms are dying, similar lesions can be demonstrated in other lobes. I have produced similar histologic lesions with cell free extracts of adult heartworms. The resultant lung injury is typical of adult respiratory distress syndrome. During these critical times of natural or induced worm death, the lung develops severe periarteritis, interstitial edema, and acute inflammatory interstitial disease. The ciliated bronchial columnar epithelia are damaged and undergo necrosis. The shear forces on endothelial cells during high flow and increased permeability contribute to increased capillary bed damage, alveolar flooding, and resulting fibrosis (Fig. 119–9). This contributes to decreased areas of gas exchange and promotes fibrosis, which further increases pulmonary vascular resistance. Unfortunately, the microvascular disease cannot be radiographically evaluated and only in dogs in which the disease is extreme or the exercise pattern of the dog has exacerbated the right-sided heart strain will the typical pattern of cor pulmonale be demonstrated. The microvascular lesion of fibrosis of pulmonary capillary bed is not reversible.

PATHOLOGY IN THE CAT

The general pulmonary arterial pathology in the cat is similar to that in the dog.[32–34] Muscular hypertrophy, villus endarteritis, and cellular infiltrates of the adventitia are typically more severe in the caudal pulmonary arteries. Typical of the reaction of the cat, the smaller arteries develop severe muscular hypertrophy. The host's response to the parasite is intense, as shown radiographically by enlarged pulmonary arteries that develop within 1 week of transplantation.[5, 20, 35] Histologically, much of the reaction is periarteriolar inflammation[34] (see Fig. 119–6).

The cause of the acute crisis in the cat is lung injury resulting in respiratory distress, most often associated with the death of an adult heartworm. The lung can become

acutely edematous, and respiratory failure, not heart failure, becomes the life-threatening event.[34, 36]

Embolization of pulmonary arteries can be a contributing factor to initiation of clinical signs. Although pulmonary hypertension does occasionally occur, right-axis electrocardiographic (ECG) changes, radiographic evidence of right-sided hypertrophy, and right-sided heart failure are infrequent, indicating that severe cor pulmonale is uncommon in the cat with heartworms.[37–39] In chronic cases, perivascular reaction and evidence of thrombus formation with re-canalization are noted and cardiac changes are minimal. Obstruction of blood flow, especially to the caudal pulmonary arteries, causes acute signs, and the lung lobe involved becomes hemorrhagic with areas of edema. If the cat survives the initial embolic lesion, re-canalization around the obstruction occurs rapidly and the lung is markedly improved within days.[34, 36]

Post-caval syndrome with ascites and right-sided heart failure will occur in rare cases with very high worm burdens. Hemoglobinuria has not been a consistent finding in cats with heartworms. Poor venous return and tricuspid insufficiency rather than cor pulmonale are considered the pathogenic mechanisms of this syndrome in cats.

The hallmark of the respiratory distress in the cat is the acute lung injury, resulting in a generalized respiratory failure. The inflammation is observed even in lung lobes not associated with embolization. Thus, the disease is not a simple obstructive disease associated with blocking of blood flow. The lesions are acute and inflammatory, usually with interstitial edema leading to alveolar flooding. The type 1 alveolar epithelial cell is often disrupted. If the cat survives the insult, the result of the acute lung injury is a type 2 alveolar cell hyperplasia[34] (Fig. 119–10).

CLINICAL SIGNIFICANCE OF DIROFILARIASIS

FELINE HEARTWORM DISEASE

If the course of a *D. immitis* infection is evaluated chronologically, the changing nature of the disease is evident. When

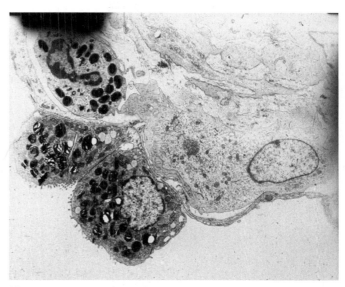

Figure 119–10. Transmission electron microscopy of cat lung shows a type 2 cell pneumocyte proliferation (cells with surfactant granules in air space) that is typical of repair of acute lung injury.

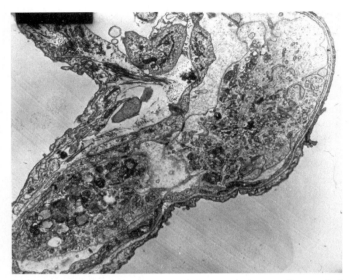

Figure 119–11. Transmission electron microscopy of a cat pulmonary bed shows a large pulmonary intravascular macrophage that is adhered by electron-dense adhesion sites to the endothelial cell. This is a major phagocytic cell in the cat and is not present in dogs or humans.

the parasite first arrives in the animal's lungs as early as 100 days after being infected by a mosquito, the lung response is intense inflammation, and "asthma-like" symptoms may develop.[40] The cat has specialized macrophages (designed to envelop and digest foreign materials) in the capillary beds of the lung that are not present in the dog[41] (Figs. 119–11 and 119–12). After the mature parasite develops, the clinical signs may be intermittent or absent. The parasite seems to be able to suppress the macrophage function in the lung.[41] The cat will have classic radiographic and histologic findings of feline heartworms but may not show clinical signs. However, at the time of worm death, suppressed macrophage function is decreased, the lungs become extremely inflamed, and the specialized macrophages may become important in the intense reaction. The result is a non-functioning lung and an acute respiratory distress syndrome. This reaction can occur as the result of even a single worm burden. After the removal of dead heartworms, there may be continued inflammatory lung disease in some cats.[20]

The disease associated with feline heartworm infection is a moving target, with the pathology, and resulting clinical signs, dependent on the stage of the life cycle involved. Early arrival of L5 larvae results in classic asthma-like radiographic and clinical signs. After the adult parasite develops, the pulmonary parenchymal changes and even enlarged caudal pulmonary arteries on ventrodorsal radiographs may decrease.[42] Immunosuppression of the macrophage population in cats after transplantation of live worms would suggest a protective mechanism for the host-parasite relationship while the worm is alive. The death of the parasite is associated with acute lung injury. The diffuse nature of the lung disease, lack of infarction of lung, and capacity of the cat to react to the death of even one heartworm reflects the hypothesis that death of heartworms induces acute respiratory distress syndrome.

CANINE HEARTWORM DISEASE

The pathology in the lung and major pulmonary arteries can cause a very wide variety of clinical signs. The majority of sedentary dogs with heartworm disease are asymptomatic at the time of diagnosis. Although there have been attempts to classify heartworm disease into classes based on clinical signs, the resultant prognosis cannot be predicted (Tables 119–3 to 119–5).

The degree of lung pathology is influenced by the host response to the parasite, and there is not a consistent relationship between the number of the adult heartworms and the severity of the disease (Fig. 119–13). Thus, a dog with severe radiographic lesions and classic cor pulmonale may not have a heavy worm burden. About one third of the dogs with spontaneously occult heartworms have no microfilariae because after being released they are destroyed. The lungs often reflect a severe pulmonary reaction, typical of eosinophilic pneumonitis, and granulomas may even develop.[23, 43, 44] This diffuse intense pulmonary reaction is often reversible when compared with classic cor pulmonale right-sided heart failure (Fig. 119–14).

Although there have not been consistent correlations between worm numbers and clinical signs when the worms are alive, there is a clinical pattern between the number of worms dying and the rapidity of death. Dogs with minimal

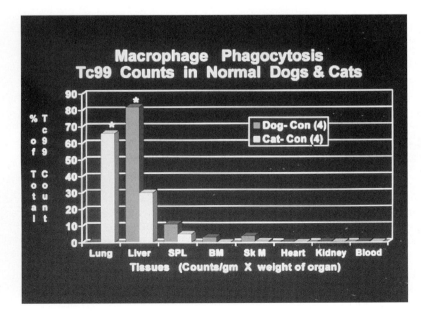

Figure 119–12. The major phagocytic organ is the liver in the dog and lung in the cat. Spleen (SPL), bone marrow (BM), skeletal muscle (SKM), heart, kidney, and blood have minor evidence of phagocytic activity.

TABLE 119–3. COMMERCIAL ADULT HEARTWORM ANTIGEN TEST KITS

	MANUFACTURER	FORMAT	TYPE OF TEST	SEMIQUANTITATIVE	TYPE OF SAMPLE
ITC Gold	Synbiotics	Membrane	Immunochromatographic	No	Plasma, serum, blood
SNAP	Idexx Laboratories	Membrane	ELISA	Yes	Plasma, serum, blood
UNI-TEC CHW	Synbiotics	Membrane	ELISA	No	Plasma, serum, blood
ASSURE/CH	Synbiotics	Wand	ELISA	No	Plasma or serum
PetChek	Idexx Laboratories	Microwell	ELISA	No/OD	Plasma or serum
DiroCHEK	Synbiotics	Microwell	ELISA	No/OD	Plasma or serum
VetRED	Synbiotics	Well (card)	Hemagglutination	No	Blood

ELISA = enzyme-linked immunosorbent assay; OD = optical density can be reported when an automated plate reader is used.
From McTier TL, McCall JW, Supakorndej N: Features of adult heartworm antigen test kits. In: Proceedings of the 1995 Heartworm Symposium, American Heartworm Society, Washington, DC, 1995, pp 115–120.

clinical signs and radiographic lesions can be at great risk if a large worm mass is killed quickly.

Thus, classification of heartworm disease is helpful but caution should be used in application to client communications relative to prognosis. Regardless of clinical signs, a high antigen load can be associated with large worm burdens and a staged kill of adults should be advised. The relationship between high antigen load and large numbers of adult female heartworms is not consistent but clinically can be used as an indication for caution.[45] Dogs with very diffuse interstitial and bronchial infiltrates on thoracic radiographs may require treatment for eosinophilic pneumonitis before attempting adulticidal therapy. Many of these dogs are brought to the veterinarian because of severe coughing, and peripheral eosinophilia and basophilia may or may not be present (Fig. 119–14). Prednisolone therapy using a tapering dosing should be completed 5 to 7 days before adulticidal therapy.

Cardiac signs of severe heartworm disease include exercise intolerance or preload complications of ascites. The exercise intolerance is often noted in physically active dogs. Right ventricular hypertrophy, enlarged pulmonary arterial segments on ventrodorsal radiographs, and right-axis deviation on an ECG are associated in dogs with markedly increased pulmonary vascular resistance. Historically, dogs that continue to exercise with active heartworm infections can induce irreversible pulmonary arterial lesions of the intima and fibrosis of pulmonary capillary beds even with low worm burdens (Figs. 119–15 and 119–16). In a working breed dog in which performance is a key issue, immediate cessation of activities that increase the cardiac output is an initial recommendation. The inability of the right ventricle to force enough blood through the pulmonary capillary bed to provide the left ventricle with preload necessary for adequate cardiac output to systemic circulation is key in the exercise intolerance. However, cardiac failure as a cause of death associated with embolization and death of the heart-

worms is uncommon. Respiratory failure rather than decreases in cardiac output is critically involved in post-adulticidal complications.

Ascites associated with heartworms can be from cor pulmonale right-sided failure, chronic post-caval syndrome, or acute post-caval syndrome. Classically, the radiographic pattern is that of severe disease and, depending on the severity of the damage, may or may not be reversible. Dogs with post-caval syndrome usually have a large worm burden (see Fig. 119–13). The closure of the tricuspid valve is altered by the physical presence of the worms, and the clinical signs are a combination of post-caval stagnation and metabolic consequence of hepatic congestion.[46] Clinically, chronic post-caval syndrome and cor pulmonale right-sided failure present as ascites of weeks to months in duration that may have abated with cage rest. Echocardiography is useful in determining the location of heartworms and competency of the tricuspid valve.[47] In the post-caval syndromes, physical removal of the heartworms with a forceps, retrieval basket, or other instruments has been very successful.[48] However, paramount in the operation should be the realization that fragmentation of adult worms or even crushing of several worms can result in rapid death of the dog from cardiac failure[49, 50] and acute respiratory distress syndrome.[34] Most dogs with caval syndromes are in their first or second season of exposure in endemic areas that often have heavy mosquito seasons. Experimentally, a dog already infected with an active adult infection exposed to 200 L3 larvae will usually not develop a large worm burden. The heartworm-naive dog is at greatest risk for caval syndromes where it can be bitten by many mosquitoes, each having a maximum of L3 larvae over a 3-month time frame (before the dog has the opportunity to initiate immunity to subsequent L3 larvae exposure).

DIAGNOSIS

Demonstration of the microfilaria of *D. immitis* in a blood sample is successful with concentration techniques (modified Knotts' and filter tests) in about 60 per cent of dogs and less than 10 per cent of cats with heartworms (see Table 119–4). Because of the survival of microfilariae after adult worms have died, a small percentage of dogs can have microfilaremia but no adult worm in the heart. In addition, puppies born to bitches with high microfilarial counts can have a transient microfilaremia, which cannot become an adult infection. Amicrofilaremia (occult infection) can be caused by immature (<6 month old) worms, single worm infections, unisex infections, host immunologic reactions to microfilariae, and iatrogenic production of occult disease. The monthly preventative medications will induce embryo stasis in the female heartworm; and after 6 months of medication

TABLE 119–4. DIAGNOSTIC TESTING FOR DIROFILARIASIS

1. Complete blood cell count
2. Concentration microfilaria test
3. Thoracic radiographs
4. Fecal examination
5. Electrocardiogram
6. Immunofluorescence—microfilarial antibody cuticle vs. somatic antigen source
7. Enzyme-linked immunosorbent assay—adult antibody (cat only)
8. Adult antigen
9. Tracheal wash
10. Arteriogram

TABLE 119–5. PARAMETERS USED TO CLASSIFY SEVERITY OF HEARTWORM DISEASE

	CLASS 1—SUBCLINICAL	CLASS 2—MODERATE	CLASS 3—SEVERE
Diagnosis of adults	Negative or "weak" positive result on semiquantitative test for HW Ag If Ag test negative: positive Knott test	Positive result on test for HW Ag Knott test may be positive or negative	Positive test for circulating HW Ag; Usually highly positive when using a semiquantitative test Knott test may be positive or negative
History	No clinical signs	Mild to moderate exercise intolerance Occasional cough with exercise	Marked exercise intolerance, weight loss Increased respiratory rate at rest, persistent cough
Physical examination	Good general condition	Good/fair general condition	Fair to poor general condition; evidence of right-sided heart failure: (ascites, jugular venous distention)
Electrocardiography	Normal	Normal ± Evidence of RVH	Right ventricular hypertrophy Right-axis shift or RBBB Arrhythmias (VPC, A. Fib.)
Thoracic radiography	Normal cardiac silhouette; ± mildly enlarged pulmonary arteries; ± mild pulmonary parenchymal infiltrate	Moderate enlargement of the right ventricle and main pulmonary artery; moderate enlargement of the caudal pulmonary arteries with evidence of truncation and tortuosity; diffuse perivascular parenchymal infiltrates	Right ventricular and right atrial enlargement Enlarged main pulmonary artery; enlarged, tortuous, and truncated lobar pulmonary arteries; diffuse perivascular pulmonary parenchymal infiltrates with evidence of PTE
Laboratory data	Normal	± moderate anemia (PCV 20–30%) Mild to moderate proteinuria common	Anemia common (PCV <20%) Significant elevations in hepatic enzymes and/or blood urea nitrogen and creatinine; moderate to severe proteinuria common
Prognosis	Good	Good/fair	Guarded

Overlap between categories is common. All abnormalities need not be present to assign a patient to a given category. Classification of older dogs and dogs weighing less than 10 kg should be biased toward the higher class. It should be emphasized that these simply represent guidelines for classification.
RVH = right ventricular hypertrophy; HW Ag = heartworm antigen; RBBB = right bundle branch block; VPC = ventricular premature complex; A. Fib. = atrial fibrillation; PCV = packed cell volume; PTE = pulmonary thromboembolism.

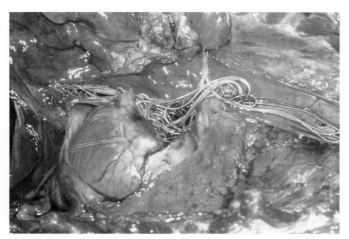

Figure 119–13. Post-caval syndrome can be acute or chronic. This dog had a history of ascites of 4 months' duration that abated when the dog was cage rested.

in a heartworm-positive dog, an occult status has been demonstrated in most dogs. Antigen testing is necessary to determine the heartworm status of a dog on monthly preventative medication.[51, 52]

Historically, in the dog, enzyme-linked immunosorbent assay (ELISA) methodology to detect dog antibody against adult heartworm proteins did not have the specificity for routine screening (see Table 119–3). The number of false-positive results was unacceptable in low incidence areas and in dogs on preventative medications. The commercial antigen detecting methods with almost 100 per cent specificity and with sensitivity typically over 85 per cent have become the screening methods of choice. The microfilarial detection concentration tests in natural infections have (5 to 60 per cent) typically 40 per cent false-negative results and the

occasional false-positive result. Although the majority of the antigen detection methods are evaluating for the presence of a glycoprotein present in many areas of the adult parasite, most of the product in circulation is released from the adult female reproductive tract.[5, 51, 52] When 1 to 2 worms were present, approximately 50 per cent of results were falsely negative. Less than 10 per cent were negative when 3 to 5 worms were present, and no false-negative results were noted when more than 20 worms were present. The comparison of testing methods is difficult because of the constant modifications and improvements in kits and methods. Historically, the laboratory-based microwell titer methods on serum or plasma have been more sensitive than "in hospital" kits in animals with low antigen loads, and discordant results between different testing methods are not uncommon in such cases. The antigen technology also allows antigen load as an estimate of worm burden and evaluates efficacy of adulticide as concentrations decrease to negative 10 to 12 weeks after therapy. The detection of circulating antigen is based on a laboratory-derived antibody binding to an adequate amount of circulating heartworm antigen. The maturity and number of females influence the amount of antigen. Immature worms and low worm burdens (especially in the cat) will be antigen negative even when worms are present in the pulmonary arteries and clinical signs are present.[55, 56]

Thoracic radiography can be a screening tool for dogs and cats with suggestive clinical signs of heartworm disease. The pulmonary arteries can be tortuous and enlarged in dogs with an enlarged pulmonary arterial segment at the 1 o'clock position on a ventrodorsal view. Right ventricular enlargement may not be noted if the hypertrophy has not been induced by physical activity or severe vascular lesions (see Figs. 119–14 and 119–15). The pulmonary parenchymal changes can be diffuse in the early L5 larval infection but can also become granulomatous in chronic severe infections.[39, 57] In the cat, cardiac changes are rare, and even an

CV

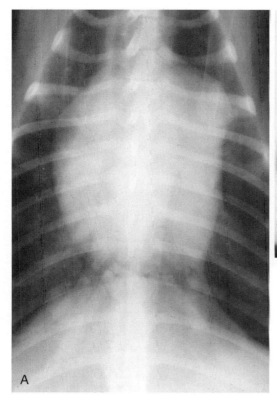

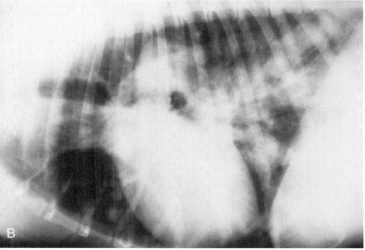

Figure 119–14. A, Typically described, heartworm disease in the dog has a reverse D appearance and the pulmonary arterial segment is visible at the 1 o'clock position on the ventrodorsal view. The caudal pulmonary arteries are enlarged and blunted beyond the edge of the cardiac border. B, On the lateral view, there is cardiomegaly, increased sternal contact, and loss of anterior space.

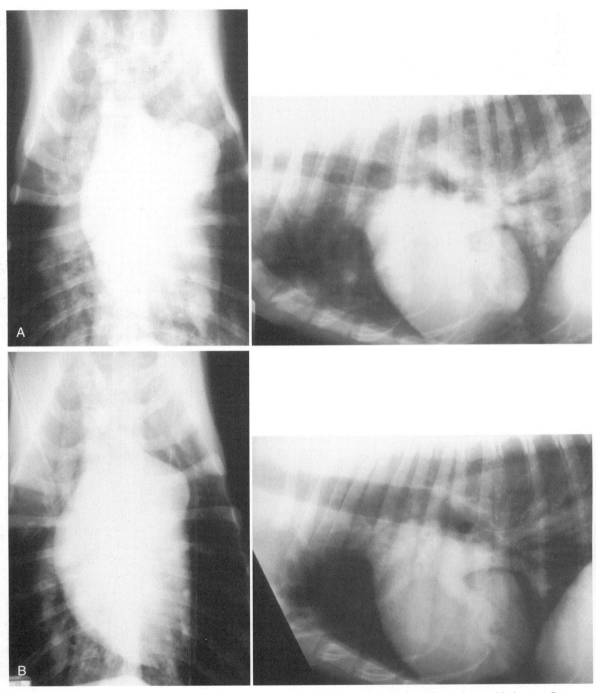

Figure 119–15. Thoracic radiographs, ventrodorsal and lateral, before *(A)* and after *(B)* corticosteroid therapy. Severe pulmonary parenchymal lung disease *(A)* can often be confused with thromboembolic disease. Although the disease is severe, after 5 days of systemic glucocorticoids the pulmonary changes were markedly reduced *(B)*.

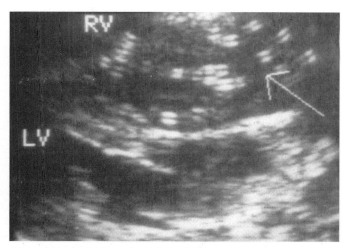

Figure 119–16. Echocardiography will demonstrate heartworms in both dogs and cats as double parallel lines (equal signs) because the cuticle is hyperechoic when it is in the beam.

enlarged pulmonary arterial segment on the ventrodorsal view is not visible beyond the cardiac shadow. Enlarged caudal pulmonary arteries are the most consistent lesion in cats with heartworms. Severe lung parenchymal changes may obscure the vascular pattern. A fluid density lung lobe is associated with acute signs in cats and may be confused with a consolidating pneumonia.[38]

Echocardiograms are diagnostic with typical "double parallel" white lines in the pulmonary arteries or right ventricles of dogs or cats[58, 59] (see Fig. 119–16). Echocardiography is especially useful in diagnosis of post-caval syndrome and ascitic conditions associated with heartworm disease.[60] In the dog, heartworms spend most of the time in the pulmonary arteries and are difficult to detect but significant when observed. In caval syndrome, the appearance of a mass of heartworms flipping in and out of the right ventricle and atrium is characteristic. The ECG will only have the typical right-axis deviation and deep S waves if there is significant right ventricular hypertrophy. Tracheal cytology is usually nonspecific and is rarely positive for bacteria in either the dog or cat. An eosinophilic cytology is usually a stage-specific reaction typical of early L5 larval infection, initial production of microfilariae, and destruction of microfilariae.

PRE-TREATMENT EVALUATION

After a diagnosis of heartworm infection, the therapeutic plan should include a pre-treatment evaluation to (1) discover subclinical or concomitant diseases, (2) anticipate complications of therapy, and (3) predict the reversibility of the disease. This evaluation is greatly influenced by the owner's anticipation of the dog's activity after therapy.

HISTORY AND PHYSICAL EXAMINATION

In addition to questions about the dog's general health, specific questions should include (1) water consumption and urination habits; (2) daily physical activity patterns; (3) changes in appetite or body weight; (4) vomiting, regurgitation, or diarrhea; and (5) history of all medications administered in the past year. Specific cardiopulmonary questions should identify exercise tolerance, coughing, hemoptysis,

collapse, seizures, abdominal enlargement, cyanosis, dyspnea, or epistaxis.

A careful physical examination rarely reveals the severity of heartworm disease. Tricuspid insufficiency may be auscultated in severe cases and caval syndromes. Mitral valvular insufficiency, pericardial tamponade, and cardiomyopathy must be differentiated in dogs with signs compatible with heartworm disease. With severe acute pulmonary thromboembolism, heart sounds are unusually loud, a split second heart sound can be heard, the pulse is bounding, and the dog will appear anxious and dyspneic.

CLINICAL PATHOLOGY

Results of the complete blood cell count, serum chemistry profile, and urinalysis of heartworm-infected dogs are usually normal. Justification of these tests is to rule out subclinical disease, which would change the therapeutic plan. In experimental infections, dogs and cats with heartworms may develop transient changes in the complete blood cell count associated with stages of the infection. Eosinophilia ($>1,200/\mu L$) is a common finding in many parasitic and dermatologic diseases. Eosinophilia and basophilia suggest occult heartworms and inflammatory lung disease. One third of dogs with heartworms have a moderate anemia, low serum iron concentration, and low iron-binding capacity, typical of chronic infection. Chronic anemia, hemolysis, and moderate reticulocytosis, typical of a microangiopathic hemolysis, are noted in dogs with severe cases. Heartworms increase platelet consumption. Mean platelet volume is often at the high normal range. Thrombocytopenia is especially associated with heartworm death and disseminated intravascular coagulation.

Some dogs with heartworm disease have increased total protein concentrations, but hypoalbuminemia is a critical concern, if present. Hypoalbuminemia can be associated with glomerular disease, hepatic failure, or protein-losing enteropathy. A patient whose urinalysis showed an elevated protein level should be screened further by determining the urine protein/creatinine ratio. Dogs with glomerular disease losing albumin also lose antithrombin III, and thus are at greater risk for thromboembolism associated with adulticidal therapy. Dogs with significant proteinuria should have a kidney biopsy to differentiate glomerulonephritis from amyloidosis. Although, on occasion, a dog with significant protein loss will improve after adulticidal therapy, dogs with amyloidosis should be considered to have a chronic progressive kidney disease; and usually therapeutic plans for heartworm disease are suspended. Early in the course of these glomerular diseases, renal filtration and concentration functions are maintained, resulting in normal blood urea nitrogen level and concentrated urine specific gravity when challenged. Other causes of renal failure may alter the therapy for heartworm disease. Evaluation of hepatic function has been historically emphasized because of the hepatotoxic nature of thiacetarsamide.[2, 3] Prediction of which normal dog will get ill associated with this therapy cannot be determined based on testing. However, dogs are at risk of toxicity with compromised liver function, as evidenced by low serum albumin concentration, abnormal serum levels of bile acids, or elevated levels of ammonia in the blood. Increased liver enzyme activity in serum has not been predictive but provides a baseline if illness does occur during therapy. Use of melarsomine, which is less hepatotoxic, has decreased much of the concern of liver function testing before heartworm therapy.

CV

ELECTROCARDIOGRAPHY

Most dogs with heartworm disease have a normal ECG. If the dog is physically active and frequently attempts to generate increased cardiac output, the drive for right ventricular hypertrophy will generate a thickened right ventricular free wall and interventricular septum, resulting in a right-axis deviation (>100 degrees). Increased cardiac output causes the pulmonary arterial lesions to become more reactive and increases the severity of cor pulmonale. Although most dogs with significant right ventricular hypertrophy have pulmonary hypertension and increased pulmonary vascular resistance, some dogs with increases in pulmonary vascular resistance have normal ECGs because of their relative inactivity. Because the ECG reflects muscle mass, some dogs with dilated right ventricles and enlargement of right ventricles on radiographs may have normal ECGs.[3] Holter monitoring of dogs may reflect that during exercise, S-wave, ST-segment, and T-wave changes may occur with acute cor pulmonale. The abnormal vessel responsiveness of heartworm-infected dogs may show stress to hearts during exercise that is not recorded at rest.[61]

The ECG cannot be used to rule out heartworm disease. Classically, dogs presented with ascites associated with heartworms should have an abnormal ECG, reflecting a right ventricular hypertrophy pattern and/or an enlarged right ventricle on thoracic radiographs. However, the lack of or the degree of ECG changes does not correlate with heartworm numbers nor the prognosis for complications during therapy. A dog can have a large worm burden, which could provide a major complication when killed, yet have a normal ECG during evaluation.

THERAPY FOR HEARTWORM INFECTIONS IN DOGS

The therapeutic plan (Tables 119–6 to 119–8) after clinical evaluation includes adulticidal therapy, post-adulticide monitoring, microfilarial assessment and treatment, preventative medications, post-adulticidal efficacy evaluation, and re-evaluation of heartworm status 6 months to 1 year after initiation of therapy.

ADULTICIDES

Adulticidal therapy eliminates the adult parasite and allows the host to repair the damage where fibrosis has not occurred. The death of worms in both dogs and cats is associated with the most severe parenchymal lung injury and is proportional to the worm mass and rapidity of worm death.[34] The alternative of not treating the infection allows continued damage to the cardiovascular system, with the worms dying spontaneously and creating staged acute lung

TABLE 119–6. THERAPY FOR CANINE HEARTWORM DISEASE

1. Pre-treatment evaluation
2. Adulticide: 4–6 weeks of restricted exercise
3. Microfilaricide: 3 weeks after adulticide
4. Initiation of monthly macrolide
5. Post-microfilaricide microfilaria assay: 2 weeks
6. Antigen assay: 4–6 months after adulticide
7. Evaluation of heartworm status: 6–12 months

injury. The organic arsenical compounds thiacetarsamide and melarsomine are the only Food and Drug Administration (FDA)–approved adulticides. Regardless of the product administered, immature worms (4 to 6 months old) and female worms are more resistant to adulticides.[62, 63]

Thiacetarsamide

Thiacetarsamide (Caparsolate) has been used for many years with different vehicles and with varied dose recommendations (Table 119–9). However, consistent results have been lacking because of variable drug metabolism by individual dogs and age of worms being treated.[3] The drug must be stored under refrigeration, must be protected from light, and is caustic if administered subcutaneously. Because efficacy is directly related to blood concentrations after the end of a series of injection,[5] timing of dosing is an additional variable. The initial two doses should be administered not more than 10 hours apart to enhance the cumulative effects, and the overnight interval should not be more than 14 hours. Concomitant administration of glucocorticoids will decrease the efficacy of adulticidal activity. Hepatotoxic effects cannot be predicted in normal dogs, and the elevation of hepatic enzymes is common and does not preclude continuation of therapy. Vomiting after administration is common, and feeding 1 hour before injection is recommended. Icterus and persistent vomiting are indications to halt treatment. If treatment is interrupted for more than 18 hours, the total series of injections must be repeated. A single pre-treatment injection of thiacetarsamide to "prime the liver" for metabolism may result in enhanced metabolism that decreases therapeutic blood levels and efficacy. The importance of consistent blood concentrations was demonstrated when I removed worms 2 hours after the end of the fourth injection, rinsed the worms, and successfully transplanted them into other dogs with no death of worms. The dog should be monitored carefully during the first 2 to 3 days for hepatotoxicity. The microhematocrit tube will become yellow before the dog becomes clinically icteric. A 10 per cent higher dose has been associated with increased efficacy; however, toxicity is also more likely. Six injections over a 3-day period have been recommended but no improvement in adult worm kill occurs. Because of the caustic nature of the product, intravenous administration should be with a butterfly catheter or a different needle than was used to fill the syringe. If any extravasation is suspected, the area should be infiltrated with corticosteroids and Ringer's solution. Topical dimethyl sulfoxide should be applied for 24 hours. Severe edema, pain, and necrosis can result from even small amounts of extravascular thiacetarsamide.[2, 3, 62–64]

Because of the poor efficacy of thiacetarsamide against young worms, and especially female worms, this product has produced all female worm burdens, which, if microfilaremic previously, became occult, giving the illusion of successful treatment. Post-adulticidal antigen testing 4 months after adulticidal administration is required to document a successful therapy.

Melarsomine

Melarsomine (Immiticide) is effective at the recommended dose (Table 119–10) against both immature and mature heartworms. Melarsomine is distributed as a lyophilized powder in 50-mg vials that when rehydrated and refrigerated in the dark is stable for 24 hours. In addition to added

TABLE 119-7. DRUGS COMMONLY USED TO TREAT HEARTWORM DISEASE

DRUG/INTERVENTION	INDICATION	DOSAGE	COMPLICATIONS
Prednisolone	PTE Eosinophilic pneumonitis	1–2 mg/kg divided PO bid taper after clinical response	Potential to decrease adult worm kill, gastrointestinal ulceration
Heparin	PTE prevention and therapy of DIC	50–100 IU/kg SQ tid or dose sufficient to increase APTT to one and one-half to two times baseline, start 2 weeks before adulticide therapy and continue as long as 4 weeks after completion	Spontaneous hemorrhage
Melarsomine	Adulticide	2.5 mg/kg IM two injections 24 hours apart or 1 injection followed ≥30 days later by two injections 24 hours apart	Mild, local cellulitis, excessive salivation; PTE after worm death
Thiacetarsamide	Adulticide	2.2 mg/kg IV, two injections per day for 2 consecutive days, 8 hours between injections on the same day, no more than 15 hours between third and fourth injections	Severe cellulitis associated with extravasation; acute hepatic and/or renal dysfunction; PTE after adult worm death
Supplemental oxygen	PTE, CHF Pulmonary hypertension	40% Fio$_2$ via nasal insufflation or cage	Long-term exposure to 100% Fio$_2$ may cause lung injury
Hydralazine*	Pulmonary hypertension, CHF	0.5 mg/kg PO initial dose titrated to 0.5–2.0 mg/kg PO bid	Systemic hypotension Pulmonary hypertension Gastrointestinal: anorexia, vomiting
Diltiazem*	Pulmonary hypertension, CHF	1.0–1.5 mg/kg PO tid	Systemic hypotension
Digoxin†	Heart failure, supraventricular tachyarrhythmias	0.22 mg/M^2 PO bid or 0.005–0.01 mg/kg PO bid	Gastrointestinal: anorexia, vomiting Cardiac: ventricular arrhythmias, bradyarrhythmias
Furosemide‡	CHF	0.5–2.0 mg/kg PO sid-tid	Hypovolemia, electrolyte and acid-base abnormalities
Aspirin§	PTE—pre-treatment	3–10 mg/kg PO sid	Gastrointestinal ulceration, bleeding
Angiotensin-converting inhibitor	Severe hypertension and RVH		Renal complications
Cage confinement	Ascites Right-sided heart failure	30 days	Owner compliance

CHF = congestive heart failure; PTE = pulmonary thromboembolism; M^2 = body surface area in meter squared; DIC = disseminated intravascular coagulation; APTT = activated partial thromboplastin time; RVH = right ventricular hypertrophy.

*Data regarding the response to vasodilators is sparse and somewhat conflicting; individual variation is marked and caution should be taken not to cause systemic hypotension. This is especially important when using these drugs in combination with a diuretic.

†The efficacy of digoxin in severe heartworm disease is controversial; conservative dosing with frequent monitoring of serum digoxin levels is prudent; if ascites is present, an estimate of patient weight without ascites should be the basis for dosing.

‡High doses of diuretic should be avoided.

§The American Heartworm Society does not recommend the routine use of aspirin in dogs with heartworm disease.

efficacy, melarsomine is safer during the initial treatment period compared with thiacetarsamide. Compared with thiacetarsamide, melarsomine is significantly more expensive in large dogs. Because of the greater efficacy in dogs with large worm burdens, the complications of thromboembolism are greater. The dosing can be altered to avoid the significant acute lung injury by giving a single intramuscular injection and delaying the two injections over 24 hours to a later date, usually 1 month. The three-dose approach allows a staged kill in dogs with large worm burdens or severe cardiopulmonary disease. Melarsomine is rapidly absorbed from the intramuscular injection site and is rapidly eliminated as the unchanged drug and a major metabolite in the feces and a minor metabolite in urine. The drug should be administered deeply into the epaxial lumbar muscles. This site is recommended because of the good vascular supply and lymphatic drainage and the minimal clinical signs associated with the occasional local reaction. About one third of dogs demonstrate some degree of local pain, swelling, soreness on movement, and, on occasion, sterile abscessation. Injection site reactions regress within 6 to 12 weeks, and local fibrosis is uncommon. An increase in creatine kinase activity is noted in some dogs. A reaction after the initial injection may not be noted at other injection sites. Manufacturer recommendations as to needle size and site should be closely considered. Care to avoid depositing the product too close to transverse or dorsovertebral processes is important. Hepatic and renal

toxicity have not been noted when recommended doses are administered.[65-67] Complications are related to death of heartworms, and a staged kill will decrease this possibility. Although staging of dogs based on clinical signs is an initial step, it is imperative to emphasize that inactive dogs with minimal signs can still harbor significant worm burdens that at worm death can produce life-threatening severe lung injury.

Levamisole

Levamisole administered at an oral dose of 10 to 12 mg/kg per day for 30 days has been demonstrated to kill male worms and older female worms. The complications of drug toxicity and migration of adult worms, however, make this a poor choice as an adulticide. The use of this therapy does induce a microfilaria-negative dog and thus has been misrepresented as an "effective alternative" to arsenic compounds.[3]

MACROLIDES

Ivermectin combined with pyrantel (Heartgard Plus) has demonstrated a slow but significant adulticidal activity.[68] This product administered (6 μg/kg ivermectin with 5 mg/kg of pyrantel) for 16 consecutive months provided a significant

TABLE 119–8. SELECTED CANINE AND FELINE PARASITICIDES*†

DRUG	PROPRIETARY NAME	FORMULATIONS	DOSAGE	INDICATIONS	NOTES
Diethylcarbamazine	Carbam, Filaribits, Filaribits-Plus, several other formulations	Tablet, chewable tablet (various sizes), liquid	3 mg/lb daily for heartworm prevention and aid in control of gastrointestinal parasites; treatment of gastrointestinal parasites requires higher dosage	For prevention of heartworm (*Dirofilaria immitis*) infections and to aid in the treatment or control of *Toxocara canis* and *Toxascaris leonina* infections in dogs	Combined with oxibendazole in some formulations
Milbemycin oxime	Interceptor	Flavored tablet	0.5 mg/kg Re-treat at 1-month intervals	For prevention of heartworm disease, control of adult hookworm (*Ancylostoma caninum*) infection, and removal and control of adult roundworms (*Toxocara canis, Toxascaris leonina*) and whipworms (*Trichuris vulpis*) in adult dogs and puppies	
Ivermectin and Pyrantel	Heartgard Plus	Flavored chewable	6 µg/kg ivermectin and 5 mg/kg pyrantel Re-treat at 1-month intervals	To prevent heartworm (*Dirofilaria immitis*) disease and to treat and control ascarid (*Toxocara canis, Toxascaris leonina*) and hookworm (*Ancylostoma caninum*) infections in dogs	
Ivermectin	Heartgard for Cats	Flavored chewable	12 µg/kg ivermectin Re-treat at 1-month intervals	To prevent heartworm (*Dirofilaria immitis*) disease and to remove and control hookworms	

*Annotated list. Not all available parasiticides or formulations are presented. Always consult label for more definitive drug information.
†Some products may have been withdrawn from the market voluntarily by the sponsor.

TABLE 119–9. CHECKLIST FOR THIACETARSAMIDE (CAPARSOLATE) ADULTICIDE THERAPY

Before initiating treatment:
1. Confirm diagnosis.
2. Perform pre-treatment evaluation.
3. Manage any concurrent problems.

Initial thiacetarsamide dose:
1. Feed 30 to 60 minutes before treatment.
2. Clip and prepare vein.
3. Prepare syringe with thiacetarsamide dose (2.2 mg/kg) and syringe with saline flush.
4. Insert butterfly needle into vein; do not tape in place. If not successful on first attempt, use another vein.
5. Flush with saline to confirm venipuncture.
6. Inject thiacetarsamide, being careful that needle does not move.
7. Flush well with saline.
8. Remove needle and apply small pressure wrap to avoid hematoma.

For remaining injections:
1. Observe for vomiting, lethargy/depression, inappetence, fever, icterus, dehydration, and bilirubinuria. If present, therapy may need to be discontinued.
2. If no signs of toxicity, feed 30 to 60 minutes before injection; note appetite.
3. Examine previous venipuncture site; choose a different site for next injection. Injections should be given in alternate legs; subsequent injections in a previously used vein are given proximal to the first site if there is no evidence of inflammation.
4. Prepare and inject as for initial dose (steps 2 to 8).

---

reduction in worm counts, and the majority of parasites found were dead and degenerating as compared with findings in untreated dogs and in dogs treated with 500 μg/kg of milbemycin (Interceptor). Histologic changes were noted in parasites that had received the ivermectin. Although the use of ivermectin and pyrantel would suggest an alternative therapy in dogs with severe heartworm disease, allowing a very slow prolonged kill over a 1-year time period, the potential for progressive pulmonary vascular and parenchymal injury associated with this extremely slow kill has not been evaluated. Monthly administration of ivermectin provides an alternative therapeutic plan in dogs with other clinical diseases that preclude arsenical products. In addition, this approach after 6 months will eliminate the microfilaremia and remove the dog as a reservoir in the environment.

TABLE 119–10. CHECKLIST FOR MELARSOMINE (IMMITICIDE) ADULTICIDE THERAPY

Before initiating treatment:
1. Confirm diagnosis.
2. Perform pre-treatment evaluation and management.
3. Determine class (severity) of disease.
4. Determine Immiticide treatment regimen.

Standard treatment regimen (for class 1 and most class 2 dogs):
1. Draw 2.5 mg/kg of Immiticide into a syringe; attach a fresh, sterile 23-gauge needle: 1 inch (2.5 cm) long for dogs <10 kg or 1.5 inch (3.75 cm) long for dogs >10 kg.
2. Give by deep intramuscular injection into lumbar (epaxial) musculature in the L3 to L5 region; avoid subcutaneous leakage.
3. Repeat steps 1 and 2 at 24 hours after first dose; use opposite side for injection.
4. Enforced rest for 4 to 6 weeks minimum; symptomatic treatment as needed.

Alternate treatment regimen (for class 3 and some class 2 dogs):
1. Symptomatic treatment as needed; enforced rest.
2. When condition is stable, administer one dose of 2.5 mg/kg as described above in the standard treatment regimen.
3. Continue enforced rest and symptomatic treatment as needed.
4. One month later, administer two more doses, 24 hours apart, according to the standard treatment regimen.

SURGICAL REMOVAL

Surgical removal of heartworms has been performed for caval syndrome using forceps and a jugular venotomy[48] (Fig. 119–17). Direct removal of worms from the right ventricle, right atrium, and pulmonary arteries through a thoracotomy or with flexible forceps through the jugular vein is an expensive but attractive alternative in heavily parasitized dogs in which the risks of acute lung injury and thromboembolism are severe.[3, 69, 70] Care must be maintained not to crush or break the worms during removal, and chemotherapy is still required to remove residual worms.

MICROFILARICIDE THERAPY

Ivermectin and milbemycin are effective microfilaricidal drugs that are safe when administered to heartworm-negative dogs.[62] Reactions can be assumed to be associated with microfilarial death. Although it is generally assumed that dogs that have occult disease at the time of heartworm diagnosis do not require microfilaricide, on occasion, dogs receiving arsenical products will become microfilaremic. Dithiazanine iodide is effective when absorbed and eliminates adult heartworms; however, although it is the only FDA-approved drug for removal of microfilariae it is not currently available. There is no pathologic process associated with live microfilariae, and eliminating microfilariae before initiating adulticidal therapy has not been of benefit. Microfilarial size (>6 μm × >290 μm) dictates that these organisms must actively "swim" though capillary beds when alive. However, as they die, they become emboli in capillary beds throughout the body that must be phagocytized and removed over a period of several weeks. A moderately heavy microfilarial load in a 20-lb dog represents over 24 million such areas. Treatment of microfilariae is usually done 3 to 4 weeks after the last adulticidal therapy.[2, 3, 62] Rapid death of a large number of microfilariae with any agent will result in circulatory collapse, lethargy, retching, and shock. Less severe signs may only include lethargy, salivation, defecation, and tachycardia.[64] Most dogs that have the reaction are small dogs (<20 lb) and have large numbers of microfilariae (>40,000/mL), and the reaction occurs within 3 to 8 hours. Initiation of glucocorticoid therapy (prednisolone sodium succinate) and intravenous administration of lactated Ringer's solution usually avoids serious consequences. After a

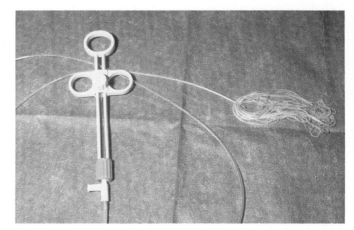

Figure 119–17. If heartworms are physically removed, care must be taken to ensure that heartworms are not crushed or broken because immediate shock often occurs.

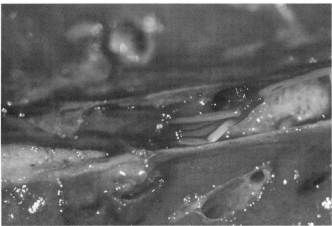

Figure 119–18. Although the death of heartworms in dogs is often considered a thromboembolic disease blocking arteries, the severe diffuse lung parenchymal damage is the critical life-threatening aspect of the event. Note the severe edema of the lung parenchyma both proximal and distal to the dying heartworm.

microfilaricide is administered, dogs should be observed for complications for 8 hours. Because of the inflammation associated with the death of microfilariae in all areas of the body, inflammatory granulomas can be found on biopsy samples of organs (e.g., brain, lung, lymph node, liver) for up to 1 month after microfilaricide therapy. Elevation of hepatic enzymes for 6 weeks has been associated with the continued inflammatory process.

Ivermectin has been administered in a single oral dose of 50 μg/kg as an effective microfilaricide and can be safely administered at this dose to collies. A common practice is to use the cattle product and dilute 1 mL of ivermectin (10 mg/mL) in 9 mL of propylene glycol and administer the mixture orally, 1 mL/9 lb of body weight. Milbemycin oxime at the current preventative dose (.5 mg/kg) is microfilaricidal and can be used as an alternative to ivermectin. Although microfilarial death is often rapid, most dogs are re-checked for the presence of microfilariae at 10 days to 2 weeks and repeatedly dosed every 2 weeks until they are negative for microfilariae. An added benefit of these two products is that they are preventative in their activity.

Other microfilaricidal drugs include levamisole and fen-thion. Levamisole (Levasol) at a single daily dose of 5 mg/lb/d for 7 to 14 days has been successfully used to eliminate microfilariae. The drug is rapidly absorbed and must be given with food. Vomiting, seizures, tremors, diarrhea, dementia, and bizarre behavior can develop. The tablet should not be crushed or crumbled because enhanced gastric absorption will increase toxicity. Fenthion (Spotton) has been used to eliminate microfilariae at a topical dose of 7 mg/lb once a week for up to three treatments.

POST-ADULTICIDAL COMPLICATIONS

The most serious complication of heartworm therapy occurs 2 to 3 weeks after adulticide administration. Acute lung injury is compounded by endothelial sloughing, pulmonary vascular obstruction, and intense platelet activation.[3] Dyspnea after adulticide therapy in dogs should be considered an emergency. Nasal oxygen and glucocorticoids are required to stabilize damaged lung parenchymal damage. Although the dogs may appear in shock, the cardiac output is usually maintained. Large volumes of intravascular colloids should not be administered, and central venous pressure must be carefully monitored. If significant pulmonary embolization with vascular occlusion has occurred, large volumes of fluids will increase end-diastolic right ventricular pressure, resulting in poor perfusion of the right ventricular free wall and myocardial failure.[71] Many dogs with severe thromboembolism have significant dyspnea and hypoperfused caudal lung lobes (Fig. 119–18). Most dogs with dying heartworms have significant activation of platelets[72] (Figure 119–19), which cannot be blocked with extremely high doses of aspirin. Thrombocytopenia (<100,000/μL) is common 2 to 3 weeks after adulticide administration in asymptomatic dogs with heartworms. If platelet counts below 100,000/μL are noted, dogs should be screened for disseminated intravascular coagulation. In the absence of disseminated intravascular coagulation, many dogs will respond to oxygen and glucocorticoid therapy within 24 hours. Because of the fragile nature of the capillary beds of the lungs, complete rest should be maintained[73] (Fig. 119–20).

After 24 hours of supplemental oxygen, partial pressures of oxygen below 70 mmHg reflect severe diffuse lung injury and often a poor prognosis. Heparin therapy, warfarin derivatives, and clot-lysing agents are ineffective. Slow-release

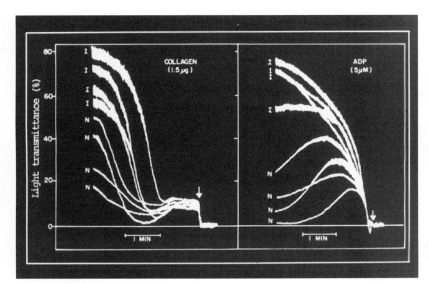

Figure 119–19. Platelet activation is noted in dogs with heartworm disease (HWI). Aspirin has not been successful in blocking the aggregation response even at high doses.

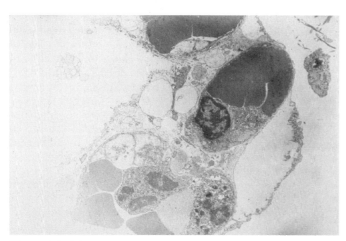

Figure 119–20. Transmission electron microscopy shows focal edema of alveolar area. Alveolar septal edema is noted by separation of endothelial cell from pneumocyte, and alveolar hemorrhage has occurred. This is typical of all dogs after heartworm death.

Anti-thrombotic agents have a potential benefit of reducing the severity of vascular lesions and blocking vasoconstrictive events. Aspirin may decrease myointimal proliferation from living worms after thiacetarsemide. These results have not been verified. Platelet activation cannot be blocked in dogs with heartworms after aspirin and dipyridamole therapy. The American Heartworm Society does not endorse anti-thrombotic therapy for routine treatment of heartworm disease in dogs.

Early aggressive intervention with glucocorticoids continues to provide the best clinical approach during the post-adulticidal period. Low alternate-day doses of corticosteroids have been advocated to treat the periarteritis in heartworm dogs, and these agents have definite indications in dogs with severe eosinophil pneumonitis.

The first 3 weeks are critical after adulticide. Residual worm fragments in small pulmonary arteries can be demonstrated for up to 6 weeks. Strict exercise restriction and maintaining a low cardiac output is important to facilitate lung repair rather than encourage fibrosis.[36, 41, 74, 75] The reversibility of pathology cannot be predicted based on initial radiographic pattern. Dogs with significant elevations in pulmonary vascular resistance at presentation have irreversible morphologic changes in the pulmonary beds. An intense response of the dog to worm death may alter the initial clinical impression that the disease state was mild. Because some of the cardiovascular response to heartworm disease is

calcium heparin (not commercially available in the United States) given subcutaneously did demonstrate some beneficial effects in severe heartworm infections, with a mortality of 2.5 per cent compared with 26 per cent in dogs receiving antiplatelet drugs[73] (Fig. 119–21).

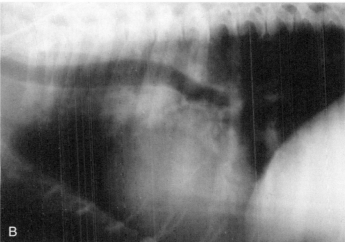

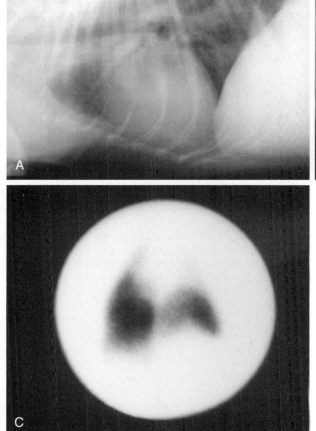

Figure 119–21. Lateral radiographs demonstrate that the thromboembolic disease is commonly associated with adulticidal therapy (A) and can cause severe embolization and occlusion of blood flow causing hypoperfusion of caudal lung lobes (B). These severe cases frequently have severe occlusion of blood flow, as demonstrated by hypoperfusion of caudal lung using gamma camera technique. Note lack of radioactivity in right caudal lung lobe from total occlusion (C).

vasoactive, not mechanical, and removal of the heartworms encourages repair, not fibrosis, most owners report clinical improvement after the successful removal of heartworms.

EVALUATION OF ADULTICIDAL THERAPY

A serologic assay for circulating adult heartworm antigen should be negative 5 to 6 months after successful adulticidal therapy.[3, 64] Many dogs will be negative as early as 4 months after therapy,[76] but testing can be delayed to avoid re-testing issues if positive.[77] If a positive test is reported, additional adulticidal therapy is usually delayed for 6 months to ensure that worms are older and more susceptible to arsenical compounds. If the dog has been administered monthly macrolides as preventative medication after adulticide, re-infection is uncommon. The decision to re-administer arsenical compounds depends on the dog's general health and activity. Athletic and performance dogs should be re-treated. Maintaining the dogs on Heartgard Plus to slowly kill residual adult worms over the next year is an alternative that may be considered in sedentary dogs.[77]

HEARTWORM PREVENTION

With current preventatives, which are 100 per cent efficacious and totally safe, a heartworm infection represents the absence of adequate veterinary care, as in mongrel dog populations, or the lack of adequate client compliance. The immunity of a dog or cat to heartworm disease is not permanent, and re-infection of a dog successfully treated but not placed on preventative medications is common in endemic areas. Dog and cat owners often need little inducement to use preventative medications when presented with the medical and financial consequences of treating an infection rather than prevention. The increased awareness of the general population via the popular media has alleviated the apparent self-promotional aspects of encouraging the owners to use preventative medications.

For a dog or cat to get heartworms, any one of several different species of mosquito has to bite a reservoir host with microfilariae (usually a dog, coyote, or fox), the mosquito has to live in a warm enough environment for the larvae to develop, and then that mosquito has to be willing to feed on the animal getting infected (e.g., dog, cat, ferret, fox, coyote, human). The feeding pattern of the mosquito dictates the incidence of infection in alternate hosts like ferrets and cats, not the rate of infection in the mongrel dog population. Research has revealed that the feeding preferences of different species of mosquitoes influence the alternate host disease.[78, 79]

Because the mosquito has to allow the microfilariae to migrate and develop in a warm moist environment, models have been developed to determine the area of the country where a mosquito, during its average life span of about 30 days, will be exposed to enough heat units to complete its part of the cycle.[80] In regions where average daily temperatures remain at or below about 62°F (17°C) from late fall to early spring, insufficient heat is available for the infective larvae to mature in the mosquito. This assumes that mosquitoes live in the environment and do not overwinter in warmer areas. However, this has led some to suggest that transmission is limited to only a few months in the most northern part of the United States and that year-round transmission is possible only in the far southern edges of the continental United States. Based on this model and considering only the prevention of heartworms, monthly preventative therapy would only be necessary from June through October or November in most of the country and from April through November or December for animals in the most southern third of the United States. Year-round monthly preventive therapy is often still considered prudent in many areas on the assumption of increased owner compliance, increased efficacy with year-round therapy if several doses are missed, and the combination of heartworm medications with other agents for continued control of fleas or intestinal parasites.

Preventative therapy should be initiated at 6 to 8 weeks of age and continued for the life of the animal in endemic areas. No tests are necessary at this age, and even if microfilariae were noted, the microfilariae would represent microfilariae that crossed the placenta from the bitch, and these would not develop into adults with or without the presence of preventative medication.[3, 61] Dogs presented at 6 months of age or older with no previous history of preventative medication should be evaluated with an antigen test and microfilarial assay. The owner should be advised that immature adults or pre-cardiac stages could still be present at this time, the testing may be negative, and adult heartworms may develop over the next several months while on preventative medication. The ability of macrolides administered for 1 year to kill 4-month-old larvae is an additional argument for year-round preventative medication.[81]

Three drugs are available for preventing cardiac stages of the adult heartworm: ivermectin, milbemycin oxime, and diethylcarbamazine (see Table 119–8). Ivermectin is effective in preventing heartworm infection if given monthly in doses of 2.7 μg/lb once every 30 days and is safe in collies. Ivermectin in doses of 23 μg/lb (frequently used microfilaricidal doses) has been safely used in susceptible collies. Milbemycin oxime is effective for preventing heartworm infection, and doses of 227 μg/lb once every 30 days are protective against infections. Milbemycin oxime is safe in collies; however, at the 227 μg/lb preventative dose, it has microfilaricide activity, and shock reactions can occur in dogs with large numbers of circulating microfilariae. The monthly medications are described as blocking the maturation of L3 and L4 larvae and affecting infections acquired during the past month. However, the actual death of the migrating larvae is delayed, and continued migration and maturation may occur for several more months. The continued survival of the larvae after the 30-day dosing explains why both dogs and cats can develop antibody titers when exposed to L3 larvae, although neither adult worms nor a positive antigenemia develops. The macrolides have varying degrees of activity against microfilariae, with the preventative dose of milbemycin oxime being filaricidal. However, because of activity on the reproductive tract of the adult parasites, most female heartworms develop embryo stasis after administration of 6 months of preventative macrolide medication. In most dogs, this induced occult status of the infection is not reversed when the preventative is not administered for another 6 months.[52, 82] Therefore, dogs that are presented for evaluation of heartworm status and are on a monthly heartworm preventative should be evaluated with an antigen assay.

Diethylcarbamazine (DEC) has been used for over 30 years for prevention of heartworm disease. An oral dose of 1.4 mg/lb of the active drug (3 mg/lb of the 50 per cent citrate) once per day will affect the L3 to L4 larval molt. Because this molt is 9 to 12 days after infection, DEC is administered year round or in colder climates 1 month before the mosquito season and discontinued 1 to 2 months after a killing frost. Although the medication is given daily, occasional failures occur and efficacy is not 100 per cent. Before starting DEC prevention and even after a lapse of therapy of as short as 3 days, a test for microfilariae is recommended. If DEC is administered to dogs with high numbers of microfilariae, an acute hypovolemic shock reaction may occur within 1 hour of administration.[3, 62] Immediate initiation of large volumes of intravenous fluids and glucocorticoid is usually successful. On occasion, disseminated intravascular coagulation and severe vasculitis will result in death. Microfilarial testing of dogs after a lapse of 3 days of therapy is done to detect dogs that have had adult heartworms for the past several months and in which the 3 days have allowed the addition of enough microfilariae that have not been previously exposed to DEC to initiate a reaction. Dogs presented for lapses of DEC therapy can be safely placed on macrolides for 1 year to retroactively eliminate infections acquired over the previous 3 to 4 months. Yearly evaluation of dogs on DEC should use both microfilaria testing and antigen testing. Dogs with occult heartworm disease may be given DEC, and therapy for dogs discovered to have heartworms while on daily doses of DEC can be safely continued as long as it is done daily during adulticidal therapy.[64] No reproductive abnormalities caused by DEC have been substantiated. The combination product of DEC and oxibendazole (Filaribits-Plus) has been marketed for use as a preventative for heartworms and hookworms in dogs. In a small percentage of dogs, acute and chronic hepatitis has developed, which may be irreversible and fatal even after only several doses. It is suggested that this product not be given to any breeds with histories of hepatic disease (e.g., Doberman, West Highland white, Bedlington terriers), to dogs with a history of hepatic disease, or to dogs being administered any hepatotoxic drugs (e.g., phenobarbital, anticonvulsants with phenobarbital metabolites, corticosteroids).

Moxidectin, a macrolide product not marketed, is a safe and 100 per cent preventative agent at 1.4 µg/lb given monthly or bimonthly up to 2 months' post infection. With some microfilaricidal effects at the preventative dose, there is no adverse reaction at 6.8 µg/lb the microfilaricidal dose.

Periodic re-testing of dogs is recommended. Heartworm antigen and microfilaria tests are recommended after 1 year to confirm a heartworm-negative status. Questions of when and how often to re-test contrast the 100 per cent efficacy of a product when re-testing would be unnecessary but for real world owner compliance estimated to be in the 50 per cent range. Annual re-testing is based on local practice standards, reliability of the client compliance, and product efficacy. If a dog is found to be antigen positive and is on monthly preventative medication, it is prudent to re-test the dog. Monthly preventative agents have 100 per cent efficacy, even when occasional months are missed. Positive antigen tests assume lack of owner compliance or underdosing because of weight change. Dogs on DEC should be tested by both microfilarial concentration methods and antigen testing.

CLINICAL ASPECTS OF FELINE HEARTWORM DISEASE

The clinical signs and diagnostic approach for heartworm disease are different in the cat as compared with those in the dog. New techniques and methodologies have now made the cat owner and veterinarian better able to be aware of this potentially severe disease.

RISK FACTORS

Cats are at risk of heartworm disease if there are dogs in the area with heartworms. There is no age predilection to *D. immitis* infection in cats, and a wide age range of clinically infected cats is reported (6 months to 17 years). Indoor and outdoor cats have been presented for feline heartworm disease.[16, 38, 83] In a clinical survey of 215 cats presented for coughing, vomiting, or dyspnea, 11 per cent of the antibody-positive cats were reported to be 100 per cent indoors and 35 per cent were reported to be less than 10 per cent outdoors.[84] The infection of indoor cats may reflect an altered feeding pattern of the vector or an increased susceptibility of a heartworm-naive cat to infection.[17]

Males are more susceptible than females in experimental and clinical cases and harbor a higher worm burden when infected.[12, 16] Feline leukemia virus infection is not a predisposing factor, and heartworms are not a common incidental finding.[85, 86]

CLINICAL SIGNS

Clinical signs are dependent on the stage of the heartworm life cycle. Infected cats may die acutely, exhibit chronic signs, or be asymptomatic (Table 119–11). Arrival of immature heartworms in the lungs and death of adults are the stages most likely to be associated with early clinical signs. The initial arrival (as early as 100 days after infection) of the L5 larvae in the distal pulmonary arteries induces a diffuse pulmonary infiltrate and signs typical of "eosinophilic pneumonitis."[7, 20, 86, 87] The initial respiratory clinical signs the owner may report as coughing, occur most frequently in the 4 to 7 months after the exposure. At this time, because the worms are immature, antigen tests are negative. After the initial host response, the signs may abate and become subclinical for a period of time. Based on cardiopulmonary changes and experimental studies, most heartworm cats even with severe heartworm disease are asymptomatic once the infection becomes established.[7, 86, 88] Subsequent death of adult heartworms may cause additional severe signs. In acute cases, death may be so rapid as to preclude diagnosis or treatment. Sudden death has been attributed to pulmonary congestion, edema, circulatory collapse, and respiratory failure from acute pulmonary arterial infarction and acute lung injury.[7] Acute collapse may occur with or without previous clinical signs, and one worm can be the cause. Cats that die of heartworm infection can be clinically normal 1 hour before death.[16] All cats with peracute death in heartworm endemic areas should be examined for heartworm disease. The worms in the acute syndrome can be in the distal (usually caudal) pulmonary arteries.

TABLE 119–11. CLINICAL SIGNS OF FELINE HEARTWORM DISEASE

CHRONIC SIGNS	ACUTE SIGNS
Coughing*	Convulsions
Dyspnea*	Vomiting/diarrhea
Vomiting*	Collapse
Lethargy	Blindness
Weight loss	Anorexia
Chylothorax	Tachycardia
	Syncope

*Most common presentation.

Although less common, the aberrant locations of immature L5 larvae or adult worms have been associated with neurologic signs.[89] Seizures, head tilt, blindness, ataxia, and acute vestibular syndrome have been recorded.[16, 90] Presentation of acute posterior paresis from an aortic location has been rarely observed. The novelty of unusual presentations of cats with feline heartworm disease has jaded the literature relative to the true nature of the spontaneous disease.

HISTORY

The most common historical complaints in cats with clinical signs are coughing, dyspnea, vomiting, lethargy, anorexia, and weight loss[16, 83, 90] (see Table 119–11). In a clinical survey of 215 cats presented to 15 practices in the southeastern United States for signs of feline heartworm disease, the antibody-positive cats (92) were presented for coughing (39 per cent), vomiting (24 per cent), or vomiting and respiratory signs (34 per cent).[35]

Vomiting of food and/or foam (rarely bile stained) tends to be sporadic and usually unrelated to eating. The etiology of vomiting in heartworm cats is unknown, although the release of inflammatory mediators from the lungs that stimulates the chemoreceptor trigger zone has been hypothesized.[16] Supporting this concept is the clinical observation that low doses of corticosteroids (2.5 to 5 mg of prednisolone every other day) usually prevent the vomiting. Retching and severe paroxysmal vomiting is unusual. Heartworm disease should be included in the differential diagnosis of chronic emesis in the cat.

Coughing and intermittent dyspnea are common; hemoptysis is less common. Severe paroxysmal coughing attacks, with periods of normalcy (days to weeks), occur. Coughing is usually temporarily corticosteroid responsive, with exacerbation and acute dyspnea still a risk. Chylothorax has been noted but is not common.

The clinical presentation, radiographic pattern, and response to therapy often lead to a tentative diagnosis of bronchial asthma.[16, 91] The acute dyspnea may be a result of acute lung injury especially associated with worm death. On occasion, occlusion of a pulmonary artery (right caudal being the most common) is accompanied by a radiographic appearance of lung lobe consolidation and the development of life-threatening acute dyspnea.[92–94]

The non-specific clinical signs are consistent with those of many feline diseases. Anorexia and/or lethargy can be the only presenting signs in cats with heartworms. In these cases, heartworm disease is often an incidental finding on thoracic radiographs during diagnostic screening. Cats with worms found in abnormal locations may have signs attributable to local pathology. Neurologic signs are uncommon but can occur in infected cats with or without worms in the central nervous system.

The residual damage associated with feline heartworm disease is difficult to document clinically or experimentally. There are few long-term studies.[7] I have evaluated clinical cats with feline heartworm disease 1 to 2 years after the cats become antibody negative that continue to have radiographic evidence of peribronchial disease and require corticosteroid therapy to prevent coughing. The relationship with bronchial asthma after elimination of the heartworms remains unanswered. Proteins of excretory/secretory materials from heartworms have been associated with increased lymphocyte cytokine production and increased immunoglobulin response to vaccine challenge in cats.[95]

PHYSICAL EXAMINATION

The physical examination is usually normal in *D. immitis*–infected cats. A systolic murmur over the tricuspid valve area and occasionally a gallop rhythm can be present, but, as a general rule, these findings are uncommon. In cats presented with murmurs, only 9 per cent were positive for heartworms. Harsh lung sounds (dry rales) are the most frequent abnormal auscultatory finding and can be present in cats without respiratory signs. Ascites, chylothorax, exercise intolerance, and signs of right-sided heart failure are rare. There does not seem to be a correlation between the clinical signs, physical findings, and radiographic findings.

DIAGNOSIS

Unlike the diagnostic approach in dogs, the diagnostic modalities are less clearly defined and none are without exception. If one defines feline heartworm disease related to the life cycle, diagnostic findings can change chronologically (Figs. 119–22 to 119–27).

Complete Blood Cell Counts

Routine complete blood cell counts may demonstrate a mild anemia (hematocrit: 23–33 per cent), occasionally nucleated red blood cells, and basophilia (rare). Anemia in about one third of infected cats is non-regenerative, as in heartworm-positive dogs. Peripheral eosinophilia is an inconsistent finding even on serial samples in the same cat and is dependent on the stage of the infective larvae. The eosinophilia typically occurs 4 to 7 months after infection and intermittently thereafter.[7, 97, 98] The absence of eosinophilia does not exclude a diagnosis of feline heartworms. Cytology of bronchial alveolar lavage fluid may contain eosinophils without the presence of a peripheral eosinophilia. As in the dog, the presence of basophilia is highly suggestive of heartworm disease.[35, 84]

Tracheal Cytology

The finding of eosinophils on cytologic evaluation of tracheal lavage fluid is common in cats with heartworm disease, asthma, and parasitic lung diseases and in healthy

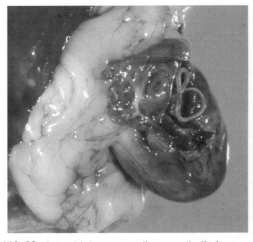

Figure 119–22. Cats with heartworm disease typically have one to three worms found as adults in pulmonary arteries and right ventricle.

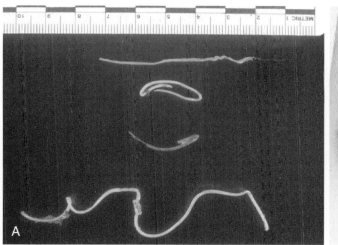
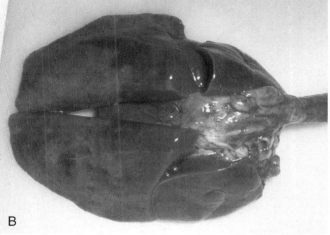

Figure 119–23. Associated with heartworm death (A), one adult female and one degenerating male worm; the reaction of the entire lung parenchyma is an intense inflammatory response (B).

CV

cats.[96] In feline heartworm disease, the presence of eosinophils in the tracheal lavage fluid seems to occur 4 to 7 months after L3 larval infection and often may not be present later in the infection even when adult worms are present. Tracheal cytology typical of chronic inflammation may be present after the eosinophilic reaction resolves. Careful fecal examination should be performed before the lavage. Fecal flotation and direct smears may reveal the large operculated egg of *Paragonimus kellicotti* or the larvae of *Aelurostrongylus abstrusus*.

Blood Chemistries and Urinalysis

Results of blood chemistries and urinalysis are usually normal. Hyperglobulinemia is neither consistent nor predictable and should not be used to rule out feline heartworm disease. Proteinuria has not been associated with feline heartworm disease.[16, 94]

Detection of Microfilariae

Experimental infections produced by L3 larvae or transplantation of adults usually result in a microfilaremia of short duration and low numbers.[12] Concentration tests such as Knott tests or millipore filter techniques are best. In North and South America, the only filarial disease of cats is heartworm infection; therefore, any microfilariae observed should be considered *D. immitis*.

Serology

The confusion over the interpretation of the different tests and the variability of the methodology of individual laboratories has caused the practicing veterinarian problems in making a definitive diagnosis. With the high incidence of occult disease in the cat, the use of serology is a valuable asset.

Three serologic methods have been used to assess feline

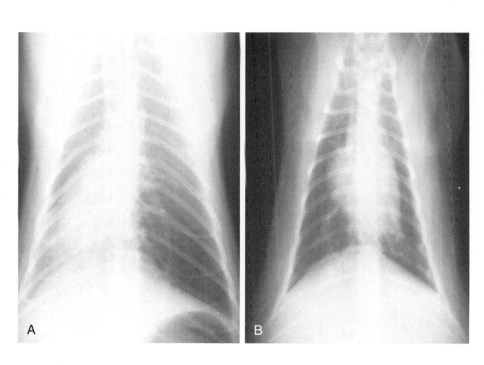

Figure 119–24. Ventrodorsal radiograph of a cat presented for acute dyspnea. The left caudal lung is edematous on presentation (A) but responds to 2 days of corticosteroid and oxygen therapy (B), at which time the enlarged caudal lobar arteries can be visualized.

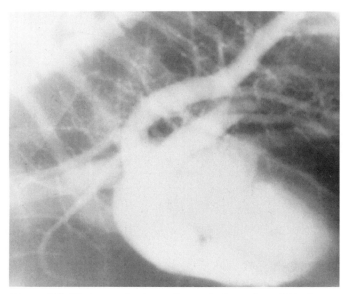

Figure 119–25. A non-selective angiogram in the cat is useful in demonstrating abnormal pulmonary arteries and requires no special equipment.

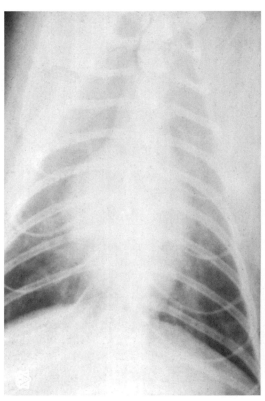

Figure 119–27. Many of the cats with early lesions of heartworm disease do not have enlarged pulmonary arteries, and only a diffuse infiltrative lung disease will be observed.

heartworm disease: immunofluorescence for microfilarial antibody, detection of host antibody against adult, and adult antigen detection by ELISA and colloid gold.

Immunofluorescence Testing. Application of the canine immunofluorescence test (detecting antibodies to microfilarial cuticular antigen) was useful in early research and

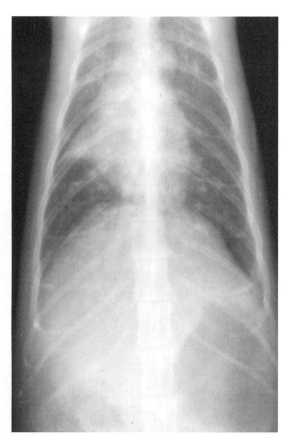

Figure 119–26. Many cats with heartworms continue to have clinical signs typical of asthma years after heartworm disease and may have peribronchial infiltration noted through the lung. In this cat, a collapsed right middle lung lobe, an occasional finding, is observed.

approximately diagnostic in about 33 per cent of cats with adult heartworms, but the presence of immature or sterile worms, worms of only one sex, or the absence of host response to antigen does not produce a diagnostic titer.[16, 99] These assays have been helpful in researching the biology of the parasite-host interaction but have limited application to clinical diagnostics. Use of anti–*D. immitis* antibody to somatic antigens has been re-introduced but has not been independently validated.

Antibody Detection. The detection of feline antibodies to adult heartworm antigen has advantages over antigen testing in cats that demonstrate clinical signs consistent with feline heartworm disease. Initial concerns related to false-positive results from cross-reactivity have not been observed. Initial studies of cats that have eliminated the adult parasite naturally or after adulticide reveals that a negative titer develops when the host antibody gradually decreases to negative concentrations (4 to 6 months). The antibody denotes a method of analysis; therefore, antigen preparation, antibody sources, and techniques can vary between diagnostic laboratories; and titers may differ accordingly. Because the antibody being detected is produced by the cat in response to the early migration of the L3 or L4 larvae, positive titers are detected 2 to 3 months after a successful infection on about 50 per cent of cats and is consistently positive by 5 months.[56, 84, 100, 101] Detection of antibodies in symptomatic cats does confirm a successful infection of the L3–L4 larval stages.

With the use of macrolides as preventative medication, the larvae in a cat can initiate a positive antibody response and then can be killed by the macrolide, leading to an antibody-positive but heartworm-negative outcome. Additionally, the death of adult heartworms may produce a strong antibody response after release of large amounts of antigen. Some of the highest titers are associated with severe clinical signs in cats in which the worms have died and in which the disease may be resolving.[84] In rare cases, the antibody test result can be negative even in the presence of adult worms. Of the different antibody tests currently available, there are differences in the antibody that each appears to quantitate. There appears to be no correlation between antibody levels and the number of worms or severity of disease in the initial studies based on antibody titers by Animal Diagnostics, Inc., St. Louis, Missouri. Detection of high concentrations of antibody to recombinant heartworm antigen by Heska Co., Fort Collins, Colorado, has been noted in some cats with larger adult worm burdens.[102] I have observed confirmed cases of heartworms that are antibody negative by all current assays. Early evidence suggests that during an active heartworm infection, the currently available antibody detection methods are triggered by different antigens; thus, discordant results between two antibody testing methods should not surprise the veterinarian. Serial testing frequently yields a negative test result that becomes positive 1 to 3 months later. Based on initial impressions, after an L3 larval infection, the polyclonal antibody detected by Animal Diagnostics is noted 1 to 2 months before the antibody detected by Heska Co. Although this indicates early infection, neither test result indicates adult infection.

A positive antibody result shows that the cat has been successfully infected with L3 larvae, that an L4 larval molt has occurred, and that the larvae have lived at least 2 to 3 months and may or may not have developed into adult heartworms.[12, 56] The duration of continued antibody response in a cat with a chronic adult infection (i.e., a cat with a 2-year heartworm infection) cannot be confirmed using all testing methods at this time. Because the antibody detection is specific for feline antibody, these methods cannot be used in other species.

Antigen Testing. Heartworm antigen detection tests utilizing blood or serum have been successful in dogs and have been positive in cats within days of transplantation of mature adult worms from dogs into cats.[39] Because the antigen being detected is derived primarily from the adult female reproductive tract, immature infections, a low worm burden, male-only infections, or sexually immature worms will not produce enough antigen to be detected. The elimination of the adult parasite will also cause a negative antigen test result.[5]

Cats may develop positive antigen tests 8 months after the experimental infections with large numbers of L3 larvae.[5, 12] However, clinical cats and experimentally infected cats with active heartworm disease and high antibody titers can be negative on antigen testing.[5] The low heartworm numbers in clinical infections and the clinical signs associated with immature worms make it prudent to consider a positive antigen test diagnostic but not to rule out heartworms based on a negative result of an antigen test. Most cats with heartworm disease are antigen negative. Of the different assays for antigen in the blood, each should be reviewed for strengths and weaknesses. Data would support the basic consideration that a microwell titer technology on serum is the best to detect low antigen concentrations.

Electrocardiography

Although subtle signs of right ventricular enlargement are occasionally noted (with unipolar chest leads) a right-axis vector (>120 degrees) on a standard six-lead ECG is rare.

Ectopic ventricular beats and other arrhythmias have been infrequently noted after adulticide in asymptomatic cats.

Radiography

The pulmonary parenchymal changes are non-specific and can change rapidly in infected cats.[39, 86, 88, 103] The lung lesions include diffuse or coalescing infiltrates, perivascular densities, and lung atelectasis. The most distinctive radiographic sign is enlarged pulmonary arteries with ill-defined margins, most prominent in the caudal lung lobes on the ventrodorsal view. Blunting and tortuosity of the pulmonary arteries are occasionally seen but are not as common in cats as in dogs. An enlarged main pulmonary arterial segment extending beyond the cardiac border on the ventrodorsal or dorsoventral view is not a classic feature of feline heartworm disease. The enlargement of the caudal pulmonary artery may disappear over a period of several months. Some cats with heartworm disease have normal radiographs. Severe infiltrative disease may also inhibit visualization of the pulmonary arteries. After an acute episode, a lung lobe (left caudal, right caudal, right middle) may appear consolidated. The pulmonary interstitial edema and hemorrhage is often corticosteroid responsive. Atelectasis of the right middle lung lobe appears to be less likely to resolve and may become permanent.

Arteriograms as a diagnostic tool may demonstrate the enlarged pulmonary arteries and embolus.[39] A non-selective angiocardiogram is a simple and safe method of confirming a tentative diagnosis of heartworms. A radiographic exposure 5 to 6 seconds after injection of a contrast material into the jugular vein will provide good visualization of the pulmonary vasculature and on occasion the presence of worms. There does not seem to be a correlation between the severity of lesions based on angiocardiogram and the severity of clinical signs or post-adulticide reaction. Because of the changing nature of the disease over time, repeated radiographs are often necessary.

Echocardiography

Parallel hyperechoic lines, representing an image from the heartworm cuticle, may be observed in the pulmonary arteries, right ventricle, or, rarely, the right atria.[104, 105] These lines are generally not over 0.5 to 1 cm in length because of the angle of the probe and curved nature of the worms in the heart. Heartworms in the most distal pulmonary arteries often cannot be visualized. Echocardiography is useful to confirm a tentative diagnosis of heartworms.[59] The right parasternal view gives the best view of the pulmonary outflow tract,[58] the most common location of the adult worm.

DIFFERENTIAL DIAGNOSIS

In the cat with respiratory signs, heartworm disease must be differentiated from *Aelurostrongylus abstrusus* or *Paragonimus kellicotti* infection, asthma, cardiomyopathy, and other diseases associated with dyspnea (e.g., pyothorax, pleural effusion, pneumothorax, feline infectious peritonitis [FIP], lymphosarcoma, anemia). Although each in various stages can mimic the clinical and radiographic pulmonary parenchymal changes, the pulmonary arterial changes of heartworm disease are unique, if present, and can be enhanced by use of contrast agents. The changing clinical and radiographic pattern of disease makes the diagnosis difficult,

CV

and over the time course of the disease there will be differences in diagnostic results. The peripheral eosinophilia, eosinophilic tracheal cytology, and chronic cough of the cat with feline heartworm disease is consistent with a diagnosis of "bronchial asthma." However, an apparent higher incidence of asthma has not been reported in heartworm endemic areas.

CLINICAL MANAGEMENT OF FELINE HEARTWORM DISEASE

After the diagnosis of feline heartworm disease, the veterinarian and client are in a lose-lose proposition. Conservative management of adult worms allow them to die spontaneously over months to years with the risk of chronic problems and/or an acute crisis. The aggressive approach is to use an adulticide to eliminate the worms and risk the severe consequences of acute complications associated with the worm(s) dying at one time. Because of the dire consequences of management of feline heartworm disease, preventative medication for cats is recommended if heartworm-infected dogs are in the area.

THERAPY FOR HEARTWORM-POSITIVE CATS

Owners' attitudes dictate the approach to therapy. Because cats with heartworm disease are often asymptomatic or demonstrate only chronic vomiting or intermittent respiratory signs, the owner must be reminded that this is a serious disease. Owners should be reminded that spontaneous acute complications and death do occur in a small percentage of cats with heartworms.

No relationship has been detected between the clinical signs and risk of acute complications. Because the adult heartworm has a shortened longevity in the cat compared with the dog, the possibility of spontaneous recovery should also be discussed. Although the natural death of the adult worms can be associated with severe respiratory signs, most cats will recover without severe complications. Cats managed conservatively by intermittent corticosteroid therapy still are at risk for acute signs. In the cat with recurrent dyspnea that is life threatening or with clinical signs that are unacceptable to the owner, adulticidal therapy has been used safely and should be considered.

ADULTICIDAL THERAPY

Treatment of feline heartworm disease with thiacetarsamide sodium (1 mg/lb IV, bid for 2 days) is tolerated by cats without immediate complications of hepatotoxicity or renal toxicity. Concerns as to a direct acute lung injury from thiacetarsamide in normal cats causing pulmonary edema and respiratory failure[106] could not be reproduced in studies in 12 normal cats.[107] The use of ketamine as a sedative to aid in careful administration of thiacetarsamide is recommended in active cats. There are reports of acute symptoms after thiacetarsamide injection, but slow injections have not caused acute collapse in normal healthy cats in my experience. Although the presence of circulating microfilaria is uncommon, ivermectin has been used successfully as a microfilaricide.

POST-ADULTICIDAL COMPLICATIONS

Complications after therapy are usually related to acute lung injury associated with dying heartworms. Sudden death from respiratory failure can occur especially within the first 10 days after adulticide administration. Embolization can induce severe lung injury, hemoptysis, and dyspnea. Severe thrombocytopenia and disseminated intravascular coagulation have not been noted. Based on the assumption that heartworm mass is related to antigen load, a cat with a "strong positive" antigen test would be more likely to develop post-adulticide complications. Worm death most often affects the caudal lung lobes, and thoracic radiographs may demonstrate a lung lobe with increased density. Oxygen therapy is indicated if dyspnea occurs. High doses of corticosteroids (1 to 2 mg/lb of prednisolone three times a day) with careful intravenous fluid therapy can support the cat through the crisis. The routine use of corticosteroids is not recommended before or after therapy with thiacetarsamide in cats. Use of aspirin is not indicated in feline heartworm disease.[108] Because of the potential protective effects of ketamine as a serotonin antagonist, a single intramuscular injection of ketamine has been recommended before administration of the first dose of thiacetarsamide. The acute nature of the post-adulticide reaction dictates that the cat be under 24-hour per day observation, especially during the first 2 weeks. The clinical and radiographic signs of acute embolization can resolve over 1 to 2 days. However, death can occur before therapy can be instituted. The client should be aware that the risk of complications in the cat seems to be greater than in the dog. The severity of a post-adulticidal reaction poses a dilemma for the veterinarian, and the risk of post-adulticide complications is probably greater than the risk of spontaneous death in the asymptomatic, heartworm-infected cat. The advantage of treating a cat is being able to observe the cat while the worms are dying compared with waiting for spontaneous death of worms. However, adulticidal therapy in one study did not increase mean survival time in cats administered an adulticide compared with conservative therapy.[83] Owners should be advised that 30 per cent of cats receiving adulticidal therapy will have a life-threatening crisis within 3 weeks of therapy.[16]

EFFICACY OF TREATMENT

The efficacy of thiacetarsamide cannot be evaluated because of the occult nature of the disease. Current research seems to indicate that the adulticide is effective, and clinical signs usually abate during the initial weeks after thiacetarsamide.[3] Based on data in dogs, immature worms are probably resistant to thiacetarsamide. If a cat was antigen positive before therapy, the antigen test should be negative 12 weeks after successful adulticide therapy. Data on immiticide use in feline heartworm disease is limited,[109] but anecdotal reports would advise against using the dog protocol.

SURGICAL THERAPY

Removal of heartworms by jugular venotomy has been used successfully with an endoscopic basket[110] and by wrapping the heartworms with horsehair brushes or Swan-Ganz balloon flotation catheters. More invasive is a thoracotomy and removal of the heartworms by right ventricular incision or pulmonary arteriotomy. Invasive surgery should be reserved for cats in which heartworms have been visualized by echocardiography.[111]

CONSERVATIVE THERAPY

The owner should be educated as to the nature of the peracute signs of heartworm disease. Alternate-day prednisolone therapy (1–2 mg/lb) has been used successfully to prevent clinical signs of coughing and vomiting. Progression of radiographic lesions has been observed during corticosteroid therapy. Acute respiratory distress and death have occurred in cats on conservative glucocorticoid therapy. An emergency dose of oral or injectable glucocorticoid should be dispensed to the owner to be administered if collapse or dyspnea is noted. The onset of acute respiratory signs in a cat with heartworms is a true emergency requiring immediate care. The radiographic signs of severe lung pathology should not be overinterpreted as "consolidation or pneumonia." The initiation of intranasal oxygen therapy, cage rest, small volumes of intravenous fluids, and injectable prednisolone (100–250 mg prednisolone sodium succinate) has resulted in clinical improvement and resolution of radiographic signs within 24 hours of presentation in cats with life-threatening dyspnea and collapse.

Subtle respiratory signs should be treated aggressively in heartworm-positive cats. Serial antibody testing (at 6-month intervals) can be used to assess the heartworm status. Generally, cats that have eliminated the adult infection will be antibody negative 6 to 9 months after all adult worms are removed.

PREVENTATIVE MEDICATION

In endemic areas with vector populations (dogs) providing the mosquito with a reservoir, the incidence of heartworms in cats and the dire consequences of the infection indicate that preventive medication is warranted. Studies in most endemic areas indicate an infection rate, based on necropsy data, of 2.5 per cent to 16 per cent, with a median of 7 per cent.[13] The antibody test results have been reported as 15 to 35 per cent, positive, reflecting successful infection of L3 larvae, molting of L4 larvae, and survival for at least 2 to 3 months.[112, 113] Of 215 cats presented to 15 practices in southeastern United States for vomiting or respiratory signs, 43 per cent were antibody positive and 11 per cent were 100 per cent indoors and 35 per cent were less than 90 per cent outdoors. One third of cats with feline heartworm disease are considered indoor cats by their owners.[100–102]

Ivermectin (10 mg/lb)[114] and milbemycin (227 mg/lb)[115] administered orally once a month safely prevent heartworm infections in cats. Heartgard for Cats (25 μg/kg of ivermectin) has been marketed for use in cats. In endemic areas, it is suggested that preventative medication be administered at 4 to 6 weeks of age and continued for the life of the cat. Although heartworm disease may be of low incidence in many areas, the high rate of complications associated with feline heartworm disease makes preventative medication an attractive alternative.

Because current antigen testing is inconsistent in cats, especially those with a low worm burden, antigen testing before instituting preventative therapy in an adult cat would not seem to be cost effective. Use of antibody testing would be positive if the cat had been successfully infected and the heartworm had lived at least 2 to 3 months, but it does not equate with status of adult infections. Furthermore, a heartworm-positive cat even with microfilariae can be safely administered Heartgard for Cats.[114] Regardless of the results of any of the serodiagnostics, a cat can be safely placed on preventative medication. The diagnostics would aid the owner and veterinarian in knowing the risk of infection in the cat. If either antigen or antibody positive, additional diagnostics could be pursued.

The status of diagnostics before preventative medication will continue to evolve as diagnostic modalities become more refined. After a cat has been on preventative medication and if exposed to L3 larvae, the larvae may live long enough to induce a positive antibody response but an infection with adult worms would not develop. The antibody test would have limited application in yearly re-checks of cats.

Although heartworm disease can be self-limiting in many cats, the potential for it to initiate inflammatory lung disease and predispose to continued respiratory disease may prove to be adequate indications for use of preventative medications in cats in endemic areas.

REFERENCES

1. Travassos LP: Notas helmintolicas. Brazil-Med 35:67, 1921.
2. Atwell RB, Boreham PFL (eds): Dirofilariasis. Queensland, Australia, CRC Press, 1988.
3. Rawlings CA: Heartworm Disease in Dogs and Cats. Philadelphia, WB Saunders, 1986.
4. Slocombe JOD, Surgeoner CA, Srivastava B: Determination of heartworm transmission period and its use in diagnosis and control. In Otto GF (ed): Proceedings of the Heartworm Symposium '89, Charleston, SC. Washington, DC, American Heartworm Society, 1989, pp 19–26.
5. McCall JW, Guerrero J, Supakorndej P, et al: Evaluation of the accuracy of antigen and antibody tests for detection of heartworm infection in cats (abstract). In: Proceedings of the Heartworm Symposium '98. Orlando, FL, American Heartworm Society, 1998, p 32.
6. McCall JW, McTier TL Supakorndej N, et al: Clinical prophylactic activity of macrolides on young adult heartworms. In Soll MD, Knight DH (eds): Proceedings of the Heartworm Symposium '95, Auburn, Alabama. Batavia, IL, American Heartworm Society, 1995, pp 187–195.
7. Dillon AR, Brawner WR, Grieve RB, et al: The chronic effects of experimental Dirofilaria immitis infection in cats. Vet Med Surg 2:72–77, 1987.
8. Dillon AR, Brawner WR, Hanrahan L: Influence of number of parasites and exercise on the severity of heartworm disease in dogs. In Soll MD, Knight DH (eds): Proceedings of the Heartworm Symposium '95, Auburn, Alabama. Batavia, IL, American Heartworm Society, 1995, p 113.
9. Donahoe JM: Experimental infection of cats with D. immitis. J Parasitol 61:599–605, 1975.
10. Fowler JL, Matsuda K, Fernau RC: Experimental infection of the domestic cat with D. immitis. JAVMA 8:79–80, 1972.
11. Mansour AE, McCall JW, McTier TL, et al: Epidemiology of feline dirofilariasis: Infections induced by simulated natural exposure to Aedes aegypti experimentally infected with heartworms. In Soll MD, Knight DH (eds): Proceedings of the Heartworm Symposium '95, Auburn, Alabama. Batavia, IL, American Heartworm Society, 1995, pp 87–95.
12. McCall JW, Nonglak S, Ryan W, et al: Utility of an ELISA-based antibody test for detection of heartworm infection in cats. In Soll MD, Knight DH (eds): Proceedings of the Heartworm Symposium '95, Auburn, Alabama. Batavia, IL, American Heartworm Society, 1995, pp 127–133.
13. Ryan WG, Newcomb KM: Prevalence of feline heartworm disease—a global review. In Soll MD, Knight DH (eds): Proceedings of the Heartworm Symposium '95, Auburn, Alabama. Batavia, IL, American Heartworm Society, 1995, pp 79–86.
14. Hayasaki M: Re-migration of fifth-stage juvenile Dirofilaria immitis into pulmonary arteries after subcutaneous transplantation in dogs, cats, and rabbits. J Parasitol 82:835–837, 1996.
15. Donahoe JM, Kneller SK, Lewis RD: In vivo pulmonary arteriography in cats infected with D. immitis. J Am Vet Radiol Soc 17:147–151, 1976.
16. Dillon AR: Feline heartworms: More than just a curiosity. Vet Forum, December 1995, pp 18–26.
17. Genchi C, Di Sacco B, Cancrin G, et al: Epizootiology of canine and feline heartworm infections in Northern Italy: Possible mosquito vectors. In Soll MD, Knight DH (eds): Proceedings of the Heartworm Symposium '95, Auburn, Alabama. Batavia, IL, American Heartworm Society, 1995, pp 39–46.
18. Labarthe N, Serrão ML, Melo YF, et al: Heartworm in the state of Rio de Janeiro, Brazil (abstract). In: State of the Heartworm Symposium '98, Orlando, FL. Batavia, IL, The American Heartworm Society, 1998, p 18.
19. Elkins AD, Kadel W: Feline heartworm disease and its incidence in western Kentucky. Comp Small Anim Pract 10:585–590, 1988.
20. Wong MM, Pedersen NC, Cullen J: Dirofilariasis in cats. J Am Anim Hosp Assoc 19:855–864, 1983.
21. Calvert CA, Rawlings CA: Pulmonary manifestations of heartworm disease. Vet Clin North Am 15:991, 1985.

CV

22. Thrall DE, Losonsky JM: A method of evaluating canine pulmonary circulating dynamics from survey radiographs. J Am Anim Hosp Assoc 12:457, 1976.

23. Wong MM: Experimental occult dirofilariasis in dogs with special reference to immunological responses and its relationship to "eosinophilic lung" in man. Southeast Asian J Trop Med Public Health 5:480, 1974.

24. Knight DH: Heartworm diseases. In Kirk RW, Bonagura J (eds): Current Therapy XII. Philadelphia, WB Saunders, 1995.

25. Atwell RB, Sutton RH, Buoro IB: Early pulmonary lesions caused by dead Dirofilaria immitis in dogs exposed to homologous antigens. Br J Exp Pathol 67:395–405, 1986.

26. Kaiser L, Williams JF, Meade EA, et al: Altered endothelial cell mediated arterial dilation in dogs with D. immitis infection. Am J Physiol 253:H1325–H1329, 1987.

27. Kaiser L, Lamb VL, Tithof PK, et al: Dirofilaria immitis: Do filarial cyclooxygenase products depress endothelium-dependent relaxation in in vitro rat aorta. Exp Parasitol 75:159–167, 1992.

28. Owhashi M, Fulaki S, Kilagaw K, et al: Molecular cloning of characterization of novel neutrophil chemotactic factor from filarial parasite. Mol Immunol 30:1315–1320, 1993.

29. Collins JM, Williams JF, Kaiser L: Dirofilaria immitis: Heartworm products contract rat trachea in vitro. Exp Parasitol 78:76–85, 1994.

30. Atwell R, Tarish J: Effect of oral, low-dose prednisolone on extent of pulmonary pathology associated with dead Dirofilaria immitis in a canine lung model. In Soll MD, Knight DH (eds): Proceedings of the Heartworm Symposium '95, Auburn, Alabama. Batavia, IL, American Heartworm Society, 1995, pp 103–111.

31. Boudreaux MK, Dillon AR: Platelet function, antithrombin-III activity, and fibrinogen concentration in heartworm-infected and heartworm-negative dogs treated with thiacetarsamide. Am J Vet Res 52:1986–1991, 1991.

32. Byerly CS, Donahoe JMR, Todd KS: Histopathologic changes in cats experimentally infected with Dirofilaria immitis. In Otto GF (ed): Proceedings of Heartworm Symposium. Bonner Springs, KS, Veterinary Medicine Publishing Co, 1977.

33. McCracken MD, Patton S: Pulmonary arterial changes in feline dirofilariasis. Vet Pathol 30:64–69, 1990.

34. Dillon AR, Warner AE, Molina RM, et al: Pulmonary parenchymal changes in dogs and cats after experimental transplantation of dead Dirofilaria immitis. In Soll MD, Knight DH (eds): Proceedings of the Heartworm Symposium '95, Auburn, Alabama. Batavia, IL, American Heartworm Society, 1995, pp 97–101.

35. Dillon AR: Feline dirofilariasis. In Atwell RB, Boreham PFL (eds): Dirofilariasis. Queensland, Australia, CRC Press, 1988, pp 205–215.

36. Dillon AR, Warner AE, Molina R: Dirofilaria immitis infection in dogs and rats results in pulmonary airway epithelial and microvascular injury. J Vet Intern Med 7:119, 1993.

37. Calvert CA, Mandell CP: Diagnosis and management of feline heartworm disease. JAVMA 180:5650–5652, 1982.

38. Dillon AR: Feline heartworm disease. Vet Clin North Am 14:1185–1199, 1984.

39. Rawlings CA: Pulmonary arteriography and hemodynamics during feline heartworm disease. J Vet Intern Med 4:285, 1990.

40. Holmes RA, Clark JN, Casey HW, et al: Histopathologic and radiographic studies of the development of heartworm pulmonary vascular disease in experimentally infected cats. In Soll MD (ed): Proceedings of the Heartworm Symposium '92. Batavia, IL, American Heartworm Society, 1992, pp 81–89.

41. Dillon AR, Warner A, Hudson J, et al: Role of PIM in inflammatory lung disease of cats and dogs. J Vet Intern Med 10:162, 1996.

42. Selcer BA, Newell SM, Mansour MS, McCall JW: Radiographic and 2-D echocardiographic findings in eighteen cats experimentally exposed to D. immitis via mosquito bites. Vet Radiol Ultrasound 37:3744, 1996.

43. Calvert CA, Losonsky JM: Occult heartworm disease–associated allergic pneumonitis. JAVMA 186:1097, 1985.

44. Confer AW, et al: Four cases of pulmonary nodular eosinophilic granulomatosis in dogs. Cornell Vet 73:41, 1983.

45. Courtney CH, Zeng Q-Y: Predicting heartworm burdens with a heartworm antigen test kit. J Am Anim Hosp 23:387–390, 1987.

46. Ishahara K, et al: Clinicopathological studies in canine dirofilarial hemoglobulinuria. Jpn J Vet Sci 40:525, 1978.

47. Atkins CE: Pathophysiology of heartworm caval syndrome: Recent advances. In Otto GF (ed): Proceedings of the Heartworm Symposium '89. Charleston, SC. Washington, DC, American Heartworm Society, 1989, pp 27–31.

48. Jackson RF, et al: Surgical treatment of the caval syndrome of canine heartworm disease. JAVMA 171:1065–1069, 1977.

49. Lillibridge CD, Rudin W, Philipp MT: Dirofilaria immitis: Ultrastructural localization, molecular characterization, and analysis of the expression of p27, a small heat shock protein homolog of nematodes. Exp Parasitol 83:30–45, 1996.

50. Kitagawa H, Sasaki Y, Ishihara K, et al: Heartworm migration toward right atrium following artificial pulmonary arterial embolism or injection of heartworm body fluid. Jpn J Vet Sci 52:591–599, 1990.

51. McTier TL, McCall JW, Supakorndej N: Features of adult heartworm antigen test kits. In Soll MD, Knight DH (eds): Proceedings of the Heartworm Symposium '95, Auburn, Alabama. Batavia, IL, American Heartworm Society, 1995, pp 115–120.

52. Lok JB, Harpaz T, Knight DH: Abnormal patterns of embryogenesis in Dirofilaria immitis treated with ivermectin. J Helminthol 62:175–180, 1988.

53. Weil GJ, Malone MS, Powers KG, et al: Monoclonal antibodies to parasite antigens found in the serum of Dirofilaria immitis–infected dogs. J Immunol 134:1185–1191, 1985.

54. Hoover JP, Campbell GA, Fox JC, et al: Comparison of eight diagnostic blood tests for heartworm infection in dogs. Canine Pract 21:11–19, 1996.

55. McTier TL, McCall JW, Dzimianski MT, et al: Epidemiology of heartworm infection in beagles naturally exposed to infection in three southeastern states. In Soll MD (ed): Proceedings of the Heartworm Symposium '92, Austin, Texas. Batavia, IL, American Heartworm Society, 1992, pp 47–57.

56. McTier TL, Supakorndej N, McCall JW, et al: Evaluation of ELISA-based adult heartworm antigen test kits using well-defined sera from experimentally and naturally infected cats. Am Assoc Vet Parasitol, 38:37, 1993.

57. Calvert CA, et al: Comparison of radiographic and electrocardiographic abnormalities in canine heartworm disease. Vet Radiol 27:2, 1986.

58. Venco L, Morini S, Ferrari E, et al: Technique for identifying heartworms in cats by 2D echocardiography (abstract). In: Proceedings of the Heartworm Symposium '98. Orlando, FL, American Heartworm Society, 1998, p 23.

59. Genchi C, Kramer L, Venco L, et al: Comparison of antibody and antigen testing with echocardiography for the detection of heartworm (Dirofilaria immitis) in cats (abstract). In: Proceedings of the Heartworm Symposium '98. Orlando, FL, American Heartworm Society, 1998, p 40.

60. Atkins CE, Keene BW, McGuirk SM: Pathophysiologic mechanism of cardiac dysfunction in experimentally induced heartworm caval syndrome in dogs: An echocardiographic study. Am J Vet Res 49:403–410, 1988.

61. Miller MS: The electrocardiogram of dogs with heartworm infection: Clinical report and review of the literature. Semin Vet Med Surg 2:28, 1987.

62. American Heartworm Society: Recommended procedures for the diagnosis, prevention, and management of heartworm (Dirofilaria immitis) infection in dogs. In Soll MD, Knight DH (eds): Proceedings of the Heartworm Symposium '95, Auburn, Alabama. Batavia, IL, American Heartworm Society, 1995, pp 303–308.

63. Rawlings CA, Raynaud JP, Lewis RE, et al: Pulmonary thromboembolism and hypertension after thiacetarsamide vs melarsomine dihydrochloride treatment of Dirofilaria immitis infection in dogs. Am J Vet Res 54:920–925, 1993.

64. Blair LS, et al: Efficacy of thiacetarsamide in experimentally infected dogs at 2, 4, 6, 12, or 24 months post-infection with Dirofilaria immitis. In Otto GF (ed): Proceedings of the Heartworm Symposium '86. Washington, DC, American Heartworm Society, 1986, p 71.

65. Kitagawa H, Sasaki Y, Kumasaka J, et al: Clinical and laboratory changes after administration of milbemycin oxime in heartworm-free and heartworm-infected dogs. Am J Vet Res 54:520–526, 1993.

66. Miller MW, Keister DM, Tanner PA, et al: Clinical efficacy of melarsomine dihydrochloride (RM340) and thiacetarsamide in dogs with moderate (class 2) heartworm disease. In Soll MD, Knight DH (eds): Proceedings of the Heartworm Symposium '95, Auburn, Alabama. Batavia, IL, American Heartworm Society, 1995, pp 233–241.

67. Case JL, Tanner PA, Keister DM: A clinical field trial of melarsomine dihydrochloride (RM340) in dogs with severe (class 3) heartworm disease. In Soll MD, Knight DH (eds): Proceedings of the Heartworm Symposium '95, Auburn, Alabama. Batavia, IL, American Heartworm Society, 1995, pp 243–250.

68. McCall JW, Ryan WG, Roberts RE, et al: Heartworm adulticidal activity of monthly prophylactic doses of ivermectin (6 μg/kg) and pyrantel given to dogs (abstract). In: State of the Heartworm Symposium '98. American Heartworm Society, 1998, p 45.

69. Kuntz CA, Smith-Carr S, Huber M, et al: Use of a modified surgical approach to the right atrium for retrieval of heartworms in a dog. JAVMA 208:692–694, 1996.

70. Morini S, Venco L, Fagioli P, et al: Surgical removal of heartworms vs. melarsomine treatment of naturally infected dogs with high risk of thromboembolism (abstract). In: State of the Heartworm Symposium '98. Orlando, FL, American Heartworm Society, 1998, p 49.

71. Boudreaux MK, Dillon AR, Ravis WR, et al: Effects of treatment with aspirin or aspirin/dipyridamole combination in heartworm-negative, heartworm-infected, and embolized heartworm-infected dogs. Am J Vet Res 2:1992–1999, 1991.

72. Rawlings CA, et al: An aspirin-prednisolone combination to modify postadulticide lung disease in heartworm-infected dogs. Am J Vet Res 45:2371, 1984.

73. Vezzoni A, Genchi C: Reduction of post-adulticide thromboembolic complications with low dose heparin therapy. In Otto GF (ed): Proceedings of the Heartworm Symposium '89, Charleston, SC. Washington, DC, American Heartworm Society, 1989, pp 73–83.

74. Fukami N, Hagio M, Okano S, et al: Influence of exercise on recovery of dogs following heartworm adulticide treatment with melarsomine (abstract). In: State of the Heartworm Symposium '98. Orlando, FL, American Heartworm Society, 1998, p 47.

75. Dillon AR, Brawner WR, Hanrahan L: Influence of number of D. immitis and exercise on the severity of heartworm disease in the dog. J Vet Intern Med 10:195–195, 1996.

76. Tanner PA, Keister DM: Final efficacy results of immiticide used to treat dogs with severe heartworm disease. J Vet Intern Med 8:176, 1994.

77. LeSage G, Freeman KP: Critical use of heartworm antigen titers. Canine Pract 20:6–9, 1994.

78. Rawlings CA, Tackett RL: Postadulticide pulmonary hypertension of canine heartworm disease: Successful treatment with oxygen and failure of antihistamines. Am J Vet Res 51:1565–1569, 1990.

79. Keister DM, Tanner PA, Meo NJ: Immiticide—review of discovery, development, and utility. In Soll MD, Knight DH (eds): Proceedings of the Heartworm Symposium '95, Auburn, Alabama. Washington, DC, American Heartworm Society, 1995, pp 201–219.

80. Knight DH, Lok JB: Seasonal timing of heartworm chemoprophylaxis in the

United States. *In* Soll MD, Knight DH (eds): Proceedings of the Heartworm Symposium '95, Auburn, Alabama. Washington, DC, American Heartworm Society, 1995, pp 37–42.

81. McCall JW, McTier TL, Ryan WG, et al: Evaluation of ivermectin and milbemycin oxime efficacy against *Dirofilaria immitis* infections of three and four months' duration in dogs. JAVMA 57:1189–1192, 1996.

82. Lok JB, Knight DH, Selavka CM, et al: Studies of reproductive competence in male *Dirofilaria immitis* treated with milbemycin oxime. Trop Med Parasitol 46:235–240, 1995.

83. Atkins CE, DeFrancesco TD, Miller M, et al: Prevalence of heartworm infection in cats with cardiorespiratory abnormalities (abstract). J Vet Med 10:161, 1996.

84. Dillon AR, Brawner WR, Robertson CK, et al: Feline heartworm disease: Correlations of clinical signs, serology, and other diagnostics: Results of a multicenter study (abstract). *In:* State of the Heartworm Symposium '98. Orlando, FL, American Heartworm Society, 1998, p 36.

85. Dillon AR: Feline heartworm disease: Clinical evaluation. *In* Otto GF (ed): Proceedings of Heartworm Symposium '83. Bonner Springs, KS, Veterinary Medicine Publishing Co, 1983, pp 31–33.

86. Holmes RA, Clark JN, Casey HW, et al: Histopathologic and radiographic studies of the development of heartworm pulmonary vascular disease in experimentally infected cats. *In* Soll MD (ed): Proceedings of the Heartworm Symposium '92. Batavia, IL, American Heartworm Society, 1992, p 89.

87. Schafer M, Berry CR: Cardiac and pulmonary artery mensuration in feline heartworm disease. Vet Radiol Ultrasound 36:499–505, 1995.

88. Selcer BA, Newell SM, Mansour MS, et al: Radiographic and 2-D echocardiographic findings in eighteen cats experimentally exposed to *D. immitis* via mosquito bites. Vet Radiol Ultrasound 37:3744, 1996.

89. Donahoe JM, Holzinger EA: *D. immitis* in the brains of a dog and a cat. JAVMA 164:518–519, 1974.

90. Cusick PK, Todd KS, Blake JA, et al: *D. immitis* in the brain and heart of a cat from Massachusetts. J Am Anim Hosp Assoc 12:490–491, 1976.

91. Holmes RA: Feline heartworm disease. Compend Contin Ed Vet Pract 15:687–695, 1993.

92. Dillon AR, Warner AE, Molina RM, et al: Pulmonary parenchymal changes in dogs and cats after experimental transplantation of dead *Dirofilaria immitis*. *In* Soll MD, Knight DH (eds): Proceedings of the Heartworm Symposium '95, Auburn, Alabama. Batavia, IL, American Heartworm Society, 1995, pp 97–101.

93. Benard MA: Acute dirofilarial death. Can Vet J 11:190–191, 1978.

94. American Heartworm Society: Guidelines for the diagnosis, treatment, and prevention of heartworm (*Dirofilaria immitis*) infection in cats. *In* Soll MD, Knight DH (eds): Proceedings of the Heartworm Symposium '95, Auburn, Alabama. Batavia, IL, American Heartworm Society, 1995, pp 309–312.

95. Zeidner NS, Belasco DL, Dreitz MJ, et al: Gliding bacterial adjuvant stimulates feline cytokines in vitro and antigen-specific IgG in vivo. Vaccine 13:1294–1299, 1995.

96. Padrid P, Feldman BF, Funk K, et al: Cytologic, microbiologic, and biochemical analysis of bronchoalveolar lavage fluid obtained from 24 healthy cats. Am Vet Res 52:1300–1307, 1991.

97. Kobayashi Y, Awakura T, Shimada A, et al: Dirofilariasis in a cat with eosinophilic interstitial nephritis. J Jpn Vet Med Assoc 45:862–864, 1992.

98. Dillon AR, Sakas PS, Buxton BA, et al: Indirect immunofluorescence testing for diagnosis of occult *Dirofilaria immitis* infection in three cats. JAVMA 180:80–82, 1982.

99. Ryan WG, Gross SJ, Soll MD: Diagnosis of feline heartworm infection. *In* Soll MD, Knight DH (eds): Proceedings of the Heartworm Symposium '95, Auburn, Alabama. Batavia, IL, American Heartworm Society, 1995, pp 121–126.

100. Prieto C, Venco L, Simon F, et al: Feline heartworm (*Dirofilaria immitis*) infection: Detection of specific IgG for the diagnosis of occult infections. Vet Parasitol 70:209–217, 1997.

101. Miller MW, Zoran DL, Relford RL, et al: Seroprevalence of antibodies to *Dirofilaria immitis* in asymptomatic cats in the Bryan/College Station area of Texas (abstract). *In:* State of the Heartworm Symposium '98. Orlando, FL, American Heartworm Society, 1998, p 37.

102. Donoghue AR, Piché CA, Radecki SV, et al: Effect of prophylaxis on heartworm antibody levels in cats receiving trickle experimental infections of *Dirofilaria immitis* (abstract). *In:* State of the Heartworm Symposium '98, American Heartworm Society, 1998, p 33.

103. Zanotti S, Kaplan P: Feline dirofilariasis. Compend Contin Ed Vet Pract 11:1005–1015, 1989.

104. DeFrancesco TD, Atkins CE, Meurs K: Diagnostic utility of echocardiography in heartworm disease (abstract). J Vet Intern Med 11:141, 1997.

105. Venco L, Ghelfi E, Calzolari D, et al: Diagnostic techniques (radiography, electrocardiography, ultrasound) in heartworm disease in cats. Vet Cremona 10:23–27, 1996.

106. Turner JL, Lees GE, Brown SA, et al: Thiacetarsamide in healthy cats: Clinical and pathological observations. J Am Anim Hosp Assoc 27:275–280, 1991.

107. Dillon R, Cox N, Brawner B, et al: The effects of thiacetarsamide administration to normal cats. *In* Soll MD, Knight DH (eds): Proceedings of the Heartworm Symposium '95, Auburn, Alabama. Batavia, IL, American Heartworm Society, 1995, pp 133–137.

108. Rawlings CA, Farrell RL, Mahood RM: Morphologic changes in the lungs of cats experimentally infected with *Dirofilaria immitis:* Response to aspirin. J Vet Intern Med 4:292–300, 1990.

109. Brown WA, Thomas WP: Surgical treatment of feline heartworm disease (abstract). *In:* Proceedings of the 16th ACVIM Forum. San Diego, CA, 1998, p 88.

110. Borgarelli M, Venco L, Piga PM, et al: Surgical removal of heartworms from the right atrium of a cat. JAVMA 211:68–69, 1997.

111. Venco L, Borgarelli M, Ferrari E, et al: Surgical removal of heartworms from naturally infected cats (abstract). *In:* Proceedings of the Heartworm Symposium '98. Orlando, FL, American Heartworm Society, 1998, p 50.

112. Piché CA, Radecki SV, Donoghue AR: Results of antibody and antigen testing for feline heartworm infection at HESKA Veterinary Diagnostic Laboratories (abstract). *In:* Proceedings of the Heartworm Symposium '98. Orlando, FL, American Heartworm Society, 1998, p 34.

113. Watkins BF, Torc M: Results found using the Animal Diagnostics' heartworm antibody test (abstract). *In:* Proceedings of the Heartworm Symposium '98. Orlando, FL. American Heartworm Society, 1998, p 35.

114. Longhoffer SL, Daurio CP, Plue RE, et al: Ivermectin for prevention of feline heartworm disease. *In* Soll MD, Knight DH (eds): Proceedings of the Heartworm Symposium '95, Auburn, Alabama. Batavia, IL, American Heartworm Society, 1995, pp 177–182.

115. Stewart VA, Blagburn BL, Hendrix CM, et al: Milbemycin oxime as an effective preventative of heartworm (*Dirofilaria immitis*) infection in cats. *In:* Soll MD, Knight DH (eds): Proceedings of the Heartworm Symposium '95, Auburn, Alabama. Batavia, IL, American Heartworm Society, 1995, pp 126–131.

CV

CHAPTER 120

PERIPHERAL VASCULAR DISEASE

Philip R. Fox, Jean-Paul Petrie, and Peter F. Suter

Peripheral vessels (e.g., arteries, arterioles, capillaries, venules, veins, and lymphatics) directly or indirectly affect many disease processes. Vascular disorders may be associated with a lesion or condition that originates in a particular tissue or organ but subsequently spreads to involve adjacent vessels. In other cases, vessels themselves develop pathology that secondarily affects surrounding tissues. Many peripheral vascular diseases identified in humans also occur in dogs and cats, although their clinical identification is frequently overlooked. To better portray the scope of organic, functional, occlusive, and nonocclusive vascular diseases, a classification scheme by location has been proposed (Table 120–1).

DISEASES OF ARTERIES

OCCLUSIVE ARTERIAL DISEASES

Arterial occlusion typically results from organic (morphologic) obstruction (Fig. 120–1). The most common causes include trauma, thrombi, emboli, arteritis, and degenerative lesions such as atherosclerosis. Most emboli constitute blood clots that have broken free from a site of thrombus formation

TABLE 120–1. PERIPHERAL VASCULAR DISEASES

Diseases of arteries and arterioles
  Organic forms
    Occlusive diseases
      Arterial embolism
      Arterial thrombosis
      Angiitis, vasculitis
      Posttraumatic vascular disorders
      Diabetic arteriopathy
    Nonocclusive diseases
      Arteriovenous fistula
      Arterial aneurysm
      Arterial calcification
      Arteriosclerosis, hyalinosis, amyloidosis
      Atherosclerosis, atheromatosis angiitis, vasculitis
  Functional forms
    Vasospasm, traumatic, toxic
Diseases of veins
  Phlebectasia
  Varicosis
  Phlebitis
  Thrombophlebitis
Diseases of capillaries
  Lymphangitis
  Lymphatic atrophy
  Lymphedema
  Lymphangiectasia
  Hypoplasia, aplasia, hyperplasia
Tumors of peripheral blood vessels
  Angioma, hemangioma, vascular hematoma, hemangiosarcoma

(thromboemboli). Emboli can also consist of tissue particles, fat droplets, gas, clumps of bacteria, fibrin, parasites (e.g., heartworms), tumor, or foreign bodies. Entrapped emboli may themselves become thrombogenic. Lesions can acutely or gradually occlude the arterial lumen, as with mural or extramural hematomas, extramural masses (neoplasms, abscesses), increased pressure exerted on surrounding tissue (compartmental syndrome), or intimal tears forming valve-like structures.[1–3]

The consequences of arterial occlusion may be minimal, but in other cases occlusion induces tissue hypoxemia, ischemia, neuropathy, and eventually tissue necrosis (infarction). The outcome depends on the location, extent, and time course of occlusion and the presence or subsequent development of collateral blood supply. Infarcts are uncommon compared with the high frequency of traumatic vascular injuries, probably because of the rich supply of collateral limb and organ vessels. Exceptions include the kidneys (Fig. 120–2) and tissues supplied by endarteries, which have no connections to collateral vascular beds.

Systemic Arterial Thromboembolism in Cats
(see Chapter 117)

Systemic Arterial Thrombosis and Thromboembolism in Dogs

Hemostasis is a complex mechanism that involves blood vessels, platelets, and coagulation proteins, as well as naturally occurring anticoagulants and platelet inhibitors. An imbalance of the hemostatic system can lead to either thrombosis or hemorrhage. Most thrombi represent aggregations of platelets and fibrin with entrapped blood cells, form in the left side of the heart, and result in dislodgment (thromboembolism) with subsequent distal vascular occlusion. The terminal aorta is the most common site for systemic embolism (see Fig. 120–1B), although other peripheral arteries may be affected.

Arterial thrombosis requires one or more inciting local or systemic conditions: (1) vascular endothelial damage, (2) sluggish blood flow (prestasis, stasis, or disrupted flow patterns), and (3) changes in blood constituents (especially platelets, coagulation proteins, and/or coagulation inhibitors) causing a hypercoagulable state.[4] Vascular endothelial injury most commonly results from inflammation, infection, bacterial endocarditis, trauma, or aberrant parasite migration such as in dirofilariasis. Thrombosis may be favored by conditions such as tumors or compressive lesions that reduce blood flow or cause stasis.

Hypercoagulable states (Table 120–2) have become increasingly recognized for their role in thrombogenesis.[4] Pri-

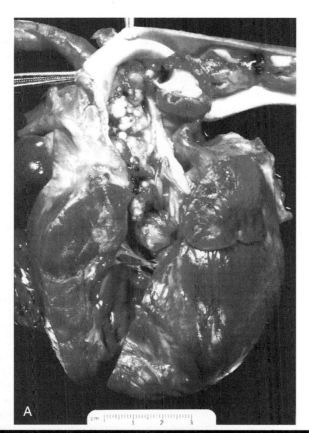

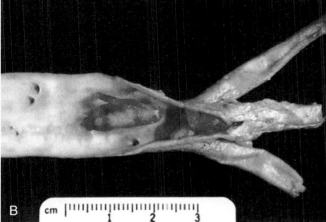

Figure 120–1. *A*, Gross heart dissected to illustrate the left ventricular outflow tract, from a dog that experienced acute posterior paresis. An extensive pedunculated mass (tumor) is present from the sinus of Valsalva and extending through the ascending aorta. *B*, Distal aorta from this dog containing a saddle embolus.

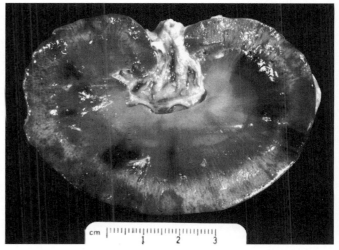

Figure 120–2. Kidney from the dog in Figure 120–1. There is extensive, acute hemorrhage associated with renal infarction.

CV

(AT-III, protein C, protein S) are being vigorously investigated for their potential thromboembolic roles.[4] Platelet activation may be initiated by a variety of stimuli. Platelets irreversibly aggregate in response to adenosine diphosphate (ADP), thrombin, and collagen. Species differences exist in platelet response to arachidonic acid, 5-hydroxytryptamine, and platelet-activating factor.[13,14] Thrombosis secondary to sodium heparin therapy has also been reported in humans, with autoantibodies directed against the circulating heparin complex resulting in platelet aggregation, thrombocytopenia, and thrombosis.[15]

The pathologic state disseminated intravascular coagulation (DIC) may complicate many disease processes and can be triggered by many factors. These include (1) activation of the intrinsic coagulation pathway by antigen–antibody

TABLE 120–2. CAUSES AND PREDISPOSING FACTORS OF THROMBOSIS AND THROMBOEMBOLISM

Vascular disorders (endothelial and/or wall injury)
Arteriosclerosis (hyalinosis, amyloidosis)
Artherosclerotic vascular disease
Vasculitis (angiitis), phlebitis, arteritis
Suppurative, septicemic, or granulomatous processes
Parasitism (aberrant dirofilariasis)
Catheterization, indwelling catheters
Injection of irritating or hypertonic substances
Neoplasia
Abscesses
Slowed or disrupted blood flow
Hypovolemia
Shock
Congestive heart failure
Bacterial endocarditis (heart valve vegetations)
Vascular incarceration or compression
Hypercoagulability, changes in blood constituents (proteins C and S, antithrombin III, homocysteine)
Cushing's syndrome
Protein-losing enteropathy
Renal amyloidosis, glomerulopathies
Disseminated intravascular coagulation (DIC)
Polycythemia
Platelet disorders, thrombocytosis
Immune hemolytic anemia
Dehydration and/or hyperviscosity
Thromboembolism
Septic, nonseptic emboli
Extraneous foreign material (hair, catheter fragments, foreign bodies)

mary hypercoagulable states include congenital abnormalities of hemostasis and remain poorly characterized in animals. In contrast, secondary hypercoagulable states have long been recognized as predisposing risk factors for thrombosis.[4] Systemic or metabolic diseases such as glomerulopathy, nephrotic syndrome, hyperadrenocorticism, neoplasia, and protein-losing enteropathy have been associated with thromboembolism.[5–12] Destruction of red blood cells in immune-mediated hemolytic anemia releases thrombogenic substances, and pulmonary thromboembolism may accompany this condition.[9] Antithrombin III (AT-III) has been identified in the pathogenesis of nephrotic syndrome.[6] Disruptions of naturally occurring anticoagulants and cofactors complexes, particulate or colloidal substances, or endothelial injury; (2) activation of the extrinsic coagulation pathway by thromboplastic substances; and (3) direct activation of prothrombin (factor X).[16] After the coagulation system has been activated, both thrombin and plasmin circulate systemically. Thrombin cleaves fibrinopeptides from fibrinogen into fibrin monomers, which polymerize to fibrin clots and lead to microvascular thrombosis. Circulating levels of proteins C and S, vitamin K-dependent factors, may be reduced in DIC and contribute to the development of coagulation abnormalities.[4] Alternatively, the general proteolytic enzyme plasmin cleaves fibrinogen into fibrin degradation products. These may interfere with platelet function and result in hemorrhage. Once a DIC process has been triggered, it may self-perpetuate. Paradoxically, hypercoagulability may cause both a bleeding tendency and thrombosis to coexist.

History

Acute arterial occlusion is usually indicative of significant systemic, metabolic, or cardiovascular disease. Prompt diagnosis and identification of the etiology, are enhanced by an insightful history, complete physical examination, and appropriate diagnostic tests. Some animals have a history of intermittent claudication, whereas in others acute paresis or paralysis is the major presenting sign. Acute arterial occlusion results in extreme hindlimb pain and general distress. In some cases the animal may present with an unsteady gait, lameness, progression to stumbling, weakness, or collapse in the hindquarters. Other potential signs include weight loss, exercise intolerance, hindlimb licking or chewing, and hypersensitivity over the lumbosacral region and the hindlimbs. Acute complete arterial occlusion may cause posterior paresis, extreme hindlimb pain, and general distress.[17] Other signs attributable to systemic or metabolic diseases may sometimes be detected.

Clinical Signs and Physical Examination

Microthrombus formation is common, particularly after trauma or surgery. However, rapid clot lysis and abundant collateral circulation usually result in absence of outward clinical signs. Clinical presentation is often variable because (1) most thrombotic events are secondary to an underlying disorder, (2) the sites and degree of arterial occlusion change, and (3) thrombi can simultaneously form at multiple sites. For example, signs referable to an underlying primary disease (e.g., endocarditis, hemolysis, hemorrhage, dirofilariasis, renal disease) may combine with signs caused by arterial occlusion of the limbs, kidneys, and intestines.

Manifestations of acute arterial occlusion reflect the physiologic consequences of the organ supplied by the involved artery. Acute, complete arterial occlusion causes rapid ischemic injury. This is largely due to release of vasoactive substances by the clot, which induces vasoconstriction and reduces collateral circulation. A substantial component of tissue injury may occur after reperfusion of ischemic tissue. In addition to acute effects, long-term injury may take days or weeks, as with postischemic muscle fibrosis and neuromyopathy after distal arterial embolism.[17,18]

The type and severity of clinical signs depend on (1) the location, size, and number of thrombi; (2) the completeness and time frame of vascular occlusion; (3) the age, composition, and organization of the thrombus; (4) whether the clot is infected or sterile; (5) whether the event is solitary or repeated; (6) the adequacy of compensatory mechanisms (e.g., collateral vessel recruitment, vasodilatation, clot lysis, and restoration of blood flow); (7) the effects of vasoactive chemicals elaborated by the clot on collateral vessels (i.e., vasoconstriction); and (8) related complications (tissue necrosis, local infection, hyperesthesia).

Classic signs of acute arterial limb occlusion are the seven "Ps," namely pain, paleness, paresthesia, pulselessness, polar (cold), paresis or paralysis, and prostration. The site most frequently diagnosed with peripheral thrombosis is the distal aorta (often referred to as "saddle" thromboembolism). Aortic thromboembolism has been reported in dogs with bacterial endocarditis, aberrant heartworm migration, neoplasia, and renal amyloidosis.[5,12,18] Occasionally, only one limb is affected.

Physical examination may reveal cool distal limbs and swollen muscles. Segmental and pedal reflexes may be depressed. Hypersensitivity over the lumbar spine may exist. A slow onset and progressive peripheral neuropathy after trauma may be associated with ischemia of peripheral nerves. Arterial thrombosis of a front limb may also occur. Clinical signs are usually less severe than those described for posterior limb thrombosis.

In the central nervous system, arterial occlusion is rarely diagnosed. For signs to be recognizable, several arteries have to be occluded simultaneously, as can occur in severe atherosclerosis or with embolization after arterial catheterization. Cerebrovascular occlusions may lead to sudden disorientation, weakness, anisocoria, and hemiamaurosis. Infarction may follow thromboembolism to a localized area of the brain. *Stroke* is a generic term denoting any acute, nonconvulsive, focal neurologic deficit stemming from cerebrovascular disease. The classic presentation includes hemiparesis, but a broad spectrum of neurologic injuries may result. Neurologic signs depend on the site, extent, and time course of vascular occlusion. In a series of 17 affected dogs, cerebrovascular disease was associated with coagulopathy, metastatic brain tumor, trauma, sepsis, atherosclerotic thrombus, unknown cause, and vascular malformation.[19] A cerebellar infarction caused by meningeal arterial thrombosis has also been described.[20] We have occasionally observed neurologic signs related to stroke in cats associated with severe systemic hypertension. Affected animals usually present acutely blind and show signs of retinal hemorrhage and detachment.

With endocarditis, a heart murmur of mitral or aortic insufficiency may be auscultated. Bacterial embolization from these valves may cause a systemic shower of emboli, which frequently affect abdominal organs, especially the kidneys and small intestines. Complete occlusion of renal arcuate arteries causes localized infarction, which usually goes unnoticed. These vessels are endarteries without collateral circulation. However, complete unilateral or bilateral renal arterial occlusion invariably causes severe renal infarction. Affected dogs are depressed and may exhibit an arched back, sublumbar pain, and hematuria.

Acute occlusion of several mesenteric arteries may cause initial gastric hyperactivity. This may be followed by ileus and intestinal infarction. Sudden anorexia, vomiting, bowel evacuation, and abdominal pain may be present. Feces may contain blood. With bowel infarction, bloody diarrhea, severe signs of an acute abdomen, and shock may develop.

Diagnosis

When peripheral arterial thrombosis is suspected, a survey thoracic radiograph is indicated to evaluate cardiac size and shape and to assess for pulmonary changes including edema, thrombosis, or dirofilariasis. Chest and abdominal radiographs should be evaluated for orthopedic lesions, which could result in posterior paresis. In addition, radiographs of the pelvic and hindlimb region may be indicated to check for masses that could exert pressure on the aorta and for periosteal reactions in the sublumbar area. Doppler echocardiography may be useful for identifying vascular disturbances.

Laboratory data may help characterize the underlying primary disease. Coagulation profiles are variable. Some cases of glomerulopathies and hypoproteinemia have been associated with reduced levels of antithrombin III.[11] Assessment of protein C and protein S levels should be considered when these tests are available. A clinical pathology database is also advised to evaluate and detect renal or hepatic disease, dirofilariasis, DIC, and systemic and metabolic disorders. Blood cultures are indicated if endocarditis, bacteremia, or sepsis is suspected.

Diagnostic confirmation usually requires proof of a vascular occlusion. This can be accomplished with an arteriogram or diagnostic ultrasonography.[21,22] The arteriogram can indicate the exact location of the thrombus or illustrate the extent of vascular occlusion and collateral vascular supply (Figs. 120–3 and 120–4). Furthermore, radiolucent emboli such as heartworms may be outlined when present as longitudinal filling defects. Selective catheterization is performed

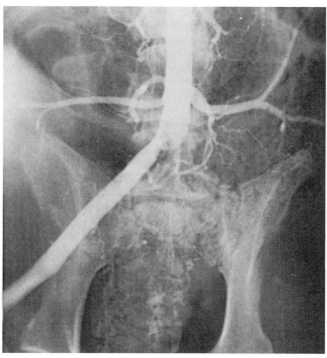

Figure 120–4. Aortogram of a 7-year-old Saint Bernard dog with a saddle thrombus at the aortic trifurcation associated with a chondrosarcoma located in the vicinity of the terminal aorta. The owner had observed four episodes of pain and weakness in the hindlimbs that developed gradually when the dog was taken for a walk. At the beginning of the walk, the dog was normal. If the dog was forced to continue walking after the signs of pain and lameness had appeared, it collapsed. After resting for a few moments the dog was able to walk again. On clinical examination the femoral pulse was difficult to feel, and the periphery of the hindlimbs was cool. Pain could be elicited when the pelvic area was palpated. Aortography was performed and a radiograph was taken 4 seconds after the beginning of the injection of contrast medium. On the aortogram the common origin of the internal iliac arteries and the left external iliac artery contain no contrast medium, suggesting that they have been occluded completely. A partial occlusion has reduced the flow of contrast medium into the right external iliac artery. Some collateral blood supply to the hind limbs probably occurs via the seventh lumbar artery. Anticoagulation therapy was instituted, but it failed to provide relief and the dog underwent euthanasia at the request of the owner.

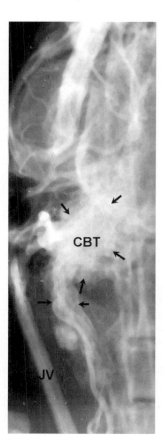
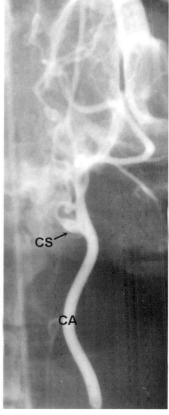

Figure 120–3. Two ventrodorsal angiograms of a dog with a carotid body tumor. The left panel demonstrates a late arterial-venous phase after injection of contrast medium into the right common carotid artery. There is a tumor "blush" with contrast medium opacifying vessels feeding the carotid body tumor (CBT, arrows). Venous return is observed via the jugular vein (JV). The angiogram in the right panel is a useful comparison and was taken after injection of contrast material into the left common carotid artery (CA). Normal flow is observed and the carotid sinus (CS), an area for sensing blood pressure, is evident. (Courtesy of John Bonagura, DVM.)

by injecting radiocontrast agent at 0.5 to 1 mL/kg through a catheter introduced through the carotid or femoral artery and directed into the desired region using fluoroscopic guidance. Alternative imaging methods are becoming available at some referral or research institutions, including thermography and perfusion scans.[23]

Differential Diagnoses

Differential diagnoses include trauma; peripheral neuropathy; spinal, pelvic, or vascular tumors; infections; toxoplasmosis; degenerative myelopathy, interventricular disk protrusion; fibrocartilaginous embolic myelopathy; and the cauda equina compression syndrome. Radiographs should be systematically evaluated for signs related to these disorders.

Therapy

For management of associated primary diseases, the reader is referred to respective chapters in this textbook (see also Chapter 117). Therapies should be directed toward the underlying disease or cause of thrombosis whenever possible. When diagnosed early, especially within 8 to 12 hours, some thrombi may be physically removed by embolectomy or by resection anastomosis. In most cases, however, these procedures are associated with high morbidity or mortality. Analgesics can be used for pain. Fluid therapy should be initiated to correct acid-base or electrolyte abnormalities and dehydration. Colloids such as dextran and hetastarch have been used for their rheologic properties, to reduce platelet aggregation, and to decrease the relative concentration of clotting factors.[24] The most important step in treatment of DIC is elimination of the underlying pathologic condition or triggering mechanisms and the conditions that promote this hypercoagulable state. Anticoagulants are usually advocated, although there is controversy about their efficacy.

Heparin is the drug most commonly chosen to prevent clot propagation. Effects vary considerably from case to case, and the dose must be individualized. The goal is to stop or retard thrombus growth with the lowest effective dose without causing a bleeding tendency. In practice, this is often difficult to achieve. Heparin potentiates the action of plasma AT-III (the primary action of AT-III is inactivation of thrombin and factors XII, XI, X, and IX). This reduces the tendency for intravascular coagulation and thrombosis. Heparin does not prevent platelet aggregation or cause thrombolysis. In diseases associated with reduced AT-III (e.g., nephrotic syndrome), heparin can be administered with fresh-frozen plasma to supply clotting factors including AT-III. Many heparin treatment regimens have been advocated, although there are few clinical data concerning efficacy. Low-dose heparin (5 to 10 IU/kg constant-rate intravenous infusion or 75 to 150 IU/kg subcutaneously every 6 to 8 hours) has frequently been used. Monitoring by activated partial thromboplastin time (APTT) is necessary to adjust the dose so that the APTT is prolonged from 1.5 to 2 times normal. In the event of severe hemorrhage, heparin can be neutralized by protamine sulfate administration. Heparin is ideally continued until the hypercoagulable state is resolved or bleeding complications occur.

Oral anticoagulant therapy (warfarin, cat, 0.25 to 0.5 mg q24h; dog, 0.1 to 0.2 mg/kg q24h) may be considered in some cases. When initiated, it is overlapped with heparin therapy for 3 or 4 days. The coumarin dose is titrated by monitoring clotting time, but there is little information about dose and efficacy, particularly in dogs. Inhibitors of platelet function have also been suggested. Aspirin inhibits cyclooxygenase, leading to decreased thromboxane A_2 synthesis. This renders platelets nonfunctional by preventing their aggregation. For example, low-dose aspirin administration (0.5 to 3.5 mg/kg every 12 hours) significantly decreases canine platelet aggregation.[25,26] Aspirin is not advocated during acute DIC or with thrombocytopenia.

Thrombolytic agents such as streptokinase, urokinase, and tissue plasminogen activator are potent activators of fibrinolysis. They transform plasminogen to plasmin, are expensive, and have been used thus far with limited success in veterinary medicine.[27–29]

Prognosis

The prognosis depends on the etiology, extent and severity of occlusion, presence or absence of local complications (ischemic neuromyopathy, ulcers), and concurrent embolization to visceral organs. Even in cases with spontaneous recovery, relapses must be expected. Rapid diagnosis and treatment are essential to avoid severe or even irreversible tissue injury.

NONOCCLUSIVE ARTERIAL DISEASES

Causes of nonocclusive arterial diseases include trauma, arterial aneurysms, arteriovenous fistulas, arteriosclerosis, angiitis (vasculitis), and functional abnormalities. Some nonocclusive diseases can become secondarily occlusive (e.g., arteriosclerosis). Degenerative arterial wall abnormalities can occur with metabolic, traumatic, toxic, or infectious conditions. Mild to moderate degenerative arterial wall changes often occur in old dogs and cats.

Arterial Aneurysm

An arterial aneurysm is defined as a circumscribed dilatation of an arterial wall or a blood-containing swelling connecting directly with the lumen of an artery. Arterial aneurysms are rare in dogs and cats and only isolated cases have been reported.[30,31] Aneurysms can be categorized on the basis of their shape (saccular or fusiform), etiology (atherosclerotic, mycotic, inflammatory, arteritis, traumatic, congenital, dissecting) or their histologic appearance. Two major histologic classes of aneurysms are true aneurysms (aneurysma verum) and false aneurysms (aneurysma spurium).

True Aneurysm

A true aneurysm is a vascular dilatation caused by a weakened arterial or venous wall with subsequent widening of the vascular lumen. Histologically, true aneurysms involve the entire arterial wall and contain three microscopic arterial layers. Aneurysms may result from destruction of the media and/or the elastic fibers of large arteries by inflammatory or degenerative processes. Traumatic aneurysms can be true aneurysms or pseudoaneurysms, depending on their etiology and histologic appearance. In dogs, aneurysms have been found in the aorta that were caused by migrating larvae of *Spirocerca sanguinolenta* (formerly, *S. lupi*)[32] (Fig. 120–5). Aneurysms have also been shown to result from turbulent blood flow with arteriovenous fistulas. Dissecting aneurysms are associated with a biochemical or mechanical defect involving the arterial media.

Peripheral aneurysms appear as soft, warm, pulsating bulges. Occasionally, a "machinery" murmur can be auscultated over these areas (see Arteriovenous Fistulas). Clinical signs are frequently absent or vague. If spontaneous vascular rupture occurs, pain, signs of anemia and shock, and pleural or mediastinal effusion may be present. Exsanguination resulting from aneurysmal rupture is rare.

Spurious (Pseudo) Aneurysm

Spurious aneurysms, also known as pseudoaneurysms, are caused by localized disruption of the native artery. Their histologic appearance includes arterial walls that are formed by fibrous tissue. One cause of spurious aneurysms is a hematoma that communicates with an arterial lumen resulting from venipuncture.[33] Traumatic spurious aneurysms are probably more common than is usually realized. Clinical signs may include lameness, persistent pain, and deep muscular swelling unresponsive to local therapeutic measures, antibiotics, or glucocorticosteroids. Pitting peripheral edema may be present and neither blood nor pus can be aspirated from the swelling. The diagnosis of spurious aneurysms may be suspected from physical examination. Survey radiographs may indicate soft tissue swelling. Diagnostic confirmation has classically relied on arteriography, which illustrates a

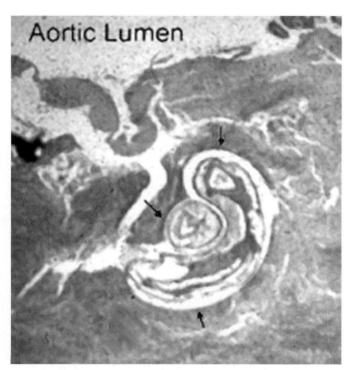

Figure 120–5. Photomicrograph of a canine aorta. The intima and media have been disrupted by the presence of the subtropical-tropical parasite *Spirocerca sanguinolenta* (formerly *S. lupi*). The parasite is seen in cross section (arrows). The aortic lumen is at the top of the figure. (Courtesy of John Bonagura, DVM.)

nodular exudation of contrast medium at the arterial defect. Doppler echocardiography, especially color flow Doppler imaging, aids in identification by depicting blood flow and turbulence. Additional diagnostics tests include computed tomography, radionuclide angiography, and surgical exploration. The differential diagnosis includes chronic infection, obstruction of a deep vein, and abscessation. In spurious aneurysm, however, pyrexia and neutrophilia are not encountered. The prognosis is favorable if surgical vascular repair can be accomplished.

Arteriovenous Fistulas (Arteriovenous Malformations)

Arteriovenous (A-V) fistula is an abnormal communication between an artery and vein that bypasses the capillary network. The true incidence is unknown, although A-V fistulas are reported uncommonly in dogs and rarely in cats. Centrally located anomalies may occur between the cardiac chambers (e.g., ventricular septal defect) or between the great vessels (e.g., patent ductus arteriosus), and these are reviewed in Chapter 112. In this section, only peripheral A-V malformations (A-V fistulas) are discussed.

Congenital A-V fistulas are rare and are caused by arrest or misdirection of the embryologic vascular differentiation. The persistence of primitive equipotential capillaries (primary anlage) and the subsequent failure of the existing anastomotic embryologic channels to differentiate into arteries or veins are responsible for the persistence of their abnormal communications. Terminology applied to congenital A-V fistulas has been a source of confusion (e.g., hemangioma racemosum, Park-Weber syndrome, hemangioma cavernosum, strawberry birthmark, nevus angiectasis, cirsoid aneurysm, congenital A-V aneurysm).

The most common cause of an acquired A-V fistula is blunt or penetrating trauma including iatrogenic trauma.[34] The latter is often related to venipuncture and accidental perivascular injection of irritating substances such as thiobarbiturates.[35] Additional causes include neovascularized tumors of the neck area (carotid body tumor, thyroid tumor), spontaneous aneurysmal rupture, mass ligature of arteries and veins, and erosion of contiguous vessel walls by infection or arteriosclerosis.[36] Although uncommon, most A-V fistulas involve the extremities. However, they may occur anywhere in the body—the neck, spinal cord, flank, head, brain, abdomen, liver, and lung—and they have been recorded as a complication of mass ligation of arteries and veins during closed castration.[37-39] Irrespective of etiology and location, A-V fistulas cause similar altered blood flow dynamics and may act as a potent stimulus for the development of an extensive collateral circulation. Cardiovascular responses to the altered flow dynamics have been studied extensively in experimental dogs.[40]

An A-V fistula creates two competing circulatory pathways. One is the normal arterial-capillary-venous system; the other is the new system with reduced peripheral resistance. The A-V fistula creates a low-pressure conduit for systemic circulation to be diverted to the venous system because of the pressure gradient from arteries to veins. Fistulas with large shunts may result in arterial hypotension and reduced peripheral vascular resistance, venous hypertension, increased cardiac preload, elevated heart rate, pulmonary hypertension, and potentially high-output heart failure. The communicating shunt increases venous pressure, venous blood oxygen saturation, and the diameter and number of anastomotic arteries and veins. Eventually, an ectasia of the feeding artery and aneurysmal sacs in the venous area of the A-V communications may develop. Histologic changes occur in affected vessels so that arteries begin to look more like veins (venification) and veins like arteries (arterialization). The rapid runoff of blood through the A-V fistula into the capacitant venous circulation causes turbulence and, potentially, sound (*bruit*).[42]

Shunted blood flow through a large fistula can be so great that retrograde flow from a distal artery into the fistula occurs. Arterial blood supply to the tissues distal to the A-V fistula may become compromised by competition with the fistula and secondary venous hypertension, resulting in stagnation of venous blood flow in the dilated veins or even reversal of blood flow in a distal rather than proximal direction. Local edema and ischemia followed by tissue necrosis, ulceration, or organ dysfunction may ensue. In large and mostly centrally located fistulas, the central blood dynamics also become affected. Large flow volumes across the A-V fistula compromise the blood supply to other regions of the body by shifting blood into the capacitant venous circulation. Owing to compensatory reactions, the blood volume, heart rate, and cardiac contractions increase. Augmented cardiac output and gradual expansion of the blood volume partially restore the blood supply to deprived tissues. Eventually, however, the increased venous return (increased preload) and elevated cardiac workload may induce high-output heart failure.[41]

The hemodynamic effect of the fistula and degree of collateral vessel development are related to several factors including fistula location, type and diameter of involved vessels, duration of shunt flow, and the number and distensibility of involved vessels. Collateral development is a continuous process. Collateral circulation develops mostly from preexisting, unused arterial communications.

CV

Clinical history and signs vary according to the location, size, duration, etiopathology, and topography of the fistula. Small A-V fistulas of the extremities are noticed by the owners as painless, easily compressible, warm bulges. Sometimes they are detected incidentally during routine clinical examination. With medium-sized or large fistulas of the extremities, a continuous palpable thrill and pulsation, along with a machinery murmur, can be detected. The leg or region distal to the fistula may be swollen and warmer or colder than the proximal area (sometimes with severe local ischemia), painful, and affected by pitting or secondary inflammatory edema. Lameness, cyanosis, and/or therapy-resistant toe ulcers, sometimes with severe local ischemia, scab formation, or even gangrene, can occasionally occur distal to the fistula. In the dilated superficial veins, a faint pulsation may be felt (Fig. 120–6). Pulse and heart rate are increased in medium-sized to large fistulas. In the feeding arteries a water hammer pulse is often present. Animals with high-output heart failure may develop a cardiac murmur of mitral regurgitation and moist lung sounds indicating pulmonary edema.

When firm pressure is applied proximal to the A-V fistula or the feeding artery is compressed, the thrill and bruit disappear and pulse and heart rate may drop as a result of diminished venous return and reduced cardiac output. This is referred to as Branham's bradycardia sign, and the maneuver is called the Branham or Nicoladoni–Branham test. Together with the local thrill or fremitus and the bruit, *Branham's sign* is pathognomonic for A-V fistulas.

Other signs have been reported and vary with respect to location and hemodynamic alterations caused by the A-V fistula as follows. An A-V fistula in the orbit caused exophthalmos.[42] Recurrent bleeding from the mouth was observed in an A-V fistula of the tongue.[38] Restless behavior and lethargy followed by progressive seizures and hemiparesis were present in a 10-year-old mixed breed dog with a subcortical cerebral A-V malformation.[43] An A-V fistula of the spinal cord at the thoracolumbar junction in a 10-month-old female Australian shepherd dog caused a deteriorating hindlimb ataxia, difficulty in getting up and down, hypersensitivity over the lumbosacral region, and, after 3 months, urinary incontinence.[44] Cardiomegaly and pulmonary overcirculation were detected radiographically in a dog with a postsurgical A-V fistula, and these changes regressed after the fistula was surgically closed.[37] An A-V fistula was found surgically in the jejunum of an 8-month-old dog with persistent anemia and melena.[45] A-V fistulas in tumors have been recognized because of the strong pulsation and fremitus detectable during palpation of the tumor mass.[34] Auscultation of the tumor mass may reveal a machinery-type murmur or bruit.

A-V fistulas of the liver connect the hepatic artery to the portal vein and cause portal hypertension or even reversal of the blood flow in the portal vein.[46] Abdominal distention caused by low-protein ascites is a major clinical sign. Furthermore, as a result of a hepatofugal blood flow, portosystemic collateral vessels and signs of hepatoencephalopathy may develop.[47] A-V fistulas of the liver and associated vasculature can often be differentiated from portosystemic shunts using abdominal ultrasonography and color Doppler imaging techniques.[48]

Pulmonary A-V fistulas can lead to respiratory distress and cyanosis. Survey thoracic radiographs of animals with large fistulas may indicate cardiomegaly, a prominent aortic arch, a hypervascular lung field, and an increased interstitial or patchy pulmonary radiodensity indicating pulmonary congestion or edema, respectively.

Angiography is used preoperatively to evaluate fistula anatomy and location, help direct surgical strategies, and suggest the prognosis. This information may also help guide a surgeon to preserve arterial blood supply and direct proper venous drainage distal to the fistula after radical excision of the lesion. With this technique, a small cut-down is made over the affected area. To perform angiography, a catheter or suitable needle-catheter combination is introduced into the vessel. If the fistula is located in the proximal third of the limb, in the trunk, or in an internal organ, selective catheterization of the feeding vessel at its origin from the aorta or the carotid artery should be attempted under image-intensified fluoroscopic control. For A-V fistulas located in the distal two thirds of a limb, the contrast medium is injected into the brachial or femoral artery. The correct position of the catheter is checked with a test injection of 2 to 5 mL of a contrast medium. A suitable intravenous contrast agent is then injected. For small fistulas, 3 to 4 mL is used. Large fistulas may require 15 to 20 mL of contrast medium. Several radiographs should be obtained in rapid sequence beginning at the time of the contrast medium injection to outline both arteries and veins. Application of a tourniquet may facilitate the outlining of multiple congenital small fistulas at different locations in the limb.

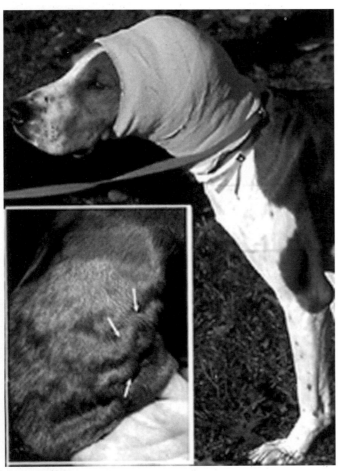

Figure 120–6. Coon dog with an arteriovenous fistula of the ear. The dog was presented for severe bleeding caused by trauma to large distended veins (inset, arrows). A continuous murmur was auscultated over the ear and Doppler studies demonstrated continuous arterial-to-venous flow. Venous distention is secondary to direct transmission of arterial pressure and marked increases in flow. (Courtesy of S. E. Johnson, DVM and J. Bonagura, DVM.)

The absence of a normal capillary phase and premature outlining of the veins are typical arteriographic findings in shunting lesions. It is important to try to identify the barely visible distal continuation of the artery feeding the fistula. The differential diagnoses of A-V fistulas include neoplasms, varices, abscesses, cystic skin lesions, aneurysms, lymphedema, and scars.

Diagnostic ultrasonography, especially color Doppler imaging, has been clinically useful in humans for identifying and localizing A-V fistulas.[46] Findings included the presence of focal, intra-arterial flow at the fistula site throughout the cardiac cycle, turbulent pulsatile venous flow at the fistula site, and nonpulsatile venous flow proximal to the fistula. The communication between artery and vein may be identified. Doppler echocardiography has been similarly applied in veterinary medicine to diagnose and evaluate traumatic, hepatic, and pulmonary arterial A-V fistulas in dogs (Fig. 120–7).[48-50]

The treatment of A-V fistulas has historically been surgical.[51] Small lesions can be controlled temporarily by pressure wraps. Careful ligation of all proximal and distal arteries feeding the fistula, ligation of the draining veins (so-called quadruple ligation), and complete excision of the A-V collaterals with the venous aneurysmal sacs have been advocated. If relapse occurs after an initial careful resection or if multiple fistulas are present, a wide excision of the involved area(s) or limb amputation may be the only alternative. Animals with large A-V fistulas have substantially increased blood volume. Sudden shunt closure is followed by an immediate increase in blood pressure and a vagally mediated bradycardia.

Surgical approaches can often be technically difficult, mutilating, and hazardous and have a high failure rate with residual clinical symptoms.[52] In human medicine, arterial embolization techniques have been used successfully to occlude A-V fistulas.[52,53] Embolization has been achieved with selective or superselective injection of biodegradable substances (muscle tissue, gelatin sponge) or nonresorbable material (silicone microspheres, polyvinyl alcohol foam, isobutyl-2-cyanoacrylate, or special embolization wire coils). These techniques may be viable for selected veterinary cases.

The prognosis for animals with small A-V fistulas is often good. Morbidity is highest with centrally located A-V fistulas, with fistulas that cause organ dysfunction, and with large fistulas that induce a high cardiac output. There is an inherent tendency of collateral vascular flow to increase continuously.

Arteriosclerosis and Atherosclerosis

Arteriosclerosis is defined as chronic arterial wall change consisting of hardening, loss of elasticity, and luminal narrowing. It results from proliferative and degenerative vascular changes, not inflammation.[54] Arteriosclerotic lesions are common incidental findings in old dogs and cats.[55,56] They are typically mild and usually unimportant to health and survival. Thrombosis is rarely a complication of such microscopic lesions and their functional significance is not known. Similar arteriosclerotic changes are seen in peripheral arteries including aorta and cerebral, renal, and spinal arteries.[54] Some exceptions do occur, especially related to hyaline degeneration of intramural coronary arteries. Intramural coronary arteriosclerosis is particularly common in aged dogs with heart failure associated with endocardiosis. Intramural coronary artery fibrosis, hyalinosis, and amyloidosis were found in 26.4 per cent of old dogs undergoing necropsy.[57] Extensive nonthrombotic, nonatherogenic stenosis of extramural coronary arteries was described in two adult male Labrador retriever dogs with congestive heart failure.[58] Disease of extramural arteries is less common but not rare. Endothelial aortic plaque formation caused by arteriosclerosis was present in 77.8 per cent of 58 dogs brought to a small animal clinic in Helsinki for euthanasia.[59] Some of these arteriosclerotic changes were associated with clinical signs. Spontaneous arteriosclerosis, with a predilection for renal vasculature, has also been demonstrated in 15- to 20-month-old greyhounds.[60]

Atherosclerosis refers to the deposition of different classes of serum lipids within the arterial wall and is considered a form of arteriosclerosis.[57] Histologically, the inner sections of arterial wall (intima and inner media) are thickened by deposits of plaque containing cholesterol, lipoid material, focal calcification, and lipophages.[61,62] There can be widespread involvement of arteries from many organs. Affected vessels often appear grossly thickened (Fig. 120–8), yellow-white, and may have narrowed lumina. The risks of arterial occlusion are highest in arteries containing lipoid plaques (atheromas). Atheromas are only rarely formed in dogs with arteriosclerosis. However, they are a feature of atherosclerosis and are sometimes referred to as arterial xanthomatosis. Atherosclerosis has been detected in older dogs as a consequence of hypercholesterolemia and lipidemia associated with thyroid atrophy.[57] The term "atherosclerosis" is used as defined by Liu et al., namely a thickening of the inner arterial wall in association with lipid deposits. Unlike the disease in humans, however, canine atherosclerosis is uncommonly associated with extensive plaque formation, arterial calcification, or thrombosis. A predisposition for spontaneous atherosclerosis was reported in old, obese, dogs with atrophied thyroid glands and hypothyroidism.[57] This observation is in accordance with experiments in which atherosclerosis could be induced in thyroidectomized dogs fed

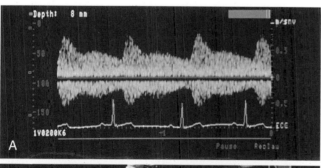

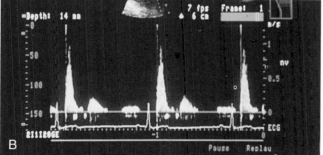

Figure 120–7. Pulsed wave Doppler recordings from a 5-year-old female golden retriever dog with traumatic A-V fistula. *A,* Doppler interrogation of a large, pulsatile, dilated vessel associated with the right radial artery identified by color flow Doppler at the medial right brachium. Notice the continuous flow best seen during diastole. *B,* Pulsed Doppler flows recorded from the normal left radial artery in the same dog.

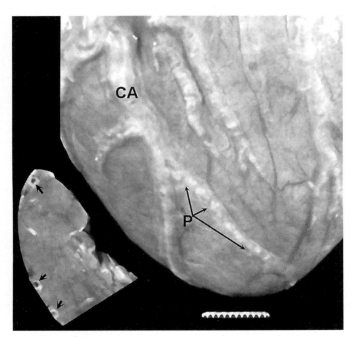

Figure 120–8. Coronary atherosclerosis of extramural coronary arteries in a dog with severe hypercholesterolemia (>650 mg/dL) caused by hypothyroidism. Epicardial coronary arteries are evident. A larger epicardial branch is labeled (CA). Note numerous light plaques (P) within the arteries that represent deposition of lipid. The lower left portion of the figure shows a cut segment of myocardium. The lumina of the subepicardial arteries are also surrounded by a concentric layer of lipid. (Courtesy of John Bonagura, DVM.)

large quantities of cholesterol or cholic acids.[63,64] The spontaneous disease mainly affects male and spayed female dogs. An increased prevalence in miniature schnauzers, Doberman pinschers, and Labrador retrievers has been reported.[57] Hypertension caused by renal disease seems to accelerate the development of stenotic lesions.[59] Atherosclerosis has not been described in cats. Stenotic arterial lesions may develop. They are most common and severe in the extramural and intramural coronary arteries, where infarction can result. Other commonly affected vessels include the carotid and renal arteries. Severe lesions associated with infarcts have been found in the cerebral arteries.[65] The distribution and severity of arterial lesions and thyroid atrophy are typically associated with clinical signs of lethargy, anorexia, weakness, dyspnea, collapse, heart failure, vomiting, disorientation, blindness, circling, and coma.[57,65] Recorded electrocardiographic abnormalities included atrial fibrillation, notched QRS complexes, and ST segment elevation. Laboratory abnormalities include hypercholesterolemia, lipidemia, low serum triiodothyronine (T_3) and thyroxine (T_4) values, elevated blood urea nitrogen (BUN) (often associated with renal infarction) and liver enzymes, and high alpha$_2$ and beta fractions in the protein electrophoresis.

The prognosis for dogs with clinical signs related to stenosing atherosclerosis is poor. Potential treatments include thyroid replacement drugs, antihypertensive medication, blood cholesterol–reducing agents, and a low-cholesterol diet. Treatment strategies have not been tested in dogs, and severe lesions are essentially irreversible. Not all dogs with hypothyroidism develop atherosclerosis. Only those referred to as "hyperresponders," in which increased levels of very-low-density beta-lipoproteins are found, are prone to develop atherosclerosis and plaques. Blood levels of low-density lipoproteins may be increased in these dogs because lipopro-

tein receptors are reduced and lipoid removal by the tissues is decreased. The elevated lipoprotein concentrations account for arterial lipoid deposits.[65]

Vasculitis, Angiitis

The terms vasculitis and angiitis refer to the pathologic syndrome that is characterized by vascular inflammation and necrosis. Although there have been many reported causes of vasculitis, there are only a few histologic manifestations of the disease. Vasculitis can occur in toxic, immune-mediated, infectious, inflammatory, and neoplastic disorders. Blood vessels of any type in any organ can be affected, resulting in a wide variety of clinical signs. The clinical spectrum of disease varies from a primary disease involving the blood vessels exclusively to minor histologic alterations. The nonspecific nature of histologic lesions, coupled with the plethora of clinical presentations, makes the diagnosis of primary vasculitis quite challenging. The clinical consequences of vasculitis depend on the size, number, and type of blood vessels affected in addition to the degree and duration of obstruction.[66]

Histologically, vasculitis is characterized by the presence of inflammatory cells within and around blood vessel walls. Vascular injury is associated with necrosis and degeneration of endothelial and smooth muscle cells and fibrin deposition. A collection of fibrin, immunoglobulins, complement, and platelets may appear by light microscopy as eosinophilic material within the vessel wall and lumen and is referred to as *fibrinoid*. Eosinophilia secondary to degeneration of collagen and smooth muscle can also be present within the vessel wall.[67] The vascular wall lesions already described distinguish vasculitis from perivascular inflammation. Vasculitides have been classified on the basis of specific inflammatory cell infiltrates.[67,68] These may include neutrophils, lymphocytes, or macrophages. As the disease becomes chronic or begins to resolve, predominant cell populations may change.

Vasculitis may develop from within a vessel as a result of infectious, immune-mediated, or toxic injury or by extension from adjacent areas of inflammation. Infectious agents can injure endothelial cells directly or through the production of endotoxins and exotoxins. The exact mechanism of endothelial injury is not known but involves the formation of oxygen free radicals, local inflammatory mediators, and the recruitment of inflammatory cells.[69] Exposure of the subendothelial collagen by endothelial damage results in the activation of Hageman's factor and the subsequent activation of the complement, kinin, and plasmin systems. These lead to increased vascular permeability and inflammation.

Type III hypersensitivity reactions can cause necrotizing vasculitis resulting from the deposition of immune complexes within the vessel walls. Activation of the complement cascade may attract neutrophils, cause immune complex phagocytosis, and result in the release of lysosomal enzymes and oxygen free radicals, thereby leading to further inflammation and necrosis. In the chronic state this reaction becomes diminished and the neutrophilic inflammation is replaced by mononuclear cells. Immune complex reactions of this type can occur in many disease conditions such as primary immune-mediated disease or be secondary to infectious disease. Identification of immune complex activity can be misleading because immune complexes are rapidly cleared from the circulation and may reflect the chronicity of certain lesions.[68,70] In humans, the discovery of antineutrophil cytoplasmic autoantibodies (specific for antigens in neutrophil granules and monocyte lysosomes) has allowed further identification of immune-mediated processes in which immune complexes were suspected but not identified.[67]

Cell-mediated immunopathogenic mechanisms are initiated in the blood vessel wall. This type of vasculitis is characterized by accumulations of lymphocytes and macrophages within vascular walls. Myocyte necrosis results in fibrinoid degeneration, endothelial hyperplasia, and occasionally thrombosis. A granulomatous-type reaction of the vessel wall can result, particularly in chronic cases. These changes may be accompanied by hemorrhage and ischemic changes in surrounding tissues.[70]

The etiology of secondary vasculitides is, by definition, known and classifications are based accordingly. These conditions usually result from infectious diseases such as feline infectious peritonitis, canine coronavirus infection, parvovirus infection (rare), Rocky Mountain spotted fever, leishmaniasis, and dirofilariasis. They may also occur in drug reactions and in immunopathogenic connective tissue and collagen diseases such as systemic lupus erythematosus and rheumatoid arthritis.

Microscopic Necrotizing Vasculitis

Microscopic necrotizing vasculitis (MNV) refers to a large, heterogeneous group of clinical syndromes that share similar histologic properties. Hypersensitivity vasculitis is often referred to in dermatologic manifestations and is often clinically distinct from the multisystemic form of necrotizing vasculitis termed juvenile polyarteritis syndrome (JPS), reported in young beagle dogs.[71,72] There is less distinction between JPS and the syndromes described as idiopathic steroid-responsive vasculitides, which can be manifest as multisystemic or localized disease.[73,74] Lesions affect mainly arterioles, capillaries, and venules.

Clinical abnormalities of MNV are often associated with phasic pyrexia, listlessness, and anorexia. In some cases lymphadenopathy, myalgia, epistaxis, drooling, sneezing, and arthralgia may occur. In addition to the generalized signs, manifestations of specific organ lesions may occur.[75] The most common presenting clinical signs in small animals are dermatologic lesions. Hemorrhagic maculae resembling circular petechiae and ecchymoses are common. Other lesions seen include wheals, urticaria, purpura, nodules, bullae, necrosis, and ulcers. In many cases the skin lesions are associated with pain and/or pruritus. Less frequently encountered lesions include ulcers at the mucocutaneous junctions or of the mucous membranes, especially located on the head (external ear canal and pinnae, face), bony prominences of the limbs and the footpads, and pitting edema involving dependent areas such as limbs, ventral trunk, head, and scrotum.[70,71]

Internal organ involvement with MNV frequently goes undiagnosed. This is because clinical signs are vague, there is often simultaneous multiorgan involvement, or organ manifestations are confused with those of infectious, degenerative, or traumatic conditions (e.g., pneumonia, glomerulonephritis, arthritis, spinal or neuromuscular conditions). The clinicopathologic findings of primary MNV vary according to severity, duration, and specific organ. Lymphopenia, eosinopenia, hypoalbuminemia, hyperglobulinemia, and hyperfibrinogenemia occur commonly. Less consistent findings include leukocytosis with a left shift and toxic neutrophils,[25] leukopenia, neutropenia, monocytosis, a mild normocytic, normochromic anemia, and thrombocytopenia. Serum liver enzymes and triglycerides are often elevated.[66,68]

An idiopathic cutaneous and renal glomerular vasculopathy has been described in kenneled and racing greyhounds with many characteristics similar to those of MNV.[76] It is characterized by fibrinoid arteritis, thrombosis, and infarction with deep, slowly healing skin ulcers and peracute renal glomerular necrosis with a predilection for afferent arterioles.

Diagnostic confirmation requires histologic examination of skin, organ, or lymph node biopsy specimen and exclusion of other immune-mediated disease. Special immunologic tests have been recommended to demonstrate a low or high concentration of complement, C3, and elevated levels of circulating immune complexes. The history may be helpful if drug hypersensitivity is suspected.

Primary periarteritis, or polyarteritis, a necrotizing vasculitis affecting small and medium-sized muscular arteries, has been identified in colonies of beagles.[69,77,78] This polyarteritis occurs in two forms. One form occurs mainly in young beagles, in which arteritis affects major branches of coronary arteries almost exclusively. Clinical signs are usually absent. A second form of polyarteritis is associated with vague multisystemic signs (fever, depression, anorexia, neutrophilia, decreased albumin-to-globulin ratio), a stiff gait, and/or pain on abdominal palpation (beagle pain syndrome). The signs are associated with vascular lesions including disseminated, focal, or diffuse intimal thickening and acute, fibrinoid necrosis of the media resulting in occlusion and thrombosis.

The differential diagnosis includes pemphigus vulgaris and foliaceus, bullous pemphigoid; systemic lupus erythematosus; dirofilariasis; specific infectious diseases; chronic neoplasia; and cold hemagglutination disease. The prognosis is usually favorable.

Many therapies have been advocated. Administration of all unnecessary drugs should be discontinued. In many cases immunosuppressive dosages of glucocorticoids with or without an antibiotic have been used successfully. Cyclophosphamide may be administered if that fails. Dogs with lesions involving only the skin can be given sulfasalazine (Azulfidine) at an initial dose of 22 mg per pound (49 mg/kg) every 8 hours.[66] Dosage frequency can be decreased after lesions improve, from three times to twice a day and, later, to once a day. Dogs receiving sulfasalazine should be observed for side effects such as fever, keratoconjunctivitis, and hematologic abnormalities.

Polyarteritis Nodosa

Polyarteritis nodosa (PAN) is a rare polysystemic disease associated with a necrotizing vasculitis of unknown cause. The disease affects predominantly segments and bifurcations of small and medium-sized muscular arteries. In humans PAN is classified among immune-mediated collagen disorders and derives its name from purpural lesions that are palpable in the subcutaneous tissue. In contrast, palpable nodules are not a regular feature of PAN in animals.[79,80] The vascular lesions consist of intimal proliferation, vessel wall degeneration, necrosis, and thrombosis in all stages of development. PAN leads to a loss of vessel wall integrity, petechial and ecchymotic hemorrhages, focal areas of tissue infarction and necrosis, aneurysm formation, nodular swelling, and thickening of the major arteries. Target tissues of canine PAN include the kidneys, skin, mucous membranes, adrenals, meninges, gastrointestinal tract, connective tissue, and myocardium.[81] The lungs are usually spared.

The clinical presentation includes systemic signs (pyrexia,

lethargy, reluctance to walk, vague pain, or weight loss) and a wide spectrum of organ system abnormalities (linear skin ulceration, ulceration of mucous membranes, nasal discharge, spinal pain, and signs of cardiac and/or renal failure).[2] Clinicopathologic findings may include leukocytosis with a left shift and proteinuria.

The main differential diagnoses are hypersensitivity angiitis and idiopathic polyarteritis. The diagnosis is confirmed by histologic examination of a skin biopsy specimen. The prognosis is guarded to poor. Treatment includes glucocorticoids and/or cyclophosphamide.

Lymphomatoid Granulomatosis and Miscellaneous Vasculitides

Lymphomatoid granulomatosis and other unclassified vasculitides are characterized by a polymorpholymphocytoid, plasmacytoid, and histiocytoid granulomatous infiltration around blood vessels. Pulmonary nodular lesions of variable size caused by lymphomatosis were first described in dogs.[82] Infarction, necrosis, and cavitation occur in some of the masses. The bronchial lymph nodes can be slightly to greatly enlarged, and pulmonary thrombosis is common. The etiology of this rare condition is unknown. Occasionally, similar lesions are associated with eosinophilic pneumonitis in occult dirofilariasis, although they can also occur outside endemic areas of dirofilariasis. An immune-mediated cause is likely because in some cases large amounts of immunoglobulins G and M can be demonstrated in plasma cells and macrophages.[83] The differential diagnosis is that of primary or secondary neoplasia, with which this condition is often confused. Diagnosis is rarely made clinically and requires histologic examination of biopsy material. The prognosis is usually poor. In some patients multicentric lymphosarcoma may develop at a later date. Surgery or treatment with glucocorticoids and immunosuppressive drugs is only temporarily effective.

FUNCTIONAL FORMS OF ARTERIAL DISEASES

Vasospasm

Vasospasm is a common response to blunt and perforating vascular trauma and may also result from perivascular injection of irritating substances. When this occurs, tissue injury and vasospasm can be minimized by local infiltration with procaine hydrochloride or lidocaine. Uncommonly, vasospasm occurs in association with spontaneous arterial rupture (e.g., ruptured cerebral aneurysm or stroke). Angiography is usually required for confirmation. Vasospasm may be elicited by exotoxins. The best known example is ergotism. The differential diagnosis of vasospasm is that of thrombosis caused by vasculitis (see later in this chapter).

DISEASES OF VEINS

Diseases of the venous system are usually of minor clinical importance in dogs and cats despite the fact that veins are commonly affected by or involved in trauma, thromboembolism, edema, local inflammation, and septic processes. Common venous disorders include traumatic injuries, superficial and deep phlebitis and thrombosis (thrombophlebitis), pulmonary embolism, venous compression syndromes, varices, and ulcers.

Varicosis and ulceration are rare in dogs and cats and,

when detected, often accompany arteriovenous fistulas. Cutaneous phlebectasia is a benign lesion sometimes erroneously called telangiectasis. It is reported almost exclusively in dogs with spontaneous or iatrogenic Cushing's syndrome.[84] Phlebectasia is an abnormal dilatation, extension, or reduplication of veins or capillaries or a combination of these changes. No specific treatment is required.

Venous perforation or *blunt trauma* is usually well tolerated. Rapid clotting results in venous occlusion. If venous occlusion or severance is severe, edema and cyanosis are usually temporary because of good collateral circulation. If all veins draining an area are compromised, edema and necrosis can ensue. Fat tissue is particularly vulnerable to necrosis. Blunt trauma has been associated with caudal vena caval obstruction or kinking of the intrathoracic caudal vena cava and ascites.[85]

Thrombosis is common after blunt trauma and perforating injuries, particularly with venipuncture or prolonged venous catheterization (Fig. 120–9). Phlebitis is a major cause of intimal damage leading to thrombosis. The thrombosis is usually of little local consequence. However, emboli may be carried to the lung and cause pulmonary thromboembolism. In most animals, blood clots carried to the lung are rapidly lysed and cause no problems. However, when inflammatory diseases, dehydration, or circulatory failure occurs, clot formation may continue in the pulmonary vessels and lead to vascular occlusion, severe dyspnea, pain, and death.[10] In infectious thrombophlebitis, bacterial emboli may be carried

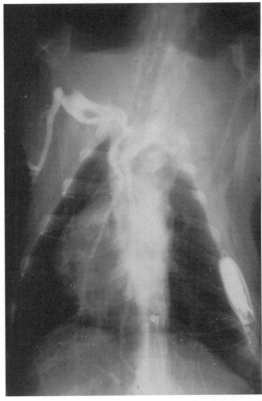

Figure 120–9. Angiogram of a dog with a cranial vena caval thrombus. The animal developed lymphedema of the neck, face, and front legs 1 week after a transvenous pacemaker lead had been inserted through the jugular vein to facilitate temporary cardiac pacing for complete heart block. Contrast medium was injected into an accessory cephalic vein with the animal positioned in sternal recumbency. There is extensive collateral circulation, but filling of the cranial vena cava is not identified. An epicardial electrode is visible in the cardiac apex and the pulse generator can be seen subcutaneously in the left lateral thorax. (Courtesy of Nancy Morris, DVM.)

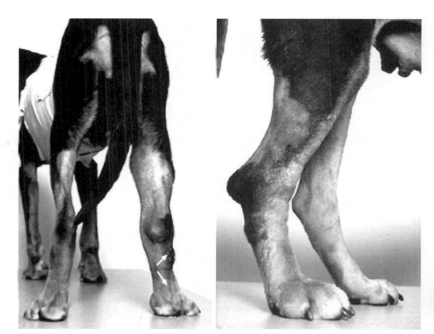

Figure 120–10. Caudal (left) and lateral (right) views of the right rear limb of a young dog with severe edema caused by thrombophlebitis. The problem developed after placement of saphenous vein catheter. The limb is markedly swollen and edema fluid (arrows) is leaking through a small ulcer in the skin. Thrombosis of the vein prevents venous drainage and increases lymphatic fluid formation. (Courtesy of John Bonagura, DVM.)

to the lungs and cause thromboembolic pneumonia. Spontaneous venous thrombosis is rare, although portal vein thrombosis has been reported. Clinical signs include ascites, peripheral pitting edema, and portosystemic shunting.[56]

Phlebitis can result from a local inflammatory process extending to the veins or can originate from a venous intimal lesion. Common causes of venous intimal lesions are perivenous injection of irritating drugs, infusion of large amounts of fluid, and long-term use of intravenous catheters. Infusion-related phlebitis occurs in three forms: (1) chemical (injury of vein by irritating drugs), (2) physical (trauma to the intima by catheters, needles, hypertonicity, or particulate matter in infused fluids), and (3) microbial (infected fluids, skin, or catheter tip). The resulting sterile or septic thrombophlebitis usually remains localized with pain, swelling, and exudation (Fig. 120–10). Patients with serious illnesses or compromised immune systems, however, may develop septic complications such as thromboembolic pneumonia or endocarditis.

In cases of venous occlusion, clinical signs depend on the anatomic location, extent, and duration of the obstruction. Acute obstruction of centrally located and deep veins causes edema, cyanosis, discomfort, and venous dilatation distal to the obstruction site. Obstruction of the cranial vena cava causes edema in the neck, head, front limbs, and dependent portions of the chest wall (Fig. 120–11). Pleural effusion commonly results from venous obstruction. Clinical disorders of the intrathoracic caudal vena cava occasionally occur in dogs (Fig. 120–12).[35] Obstructions of the renal or pelvic area cause edema of the hindlimbs and the scrotum. The clinical signs depend on the collateral vessel reserve and capacity of regional lymphatics. In addition to thrombosis, common causes of venous obstruction include invasive malignant processes and venous compression by abscesses, hematomas, tumors, and lymphadenopathy. A number of tumors have a tendency for venous invasion, including chemodectomas, adrenal tumors, and hemangiosarcomas. Angiography may indicate the occlusive or compressive lesion and/or highlight increased collateral circulation (Fig. 120–13). Diagnostic ultrasonography can often detect masses or flow disturbances.

The prognosis and therapy of venous obstruction depend on the primary disease. These are discussed in various chapters throughout this textbook.

DISEASES OF THE PERIPHERAL LYMPHATICS

Lymphatics originate within the interstitium as specialized endothelium-lined capillaries and transport fluid, solutes, and

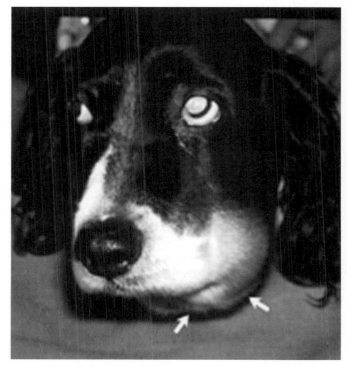

Figure 120–11. Marked intermandibular edema (arrow) in a dog with so-called cranial (anterior) mediastinal syndrome caused by a large mediastinal mass that obstructed the cranial vena cava. (Courtesy of Drs. John Bonagura and Richard Eaton-Wells.)

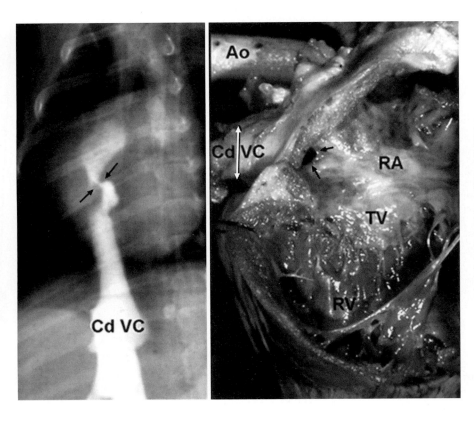

Figure 120–12. Acquired stenosis (fibrosis) of the caudal vena cava in an older dog. The left panel shows an angiogram of the caudal vena cava (Cd VC), which demonstrates a severe narrowing of the dye column (arrows) at the venous entry into the caudal right atrium. The right panel is a postmortem view of the heart taken from the right lateral perspective. The right atrial and ventricular walls have been retracted to demonstrate the stenotic, caval orifice (small arrows). Compare this opening with the diameter of the caudal vena cava (to the left, large vertical arrow). The right ventricle (RV), tricuspid valve (TV), right atrium (RA), and descending aorta (Ao) are shown. (Courtesy of John Bonagura, DVM, and Matthew W. Miller, DVM.)

macromolecular particles back into the venous system.[87–98] Unlike blood vessels, lymphatic vessels contain a discontinuous basement membrane and lack intercellular tight junctions. Lymphatic vessels increase in diameter as lymph flows centrally, passing through lymph nodes or directly into larger lymphatic ducts.[87] The thoracic duct is the common duct for all lymph flow with the exception of that of the right lymphatic duct, which drains the right side of the head and neck and right forelimb. The thoracic duct empties into the brachycephalic vein or the left subclavian vein. Lymph flow relies on both extrinsic and intrinsic factors. Extrinsic factors include movement of adjacent skeletal muscles and organs. Intrinsic factors involve smooth muscle contraction in the lymphatic vessel wall. Smooth muscle contraction is regulated by the distention of the vessel, humoral mediators, and the sympathetic nervous system. Unidirectional flow is maintained through the presence of valves in the larger lymphatic vessels and collecting ducts. No valves are present in the lymphatic capillaries or lymph nodes.[89] Anchoring filaments are present to provide structural support to the capillaries, and when interstitial fluid pressure rises, they tighten to widen intercellular spaces and prevent collapse of the lymphatic capillary.

Permeability of the lymphatic endothelium is partially controlled by local interstitial pressures. As interstitial fluid pressure rises, intercellular junctions begin to open and fluid enters the lymphatic capillaries. The exact mechanism of lymph formation is controversial and is dependent on Starling's forces and the passive diffusion of fluid from the interstitial space.[88] Lymph formation is an active process in which extrinsic compressive forces push water out of lymphatic capillaries, leaving larger macromolecules within the lumen. This concentrated lymph then acts as an osmotic force to draw fluid into the terminal lymphatics. Return of the lymph fluid to the interstitium is impeded by the flaplike arrangement of intercellular clefts.[90]

In addition to its transport function, the lymph system plays a major role in host defense. It serves as a filtering system to impede the spread of microorganisms and neoplastic cells. The cellular components, in particular the lymphocytes, are indispensable for immunologic reactions and antibody formation.

Lymphatic disorders can be subdivided into those of internal organs, such as intestinal lymphangiectasis, and peripheral lymphatic disorders. Several lymphatic diseases have been recognized in animals including lymphedema, intestinal

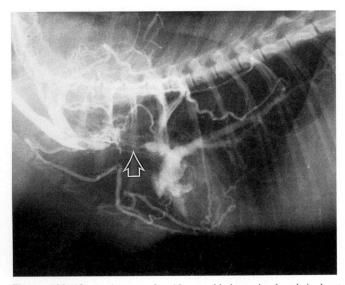

Figure 120–13. Angiogram of a 10-year-old domestic short-haired cat who presented with pleural effusion and edema of the head and neck. Radiocontrast dye was injected into the external jugular vein. There is interruption of venous return in the cranial vena cava (arrow) caused by compression and obstruction of this vessel by a mediastinal tumor. Note the prominent collateral venous network.

lymphangiectasia, chylothorax, lymphadenitis, lymphocysts, lymphoma, lymphangioma, and lymphangiosarcoma. Types and causes of peripheral lymphatic disorders are summarized in Table 120–3.

INFLAMMATORY LYMPHATIC DISORDERS (LYMPHANGITIS AND LYMPHADENITIS)

Lymphangitis and lymphadenitis are often secondary to local inflammation, particularly involving the skin, mucous membranes, and subcutaneous tissues. Lymphangitis can also result from bacterial or fungal infection or adjacent neoplastic and inflammatory disease. Lymphatics may be affected and occluded as they drain inflammatory agents and their by-products from tissue spaces. In lymph nodes, microorganisms are phagocytized and inactivated or killed by humoral and cellular mechanisms. During this process, lymph nodes may become obstructed, enlarged, warm, and painful. When limbs are affected, lameness may be accompanied by a warm, painful, and local swelling. Pyrexia, anorexia, and depression are common and leukocytosis may be present with acute, severe lymphangitis.

Lymphangitis may become chronic when associated with a granulomatous or static lesion such as a foreign body or with unsuccessfully treated acute inflammation. Persistence of inflammatory edema results in mesenchymal cell proliferation, which in turn can cause irreversible thickening of skin and subcutis.

The prognosis is favorable with early and appropriate treatment. Therapy consists of moist, warm, local compresses or soaks, which reduce swelling and promote drainage. Aggressive local and systemic antibiotic therapy usually promotes recovery in animals with fever and anorexia. Bacterial culture and sensitivity testing should be performed if acute lymphangitis fails to respond to treatment and in cases of chronic lymphangitis. Surgical exploration is indicated if fistulous tracts or abscesses are present or if a foreign body is suspected.

TABLE 120–3. ETIOLOGIES OF PERIPHERAL LYMPHATIC DISORDERS

Lymphangitis, lymphedema, lymphadenitis, lymphadenopathy
  Infection
  Neoplasia
  Reactive hyperplastic disease
  Granuloma
Lymphedema
  Primary—developmental abnormality of lymph vessels
    Hypoplasia
    Aplasia
    Lymphangiectasia
    Hyperplasia
  Secondary—acquired occlusion or loss of lymphatic pathways
    Surgical excision of lymphatics or lymph nodes
    Posttraumatic lymphangiopathy
    Neoplastic invasion
    Extrinsic compression of lymph vessels or tissue
    Acute obstructive lymphadenitis
    Chronic sclerosing lymphadenitis and lymphangitis
    Lymphatic atrophy with interstitial fibrosis
    Radiation therapy
Lymphocysts
  Cystic hygroma, lymphoceles, pseudocyst
Lymphangiomas
Lymphangiosarcomas

LYMPHEDEMA

Lymphedema refers to an accumulation of fluid in the interstitial space secondary to abnormal lymphatic drainage.[87] This term should not be used for other forms of edema, such as circulatory edema related to venous obstruction or generalized edema related to hypoproteinemia. Lymphedema may result when capillary filtration exceeds the resorptive capacity of the veins and lymphatics. The protein-rich fluid (2 to 5 g/dL) causes a high osmotic gradient and exacerbates fluid accumulation.[88] Numerous classification schemes have been used to categorize lymphedema.[67] One commonly used scheme based on etiology[91] divides lymphedema into six etiologic categories: overload, inadequate collection into lymphatic capillaries, abnormal lymphatic contractility, insufficient lymphatics, lymph node obstruction, and main lymphatic ductal defects. More traditionally, primary lymphedema refers to an abnormality of the lymphatic vessels or lymph nodes. Secondary lymphedema refers to conditions caused by a disease in the lymphatic vessels or lymph nodes that began in a different tissue. Secondary lymphedema can occur as a result of neoplasia, surgery, trauma, parasites, or infection and is more common than primary lymphedema.

Primary Lymphedema

Primary lymphedema can result from three principal morphologic abnormalities: (1) aplasia (absence of the lymph vessels or lymph nodes), (2) hypoplasia (lymph vessels or nodes deficient in size and number), and (3) hyperplasia (a diffuse increase in size and number).[91] These abnormalities are confined to the cutis and subcutis, sparing deeper tissues.

Lymphedema caused by aplasia, hypoplasia, or dysplasia of proximal lymph channels and/or popliteal lymph nodes occurs most often in the hindlimbs of young dogs (Figs. 120–14 and 120–15). The edema can be transient, observed only during the juvenile period, or permanent. Mild cases are restricted to the hindlimbs, whereas severe cases may progress to whole body edema.[92–95] Although the condition is frequently bilateral, one limb is often more swollen than the other.[96] A number of cases of suspected congenital lymphedema have been reported.[93–96] Affected breeds include bulldogs, poodles, Old English sheepdogs, and Labrador retrievers, although it is not clear whether these breeds are at increased risk.

The history may identify chronic limb swelling since birth or edema appearing later in life. The swelling represents a pitting edema of varying magnitude that is neither too warm nor cold. The edema is not usually accompanied by lameness or pain unless there is massive enlargement or cellulitis. Growth and activity are usually normal, but rest and limb massage do not typically reduce the severity of edema. Total plasma protein, serum protein electrophoresis, hemogram, and blood chemistry are generally unremarkable. The diagnosis of primary lymphedema is based on history (age of onset, disease progression, affected limbs, and distribution of edema) and clinical signs. Previous surgery, trauma, or infections should also be noted. Radiographic lymphography may be needed to confirm the diagnosis in subtle cases and is helpful in determining the morphology of anomalous lymphatic systems (see Fig. 120–15).

The prognosis for resolution of congenital lymphedema is guarded. Occasionally, dogs who develop hindlimb edema during the neonatal period may improve spontaneously. More frequently, dogs with severe edema of the limbs and trunk succumb during the first few weeks after birth.[92] In

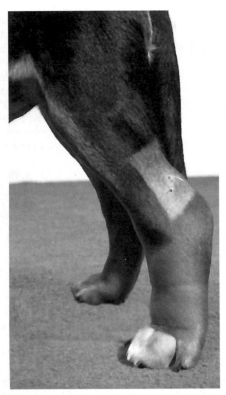

Figure 120–14. Marked, nonpainful edema of the left rear limb in a young dog with congenital lymphatic dysplasia. (Courtesy of John Bonagura, DVM.)

long-standing untreated lymphedema, a mesenchymal response leads to permanent induration of the edematous region. Complications such as abrasions and infection often develop. Dogs with primary lymphedema should not be used for breeding. Test matings of dogs with congenital lymphedema support the hypothesis of autosomal dominant inheritance with variable expression.[96]

Secondary Lymphedema

Persistent lymphedema occurs only after destruction or blockage of a considerable number of major lymph channels or several sequential lymph nodes with their afferent or efferent lymphatics.[87] Factors that can delay or prevent edema formation include opening of collateral vessels, re-routing of lymph flow through peripheral lymphaticovenous anastomoses and perilymphatic routes of lymph drainage, and increased venous fluid uptake. Secondary lymphedema is often related to a combination of lymphatic and venous obstruction. Inhibited venous return increases lymphatic flow by disturbing Starling's equilibrium of tissue fluid formation. This overloads the lymphatic capillaries and results in the accumulation of fluid in the interstitial space.[97] Distal lymphatics may become more distended, causing loss of valvular competence, stagnation of lymph flow, mural insufficiency, and further accumulation of proteinaceous fluid in subcutaneous tissues. Other common etiologies include posttraumatic or postsurgical interruption of lymphatics, excision of lymph nodes containing neoplastic metastases, and blockage of lymph nodes and lymph vessels by compression or invasive neoplasms. Lymphedema secondary to local neoplasia is usually a sign of a widely disseminated and highly invasive malignant process. Several causes of secondary lymphedema have been summarized in Table 120–3.

Clinical signs associated with secondary lymphedema vary depending on the underlying systemic causes. Lymphedema may be localized to the periphery of an extremity (Fig. 120–16) or extend proximally to the subcutaneous tissues (Fig. 120–17).[98] The location and severity of obstruction determine the extent of edema formation. For example, sublumbar or intrapelvic obstruction induces bilateral hindlimb edema and edema of the thighs and external genitalia. Mediastinal masses and thrombosis of the cranial vena cava induce bilateral edema of the front limbs and tissue of the ventral thorax, neck, and head. The clinician must palpate all lymph nodes carefully for enlargement and pain. With bilateral hindlimb edema, it is important to perform rectal or abdominal palpation to assess sublumbar lymph nodes. The prostate and anal region or mammary glands and vaginal area should be carefully inspected for neoplasms, which can lead to obstructive intrapelvic processes. Intrapelvic masses should be suspected in all dogs with hindlimb edema and vague signs of sublumbar pain, discomfort during ambula-

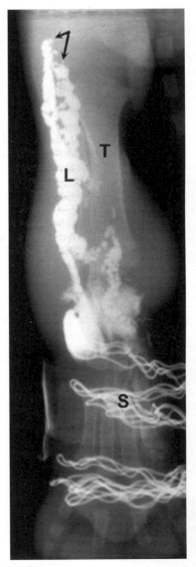

Figure 120–15. Lymphangiogram of a young dog with lymphatic dysplasia. After cannulation of a distal lymphatic vessel, contrast medium was infused into the lymphatic system. Note the dilated, tortuous, lymphatic channels (L) that end blindly at the stifle (arrows). T = tibia; S = radiopaque surgical sponges. (Courtesy of C. Wendy Myer, DVM, and John Bonagura, DVM.)

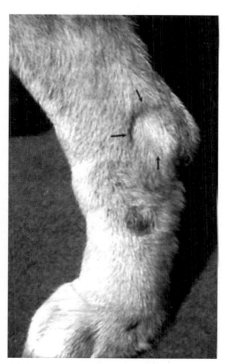

Figure 120-16. Pitting edema in a dog with a caudal lumbar mass. The edema was caused by either obstruction of venous return in the rear limbs or obstruction of lymphatic drainage. Tissue fluid was deformed by light digital pressure, resulting in a visible subcutaneous "pit" in the rear limb (arrows). (Courtesy of John Bonagura, DVM.)

tion, or difficulties with defecation or urination. Depending on the type and extent of underlying systemic illness, limb edema may be the only detectable abnormality or may be accompanied by fever, anorexia, and weight loss. Clinicopathologic findings depend on the underlying primary disorder.

Diagnosis is based largely on history and clinical examination and is facilitated by diagnostic imaging. Survey radiographs should be taken of suspicious areas, which often include the pelvis or cranial thorax. In a substantial number of cases, soft tissue masses or destructive bony lesions can be detected. Ultrasonography can provide valuable information about soft tissue masses and readily identifies enlarged lymph nodes and other structures. Specialized radiographic contrast studies may be indicated if the diagnosis remains unclear.

Lymphography is often relied upon for definitive diagnosis. With indirect lymphography, a contrast agent is infused into the tissues adjacent to the lymphatics.[99] The contrast medium is then selectively absorbed and transported through the lymphatic channels. Direct lymphography is more challenging unless lymphangiectases have formed but provides superior results. The identification of lymphangiectases is facilitated in milder cases by subcutaneous injection of vital dyes (e.g., 3 per cent Evan's blue dye or 11 per cent patent blue violet) into the toe webs. By selective resorption of these dyes, the main lymphatic channels proximal to the metacarpus or metatarsus become grossly outlined. Selective lymphatic cannulation requires aseptic cut-down over the lymphatic region of interest; the lymphatic vessel is then cannulated with a 27- or 30-gauge needle, small plastic tubing, or a special lymphatic cannula.[99] An iodine-containing soluble contrast medium such as sodium and meglumine diatrizoate (Renografin, Hypaque) is injected slowly

into the vessel. Because water-soluble contrast media diffuse rapidly through lymphatic walls into surrounding tissues, the radiographic detail is blurred unless radiographs are taken shortly after dye injection. After the cut-down for lymphangiography, abnormal lymphatic vessels that have taken up vital dye are sometimes recognized. In some cases the lymphatics are hypoplastic throughout their course. When aplastic, lymphatics suitable for cannulation and injection of radiocontrast agent may not be found. Failure to outline a lymph node after lymphography is not absolute proof of its absence.[87] Lymphographic features of primary lymphedema include lymph node aplasia and small lymphatics that end blindly or anastomose into collateral vessels around (instead of into) lymph nodes where they would be normally found.

Lymphoscintigraphy is an alternative approach for imaging peripheral lymphatics. This technique requires a gamma-camera system and intradermal injection of high-molecular-weight radiolabeled colloids.[100] Such equipment and specialized training are not widely available.

Differential diagnoses for dogs with edema confined to one limb include inflammation, trauma, vascular obstruction, hemorrhage, cellulitis, phlebitis, and A-V fistula. Diagnostic considerations for dogs with edema involving both forelimbs include thrombosis of the cranial vena cava or compression or invasion of the vein by a mediastinal mass. With the latter, edema usually involves the head and neck regions as well as the limbs. Causes of only bilateral hindlimb edema include obstruction of sublumbar lymph nodes by neoplastic infiltration. If all four limbs are involved, the differential diagnoses should include hypoproteinemia, congestive heart failure, renal failure, and portal hypertension. The close association of lymphatic and venous structures can make it difficult to distinguish between lymphatic and venous obstruction, and both can occur at the same time. Ulceration, dermatitis, cyanosis, weeping varices, and/or fat necrosis are signs of venous obstruction rather than lymph stasis.

Therapy is usually unrewarding. In the early stages of lymphedema medical management is directed to maintaining the patient's comfort and reducing swelling. Infectious disorders require long-term antimicrobial therapy. Some neoplas-

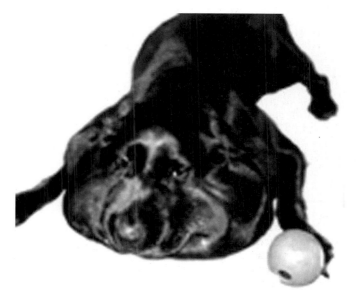

Figure 120-17. Severe subcutaneous edema in a Labrador retriever with tight congenital tricuspid valve stenosis. The stenosis resulted in severe systemic venous hypertension. (Courtesy of John Bonagura, DVM, and Richard Bell, DVM.)

CV

tic conditions may benefit from chemotherapy or radiation therapy. Long-term heavy bandage application (e.g., Robert Jones splint) may encourage lymphatic flow and reduce subcutaneous lymph accumulation. Local topical skin care and intermittent antibiotic therapy are helpful in reducing cellulitis. With the exception of isolated instances, pharmacologic therapies are generally unrewarding. Coumarin has been advocated to reduce high-protein edema in humans by stimulating macrophages, promoting proteolysis, and enhancing absorption of protein fragments.[101] After reduction of interstitial fluid with diuretic therapy, residual interstitial space proteins may cause tissue injury,[99] and thus long-term diuretic administration may be contraindicated. Surgical options may include (1) procedures to facilitate lymph drainage from affected limbs (lymphangioplasty, bridging procedures, shunts, omental transposition) and (2) procedures to excise abnormal tissue.[34] Surgical excision of the subcutaneous edematous tissue should be staged to decrease devascularization.[99] Short-term administration of anti-inflammatory agents or diuretics, bandaging, and physical therapy may be helpful in cases of traumatic and postsurgical induced lymphedemas.

LYMPHANGIOMA, LYMPHANGIOSARCOMA

Lymphangiomas are benign tumors of lymphatic capillaries and are thought to develop when primitive lymphatic sacs fail to establish venous communication.[102] The lesions present as large, fluctuant masses in the subcutaneous, fascial, mediastinal, and retroperitoneal spaces.[103] Lymphangioma was diagnosed on the metacarpal pad of a dog with persistent lameness and ulceration.[104] Lymphangiomas usually consist of dilated cystic, fluid-filled cavities lined by flattened endothelial cells and focal lymphoid aggregates and subdivided by multiple septa. They are bound externally by a fairly thick connective tissue wall and are filled with translucent or blood-tinged sterile fluid with a variable protein content (1.3 to 4.5 g/dL). Lymphangiomas are often noticed incidentally. In other cases, lymphangiomas exert pressure on surrounding structures and may interfere with muscle function, breathing (compression of the trachea), urination, or intestinal function. Lymph may ooze to the skin surface through single or multiple fistulous tracts. Differential diagnoses include other space-occupying masses such as abscesses, enlarged lymph nodes, neoplasms, and congenital cysts of nonlymphogenic origin. The prognosis is usually good after appropriate surgical excision, marsupialization, or radiation therapy.[105] The risk of recurrence is high with any of these treatment modalities because of inability to identify distinct boundaries.

Lymphangiosarcoma originates from lymphatic endothelial cells.[106] It is a rare malignant tumor in dogs and cats, although it is frequently reported secondary to chronic lymphedema in humans.[107,108] A breed or sex predisposition has not been detected, but medium to large breeds may be at highest risk, and both young and older animals are affected.[106,109] Metastasis occurs commonly in most dogs, although an isolated case without metastasis has been reported.[106,110] Clinical signs include pitting edema of the extremities, inguinal region, and axilla. Associated chylous effusions (pleural, abdominal, subcutaneous) have been reported.[111–113] Diagnosis requires biopsy confirmation. Surgical excision is difficult and the prognosis is poor.

REFERENCES

1. Comerota AJ, et al: Acute arterial occlusion. *In* Young JR, et al (eds): Peripheral Vascular Diseases. St. Louis, CV Mosby, 1996, p 273.
2. Fuster V, Verstraete M (eds): Thrombosis in Cardiovascular Disorders. Philadelphia, WB Saunders, 1992.
3. Whigham HM, et al: Aortic foreign body resulting in ischemic neuromyopathy and development of collateral circulation in a cat. JAVMA 213:829, 1998.
4. Bick RL, et al: Syndromes of thrombosis and hypercoagulability. Congenital and acquired cases of thrombosis. Med Clin North Am 82:409, 1998.
5. Ihle SL, et al: Probable recurrent femoral artery thrombosis in a dog with intestinal lymphosarcoma. JAVMA 208:240, 1996.
6. Ritt MG, et al: Nephrotic syndrome resulting in thromboembolic disease and disseminated intravascular coagulation in a dog. J Am Anim Hosp Assoc 33:385, 1997.
7. Dibartola SP, et al: Clinicopathologic findings in dogs with renal amyloidosis: 59 cases (1976–1986). JAVMA 195:358, 1989.
8. Nichols R: Complications and concurrent disease associated with canine hyperadrenocorticism. Vet Clin North Am Small Anim Pract 27:309, 1997.
9. Klein MK, et al: Pulmonary thromboembolism associated with immune-mediated hemolytic anemia in dogs. Ten cases (1982–1987). JAVMA 195:246, 1989.
10. LaRue MJ, et al: Pulmonary thromboembolism in dogs: 47 cases (1986–1987). JAVMA 197:1368, 1990.
11. Cook AK, et al: Clinical and pathological features of protein-losing glomerular disease in the dog: A review of 137 cases (1985–1992). J Am Anim Hosp Assoc 32:313, 1996.
12. Greene RA, et al: Hypoalbuminemia-related platelet hypersensitivity in two dogs with nephrotic syndrome. JAVMA 186:485, 1985.
13. Meyers KM: Reaction of platelets from food-producing, companion and laboratory animals. *In* Holmsen H (ed): Platelet Response and Metabolism, Vol 1. New York, CRC Press, 1987, p 209.
14. Harker LA: Platelets in thrombotic disorders: Quantitative and qualitative platelet disorders predisposing to arterial thrombosis. Semin Hematol 35:241, 1998.
15. Murphy KD, et al: Heparin-induced thrombocytopenia and thrombosis syndrome. Radiographics 18:111, 1998.
16. Meyers K, et al: Platelets and coagulation. Adv Vet Sci Comp Med 36:87, 1991.
17. Fox PR: Feline myocardial diseases. *In* Fox PR (ed): Canine and Feline Cardiology. New York, Churchill Livingstone, 1988, p 454.
18. Van Winkle TJ, et al: Clinical and pathological features of aortic thromboembolism in 36 dogs. J Vet Emerg Crit Care 3:13, 1993.
19. Joseph RJ: Canine cerebrovascular disease: Clinical and pathological findings in 17 cases. J Am Anim Hosp Assoc 24:569, 1988.
20. Bagely RS, et al: Cerebellar infarction caused by arterial thrombosis in a dog. JAVMA 192:785, 1988.
21. Reimer P, et al: Non-invasive imaging of peripheral vessels. Eur Radiol 8:858, 1998.
22. Tithof PK: Ultrasonographic diagnosis of aorto-iliac thrombosis. Cornell Vet 75:540, 1985.
23. Kraus KH, et al: Use of thermography in the diagnosis of aortic thrombosis in a dog. J Am Anim Hosp Assoc 22:489, 1986.
24. Smiley LE: The use of hetastarch for plasma expansion. Probl Vet Med 4:652, 1992.
25. Rackear D, et al: The effect of three different dosages of acetylsalicylic acid on canine platelet aggregation. J Am Anim Hosp Assoc 24:23, 1988.
26. Grauer GF, et al: Effects of low-dose aspirin and specific thromboxane synthetase inhibition on whole blood platelet aggregation and adenosine triphosphate secretion in healthy dogs. Am J Vet Res 53:1631, 1992.
27. Killingworth CR, et al: Streptokinase treatment of cats with experimentally induced aortic thrombosis. Am J Vet Res 47:1351, 1986.
28. Clare AC, et al: Use of recombinant tissue-plasminogen activator for aortic thrombolysis in a hypoproteinemic dog. JAVMA 212:539, 1998.
29. Ramsey CC, et al: Use of streptokinase in four dogs with thrombosis. JAVMA 209:780, 1996.
30. Bevilacqua G, et al: Spontaneous dissecting aneurysm of the aorta in a dog. Vet Pathol 18:273, 1981.
31. Chalifoux A, et al: Case report. Thrombo-aneurysm of the left subclavian artery in a dog. Can Vet J 13:146, 1972.
32. Hamir AN: Perforation of the thoracic aorta in a dog associated with *Spirocerca lupi* infection. Aust Vet J 61:64, 1984.
33. Stetter MD, et al: Femoral artery pseudoaneurysm in a monkey. JAVMA 201:1091, 1992.
34. Bouayad H, et al: Peripheral acquired arteriovenous fistula: A report of four cases and literature review. J Am Anim Hosp Assoc 23:205, 1987.
35. Turner BM: Acquired arteriovenous fistula in a dog following perivascular injection of thiopentone sodium. J Small Anim Pract 28:301, 1987.
36. Hopper PE, et al: Carotid body tumor associated with an arteriovenous fistula in a dog. Compend Contin Vet Med Educ 5:68, 1993.
37. Aiken SW, et al: Acquired arteriovenous fistula secondary to castration in a dog. JAVMA 202:965, 1993.
38. Franczuski D, et al: Arteriovenous fistula in the tongue of a dog: A case report. J Am Anim Hosp Assoc 22:355, 1986.
39. Moore PF, et al: Hepatic lesions associated with intrahepatic arterioportal fistulas. Vet Pathol 23:57, 1986.
40. Hollman E: Reflection on arteriovenous fistulas. Ann Thorac Surg 11:176, 1971.
41. Bolton GR, et al: Arteriovenous fistula of the aorta and caudal vena cava causing congestive heart failure in a cat. J Am Anim Hosp Assoc 12:463, 1976.

42. Rubin LF, et al: Arteriovenous fistula of the orbit in a dog. Cornel Vet 55:471, 1965.
43. Hause WR, et al: Cerebral arteriovenous malformation in a dog. J Am Anim Hosp Assoc 18:601, 1982.
44. Cordy DR: Vascular malformations and hemangiomas of the canine spinal cord. Vet Pathol 16:275, 1979.
45. Gelens HJ, et al: Arteriovenous fistula of the jejunum associated with gastrointestinal hemorrhage in a dog. JAVMA 202:1867, 1993.
46. Rogers WA, et al: Intrahepatic arteriovenous fistulas in a dog resulting in portal hypertension, portocaval shunts, and reversal of portal blood flow. J Am Anim Hosp Assoc 28:53, 1992.
47. Schermerhorn T, et al: Suspected microscopic hepatic arteriovenous fistulae in a young dog. JAVMA 211:70, 1997.
48. Baily MQ, et al: Ultrasound findings associated with congenital hepatic arteriovenous fistulas in 3 dogs. JAVMA 192:1009, 1988.
49. Igidbashian DO, et al: Iatrogenic femoral arteriovenous fistula: Diagnosis with color flow Doppler imaging. Radiology 170:749, 1989.
50. Jacobs GJ, et al: Diagnosis of right coronary artery to right atrial fistula in a dog using two-dimensional echocardiography. J Small Anim Pract 37:387, 1996.
51. Davidovic L, et al: Post-traumatic AV fistulas and pseudoaneurysms. J Cardiovasc Surg 38:645, 1997.
52. Ford EG, et al: Peripheral congenital arteriovenous fistulae: Observe, operate, or obturate. J Pediatri Surg 27:714, 1992.
53. Weber J, et al: Techniques and results of therapeutic catheter embolization of congenital vascular defects. Int Angiol 9:214, 1990.
54. Kelly DF, et al: Classification of naturally occurring arterial disease in the dog. Toxicol Pathol 17:77, 1989.
55. Lefborn BK, et al: Mineralized arteriosclerosis in a cat. Vet Radiol Ultrasound 37:420, 1996.
56. Mohr FC, et al: Arteriosclerosis in a cat. Vet Pathol 24:466, 1987.
57. Liu SK, et al: Clinical and pathologic findings in dogs with atherosclerosis: 21 cases (1970–83). JAVMA 189:227, 1986.
58. Kelly DF, et al: Arteriosclerosis of extramural coronary arteries in Labradors with congestive heart failure. J Small Anim Pract 33:437, 1992.
59. Valtonen MH, et al: Cardiovascular disease and nephritis in dogs. J Small Anim Pract 13:687, 1972.
60. Bjotvedt G: Spontaneous renal arteriosclerosis in greyhounds. Canine Pract 13:16, 1986.
61. Basha BJ, et al: Atherosclerosis: An update. Am Heart J 131:1192, 1996.
62. Kagawa Y, et al: Systemic atherosclerosis in dogs: Histopathological and immunohistochemical studies of atherosclerotic lesions. J Comp Pathol 118:195, 1998.
63. McAllister WB, et al: Vascular lesions in the dog following thyroidectomy and viosterol feeding. Yale J Biol Med 22:651, 1950.
64. Rogers WA, et al: Lipids and lipoproteins in normal dogs and in dogs with secondary hyperlipoproteinemia. JAVMA 166:1092, 1975.
65. Patterson JS, et al: Neurologic manifestations of cerebrovascular atherosclerosis associated with primary hypothyroidism in a dog. JAVMA 186:499, 1985.
66. Crawford MA, Foil CS: Vasculitis: Clinical syndromes in small animals. Compend Contin Vet Med Educ 11:400, 1989.
67. Jennette JC, et al: Small-vessel vasculitis. N Engl J Med 337:1512, 1997.
68. Randell MG, et al: Immune-mediated vasculitis in five dogs. JAVMA 183:207, 1983.
69. Hogenesch H, et al: Interleukin-6 activity in dogs with juvenile polyarteritis syndrome: Effect of corticosteroids. Clin Immunol Immunopathol 77:107, 1995.
70. Robinson WF, et al: The cardiovascular system. in Jubb KVF, et al (eds): Pathology of Domestic Animals, 4th ed, Vol 1. San Diego, Academic Press 1993, p 51.
71. Rachofsky MA, et al: Probable hypersensitivity vasculitis in a dog. JAVMA 194:1592, 1989.
72. Scott-Moncrieff JCR, et al: Systemic necrotizing vasculitis in nine young beagles. JAVMA 201:1553, 1992.
73. Meric SM, et al: Necrotizing vasculitis of the spinal pachyleptomeningeal arteries in three Bernese Mountain Dogs. JAVMA 22:459, 1986.
74. Turk JR, et al: Necrotizing pulmonary arteritis in a dog with patent ductus arteriosus. J Small Anim Pract 22:603, 1981.
75. Hoff EJ, et al: Case report: Necrotizing vasculitis in the central nervous systems of two dogs. Vet Pathol 18:219, 1981.
76. Carpenter JL, et al: Idiopathic cutaneous and renal glomerular vasculopathy of greyhounds. Vet Pathol 25:401, 1988.
77. Albassam MA, et al: Polyarteritis in a beagle. JAVMA 194:1595, 1989.
78. Snyder PW, et al: Pathologic features of naturally occurring juvenile polyarteritis in beagle dogs. Vet Pathol 32:237, 1995.
79. Curtis R, et al: Polyarteritis in a cat. Vet Rec 105:354, 1979.
80. Carpenter JL, et al: Polyarteritis nodosa and rheumatic heart disease in a dog. JAVMA 192:929, 1988.
81. Kelly DF, et al: Polyarteritis in the dog: A case report. Vet Rec 92:363, 1973.
82. Lucke VM, et al: Lymphomatoid granulomatosis of the lung in young dogs. Vet Pathol 16:405, 1979.
83. Von Rotz A, et al: Eosinophilic granulomatous pneumonia in a dog. Vet Rec 118:631, 1986.
84. Scott DW: Cutaneous phlebectasias in cushingoid dogs. J Am Anim Hosp Assoc 21:351, 1985.
85. Cornelius L, Mahaffey M: Kinking of the intrathoracic caudal vena cava in five dogs. J Small Anim Pract 26:67, 1985.
86. Willard MD, et al: Obstructed portal venous flow and portal vein thrombosis in a dog. JAVMA 194:1449, 1989.
87. Witte CL, et al: Disorders of lymph flow. Acad Radiol 2:324, 1995.
88. Fossum TW, et al: Lymphedema. Etiopathogenesis. J Vet Intern Med 6:283, 1992.
89. Kobayashi MR, et al: Lymphedema. Clin Plast Surg 14:303, 1987.
90. Johnston MG, et al: Quantitative approaches to the study of lymphatic contractile activity in vitro and in vivo: Potential role of this dynamic "lymph pump" in the re-expansion of the vascular space following hemorrhage. Lymphology 19:45, 1986.
91. Browse NL, et al: Lymphoedema: Pathophysiology and classification. J Card Surg 26:91, 1985.
92. Ladds PW, et al: Lethal congenital lymphedema in bulldog pups. JAVMA 159:81, 1971.
93. Leighton RL, et al: Primary lymphedema of the hind limb in the dog. JAVMA 174:369, 1979.
94. Davies AP, et al: Primary lymphedema in three dogs. JAVMA 174:1316, 1979.
95. Gill J, et al: Primary lymphedema in a dog—A case report. J Small Anim Pract 23:13, 1982.
96. Patterson DF, et al: Congenital hereditary lymphedema in the dog. Part I. Clinical and genetic studies. J Med Genet 4:145, 1967.
97. Carmichael NG, et al: Secondary lymphedema in a dog. J Small Anim Pract 27:335, 1986.
98. Farnsworth R, et al: Subcutaneous accumulation of chyle after thoracic duct ligation in a dog. JAVMA 208:2016, 1996.
99. Fossum TW, et al: Lymphedema. Clinical signs, diagnosis, and treatment. J Vet Intern Med 6:312, 1992.
100. Weissleder H, et al: Lymphedema: Evaluation of qualitative and quantitative lymphoscintigraphy in 238 patients. Radiology 167:729, 1988.
101. Casley-Smith JR, et al: The pathophysiology of lymphedema and action of benzo-pyrones in reducing it. Lymphology 21:190, 1988.
102. Stambaugh JE, et al: Lymphangioma in four dogs. JAVMA 173:759, 1978.
103. Fossum TW, et al: Generalized lymphangiectasis in a dog with subcutaneous chyle and lymphangioma. JAVMA 197:231, 1990.
104. Danielson F: Lymphangioma in the metacarpal pad of a dog. J Small Anim Pract 39:295, 1998.
105. Turrel JM, et al: Response to radiation therapy of recurrent lymphangioma in a dog. JAVMA 193:1432, 1988.
106. Rudd RG, et al: Lymphangiosarcoma in dogs. J Am Anim Hosp Assoc 25:695, 1989.
107. Eby CS, et al: Lymphangiosarcoma: A lethal complication of chronic lymphedema. Arch Surg 94:223, 1967.
108. Woodward AH, et al: Lymphangiosarcoma arising in chronic lymphadenematous extremities. Cancer 30:562, 1972.
109. Sagartz JE, et al: Lymphangiosarcoma in a young dog. Vet Pathol 33:353, 1996.
110. Walsh KM, Abbott DP: Lymphangiosarcoma in two cats. J Comp Pathol 94:611, 1984.
111. Myers NC, et al: Chylothorax and chylous ascites in a dog with mediastinal lymphangiosarcoma. J Am Anim Hosp Assoc 32:263, 1996.
112. Gores BR, et al: Chylous ascites in cats: Nine cases (1978–1993). JAVMA 205:1161, 1994.
113. Fossum TW, et al: Lymphangiosarcoma in a dog presenting with massive head and neck swelling. J Am Anim Hosp Assoc 34:301, 1998.

CV

INDEX

Note: Page numbers in *italics* refer to illustrations; page numbers
followed by t indicate tables.

AB blood group system, 353, *353,* 1798
Abdomen, distention of, 137–139, *138*
    liver disease and, 1273t, 1276
    fluid in. See *Ascites.*
Abducens nerve, anatomy of, 664t
    examination of, 562–566, *564,* 567t
Abelcet, for blastomycosis, 462
    for fungal infection, 456, 475t
Abortion, induced, 1544–1548, *1547*
    spontaneous, 1527–1528, 1592
Abrus precatorius, toxicity of, 364–365
Abscesses, of anal sacs, 1266–1267
    of brain, 556, 583, 591
    of dental pulp, 1135, 1136
    of liver, 1337
        ultrasonography of, 1292
    of lung, 1065, 1065t
    of prostate, 1692–1693
    of skin, 36–37, 39, 391t, 398–399
    of spleen, 1858
    periodontal, 1129
    subcutaneous, 63, 65
Abyssinian, renal amyloidosis in, 1699t, 1700,
    1982t
Acanthamoeba infection, polysystemic, 416
Acanthomatous epulis, 1114, *1115,* 1117
Acanthosis nigricans, 1994t
Acarbose, for diabetes, 1448
Acariasis. See *Mite infestation.*
Accelerated idioventricular rhythms, 816
Accessory nerve, anatomy of, 664t
    examination of, 563, 567t
Acemannan, for feline immunodeficiency virus
        infection, 437, 437t
    for feline leukemia virus infection, 430
Acepromazine, as tranquilizer, in heart failure,
        733–734
    in lung infection, 1065t
    in pulmonary edema, 1065t, 1082
    cardiac effects of, echocardiography of, 842–
        843, 845t
    for tick paralysis, 673
    for vascular neuropathy, 679
Acetaminophen, 318
    for pain, 24t, 25
    toxicity of, to liver, 1327, 1331–1332
Acetic acid, in ear cleansing, for otitis externa,
        989t, 994, 996
Acetylcholine, in gastric acid secretion, 1156,
    1156
    receptors of, in myasthenia gravis, 675–676
N-Acetylcysteine, for acetaminophen toxicity, to
        liver, 1332
    for hemolytic anemia, 1802
Achalasia, cricopharyngeal, 1145, 1976t, 1985t
    esophageal, vs. idiopathic megaesophagus,
        1149

Achondroplasia, 1975t, 1983t
    and dwarfism, 1898
    maxillofacial development in, 1123–1124
    narrow pelvic canal in, and dystocia, 1534
Acid citrate dextrose, in blood storage, 350, 350t
Acidophil cell hepatitis, 1306–1307, 1330–1331
Acidosis, fluid therapy in, 330t
    hyperkalemia in, 342
    in renal disease, prevention of, diet in, 270
    metabolic, in renal failure, acute, 1624, 1629
        chronic, 1640, 1652
    renal tubular, 1707–1708, 1709t
        and hyperchloremia, 234
    respiratory, blood gas analysis in, 1039
Aciduria, 1605
    renal tubular disorders and, 1704–1706, 1709
Acinar atrophy, pancreatic, and exocrine
        insufficiency, 1355, *1355,* 1359
Acoustic reflex testing, in deafness, 1001
Acquired immunodeficiency syndrome (AIDS),
        cat scratch disease with, 382, 386
Acral mutilation, 669, 1994t
Acrodermatitis, 48, 1994t, 1995t
Acromegaly (hypersomatotropism), 1370–1373,
        1370–1373
    and cardiomyopathy, 914
    and obesity, 71
    polyphagia with, 105
Acrylamide, toxicity of, to peripheral nerves,
        673t
ACTH. See *Adrenocorticotropic hormone.*
Actigall, for cholangiohepatitis, 1310
    for liver disease, 1304
Actinic dermatitis, and carcinoma, client
        information on, 1926
    of pinna, 988–991, 989t
Actinic keratosis, and nasal carcinoma, 1019,
        1020
Actinomycosis, 391t, 395
    and enteritis, 1219
    and meningitis, spinal, 616
Actisite, for periodontitis, 1132
Acupuncture, 366–373
    diagnosis in, 366–367, *367*
    for intervertebral disk disease, *370,* 373, 634
    for pain, 25
    in cancer management, 374–375, 375t
    in small animal practice, *370–372,* 370–373
    meridians in, 367–369, *368*
    working mechanism of, 369–370
Acutrim, for urinary dysfunction, 320, 1739t
Acyclovir, for feline herpesvirus infection, 447
Addison's disease, 1488–1498. See also
        Hypoadrenocorticism.
Adenine arabinoside, for feline infectious
        peritonitis, 441
Adenitis, sebaceous, 48

Adenocarcinoma. See *Carcinoma.*
Adenocard, for arrhythmia, 826t, 828t, 831–832
Adenoma, of rectum, 1260–1262
    parathyroid. See *Hyperparathyroidism.*
    perianal, 1267–1268
    pituitary, 584t
        and hyperadrenocorticism, 1462
    rectal, 1254, *1254*
Adenomatous polyposis coli gene, in
        carcinogenesis, 478–479
Adenosine, for arrhythmia, 826t, 828t, 831–832
Adenosine triphosphatase, in heart failure, 704t
Adenovirus infection, and hepatitis, 419, 419t,
        1306, 1330
    and tracheobronchitis, 419t, 419–420
Adhesins, in periodontal disease, 1128
Adrenal glands, anatomy of, 1488
    disorders of, neurologic signs of, 551
    hyperfunction of, 1460–1487. See also *Hypera-
        drenocorticism.*
    hypofunction of, 1488–1498. See also *Hypoad-
        renocorticism.*
    hypoplasia of, 1986t
    steroid production in, 307–308, *308*
Adrenergic receptors, drugs blocking. See *Beta
        blockers.*
    steroid effects on, 311
Adrenocorticotropic hormone, ectopic production
        of, paraneoplastic, 503
    in hyperadrenocorticism, 1486
        in stimulation test, *1469,* 1469–1471, 1470t,
            1485
    in hypoadrenocorticism, 1489, 1496, 1498
        in stimulation test, 1495, 1498
    in steroid production, 307, *308*
Adriamycin. See *Doxorubicin.*
Advantage, in flea control, client information on,
    1971
Aelurostrongylus abstrusus infestation, of lung,
    1065t, 1070
Afghan hound, myelopathy in, 1991t
Afterload, in cardiac output, 693
    in heart failure, assessment of, 708
Agalactia, 1538
Agar-disk diffusion test, 303
Agglutination tests, in hemolytic anemia,
        immune-mediated, *1795,* 1795–1796
Aggression, glucocorticoids and, 316
    in cats, 160t, 160–162, *161,* 1597, 1597t
    in dogs, 156–158, *157,* 158t
    sleep-associated, 152
Aging, and adverse drug reactions, 322–323
    and deafness, 1001
    and drug disposition, 296
    and tremors, 141
Aglepristone, in abortion induction, 1545
AIDS, cat scratch disease with, 382, 386

IND

IND

IND

IND

IND

IND

IND

IND

IND

IND

Ketoconazole, for blastomycosis, 460–461
for coccidioidomycosis, 467
for cryptococcosis, 471
for dermatophytosis, 49
for epidermal dysplasia, in West Highland
white terrier, 48
for fungal infection, 456–457, 475t
for histoplasmosis, 464
for hyperadrenocorticism, 1481–1482, 1486
for *Malassezia* infection, in dermatitis, 50
in otitis, 990t, 996
Ketones, in urinalysis, 1605–1606
Ketoprofen, for fever, 9
for pain, 24t
Key-Gaskell syndrome, and megaesophagus,
1150t, 1151
Kidney(s). See also *Renal.*
amyloidosis of, 1667–1674. See also *Amyloidosis.*
disorders of, and adverse drug reactions, 323t,
324
and anemia, 1808
and cachexia, 74
and diabetes insipidus. See *Diabetes insipidus.*
and hyperchloremia, 234
and hyperlipidemia, 290
and hypokalemia, 225, *226,* 227
and hyponatremia, 222t, 222–223, *224,*
1644, 1651
and polyuria, 85t, 85–89, *86,* 87t, 88t
and proteinuria, 100–102, *101*
congenital, in cats, 1982t
in dogs, 1996t
dextran and, 333
diabetes mellitus and, 1458–1459
diet in, 269–271, 271t, 272t, 273–274
evaluation of, biopsy in, 1612–1613, *1613*
clinical, 1600–1601, *1601*
glomerular function tests in, 1601–1603,
1602, 1602t
microbiologic, 1610–1611
radiography in, 1611–1612
tubular function tests in, 1603–1605,
1604t
ultrasonography in, 1612
urinalysis in, 1605–1610, 1606t, *1606–
1611,* 1607t
familial, 1698–1703, 1699t
hypertension and, with hyperadrenocorticism, 1466
in heart failure, 702t, 703
in hyperkalemia, 228, *229*
in hyperthyroidism, 1402, 1403t, 1404
in multiple myeloma, 516–517, 519
skin lesions with, 28
with dirofilariasis, 947
erythropoietin production in, in polycythemia,
203, 204
glomerular function in, 1662–1663, *1663*
glomerular inflammation in, 1663–1676. See
also *Glomerulonephritis.*
in bilirubin metabolism, 211
in drug elimination, 297
infarction of, 964, *965*
inflammation of, hyperadrenocorticism and,
1482
lymphoma of, 508, 508t
steroid effects on, 311
toxicity to, amphotericin B and, 455–456,
1616
chemotherapy and, 487, 487t
ethylene glycol and, client information on,
1965
furosemide and, in heart failure, 715–716

Kidney(s) *(Continued)*
transplantation of, 1632, 1659t, 1659–1660
tubular disorders in, 1704–1709, 1709t. See
also *Renal tubules.*
tumors of, 542
vascular disorders in, and hypertension, 180–
182, *181*
Kitten. See *Neonate.*
Klebsiella infection, antibiotics for, 303,
305–306
Knee, synovitis of, 1883–1885
Krabbe type globoid cell leukodystrophy, 589,
590t, 1980t, 1992t
and peripheral neuropathy, 670
genetics in, 3t
spinal cord demyelination in, 627–628
Krebs-Henseleit cycle, 1286, *1286*

Labetalol, for arrhythmia, 827
Labor. See *Parturition.*
Labrador retriever, myopathy in, 688–689, 1993t
Lacrimal punctum, imperforate, 1988t
Lactase, deficiency of, 1197
Lactate, elevated blood level of, paraneoplastic,
499
Lactate dehydrogenase, in liver disease, 1283
in pleural effusion, 1105
Lactation, disorders of, 1538
in neonatal nutrition, 241–244, 243t
in pseudopregnancy, 1526
management of, 1596
Lactitol, for hepatic encephalopathy, 1333
Lactose, intolerance to, 253
Lactulose, for constipation, 132
for hepatic encephalopathy, 1333, 1334t
for portosystemic shunt, congenital, 1314,
1315
Laminectomy, for intervertebral disk disease,
1919
Lanoxin. See *Digoxin.*
Lansoprazole, for gastric ulcers, 1168
Laparoscopy, for liver biopsy, 1296t, 1297
Large intestine. See *Colon.*
Larva migrans, zoonotic infection and, 386–387
Larvae, in chigger infestation, and pruritus, 33t
in heartworm disease, 937, *937, 938,* 958–
959. See also *Dirofilariasis.*
Laryngitis, 1030
Larynx, disorders of, 1029–1031
hypoplasia of, 1981t, 1994t
paralysis of, congenital, 1994t
in Dalmatian, with polyneuropathy, 668
nerve degeneration and, 669
physiology of, 1025, 1026
Lasalocid, toxicity of, to peripheral nerves, 673t
Lasix. See *Furosemide.*
Lassitude, 10
Latissimus dorsi muscle, in surgery, for
cardiomyopathy, 885
Lavage, bronchoalveolar, 1038
in tracheal disorders, 1042
for pyothorax, 1106–1107
Laxatives, 131, 132t
over-the-counter, 319–320
Lead, accumulation of, in bone, 1909, *1910*
toxicity of, 361–362
and megaesophagus, 1150t
to central nervous system, 586
to peripheral nerves, 673t
Leflunomide, for arthritis, 1884–1885
Legg-Calvé-Perthes disease, 1873, *1874,* 1984t
Leiomyoma, of stomach, 1176, 1177
Leiomyosarcoma, colorectal, 1253–1254

Leishmaniasis, and arthritis, 1878–1879
and hypopigmentation, 57
polysystemic, 410t, 415
skin lesions in, 28
Lenses, cataracts of, and vision loss, 17, 17t
congenital, 1977t, 1987t
diabetes and, 985, 1458
systemic disease and, 985
congenital defects of, 1977t, 1978t, 1987t,
1988t
Lente insulin, for diabetes mellitus, 1451–1452
Lenticonus, 1988t
Leprosy, 393, 394
Leptospirosis, 391t, 397–398
and anemia, 199
and renal failure, 1617, 1622, 1631
of liver, 1307, 1337
zoonotic, 384t
Lethargy, 10
Leucine, in diet, 239t
Leukemia, and anemia, 1814–1815
and thrombopoietic disorders, 1823
lymphoblastic, acute, 514, *514,* 1854, *1854*
chronic, 1855, *1855*
lymphocytic, *514,* 514–515
myeloid, *1853,* 1853–1854, *1854*
nonlymphoid, 515t, 515–516
of granular lymphocytes, 1854–1855, *1855*
undifferentiated, acute, 1854
Leukemia virus infection, feline, 424–432
and anemia, aplastic, 1813
non-regenerative, 1810t, 1810–1811
and enteritis, 1217
and lymphoma, 508t, 509
and lymphopenia, 1851
and rectal cancer, 1261
and urinary incontinence, 1742
client information on, 1957
diagnosis of, 425–426
epidemiology of, 424–425
management of, 428–432
pathogenesis of, 426–427
prevention of, 427–428, *429*
screening for, in blood donors, 349
Leukocyte adhesion protein deficiency, in
granulocytopathy syndrome, 1850, 1990t
Leukocyte esterase reaction, in urinalysis, 1606
Leukocytes, 1842–1855. See also specific types,
e.g., *Neutrophils.*
changes in, in disease prognosis, 1852
in brain inflammation, 591–592
in cerebrospinal fluid, 574, 574t
in urinary tract infection, *98,* 99, 1607, *1607,*
1607t, 1678, 1680
inclusions in, 1846–1848, *1846–1848*
production of, 1842
Leukocytosis, in hemolytic anemia, 1794
in hyperthyroidism, 1403, 1403t
of brain, 591–592
paraneoplastic, 504–505
Leukoderma, 55–57, *56*
Leukodystrophy, globoid cell, 589, 590t, 1980t,
1992t
and peripheral neuropathy, 670
genetics in, 3t
spinal cord demyelination in, 627–628
metachromatic, 589, 590t, 1980t
Leukoencephalomyelopathy, in rottweilers, 589,
636
Leukogram, stress, 1844
Leukotrichia, 55–57, *56*
Leukotrienes, in inflammation, steroid effects on,
310
Levamisole (Levasol), for dirofilariasis, 949, 952
for lungworm infestation, 1070, 1071

Lung(s) *(Continued)*
  mineralization of, 1088
  parasitosis of, 1065t, 1068–1071, *1069*, 1083–1084
  thromboembolism in, 1078–1080, *1079, 1080*
    hyperadrenocorticism and, 1483
  trauma to, *1083*, 1084–1088, *1085*
  tumors of, bronchoscopy of, 1038t
    in malignant histiocytosis, 1078
    lymphomatous, *1077*, 1077–1078
    metastatic, 1075–1077, *1076, 1077*
      from oral cancer, 1114–1115
    primary, 1073–1075, *1074, 1075*
Lungworm infestation, 1068–1071, *1069*
  of trachea, *1044*, 1044–1045
Lupus, discoid, 55, 57
Lupus erythematosus, systemic, and megaesophagus, 1150t
  arthritis in, 78, 80, 1882
    treatment of, 1883–1885
  hypopigmentation in, 57
  lungs in, 1072
  skin lesions in, 29
Lutalyse. See *Prostaglandins.*
Luteal phase, in estrous cycle, *1510*, 1510–1514, *1514, 1515*
Luteinization, pre-ovulatory, 1511
Luteinizing hormone, in estrous cycle, 1510–1516, *1511, 1514, 1515*, 1520, 1522, 1589
  and timing of artificial insemination, 1575–1576, *1576*
Lym Dyp (lime sulfur), for mange, notoedric, 61
Lyme disease. See *Borreliosis.*
Lymph nodes, evaluation of, in hypercalcemia, 1388
Lymphadenitis, 977, 977t
Lymphadenopathy, hilar, fungal infection and, 1067–1068
  lymphoma and, 1077, *1077*
  with bronchial compression, 1059–1060, *1060*
  mediastinal, 1095t, 1096, *1096*
Lymphangiectasia, of small intestine, *1229*, 1229–1230, *1230*
  and nutrient delivery blockade, 1198
  congenital, 1976t, 1985t
  with chylothorax, 1107, *1107*
Lymphangioma, 980
Lymphangiosarcoma, 980
Lymphangitis, 977, 977t
Lymphatic system, congenital disorders of, 1989t, 1990t
  fluid dynamics in, 326
  in tumor metastasis, 481, 483
  peripheral, anatomy of, 975–976
    disorders of, 976–977, 977t
Lymphedema, congenital, 1979t, 1990t
  peripheral, 977t, 977–980, *978, 979*
Lymphoblastic leukemia, acute, 514, *514*, 1854, *1854*
  chronic, 1855, *1855*
Lymphocytes, granular, leukemia of, 1854–1855, *1855*
  in colonic mucosal immunity, 1239
  in feline immunodeficiency virus infection, 434
  in glomerulonephritis, 1663–1664
  in inflammation, steroid effects on, 310–311
  in lymphoma, cutaneous, 49
  in mycosis fungoides, 508, *508*
  in skin lesions, in cytology, 53
  in small intestinal immune response, 1195–1196, *1196*
  with plasma cells, in gastritis, chronic, 1162, 1163

Lymphocytic choriomeningitis, zoonotic, 384t
Lymphocytic leukemia, *514*, 514–515
Lymphocytic portal hepatitis, 1309
Lymphocytic-plasmacytic colitis, 1247–1248, *1248*, 1248t, 1249t
Lymphocytic-plasmacytic enteritis, 1227–1228
Lymphocytic-plasmacytic infiltrates, in gastritis, 1162–1163
Lymphocytic-plasmacytic splenitis, 1858t, 1859
Lymphocytic-plasmacytic synovitis, 78–80
  of knee, 1883–1885
Lymphocytosis, 1850–1851, 1851t
Lymphography, 979
Lymphoma, 507–514
  and cachexia, 499
  Burkitt's, 481
  classification of, 507, 507t, 508t
  client information on, 1923
  cutaneous, 528
    T-cell, 49, 508, *508*
  diagnosis of, 508–510, *509*, 510t
  epitheliotrophic, 42
  etiology of, 507
  feline immunodeficiency virus infection and, 435, *436*
  hepatic, ultrasonography of, 1292
  mediastinal, 508, *508*, 508t, 509t, 1095–1096, *1095*
  of brain, primary, 584t
  of kidney, 542
  of lung *1077*, 1077–1078
  of pharynx, 1029
  prognosis of, 512–514, *513*, 513t
  signs of, 507–508, *508*
  treatment of, 510–512, 511t, *512*
Lymphomatoid granulomatosis, 974, 1072, 1077–1078
Lymphopenia, 1851, 1851t
  in hyperthyroidism, 1403, 1403t
  in stress leukogram, 1844
Lymphosarcoma, of colon, 1253–1254
  of rectum, 1253–1254, 1260–1262
  of small intestine, 1234, *1235*
  of stomach, 1176, 1177
Lynxacarus radovskyi mite infestation, 59t, 61
Lysine, in diet, 239t
Lysodren. See *o,p'-DDD.*
Lysosomal glucosidase deficiency, 1290, 1992t
Lysosomal storage diseases, 589, 590t, 1980t, 1992
  leukocyte inclusions in, 1847, *1847*

Machinery murmurs, 172–174
Macrocytosis, familial, 1990t
  in hemolytic anemia, 1791t
Macroglobulinemia, Waldenström's, 516, 517
Macrophages, in feline immunodeficiency virus infection, 434
  in hyperthermia, 7, 7t, 8
  in inflammation, steroid effects on, 311
  in lung, in dirofilariasis, 942, *942*
  in skin lesions, 53
Magnesium, blood level of, decreased, 232–233, 346
    diuretics and, in heart failure, 716
    renal tubular dysfunction and, 1706
    elevated, 233, 346
      in renal failure, 1643
  functions of, 232
  in diet, 239t
    in calcium oxalate urolithiasis, 1727
    in heart disease, 265t
Magnesium ammonium phosphate urolithiasis, in cats, 1711–1712, *1712, 1713*, 1723t, 1730t, 1730–1732, 1731t

Magnesium ammonium phosphate urolithiasis *(Continued)*
  in dogs, 1758t, 1760–1763
    with calcium oxalate lithiasis, 1765–1766, *1766*, 1770, *1771*
Magnesium chloride, in cardiopulmonary resuscitation, 192t, 193
Magnesium sulfate, for torsades de pointes, 815
  for ventricular arrhythmia, with hypotension, 184t
Magnetic resonance imaging, in congenital heart disease, 741
  in hyperadrenocorticism, 1473, *1474, 1475*
  of bone disorders, 1891
  of brain, 576
  of nasal cavity, 1012–1013, *1016*
  of pericardial effusion, 931
Malabsorption, and diarrhea, 125–126
  in pancreatic exocrine insufficiency, 1208, 1358
  of fat, medium-chain triglycerides for, 259
  signs of, 1203, 1205
  small intestinal disorders and, 1200, 1200t, 1201
Malamute, atopic dermatitis in, with zinc deficiency, 48–49
  polyneuropathy in, 667–668
  renal dysplasia in, 1699t, 1700
Malassezia infection, and dermatitis, with crusting, 49–50
  with pruritus, 32, 33t, 34, 34t
  and hyperpigmentation, 58
  and otitis externa, 990t, 993, 994, 996
  and skin erosion, 40, 42
  in epidermal dysplasia, in West Highland white terrier, 48
Malassimilation. See *Malabsorption.*
Malnutrition, anorexia and, 102–103
  in neonate, 244
  in pancreatic exocrine insufficiency, 1358
  in renal failure, 1648, *1648*
  with cachexia, 73
Malocclusion, *1123*, 1124–1126, *1125, 1126*
Maltese dog, bile acids in, postprandial, 1289
  encephalitis in, 598
Mammary glands, absence of, 1980t
  disorders of, postparturient, 1538
  examination of, in infertility, 1558
  hyperplasia of, fibroadenomatous, 1591–1592, *1592, 1593*
  in lactation, disorders of, 1538
    in neonatal nutrition, 241–244, 243t
    in pseudopregnancy, 1526
  management of, 1596
  tumors of, 544–545
    after sterilization, 1542, *1542*
    client information on, 1928
Mandible, articulation of, with temporal bone, instability of, 1868
  development of, deciduous teeth in, 1123
  dropped, in trigeminal neuropathy, 582
  giant cell granuloma of, central, 1905
  osteopathy of, with cranial osteopathy, 1898, *1900, 1901*, 1983t
Manganese, in diet, 239t
  in orthopedic developmental disorders, 248
Mange, 59t, 61. See also *Mite infestation.*
  of pinna, 988, 989t
Mannitol, for cerebral edema, 147
  after portosystemic shunt ligation, 1314
  in hepatic failure, 1302t
    traumatic, 579–580
    with inflammation, 593t
  for intracranial pressure elevation, 577
  for renal failure, 1627

Nervous system (*Continued*)
and tremors, 139–141, *140*, 606–607
and weakness, 12
anoxia and, 586
as signs of systemic disease, 548–551, 549t, *550*
congenital, in cats, 1979t–1980t
in dogs, 1991t–1993t
degenerative, 607
diabetes and, 1458
in constipation, 129, 130, 130t, *131*
in hypothyroidism, 1421–1422
in renal failure, 1624
lead toxicity and, 361–362, 586
paraneoplastic, 506, 506t
pupillary examination in, 657–661, *658, 659t, 660t, 661*
rabies and, 419t, 422–423, 449–450, 594–595
in heart failure, compensatory mechanisms in, 699–701, 700t
in pain perception, 20–21
in pruritus, 31–32
inflammation of. See also *Meningitis* and *Meningoencephalitis*.
borna disease virus and, 450–451
multifocal, 603–606, 604t, *605, 606*
metabolic disease of, 607
peripheral, disorders of, 662–681
and fecal incontinence, 1268, 1268t, 1269
developmental, 666–671
evaluation of, 662–665, 663t, 664t
hypothyroidism and, 671–672
in acquired demyelinating neuropathy, 674
in botulism, 672
in brachial plexus neuritis, 674–675
in chronic relapsing neuropathy, 674
in dancing Doberman disease, 679–680
in diabetes mellitus, 671
in distal denervating disease, 679
in distal symmetric polyneuropathy, 679
in dysautonomia, 680
in myasthenia gravis, 675–676
in paraneoplastic syndromes, 677–678
in polyradiculoneuritis, 673–674
in renal failure, 1638t, 1638–1639
in sensory ganglioneuritis, 675
in tick paralysis, 672–673
mechanisms of, 665–666
toxic, 673, 673t
vascular disorders and, 678–679
inflammation of, idiopathic, facial, 680–681
trigeminal, 680
structure of, 662, *662*
trauma to, 678
tumors of, 676–677
vestibular dysfunction in, idiopathic, 681
toxicity to, 607
plants and, 365
tumors of, 556, 607
vascular disease of, 607
Nettles, toxicity of, 365
Neupogen. See *Granulocyte colony-stimulating factor*.
Neural tube, closure of, defects of, 1979t, 1980t, 1991t
Neuralgia, glossopharyngeal, 1029
Neurilemoma, 677
Neurinoma, 677
Neuritis, facial, idiopathic, 680–681
of brachial plexus, 674–675
optic, and anisocoria, 660t
trigeminal, idiopathic, 680
Neuroaxonal dystrophy, 589, 642, 1980t, 1992t

Neuroblastoma, peripheral, 677
Neurofibroma, 677
Neurofibrosarcoma, 677
Neuroma, after tail docking, and pruritus, 33t
Neuromuscular junction, disorders of, and regurgitation, 115, 117t
paraneoplastic, 506, 506t
Neuronopathy, progressive, in cairn terrier, 666, 1992t
Neurons, congenital disorders of, 1992t
Neurotensin, 1501–1502
Neurotoxins, endogenous, 549t, 550–551
Neutering. See *Sterilization*.
Neutropenia, 1848t, 1848–1849
chemotherapy and, 485–486, *486*
Neutrophilia, 1842–1844, *1844*, 1844t, *1845*
estrogen-induced myelotoxicity and, 1849, *1849*
in pyometra, with cystic endometrial hyperplasia, 1550
Neutrophils, granulation of, anomalous, 1847t, 1978t
hypersegmentation of, 1845–1846
in gastritis, 1160
in inflammation, 1844–1845, *1845*
in inflammatory bowel disease, 1249
in skin lesions, in cytology, 53
in stress leukogram, 1844
in synovial fluid, in joint inflammation, 79, 80
inclusions in, 1846–1848, *1846–1848*
inherited defects of, *1849*, 1849–1850
morphologic abnormalities of, 1845, *1845*
pools of, 1842, *1843*
production of, 1842
transfusion of, 351
Nevi, 36, 1982t, 1995t
Newborn. See *Neonate*.
Niacin, in diet, 239t, 239–240
Niclosamide, for intestinal parasitosis, 1221t
Nicotine, toxicity of, 357, 365
Nictitating membrane, protrusion of, systemic disease and, 984
Niemann-Pick disease, and peripheral neuropathy, 670–671
Nifedipine, for arrhythmia, 830, 831
Nifurtimox, for trypanosomiasis, 410t, 416
Nightshade, toxicity of, 364
Nitrates, for heart failure, 724–726
Nitric oxide, in heart failure, 701
Nitrofurantoin, dosage of, in renal failure, 1649t
Nitrogen, in dietary protein, 237
metabolism of, disorders of, and aminoaciduria, 1704–1705
and uricaciduria, 1705–1706
and xanthinuria, 1706
urea. See *Urea nitrogen*.
Nitroglycerin, for heart failure, 724–725
Nitroprusside, for cardiomyopathy, dilated, 884
for heart failure, 725–726
with mitral insufficiency, 794
Nitroscanate, for intestinal parasitosis, 1221t
Nizatidine, for gastric motility disorders, 1176
for gastric ulcers, 1168
for gastrinoma, 1506, 1506t
Nizoral. See *Ketoconazole*.
Nocardiosis, 391t, 395
and meningitis, spinal, 616
Nociception, 20–21. See also *Pain*.
Nocturia, 89, 90
in renal failure, 1637
Nodular dermatofibrosis syndrome, 28
Nodular hyperplasia, adrenocortical, and hyperadrenocorticism, 1461–1462
of liver, 1319–1320
Nodular panniculitis, sterile, 36, 37

Nodules, in histiocytosis, 36
of pinna, 987t, 991–992
Nolvasan (chlorhexidine), for anal sacculitis, 1266
for oral disorders, with renal failure, 1629, 1630t
for otitis externa, 989t, 994
Nonsteroidal anti-inflammatory drugs, and stomach ulcers, 1165–1166
for degenerative joint disease, 1865–1866
for fever, 9
for pain, 24, 24t, 25
Norepinephrine, for hypotension, 184t
Normosol-R, in fluid therapy, 328, 329t, 330t
Norpace, for arrhythmia, 825, 825t, 826t, 828t
Norvasc (amlodipine), for arrhythmia, 824t, 830, 831
for hypertension, 182
in renal failure, 1653–1654
Norwegian Forest cat, glycogen storage disease in, 671
Nose, 1003–1023. See also *Nasal cavity*.
Nostrils, agenesis of, 1981t
congenital stenosis of, 1994t
Notoedres cati infestation, 59t, 61
of pinna, 988, 989t
Novartis (desoxycorticosterone), for hypoadrenocorticism, 1496–1498
after adrenalectomy, 1487
NPH insulin, for diabetes mellitus, 1451–1452
Nuclear transcription factors, genetic defects of, and cardiomyopathy, 877
in carcinogenesis, 478, 479t
Nucleus pulposus. See *Disks, intervertebral*.
Nutmeg, toxicity of, 365
Nutrition. See *Diet*.
Nymphomania, 1595
Nyquist limit, in echocardiography, 841, *842*
Nystagmus, congenital, 1978t
in cranial nerve examination, 565, 567t
Nystatin, for otitis externa, 990t, 995

Obesity, 70–72, *71*
after prepubertal gonadectomy, 70, 1540
and pulmonary disorders, 1088
in heart disease, 71, 266
Obturator muscle, transfer of, in perineal herniorrhaphy, 1260
Obturator nerve, injury to, signs of, 663t
Occlusion, dental, *1123–1126*, 1124–1126
Octreotide, for gastrinoma, 1506, 1506t
for pancreatic islet cell tumors, 1434t, 1435t, 1437, *1437*
Oculomotor nerve, anatomy of, 664t
examination of, 562–565, *564*, 567t
palsy of, and anisocoria, 660t
Odontoid process, in atlantoaxial subluxation, *615*, 615–616, *616*, 1984t
Odontoma, 1114
Oleander, toxicity of, 365
Olfactory function, 562
impaired, and anorexia, 103
Olfactory nerve, anatomy of, 664t
Oligodendroglioma, 584t, 585t
Oligodontia, 1122
Oligozoospermia, 1579
Oliguria, in renal failure, 1623
Ollulanus tricuspis infestation, and gastritis, 1164–1165
Omega-3 fatty acids, in fish oil, for hyperlipidemia, 289
for renal failure, 1646–1647, 1647t, 1658
Omeprazole, for esophagitis, 1148, 1149

IND

IND

IND

IND

IND